BMA

D1759467

WITHDRAWN
FROM LIBRARY

BRITISH MEDICAL ASSOCIATION

1002359

Interventional Cardiology
Principles and Practice
Second Edition

Edited by

George D. Dangas, MD, PhD, FACC, FSCAI, FESC, FAHA
Professor of Medicine
Director, Cardiovascular Innovation
Mount Sinai Medical Center
New York, NY
USA

Carlo Di Mario, MD, PhD, FRCP, FACC, FSCAI, FESC
Consultant Cardiologist
Royal Brompton Hospital
Professor of Clinical Cardiology
National Heart & Lung Institute Imperial College London
London
UK

Nicholas N. Kipshidze, MD, PhD, FACC, FESC, FSCAI
Professor of Medicine and Surgery
Consultant Cardiologist
N. Kipshidze Central University Hospital
Tbilisi, Georgia
Director,
New York Cardiovascular Research,
New York, NY
USA

Associate Editors

Peter Barlis and Tayo Addo

Foreword by

Patrick W. Serruys, MD, PhD

WILEY Blackwell

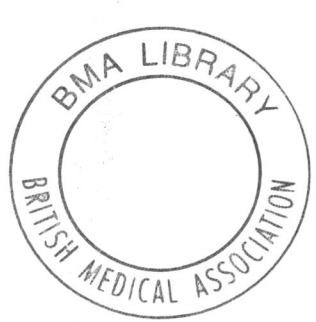

BMA LIBRARY
BRITISH MEDICAL ASSOCIATION

This edition first published 2017 © 2011, 2017 by John Wiley & Sons, Ltd

Registered Office
John Wiley & Sons, Ltd, The Atrium, Southern Gate, Chichester, West Sussex, PO19 8SQ, UK

Editorial Offices
9600 Garsington Road, Oxford, OX4 2DQ, UK
1606 Golden Aspen Drive, Suites 103 and 104, Ames, Iowa 50010, USA

For details of our global editorial offices, for customer services and for information about how to apply for permission to reuse the copyright material in this book please see our website at www.wiley.com/wiley-blackwell.

The right of the author to be identified as the author of this work has been asserted in accordance with the UK Copyright, Designs and Patents Act 1988.

All rights reserved. No part of this publication may be reproduced, stored in a retrieval system, or transmitted, in any form or by any means, electronic, mechanical, photocopying, recording or otherwise, except as permitted by the UK Copyright, Designs and Patents Act 1988, without the prior permission of the publisher.

Designations used by companies to distinguish their products are often claimed as trademarks. All brand names and product names used in this book are trade names, service marks, trademarks or registered trademarks of their respective owners. The publisher is not associated with any product or vendor mentioned in this book. It is sold on the understanding that the publisher is not engaged in rendering professional services. If professional advice or other expert assistance is required, the services of a competent professional should be sought.

The contents of this work are intended to further general scientific research, understanding, and discussion only and are not intended and should not be relied upon as recommending or promoting a specific method, diagnosis, or treatment by health science practitioners for any particular patient. The publisher and the author make no representations or warranties with respect to the accuracy or completeness of the contents of this work and specifically disclaim all warranties, including without limitation any implied warranties of fitness for a particular purpose. In view of ongoing research, equipment modifications, changes in governmental regulations, and the constant flow of information relating to the use of medicines, equipment, and devices, the reader is urged to review and evaluate the information provided in the package insert or instructions for each medicine, equipment, or device for, among other things, any changes in the instructions or indication of usage and for added warnings and precautions. Readers should consult with a specialist where appropriate. The fact that an organization or Website is referred to in this work as a citation and/or a potential source of further information does not mean that the author or the publisher endorses the information the organization or Website may provide or recommendations it may make. Further, readers should be aware that Internet Websites listed in this work may have changed or disappeared between when this work was written and when it is read. No warranty may be created or extended by any promotional statements for this work. Neither the publisher nor the author shall be liable for any damages arising herefrom.

Library of Congress Cataloging-in-Publication Data

Names: Dangas, George D., editor. | Di Mario, Carlo, editor. | Kipshidze,
    Nicholas N., editor.
Title: Interventional cardiology : principles and practice / edited by George
    D. Dangas, Carlo Di Mario, Nicholas N. Kipshidze ; foreword by Patrick W.
    Serruys.
Other titles: Interventional cardiology (Di Mario)
Description: Second edition. | Chichester, West Sussex ; Ames, Iowa : John
    Wiley & Sons, Inc., 2017. | Includes bibliographical references and index.
Identifiers: LCCN 2016018228 (print) | LCCN 2016018438 (ebook) | ISBN
    9781118976036 (cloth) | ISBN 9781118975930 (pdf) | ISBN 9781118976067
    (epub)
Subjects: | MESH: Cardiovascular Diseases–therapy | Cardiac Surgical
    Procedures | Cardiovascular Diseases–diagnosis
Classification: LCC RD598 (print) | LCC RD598 (ebook) | NLM WG 166 | DDC
    617.4/12–dc23
LC record available at https://lccn.loc.gov/2016018228

A catalogue record for this book is available from the British Library.

Wiley also publishes its books in a variety of electronic formats. Some content that appears in print may not be available in electronic books.

Cover image: Courtesy of the Editors and Associate Editors.

Set in 9/11pt Minion by SPi Global, Pondicherry, India
Printed and bound in Singapore by Markono Print Media Pte Ltd

1   2017

Contents

About the Companion Website

Don't forget to visit the companion website for this book:

www.wiley.com/go/dangas/cardiology

There you will find valuable material designed to enhance your learning, including:
- 19 procedural videos illustrating key procedures
- More than 400 interactive multiple choice questions

Scan this QR code to visit the companion website:

Contributors

Alexandre A.C. Abizaid, MD, PhD
Director, Invasive Cardiology Department
Instituto Dante Pazzanese de Cardiologia (IDPC);
Hospital do Coração—Associação do Sanatório Sírio (HCor);
Hospital Israelita Albert Einstein
São Paulo, Brazil

Tayo Addo, MD
Associate Professor of Medicine
University of Texas Southwestern Medical Center
Dallas, TX, USA

Flavio Airoldi, MD
Director
Interventional Cardiology Unit
IRCCS Multimedica
Sesto San Giovanni, Italy

Dominick J. Angiolillo, MD, PhD
Department of Medicine, Division of Cardiology
University of Florida College of Medicine—Jacksonville
Jacksonville, FL, USA

Kaleab N. Asrress, MA, PhD, MRCP
Department of Cardiology
St. Thomas' Hospital;
King's College London British Heart Foundation Centre of
Excellence
The Rayne Institute, St. Thomas' Hospital
London, UK

Zoë Astroulakis, MBBS, MRCP, PhD
Consultant in Interventional Cardiology
Department of Cardiology, St George's Hospital
London, UK

Usman Baber, MD, MS
Director of Clinical Biometrics
Cardiovascular Institute Assistant Professor of Medicine
Icahn School of Medicine at Mount Sinai
New York, NY, USA

Stephen Balter, PhD
Professor of Radiology and Medicine
Columbia University Medical Center
New York, NY, USA

Subhash Banerjee, MD
Chief of Cardiology
VA North Texas Health Care System;
Professor of Medicine
University of Texas Southwestern Medical Center
Dallas, TX, USA

Adrian P. Banning, MBBS, MD, FRCP, FESC
Consultant Cardiologist
Oxford Heart Centre, Oxford University Hospitals
John Radcliffe Hospital
Oxford, UK

Vinayak N. Bapat, MBBS, MS, FRCS.CTh
Department of Cardiology and Cardiothoracic Surgery
St Thomas' Hospital;
King's College London British Heart Foundation Centre of Excellence
The Rayne Institute, St. Thomas' Hospital
London, UK

Peter Barlis, MBBS, MPH, PHD, FACC, FESC, FRACP
Professor of Medicine
Faculty of Medicine, Dentistry & Health Sciences
The University of Melbourne
Victoria, Australia

Jonathan A. Batty, BSc, MBChB
Institute of Cellular Medicine
Newcastle University;
The Royal Victoria Infirmary
Newcastle upon Tyne NHS Foundation Trust
Newcastle upon Tyne, UK

William Beckerman, MD
Resident in Vascular Surgery
Division of Vascular Surgery
Icahn School of Medicine at Mount Sinai
New York, NY, USA

Stefan C. Bertog, MD
CardioVascular Center Frankfurt
Frankfurt, Germany

Johan L.M. Björkegren, MD, PhD
The Zena and Michael A. Wiener Cardiovascular Institute
and the Department of Genetics & Genomic Sciences
Institute of Genomics and Multiscale Biology
Icahn School of Medicine at Mount Sinai
New York, NY, USA

Carlo Briguori, MD, PhD, FACC, FSCAI
Chief of Interventional Cardiology
Laboratory of Interventional Cardiology and Department of Cardiology
Clinica Mediterranea
Naples, Italy

Emmanouil S. Brilakis, MD, PhD
Minneapolis Heart Institute
Minneapolis, MN, USA;
Professor of Medicine
University of Texas Southwestern Medical Center
Dallas VA Medical Center
Dallas, TX, USA

Eric Brochet, MD
Cardiologist
Echocardiography Laboratory
Department of Cardiology
Hôpital Bichat-Claude Bernard
Paris, France

Giuseppe Bruschi, MD, FESC
Department of Cardiology and Cardiothoracic Surgery
Niguarda Ca' Granda Hospital
Milan, Italy

Gill Louise Buchanan, MBChB
Department of Cardiology
North Cumbria University NHS Trust
Carlisle, UK

David A. Burke, MD
Division of Cardiovascular Medicine, Department of Medicine
Beth Israel Deaconess Medical Center
Harvard Medical School
Boston, MA, USA

Allison K. Cabalka, MD
Division of Pediatric Cardiology
Mayo Clinic College of Medicine
Rochester, MN, USA

Gianluca Caiazzo, MD, PhD
Division of Cardiology, Department of Medical and Surgical Sciences
Magna Graecia University
Catanzaro, Italy;
National Institute of Health Research (NIHR)
Royal Brompton & Harefield NHS Foundation Trust
London, UK

Adriano Caixeta, MD, PhD
Interventional Cardiologist
Hospital Israelita Albert Einstein;
Professor of Medicine
Universidade Federal de São Paulo,
São Paulo, Brazil

Davide Capodanno, MD, PhD
Associate Professor of Cardiology
University of Catania;
Interventional Cardiologist
Ferrarotto Hospital
Catania, Italy

Piera Capranzano, MD
Cardiovascular Department
Ferrarotto Hospital, University of Catania
Catania, Italy

Alain Carpentier, MD, PhD
Hôpital Européen Georges-Pompidou
Paris, France

Fausto Castriota, MD
Maria Cecilia Hospital
GVM Care & Research
Cotignola, Italy

Charles E. Chambers, MD
Professor of Medicine and Radiology
Penn State Hershey Medical Center
Hershey, PA, USA

Kasey Chaszczewski, MD
Rush University Medical Center
Chicago, IL, USA

Gailing Chen, MD
Sinai Center for Thrombosis Research
Cardiac Catheterization Laboratory
Baltimore, MD, USA

Bernard Chevalier, FESC
Institut Cardiovasculaire Paris Sud
Hôpital Privé Jacques Cartier, Massy;
Hôpital Privé Claude Galien
Quincy, France

Alaide Chieffo, MD
Consultant Interventional Cardiologist
Interventional Cardiology Unit
San Raffaele Scientific Hospital
Milan, Italy

Georgios E. Christakopoulos, MD
Research Fellow
VA North Texas Health Care System;
University of Texas Southwestern Medical Center
Dallas, TX, USA

Bimmer E.P.M. Claessen, MD, PhD
Department of Cardiology
Academic Medical Center—University of Amsterdam
Amsterdam, The Netherlands

Rachel E. Clough, MD
University Heart Center Rostock
Department of Internal Medicine
Cardiology, Pulmonology, Intensive Care Medicine
Rostock School of Medicine
Rostock, Germany

Antonio Colombo, MD
Interventional Cardiology Unit
San Raffaele Scientific Hospital
Milan, Italy

Paola Colombo, MD, PhD
Department of Cardiology and Cardiothoracic Surgery
Niguarda Ca' Granda Hospital
Milan, Italy

Christopher J. Cooper, MD
Department of Medicine, Cardiovascular Medicine
University of Toledo
Toledo, OH, USA

J. Ribamar Costa, Jr., PhD
Chief of the Medical Section of Coronary Intervention of the Instituto Dante
Pazzanese de Cardiologia (IDPC);
Hospital do Coração—Associação do Sanatório Sírio (HCor)
São Paulo, Brazil

Pedro R. Cox-Alomar, MD, MPH, FACC
Interventional Cardiology Fellow
Division of Cardiology
University of Florida College of Medicine
UF Health Medical Center
Jacksonville, FL, USA

Alberto Cremonesi, MD
Maria Cecilia Hospital
GVM Care & Research
Cotignola, Italy

George D. Dangas, MD, PhD, FACC, FSCAI, FESC, FAHA
Professor of Medicine
Director, Cardiovascular Innovation
Department of Cardiology
Mount Sinai Medical Center
New York, NY
USA

Justin Davies, BSc, MBBS, MRCP, PhD
Imperial College London
London, UK

Giovanni Luigi De Maria, MD
Oxford Heart Centre, Oxford University Hospitals
John Radcliffe Hospital
Oxford, UK

Ian del Conde, MD, FACC
Miami Cardiac and Vascular Institute
Miami, FL, USA

Carlo Di Mario, MD, PhD, FRCP, FACC, FSCAI, FESC
Consultant Cardiologist
National Institute of Health Research (NIHR)
Royal Brompton & Harefield NHS Foundation Trust, London;
Professor of Clinical Cardiology
National Heart & Lung Institute Imperial College London
London, UK

Michael Donahue, MD
Interventional Cardiologist
Laboratory of Interventional Cardiology and Department of Cardiology
Clinica Mediterranea
Naples, Italy

Jennifer Drury
Physician Assistant
Lenox Hill Heart and Vascular Institute
New York, NY
USA

Gregory Ducrocq, MD
Hôpital Bichat-Claude Bernard
Paris, France

Joseph R. Dunford, MRes
Institute of Cellular Medicine
Newcastle University
Newcastle upon Tyne, UK

Mackram F. Eleid, MD
Division of Cardiovascular Diseases
Mayo Clinic College of Medicine
Rochester, MN, USA

Sebastian Ewen, MD
Klinik für Innere Medizin III
Universitätsklinikum des Saarlandes
Homburg-Saar, Germany

Fabrice Extramiana, MD
Hôpital Bichat-Claude Bernard
Paris, France

Enrico Fabris, MD
Interventional Cardiologist
National Institute of Health Research (NIHR)
Royal Brompton & Harefield NHS Foundation Trust, London;
NHLI Imperial College London
London, UK;
Cardiovascular Department
Ospedali Riuniti and University of Trieste
Trieste, Italy

Peter L. Faries, MD, FACS
The Franz W. Sichel Professor of Surgery
Chief, Division of Vascular Surgery
Professor of Surgery & Radiology
Icahn School of Medicine at Mount Sinai
New York, NY, USA

Amir-Ali Fassa, MD
La Tour Hospital
Geneva, Switzerland

Ted Feldman, MD, FESC, FACC, MSCAI
Director, Cardiac Catheterization Laboratories
Evanston Hospital
NorthShore University HealthSystem
Evanston, IL, USA

Pim J. de Feyter, MD, PhD, FESC, FACC
Professor of Cardiac Imaging
Departments of Cardiology and Radiology
Erasmus MC University Medical Center
Rotterdam, The Netherlands

Farzan Filsoufi, MD
Professor
Department of Cardiovascular Surgery
Icahn School of Medicine at Mount Sinai
New York, NY
USA

Thomas J. Ford, MBChB
Department of Cardiology
St. George Hospital;
Faculty of Medicine
University of New South Wales
Sydney, New South Wales
Australia

Anna Franzone, MD
Department of Cardiology
Bern University Hospital
Bern, Switzerland

Sameer Gafoor, MD
CardioVascular Center Frankfurt
Frankfurt, Germany;
Swedish Medical Center
Seattle, WA, USA

Gyula Gál, MD
Department of Radiology, Section of Neuroradiology
Odense University Hospital
Odense, Denmark

Giuseppe Gargiulo, MD
Cardiovascular Department
Ferrarotto Hospital
University of Catania
Catania, Italy

Philippe Garot, FESC
Institut Cardiovasculaire Paris Sud
Hôpital Privé Jacques Cartier, Massy;
Hôpital Privé Claude Galien
Quincy, France

Philippe Généreux, MD
Clinical Instructor
Division of Cardiology
Center for Interventional Vascular Therapy
Columbia University Medical Center
New York, NY, USA

Bernard J. Gersh, MBChB, DPhil, FACC
Professor of Medicine
Mayo Clinic and Mayo Clinic College of Medicine
Rochester, MN, USA

Anthony Gershlick, MBBS, BSc, FRCP
University of Leicester
Leicester, UK

Joanna Ghobrial, MD, MS
Division of Cardiovascular Medicine
Department of Medicine
Beth Israel Deaconess Medical Center
Harvard Medical School
Boston, MA, USA

Shane Gieowarsingh, MBBS, MET
Maria Cecilia Hospital
GVM Care & Research
Cotignola, Italy

Apoorva Gogna, MBBS, FRCR
Consultant, Interventional Radiology
Singapore General Hospital
Singapore

Iris Q. Grunwald, MD, PhD
Post Graduate Medical Institute
Anglia Ruskin University
Chelmsford, UK;
Southend University Hospital
Southend-on-Sea, UK

Mayra Guerrero, MD, FACC, FSCAI
NorthShore University HealthSystem
Evanston, IL, USA

Leonardo Guimarães, MD
Interventional Cardiologist
Hospital Israelita Albert Einstein;
Universidade Federal de São Paulo
São Paulo, Brazil

Karthik Gujja, MD, MPH
Assistant Professor of Medicine
Icahn School of Medicine at Mount Sinai;
Assistant Director of Endovascular Fellowship
The Zeta and Michael A. Weiner Cardiovascular Institute
Icahn School of Medicine at Mount Sinai
New York, NY, USA

Paul A. Gurbel, MD
Director, Inova Center for Thrombosis
Research and Drug Development
Inova Heart and Vascular Institute
Falls Church, VA, USA

Steven T. Haller, PhD
Department of Medicine
Cardiovascular Medicine
University of Toledo
Toledo, OH, USA

Umair Hayat
Melbourne Medical School
Faculty of Medicine, Dentistry and Health Sciences
The University of Melbourne
Victoria, Australia

Carl Hayward, MB, BChir, MRCP, MA
Cardiology Research Fellow
National Institute of Health Research (NIHR)
Royal Brompton & Harefield NHS Foundation Trust
London, UK

José P.S. Henriques, MD, PhD
Department of Cardiology
Academic Medical Center—University of Amsterdam
Amsterdam, The Netherlands

Ziyad M. Hijazi, MD, MPH, MSCAI
Professor of Pediatrics
Weill Cornell Medicine
Chair, Department of Pediatrics
Sidra Medical and Research Center
Doha, Qatar

Jonathan M. Hill, MD
Department of Cardiology
King's College Hospital NHS Foundation Trust
London, UK

Dominique Himbert, MD
Cardiologist
Department of Cardiology
Hôpital Bichat-Claude Bernard
Paris, France

Ilona Hofmann, MD
CardioVascular Center Frankfurt
Frankfurt, Germany

Ciro Indolfi, MD
Division of Cardiology, Department of Medical
and Surgical Sciences
Magna Graecia University
Catanzaro, Italy

Farouc Amin Jaffer, MD, PhD
Associate Professor
Cardiology Division
Massachusetts General Hospital, Harvard Medical School
Boston, MA, USA

Amit Jain, MD
Lenox Hill Heart and Vascular Institute
New York, NY, USA

Hillary Johnston-Cox, MD, PhD
The Zena and Michael A. Wiener Cardiovascular Institute
and the Department of Genetics & Genomic Sciences
Institute of Genomics and Multiscale Biology
Icahn School of Medicine at Mount Sinai
New York, NY, USA

Brandon M. Jones, MD
Fellow in Cardiovascular Medicine
and Interventional Cardiology
Robert and Suzanne Tomsich Department
of Cardiovascular Medicine
Cleveland Clinic
Cleveland, OH, USA

Samir R. Kapadia, MD
Director, Sones Cardiac Catheterization Laboratory
Section Head, Interventional Cardiology
Professor of Medicine
Robert and Suzanne Tomsich Department of Cardiovascular Medicine
Cleveland Clinic
Cleveland, OH, USA

Vishal Kapur, MD, FACC
Assistant Professor of Cardiology
The Zena and Michael A. Wiener Cardiovascular Institute
Icahn School of Medicine at Mount Sinai
New York, NY, USA

Barry T. Katzen, MD
Miami Cardiac and Vascular Institute
Miami, FL, USA

Upendra Kaul, MD, DM, FCSI, FSCAI, FACC, FAMS
Executive Director and Dean Cardiology
Fortis Escorts Heart Institute
New Delhi, India

Damien Kenny, MB, MD, FACC, FSCAI
Consultant Cardiologist
Our Lady's Children's Hospital
Dublin, Ireland

Ismail Dogu Kilic, MD
Department of Cardiology
Pamukkale University Hospitals
Denizli, Turkey

Annapoorna S. Kini, MD
The Zena and Michael A. Wiener Cardiovascular Institute
The Marie-Josée and Henry R. Kravis Cardiovascular
Health Center
Icahn School of Medicine at Mount Sinai
New York, NY, USA

Jacob S. Koruth, MD
Director, Experimental Lab
Helmsley Electrophysiology Center;
Assistant Professor of Medicine and Cardiology
Mount Sinai Hospital
New York, NY, USA

Jason C. Kovacic, MD, PhD
The Zena and Michael A. Wiener Cardiovascular Institute
The Marie-Josee and Henry R. Kravis Cardiovascular Health Center
Icahn School of Medicine at Mount Sinai
New York, NY, USA

Prakash Krishnan, MD, FACC, FSCAI
Assistant Professor of Medicine-Cardiology and Radiology
Icahn School of Medicine at Mount Sinai;
Director of Endovascular Services
The Zena and Michael A. Weiner Cardiovascular Institute
Icahn School of Medicine at Mount Sinai
New York, NY, USA

Amar Krishnaswamy, MD
Associate Program Director, Interventional Cardiology
Robert and Susan Tomsich Department of Cardiovascular Medicine
Cleveland Clinic
Cleveland, OH, USA

Anna Luisa Kühn, MD, PhD
Department of Radiology
University of Massachusetts Medical School
Worcester, MA, USA

Vijay Kunadian, MBBS, MD, FRCP, FESC, FACC
Institute of Cellular Medicine
Faculty of Medical Sciences, Newcastle University
Newcastle upon Tyne;
Freeman Hospital Newcastle upon Tyne Hospital NHS Foundation Trust
Newcastle upon Tyne, UK

Paul S. Lajos MD, RPVI
Associate Chief of Vascular Surgery
Mount Sinai Queens;
Division of Vascular Surgery
Assistant Professor of Surgery & Radiology
Department of Surgery
The Mount Sinai Hospital
Icahn School of Medicine at Mount Sinai
New York, NY, USA

Omosalewa O. Lalude, MBBS, FACC
Medical Director, Adult Cardiac Imaging
Memorial Healthcare System
Hollywood, FL, USA

Azeem Latib, MBBCh
Interventional Cardiologist
Interventional Cardiology Unit
San Raffaele Scientific Institute
Milan, Italy

Thierry Lefevre, FESC, FSCAI
Institut Cardiovasculaire Paris Sud
Hôpital Privé Jacques Cartier
Massy;
Hôpital Privé Claude Galien
Quincy, France

Stamatios Lerakis, MD, PhD
Professor of Medicine (Cardiology), Radiology and Imaging Sciences
Adjunct Professor of Biomedical Engineering
Emory University School of Medicine and Georgia Institute of Technology
Director of Imaging for the Emory Structural and Valve Heart Center
Director of Cardiac MRI at Emory University Hospital and Emory Clinic
Atlanta, GA, USA

Fang Liu, MD
Sinai Center for Thrombosis Research
Cardiac Catheterization Laboratory
Baltimore, MD, USA

Yves Louvard, FSCAI
Institut Cardiovasculaire Paris Sud
Hôpital Privé Jacques Cartier
Massy;
Hôpital Privé Claude Galien
Quincy, France

Barry Love, MD
Assistant Professor of Pediatrics and Medicine
Icahn School of Medicine
Mount Sinai Medical Center
New York, NY, USA

Akiko Maehara, MD
Columbia University Medical Center;
Cardiovascular Research Foundation
New York, NY, USA

Felix Mahfoud, MD
Klinik für Innere Medizin III
Universitätsklinikum des Saarlandes
Homburg-Saar, Germany;
Harvard-MIT Biomedical Engineering
Institute of Medical Engineering and Science
Cambridge, MA, USA

Francesco Maisano, MD, FESC
Division of Cardiac and Vascular Surgery
University Hospital Zurich
Zurich, Switzerland

C.N. Manjunath, MD, DM
Professor and Head of Department of Cardiology
Sri Jayadeva Institute of Cardiovascular Sciences and Research
Bangalore, India

Michael L. Marin, MD, FACS
The Jacobson Professor of Surgery
Chairman, Department of Surgery
Icahn School of Medicine at Mount Sinai
Surgeon-In-Chief
Mount Sinai Health System
New York, NY, USA

Predrag Matic, MD
CardioVascular Center Frankfurt
Frankfurt, Germany

Alessio Mattesini, MD
Department of Heart and Vessels
AOUC Careggi
Florence, Italy

Roxana Mehran, MD
Department of Cardiology
Mount Sinai Medical Center
New York, NY, USA

Marco G. Mennuni, MD
Interventional Cardiologist
Department of Cardiology
Humanitas Research Hospital
Rozzano, Milan, Italy

Béla Merkely, MD, PhD, DSc
Chairman and Director
Heart and Vascular Center, Semmelweis University
Budapest, Hungary

Stephanie Mick, MD
Department of Cardiovascular Surgery
Cleveland Clinic
Cleveland, OH, USA

Gary S. Mintz, MD
Chief Medical Officer
Columbia University Medical Center;
Cardiovascular Research Foundation
New York, NY, USA

Werner Mohl, MD, PhD
Professor of Surgery
Department of Cardiac Surgery
Medical University of Vienna
Vienna, Austria

Levente Molnár, MD
Assistant Lecturer
Semmelweis University
Budapest, Hungary

Nagaraja Moorthy, MD, DM
Assistant Professor
Department of Cardiology
Sri Jayadeva Institute of Cardiovascular Sciences and Research
Bangalore, India

Katarzyna Nasiadko, MD, MHA
Research Assistant
Icahn School of Medicine at Mount Sinai
New York, NY, USA

Martin K.C. Ng, PhD, MBBS
University of New South Wales Medical School,
The University of Sydney;
Department of Cardiology, Royal Prince Alfred Hospital
Sydney, New South Wales
Australia

Christoph A. Nienaber, MD, PhD
University Heart Center Rostock, Department
of Internal Medicine I
Cardiology, Pulmology, Intensive Care Medicine
Rostock School of Medicine
Rostock, Germany

Sukhjinder Nijjer, BSc, MBChB, MRCP, PhD
Hammersmith Hospital
Imperial College Healthcare NHS Trust
London, UK

Kevin O'Gallagher, BA, MBBS, MRCP
Registrar in Interventional Cardiology
Department of Cardiology, King's College Hospital NHS Foundation Trust
London, UK

Peter O'Kane, MD
Dorset Heart Centre
Royal Bournemouth Hospital
Bournemouth, UK

Yoshinobu Onuma, MD
Research Fellow
Thoraxcenter
Erasmus Medical Center
Rotterdam, The Netherlands

Dagmar Ouweneel, MSc
Department of Cardiology
Academic Medical Center—University of Amsterdam
Amsterdam, The Netherlands

Jorge G. Panizo, MD
Helmsley Electrophysiology Center
Mount Sinai Hospital
New York, NY, USA

Ankit Parikh, MD
Emory University School of Medicine
Atlanta, GA, USA

Sahil A. Parikh, MD, FACC, FSCAI
Assistant Professor of Medicine
Case Western Reserve University School of Medicine
Director, Center for Research and Innovation
Director, Interventional Cardiology Fellowship Program
Director, Experimental Interventional Cardiology Laboratory
University Hospitals Case Medical Center, Harrington Heart & Vascular Institute
Cleveland, OH, USA

Fernando Pastor, MD
Medical Director & Director Cardiac Catheterizations
Laboratory
Instituto Cardiovascular Cuyo
Sanatorio La Merced
Villa Mercedes, Argentina

Hitesh C. Patel, BSc, MB, BS, MRCP
Cardiology Research Fellow
National Institute of Health Research (NIHR)
Royal Brompton & Harefield NHS Foundation Trust
London, UK

Femi Philip, MD
Division of Cardiovascular Medicine
University of California, Davis Medical Center
Sacramento, CA, USA

Raffaele Piccolo, MD
Department of Cardiology
Bern University Hospital
Bern, Switzerland

Michele Pighi, MD
National Institute of Health Research (NIHR)
Royal Brompton & Harefield NHS Foundation Trust
London, UK

Duane S. Pinto, MD, MPH
Division of Cardiovascular Medicine
Department of Medicine
Beth Israel Deaconess Medical Center
Harvard Medical School
Boston, MA, USA

Stuart J. Pocock, PhD
Professor and Chair
London School of Hygiene and Tropical Medicine
University of London
London, UK

Abhiram Prasad, MD, FRCP, FESC, FACC
Professor of Interventional Cardiology
St George's, University of London
London, UK

Patrizia Presbitero, MD
Senior Consultant in Interventional Cardiology
Department of Cardiology
Humanitas Research Hospital
Rozzano, Milan, Italy

Francesca Pugliese, MD
Erasmus MC University Medical Center
Rotterdam, The Netherlands

Gopi Punukollu, MD
Interventional Cardiology
Lenox Hill Hospital (North Shore LIJ)
New York, NY, USA

Robert Pyo, MD
Montefiore Medical Center
Albert Einstein College of Medicine
New York, NY, USA

Simon R. Redwood, MB, BS, MD, FRCP, FACC
Professor of Interventional Cardiology
Consultant Interventional Cardiologist
Department of Cardiology
St. Thomas' Hospital;
King's College London British Heart Foundation Centre of Excellence
The Rayne Institute, St Thomas' Hospital
London, UK

Markus Reinartz, MD
CardioVascular Center Frankfurt
Frankfurt, Germany;
Herz-Jesu-Krankenhaus
Dernbach, Germany

Charanjit S. Rihal, MD, MBA
Division of Cardiovascular Diseases
Mayo Clinic College of Medicine
Rochester, MN, USA

Jason H. Rogers, MD
Director, Interventional Cardiology
Division of Cardiovascular Medicine
University of California, Davis Medical Center
Sacramento, CA, USA

Robert J. Rosen, MD
Lenox Hill Heart and Vascular Institute
New York, NY, USA

Cristina Sanina, MD
Postdoctoral Fellow, ISCI
University of Miami Miller School of Medicine
Miami, FL, USA

Saurabh Sanon, MD, FACC
Division of Cardiovascular Diseases
Mayo Clinic College of Medicine
Rochester, MN, USA

Mohammad Sarraf, MD
NorthShore University HealthSystem
Evanston, IL, USA

Mikkel Malby Schoos, MD, PhD
Department of Cardiology
Zealand University Hospital
Denmark

P. Christian Schulze, MD, PhD
Department of Internal Medicine I
Division of Cardiology, Angiology
Pneumology and Intensive Medical Care
Friedrich-Schiller-University Jena
Jena, Germany

Gioel Gabrio Secco, MD, PhD
Interventional Cardiologist
Department of Cardiology
Santi Antonio e Biagio e Cesare Arrigo Hospital
Alessandria, Italy

Roberta Serdoz, MD
National Institute of Health Research (NIHR)
Royal Brompton & Harefield NHS Foundation Trust, London;
NHLI Imperial College London
London, UK

Patrick W. Serruys, MD, PhD
Faculty of Medicine
National Heart & Lung Institute
Imperial College London
London, UK

Samin K. Sharma, MD
The Zena and Michael A. Wiener Cardiovascular Institute
The Marie-Josée and Henry R. Kravis Cardiovascular Health Center
Icahn School of Medicine at Mount Sinai
New York, NY, USA

Mehdi H. Shishehbor, DO, MPH, PhD
Director, Endovascular Services
Associate Program Director
Interventional Cardiology
Heart & Vascular Institute
Cleveland Clinic
Cleveland, OH, USA

Horst Sievert, MD, PhD
CardioVascular Center Frankfurt
Frankfurt, Germany;
Anglia Ruskin University
Chelmsford
Essex, UK

Ulrich Sigwart
Emeritus Professor
Geneva University Hospitals
Geneva, Switzerland

Dimytri Alexandre Siqueira, MD, PhD
Dante Pazzanese Institute of Cardiology
São Paulo, Brazil

Alex Sirker, MA (Cantab), MB, BChir, MRCP, PhD
Consultant in Interventional Cardiology
Department of Cardiology, UCLH and St Bartholomew's Hospital
London, UK

Steven R. Steinhubl, MD
Scripps Translational Science Institute
San Diego, CA, USA

Neil Swanson, MBChB
University of Leicester
Leicester, UK

Corrado Tamburino, MD, PhD
Professor of Cardiology
University of Catania;
Director, Cardio-Thoracic-Vascular Department
Ferrarotto Hospital
Catania, Italy

Manish Taneja, MBBS, FRCR
Specialist in Interventional Radiology and Interventional Neuroradiology
Raffles Hospital, Singapore

Udaya S. Tantry, PhD
Director, Thrombosis Research Lab
Inova Center for Thrombosis Research and Drug Development
Inova Heart and Vascular Institute
Falls Church, VA, USA

Arthur Tarricone, BS
Senior Associate Researcher
Icahn School of Medicine at Mount Sinai
New York, NY, USA

Vikas Thondapu
Melbourne Medical School
Faculty of Medicine, Dentistry and Health Sciences
The University of Melbourne
Victoria, Australia

Matthew I. Tomey, MD
Assistant Professor of Medicine (Cardiology)
The Zena and Michael A. Wiener Cardiovascular Institute, and The Marie-Josée and Henry R. Kravis Cardiovascular Health Center
Icahn School of Medicine at Mount Sinai
New York, NY, USA

Tim Tsay
Melbourne Medical School
Faculty of Medicine, Dentistry and Health Sciences
The University of Melbourne
Victoria, Australia

E. Murat Tuzcu, MD
Professor of Medicine, Interventional Cardiology
Chief Academic Officer
Chief, Department of Cardiovascular Medicine
Cleveland Clinic
Abu Dhabi, United Arab Emirates

Alec Vahanian, MD, FESC, FACC
Head of Cardiology
Hôpital Bichat-Claude Bernard
Paris, France

Laura Vaskelyte, MD
CardioVascular Center Frankfurt
Frankfurt, Germany

Gerald S. Werner, MD, PhD, FACC, FSCAI, FESC
Professor of Cardiology and Director
Medizinische Klinik I (Cardiology & Intensive Care)
Klinikum Darmstadt GmbH
Darmstadt, Germany

Jose M. Wiley, MD, MPH, FACC, FACP, FSCAI
Associate Professor of Clinical Medicine
Albert Einstein College of Medicine
Director of Endovascular Interventions
Division of Cardiology
Montefiore Einstein Center for Heart & Vascular Care
Bronx, NY, USA

Stephan Windecker, MD
Department of Cardiology
Bern University Hospital
Bern, Switzerland

Kun Xiang, MD, PhD
Department of Medicine, Cardiovascular Medicine
University of Toledo
Toledo, OH, USA

Luiz Fernando Ybarra, MD
Interventional Cardiologist
Hospital Israelita Albert Einstein;
Universidade Federal de São Paulo
São Paulo, Brazil

Gregory W. Yost, DO
Department of Cardiology
Geisinger Medical Center
Danville, PA, USA

Mark Shipeng Yu, MD
Department of Medicine, Cardiovascular Medicine
University of Toledo
Toledo, OH, USA

Foreword

The development of interventional cardiology has followed the evolutionary trend of internal medicine. After World War II and during the latter part of the twentieth century, the number of subspecialties in the field of Internal Medicine exploded. The "Great Internal Medicine" became Cardiology, Pneumonology, Gastroenterology, Endocrinology, and so on.

Interventional cardiology was originally created by Andreas Grüntzig when, for the first time in a conscious patient, he applied the technique of percutaneous transluminal angioplasty: the whole intervention consisted of "inflating" a balloon inside the narrowed section of a coronary artery. It took almost two decades to diversify the approach of the percutaneous treatment of coronary artery disease with devices such as directional atherectomy, rotational atherectomy, and stenting.

The ground-breaking work in congenital treatment, the first pulmonary balloon angioplasty, the first closure of an atrial septum defect, almost went unnoticed by the "mature" interventional cardiologist. It was not until Alain Cribier's pioneering work that the field of adult valvular intervention ushered in the specialty of interventional cardiology outside the coronary arteries.

In the 1990s the term TCT was coined (transcatheter treatment) and this further evolved into the concept of percutaneous coronary intervention (PCI), which today englobes and comprises intracranial treatment, carotid treatment, aortic arch reconstruction, descending aorta, femoral, popliteal, pedal artery, most of the congenital abnormalities including ASD, VSD, patent ductus arteriosus, and also left atrial appendage and most recently the extraordinary explosion of devices to treat aortic stenosis, aortic regurgitation, and mitral valve stenosis … as well as others such as the alcoholization of the interventricular septum in hypertrophic cardiomyopathy.

As a consequence of this diversification, we see highly specialized doctors in interventional cardiology, who dedicate their time to total chronic occlusion, bifurcation, aortic stenosis with TAVR, mitral clips, mitral valve replacement, and so on.

What is striking is that the development of a highly specialized subspecialty requires an in-depth knowledge of very specific details to efficiently and safely perform these interventions. For instance, the transseptal punctures for left appendage closure or clip implantation are quite different and necessitate 3D imaging online with precise measurement in 3D dimension of the site of the puncture, which has to be a few millimeters below, above, at the back, in the front of the septum, and so on. Thus, the new generation gets involved in a very granular analysis of the syndromes, techniques, type of lesion, and type of imaging, and may, at some point, lose the "helicopter view of the field." Therefore we must commend the editors of the second edition of the *Interventional Cardiology* for having a very broad and wide description of the field, which is an increasingly challenging endeavor.

It would be easy to be laudative about the content. It is apparent that all the authors have done their utmost to cover the field. It is always very challenging to start and maintain a so-called "textbook." In my personal experience as an editor/co-editor of 42 (text) books; I can frankly say that a textbook in the field is a most exacting activity, in the sense that only a few great names have been able to repeat the experience multiple times during their lifetime and their textbook became such a historical entity that the baton was taken up by other people.

So once more I can only congratulate the editors for having conceived, constructed, and finalized the expanded second edition of this textbook. A textbook is a matter of endurance and repetition, and while it might be easy to criticize the content, the real question is this: will these three magnificent editors be able to continue the work of updating their textbook throughout their careers, because that's what really gives a sense of purpose to a textbook. I sincerely hope that they will.

Patrick W. Serruys, MD, PhD
January 2016

Preface

There is no doubt that our specialty has been expanding in every direction at a fast pace in recent years. Just in the 5 years since publication of the first edition of *Interventional Cardiology*, almost its entire content has been revised extensively. The updated edition includes not only current data and critical new information on the most important subjects, but also introduces new subspecialties that have been developing in the intervening years. Additionally, specialists from other areas of medicine and surgery are taking part in the treatment of patients with interventional, percutaneous, minimally invasive methods and techniques. The technological advances are vast and highlight the overall growth of cardiovascular interventions.

In this edition, we have been fortunate to have a group of internationally recognized authorities in many fields contributing chapters describing the use of these techniques in a wide range of cardiovascular diseases.

Accordingly, we have expanded considerably the second edition of this textbook to cover four major sections: coronary interventions, interventional pharmacology, structural heart interventions, and endovascular therapy. We believe that the reader will find this approach useful and practical. Each section includes key subjects presented in an organized way: starting with the pathophysiological background and relevant pathology, followed by mechanisms of treatment, device description, procedural techniques, follow-up care, risks, contraindications, and complications, where applicable. The inclusion of multiple choice questions with each online chapter allows both self-assessment as well as completion of accredited learning hours.

The modular presentation of this textbook, both as a printed book, and as an e-book CD-ROM or web-based program reflects the efforts of the publisher and the editors to reach out to many generations of physicians in training. The evolution of specialty certification and recertification has indeed made life learning a reality in our era. Therefore, the present textbook must also fulfill the quest to approach the new and tech-savvy learner, those ahead of an initial certification examination, those in advanced clinical practice who need practical instruction for a certain specialized subject, as well as those who have been practicing for a long time and need to refresh their knowledge with or without a recertification examination ahead of them. We have tried our best, and we certainly hope the reader will concur.

George D. Dangas
Carlo Di Mario
Nicholas N. Kipshidze

Acknowledgments

In a time when interventional cardiology has become too complex to be mastered by one or even three individuals, we decided to involve the best scholars in the field to cover the various topics of this book: without their help we could not have achieved this final result.

Our masters have taught us more than to push catheters. They made us love our profession and love teaching: we are delighted that many of them also contributed to this textbook.

Our Fellows have told us with their questions and doubts that not everything can be found in the many existing textbooks and the Internet. They inspired us to embark on this endeavor and acted as a continuous source of inspiration to draw enough attention to practical details.

Finally, we have neglected our spouses and children to spend long hours in front of a computer screen. We are confident that our wives already understand us and we hope one day our children will see this textbook on the shelves of the family library, read some pages, and forgive us.

George D. Dangas
Carlo Di Mario
Nicholas N. Kipshidze

PART I

Principles and Techniques

CHAPTER 1

Atherogenesis and Inflammation

Umair Hayat[1], Vikas Thondapu[1], Tim Tsay[1], and Peter Barlis[2]

[1] Melbourne Medical School, The University of Melbourne, Australia
[2] The University of Melbourne, Australia

Atherosclerosis and its clinical consequences are the leading cause of death in Western nations [1]. Several factors have been implicated in the evolution, progression, and destabilization of atherosclerotic plaque highlighting its multifaceted nature. Atherosclerosis, now considered a chronic inflammatory disease, begins at a young age and progresses slowly for decades [2–4]. The clinical symptoms of atheroma occur in adults and usually involve plaque rupture and thrombosis [5–7].

While several advances have helped curb some of the complications resulting from atherosclerosis, this disease still represents an ongoing challenge with several new insights raising optimism that help to improve clinical outcomes is at hand. This chapter reviews the pathogenesis of atherosclerosis and the inflammatory cascades leading to plaque progression and destabilization. New coronary imaging modalities and developments in computer modeling are critiqued as tools to help improve the understanding of cardiovascular diseases.

Pathogenesis of atherosclerosis

Atherosclerosis is an inflammatory fibro-proliferative process in which plaque forms in the intima, bringing about stenosis or thrombosis and hence ischemia [8–10]. Though the exact initiator of plaque formation remains unknown, there is a general consensus that the triggering episode is endothelial damage, which could be caused by factors such as cigarette smoke toxins, hypertension, or immune injury [4,11–15]. Damaged cells become more permeable, ultimately causing subendothelial macrophages to consume circulating low density lipoproteins (LDL) which are altered in the intima to induce further endothelial damage [8,9,16]. More macrophages are then recruited, after which they remain in the intima as lipid-rich foam cells [9,10,17–19]. Meanwhile, in an attempt to restore endothelial function, smooth muscle cells migrate from the media to the intima to proliferate and generate a connective tissue matrix to cap the lipid core, further thickening the lesion [8,19,20]. Plaques enlarge as the process becomes chronic, classified as stable or unstable (Figures 1.1 and 1.2), either of which can lead to clinical sequelae [8,17,21].

Clinical features

The first indication of coronary artery disease (CAD) may be sudden death, or patients can present with silent ischemia, stable angina, or an acute coronary syndrome (ACS) [22]. ACSs comprise a range of syndromes resulting from atherosclerotic plaque disruption or rupture and are divided into unstable angina (UA), non-ST-elevation myocardial infarction (NSTEMI), and ST-elevation myocardial infarction (STEMI) [21,23,24]. An unstable plaque, characterized by a large lipid core covered by a thin and unstable fibrous cap, is prone to rupture [21,25–27]. The sudden rupture can cause thrombus formation, in turn leading to ACS (Figure 1.2) [26,28,29]. Conversely, a stable plaque has a thick fibrous cap which is not easily ruptured (Figure 1.1), causing the chronic condition of stable angina through episodes of ischemia experienced upon physical exertion [25,27,30].

Consequences of atherosclerosis

The risk of major thrombotic and thromboembolic complications of atherosclerosis appears to be related more to the stability of atheromatous plaques than to the extent of disease [31,32]. Stable angina is associated with smooth fibrous coronary artery plaques (stable plaque), whereas unstable angina, acute myocardial infarction (AMI), and sudden cardiac death are almost invariably associated with destabilization of plaques [29]. Similarly, in patients with carotid artery atherosclerotic disease, plaque irregularity and rupture are closely associated with cerebral ischemic events, and patients with irregular or ulcerated plaque demonstrate a higher risk of ischemic stroke irrespective of the degree of luminal stenosis [33].

Much attention has been placed on trying to identify plaques at high risk of disruption leading to thrombosis. Such "vulnerable plaques" have also been areas of intense research using novel intracoronary imaging modalities: optical coherence tomography (OCT) [6,29]. OCT offers the advantages over intravascular ultrasound or angiography of ultra-high resolution and superiority in imaging the vessel wall and lumen interface [34–36].

Interventional Cardiology: Principles and Practice, Second Edition. Edited by George D. Dangas, Carlo Di Mario, and Nicholas N. Kipshidze.
© 2017 John Wiley & Sons, Ltd. Published 2017 by John Wiley & Sons, Ltd.

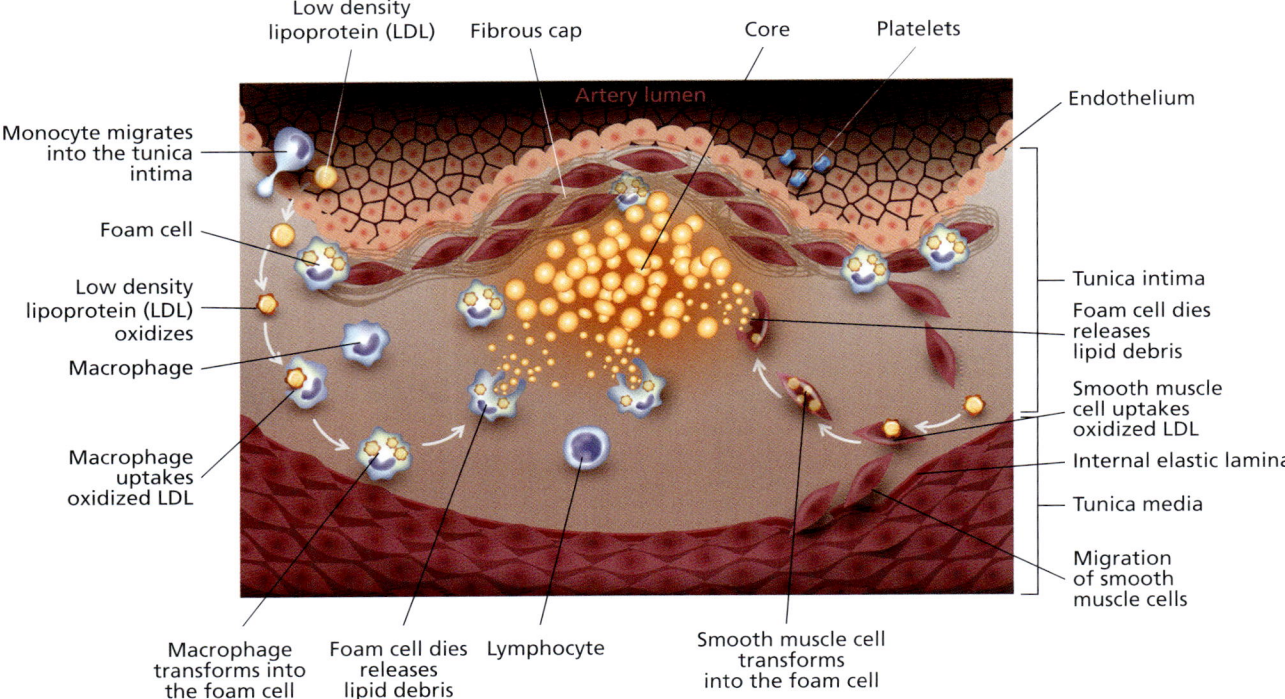

Figure 1.1 Stable atherosclerotic plaque characterized by the presence of a low inflammatory infiltrate. This type of lesion is constituted by a lipid core (extracellular lipid, cholesterol crystals, and necrotic debris) covered by a *thick* fibrous cap consisting principally of smooth muscle cells (SMC) in a collagenous–proteoglycan matrix, with varying degrees of infiltration by macrophages and T lymphocytes. HDL, high density lipoprotein.

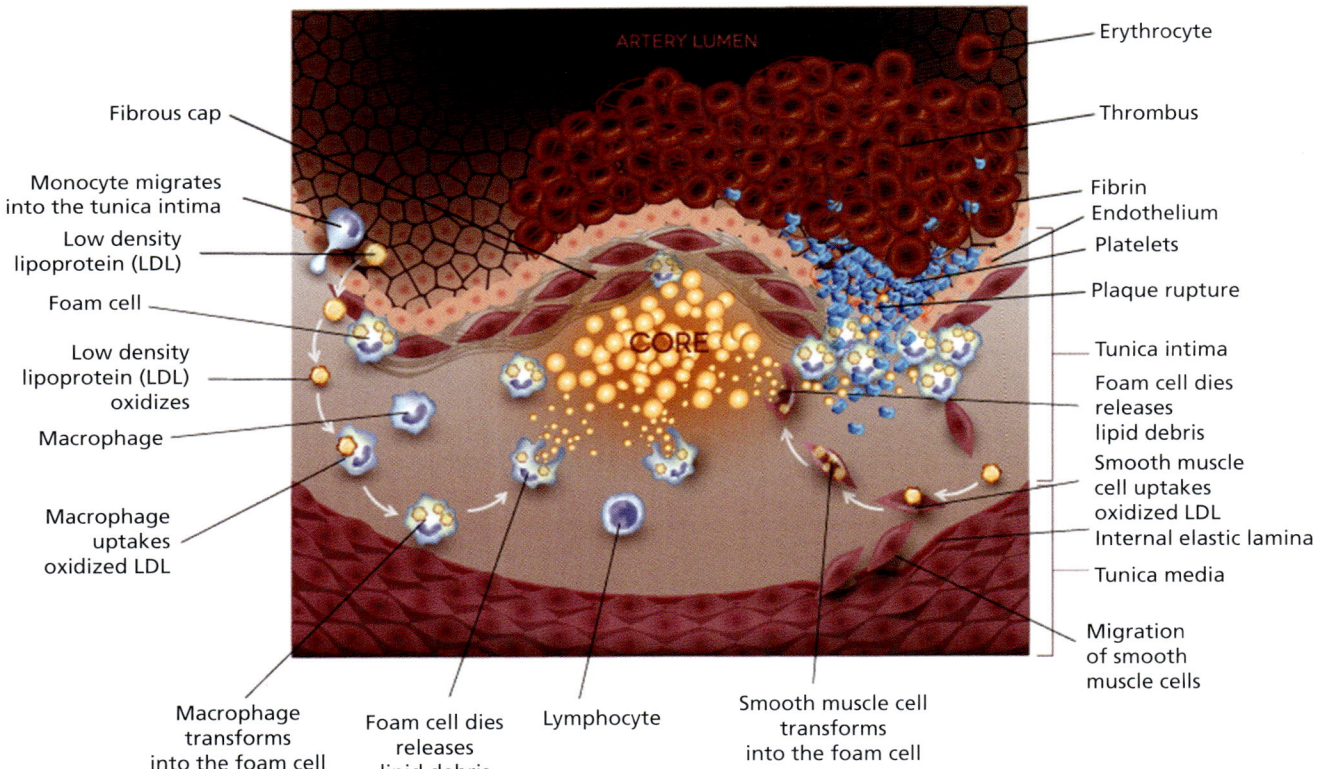

Figure 1.2 Unstable atherosclerotic plaque characterized by the presence of a *thin* fibrous cap rich in inflammatory macrophagic foam cells and T lymphocytes. Rupture of the fibrous cap at the shoulder region has resulted in thrombus formation.

Considerable data exist to sustain the hypothesis that several morphologic and molecular markers identifying unstable plaques could be expressed during plaque vulnerability. As shown by a number of anatomical and clinical studies, these vulnerable plaques are more often associated with rupture and thrombosis than stable plaques covered by a thin fibrous cap and show an extensive inflammatory infiltrate [28,37].

Unlike the stable plaque that shows a chronic inflammatory infiltrate, the vulnerable and ruptured plaque is characterized by features of acute inflammation [37,38]. There are a large number of studies showing that "active" inflammation mainly involves T lymphocytes and macrophages which are activated toward a pathway of inflammatory response, secrete cytokines and lytic enzymes which in turn cause thinning of the fibrous cap, predisposing to plaque rupture. Recent research has furnished new insight into the molecular mechanisms that cause transition from a stable to an unstable phase of atherosclerosis and points to inflammation as the playmaker in the events leading to plaque destabilization and suggest that alterations in shear stress may also play a pivotal part [39,40].

A current challenge is to identify morphological and molecular markers able to discriminate stable plaques from vulnerable ones allowing the stratification of "high risk" patients for acute cardiac and cerebrovascular events before clinical syndromes develop. Bearing this aim in mind, this chapter focuses on cellular and molecular mechanisms affecting plaque progression and serum markers correlated to plaque inflammation.

Insights from coronary imaging

Traditionally, coronary angiography has been the gold standard to detect extent and severity of CAD. These findings form the foundation of the interventionist's clinical decision-making process and whether to proceed to percutaneous therapy. It is widely acknowledged, however, that angiography has several limitations. First, it maintains a relatively low image resolution. Second, it represents a luminogram of the artery and stenosis. Therefore little detail is provided as to the composition of the underlying plaque causing the stenosis and, finally, it is a 2D imaging method used to assess what are complex 3D structures.

Intravascular ultrasound

Intravascular ultrasound (IVUS) utilizes ultrasound waves that reflect off vascular tissues to yield real-time images [41,42]. While angiography only portrays a luminal silhouette [41], IVUS, with a resolution of 100–150 µm, captures details not retrievable with angiography—cross-sections of the lumen and vessel wall, even a differentiation of its layers [43–46]. Thus, IVUS enables study of the atherosclerotic process through the visualization of plaque in the vessel wall [41,47–49]. Indeed, the technology has demonstrated a greater prevalence of atherosclerosis than initially claimed with angiography [44].

Optical coherence tomography

OCT, the optical analog of IVUS, employs the reflection of near-infrared (NIR) light instead of sound. Initially applied in ophthalmology, advancement in the technology has now enabled OCT to capture non-transparent tissues such as coronary vessels [50,51]. OCT offers real-time, *in vivo* and *in situ* cross-sectional imaging of vascular structures with a resolution 10-fold that of IVUS (15 µm versus 150 µm) and a penetration depth similar to that of histology [34,43,50–53].

By virtue of its superior resolution, OCT can provide near-histological analysis of atherosclerotic plaques in real time (Figure 1.3). OCT definition of thin cap fibroatheroma (TCFA) follows the findings of autopsy studies of sudden death patients that had revealed the presence of fibrous caps <65 µm in the majority of plaques that had ruptured. These thin ruptured caps were also found to have an infiltrate of macrophages [54]. Whereas OCT is well placed in precisely defining the thinness of fibrous cap, macrophage infiltration seen as punctate, signal-rich spots at the junction of fibrous cap and lipid pool has been described less consistently. Previous autopsy studies had also shown that plaque rupture, erosion, and calcified nodules were the three leading underlying mechanisms for luminal thrombosis with a frequency of 65%, 30%, and 5%, respectively [25]. In recent years OCT has enabled this type of information to be obtained *in vivo* and has confirmed similar prevalence of plaque morphologies in patients presenting with STEMI and NSTEMI [55].

Plaque rupture on OCT is identified by a clear-cut disruption in the signal-rich thin fibrous cap overlying a signal-poor necrotic core resulting in extrusion of highly thrombogenic material into the lumen. Plaque erosion on the other hand is identified by the presence of luminal thrombus adjacent to a plaque that has an irregular but intact, thicker fibrous cap. Such plaques are mostly devoid of necrotic core. Calcified nodules are the least common etiology in ACS and are less well defined. They are recognized by sharp nodules protruding into the lumen causing discontinuation of the fibrous cap (Figure 1.4).

In patients with stable CAD, coronary imaging can provide lesion level information and help to show the changes in plaque microstructure in response to pharmacotherapies. Kataoka *et al.* [56] evaluated 293 and 122 lipid and fibrous plaques in 280 stable statin-treated patients with CAD and reported that patients with LDL-C levels <50 mg/dL were less likely to have lipid plaques, and had more features of plaque stability such as thicker fibrous caps and smaller lipid arcs.

The vulnerable plaque

Atherosclerotic lesions, according to the classification of the American Heart Association modified by Virmani *et al.* [29], are divided in two groups: (i) non-atherosclerotic intimal lesions and (ii) progressive atherosclerotic lesions which include stable, vulnerable, and thrombotic plaques.

The different pathologic characterization of atherosclerotic lesions largely depends on the thickness of the fibrous cap and its grade of inflammatory infiltrate, which is in turn largely constituted by macrophages and activated T lymphocytes. Typically, the accumulating plaque burden is initially accommodated by an adaptive positive remodeling with expansion of the vessel external elastic lamina and minimal changes in lumen size [57,58]. The plaque contains monocyte-derived macrophages, smooth muscle cells, and T lymphocytes. Interaction between these cells types and the connective tissue appears to determine the development and progression of the plaque itself, including important complications such as thrombosis and rupture.

The lesions classified as vulnerable or TCFA identify a plaque prone to rupture and thrombosis characterized by a large necrotic core containing numerous cholesterol clefts. The overlying cap is thin and rich in inflammatory cells, macrophages, and T lymphocytes with few smooth muscle cells [28,29,59]. Burke *et al.* [54] identified a cut-off value for cap thickness of 65 µm to define a vulnerable coronary plaque. Despite the predominant hypothesis

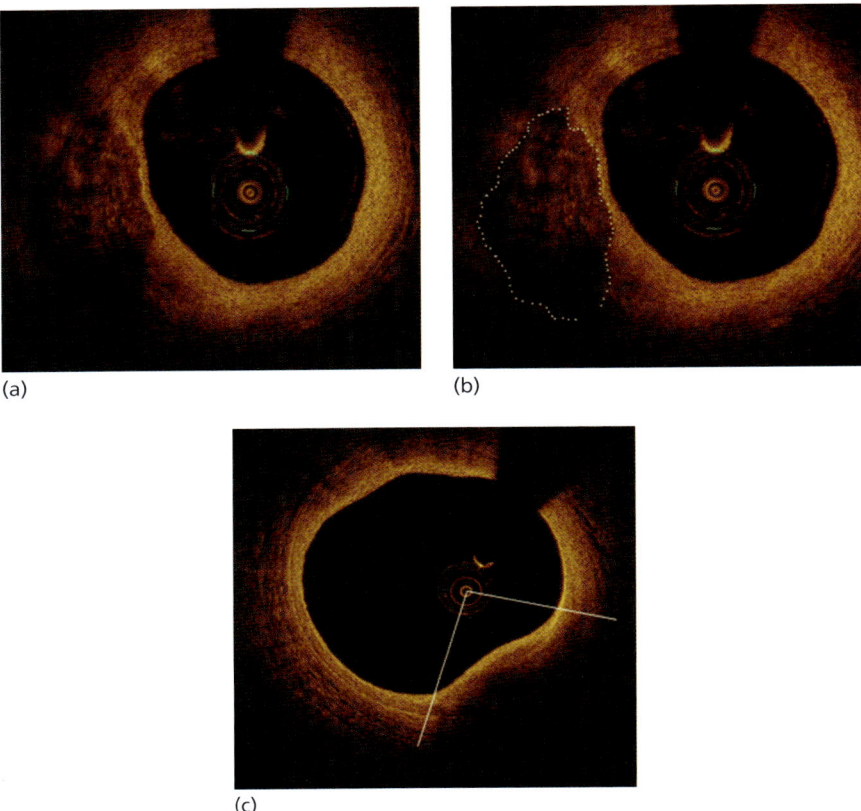

Figure 1.3 Stable coronary plaques seen on optical coherence tomography (OCT). (a) Calcified plaque is seen at 7- to 10 o'clock position. It is characterized by sharply delineated borders and heterogeneous core. (b) Calcified plaque is outlined with white dotted line. (c) Lipid-rich plaque marked by white lines. It is characterized by dark, signal-poor core with ill-defined margins and a bright thick fibrous cap (>65 µm). As the light rapidly attenuates through the necrotic core, OCT cannot be used to measure the depth of such plaques.

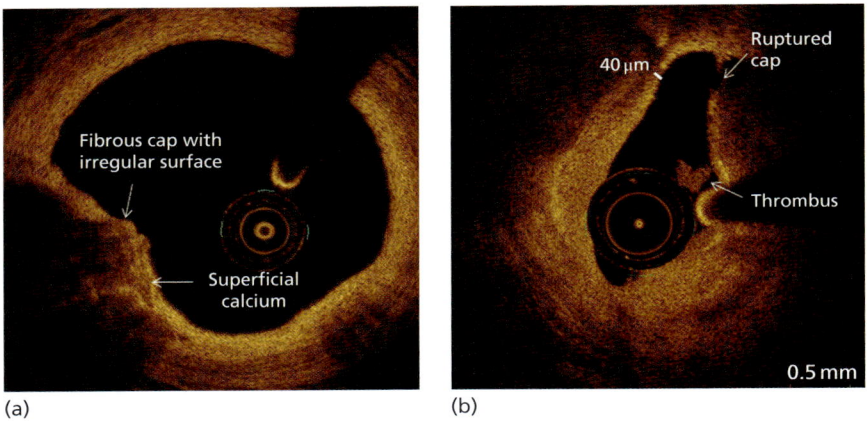

Figure 1.4 Unstable coronary plaques seen on OCT. (a) Plaque erosion: intact fibrous cap with irregular luminal surface and superficial calcium. (b) Plaque rupture with luminal thrombus. At the 11 o'clock position a thin cap fibro-atheroma (TCFA) is seen (fibrous cap thickness measured 40 µm, marked with small white bar).

focusing on the responsibility of a specific vulnerable atherosclerotic plaque rupture [5,7] for acute coronary syndromes, some pathophysiologic, clinical, and angiographic observations seem to suggest the possibility that the principal cause of coronary instability is not to be found in the vulnerability of a single atherosclerotic plaque, but in the presence of multiple vulnerable plaques in the entire coronary tree, correlated with the presence of a diffuse inflammatory process [37,38,60,61].

Within this context, recent angiographic studies have demonstrated the presence of multiple vulnerable atheromatous plaques in patients with unstable angina [20,62] and in those affected by transmural myocardial infarction [61]. Recently, by means of flow cytometry Spagnoli *et al.* [38] have demonstrated the presence of an activated and multicentric inflammatory infiltrate in the coronary vessels of individuals who died of AMI. Similar results have been obtained by Buffon *et al.* [60], who, through the determination of the neutrophil myeloperoxidase activity, have proved the presence of a diffuse inflammation in the coronary vessels in individuals affected by unstable angina. These results have been confirmed by a morphological study which demonstrated the presence of a high inflammatory infiltrate constituted by macrophages and T lymphocytes activated in the whole coronary tree, also present in the stable plaques of individuals who died of AMI. These plaques showed a two- to fourfold higher inflammatory infiltrate than aged-matched individuals dying from non-cardiac causes with chronic stable angina (SA) or without clinical cardiac history (CTRL), respectively [37]. Moreover, it has also been demonstrated that activated T lymphocytes infiltrate the myocardium both in the peri-infarcted area and in remote unaffected myocardial regions in patients who died of a first myocardial infarction [63].

The simultaneous occurrence of diffuse coronary and myocardial inflammation in these patients further supports the concept that both coronary and myocardial vulnerabilities concur in the pathogenesis of fatal AMI.

AMI—at least associated with unfavorable prognosis—is therefore likely to be the consequence of a diffuse "active" chronic inflammatory process which determines the destabilization of both the entire coronary tree and the whole myocardium, not only the part of it affected by infarction. The causes of the diffuse inflammation associated with myocardial infarction are scarcely known. The presence of activated T lymphocytes suggests the "*in situ*" presence of an antigenic stimulus which triggers adaptive immunity.

Role of inflammation in the natural history of atherosclerosis
Inception of the plaque
Endothelium injury has been proposed to be an early and clinically relevant pathophysiologic event in the atherosclerotic process [4,32]. Patients with endothelial dysfunction have an increased risk for future cardiovascular events including stroke [64]. Endothelial dysfunction was described as the ignition step in atherogenesis. From this point on, an inflammatory response leads to the development of the plaque.

Endothelial damage can be caused by physical and chemical forces, by infective agents or by oxidized LDL (ox-LDL). Dysfunctional endothelium expresses P-selectin (stimulation by agonists such as thrombin) and E-selectin (induced by IL-1 or TNF-α). Expression of intercellular adhesion molecule-1 (ICAM-1) both by macrophages and endothelium and vascular adhesion molecule-1 (VCAM-1) by endothelial cells is induced by inflammatory cytokines such as interleukin-1 (IL-1), tumor necrosis factor-1 (TNF-α), and γ-interferon (IFNγ).

Monocytes recalled in the subintimal space ingest lipoproteins and morph into macrophages. These generate reactive oxygen species (ROS), which convert ox-LDL into highly oxidized LDL. Macrophages upload ox-LDL via scavenger receptors until foam cells form. Foam cells with leukocytes migrate at the site of damage and generate the fatty streak. The loss of biologic activity of endothelium determines nitric oxide (NO) reduction together with increased expression of prothrombotic factors, proinflammatory adhesion molecules cytokines, and chemotactic factors. Cytokines may decrease NO bioavailability increasing the production of ROS. ROS

reduces NO activity both directly, reacting with endothelial cells, and indirectly via oxidative modification of eNOS or guanylyl cyclase [65]. Low NO bioavailability can upregulate VCAM-1 in the endothelial cell layer that binds monocytes and lymphocytes in the first step of invasion of the vascular wall, via induction of nuclear factor κB (NFκB) expression [66]. In addition, NO inhibits leukocyte adhesion [67] and NO reduction results in induction of monocyte chemotactic protein-1 (MCP-1) expression which recruits monocytes [68]. NO is in a sensitive balance with endothelin-1 (ET-1) regulating vascular tone [69]. Plasma ET-1 concentrations are increased in patients with advanced atherosclerosis and correlate with the severity of the disease [70,71]. In addition to its vasoconstrictor activity, ET-1 also promotes leukocyte adhesion [72] and thrombus formation [73]. Dysfunctional endothelium expresses P-selectin (stimulation by agonists such as trombin) and E-selectin (induced by IL-1 or TNF-α) [74]. The expression of both ICAM-1 by macrophages and endothelium, and VCAM-1 by endothelial cells is induced by inflammatory cytokines such as IL-1, TNF-α, and IFNγ. Endothelial cells also produce monocyte chemotactic protein-1 (MCP-1), monocyte colony-stimulating factor, and IL-6 which further amplify the inflammatory cascade [75]. IL-6 production by smooth muscle cells represents the main stimulus for C-reactive protein (CRP) production [3]. Recent evidence suggests that CRP may contribute to the proinflammatory state of the plaque both mediating recruitment of monocytes and stimulating monocytes to release IL-1, IL-6, and TNF-α [76]. The damaged endothelium allows the passage of lipids into the subendothelial space. Fatty streaks represent the first step in the atherosclerotic process.

Evolving fibro-atheromatous plaque
The atheroma evolution is modulated by innate and adaptive immune responses [3,77,78]. The most important receptors for innate immunity in atherothrombosis are the scavenger receptors and the toll-like receptors (TLRs) [79]. Adaptive immunity is much more specific than innate immunity but may take several days or even weeks to become fully mobilized. It involves an organized immune response leading to generation of T- and B-cell receptors and immunoglobulins, which can recognize foreign antigens [80].

Stable plaque
Macrophages take up lipid deposited in the intima via a number of receptors, including scavenger receptor-A, and CD36. Deregulated uptake of modified LDL through scavenger receptors leads to cholesterol accumulation and "foam cell" formation. The lipid laden macrophages (foam cells) forming the fatty streak secrete proinflammatory cytokines that amplify the local inflammatory response in the lesion, matrix metalloproteinases (MMPs), tissue factor into the local matrix, as well as growth factors, which stimulate the smooth muscle replication responsible for lesion growth. Macrophages colony-stimulating factor (M-CSF) acts as the main stimulator in this process, next to granulocyte–macrophage stimulating factor (MGGM-CSF) and IL-2 for lymphocytes [81]. Lymphocytes enter the intima by binding adhesion molecules: VCAM-1, P-selectin, ICAM-1, MCP-1 (CCL2), IL-8 (CxCL8) [75]. Such infiltrate constituted mainly by CD4+ T lymphocytes recognize antigens bound to MHC class II molecules involved in antigen presentation to T lymphocytes thus provoking an immune response [2]. The major histocompatibility complex molecules (MHC II) are expressed by endothelial cells, macrophages, and vascular smooth muscle cells in proximity to activated T lymphocytes in the atherosclerotic plaque. Proinflammatory cytokines manage a central transcriptional control

point mainly mediated by NFκB. Macrophage/foam cells produce cytokines that activate neighboring smooth-muscle cells (SMCs), resulting in extracellular matrix production [2].

Repeated inflammatory stimuli induce foam cells to secrete growth factors that induce proliferation and migration of SMCs into the intima. The continuous influx of cells in the subintimal space convert the fatty streak in a more complex and advanced lesion in which inflammatory cells (monocytes/macrophages, lymphocytes), SMCs, necrotic debris mainly resulting from cell death, ox-LDL elicit a chronic inflammatory response by adoptive immune system. SMCs form a thick fibrous cap that cover the necrotic core and avoid the exposition of thrombogenic material to the bloodstream. The volume of lesion grows and protrudes into the arterial lumen causing variable degrees of lumen stenosis. These lesions are advanced complicated "stable" atherosclerotic lesions, asymptomatic and often unrecognized [82,83].

Vulnerable plaque: a shift toward Th1 pattern

Early phases of the plaque development are characterized by an acute innate immune response against exogenous (infectious) and endogenous non-infectious stimuli. Specific antigens activate adaptive immune system leading to proliferation of T and B cells. A first burst of activation might occur in regional lymph nodes by dendritic cells (DCs) trafficking from the plaque to the lymph node. Subsequent cycles of activation can be sustained by interaction of activated/memory T cells re-entering in the plaque by selective binding to endothelial cell surface adhesion molecules with plaque macrophages expressing MHC class II molecules. In this phase of the atherogenic process the selective recruitment of a specific subtype of CD4$^+$ cells play a major part in determining the future development of the lesion. Two subtypes of CD4$^+$ cells have a juxtaposed role: Th1 and Th2 cells [84].

Th1 cells secreting proinflammatory cytokines, such as IFNγ, promote macrophage activation, inflammation, and atherosclerosis, whereas Th2 cells (cytokine pattern IL-4, IL-5, and IL-10) mediate antibody production and generally have anti-inflammatory and antiatherogenic effects [64]. Therefore the switch to a selective recruitment of Th1 lymphocyte represents a key point toward plaque vulnerability and disruption. T cells in the plaque may encounter antigens such as ox-LDL. Moreover, T-cell response can be triggered by heat shock proteins of endogenous or microbial origin [85]. It is still unknown why the initial inflammatory response becomes a chronic inflammatory condition. However, when the plaque microenvironment triggers the selective recruitment and activation of Th1 cells they in turn determine a potent inflammatory cascade.

The combination of IFNγ and TNF-α upregulates the expression of fractalkine (CX3CL1) [86]. IL-1 and TNFα-activated endothelium express also fractalkine (membrane bound form) which directly mediates the capture and adhesion of CX3CR1 expressing leukocytes providing a further pathway for leukocyte activation [87]. This cytokine network promotes the development of the Th1 pathway which is strongly proinflammatory and induces macrophage activation, superoxide production, and protease activity.

Role of inflammation as vulnerability factor

Homeostasis of plaque "microenvironment" (i.e., the balance between cell migration and cell proliferation, extracellular matrix production and degradation, macrophages and lymphocytes interplay) appears strictly related to the transition of a stable plaque into a vulnerable one.

A limited number of T cells, following the Th1 pathway, initiates the production of large amounts of molecules downstream in the cytokine cascade orchestrating the transition from the stable to unstable plaque [77,88].

Within the plaque, inflammatory cells such as foam cells and monocyte-derived macrophages are induced to produce matrix-degrading enzymes, cytokines, and growth factors strictly implicated in extracellular matrix homeostasis. In particular, cytokines such as INFγ suppress collagen synthesis, a major component of the fibrous cap [75]. Moreover, infiltration of mononuclear cells results in release of proteases which causes plaque disruption [89]. The production of ROS within the atherosclerotic plaque has important implications for its structural integrity [65]. Deregulated oxidant production has the potential to promote the elaboration and activation of matrix degrading enzymes in the fibrous cap of the plaque. Moreover, impaired NO function coupled with oxidative excess can activate MMPs [90], namely MMP-2 and MMP-9, which weaken the fibrous cap. Another mechanism that can determine the thinning of the fibrous cap is the apoptosis of smooth muscle cells. In fact, there is evidence for extensive apoptosis of SMCs within the cap of advanced atherosclerosis, as well as those cultured from plaques [32,91].

A very important role, not yet well studied, is that of dendritic cells, namely cells specialized in antigen presentation with a key role in the induction of primary immune response and in the regulation of T-lymphocyte differentiation, as well as in mechanisms of central and peripheral tolerance aiming at the elimination of T lymphocytes that are potentially self-reactive toward self-antigens [92,93]. A characteristic of dendritic cells is also the ability to polarize T-cell responses toward a T-helper phenotype (Th1) in response to bacterial antigens. Molecules expressed by activated T lymphocytes, like CD40L, OX40, stimulate the release from dendritic cells of chemokines (fractalkines) able to attract other lymphocytes toward the inflammation site, amplifying the immune response [94].

Patients with ACS are characterized by the expansion of an unusual subset of T cells, CD4$^+$CD28^{null} T cells, with functional activities that predispose for vascular injury [95,96]. CD4$^+$CD28^{null} T cells are a population of lymphocytes rarely found in healthy individuals. Disease-associated expansions of these cells have been reported in inflammatory disorders such as rheumatoid arthritis. CD4$^+$CD28^{null} T cells are characterized by their ability to produce high amounts of IFNγ [96]. Equally importantly, CD4$^+$CD28^{null} T cells have been distinguished from classic Th cells by virtue of their ability to function as cytotoxic effector cells. Possible targets in the plaque are SMCs and endothelial cells, as recently shown [97]. *In vivo*, CD4$^+$CD28^{null} cells have a tendency to proliferate with the frequent emergence of oligoclonality, raising the possibility of continuous antigenic stimulation, as it is the case in certain autoimmune disorders and in chronic infections. The demonstration of oligoclonality within the CD4$^+$CD28^{null} T-cell subsets and sharing of T-cell receptor sequences in expanded T-cell clones of patients with ACS strongly support the notion that these cells have expanded and are activated in response to a common antigenic challenge [98]. CD4$^+$CD28^{null} T cells are long-lived cells. Clonality and longevity of these cells are associated with defects in apoptotic pathways [99]. Moreover, CD28 is relevant for the expansion of naïve T cells, thus the absence of this molecule contributes to the senescence of lymphocytes. The excessive expansion of a pool of senescent T lymphocytes might compromise the efficacy of the immune responses direct against exogenous antigens as well as determinate autoimmune responses.

Recently, a subpopulation of T CD4+ cells, expressing IL-2 receptor, CD25 membrane marker, has been pointed out. Such lymphocytes represent 7–10% of T CD4+ cells and their homeostasis is due to some co-stimulatory molecules, such as CD28 receptor expressed by T cells and B7 molecules expressed by dendritic cells [100]. The current knowledge of the role of this specific subset of T cells in human atherogenesis is still incomplete, even though a very recent study carried out on mice has demonstrated an antiatherogenic effect of T CD4+CD25+ cells [101].

Th1 cells and T regulatory 1 cells have been demonstrated to play opposite roles in rupture of atherosclerotic lesion. The role of novel subset of T regulatory cells, known as CD4+CD25+Foxp3+ T cells, has been recently studied in CAD. Han *et al.* [102] found that the reduction of CD4+CD25+Foxp3+ T lymphocytes was consistent with the expansion of Th1 cells in patients with unstable CAD. The reversed development between CD4+CD25+ Tregs and Th1 cells might contribute to plaque destabilization.

Serum markers correlated to plaque inflammation

In recent years, a number of studies have correlated different serologic biomarkers with cardiovascular disease [4,103] leading to a rapid increase in the number of biomarkers available (Table 1.1). These biomarkers are useful in that they can identify a population at risk of an acute ischemic event and detect the presence of so-called vulnerable plaques and/or vulnerable patients [104,105]. Ideally, a biomarker must have certain characteristics to be a potential predictor of incident or prevalent vascular disease. Measurements have to be reproducible in multiple independent samples, the method for determination should be standardized, variability controlled, and the sensitivity and specificity should be good. In addition, the biomarker should be independent from other established risk markers, substantively improve the prediction of risk with established risk factors, be associated with cardiovascular events in multiple population cohorts and clinical trials, and the cost of the assays has to be acceptable. Finally, to be clinically useful a biomarker should correctly reflect the underlying biological process associated with plaque burden and progression.

Traditional biomarkers for cardiovascular risk include LDL cholesterol and glucose. However, 50% of heart attacks and strokes occur in individuals who have normal LDL cholesterol, and 20% of major adverse events occur in patients with no accepted risk factors [106]. Therefore, in light of changing atherosclerotic models, vulnerable blood may be better described as blood that has an increased level of activity of plasma determinants of plaque progression and rupture.

In this context, proposed biomarkers fall into nine general categories: inflammatory markers, markers for oxidative stress, markers of plaque erosion and thrombosis, lipid-associated markers, markers of endothelial dysfunction, metabolic markers, markers of neovascularization, and genetic markers. The last six biomarker categories are not treated in this chapter but only listed in Table 1.1. Some of these markers may indeed reflect the natural history of atherosclerotic plaque growth and may not be directly related to an increased risk of cardiovascular events. On the contrary, other markers are more related to complex plaque morphological features and may reflect an active process within the plaque which is in turn related to the onset of local complications and onset of acute clinical events.

However, it is important to emphasize that, in any individual patient, it is not yet clear how these biomarkers relate to quantitative risk of major adverse cardiovascular events. The best outcomes may be achieved by a panel of markers that will capture all of the different processes involved in plaque progression and plaque rupture, and that will enable clinicians to quantify an individual patient's true cardiovascular risk. In all likelihood, a combination of genetic (representing heredity) and serum markers (representing the net interaction between heredity and environment) will ultimately be the ones that should be utilized in primary prevention. Finally, different non-invasive and invasive imaging techniques may be coupled with biomarkers detection to increase the specificity, sensitivity, and overall predictive value of each potential diagnostic technique.

Markers of inflammation

Markers of inflammation include CRP, inflammatory cytokines soluble CD40L (sCD40L), soluble vascular adhesion molecules (sVCAM), and TNF.

CRP is a circulating pentraxin that has a major role in the human innate immune response [107] and provides a stable plasma biomarker for low grade systemic inflammation. CRP is produced predominantly in the liver as part of the acute phase response. However, CRP is also expressed in SMCs within diseased atherosclerotic arteries [108] and has been implicated in multiple aspects of atherogenesis and plaque vulnerability, including expression of adhesion molecules, induction of NO, altered complement function, and inhibition of intrinsic fibrinolysis [109]. CRP is considered to be an independent predictor of unfavorable cardiovascular events in patients with atherosclerotic disease. Beyond the ability of CRP to predict risk among both primary and secondary prevention patients, interest in it has increased with the recognition that statin-induced reduction of CRP is associated with less progression in adverse cardiovascular events that is independent of the lipid-associated changes [110] and that the efficacy of statin therapy may be related to the underlying level of vascular inflammation as detected by high-sensitivity CRP (hs-CRP). Among patients with stable angina and established CAD, plasma levels of hs-CRP have consistently been shown associated with recurrent risk of cardiovascular events [111,112]. Similarly, during acute coronary ischemia, levels of hs-CRP are predictive of high vascular risk even if troponin levels are non-detectable, suggesting that inflammation is associated with plaque vulnerability even in the absence of detectable myocardial necrosis [113,114]. Despite these data, the most relevant use of hs-CRP remains in the setting of primary prevention. To date, over two dozen large-scale prospective studies have shown baseline levels of hs-CRP to independently predict future myocardial infarction, stroke, cardiovascular death, and incidence of peripheral arterial disease [115,116]. Moreover, eight major prospective studies have had adequate power to evaluate hs-CRP after adjustment for all Framingham covariates, and all have confirmed the independence of hs-CRP [117]. Despite this evidence, it is important to recognize that there remain no firm data to date that lowering CRP levels per se will lower vascular risk. Further, as with other biomarkers of inflammation, it remains controversial whether CRP has a direct causal role in atherogenesis [118], and ongoing work with targeted CRP-lowering agents are required to fully test this hypothesis. However, the clinical utility of hs-CRP has been well established, and on the basis of data available through 2002, the Centers for Disease Control and Prevention and the American Heart Association endorsed the use of hs-CRP as an adjunct to global risk prediction, particularly among those at "intermediate risk" [119]. Data available since 2002 strongly reinforce these recommendations and suggest

Table 1.1 Serologic markers of vulnerable plaque/patient.

Reflecting metabolic and immune disorders	Reflecting hypercoagulability	Reflecting complex atherosclerotic plaque
Abnormal lipoprotein profile (i.e., high LDL, low HDL, lipoprotein [a], etc.)	Markers of blood hypercoagulability (i.e., fibrinogen, D-dimer, factor V Leiden)	*Morphology/structure* • Cap thickness • Lipid core size • Percentage stenosis • Remodeling (positive vs. negative) • Color (yellow, red) • Collagen content vs. lipid content • Calcification burden and pattern • Shear stress
Non-specific markers of inflammation (hs-CRP, CD40L, ICAM-1, VCAM, leukocytosis and other immuno-related serologic markers which may not be specific for atherosclerosis and plaque inflammation)	Increased platelet activation and aggregation (i.e., gene polymorphism of platelet glycoproteins IIb/IIIa, Ia/IIa, and Ib/IX)	
Serum markers of metabolic syndrome (diabetes or hypertriglyceridemia)	Increased coagulation factors (i.e., clotting of factors V, VII, VIII, XIII, von Willebrand factor)	*Activity/function* • Plaque inflammation (macrophage density, rate of monocyte and activated T-cell infiltration) • Endothelial denudation or dysfunction (local nitric oxide production, anti/procoaugulation properties of the endothelium) • Plaque oxidative stress • Superficial platelet aggregation and fibrin deposition • Rate of apoptosis (apoptosis protein markers, microsatellite) • Angiogenesis, leaking vasa vasorum, intraplaque hemorrhage • Matrix metalloproteinases (MMP-2, -3, -9) • Microbial antigens (*Chlamydia pneumoniae*) Temperature
Specific markers of immune activation (i.e., anti-LDL antibody, anti-HSP antibody	Decreased anticoagulation factors (i.e., proteins S and C, thrombomodulin, antithrombin III)	
Markers of lipid peroxidation (i.e., ox-LDL and ox-HDL)	Decreased endogenous fibrinolysis activity (i.e., reduced tissue plasminogen activator, increased type I PAI, PAI polymorphisms)	
Homocysteine	Prothrombin mutation (i.e., G20210A)	
PAPP-A	Thrombogenic factors (i.e., anticardiolipin antibodies, thrombocytosis, sickle cell disease, diabetes, hypercholesterolemia)	
Circulating apoptosis markers (i.e., Fas/Fas ligand)	Transient hypercoagulability (i.e., smoking, dehydration, infection)	*Pan arterial* • Transcoronary gradient of vulnerability biomarkers • Total calcium burden • Total coronary vasoreactivity • Total arterial plaque burden (intima media thickness)
ADMA/DDAH/ Circulating NEFA		

ADMA, asymmetric dimethylarginine; CRP, C-reactive protein; DDAH, dimethylarginine dimethylaminohydrolase; HDL, high density lipoprotein; HSP, heat shock protein; ICAM, intercellular adhesion molecule; LDL, low density lipoprotein; NEFA, non-esterified fatty acids; PAI, plasminogen activator; PAPP-A, pregnancy-associated plasma protein A; VCAM, vascular adhesion molecule.

expansion to lower risk groups, as well as those taking statin therapy. Perhaps most importantly, data for hs-CRP provides evidence that biomarkers beyond those traditionally used for vascular risk detection and monitoring can have important clinical roles in prevention and treatment.

Cellular adhesion molecules can be considered potential markers of vulnerability because such molecules are activated by inflammatory cytokines and then released by the endothelium [120]. These molecules represent the one available marker to assess endothelial activation and vascular inflammation. The Physicians' Health Study evaluated more than 14,000 healthy subjects and demonstrated ICAM-1 expression positive correlation with cardiovascular risk and showed that subjects in the higher quartile of ICAM-1 expression showed 1.8 times higher risk than subjects in the lower quartile [121]. Furthermore, soluble ICAM-1 and VCAM-1 levels showed a positive correlation with atherosclerosis disease burden [122]. IL-6 is expressed during the early phases of inflammation and it is the principal stimulus for CRP liver production. In addition, CD40 ligand, a molecule expressed on cellular membrane, is a TNFα homologue which stimulates activated macrophages proteolytic substances production [123]. CD40 and CD40L have been found on platelets and several other cell types in functional-bound and soluble (sCD40L) forms. Although many platelet-derived factors have been identified, recent evidence suggests that CD40L is actively involved in the pathogenesis of ACS. CD40L drives the inflammatory response through the interaction between CD40L on activated platelets and the CD40 receptor on endothelial cells. Such interactions facilitate increased expression of adhesion molecules on the surface of endothelial cells and release of various stimulatory chemokines. These events, in turn, facilitate activation of circulating monocytes as a trigger of atherosclerosis. Beyond known proinflammatory and thrombotic properties of CD40L, experimental evidence suggests that CD40L-induced platelet activation leads to the production of reactive oxygen and nitrogen species, which are able to prevent endothelial cell migration and angiogenesis [124]. As a consequence of inhibiting endothelial cell recovery, the risk of subsequent coronary events may be greater. Clinical studies have supported the involvement of CD40L in ACS and the prognostic value in ACS populations. Levels of sCD40L have been shown to be an independent predictor of adverse cardiovascular events after ACS [125], with increased levels portending a worse prognosis [126]. Importantly, specific therapeutic strategies have shown to be beneficial in reducing risk associated with sCD40L [127]. IL-18 is a proinflammatory cytokine mostly produced by monocytes and macrophages, which acts synergistically with IL-12 [105]. Both these interleukins are expressed in the atherosclerotic plaque and they stimulate IFNγ induction which, in its turn, inhibits collagen synthesis, preventing a thick fibrous cap formation and facilitating plaque destabilization. Mallat *et al.* [128] examined 40 stable and unstable atherosclerotic plaques obtained from patients undergoing carotid endarterectomy and highlighted how IL-18 expression was higher in macrophages and endothelial cells extracted from unstable rather than stable lesions and it correlated with clinical (symptomatic plaques) and pathological (ulceration) signs of vulnerability.

Pregnancy-associated plasma protein-A (PAPP-A) is a high molecular weight, zinc-binding metalloproteinase, typically measured in women's blood during pregnancy and later found in macrophages and SMCs inside unstable coronary atherosclerotic plaques. This protease cleaves the bond between insulin like growth factor-1 (IGF-1) and its specific inhibitor (IGFBP-4 e IGFBP-5), increasing free IGF-1 levels. IGF-1 is important for monocytes–macrophages chemotaxis and activation in the atherosclerotic lesion, with consequent proinflammatory cytokine and proteolytic enzyme release, and stimulates endothelial cell migration and organizational behavior with consequent neoangiogenesis. Hence, IGF-1 represents one of the most important mediators in the transformation of a stable lesion into an unstable one [129]. Bayes-Genis *et al.* [130] demonstrated that PAPP-A is more often expressed in the serum of patients with acute coronary syndromes (UA, MI), than subjects presenting with SA. In particular, PAPP-A serum levels >10 mIU/L recognize patient vulnerability with a specificity of 78% and a sensitivity of 89%. It has also been demonstrated that PAPP-A histological expression is higher in complex, vulnerable/ruptured carotid plaques than stable lesions [131]. As PAPP-A serum levels can be easily measured today by means of enzyme-linked immunosorbent assay (ELISA), this protease could represent an easily quantifiable marker of vulnerability, with a reproducible method, allowing the identification of a patient subgroup with a high cerebrovascular risk before its clinical manifestation.

Jaffer *et al.* [132] have published a detailed review on different techniques for detection of vulnerable plaque based on several biomarkers that have been implemented in recent years. In this context, plaques with active inflammation can be identified directly by extensive macrophage accumulation [133]. Possible intravascular diagnostic techniques [134] based on inflammatory infiltration determination within the plaque include thermography [135], contrast-enhanced MRI [136], fluorodeoxyglucose positron emission tomography [137], and immunoscintigraphy [138]. In addition, non-invasive techniques include MRI with superparamagnetic iron oxide [139,140] and gadolinium fluorine compounds [141,142].

Oxidative stress markers

Oxidative stress has a very important role in atherogenesis. Evidence shows that activation of vascular oxidative enzymes leads to lipid oxidation, foam cell formation, expression of vascular adhesion molecules and chemokines, and ultimately atherogenesis. Myeloperoxidase (MPO) is a heme peroxidase that is present in and secreted by activated phagocytes at sites of inflammation. MPO can generate several reactive, oxidatively derived intermediates, all mediated through a reaction with hydrogen peroxide, to induce oxidative damage to cells and tissues [143]. Oxidation products

from MPO are found at significantly increased rates (up to 100-fold higher than circulating LDL) on LDL isolated from atherosclerotic lesions [144] and lead to accelerated foam cell formation through nitrated apoB-100 on LDL and uptake by scavenger receptors [145]. Accumulating evidence suggests that MPO may have a causal role in plaque vulnerability [146]. Sugiyama *et al.* [147] showed that advanced ruptured human atherosclerotic plaques, derived from patients with sudden cardiac death, strongly expressed MPO at sites of plaque rupture, in superficial erosions and in the lipid core, whereas fatty streaks exhibited little MPO expression. In addition, MPO macrophage expression and HOCl were highly co-localized immunochemically in culprit lesions of these patients. Several inflammatory triggers, such as cholesterol crystals and CD40 ligand, induced release of MPO and HOCl production from MPO-positive macrophages *in vitro*. Consistent with the potential role for MPO in the atherosclerotic process, genetic polymorphisms resulting in MPO deficiency or diminished activity are associated with lower cardiovascular risk, although the generalizability of these findings is uncertain [148]. In parallel with the effects of MPO on nitric oxide, LDL oxidation, and presence within ruptured plaques, several recent clinical studies have suggested that MPO levels can provide diagnostic and prognostic data in endothelial function, angiographically determined CAD, and ACSs. In a case–control study of 175 patients with angiographically determined CAD, Zhang *et al.* [149] showed that the highest quartiles of both blood and leukocyte MPO levels were associated with odds ratios of 11.9 and 20.4, respectively, for the presence of CAD compared with the lowest quartiles. Brennan *et al.* [150] obtained MPO levels in the emergency department in 604 patients presenting with chest pain but no initial evidence of myocardial infarction, and showed that MPO levels predicted the in-hospital development of myocardial infarction, independent of other markers of inflammation, such as CRP. In addition, they showed that MPO levels were strong predictors of death, myocardial infarction, and revascularization 6 months after the initial event. Current data suggest that MPO can serve as both a marker of disease, providing independent information on diagnosis and prognosis of patients with chest pain, and also as a potential marker for assessment of plaque progression and destabilization at the time of acute ischemia.

Biomechanical stress as a trigger for plaque progression and rupture

Despite the exposure of the entire coronary tree to the *systemic* risk factors and inflammation, spatial distribution of atherosclerotic plaques is often a *focal* phenomenon [151]. Vascular endothelium is subjected to complex mechanical stresses resulting from its 3D geometry, vessel curvatures, and cardiac motion. These mechanical strains in combination with fluid frictional forces or shear stress gradients inside the arteries can lead to a number of structural and humoral changes in endothelial cells [39,152]. High wall shear stress (>15 dyne/cm²) has been found to induce endothelial quiescence and an atheroprotective gene expression profile, whereas low shear stress (<4 dyne/cm²) stimulates an atherogenic phenotype [152]. It has been shown that the plaques and wall thickenings are localized mostly on the outer wall of one or both daughter vessels at bifurcations and along the inner wall of curved segments [151]. In the Prediction study, Stone *et al.* [153] studied the natural history of plaques in 506 patients with ACS treated with percutaneous coronary intervention, and used reconstructed coronary models from angiography and IVUS. A total of 74% patients had follow-up studies at 6–10 months to relate the effects of local hemodynamic milieu on plaque changes. Authors reported that decrease in lumen area

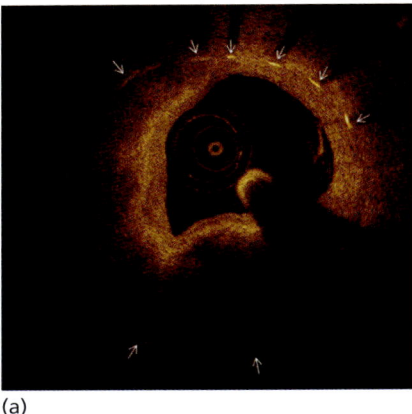
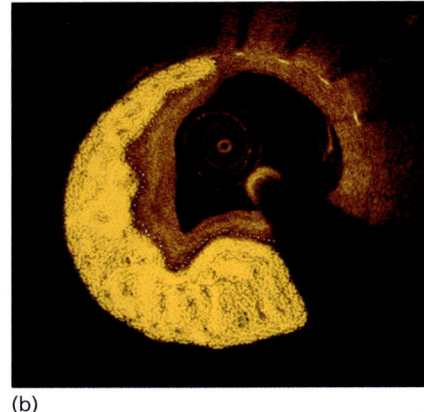

(a)   (b)

Figure 1.5 Neoatherosclerosis seen on OCT. (a) Neointimal hyperplasia inside the stent. A uniform layer of neointima is seen covering the stent struts (white arrows) from the 12 to 4 o'clock position. Remainder of the stent circumference is covered by an irregular, very thick tissue layer containing dark, signal-poor core consistent with lipid pool and signal-rich, thick fibrous cap. (b) Lipid/necrotic core in the neoatherosclerotic plaque is highlighted in yellow.

was independently predicted by baseline large plaque burden and low endothelial shear stress [153]. Other investigators have reported that high wall shear stress is associated with transformation of plaques into high risk phenotypes prone to instability and rupture [154,155].

Neoatherosclerosis

The neointimal tissue inside the stents is subject to similar atherogenic forces as the native vessels [156,157]. Neoatherosclerosis is the development of atherosclerosis within this neointima. Histologically, it is recognized by the presence of clusters of lipid-laden foamy macrophages within the neointima with or without necrotic core formation [157,158]. On OCT it is seen as areas of heterogeneous appearance within the neointima with low-intensity lipid-laden regions or well demarcated calcification within stents (Figure 1.5) [159,160]. Although the exact pathogenesis of this phenomenon is yet to be proven, inflammation and endothelial dysfunction have been shown to have a fundamental role [157,158,161]. It has been reported in autopsy and *in vivo* imaging studies that neoatherosclerosis occurs at an earlier stage and with higher frequency in DES than BMS [157,162]. It is thought to be one important mechanism for late stent failure including in-stent restenosis and very late stent thrombosis [156,158,163].

Future challenges in the treatment of vulnerable plaques

With the concept of "vulnerable" plaque not nearly as straightforward as once thought, there are challenges to creating a therapeutic strategy for assessing the risk of rupture of vulnerable plaques in asymptomatic patients.

First, there must be an ability to identify the vulnerable plaque with non-invasive or invasive techniques. It has been demonstrated that coronary plaque composition can be studied with invasive and non-invasive imaging techniques, allowing real-time analysis and *in vivo* plaque characterization including the identification of TCFA. However, the severity of the inflammatory infiltration of the cap, which certainly has a major role in plaque disruption, cannot be accurately evaluated even with the most advanced *in vivo* imaging techniques. Moreover, dynamic plaque changes, such as abrupt

intra-plaque hemorrhages from vasa vasorum which may be fundamental in predicting the potentiality of a plaque to rupture, will be extremely difficult to identify with real-time imaging techniques. Nevertheless, some promising work has been done in this regard in the SECRITT trial introducing the concept of sealing the non-obstructive, high risk IVUS and OCT-derived TCFA, using a dedicated nitinol self-expanding vShield device. Authors reported an interesting observation of neocap formation in the shielded plaques with an increase in the average cap thickness from $48 \pm 12\,\mu m$ at baseline to $201 \pm 168\,\mu m$ at 6 months' follow-up [164]. It is hoped that this study may provide the foundation for larger scale trials in future.

A second challenge is that a lesion-specific approach requires that the number of vulnerable plaques in each patient needs to be known and the number of such lesions need to be limited. That is not the case, however. Several pathological studies indicate the presence of multiple "lipid-rich" vulnerable plaques in patients dying after ACS or with sudden coronary death [37,61]. Further complicating the issue, coronary occlusion and myocardial infarction usually evolve from mild to moderate stenosis—68% of the time, according to an analysis of data from different studies.

The third and fourth challenge is that the natural history of the vulnerable plaque (with respect to incidence of acute events) has to be documented in patients treated with patient-specific systemic therapy, and the approach has to be proven to significantly reduce the incidence of future events relative to its natural history. At this time, neither is documented nor proved.

Fifth, we believe that at the current stage it is not possible to know which vulnerable plaques will never rupture. Although we suspect it is the vast majority of them, we may have to shift to a more appropriate therapeutic target. In addition, targeting not only the vulnerable plaque but also the vulnerable blood (prone to thrombosis) and/or vulnerable myocardium (prone to life-threatening arrhythmia) may be also important to reduce the risk of fatal events.

Conclusions

Atherosclerosis is now recognized as a diffuse and chronic inflammatory disorder involving vascular, metabolic, and immune system with various local and systemic manifestations. A composite vulnerability index score comprising the total burden of atherosclerosis and vulnerable plaques in the coronary, carotid, aorta, and femoral arteries, together with blood vulnerability factors, should be the ideal method of risk stratification. Obviously, such index is hard to achieve with today's tools. A future challenge is to identify patients at high risk of acute vascular events before clinical syndromes develop. At present, aside from imaging modalities such as IVUS, virtual histology, magnetic resonance, and local Raman spectroscopy that could help to identify vulnerable plaques, highly sensitive inflammatory circulating markers such as hsCRP, cytokines, PAPP-A, pentraxin-3, LpPLA2 are currently the best candidates for diffuse active plaque detection. In order to achieve this aim a coordinated effort is needed to promote the application of the most promising tools and to develop new screening and diagnostic techniques to identify the vulnerable patient.

Interactive multiple choice questions are available for this chapter on www.wiley. com/go/dangas/cardiology

References

1 Lloyd-Jones D, Adams R, Carnethon M, *et al.* Heart disease and stroke statistics—2009 update: a report from the American Heart Association Statistics Committee and Stroke Statistics Subcommittee. *Circulation* 2009; **119**(3): 480–486.

2 Libby P. Inflammation in atherosclerosis. *Nature* 2002; **420**(6917): 868–874.

3 Hansson GK, Libby P, Schonbeck U, Yan ZQ. Innate and adaptive immunity in the pathogenesis of atherosclerosis. *Circ Res* 2002; **91**(4): 281–291.

4 Ross R. Atherosclerosis: an inflammatory disease. *N Engl J Med* 1999; **340**(2): 115–126.

5 Fuster V, Badimon L, Badimon JJ, Chesebro JH. The pathogenesis of coronary artery disease and the acute coronary syndromes (1). *N Engl J Med* 1992; **326**(4): 242–250.

6 Falk E, Shah PK, Fuster V. Coronary plaque disruption. *Circulation* 1995; **92**(3): 657–671.

7 Davies MJ. Stability and instability: two faces of coronary atherosclerosis. The Paul Dudley White Lecture 1995. *Circulation* 1996; **94**(8): 2013–2020.

8 Davis NE. Atherosclerosis: an inflammatory process. *J Insur Med* 2005; **37**(1): 72–75.

9 Ross R. Cell biology of atherosclerosis. *Ann Rev Physiol* 1995; **57**: 791–804.

10 Spagnoli LG, Bonanno E, Sangiorgi G, Mauriello A. Role of inflammation in atherosclerosis. *J Nuclear Med* 2007; **48**(11): 1800–1815.

11 Alexander RW. Theodore Cooper Memorial Lecture. Hypertension and the pathogenesis of atherosclerosis. Oxidative stress and the mediation of arterial inflammatory response: a new perspective. *Hypertension* 1995; **25**(2): 155–161.

12 Chyu KY, Shah PK. Can we vaccinate against atherosclerosis? *J Cardiovasc Pharmacol Ther* 2014; **19**(1): 77–82.

13 Davignon J, Ganz P. Role of endothelial dysfunction in atherosclerosis. *Circulation* 2004; **109**(23 Suppl 1): Iii27–32.

14 Powell JT. Vascular damage from smoking: disease mechanisms at the arterial wall. *Vasc Med* 1998; **3**(1): 21–28.

15 Sherer Y, Shoenfeld Y. Mechanisms of disease: atherosclerosis in autoimmune diseases. *Nat Clin Pract Rheum* 2006; **2**(2): 99–106.

16 Pentikainen MO, Oorni K, Ala-Korpela M, Kovanen PT. Modified LDL: trigger of atherosclerosis and inflammation in the arterial intima. *J Intern Med* 2000; **247**(3): 359–370.

17 Berliner JA, Heinecke JW. The role of oxidized lipoproteins in atherogenesis. *Free Radic Biol Med* 1996; **20**(5): 707–727.

18 Boyle JJ. Macrophage activation in atherosclerosis: pathogenesis and pharmacology of plaque rupture. *Curr Vasc Pharmacol* 2005; **3**(1): 63–68.

19 Rudijanto A. The role of vascular smooth muscle cells on the pathogenesis of atherosclerosis. *Acta Med Indones* 2007; **39**(2): 86–93.

20 Weissberg PL. Vascular smooth muscle cells. In Warrell DA, Cox TM, Firth JD, Benz EJ Jr, eds. *Oxford Textbook of Medicine*, 4th edn. Oxford: Oxford University Press; 2005.

21 Naghavi M, Libby P, Falk E, *et al.* From vulnerable plaque to vulnerable patient: a call for new definitions and risk assessment strategies: Part I. *Circulation* 2003; **108**(14): 1664–1672.

22 Theroux P, Fuster V. Acute coronary syndromes: unstable angina and non-Q-wave myocardial infarction. *Circulation* 1998; **97**(12): 1195–1206.

23 Alpert JS, Thygesen K, Antman E, Bassand JP. Myocardial infarction redefined: a consensus document of The Joint European Society of Cardiology/American College of Cardiology Committee for the redefinition of myocardial infarction. *J Am Coll Cardiol* 2000; **36**(3): 959–969.

24 Sami S, Willerson JT. Contemporary treatment of unstable angina and non-ST-segment-elevation myocardial infarction: Part 1. *Texas Heart Inst J* 2010; **37**(2): 141–148.

25 Finn AV, Nakano M, Narula J, Kolodgie FD, Virmani R. Concept of vulnerable/unstable plaque. *Arterioscler Thromb Vasc Biol* 2010; **30**(7): 1282–1292.

26 Kolodgie FD, Burke AP, Farb A, *et al.* The thin-cap fibroatheroma: a type of vulnerable plaque: the major precursor lesion to acute coronary syndromes. *Curr Opin Cardiol* 2001; **16**(5): 285–292.

27 van der Wal AC, Becker AE. Atherosclerotic plaque rupture: pathologic basis of plaque stability and instability. *Cardiovasc Res* 1999; **41**(2): 334–344.

28 Virmani R, Burke AP, Farb A, Kolodgie FD. Pathology of the vulnerable plaque. *J Am Coll Cardiol* 2006; **47**(8 Suppl): C13–18.

29 Virmani R, Kolodgie FD, Burke AP, Farb A, Schwartz SM. Lessons from sudden coronary death: a comprehensive morphological classification scheme for atherosclerotic lesions. *Arterioscler Thromb Vasc Biol* 2000; **20**(5): 1262–1275.

30 Shi H, Wei L, Yang T, Wang S, Li X, You L. Morphometric and histological study of coronary plaques in stable angina and acute myocardial infarctions. *Chinese Med J* 1999; **112**(11): 1040–1043.

31 Ambrose JA, Tannenbaum MA, Alexopoulos D, *et al.* Angiographic progression of coronary artery disease and the development of myocardial infarction. *J Am Coll Cardiol* 1988; **12**(1): 56–62.

32 Group LS. Long-term effectiveness and safety of pravastatin in 9014 patients with coronary heart disease and average cholesterol concentrations: the LIPID trial follow-up. *Lancet* 2002; **359**(9315): 1379–1387.

33 Spagnoli LG, Mauriello A, Sangiorgi G, *et al.* Extracranial thrombotically active carotid plaque as a risk factor for ischemic stroke. *JAMA* 2004; **292**(15): 1845–1852.

34 Jang IK, Bouma BE, Kang DH, *et al.* Visualization of coronary atherosclerotic plaques in patients using optical coherence tomography: comparison with intravascular ultrasound. *J Am Coll Cardiol* 2002; **39**(4): 604–609.

35 Jang IK. Optical coherence tomography or intravascular ultrasound? *J Am Coll Cardiol Intv* 2011; **4**(5): 492–494.

36 Bezerra HG, Attizzani GF, Sirbu V, *et al.* Optical coherence tomography versus intravascular ultrasound to evaluate coronary artery disease and percutaneous coronary intervention. *J Am Coll Cardiol Intv* 2013; **6**(3): 228–236.

37 Mauriello A, Sangiorgi G, Fratoni S, *et al.* Diffuse and active inflammation occurs in both vulnerable and stable plaques of the entire coronary tree: a histopathologic study of patients dying of acute myocardial infarction. *J Am Coll Cardiol* 2005; **45**(10): 1585–1593.

38 Spagnoli LG, Bonanno E, Mauriello A, *et al.* Multicentric inflammation in epicardial coronary arteries of patients dying of acute myocardial infarction. *J Am Coll Cardiol* 2002; **40**(9): 1579–1588.

39 Chatzizisis YS, Coskun AU, Jonas M, Edelman ER, Feldman CL, Stone PH. Role of endothelial shear stress in the natural history of coronary atherosclerosis and vascular remodeling: molecular, cellular, and vascular behavior. *J Am Coll Cardiol* 2007; **49**(25): 2379–2393.

40 Corban MT, Eshtehardi P, Suo J, *et al.* Combination of plaque burden, wall shear stress, and plaque phenotype has incremental value for prediction of coronary atherosclerotic plaque progression and vulnerability. *Atherosclerosis* 2014; **232**(2): 271–276.

41 Garcia-Garcia HM, Costa MA, Serruys PW. Imaging of coronary atherosclerosis: intravascular ultrasound. *Eur Heart J* 2010; **31**(20): 2456–2469.

42 Bezerra HG, Costa MA, Guagliumi G, Rollins AM, Simon DI. Intracoronary optical coherence tomography: a comprehensive review clinical and research applications. *J Am Coll Cardiol Intv* 2009; **2**(11): 1035–1046.

43 Barlis P. Use of optical coherence tomography in interventional cardiology. *Interv Cardiol* 2009; **1**(1): 63–71.

44 Tuzcu EM, Kapadia SR, Tutar E, *et al.* High prevalence of coronary atherosclerosis in asymptomatic teenagers and young adults: evidence from intravascular ultrasound. *Circulation* 2001; **103**(22): 2705–2710.

45 Kawano S, Yamagishi M, Hao H, Yutani C, Miyatake K. Wall composition in intravascular ultrasound layered appearance of human coronary artery. *Heart Vessels* 1996; **11**(3): 152–159.

46 Gussenhoven EJ, Essed CE, Lancee CT, *et al.* Arterial wall characteristics determined by intravascular ultrasound imaging: an in vitro study. *J Am Coll Cardiol* 1989; **14**(4): 947–952.

47 Schoenhagen P, White RD, Nissen SE, Tuzcu EM. Coronary imaging: angiography shows the stenosis, but IVUS, CT, and MRI show the plaque. *Cleveland Clin J Med* 2003; **70**(8): 713–719.

48 Schoenhagen P, Nissen SE. Assessing coronary plaque burden and plaque vulnerability: atherosclerosis imaging with IVUS and emerging noninvasive modalities. *Am Heart Hosp J* 2003; **1**(2): 164–169.

49 Losordo DW, Rosenfield K, Kaufman J, Pieczek A, Isner JM. Focal compensatory enlargement of human arteries in response to progressive atherosclerosis: in vivo documentation using intravascular ultrasound. *Circulation* 1994; **89**(6): 2570–2577.

50 Fujimoto JG, Pitris C, Boppart SA, Brezinski ME. Optical coherence tomography: an emerging technology for biomedical imaging and optical biopsy. *Neoplasia* 2000; **2**(1–2): 9–25.

51 Suter MJ, Nadkarni SK, Weisz G, et al. Intravascular optical imaging technology for investigating the coronary artery. *JACC Cardiovasc Imag* 2011; **4**(9): 1022–1039.

52 Ferrante G, Presbitero P, Whitbourn R, Barlis P. Current applications of optical coherence tomography for coronary intervention. *Int J Cardiol* 2013; **165**(1): 7–16.

53 Regar E, Ligthart J, Bruining N, van Soest G. The diagnostic value of intracoronary optical coherence tomography. *Herz* 2011; **36**(5): 417–429.

54 Burke AP, Farb A, Malcom GT, Liang YH, Smialek J, Virmani R. Coronary risk factors and plaque morphology in men with coronary disease who died suddenly. *N Engl J Med* 1997; **336**(18): 1276–1282.

55 Higuma T, Soeda T, Abe N, et al. A combined optical coherence tomography and intravascular ultrasound study on plaque rupture, plaque erosion, and calcified nodule in patients with ST-segment elevation myocardial infarction: incidence, morphologic characteristics, and outcomes after percutaneous coronary intervention. *J Am Coll Cardiol Intv* 2015; **8**(9): 1166–1176.

56 Kataoka Y, Hammadah M, Puri R, et al. Plaque microstructures in patients with coronary artery disease who achieved very low low-density lipoprotein cholesterol levels. *Atherosclerosis* 2015; **242**(2): 490–495.

57 Galis ZS, Sukhova GK, Lark MW, Libby P. Increased expression of matrix metalloproteinases and matrix degrading activity in vulnerable regions of human atherosclerotic plaques. *J Clin Invest* 1994; **94**(6): 2493–2503.

58 Schwartz RS, Topol EJ, Serruys PW, Sangiorgi G, Holmes DR Jr. Artery size, neointima, and remodeling: time for some standards. *J Am Coll Cardiol* 1998; **32**(7): 2087–2094.

59 Virmani R, Kolodgie FD, Burke AP, et al. Atherosclerotic plaque progression and vulnerability to rupture: angiogenesis as a source of intraplaque hemorrhage. *Arterioscler Thromb Vasc Biol* 2005; **25**(10): 2054–2061.

60 Buffon A, Biasucci LM, Liuzzo G, D'Onofrio G, Crea F, Maseri A. Widespread coronary inflammation in unstable angina. *N Engl J Med* 2002; **347**(1): 5–12.

61 Goldstein JA, Demetriou D, Grines CL, Pica M, Shoukfeh M, O'Neill WW. Multiple complex coronary plaques in patients with acute myocardial infarction. *N Engl J Med* 2000; **343**(13): 915–922.

62 Garcia-Moll X, Coccolo F, Cole D, Kaski JC. Serum neopterin and complex stenosis morphology in patients with unstable angina. *J Am Coll Cardiol* 2000; **35**(4): 956–962.

63 Abbate A, Bonanno E, Mauriello A, et al. Widespread myocardial inflammation and infarct-related artery patency. *Circulation* 2004; **110**(1): 46–50.

64 Widlansky ME, Gokce N, Keaney JF Jr, Vita JA. The clinical implications of endothelial dysfunction. *J Am Coll Cardiol* 2003; **42**(7): 1149–1160.

65 Stocker R, Keaney JF Jr. Role of oxidative modifications in atherosclerosis. *Physiol Rev* 2004; **84**(4): 1381–1478.

66 Khan BV, Harrison DG, Olbrych MT, Alexander RW, Medford RM. Nitric oxide regulates vascular cell adhesion molecule 1 gene expression and redox-sensitive transcriptional events in human vascular endothelial cells. *Proc Nat Acad Sci U S A* 1996; **93**(17): 9114–9119.

67 Kubes P, Suzuki M, Granger DN. Nitric oxide: an endogenous modulator of leukocyte adhesion. *Proc Nat Acad Sci U S A* 1991; **88**(11): 4651–4655.

68 Zeiher AM, Fisslthaler B, Schray-Utz B, Busse R. Nitric oxide modulates the expression of monocyte chemoattractant protein 1 in cultured human endothelial cells. *Circ Res* 1995; **76**(6): 980–986.

69 Teplyakov AI. Endothelin-1 involved in systemic cytokine network inflammatory response at atherosclerosis. *J Cardiovasc Pharmacol* 2004; **44**(Suppl 1): S274–275.

70 Lerman A, Edwards BS, Hallett JW, Heublein DM, Sandberg SM, Burnett JC Jr. Circulating and tissue endothelin immunoreactivity in advanced atherosclerosis. *N Engl J Med* 1991; **325**(14): 997–1001.

71 Dang A, Wang B, Li W, et al. Plasma endothelin-1 levels and circulating endothelial cells in patients with aortoarteritis. *Hypertens Res* 2000; **23**(5): 541–544.

72 McCarron RM, Wang L, Stanimirovic DB, Spatz M. Endothelin induction of adhesion molecule expression on human brain microvascular endothelial cells. *Neurosci Lett* 1993; **156**(1–2): 31–34.

73 Halim A, Kanayama N, el Maradny E, Maehara K, Terao T. Coagulation in vivo microcirculation and in vitro caused by endothelin-1. *Thromb Res* 1993; **72**(3): 203–209.

74 Feletou M, Vanhoutte PM. Endothelial dysfunction: a multifaceted disorder (The Wiggers Award Lecture). *Am J Physiol Heart Circ Physiol* 2006; **291**(3): H985–1002.

75 Hansson GK, Libby P. The immune response in atherosclerosis: a double-edged sword. *Nat Rev Immunol* 2006; **6**(7): 508–519.

76 Verma S, Devaraj S, Jialal I. Is C-reactive protein an innocent bystander or proatherogenic culprit? C-reactive protein promotes atherothrombosis. *Circulation* 2006; **113**(17): 2135–2150; discussion 2150.

77 Hansson GK. Inflammation, atherosclerosis, and coronary artery disease. *N Engl J Med* 2005; **352**(16): 1685–1695.

78 Binder CJ, Chang MK, Shaw PX, et al. Innate and acquired immunity in atherogenesis. *Nat Med* 2002; **8**(11): 1218–1226.

79 Cook DN, Pisetsky DS, Schwartz DA. Toll-like receptors in the pathogenesis of human disease. *Nat Immunol* 2004; **5**(10): 975–979.

80 Nilsson J, Hansson GK, Shah PK. Immunomodulation of atherosclerosis: implications for vaccine development. *Arteriosclerosis Thromb Vasc Biol* 2005; **25**(1): 18–28.

81 Clinton SK, Underwood R, Hayes L, Sherman ML, Kufe DW, Libby P. Macrophage colony-stimulating factor gene expression in vascular cells and in experimental and human atherosclerosis. *Am J Pathol* 1992; **140**(2): 301–316.

82 Fuster V. Lewis A. Conner Memorial Lecture. Mechanisms leading to myocardial infarction: insights from studies of vascular biology. *Circulation* 1994; **90**(4): 2126–2146.

83 Libby P. Coronary artery injury and the biology of atherosclerosis: inflammation, thrombosis, and stabilization. *Am J Cardiol* 2000; **86**(8B): 3J–8J; discussion 8J–9J.

84 Constant SL, Bottomly K. Induction of Th1 and Th2 CD4+ T cell responses: the alternative approaches. *Annu Rev Immunol* 1997; **15**: 297–322.

85 Benagiano M, D'Elios MM, Amedei A, et al. Human 60-kDa heat shock protein is a target autoantigen of T cells derived from atherosclerotic plaques. *J Immunol* 2005; **174**(10): 6509–6517.

86 Ludwig A, Berkhout T, Moores K, Groot P, Chapman G. Fractalkine is expressed by smooth muscle cells in response to IFN-gamma and TNF-alpha and is modulated by metalloproteinase activity. *J Immunol* 2002; **168**(2): 604–612.

87 Fong AM, Robinson LA, Steeber DA, et al. Fractalkine and CX3CR1 mediate a novel mechanism of leukocyte capture, firm adhesion, and activation under physiologic flow. *J Exp Med* 1998; **188**(8): 1413–1419.

88 Benagiano M, Azzurri A, Ciervo A, et al. T helper type 1 lymphocytes drive inflammation in human atherosclerotic lesions. *Proc Nat Acad Sci* 2003; **100**(11): 6658–6663.

89 Garcia-Touchard A, Henry TD, Sangiorgi G, et al. Extracellular proteases in atherosclerosis and restenosis. *Arterioscler Thromb Vasc Biol* 2005; **25**(6): 1119–1127.

90 Uemura S, Matsushita H, Li W, et al. Diabetes mellitus enhances vascular matrix metalloproteinase activity: role of oxidative stress. *Circ Res* 2001; **88**(12): 1291–1298.

91 Geng YJ, Wu Q, Muszynski M, Hansson GK, Libby P. Apoptosis of vascular smooth muscle cells induced by in vitro stimulation with interferon-gamma, tumor necrosis factor-alpha, and interleukin-1 beta. *Arterioscler Thromb Vasc Biol* 1996; **16**(1): 19–27.

92 Adams S, O'Neill DW, Bhardwaj N. Recent advances in dendritic cell biology. *J Clin Immunol* 2005; **25**(3): 177–188.

93 Lanzavecchia A, Sallusto F. Regulation of T cell immunity by dendritic cells. *Cell* 2001; **106**(3): 263–266.

94 Kanazawa N, Nakamura T, Tashiro K, et al. Fractalkine and macrophage-derived chemokine: T cell-attracting chemokines expressed in T cell area dendritic cells. *Eur J Immunol* 1999; **29**(6): 1925–1932.

95 Liuzzo G, Kopecky SL, Frye RL, et al. Perturbation of the T-cell repertoire in patients with unstable angina. *Circulation* 1999; **100**(21): 2135–2139.

96 Liuzzo G, Vallejo AN, Kopecky SL, et al. Molecular fingerprint of interferon-gamma signaling in unstable angina. *Circulation* 2001; **103**(11): 1509–1514.

97 Nakajima T, Schulte S, Warrington KJ, et al. T-cell-mediated lysis of endothelial cells in acute coronary syndromes. *Circulation* 2002; **105**(5): 570–575.

98 Liuzzo G, Goronzy JJ, Yang H, et al. Monoclonal T-cell proliferation and plaque instability in acute coronary syndromes. *Circulation* 2000; **101**(25): 2883–2888.

99 Vallejo AN, Schirmer M, Weyand CM, Goronzy JJ. Clonality and longevity of CD4 + CD28null T cells are associated with defects in apoptotic pathways. *J Immunol* 2000; **165**(11): 6301–6307.

100 Shimizu J, Yamazaki S, Takahashi T, Ishida Y, Sakaguchi S. Stimulation of CD25(+)CD4(+) regulatory T cells through GITR breaks immunological self-tolerance. *Nat Immunol* 2002; **3**(2): 135–142.

101 Ait-Oufella H, Salomon BL, Potteaux S, et al. Natural regulatory T cells control the development of atherosclerosis in mice. *Nat Med* 2006; **12**(2): 178–180.

102 Han SF, Liu P, Zhang W, et al. The opposite-direction modulation of CD4 + CD25+ Tregs and T helper 1 cells in acute coronary syndromes. *Clin Immunol* 2007; **124**(1): 90–97.

103 Naghavi M, Libby P, Falk E, *et al.* From vulnerable plaque to vulnerable patient: a call for new definitions and risk assessment strategies: Part II. *Circulation* 2003; **108**(15): 1772–1778.

104 Fuster V, Fayad ZA, Moreno PR, Poon M, Corti R, Badimon JJ. Atherothrombosis and high-risk plaque: Part II: approaches by noninvasive computed tomographic/magnetic resonance imaging. *J Am Coll Cardiol* 2005; **46**(7): 1209–1218.

105 Fuster V, Moreno PR, Fayad ZA, Corti R, Badimon JJ. Atherothrombosis and high-risk plaque: part I: evolving concepts. *J Am Coll Cardiol* 2005; **46**(6): 937–954.

106 Tsimikas S, Willerson JT, Ridker PM. C-reactive protein and other emerging blood biomarkers to optimize risk stratification of vulnerable patients. *J Am Coll Cardiol* 2006; **47**(8 Suppl): C19–31.

107 Du Clos TW. Function of C-reactive protein. *Ann Med* 2000; **32**(4): 274–278.

108 Calabro P, Willerson JT, Yeh ET. Inflammatory cytokines stimulated C-reactive protein production by human coronary artery smooth muscle cells. *Circulation* 2003; **108**(16): 1930–1932.

109 Verma S, Wang CH, Li SH, *et al.* A self-fulfilling prophecy: C-reactive protein attenuates nitric oxide production and inhibits angiogenesis. *Circulation* 2002; **106**(8): 913–919.

110 Ridker PM, Cushman M, Stampfer MJ, Tracy RP, Hennekens CH. Inflammation, aspirin, and the risk of cardiovascular disease in apparently healthy men. *N Engl J Med* 1997; **336**(14): 973–979.

111 Haverkate F, Thompson SG, Pyke SD, Gallimore JR, Pepys MB. Production of C-reactive protein and risk of coronary events in stable and unstable angina. European Concerted Action on Thrombosis and Disabilities Angina Pectoris Study Group. *Lancet* 1997; **349**(9050): 462–466.

112 Ridker PM, Rifai N, Pfeffer MA, *et al.* Inflammation, pravastatin, and the risk of coronary events after myocardial infarction in patients with average cholesterol levels. Cholesterol and Recurrent Events (CARE) Investigators. *Circulation* 1998; **98**(9): 839–844.

113 Lindahl B, Toss H, Siegbahn A, Venge P, Wallentin L. Markers of myocardial damage and inflammation in relation to long-term mortality in unstable coronary artery disease. FRISC Study Group. Fragmin during Instability in Coronary Artery Disease. *N Engl J Med* 2000; **343**(16): 1139–1147.

114 Liuzzo G, Biasucci LM, Gallimore JR, *et al.* The prognostic value of C-reactive protein and serum amyloid a protein in severe unstable angina. *N Engl J Med* 1994; **331**(7): 417–424.

115 Ridker PM, Rifai N, Rose L, Buring JE, Cook NR. Comparison of C-reactive protein and low-density lipoprotein cholesterol levels in the prediction of first cardiovascular events. *N Engl J Med* 2002; **347**(20): 1557–1565.

116 Ridker PM, Stampfer MJ, Rifai N. Novel risk factors for systemic atherosclerosis: a comparison of C-reactive protein, fibrinogen, homocysteine, lipoprotein(a), and standard cholesterol screening as predictors of peripheral arterial disease. *JAMA* 2001; **285**(19): 2481–2485.

117 Pai JK, Pischon T, Ma J, *et al.* Inflammatory markers and the risk of coronary heart disease in men and women. *N Engl J Med* 2004; **351**(25): 2599–2610.

118 Hirschfield GM, Gallimore JR, Kahan MC, *et al.* Transgenic human C-reactive protein is not proatherogenic in apolipoprotein E-deficient mice. *Proc Nat Acad Sci U S A* 2005; **102**(23): 8309–8314.

119 Pearson TA, Mensah GA, Alexander RW, *et al.* Markers of inflammation and cardiovascular disease: application to clinical and public health practice: a statement for healthcare professionals from the Centers for Disease Control and Prevention and the American Heart Association. *Circulation* 2003; **107**(3): 499–511.

120 Davies MJ, Gordon JL, Gearing AJ, *et al.* The expression of the adhesion molecules ICAM-1, VCAM-1, PECAM, and E-selectin in human atherosclerosis. *J Pathol* 1993; **171**(3): 223–229.

121 Ridker PM, Rifai N, Stampfer MJ, Hennekens CH. Plasma concentration of interleukin-6 and the risk of future myocardial infarction among apparently healthy men. *Circulation* 2000; **101**(15): 1767–1772.

122 Peter K, Nawroth P, Conradt C, *et al.* Circulating vascular cell adhesion molecule-1 correlates with the extent of human atherosclerosis in contrast to circulating intercellular adhesion molecule-1, E-selectin, P-selectin, and thrombomodulin. *Arterioscler Thromb Vasc Biol* 1997; **17**(3): 505–512.

123 Libby P, Aikawa M. New insights into plaque stabilisation by lipid lowering. *Drugs* 1998; **56**(Suppl 1): 9–13; discussion 33.

124 Urbich C, Dernbach E, Aicher A, Zeiher AM, Dimmeler S. CD40 ligand inhibits endothelial cell migration by increasing production of endothelial reactive oxygen species. *Circulation* 2002; **106**(8): 981–986.

125 Varo N, de Lemos JA, Libby P, *et al.* Soluble CD40L: risk prediction after acute coronary syndromes. *Circulation* 2003; **108**(9): 1049–1052.

126 Heeschen C, Dimmeler S, Hamm CW, *et al.* Soluble CD40 ligand in acute coronary syndromes. *N Engl J Med* 2003; **348**(12): 1104–1111.

127 Semb AG, van Wissen S, Ueland T, *et al.* Raised serum levels of soluble CD40 ligand in patients with familial hypercholesterolemia: downregulatory effect of statin therapy. *J Am Coll Cardiol* 2003; **41**(2): 275–279.

128 Mallat Z, Corbaz A, Scoazec A, *et al.* Expression of interleukin-18 in human atherosclerotic plaques and relation to plaque instability. *Circulation* 2001; **104**(14): 1598–1603.

129 Bayes-Genis A, Conover CA, Schwartz RS. The insulin-like growth factor axis: a review of atherosclerosis and restenosis. *Circ Res* 2000; **86**(2): 125–130.

130 Bayes-Genis A, Conover CA, Overgaard MT, *et al.* Pregnancy-associated plasma protein A as a marker of acute coronary syndromes. *N Engl J Med* 2001; **345**(14): 1022–1029.

131 Sangiorgi G, Mauriello A, Bonanno E, *et al.* Pregnancy-associated plasma protein-a is markedly expressed by monocyte-macrophage cells in vulnerable and ruptured carotid atherosclerotic plaques: a link between inflammation and cerebrovascular events. *J Am Coll Cardiol* 2006; **47**(11): 2201–2211.

132 Jaffer FA, Libby P, Weissleder R. Molecular and cellular imaging of atherosclerosis: emerging applications. *J Am Coll Cardiol* 2006; **47**(7): 1328–1338.

133 Constantinides P. Cause of thrombosis in human atherosclerotic arteries. *Am J Cardiol* 1990; **66**(16): 37 g–40 g.

134 Fayad ZA, Fuster V. Clinical imaging of the high-risk or vulnerable atherosclerotic plaque. *Circ Res* 2001; **89**(4): 305–316.

135 Stefanadis C, Toutouzas K, Tsiamis E, *et al.* Thermal heterogeneity in stable human coronary atherosclerotic plaques is underestimated in vivo: the "cooling effect" of blood flow. *J Am Coll Cardiol* 2003; **41**(3): 403–408.

136 Ruehm SG, Corot C, Vogt P, Kolb S, Debatin JF. Magnetic resonance imaging of atherosclerotic plaque with ultrasmall superparamagnetic particles of iron oxide in hyperlipidemic rabbits. *Circulation* 2001; **103**(3): 415–422.

137 Lederman RJ, Raylman RR, Fisher SJ, *et al.* Detection of atherosclerosis using a novel positron-sensitive probe and 18-fluorodeoxyglucose (FDG). *Nucl Med Commun* 2001; **22**(7): 747–753.

138 Ciavolella M, Tavolaro R, Taurino M, *et al.* Immunoscintigraphy of atherosclerotic uncomplicated lesions in vivo with a monoclonal antibody against D-dimers of insoluble fibrin. *Atherosclerosis* 1999; **143**(1): 171–175.

139 Schmitz SA, Coupland SE, Gust R, *et al.* Superparamagnetic iron oxide-enhanced MRI of atherosclerotic plaques in Watanabe hereditable hyperlipidemic rabbits. *Invest Radiol* 2000; **35**(8): 460–471.

140 Schmitz SA, Taupitz M, Wagner S, *et al.* Iron-oxide-enhanced magnetic resonance imaging of atherosclerotic plaques: postmortem analysis of accuracy, interobserver agreement, and pitfalls. *Invest Radiol* 2002; **37**(7): 405–411.

141 Yuan C, Kerwin WS. MRI of atherosclerosis. *J Magn Reson Imaging* 2004; **19**(6): 710–719.

142 Yuan C, Kerwin WS, Ferguson MS, *et al.* Contrast-enhanced high resolution MRI for atherosclerotic carotid artery tissue characterization. *J Magn Reson Imaging* 2002; **15**(1): 62–67.

143 Vasilyev N, Williams T, Brennan ML, *et al.* Myeloperoxidase-generated oxidants modulate left ventricular remodeling but not infarct size after myocardial infarction. *Circulation* 2005; **112**(18): 2812–2820.

144 Hazen SL, Heinecke JW. 3-Chlorotyrosine, a specific marker of myeloperoxidase-catalyzed oxidation, is markedly elevated in low density lipoprotein isolated from human atherosclerotic intima. *J Clin Invest* 1997; **99**(9): 2075–2081.

145 Podrez EA, Febbraio M, Sheibani N, *et al.* Macrophage scavenger receptor CD36 is the major receptor for LDL modified by monocyte-generated reactive nitrogen species. *J Clin Invest* 2000; **105**(8): 1095–1108.

146 Hazen SL. Myeloperoxidase and plaque vulnerability. *Arterioscler Thromb Vasc Biol* 2004; **24**(7): 1143–1146.

147 Sugiyama S, Okada Y, Sukhova GK, Virmani R, Heinecke JW, Libby P. Macrophage myeloperoxidase regulation by granulocyte macrophage colony-stimulating factor in human atherosclerosis and implications in acute coronary syndromes. *Am J Pathol* 2001; **158**(3): 879–891.

148 Asselbergs FW, Tervaert JW, Tio RA. Prognostic value of myeloperoxidase in patients with chest pain. *N Engl J Med* 2004; **350**(5): 516–518; author reply 518.

149 Zhang R, Brennan ML, Fu X, *et al.* Association between myeloperoxidase levels and risk of coronary artery disease. *JAMA* 2001; **286**(17): 2136–2142.

150 Brennan ML, Penn MS, Van Lente F, *et al.* Prognostic value of myeloperoxidase in patients with chest pain. *N Engl J Med* 2003; **349**(17): 1595–1604.

151 Asakura T, Karino T. Flow patterns and spatial distribution of atherosclerotic lesions in human coronary arteries. *Circ Res* 1990; **66**(4): 1045–1066.

152 Malek AM, Alper SL, Izumo S. Hemodynamic shear stress and its role in atherosclerosis. *JAMA* 1999; **282**(21): 2035–2042.

153 Stone PH, Saito S, Takahashi S, *et al.* Prediction of progression of coronary artery disease and clinical outcomes using vascular profiling of endothelial shear stress and arterial plaque characteristics: the PREDICTION Study. *Circulation* 2012; **126**(2): 172–181.

154 Samady H, Eshtehardi P, McDaniel MC, *et al.* Coronary artery wall shear stress is associated with progression and transformation of atherosclerotic plaque and arterial remodeling in patients with coronary artery disease. *Circulation* 2011; **124**(7): 779–788.

155 Gijsen FJ, Wentzel JJ, Thury A, *et al.* Strain distribution over plaques in human coronary arteries relates to shear stress. *Am J Physiol Heart Circ Physiol* 2008; **295**(4): H1608–H1614.

156 Finn AV, Otsuka F. Neoatherosclerosis: a culprit in very late stent thrombosis. *Circ Cardiovasc Interv* 2012; **5**(1): 6–9.

157 Nakazawa G, Otsuka F, Nakano M, *et al.* The pathology of neoatherosclerosis in human coronary implants bare-metal and drug-eluting stents. *J Am Coll Cardiol* 2011; **57**(11): 1314–1322.

158 Park SJ, Kang SJ, Virmani R, Nakano M, Ueda Y. In-stent neoatherosclerosis: a final common pathway of late stent failure. *J Am Coll Cardiol* 2012; **59**(23): 2051–2057.

159 Yonetsu T, Kato K, Kim SJ, *et al.* Predictors for neoatherosclerosis: a retrospective observational study from the optical coherence tomography registry. *Circ Cardiovasc Imaging* 2012; **5**(5): 660–666.

160 Habara M, Terashima M, Suzuki T. Detection of atherosclerotic progression with rupture of degenerated in-stent intima five years after bare-metal stent implantation using optical coherence tomography. *J Invasive Cardiol* 2009; **21**(10): 552–553.

161 Inoue K, Abe K, Ando K, *et al.* Pathological analyses of long-term intracoronary Palmaz-Schatz stenting: Is its efficacy permanent? *Cardiovasc Pathol* 2004; **13**(2): 109–115.

162 Nakazawa G, Vorpahl M, Finn AV, Narula J, Virmani R. One step forward and two steps back with drug-eluting-stents: from preventing restenosis to causing late thrombosis and nouveau atherosclerosis. *J Am Coll Cardiol Cardiovasc Imaging* 2009; **2**(5): 625–8.

163 Kang SJ, Lee CW, Song H, *et al.* OCT analysis in patients with very late stent thrombosis. *J Am Coll Cardiol Cardiovasc Imaging* 2013; **6**(6): 695–703.

164 Wykrzykowska JJ, Diletti R, Gutierrez-Chico JL, *et al.* Plaque sealing and passivation with a mechanical self-expanding low outward force nitinol vShield device for the treatment of IVUS and OCT-derived thin cap fibroatheromas (TCFAs) in native coronary arteries: report of the pilot study vShield Evaluated at Cardiac hospital in Rotterdam for Investigation and Treatment of TCFA (SECRITT). *EuroIntervention* 2012; **8**(8): 945–954.

CHAPTER 2

The Essentials of Femoral Vascular Access and Closure

Ted Feldman and Mohammad Sarraf

NorthShore University HealthSystem, Evanston, IL, USA

While we are often preoccupied with the coronary and cardiac complications of catheterization and intervention, it is femoral access complications that occur more frequently, and which are certainly more recognized and remembered by patients. The incidence of local vascular complications that are considered major, as defined by the need for prolonged hospitalization, transfusion, or vascular surgery, ranges between 1% and 1.5% in diagnostic catheterization procedures, and typically between 3% and 5% in interventional procedures. More recently, refinements in techniques and antithrombotic regimes have reduced femoral vascular complications in interventional procedures to 2–3%, but they still remain frequent adverse events [1–3]. Risk factors for vascular complications include advanced age, female gender, low body surface area (BSA), aggressive antithrombin or antiplatelet agent use (e.g. GP IIb/IIIa inhibitors), emergent procedures, vascular disease, vessel size, sheath size, and puncture location [1,4]. The subjects of femoral access and management of femoral puncture after sheath removal are of vital importance in cardiac catheterizations and interventions, especially in patients with high risk of complications.

Femoral access

Anatomy

A good understanding of some key features of the local anatomy is essential for both optimal access and ideal management of the puncture site. Careful attention to access and careful evaluation of the access site are fundamental to reduce sheath insertion trauma and lead to uncomplicated sheath removal and the safe use of vascular closure devices.

It is important to puncture at the level of the common femoral artery. This allows compression of the vessel against the femoral head at the time of sheath removal. Punctures below the common femoral arterial bifurcation (hence in the profunda femoris or the superficial femoral artery) are over soft tissue and are difficult to compress (Figures 2.1 and 2.2). Such punctures have been shown to be associated with increased risk of pseudoaneurysms and arteriovenous fistula formation [5,6]. Punctures above the inguinal ligament (hence in the external iliac artery) are in the retroperitoneal space which also represents an incompressible space. Such high punctures are associated with increased risk of retroperitoneal bleeding [6–8].

Landmarks on fluoroscopy are useful for identifying the position of the common femoral artery. About 75–80% of the common femoral bifurcation is at or below the inferior border of the femoral head and 95% is at or below the mid femoral head [5,9]. While the inguinal ligament is not visualized under fluoroscopy, the deep circumflex iliac artery is commonly used as a surrogate marker of the upper border of the common femoral artery because it is the last arterial branch of the external iliac artery before the external iliac courses under the inguinal ligament and becomes the common femoral artery (Figure 2.1). The deep circumflex iliac artery arises from the lateral aspect of the external iliac artery nearly opposite the origin of the inferior epigastric artery. It ascends obliquely laterally behind the inguinal ligament, contained in a fibrous sheath formed by the junction of the transversalis fascia and iliac fascia, to the anterior superior iliac spine. Puncture above the most inferior border of the course of the deep circumflex iliac artery has been associated with increased risk of retroperitoneal hemorrhage. This landmark is above the most superior border of the acetabulum in most patients [6].

Puncture technique

The basic technique of arterial access has changed very little since it was initially introduced by Seldinger [10]. Puncture of the common femoral artery is basically unchanged, save that the original concept used a through and through puncture and withdrawal of needle into the arterial lumen, while our current approach ideally punctures only the anterior surface of the femoral artery.

However, the technique can be substantially improved by using fluoroscopy of bony landmarks to identify the likely course of the common femoral artery followed by confirmation with femoral angiography after sheath insertion [11]. A point of entry into the common femoral artery at the mid femoral head or slightly above is ideal. The femoral skin crease, which is a very commonly used landmark for puncture, is distal to the common femoral bifurcation in 72% of cases [12]. Generally speaking, younger patients have a mid femoral head location relatively close or slightly above the femoral crease. Older patients have a femoral head significantly above the femoral crease, since the crease tends to sag with age. Obese patients may have two or sometimes even three femoral creases.

Interventional Cardiology: Principles and Practice, Second Edition. Edited by George D. Dangas, Carlo Di Mario, and Nicholas N. Kipshidze.
© 2017 John Wiley & Sons, Ltd. Published 2017 by John Wiley & Sons, Ltd.

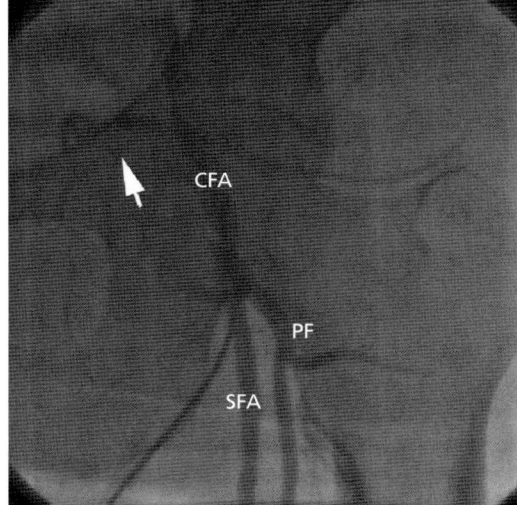

Figure 2.1 Femoral artery angiogram taken after sheath insertion. The sheath has been inserted into the superficial femoral artery (SFA). The profunda femoris or deep femoral artery is labeled PF. The sheath terminates in the common femoral artery (CFA). The arrow denotes the lower margin of the curve of the deep circumflex iliac artery. This lower border of the curve courses along the inguinal ligament. Punctures above this landmark are usually adjacent to the retroperitoneal space and poses a high risk for bleeding complications.

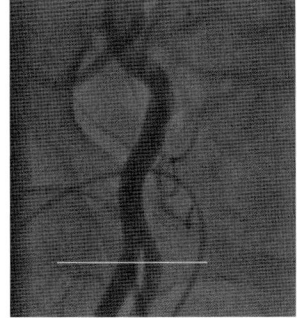 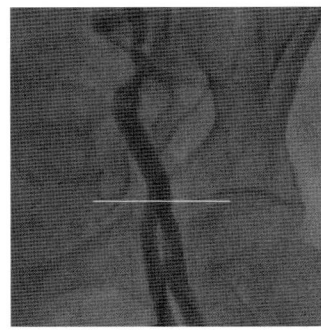

Figure 2.2 Bilateral femoral artery angiograms. On the left panel, a line is drawn through the level of the mid femoral head. This is normally an ideal location for puncture. In this case, however, the femoral artery bifurcation is above the mid femoral head and the sheath can be seen entering the deep femoral artery. The right panel shows the left femoral angiogram. A line is drawn at the level of the top of the femoral head, showing a remarkably high bifurcation in this patient. Even though the sheath insertion on this side is just below the top of the femoral head, it is also in the deep femoral artery. Although this puncture is compressible over the femoral head, the branch is relatively smaller than the common femoral artery and less well suited for use of closure devices.

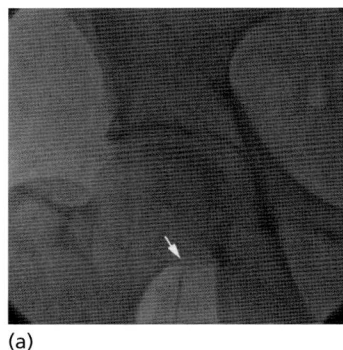 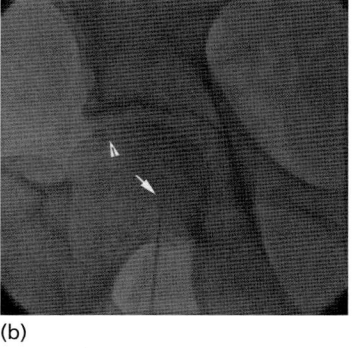 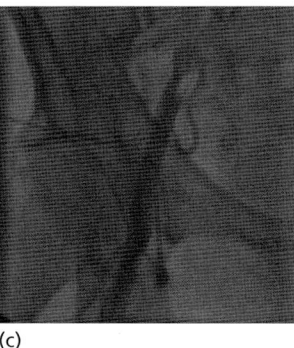

(a)　　　　　　　　　　(b)　　　　　　　　　　(c)

Figure 2.3 (a) shows a fluoroscopic image recorded prior to puncture. The 18 g thin wall needle has been laid on the skin at the point of anticipated femoral puncture based on palpation. The arrow shows the tip of the needle. Fluoroscopy demonstrates that the needle is at the lower border of the femoral head. This is an ideal location for skin entry as the needle will puncture the femoral artery superior to this point. (b) shows the needle advanced until the pulsation of the femoral artery is felt to be transmitted through the needle. The arrow shows the position of the needle. This is just below the mid femoral head and is an ideal "landing zone" for puncture. The majority of patients' femoral artery bifurcation will be below this point and the probability of common femoral artery entry is high. The arrowhead pointing upward shows the location of the skin crease. In (c) sheath angiography demonstrates that the entry point is in the common femoral artery above the line of the mid femoral head. This is higher than ideal but represents a good entry point for the sheath. Just above the sheath entry site, the U-shaped branch of the external iliac artery denotes the location of the inguinal ligament and the division between the common femoral artery and the retroperitoneal iliac vessel. This branch is the deep circumflex iliac artery.

The technique of puncture requires multiple small steps to be optimized. Before local anesthesia is given, a clamp or needle can be laid at the point where the pulse is most easily felt, just above the femoral crease. Fluoroscopy can be used to locate the position of the needle relative to the center of the femoral head (Figure 2.3). Local anesthesia can thus be given accordingly. After local anesthesia is given, the needle is advanced to a point just above the arterial wall, using palpation as a guide. At this point, it is useful to fluoroscope the location of the needle once again. This is the last chance to adjust the puncture to enter the common femoral artery in the ideal landing zone. This method is not often adhered to, but in the long run is very worthwhile and justifies the few seconds of extra time at the beginning of the procedure. Meanwhile, this is also the time to observe the behavior of the needle that is placed close to the femoral artery. If the needle is moving up and down, it is indirect evidence of puncturing the anterior wall of the common femoral artery. However, if the needle is moving side to side, it is indirect evidence of puncturing the lateral or medial side of the common femoral artery. Therefore, the operator can still adjust the angle of attack to the femoral artery.

Once the sheath has been inserted, a sheath angiogram should be performed. Using an AP projection best preserves the relationship between the puncture site and the lower border of the inferior epigastric artery, but may have overlap of the femoral bifurcation. A 20° ipsilateral angulation of the image intensifier will expose the entry point of the sheath, as well as the femoral bifurcation [6]. It can thus be determined whether the common femoral artery has in fact been entered, and whether there is atherosclerosis, calcification, or angulation of the puncture site. It is our practice to obtain the sheath angiogram at the beginning of the procedure, so that decisions about closure and sometimes anticoagulation can be made before the procedure is performed. If the sheath has been inserted into the branch vessels below the bifurcation, this will often have an impact on ultimate sheath size, for example in the setting of bifurcation or chronic total occlusion intervention, and can impact the choice of anticoagulation. When the puncture is above the most inferior border of the inferior epigastric artery, it is likely that the retroperitoneal space has been entered with the sheath. In this instance, an option is to defer intervention until a later time. Full anticoagulation with the sheath in this location greatly increases the risk of retroperitoneal bleeding, which is one of the worst and more difficult local complications to manage.

Ultrasound guided femoral access

Ultrasound guided vascular access has gained attention by catheterization laboratories for arterial access, especially for large bore vascular access. The main advantage of ultrasound guided access is to identify the anatomy of the vessels and the relationship between the artery and the vein. Ultrasound guided access helps to select the puncture site more precisely. The major landmarks should be identified by conventional fluoroscopy. By using a sterile plastic cover, the probe is positioned over the point of maximal pulsation to scan the femoral artery and vein. The scanning should start from the point of maximal pulse with cranial to caudal movement of the probe perpendicular to the skin until the bifurcation site is accurately identified. The appearance of femoral artery is a pulsatile circle, with thicker and more prominent delineation of the arterial walls. Sometimes, the calcification of the vessels or plaques inside the artery can be identified, which helps to avoid entering these areas. Identification of femoral artery versus vein is easily achieved by gentle pressure with the vascular probe; the artery is not compressible and the pulsations become more apparent. It is noteworthy that pulsation of the vessels can be misleading in patients with severe tricuspid regurgitation. The artery should be imaged in the center of the image, and the needle should be gently approached. The reverberation artifact of the needle helps to identify the path of the needle to the artery. When the needle enters the artery, the rest of the procedure follows the standard procedure for vascular access. Sometimes, the vein runs medial and posterior to the artery. Using ultrasound can occasionally be useful to avoid entering artery before venous access and prevent other complications such as arteriovenous fistulae.

Femoral access closure
Manual compression
Manual compression has been the standard for sheath removal for decades. Classically, after diagnostic catheterizations the technique involves sheath removal after normalization of the activated clotting time (ACT) to <160–180 seconds and direct digital pressures with fingers positioned over the arterial puncture site and one to two fingerbreadths more proximally. The manual pressure should be applied with enough force to allow for a faint palpable distal pulse. Pressure is held for 10–15 minutes, during which hemostasis should be achieved, after which the patient is kept under bed rest for 4–6 hours.

The use of larger arterial sheaths, more intensive anticoagulation, and antiplatelet regimes associated with coronary and cardiac interventions have led to the need for more prolonged direct pressure to achieve hemostasis and more prolonged bed rest prior to ambulation. A variety of mechanical manual compression aids, such as the Femostop (Radi Medical System, Sweden) and Compressar C-clamp (Advanced Vascular Dynamics, Portland, OR), have been developed to relieve the requirement for staff to physically apply prolonged direct digital pressure. A number of studies have compared such devices with direct manual pressure, with most studies finding lower vascular complications with mechanical compression devices [13–15] although a small study (90 subjects) found better results with direct manual pressure [16].

Clamp devices provide compression without the need to have someone using direct manual pressure. While clamps may be less demanding on personnel, they do not obviate the need for careful supervision of the compression process. If clamps are applied with too much pressure or left in place for too long, they can result in arterial or venous thrombosis. If applied without adequate pressure, bleeding can result. The Femostop (RADI Medical) uses an inflatable bubble to apply pressure to the puncture site. This is our preferred device for compression in fully anticoagulated patients with failed suture closure or large caliber arterial or venous sheaths. The bubble is clear, so the puncture site can be observed directly. The pressure is regulated with a blood pressure cuff bulb. Near systolic pressure (usually 10 mm less than systolic blood pressure) can be applied for 15–30 minutes, and then the pressure can be decreased 10–15 mmHg every 10–20 minutes.

Even with interventional procedures, there have been some remarkable experiences with ambulation as early as 2 hours after simple manual compression. With the use of bivalirudin, in a study of 100 patients, after a mean manual compression time of 13 minutes, patients were able to ambulate at a mean duration of 2 hours and 23 minutes after sheath removal [17]. Even using heparin, there are various studies suggesting ability to ambulate after 2 hours. Using a regime of a standard heparin dose of 5000 IU and 6 Fr guiding catheters, two studies involving 359 and 907 patients were able to have sheaths removed immediately, with a mean compression time of around 10 minutes and successful early ambulation within 2 hours with no significant excess in puncture site complications [18,19]. A study with more aggressive anticoagulation (ACT to 300 seconds) and subsequent sheath removal when ACT is less than 150 seconds showed no difference in site complications between patients ambulating at 2 hours compared to 4 or 6 hours. In this latter study, there are also similar results in a subgroup of patients who received GP IIb/IIIa inhibitors [20]. Thus, manual compression is clearly an acceptable form of puncture site management in all patients.

Table 2.1 Types of closure devices.

	Manufacturer	CE Mark	US Approval	Status
Plugs				
AngioSeal	St. Jude Medical	+	+	
Exoseal	Cordis	+	+	Not used frequently in the USA
Femoseal	St. Jude Medical	+	−	
Suture devices				
ProGlide	Abbott	+	+	
ProStar	Abbott	+	+	
Superstich	Sutura	+	+	
Staples/clips				
StarClose	Abbott	+	+	
Angiolink	Medtronic	+	+	
Liquid/gel				
Duett	Vascular Solutions	+	+	
Mynx	Access Closure	+	+	

Vascular closure devices

A variety of vascular closure devices have been developed to enhance vascular closure without need for prolonged compression. These are deployed at the conclusion of the cardiac catheterization procedure and can be used despite an elevated ACT. Closure devices are classified into four major categories: sutures, plugs, glues, and topical patches (Table 2.1). The current FDA-approved devices in most common use in the USA are the AngioSeal (Datascope Inc), Perclose, ProStar, and StarClose (Abbott Vascular, Redwood City CA). Hemostatic patches are also approved for use in the USA (Figure 2.4).

AngioSeal

The AngioSeal device consists of a rectangular absorbable copolymeric anchor deployed intravascularly against the arterial wall which is attached by an absorbable Dexon traction suture to an extravascular collagen plug applied to the outside of the arterial wall. The AngioSeal assembly consists of a carrier system with the anchor, collagen plug, and traction suture compacted at the distal end. There is a delivery sheath with a modified locator dilator which identifies when the sheath is intravascular. After cardiac catheterization, the working sheath is changed over to the AngioSeal delivery sheath. Once the delivery sheath is intravascular, as indicated by pulsatile flow in the arteriotomy locator system of the dilator, the dilator and wire are removed. The carrier is then advanced into the sheath, locks in place with the sheath, and then the entire assembly is withdrawn until resistance is felt. This indicates apposition of the anchor on the luminal arterial wall. Further withdrawal releases the collagen plug on the external surface of the artery, followed by a tamper tube. The

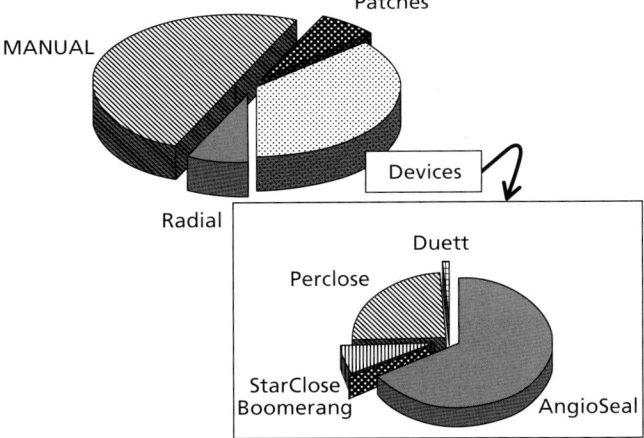

Figure 2.4 Use of vascular closure approaches in the United States.

tamper tube is used to compress the plug over the wire, followed by removal of the tamper tube and cutting of the suture, which are external to the patient. Currently, the AngioSeal is available in two sizes: 6 and 8 Fr. Deployment success rates ranged from 92% to 98%, and hemostasis success ranged from 84% to 97% [21].

Perclose

The Perclose device is a suture-mediated system which has undergone a steady evolution which included the Techstar device, Closer S 6 Fr, and the current ProGlide 6 Fr system. It incorporates two needles in the proximal compartment of the device and a catheter that houses the suture (Figure 2.5). The working sheath is exchanged over a wire for the Perclose device. The device is advanced until return of pulsatile blood in the locator, indicating appropriate intravascular placement. A lever is pulled to open the "feet," and the device is withdrawn until resistance is felt, indicating apposition of the foot processes and suture catch plates against the inner vessel wall. A plunger is depressed, forcing the needles through the outer vessel wall into the suture catch plates. The catch plates are attached to the ends of the suture. Retraction of the plunger withdraws the needles and the attached sutures through the skin. With the current ProGlide system, the device incorporates a non-absorbable polypropylene monofilament with pre-tied knot that is tightened and the vascular access site closed using a pusher device. One significant advantage of the Perclose system is to maintain access to the vessel during deploying the device by using the guidewire before withdrawing the device. Therefore the wire can be reintroduced via the device after the needle and suture deployment, and the wire removed after confirmation of adequate hemostasis. This feature is unique among the closure approaches. In most series, the device is successfully deployed in 89–100%, with hemostasis success seen in 86–99%. The Prostar device is a Perclose-based suture mediated device, which allows for closure of larger arteriotomy. It comes in 8 or 10 Fr and can incorporate one or two sutures (associated with two or four needles, respectively).

StarClose

StarClose is a device that applies a 4-mm low profile nitinol clip entirely on the external surface of the artery with no permanent intravascular component (Figures 2.6 and 2.7). The tines of the clip grasp the arterial tissue and close the arteriotomy in a purse string fashion. The device consists of the clip applier and a proprietary

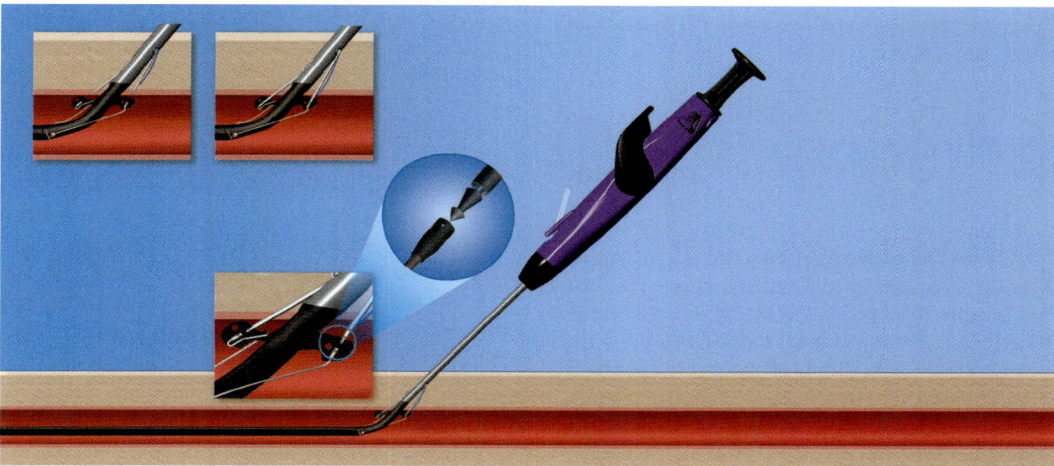

Figure 2.5 The Perclose ProGlide device is used to deliver sutures through the puncture to close the arteriotomy site. The small insets of the upper left of the figure show feet that are opened inside the artery, and the mechanism by which needles are driven from the handle of the device into the feet to capture the sutures. The sutures are then withdrawn using the needles, and a pre-tied knot is pushed through the skin to the top of the arteriotomy site on the outside of the artery.

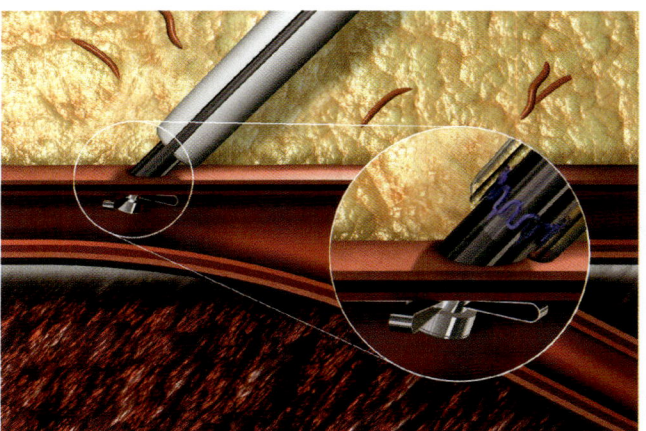
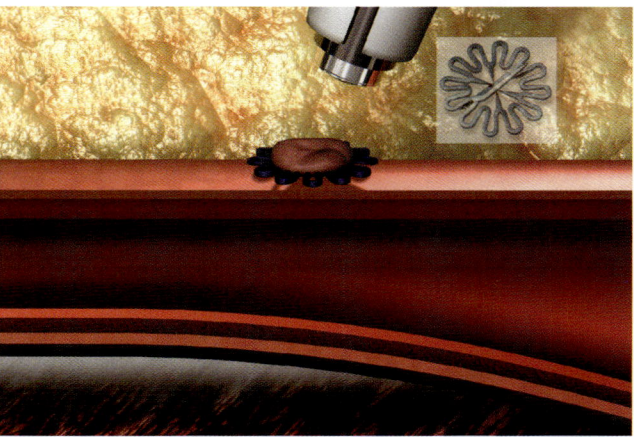

Figure 2.6 The StarClose device is delivered through a special sheath provided with the device. After the device is loaded into the artery, nitinol wings are opened within the artery and pulled back to capture the inner arterial wall. The clip device, shown on the left part of the figure, is then advanced to the outside surface of the artery. When a clip is fired, it inverts and the tines of the clip capture the arteriotomy and force it closed. This device is unique in that what is left behind is entirely extra-arterial.

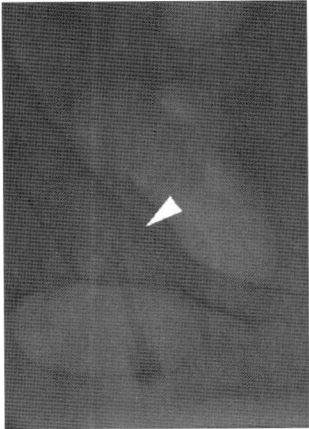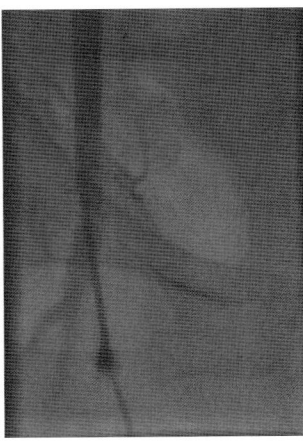

Figure 2.7 Femoral angiogram 1 year after closure with the StarClose device. The arrowhead on the left shows the device, and on the right contrast injection demonstrates the insertion site of the re-puncture. The device is entirely extravascular.

6 Fr sheath. After conclusion of cardiac catheterization, the working sheath is changed over a wire to the proprietary sheath, with further blunt dissection during the process to ease subsequent advancement of the 12 Fr clip applier through the skin and subcutaneous tissue. The clip applier has a vessel locator, which is inserted into the sheath, until the clip applier snaps into the sheath. A button is depressed which deploys small flexible nitinol wings at the end of the vessel locator, inside the artery. The entire assembly is withdrawn until resistance is felt, indicating apposition of the wings against the inner vessel wall. The sliding element with the attached clip is then depressed splitting the sheath and applies the clip to the arterial wall at the end of the assembly. At this stage, it is very important to ensure that the skin does not block the "splitter." It is reasonable therefore to nick the skin after the proprietary sheath is placed. The procedure is completed by release of the clip using a button "trigger." In the CLIP trial, which compared the StarClose with manual compression, device success was 87%, with no difference in complications between the groups [22].

Exoseal, Femoseal

Exoseal (Cordis, Bridgewater, NJ) is a passive closure device that consists of deployment of a polyglycolic acid plug (absorbed within 90 days) over the arteriotomy site for hemostasis. The system is delivered through 5–7 Fr sheaths. The minimum diameter of the femoral artery is 5 mm for closure. Time to achieve hemostasis and ambulation appears to be lower than with manual compression. Access through the same site requires a delay of at least 30 days.

Femoseal (St. Jude Medical Systems, Uppsala, Sweden) comprises a bioabsorbable polymer anchor plate that remains inside the artery and an outer disk. After procedural sheath removal, the anchor seal is deployed within the artery while the outer locking disk is placed on the outer wall of the artery. The arteriotomy is sandwiched between the two disks and held together by a bioabsorbable multifilament.

Hemostatic patches

Hemostatic patches were originally designed for military purposes to achieve temporary arterial hemostasis in the battlefield. The mechanisms of action include causing vasoconstriction, creation of a positively charged environment, which attracts negatively charged

red blood cells and platelets, or direct promotion of rapid coagulation [23–25]. Available patches include: Syvek Patch using poly-N-glucosamine (Marine Polymer Technologies, Danvers, MA); Neptune pad using calcium alginate (Biotronik, Bulach, Switzerland); Closure PAD (Medtronic, Santa Rosa, CA); Chito-Seal using chitosan gel (Abbott Vascular, Redwood, CA); SafeSeal using a microporous polysaccharide (Possis Medical, Minneapolis MN, formerly Stasys Patch, St. Jude Medical, St. Paul, MN); and D-Stat Dry using thrombin (Vascular Solutions, Minneapolis, MN) (Table 2.1) [23].

Hemostatic patches allow sheath removal in anticoagulated patients, with ACT as high as 300 seconds [24]. Studies on hemostatic patches have generally demonstrated shorter time to hemostasis and ambulation. However, a period of manual compression is generally required and may be longer than the recommended compression times from manufacturers [25–27]. It is likely a combination of both hemostatic properties of the patch and manual compression that leads to hemostasis. There are no consistent data demonstrating reduction in vascular complications with the use of hemostatic patches over manual compression. Neither the Syvek patch nor Chito-Seal has been shown to reduce vascular complications over manual compression in a review of cases registered with the American College of Cardiology-National Cardiovascular Data Registry (ACC-NCDR) [28]. D-Stat Dry used after diagnostic procedures reduced vascular complications compared to manual compression in a series utilizing a historical control [25], but no direct comparisons have been performed. As the complication rate from vascular puncture in general appears to be declining with time, direct comparisons are necessary to clearly demonstrate decreased complication rates using these patches [4]. There are now several other patches available.

Evidence-based issues for vascular closure devices

The design goals of active vascular closure devices (as replacement of manual compression for management of femoral arterial sheath removal) would include reduction in hemostasis and ambulation times with associated improved patient comfort and reduction in hemorrhagic vascular complications. As experience with this family of devices has grown it is clear that hemostasis and ambulation times can be decreased, but the reduction of vascular complications has not been as well shown. There are real concerns for the potential to increase rare but serious complications such as infection, arterial occlusion, distal embolization, and arterial wall injury with pseudoaneurysm. In addition, bleeding complications, should they occur, could potentially be more severe than seen with manual compression because manual compression requires normalization of ACT prior to sheath removal while vascular closure devices can be deployed at elevated ACT [4]. In a review of case series of AngioSeal and Perclose, the reported incidence of such complications include: infection 0.6%; pseudoaneurysm or arteriovenous fistula 0.6–1%; and occlusion or embolism 0.2–0.4% [21]. In a review of 4 years of cardiac catheterizations and interventions at the Mayo Clinic between 2000 and 2003, during which vascular closure devices were used in 1662 patients, the incidence of device-related infection was 0.24% [29].

There are numerous randomized and non-randomized comparisons of vascular closure devices and manual compression. There is significant heterogeneity between the trials in inclusion criteria and definitions of outcomes. Three meta-analyses have reviewed the studies involving collagen plug devices (AngioSeal and VasoSeal) and suture devices (Perclose) [28,30]. Use of vascular closure devices is associated with significant reductions in time to hemostasis (by 17 minutes), time to ambulation (by up to 11 hours) and time to discharge (by 0.6 days) [31]. However, in these analyses in both diagnostic and interventional settings, there is no substantial difference (benefits or harms) in vascular complications by the vascular closure devices, except for the VasoSeal device, which has been associated with increased vascular complications in two of the meta-analyses [30,32]. There are a number of limitations to assessing the relative rates of complications with manual compression and vascular closure devices. First, some trials have required femoral angiography, and higher risk patients may be eliminated from the trials, because of small caliber femoral vessels, atherosclerosis of the puncture site, or calcification. In addition, many of the trials have rigorous protocol specifications for the manner in which the closure devices are used, but generally give no guidance regarding manual compression methods, which can be highly variable. In some institutions, there are sheath removal teams who become quite expert at sheath removal, manual compression, and puncture site management. It is difficult to make comparisons between these programs and lower volume programs, or programs where new trainees are relegated to the task of sheath removal and manual compression.

The largest registry study of femoral hemostasis comes from the ACC-NCDR [33]. From this registry, the outcomes of 166,680 patients who underwent diagnostic and interventional cardiac catheterizations in 2001 were evaluated, with suture devices used in 25,495 cases, collagen-plug devices used in 28,160 cases, while the rest underwent manual compression. In the overall multivariate analysis, use of collagen plug devices was associated with reduced bleeding in diagnostic catheterization (odds ratio 0.68) and both types of closure devices were associated with reduced risk of pseudoaneurysm formation in diagnostic and interventional procedures (odds ratio 0.46–0.52). It is possible that among individual operators who develop special expertise with a particular closure device, there is potential to achieve improved success rates with lower complication rate [34].

What then are the advantages of vascular closure devices? Unquestionably, the complete avoidance of compression with immediate hemostasis and early ambulation improves patient satisfaction [35]. This alone can justify the use of these devices in many cases. However, with no clear difference in complication rates, possibly the strongest benefit may be an early (same-day) discharge of patients after percutaneous coronary intervention that could result from early ambulation [4,36]. Over the past 5 years, major vascular complications have decreased among patients undergoing percutaneous coronary intervention in the Northern New England Cardiovascular Disease Study Group. In their database, with 36,631 patients undergoing percutaneous coronary intervention, arterial complications decreased from 3.37% in 2002 to 1.98% in 2006 [30]. Whether this reflects more careful attention to needle puncture and sheath insertion, improved management of anticoagulation, better manual compression, or optimized use of closure devices cannot be ascertained without a randomized trial. Such a trial would require such a large population that is unlikely ever to be performed.

Vascular closure devices shorten the time to hemostasis and ambulation, compared with manual compression, but the aggregate of reports are mixed regarding the potential for closure devices to increase or decrease the risk of vascular complications. In a recent study of patients undergoing diagnostic coronary angiogram with a 6 Fr system, the vascular closure devices were not inferior to manual pressure. There were no increased risks of vascular complications; however, it is important to note that in this study the patients did not undergo any coronary interventions so the results should be considered in the context of diagnostic angiography. This study compared FemoSeal (St Jude Medical) with ExoSeal (Cordis). ExoSeal is not frequently used in the USA, and FemoSeal is only currently available in Europe [37].

Preclosure for large arterial sheaths

Large bore arterial sheaths (12–14 Fr) can be required for certain interventions such as retrograde balloon aortic valvuloplasty or, more recently, retrograde transcatheter aortic valve replacement (14–24 Fr). Such large bore arterial sheaths are historically associated with need for prolonged compression to achieve hemostasis, prolonged bed rest prior to mobilization (up to 12–24 hours in certain cases), and high risk of recurrent bleeding and need for transfusion. Transfusion rates after manual compression following balloon aortic valvuloplasty have been in the range of 25%. Preclosure is a technique using the Perclose or ProStar device to "preload" the suture around the puncture site prior to access with the large bore sheath to allow for subsequent suture closure at removal of the large arterial sheath. After puncture, a standard 6–8 Fr sheath is inserted and subsequently exchanged over the wire to introduce a Perclose or ProStar device. Deployment of the needle is performed with the standard manner to preload the suture around the arteriotomy. The suture is not tightened. A wire is reintroduced into the device over which an exchange is made with the subsequent large bore arterial sheath. At completion of the procedure requiring the large bore sheath, the sheath is removed and closure performed by tightening of the preloaded sutures. With this technique, a 6-Fr Perclose system had been successful in closing 12 Fr arteriotomies and a 10 Fr ProStar system had been successful in closing 14 Fr arteriotomies. In a non-randomized comparison, this technique had been successful in significantly reducing length of hospital stay and almost eliminating the need for blood transfusions after retrograde arterial balloon aortic valvuloplasty [38,39]. Although there are no commercially available closure devices for larger than 14 Fr sheath size, most operators have adopted approaches to utilize preclosure. Several novel devices for large vessel closure are under development. There are mainly three approaches of new technology to manage percutaneous closure following large bore vascular access: suture-based, suture and plug/sealant, and ipsilateral/contralateral graft placement. There are a number of products under investigation that are not available on the market yet.

Arterial access management for transcatheter aortic valvular replacement

In our catheterization laboratory, we use a standard approach for patients requiring transcatheter aortic valvular replacement (TAVR). This approach starts before the patient comes to the catheterization laboratory by meticulous attention to the aorto-iliac and femoral artery anatomy on pre-TAVR CT angiography. Understanding the location of calcifications of these vessels, tortuosity, diameter, and the presence of prior bypass grafts and/or stents is invaluable. The location of femoral bifurcations relative to the femoral head can be assessed.

We start the procedure with the contralateral access site (non-TAVR sheath) using a micropuncture needle with iterative usage of fluoroscopy. After placing a 7-Fr sheath in the contralateral artery, a JR4 or internal mammary artery catheter is used to cross into the ipsilateral common iliac artery with a wire (J tipped guidewire, angled glide wire, Wholly wire). The tip of the catheter is placed in the terminal portion of the ipsilateral external iliac artery and a cine angiogram of the ipsilateral common femoral artery is performed. A V18 guidewire is passed through the crossover catheter across the distal abdominal aortic bifurcation to the terminal segment of superficial femoral artery on the side in which the large caliber TAVR sheath will be placed. This wire is used for a possible usage of crossover balloon technique should major vascular complications occur with the TAVR sheath [40,41]. Ultrasound guidance is used as the preferred method for vascular access in some centers. It has the advantage of showing areas of calcification as well as the level of the femoral bifurcation, and better insures a puncture of the anterior wall of the common femoral artery.

At this point the ipsilateral common femoral artery is punctured for the TAVR sheath. The crossover angiogram is used as a roadmap for micropuncture. An injection through the crossover catheter can be used to verify the entry point of the needle in the common femoral artery (Figure 2.8). If we are not satisfied with the location of the femoral access, we withdraw the microcatheter and hold pressure for several minutes. Some operators prefer a pigtail from the contralateral access site. The terminal circle of the pigtail is placed over the target puncture site of the femoral head en face, to be used as a target for ipsilateral femoral access. A regular J tipped guidewire is placed in the microcatheter, and the microcatheter is removed. A 6 or 7 Fr dilator is placed over the wire to enlarge the arteriotomy prior to preclosure. Some operators recommend dissecting the subcutaneous tissue before 7 Fr dilator is removed for easier access to the vessel wall. Next we use two ProGlide devices for preclosure of the arteriotomy, the first placed at the 10 o'clock position and the second device at 2 o'clock. After the second ProGlide device is deployed a stiff Amplatzer guidewire is passed through the second ProGlide. An alternative to ProGlide device is using one or two ProStar closure devices.

Serial dilatation of the arteriotomy is not necessary, because most TAVR devices currently require 14–20 Fr arterial sheaths. We sometimes use a 14 Fr dilator (and sometimes a 14 Fr sheath) before inserting the TAVR sheath. After completion of TAVR procedure, an Amplatz Superstiff or Extrastiff wire is placed through the TAVR sheath. The first operator ties down the arteriotomy with the first ProGlide closure device with a knot pusher, while the second

operator carefully removes the TAVR sheath over the guidewire. An immediate assessment of the bleeding is a direct indication of the success of the closure device. Frequently, the first preclosure device successfully closes the arteriotomy with minimal bleeding. Subsequently, by using the knot pusher, the second preclosure knot is pushed down over the wire. Until this point, the wire is still left in place in case homeostasis is not achieved. In some cases, a third or sometimes even fourth ProGlide closure device may be necessary. When homeostasis is achieved, the wire can be removed and both knots tied down again by the knot pushers. We always perform a final femoral angiogram with digital subtraction via contralateral access, with either a pigtail above the aortic bifurcation, or via a catheter over the crossover wire. This latter approach requires placing a Toughy connector on the hub end of the catheter. If there is any contrast extravasation or stenosis of the access site, it can be managed with a crossover balloon (Figure 2.9). If the results are satisfactory, the V18 wire is removed and the contralateral femoral artery is closed.

The crossover balloon technique can also be used just before withdrawal of TAVR sheath under a controlled and safe environment. The TAVR sheath is withdrawn to the common femoral artery over the stiff wire. Using a peripheral 8–10 mm balloon over the 0.018 inch crossover wire, the balloon is placed in the terminal segment of the external iliac artery or proximal segment of the common femoral artery inflated to 1–2 atm. This creates proximal control and hemostasis with a non-traumatic occlusion of the vessel during sheath removal and knot delivery.

Large bore venous sheath management

Currently, the most common indications for using large sheaths in the common femoral vein are shunt closure, left atrial appendage occlusion, paravalvular leak closure, and MitraClip. Some devices such as percutaneous left ventricular assist devices can also require large access to the venous system; however, more frequently, patients who require percutaneous left ventricular assist devices may have to leave the catheterization laboratory with the device in place, in which case there is a long delay before sheath removal and closure devices should not be used because of the high risk of infection.

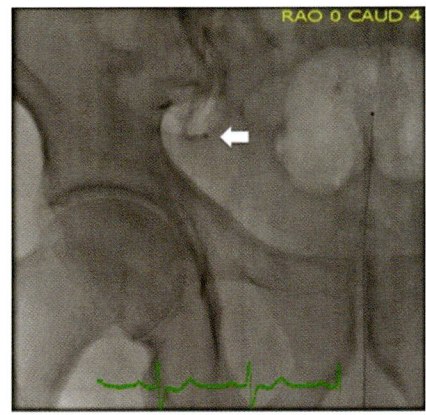 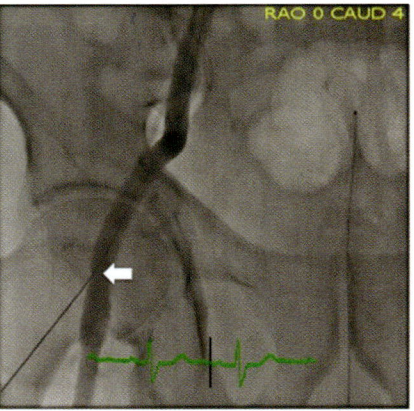

Figure 2.8 Left panel: The white arrow shows the tip of a left internal mammary artery catheter that has been passed from the left femoral artery access over the top of the aortic bifurcation and into the right external iliac artery. This crossover catheter is used for angiography and delivery of a protective crossover wire. Right panel: Micropuncture needle having entered the right common femoral artery at the level of the white arrow. A micropuncture wire can be seen going retrograde in the right iliac and femoral system. Injection through the crossover catheter demonstrates the entry point of the micropuncture needle in the common femoral artery.

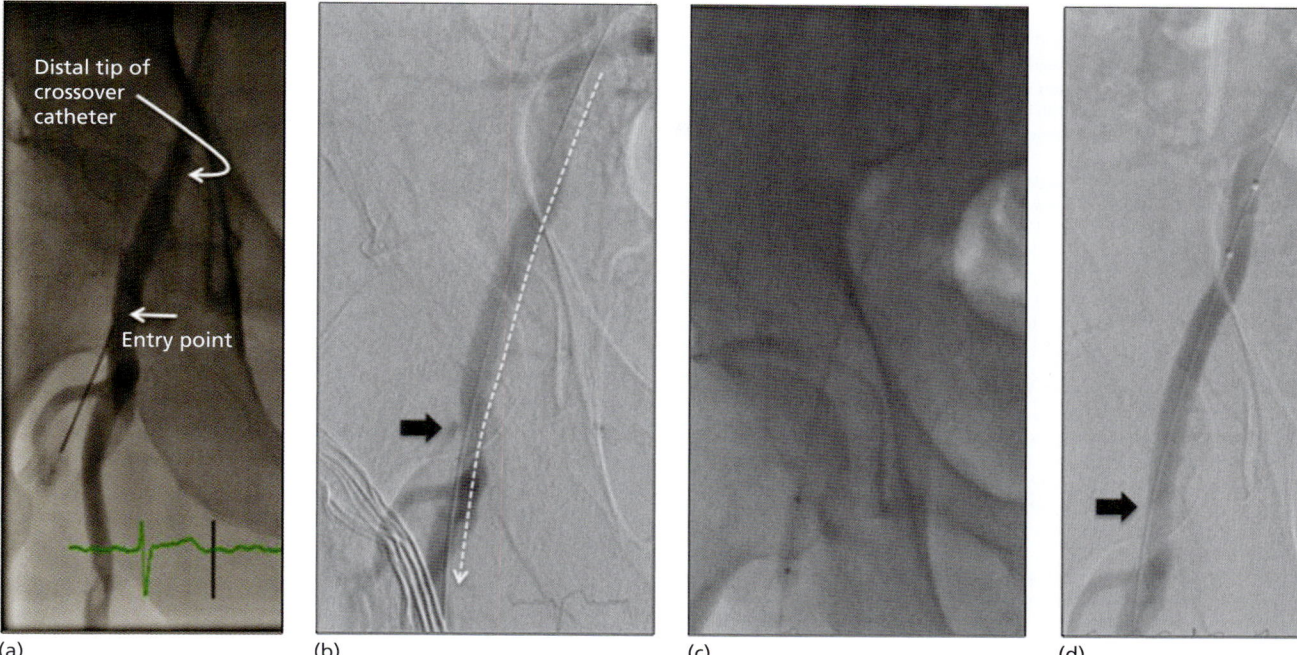

Figure 2.9 Following the completion of the procedure, crossover angiography can be used to assess the adequacy of femoral closure.
(a) Needle entry at the beginning of the procedure. The entry point of the needle is in the lower one-third of the femoral head, below the lower border of the inferior epigastric artery and above the bifurcation of the common femoral artery, in the ideal landing zone for sheath insertion.
(b) Extravasation of contrast after percutaneous closure of the large sheath entry point. The black arrow shows the contrast extravasation. The dotted white arrow shows course of a 0.018 inch crossover wire. The angiogram was taken with a pigtail positioned at the distal aorta above the iliac bifurcation. (c) A balloon passed over the crossover wire and inflated at 2 atm at the site of contrast extravasation and bleeding.
(d) Complete sealing of the artery at the closure site. The contrast injection was through the shaft of the balloon catheter, around the 0.018 inch wire, via a Toughy connector on the back end of the balloon catheter.

The strategy for managing large sheaths in the venous system is easier than for arterial punctures because of the lower pressure of the venous system. After the access is carefully obtained by a regular 18-gauge needle, we place a 7 Fr dilator in the vein. Blunt dissection of subcutaneous tissue facilitates delivery of larger sheaths. The sheath is inserted in the standard manner. After completion of the procedure, we use a "figure of 8" suture for hemostasis. For this technique, we use a 0 silk suture and we start from the distal edge of the access site, below the insertion of the sheath through the skin. The orientation of the needle entry can be either from medial to lateral or vice versa. When the needle is withdrawn from the skin, we use the same needle on the more proximal segment of the sheath, superior to the sheath insertion, with same the same direction of passage (medial to lateral or vice versa). After cutting off the needle, we take one end of the suture line and wrap around the other end three times, and finally tie down over the skin, while the sheath is still through the skin. The first operator keeps active force on the suture over the sheath as the second operator removes the sheath from the skin. Finally, the reinforcing knots will be placed. Very rarely do we see any ongoing oozing from the venous access site by using this simple and cost-effective technique [42].

antithrombotic and antiplatelet regimens, and reductions in access size have reduced ambulation times and the risks of complications. Vascular closure devices have further significantly improved hemostasis and ambulation times, and current data suggest they are mostly safe. However, there is no unequivocal evidence to suggest they reduce vascular complications in either diagnostic or interventional subgroups. Experience and expertise with whichever technique for femoral access site management one chooses are the best ways to minimize complications.

Just as important as management of vascular closure, careful attention to obtaining vascular access is important. Careful assessment of bony landmarks by fluoroscopy prior to femoral access will maximize the chance of sheath insertion into the common femoral artery with reductions in complications. Similarly, routine femoral angiography after femoral access to confirm sheath position is useful not only for assessing suitability of applications of vascular closure device, but also for assessing the risks of bleeding with use of antithrombotics which can affect interventional decision making. Femoral vascular access and closure approaches have been greatly refined by the demands of TAVR, with CT assessment for procedure planning, the use of micropuncture and ultrasound, and crossover techniques.

Conclusions

Proper management of femoral access is vital in reducing the femoral vascular adverse events, which are the most common complications in cardiac catheterizations and interventions. Refinements in

Interactive multiple choice questions are available for this chapter on www.wiley. com/go/dangas/cardiology

References

1 Piper WD, Malenka DJ, Ryan TJ Jr, *et al.* Predicting vascular complications in percutaneous coronary interventions. *Am Heart J* 2003; **145**: 1022–1029.

2 Lincoff AM, Bittl JA, Harrington RA, *et al.* Bivalirudin and provisional glycoprotein IIb/IIIa blockade compared with heparin and planned glycoprotein IIb/IIIa blockade during percutaneous coronary intervention: REPLACE-2 randomized trial. *JAMA* 2003; **289**: 853–863.

3 Waksman R, King SB 3rd, Douglas JS, *et al.* Predictors of groin complications after balloon and new-device coronary intervention. *Am J Cardiol* 1995; **75**: 886– 889.

4 Dauerman HL, Applegate RJ, Cohen DJ. Vascular closure devices: the second decade. *J Am Coll Cardiol* 2007; **50**: 1617–1626.

5 Kim D, Orron DE, Skillman JJ, *et al.* Role of superficial femoral artery puncture in the development of pseudoaneurysm and arteriovenous fistula complicating percutaneous transfemoral cardiac catheterization. *Cathet Cardiovasc Diagn* 1992; **25**: 91–97.

6 Sherev DA, Shaw RE, Brent BN. Angiographic predictors of femoral access site complications: implication for planned percutaneous coronary intervention. *Catheter Cardiovasc Interv* 2005; **65**: 196–202.

7 Ellis SG, Bhatt D, Kapadia S, Lee D, Yen M, Whitlow PL. Correlates and outcomes of retroperitoneal hemorrhage complicating percutaneous coronary intervention. *Catheter Cardiovasc Interv* 2006; **67**: 541–545.

8 Farouque HM, Tremmel JA, Raissi Shabari F, *et al.* Risk factors for the development of retroperitoneal hematoma after percutaneous coronary intervention in the era of glycoprotein IIb/IIIa inhibitors and vascular closure devices. *J Am Coll Cardiol* 2005; **45**: 363–368.

9 Schnyder G, Sawhney N, Whisenant B, Tsimikas S, Turi ZG. Common femoral artery anatomy is influenced by demographics and comorbidity: implications for cardiac and peripheral invasive studies. *Catheter Cardiovasc Interv* 2001; **53**: 289–295.

10 Seldinger SI. Catheter replacement of the needle in percutaneous arteriography: a new technique. *Acta Radiol* 1953; **39**: 368–376.

11 Turi ZG. Optimizing vascular access: routine femoral angiography keeps the vascular complication away. *Catheter Cardiovasc Interv* 2005; **65**: 203–204.

12 Grier D, Hartnell G. Percutaneous femoral artery puncture: practice and anatomy. *Br J Radiol* 1990; **63**: 602–604.

13 Pracyk JB, Wall TC, Longabaugh JP, *et al.* A randomized trial of vascular hemostasis techniques to reduce femoral vascular complications after coronary intervention. *Am J Cardiol* 1998; **81**: 970–976.

14 Semler HJ. Transfemoral catheterization: mechanical versus manual control of bleeding. *Radiology* 1985; **154**: 234–235.

15 Bogart MA. Time to hemostasis: a comparison of manual versus mechanical compression of the femoral artery. *Am J Crit Care* 1995; **4**:149–156.

16 Benson LM, Wunderly D, Perry B, *et al.* Determining best practice: comparison of three methods of femoral sheath removal after cardiac interventional procedures. *Heart Lung* 2005; **34**: 115–121.

17 Ormiston JA, Shaw BL, Panther MJ, *et al.* Percutaneous coronary intervention with bivalirudin anticoagulation, immediate sheath removal, and early ambulation: a feasibility study with implications for day-stay procedures. *Catheter Cardiovasc Interv* 2002; **55**: 289–293.

18 Koch KT, Piek JJ, de Winter RJ, *et al.* Two hour ambulation after coronary angioplasty and stenting with 6 F guiding catheters and low dose heparin. *Heart* 1999; **81**: 53–56.

19 Koch KT, Piek JJ, de Winter RJ, Mulder K, David GK, Lie KI. Early ambulation after coronary angioplasty and stenting with six French guiding catheters and low-dose heparin. *Am J Cardiol* 1997; **80**: 1084–1086.

20 Vlasic W, Almond D, Massel D. Reducing bedrest following arterial puncture for coronary interventional procedures—impact on vascular complications: the BAC Trial. *J Invasive Cardiol* 2001; **13**: 788–792.

21 Hoffer EK, Bloch RD. Percutaneous arterial closure devices. *J Vasc Interv Radiol* 2003; **14**: 865–885.

22 Hermiller JB, Simonton C, Hinohara T, *et al.* The StarClose Vascular Closure System: interventional results from the CLIP study. *Catheter Cardiovasc Interv* 2006; **68**: 677–683.

23 Van Den Berg JC. A close look at closure devices. *J Cardiovasc Surg (Torino)* 2006; **47**: 285–295.

24 Nader RG, Garcia JC, Drushal K, Pesek T. Clinical evaluation of SyvekPatch in patients undergoing interventional, EPS and diagnostic cardiac catheterization procedures. *J Invasive Cardiol* 2002; **14**: 305–307.

25 Applegate RJ, Sacrinty MT, Kutcher MA, *et al.* Propensity score analysis of vascular complications after diagnostic cardiac catheterization and percutaneous coronary intervention using thrombin hemostatic patch-facilitated manual compression. *J Invasive Cardiol* 2007; **19**: 164–170.

26 Najjar SF, Healey NA, Healey CM, *et al.* Evaluation of poly-N-acetyl glucosamine as a hemostatic agent in patients undergoing cardiac catheterization: a double-blind, randomized study. *J Trauma* 2004; **57**: S38–S41.

27 Palmer BL, Gantt DS, Lawrence ME, Rajab MH, Dehmer GJ. Effectiveness and safety of manual hemostasis facilitated by the SyvekPatch with one hour of bedrest after coronary angiography using six-French catheters. *Am J Cardiol* 2004; **93**: 96–97.

28 Tavris DR, Dey S, Albrecht-Gallauresi B, *et al.* Risk of local adverse events following cardiac catheterization by hemostasis device use—phase II. *J Invasive Cardiol* 2005; **17**: 644–650.

29 Sohail MR, Khan AH, Holmes DR Jr, Wilson WR, Steckelberg JM, Baddour LM. Infectious complications of percutaneous vascular closure devices. *Mayo Clin Proc* 2005; **80**(8): 1011–105.

30 Koreny M, Riedmuller E, Nikfardjam M, Siostrzonek P, Mullner M. Arterial puncture closing devices compared with standard manual compression after cardiac catheterization: systematic review and meta-analysis. *JAMA* 2004; **291**: 350–357.

31 Nikolsky E, Mehran R, Halkin A. *et al.* Vascular complications associated with arteriotomy closure devices in patients undergoing percutaneous coronary procedures: a meta-analysis. *J Am Coll Cardiol* 2004; **44**: 1200–1209.

32 Vaitkus PT. A meta-analysis of percutaneous vascular closure devices after diagnostic catheterization and percutaneous coronary intervention. *J Invasive Cardiol* 2004; **16**: 243–246.

33 Tavris DR, Gallauresi BA, Lin B, *et al.* Risk of local adverse events following cardiac catheterization by hemostasis device use and gender. *J Invasive Cardiol* 2004; **16**: 459–464.

34 Warren BS, Warren SG, Miller SD. Predictors of complications and learning curve using the Angio-Seal closure device following interventional and diagnostic catheterization. *Catheter Cardiovasc Interv* 1999; **48**: 162–166.

35 Duffin DC, Muhlestein JB, Allisson SB, *et al.* Femoral arterial puncture management after percutaneous coronary procedures: a comparison of clinical outcomes and patient satisfaction between manual compression and two different vascular closure devices. *J Invasive Cardiol* 2001; **13**: 354–362.

36 Rickli H, Unterweger M, Sutsch G, *et al.* Comparison of costs and safety of a suture-mediated closure device with conventional manual compression after coronary artery interventions. *Catheter Cardiovasc Interv* 2002; **57**: 297–302.

37 Schulz-Schüpke S, Helde S, Gewalt S, *et al.*; Instrumental Sealing of Arterial Puncture Site—CLOSURE Device vs Manual Compression (ISAR-CLOSURE) Trial Investigators. Comparison of vascular closure devices vs manual compression after femoral artery puncture: the ISAR-CLOSURE randomized clinical trial. *JAMA* 2014; **312**(19): 1981–1987.

38 Feldman T. Percutaneous suture closure for management of large French size arterial and venous puncture. *J Interven Cardiol* 2000; **13**: 237–241.

39 Solomon LW, Fusman B, Jolly N, Kim A, Feldman T. Percutaneous suture closure for management of large French size arterial puncture in aortic valvuloplasty. *J Invasive Cardiol* 2001; **13**: 592–596.

40 Perlowski A, Salinger MH, Justin P, Levisay, Feldman T. Femoral access for TAVR: techniques for prevention and endovascular management of complications. In Dieter RS, Dieter RA Jr, Dieter RA III (eds) *Endovascular Interventions: A Case-Based Approach*. Springer, NY: 2014; 859–874.

41 Genereux P, Kodali S, Leon MB, *et al.* Clinical outcomes using a new crossover balloon occlusion technique for percutaneous closure after transfemoral aortic valve implantation. *JACC Cardiovasc Interv* 2011; **4**(8): 861–867.

42 Cilingiroglu M, Salinger M, Zhao D, Feldman T. Technique of temporary subcutaneous "figure-of-eight" sutures to achieve hemostasis after removal of large-caliber femoral venous sheaths. *Catheter Cardiovasc Intervent* 2011; **78**: 155–160.

CHAPTER 3

Radial Artery, Alternative Arm Access, and Related Techniques

Thomas J. Ford[1,2], Martin K.C. Ng[3,4], Vikas Thondapu[5], and Peter Barlis[5]

[1] St. George Hospital, Sydney, Australia
[2] University of New South Wales, Sydney, Australia
[3] University of New South Wales Medical School, The University of Sydney, Australia
[4] Royal Prince Alfred Hospital, Sydney, Australia
[5] The University of Melbourne, Australia

The last decade has seen a paradigm shift in access site practice with an extraordinary uptake of radial artery access for both coronary angiography and interventional cardiac procedures [1]. While we are most often concerned about the coronary and cardiac complications of catheterization and intervention, vascular access complications are more common and carry prognostic importance for patients. The benefits of the radial artery as an access site for catheterization is primarily because of its superficial compressible location allowing early effective hemostasis and mobilization. The uptake of transradial access (TRA) is a triumph of contemporary evidence-based medicine as multiple large trials have challenged previous dogma about TRA causing increased risk of stroke and hand ischemia [2].

Rationale for transradial access

Ischemic complications of percutaneous coronary intervention (PCI) have reduced over time through developments in anticoagulants, antiplatelet therapy, and coronary stents coupled with procedural improvements [3]. Non-ischemic complications of PCI have increasingly been the focus of attention—namely those involving vascular access and bleeding. TRA reduces vascular access complications allowing early ambulation, improved comfort, reduced bleeding risk, shorter hospital stay, and reduced cost [4]. While the definition of major bleeding varies widely, access site hematomas large enough to require transfusion are inexorably linked to worse short-term and long-term clinical outcomes and this relationship is thought to be causal [5,6]. Pharmacological developments that result in reduced bleeding complications have been associated with reductions in mortality [7]. If the relationship between bleeding and mortality is causal, any method of reducing bleeding, including procedural advances, will also reduce mortality. This hypothesis was supported by a subgroup analysis of the multicenter randomized RIVAL study of radial vs. femoral PCI in acute coronary syndrome (ACS) showing a reduction in primary outcome (death, myocardial infarction, stroke, or major bleeding) in the highest volume radial centers and in patients with ST-elevation myocardial infarction [8]. The MATRIX study is the largest trial to date (n = 8404) comparing radial with femoral access for PCI in patients

with ACS. Radial artery PCI reduced the rate of net adverse clinical event (death, myocardial infarction, stroke, or major bleeding) by 17% (9.8% vs. 11.7% of patients; 0.83, 0.73–0.96; p = 0.0092) [9]. Mortality was reduced with radial PCI by 28% (1.6% vs. 2.2% of patients; 0.72, 0.53–0.99; p = 0.045). This is consistent with the updated meta-analysis of all trials, which shows highly significant benefits of radial access in a population with ACS for major adverse cardiac events (MACE) by 14% (6.0% vs. 7.0% of patients; 0.86, 0.77–0.95; p = 0.0051) and mortality by 28% (1.8% vs. 2.5%; 0.72, 0.6–0.88; p = 0.0011) [9].

Radial anatomy

Arterial supply to the upper limb begins as the axillary artery before it reaches the lower border of teres major becoming the brachial artery—the main blood arterial supply to the arm. This bifurcates 1–2 cm distal to the intercondylar line of the humerus (proximal border of the antecubital fossa) into the radial and ulnar arteries (Figure 3.1).

Preprocedural considerations

There are several relative contraindications to TRA (Box 3.1). The modified Allen's test is often performed prior to TRA to demonstrate patency of ulnopalmar arches because of the theoretical risk of hand ischemia in the event of radial artery occlusion (RAO). The generous redundant vascularization of the hand by the radial, ulnar, and interosseous arteries provides excellent protection against digital ischemia which is almost never seen even in instances of RAO after catheterization [10]. The test involves compression of both the radial and ulnar arteries while blood is expelled from the hand by forced fist clenching. After opening the hand, ulnar artery compression is released and the amount of time to achieve maximal palmar blush is measured. "Normal" response times vary but a common contemporary definition regards within 5 seconds as normal, 6–10 seconds as intermediate, and greater than 10 seconds as abnormal [11]. Plethysmography using a thumb pulse oximeter trace can be used to increase objectivity and diagnostic accuracy of the test (Barbeau test) [12].

Interventional Cardiology: Principles and Practice, Second Edition. Edited by George D. Dangas, Carlo Di Mario, and Nicholas N. Kipshidze.
© 2017 John Wiley & Sons, Ltd. Published 2017 by John Wiley & Sons, Ltd.

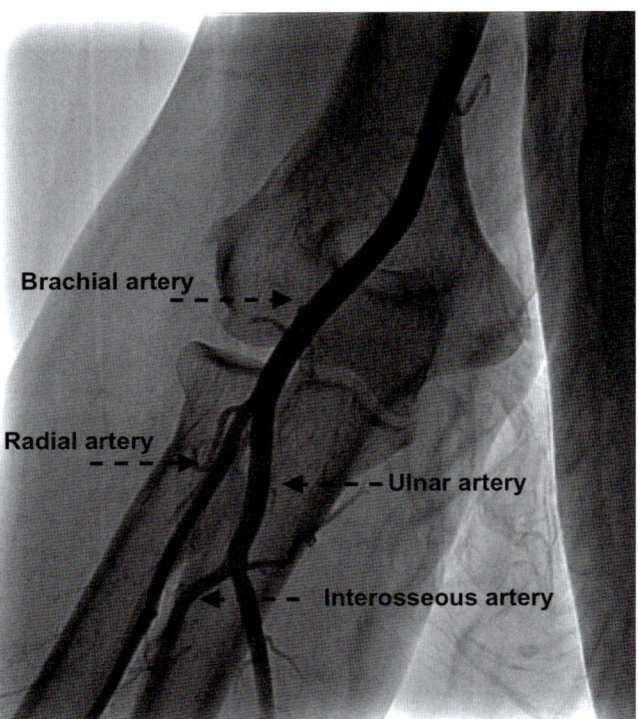

Figure 3.1 The forearm and hand benefit from a dual blood supply resulting from the radioulnar anastomosis in the hand via superficial and deep palmar arches.

Box 3.1 Transradial approach—relative contraindications

Absent radial pulse
Severe vasospastic disease (e.g., Raynaud's, CREST)
Arteriovenous fistula for dialysis (current or planned)
Requirement for radial artery aortocoronary bypass conduit

CREST, syndrome of calcinosis, Raynaud's phenomenon, esophageal dysmotility, sclerodactyly, and telangectasia.

The ability of these tests to reliably predict those at significant risk of ischemic hand complications is hotly debated [13–15]. There are only a few isolated case reports of distal hand ischemia and gangrene following TRA and these patients often had normal Allen's tests and were most likely caused by distal embolization [16,17]. The paradigm is shifting away from testing ulnar artery patency, with solid clinical evidence supporting the safety of TRA across the full spectrum of Allen's test results [11]. Almost one-quarter of operators worldwide now forgo assessment of ulnopalmar arterial supply prior to TRA while high-volume radial centers in the UK have shown this approach to be safe and without ischemic sequelae [18,19].

Right vs. left radial approach

The right-sided controls in the catheterization laboratory lend themselves to a right radial approach, which is generally preferred by both patient and operator [13]. Nevertheless, the left radial approach (LRA) can offer a favorable approach because of direct takeoff of the left subclavian artery from the aortic arch, providing better guide support akin to the femoral approach [20]. In shorter elderly patients, the LRA approach may be favorable with less subclavian tortuosity easing catheter passage into the aorta. LRA has recently been shown to be as effective as the right radial with an improved radiation safety profile to the operator [21]. Other considerations for LRA include bypass graft studies involving angiography of the left internal mammary artery and possible future need for a bypass conduit from the non-dominant hand. Importantly, in patients with previous bypass surgery LRA coronary angiography is a feasible alternative but is associated with increased contrast use, procedure time, and operator radiation exposure compared with transfemoral angiography [22].

Ulnar and brachial approach

Ulnar artery access has been used as a feasible alternative for coronary angiography and PCI, although compared with first-line TRA it is inferior with increased crossover rates to TRA. Nevertheless, in terms of access complications it was comparable to radial including comparable rates of large hematomas with no cases of ulnar nerve damage or hand ischemia [23]. The path of the ulnar artery is deeper and less centered over bone and thus does not lend itself to compressive hemostasis as readily as the radial. The brachial approach is usually reserved as a third or fourth line access site because of higher risk of major access complications than TRA: thrombosis, dissections, and median nerve injury [24].

Gaining radial access

Careful vessel palpation and planning is key to successfully gaining access and minimizing inherent risk of spasm with multiple punctures. The artery should be punctured 1–2 cm proximal to the radial styloid in order to avoid the tortuous distal radial artery and its smaller branches. Repeat procedures or attempts can be performed more proximally if required. A small quantity of 2% lidocaine is useful for anesthetic and can be mixed with a small amount of subcutaneous nitroglycerin in patients whose pulse is low volume. There are two main techniques for arterial puncture: a traditional Seldinger technique ("through-and-through" puncture) and a modified Seldinger technique ("anterior only" puncture). In the traditional Seldinger technique a needle with an overlying Teflon-coated cannula sheath is used to puncture the artery at approximately 30°. A flash of blood indicates anterior arterial wall puncture, and the needle is advanced through the posterior radial artery wall. After removal of the needle, a 0.021-inch guidewire is placed in the hub of the Teflon cannula and the entire system is withdrawn backwards until pulsatile flow occurs into the hub of the Teflon cannula indicating luminal cannula sheath position. The guidewire can be advanced and subsequently the hydrophilic introducer sheath inserted over the guidewire.

The modified Seldinger technique uses a short 21-gauge bore needle with an anterior-only puncture technique. After puncture of the anterior wall of the radial artery, a 0.021-inch guidewire is advanced into the artery allowing removal of the needle and sheathing over the guidewire.

An elegant randomized trial showed the traditional Seldinger technique (double wall puncture) to be a more reliable way to obtain radial artery access with greater success rates, shorter procedure time, and shorter time to gain access. Importantly, there were no differences in procedure-related complications such as radial hematoma or radial artery obstruction [25].

Navigating common anatomic problems

While various anomalies in radial, brachial, and axillary arterial circulation are common, knowledge of just three major anatomic variations is important as they determine most radial procedural failures [26]. With experience these can often be negotiated; however, where this is not possible the asymmetrical nature of forearm vasculature leaves contralateral radial access and the femoral approach as equally plausible options [27].

High radial–ulna bifurcation ("high take-off")

High-origin radial arteries (defined by their origin above the antecubital fossa) are the most commonly encountered radial artery anomaly, occurring in 7% of patients undergoing radial angiography. These present problems during angiography because of their small caliber and often tortuous course making them prone to spasm. Nevertheless, in experienced hands (and with frequent use of 5 Fr catheters and hydrophilic wires) the procedure can be completed transradially in over 95% of cases [26].

Radial artery loops

This is the most common cause of transradial failure for experienced radial operators [28]. Radial artery loops involve a retrograde loop in the radial artery proximally toward the brachial bifurcation before heading down to the forearm. Navigating the loop is made more challenging by the invariable association with a recurrent (accessory) radial artery, which typically is a small caliber vessel with a straight path up the arm from the apex of the loop. After defining the loop with angiography, small loops can often be navigated with a coronary wire or a soft-tipped hydrophilic wire looped into the brachial artery. Wire passage alone can straighten the loop; alternatively, a buddy wire or small caliber catheter can be exchanged allowing passage of a 0.035-inch wire with gentle traction allowing the loop to be straightened and permitting the procedure to be completed in over two-thirds of cases (Figure 3.2) [28].

Tortuous radial arteries

Radial tortuosity defined by the presence of a bend of more than 90° in the contour of the vessel occurs in around 2% of cases and is often associated with severe spasm [29]. With any resistance to wire passage, the vessel should be mapped using angiography and these angulated segments can usually be crossed using a hydrophilic or coronary wire in the majority of cases. Balloon assisted tracking (BAT) can be used facilitating non-traumatic navigation through challenging anatomic situations including severe tortuosity, resistant spasm, small caliber radial artery, and complex loops. In this technique, an inflated percutaneous transluminal coronary angioplasty (PTCA) balloon is partially protruded through the distal end of a guide (or diagnostic catheter) and deployed at 6 atmospheres. The entire assembly is then advanced over a non-traumatic PTCA guidewire and steered through the challenging segment [30].

Other barriers

After navigation to the subclavian artery, two further barriers to TRA include a tortuous subclavian system or a distal insertion of the subclavian into aorta (arteria lusoria). Risk factors for subclavian

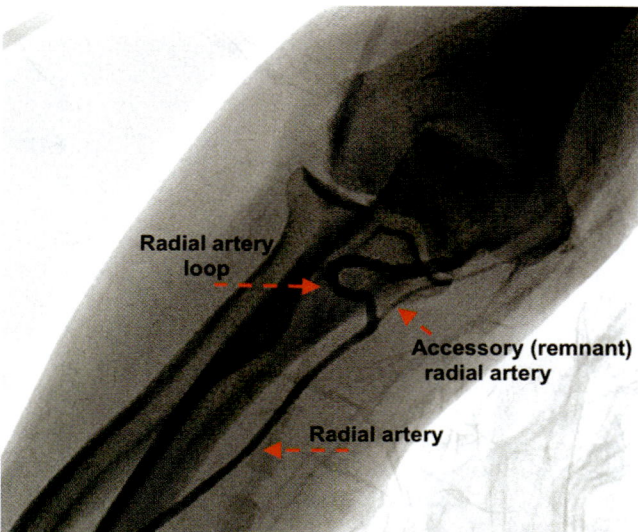

Figure 3.2 Radial artery loop with typical appearance of accessory radial artery from apex of loop.

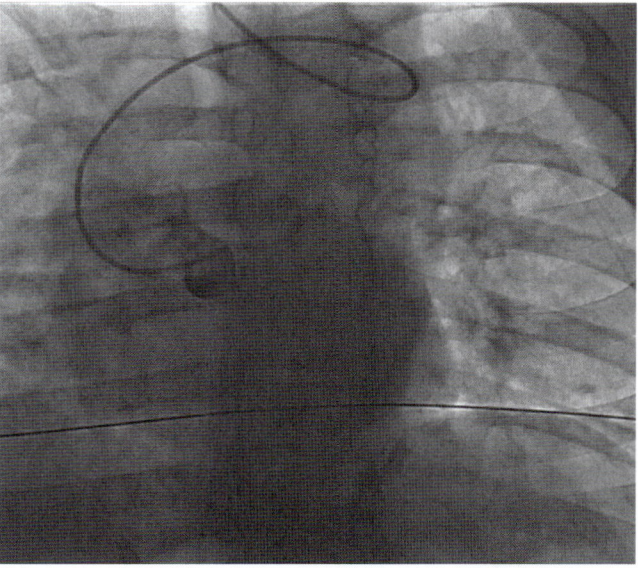

Figure 3.3 Retroesophageal right subclavian artery (RORSA). Note subclavian insertion into distal aortic arch in a young patient with acute ST elevation myocardial infarction.

tortuosity include hypertension, female gender, older age, smoker, short stature, and high body mass index [31]. A deep breath held in inspiration normally facilitates a straightening of the passage into the ascending aorta allowing correct catheter orientation in the ascending aorta. In very rare cases (0.29%), the right subclavian artery enters very distally into the aortic arch or descending aorta. While it is technically feasible to negotiate the retroesophageal right subclavian artery (RORSA; Figure 3.3), early identification of this issue with conversion to an alternative access site is advised to avoid unnecessarily long procedures with excessive radiation exposure [32].

Complications of transradial access

Spasm

The radial artery is a muscular small-caliber vessel allowing only limited clearance for catheter passage. Resultant mechanical friction combined with circulating catecholamines can trigger α_1-adrenoreceptors leading to arterial vasospasm. Catheters can become difficult to manipulate and torque potentially abetting more spasm (Table 3.1). This phenomenon occurs in around 15% of cases but the incidence varies widely (2–30%) according to center and definition used [33]. While spasm is usually painful for both the patient and operator, its incidence is reduced with increasing operator experience [34], adequate procedural sedation (opiate/anxiolytic) [35], and administration of a "spasmolytic cocktail" after sheath insertion [35,36]. This usually consists of a combination of calcium channel blockers (e.g., verapamil 2.5–5 mg) and/or nitrates (e.g., nitroglycerin 0.1–0.4 mg) given directly into the radial artery sheath. Intravascular imaging studies show the luminal area increases by 44% after 3 mg intra-arterial verapamil with only a moderate blood pressure reduction and no significant change in heart rate [37]. Intra-arterial lidocaine should be avoided as it causes paradoxical vasoconstriction [38]. Intra-arterial heparin administration may be painful so can either be given intravenously, or it can be given intra-arterially with the "cocktail" after dilution with saline or blood from the sheath to reduce arterial irritation and burning.

Table 3.1 Complications of transradial access.

Common	Uncommon
Spasm	Arterial injury (dissection/perforation/eversion/laceration)
Hematoma (forearm)	Compartment syndrome
Radial artery occlusion	Catheter entrapment
	Transient vocal cord paralysis
	Atheroembolism/thromboembolism

Hematoma

Unlike bleeding from femoral access, hematoma formation in the forearm is usually visible during the procedure and very seldom requires a blood transfusion [10]. Forearm hematomas can be classified according to the EASY classification by Bertrand: Grades I and II relate to puncture site bleeding whereas Grades III and IV relate to intramuscular bleeding (Figure 3.4) [39]. TRA is rarely associated with severe access-related bleeding complications;

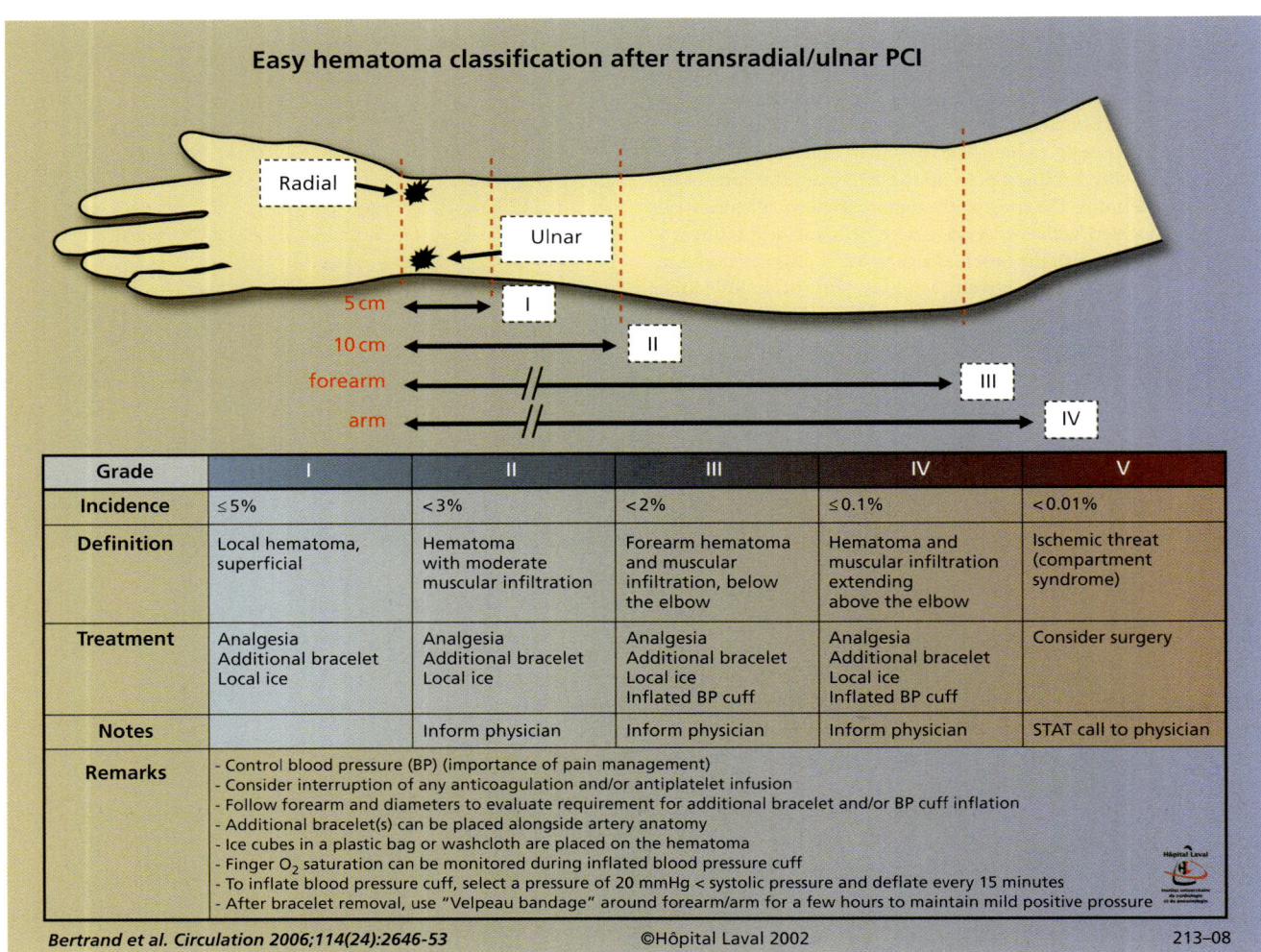

Grade	I	II	III	IV	V
Incidence	≤5%	<3%	<2%	≤0.1%	<0.01%
Definition	Local hematoma, superficial	Hematoma with moderate muscular infiltration	Forearm hematoma and muscular infiltration, below the elbow	Hematoma and muscular infiltration extending above the elbow	Ischemic threat (compartment syndrome)
Treatment	Analgesia Additional bracelet Local ice	Analgesia Additional bracelet Local ice	Analgesia Additional bracelet Local ice Inflated BP cuff	Analgesia Additional bracelet Local ice Inflated BP cuff	Consider surgery
Notes		Inform physician	Inform physician	Inform physician	STAT call to physician
Remarks	- Control blood pressure (BP) (importance of pain management) - Consider interruption of any anticoagulation and/or antiplatelet infusion - Follow forearm and diameters to evaluate requirement for additional bracelet and/or BP cuff inflation - Additional bracelet(s) can be placed alongside artery anatomy - Ice cubes in a plastic bag or washcloth are placed on the hematoma - Finger O$_2$ saturation can be monitored during inflated blood pressure cuff - To inflate blood pressure cuff, select a pressure of 20 mmHg < systolic pressure and deflate every 15 minutes - After bracelet removal, use "Velpeau bandage" around forearm/arm for a few hours to maintain mild positive pressure				

Bertrand et al. Circulation 2006;114(24):2646-53 ©Hôpital Laval 2002 213–08

Figure 3.4 Transradial hematoma classification system. Source: Bertrand 2010 [39]. Reproduced with permission of John Wiley & Sons.

however, their prompt identification allows targeted therapy at the point of pain or swelling including BP cuff inflation at 20 mmHg below the systolic pressure for 15 minutes to stop bleeding and reduce forearm pressure.

Compartment syndrome

This limb-threatening emergency is fortunately extremely rare (incidence <0.01%) [40]. It usually relates to hematoma formation but can occur in its absence [41]. Characterized by forearm pain and swelling, disastrous sequelae can usually be avoided by prompt recognition and cessation of local bleeding by [42]:

1 Cessation of anticoagulants (and/or reversal)
2 Pain and blood pressure control
3 Transient external compression (BP cuff).

Artery dissection or perforation

In the absence of wire resistance in the arm, systematic fluoroscopy is not necessary until the subclavian artery is reached. It should be commenced prior to entering the brachiocephalic artery to avoid inadvertent wiring of the right carotid, vertebral, or distal mammary artery. Where wire resistance is encountered, angiography should allow the operator to identify and often overcome the problem. If the wire is pushed against resistance, vessel dissection

or perforation can ensue. Brachial or radial artery perforation is rare (incidence around 0.05%) while angiographic images may be dramatic, rather than aborting the procedure the literature supports careful attempts to recross with a soft angioplasty wire (0.014 inch) [10]. Once crossed, guide catheters can be used to complete the PCI while the catheter will usually seal the dissection or perforation. This avoids the potential for large hematoma formation and compartment syndrome which may ensue if the procedure is aborted (Figure 3.5) [29].

This important complication of transradial access occurs in approximately 5% of cases [24,43,44]. For the anatomic reasons already described, RAO is almost always clinically silent. Nevertheless, patency of the artery is important for future TRA, while the radial artery can also be used as a hemodialysis fistula or bypass conduit, hence operators should consider the significance of this complication for each individual patient. The reported incidence varies according to the method used to detect RAO; however, the use of periprocedural anticoagulation with heparin or its analogues significantly reduces its occurrence [45]. Smaller diameter sheaths and catheters with careful hemostasis techniques are also protective against occlusion [46]. Up to half of early occlusions spontaneously recannalize within 1 month [47].

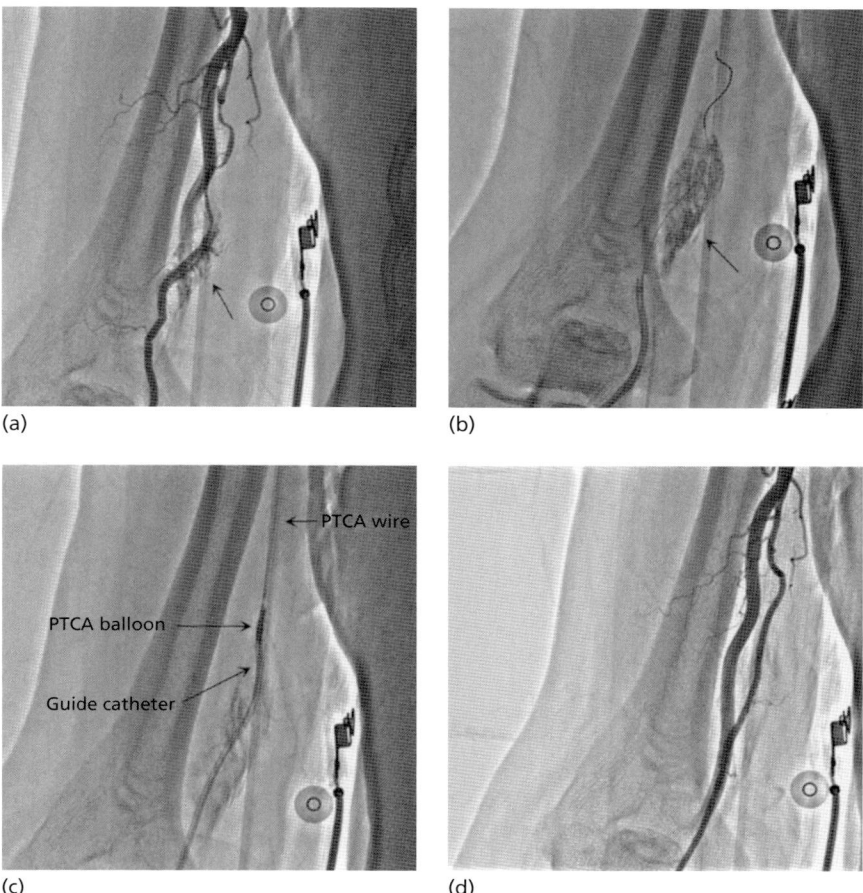

(a)   (b)

(c)   (d)

Figure 3.5 (a) Guidewire induced perforation of radial access. (b) A soft tip 0.014-inch percutaneous transluminal coronary angioplasty (PTCA) guidewire crossed the perforated segment (arrow). (c) Successful use of balloon assisted tracking (BAT) technique to navigate a 6 Fr guide catheter through the perforated segment (arrow). (d) Post procedure injection revealed proper sealing of perforation and no extravasation. System. Source: Patel *et al.* 2013 [29]. Reproduced with permission of John Wiley & Sons.

Table 3.2 Common diagnostic and guide catheter shapes for TRA.

Universal diagnostic	Diagnostic	Universal guide	Guide (left)	Guide (right)
Tiger II (Tig)	Judkins left 3.5	IKARI left	EBU/XB 3.5	Judkins right 4.0
Kimny	Judkins right 4.0	MAC 30/30	Judkins left	Amplatz right
Jacky		Kimny	Amplatz left	Amplatz left
			IKARI left	IKARI right

Techniques for radial artery hemostasis

There are many similar devices developed to achieve hemostasis following TRA catheterization. The crux of most designs is a band around the wrist enabling discrete pressure over the radial artery while ulnar flow is left unimpeded. The TR band (Terumo, Tokyo, Japan) is a transparent band allowing puncture site visualization while air is titrated into a sack compressing the radial artery. It compares favorably in a non-randomized comparison with the HemoBand (HemoBand, Portland, OR), the latter associated with higher rates of RAO (7.2% vs. 3.2% at 30 days; p = 0.04) [48]. If compression is too aggressive, a no-flow state occurs and is the biggest predictor of subsequent RAO [47]. The technique of "patent hemostasis" to preserve antegrade flow is the preferred method of radial artery closure. RAO is minimized by using either plethysmography (Barbeau test) or mean arterial pressure (via TR band attached to sphygmomanometer) to achieve hemostasis while preserving antegrade flow [46,49].

Basic catheter selection

There are an increasing number of catheters specifically designed for radial access (Table 3.2); however, the majority of operators worldwide still prefer standard femoral shapes for TRA procedures [13]. When compared with the femoral approach, a shorter curve of the Judkins left catheter 3.5 is preferable and often requires more manipulation from the radial approach. The 0.035-inch wire may be advanced into the cusp of interest to direct the catheter; subsequently the wire can be kept inside the catheter tip to facilitate torqueing and prevent the catheter curling back up the aorta. Gentle advancement with counterclockwise rotation can assist in selectively engaging the left main ostium with a Judkins left catheter. A J-wire should be used to change to the Judkins right coronary catheter; a long length exchange J-wire should be used to keep the position in the ascending aorta in cases with significant subclavian or aortic tortuosity. Technique to engage the right coronary artery with a Judkins right catheter is similar to the femoral approach where withdrawal occurs with clockwise torque.

One advantage of TRA is the opportunity to use a universal catheter shape incorporating end and side holes facilitating left and right coronary angiography and left ventriculography with a single catheter. The Tiger II catheter (Terumo, Sommerset, NJ) is the most commonly used universal catheter shape; however, the Kimny (Boston Scientific, Natick, MA) and other similar designs are in use [13]. Caveats of the universal catheter approach include the learning curve from traditional femoral shapes, potential for non-coaxial engagement, poor artery opacification, "deep-throating" coronary arteries with inherent risk of ostial trauma and vessel dissection. Potential benefits include reduction in catheter exchanges, spasm, and procedure time, particularly beneficial in the setting of ST-elevation myocardial infarction (STEMI).

Common guides for TRA left coronary angiography include EBU/XB 3/3.5/4, while right coronary guides include JR4, AL0.75/1. For most angioplasties, 6 Fr equipment is sufficient; however, where two stent techniques or large thrombectomy devices are required a 7-Fr approach can be used utilizing sheathless guiding catheters. These feature combined hydrophilic coating with inner dimensions larger than 7 Fr but smaller outer profile than a conventional 6 Fr introducer sheath. They are useful in patients with severe spasm and those with small arteries enabling complex transradial PCI that would not be feasible using conventional techniques.

Conclusions

The access site is a major determinant of successful angiography and PCI as well as a predictor of procedural complications. Radial access has evolved over the last three decades to emerge as the safest access site with clear advantages over the femoral approach. There is a weight of clinical evidence supporting TRA for physician-oriented hard clinical endpoints including bleeding, vascular complications, and MACE. For the authors' patients, TRA is preferred with better functional outcomes allowing early mobilization and discharge. For hospitals and governments there are cost-saving implications. The exponential rise of TRA is clear and here to stay.

Interactive multiple choice questions are available for this chapter on www.wiley.com/go/dangas/cardiology

References

1 Feldman DN, Swaminathan RV, Kaltenbach LA, *et al.* Adoption of radial access and comparison of outcomes to femoral access in percutaneous coronary intervention: an updated report from the national cardiovascular data registry (2007–2012). *Circulation* 2013; **127**: 2295–2306.

2 Karrowni W, Vyas A, Giacomino B, *et al.* Radial versus femoral access for primary percutaneous interventions in ST-segment elevation myocardial infarction patients: a meta-analysis of randomized controlled trials. *JACC Cardiovasc Interv* 2013; **6**: 814–823.

3 Singh M, Rihal CS, Gersh BJ, *et al.* Twenty-five-year trends in in-hospital and long-term outcome after percutaneous coronary intervention: a single-institution experience. *Circulation* 2007; **115**: 2835–2841.

4 Hamon M, Pristipino C, Di Mario C, *et al.* Consensus document on the radial approach in percutaneous cardiovascular interventions: position paper by the European Association of Percutaneous Cardiovascular Interventions and Working Groups on Acute Cardiac Care and Thrombosis of the European Society of Cardiology. *EuroIntervention* 2013; **8**: 1242–1251.

5 Chhatriwalla AK, Amin AP, Kennedy KF, *et al.* Association between bleeding events and in-hospital mortality after percutaneous coronary intervention. *JAMA* 2013; **309**: 1022–1029.

6 Kwok CS, Rao SV, Myint PK, *et al.* Major bleeding after percutaneous coronary intervention and risk of subsequent mortality: a systematic review and meta-analysis. *Open Heart* 2014; **1**: e000021.

7 Stone GW, Witzenbichler B, Guagliumi G, *et al.* Bivalirudin during primary PCI in acute myocardial infarction. *N Engl J Med* 2008; **358**: 2218–2230.

8 Jolly SS, Yusuf S, Cairns J, *et al.* Radial versus femoral access for coronary angiography and intervention in patients with acute coronary syndromes (RIVAL): a randomised, parallel group, multicentre trial. *Lancet* 2011; **377**: 1409–1420.

9 Valgimigli M, Gagnor A, Calabró P, *et al.* Radial versus femoral access in patients with acute coronary syndromes undergoing invasive management: a randomised multicentre trial. *Lancet* 2015; **385**: 2465–2476.

10 Dandekar VK, Vidovich MI, Shroff AR. Complications of transradial catheterization. Cardiovascular revascularization medicine: including molecular interventions. *Cardiovasc Revasc Med* 2012; **13**: 39–50.

11 Valgimigli M, Campo G, Penzo C, *et al.* Transradial coronary catheterization and intervention across the whole spectrum of Allen test results. *J Am Coll Cardiol* 2014; **63**: 1833–1841.

12 Barbeau GR, Arsenault F, Dugas L, Simard S, Lariviere MM. Evaluation of the ulnopalmar arterial arches with pulse oximetry and plethysmography: comparison with the Allen's test in 1010 patients. *Am Heart J* 2004; **147**: 489–493.

13 Bertrand OF, Rao SV, Pancholy S, *et al.* Transradial approach for coronary angiography and interventions: results of the first international transradial practice survey. *JACC Cardiovasc Interv* 2010; **3**: 1022–1031.

14 Gilchrist IC. Is the Allen's test accurate for patients considered for transradial coronary angiography? *J Am Coll Cardiol* 2006; **48**: 1287; author reply 8.

15 Hildick-Smith D. Use of the Allen's test and transradial catheterization. *J Am Coll Cardiol* 2006; **48**: 1287; author reply 8.

16 Bertrand OF, Carey PC, Gilchrist IC. Allen or no Allen: that is the question! *J Am Coll Cardiol* 2014; **63**: 1842–1844.

17 Ayan M, Smer A, Azzouz M, Abuzaid A, Mooss A. Hand ischemia after transradial coronary angiography: resulting in right ring finger amputation. *Cardiovasc Revasc Med* 2015; **16**: 367–369.

18 Shah AH. Allen's test: does it have any significance in current practice? *J Invasive Cardiol* 2015; **27**: E70–E73.

19 Ghuran AV, Dixon G, Holmberg S, de Belder A, Hildick-Smith D. Transradial coronary intervention without pre-screening for a dual palmar blood supply. *Int J Cardiol* 2007; **121**: 320–322.

20 Norgaz T, Gorgulu S, Dagdelen S. A randomized study comparing the effectiveness of right and left radial approach for coronary angiography. *Catheter Cardiovasc Interv* 2012; **80**: 260–264.

21 Kado H, Patel AM, Suryadevara S, *et al.* Operator radiation exposure and physical discomfort during a right versus left radial approach for coronary interventions: a randomized evaluation. *JACC Cardiovasc Interv* 2014; **7**: 810–816.

22 Michael TT, Alomar M, Papayannis A, *et al.* A randomized comparison of the transradial and transfemoral approaches for coronary artery bypass graft angiography and intervention: the RADIAL-CABG Trial (RADIAL Versus Femoral Access for Coronary Artery Bypass Graft Angiography and Intervention). *JACC Cardiovasc Interv* 2013; **6**: 1138–1144.

23 Hahalis G, Tsigkas G, Xanthopoulou I, *et al.* Transulnar compared with transradial artery approach as a default strategy for coronary procedures: a randomized trial. The Transulnar or Transradial Instead of Coronary Transfemoral Angiographies Study (the AURA of ARTEMIS Study). *Circ Cardiovasc Interv* 2013; **6**: 252–261.

24 Kiemeneij F, Laarman GJ, Odekerken D, Slagboom T, van der Wieken R. A randomized comparison of percutaneous transluminal coronary angioplasty by the radial, brachial and femoral approaches: the Access study. *J Am Coll Cardiol* 1997; **29**: 1269–1275.

25 Pancholy SB, Sanghvi KA, Patel TM. Radial artery access technique evaluation trial: randomized comparison of Seldinger versus modified Seldinger technique for arterial access for transradial catheterization. *Catheter Cardiovasc Interv* 2012; **80**: 288–291.

26 Lo TS, Nolan J, Fountzopoulos E, *et al.* Radial artery anomaly and its influence on transradial coronary procedural outcome. *Heart* 2008; **95**: 410–415.

27 Rodriguez-Niedenfuhr M, Vazquez T, Nearn L, Ferreira B, Parkin I, Sanudo JR. Variations of the arterial pattern in the upper limb revisited: a morphological and statistical study, with a review of the literature. *J Anat* 2001; **199**: 547–566.

28 Louvard Y, Lefevre T. Loops and transradial approach in coronary diagnosis and intervention. *Catheter Cardiovasc Interv* 2000; **51**: 250–252.

29 Patel T, Shah S, Pancholy S, *et al.* Working through complexities of radial and brachial vasculature during transradial approach. *Catheter Cardiovasc Interv* 2014; **83**: 1074–1088.

30 Patel T, Shah S, Pancholy S, Rao S, Bertrand OF, Kwan T. Balloon-assisted tracking: a must-know technique to overcome difficult anatomy during transradial approach. *Catheter Cardiovasc Interv* 2014; **83**: 211–220.

31 Cha KS, Kim MH, Kim HJ. Prevalence and clinical predictors of severe tortuosity of right subclavian artery in patients undergoing transradial coronary angiography. *Am J Cardiol* 2003; **92**: 1220–1222.

32 Abhaichand RK, Louvard Y, Gobeil JF, Loubeyre C, Lefevre T, Morice MC. The problem of arteria lusoria in right transradial coronary angiography and angioplasty. *Catheter Cardiovasc Interv* 2001; **54**: 196–201.

33 Kristic I, Lukenda J. Radial artery spasm during transradial coronary procedures. *J Invasive Cardiol* 2011; **23**: 527–531.

34 Ball WT, Sharieff W, Jolly SS, *et al.* Characterization of operator learning curve for transradial coronary interventions. *Circ Cardiovasc Interv* 2011; **4**: 336–341.

35 Deftereos S, Giannopoulos G, Raisakis K, *et al.* Moderate procedural sedation and opioid analgesia during transradial coronary interventions to prevent spasm: a prospective randomized study. *JACC Cardiovasc Interv* 2013; **6**: 267–273.

36 Varenne O, Jegou A, Cohen R, *et al.* Prevention of arterial spasm during percutaneous coronary interventions through radial artery: the SPASM study. *Catheter Cardiovasc Interv* 2006; **68**: 231–235.

37 Edmundson A, Mann T. Nonocclusive radial artery injury resulting from transradial coronary interventions: radial artery IVUS. *J Invasive Cardiol* 2005; **17**: 528–531.

38 Abe S, Meguro T, Endoh N, *et al.* Response of the radial artery to three vasodilatory agents. *Catheter Cardiovasc Interv* 2000; **49**: 253–6.

39 Bertrand OF. Acute forearm muscle swelling post transradial catheterization and compartment syndrome: prevention is better than treatment! *Catheter Cardiovasc Interv* 2010; **75**: 366–368.

40 Tizon-Marcos H, Barbeau GR. Incidence of compartment syndrome of the arm in a large series of transradial approach for coronary procedures. *J Interv Cardiol* 2008; **21**: 380–384.

41 Araki T, Itaya H, Yamamoto M. Acute compartment syndrome of the forearm that occurred after transradial intervention and was not caused by bleeding or hematoma formation. *Catheter Cardiovasc Interv* 2010; **75**: 362–365.

42 Caputo RP, Tremmel JA, Rao S, *et al.* Transradial arterial access for coronary and peripheral procedures: executive summary by the Transradial Committee of the SCAI. *Catheter Cardiovasc Interv* 2011; **78**: 823–839.

43 Stella PR, Kiemeneij F, Laarman GJ, Odekerken D, Slagboom T, van der Wieken R. Incidence and outcome of radial artery occlusion following transradial artery coronary angioplasty. *Cathet Cardiovasc Diagn* 1997; **40**: 156–158.

44 Zankl AR, Andrassy M, Volz C, *et al.* Radial artery thrombosis following transradial coronary angiography: incidence and rationale for treatment of symptomatic patients with low-molecular-weight heparins. *Clin Res Cardiol* 2010; **99**: 841–847.

45 Plante S, Cantor WJ, Goldman L, *et al.* Comparison of bivalirudin versus heparin on radial artery occlusion after transradial catheterization. *Catheter Cardiovasc Interv* 2010; **76**: 654–658.

46 Pancholy S, Coppola J, Patel T, Roke-Thomas M. Prevention of radial artery occlusion-patent hemostasis evaluation trial (PROPHET study): a randomized comparison of traditional versus patency documented hemostasis after transradial catheterization. *Catheter Cardiovasc Interv* 2008; **72**: 335–340.

47 Sanmartin M, Gomez M, Rumoroso JR, *et al.* Interruption of blood flow during compression and radial artery occlusion after transradial catheterization. *Catheter Cardiovasc Interv* 2007; **70**: 185–189.

48 Pancholy SB. Impact of two different hemostatic devices on radial artery outcomes after transradial catheterization. *J Invasive Cardiol* 2009; **21**: 101–104.

49 Cubero JM, Lombardo J, Pedrosa C, *et al.* Radial compression guided by mean artery pressure versus standard compression with a pneumatic device (RACOMAP). *Catheter Cardiovasc Interv* 2009; **73**: 467–472.

CHAPTER 4

Optimal Angiographic Views for Coronary Angioplasty

Gioel Gabrio Secco[1] and Carlo Di Mario[2]

[1] Santi Antonio e Biagio e Cesare Arrigo Hospital, Alessandria, Italy

[2] National Institute of Health Research (NIHR), Royal Brompton & Harefield NHS Foundation Trust, London, and National Heart & Lung Institute, Imperial College London, UK

Angiography has been the keystone tool to assess coronary anatomy, leading to the development of largely applied revascularization techniques such as coronary artery bypass graft (CABG) and percutaneous coronary intervention (PCI). When CABG was the only revascularization strategy, the main scope of angiography was to detect the presence of significant stenosis and to provide information on vessel distality and contrast run-off. There was no need to be parsimonious with contrast because no further angiographic procedures were being planned. However, with the development of PCI, angiography has become far more important. In addition to clearly demonstrating the entire length of all epicardial arteries, the focus is to identify the anatomy of the lesion including its extension and the relationship with side branch vessels in order to allow correct planning of the revascularization strategy. The number of views and contrast use is restricted to the minimum required in anticipation of further contrast requirement during intervention. Therefore, angioplasty-focused projections should be favored in view of standard acquisitions, carefully selecting the more informative views in order to avoid foreshortening or overlapping of the diseased vessels.

The main limitation of angiography is that it can only provide a limited analysis of lumen profile without providing in-depth information about vessel wall characteristics or the composition of coronary lesions. New intracoronary imaging techniques have been developed to overcome these limitations. Intravascular ultrasound (IVUS) was the first intracoronary imaging modality introduced in interventional cardiology in the early 1990s, followed more than a decade after by optical coherence tomography (OCT), a near-infrared light-based technology. The use of ultrasound reflectance and near-infrared light allows IVUS and OCT to provide information about intravascular anatomy with a level of detail far exceeding that achieved from conventional angiography.

Catheter selection

Since the first human cardiac catheterization, performed by Forssmann in 1929, access site approach and angioplasty equipment have undergone considerable evolution. Miniaturization and refinement of materials have been among the most important goals, allowing interventionalists to perform more complex procedures and resolving most of the percutaneous limitations. The size of sheath, catheter, balloon, and stent delivery systems has been dramatically reduced in the last few years. From 9 French (Fr) devices used by Gruentzig in the late 1970s [1], now most PCI can be safely performed with a 6 Fr guiding catheter [1]. Contemporary diagnostic catheters are preshaped to facilitate intubation of the coronary ostia, in most cases with only minimal catheter manipulation. These smaller catheters appear of particular interest in the "transradial era" where transradial PCI has emerged as a gold standard in many centers replacing the transfemoral route in daily practice. The lack of back-up support offered by smaller catheters can be partially compensated by extra-stiff wires for the cannulation of the ostium and the use of extra-support guidewire or "mother and child" systems during the intervention. Moreover, the flexible tips facilitate the deep intubation of the target vessel and reduce the risk of vessel damage. Access site, sizing of the ascending aorta, and origin and take off of the target artery strictly condition the selection of the ideal curve for the catheter.

Left coronary

Judkins curve catheters are used most widely. Judkins left (JL) 4 would suit the anatomy of most patients although downsizing to JL3.5 may be required in patients with a smaller diameter aorta such as women. If the aortic root is dilated, JL4.5, JL5, or even JL6 with longer secondary curves may be required. Selective intubation can be encountered when there is a short left main stem (LMS) or separate origin of the left anterior descending (LAD) and circumflex (Cx) arteries, which may necessitate selecting a catheter with an upwards pointing tip (e.g., JL3.5) for intubation of the LAD and a more horizontal tip (e.g., JL4) for intubation of the Cx.

Right coronary

The take off of the right coronary artery (RCA) varies more than the left. A Judkins right (JR) 4 curve is most often used successfully. High anterior origin of the RCA may necessitate the use of an Amplatz right or left curve if a JR is unsuccessful.

Radial approach

The same curves suit most patients during left radial intervention, while a 0.5 downsizing of the left curve (e.g., to JL3.5 if JL4 would have been suitable from the femoral approach) is generally required when using the right arm. A Barbeau, Tiger, or Ikari catheter suitable for both the left and right coronaries can also be used from the right radial approach.

Interventional Cardiology: Principles and Practice, Second Edition. Edited by George D. Dangas, Carlo Di Mario, and Nicholas N. Kipshidze.
© 2017 John Wiley & Sons, Ltd. Published 2017 by John Wiley & Sons, Ltd.

Coronary intubation

The left anterior oblique (LAO) view is most useful for intubation of the left and right coronary arteries, because the left and right coronary sinuses are maximally separated and there is minimal overlap between the ostia and the coronary sinuses (Figure 4.1). For intubation of the left system the J-wire is advanced up to just above the aortic leaflets. The catheter is advanced over the wire and when the tip nears the aortic sinuses the J-wire is withdrawn to allow it to approach close to or intubate the coronary ostium. Slow J-wire withdrawal is recommended to avoid the catheter tip flicking into the ostium which can cause dissection, plaque dislodgement, or spasm, and also to avoid sucking air into the proximal catheter hub. The right coronary is intubated by advancing the JR catheter over the J-wire until the tip is just above the aortic leaflets. The wire is then withdrawn into the distal catheter to facilitate manipulation. Gentle counterclockwise rotation aiming the catheter tip toward the left with concomitant withdrawal is usually required. Gentle movements are emphasized to avoid sudden or deep intubation, which can precipitate spasm. Before proceeding to inject dye the pressure trace is checked. The pressure trace can be damped or ventricularized indicating the possibility of ostial right or LMS disease, spasm, complete occlusion of a non-dominant RCA, or that the catheter tip is abutting the vessel wall. Forceful contrast injection during any of these scenarios could result in dissection or plaque dislodgement. Contrast injection with an occlusive catheter with contrast remaining at the end of the injection, for instance holding up into the conus branch, should also be avoided because this can precipitate ventricular fibrillation. Spasm can be reversed with intracoronary nitrate, for example isosorbide dinitrate (ISDN) 100–200 μg. Rapid

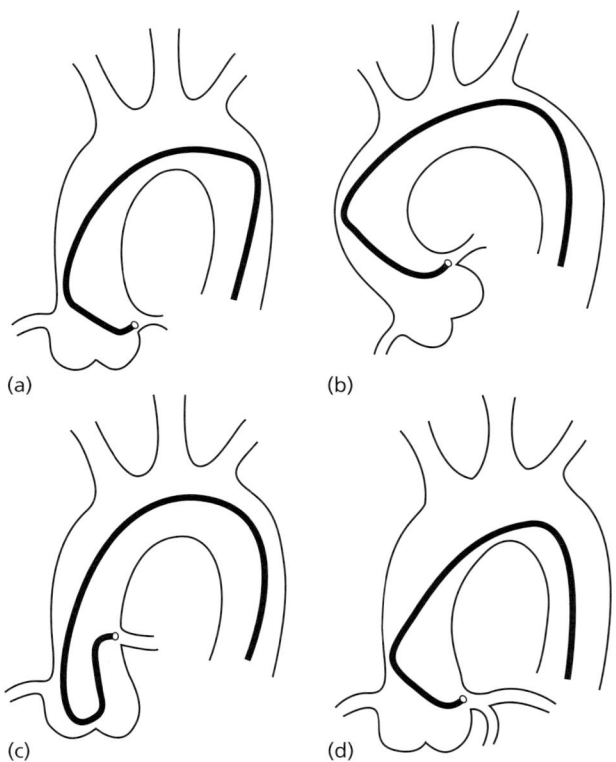

Figure 4.1 Guiding catheter selection for left coronary artery.
(a) Normal: JL4. (b) Dilated root: JL5, VL4, GL4, EBU. (c) Superior origin: AL3, VL4, GL4, EBU, Champ. (d) Short left main: JL4 short tip, JL3.5.

but gentle catheter withdrawal is indicated until the coronary ostium is extubated or the pressure trace normalizes. A small dose of intracoronary nitrate can be required to counteract any coronary vasospasm (e.g., ISDN 100–500 μg depending on the blood pressure). On occasion, smaller (e.g., 5F or 4F) catheters are required to avoid damping caused by spasm in hyper-reactive arteries or when there is ostial plaque.

The active support offered by deep intubation is frequently used also during interventions. However, this technique presents several relative limitations. The obstruction of flow during deep cannulation can induce severe ischemia, not always prevented by the presence of side holes [2]. Moreover, there is a potential risk of air embolism because of aspiration of air through the Y-connector while the catheter is damped inside the artery with a low back pressure. In any case, if the guide catheter is advanced coaxial with gentle rotation over the rail offered by a previously inserted wire and balloon, the risk of vessel damage is extremely low. A balloon can also be inflated at low pressure in the artery to stabilize the system while pushing the guiding catheter.

Diagnostic angiography
Left-sided views

The first view is chosen to identify LMS disease. Either a postanterior (PA) view with minimal angulation to the right to project the catheter tip off the spine or a LAO caudal (the so-called spider) view, are used most often. At least three to four perpendicular views are required to visualize the left coronary tree (Table 4.1 shows the most widely used combinations of views). In many patients these views would suffice, potentially even when proceeding immediately to angioplasty. However, because of variations in patient anatomy such as increased overlap caused by prominent tortuosity, displacement, or rotation of the heart axis in the chest (e.g., when there is normal anatomic variation, chest wall deformity, previous cardiothoracic surgery, or lung pathology), modification of views or additional views are sometimes required. When a lesion is identified, additional views can be indicated depending on how well the affected coronary segment has been visualized (Table 4.2).

Right-sided views

Two perpendicular views are advocated for the RCA, usually LAO and right anterior oblique (RAO). However, it is frequently impossible to exclude disease at or beyond the crux without an additional view with cranial angulation (e.g., PA cranial or LAO cranial).

Lesion-specific approach
Optimal views for each coronary segment

Views that reliably demonstrate the full length of each coronary segment while minimizing foreshortening and overlap for the left coronary arteries are shown in Figures 4.2 and 4.3(a). However, because of the wild degree of variation in human anatomy there are no views that will in all cases demonstrate clearly a lesion in a particular coronary segment. An example of a patient where the lesion was only clearly demonstrated after further adjustment of the gantry to unusual angles is shown in Figure 4.4.

Left main stem

Lesions in the ostium or mid segment of the LMS are often best seen in the anteroposterior (AP) cranial view. The straight AP view with only slight rightward angulation to project the catheter tip off

Table 4.1 Angiographic projections and optimal visualization of left and right coronary artery segments.

Coronary artery segment	LAO 40–50° Caudal 25–40° (spider)	AP RAO 5–15° Caudal 30°	RAO 30–45° Caudal 30–40°	AP/RAO 5–10° Cranial 35–45°	LAO 35–40° Cranial 25–35°	Lateral ± Caudocranial 10–30°	LAO 45–60°	RAO 30–45°
LM ostium	++	+	+	+++	+++	−	−	−
LM bifurc	+++	+++	++	−	−	−	−	−
LAD prox	++	++	+++	++	++	+	−	−
LAD mid	−	+	+	+++	++	++	−	−
LAD dist	+	+	+++	+	−	+++	−	++
LAD/DG	++	+	−	++	+++	−	−	−
LCX prox	+	+++	+++	−	−	−	−	−
LCX dist	+	+	++	+++	++	+	++	−
OM bifurc	++	+++	++	−	−	−	+	−
RCA prox	−	−	−	+	+++	−	++	−
RCA mid	−	−	−	−	+	+++	++	+++
RCA dist/crux	−	−	−	+++	+++	−	++	−
PDA	−	−	−	+++	++	−	+	++
PLV	+	−	−	+++	++	+	+	−
LIMA anast	+	−	−	−	−	+++	−	−

− not recommended; + occasionally useful; ++ very useful;: +++ ideal.

AP, anteroposterior; LAD, left anterior descending; LAO, left anterior oblique; LCX, left circumflex; LIMA, left internal mammary artery; OM, obtuse marginal; PDA, posterior descending artery; PLV, posterior left ventricular; RAO, right anterior oblique; RCA, right coronary artery.

the spine is sometimes advocated but may not be optimal because the ostium of the LMS can be projected over the left coronary sinus. The ostium of the LMS can also be seen clearly in an LAO caudal view (30–50° left; 25–40° caudal), which will also demonstrate the mid LMS and can sometimes be the only view to clearly separate the LMS bifurcation. In this view, also known as the "spider view," the picture can be grainy and of poor quality particularly when angulation is steep and in obese patients. The image can be optimized by positioning the LMS in the center of the field and reducing image contrast by blanking the field from the 12 o'clock to the 3 o'clock position. A small test injection before acquisition is sensible because a more horizontal axis of the heart can require steeper caudal angulation and occasionally overlap at the LMS bifurcation can be separated by rotating more steeply to the left or toward AP caudal.

Left anterior descending

Separation of the bifurcation of the LMS in the LAO caudal view also shows the ostium of the LAD clearly as well as the proximal LAD and frequently also the origin of the first diagonal. For these reasons the LAO caudal view is useful for wiring the proximal LAD

or for stent positioning at the ostium of the LAD, but if possible it should be avoided as a working view because X-ray attenuation caused by the highly angled projection through the spine results in higher X-ray doses. Working views for the LAD ostium include RAO caudal and RAO cranial, although in the latter more than 30° of rightward angulation are sometimes required to move the circumflex off the region of interest. Although the RAO cranial view can clearly demonstrate lesions in the proximal and mid LAD this is not the ideal working view because steep >40° rightward angulation is required to eliminate overlap with diagonals and wide diaphragmatic excursion during breathing causes highly variable contrast ratio in the field of view. Simply moving the gantry from AP to AP cranial elongates the proximal LAD and separates the diagonals to the right of the screen. A rightward tilt of <5° may be required to separate the proximal segment from the spine and the catheter in order to produce an excellent standard working view for the proximal and mid LAD unaffected by movement of the diaphragm. For diagnostic purposes, the ostia of the diagonals may be better seen in the LAO cranial view. However, LAO cranial is seldom used as a working view because a deep breath hold is

Table 4.2 Popular view combinations for diagnostic angiography with benefits and limitations of each view.

View	Good for visualizing	Limitations
Combination 1		
AP (5–10° RAO)	LMS (ostium and main shaft)	Overlap on LMS bifurcation and sometimes LMS ostium with left coronary sinus
Lateral	Mid and distal LAD, mid Cx	Potentially high radiation dose to operator, usually limited view of proximal LAD, patient's arms need to be above head to visualize posterior arteries, often overlap diagonals/LAD
RAO cranial	Proximal and mid LAD, distal Cx	Test injections can be required to adjust angulation to ensure diagonals are above LAD, overlap with dominant Cx, and position of the diaphragm
RAO caudal	Circumflex and distal LAD	
Combination 2		
LAO caudal	LMS bifurcation, proximal LAD and proximal circumflex	Potentially a higher radiation dose to the patient, poor quality images sometimes in large patients
LAO cranial	Mid LAD, origin of diagonals, proximal and mid Cx	Patient required to hold in inspiration during acquisition to elongate the proximal LAD
AP cranial	Proximal and mid LAD, distal Cx	Steep cranial angulation required can be a problem for patients with cervical spine fixation
RAO caudal	Circumflex and distal LAD, sometimes LAD ostium	

AP, anteroposterior; Cx, circumflex; LAD, left anterior descending; LAO, left anterior oblique; LMS, left main stem; RAO, right anterior oblique.

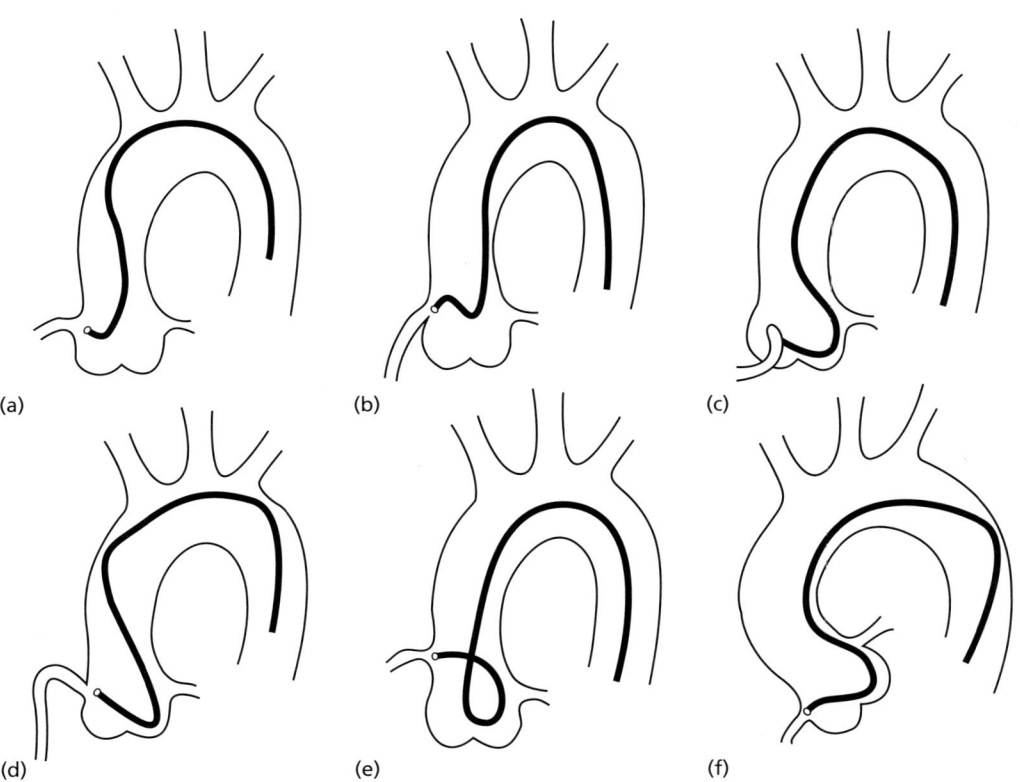

(a) (b) (c)

(d) (e) (f)

Figure 4.2 Guiding catheter selection for right coronary artery. (a) Normal: JR4. (b) Inferior orientation: modified right Amplatz. (c) Anterior origin (right cusp): Multipurpose. (d) Shepherd's crook: Arani 75°, Champ. (e) Superior origin: MAC, Champ, Multipurpose. (f) Dilated root: AL2.

required to reduce foreshortening and reduce projection of the diaphragm over the proximal and mid LAD. The body habitus of some patients also requires steep leftward angulation to project the LAD off the spine. An alternative but much less frequently used working view for lesions in the proximal and mid LAD is the left lateral. If the only vessel of interest is the LAD it is not necessary to ask patients to remove their arms from the field of view by keeping them above their heads, as this requirement is often uncomfortable and can be impossible for the elderly and patients with arthritis or old shoulder injuries.

Panning is usually required in the RAO cranial and LAO cranial views to demonstrate the distal LAD. Smooth slow panning allows

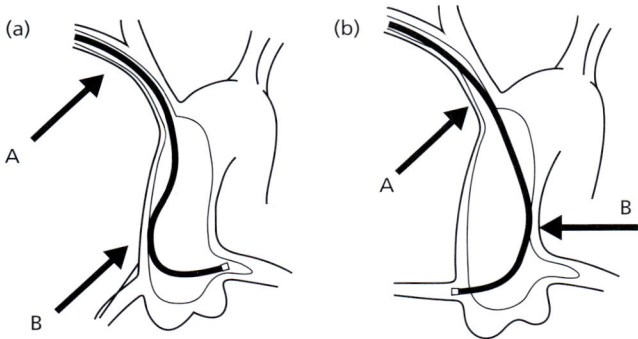

Figure 4.3 Ikari catheters for radial approach. (a) Ikari left. (b) Ikari right. Curve A to fit angle of brachiocephalic artery; straight portion B to generate strong back-up force supported by opposite site of the aorta wall.

the X-ray generator to adjust automatically to changes in X-ray attenuation. The lateral view is a good alternative for demonstrating the distal LAD around the apex but can also require controlled movement of the table during the acquisition toward the floor and/or in the direction of the head. The RAO caudal view can include the distal LAD without the requirement for table movement or being affected by diaphragmatic movement.

Circumflex

The circumflex ostium can be clearly seen together with the LMS bifurcation in the LAO caudal view. Occasionally, eccentric ostial lesions not clearly seen in other views can be delineated in the RAO cranial view although steep angulation may be required. The RAO caudal is the most useful diagnostic view for the circumflex and can clearly define lesions in the ostium, proximal, and mid vessel as well as the bifurcations and obtuse marginals. To obtain a working view with improved image quality by eliminating overlap with the diaphragm and reduced X-ray attenuation the view can be modified to AP caudal with only 10–15° rightward angulation.

The proximal and mid circumflex territory can also be viewed in the left lateral. A drawback of this view is that the patient has to remove their arms from the field of view by elevation above their head. Even young patients without arthritis can find this difficult to maintain for prolonged periods. Additional caudal angulation can be required to reduce overlap with marginal vessels. RAO or LAO with cranial angulation can be required to view lesions in the distal circumflex when the RAO caudal is suboptimal. If the circumflex is dominant, the LAO cranial or AP cranial views may open up the distal bifurcation and elongate the posterior descending artery (PDA).

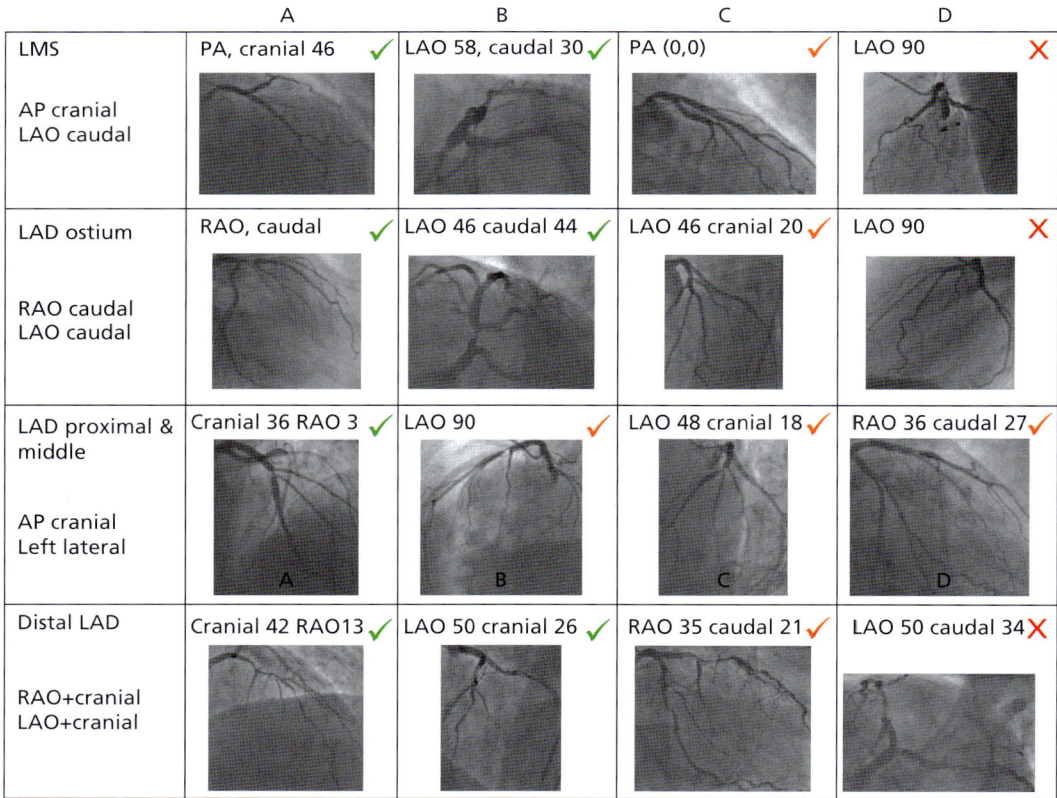

Figure 4.4 Optimal angiographic views for specific segments of the left anterior descending artery are indicated with a green tick mark. Some views that may be useful but are not generally recommended are indicated with an orange tick mark and inadequate views with a red cross.

Right coronary artery

Views that reliably demonstrate the full length of each coronary segment while minimizing foreshortening and overlap for the RCA are shown in Figure 4.3. Usually, the only two views required to demonstrate lesions in the proximal, mid, and distal RCA are LAO and RAO, because of the absence of side branches in these segments. Ostial lesions in the RCA are often detected in LAO but can be significantly foreshortened in this view. If stent placement is being considered, finding the least foreshortened segment can facilitate accurate positioning at ostium. The ostial segment and proximal RCA often lay perpendicular to the X-ray beam in the AP cranial and LAO caudal views, despite variation in the origin of the RCA toward anterior or posterior. The lateral view with cranial angulation can identify occasional highly eccentric ostial lesions not clearly seen in other views. The lateral view can also occasionally help to better delineate lesions in a highly tortuous mid RCA or when right ventricular branches overlap the main vessel.

The distal RCA, PDA, and posterior left ventricular (PLV) branches lie posterior to the heart and require cranial angulation (in LAO) or caudal angulation (in RAO or AP) to be visualized without overlap. Many operators routinely include a third view, either AP cranial or LAO cranial, in addition to LAO and RAO as standard during diagnostic imaging.

Vein grafts

An operative report describing graft number and insertions is imperative to reduce the chances of missing a graft as well as to reduce fluoroscopy dose and procedure time spent hunting for an unknown number of grafts. An aortogram can be helpful for graft localization, potentially saving time and contrast, but it is not a panacea, because grafts can sometimes opacify only if the pigtail catheter is positioned at the level of the graft origin, if at all, when the take off is vertical and/or flow is slow. The insertions of vein grafts can vary substantially, in particular after redo bypass surgery. A rule of thumb is that the aorto-ostial insertions of vein grafts to the left coronary system tend to arise lower and more anterior for grafts to an anterior artery (e.g., LAD) and progressively more superior and leftward as the insertion site moves more toward left lateral (e.g., diagonal, intermediate, obtuse marginal, AV circumflex). In the RAO view, left-sided grafts can be intubated by pointing the catheter toward the right of the screen. Right-sided grafts can be found in LAO by dragging the catheter pointing to the left of the screen along the ascending aorta starting above the RCA ostium. A patent graft with slow flow may only partially opacify and thus appear occluded if intubated with a catheter tip that is angulated toward the wall of the graft, for example vertical origin of vein grafts to the RCA intubated with a JR catheter. In these instances a coaxially aligned catheter, for example a multipurpose or right coronary bypass (RCB) catheter for a right-sided graft and a multipurpose or left coronary bypass (LCB) for left-sided grafts, should be used to clarify whether or not a graft is occluded. The views are selected according to the native coronary segment where the graft inserts. Two perpendicular views are required.

Left internal mammary artery grafts

The left internal mammary artery (LIMA) graft is usually prognostically the most important. Selective intubation of the LIMA with demonstration of the entire length of the graft and native vessel including any lesions and collateral supply is the standard. The origin of the left subclavian artery is usually engaged in the AP view.

An 0.035-inch J-wire is used to lead before the catheter is advanced over it to reduce the risk of trauma to the vessels. If difficulty is encountered with an abnormal aortic arch, severe tortuosity, or stenosis the following steps can be tried: intubation of the left subclavian may be easier in the LAO view; making use of non-selective contrast injections to delineate the anatomy; using a JR rather than an internal mammary artery (IMA) catheter to engage the left subclavian and exchanging it via a 300-cm J-wire for an IMA catheter if necessary once the catheter is beyond the origin of the LIMA; and making use of a 0.035-inch steerable hydrophilic J-wire if extreme tortuosity is preventing passage of the standard J-wire. Once the catheter tip is near the ostium of the LIMA, the AP view is most useful for engagement. If the JR catheter tip appears too horizontal during gentle withdrawal or too short to engage the ostium of the LIMA, an IMA catheter can be used or sometimes the even more acute hook of a Bartorelli-Cozzi (BC) catheter. Before contrast injection—including test injections—it is important to remember to check that the pressure tracing does not indicate wedging of the catheter tip against the vessel wall. If selective intubation via the femoral route proves elusive despite multiple attempts, the left radial route can offer a safer alternative. A drawback of the left radial route is that right internal mammary artery (RIMA) grafts cannot be engaged, although successful intubation of the LIMA via the right radial route has been previously described [3]. The first angiographic view for the LIMA requires panning from origin to the distal LAD. The views that best show the insertions are RAO cranial and left lateral. Collateral filling of other vessels should also be documented. Intubation to the diaphragm of a pedicle RIMA graft follows the same principles as for the LIMA, but with even greater care in view of the close proximity of the right internal carotid artery.

Coronary variants

Aberrant coronary anatomy occurs infrequently and the prevalence of <1.3% is remarkably consistent in different series of patients attending for angiography [4]. Some anomalies are easy to identify, such as abnormal origin of RCA (Figure 4.5) but others can be more subtle, such as anomalous non-dominant circumflex (Figure 4.6). The culprit lesion can be missed if the aberrant anatomy is not identified (Figures 4.7 and 4.8). Systematic review to identify areas of the myocardium for which a vascular supply has not been demonstrated is helpful in this respect and also for identifying occlusions (Figure 4.8). Once it is known which vessel is anomalous, a review of the images can identify ghosting of the vessel. If there are no clues as to the origin, a systematic search starting with the most common variant is required. The diagnostic catheter shape needs to be changed as required to reach the wall of the aortic root in the area of interest. The most common coronary anomaly is an absent LMS. A slightly smaller curve catheter is required to intubate the LAD selectively (e.g., JL3.5 if JL4 preferentially and exclusively intubates the Cx). The Cx arising from the right coronary sinus can often be cannulated using the JR4 catheter, but a steep take off can require a multipurpose catheter whereas a posterior or high anterior origin can require an AR or AL shape. If the RCA arises from the left side separately from the LMS an AL1 or multipurpose catheter is most likely to be successful.

Once the anomalous coronary vessel has been intubated the standard views are often sufficient for the mid and distal vessel if the heart has a normal position and orientation (Figures 4.2 and 4.3), while the views for the proximal vessel and ostium may need to be modified depending on the origin and course.

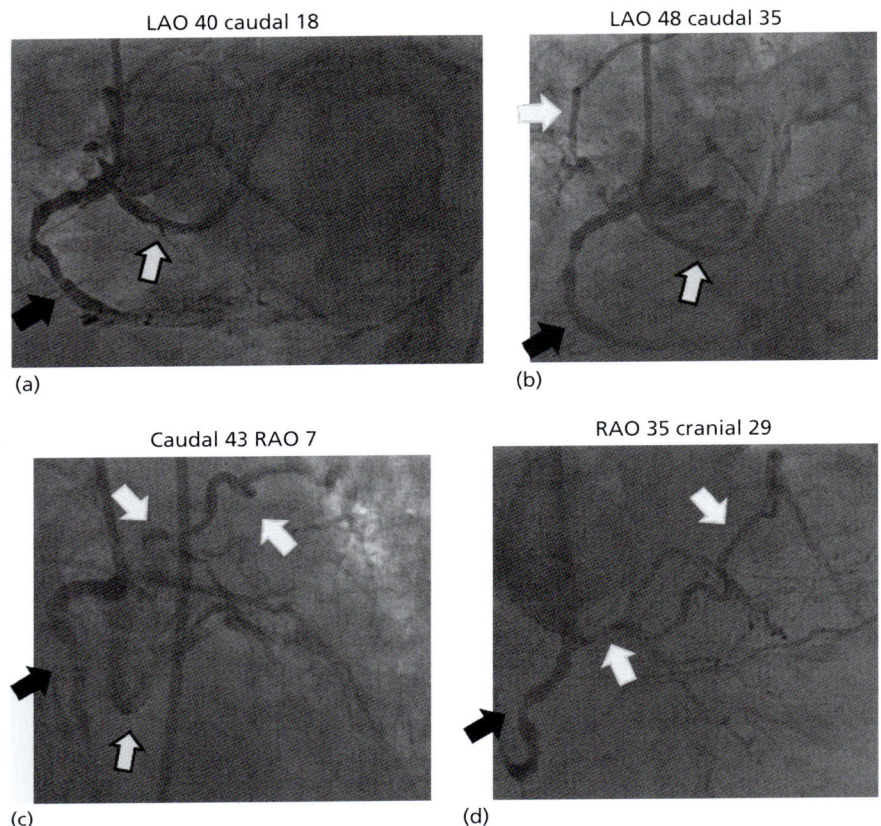

Figure 4.5 This 80-year-old obese female was admitted for angiography following a recent worsening of angina. She had a previous history of myocardial infarction. Preceding this presentation her angina symptoms had been stable for many years and were not previously investigated with angiography. A coronary ostium could not be engaged at the left aortic sinus. The left anterior descending (LAD), circumflex, and right coronary arteries originated from a single right-sided ostium. The right coronary artery (RCA) (black arrows, a–d) was occluded distally. The left anterior descending (LAD) (white arrows, a–c) was critically stenosed proximal to a large diagonal and the circumflex (gray arrows, b–d) was critically stenosed mid course. The catheter partially obscures the LAD in (a) and the circumflex in (d).

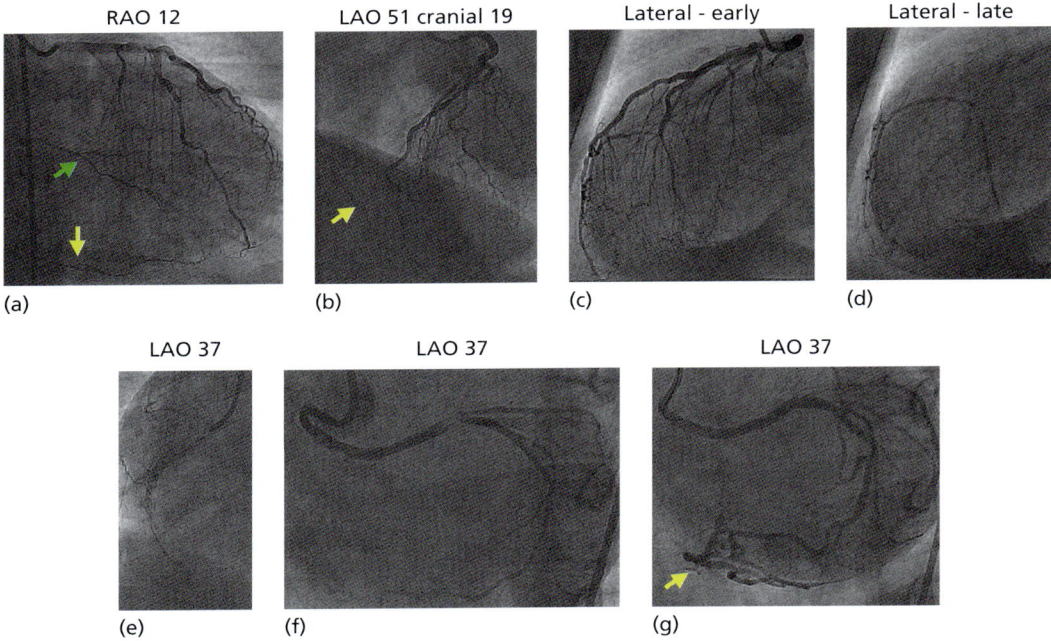

Figure 4.6 These views were taken during primary angioplasty performed in a 41-year-old male who presented with an acute inferolateral myocardial infarction. No antegrade perfusion was evident in the circumflex territory (a to d), although retrograde collaterals to an obtuse marginal branch were seen in some views (green arrow, a). The right coronary artery (RCA) was occluded and filled retrogradely via the left anterior descending (LAD) (yellow arrow, a and b; d and e). The culprit lesion was in an aberrant circumflex arising from the right sinus (f). Following aspiration thrombectomy and stent deployment it was evident that the aberrant circumflex provided the principal collateral supply to a chronically occluded dominant RCA (yellow arrow, g).

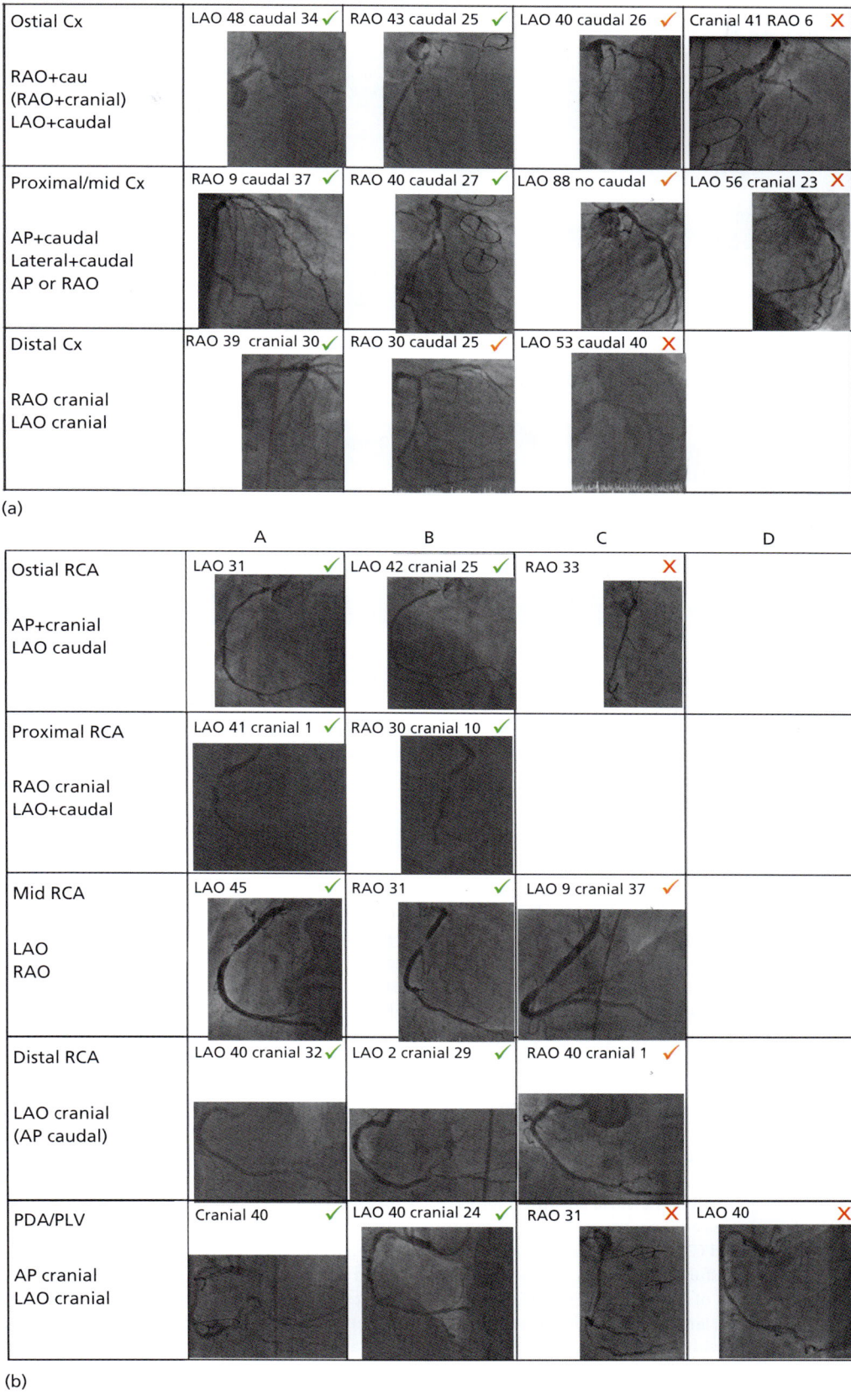

Figure 4.7 Optimal angiographic views for specific segments in the circumflex and right coronary are indicated with a green tick mark. Some views that may be useful but are not generally recommended are indicated with an orange tick mark and inadequate views with a red cross.

Conventional views:

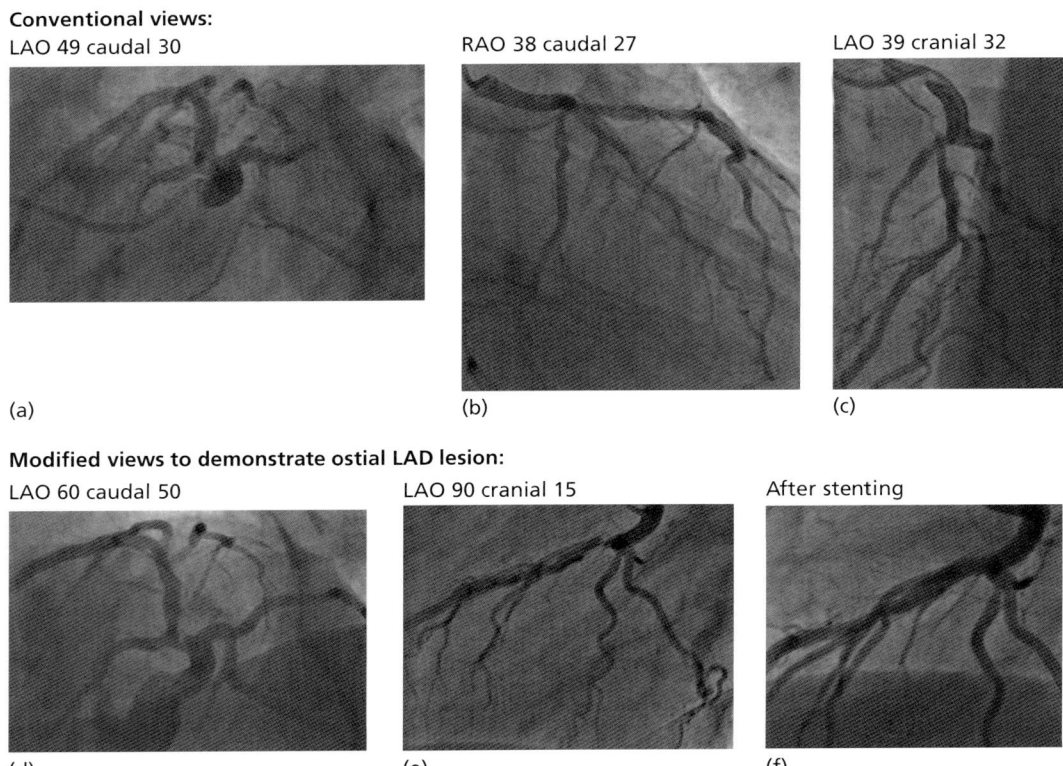

LAO 49 caudal 30

(a)

RAO 38 caudal 27

(b)

LAO 39 cranial 32

(c)

Modified views to demonstrate ostial LAD lesion:

LAO 60 caudal 50

(d)

LAO 90 cranial 15

(e)

After stenting

(f)

Figure 4.8 This 47-year-old male with known coronary disease presented with deteriorating angina and reversible ischemia in the anterior territory on perfusion imaging. Conventional views (a–c) raised suspicion of a lesion in the left anterior descending (LAD) ostium due to haziness (a) but were limited by overlap at the ostium of the LAD due to unusual tortuosity (a). Unusual modification including a steep spider view and a lateral view with cranial angulation were required to delineate the lesion (d, e). The final angiographic result is shown after stenting (f).

Chronic total occlusion

Chronic total occlusions (CTO) affect almost 20–30% of patients with coronary artery disease undergoing angiography [5,6]. Recent advancement in materials such as guidewires, microcatheters, and crossing devices has increased the success rate of CTO percutaneous recanalization from 50–60% [7,8] to 70–80% [9–11], with peaks above 90% for a few highly specialized centers [12–14]. The lack of a general consensus regarding the usefulness of CTO recanalization together with the difficulty of the procedure have partially affected the development of CTO-PCI in daily practice. Two large registries in the USA addressed the benefit of CTO recanalization procedure on long-term survival leading to conflicting results, negative in the first [15] and positive only for LAD recanalization in the other [16]. However, they both included patients treated with plain balloon angioplasty alone suffering from a high percentage of re-occlusion. More recent studies, conducted in the drug-eluting stent (DES) era, showed that successful recanalization is associated with improved long-term survival and reduced need for surgical revascularization at follow-up compared with failed CTO procedure. Moreover, it has been recently shown that successful recanalization provided a significant improvement in quality of life, with less physical activity limitation, rarer angina episodes, and higher treatment satisfaction when compared with patients with failed procedure [17]. These positive findings have led to a rapid increase in percutaneous CTO procedures. However, when approaching these complex interventions the selection of the correct angiographic views, especially during retrograde recanalization, is pivotal.

The correct imaging of a coronary occlusion requires acquisitions in multiple views and the acquisition must be prolonged enough to visualize the distal segments eventually filled by collaterals. A dual injection performed using low magnification, so that the entire coronary tree is visualized, is generally recommended. The injections should be performed at the beginning of the procedure because wire and catheter advancement might impair the ipsilateral collaterals flow, thus resulting in a collateral or preferential collateral shift to the retrograde collaterals. Moreover, initial careful evaluation of the collaterals provides important information in choosing the most appropriate one and alerts the operator to the risk for ischemia and hemodynamic or electrical instability if the collateral becomes occluded [18]. Coronary collaterals are a network of nascent microvessels, which, in case of coronary occlusion, grow in favor of a viable distal myocardium. The most widely used method to assess coronary collaterals is angiography using the view with the least foreshortening of the collateral connection. Collaterals' anatomic pathways are generally summarized in four categories: septal, intra-arterial (bridging), epicardial with proximal take off (atrial branches), and epicardial with distal take off [19]. The size of the collateral connection (CC) diameter is classified according to Werner *et al.*: CC0, no continuous connection between donor and recipient artery; CC1, continuous, threadlike connection; and CC2, continuous, small side branch-like size of the collateral through its course [20].

The treatment of CTO often involves the X-ray gantry being maintained in one working view, with occasional rotation in an orthogonal and equally fixed view, so the same skin and body segments are therefore exposed to the majority of the radiation dose. Given that, a careful evaluation of radiation-induced skin injury should be performed and the most recent recommendation from the EuroCTO consensus document should be strictly followed [21].

Multi-slice computed tomography can provide additional information regarding the plaque characterization, tortuosity, and length of the occluded artery. Moreover, 3D reconstruction integrated with 2D angiographic images during CTO intervention helps identify the best projection giving a directional guide for the missing angiographic segment [22].

Ventriculography

Knowledge of ventricular function is essential to interpreting the clinical relevance of coronary disease and planning appropriate treatment. Many patients have a contemporary assessment of left ventricular function by non-invasive testing, which provides similar or superior definition of the left ventricular cavity volume and global and regional wall motion, with the advantage that most of them can also dynamically study wall thickness and tissue characteristics (echocardiography, magnetic resonance imaging, nuclear imaging, and multidetector CT), when attending for coronary angiography [23]. These modalities provide more information on the function and morphology of the left ventricle than conventional ventriculography and can obviate the need for further assessment. Ventriculography should be performed in the catheter laboratory if left ventricular function has not been assessed recently. The RAO view is standard, although an additional LAO view could be considered if assessment of the postero-lateral wall, usually supplied by the circumflex, is likely to influence management.

Interactive multiple choice questions are available for this chapter on www.wiley.com/go/dangas/cardiology

References

1 Secco GG, Agostoni PF. Coronary interventions: 5F versus 6F to 7F. In Bertrand O, Rao S. (eds) *Best Practice for Transradial Approach in Diagnostic Angiography and Intervention*. Wolters Kluwer: 2015.

2 Di Mario C, Ramasami N. Techniques to enhance guide catheter support. *Catheter Cardiovasc Interv* 2008; **72**: 505–512.

3 Cha KS, Kim MH. Feasibility and safety of concomitant left internal mammary arteriography at the setting of the right transradial coronary angiography. *Catheter Cardiovasc Interv* 2002; **56**(2): 188–195.

4 Angelini P, Velasco JA, Flamm S. Coronary anomalies: incidence, pathophysiology, and clinical relevance. *Circulation* 2002; **105**(20): 2449–2454.

5 Puma JA, Sketch Jr MH, Tcheng JE, *et al*. Percutaneous revascularization of chronic coronary occlusions: an overview. *J Am Coll Cardiol* 1995; **26**: 1–11.

6 Aziz S, Ramsdale DR. Chronic total occlusions: a stiff challenge requiring a major breakthrough. Is there light at the end of the tunnel? *Heart* 2005; **91**: 42–48.

7 Tsujita K, Maehara A, Mintz GS, *et al*. Intravascular ultrasound comparison of the retrograde versus antegrade approach to percutaneous intervention for chronic total coronary occlusions. *JACC Cardiovasc Interv* 2009; **2**: 846–854.

8 Di Mario C, Barlis P, Tanigawa J, *et al*. Retrograde approach to coronary chronic total occlusions: preliminary single European centre experience. *EuroIntervention* 2007; **3**: 181–187.

9 De Felice F, Fiorilli R, Parma A, *et al*. 3-year clinical outcome of patients with chronic total occlusion treated with drug-eluting stents. *JACC Cardiovasc Interv* 2009; **2**: 1260–1265.

10 Aziz S, Stables RH, Grayson AD, *et al*. Percutaneous coronary intervention for chronic total occlusions: improved survival for patients with successful revascularization compared to a failed procedure. *Catheter Cardiovasc Interv* 2007; **70**: 15–20.

11 Lee NH, Seo HS, Choi JH, *et al*. Recanalization strategy of retrograde angioplasty in patients with coronary chronic total occlusion: analysis of 24 cases, focusing on technical aspects and complications. *Int J Cardiol* 2010; **144**(2): 219–229.

12 Morino Y, Kimura T, Hayashi Y, *et al*. J-CTO Registry Investigators. In-hospital outcomes of contemporary percutaneous coronary intervention in patients with chronic total occlusion insights from the J-CTO Registry (Multicenter CTO Registry in Japan). *JACC Cardiovasc Interv* 2010; **3**: 143–151.

13 Kimura M, Katoh O, Tsuchikane E, *et al*. The efficacy of a bilateral approach for treating lesions with chronic total occlusions the CART (controlled antegrade and retrograde subintimal tracking) registry. *JACC Cardiovasc Interv* 2009; **2**: 1135–1141.

14 Syrseloudis D, Secco GG, Barrero EA, *et al*. Increase in J-CTO lesion complexity score explains the disparity between recanalisation success and evolution of chronic total occlusion strategies: insights from a single-centre 10-year experience. *Heart* 2013; **99**: 474–479.

15 Prasad A, Rihal CS, Lennon RJ, *et al*. Trends in outcomes after percutaneous coronary intervention for chronic total occlusions: a 25-year experience from the Mayo Clinic. *J Am Coll Cardiol* 2007; **49**: 1611–1618.

16 Suero JA, Marso SP, Jones PG, *et al*. Procedural outcomes and long-term survival among patients undergoing percutaneous coronary intervention of a chronic total occlusion in native coronary arteries: a 20-year experience. *J Am Coll Cardiol* 2001; **38**: 409–414.

17 Borgia F, Viceconte N, Ali O, *et al*. Improved cardiac survival, freedom from mace and angina-related quality of life after successful percutaneous recanalization of coronary artery chronic total occlusions. *Int J Cardiol* 2012; **161**: 31–38.

18 Galassi A, Grantham A, Kandzari D, *et al*. Percutaneous treatment of coronary chronic total occlusion. Part 2: Technical approach. *Radcliffe Cardiol* 2014; **9**(3): 201–207.

19 Rockstroh J, Brown BG. Coronary collateral size, flow capacity, and growth: estimates from the angiogram in patients with obstructive coronary artery disease. *Circulation* 2002; **104**: 2012–2017.

20 Werner GS, Ferrari M, Heinke S, *et al*. Angiographic assessment of collateral connections in comparison with invasively determined collateral function in chronic coronary occlusions. *Circulation* 2003; **107**: 1972–1977.

21 Di Mario C, Werner GS, Sianos G, *et al*. European perspective in the recanalisation of Chronic Total Occlusions (CTO): consensus document from the EuroCTO Club. *EuroIntervention* 2007; **3**: 30–43.

22 Magro M, Schultz C, Simsek C, *et al*. Computed tomography as a tool for percutaneous coronary intervention of chronic total occlusions. *EuroIntervention* 2010; **6**(Suppl G): 123–131.

23 Di Mario C, Sutaria N. Coronary angiography in the angioplasty era: projections with a meaning. *Heart* 2005; **91**: 968–976.

CHAPTER 5

Material Selection

Sahil A. Parikh[1], Michele Pighi[2], and Carlo Di Mario[2,3]

[1] Harrington Heart & Vascular Institute, Case Western Reserve University School of Medicine, Cleveland, OH, USA

[2] National Institute of Health Research (NIHR), Royal Brompton & Harefield NHS Foundation Trust, London, UK

[3] National Heart & Lung Institute, Imperial College London, UK

Legend has it that the first coronary angioplasty balloons were made by Andreas Gruentzig and his wife in a kitchen. They were very bulky, difficult to position as there was no guidewire lumen, and too compliant to safely expand resistant lesions in coronary arteries. Further understanding and development in manufacturing techniques and evolution of materials have reduced the profile of angioplasty balloons while increasing their robustness, deliverability, reliability, and safety profile. Similarly, workhorse guidewires have been developed with improvements in torque and force transmission while having more durable and less traumatic but shapeable tips. Specialty guidewires have been developed for the treatment of specific lesion types including chronic total occlusions. A wide range of guide catheters, guidewires, and angioplasty balloons are now available, and continue to evolve to overcome variations in anatomy, changes in vascular access, and evolution in technique. The appropriate selection and safe and optimal use of these devices can reduce procedural time and increase procedural success and safety with hopes of improving clinical outcomes.

Guide catheter selection
Functional design of modern guide catheters

Guide catheters permit safe intubation of the coronary ostia, accurate hemodynamic monitoring, injection of contrast, and passage of guidewires, balloons, and stents. The clinical, anatomic, and angiographic scenario must be considered when selecting the size, shape, and length of a guide catheter. Modern catheters have a soft tip to reduce the risk of vessel trauma during intubation or manipulation. The wall consists of an outer layer which retains a predefined curve and increases shaft stiffness to provide backup support during intervention, a middle layer of wire braid to increase kink resistance, improve torque transmission, and shaft radiopacity, and a smooth lubricated inner layer to facilitate the transit of equipment. Guide catheters have thinner walls than diagnostic catheters to increase inner lumen size and can be easily damaged by excessive rotation (Table 5.1).

When difficulty is encountered in engaging the coronary ostia, one must first consider whether the guide catheter shape is appropriate. The use of a supportive 0.035 inch guidewire within the catheter can facilitate manipulation. Similarly, deep inspiration by the patient can facilitate coronary intubation. In the case of excessive vascular tortuosity or calcification, the use of a peripheral sheath long enough to straighten the most tortuous arterial segments can improve guide catheter maneuverability. The optimal view for left and right coronary intubation is the left anterior oblique because in most patients it offers the least superimposition of the coronary ostia with the left and right aortic sinuses.

Size requirements

The advantages and disadvantages of smaller and larger catheter sizes are listed in Table 5.2. Routine angioplasty using 5 French (Fr) guiding catheters may be ideal when direct stenting is planned, but not all stents are deliverable through a 5 Fr guide and most bifurcation techniques are not applicable [1]. The general standard is a 6 Fr (2.00 mm external diameter) guide catheter which permits radial access, allows active engagement ("deep seat"), accommodates two modern rapid exchange balloons or a 1.50 or 1.75 mm rotational atherectomy burr, and uses less contrast than larger catheter diameters. For bifurcation techniques requiring the simultaneous insertion of two stents (Crush, V stenting), 7 Fr (2.33 mm diameter) guides are required. These are necessary for advanced techniques that require two over the wire (OTW) catheters and facilitate the insertion of rotational atherectomy burrs greater than 1.75 mm. For rotational atherectomy burrs greater than 2.0 mm in diameter and complex techniques requiring multiple wires, balloons, and/or stents, 8 Fr (2.66 mm diameter) guides are used. The use of guide catheters greater than 8 Fr is extremely rare in contemporary coronary intervention.

Shape relection

Selection of guide catheter shape is critical to allow positioning of the catheter coaxially with the proximal segment of the artery, to reduce the risk of catheter-induced vessel trauma, and optimize support during intervention. When selecting the shape of the catheter, the following factors should be considered: the curve and fit of the diagnostic catheter; size of the aortic root; origin and take off of the artery; location and complexity of the lesion; and the devices likely to be utilized during intervention.

Shape selection for the left coronary system

Shapes for commonly used guide catheters for the left coronary system are shown in Figure 5.1. The curve sizes of different shapes have been largely standardized and the comparable curve sizes used most commonly are shown in Table 5.3.

Interventional Cardiology: Principles and Practice, Second Edition. Edited by George D. Dangas, Carlo Di Mario, and Nicholas N. Kipshidze.
© 2017 John Wiley & Sons, Ltd. Published 2017 by John Wiley & Sons, Ltd.

Table 5.1 Guide catheter inner lumen size by manufacturer and outer lumen size.

Guide/manufacturer		Outer lumen size (French)			
		5	6	7	8
Launcher/Medtronic	Inner lumen (in)	0.058	0.071	0.081	0.090
Vista Brite Tip/Cordis		0.056	0.070	0.078	0.088
Mach1/Boston Scientific		NA	0.070	0.081	0.091
Viking/Guidant Abbott		NA	0.068	0.078	0.091
Wiseguide/Boston Scientific		NA	0.066	0.076	0.086

Table 5.2 The advantages and disadvantages of smaller versus larger catheter diameters have to be weighed when selecting catheter size.

Smaller diameter	Larger diameter
Advantages	
Smaller puncture	Increased torque
Small vessel access	Increased support
Less traumatic radial access	Improved visualization
Allows deeper engagement without significant damping	Allows two balloon/stent strategy
Disadvantages	
Less torque	Larger puncture: increased access site trauma /recovery time
Reduced visualization	Pressure damping
Less support	Increased contrast use
Difficult or impossible to use two balloon/stent strategy	

For the left coronary artery, catheters with a smaller curve will point upward and selectively engage to left anterior descending (LAD) and a larger curve will selectively engage and provide better support for the circumflex. The tip of Amplatz Left (AL) guides tend to point downward and are useful to selectively engage the circumflex in situations where there is a short or absent left main.

The shape of the guide catheter is an important component of the backup or support system that allows delivery of devices to the target lesion. Changing the guide catheter to improve support in the middle of a procedure can be problematic, and therefore careful consideration of guide support prior to intervention is critical. It is also important to appreciate that selection of a guide with optimal backup may obviate the need for stiffer wires or balloons, with a corresponding reduction in cost and procedure time. Although Judkins Left (JL) curves are commonly used for diagnostic intervention, these guide shapes provide less support than "backup" guides which provide contralateral aortic wall support such as the XB, EBU-, or Q-type curves. Because of the secondary curve on the JL, the tip may be withdrawn from the coronary ostium when resistance is encountered. XB/EBU/Q/ Voda or similar curves provide comparatively more support with minimally increased risk of damage to the coronary ostia. AL curves are required in certain situations, but should only be used by experienced operators in view of the increased risk of iatrogenic dissection. Techiques to obtain support other than the passive support allowed by the guide catheter shape are discussed later in this chapter.

Shape selection for the right coronary system

Shapes and sizes of commonly used guide catheters for the right coronary system are shown in Figure 5.2. The take off of the right coronary artery tends to vary more than that of the left coronary. If the take off is transverse, the most commonly used guide would probably be a Judkins Right (JR) 4. With a superiorly directed take off, a JR, Hockeystick, EBU-R, or Amplatz R or L are more suitable. Inferiorly directed take offs can be cannulated with a multipurpose or SLS catheter. Although the JR shape does not provide much active support, the guide can often be actively engaged more deeply to augment support if required via "deep seating" by advancing and clockwise rotating the guide.

Length

The standard length of a coronary guide catheter is 100 cm. Occasionally, shorter lengths (85 or 90 cm) are required to reach for distal lesions (e.g., lesions reached via the left internal mammary artery (LIMA), sequential saphenous vein grafts (SVGs), or retrograde approach to chronic total occlusions (CTO)). Longer lengths (110–115 cm) are required for unusually tall patients or severely tortuous aorto-iliac vessels. The use of a long sheath and of longer balloon catheters (>145 cm) has partially overcome this problem but stent delivery catheters remain 135 cm.

Side holes or not?

Side holes help to maintain coronary perfusion when there is the likelihood of ostial obstruction by the guide catheter that results in pressure dampening. This can occur when using a larger guide caliber, in the presence of aorto-ostial disease, non-coaxial engagement, and in small caliber arteries encountered in smaller patients. Side holes can reduce contrast opacification of the arteries with a consequent reduction in image quality and increased overall contrast dye utilization. The persistence of aortic pressure morphology can mask severe catheter-induced pressure dampening which is of

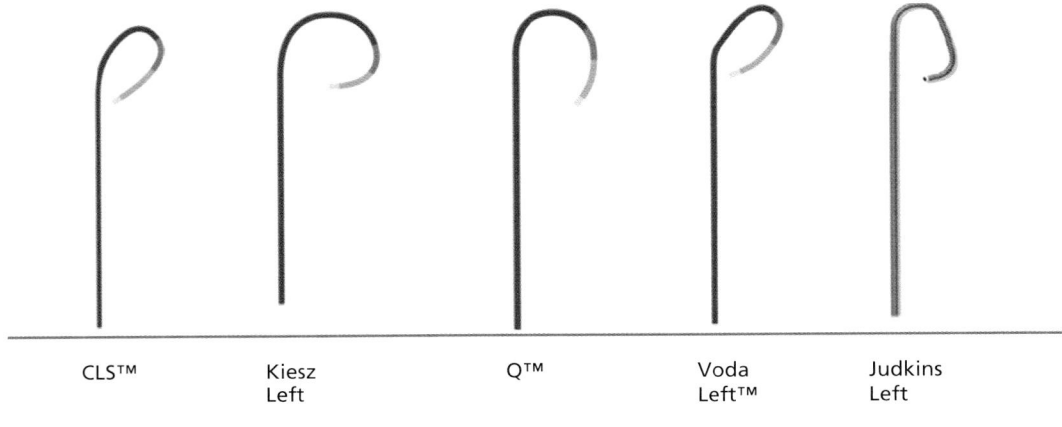

Figure 5.1 Shapes of a selection of guide catheters for the left coronary system.

Table 5.3 Comparability of curve sizes for different shapes of left sided guide catheters.

	AL (Amplatz) Curve	CLS or XB Curve	JL (Judkins Left) Curve	Q Curve	VL (Voda Left) Curve
Normal	AL 1	XB 4.0 or 3.5	JL 4	Q 4	VL 4
Dilated	AL 2	XB 4.0 or 4.5	JL 4.5	Q 4.5	VL 5
Narrow	AL 0.75	XB 3.0 or 3.5	JL 3.5	Q 3.5	VL 3

importance for measuring fractional flow reserve and may not always protect from hydraulically induced vessel dissection [2].

Variation in access site

The same guide catheters can be used for transradial access as well as transfemoral access. Dedicated transradial guide catheters include the Barbeau, Ikari, and brachial/radial curves. Such curves can be used for access to either the left or right coronary system and provide support against the contralateral aortic wall (Figure 5.3).

Vein grafts

Both right- and left-sided vein grafts with a transverse origin can often be cannulated with a JR4 guide catheter; however, guide support can be suboptimal. If the vein graft points downwards (inferior or vertical such as often for right coronary artery (RCA) grafts), coaxial engagement may be difficult with a JR guide. A multipurpose or RCB guide is usually coaxially aligned when the take off is inferior and would also offer good support if required. Left-sided vein grafts lesions can also often be attempted with a JR guide or, if more support is needed, with an Amplatz or Hockeystick guide catheter. If the ascending aorta is large or dilated, a guide with a more pronounced secondary curve is frequently required such as the left coronary bypass (LCB) or an Amplatz shape may be selected.

Left and right internal mammary arteries

Although the LIMA can often be reached with a JR guide, the more acute primary angle and longer tip of an internal mammary artery (IMA) guide may be required. Short-tip hook-shaped IMA catheters can occasionally be required to intubate a very steep take off angle. Sometimes, because of subclavian stenosis or extreme tortuosity, the IMA can only be selectively cannulated via the left radial approach.

Gastroepiploic artery grafts

In an attempt to simulate the longevity of IMA grafts and overcome the problem of reaching the distal RCA, the gastroepiploic artery (GEA) is sometimes used as an *in situ* graft to the posterior or inferior surface of the heart (RCA, posterior descending artery, posterior left ventricular) [3]. The GEA can be cannulated using catheters designed for abdominal vascular intervention such as Cobra or Simmons catheters [4]. The celiac trunk is accessed from the abdominal aorta in the direction of the common hepatic artery (the other branch being the splenic artery) (Figure 5.4). The gastro-duodenal artery arises in an inferior direction and gives off the pancreatico-duodenal branch beyond which it becomes the GEA, which passes through the diaphragm to reach the inferior wall of the heart (Figure 5.4). Anastomotic stenoses require percutaneous treatment [5].

Support

Complex anatomic situations including tortuosity, calcification, or diffuse atherosclerosis frequently require escalating degrees of backup support. The components of the "backup" support intrinsic to an angioplasty system includes the guide catheter, guidewire(s), and balloon(s) in the target artery. The components can be changed individually or in combination as demanded by the difficulties that are encountered. Hybrid strategies using more complex wire and/or balloon-based techniques are sometimes required to overcome more challenging anatomy.

Guide catheter support

The role of shape selection has been discussed. Guide catheter support is either passive or active. Passive support is provided by a large diameter catheter positioned optimally in the coronary ostium

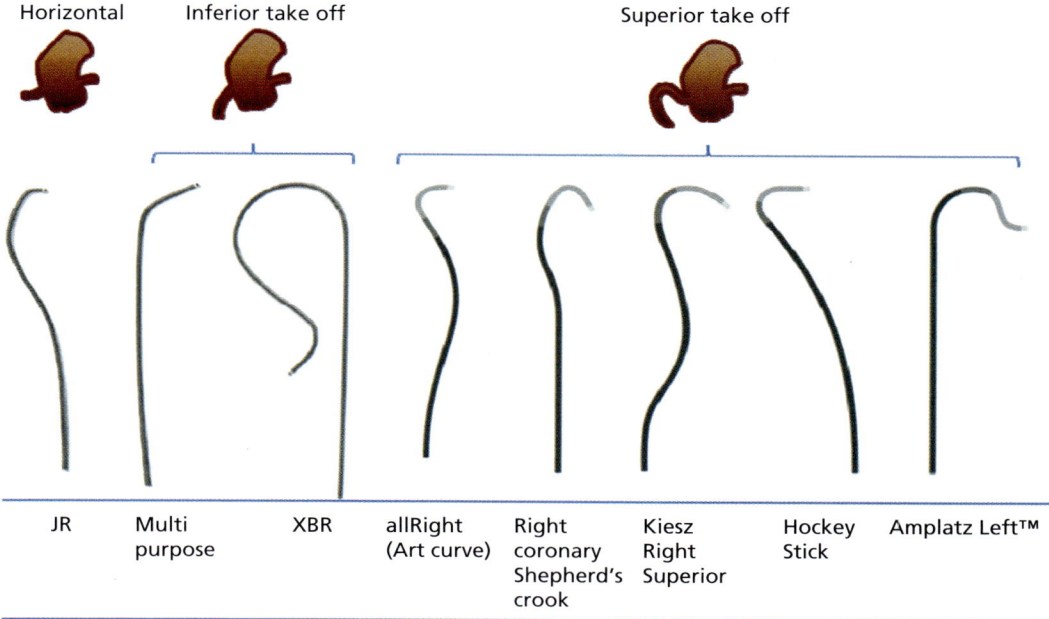

Figure 5.2 Shapes of commonly used guide catheters for the right coronary system.

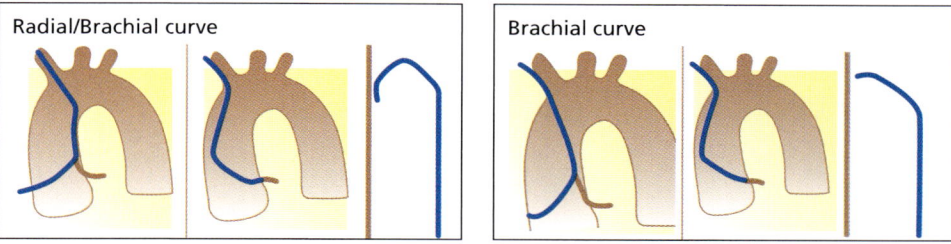

Figure 5.3 The Barbeau and radial/brachial curve catheters can be used via the radial route and have a "one size fits all" design for intervention to either the left or right coronary systems. (Diagram courtesy of Cordis International.)

whereas active support is provided by judiciously advancing a small diameter catheter to deeply intubate an epicardial artery.

Passive support

Although 6 Fr guide catheters are successfully used for most cases of angioplasty, larger catheters are required when complex lesions are encountered such as bifurcation stenting or CTO [6] (Figure 5.5).

Active support

Guide catheters smaller than 6 Fr can be advanced over the guidewire and balloon catheter shaft to sub-selectively engage the proximal or mid segment of an artery (Figure 5.5). This technique is also referred to as active engagement or "deep seating" of the guide catheter. The risk of damage to the artery can be minimized by ensuring that the catheter is advanced coaxially over a balloon already inside the vessel. Stabilization of the system while advancing the guide catheter is sometimes required and can be achieved by inflating a balloon within the artery. When considering the use of active support, it is important to bear in mind that deep engagement of large arteries can cause profound ischemia. The use of side holes may not prevent and may even delay detection of catheter-induced ischemia. A further risk is that of air embolism following aspiration through the Y-connector while the back pressure in the guide catheter is reduced as a result of damping inside the artery. Despite these risks,

for a skilled operator capable of rapidly advancing and withdrawing catheters, active support offers an efficient solution in most cases.

Hybrid support

Several additional strategies have been described based upon the concept of inserting an additional device, wire, balloon, or other catheter specifically to augment support when active and/or passive support of the guide catheter proves insufficient (Figure 5.6).

Wire support

The buddy wire technique refers to the passage of a second or third guidewire distal to a target lesion to provide additional support for delivery of angioplasty equipment. This is a commonly used strategy for crossing difficult lesions with a balloon or a stent [7]. The additional wire provides a rail that facilitates advancement across calcification, tortuosity, or recently deployed stents. The wire facilitates active engagement of the guide catheter and can straighten tortuosity when a supportive wire is used. This technique is also the first essential step for the distal anchor balloon technique. Although it can at first appear to be counterintuitive, advancing an additional wire into a branch that lies proximal to the target lesion may increase support only slightly, but sufficiently to allow passage of a balloon, stent, or additional wire along the first wire into the tortuous distal vessel (Figure 5.6) [8].

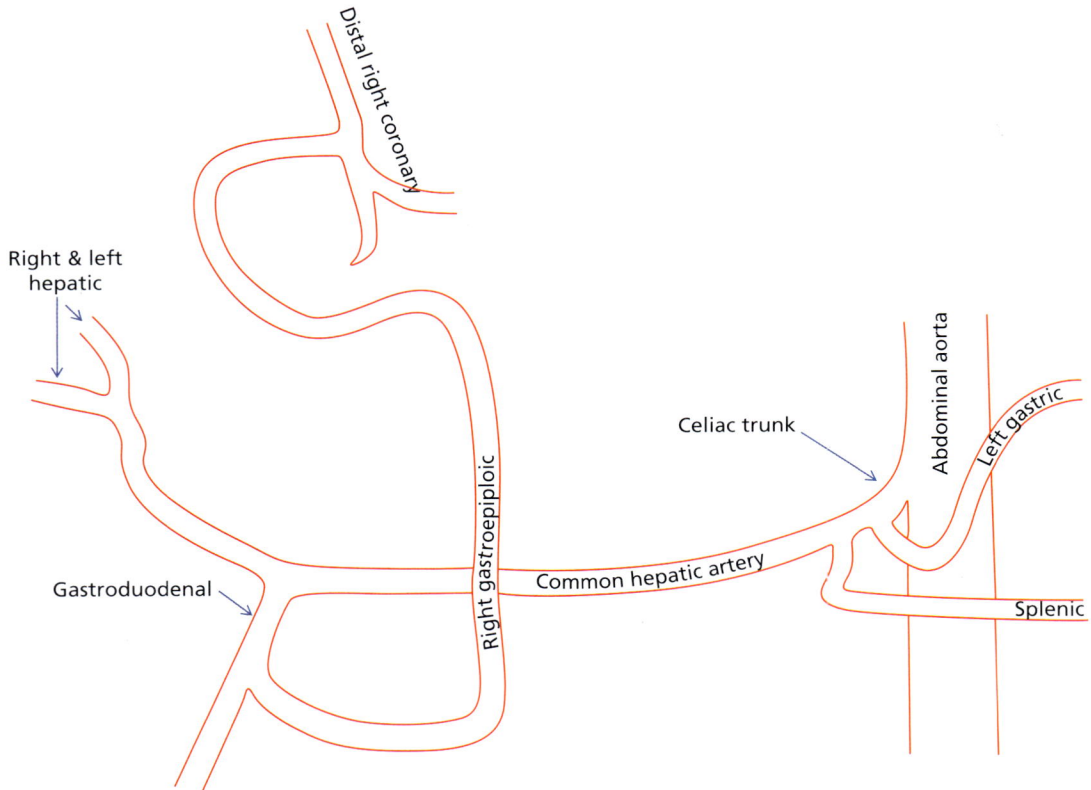

Figure 5.4 Vascular anatomy of a pedicle graft of the right gastroepiploic artery to right coronary artery.

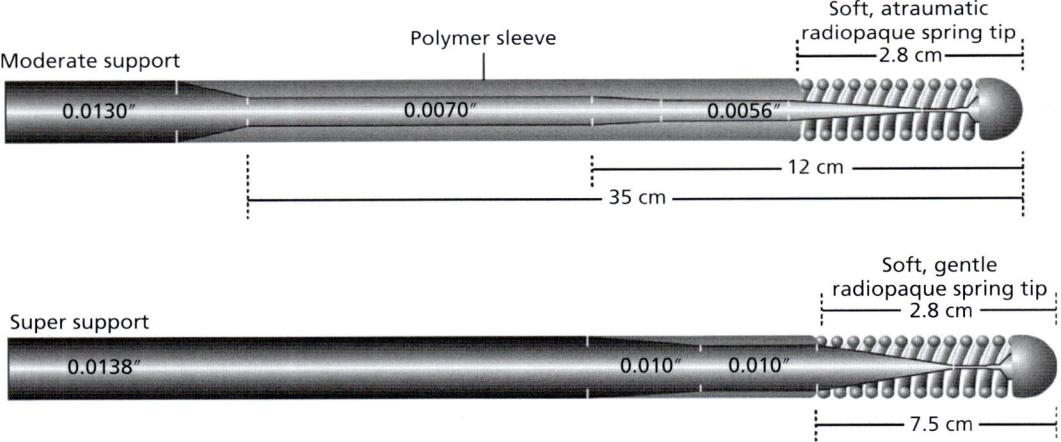

Figure 5.5 Approaches to increase guide catheter support for treating complex lesions.

The risks of deep engagement or the delays and potential difficulties of upgrading the guide catheter can then be avoided. A floppy, steerable wire can advance easily and be exchanged using an OTW catheter for a wire with a supportive shaft but soft flexible tip. The use of stiff hydrophilic wires as a "buddy wire" is discouraged because of the risk of perforation. Occasionally, if support from the guide and an additional wire still proves insufficient, additional techniques are needed and are delineated subsequently.

Anchor balloon technique

Inflation of an adequately sized balloon at low pressure (3–6 atmospheres) in a proximal branch can augment support by anchoring the guide catheter to the vessel and the branch (Figure 5.6) [9]. Low inflation pressures are essential to reduce the risk of dissection or damage to a small right ventricular branch or diagonal/marginal branch. In these branches, ischemia resulting from prolonged inflation is well tolerated. The technique is mostly used in treating CTO and requires a large guide catheter.

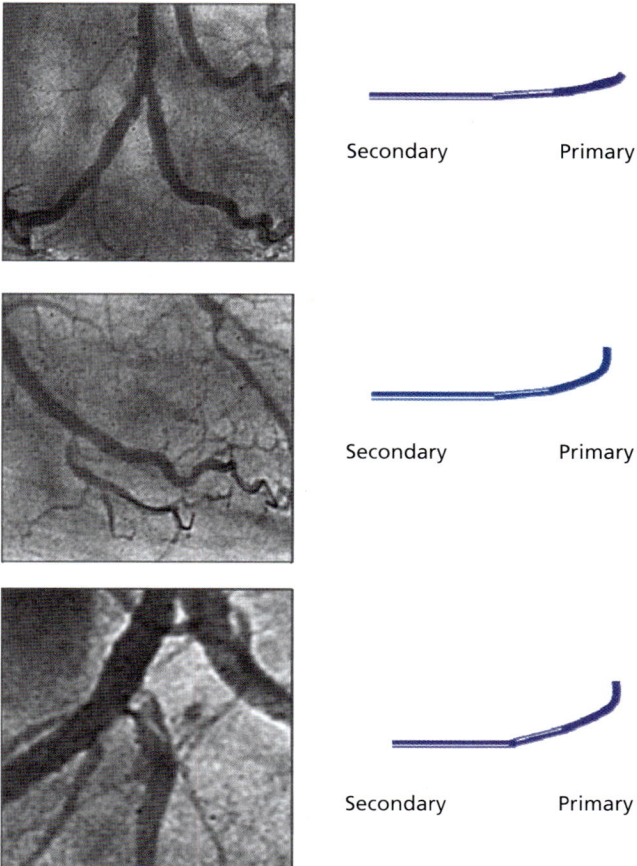

Figure 5.6 "Intraluminal" hybrid support techniques that can be used to substantially augment guide catheter support when treating complex lesions.

Another strategy that can be tried when a buddy wire does not resolve problems in tracking a stent to a target lesion because of tortuosity or calcification of the proximal segment, is to advance over the buddy wire a balloon optimally sized to match the diameter of the distal vessel (Figure 5.6). The balloon is positioned distal to the lesion and inflated at low pressure allowing enough space for the stent to be fully advanced across the target stenosis. It is imperative to remember that the distal anchoring balloon must be deflated and removed before the stent is deployed. In addition to providing extra support, the shaft of the distal balloon also acts as a rail to facilitate stent advancement. The operator needs to be experienced enough to anticipate when the force required may detach the stent from the balloon. Additional strategies can then be considered such as the need for better lesion preparation or the insertion of a sub-selectively engaged guiding catheter around the most tortuous segment, using the guide already in place or a 5 Fr in 6 or 7 Fr strategy as outlined in the next section (Figure 5.5).

Adjunctive techniques
Double coaxial guiding catheter technique (also known as mother–child)

By placing one guide catheter inside another, the advantages of the passive support provided by a large guide catheter are combined with the ability to actively engage the smaller catheter into the target vessel (Figure 5.5) [10]. Compatibility of different guide catheter lengths and diameter is a limiting factor. Mainly a 6 Fr, 110 cm long "child" guide catheter is combined within an 85 or 90 cm 7 or 8 Fr "mother" guide catheter. A greater difference between the lengths of the "mother" and "child" catheters, however, enables more flexibility because it permits further advancement of the "child" catheter into the artery. The "mother" catheter shape is selected to cannulate the ostium of the target vessel and is inserted first. In contrast, a straight "child" catheter, with a soft atraumatic tip, is desirable. If an unusual shape is required for the "mother" catheter that is not available in a short length, the solution is to cut the distal end of a 100 cm guiding catheter of the selected shape and insert within it a smaller valved sheath. Leakage from an insufficiently tight seal can affect the quality of contrast injections. A further risk is the potential for air trapping within the sheath and subsequent inadvertent intracoronary air embolism.

This is an advanced technique that has been used for treating CTO, but may very occasionally also be useful in other situations where a very high level of backup is required, such as when one encounters extreme coronary tortuosity often combined with calcification. It may also be useful for example when a 7 or 8 Fr guide is too large to engage ostial disease or a critically diseased vessel and other situations where deep engagement of the guide is undesirable. The smaller guide can then be engaged into the vessel ostium, whereas the larger guide adds passive backup to the system. Relative adjustments of the positions of the two guide tips can help to achieve optimal orientation of the tip of the "daughter" catheter.

When using this technique care has to be taken not to damage the proximal arterial segment.

Guide catheter extensions

Over the past few years technology evolution has allowed the introduction of new devices, called guide catheter (GC) extensions, specially designed to address the problem of support in the treatment of unfavorable tortuous coronary anatomy and complex, heavily calcified, and often distally located lesions, which otherwise may have been considered unsuitable for percutaneous coronary intervention (PCI). GC extensions include early OTW devices such as 5 Fr-in-6 Fr Heartrail II® and 4 Fr-in-6 Fr Kiwami® catheters (Terumo, Tokyo, Japan), and more recent rapid exchange GuideLiner® (Vascular Solutions, Maple Grove, MN, USA) and Guidezilla™ (Boston Scientific, Marlbourough, MA, USA).

The Heartrail II® "five-in-six catheter system" comprises a flexible-tipped, long (120 cm) 5 Fr catheter advanced through a standard 6 Fr guiding catheter to deeply intubate the target vessel. This system uses the target vessel itself to provide the extra backup support required for stent delivery. Furthermore, the absence of a primary curve and the flexibility of its tip permit the "child" catheter to remain coaxial with the target vessel, thereby minimizing the risk of catheter-induced coronary dissection. Use of this system has been shown to be useful in the treatment of CTO cases where such increased backup support is important. However, its use requires removal of the Y-connector, making the procedure more demanding [11].

Kiwami® 4 Fr-in-6 Fr catheter measures 120 cm, 1.43 mm (outer diameter) 1.27 mm (inner diameter); the inner layer is coated with polytetrafluoroethylene (PTFE) and the surface is coated with a hydrophilic surface up to 15 cm from the tip of the catheter. The backstream prevention valve (Terumo) is connected to the guide catheter of 6 or 7 Fr. The conventional Y-connector is attached to Kiwami® (child) which was inserted in the 6 or 7 Fr (mother) catheter. Because the effective length of Kiwami® is 120 cm, the projected length from the mother catheter differs depending on the length of mother catheter used [12]. While the 4 Fr-in-6 Fr Kiwami® catheter probably is the most deliverable among the GC extensions, it has the smallest lumen (0.050 inch) and has the highest risk of air embolism [13].

The GuideLiner® catheter is a coaxial device mimicking the "mother–child" technique. The device is mounted on a monorail system, which extends the guide catheter and enables deep intubation of the coronary artery to achieve extra support and improve coaxial alignment. It has a distal end of 20 cm, consisting of a flexible extension with a radiopaque marker situated 2.7 mm from the tip and a coaxial exchange system 20 cm from the tip, joined to a 125 cm compact metal hypotube by means of a ring ("collar", made of metal in the first version and replaced by a lubricious polymer in the V2 version), which can be deployed through the existing Y-adapter for rapid exchange delivery. The device is available in three sizes: 5-in-6 (0.056 inch internal diameter (ID)), 6-in-7 (0.062 inch ID), and 7-in-8 (0.071 inch ID). Its monorail design permits rapid exchange and offers important advantages over its predecessors, the "five-in-six mother and child" catheters Heartrail II®, which had a coaxial system that made their utilization more demanding [11]. Furthermore, rapid exchange helps with deployment through the existing hemostatic valve without extending the guiding catheter length, and so does not limit the useable length of balloons and wires. De Man et al. [14], published results from the Twente GuideLiner Registry identifying three primary indications for the use of the device: improvement of back-up and facilitated stent delivery (59%), more selective contrast injection (13%), and improvement of alignment of the guide (29%). Morever, they found a device and procedural success rate of 93% and 91%, respectively, without major complications and a small incidence of minor complications (3%). The safety and efficacy of utilizing the GuideLiner monorail catheter to treat complex lesions was confirmed in a recent experience published by Chang et al. showing good performance of the device in the settings of bypass graft intervention, bifurcation lesions, and chronic total occlusions. On the basis of the presented data, the authors suggested the following tips and tricks for a safe and effective use of this device:

- In case of non-coaxial alignment of the coronary ostium and extreme proximal vessel tortuosity (e.g., the "shepherd's crook"), a balloon inflated distally can be used to "attract" the GuideLiner and facilitate intubation of the coronary artery.
- The placement of a balloon that can also be used for lesion predilatation (i.e., matching the diameter of the target artery or slightly undersized) prior to intubation with the GuideLiner is always recommended (to improve support and to reduce the chance of damaging the ostium and the proximal vessel by acting as centering rail).
- The positioning of the transition zone of the GuideLiner in a straight part of the descending aorta rather than at the aortic arch, typically by gently withdrawing and rotating the GuideLiner helps in avoiding occasional difficulties in the advancement of coronary stents across the rapid exchange transition zone. This problem was solved, in the last verison of the device GuideLiner catheter (V2), by replacing the metal transition zone with a lubricious polymer.

The most recent GC extension available on the market is the Guidezilla™. The device is mounted on a monorail system, which extends the guide catheter and enables deep intubation of the coronary artery. It is made of a distal end of 25 cm covered by a hydrophilic polymer, joined to a 120-cm compact metal hypotube. The distal flexible extension consists of a pair radiopaque markers, the first situated 2 mm from the tip and the second 3 mm from the transition collar. The device is available in one size 5-in-6 and compatible with guide catheter ≥6 Fr.

Guidewire selection

Guidewires are required to cross the target lesion and to provide support for the delivery of balloons, stents, and other devices while at the same time minimizing the risk of vessel trauma. A guidewire needs to be steerable, visible, flexible, lubricious, and supportive. There is no single wire that has the perfect combination of these characteristics for all situations. Variation in guidewire components have produced a wide range of wires. Wire selection depends on which characteristics are thought to optimally facilitate angioplasty for a given clinical and angiographic scenario.

Guidewires typically come in two basic lengths ranging from 180–195 cm for rapid exchange (Rx) use to 300 cm for OTW use. They consist of a central core of stainless steel or nitinol alloy that makes up the proximal section of the wire, approximately 145 cm long, and which tapers toward a distal tip, a distal section measuring 35–40 cm has a further outer covering of either a fine coil spring consisting of tungsten, platinum or stainless steel, or a polymer coating loaded with a material such as tungsten to improve radioopacity, and the tip often has a lubricious coating that is either hydrophobic or hydrophilic (Figure 5.7). Using stainless steel as the core material improves the steerability and torque control, but steel wires can be deformed by tortuosity and cannot be reshaped. A nitinol core also offers excellent torque control, but the wire will retain its shape and can be reshaped if deformed. Increasing the

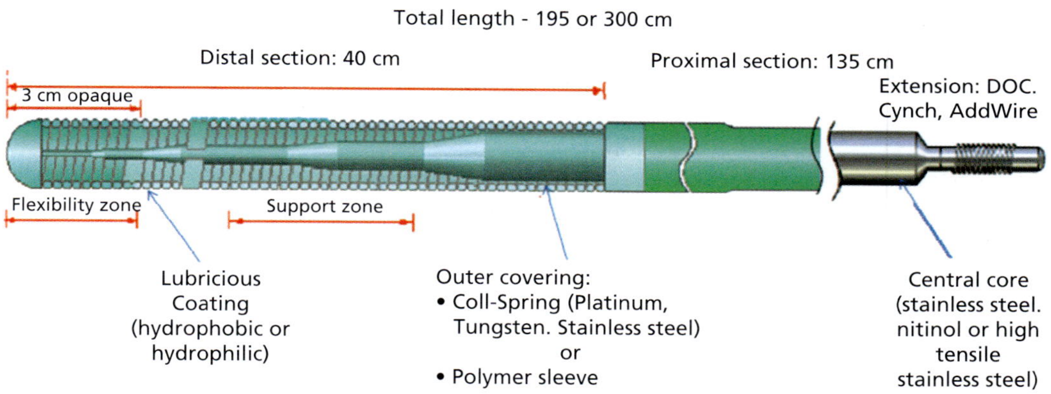

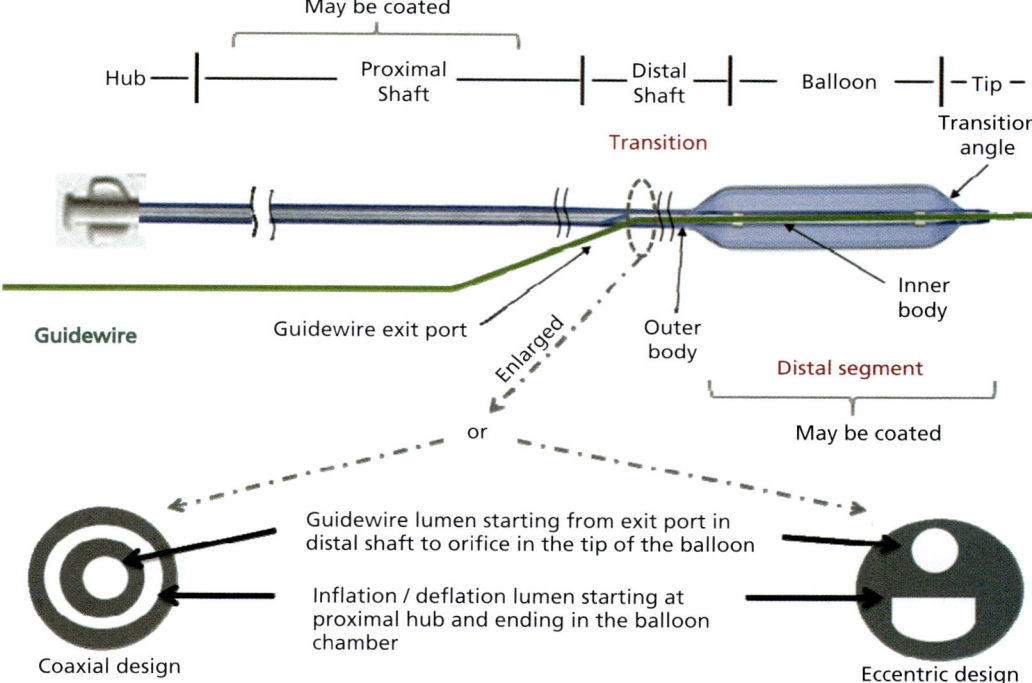

Figure 5.7 Components of guidewire design.

Figure 5.8 The components of a rapid exchange balloon catheter.

core diameter increases shaft support (Figure 5.8). There is often a short transition zone between the tapered distal segment whereas some wires have a very gradually tapering central core, which tends to track better around tortuous anatomy and prolapse less when there is extreme angulation (Figure 5.8). Features of the functional design of guidewires are listed in Table 5.4. Guidewires can be classified into general purpose or "workhorse" and dedicated wires (Table 5.5).

Workhorse guidewires typically possess soft tips, but the amount of shaft support varies (Table 5.5). Although some wires have preshaped tips, the tip stiffness can be increased by heating during the preshaping process so the angle may not match the anatomy. Guidewire shaping can be achieved in many ways including curling the shaping ribbon of the wire over the side of the introducer needle, advancing the wire through the introducer tip and bending it gently outside of the introducer needle tip, or curling it with a finger. It does not matter which method is used to

shape the wire tip, provided that it is done without damaging the wire. As a result, preshaping rarely offers an advantage except perhaps for polymer-coated wires, which can be difficult to shape, or in the case of certain CTO wires. When shaping the tip of a wire, the primary curve should match the greatest angle to be negotiated, whereas the secondary curve is chosen to match the size of the vessel (Figure 5.9).

Hydrophilic wires are not recommended as a first choice for general purpose use, because the highly lubricious tip can easily slip beneath a plaque and create a dissection during insertion. These wires also have a higher tendency to migrate distally and increase the risk of perforation, give less tactile feedback, and have lower visibility. Highly tortuous vessels require a flexible lubricious wire in the first instance (e.g., BMW Universal, WhisperMS, Choice floppy), which can then be exchanged via an OTW balloon for a more supportive wire (e.g., Choice extra support, Mailman, Ironman, Grand Slam, Platinum Plus). When

Table 5.4 The selection of a guidewire depends on the characteristics required to deal with lesion complexity or particular vessel characteristics. The characteristics of guidewires can be altered by modifying specific components during the production process.

Flexibility	Flexible wires can better negotiate severe tortuosity or angulation without deformation	Shaft core material (nitinol offers greater flexibility and shape retention), core thickness (thinner core = more flexible)
Support	Improved equipment delivery when hampered by angulation, tortuosity, lesion severity, calcification	Shaft core material, core thickness
Steerability is a function of:		
• torque transmission	1 : 1 transmission of torque to the tip is the ideal	Core materials are chosen for having good torque transmission, which is also improved by a thicker core with more gradual distal taper
• tip shape ability	Importance increases as lesion complexity increases	Nitinol is more difficult to shape, but can be reshaped; steel is easier to shape but can be ruined by being deformed
Lubricity	Can ease wire passage in tight, calcified, severely tortuous lesions	Tip or distal segment coating with silicon, hydrophilic coating, or polymer coating: "plastic jacketed" wires are the most lubricious but also the most dangerous; when combined with a stiff tip long dissections can be inadvertently created: • hydrophilic requires water for activation • hydrophobic does not require water for activation, allows feedback from distal tip so that excessive friction when creating a subintimal dissection or going below stent struts can be detected
Tendency to prolapse	Can be important when negotiating angles >75°	A gradually tapering core with a smooth transition toward the tip improves support and tracking around bends; abrupt tapers and floppy cores are more likely to prolapse
Visibility	The level of visibility becomes more important in obese patients or when angled working views are required	Lubricious polymer-coated nitinol wires can be difficult to see, platinum, steel, or tungsten markers at distal tip
Tactile feedback	Provides the operator with essential non-visual information, allows "palpation" of the lesion at the distal wire tip	Hydrophylic wires provide poor tactile feedback; hydrophobic wires provide more feedback
Tip stiffness	A soft gentle tip is essential for all "workhorse" wires; to reduce the risk of vessel trauma; stiffer tips are required for dedicated CTO wires	More gradual distal taper, distal core material (e.g., high tensile steel)

additional support is required, guidewires can be exchanged for those with greater shaft support if required or, more frequently, a second wire can be placed alongside the initial wire to facilitate equipment passage. This so-called "buddy" wire can behave as an additional as previously discussed.

The handling characteristics of different wires vary substantially and even the same wire can have a very different "feel" under different circumstances. For example, wires frequently perform differently and offer different tactile feedback in more complex lesion subsets including those with diffuse disease with heavy calcification or angulation. Inexperienced operators often progress more confidently by becoming familiar with one

workhorse wire used for most cases. Nitinol wires are more forgiving and can be reshaped. An important principle is never to push when the wire bends or buckles, but rather to withdraw and rotate before gently re-advancing it. Learning how to exchange a wire using OTW balloons or microcatheters is an essential skill before tackling complex lesions. More complex angioplasty will also provide an opportunity to gain familiarity with an expanded range of wires.

Dedicated wires for treating CTO have stiffer tips. Tip stiffness is measured in grams of forward pressure required to flex the tip. Specialty wires are listed in Table 5.5 and are discussed in other chapters. Over the last two decades, technologies used for

Table 5.5 Classification of guidewires.

Product name	Core material	Rail support	Radio-paque tip length (cm)	Tip type	Tip style	Tip tapering	Tip stiffness	Tip load (g)	Tip coating type
Workhorse wires									
Hi-Torque BMW Universal	Elastine Nitinol	Moderate	3	Polymer/Spring coil	Shaping ribbon	Non-tapered (0.014")	Soft	0.7	Hydrophilic
CholCE Floppy	Stainless steel	Light	3	Polymer/Spring coil	Core-to-tip	Non-tapered (0.014")	Soft	0.8	Hybrid (distal 3 cm uncoated)
Runthrough NT	Stainless steel/Nitinol	Light	3	Stainless steel coils	Shaping ribbon	Non-tapered (0.014")	Soft	1.0	Hydrophilic
Asahi Soft	Tru Torque Steel	Moderate	3	Spring coil	Core-to-tip	Non-tapered (0.014")	Soft	0.7	Hydrophobic
Hi-Torque Floppy II	Stainless steel	Moderate	2/30	Spring coil	Shaping ribbon	Non-tapered (0.014")	Soft	0.4	Hydrophilic/hydrophobic
PROWATER (Rinato)	Tru Torque Steel	Moderate	3	Spring coil	Core-to-tip	Non-tapered (0.014")	Soft	0.8	Hydrophilic
Extra support wires									
HT Iron Man	Stainless steel	Extra support	3	Spring coil	Core-to-tip	Non-tapered (0.014")	Soft	1.0	Hydrophobic
Grand Slam	Tru Torque Steel	Extra support	4	Spring coil	Core-to-tip	Non-tapered (0.014")	Soft	0.7	Hydrophilic
HT BHW	Elastine/Nitinol	Extra support	4.5	Spring coil	Shaping ribbon	Non-tapered (0.014")	Soft	0.7	Hydrophilic
HT Extra S'Port	Stainless steel	Extra Support	3	Spring coil	Core-to-tip	Non-tapered (0.014")	Soft	0.9	Hydrophobic
Hi-Torque Whisper ES	Durasteel	Extra Support	3	Polymer over coils	Core-to-tip	Non-tapered (0.014")	Soft	1.2	Hydrophilic
CholCE Extra Support	Stainless steel	Extra Support	3	Polymer/Spring coils	Core-to-tip	Non-tapered (0.014")	Soft	0.9	Hybrid (distal 3 cm uncoated)
Lubricious/tortuous/subtotal/CTO lesions wires									
Hi-Torque Whisper LS	Durasteel	Light	3	Polymer over coils	Core-to-tip	Non-tapered (0.014")	Soft	0.8	Hydrophilic
Hi-Torque Whisper MS	Durasteel	Moderate	3	Polymer over coils	Core-to-tip	Non-tapered (0.014")	Soft	1.0	Hydrophilic

(Continued)

Table 5.5 (Continued)

Product name	Core material	Rail support	Radiopaque tip length (cm)	Tip type	Tip style	Tip tapering	Tip stiffness	Tip load (g)	Tip coating type
Hi-Torque Pilot 50	Durasteel	Moderate	3	Polymer over coils	Core-to-tip	Non-tapered (0.014″)	Intermediate	1.5	Hydrophilic
Fielder/Fielder FC	Tru Torque Steel	Moderate	3	Polymer over coils	Core-to-tip	Non-tapered (0.014″)	Soft	1.0/0.8	Hydrophilic
Fielder XT	Tru Torque Steel	Moderate	16	Polymer over coils	Core-to-tip	Non-tapered (0.009″)	Soft	0.8	Hydrophilic
Sion	Tru Torque Steel	Moderate	3	Spring coil	Core-to-tip	Non-tapered (0.014″)	Soft	0.7	Hydrophilic
Sion Blu	Tru Torque Steel	Moderate	3	Spring coil	Core-to-tip	Non-tapered (0.014″)	Soft	0.5	Hydrophilic (except very distal tip)
Miracle 3/4.5/6/12	Tru Torque Steel	Moderate	11	Spring coil	Core-to-tip	Non-tapered (0.014″)	Intermediate (3/4.5), Stiff (6/12)	3.0/4.5/ 6.0/12.0	Hydrophilic
Conquest	Tru Torque Steel	Moderate	20	Spring coil	Core-to-tip	Non-tapered (0.014″)	Stiff	9.0	Hydrophobic
Conquest (Confianza) Pro	Tru Torque Steel	Moderate	20	Spring coil	Core-to-tip	Non-tapered (0.014″)	Stiff	9.0	Hydrophilic (except distal tip)
Conquest (Confianza) Pro 12	Tru Torque Steel	Moderate	20	Spring coil	Core-to-tip	Non-tapered (0.014″)	Stiff	12.0	Hydrophilic (except very distal tip)
GAIA First	Stainless Steel	Moderate	15	Polymer over coils	Core-to-tip	Tapered (0.014-0.010″)	Soft	1.7	Hydrophilic
GAIA Second	Stainless Steel	Moderate	15	Polymer over coils	Core-to-tip	Tapered (0.014-0.011″)	Soft	3.5	Hydrophilic
GAIA Third	Stainless Steel	Moderate	15	Polymer over coils	Core-to-tip	Tapered (0.014-0.012″)	Soft	4.5	Hydrophilic

3.0 × 20 mm Test length	Balloon junction (prox. seal OD)	Proximal shoulder (2/3)	Distal profile (1 mm)	Tip seal (xing profile)	Tip entry profile	Tip I.D.
Cross Sail	0.037″	0.031″	0.031″	0.024″	0.019″	0.0155″
Maverick	0.038″	0.034″	0.033″	0.026″	0.018″	0.0156″

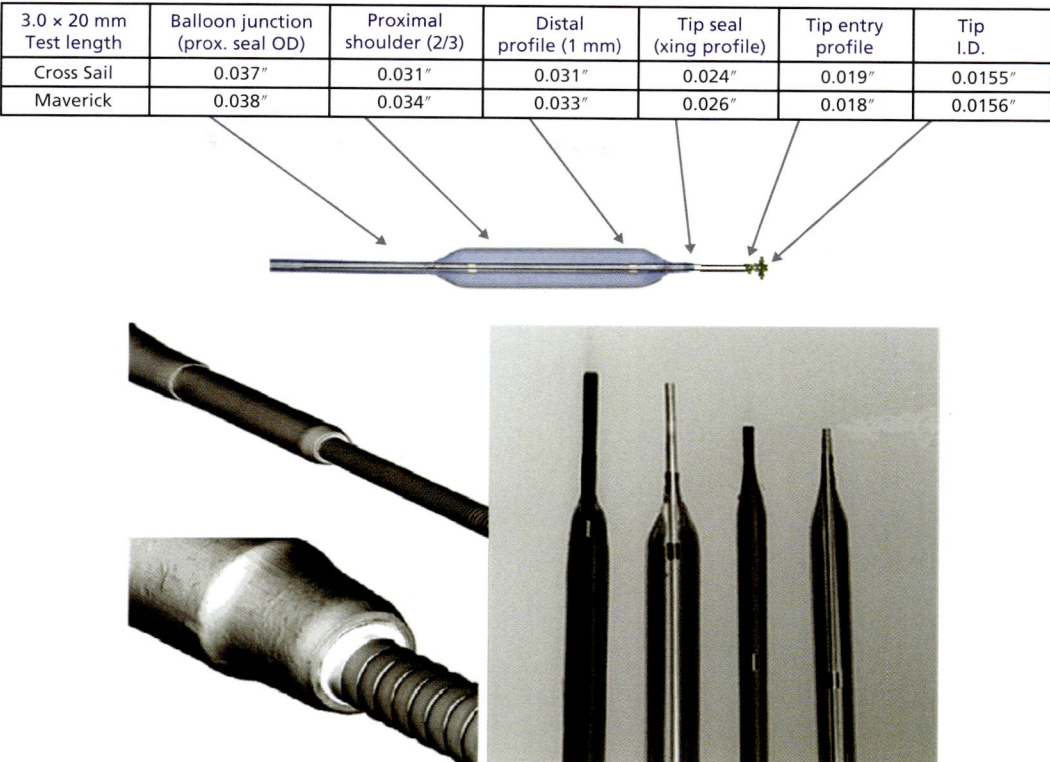

Figure 5.9 Distal tip styles and components contributing to the crossing profile of balloon catheters.

CTO recanalization have emerged with the production of wires specially developed to satisfy the demands of operators involved in this challenging field. The development of new interventional recanalization techniques has been followed by a concomitant increase in the number of specialized wires, mostly produced by Asahi (Asahi Intecc, Japan) for specific applications:

- Drilling technique (Miracle family)
- Penetration techinique (Conquest family)
- Sliding technique (Fielder family)
- Deflection and rotation techniques (Gaia family).

In particular, the development over the last 5 years of the new Sion (Sion, Sion Blue, and Sion Black, Asahi Intecc, Japan) and Gaia wire families (first, second, and third, Asahi Intecc, Japan) have expanded the interventional toolbox for CTO. The Sion wire is currently the gold standard for epicardial collateral tracking, because of its unique trackability which enables the wire to follow most collateral bends. Using this innovative wire, epicardial connections are successfully utilized in almost 35% of retrograde cases in contemporary series from Japan [15,16]. It uses a composite core technology that includes multiple wire components to enhance durability and torque transmission. The tip of the wire can be shaped and successfully retain its shape through collateral tracking. This technology allowed the introduction in contemporary CTO practice of new interventional strategies such as the septal "surfing" technique, which utilizes septal collateral connections between the left and right coronary arteries. A polymer jacketed soft guidewire, traditionally the Fielder FC wire and more recently the Sion Black wire with composite core technology, is advanced to the septal branch supported by a microcatheter. The wire is steered toward the septal branch and kept in constant motion, forward and backward, in an attempt to engage the distal true lumen of the occluded epicardial artery. Septal "surfing" is the norm for investigating septal connections and is further reviewed elsewhere in this book. While wire "exits" or microperforations occur frequently, they rarely result in clinical sequelae. Nevertheless, because of technical complexity, septal surfing should only be used by operators considerably experienced in the retrograde approach.

Gaia wires also feature the composite core technology. They present a unique trackability and 1/1 guidewire motion. These wires allowed a new approach to the manipulation of a CTO, with the "rotation and deflection" principle, representing a breakthrough in these complex lesions. The wires are preshaped and do not lose their shape while being rotated through the body of the occlusion. Their application remains primarily in the complex CTO subset.

Balloon catheters

Balloon catheters remain an important tool in interventional cardiology despite the advent of adjunctive devices such as stents. When Gruentzig first introduced coronary angioplasty balloons, the correct choice of balloon diameter and length, compliance, pressure, and duration of inflation were the key ingredients for a successful PCI and reflected the experience and quality of individual operators. However, in today's era of direct stent deployment, sometimes without pre- or post-dilatation, high quality angioplasty technique has been minimized. Nevertheless, the experienced operator recognizes that balloon angioplasty confers not only important acute gain, but also assists in estimation of lesion diameter and length for the selection of stents, can facilitate exchange after wire

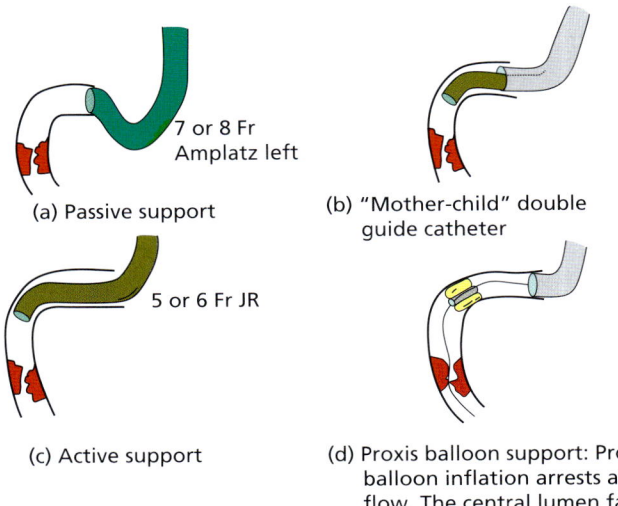

Figure 5.10 Support can be increased by increasing core diameter.

(a) Passive support — 7 or 8 Fr Amplatz left

(b) "Mother-child" double guide catheter

(c) Active support — 5 or 6 Fr JR

(d) Proxis balloon support: Proximal balloon inflation arrests antegrade flow. The central lumen facilitates passage of guidewire and stent balloon to treat the target lesion

crossing (OTW), and holding the guide catheter in place when greater support is required (anchor balloon in side branches or proximal–distal to the lesion in the main vessel). Moreover, with the advent of drug-coated balloons, angioplasty balloons are again able to deliver more than acute gain from vessel dilatation, but also deliver adjunctive pharmacotherapy to mitigate neointimal hyperplasia and reduce restenosis.

Anatomy of a balloon catheter

The anatomy of an angioplasty balloon from proximal to distal consists of a hub, a proximal shaft, and a distal shaft. It has a cylindrical body with proximal and distal conical tapers and a distal tip (Figure 5.10). Early balloon catheters had a fixed wire proximal to the balloon, as dual lumen catheters were typically bulky and difficult to advance into the coronary circulation. Contemporary balloon catheters are dual lumen with separate ports for the guidewire and balloon inflation. OTW balloons have a lumen for the guidewire extending along the length of the catheter, a feature very useful and sometimes essential for procedures requiring wire exchange without re-wiring a vessel such as in the treatment of CTO, crossing of very tortuous lesions, advancement of poorly steerable wires such as those for rotational atherectomy. The principle of the Monorail or rapid exhange technique is that the wire lumen is limited to a short segment (20–30 cm) at the distal tip which allows the rapid exchange of balloons with no need for long wires or wire extensions. The shaft of the catheter only contains a lumen for balloon inflation and deflation (i.e., can be thinner) and often consists of a reinforced hollow metal tube providing great pushability. OTW balloons are typically touted for their superior support but require two operators for optimal control, whereas monorail systems dominate the market and permit a single operator to control all devices.

The parameters considered when selecting a balloon are balloon diameter, length, and compliance, although occasionally the shaft diameter, length, and crossing profile are also important considerations (e.g., bifurcation techniques using smaller bore guides, retrograde recanalization of CTO, very tall patients, extreme tortuosity, or target lesion distance from the access site as in peripheral vascular interventions).

Balloon diameter is normally selected to match the vessel size with balloon to artery ratios of 1 : 1 in general. Vessel size can be measured using quantitative coronary angiography (QCA)

or intravascular imaging such as intravascular ultrasound (IVUS) or optical coherence tomography (OCT). Aiming for a balloon to reference vessel ratio of 0.9 : 1.1 is typical. For pre-dilatation, "undersizing" may be acceptable whereas for post-dilatation balloon to vessel ratios are typically >1 : 1. For long tapering lesions, the diameter of the vessel at the distal end of the segment to be dilated is typically used as the reference vessel diameter for balloon selection. An appropriately sized balloon for postdilatation is a critical step to achieve better expansion and apposition when the initial balloon deployment fails, despite the high pressures allowed by modern stent delivery balloons, to fully expand the stent.

Balloon length is selected depending upon lesion and stent length. Especially after the introduction of drug eluting stents when the principle is to avoid injuring segments that will not be covered by stents, a situation known as geographic miss, smaller balloons tend to be used for predilatation, just aiming to create a passage for stent insertion and exclude the presence of truly undilatable lesions [8]. Postdilatation balloons should be shorter than the stent and short balloons are recommended for postdilating resistant lesions.

The first angioplasty balloons were composed of flexible polyvinyl chloride (PVC), a material characterized by great compliance. Subsequent generations were made of cross-linked polyethylene, polyethylene terephthalate (PET), nylon, Pebax, and polyurethane. Most modern balloons allow controlled limited expansion, burst resistance up to high pressure, and have a low crossing profile. The tip style (tapering, length, flexibility) varies substantially among different balloons, and is one of the factors contributing to a successful crossing (Figure 5.11). Compliant balloons show a linear increase in diameter with increasing inflation pressure whereas the diameter increase tends to plateau in semi- or non-compliant balloons until reaching the rated burst pressure. More compliant balloons have a limited pressure range whereas non-compliant balloons have a limited diameter range and are useful for treating resistant lesions requiring high pressure inflation or postdilatation. Semi-compliant balloons fall between these two extremes and tend to be multipurpose "workhorse" balloons. Familiarity with the compliance charts of balloons is necessary to reduce the risk of trauma to the healthy vessel or of exceeding the vessel elasticity and induce dramatic vessel ruptures. Terms encountered on these charts include the following:

1 Nominal: the pressure at which the balloon reaches its nominal diameter (diameter on the label);
2 Rated burst pressure: the pressure below which *in vitro* testing has shown that 99.9% of the balloons will not burst with 95% confidence;
3 Mean burst pressure: the mathematical mean pressure at which a balloon bursts.

Wall stress within a cylindrical balloon can be represented by the following equations:

$$\sigma_{radial} = pd/2t$$

$$\sigma_{axial} = pd/4t$$

where σ_{radial} = radial stress, σ_{axial} = axial or longitudinal stress, p = pressure, d = diameter, and t = wall thickness. It can be seen that wall stress is linearly proportional to diameter which means that higher dilatation pressure is possible with smaller diameter balloons. Furthermore, axial stress is half of radial stress which means that balloon rupture is usually longitudinal rather than circumferential and therefore less likely to result in vessel trauma.

Balloons have proximal and distal radiopaque markers to allow positioning (one central marker for some small diameter balloons). Rewrap refers to the ability of the balloon to regain its original folded state following deflation. Deflation and rewrapping can take time when large and long balloons are used. Rewrapping is essential to allow safe withdrawal of the balloon into the catheter. Stent deployment balloons tend to rewrap less well, have more variable expansion characteristics, and should ideally not be used for post-dilatation. Balloon catheters may also be used to augment support when treating complex lesions.

The past decade has heralded the development of several specialty balloons including cutting balloons, focal force balloons, and drug-coated balloons (Figure 5.12) with specific applications for each type of balloon.

The cutting balloon is marketed by Boston Scientific (Malborough, MA, USA) as the "Flextome." The balloon has three blades equally spaced about its circumference which come into contact with the arterial wall and score the vessel wall. The balloon is specifically indicated for discrete lesions with resistance to conventional balloon angioplasty without heavy calcification. This balloon is frequently used to dilate highly resistant lesions, particularly fibrotic lesions.

Focal force balloons such as the Angiosculpt (Spectranetics, Inc, Colorado Springs, CO, USA) and the Chocolate (TriReme Medical,

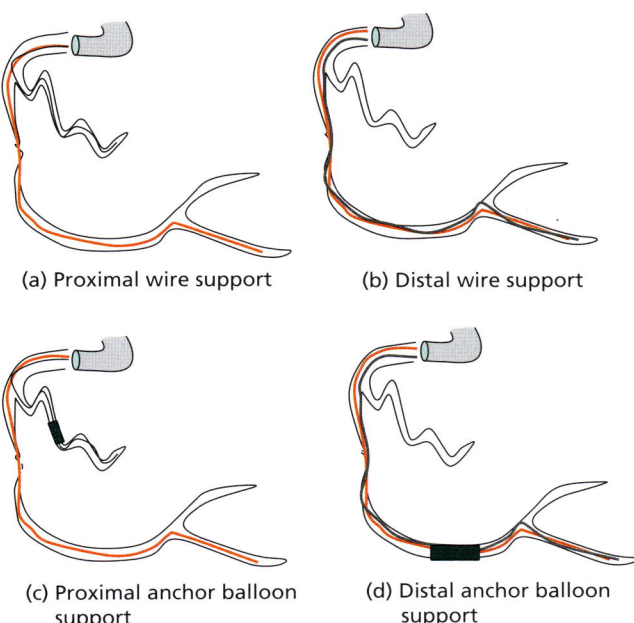

(a) Proximal wire support

(b) Distal wire support

(c) Proximal anchor balloon support

(d) Distal anchor balloon support

Figure 5.11 The primary curve is shaped to fit the tightest angle to be wired and the secondary curve to reflect vessel size.

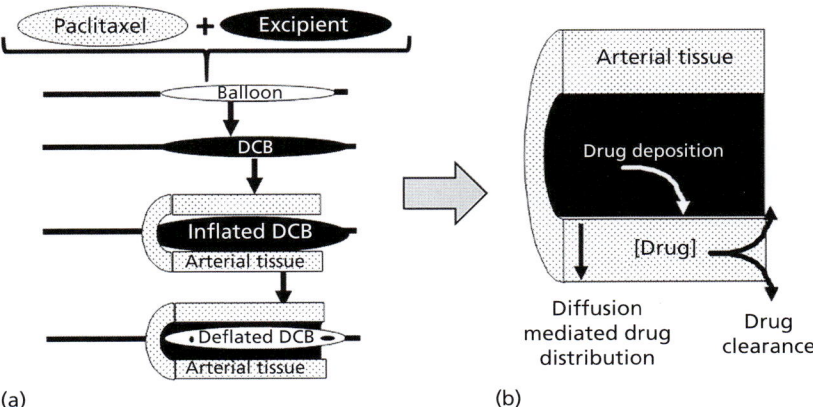

(a)   (b)

Figure 5.12 Drug-coated balloons and arterial drug delivery: mechanism of action. (a) Drug-coated balloons are comprised of a drug such as paclitaxel admixed with an excipient that helps bind the drug to an angioplasty balloon catheter. When the balloon is inflated, the bonds between the drug and excipient and the balloon are broken depositing a layer of drug and excipient on to the arterial surface. (b) Endovascular drug administration results in adluminal drug entering arterial tissue via diffusion mediated transport. The balance between the steady state diffusion mediated drug distribution and drug clearance results in the ultimate arterial drug concentration. This drug concentration is directly related to the efficacy of the drug.

Pleasanton, CA, USA) have recently established a niche in the market for treatment of resistant lesions. The Angiosculpt is a non-compliant balloon with three nitinol wires or elements spiraling from the tip to the shaft transition. The function and application is similar to a cutting balloon; however, the degree of vascular injury imparted is thought to be less than the Flextome balloon. Developed for both coronary and peripheral vascular applications, the Angiosculpt is similarly used in highly resistant lesions when conventional balloons are unable to dilate the vessel. Another focal force balloon is the Chocolate balloon which is a traditional semi-compliant balloon within a nitinol cage. When the balloon is inflated, the cage restrains the balloon expansion, and the balloon protrudes from between the struts of the nitinol cage applying focal pressure to discrete areas of the plaque. Theoretically, this will result in more controlled plaque fracture. These balloons are frequently applied in vessels where stenting is inadvisable (side branches) or not possible (small vessels). Lesion preparation is felt to also be better with focal force balloons [17].

Conclusions

A good operator will have a thorough knowledge of the advantages and limitations of each specific piece of equipment, familiarity with their specific characteristics and modalities of use, and a preparedness to change to an alternative strategy or strategies if required.

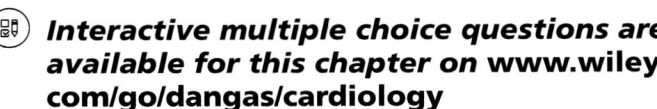

Interactive multiple choice questions are available for this chapter on www.wiley. com/go/dangas/cardiology

References

1 Hamon M, Sabatier R, Zhao Q, Niculescu R, Valette B, Grollier G. Mini-invasive strategy in acute coronary syndromes: direct coronary stenting using 5 Fr guiding catheters and transradial approach. *Catheter Cardiovasc Interv* 2002; **55**(3): 340–343.

2 de Bruyne B, Stockbroeckx J, Demoor D, Heyndrickx GR, Kern MJ. Role of side holes in guide catheters: observations on coronary pressure and flow. *Cathet Cardiovasc Diagn* 1994; **33**(2): 145–152.

3 Pym J, Brown P, Pearson M, Parker J. Right Gastroepiploic-to-coronary artery bypass: the first decade of use. *Circulation* 1995; **92**(9): 45–49.

4 Isshiki T, Yamaguchi T, Nakamura M, et al. Postoperative angiographic evaluation of gastroepiploic artery grafts: technical considerations and short-term patency. *Cathet Cardiovasc Diagn* 1990; **21**(4): 233–238.

5 Alam M, Safi AM, Mandawat MK, et al. Successful percutaneous stenting of a right gastroepiploic coronary bypass graft using monorail delivery system: a case report. *Catheter Cardiovasc Interv* 2000; **49**(2): 197–199.

6 Colombo A, Mikhail GW, Michev I, et al. Treating chronic total occlusions using subintimal tracking and reentry. The STAR Technique. *Catheter Cardiovasc Interv* 2005; **64**(4): 407–411.

7 Jafary FH. When one won't do it, use two—double 'buddy' wiring to facilitate stent advancement across a highly calcified artery. *Catheter Cardiovasc Interv* 2006; **67**(5): 721–723.

8 Hamood H, Makhoul N, Grenadir E, Kusniec F, Rosenschein U. Anchor wire technique improves device deliverability during PCI of CTOs and other complex subsets. *Acute Cardiac Care* 2006; **8**(3): 139–142.

9 Fujita S, Tamai H, Kyo E, et al. New technique for superior guiding catheter support during advancement of a balloon in coronary angioplasty: the anchor technique. *Catheter Cardiovasc Interv* 2003; **59**(4): 482–488.

10 Takahashi S, Saito S, Tanaka S, et al. New method to increase a backup support of a 6 French guiding coronary catheter. *Catheter Cardiovasc Interv* 2004; **63**(4): 452–456.

11 Mamas MA, Eichhöfer J, Hendry C, et al. Use of the Heartrail II catheter as a distal stent delivery device: an extended case series. *EuroIntervention* 2009; **5**(2): 265–271.

12 Hiwatashi A, Iwabuchi M, Yokoi H, et al. PCI using a 4-Fr "child" guide catheter in a "mother" guide catheter: Kyushu KIWAMI* ST registry. *Cathet Cardiovasc Intervent* 2010; **76**(7): 919–923.

13 Fraser DG, Mamas MA. Guide catheter extensions: where are they taking us? *EuroIntervention* 2012; **8**(3): 299–301.

14 de Man FHAF, Tandjung K, Hartmann M, et al. Usefulness and safety of the GuideLiner catheter to enhance intubation and support of guide catheters: insights from the Twente GuideLiner registry. *EuroIntervention* 2012; **8**(3): 336–344.

15 Yamane M, Muto M, Matsubara T, et al. Contemporary retrograde approach for the recanalisation of coronary chronic total occlusion: on behalf of the Japanese Retrograde Summit Group. *EuroIntervention* 2013; **9**(1): 102–109.

16 Tsuchikane E, Yamane M, Mutoh M, et al. Japanese multicenter registry evaluating the retrograde approach for chronic coronary total occlusion. *Cathet Cardiovasc Intervent* 2013; **82**(5): E654–661.

17 Kleber FX, Mathey DG, Rittger H, Scheller B. German Drug-eluting Balloon Consensus Group. How to use the drug-eluting balloon: recommendations by the German consensus group. *EuroIntervention* 2011; **7**(Suppl K): 125–128.

CHAPTER 6

Physiologic Assessment in the Cardiac Catheterization Laboratory: CFR, FFR, iFR, and Beyond

Sukhjinder Nijjer[1] and Justin Davies[2]

[1] Hammersmith Hospital, Imperial College Healthcare NHS Trust, London, UK
[2] Imperial College London, London, UK

Coronary angiography is the current gold standard in quantifying the presence of epicardial coronary disease but has well-known limitations driven by the difficulties of assessing three-dimensional structures using two-dimensional approaches.

Although intravascular imaging provides insight into the levels of atheroma in a coronary artery, there is a disconnect between stenosis appearance and the flow limitation it imposes. Physiologic interrogation provides not only determination of flow limitation, but stratification of risk and the potential value from revascularization. Conceptually, physiologic assessment should improve outcomes by focusing revascularization where the gain is greatest.

Measuring coronary flow remains the ultimate aim of all physiologic parameters, including those that estimate flow based by measuring pressure only.

This chapter reviews the basic principles of coronary physiology and their clinical application in the cardiac catheterization laboratory. Specifically, CFR, FFR, iFR, and IMR are discussed in detail.

Impact of a stenosis upon coronary flow

Every coronary stenosis imposes a degree of resistance to flow in the epicardial vessel. Coronary autoregulation, working through a variety of paracrine and neural factors, responds by microcirculatory vasodilatation. This maintains normal resting coronary flow up to a stenosis diameter of 85%, at the expense of distal coronary pressure (Figure 6.1) [1]. Distal pressure falls as a result of kinetic energy loss from viscous friction, turbulence, and flow separation across the stenosis, producing a resting trans-stenotic pressure gradient which increases with increasing stenosis severity (Figure 6.2). The degree of gradient at rest is therefore a marker of the physiologic impact of the stenosis upon the microcirculation.

Because of limitations in pressure wire technology, with bulky catheters with low fidelity cycle averaged traces, it was not practically possible to make detailed assessment of stenosis significance under resting conditions. Instead, hyperemia was sought, with the aim to increase flow and therefore increase the measurable gradient across a given stenosis to more easily distinguish mild, moderate, and severe stenoses. Typically, adenosine, ATP, papaverine, or balloon occlusion can be used to induce varying degrees of hyperemia. This reduces microcirculatory resistance and increases coronary flow but does so in a non-uniform manner. Trivial and mild stenoses demonstrate the greatest increase in flow in response to hyperemic stimulus. With stenoses over 30% a reduction in hyperemic flow is observed while a more marked reduction is evident in stenoses over 50% (Figure 6.1).

As stenoses cause natural microcirculatory vasodilatation, the vasodilator reserve, which is the capacity to respond to a hyperemic stimulus by increasing flow, falls with increasing stenosis severity. It follows that severe stenoses that genuinely limit flow will have an impaired response to hyperemia and with increasing severity there is less additional gain in the gradient observed above that evident at rest.

The degree of pressure loss or gradient observed with these stenoses will be dependent upon the geometry of the stenosis; if turbulence is minimal, flow can escalate significantly with little pressure loss. If turbulence predominates, pressure loss is exacerbated even if flow is increasing significantly and there is no true "flow limitation." In long lesions, a great deal of resistance can cause considerable pressure loss alongside a failure to increase flow in response to hyperemia.

For each stenosis, coronary flow and pressure have a curvilinear relationship in which curve steepness is directly related to stenosis severity (Figure 6.3). The greater stenosis severity, the greater the imposition on trans-stenotic flow and the larger the detectible pressure gradient. In such stenoses, trivial increases in flow over the resting state are expected with a considerable resting pressure gradient. In milder stenoses, resting gradients can be small but become larger if the trans-stenotic flow is increased considerably. It follows that such stenoses are non-flow-limiting despite the detectible pressure gradient.

The capacity to increase flow is a marker of microcirculatory function in the absence of epicardial disease, or a combined marker of epicardial and microcirculatory resistance when a stenosis is present. If flow can be made to increase significantly across a stenosis, then it is likely that microcirculatory function must be intact even if

Interventional Cardiology: Principles and Practice, Second Edition. Edited by George D. Dangas, Carlo Di Mario, and Nicholas N. Kipshidze.
© 2017 John Wiley & Sons, Ltd. Published 2017 by John Wiley & Sons, Ltd.

not entirely normal. Microcirculatory vasodilatation is related to size of the tissue bed and the demand placed. If vasodilatation cannot compensate for the stenosis, distal flow diminishes and ischemia under resting conditions would result.

Fundamentals of practical physiologic assessment

Physiologic assessment requires the use of adequately sized guiding catheters to engage the vessel of interest. Catheters of 6 Fr are suitable. Caution is required to ensure there is no damping of the pressure signal after engagement, because this will compromise all measurements. Catheters with side holes should be avoided; although the side hole can improve the appearance of the pressure trace, there remains a relative ostial obstruction. In the event of pressure damping or the presence of important ostial disease, it is appropriate to perform measurements with the guiding catheter disengaged. However, this obviates the possibility of using intracoronary vasodilators or injectants for thermodilution.

Essential to all invasive coronary physiologic assessment is the use of heparin to prevent thrombosis upon the wire; typically 70–100 IU/kg is administered before any wires are placed.

A further essential step is to provide adequate intracoronary nitrates (200–300 µg). Nitrates do *not* create a long-lasting hyperemic

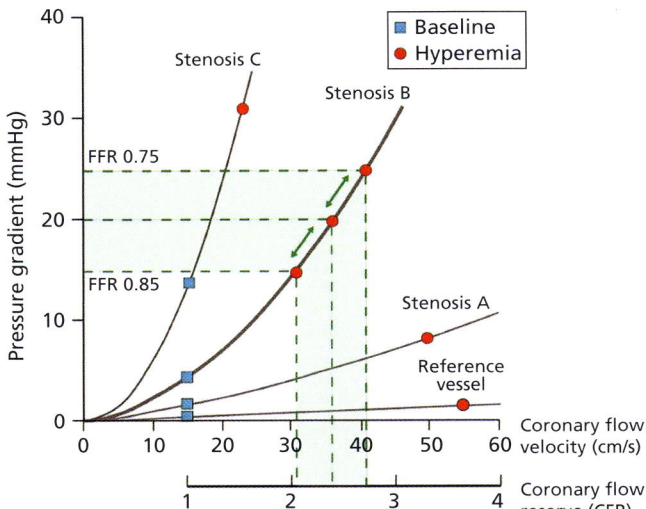

Figure 6.3 The curvilinear relationship between pressure and flow is unique for each stenosis. Pressure drop across a stenosis is determined by $\Delta P = Fv + Sv^2$ (where F is friction losses and S is separation losses). This produces curvilinear relationship unique to any stenosis; the steepness of the curve reflects the severity of the lesion (e.g., reference vessel, stenosis A, B, C). Increasing the flow velocity across a stenosis will alter the pressure gradient observed. In stenosis A, there is a large resting pressure gradient that is accentuated during hyperemia with little increase in flow. In stenosis B, increasing the concentration of hyperemic agent (depicted as arrows) will increase flow velocity to generate a larger gradient; as resting flow is unchanged, CFR and FFR will move in opposite directions. In even milder stenoses, such as A, large escalations of flow velocity from a relatively low resting value could create a large pressure gradient; in these situations, pressure does not reflect the change in flow. Source: Adapted by permission from Macmillan Publishers Ltd: *Nat Rev Cardiol*, van de Hoef TP, *et al.* Fractional flow reserve as a surrogate for inducible myocardial ischaemia, 10, 439–452, copyright 2013.

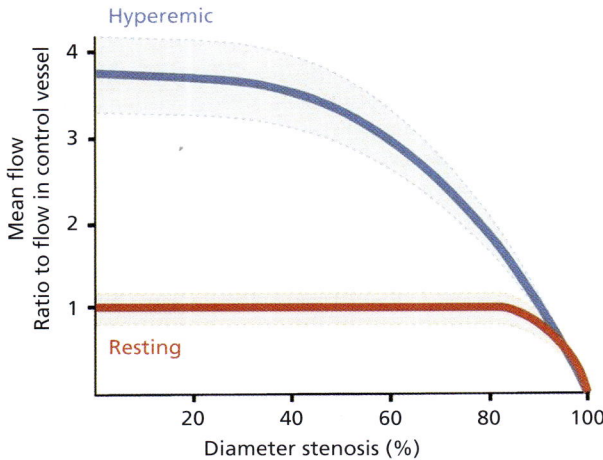

Figure 6.1 Behavior of resting and hyperemic flow in relation to stenosis severity. Resting flow is remarkably preserved despite worsening stenosis severity—up to 85% diameter stenosis by formal measurement. Hyperemic flow starts falling when stenoses are 30% but falls significantly once stenoses are 50%. Source: Adapted from Gould *et al.* 1974 [1].

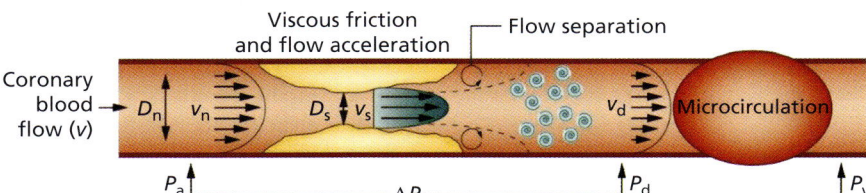

Figure 6.2 The flow of blood across a coronary stenosis. Pressure gradients across stenoses are due to both viscous and separation losses. Pressure is lost owing to viscous friction along the stenosis (Poiseuille's law). Flow also accelerates as it passess through the narrowed segment, causing pressure loss as pressure is converted into kinetic energy (Bernoulli's law). Flow separation and the formation of eddies prevent complete pressure recovery at the exit of the stenosis. Measurement of intracoronary hemodynamics includes proximal perfusion pressure (P_a), coronary pressure and flow velocity distal to the stenosis (P_d and V_d, respectively), and the venous pressure (P_v), which is typically assumed to be negligible. ΔP is the difference between P_d and P_a. Normal diameter (D_n), stenosis diameter (D_s), proximal velocity (V_n), and stenosis velocity (V_s) are indicated. Source: Reprinted by permission from Macmillan Publishers Ltd: *Nat Rev Cardiol*, van de Hoef TP, *et al.* Fractional flow reserve as a surrogate for inducible myocardial ischaemia, 10, 439–452, copyright 2013.

effect but remove wire-related and guide-related vessel spasm and ensure epicardial resistance is minimized. This enables accurate physiologic assessment; readings without nitrates should be repeated, as even a small degree of distal wire spasm will raise distal coronary pressure while more proximal spasm will make distal assessment appear worse.

Hyperemia

Hyperemia is believed to occur in two stages. Agents primarily achieve maximal hyperemia through their vasodilator action on microvascular smooth muscle cells (an endothelium-independent response). The resultant increase in blood flow is thought to stimulate shear stress-induced endothelial nitric oxide release, which promotes further vasodilatation of the microcirculation (flow-mediated dilatation) and increase in blood flow (an endothelium-dependent response). Therefore the response to hyperemic agents will integrate a change in coronary blood flow and microvascular function but alone cannot distinguish between components.

Non-specific agents such as adenosine and papaverine are commonly used to induce maximal hyperemia for assessment of indices such as coronary flow reserve (CFR), fractional flow reserve (FFR), and index of microcirculatory resistance (IMR). The dose of adenosine is accepted as 140 µg/kg/min when given as a central venous infusion (e.g., femoral vein); ATP can be given as an alternative. The hyperemic effect is typically observed after 30 seconds and infusions should continue for 1–2 minutes to observe for stable hyperemia. Side effects include relative hypotension, a central chest discomfort or burning, dyspnea, and bronchospasm. It should be avoided in patients with severe brittle asthma. Short-lived atrioventricular conduction delay is frequent. It is common to seek peripheral veins to avoid additional femoral venous puncture; there are data to support this approach but hyperemia can become more variable with a longer time course [2].

For intracoronary dosing, clinical practice remains variable. Early validation work was performed using considerably lower doses than found in clinical practice today. Accepted intracoronary doses of adenosine or ATP are 80–120 µg in the left coronary system and 40 µg in right coronary artery; these typically produce hyperemia lasting 5–10 seconds [3]. Caution is required in ensuring pressure ports are closed to ensure appropriate pressure traces can be recorded.

Papaverine is an alternative intracoronary agent that achieves a longer lasting hyperemia of 30–60 seconds which permits pullback assessments at the cost of transient QT prolongation and rare trigger ventricular tachycardia or torsarde de pointes [3]. It is typically used when adenosine is not available (15–20 mg in the left coronary artery; 10–12 mg in the right coronary artery) [3].

Newer alternatives include regadenoson, a selective A_{2A} receptor agonist which has been approved for use in myocardial perfusion imaging. Given as a single bolus into a peripheral vein using a weight-unadjusted dose (400 µg over 10 seconds), regadenoson achieves a peak flow velocity after 1 minute and declines thereafter [4]. However, the duration of hyperemia is very variable among patients, making pullback and multi-vessel assessment unreliable and inconsistent. Side effects include adenosine-like effects with hypotension, chest discomfort, and flushing. Third-degree heart block has also occurred.

Alternatives to achieve increased flow include the use of contrast—which in some settings can have a similar effect to that of other intracoronary hyperemic agents [5]. Caution is required as the hyperemic effect is variable between injections, very short-lived, and can contribute to considerable contrast burden. Furthermore, it remains unclear what the threshold for treatment should be; small studies have limited power to determine cut-offs while larger ones are not helpful if different types and volumes of contrast are used. As the hyperemia is submaximal, changing volumes can lead to different pressure ratios and uncertainty.

Coronary flow reserve and relative CFR

The concept of CFR is to compare the flow at rest with that measured under hyperemia. CFR is derived from the ratio of steady state maximal hyperemic flow to resting flow in a given artery [6]. Conceptually simple, CFR can be measured invasively using intracoronary wires capable of measuring coronary flow velocity (using a piezo-electric Doppler; Figure 6.4) or apply thermodilution

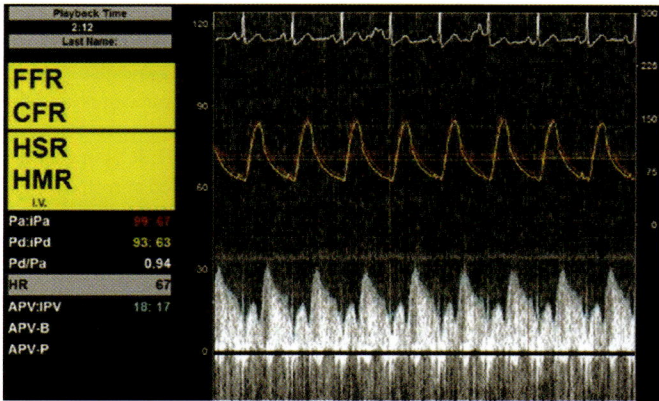

Baseline recording of pressure and flow velocity

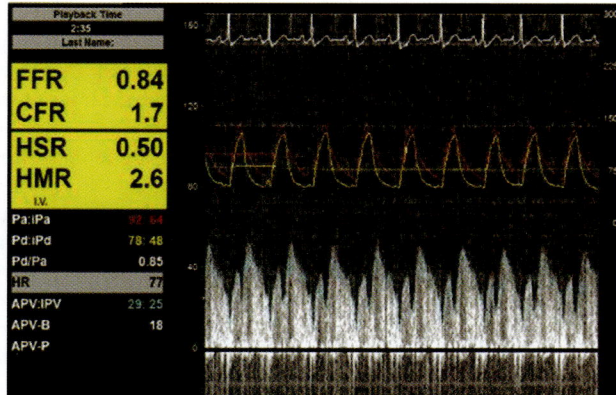

Recording during hyperemia - adenosine 140 µg/kg/min

Figure 6.4 Physiologic interrogation in the catheter laboratory. Left panel shows baseline data at rest. There is trivial resting gradient (Pd/Pa 0.94). Note the spectral Doppler trace has the majority of flow in diastole; also note the digital tracking has been optimized to avoid extraneous noise. Right panel shows data after hyperemia. CFR is calculated as the ratio of average peak velocity (APV) at maximal hyperemia to baseline. In this case, FFR and HSR are negative suggesting no significant limitation on flow; CFR is low—which will be partly caused by the stenosis and partly caused by microvascular disease.

principles (using wires with a thermistor). It can also be measured during non-invasive testing using positron emission tomography (PET) derived quantification of regional myocardial blood flow or by transthoracic echocardiographic assessment of coronary blood flow. Comparison with non-invasive functional imaging techniques has shown that a CFR <2.0 strongly correlates with ischemia in the subtended territory [7]. Extensive prognostic data that strongly suggest that events are low if flow can elevate greater than twice that measurable at rest [8].

Relative CFR (rCFR) indexes the CFR value of the interrogated vessel by that of a normal unobstructed reference vessel in the same patient, provided that at least one vessel is available [6]. Accordingly, a normal rCFR is between 0.65 and 1.0. An important limitation is that of potential collateralization between coronary territories in the presence of a severe stenosis can alter the values. As vasodilators cause indiscriminate microcirculatory vasodilatation, then flow in the reference vessel can be significantly higher than if the stenosis in the neighboring territory was absent. Consequently, the CFR in the reference vessel may be supra-normal, causing overestimation of the significance of the stenosed territory. Alternatively, an inadequate hyperemic response in the "reference" territory would lead to underestimation of the importance of the stenosed vessel.

Practical approaches to measuring CFR

CFR is calculated using either Doppler flow velocity or thermodilution. Doppler flow velocity traces are acquired using a piezoelectric tipped guidewire to elicit spectral traces; average peak flow velocity (APV) is determined by digital tracking (Figure 6.4) and CFR is computed using the ratio of APV at rest and hyperemia. Epicardial resistance must be stabilized using intracoronary nitrates, ensuring a constant surface area which allows flow velocity to be directly proportional to flow.

Added care and attention is required to ensure the flow sensor is coaxial within the vessel. Not only must the Doppler signal be dense, but the automated digital tracing around the Doppler flow velocity signal must also be fully optimized. Inadequate tracking will impair CFR calculation and any phasic analysis. When stenoses are highly obstructive, acquisition of high quality traces is challenging.

The principle of thermodilution is based upon the concept that transit time of an intracoronary injectate, derived from a thermodilution curve, is inversely proportional to flow [2]. CFR can therefore be derived as the ratio of the mean transit time of an intracoronary injectate at baseline and maximal hyperemia. Dedicated pressure wires with a temperature sensor can detect the transit time of a handheld 3–4 mL intracoronary injectate of room temperature saline [9–11]. The shaft of this wire, on which the temperature-dependent electrical resistance is monitored, acts as a proximal thermistor. The distal pressure sensor also allows simultaneous high fidelity temperature measurements. Multiple injectants are typically performed to take an averaged thermodilution curve. Thermodilution techniques require for a standardized volume of injectant, given at a standard speed and force, followed by a standard flush time. Changing these parameters can lead to subtle changes in the thermodilution patterns observed. The need to inject means intravenous hyperemia is required.

Clinical interpretation of CFR

In the absence of an epicardial stenosis, CFR is a measure of microvascular reserve and the capacity to respond to an exogenous vasodilator. In the presence of an epicardial stenosis, CFR provides a marker of flow obstruction; values below 2 are considered flow limiting. When used alone, CFR cannot estimate the relative contribution of microvascular dysfunction and epicardial stenosis because it inherently combines both. CFR may be used alongside another hyperemic index such as FFR; however, there may be similar concern that inadequate hyperemia can lead to misclassification of stenosis significance. Discrepancy between FFR and CFR occurs in 30–60% of cases. Typically, the pressure-based index has been considered correct since the availability of FAME study data, although alternative explanations should be considered as pressure is being used to estimate flow.

When CFR is low, and FFR is above the treatment threshold, it can be interpreted that that there is a non-flow limiting stenosis with microvascular dysfunction. However, as FFR is reliant upon achieving adequate hyperemia, then a non-significant value may not be accurate. In this case, alternative hyperemic approaches should be sought: papaverine may overcome resistance to adenosine. Alternatively, a resting index such as the instantaneous wave-free ratio (iFR) may help. Since the resting index relies upon the natural response of the circulation to the stenosis it is not reliant on the response to the exogenous agent. A truly significant stenosis will cause resting pressure loss even if the response to a hyperemic agent is incomplete. If the iFR is positive, then it suggests, together with the low CFR, that the flow limitation is genuine and that a high FFR is caused by a lack of microcirculatory response to adenosine. If the iFR is negative, it suggests that the epicardial resistance offered by the stenosis is small and predominantly microvascular disease is present.

An alternative discrepancy is that CFR may be high, suggesting there is no difficulty in escalating flow when required, while FFR may be strongly significant, suggesting a flow limitation. This situation occurs because high flow velocities across even trivial stenoses can generate turbulence and energy loss that is detectible as pressure loss, despite the capacity to increase flow. Should a resting index such as iFR be negative, it suggests little impact of the epicardial stenosis. Alternatively, a combined pressure and flow velocity parameter such as the hyperemic stenosis resistance (HSR) may help (Figures 6.4 and 6.5).

Hyperemic stenosis resistance and basal stenosis resistance

The pressure–flow velocity relationships of a stenosis can be described by the gradient of the curve and this is encapsulated by HSR and basal stenosis resistance (BSR). Both measures use the translesional pressure gradient and index it by the flow velocity distal to the stenosis (Pa-Pd/flow velocity) [12]. HSR is measured under hyperemic conditions, while BSR is measured at rest; application of both enable elucidation of the relative contributions of epicardial and microvascular resistance to impaired coronary flow. Both are accurate surrogates for mycardial ischemia [12–14]. Stenoses with hyperemic resistance over 0.80 mmHg/cm/s or resting resistance over 0.66 mmHg/cm/s are likely to be causing ischemia [13,14].

As both HSR and BSR include both pressure and flow measurements, the difficulties posed by CFR or FFR measurement are resolved. High flow situations causing pressure loss due to Bernouli's principle are readily detected; similarly microvascular disease limiting flow increases without epicardial limitation can be determined.

The specific value of these parameters is that they remove the likelihood of false positive pressure gradients that can occur when

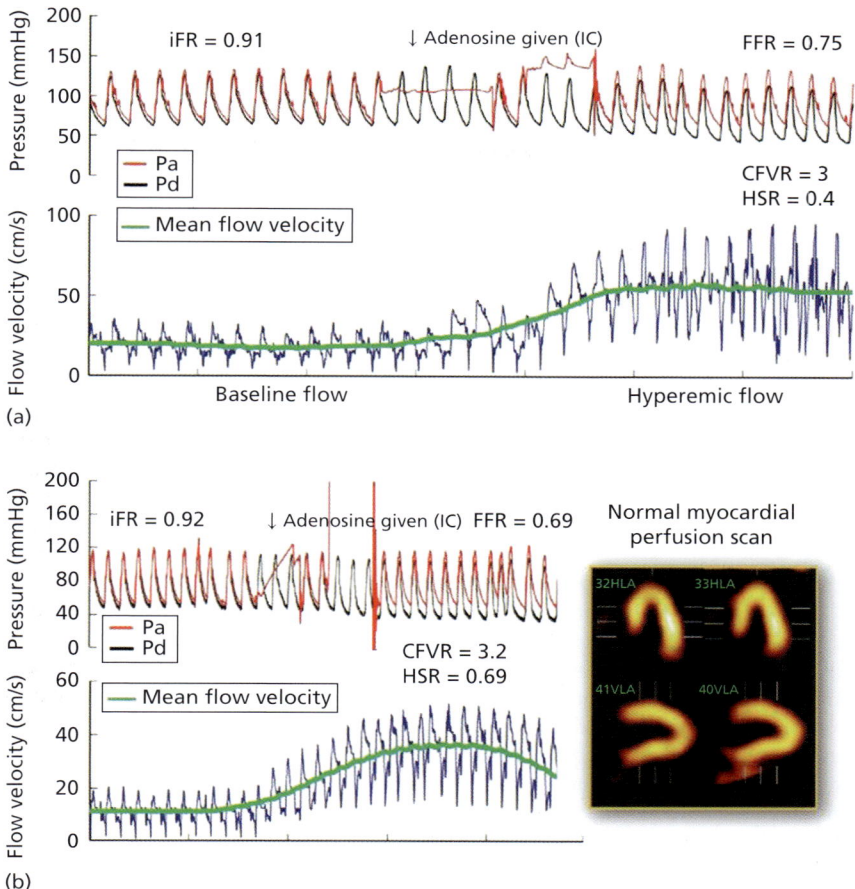

Figure 6.5 Examples of cases in which low FFR values are generated by high magnitudes of hyperemic flow. In both cases, baseline instantaneous wave-free ratio (iFR), coronary flow velocity reserve (CFVR), and hyperemic stenosis resistance index (HSR) were normal, indicating a mild, not flow-limiting stenosis. In (b) a SPECT myocardial perfusion scan also confirms the absence of myocardial ischemia. In these cases, hyperemic pressure is not reflecting flow and is not representative of ischemia. Source: Petraco *et al.* 2014 [39]. Reproduced with permission of Wolters Kluwer Health.

coronary flow increases significantly across an otherwise mild non-flow-limiting stenosis. As predicted by the curvilinear relationship between pressure and flow, even a trivial narrowing can generate a considerable pressure gradient if the flow increases dramatically and this can occur particularly in proximal lesions in vessels subtending a large territory (such as the left anterior descending; LAD) with a microcirculation that is particularly response to exogenous vasodilators (Figure 6.5). First, the large response to a vasodilator suggests there is considerable vasodilatory reserve within the microcirculation which has not had to adapt to flow-limiting stenosis. Second, the fact that flow can elevate significantly across the stenosis suggests it cannot be flow limiting. Using a pressure-only index, under conditions of hyperemia, a large gradient manifest in this manner ("false positive") would be indistiguisable from a "true positive" value. By measuring both the gradient and the actual flow, both HSR and BSR resolve this difficulty and give a highly accurate representation of the significance of a stenosis.

In modern clinical practice, HSR and BSR can be acquired using a combined pressure and flow velocity guidewire, which features both a pressure sensor and a piezo-electric crystal capable of measuring Doppler flow velocity. As with CFR, optimized flow signals are required and familiarity with wire handling. Advances in the commercially available consoles can facilitate use of these parameters but, until then, HSR and BSR remain in the research domain.

Fractional flow reserve

Fractional flow reserve (FFR) is a reference standard for coronary physiology in the catheter laboratory. It is used routinely in clinical practice and is supported by a large volume of research data. FFR, as a concept, is defined as the maximum myocardial blood flow in the presence of an epicardial stenosis divided by the theoretical maximum flow in the absence of a stenosis (maximum flow when the vessel is normal) in a given artery [1–3,15]. In clinical practice, FFR does not measure flow, instead measuring intracoronary pressure [15]. As pressure and flow are not linearly related, a direct relationship can only be inferred if coronary microcirculatory resistance is constant (and minimal) as is theoretically the case during maximal arteriolar vasodilatation [15]. Hyperemic agents such as adenosine, papaverine, ATP, or regadenoson are used to reduce resistance and increase coronary flow, thereby magnifying a trans-stenotic pressure gradient that is often present at rest [15]. FFR is therefore defined in the catheter laboratory as a ratio of the distal and proximal coronary pressures (Pd/Pa) during stable hyperemia averaged over 3–5 complete cardiac cycles.

When administering vasodilators, it is appropriate to observe the change in the Pd/Pa ratio as it may fluctuate before settling during a period of stable hyperemia [16]. When using short-lived intracoronary vasodilators, the lowest Pd/Pa ratio achieved can be used. Caution should be exercised when relying upon automated device calculation, as the lowest value may be spurious, such as calculated during arterial port opening, an ectopic beat, or a cardiac pause [15].

Conceptually, a vessel with FFR of 0.80 has 80% of the blood flow it should have if the stenosis was absent. Theoretically, if a stenosis was removed from that vessel, the FFR should be 1.0. For FFR to be correct the resistance imposed by the microcirculation and any collaterals must be entirely stable and flow across the stenosis maximal. If higher flow across the stenosis can be achieved, or if the microcirculation resistance can be lower, then the severity of the stenosis will be underestimated and the calculated value of FFR will be overestimated (e.g., 0.85 when it should be 0.76).

Consideration of right atrial pressure

Outflow of blood from capillaries into the venous circulation contributes to resistance; and this was accounted for by the original definition of FFR (FFRmyo = Pd–Pv/Pa–Pv) [17]. To simplify FFR and its increase adoption, venous pressure is typically assumed to be zero. If zero, Pv can be removed from the equations calculating FFR. However, typical venous pressures of 2–8 mmHg are reported during hyperemia and patients with cardiac impairment can have higher values [18]. The implications are that stenosis severity may be underestimated, particularly if venous pressure is elevated [19]. While the effects may be diluted in population samples, for individual patients the effects and the change in categorization can be marked and measurement of right atrial pressure should be considered.

Stenosis-specific assessment

In modern practice, FFRmyo (total flow through the myocardial bed, including collateral flow) and FFRcor (quantification of flow limitation caused by stenosis) are considered the same. FFRcor requires coronary wedge pressure (Pw)—measured during balloon occlusion of a stenosis—to estimate the flow contribution from collateral vessels. Pd–Pw/Pa–Pw is required for FFR to provide stenosis specific information, and it is known that the simplified FFRmyo underestimates FFRcorr [17,20]. However, for practical reasons when assessing an intermediate stenosis the risks of balloon inflation may be undesirable, and therefore a balloon occlusion measurement is rarely performed.

Thresholds for significance and evidence to support

A cut-off FFR value of <0.75 across an epicardial stenosis is accepted to be indicative of myocardial ischemia. There is a close correlation between FFR <0.75 and different non-invasive indices of reversible myocardial ischemia [21]. While there may be discrepancy with individual functional tests, when multiple tests are performed agreement is more likely; early work suggests FFR ≤0.75 detects 97% of ischemia [21]. Meta-analytical work suggests the match with non-invasive testing is typically 70% [22]. The DEFER study demonstrated it was clinically safe to defer revascularization with FFR values over 0.75, although the study was small and the number of points in the intermediate range even smaller [9].

FFR values over 0.80 have over 90% sensitivity of excluding ischemia. The FAME and FAME II studies both used a 0.80 threshold, ostensibly to ensure potentially ischemic stenoses were not missed. FAME randomized patients to either FFR-guided revascularization in multivessel disease or an angiographic approach where all stenoses ≥50% were stented; FFR reduced the number and length of stents placed and reduced the number of lesions considered significant (Figure 6.6) [10]. This led to an improvement in composite outcomes of death, myocardial infarction (MI), and repeat revascularization [10]. FAME II randomized those patients with confirmed FFR ≤0.80 to PCI with optimal medical therapy or optimal medical therapy alone. Two-year follow-up suggested the composite of death, non-fatal MI, and revascularization was significantly lower with PCI than medical therapy when peri-procedural events were excluded, although the majority of the events were urgent revascularization and the trial was stopped early which could overestimate the benefits (Figure 6.6) [11].

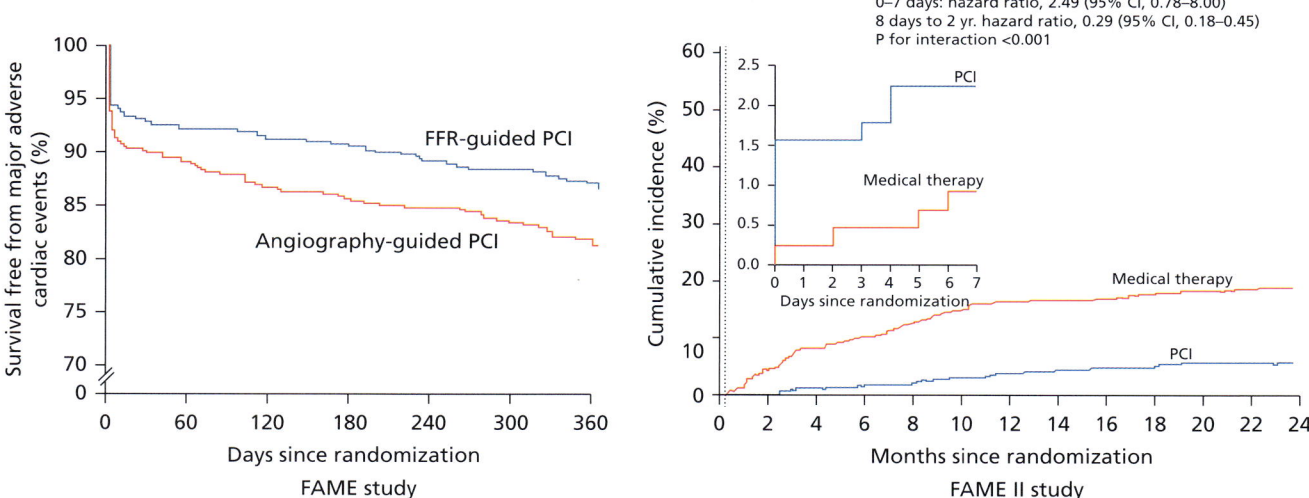

Figure 6.6 Results of FAME and FAME II studies. FAME randomized patients with multivessel disease to a FFR or angiographic guided approach; stenoses with FFR >0.80 were deferred. FAME II randomized patients with a stenosis found to have an FFR ≤0.80 to PCI with optimal medical therapy (OMT) or to OMT alone.

Therefore, it is typical for revascularization to be offered when stenoses have FFR ≤0.75, while deferral is more likely when FFR >0.80. For values in the "gray zone" (between 0.75 and 0.80), clinical judgment is required, combining knowledge of the patient's clinical presentation, other investigations, and the impact of natural variability [23]. It is common practice to give additional doses of hyperemic agent when values are close to the threshold: higher doses can give confidence that maximal hyperemia has been achieved, but as flow is not being directly measured, caution is required because some changes result from the hemodynamic disturbance of higher doses.

An area of great potential remains the use of FFR during routine clinical angiography rather than at the time of coronary intervention. Greater utility can be gained by performing multivessel physiologic assessment at the time of angiography to objectively delineate the clinical significance of any coronary atheroma. Studies suggest there could be significant changes in medical decision making with the additional information [24,25].

Clinical technique for assessment of FFR

FFR is measured using pressure-tipped guidewires (pressure wire) [3]. The pressure wire is introduced through a standard guiding catheter and positioned distal to the coronary stenosis being investigated under fluoroscopic guidance. Prior to passing the wire past the stenosis, effort should be made to ensure that the distal pressure trace (Pd) is equalized or "normalization" with aortic pressure trace (Pa) at the origin of the vessel (left main stem or osmium of the right coronary artery) (Figure 6.7). If ostial stenosis is suspected, the wire will require normalization in the aorta. Measurements should be made with the needle-introducer fully closed to avoid minor pressure drift. Once the wire is passed past the stenosis, it is recommended that sensor is at least 2–3 vessel diameters away from the stenosis to reduce the impact of pressure recovery phenomena. Pd and Pa traces are displayed continuously, and either intravenous or intracoronary hyperemic vasodilator should be administered; FFR is then taken during a period of stability.

When there is diffuse disease, it is possible to move the pressure wire backwards by applying gentle traction to bring the sensor to the vessel osmium. This permits estimation of areas of large pressure drops if performed while continuous hyperemia is achieved—most easily with an intravenous infusion of adenosine.

The sensor should always be returned to the vessel ostium after assessment to exclude the presence of significant pressure wire or hemodynamic system drift which would make the measurement unreliable. Values of drift over 2 mmHg suggest the measurement should be repeated.

Caution is required when there are large hemodynamic shifts in aortic pressures caused by central adenosine infusions. Large falls in proximal aortic pressure cannot account for a significant proportion of the change in distal coronary pressure and can alter the FFR results. Caution should taken to ensure ratios are calculated during stable hyperemia to match the original validation work. In some

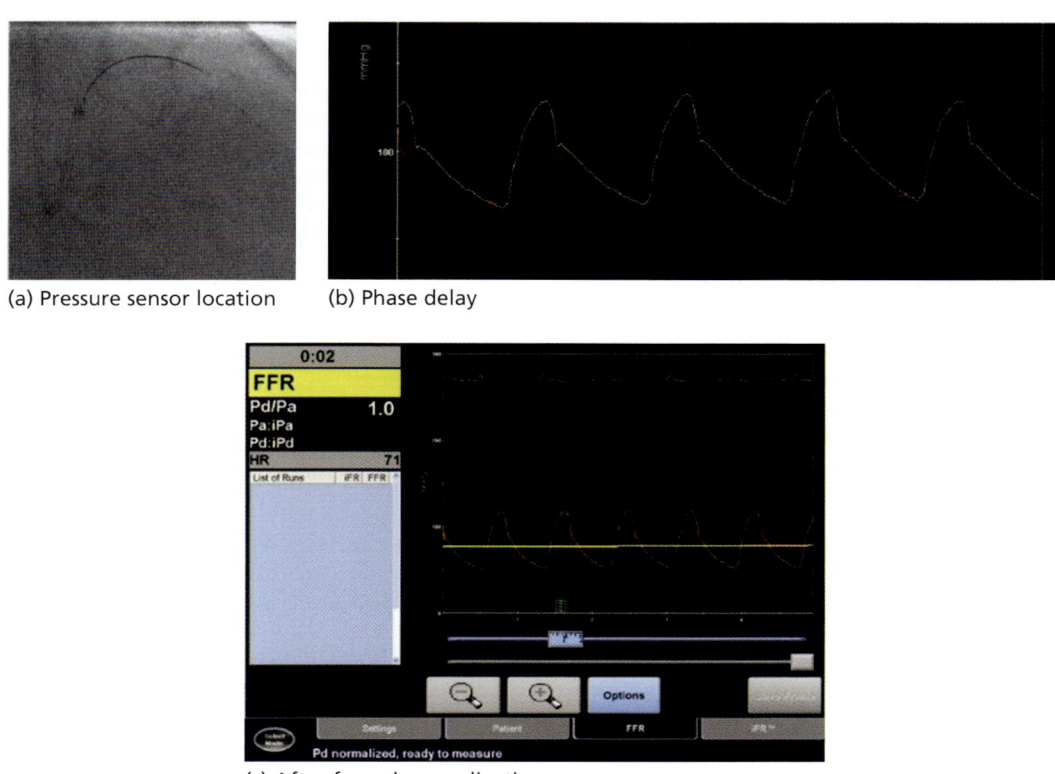

(a) Pressure sensor location   (b) Phase delay

(c) After formal normalization

Figure 6.7 Active and phasic normalization. (a) The pressure wire sensor should be normalized at the ostium of the vessel. For most pressure wires the sensor is at the junction of the radiopaque marker. (b) There is a phase delay between proximal aortic pressure (Pa, red) and distal wire pressure (Pd, yellow); while the Pd/Pa ratio over the whole cycle is 1.0, during the wave-free period in diastole, the ratio is an erroneous 1.08 at the ostium. Therefore any measurements taken would be erroneous. (c) After the formal normalization process, the Pd and Pa are now aligned.

situations, the lowest FFR value can occur during the initial peak hyperemic phase causing a change in classification of stenosis significance [15]. Prolonged intravenous infusions of adenosine can cause paradoxical vasoconstriction of the microcirculation and the whole trace should be observed for a reliable value [26,27].

Clinical applications of FFR

FFR has been widely assessed in a number of different settings to assist clinical decision making. There are clinical studies utilizing FFR for the assessment of left main stem disease [28,29], side branch vessels, and for guiding surgical graft placement [30]. There remains limited data for the use of FFR within surgical grafts [31]. FFR has been used in patients with acute coronary syndromes with reasonable reproducibility, despite concerns that the microvasculature is not optimally responsive to adenosine shortly after infarction.

A number of studies have sought to correlate intravascular ultrasound (IVUS) or optical coherence tomography (OCT) parameters with FFR. Overall, the thresholds determined will be dependent upon the underlying population and the distribution of the FFRs studied. Although this avenue of research remains attractive to those wishing to minimize vessel instrumentation, tools, intracoronary imaging, and physiology offer complementary not mutually exclusive information to aid clinical decisions.

Instantaneous wave-free ratio

The instantaneous wave-free ratio (iFR) is a resting index of stenosis severity that quantifies the impact a stenosis upon the coronary circulation [32]. A pressure-only index, it is measured during the wave-free period in diastole. The wave-free period was determined using wave-intensity analysis, and is a period where the conflicting forces that control blood flow are quiescent, and microcirculatory resistance is at its lowest compared to whole cardiac cycle. As such, pressure and flow are linearly related over the wave-free period, enabling a resting pressure index to assess stenosis severity without the need of an exogenous vasodilator [32,33].

IFR is calculated in the same manner as FFR or other pressure-based approaches. Once the pressure sensor beyond the stenosis in question, iFR can be calculated as a single heart beat calculation, or an average over five heart beats. Initial commercial systems have required ECG monitoring to determine the correct phase in the cardiac cycle, but newer pressure-only algorithms remove this need.

The wave-free period is not significantly affected by beat-to-beat variability or atrial arrhythmias. Heart rates typical for performing physiologic assessment (40–130 bpm). Algorithms within the commercial consoles are capable of excluding inappropriate beats with a wide variability.

IFR can be plotted throughout the vessel during gentle pressure wire pullback to identify focal and diffuse disease throughout the vessel. The degree of information observed will depend partly upon the speed of pullback; 20–30 seconds typically suffices. As this information is acquired at rest, the degree of flow interaction that can occur between mutliple stenoses during hyperemia is minimized [34]. This provides an additional advantage of an iFR-pullback approach, because it becomes possible to predict the hemodynamic effect of removing a stenosis (Figure 6.8) [35]. The residual resting gradients typically remain the same after coronary intervention because resting flow velocity changes little. In contrast, hyperemic pullbacks, while they can identify areas of high pressure gradient, cannot predict the hemodynamic impact of stenting because hyperemic pressure gradients change after the removal of a stenosis. This

novel additional information can facilitate a more physiologically guided coronary intervention than hitherto possible.

It is also possible to measure iFR during administration of a vasodilator such as adenosine. While this has consistently produced lower iFR values, many even lower than FFR, because the stability of resistance is unchanged there is no significant incremental diagnostic yield. It appears the information available at rest is sufficient. If used, a much lower threshold (0.66 for ischemia) must also be applied.

IFR in clinical trials

IFR has been compared with FFR in a number of studies, notably the ADVISE family of studies [32,36,37]. The degree of classification match is strongly dependent upon the distribution of lesions included with clinical cohorts demonstrating 80–88% match. The limit of match is driven by the capacity for FFR to match itself when repeated. This varies according to the technique and analysis route chosen but can be as much as 15% change in classification match when FFR is close to its threshold. When compared with third party markers of ischemia, including HSR, CFR, SPECT, and PET imaging, iFR and FFR are equal in their capacity to detect ischemia (Figure 6.9) [33,38–41].

Clinical outcome studies are underway in very large randomized controlled trials: DEFINE-FLAIR and the iFR-Swedeheart studies will compare clinical outcomes when patients undergo revascularization based upon either iFR or FFR.

Practical considerations of iFR measurement

When performing resting physiologic assessment, a rigorous standardized approach is necessary, encapsulated by the "3Ns": nitrates, normalize, and no touch.

First is to administer intracoronary nitrates. Nitrates are required for all physiologic assessment to stabilize epicardial resistance, since the introduction of the pressure wire will cause a highly variable degree of spasm not always evident upon angiography. Typically, 300 µg is sufficient and this should be administered as soon as the guiding catheter is engaged, before the pressure wire is passed into the vessel. If time has elapsed between the last administration and a recording, it is usual to re-administer the nitrate. Nitrates do not cause significant or long-lived hyperemia; any increase in flow has returned to baseline within 30 seconds.

Second, "normalization" of the pressure wire at the vessel ostium is strongly recommended prior to passing the wire into the vessel in question. This should be performed with the introducer needle removed. Active normalization will not only ensure the pressure ratios are 1.0, but also ensure there is no time delay between proximal and distal pressure tracings. This is pertinent for phasic pressure analysis such as iFR, as time offsets will generate incorrect calculation (Figure 6.7).

Third, once the wire has been positioned in the location for measurement, there should be no further touching of the pressure wire. For optimal resting assessment, additional contrast injections should be avoided just prior to measurement of the index. If a contrast injection is necessary, it would be appropriate to wait 20 seconds to allow the impact of submaximal hyperemia to subside.

In the post-PCI state, either after ballooning or stenting, resting flow states have typically resumed by the time the balloon is withdrawn and the catheters have been flushed. In practical terms, there is no delay in the time required to make a resting measurement.

Other concerns that patient anxiety or conscious state affect resting measurements has not been found in practice. The ADVISE family of studies were all performed in typical patients attending the catheter laboratory without a specific protocol for sedation.

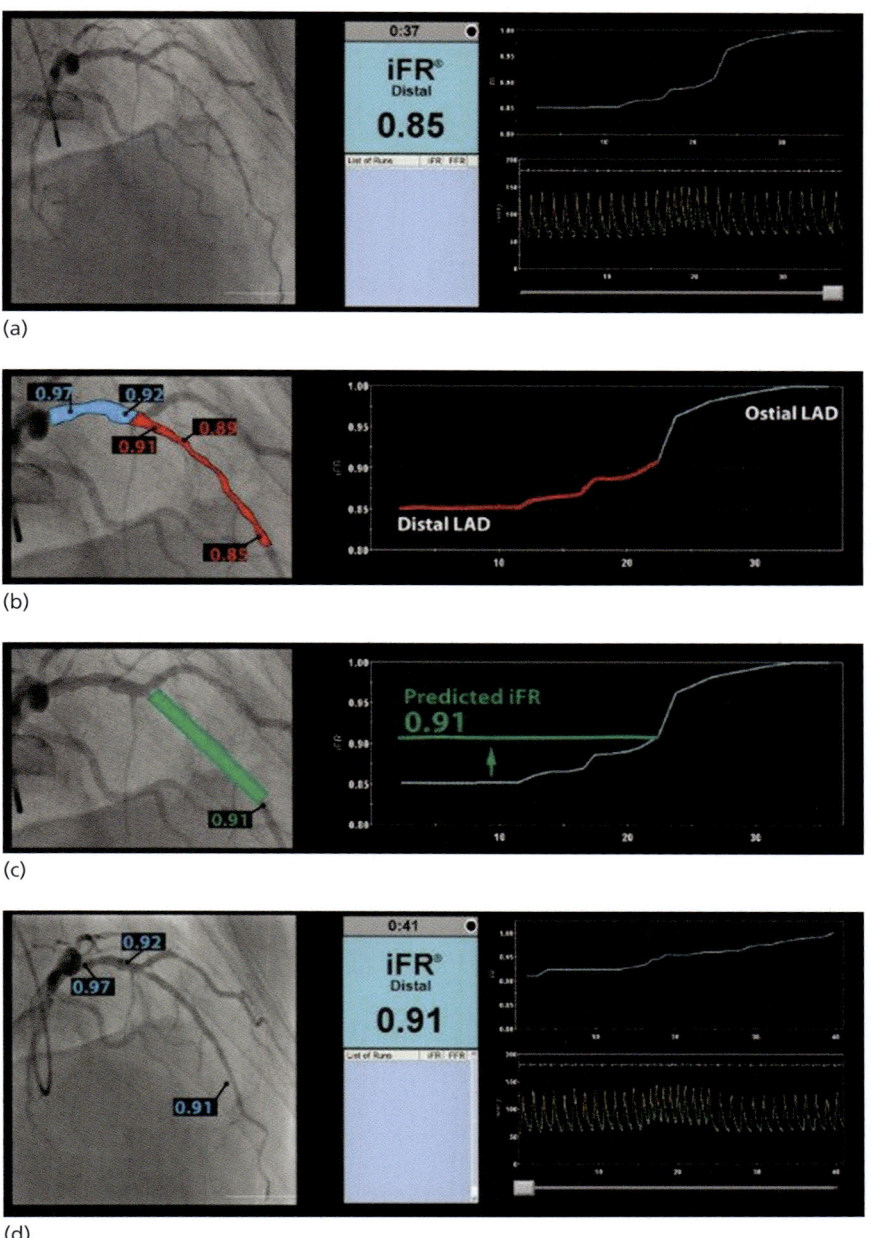

Figure 6.8 iFR pullback can be used to predict post-PCI iFR values. (a) The left anterior descending (LAD) has a moderate proximal stenosis and a long segment of moderate-to-severe disease. iFR is positive for ischemia. (b) The live beat-to-beat iFR-pullback suggests the proximal stenosis contributes 0.05 iFR units while the mid-vessel disease is 0.06. (c) Removing the mid-vessel disease is predicted to give an iFR of 0.91, above the treatment threshold. (d) Repeat iFR post-stenting the mid-vessel disease confirms an iFR of 0.91; pullback shows that proximal disease continues to contribute 0.05 pressure drop and can be deferred.

IFR has attraction in simplifying stenosis assessment by removing the absolute need for a vasodilator. This likely reduces cost, time, and patient discomfort from vasodilators. There is potential use in patients who cannot be given a vasodilator, such as those with allergy, severe airways disease, or with conditions that cannot tolerate hypotension—including aortic stenosis. Multivessel assessment and physiologically planned coronary intervention with assessment after intervention provide further potential scenarios.

Assessment of coronary microvascular function

The functional state of the coronary microcirculation has a strong prognostic role [4] and assessment of coronary microvascular function can assist in risk stratification of patients. Current approaches rely upon indirect assessment of the microcirculation: assessing a change in coronary flow in response to a specific agonist that evokes differential microvascular responses. Agonists are either endothelium-dependent (requiring an intact endothelium to

Study	No. of stenoses	Reference standard	p	Hyperemia (FFR) BETTER ← → Resting (iFR) BETTER
CLARIFY	51	Hyperemic stenosis resistance	ns	
Van de Hoef et al.	85	Myocardical perfusion	ns	
Sen et al.	120	Hyperemic stenosis resistance	<0.01	
JUSTIFY-CFR	216	Coronary flow reserve	<0.01	
De Ward et al.	49	Positron emisson tomography	ns	

Difference in accuracy (%)

Figure 6.9 iFR and FFR compared with ischaemic parameters. Adenosine-free instantaneous wave-free ratio (iFR) has equivalent diagnostic accuracy to adenosine-mediated fractional flow reserve (FFR). In multiple studies where both parameters are compared to a third-party parameter of ischemia, including the gold standard of positron emission tomography (PET), there is no difference in the accuracy of either pressure index to detect ischemia.

function, such as acetylcholine, substance P, and bradykinin) or endothelium-independent (such as nitrate and nitroprusside) [42]. The level of change in coronary blood flow in response to a given agonist is inversely proportional to the functional state of the microcirculation.

Research approaches to assessing coronary microvascular function

The basic principle requires determination of blood flow in response to a microvascular agonist. Flow can derived from the product of the cross-sectional area of the vessel and the average velocity of the fluid within: flow = $(\pi D2/4) \times (0.5 \times APV)$, where D is the diameter of the vessel measured using quantitative coronary angiography and APV is the average peak velocity measured using a Doppler guidewire. Vessel diameter measurements should be rigorously performed, over a 5-mm segment approximately 2.5 mm distal to the Doppler sensor. Following acquisition of baseline coronary flow, measurements should be repeated after delivery of the agonist, either as a continuous infusion through a guiding catheter together with an infusion pump or as an intracoronary bolus. The change in flow can be quantified as percentage change compared with baseline or hyperemic flow. The potential for error, from diameter measurements or inadequate flow velocity envelopes, is significant and care is required.

IMR: a clinical tool to assess microvascular function

IMR measures the resistance of coronary microvacular vessels and is derived from application of Ohm's law (that the potential difference across an ideal conductor is proportional to the current through the conductor) [43]. By neglecting the influence of venous pressure, IMR is determined by dividing hyperemic distal coronary pressure (Pd) by hyperemic flow; since it is typically derived using thermodilution techniques, it is readily calculated by the product of Pd with transit time (Tmn) under hyperemia [43]. A brisk injectant of 3 mL saline at room temperature should be used to determine transit times under maximal hyperemia, typically achieved using intravenous adenosine infusions (Figure 6.10).

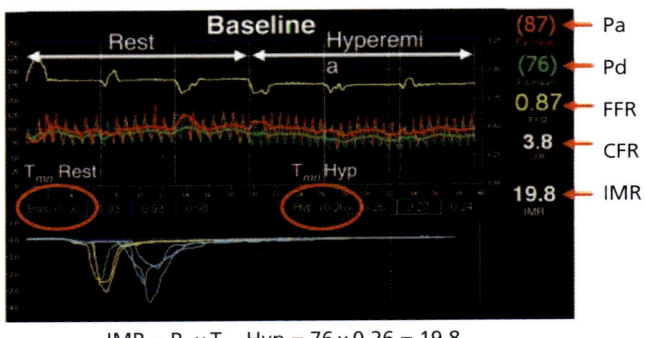

$$IMR = P_d \times T_{mn}Hyp = 76 \times 0.26 = 19.8$$

Figure 6.10 IMR calculation. A combined pressure–temperature guidewire is used to obtain mean Pd and mean distal coronary blood flow (based on the principles of thermodilution in response to a 3 mL handheld intracoronary injection of room temperature saline). IMR is derived from the ratio of mean P_d (green circle) and mean distal coronary flow at maximal hyperemia. Distal coronary flow is inversely proportional to the mean transit time (T_{mn}) of the injectate. Therefore $IMR = P_d : 1/T_{mn} = P_d \times T_{mn}$.

IMR correlates significantly with true microcirculatory resistance measured in an open-chested pig model. In the presence of an epicardial stenosis, coronary wedge pressure should be included in the calculation (IMR = Pa × hyperemic mean transit time × [(Pd–Pw)/(Pa–Pw)]); this is particularly important in significant stenoses with an FFR ≤0.60 where the likelihood of collateral flow is high. Mathematical derivation of Pw is also possible based upon the statistical relationship between FFRcorr and FFRmyo; IMR can therefore be calculated as:

$$IMR_{calc} = Pa \times T_{mn}Hyp \times \left(1.35 \times P_d / P_a - 0.32\right)[20].$$

No threshold has been formally accepted and IMR can be considered a relative rather than absolute index. However, values below 25 have been found in two small healthy populations with normal angiographic appearance to vessels [44]. After ST-segment elevation myocardial infarction (STEMI), patients with high IMR values (>40) are more likely to have raised cardiac enzymes, less cardiac recovery on non-invasive imaging, and evidence of microvascular obstruction on magnetic resonance imaging [45]. Values below 40 are associated with lower rates of death or rehospitalization for congestive heart failure or death alone. Active research is seeking adjunctive approaches to minimize microvascular dysfunction during STEMI and after elective intervention in stable patients as assessed by IMR. There may also be utility in using high IMR values to diagnose microvascular dysfunction as the cause of angina in patients with otherwise normal appearing coronary vessels.

Interactive multiple choice questions are available for this chapter on www.wiley.com/go/dangas/cardiology

References

1 Gould KL, Lipscomb K, Hamilton GW. Physiologic basis for assessing critical coronary stenosis: instantaneous flow response and regional distribution during coronary hyperemia as measures of coronary flow reserve. *Am J Cardiol* 1974; **33**(1): 87–94.

2 Seo MK, Koo BK, Kim JH, *et al.* Comparison of hyperemic efficacy between central and peripheral venous adenosine infusion for fractional flow reserve measurement. *Circ Cardiovasc Interv* 2012; **5**(3): 401–405.

3 Kern MJ, Lerman A, Bech JW, *et al.* Physiological assessment of coronary artery disease in the cardiac catheterization laboratory a scientific statement from the American Heart Association Committee on Diagnostic and Interventional Cardiac Catheterization, *Council on Clinical Cardiology. Circulation* 2006; **114**(12): 1321–1341.

4 Nair PK, Marroquin OC, Mulukutla SR, *et al.* Clinical utility of regadenoson for assessing fractional flow reserve. *JACC Cardiovasc Interv* 2011; **4**(10): 1085–1092.

5 De Bruyne B, Pijls NHJ, Barbato E, *et al.* Intracoronary and intravenous adenosine 5′-triphosphate, adenosine, papaverine, and contrast medium to assess fractional flow reserve in humans. *Circulation* 2003; **107**(14): 1877–1883.

6 Gould KL, Kirkeeide RL, Buchi M. Coronary flow reserve as a physiologic measure of stenosis severity. *J Am Coll Cardiol* 1990; **15**: 459–474.

7 Miller DD, Donohue TJ, Younis LT, *et al.* Correlation of pharmacological 99mTc-sestamibi myocardial perfusion imaging with poststenotic coronary flow reserve in patients with angiographically intermediate coronary artery stenoses. *Circulation* 1994; **89**(5): 2150–2160.

8 Chamuleau SAJ, Tio RA, de Cock CC, *et al.* Prognostic value of coronary blood flow velocity and myocardial perfusion in intermediate coronary narrowings and multivessel disease. *J Am Coll Cardiol* 2002; **39**(5): 852–858.

9 Bech GJW, Bruyne BD, Pijls NHJ, *et al.* Fractional flow reserve to determine the appropriateness of angioplasty in moderate coronary stenosis: a randomized trial. *Circulation* 2001; **103**(24): 2928–2934.

10 Tonino PAL, De Bruyne B, Pijls NHJ, *et al.* Fractional flow reserve versus angiography for guiding percutaneous coronary intervention. *N Engl J Med* 2009; **360**(3): 213–224.

11 De Bruyne B, Fearon WF, Pijls NHJ, *et al.* Fractional flow reserve-guided PCI for stable coronary artery disease. *N Engl J Med* 2014; **371**(13): 1208–1217.

12 Siebes M, Verhoeff B-J, Meuwissen M, de Winter RJ, Spaan JAE, Piek JJ. Single-wire pressure and flow velocity measurement to quantify coronary stenosis hemodynamics and effects of percutaneous interventions. *Circulation* 2004; **109**: 756–762.

13 Meuwissen M, Siebes M, Chamuleau SAJ, *et al.* Hyperemic stenosis resistance index for evaluation of functional coronary lesion severity. *Circulation* 2002; **106**: 441–446.

14 van de Hoef TP, Nolte F, Damman P, *et al.* Diagnostic accuracy of combined intracoronary pressure and flow velocity information during baseline conditions: adenosine-free assessment of functional coronary lesion severity. *Circ Cardiovasc Interv* 2012; **5**: 508–514.

15 Echavarria-Pinto M, Petraco R, van de Hoef TP, *et al.* Fractional flow reserve and minimum Pd/Pa ratio during intravenous adenosine infusion: very similar but not always the same. *EuroIntervention* 2016; **11**(9): 1013–1019.

16 Tarkin JM, Nijjer S, Sen S, *et al.* Hemodynamic response to intravenous adenosine and its effect on fractional flow reserve assessment results of the Adenosine for the Functional Evaluation of Coronary Stenosis Severity (AFFECTS) Study. *Circ Cardiovasc Interv* 2013; **6**(6): 654–661.

17 Pijls NH, van Son JA, Kirkeeide RL, De Bruyne B, Gould KL. Experimental basis of determining maximum coronary, myocardial, and collateral blood flow by pressure measurements for assessing functional stenosis severity before and after percutaneous transluminal coronary angioplasty. *Circulation* 1993; **87**(4): 1354–1367.

18 De Bruyne B, Baudhuin T, Melin JA, *et al.* Coronary flow reserve calculated from pressure measurements in humans: validation with positron emission tomography. *Circulation* 1994; **89**(3): 1013–1022.

19 Perera D, Biggart S, Postema P, *et al.* Right atrial pressure: can it be ignored when calculating fractional flow reserve and collateral flow index? *J Am Coll Cardiol* 2004; **44**(10): 2089–2091.

20 Yong AS, Layland J, Fearon WF, *et al.* Calculation of the index of microcirculatory resistance without coronary wedge pressure measurement in the presence of epicardial stenosis. *JACC Cardiovasc Interv* 2013; **6**(1): 53–58.

21 Pijls NH, De Bruyne B, Peels K, *et al.* Measurement of fractional flow reserve to assess the functional severity of coronary-artery stenoses. *N Engl J Med* 1996; **334**(26): 1703–1708.

22 Christou MAC, Siontis GCM, Katritsis DG, Ioannidis JPA. Meta-analysis of fractional flow reserve versus quantitative coronary angiography and noninvasive imaging for evaluation of myocardial ischemia. *Am J Cardiol* 2007; **99**(4): 450–456.

23 Petraco R, Sen S, Nijjer SS, Escaned J, Francis DP, Davies JE. Fractional flow-guided coronary revascularisation: implications of its biological variability on clinical decisions. *JACC Cardiovasc Interv* 2013; **6**(3): 222–225.

24 Van Belle EV, Rioufol G, Pouillot C, *et al.* Outcome impact of coronary revascularization strategy reclassification with fractional flow reserve at time of diagnostic angiography: insights from a large French multicenter fractional flow reserve registry. *Circulation* 2014; **129**(2): 173–185.

25 Curzen N, Rana O, Nicholas Z, *et al.* Does routine pressure wire assessment influence management strategy at coronary angiography for diagnosis of chest pain? *The RIPCORD Study. Circ Cardiovasc Interv* 2014; **7**(2): 248–255.

26 Nijjer SS, Sen S, Petraco R, *et al.* Improvement in coronary haemodynamics after percutaneous coronary intervention: assessment using instantaneous wave-free ratio. *Heart* 2013; **99**(23): 1740–1748.

27 Siebes M, Chamuleau SA, Meuwissen M, Piek JJ, Spaan JA. Influence of hemodynamic conditions on fractional flow reserve: parametric analysis of underlying model. *Am J Physiol Heart Circ Physiol* 2002; **283**(4): H1462–1470.

28 Hamilos M, Muller O, Cuisset T, *et al.* Long-term clinical outcome after fractional flow reserve-guided treatment in patients with angiographically equivocal left main coronary artery stenosis. *Circulation* 2009; **120**(15): 1505–1512.

29 Yong ASC, Daniels D, De Bruyne B, *et al.* Fractional flow reserve assessment of left main stenosis in the presence of downstream coronary stenoses. *Circ Cardiovasc Interv* 2013; **6**(2): 161–165.

30 Botman CJ, Schonberger J, Koolen S, *et al.* Does stenosis severity of native vessels influence bypass graft patency? A prospective fractional flow reserve-guided study. *Ann Thorac Surg* 2007; **83**(6): 2093–2097.

31 Pijls NHJ, Botman KJ. Functional assessment of bypass grafts by fractional flow reserve. *Eur J Cardiothorac Surg* 2007; **31**(3): 381–382.

32 Sen S, Escaned J, Malik IS, *et al.* Development and validation of a new adenosine-independent index of stenosis severity from coronary wave–intensity analysis. *J Am Coll Cardiol* 2012; **59**(15): 1392–1402.

33 Sen S, Asrress KN, Nijjer S, *et al.* Diagnostic classification of the instantaneous wave-free ratio is equivalent to fractional flow reserve and is not improved with adenosine administration. Results of CLARIFY (Classification Accuracy of Pressure-Only Ratios Against Indices Using Flow Study). *J Am Coll Cardiol* 2013; **61**(13): 1409–1420.

34 Nijjer SS, Sen S, Petraco R, Mayet J, Francis DP, Davies JER. The Instantaneous wave-free ratio (iFR) pullback: a novel innovation using baseline physiology to optimise coronary angioplasty in tandem lesions. *Cardiovasc Revasc Med* 2015; **16**(3): 167–171.

35 Nijjer SS, Sen S, Petraco R, *et al.* Pre-angioplasty instantaneous wave-free ratio pullback provides virtual intervention and predicts hemodynamic outcome for serial lesions and diffuse coronary artery disease. *JACC Cardiovasc Interv* 2014; **7**(12): 1386–1396.

36 Petraco R, Escaned J, Sen S, *et al.* Classification performance of instantaneous wave-free ratio (iFR) and fractional flow reserve in a clinical population of intermediate coronary stenoses: results of the ADVISE registry. *EuroIntervention* 2013; **9**(1): 91–101.

37 Petraco R, Al-Lamee R, Gotberg M, *et al.* Real-time use of instantaneous wave-free ratio: results of the ADVISE in-practice. An international, multicenter evaluation of instantaneous wave-free ratio in clinical practice. *Am Heart J* 2014; **168**(5): 739–748.

38 Sen S, Nijjer S, Petraco R, Malik IS, Francis DP, Davies J. Instantaneous wave-free ratio: numerically different, but diagnostically superior to FFR? Is lower always better? *J Am Coll Cardiol* 2013; **62**(6): 566.

39 Petraco R, van de Hoef TP, Nijjer S, *et al.* Baseline instantaneous wave-free ratio as a pressure-only estimation of underlying coronary flow reserve: results of the JUSTIFY-CFR Study. *Circ Cardiovasc Interv* 2014; **7**(4): 492–502.

40 Van de Hoef TP, Meuwissen M, Escaned J, *et al.* Head-to-head comparison of basal stenosis resistance index, instantaneous wave-free ratio, and fractional flow reserve: diagnostic accuracy for stenosis-specific myocardial ischaemia. *EuroIntervention* 2015; **11**(8): 914–925.

41 De Waard G, Danad I, da Cunha RP, *et al.* Hyperemic FFR and baseline iFR have an equivalent diagnostic accuracy when compared to myocardial blood flow quantified by H$_2$^{15}O PET perfusion imaging. *J Am Coll Cardiol* 2014; **63**(12, Suppl): A1692.

42 Melikian N, Kearney MT, Thomas MR, Bruyne BD, Shah AM, MacCarthy PA. A simple thermodilution technique to assess coronary endothelium-dependent microvascular function in humans: validation and comparison with coronary flow reserve. *Eur Heart J* 2007; **28**(18): 2188–2194.

43 Kobayashi Y, Fearon WF. Invasive coronary microcirculation assessment. *Circ J* 2014; **78**(5): 1021–1028.

44 Melikian N, Vercauteren S, Fearon WF, *et al.* Quantitative assessment of coronary microvascular function in patients with and without epicardial atherosclerosis. *EuroIntervention* 2010; **5**(8): 939–945.

45 McGeoch R, Watkins S, Berry C, *et al.* The Index of microcirculatory resistance measured acutely predicts the extent and severity of myocardial infarction in patients with ST-segment elevation myocardial infarction. *JACC Cardiovasc Interv* 2010; **3**(7): 715–722.

CHAPTER 7

Intravascular Ultrasound and Virtual Histology: Principles, Image Interpretation, and Clinical Applications

Adriano Caixeta[1], Akiko Maehara[2], and Gary S. Mintz[2]

[1] Hospital Israelita Albert Einstein; Universidade Federal de São Paulo, São Paulo, Brazil

[2] Columbia University Medical Center and the Cardiovascular Research Foundation, New York, NY, USA

Medical uses of ultrasound came shortly after the end of World War II. However, real-time ultrasound imaging originated in the late 1960s and early 1970s when Bom *et al.* [1] pioneered the development of linear array transducers for use in the cardiovascular system. The first two-dimensional catheter imaging system was designed in 1972 using a solid-state transducer array of 32 elements arranged radially at the tip of a 9 Fr catheter [2]. By the late 1980s, Yock *et al.* [3,4] had successfully miniaturized a single-transducer system that could be placed within coronary arteries. Ever since, intravascular ultrasound (IVUS) has become an increasingly important catheter-based imaging technology providing both practical guidance for percutaneous coronary interventions (PCI) as well as many different clinical and research insights [5–10].

Coronary angiography has numerous limitations, including foreshortening and vessel overlap, high inter- and intra-observer variability when assessing lesion severity, and provides no details of plaque burden or composition. Conversely, IVUS directly images the atheroma within the vessel wall, allowing reproducible measurement of plaque size, distribution, and to some extent its composition. The application of IVUS as a prognostic tool and to guide coronary intervention is well established. IVUS has also provided new insights into the efficacy and safety of drug-eluting stent (DES). Thus, IVUS has been established as the method of choice for the serial assessment of atherosclerotic plaque burden in progression–regression trials.

Recent advances in IVUS technology permit identification of plaque composition and morphology using computed-assisted analysis of raw radiofrequency signal (e.g., virtual histology; VH). Several studies have emerged correlating these newer IVUS approaches with patient outcomes in a variety of clinical scenarios. This chapter reviews the rationale, technique, and interpretation of grayscale IVUS and VH imaging in diagnostic and therapeutic applications.

Principles of IVUS imaging

Ultrasound is acoustic energy with a frequency above human hearing. The highest frequency that the human ear can detect is approximately 20 thousand cycles per second (20,000 Hz). This is where the sonic range ends and where the ultrasonic range begins. In medical imaging, high-frequency acoustic energy is the range of millions of cycles per second (megahertz; MHz). Current IVUS catheters used in the coronary arteries have frequencies ranging 20–45 MHz and 100–200 µm axial resolution [11].

IVUS supplements angiography by providing a tomographic perspective of lumen geometry and vessel wall structure. The equipment required to perform intracoronary ultrasound consists of a catheter incorporating a miniaturized transducer and a console to reconstruct the images. The IVUS transducer converts electrical energy into acoustical energy through a piezo-electric (pressure-electric) crystalline material that expands and contracts to produce sound waves when electrically excited (i.e., a series of pulse/echo sequences or vectors). After reflection from tissue, part of the ultrasound energy returns to the transducer; the transducer then generates an electrical impulse that is converted into moving pictures [12]. All materials in the body reflect sound waves. Sound waves bounce back at various intervals depending on the type of material and the distance from the transducer. It is the variation in reflective sound waves that creates the ultrasound image on the console.

The intensity of reflected (or backscattered) ultrasound depends on a number of variables including the intensity of the transmitted signal, the attenuation of the signal by the tissue, the distance from the transducer to the target, the angle of the signal relative to the target, and the density of the tissue [5]. Several clinically relevant properties of the ultrasound image—such as the resolution, depth of penetration, and attenuation of the acoustic—are dependent on the geometric and frequency properties of the transducer. The higher the center frequency, the better the axial resolution, but the lower the depth of penetration. For coronary imaging, because the transducer is close to the vessel wall, high ultrasound frequencies are used that are centered at 20–40 MHz. The use of high ultrasound frequencies provides axial resolution between 80 and 120 µm and lateral resolution (dependent on imaging depth and beam shape) between 200 and 500 µm [5].

Equipment for IVUS examination

Two different transducer designs are commonly used yielding comparable information: mechanically rotated and electronically activated phased-array. Mechanical probes use a drive cable to rotate a single-element transducer at the tip of the catheter at 1800 rpm.

Interventional Cardiology: Principles and Practice, Second Edition. Edited by George D. Dangas, Carlo Di Mario, and Nicholas N. Kipshidze.
© 2017 John Wiley & Sons, Ltd. Published 2017 by John Wiley & Sons, Ltd.

At approximately 1° increments, the transducer sends and receives ultrasound signals providing 256 individual radial scan lines for each image. The mechanical transducer has the advantage of a simple design, greater signal-to-noise ratio, and higher temporal and spatial resolution. In electronic systems, multiple tiny transducer elements in an annular array are activated sequentially to generate the cross-sectional image [5,12].

The IVUS console contains numerous imaging controls such as zoom, gain, TGC (time-gain-compensation), gamma curves, compression and reject, and others. With both systems, still frames and video images can be digitally archived on local storage memory or a remote server using DICOM format.

Imaging artifacts

Artifacts often appear in images generated by contemporary IVUS devices and can interfere in imaging interpretation and measurements.

Ring-down

Ring-down artifacts usually appear as a series of parallel bands or halos of variables thickness surrounding the catheter obscuring near field imaging. Phased-array systems tend to have more ring-down artifacts (Figure 7.1).

Non-uniform rotational distortion

Non-uniform rotational distortion (NURD) arises from frictional forces to the rotating elements in mechanical catheters. NURD creates stretched or compacted portions of the images. Because accurate reconstruction of IVUS two-dimensional images is dependent on uniform rotation of the catheter, non-uniform rotation can create errors during IVUS measurements (Figure 7.1) [13]. For practical propose the mean lumen area tends to increase as the degree of distortion increases [14]. NURD artifacts can also occur because of bends in the catheter driveshaft or in the presence of acute bends in the artery.

Reverberations

Strong spatial tissue heterogeneity creates acoustic noise and pulse reverberations—multiple echoes reaching the transducer before the next pulse transmission to give rise to multiple copies of the anatomy (Figure 7.1). Reverberation artifacts are more common from strong echoreflectors such as stents, guidewires, guiding catheters, and calcium (especially after rotational atherectomy).

Other artifacts

A few other artifacts can also interfere in IVUS interpretation; *side lobes* and *ghost* artifacts also generated from strong echoreflectors such as calcium and stent metal [5]. In longitudinal or L-mode display, catheter motion artifacts during the pullback results in a "saw tooth" appearance (Figure 7.2).

Catheter position also has an important role in image quality. Off-axis position of the catheter can alter vessel geometry in an elliptical fashion to mislead the operator to overestimate the lumen and vessel area [15]. Axial (antegrade–retrograde) movement of the IVUS probe during the cardiac cycle scrambles consecutive image slices that can have implications for three-dimensional reconstruction and attempts to assess coronary artery compliance [16].

Image acquisition and presentation

Two important consensus documents have been published: Standards for the acquisition, measurement, and reporting of IVUS studies: a report of the American College of Cardiology Task Force on Clinical Expert Consensus Documents [12] and the Study Group on Intracoronary Imaging of the Working Group of Coronary Circulation and the Subgroup on Intravascular Ultrasound of the Working Group of Echocardiography of the European Society of Cardiology [17].

IVUS is displayed as a tomographic cross-sectional view. A longitudinal view (L-mode or long-view) can be also displayed, but this should be done only when using motorized transducer pullback. Longitudinal representation of IVUS images is useful for lengths measurements, for interpolation of shadowed deep arterial structures (i.e., external elastic membrane behind calcium or stent metal).

There are advantages and disadvantages to using manual or motorized pullback; however, motorized pullback is usually preferable. Using motorized transducer pullback allows assessment of lesion length, volumetric measurements, consistent and systematic IVUS image acquisition among different operators, and uniform and reproducible image acquisition for multicenter and serial studies [18,19].

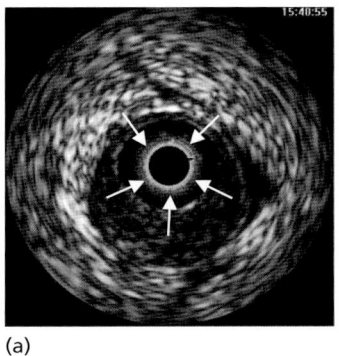 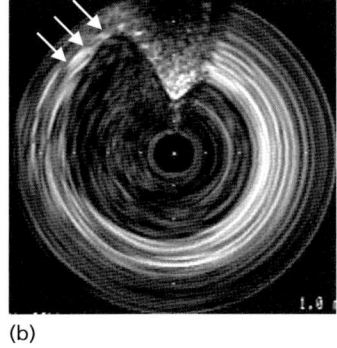 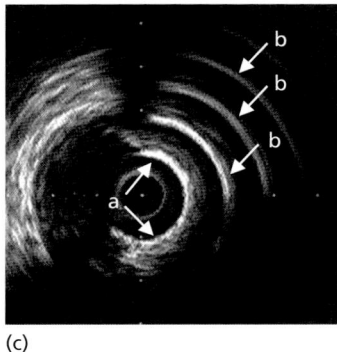

(a) (b) (c)

Figure 7.1 Three examples of artifacts. In (a), ring-down artifacts in an electronic-array system image, near-field bright halos (arrows) close to the face of the catheter can obscure the area immediately adjacent to the catheter. In (b), non-uniform rotation distortion (NURD) occurs only with mechanical systems. Part of the image is expanded causing deformation of the image in its circumferential view—the image appears elliptical (arrows). In (c), reverberations are repetitive echoes of the same structure. This is an example of reverberations from calcium. The arcs of calcium are indicated by the arrows **a**, and the false structures (reverberations) are indicated by arrows **b**.

In standard image acquisition after anticoagulation and intra-coronary nitroglycerin administration, the IVUS catheter should be placed distal to the segment of interest (at least 10 mm of distal reference), and a continuous pullback to the aorta should be recorded. The preferred pullback speed is 0.5 mm/s.

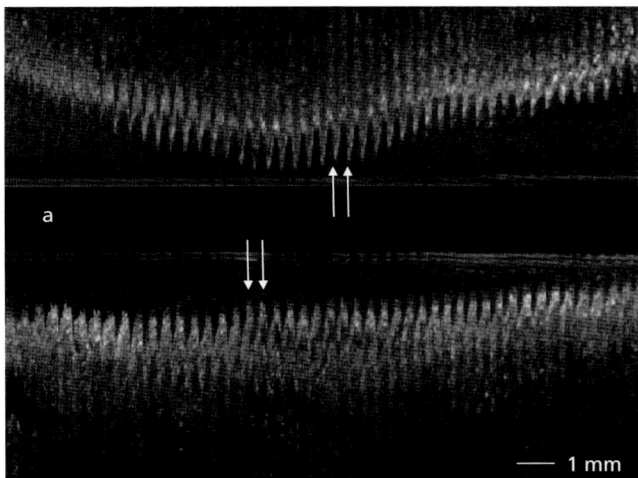

Figure 7.2 Longitudinal image reconstruction (or L-mode) is shown. There is excessive motion of the transducer **a** relative to the artery, causing zigzag or sawtooth appearance (white arrows). This artifact is more of a problem with the right and circumflex arteries, because of the wide atrioventricular groove movement between systole and diastole.

Normal artery morphology

The ultrasound appearance of normal human arteries *in vitro* and *in vivo* has been reported [3,7,20–22]. In muscular arteries such as the coronary tree there are three layers: intima, media, and adventitia. Normal intima thickness increases with age, from a single endothelial cell at birth to a mean of 60 μm at 5 years to 220–250 μm at 30–40 years of age [23]. The definition of abnormal intimal thickness by IVUS is still controversial; in general, the threshold of "normal intimal thickness" is <300 μm (0.3 mm). The innermost layer of the intima is relatively echogenic compared with the lumen and media and displayed on the screen as a single bright concentric echo. The lower ultrasound reflectance of the media is due to its homogeneous smooth muscle cells distribution and smaller amounts of collagen, elastic tissue, and proteoglycans. The thickness of media histologically averages 200 μm, but medial thinning occurs in the presence of atherosclerosis [24]. In advanced atherosclerotic disease, the media may not appear as a distinct layer around the full circumference of the vessel; media thickness of coronary arteries is inversely related to lesion thickness [25]. The intima–media border is poorly defined because the intimal layer reflects ultrasound more strongly than the media. Conversely, the media–adventitia border, consistent with the location of the external elastic membrane (EEM), is accurately defined because a step-up in echo reflectivity occurs without *blooming*. The outermost layer, the adventitia, is composed of collagen and elastic tissue; it is 300–500 μm thick. The outer border of the adventitia is also indistinct due to echo reflectivity similar to the surrounding peri-adventitial tissues [13,21]. Therefore, the normal coronary artery is either (i) "mono-layered" in cases of intimal thickness <100 μm because of a 40 MHz IVUS catheter resolution is less than 100 μm; or (ii) "three-layered" to include a bright echo from the intima, a dark zone from the media, and bright surrounding echoes from the adventitia (Figure 7.3).

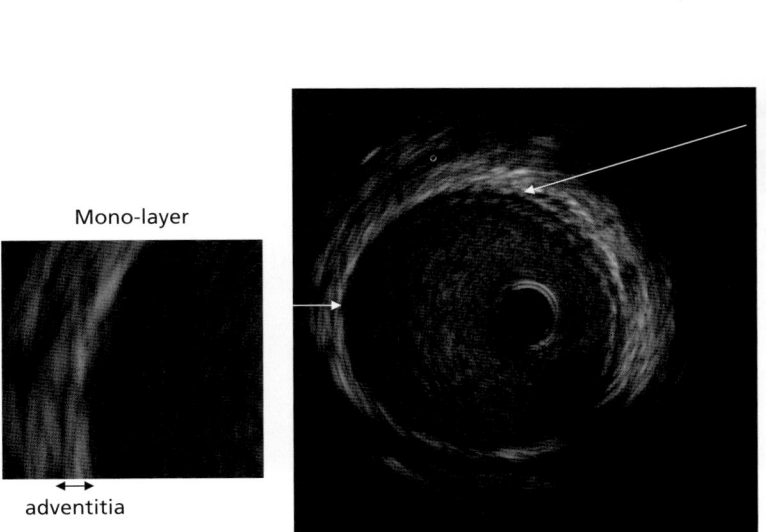

Figure 7.3 Normal coronary artery morphology in cross-sectional view. In the magnified image on the right, the bright inner layer (intima), middle echolucent zone (media), and outer bright layer (adventitia) are representative of the "three-layered" appearance of intravascular ultrasound (IVUS). In the magnified image on the left, only the outer bright adventitial layer is representative of the "mono-layered" appearance.

Quantitative analysis

In non-stented lesions there are two strong acoustic interfaces that are well visualized by ultrasound: the leading edge of the intima and the outer border of the media (or media–adventitia junction). Therefore, two cross-sectional area (CSA) measurements can be defined by IVUS: the lumen CSA and the media–adventitia CSA (or EEM CSA). The atheroma or plaque&media (P&M) complex is calculated as EEM minus lumen; the media cannot be measured as a distinct structure. Thus, complete quantification of a non-stented lesion is possible by tracing the EEM and lumen areas of the proximal reference, lesion, and distal reference; calculating derived measures (minimum and maximum EEM and lumen diameters, P&M area and thickness, and plaque burden; P&M divided by EEM); and measuring lesion length (distance between the proximal and distal reference) (Figure 7.4).

In stented vessels, the stent forms a third measurable structure (stent CSA). It appears as bright points along the circumference of the vessel. Complete quantification of a stented lesion is possible by tracing the EEM and lumen areas of the proximal and distal reference and the EEM, lumen, and stent areas of the stented lesion; calculating derived measures (minimum and maximum EEM, stent, and lumen diameters; peri-stent P&M area and thickness; and intra-stent intimal hyperplasia [IH, area and %IH]); and measuring stent length. With the use of motorized pullback, area measurements can be added to calculate volumes using Simpson's formula.

Qualitative analysis

Grayscale IVUS has some ability to differentiate plaque composition based on different echoreflectivity of the tissue. Atherosclerotic plaques are rarely homogeneous and contain a mixture of plaque components with different impedance (density). A standard approach is to compare the echointensity or "brightness" of the plaque to the surrounding adventitia that is used as a reference. Three basic types of lesions are distinguished according to plaque echogenicity: (i) "soft" or hypoechoic plaque does not reflect much ultrasound and appears dark with less echointensity compared to the adventitia (Figure 7.5); (ii) fibrous; and (iii) calcific plaques are characterized by equal or greater intensity than the adventitia. A plaque that is not so reflective as to cause shadowing is labeled "hard" or hyperechoic and is composed primarily of fibrous tissue (Figure 7.5). The presence of acoustic shadowing along with the brightest echoes and reverberations are characteristic of the presence of calcification (Figure 7.5).

Intimal hyperplasia due to in-stent restenosis often appears to have low echogenecity depending, in part, on age and adjunct therapies (i.e., brachytherapy) (Figure 7.6).

The identification of thrombus is difficult by IVUS. It may appear as lobulated hypoechoic mass within the lumen, scintillating echoes, a distinct interface between the presumed thrombus imaging and underlying plaque, and blood flow through the thrombus (Figure 7.7).

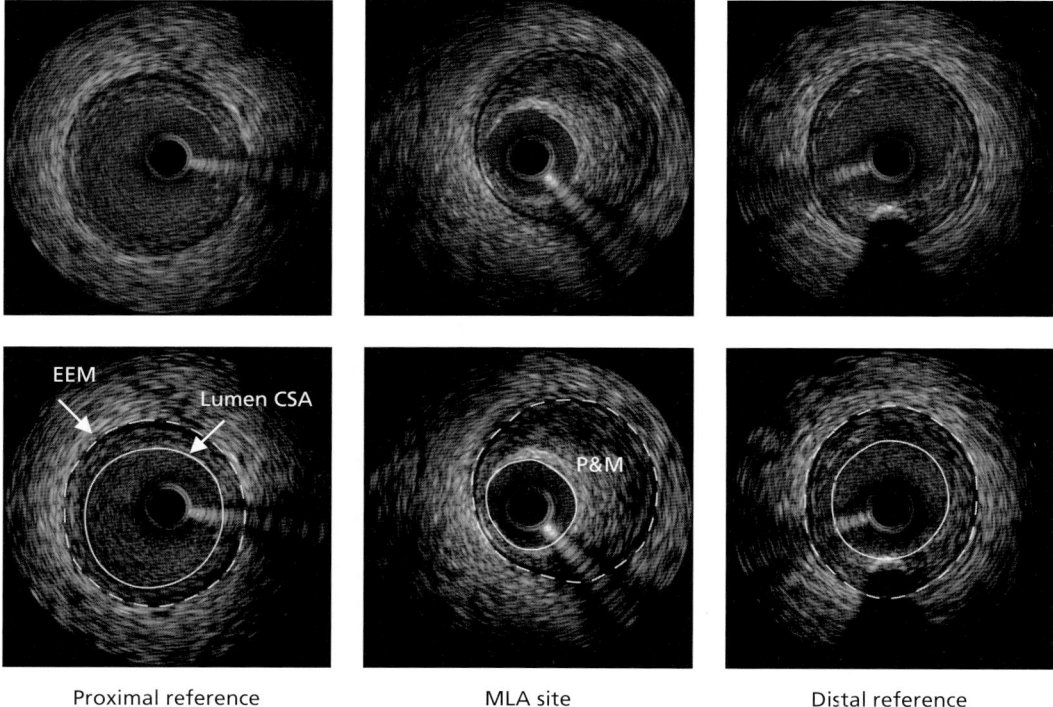

Proximal reference   MLA site   Distal reference

Figure 7.4 IVUS measurements pre-intervention in a non-stented artery. The proximal and distal reference and minimum lumen area (MLA) of the lesion are shown. The IVUS study is shown in duplicate: one unlabeled and one highlighted with lines to illustrate quantitative analysis. The dashed line highlights each external elastic membrane cross-sectional area (EEM CSA), and the solid line indicates each lumen interface (lumen CSA). The minimal lumen cross-sectional area (lumen CSA) at the lesion site is 2.1 mm². Between the EEM CSA and lumen CSA, the atheroma or plaque&media (P&M) complex is calculated.

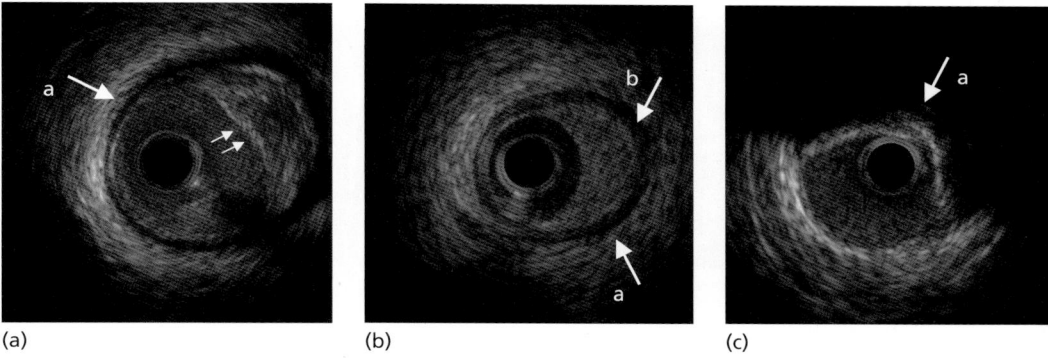

(a)   (b)   (c)

Figure 7.5 A pure soft or hypoechoic plaque is uncommon because atherosclerotic plaques are rarely homogeneous. (a) shows an example of a predominantly soft plaque—a thin fibrous cap (small arrows) and lipid core underlying it; the plaque is less bright than the adventitia **a**. In (b), fibrous plaque or hyperechoic plaque is shown. Hyperechoic plaque is as bright as or brighter than the adventitia **a** without shadowing. In this eccentric plaque, the thickness of the media behind the thickest part of the plaque **b** is an artifact caused by attenuation of the beam as it passes through the hyperechoic plaque. In reality, the media becomes thinner with increasing atherosclerosis. Note that the media behind the thinnest part of the plaque is also thinner—without artifacts. (c) shows superficial calcium—defined as calcium **a** that is closer to the intima than it is to the adventitia. Calcium shadows the deeper arterial structures; in this case, the arc of calcification is ~180°.

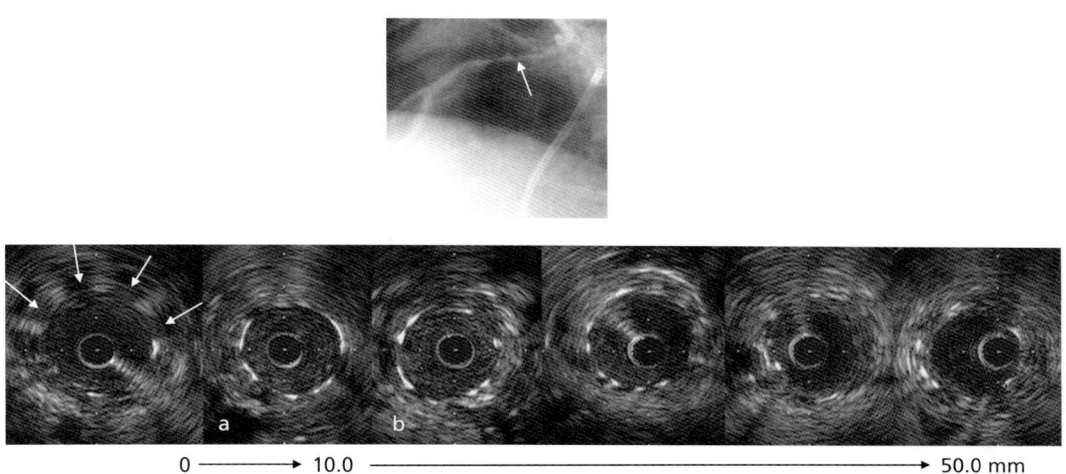

0 ——→ 10.0 ——————————————————————→ 50.0 mm

Figure 7.6 This patient presented with diffuse in-stent restenosis (white arrow on angiogram). Neointimal tissue is packed around the IVUS catheter at **a** and **b**, where the maximum amount of intimal hyperplasia occurs. There is also stent malapposition proximally (white arrows). Source: Mintz 2005 [5]. Reproduced with permission of Taylor & Francis.

Comparison of IVUS and angiography

Coronary angiography depicts the coronary anatomy as a longitudinal silhouette of the lumen. Conversely, IVUS with its tomographic perspective directly images the lumen, atheroma, and the vessel wall. Coronary angiography significantly underestimates the presence, severity, and extent of atherosclerosis compared to IVUS [19,26,27]. Furthermore, IVUS routinely shows significant atherosclerosis in angiographically "normal" segments in patients undergoing PCI [28]. This phenomenon may be explained by three major factors: (i) coronary atherosclerosis is often diffusely distributed involving long segments of the vessel containing no truly normal reference segment for comparison; (ii) complex atherosclerotic plaques are not appreciated by the two-dimensional "silhouette"; and (iii), most importantly, the presence of arterial wall remodeling [12]. In some circumstances diffuse, concentric, and symmetrical coronary disease can affect the entire length of

the vessel resulting in an angiographic appearance of a small artery with minimal luminal narrowing.

Coronary artery remodeling

Arterial remodeling of the vessel wall at the site of coronary plaques was originally described from necropsy examinations by Glagov *et al.* [29] and later validated *in vivo* by IVUS imaging [30]. "Positive," "outward," or "expansive" remodeling is defined as an increased in arterial dimensions; and "negative," "inward," or "constrictive" remodeling is defined as a smaller arterial dimension. Positive remodeling occurs as a compensatory increase in local vessel size in response to increasing plaque burden, especially during early stages of atherosclerosis [31]. An absolute reduction in lumen dimensions typically does not occur until the lesion occupies, on average, an estimated 40–50% of the area within the EEM (40–50% plaque burden) [29]. Conversely, negative remodeling has been

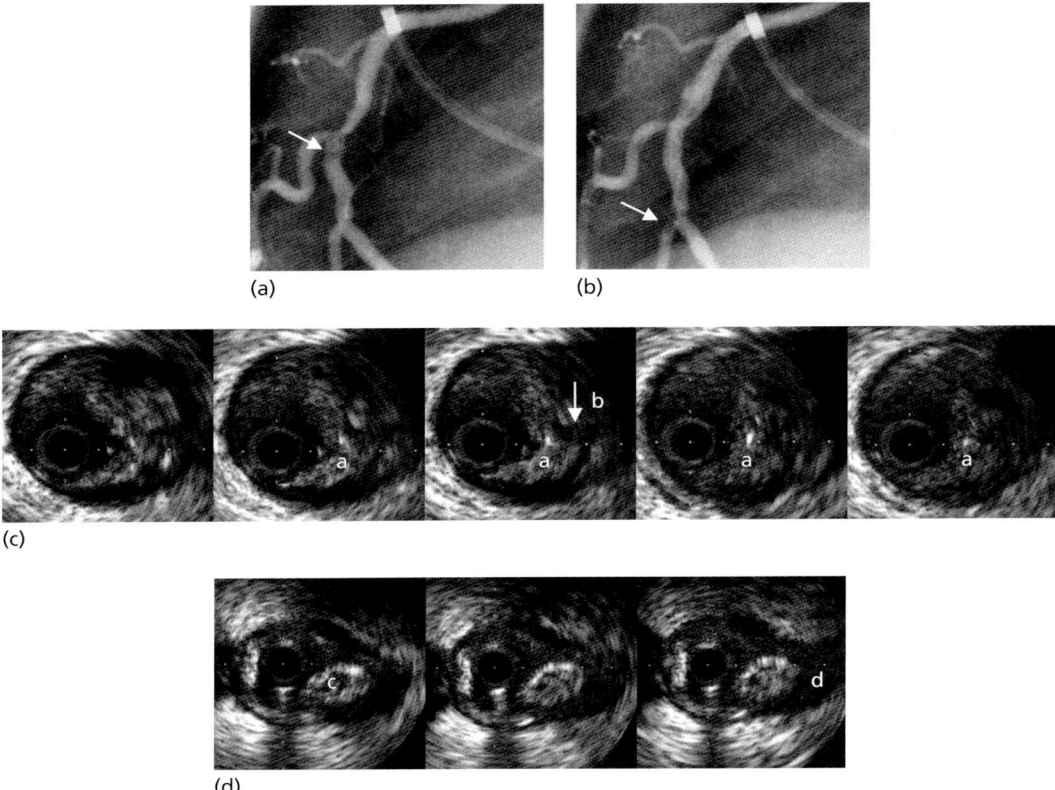

Figure 7.7 An unstable plaque before (white arrow in a) and after balloon angioplasty (b). A new post-balloon angioplasty filling defect at the origin of the acute marginal branch is shown (white arrow in b). Pre-intervention IVUS (c) shows a lobulated and penduculated thrombus **a** and a distinct interface with the underlying vessel wall **b**. Post-balloon angioplasty IVUS (d) shows the thrombus **c** that has embolized into the acute marginal branch **d**. Source: Mintz 2005 [5]. Reproduced with permission of Taylor & Francis.

implicated in the development of native significant stenosis in the absence of plaque accumulation (Figure 7.8) [32,33].

A number of definitions of remodeling have been proposed and published [12,30–36]. One definition compares the lesion EEM CSA to the average of the proximal + distal reference EEM CSA; positive remodeling is an index >1.0 and negative remodeling <1.0. A second definition defines positive remodeling as a lesion EEM greater than the proximal reference EEM, intermediate remodeling as a lesion EEM between the proximal and distal reference EEM, and negative remodeling as a lesion EEM less than the distal reference EEM. Using a third definition, arterial remodeling has been calculated by a remodeling index (lesion/reference EEM); positive remodeling is an index >1.05, intermediate remodeling is an index of 0.95–1.05, and negative remodeling is an index <0.95.

It is important to note that all of these remodeling definitions are based on a comparison of the reference EEM and lesion EEM. Accordingly, because both reference and lesion sites may have undergone quantitative changes in EEM during the atherosclerotic process, the evidence of remodeling derived from this index is relative and indirect. It depends on the definition of the reference, and the classification of an individual lesion depends on the definition used.

More recently, Inaba et al. [37], have reported a novel concept of remodeling, in which positive (RI >1.0) and negative (RI <0.88) lesion site remodeling was associated with unanticipated non-culprit lesion major adverse cardiac events in the PROSPECT study.

Unstable lesions

In patients with acute coronary syndromes, culprit lesions more frequently exhibit positive remodeling and a large plaque area; conversely, patients with a stable clinical presentation more frequently show negative remodeling and a smaller plaque area [34]. Echolucent plaques are also more common in unstable than in stable patients. In addition, unstable lesions have less calcium than stable lesions; and when present, calcific deposits in unstable lesions are small, focal, and deep [38]. Plaque ruptures can occur with varying clinical presentations although they are more often associated with acute coronary syndromes (Figure 7.9) [39]. Multiple ruptured plaques have been reported in patients with acute coronary syndromes; their prevalence, however, is the subject of controversy [40,41]. Typical IVUS features of acute myocardial infarction include plaque rupture, thrombus, positive remodeling, attenuated plaque, spotty calcification, and thin-cap fibroatheroma (Figure 7.10) [42].

Attenuated plaque is defined as hypoechoic or mixed atheroma with deep ultrasound attenuation without calcification or very dense fibrous plaque. Wu et al. [43] reported that 78% of the patients with acute myocardial infarction had attenuated plaques in the Harmonizing Outcomes With Revascularization and Stents in Acute Myocardial Infarction (HORIZONS-AMI) trial. Lee et al. [44] documented that attenuated plaque was observed in 39.6% of patients with ST-segment elevation myocardial infarction (STEMI) and 17.6% of those with non-ST-segment elevation myocardial

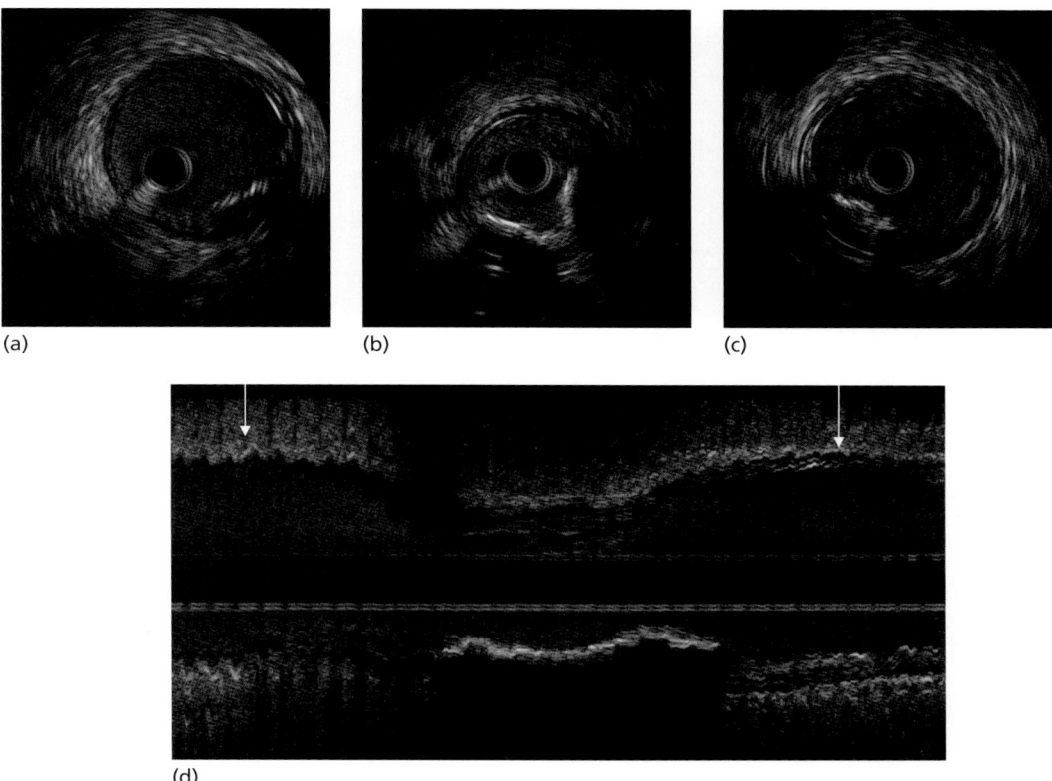

Figure 7.8 An eccentric, calcific, and small plaque accumulation leading to negative remodeling. (a) and (c) refer to proximal and distal vessel references and their respective longitudinal views (white arrows in d). In (b) notice how the vessel cross-sectional area (or EEM) is smaller than both the proximal and distal vessels. The longitudinal view depicts clearly the artery shrinkage at the lesion site.

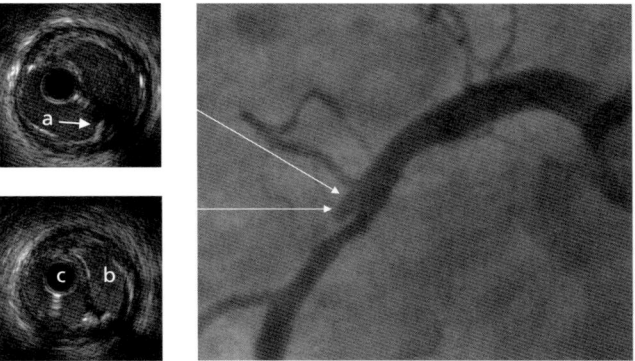

Figure 7.9 This patient presented with an acute coronary syndrome and a complex right coronary lesion (white arrows) and disrupted plaque by IVUS. The IVUS imaging run shows the residual fibrous cap **a**, the evacuated plaque cavity **b**, and the true lumen containing the catheter **c**.

infarction (NSTEMI). Plaque ruptures and attenuated plaques are considered to be unstable and have been identified in both culprit and non-culprit lesions of patients with (STEMI) [45]. Histopathologically, the vast majority of attenuated plaques correspond to either a fibroatheroma with a necrotic core or pathologic intimal thickening with a lipid pool; almost all segments with superficial echo attenuation indicated the presence of an fibroatheroma with an advanced necrotic core [46]. Most importantly,

attenuated plaque has been associated with the occurrence of microvascular obstruction after primary PCI [47], no-reflow phenomenon [43], and with late acquired stent malapposition in patients with STEMI [48].

Intermediate lesions and left main coronary artery disease

Coronary angiography underestimates stenosis severity most markedly in arteries with a 50–75% plaque burden and in patients with multivessel disease [27,49]. In patients with stable coronary artery disease, fractional flow reserve (FFR) is the well-established physiologic index to assess the functional significance of a coronary stenosis. Recent studies have used FFR ≤ 0.80 as the optimal cut-off point to guide revascularization [50,51], and have reported correlation between FFR values and anatomic parameters (specially minimum lumen area; MLA) derived from IVUS or optical coherence tomography (OCT) [52–59]. Of the IVUS-derived measurements, MLA cut-off values to predict FFR had been widely reported [60]. The correlation between MLA cut-off points and ischemic FFR threshold ranged from 2.0 to 3.9 mm^2 in non-left main coronary artery (LMCA) intermediate stenosis and from 4.5 to 5.9 mm^2 in LMCA stenosis [60]. The FIRST (Fractional Flow Reserve and Intravascular Ultrasound Relationship) study, based on a multicenter, prospective registry in the USA and Europe proposed 3.07 mm^2 as a best cut-off value to define the presence of myocardial ischemia [58]. In the largest sample-size and international multicenter study with 822 patients (881 lesions), Han *et al.* [59] found that best cut-off value of IVUS-MLA to define the functional

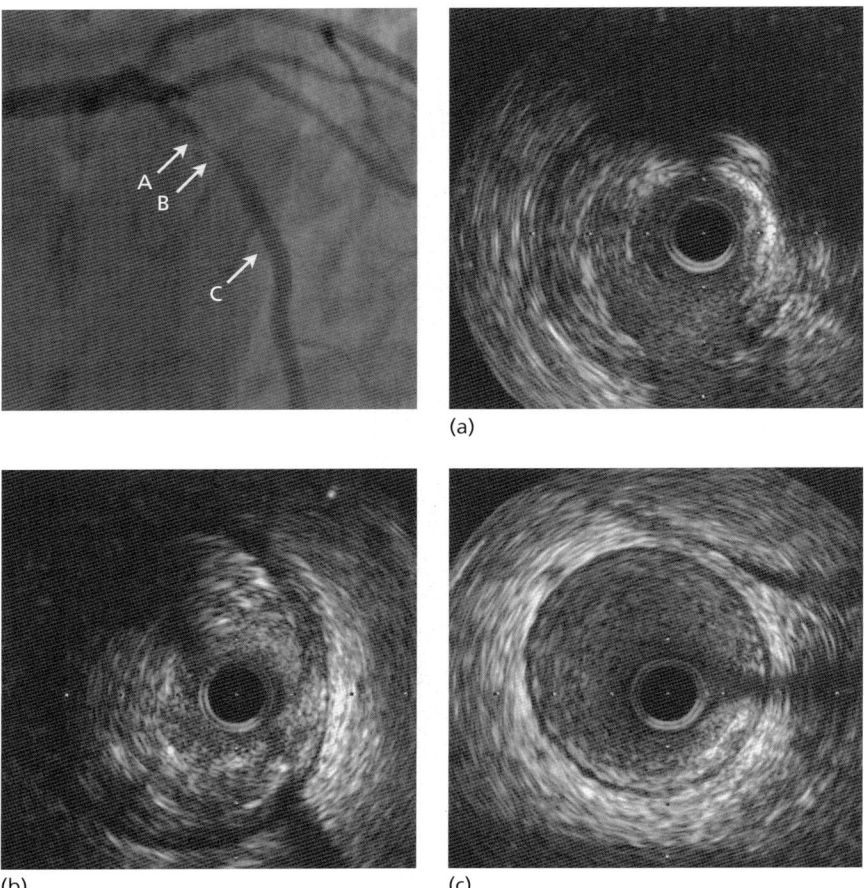

Figure 7.10 This patient presented with STEMI. Note a severe lesion in the angiogram after manual thrombectomy. The corresponding IVUS image shows the ruptured plaque cavity (a). Distal to the plaque rupture on the angiogram (b) is an echo-attenuated plaque; attenuation is defined as shadowing or attenuation of the ultrasound signal (loss of echoes) in the absence of calcification. Also note positive remodeling. Normal reference vessel with three-layer aspect (c).

significance (FFR <0.8) to be 2.75 mm², further subgroup analysis showed that ethnicity influenced on the cut-off value of MLA, it was 2.75 mm² in Asians and 3.0 mm² in Westerners. A meta-analysis of 11 studies comparing IVUS-MLA with FFR for assessment of intermediate lesions showed that the weighted overall mean MLA cut-off was 2.61 mm² in non-LMCA and 5.35 mm² in LMCA to predict a functional stenosis [61].

LMCA atherosclerosis is often underestimated by coronary angiography. Several studies have showed that a very high percentage of patients with angiographically normal LMCA have disease by IVUS [62–64]. Conversely, only that half of angiographically ambiguous LMCA stenosis had a significant stenosis, especially in ostial lesions [65]. The main reasons for the discrepancy between angiography and IVUS are the following: (i) diffuse atherosclerotic plaque involvement may lead to a lack of a normal reference segment; (ii) a short LMCA makes identification of a normal reference segment difficult; (iii) the presence of arterial remodeling; (iv) the correlation between angiography and necropsy or IVUS appears to be better in non-LMCA lesions possibly because of unique geometric issues in the LMCA [66]; and (v) significant inter- and intraobserver variability in the angiographic assessment of LMCA disease [67], especially in ostium location [68].

Other unusual lesion morphology

During coronary angiography it is common to encounter unusual appearing lesions that elude accurate characterization despite thorough examination using multiple radiographic projections. The use of IVUS allows accurate characterization of unusual morphology: filling defects, aneurysms, and spontaneous dissections. While most filling defects are true thrombi, a small percentage are highly calcified plaque (Figure 7.11) or even calcified nodules, an unusual form of vulnerable plaque.

In an IVUS analysis of 77 angiographically diagnosed aneurysms, 27% were true aneurysms (Figure 7.12), 4% were pseudoaneurysms (Figure 7.13), 16% were complex plaques, and 53% were normal arterial segments adjacent to stenoses [59].

By IVUS, a spontaneous dissection appears as a medial dissection with an intramural hematoma occupying some or all of the dissected false lumen without identifiable intimal tears and without a communication between the true and false lumens, typically in a non-atherosclerotic artery.

In-stent neoatherosclerosis has been recently described as an important mechanism of late stent failure (i.e., restenosis and stent thrombosis). The development of neoatherosclerosis appears to occur more frequently and much earlier following DES than bare

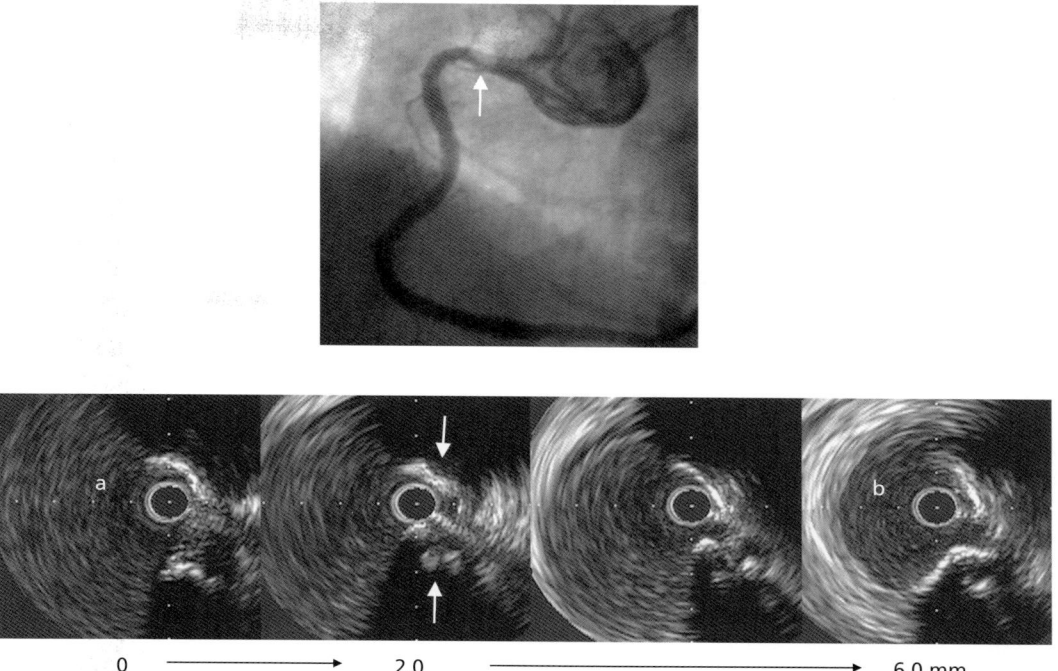

Figure 7.11 Diagnostic IVUS was performed to assess this angiographic filling defect at the proximal right coronary artery (white arrow in the angiogram). The IVUS imaging run begins at the ostium **a** of the right coronary artery to beyond the filling defect **b**. Note the calcification (white arrow in the IVUS) without lumen compromise. Source: Mintz 2005 [5]. Reproduced with permission of Taylor & Francis.

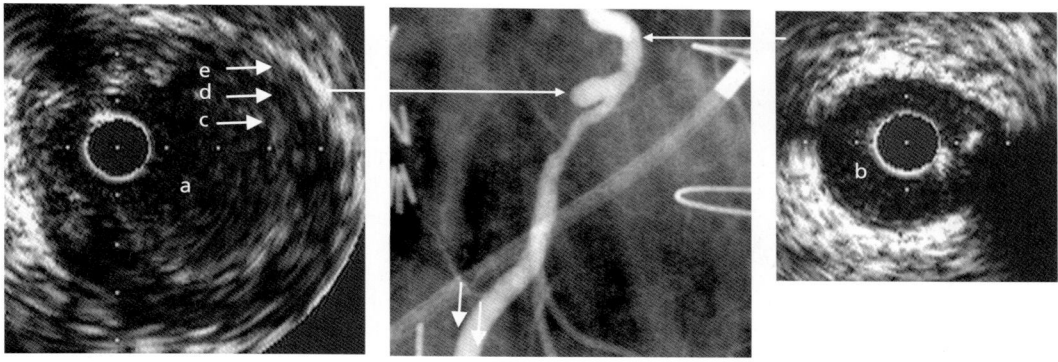

Figure 7.12 This patient presented with a true saccular aneurysm in the right coronary artery. IVUS imaging shows the aneurysm **a** and the proximal vessel **b**. Note that the intima **c**, the media **d**, and the adventitia **e** are intact, making this a true aneurysm. Source: Mintz 2005 [5]. Reproduced with permission of Taylor & Francis.

metal stent (BMS) implantation. Importantly, fibrous cap thickness negatively correlates with follow-up time, especially after DES [69].

Guidance for stent implantation
Stent sizing
Pre-interventional IVUS is performed to assess stenosis severity and plaque composition and distribution, measure reference vessel size, and measure lesion length. As a result, stent size can be chosen more accurately than solely by angiography. There are a number of paradigms that can be used. Stent size can be selected by identifying the maximum reference *lumen* diameter (proximal or distal to the lesion); it results in stent upsizing without an increase in complications. At the other extreme, stents can be sized to the "true vessel,"

"media-to-media," or mid-wall dimensions to reflect the amount of angiographically silent disease and, in most cases, the extent of positive remodeling, not just vessel size. Typically, this measurement will be larger than reference *lumen* reference and, thus, should be used only by experienced operators who understand its limitations.

IVUS measures lesion length more accurately than angiography because IVUS eliminates foreshortening, vessel tortuosity, or bend points.

Stent expansion and malapposition
IVUS studies have shown that lumen enlargement after stent implantation is a combination of vessel expansion and plaque redistribution/embolization, not plaque compression [70–72]. Plaque

reduction in patients with acute coronary syndromes is attributed to plaque or thrombus embolization. Intrusion or prolapse of plaque through the stent mesh into the lumen is more common in acute coronary syndromes and in saphenous vein graft lesions. Importantly, after stent implantation there is a significant residual plaque burden behind the stent struts that almost always measures 50–75% at the center of the lesion. Thus, the stent CSA always looks smaller than the EEM even when the stent is fully expanded.

Apposition refers to the contact between the stent struts to the arterial wall. Incomplete stent apposition is defined as one or more

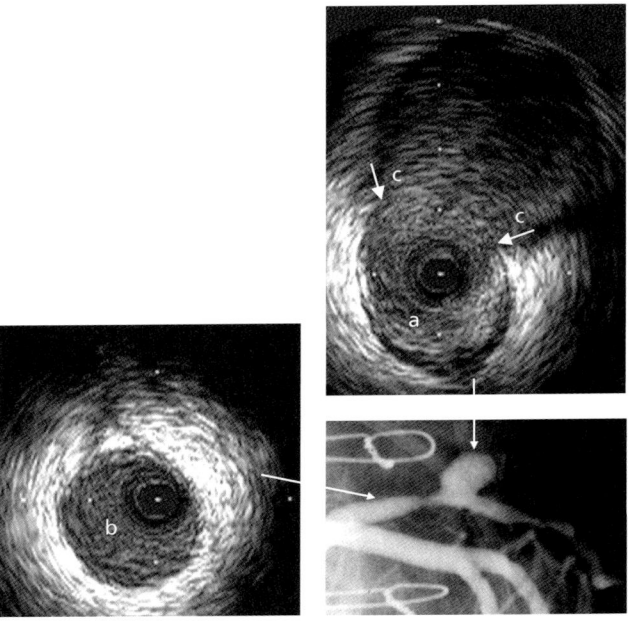

Figure 7.13 This patient underwent a previous directional coronary atherectomy of a lesion, in the left anterior descending artery, during which the artery was perforated. Follow-up catheterization showed both restenosis and a large aneurysm on angiography. The IVUS shows the body of the aneurism **a** and the eccentric proximal restenotic lesion **b**. Notice that the adventitia stops at the point of transition from the vessel to the aneurism **c**, indicating loss of vessel wall integrity and making this, in fact, a pseudoaneurysm. Source: Mintz 2005 [5]. Reproduced with permission of Taylor & Francis.

struts clearly separated from vessel wall with evidence of blood speckles behind the strut (Figure 7.14). There is no conclusive evidence suggesting that isolated acute incomplete stent apposition (in the absence of concomitant underexpansion) is associated with adverse clinical outcomes. The incidence of post-procedural incomplete stent apposition with DES has been reported comparable to that with BMS, ranging from 7.0% to 16.2% [73,74].

IVUS-guided stent implantation and predictors of restenosis and thrombosis

The two main uses of IVUS are to insure optimal stent expansion (stent CSA) and full coverage of the lesion (especially with DES implantation). In the majority of pre- DES studies, IVUS use optimized stent expansion; and the initially larger minimum stent area (MSA) achieved was associated with a lower restenosis rate [75–83]. In a meta-analysis by Parise et al. [84] evaluating 2193 patients from five randomized studies, IVUS guidance was associated with a significantly larger post-procedure angiographic minimum lumen diameter (MLD), and was also associated with a significantly lower rate of 6-month angiographic restenosis, a significant reduction in the revascularization rate, and overall major adverse cardiac events.

At the introduction of DES, the importance of optimal stent deployment was initially underestimated. Suboptimal stent expansion with both BMS and DES was a risk factor for restenosis and target vessel revascularization, but also for stent thrombosis [85–88]. Roy et al. [89] reported that IVUS guidance during DES implantation had the potential to reduce both DES thrombosis and the need for repeat revascularization. In this study, 884 patients undergoing IVUS-guided DES implantation were compared with 884 propensity-score matched patients undergoing DES implantation with angiographic guidance alone. At 30 days and at 12 months, a lower rate of definite stent thrombosis using the ARC definition was seen in the IVUS-guided group (0.5% vs. 1.4%; p = 0.046) and (0.7% vs. 2.0%; p = 0.014), respectively. At 1 year, target lesion revascularization (TLR) was also lower in the IVUS-guided group (5.1% vs. 7.2%; p = 0.07). A multicenter MAIN-COMPARE registry of LMCA interventions showed that in 201 matched pairs of the overall population, patients treated with IVUS-guided DES implantation had better 3-year survival than patients in whom IVUS was not used to guide LMCA DES implantation (4.7% vs. 16.0%, log-rank p = 0.048). Finally, a recent meta-analysis of outcomes after IVUS-guided vs. angiography-guided DES implantation in 26,503 patients enrolled in three randomized trials and 14 observational studies,

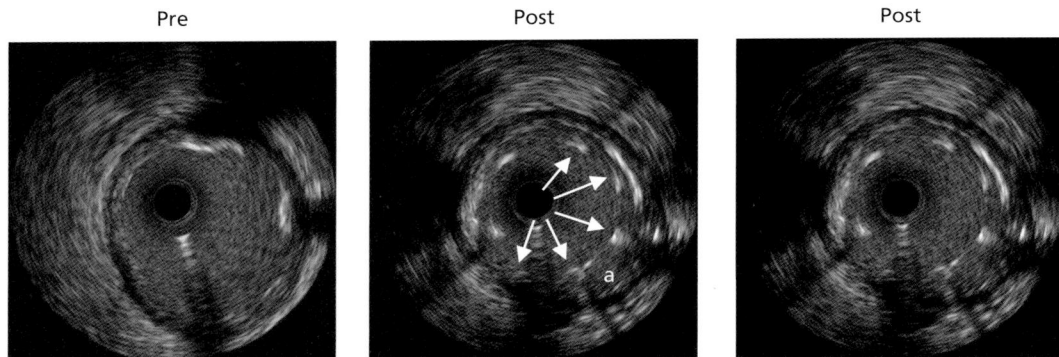

Pre | Post | Post

Figure 7.14 Acute stent malapposition. Notice the space between the stent strut and the intima and the blood speckle behind the stent struts **a**. Five stent struts are malapposed (white arrows). Because of stent malapposition, the stent area (9.4 mm²) is smaller than the lumen area (14.4 mm²). The post-stent implantation IVUS image is shown in duplicate.

demonstrated that IVUS-guided PCI was associated with a significantly lower risk of TLR (odds ratio (OR) 0.81, 95% CI 0.66–1.00; p=0.046). In addition, the risk of death (OR 0.61, 95% CI 0.48–0.79; p <0.001), MI (OR 0.57, 95% CI 0.44–0.75; p <0.001), and stent thrombosis (OR 0.59, 95% CI 0.47–0.75; p <0.001) were also decreased [90].

Complications

IVUS has a higher sensitivity than angiography in identifying complications that can occur during PCI. Angiography tends to underestimate the presence and extent of dissection. Stent edge dissections are common because the junction between stent metal and reference segment tissue is a site of compliance mismatch. Edge dissections are more common when the stent ends in a reference segment that contains: (i) both plaque and normal vessel wall; or (ii) both calcific (or hard) and soft plaque elements (Figure 7.15). Dissection may not be visible by IVUS if the true lumen is severely stenotic and the ultrasound catheter presses the flap against the arterial wall or if the dissection occurs behind a calcified plaque that prevents accurate morphologic definition. In general, the treatment of coronary dissection with stent implantation depends on the combination of angiographic assessment, flow assessment, and signs or symptoms of ischemia, and residual IVUS MLA. Treatment of dissections

should be based on IVUS findings when they show evidence: (i) reduced lumen dimensions below the threshold for an optimum result; (ii) impingement of the dissection flap on the IVUS catheter; (iii) mobility; and (iv) increased length. In general, minor edge dissections should not be treated unless they result in lumen compromise; the vast majority have healed when imaged at follow-up.

Intramural hematoma is a variant of dissection. Blood accumulates in the medial space; the EEM expands outward, and the internal elastic membrane is pushed inward to cause lumen compromise. Intramural hematomas are typically hyperechoic and crescent-shaped, with straightening of the internal elastic membrane [91]. In general, an intramural hematoma should be treated because of the propensity for propagation and lumen compromise.

Coronary perforation and rupture usually occurs with over-aggressive and/or oversized balloon dilatation although it can occur with a guidewire and stenting as well. In general, there are three distinct IVUS morphologic patterns indicating arterial rupture: (i) free blood speckle outside the EEM (Figure 7.16); (ii) extramural hematoma—an accumulation of blood outside the EEM; and (iii) less common, a new peri-adventitial echolucent interface representing contrast extravasation [3]. Acute management includes conservative strategy of monitoring to prolonged balloon inflations, covered stents, and surgery.

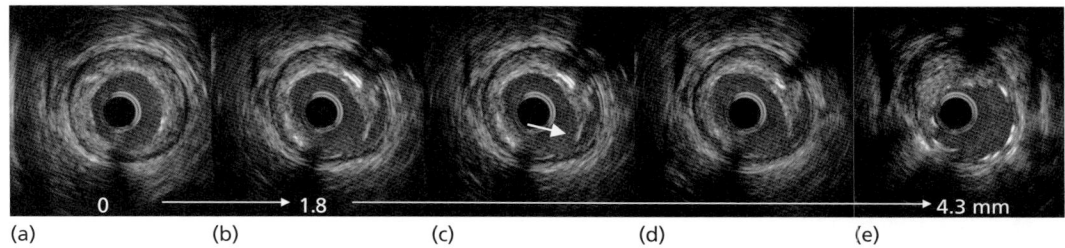

Figure 7.15 This patient presented with proximal edge dissection after coronary stenting. (a) depicts the proximal reference segment, which contains mild plaque. (e) shows the stent. Notice the tear into the lumen (arrow) and the dissection reaching the medial layer of the vessel (b, c, and d).

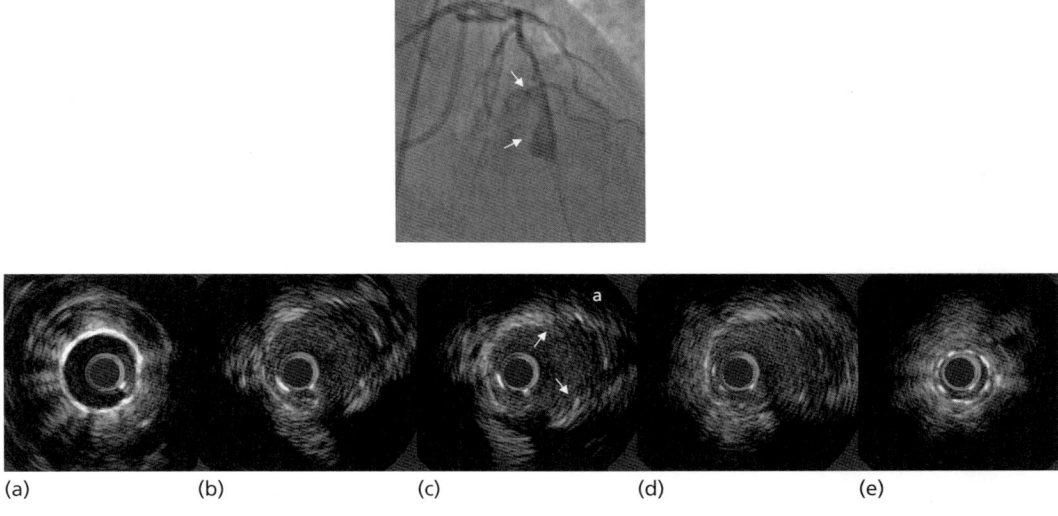

Figure 7.16 This patient presented with in-stent restenosis. After balloon dilatation, coronary perforation with myocardial contrast extravasation occurred, as seen by angiography (arrows). On IVUS, notice the small vessel with stenting at a distal site (image e) and the medial and adventitial discontinuation at the site of perforation (images b, c, and d, and arrows). Notice also an accumulation of blood outside the EEM **a**. One stent graft was implanted prior to IVUS assessment (image a), followed by an additional stent graft after IVUS assessment.

Serial IVUS studies of restenosis
Restenosis

Serial IVUS studies have shown that the main mechanism of restenosis in non-stented arteries is negative arterial remodeling (decrease in EEM area), not intimal hyperplasia [33]. Conversely, in-stent restenosis is primarily due to neointimal proliferation, not chronic stent recoil. By IVUS, %IH (IH volume divided by stent volume) has been shown to be consistent for each stent type. DES reduce restenosis by reducing IH from an average of 30% in BMS [92] to 3–5% in sirolimus-eluting stents (SES) [93,94], to 8–13% in polymer-based paclitaxel-eluting stents [95], 16% in zotarolimus-eluting stents [96], and to 6% in everolimus-eluting stents [97].

Stent underexpansion is a common finding in restenotic stents. It is the result of poor expansion at implantation, not chronic stent recoil. In an analysis of over 1000 patients with BMS restenosis, 15% had a MSA <4.5 mm^2 and 25% had a MSA of 4.5–6.0 mm^2. In addition, in 4.5% there were technical and mechanical complications of stent implantation that contributed to the restenosis. Examples of mechanical complications have included (i) missing the lesion (e.g., an aorto-ostial stenosis); (ii) stent "crush" (Figure 7.17); (iii) having the stent stripped off the balloon during the implantation procedure; or (iv) DES fracture (Figures 7.18 and 7.19) [98,99].

Acquired late stent malaposition

Late stent malapposition (LSM) is usually caused by regional vessel positive remodeling (Figure 7.20). LSM has been reported in 4–5% after BMS implantation [74,100]. Studies have suggested a higher incidence of LSM after DES (especially after first-generation DES) [101–105].

Hong *et al.* [74] showed *in vivo* that BMS implantation during primary PCI was an independent predictor of late incomplete stent apposition (ISA), but it was not linked to increased rates of adverse events at 3-year follow-up. Hoffmann *et al.* [103] studied the impact of LSM after SES implantation on 4-year clinical events. This pooled IVUS analysis from three randomized trials comparing SES with BMS showed that LSM at follow-up was more common after SES than after BMS (25% vs. 8.3%; p = 0.001); however, major adverse cardiac event free survival at 4 years was identical for those with and without LSM (11.1% vs. 16.3%, p = 0.48), and LSM was not a predictor for target lesion revascularization, target vessel failure, or late stent thrombosis during the 4-year follow-up period in either patient group.

Conversely, others have suggested that LSM can contribute to late stent thrombosis [106,107]. Cook *et al.* [107] studied 13 patients presenting with very late stent thrombosis (>1 year) after DES implantation and compared them with 144 control patients who did not experience stent thrombosis. Compared with DES controls,

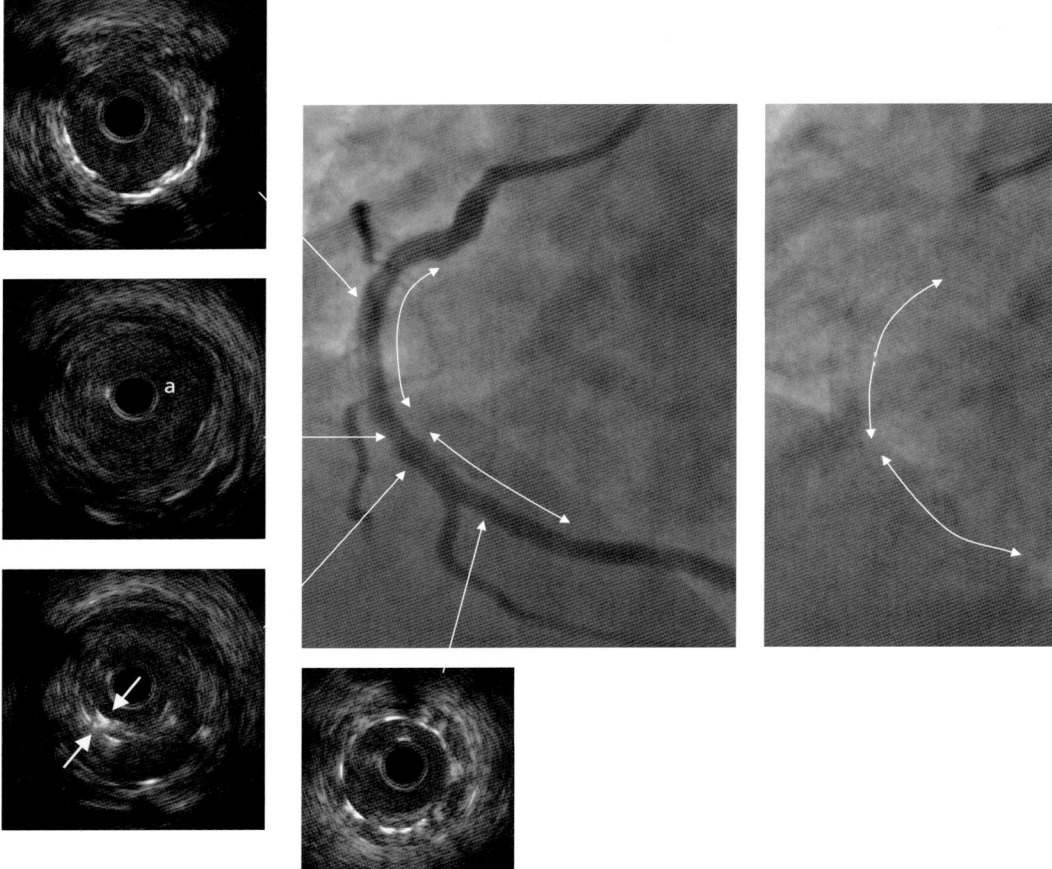

Figure 7.17 Stent crush at the right coronary artery detected at IVUS follow-up. Two stents have been implanted with a gap between them **a**. The proximal edge of the second stent has been crushed as shown on IVUS (arrows) but not on angiography.

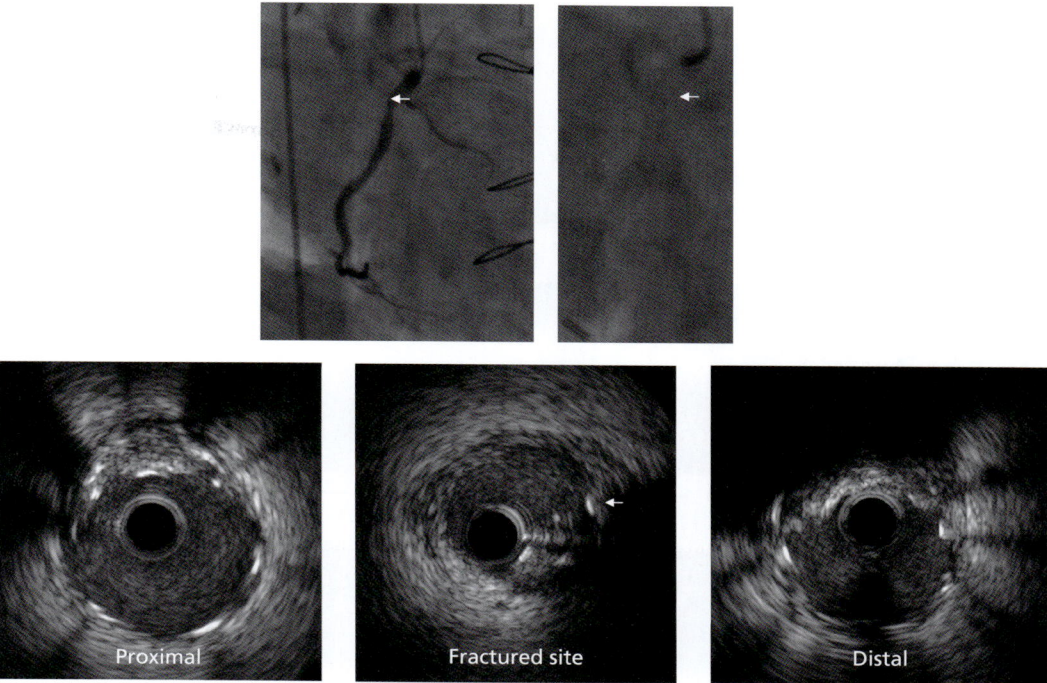

Figure 7.18 This patient presented with restenosis at follow-up after Cypher™ stent implantation in the right coronary artery (arrows on angiogram). Note the stent fracture with acquired transection on fluoroscopy. On IVUS, all stent struts are seen at proximal and distal references, whereas at the fracture site only one stent strut is seen (arrow).

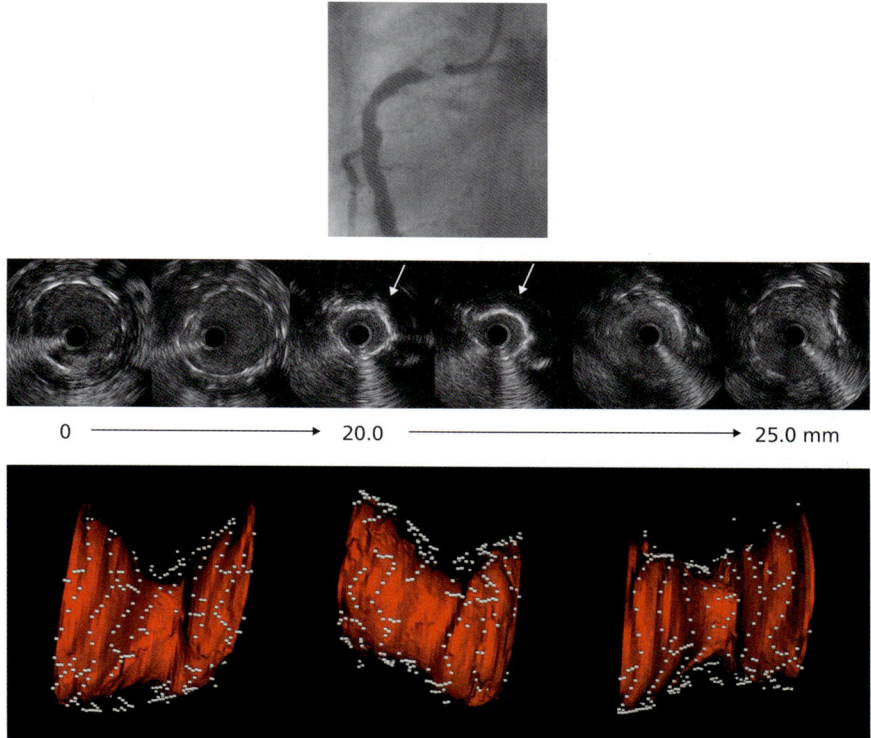

Figure 7.19 Stent fracture by coronary CT angiography and IVUS (arrows) at the ostial right coronary artery 1 year after Xience V everolimus-eluting stent.

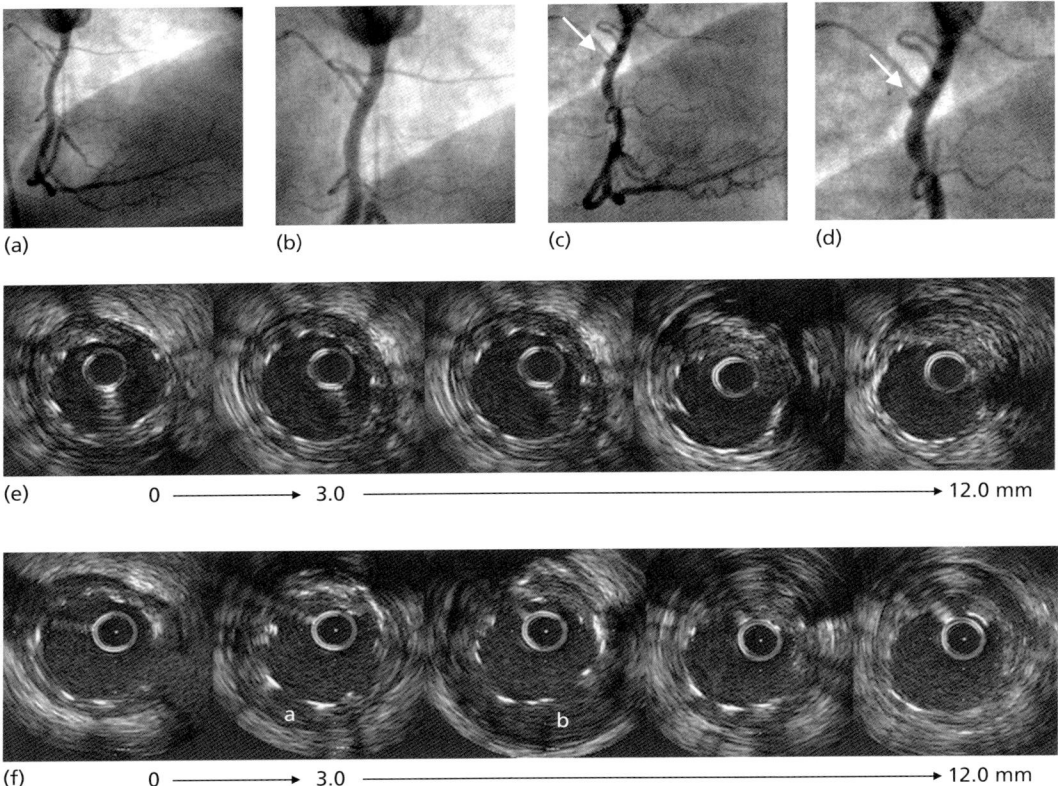

Figure 7.20 This patient underwent sirolimus-eluting stent (Cypher™) implantation in a right coronary stenosis. The final angiogram is shown in (a) and (b). At follow-up (c and d), there was a proximal and focal angiographic aneurysm (white arrows). Final (post-stent implantation) IVUS image is shown in (e), and the follow-up IVUS image is shown in (f). Note the late stent malapposition (a and b). At the site of maximum stent malapposition (b), there has been an increase in EEM CSA from 17.8 to 28.9 mm². The stent CSA (8.8 mm²) and the peri-stent P&M (8.9 mm²) have not changed. Source: Mintz GS, Weissman NJ. Intravascular ultrasound in the drug-eluting stent era. *J Am Coll Cardiol* 2006; **48**(3): 421–429.

patients with very late stent thrombosis had longer lesions and stents, more stents per lesion, and more stent overlap. Vessel cross-sectional area was significantly larger for the in-stent segment (28.6 ± 11.9 vs. 20.1 ± 6.7 mm²; p = 0.03) in very late stent thrombosis patients compared with DES controls, denoting evidence of positive arterial remodeling. Although IVUS was not performed at stent implantation in any patients of either group, incomplete stent apposition was more frequent (77% vs. 12%, p <0.001) and maximal incomplete stent apposition area was larger (8.3 ± 7.5 vs. 4.0 ± 3.8 mm²; p = 0.03) in patients with very late stent thrombosis compared with controls. Guagliumi *et al.* [108] demonstrated by combined IVUS and OCT assessments that the presence and magnitude of incomplete stent apposition were significantly higher in patients with DES thrombosis than in those without. Alfonso *et al.* [109] also identified ISA in patients with ST using IVUS and OCT (ISA was identified in 40% and 47% of patients, respectively). Kang *et al.* [110] performed OCT imaging in 33 patients with very late ST and found that in the DES group, 52% and 64% had ISA and thrombi, respectively, whereas no patients presented with ISA in the BMS group.

Flow disturbances and risk of delayed strut coverage both increase with incomplete stent apposition, especially with detachment distance >100 μm; suggesting a role of ISA in the pathogenesis of late stent thrombosis. Nevertheless, based on these studies with conflicting data, it is still speculative as to how to treat patients with IVUS or OCT findings of LSM.

Blood-free environment obtained during OCT image acquisition along with its higher axial resolution provides a sharper delineation of the stent–lumen interface compared with IVUS [105]. Several studies demonstrated that OCT is superior to IVUS in detecting ISA. Yet, OCT allows a cross-sectional and longitudinal level of assessment of strut-level analysis, which enables the diagnosis and quantification of ISA in each individual strut— and IVUS does not. Although IVUS and OCT complement each other in the identification and characterization of ISA, OCT should be preferred in clinical practice, especially in an era of bioresorbable vascular scaffold (BVS) (Figure 7.21).

Virtual histology and IVUS radiofrequency

The major limitation of IVUS is its limited spatial resolution (axial resolution of 100–200 μm and a lateral resolution of 250 μm). Although it can visualize deep structures, IVUS is not a suitable imaging modality for detecting thin fibrous cap that is one of the main components of vulnerable plaques (TCFA). Grayscale IVUS not only accurately assesses plaque composition, but atherosclerotic plaques in most cases have a complex and heterogeneous composition consisting of a mixture of plaque components [111]. These limitations have been partially overcome by analysis of the IVUS acoustic signal before demodulation and scan conversion. There are three modalities currently available: virtual histology IVUS (VH-IVUS, Volcano Therapeutics, Rancho Cordova, CA, USA), iMAP-IVUS

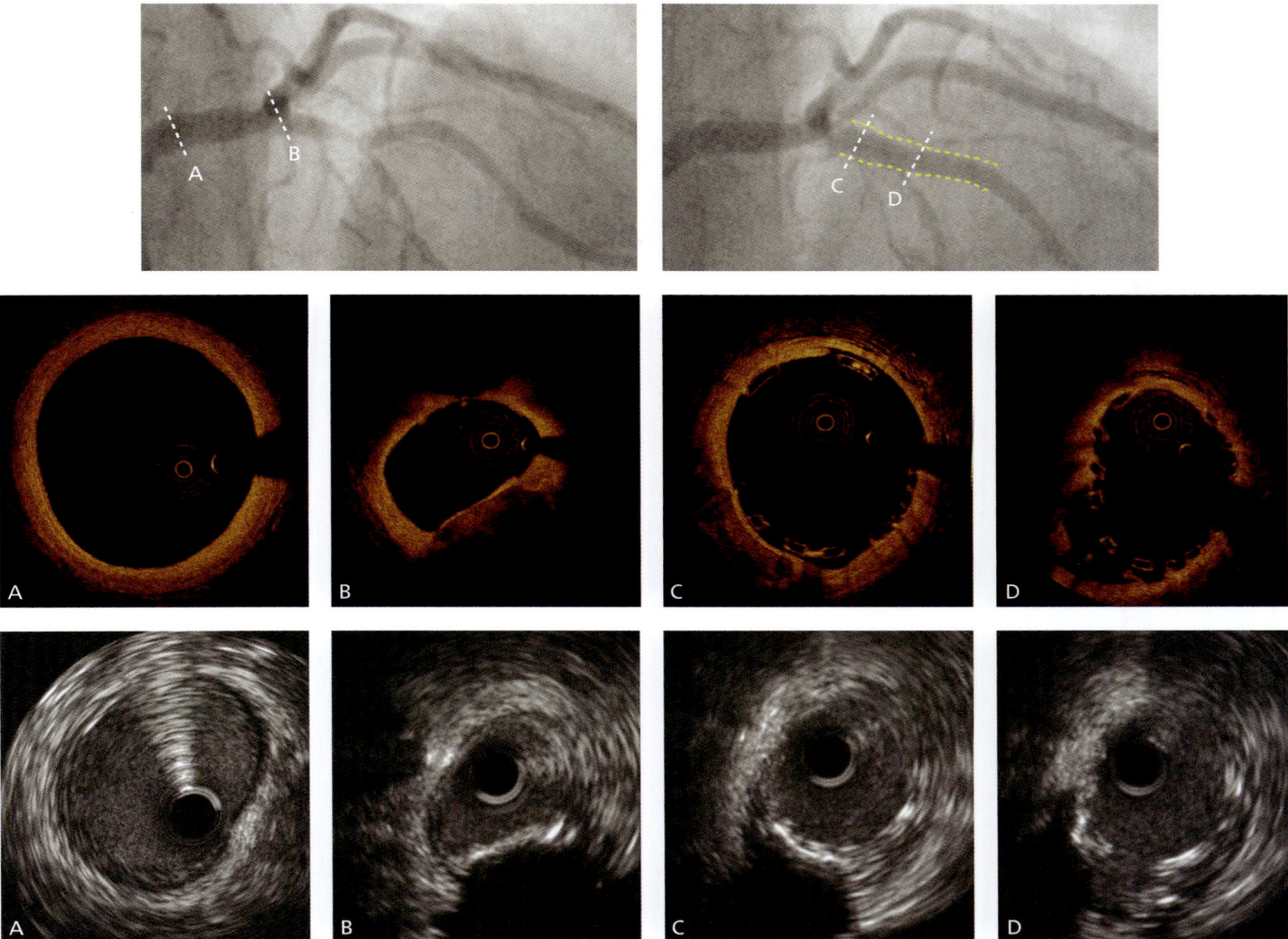

Figure 7.21 This patient underwent Absorb bioresorbable vascular scaffold implantation in proximal left anterior descending (LAD) and first diagonal. Co-registered images by optical coherence tomography (OCT) and IVUS after device implantation; OCT shows mild incomplete scaffold malappostion and dissection behind the strut at 8 o'clock (C); IVUS was unable to identify.

(Boston Scientific, Santa Clara, CA, USA), and integrated backscatter IVUS (IB-IVUS, YD, Nara, Japan).

To date, only VH-IVUS has been commercialized in the USA, utilizing a spectral radiofrequency analysis of the backscattered ultrasound signal with a classification algorithm developed from *ex vivo* coronary datasets [112]. The reported accuracies are 91% for calcified regions, 93% for fibrofatty regions, 90% for necrotic regions, and 90% for fibrous regions. VH-IVUS classified tissue as fibrous tissue (dark green), fibrofatty tissue (light green), necrotic core (red), and dense calcium (white) and lesions as pathologic intimal thickening (PIT), fibrotic, fibrocalcific, thick-cap fibroatheroma (ThFA), or thin-cap fibroatheromas (TCFA) (Figure 7.22) [113,114].

VH-IVUS data are collected with a 20-MHz, 2.9 Fr phased-array transducer catheter (Eagle Eye™ Gold, Volcano Therapeutics, Rancho Cordova, CA, USA) that acquires IVUS data that are ECG-gated.

The potential value of VH-IVUS-derived plaque types in the prediction of future adverse coronary events was evaluated in the Providing Regional Observations to Study Predictors of Events in the Coronary Tree (PROSPECT) study [115]. This 697 patients study demonstrated that non-culprit lesions associated with recurrent events were more likely than those not associated with recurrent events to be characterized by a plaque burden of ≥70%, a minimal luminal area of ≤4.0 mm^2, or to be classified as TCFAs. Conversely, non-fibroatheroma lesions were clinically stable and were rarely associated with clinical events during 3 years of follow-up [116]. In the VIVA study, Calvert *et al.* [117] analyzed 170 patients who were prospectively enrolled and underwent three-vessel VH-IVUS pre-PCI and also post-PCI in the culprit vessel. Non-culprit lesion factors associated with non-restenotic major adverse cardiac events (MACE) included VH-TCFA and plaque burden >70%. In addition, VH-TCFA, plaque burden >70%, and MLA <4 mm^2 were associated with total MACE. Thus, as shown in the PROSPECT and VIVA studies, prospective identification and characterization of atherosclerotic non-culprit lesions in the coronary arteries is feasible with VH-IVUS and is predictive of adverse cardiovascular future events.

Plaque composition detected by VH-IVUS was also associated with the occurrence of distal embolization after PCI. Several studies showed a relationship between the amount of necrotic core and distal embolization [118].

Another commercially available system (outside of the USA) is the iMAP software, which uses a 40-MHz single rotational

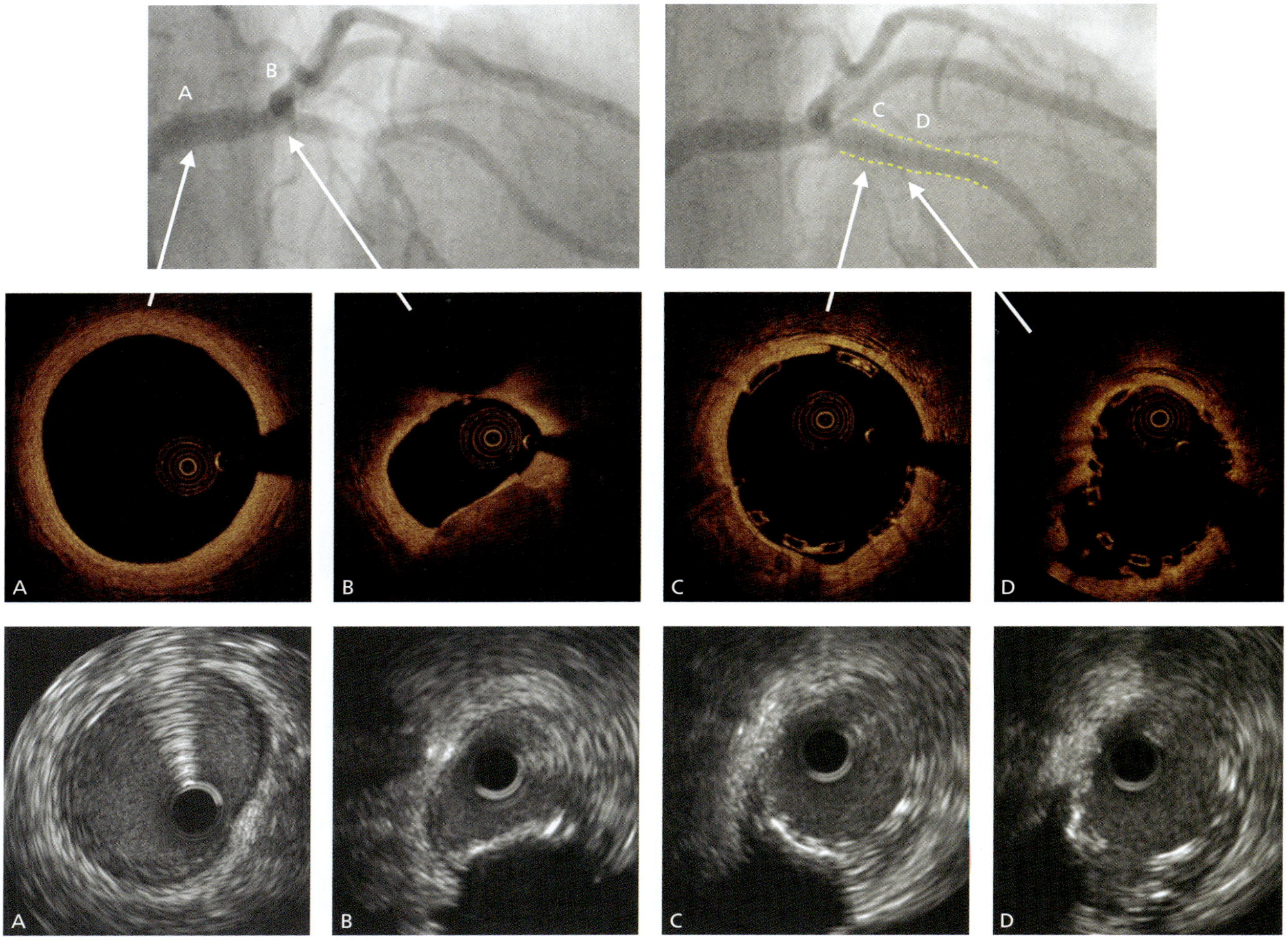

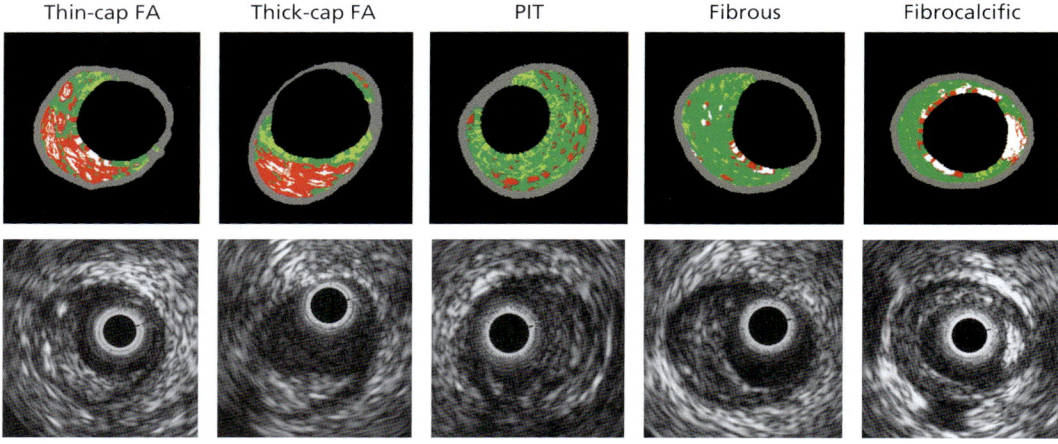

Figure 7.21 (Continued)

Figure 7.22 Five types of phenotypes documented by virtual histology IVUS (VH-IVUS). From left to right, thin cap fibroatheroma (TCFA), thick cap fibroatheroma (ThCFA), pathologic intimal thickening (PIT) and fibrocalficic plaques.

transducer (Atlantis™ SR Pro, Boston Scientific) to obtain the radiofrequency signal. iMAP uses a pattern recognition algorithm on the spectra that were obtained from fast Fourier transformation of the backscattered signals. *Ex vivo* validation demonstrated accuracies at the highest level of confidence as: 97%, 98%, 95%, and 98% for necrotic, lipidic, fibrotic, and calcified regions, respectively (Figure 7.23) [119]. Preliminary study by our group has shown that the software can appropriately identify TCFA in patients with acute

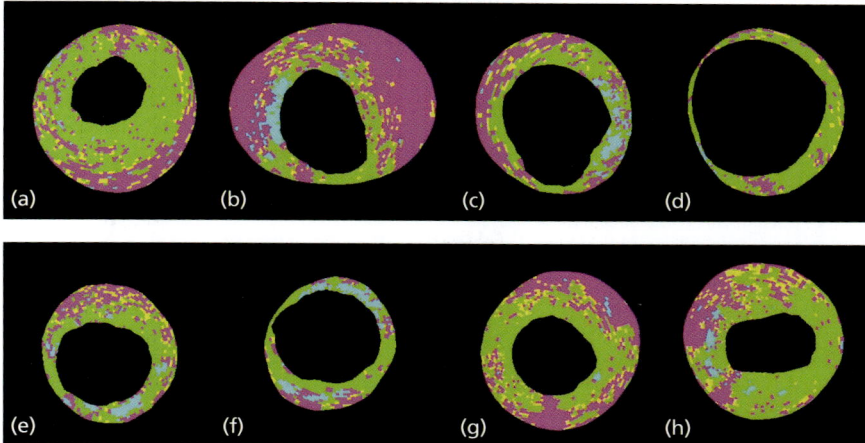

Figure 7.23 Various types of plaque composition (a–h). (a) plaques tissue composition by iMAP. Fibrotic tissue (green) and necrotic core (red) are the main tissue component (ThCFA), in which necrotic core represents 27% of total area of the plaque. (b) necrotic core abutting to the lumen with superficial calcification (from 8 to 10 o'clock; TCFA). (c) ThCFA with calcification at 3 o'clock. (d) necrotic core and fibrotic tissue. (e) mild atherosclerosis with calcification (blue). (g) and (h) Fibroatheromas.

myocardial infarction. However, it is limited by the wire artifact, which overestimates the tissue component of the necrotic core [120]. A prospective natural history study of vulnerable atherosclerotic plaque using iMAP is lacking.

Integrated backscatter (IB) analysis is another tissue classification scheme based on radiofrequency analysis of the reflected ultrasound signal. Comparison of IB-IVUS to histopathology demonstrated that the sensitivity of IB-IVUS for characterizing lipid pool, fibrosis, and calcification was 84%, 94%, and 100%, respectively, with specificity of 97%, 84%, and 100%, respectively. This system has been also shown capable to identify TFCA, and potentially be used to identify lesions with an elevated risk of myocardial infarction after PCI [121,122].

Conclusions

Grayscale IVUS provides (i) high quality, tomographic imaging of the lumen, the atheroma, and the vessel wall; (ii) incremental and more detailed qualitative and quantitative information than coronary angiography; (iii) practical guidance for percutaneous coronary intervention; and (iv) many clinical and research insights. IVUS has become an important part of DES studies, representing an effective way to understand the mechanisms, effects, and complications of stent technology. Grayscale IVUS may not accurately assess plaque composition. Variations of the traditional grayscale IVUS technique permit more detailed tissue characterization of atherosclerotic plaques. The most commonly technique used is referred to as VH-IVUS, which is based upon the radiofrequency analysis of the backscattered ultrasound signal. Development of high-definition IVUS, hybrid IVUS-OCT imaging or integration of novel techniques, including IVUS and near-infrared spectroscopy has great potential to improve our current ability to identify plaques at higher risk of rupture.

Interactive multiple choice questions are available for this chapter on www.wiley.com/go/dangas/cardiology

References

1 Bom N, Lancee CT, Honkoop J, Hugenholtz PG. Ultrasonic viewer for cross-sectional analyses of moving cardiac structures. *Biomed Eng* 1971; **6**(11): 500–503, 505. PubMed PMID: 5133281.

2 Bom N, Lancee CT, Van Egmond FC. An ultrasonic intracardiac scanner. *Ultrasonics* 1972; **10**(2): 72–76. PubMed PMID: 5017589.

3 Yock PG, Linker DT, Angelsen BA. Two-dimensional intravascular ultrasound: technical development and initial clinical experience. *J Am Soc Echocardiogr* 1989; **2**(4): 296–304. PubMed PMID: 2697308.

4 Yock PG, Linker DT, White NW, *et al.* Clinical applications of intravascular ultrasound imaging in atherectomy. *Int J Cardiac Imaging* 1989; **4**(2-4): 117–125. PubMed PMID: 2527914.

5 Mintz G. *Intracoronary Ultrasound*. Taylor & Francis, Abingdon, UK: 2005.

6 Yock PG, Linker DT. Intravascular ultrasound: looking below the surface of vascular disease. *Circulation* 1990; **81**(5): 1715–1718. PubMed PMID: 2184950.

7 Tobis JM, Mallery J, Mahon D, *et al.* Intravascular ultrasound imaging of human coronary arteries in vivo: analysis of tissue characterizations with comparison to in vitro histological specimens. *Circulation* 1991; **83**(3): 913–926. PubMed PMID: 1999040.

8 Mintz GS, Potkin BN, Cooke RH, *et al.* Intravascular ultrasound imaging in a patient with unstable angina. *Am Heart J* 1992; **123**(6): 1692–1694. PubMed PMID: 1595551.

9 Nissen SE, De Franco AC, Tuzcu EM, Moliterno DJ. Coronary intravascular ultrasound: diagnostic and interventional applications. *Coron Artery Dis* 1995; **6**(5): 355–367. PubMed PMID: 7655722.

10 Honda Y, Fitzgerald PJ. Frontiers in intravascular imaging technologies. *Circulation* 2008; **117**(15): 2024–2037. PubMed PMID: 18413510.

11 Otake H, Honda Y, Fitzgerald PJ. The role of intravascular ultrasound in percutaneous coronary intervention. In Redwood S, Curzen N, Thomas M. (eds) *Oxford Texbook of Interventional Cardiology*. Oxford University Press, Oxford, UK: 2010; 149–174.

12 Mintz GS, Nissen SE, Anderson WD, *et al.* American College of Cardiology Clinical Expert Consensus Document on Standards for Acquisition, Measurement and Reporting of Intravascular Ultrasound Studies (IVUS). A report of the American College of Cardiology Task Force on Clinical Expert Consensus Documents. *J Am Coll Cardiol* 2001; **37**(5): 1478–1492. PubMed PMID: 11300468.

13 Kimura BJ, Bhargava V, Palinski W, Russo RJ, DeMaria AN. Distortion of intravascular ultrasound images because of nonuniform angular velocity of mechanical-type transducers. *Am Heart J* 1996; **132**(2 Pt 1): 328–336. PubMed PMID: 8701894.

14 Kearney PP, Ramo MP, Spencer T, *et al.* A study of the quantitative and qualitative impact of catheter shaft angulation in a mechanical intravascular ultrasound system. *Ultrasound Med Biol* 1997; **23**(1): 87–93. PubMed PMID: 9080621.

15 Takahashi T, Honda Y, Russo RJ, Fitzgerald PJ. Intravascular ultrasound and quantitative coronary angiography. *Catheter Cardiovasc Interv* 2002; **55**(1): 118–128. PubMed PMID: 11793508.

16 Arbab-Zadeh A, DeMaria AN, Penny WF, Russo RJ, Kimura BJ, Bhargava V. Axial movement of the intravascular ultrasound probe during the cardiac cycle: implications for three-dimensional reconstruction and measurements of coronary dimensions. *Am Heart J* 1999; **138**(5 Pt 1): 865–872. PubMed PMID: 10539817.

17 Di Mario C, Gorge G, Peters R, *et al*. Clinical application and image interpretation in intracoronary ultrasound. Study Group on Intracoronary Imaging of the Working Group of Coronary Circulation and of the Subgroup on Intravascular Ultrasound of the Working Group of Echocardiography of the European Society of Cardiology. *Eur Heart J* 1998; **19**(2): 207–229. PubMed PMID: 9519314.

18 Fuessl RT, Mintz GS, Pichard AD, *et al*. In vivo validation of intravascular ultrasound length measurements using a motorized transducer pullback system. *Am J Cardiol* 1996; **77**(12): 1115–1118. PubMed PMID: 8644670.

19 Nissen SE, Yock P. Intravascular ultrasound: novel pathophysiological insights and current clinical applications. *Circulation* 2001; **103**(4): 604–616. PubMed PMID: 11157729.

20 Siegel RJ, Chae JS, Maurer G, Berlin M, Fishbein MC. Histopathologic correlation of the three-layered intravascular ultrasound appearance of normal adult human muscular arteries. *Am Heart J* 1993; **126**(4): 872–878. PubMed PMID: 8213444.

21 Nishimura RA, Edwards WD, Warnes CA, *et al*. Intravascular ultrasound imaging: in vitro validation and pathologic correlation. *J Am Coll Cardiol* 1990; **16**(1): 145–154. PubMed PMID: 2193046.

22 Gussenhoven EJ, Essed CE, Lancee CT, *et al*. Arterial wall characteristics determined by intravascular ultrasound imaging: an in vitro study. *J Am Coll Cardiol* 1989; **14**(4): 947–952. PubMed PMID: 2677088.

23 Velican D, Velican C. Comparative study on age-related changes and atherosclerotic involvement of the coronary arteries of male and female subjects up to 40 years of age. *Atherosclerosis* 1981; **38**(1-2): 39–50. PubMed PMID: 7470204.

24 Isner JM, Donaldson RF, Fortin AH, Tischler A, Clarke RH. Attenuation of the media of coronary arteries in advanced atherosclerosis. *Am J Cardiol* 1986; **58**(10): 937–939. PubMed PMID: 3776849.

25 Gussenhoven EJ, Frietman PA, The SH, *et al*. Assessment of medial thinning in atherosclerosis by intravascular ultrasound. *Am J Cardiol* 1991; **68**(17): 1625–1632. PubMed PMID: 1746464.

26 Topol EJ, Nissen SE. Our preoccupation with coronary luminology: the dissociation between clinical and angiographic findings in ischemic heart disease. *Circulation* 1995; **92**(8): 2333–2342. PubMed PMID: 7554219.

27 Fernandes MR, Silva GV, Caixeta A, Rati M, de Sousa e Silva NA, Perin EC. Assessing intermediate coronary lesions: angiographic prediction of lesion severity on intravascular ultrasound. *J Invasive Cardiol* 2007; **19**(10): 412–416. PubMed PMID: 17906342.

28. Mintz GS, Painter JA, Pichard AD, *et al*. Atherosclerosis in angiographically "normal" coronary artery reference segments: an intravascular ultrasound study with clinical correlations. *J Am Coll Cardiol* 1995; **25**(7): 1479–1485. PubMed PMID: 7759694.

29 Glagov S, Weisenberg E, Zarins CK, Stankunavicius R, Kolettis GJ. Compensatory enlargement of human atherosclerotic coronary arteries. *N Engl J Med* 1987; **316**(22): 1371–1375. PubMed PMID: 3574413.

30 Hermiller JB, Tenaglia AN, Kisslo KB, *et al*. In vivo validation of compensatory enlargement of atherosclerotic coronary arteries. *Am J Cardiol* 1993; **71**(8): 665–668. PubMed PMID: 8447262.

31 Losordo DW, Rosenfield K, Kaufman J, Pieczek A, Isner JM. Focal compensatory enlargement of human arteries in response to progressive atherosclerosis: in vivo documentation using intravascular ultrasound. *Circulation* 1994; **89**(6): 2570–2577. PubMed PMID: 8205666.

32 Nishioka T, Luo H, Eigler NL, Berglund H, Kim CJ, Siegel RJ. Contribution of inadequate compensatory enlargement to development of human coronary artery stenosis: an in vivo intravascular ultrasound study. *J Am Coll Cardiol* 1996 Jun; **27**(7):1571–6. PubMed PMID: 8636538.

33 Mintz GS, Kent KM, Pichard AD, Satler LF, Popma JJ, Leon MB. Contribution of inadequate arterial remodeling to the development of focal coronary artery stenoses: an intravascular ultrasound study. *Circulation* 1997; **95**(7): 1791–1798. PubMed PMID: 9107165.

34 Schoenhagen P, Ziada KM, Kapadia SR, Crowe TD, Nissen SE, Tuzcu EM. Extent and direction of arterial remodeling in stable versus unstable coronary syndromes : an intravascular ultrasound study. *Circulation* 2000; **101**(6): 598–603. PubMed PMID: 10673250.

35 Pasterkamp G, Wensing PJ, Post MJ, Hillen B, Mali WP, Borst C. Paradoxical arterial wall shrinkage may contribute to luminal narrowing of human atherosclerotic femoral arteries. *Circulation* 1995; **91**(5): 1444–1449. PubMed PMID: 7867185.

36 Pasterkamp G, Schoneveld AH, van der Wal AC, *et al*. Relation of arterial geometry to luminal narrowing and histologic markers for plaque vulnerability: the remodeling paradox. *J Am Coll Cardiol* 1998; **32**(3): 655–662. PubMed PMID: 9741507.

37 Inaba S, Mintz GS, Farhat NZ, *et al*. Impact of positive and negative lesion site remodeling on clinical outcomes: insights from PROSPECT. *JACC Cardiovasc Imaging* 2014; **7**(1): 70–78. PubMed PMID: 24433710.

38 Mintz GS, Pichard AD, Popma JJ, *et al*. Determinants and correlates of target lesion calcium in coronary artery disease: a clinical, angiographic and intravascular ultrasound study. *J Am Coll Cardiol* 1997; **29**(2): 268–274. PubMed PMID: 9014977.

39 Ge J, Chirillo F, Schwedtmann J, *et al*. Screening of ruptured plaques in patients with coronary artery disease by intravascular ultrasound. *Heart* 1999; **81**(6): 621–627. PubMed PMID: 10336922. Pubmed Central PMCID: 1729066.

40 Rioufol G, Finet G, Ginon I, *et al*. Multiple atherosclerotic plaque rupture in acute coronary syndrome: a three-vessel intravascular ultrasound study. *Circulation* 2002; **106**(7): 804–808. PubMed PMID: 12176951.

41 Hong MK, Mintz GS, Lee CW, *et al*. Comparison of coronary plaque rupture between stable angina and acute myocardial infarction: a three-vessel intravascular ultrasound study in 235 patients. *Circulation* 2004; **110**(8): 928–933. PubMed PMID: 15313951.

42 Hasegawa T, Ehara S, Kobayashi Y, *et al*. Acute myocardial infarction: clinical characteristics and plaque morphology between expansive remodeling and constrictive remodeling by intravascular ultrasound. *Am Heart J* 2006; **151**(2): 332–337. PubMed PMID: 16442895.

43 Wu X, Mintz GS, Xu K, *et al*. The relationship between attenuated plaque identified by intravascular ultrasound and no-reflow after stenting in acute myocardial infarction: the HORIZONS-AMI (Harmonizing Outcomes With Revascularization and Stents in Acute Myocardial Infarction) trial. *JACC Cardiovasc Interv* 2011; **4**(5): 495–502. PubMed PMID: 21596321.

44 Lee SY, Mintz GS, Kim SY, *et al*. Attenuated plaque detected by intravascular ultrasound: clinical, angiographic, and morphologic features and post-percutaneous coronary intervention complications in patients with acute coronary syndromes. *JACC Cardiovasc Interv* 2009; **2**(1): 65–72. PubMed PMID: 19463400.

45 Souza CF, Doi H, Mintz GS, *et al*. Morphological changes and clinical impact of unstable plaques within untreated segments of acute myocardial infarction patients during a 3-year follow-up: an analysis from the HORIZONS-AMI trial. *Coron Artery Dis* 2015; **26**(6): 469–475. PubMed PMID: 25919902.

46 Pu J, Mintz GS, Biro S, *et al*. Insights into echo-attenuated plaques, echolucent plaques, and plaques with spotty calcification: novel findings from comparisons among intravascular ultrasound, near-infrared spectroscopy, and pathological histology in 2,294 human coronary artery segments. *J Am Coll Cardiol* 2014; **63**(21): 2220–2233. PubMed PMID: 24681142.

47 Shiono Y, Kubo T, Tanaka A, *et al*. Impact of attenuated plaque as detected by intravascular ultrasound on the occurrence of microvascular obstruction after percutaneous coronary intervention in patients with ST-segment elevation myocardial infarction. *JACC Cardiovasc Interv* 2013; **6**(8): 847–853. PubMed PMID: 23871509.

48 Xu K, Mintz GS, Kubo T, *et al*. Long-term follow-up of attenuated plaques in patients with acute myocardial infarction: an intravascular ultrasound substudy of the HORIZONS-AMI trial. *Circ Cardiovasc Interv* 2012; **5**(2): 185–192. PubMed PMID: 22438429.

49 Waller BF. Anatomy, histology, and pathology of the major epicardial coronary arteries relevant to echocardiographic imaging techniques. *J Am Soc Echocardiogr* 1989; **2**(4): 232–252. PubMed PMID: 2697305.

50 Pijls NH, Fearon WF, Tonino PA, *et al*. Fractional flow reserve versus angiography for guiding percutaneous coronary intervention in patients with multivessel coronary artery disease: 2-year follow-up of the FAME (Fractional Flow Reserve Versus Angiography for Multivessel Evaluation) study. *J Am Coll Cardiol* 2010; **56**(3): 177–184. PubMed PMID: 20537493.

51 De Bruyne B, Fearon WF, Pijls NH, *et al*. Fractional flow reserve-guided PCI for stable coronary artery disease. *N Engl J Med* 2014; **371**(13): 1208–1217. PubMed PMID: 25176289.

52 Ben-Dor I, Torguson R, Gaglia MA Jr, *et al*. Correlation between fractional flow reserve and intravascular ultrasound lumen area in intermediate coronary artery stenosis. *EuroIntervention* 2011; **7**(2): 225–233. PubMed PMID: 21646065.

53 Stefano GT, Bezerra HG, Attizzani G, *et al*. Utilization of frequency domain optical coherence tomography and fractional flow reserve to assess intermediate coronary artery stenoses: conciliating anatomic and physiologic information. *Int J Cardiovasc Imaging* 2011; **27**(2): 299–308. PubMed PMID: 21409535. Pubmed Central PMCID: 3984934.

54 Guagliumi G, Sirbu V, Petroff C, *et al*. Volumetric assessment of lesion severity with optical coherence tomography: relationship with fractional flow. *EuroIntervention* 2013; **8**(10): 1172–1781. PubMed PMID: 23425542.

55 Gonzalo N, Escaned J, Alfonso F, *et al*. Morphometric assessment of coronary stenosis relevance with optical coherence tomography: a comparison with fractional flow reserve and intravascular ultrasound. *J Am Coll Cardiol* 2012; **59**(12): 1080–1089. PubMed PMID: 22421301.

56 Briguori C, Anzuini A, Airoldi F, *et al*. Intravascular ultrasound criteria for the assessment of the functional significance of intermediate coronary artery stenoses and comparison with fractional flow reserve. *Am J Cardiol* 2001; **87**(2): 136–141. PubMed PMID: 11152827.

57 Kang SJ, Lee JY, Ahn JM, *et al.* Validation of intravascular ultrasound-derived parameters with fractional flow reserve for assessment of coronary stenosis severity. *Circ Cardiovasc Interv* 2011; **4**(1): 65–71. PubMed PMID: 21266708.

58 Waksman R, Legutko J, Singh J, *et al.* FIRST: Fractional Flow Reserve and Intravascular Ultrasound Relationship Study. *J Am Coll Cardiol* 2013; **61**(9): 917–923. PubMed PMID: 23352786.

59 Han JK, Koo BK, Park KW, *et al.* Optimal intravascular ultrasound criteria for defining the functional significance of intermediate coronary stenosis: an international multicenter study. *Cardiology* 2014; **127**(4): 256–262. PubMed PMID: 24480866.

60 Ma YF, Fam JM, Zhang BC. Critical analysis of the correlation between optical coherence tomography versus intravascular ultrasound and fractional flow reserve in the management of intermediate coronary artery lesion. *Int J Clin Exp Med* 2015; **8**(5): 6658–6667. PubMed PMID: 26221203. Pubmed Central PMCID: 4509148.

61 Nascimento BR, de Sousa MR, Koo BK, *et al.* Diagnostic accuracy of intravascular ultrasound-derived minimal lumen area compared with fractional flow reserve— meta-analysis: pooled accuracy of IVUS luminal area versus FFR. *Catheter Cardiovasc Interv* 2014; **84**(3): 377–385. PubMed PMID: 23737441.

62 Hermiller JB, Buller CE, Tenaglia AN, *et al.* Unrecognized left main coronary artery disease in patients undergoing interventional procedures. *Am J Cardiol* 1993; **71**(2): 173–176. PubMed PMID: 8421979.

63 Gerber TC, Erbel R, Gorge G, Ge J, Rupprecht HJ, Meyer J. Extent of atherosclerosis and remodeling of the left main coronary artery determined by intravascular ultrasound. *Am J Cardiol* 1994; **73**(9): 666–671. PubMed PMID: 8166063.

64 Ge J, Liu F, Gorge G, Haude M, Baumgart D, Erbel R. Angiographically "silent" plaque in the left main coronary artery detected by intravascular ultrasound. *Coron Artery Dis* 1995; **6**(10): 805–810. PubMed PMID: 8789673.

65 Sano K, Mintz GS, Carlier SG, *et al.* Assessing intermediate left main coronary lesions using intravascular ultrasound. *Am Heart J* 2007; **154**(5): 983–988. PubMed PMID: 17967608.

66 Alfonso F, Macaya C, Goicolea J, *et al.* Intravascular ultrasound imaging of angiographically normal coronary segments in patients with coronary artery disease. *Am Heart J* 1994; **127**(3): 536–544. PubMed PMID: 8122599.

67 Isner JM, Kishel J, Kent KM, Ronan JA Jr, Ross AM, Roberts WC. Accuracy of angiographic determination of left main coronary arterial narrowing: angiographic–histologic correlative analysis in 28 patients. *Circulation* 1981; **63**(5): 1056–1064. PubMed PMID: 7471365.

68 Cameron A, Kemp HG Jr, Fisher LD, *et al.* Left main coronary artery stenosis: angiographic determination. *Circulation* 1983; **68**(3): 484–489. PubMed PMID: 6872161.

69 Kang SJ, Mintz GS, Akasaka T, *et al.* Optical coherence tomographic analysis of in-stent neoatherosclerosis after drug-eluting stent implantation. *Circulation* 2011; **123**(25): 2954–2963. PubMed PMID: 21646494.

70 Ahmed JM, Mintz GS, Weissman NJ, *et al.* Mechanism of lumen enlargement during intracoronary stent implantation: an intravascular ultrasound study. *Circulation* 2000; **102**(1): 7–10. PubMed PMID: 10880407.

71 Maehara A, Takagi A, Okura H, *et al.* Longitudinal plaque redistribution during stent expansion. *Am J Cardiol* 2000; **86**(10): 1069–1072. PubMed PMID: 11074201.

72 Prati F, Pawlowski T, Gil R, *et al.* Stenting of culprit lesions in unstable angina leads to a marked reduction in plaque burden: a major role of plaque embolization? A serial intravascular ultrasound study. *Circulation* 2003; **107**(18): 2320–2305. PubMed PMID: 12707236.

73 Ako J, Morino Y, Honda Y, *et al.* Late incomplete stent apposition after sirolimus-eluting stent implantation: a serial intravascular ultrasound analysis. *J Am Coll Cardiol* 2005; **46**(6): 1002–1005. PubMed PMID: 16168282.

74 Hong MK, Mintz GS, Lee CW, *et al.* Incidence, mechanism, predictors, and long-term prognosis of late stent malapposition after bare-metal stent implantation. *Circulation* 2004; **109**(7): 881–886. PubMed PMID: 14967732.

75 de Feyter PJ, Kay P, Disco C, Serruys PW. Reference chart derived from post-stent-implantation intravascular ultrasound predictors of 6-month expected restenosis on quantitative coronary angiography. *Circulation* 1999; **100**(17): 1777–1783. PubMed PMID: 10534464.

76 Frey AW, Hodgson JM, Muller C, Bestehorn HP, Roskamm H. Ultrasound-guided strategy for provisional stenting with focal balloon combination catheter: results from the randomized Strategy for Intracoronary Ultrasound-guided PTCA and Stenting (SIPS) trial. *Circulation* 2000; **102**(20): 2497–2502. PubMed PMID: 11076823.

77 Gaster AL, Slothuus Skjoldborg U, Larsen J, *et al.* Continued improvement of clinical outcome and cost effectiveness following intravascular ultrasound guided PCI: insights from a prospective, randomised study. *Heart* 2003; **89**(9): 1043–1049. PubMed PMID: 12923023. Pubmed Central PMCID: 1767812.

78 Schiele F, Meneveau N, Vuillemenot A, *et al.* Impact of intravascular ultrasound guidance in stent deployment on 6-month restenosis rate: a multicenter, randomized study comparing two strategies—with and without intravascular ultrasound

guidance. RESIST Study Group. REStenosis after Ivus guided STenting. *J Am Coll Cardiol* 1998; **32**(2): 320–328. PubMed PMID: 9708456.

79 Oemrawsingh PV, Mintz GS, Schalij MJ, *et al.* Intravascular ultrasound guidance improves angiographic and clinical outcome of stent implantation for long coronary artery stenoses: final results of a randomized comparison with angiographic guidance (TULIP Study). *Circulation* 2003; **107**(1): 62–67. PubMed PMID: 12515744.

80 Mudra H, di Mario C, de Jaegere P, *et al.* Randomized comparison of coronary stent implantation under ultrasound or angiographic guidance to reduce stent restenosis (OPTICUS Study). *Circulation* 2001; **104**(12): 1343–1349. PubMed PMID: 11560848.

81 de Jaegere P, Mudra H, Figulla H, *et al.* Intravascular ultrasound-guided optimized stent deployment: immediate and 6 months clinical and angiographic results from the Multicenter Ultrasound Stenting in Coronaries Study (MUSIC Study). *Eur Heart J* 1998; **19**(8): 1214–1223. PubMed PMID: 9740343.

82 Albiero R, Rau T, Schluter M, *et al.* Comparison of immediate and intermediate-term results of intravascular ultrasound versus angiography-guided Palmaz–Schatz stent implantation in matched lesions. *Circulation* 1997; **96**(9): 2997–3005. PubMed PMID: 9386168.

83 Gil RJ, Pawlowski T, Dudek D, *et al.* Comparison of angiographically guided direct stenting technique with direct stenting and optimal balloon angioplasty guided with intravascular ultrasound: the multicenter, randomized trial results. *Am Heart J* 2007; **154**(4): 669–675. PubMed PMID: 17892989.

84 Parise H, Maehara A, Stone GW, Leon MB, Mintz GS. Meta-analysis of randomized studies comparing intravascular ultrasound versus angiographic guidance of percutaneous coronary intervention in pre-drug-eluting stent era. *Am J Cardiol* 2011; **107**(3): 374–382. PubMed PMID: 21257001.

85 Cheneau E, Leborgne L, Mintz GS, *et al.* Predictors of subacute stent thrombosis: results of a systematic intravascular ultrasound study. *Circulation* 2003; **108**(1): 43–47. PubMed PMID: 12821553.

86 Fujii K, Carlier SG, Mintz GS, *et al.* Stent underexpansion and residual reference segment stenosis are related to stent thrombosis after sirolimus-eluting stent implantation: an intravascular ultrasound study. *J Am Coll Cardiol* 2005; **45**(7): 995–998. PubMed PMID: 15808753.

87 Okabe T, Mintz GS, Buch AN, *et al.* Intravascular ultrasound parameters associated with stent thrombosis after drug-eluting stent deployment. *Am J Cardiol* 2007; **100**(5): 615–620. PubMed PMID: 17697816.

88 Caixeta A, Braga VC, Mintz GS. Very late stent thrombosis with bare-metal stent: identifying severe stent malapposition and underexpansion by intravascular ultrasound. *Einstein* 2013; **11**(3): 364–366. PubMed PMID: 24136765.

89 Roy P, Steinberg DH, Sushinsky SJ, *et al.* The potential clinical utility of intravascular ultrasound guidance in patients undergoing percutaneous coronary intervention with drug-eluting stents. *Eur Heart J* 2008; **29**(15): 1851–1857. PubMed PMID: 18550555.

90 Ahn JM, Kang SJ, Yoon SH, *et al.* Meta-analysis of outcomes after intravascular ultrasound-guided versus angiography-guided drug-eluting stent implantation in 26,503 patients enrolled in three randomized trials and 14 observational studies. *Am J Cardiol* 2014; **113**(8): 1338–1347. PubMed PMID: 24685326.

91 Maehara A, Mintz GS, Bui AB, *et al.* Incidence, morphology, angiographic findings, and outcomes of intramural hematomas after percutaneous coronary interventions: an intravascular ultrasound study. *Circulation* 2002; **105**(17): 2037–2042. PubMed PMID: 11980682.

92 Hoffmann R, Mintz GS, Pichard AD, Kent KM, Satler LF, Leon MB. Intimal hyperplasia thickness at follow-up of stent size: a serial intravascular ultrasound study. *Am J Cardiol* 1998; **82**(10): 1168–1172. PubMed PMID: 9832088.

93 Moses JW, Leon MB, Popma JJ, *et al.* Sirolimus-eluting stents versus standard stents in patients with stenosis in a native coronary artery. *N Engl J Med* 2003; **349**(14): 1315–1323. PubMed PMID: 14523139.

94 Caixeta A, Leon MB, Lansky AJ, *et al.* 5-year clinical outcomes after sirolimus-eluting stent implantation insights from a patient-level pooled analysis of 4 randomized trials comparing sirolimus-eluting stents with bare-metal stents. *J Am Coll Cardiol* 2009; **54**(10): 894–902. PubMed PMID: 19712798.

95 Weissman NJ, Koglin J, Cox DA, *et al.* Polymer-based paclitaxel-eluting stents reduce in-stent neointimal tissue proliferation: a serial volumetric intravascular ultrasound analysis from the TAXUS-IV trial. *J Am Coll Cardiol* 2005; **45**(8): 1201–1205. PubMed PMID: 15837249.

96 Iqbal J, Serruys PW, Silber S, *et al.* Comparison of zotarolimus- and everolimus-eluting coronary stents: final 5-year report of the RESOLUTE all-comers trial. *Circ Cardiovasc Interv* 2015; **8**(6): e002230. PubMed PMID: 26047993. Pubmed Central PMCID: 4495878.

97 Dangas GD, Serruys PW, Kereiakes DJ, *et al.* Meta-analysis of everolimus-eluting versus paclitaxel-eluting stents in coronary artery disease: final 3-year results of the SPIRIT clinical trials program (Clinical Evaluation of the Xience V Everolimus Eluting Coronary Stent System in the Treatment of Patients With De Novo Native Coronary Artery Lesions). *JACC Cardiovasc Interv* 2013; **6**(9): 914–922. PubMed PMID: 24050859.

98 Castagna MT, Mintz GS, Leiboff BO, et al. The contribution of "mechanical" problems to in-stent restenosis: an intravascular ultrasonographic analysis of 1090 consecutive in-stent restenosis lesions. Am Heart J 2001; **142**(6): 970–974. PubMed PMID: 11717599.

99 Ohya M, Kadota K, Tada T, et al. Stent Fracture after sirolimus-eluting stent implantation: 8-year clinical outcomes. Circ Cardiovasc Interv 2015; **8**(8): e002664. PubMed PMID: 26227346.

100 Nakamura M, Kataoka T, Honda Y, et al. Late incomplete stent apposition and focal vessel expansion after bare metal stenting. Am J Cardiol 2003; **92**(10): 1217–1219. PubMed PMID: 14609603.

101 Serruys PW, Degertekin M, Tanabe K, et al. Intravascular ultrasound findings in the multicenter, randomized, double-blind RAVEL (RAndomized study with the sirolimus-eluting VElocity balloon-expandable stent in the treatment of patients with de novo native coronary artery Lesions) trial. Circulation 2002; **106**(7): 798–803. PubMed PMID: 12176950.

102 Tanabe K, Serruys PW, Degertekin M, et al. Incomplete stent apposition after implantation of paclitaxel-eluting stents or bare metal stents: insights from the randomized TAXUS II trial. Circulation 2005; **111**(7): 900–905. PubMed PMID: 15710761.

103 Hoffmann R, Morice MC, Moses JW, et al. Impact of late incomplete stent apposition after sirolimus-eluting stent implantation on 4-year clinical events: intravascular ultrasound analysis from the multicentre, randomised, RAVEL, E-SIRIUS and SIRIUS trials. Heart 2008; **94**(3): 322–328. PubMed PMID: 17761505.

104 Guagliumi G, Costa MA, Sirbu V, et al. Strut coverage and late malapposition with paclitaxel-eluting stents compared with bare metal stents in acute myocardial infarction: optical coherence tomography substudy of the Harmonizing Outcomes with Revascularization and Stents in Acute Myocardial Infarction (HORIZONS-AMI) Trial. Circulation 2011; **123**(3): 274–281. PubMed PMID: 21220730.

105 Attizzani GF, Capodanno D, Ohno Y, Tamburino C. Mechanisms, pathophysiology, and clinical aspects of incomplete stent apposition. J Am Coll Cardiol 2014; **63**(14): 1355–1367. PubMed PMID: 24530675.

106 Joner M, Finn AV, Farb A, et al. Pathology of drug-eluting stents in humans: delayed healing and late thrombotic risk. J Am Coll Cardiol 2006; **48**(1): 193–202. PubMed PMID: 16814667.

107 Cook S, Wenaweser P, Togni M, et al. Incomplete stent apposition and very late stent thrombosis after drug-eluting stent implantation. Circulation 2007; **115**(18): 2426–2434. PubMed PMID: 17485593.

108 Guagliumi G, Sirbu V, Musumeci G, et al. Examination of the in vivo mechanisms of late drug-eluting stent thrombosis: findings from optical coherence tomography and intravascular ultrasound imaging. JACC Cardiovasc Interv 2012; **5**(1): 12–20. PubMed PMID: 22230145.

109 Alfonso F, Dutary J, Paulo M, et al. Combined use of optical coherence tomography and intravascular ultrasound imaging in patients undergoing coronary interventions for stent thrombosis. Heart 2012; **98**(16): 1213–1220. PubMed PMID: 22826559.

110 Kang SJ, Lee CW, Song H, et al. OCT analysis in patients with very late stent thrombosis. JACC Cardiovasc Imaging 2013; **6**(6): 695–703. PubMed PMID: 23643282.

111 Fujii K, Hao H, Ohyanagi M, Masuyama T. Intracoronary imaging for detecting vulnerable plaque. Circ J 2013; **77**(3): 588–595. PubMed PMID: 23370454.

112 Nair A, Kuban BD, Tuzcu EM, Schoenhagen P, Nissen SE, Vince DG. Coronary plaque classification with intravascular ultrasound radiofrequency data analysis. Circulation 2002; **106**(17): 2200–2226. PubMed PMID: 12390948.

113 Rodriguez-Granillo GA, Bruining N, McFadden E, et al. Geometrical validation of intravascular ultrasound radiofrequency data analysis (Virtual Histology) acquired with a 30 MHz boston scientific corporation imaging catheter. Catheter Cardiovasc Interv 2005; **66**(4): 514–518. PubMed PMID: 16281299.

114 Nasu K, Tsuchikane E, Katoh O, et al. Accuracy of in vivo coronary plaque morphology assessment: a validation study of in vivo virtual histology compared with in vitro histopathology. J Am Coll Cardiol 2006; **47**(12): 2405–2412. PubMed PMID: 16781367.

115 Stone GW, Maehara A, Lansky AJ, et al. A prospective natural-history study of coronary atherosclerosis. N Engl J Med 2011; **364**(3): 226–235. PubMed PMID: 21247313.

116 Dohi T, Mintz GS, McPherson JA, et al. Non-fibroatheroma lesion phenotype and long-term clinical outcomes: a substudy analysis from the PROSPECT study. JACC Cardiovasc Imaging 2013; **6**(8): 908–916. PubMed PMID: 23850249.

117 Calvert PA, Obaid DR, O'Sullivan M, et al. Association between IVUS findings and adverse outcomes in patients with coronary artery disease: the VIVA (VH-IVUS in Vulnerable Atherosclerosis) Study. JACC Cardiovasc Imaging 2011; **4**(8): 894–901. PubMed PMID: 21835382.

118 Claessen BE, Maehara A, Fahy M, Xu K, Stone GW, Mintz GS. Plaque composition by intravascular ultrasound and distal embolization after percutaneous coronary intervention. JACC Cardiovasc Imaging 2012; **5**(3 Suppl): S111–118. PubMed PMID: 22421225.

119 Sathyanarayana S, Carlier S, Li W, Thomas L. Characterisation of atherosclerotic plaque by spectral similarity of radiofrequency intravascular ultrasound signals. EuroIntervention 2009; **5**(1): 133–139. PubMed PMID: 19577995.

120 Souza CF, Alves CMR, Carvalho AC, et al. iWONDER (Imaging WhOle vessel coronary tree with intravascular ultrasound and iMap* in patients with acute myocardial infarction) Study: Rationale and Study Design Revista Brasileira de Cardiologia Invasiva. 2015; **20**: 199–203.

121 Ozaki Y, Ohota M, Ismail TF, Okumura M, Ishikawa M, Muramatsu T. Thin cap fibroatheroma defined as lipid core abutting lumen (LCAL) on integrated backscatter intravascular ultrasound: comparison with optical coherence tomography and correlation with peri-procedural myocardial infarction. Circ J 2015; **79**(4): 808–817. PubMed PMID: 25740668.

122 Koga S, Ikeda S, Miura M, et al. iMap-Intravascular ultrasound radiofrequency signal analysis reflects plaque components of optical coherence tomography-derived thin-cap fibroatheroma. Circ J 2015; **79**(10): 2231–2237. PubMed PMID: 26289833.

CHAPTER 8

Optical Coherence Tomography, Near-Infrared Spectroscopy, and Near-Infrared Fluorescence Molecular Imaging

Ismail Dogu Kilic[1,2], Roberta Serdoz[2], Enrico Fabris[2,3], Farouc Amin Jaffer[4], and Carlo Di Mario[2]

[1] Department of Cardiology, Pamukkale University Hospitals, Denizli, Turkey

[2] National Institute of Health Research (NIHR), Royal Brompton & Harefield NHS Foundation Trust, London, and NHLI Imperial College London, UK

[3] Cardiovascular Department, Ospedali Riuniti and University of Trieste, Trieste, Italy

[4] Cardiology Division, Massachusetts General Hospital, Harvard Medical School, Boston, MA, USA

Optical coherence tomography

Intravascular optical coherence tomography (OCT) has emerged in recent years. This technology, originally described in the early 1990s by David Huang, was first applied in the field of ophthalmology [1] and named OCT by James Fujimoto. In 1996, Brezinski *et al.* [2] published on the possibility of imaging coronary arteries with an OCT device. Subsequent advances in OCT technology enabled faster image acquisition rates, sufficient for its *in vivo* application in humans.

OCT is a high-resolution imaging technology that employs a bandwidth in the near-infrared spectrum with wavelengths ranging from 1250 to 1350 nm to probe micrometer-scale structures in combination with advanced fiber-optics to create images. The light that illuminates the vessel is absorbed and backscattered, or reflected, by the structures in tissue at different degrees, and images are formed by measuring the magnitude and time delay of a reflected backscattered light signal in a manner analogous to intravascular ultrasound (IVUS) [3]. The speed of light (3×10^8 m/s) is several orders of magnitude faster than that of sound (1.5×10^3 m/s), and in OCT an interferometer is used to transmit the reflected light signal [4]. The interferometer shares the light source in two arms: a reference arm and a sample arm, which is directed toward the tissue. The images are created comparing the back-reflected optical signal from the two arms (interference signal). Compared with IVUS, OCT offers a 10 times higher image resolution (with an axial resolution of 10–20 μm); however, this high resolution is at the expense of reduced penetration depth into tissue and the need to create a transient blood-free field of view during imaging acquisition. The tissue penetration is limited to 1–3 mm compared to 4–8 mm achieved by IVUS.

OCT system

Early commercially available versions of the technology used time domain (TD) detection, while the second generation systems using Fourier domain (FD) has significantly improved the signal-to-noise ratio and allows high speed pullbacks with faster acquisition [5].

Time domain OCT

The M2/M2x TD-OCT Imaging System (ImageWire™ LightLab Imaging Inc., Westford, MA, USA) was the first commercially available OCT system. The first generation OCT (ImageWire™ and M2/3 OCT system; LightLab Imaging Inc.) incorporated an OCT imaging wire and an over-the-wire occlusion balloon. The OCT imaging wire had a maximum outer diameter of 0.019 inch (with a standard 0.014 inch radiolucent coiled tip) and contained a single-mode fiber-optic core within a translucent sheath. An over-the-wire low-pressure occlusion balloon with distal flush ports was used to infuse saline at approximately 0.5 mL/s to selectively displace blood during acquisition [6]. Attempts were made to switch to a non-occlusive technique for OCT image acquisition using a flexible catheter with a short monorail distal lumen, injecting manually or via a power injector through the guiding catheter. Because of the slow speed of acquisition, the automatic pullback speed had to be set between 1.0 and 3.0 mm/s, with cross-sectional images being acquired at up to 20 frames/s resulting in 7 frames/mm or pitch of 142 μm [6]; however, maximal pullback length under 20–30 mm, the maximal duration that flushing can be expected to last, was inadequate for routine use.

Fourier domain OCT

Fourier domain OCT (FD-OCT) (Dragonfly Duo™ St. Jude/LightLab Imaging Inc., and Fastview Terumo, Lunawave®) is the new generation of OCT systems which enables rapid imaging of the coronary arteries without occlusive acquisition. There are two types of FD-OCT; spectral domain OCT (SD-OCT), which relies on a broadband light source, and a spectrometer as a detector. In the latter, the light source is a wavelength-swept laser and receiver comprises single-element photodiodes. A frequency shifter is typically used to resolve otherwise degenerate positive and negative depths to the reference arm path length. These systems are also referred to as frequency domain OCT, optical frequency domain imaging (OFDI) [7]. Because of its fast acquisition mode, FD-OCT systems can acquire images of long segments maintaining good longitudinal resolution during short injections.

Interventional Cardiology: Principles and Practice, Second Edition. Edited by George D. Dangas, Carlo Di Mario, and Nicholas N. Kipshidze.
© 2017 John Wiley & Sons, Ltd. Published 2017 by John Wiley & Sons, Ltd.

Table 8.1 Comparison of optical coherence tomography systems.

	IVUS	TD-OCT	FD-OCT (St. Jude)	OFDI (Terumo)
Energy wave	Ultrasound	Near-infrared	Near-infrared	Near-infrared
Wavelegth (μm)	35–80	1.3	1.3	1.3
Axial resolution (μm)	100–150	15–20	10–15	10–20
Lateral resolution (μm)	150–300	25–40	20–30	20
Tissue penetration (mm)	4–8	1.5–2	1.5–2	1–2
Frame rate (frames/s)	30	20	180	158
Pullback speed (mm/s)	0.5–2	1–3	18–36	Up to 40

FD, Fourier domain; IVUS, intravenous ultrasound; OCT, optical coherence tomography; OFDI, optical frequency domain imaging; TD, time domain.

The optical probe is integrated into a short monorail catheter that can be advanced in the coronary artery over any conventional 0.014 inch guide wire. The catheter profile varies from 2.4 to 3.2 Fr and are compatible with 6 Fr guiding catheters (in fact, these catheters can be inserted through 5 Fr guiding catheters as well, but then the speed of contrast flushing is often inadequate). The position and number of the radiopaque markers varies among different systems. During imaging, the optical fiber probe is pulled along the catheter sheath. The FD-OCT frame rate is typically 100 frames/s, with a pullback speed of 20 mm/s, achieving 5 frames/mm or a frame pitch of 200 μm. Newer systems acquiring data at 180 frames/s markedly enabled high-speed acquisitions, adequate for 3D reconstruction, of up to 10 cm and this image segment length, sufficient for complete assessment of most vessels. However, in spite of claims of better axial resolution, the tissue penetration remains limited to 0.5–2.0 mm. Currently, available commercial systems for clinical use are the St. Jude/LightLab Imaging Inc., Westford, MA, USA and Lunawave Terumo, Tokyo, Japan. A summary of the characteristics of the OCT systems is shown in Table 8.1.

Post-processing and interpretation of Z-offset

Calibrating the system is an important phase of the OCT imaging, which is critical for accurate measurements. Although semi-automated calibration is standard with currently available systems, calibration can still be incorrect because of failed automated calibration, incorrect manual adjustment, or changes in length of the optic fiber caused by bending of the imaging wire and proximity to the vessel wall [8]. The Z-offset is a manually adjustable image calibration, critical for accurate measurements. It is the zero-point setting of the system that corrects the difference in the optical measurement between the sample and reference arms. The catheter diameter acts a reference for optimal Z-offset determination within an image frame, aligning the marks to the outer surface of the catheter. Typically, calibration is made before starting image acquisition and repeated before the automatic measurement process is started.

Artifacts

Interpretation of OCT data and their application in clinical situations is limited by image artifacts (Figure 8.1). Knowledge of these artifacts can be used to guide the operator to a better interpretation of the OCT images.

Shadowing Dense objects such as guidewires, metallic stent struts (Figure 8.1a), blood or lipid-laden macrophage accumulations rapidly attenuate or completely obstruct the OCT signal, leading to a loss of signal and no visualization behind them. Compensation algorithms attempt to reduce shadowing and improve signal from the deepest tissues [9].

Residual blood Blood contamination usually results from inadequate flushing and can be prevented by using power injection through a pump at a speed greater than the maximal coronary flow (typically, 4–6 mL/s in the left coronary and 2–4 mL/s for the right coronary artery). Residual red blood cells disturb the OCT light beam, reducing the visibility and brightness of the vessel wall (Figure 8.1b); blood swirling along the vessel wall can be mistaken for thrombus.

Motion artifacts Physiologic phenomena such as cardiac motion, vessel pulsatility, or, to a lesser extent, catheter movement and respiratory movements are associated with beam scanning or movement of the operator's hand (Figure 8.1c). "Sew-up" artifacts appear as a result of rapid vessel movement during imaging, but they are less prominent than in the much slower IVUS pullbacks and have become clinically irrelevant at the high pullback speeds of the newest OCT systems.

Non-uniform rotational distortion Imaging modalities that use a mechanically rotated endoscopic probe to scan an artery often suffer from image degradation caused by a variation in the rotational speed of rotating optical components during image acquisition [10]. This occurs in the presence of acute angulations, tight hemostatic valve, kinking of the imaging sheath, a defective catheter, or while the catheter crosses a tight stenosis.

Saturation artifact These occur when the signal from a highly reflective surface exceeds the dynamic range of the detector (Figure 8.1d). The shape of signal appears distorted as linear streaks of high and low intensities along the axial direction. Stent struts and guidewires are the most common structures to cause this artifact.

Tangential signal dropout If the imaging beam strikes the tissue with a near parallel angle, a signal-poor area with diffuse borders, covered by a thin signal-rich layer arises (Figure 8.1e), and mimics a lipid-rich plaque with a fibrous cap [11].

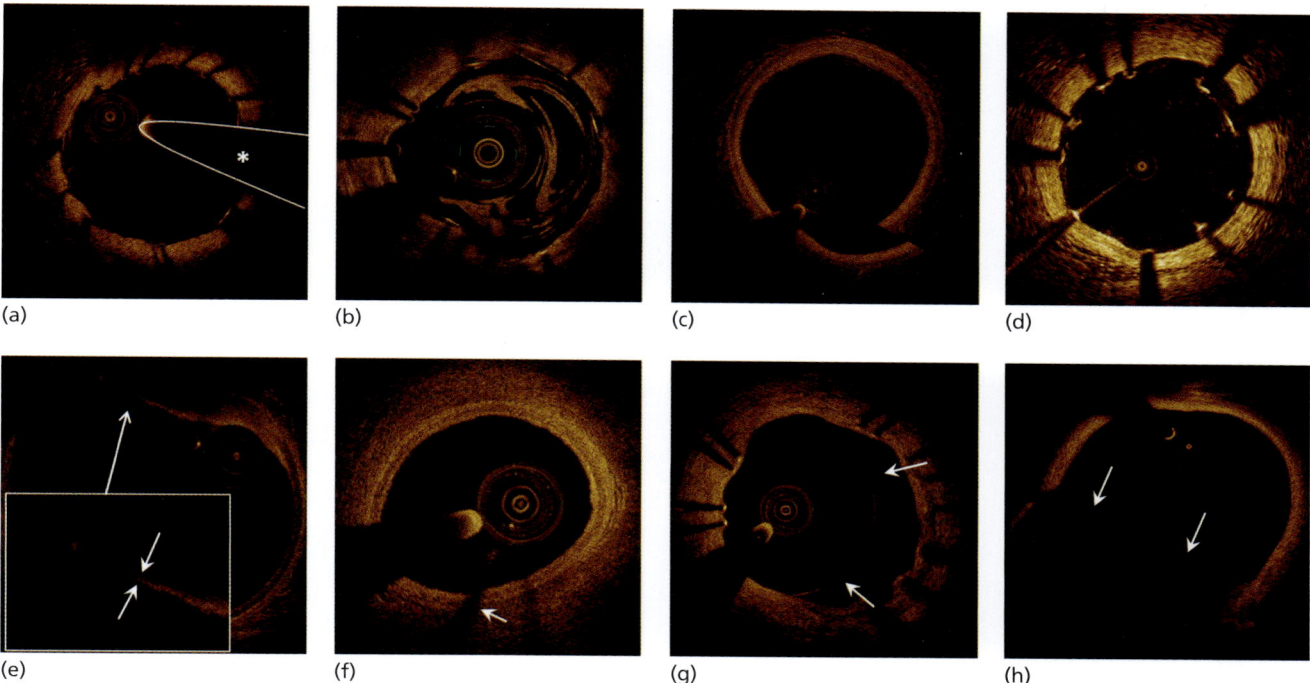

Figure 8.1 Frequent artifacts in optical coherence tomography imaging. (a) Shadowing of guidewire (asterisk) and stent struts. (b) Residual blood. (c) Motion artifact. (d) Saturation artifact. (e) Tangential signal drop-out artifact. Please note that this artifact cause a signal-rich area overlying a signal-poor region in an area of adaptive intimal thickening. (f) Bubble in the catheter causes a shadow on the vessel wall (arrow). (g) Multiple reflections. (h) Fold-over artifact.

Blooming artifact The intense signal generated by the reflection of light causes the appearance of a bright reflector maximized and dispersed along the axial direction [12]. This is most commonly caused by stent struts, which appear thicker. Unlike IVUS where the leading edge is the point used for measurements, the true edge of the strut lies somewhere in the *middle* of the blooming and this should be used in measuring the distance strut wall.

Bubble artifact These occur as a result of air bubbles in the catheter sheath. Bubbles also form in the silicon lubricant used to reduce friction between the sheath and the revolving optic fiber in TD-OCT systems [13]. Bubbles can attenuate the signal along a region of the vessel wall, and images with this artifact are unsuitable for tissue characterization (Figure 8.1f).

Multiple reflections This artifact is caused by the reflected surface of some catheters creating one or more circular line within the image (Figure 8.1g).

Strut orientation artifacts When the OCT catheter resides close to a stented artery wall, imaging metal coronary stents deployed appear as a bending of stent struts toward the imaging catheter. This so-called sunflower effect occurs when the catheter occupies an eccentric position within the vessel lumen and the struts appear as a straight line, perpendicular to the imaging light beam and obliquely oriented to the luminal wall [14]. This artifact can cause misclassification of apposed struts as malapposed. Bioabsorbable vascular scaffolds (BVS) are not susceptible to this artifact.

Fold-over artifact This artifact is more specific to FD-OCT systems. It occurs when the vessel is larger than the ranging depth, thus it is typically observed in large vessels or side branches.

Consequently, the vessel might appear to be folded over in the image (Figure 8.1h).

Normal coronary vessel anatomy

With the exception of the left main stem, coronary arteries are muscular arteries and are histologically organized into three layers. The intima consists of a lining layer of endothelial cells supported by a subendothelial layer [15], which is exceedingly thin at birth and grows progressively with age, eventually reaching OCT resolution limits [16]. In OCT, the intima can be visualized as a signal-rich luminal layer. The intimal thickens with age, and nearly all adult coronaries display an extent of intimal thickening [17]. There is no established cut-off for the identification of pathologic intimal thickening; however, some authors use, rather arbitrarily, a cut-off of 300 μm to identify intimal thickening, and above 600 μm for pathologic intimal thickening in the absence of a lipid pool or calcified region >1 quadrant [18]. The medial layer is a signal-poor region isolated from the intimal layer by an internal elastic membrane and from the adventitia by an external elastic membrane. Occasionally, these layers can be visualized as highly backscattering structures at the intima–media and media–adventitia borders [12]. The adventitia is recognized as a heterogeneous high signal outer layer.

Plaque characterization

Atherosclerotic plaque components can be categorized by utilizing various optical properties of different tissues (Figure 8.2). Fibrous plaques are identified as homogenous, highly backscattering, low attenuation lesions. However, as emitted light is absorbed by lipids (low backscattering), which leads to a high level of posterior signal attenuation, plaques appear as poor signal regions with poor delineation. Calcifications are also regions of low backscatter (signal poor), but let light filter rather than absorb it, so that they maintain

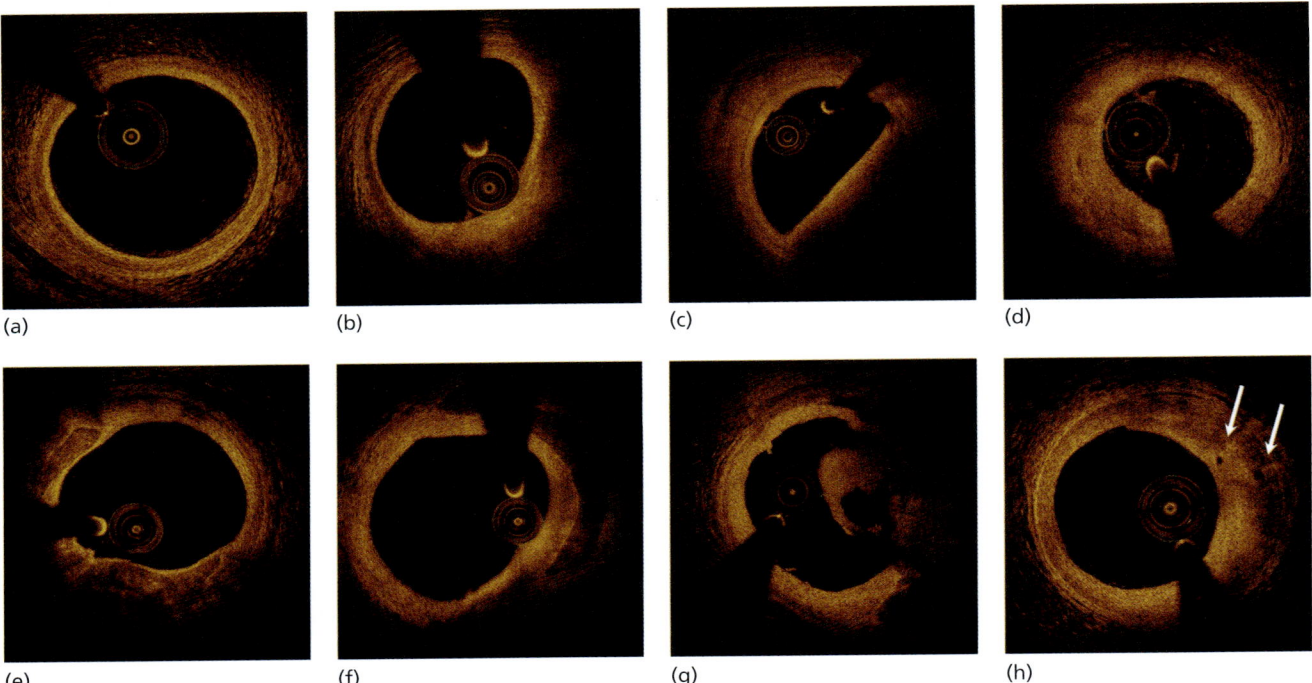

Figure 8.2 Plaque characterization with optical coherence tomography. (a) Normal coronary anatomy organized in three layers. (b) Lipid-rich plaque; note possible macrophage accumulations around 3 o'clock. (c) Lipid-rich plaque in a saphenous vein graft. (d) Fibrous plaque. (e) Calcification extending deep into the vessel wall between 4 and 11 o'clock. Outer border of the calcification cannot be delineated. (f) Calcification between 12 and 4 o'clock. (g) Thrombus protruding into the lumen. (h) Neovascularization (arrows).

well-delineated external borders. However, differentiation of signal-poor areas is not always straightforward and calcium can be misinterpreted as lipids, particularly if the calcification is situated deep in the vessel wall.

An early *ex vivo* study established a sensitivity and specificity ranging 71–79% and 97–98% for fibrous plaques, 95–96% and 97% for fibro-calcific plaques, and 90–94% and 90–92% for lipid-rich plaques with low inter-observer and intra-observer variability [19]. However, other studies showed conflicting results. For instance, in an OCT study, only 45% of atheromas were identified, with higher identification percentages in fibro-calcific and fibrous plaques of 68% and 83%, respectively [20]. Misinterpretation in this study was mainly caused by low OCT signal penetration, which precluded the detection of lipid pools or calcium behind thick fibrous caps and by misclassification of calcium deposits for lipid pools and vice versa [20]. Furthermore, artifacts such as superficial shadowing and tangential signal dropout can produce images with signal-poor regions covered by a thin signal rich layer mimicking thin-cap fibroatheromas (TCFA) [11]. Rather than relying only on subjective visual interpretations, algorithms based on the optical attenuation coefficient to classify plaques quantitatively have been proposed; however, as yet, these algorithms are not sufficiently robust to be used in the clinical setting [21].

OCT imaging can also demonstrate thrombi as protrusions or floating masses. Red and white thrombi can be identified via the differences in attenuation intensity, with red thrombi showing high attenuation and complete wall shadowing and white thrombi appearing as low attenuation intraluminal masses or layers [22].

Vulnerable plaque assessment

Imaging in acute coronary syndromes (ACS) includes ruptured plaques and histomorphologic features that can be detected by OCT (superficial lipids, fibrous cap thickness as well the presence of macrophages and neovascularization). Accurate *in vivo* detection of plaque components permits the detection of plaques at high risk of rupture. However, the limited penetration depth of OCT precludes the evaluation of remodeling as well as the calculation of plaque burden.

A semi-quantitative definition of the presence of superficial lipids in ≥2 quadrants is used to describe lipid-rich plaques in OCT studies [23]. However, low penetration depth prevents accurate evaluation of the lipid core thickness.

Pathologic studies reported that ruptured plaques harbor a thin fibrous cap being <65 μm in 95% of ruptured plaques [24]. Using OCT, the fibrous cap can be detected as a high signal homogeneous band covering the lipid-rich core. OCT was shown to provide accurate measurement of fibrous cap thickness (FCT) *ex vivo* [25]; previous studies demonstrated thinner fibrous caps in patients with ACS [23,26]. However, there is no established *in vivo* OCT "clinically important" cut-off for defining "thin" fibrous caps; current thresholds are obtained from histopathologic studies, raising concerns regarding possible tissue shrinkage during pathologic preparation [27]. A study that aimed to evaluate the relationship between FCT and plaque rupture *in vivo* found that in 95% of ruptured plaques, the thinnest FCT was <80 μm and so the investigators proposed this value as an alternative *in vivo* threshold [28].

The progression of atherosclerosis and plaque vulnerability is critically affected by macrophages. Their accretion in atherosclerotic plaques can be identified as high signal regions appearing either distinct or confluent punctate visually. With dedicated software, OCT-derived indices can be used to identify macrophages [29]. Nonetheless, macrophages should only be considered in the presence of a fibroatheroma, because there have not yet been any studies to confirm macrophages on normal vessel walls or intimal hyperplasia [12]. In addition, high speckle from microcalcifications or cholesterol crystals can also appear similar to macrophages [30].

Plaque neovascularization is considered as a feature of vulnerable plaques. These microvessels are inherently fragile and leaky, giving rise to local extravasation of plasma proteins and erythrocytes [31]. OCT reveals these vessels as small black holes in the atherosclerotic plaque [32]. The presence of these microchannels is associated with vulnerable features such as thin fibrous cap and positive remodeling [33]. In a larger study, similar results were reproduced only in culprit lesions of patients with ACS, not in non-culprit lesions of patients with ACS or in stable patients [34]. Another study found no difference in the prevalence of microchannels in ACS and non-ACS patients; however, the closest distance from the lumen to the microchannel was shorter in ACS subjects than in non-ACS [35].

OCT imaging over time can provide insights and therapeutic strategies for plaque stabilization. In an initial study, patients on preceding statin therapy were found to have a reduced incidence of ruptured plaques and a trend toward thicker fibrous caps [36]. The influence of statins on fibrous caps was further investigated in a study of 40 patients with previous myocardial infarction. FCT was found to increase in both the statin and control group over time, but more so in the statin group [37]; this was confirmed ensewhere [38]. Recently, atorvastatin therapy at 20 mg/day provided a greater increase in FCT than 5 mg [39]. In an additional study, despite comparable reduction in total cholesterol and low density lipoprotein cholesterol levels with statin therapy in ACS patients, non-culprit lesions *without* neovascularization showed greater increase in fibrous cap thickness than lesions *with* neovascularization at a 6–12 months' follow-up [40]. These important insights into the operative mechanism of statins reveal qualitative arterial wall changes explaining stabilization without significant modification of angiographic lumen dimensions and only minimal volumetric plaque changes by IVUS [41–43].

Acute coronary syndromes

The presence of a disrupted fibrous cap alongside a cavity describes plaque rupture. Plaque rupture can be observed in a variety of clinical scenarios. One study revealed that plaque rupture, TCFA, and red thrombus are more frequent in patients with ST-elevation myocardial infarction (STEMI). Additionally, the size of the ruptured cavities was greater and an aperture opposite to the flow direction was more frequent in patients with STEMI [44]. OCT also showed differences in the morphology of ruptured plaques in non-STEMI and asymptomatic coronary artery disease (CAD) [45]. Pathologic studies suggest that ruptures do not necessarily lead to ACS, and ruptures can heal and cause plaque progression. Using OCT, healed plaques can be identified as multiple layers of different optical densities overlying a large necrotic core [46].

Although plaque rupture is the most common cause of ACS, more than 20–30% of events are caused by plaque erosion, or with the presence of superficial often protruding calcific nodules shown on OCT (Figure 8.3). Indeed, OCT can detect the presence or absence of plaque disruption and categorize plaque morphology *in vivo* [47] and the characterization of these plaques could aid in the derivation of alternative treatment strategies [48].

Percutaneous coronary intervention

Angiography has been used as the gold standard to evaluate the presence, location, and severity of CAD; however, it is an analysis limited to the vessel lumen and has obvious drawbacks without offering direct information on the characteristics and composition of the coronary lesions. The widespread application of a non-occlusive technique using monorail OCT catheters, the high pullback speed allowed by newer generation FD-OCT systems, and the availability of semi-automatic measurements have made OCT a

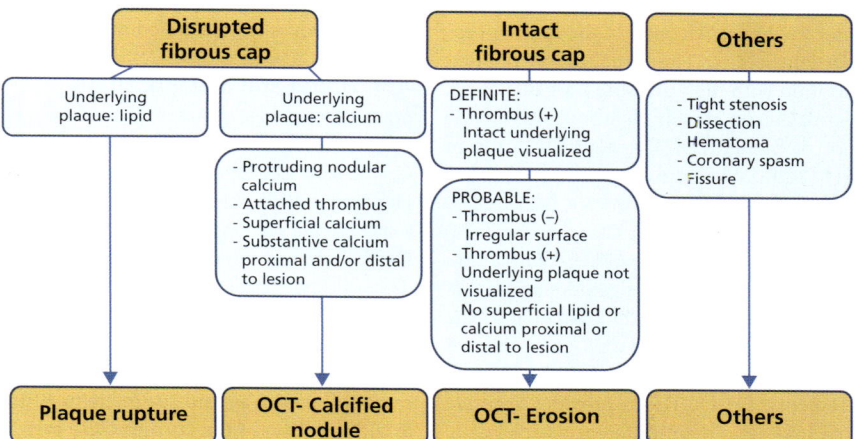

Figure 8.3 Plaque classification algorithm by optical coherence tomography (OCT). Plaque rupture is defined as the presence of fibrous cap discontinuity with a clear cavity formed inside the plaque. Definite OCT erosion is identified by the presence of attached thrombus overlying an intact and visualized plaque, whereas probable OCT erosion is defined by: (i) luminal surface irregularity at the culprit lesion in the absence of thrombus; or (ii) attenuation of underlying plaque by thrombus without superficial lipid or calcification immediately proximal or distal to the site of thrombus. The OCT calcified nodule is defined when fibrous cap disruption is detected over a calcified plaque characterized by protruding calcification, superficial calcium, and the presence of substantive calcium proximal and/or distal to the lesion. Source: Jia *et al.* 2013 [47]. Copyright (2013), with permission from Elsevier.

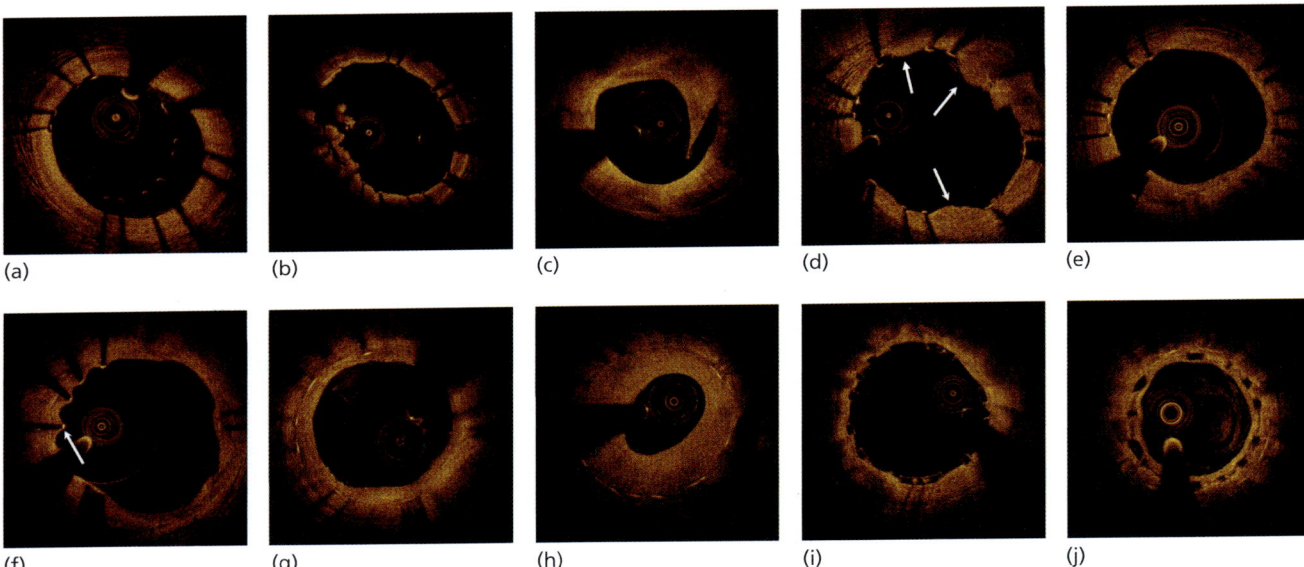

Figure 8.4 Optical coherence tomography in coronary interventions. (a) Strut malapposition. Malapposed struts can be seen between 12 and 6 o'clock. (b) Intracoronary thrombus formation during coronary intervention. (c) Edge dissection. (d) Tissue prolapse. (e) Neointimal coverage of stent struts in the follow-up. (f) Intimal coverage of malapposed struts (arrow). (g) Neointimal hyperplasia. (h) In-stent restenosis. (i) Bioabsorbable vascular scaffold (BVS). Note BVS struts are transparent to light. (j) BVS in the follow-up.

potential alternative for guidance of percutaneous coronary interventions (PCI), overcoming drawbacks of coronary angiography and avoiding the difficulties in interpretation and quantitation of IVUS (Figure 8.4). However, it is very important to understand that OCT and IVUS are not interchangeable intravascular techniques and that they have advantages, limitations, and differences in the way the procedure is guided via online measurements during the PCI procedure.

Because of the sharp delineation of lumen contours, OCT easily provides automatic lumen measurements. Accurate measurement of the reference lumen dimensions allows for optimal stent diameter selection, while the precise identification of the longitudinal extent of the atherosclerotic plaque facilitates selection of the most appropriate stent length and landing zones. The visualization of stent expansion permits optimization with high pressure post-dilatation, in the case of focal underexpansion readily demonstrated in the online lumen profile maps of modern OCT systems. In a recent study, which compared FD-OCT, IVUS, and quantitative coronary angiography [49], the mean minimum lumen diameter measured by quantitive coronary angiography (QCA) was smaller than by OCT, which was smaller than that by IVUS, a result consistent with a previous report [50]. Using a phantom model, investigators showed that mean lumen area (MLA) according to FD-OCT was equal to the actual lumen area of the phantom model while IVUS overestimated the lumen area and was less reproducible than FD-OCT. In addition to cross-sectional measurements, FD-OCT also provides accurate longitudinal measurements [51]. The main difference with IVUS, however, is the inability of OCT to measure the media-to-media diameter in most cases, with the rare exception of some distal reference segments with very small plaque burden and vessel diameter.

OCT-guided coronary intervention

Only a few studies have investigated the role of OCT guidance in PCI. Repeated examinations with OCT can be safely used to guide stent selection and improve stent expansion and apposition [52].

After full lesion predilatation, OCT pullback imaging suggested proceeding directly with stenting in 48% while in 52% advised further treatment. Out of the 207 pullback imaging after stenting, 14% suggested new stent implantation because of dissection or residual stenosis and 31% suggested further optimization with high pressure or larger sized balloon. A multicenter trial compared the outcomes of an angiographic-guided strategy with an OCT-guided strategy in 670 patients [53]; OCT disclosed adverse features requiring further interventions in 35%. OCT guidance was associated with a significantly lower risk of cardiac death or myocardial infarction at 1 year, even after adjustment of important potential confounders. However, further investigations are needed to confirm whether the use of OCT improves clinical outcomes.

Apposition and malapposition

Strut apposition is a part of optimal stent deployment criteria and is defined as the contact of the stent struts with the arterial wall. Conversely, malapposition is defined as lack of strut-wall contact. However, OCT detection of malapposition requires recognition that *only the leading edge* of the metallic stent strut is visible with OCT, therefore stent strut and polymer thickness for each type of drug-eluting stent (DES) should be considered in assessing malapposition. Incomplete strut apposition is defined as a strut-wall distance greater than the strut thickness (metal plus polymer) with the addition of a correction factor, most often ~15 μm (usually ranging between 10 and 20 μm, up to 30 μm taking into account the axial resolution of the current OCT systems) [54]. Unlike metallic stents, BVS are transparent to light, therefore the abluminal border of the struts can be easily identified and incomplete strut apposition can simply be established as the presence of struts separated from the underlying vessel wall [55].

However, the clinical implications of stent malapposition remain controversial. Ultrasound studies found conflicting results in the correlation between stent malapposition and adverse clinical events [56–58]. According to a recent OCT analysis of 356 coronary lesions that received a DES, acute stent malapposition was observed in 62% of lesions, approximately half of them being located within the stent edges [59]. Severe diameter stenosis, calcified lesions, and long stents were independent predictors of acute stent malapposition. Acute stent malapposition with a volume >2.56 mm³ differentiated malapposition that persisted at follow-up from stent malapposition that resolved. Moreover, in this study, long-term clinical outcomes of late stent malapposition detected by OCT were favorable [59]. However, segments with acute incomplete strut apposition have higher risk of delayed coverage than well-apposed segments. Acute incomplete strut apposition size (estimated as volume or maximum distance per strut) was an independent predictor of persistence of incomplete strut apposition and of delayed healing at follow-up in 66 stents of different designs [60]. Strut malapposition can cause turbulent blood flow, which in turn can trigger platelet activation and thrombosis. In fact, incomplete strut apposition in addition to delayed neointimal healing of the stent and incomplete endothelialization of the struts is a common morphologic finding in fatal cases of late and very late stent thrombosis [57,61–63]. However, biological and mechanical factors (including levels of circulating endothelial progenitor cells or regional shear stress) can also have a role in neointimal healing and differences in percentage coverage cannot always entirely explain clinically overt stent thrombosis [63].

Tissue protrusion

In OCT, plaque protrusion is characterized by a smooth surface and no signal attenuation, and thrombus protrusion by irregular surface and significant signal attenuation. Tissue protrusion is more frequently observed in the culprit lesions of acute coronary syndromes, as unstable lesions contain soft lipid tissue and thrombi; its clinical significance of tissue protrusion is not clear.

Vascular injury: dissections

OCT is a very sensitive tool in detecting micro-dissections and subclinical dissections [64]. Dissections occur more frequently when the plaque at the edge of the stent is fibro-calcific or lipid-rich than when is fibrous [65]. Nevertheless, currently there is no evidence that subclinical dissections carry adverse prognostic implications [66].

Guidance of complex lesion treatment

Bifurcations represent complex coronary lesions with high rates of acute and late stent failure. Knowing the reference diameter of the vessel distal and proximal to the side branch is critical in correct sizing of the stent and post-dilatation balloon. In both simple (one stent) or complex strategies of bifurcation stenting, OCT showed that the rate of malapposed struts is significantly higher at the side branch ostium than in the vessel side opposite to the ostium [67]. In a series of 45 lesions, OCT showed the persistence of malapposition was as high as 43%, despite consistent use of kissing balloon dilatation and proximal optimization technique [68]. The overall rate of malapposed struts was significantly higher in the lesions treated with angiography-guided than in those undergoing OCT-guided PCI [68].

The position where the guidewire re-crosses the stent struts into the side branch (i.e., proximal, mid, or distal cell) has been demonstrated to be one of the most important factors for strut apposition in the side branch ostium after balloon dilatation. Crossing to the side branch through a proximal cell provides no scaffolding of the side branch ostium and leaves many struts unapposed near the carina, reducing the strut-free side branch ostial area and current recommendations suggest attempting to re-cross the wire through the most distal cell of the main vessel stent in order to efficiently open a stent at the side branch ostium [69]. The feasibility and effectiveness of OCT-guided stent re-crossing compared with angiography guidance has been evaluated in a 52 patients [70]; the OCT-guided group showed a significantly lower number of malapposed stent struts, especially in the quadrants toward the side branch ostium (9 vs. 42%; p <0.0001).

Three-dimensional (3D) reconstruction of OCT images is also potentially useful to assess the spatial aspect of bifurcation stenting [71–75] and using 3D-OCT reconstruction, the side branch guidewire can be easily tracked. The clinical application of high quality off-line 3D-OCT to optimize side branch opening by identifying the configuration of overhanging struts in front of the side branch ostium according to the presence of the link between hoops at the carina and the appropriate distal cell for the re-crossing position has been evaluated in 22 patients [76]. This study showed that 3D-OCT confirmation of the re-crossing into the jailed side branch is feasible during PCI and helps to achieve distal rewiring and favorable stent positioning against the side branch ostium, leading to reduction in incomplete strut apposition and potentially better clinical outcomes [76]. Finally, OCT has also been used to assess the procedural success of new bifurcation stenting (i.e., dedicated side branch stents) [77].

For other complex lesions, such as chronic total occlusions, after recanalization OCT can assess extent of calcific and fibrotic changes and detect the presence of subintimal wire positions, distal dissections, and double channels.

Assessment at follow-up

The possibility to detect tissue coverage and neointima formation in DES over time is one of the most important current research applications of OCT studies investigating the underlying mechanisms implicated in stent failure, such as stent thrombosis, in-stent restenosis, and neoatherosclerosis; delayed neointimal healing has been considered a possible underlying substrate of fatal stent thrombosis [61,78]. The percentage of uncovered stent struts represented the best morphometric predictor of late DES thrombosis and the risk increases with the percentage of uncovered stent struts per section [61].

An important caveat is the inability of OCT to detect thin layers of neointima below its axial resolution and to differentiate between neointima (smooth muscle cells and matrix) and other pathologic components such as fibrin or thrombus. The latter becomes an issue at very early phases after stenting, when the prevalence of struts covered by fibrin is high. Thus, DES are completely covered with fibrin, rather than a neointima, 1–3 days after implantation, but the low discriminative power of OCT results in false coverage rates of 45–76% [79]. Moreover, fibrin coverage might persist longer with DES. The analysis of optical density might aid discriminating between neointima and fibrin [79,80]. However, as the greatest interest is to assess intimal coverage at late follow-up, when the prevalence of fibrin-covered struts is low, the practical impact of this limitation is minimal. Significant differences exist in stent strut coverage and apposition between various DES at 3–12 months post implantation and this could explain the different clinical results obtained with second generation compared with first generation DES [81]. This is possibly due to the thickness and biocompatibility of the polymer that could be responsible for triggering inflammatory reactions or the different strut thickness and cell design. The analysis of strut coverage by OCT has contributed to a better understanding of the vascular healing process after BVS implantation showing its unique potential in vascular repair, such as late lumen enlargement and plaque media reduction [82,83].

In-stent restenosis and neoatherosclerosis

OCT offers data concerning the underlying pathophysiology that contributes to in-stent restenosis (ISR), such as stent underexpansion, strut fracture, and strut distribution. OCT is additionally capable of assessing the specific lumen shape and neointimal tissue. Yet, because of reduced tissue penetration of OCT, plaque behind the stent struts is poorly visualized [84]. OCT accurately measures the percentage of neointimal volume obstruction, which is conventionally evaluated with IVUS to portray any neointimal hyperplasia inside the stents, and has become a standard in trials assessing the efficacy and safety of novel stents [85].

Various ISR tissue patterns have been defined based on optical homogeneity (homogenous, heterogeneous, and layered), restenotic tissue backscatter (high, low), visibility of microvessels, lumen shape (regular, irregular), and the existence of intraluminal components [86]. Bare metal stents are associated with homogenous patterns, whereas DES are typically associated with heterogeneous patterns [87,88]. Furthermore, hyperplastic tissue evolution into neoatherosclerosis can be evaluated by OCT; this is important, because there has been emerging data claiming the relevance of late de novo neoatherosclerosis in late ISR or thrombosis [89,90].

In ISR, OCT can also be used to precisely follow the irregular lumen contour after cutting balloon and to guide cutting balloon sizing. In particular, OCT can confirm if cutting balloons have scored the plaque up to the stent at multiple points, which greatly facilitates extrusion and lumen expansion. This is possible because metal struts are powerful enough light reflectors to be visualized through very thick plaques. Through an OCT-guided cutting balloon strategy, intimal hyperplasia was reduced from 69% to 25% in the minimal lumen area segment allowing better preparation for stent deployment or drug-eluting balloon dilatation [54].

Bioabsorbable vascular scaffolds

Bioabsorbable drug-eluting scaffolds have emerged as a potential major breakthrough for treatment of symptomatic coronary artery lesions showing unique potential in vascular repair with restoration of vasomotion, reduction of plaque thickness, and compensatory late lumen enlargement. OCT has been used since the first implants of BVS to study the vessel wall response [82,83] and the timing of the resorption process [91]. Unlike metallic stents which are powerful light reflectors and induce posterior shadowing and blooming artifacts on the vessel surface, polymeric struts of BVS are transparent to the light so that scaffold integrity, apposition to the underlying wall, and changes in the strut characteristics over time can be easily studied. OCT has been used to compare the acute performance of this new device with that of second-generation DES in the treatment of complex coronary artery disease in a real-world setting [92], as well as device-specific complications, such as BVS rupture.

Near-infrared spectroscopy

Atherosclerotic plaque formation is the consequence of inflammation and extracellular matrix formation as well as cholesterol deposition in the vasculature. This process involves the retention of highly atherogenic lipoproteins in the intima of the arterial wall. These lipoproteins accumulate and are modified further deep in the abluminal part of the intima. Altered lipids attract proteolytic enzyme-producing macrophages to their site, which engulf the lipids and leave behind a soft and unstable core that is highly abundant in foam cells and lipids [31]. Cholesterol, whether esterified or unesterified, forms the major part of the lipid core. Histologic studies as well as studies with intravascular imaging have depicted the association of the presence of lipid-laden plaques with the risk of an ACS and increased peri-interventional complications. The ability to detect lipid-rich plaques in patients is therefore of great clinical significance.

Near-infrared spectroscopy (NIRS) is widely used in many disciplines to identify the chemical composition of unknown substances. It utilizes the absorbance and reflectance of near-infrared light from an illuminated targeted area to derive the presence of the target substance. This method is a simple quick technique that provides multiconstituent analysis, and requires no sample preparation or manipulation with hazardous agents [93]. Studies have documented the ability of NIRS to accurately identify lipid-core atherosclerotic plaques in animal models or autopsy specimens and finally, after *in vivo* and *ex vivo* validation studies [94,95], the intraluminal spectroscopy catheter was developed and marketed.

System description

Initially, intracoronary NIRS was developed as an independent imaging modality, but a major drawback was the inability to provide spatial orientation to match the lipid content alongside the plaque distribution. However, current co-registered NIRS-IVUS catheters (TVC Imaging System, InfraReDx Inc, Burlington, MA, USA) provide data regarding both the vessel structure and the plaque composition.

After completion of an automatic pullback, data are processed displaying a two-dimensional map of the vessel, revealing the probability of the presence of a lipid core plaque (LCP), with the pullback position in millimeters on the x-axis and the circumferential position on the y-axis. This display is known as the "chemogram." For each pixel of 0.1 mm and 1°, length and angle respectively, the lipid core probability is calculated from the spectral data collected and semi-quantitatively coded on a color scale from 0 for red and to 1 for yellow. Whenever a pixel lacks sufficient data, for instance the guidewire is shadowing, the pixel appears black.

The block chemogram, also created from the NIRS images, combines the results for each 2-mm section of the artery to create a "virtual block" that summarizes and reflects the probability of LCP intervals. The numeric value of each block produced is the 90th percentile of all pixel values obtained in the corresponding 2-mm section of the artery in the chemogram. Here, the red coloration indicates a low probability of an LCP, whereas yellow coloration determines a higher probability of an LCP, alongside the intensity of the color reflecting the amount of cholesterol present. In isolation, the block chemogram specifically adapts a four-color scale method of analysis (red ($p < 0.57$), orange ($0.57 \leq p < 0.84$), tan ($0.84 \leq p < 0.98$) and yellow ($p \geq 0.98$)) that reflects the probability of the existence of an LCP in each 2-mm block of pullback which aids the overall visual interpretation. Spectral data are paired with corresponding IVUS frames, overall displayed as a ring around the IVUS image. The lipid core burden index (LCBI) measures the portion of pixels that exceed an LCP probability of 0.6, in all viable pixels within the scanned region, multiplied by 1000. This is a quantitative measure of the intensity of yellow pixels present on the chemogram. The LCBI values vary from 0 to 1000 and the maximum value of LCBI for any of the 4-mm segments along the analyzed segment is defined as the $maxLCBI_{4mm}$.

Potantial clinical uses
Determination of high-risk plaque

The necrotic core region has an abundance of lipid deposition and lacks mechanical stability because of the degradation of fibrous tissue and disappearance of cells. The size of the necrotic core has been significantly associated with the likelihood of plaque rupture. In a previous pathologic study of aortic plaques, ulceration and thrombosis were characteristic of plaques with >40% of their volume occupied by extracellular lipids [96]. As the lipid core increases plaque vulnerability, the NIRS can potentially be used to identify high risk plaques (Figure 8.5). It has been shown that the target lesions responsible for ACS were in most cases lipid-rich plaques; additionally, patients with ACS commonly harbored remote, non-target lipid-rich plaques [97]. In another study in patients with STEMI, $maxLCBI_{4mm} > 400$ in NIRS accurately distinguished culprit from non-culprit segments within the artery and from the lipid-rich plaque-free autopsy histology segments [98]. In a recently published prospective observational study, NIRS imaging was performed in a non-culprit coronary artery in 203 patients referred for angiography due to stable angina pectoris or ACS. It was shown that the 1-year cumulative incidence of a cardiovascular event in patients with an LCBI equal to or above the median value (43.0) was significantly higher than those with an LBCI value below the median [99].

Prevention of peri-procedural myocardial infarction and optimizing interventions Peri-procedural myocardial infarction can be related to distal embolization of LCP component, contents, and/or intracoronary thrombus. In a sub-study of COLOR (Chemometric Observation of Lipid Core Plaques of Interest in Native Coronary Arteries) registry, the cardiac biomarkers in 62 stable patients undergoing stenting were evaluated. Findings revealed that 7 out of 14 (50%) patients with a $maxLCBI_{4mm} \geq 500$ developed peri-procedural

myocardial infarction in comparison with the occurrence of this in only 2 out of 48 (4.2%) patients with a $< maxLCBI_{4mm}$ [100]. In a study by Raghunathan *et al.* [101], in which a creatinine kinase-MB increase >3 times the upper normal limit was observed in 27% of patients with a ≥ 1 yellow block as opposed to none of the patients without a yellow block within the stented lesion. Similarly, in the CANARY (Coronary Assessment by Near-infrared of Atherosclerotic Rupture-prone Yellow) trial, patients with peri-interventional myocardial infarction had higher $maxLCBI_{4mm}$ than patients without MI [102]. However, preventive measures for this situation remain uncertain. The use of a distal emboli protection device frequently resulted in embolized material retrieval during intervention in a small group of patients with LCP [103]; however, there was no benefit of this adjunctive treatment in the randomized CANARY trial.

A prospective use of NIRS in catheterization laboratories is in stent sizing to ensure adequate lesion coverage. Visual evaluation of lesions by angiography occasionally lack accuracy and using NIRS, Dixon *et al.* [104] demonstrated that in 16% of the lesions assessed in their study, the LCP extended beyond the angiographic margins of the initial target lesion. Therefore, together with the information provided by IVUS, NIRS data can be used for determining the size and length of the artery to be stented.

Guiding the effects of treatment The effects of current or novel agents that modify plaque composition can be evaluated using NIRS, because it is able to assess the lipid content over time. The YELLOW trial recruited patients with multivessel CAD undergoing PCI. After NIRS and IVUS baseline assessment, patients were randomized to either rosuvastatin 40 mg/day versus the standard of care lipid-lowering therapy. After 7 weeks of short-term intensive statin therapy, a significant reduction in the lipid content was found when measured via max $LCBI_{4mm}$ [105].

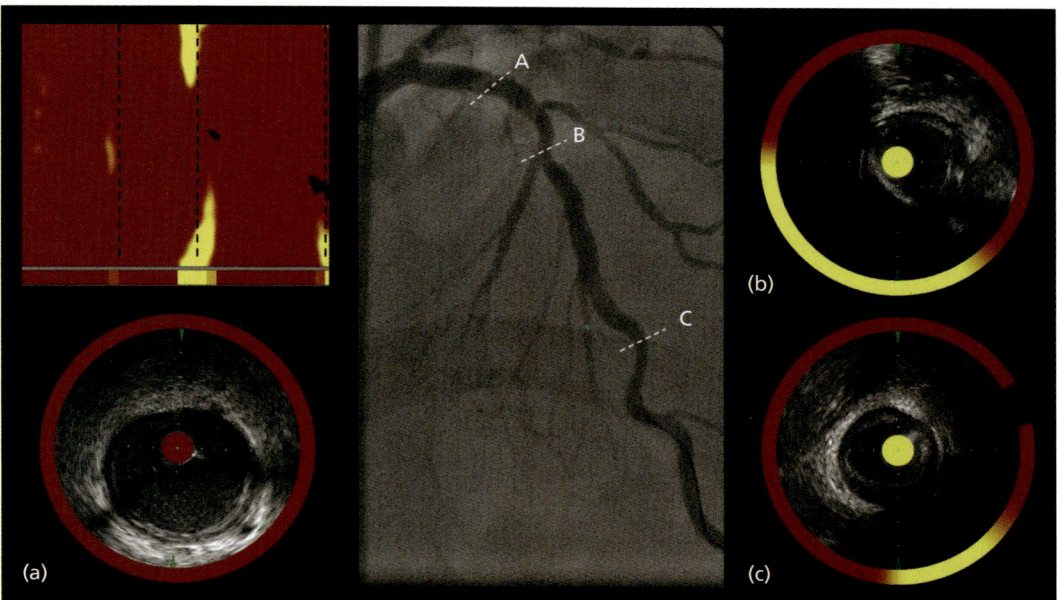

Figure 8.5 A 39-year-old man was admitted with unstable angina. Angiography showed significant lesions in right and left anterior descending arteries. After post-dilatation, near-infrared spectroscopy–intravenous ultrasound (NIRS-IVUS) imaging was performed, which revealed lipid core plaque in the mid- and distal left anterior descending (LAD) (b and c). Proximal segments were relatively disease free (a). Right coronary artery (RCA) also harbored lipid core plaques.

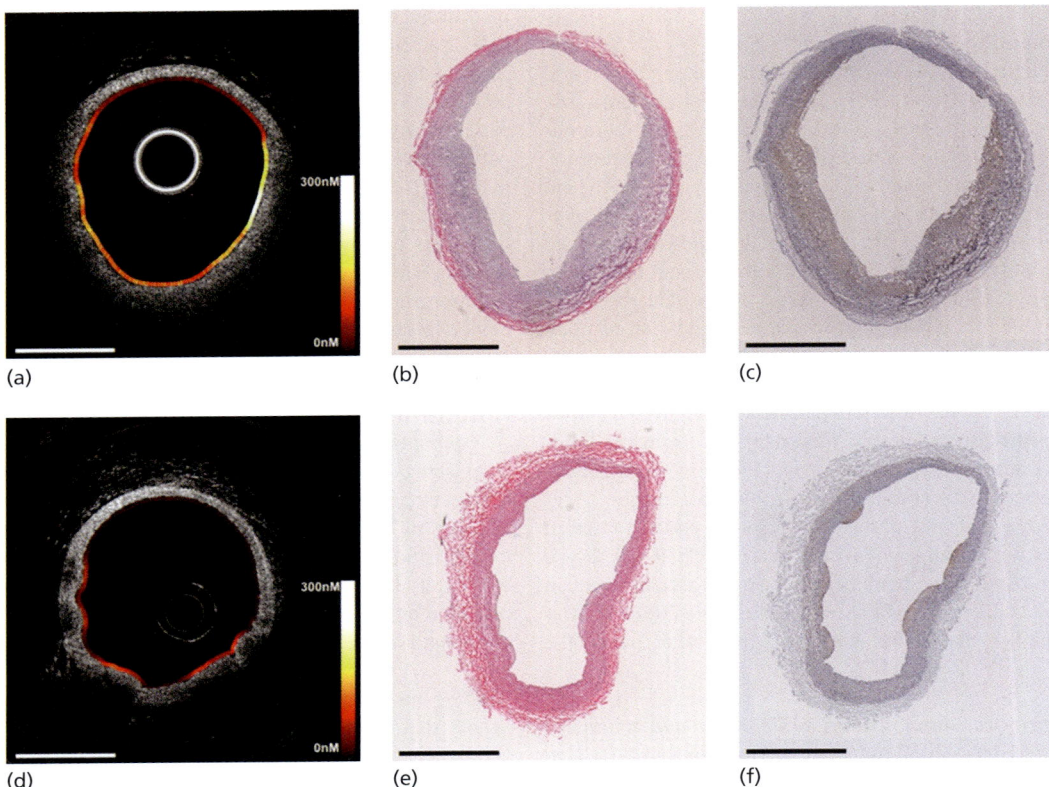

Figure 8.6 Intravascular near-infrared fluorescence molecular imaging of plaque inflammation integrated with exactly co-registered OCT. A dual-modal near-infrared fluorescence (NIRF) OCT catheter was evaluated in inflammatory atherosclerosis in the rabbit aorta, a vessel of similar caliber to the human coronary artery. Twenty-four hours after an intravenous injection of Prosense VM110, a NIRF molecular imaging agent that reports on cathepsin protease activity in atheroma, *in vivo* intravascular NIRF-OCT was performed. NIRF revealed augmented protease activity in OCT-defined atheroma, with substantial inflammation heterogeneity seen across atheroma (a,d). The OCT catheter is seen in the middle of the image; the NIRF signal intensity (representing quantitative protease inflammatory activity) is represented by a color scale bar mapped on to the luminal border. The NIRF-OCT findings were confirmed by histology (H&E, middle column b and e), and cathepsin B immunohistochemistry (right column, c and f). Source: Yoo *et al.* 2011 [110]. Reproduced with permission of Nature Publishing Group.

Ongoing trials

The prospective multicenter PROSPECT II trial aims to collect the post-PCI NIRS/IVUS data of patients with ACS and evaluate the prognostic value of LCBI >400 to evaluate in the 2-year follow-up. The Lipid-Rich Plaque Study will enroll 9000 patients presenting for a coronary angiography where an IVUS and/or NIRS evaluation is planned or could be added as part of a clinically indicated evaluation. Here, the primary outcome to be investigated is the prediction of the non-culprit lesion-related major adverse cardiac events. The IBIS-3 study aims to test the effect of high-dose rosuvastatin in improving the plaque composition of non-intervened coronary arteries as well as the progression of their necrotic core volume assessed with VH-IVUS and NIRS.

Near-infrared fluorescence molecular imaging

A limitation of current intravascular imaging approaches such as OCT or IVUS is the inability to assess specific biologic processes in the coronary arteries of living subjects. Molecular imaging is a relatively new field that aims to image specific molecules and cells involved in the pathogenesis of vascular disease, including macrophages, endothelial cell adhesion molecules, fibrin, and coagulation

factor XIII activity [106,107]. Molecular imaging requires injectable targeted imaging agents that bind a specific molecular or internalized within a cell. These agents can then be detected by an appropriate hardware imaging system, including positron-emission tomography (PET), magnetic resonance imaging (MRI), single-photon emission tomography (SPECT), ultrasound and, more recently, fluorescence imaging systems.

While PET and MRI molecular imaging approaches appear promising for large arterial beds (e.g., carotids, peripheral arteries), the smaller size of the coronary arteries dictates an intravascular-based imaging approach to achieve sufficient sensitivity and resolution. To meet this need, optical-based imaging using near-infrared fluorescence (NIRF) has evolved to serve as a promising coronary artery-targeted intravascular imaging platform. The NIR window (650–900 nm) is advantageous for fluorescence imaging as this window exhibits reduced blood absorption and scattering, and reduced background tissue autofluorescence, which serves to increase the ability to detect NIRF molecular imaging agents *in vivo*.

Over the past 7 years, several intravascular NIRF systems have been engineered, including a one-dimensional wire spectroscopic-based system, a standalone two-dimensional imaging system, and most recently, a combined NIRF-OCT imaging system [108–110]. These preclinical investigations provided the first demonstrations that inflammatory protease activity in atheroma, and fibrin deposition on stents, could be specifically imaged *in vivo* in the aorta of rabbits, which have a similar dimension to human coronary arteries. The most recent NIRF-OCT system has the further advantage of providing simultaneous anatomic information that is precisely co-registered with NIRF molecular information, which further allows quantitative NIRF imaging (Figure 8.6). Similarly to NIRF-OCT, a NIRF-IVUS catheter has been developed but has not been tested *in vivo* through blood yet [111].

Clinical translation

NIRF-OCT imaging system Recently, investigators performed the first human coronary imaging studies of patients using a clinically approved NIRF-OCT catheter [112]. While this catheter was used to detect plaque NIR autofluorescence, or NIRAF (no imaging agent was injected), the ability to safely acquired NIRF-OCT images is a major step forward in realizing intracoronary molecular imaging.

NIRF molecular imaging agents In addition to having a clinically approved catheter, clinical NIRF molecular imaging agents will be required. A promising candidate is indocyanine green (ICG), an amphiphilic molecule that has been FDA-approved for decades to study cardiac, hepatic, and retinal blood flow. In 2011, Vinegoni *et al.* [113] showed that ICG can unexpectedly target plaque macrophages and plaque lipid, and thus could be useful for clinical intracoronary NIRF molecular imaging of vulnerable plaques. This finding was recently confirmed by others [114], and recently in human carotid atheroma patients [115]. Beyond ICG, many targeted NIRF agents are expected to be available for arterial disease in the future, driven primarily by the field of cancer NIRF molecular imaging [116].

 Case Study

A 61-year-old man with a history of hypercholesterolemia presents with typical chest pain on exertion. Diagnostic angiogram showed a chronic total occlusion of the right coronary artery (RCA), in addition to critical stenoses in left circumflex (LCx), obtuse marginal (OM), and mid portion of the left anterior descending (Figure 8.7). The operator decided to proceed with coronary intervention.

He started with predilating LCx with a 2.0 × 20 mm percutaneous transluminal coronary angioplasty (PTCA) balloon, into the OM1. Lesions were, then, covered by a 2.5 × 28 mm bioresorbable vascular scaffold (BVS), which post-dilated with a 3.0 × 8 mm necrotic coreballoon in the proximal part. Angiogram showed excellent results (Figure 8.8). The operator decided to perform an optical coherence tomography (OCT) imaging to better evaluate the results with BVS. However, OCT reveals malapposed struts in the proximal part of the scaffold (Figure 8.9), which was corrected with further post-dilatation and confirmed by a second OCT pullback (Figure 8.10).

He then proceeded with the LAD intervention and implanted a 3.0 × 28 mm BVS. This was post-dilated by a 3.0 × 8 mm necrotic coreballoon at high atmospheres. Angiogram showed good results (Figure 8.11). He, again, performed an OCT pullback. Despite good angiographic results, OCT revealed a distal edge dissection, which was treated by implanting another BVS (Figure 8.12). Moreover, although blood clearance was insufficient in the proximal part, underexpansion of the BVS was evident in this segment. A second post-dilatation was performed using a 3.5 × 8 mm necrotic coreballoon.

Patient was discharged the following day without complications. Chronic total occlusion of the RCA was successfully opened in a staged procedure.

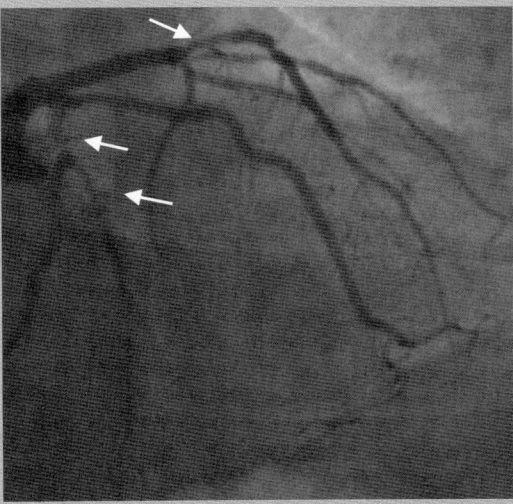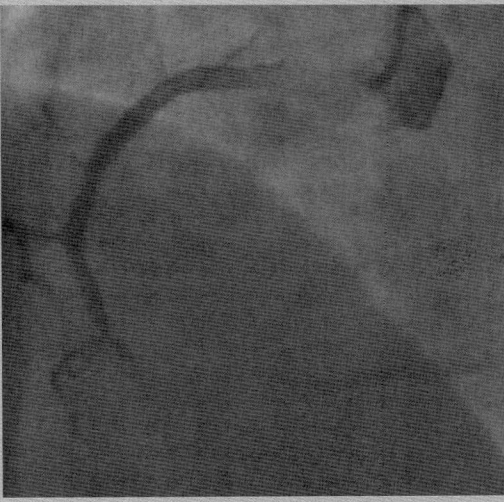

Figure 8.7 Angiogram of the left coronary system showed critical stenoses (arrows). The right coronary was totally occluded.

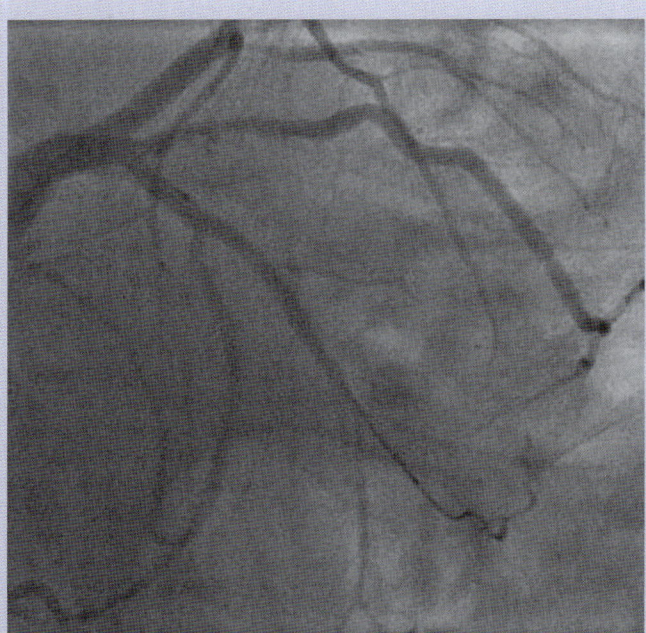

Figure 8.8 Angiogram of the LCx after intervention.

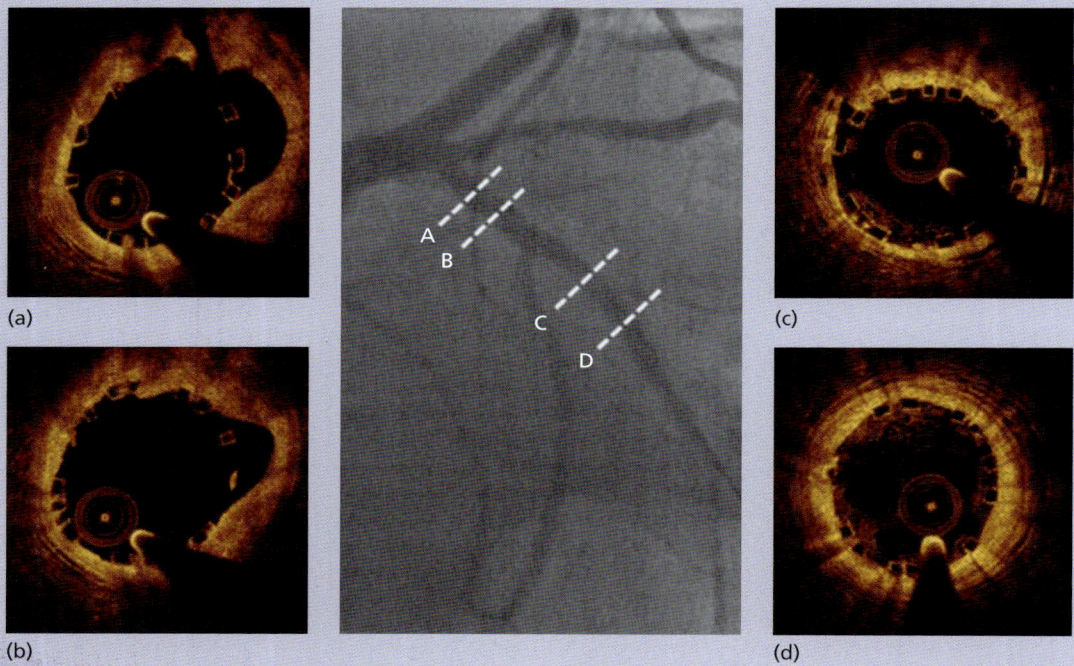

(a)

(b)

(c)

(d)

Figure 8.9 OCT showed malapposed struts in the proximal part.

Discussion

Angiography remains for the gold standard in the treatment of coronary artery disease. However, it provides limited information on the degree and extent of atherosclerosis and falls short in stent assessment. On the other hand, optical coherence tomography provides high-resolution cross-sectional images, offering additional information such as plaque characteristics, lumen measurements, strut apposition and stent expansion, presence of edge dissections.

In this case, the operator preferred an OCT imaging to optimize the results after implantation of BVS. Unlike metallic stents, which are powerful light reflectors and induce posterior shadowing and blooming artifacts on the vessel surface, polymeric struts of BVS are transparent to the light so that scaffold

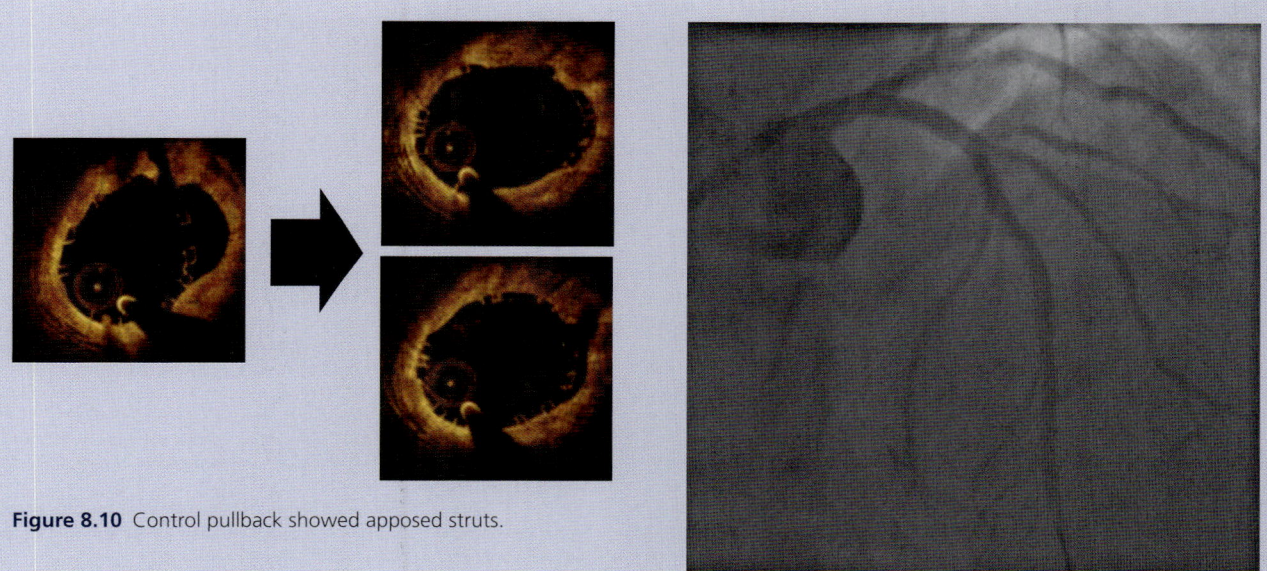

Figure 8.10 Control pullback showed apposed struts.

Figure 8.11 Angiogram after post-dilatation of the BVS.

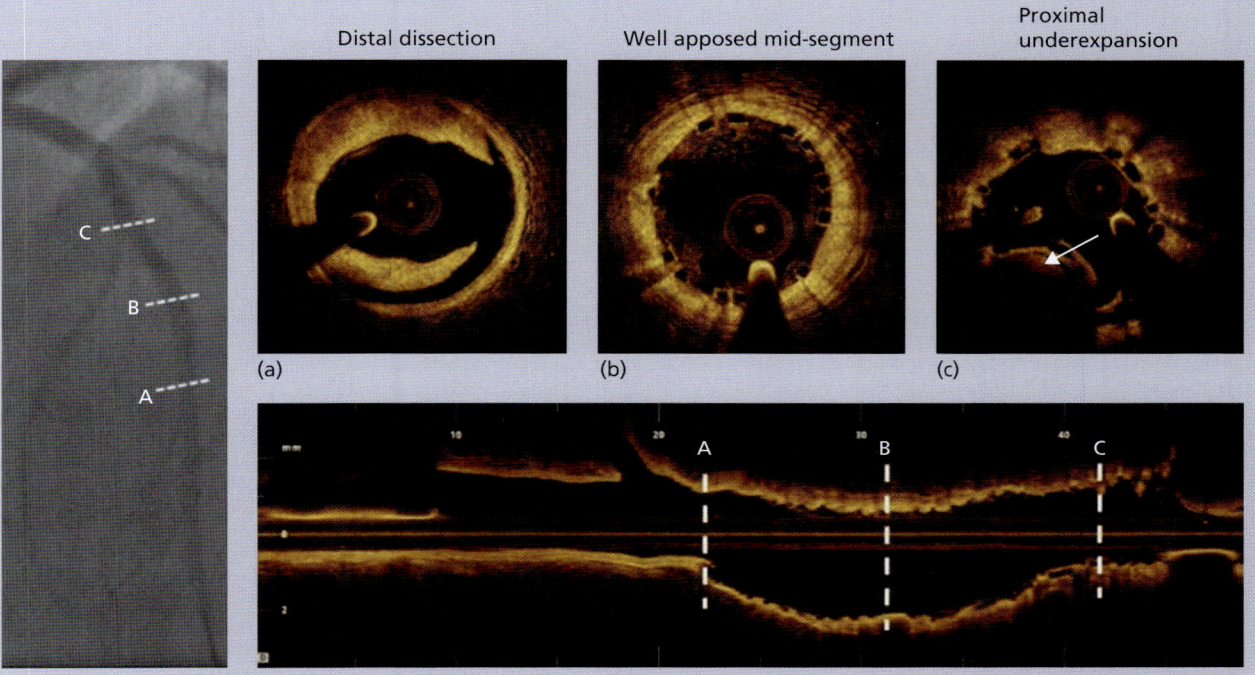

Figure 8.12 Struts were well apposed along the vessel. However, OCT revealed an edge dissection at the distal end. Moreover, BVS was underexpanded in the proximal part of the scaffold. Arrow indicates the blood artifact; note the signal attenuation.

integrity, apposition to the underlying wall, and changes in the strut characteristics over time can be easily studied. Despite conflicting results, some data suggest strut malapposition might be related to stent thrombosis. Similarly, stent underexpansion is a potential cause of stent failure. Dissections usually appear at the stent edges, but most dissections are too small to be detected by angiography. On the contrary, OCT is a sensitive tool in detecting dissections because of its high resolution. Prognostic significance of edge dissections, currently, remains to be clarified.

This case clearly illustrates OCT's help in recognizing stent malapposition, stent underexpansion, and edge dissections, which can be present despite good angiographic results.

Interactive multiple choice questions are available for this chapter on www.wiley.com/go/dangas/cardiology

References

1 Huang D, Swanson EA, Lin CP, *et al.* Optical coherence tomography. *Science* 1991; **22**: 1178–1181.

2 Brezinski ME, Tearney GJ, Bouma BE, *et al.* Imaging of coronary artery microstructure (in vitro) with optical coherence tomography. *Am J Cardiol* 1996; **77**(1): 92–93.

3 Lowe HC, Narula J, Fujimoto JG, Jang I-K. Intracoronary optical diagnostics current status, limitations, and potential. *JACC Cardiovasc Interv* 2011; **4**(12): 1257–1270.

4 Raffel OC, Akasaka T, Jang I-K. Cardiac optical coherence tomography. *Heart* 2008; **94**(9): 1200–1210.

5 Choma M, Sarunic M, Yang C, Izatt J. Sensitivity advantage of swept source and Fourier domain optical coherence tomography. *Opt Express* 2003; **11**(18): 2183–2189.

6 Gonzalo N, Tearney GJ, Serruys PW, *et al.* Second-generation optical coherence tomography in clinical practice: high-speed data acquisition is highly reproducible in patients undergoing percutaneous coronary intervention. *Rev Esp Cardiol* 2010; **63**(8): 893–903.

7 Bouma BE, Yun SH, Vakoc BJ, Suter MJ, Tearney GJ. Fourier-domain optical coherence tomography: recent advances toward clinical utility. *Curr Opin Biotechnol* 2009; **20**(1): 111–118.

8 Hebsgaard L, Christiansen EH, Holm NR. Calibration of intravascular optical coherence tomography as presented in peer reviewed publications. *Int J Cardiol* 2014; **171**(1): 92–93.

9 Foin N, Mari JM, Nijjer S, *et al.* Intracoronary imaging using attenuation-compensated optical coherence tomography allows better visualisation of coronary artery diseases. *Cardiovasc Revasc Med* 2013; **14**(3): 139–143.

10 Van Soest G, Bosch JG, van der Steen AFW. Alignment of intravascular optical coherence tomography movies affected by non-uniform rotation distortion. *Proc SPIE 6847, Coherence Domain Optical Methods and Optical Coherence Tomography in Biomedicine XII*, 684721: 2008.

11 Van Soest G, Regar E, Goderie TPM, *et al.* Pitfalls in plaque characterization by OCT: image artifacts in native coronary arteries. *JACC Cardiovasc Imaging* 2011; **4**(7): 810–813.

12 Tearney GJ, Regar E, Akasaka T, *et al.* Consensus standards for acquisition, measurement, and reporting of intravascular optical coherence tomography studies: a report from the International Working Group for Intravascular Optical Coherence Tomography Standardization and Validation. *J Am Coll Cardiol* 2012; **59**(12): 1058–1072.

13 Bezerra HG, Costa MA, Guagliumi G, Rollins AM, Simon DI. Intracoronary optical coherence tomography: a comprehensive review clinical and research applications. *JACC Cardiovasc Interv* 2009; **2**(11): 1035–1046.

14 Elahi S, Mancuso JJ, Milner TE, Feldman MD. Sunflower artifact in OCT. *JACC Cardiovasc Imaging* 2011; **4**(11): 1220–1221.

15 Waller BF, Orr CM, Slack JD, Pinkerton CA, Van Tassel J, Peters T. Anatomy, histology, and pathology of coronary arteries: a review relevant to new interventional and imaging techniques. *Part I. Clin Cardiol* 1992; **15**(6): 451–457.

16 Fulton WFM. *The Coronary Arteries: Arteriography, Microanatomy, and Pathogenesis of Obliterative Coronary Artery Disease.* C.C. Thomas; 1965.

17 Prati F, Regar E, Mintz GS, *et al.* Expert review document on methodology, terminology, and clinical applications of optical coherence tomography: physical principles, methodology of image acquisition, and clinical application for assessment of coronary arteries and atherosclerosis. *Eur Heart J* 2010; **31**(4): 401–415.

18 Radu MD, Räber L, Garcia-Garcia H, Serruys PW (eds) *The Clinical Atlas of Intravascular Optical Coherence Tomography*, 2013.

19 Yabushita H, Bouma BE, Houser SL, *et al.* Characterization of human atherosclerosis by optical coherence tomography. *Circulation* 2002; **106**(13): 1640–1645.

20 Manfrini O, Mont E, Leone O, *et al.* Sources of error and interpretation of plaque morphology by optical coherence tomography. *Am J Cardiol* 2006; **98**(2): 156–159.

21 Van Soest G, Goderie T, Regar E, *et al.* Atherosclerotic tissue characterization in vivo by optical coherence tomography attenuation imaging. *J Biomed Opt* 2010; **15**(1): 011105.

22 Kume T, Akasaka T, Kawamoto T, *et al.* Assessment of coronary arterial thrombus by optical coherence tomography. *Am J Cardiol* 2006; **97**(12): 1713–1717.

23 Jang I-K, Tearney GJ, MacNeill B, *et al.* In vivo characterization of coronary atherosclerotic plaque by use of optical coherence tomography. *Circulation* 2005; **111**(12): 1551–1555.

24 Burke AP, Farb A, Malcom GT, Liang YH, Smialek J, Virmani R. Coronary risk factors and plaque morphology in men with coronary disease who died suddenly. *N Engl J Med* 1997; **336**(18): 1276–1282.

25 Kume T, Akasaka T, Kawamoto T, *et al.* Measurement of the thickness of the fibrous cap by optical coherence tomography. *Am Heart J* 2006; **152**(4): 755.e1–4.

26 Kubo T, Imanishi T, Kashiwagi M, *et al.* Multiple coronary lesion instability in patients with acute myocardial infarction as determined by optical coherence tomography. *Am J Cardiol* 2010; **105**(3): 318–322.

27 Radu MD, Falk E. In search of vulnerable features of coronary plaques with optical coherence tomography: is it time to rethink the current methodological concepts? *Eur Heart J* 2012; **33**(1): 9–12.

28 Kimura S, Kakuta T, Yonetsu T, *et al.* Clinical significance of echo signal attenuation on intravascular ultrasound in patients with coronary artery disease. *Circ Cardiovasc Interv* 2009; **2**(5): 444–454.

29 Di Vito L, Agozzino M, Marco V, *et al.* Identification and quantification of macrophage presence in coronary atherosclerotic plaques by optical coherence tomography. *Eur Heart J Cardiovasc Imaging* 2015; **16**(7): 807–813.

30 Tanaka A, Tearney GJ, Bouma BE. Challenges on the frontier of intracoronary imaging: atherosclerotic plaque macrophage measurement by optical coherence tomography. *J Biomed Opt* 2010; **15**(1): 011104.

31 Falk E, Nakano M, Bentzon JF, Finn AV, Virmani R. Update on acute coronary syndromes: the pathologists' view. *Eur Heart J* 2013; **34**(10): 719–728.

32 Vorpahl M, Nakano M, Virmani R. Small black holes in optical frequency domain imaging matches intravascular neoangiogenesis formation in histology. *Eur Heart J* 2010; **31**(15): 1889.

33 Kitabata H, Tanaka A, Kubo T, *et al.* Relation of microchannel structure identified by optical coherence tomography to plaque vulnerability in patients with coronary artery disease. *Am J Cardiol* 2010; **105**(12): 1673–1678.

34 Tian J, Hou J, Xing L, *et al.* Significance of intraplaque neovascularisation for vulnerability: optical coherence tomography study. *Heart* 2012; **98**(20): 1504–1509.

35 Kato K, Yonetsu T, Kim SJ, *et al.* Nonculprit plaques in patients with acute coronary syndromes have more vulnerable features compared with those with non-acute coronary syndromes: a 3-vessel optical coherence tomography study. *Circ Cardiovasc Imaging* 2012; **5**(4): 433–440.

36 Chia S, Raffel OC, Takano M, Tearney GJ, Bouma BE, Jang IK. Association of statin therapy with reduced coronary plaque rupture: an optical coherence tomography study. *Coron Artery Dis* 2008; **19**(4): 237–242.

37 Takarada S, Imanishi T, Kubo T, *et al.* Effect of statin therapy on coronary fibrous-cap thickness in patients with acute coronary syndrome: assessment by optical coherence tomography study. *Atherosclerosis* 2009; **202**(2): 491–497.

38 Hattori K, Ozaki Y, Ismail TF, *et al.* Impact of statin therapy on plaque characteristics as assessed by serial OCT, grayscale and integrated backscatter-IVUS. *JACC Cardiovasc Imaging* 2012; **5**(2): 169–177.

39 Komukai K, Kubo T, Kitabata H, *et al.* Effect of atorvastatin therapy on fibrous cap thickness in coronary atherosclerotic plaque as assessed by optical coherence tomography. *J Am Coll Cardiol* 2014; **64**(21): 2207–2217.

40 Tian J, Hou J, Xing L, *et al.* Does neovascularization predict response to statin therapy? Optical coherence tomography study. *Int J Cardiol* 2012; **158**(3): 469–470.

41 Nissen SE, Tuzcu EM, Schoenhagen P, *et al.* Effect of intensive compared with moderate lipid-lowering therapy on progression of coronary atherosclerosis: a randomized controlled trial. *JAMA* 2004; **291**(9): 1071–1080.

42 Nissen SE, Nicholls SJ, Sipahi I, *et al.* Effect of very high-intensity statin therapy on regression of coronary atherosclerosis: the ASTEROID trial. *JAMA* 2006; **295**(13): 1556–1565.

43 Nicholls SJ, Ballantyne CM, Barter PJ, *et al.* Effect of two intensive statin regimens on progression of coronary disease. *N Engl J Med* 2011; **365**(22): 2078–2087.

44 Ino Y, Kubo T, Tanaka A, *et al.* Difference of culprit lesion morphologies between ST-segment elevation myocardial infarction and non-ST-segment elevation acute coronary syndrome: an optical coherence tomography study. *JACC Cardiovasc Interv* 2011; **4**(1): 76–82.

45 Shimamura K, Ino Y, Kubo T, *et al.* Difference of ruptured plaque morphology between asymptomatic coronary artery disease and non-ST elevation acute coronary syndrome patients: an optical coherence tomography study. *Atherosclerosis* 2014; **235**(2): 532–537.

46 Otsuka F, Joner M, Prati F, Virmani R, Narula J. Clinical classification of plaque morphology in coronary disease. *Nat Rev Cardiol* 2014; **11**(7): 379–389.

47 Jia H, Abtahian F, Aguirre AD, *et al.* In vivo diagnosis of plaque erosion and calcified nodule in patients with acute coronary syndrome by intravascular optical coherence tomography. *J Am Coll Cardiol* 2013; **62**(19): 1748–1758.

48 Prati F, Uemura S, Souteyrand G, *et al.* OCT-based diagnosis and management of STEMI associated with intact fibrous cap. *JACC Cardiovasc Imaging* 2013; **6**(3): 283–287.

49 Kubo T, Akasaka T, Shite J, *et al.* OCT compared with IVUS in a coronary lesion assessment: the OPUS-CLASS study. *JACC Cardiovasc Imaging* 2013; **6**(10): 1095–1104.

50 Habara M, Nasu K, Terashima M, *et al.* Impact of frequency-domain optical coherence tomography guidance for optimal coronary stent implantation in comparison with intravascular ultrasound guidance. *Circ Cardiovasc Interv* 2012; **5**(2): 193–201.

51 Liu Y, Shimamura K, Kubo T, *et al.* Comparison of longitudinal geometric measurement in human coronary arteries between frequency-domain optical coherence tomography and intravascular ultrasound. *Int J Cardiovasc Imaging* 2014; **30**(2): 271–277.

52 Viceconte N, Chan PH, Barrero EA, *et al.* Frequency domain optical coherence tomography for guidance of coronary stenting. *Int J Cardiol* 2013; **166**(3): 722–728.

53 Prati F, Di Vito L, Biondi-Zoccai G, *et al.* Angiography alone versus angiography plus optical coherence tomography to guide decision-making during percutaneous coronary intervention: the Centro per la Lotta contro l'Infarto-Optimisation of Percutaneous Coronary Intervention (CLI-OPCI) study. *EuroIntervention* 2012; **8**(7): 823–829.

54 Secco GG, Foin N, Viceconte N, Borgia F, De Luca G, Di Mario C. Optical coherence tomography for guidance of treatment of in-stent restenosis with cutting balloons. *EuroIntervention* 2011; **7**(7): 828–834.

55 Mattesini A, Pighi M, Konstantinidis N, *et al.* Optical coherence tomography in bioabsorbable stents: mechanism of vascular response and guidance of stent implantation. *Minerva Cardioangiol* 2014; **62**(1): 71–82.

56 Hong M-K, Mintz GS, Lee CW, *et al.* Late stent malapposition after drug-eluting stent implantation: an intravascular ultrasound analysis with long-term follow-up. *Circulation* 2006; **113**(3): 414–419.

57 Cook S, Wenaweser P, Togni M, *et al.* Incomplete stent apposition and very late stent thrombosis after drug-eluting stent implantation. *Circulation* 2007; **115**(18): 2426–2434.

58 Hassan AKM, Bergheanu SC, Stijnen T, *et al.* Late stent malapposition risk is higher after drug-eluting stent compared with bare-metal stent implantation and associates with late stent thrombosis. *Eur Heart J* 2010; **31**(10): 1172–1180.

59 Im E, Kim BK, Ko YG, *et al.* Incidences, predictors, and clinical outcomes of acute and late stent malapposition detected by optical coherence tomography after drug-eluting stent implantation. *Circ Cardiovasc Interv* 2014; **7**(1): 88–96.

60 Gutiérrez-Chico JL, Wykrzykowska J, Nüesch E, *et al.* Vascular tissue reaction to acute malapposition in human coronary arteries: sequential assessment with optical coherence tomography. *Circ Cardiovasc Interv* 2012; **5**(1): 20–9, S1–8.

61 Finn AV, Joner M, Nakazawa G, *et al.* Pathological correlates of late drug-eluting stent thrombosis: strut coverage as a marker of endothelialization. *Circulation* 2007; **115**(18): 2435–2441.

62 Joner M, Finn AV, Farb A, *et al.* Pathology of drug-eluting stents in humans: delayed healing and late thrombotic risk. *J Am Coll Cardiol* 2006; **48**(1): 193–202.

63 Gutiérrez-Chico JL, van Geuns RJ, Regar E, *et al.* Tissue coverage of a hydrophilic polymer-coated zotarolimus-eluting stent vs. a fluoropolymer-coated everolimus-eluting stent at 13-month follow-up: an optical coherence tomography substudy from the RESOLUTE All Comers trial. *Eur Heart J* 2011; **32**(19): 2454–2463.

64 Gonzalo N, Serruys PW, Okamura T, *et al.* Optical coherence tomography assessment of the acute effects of stent implantation on the vessel wall: a systematic quantitative approach. *Heart* 2009; **95**(23): 1913–1919.

65 Gonzalo N, Serruys PW, Okamura T, *et al.* Relation between plaque type and dissections at the edges after stent implantation: an optical coherence tomography study. *Int J Cardiol* 2011; **150**(2): 151–155.

66 Radu MD, Räber L, Heo J, *et al.* Natural history of optical coherence tomography-detected non-flow-limiting edge dissections following drug-eluting stent implantation. *EuroIntervention* 2014; **9**(9): 1085–1094.

67 Tyczynski P, Ferrante G, Moreno-Ambroj C, *et al.* Simple versus complex approaches to treating coronary bifurcation lesions: direct assessment of stent strut apposition by optical coherence tomography. *Rev española Cardiol* 2010; **63**(8): 904–914.

68 Viceconte N, Tyczynski P, Ferrante G, *et al.* Immediate results of bifurcational stenting assessed with optical coherence tomography. *Catheter Cardiovasc Interv* 2013; **81**(3): 519–528.

69 Lassen JF, Holm NR, Stankovic G, *et al.* Percutaneous coronary intervention for coronary bifurcation disease: consensus from the first 10 years of the European Bifurcation Club meetings. *EuroIntervention* 2014; **10**(5): 545–560.

70 Alegría-Barrero E, Foin N, Chan PH, *et al.* Optical coherence tomography for guidance of distal cell recrossing in bifurcation stenting: choosing the right cell matters. *EuroIntervention* 2012; **8**(2): 205–213.

71 Okamura T, Onuma Y, García-García HM, *et al.* 3-Dimensional optical coherence tomography assessment of jailed side branches by bioresorbable vascular scaffolds: a proposal for classification. *JACC Cardiovasc Interv* 2010; **3**(8): 836–844.

72 Okamura T, Yamada J, Nao T, *et al.* Three-dimensional optical coherence tomography assessment of coronary wire re-crossing position during bifurcation stenting. *EuroIntervention* 2011; **7**(7): 886–887.

73 Farooq V, Serruys PW, Heo JH, *et al.* New insights into the coronary artery bifurcation hypothesis-generating concepts utilizing 3-dimensional optical frequency domain imaging. *JACC Cardiovasc Interv* 2011; **4**(8): 921–931.

74 Farooq V, Okamura T, Onuma Y, Gogas BD, Serruys PW. Unravelling the complexities of the coronary bifurcation: is this raising a few eyebrows? *EuroIntervention* 2012; **7**(10): 1133–1141.

75 Farooq V, Gogas BD, Okamura T, *et al.* Three-dimensional optical frequency domain imaging in conventional percutaneous coronary intervention: the potential for clinical application. *Eur Heart J* 2013; **34**(12): 875–885.

76 Okamura T, Onuma Y, Yamada J, *et al.* 3D optical coherence tomography: new insights into the process of optimal rewiring of side branches during bifurcational stenting. *EuroIntervention* 2014; **10**(8): 907–915.

77 Ferrante G, Kaplan AV, Di Mario C. Assessment with optical coherence tomography of a new strategy for bifurcational lesion treatment: the Tryton Side-Branch Stent. *Catheter Cardiovasc Interv* 2009; **73**(1): 69–72.

78 Virmani R, Guagliumi G, Farb A, *et al.* Localized hypersensitivity and late coronary thrombosis secondary to a sirolimus-eluting stent: should we be cautious? *Circulation* 2004; **109**(6): 701–705.

79 Templin C, Meyer M, Müller MF, *et al.* Coronary optical frequency domain imaging (OFDI) for in vivo evaluation of stent healing: comparison with light and electron microscopy. *Eur Heart J* 2010; **31**(14): 1792–1801.

80 Malle C, Tada T, Steigerwald K, *et al.* Tissue characterization after drug-eluting stent implantation using optical coherence tomography. *Arterioscler Thromb Vasc Biol* 2013; **33**(6): 1376–1383.

81 Papayannis AC, Cipher D, Banerjee S, Brilakis ES. Optical coherence tomography evaluation of drug-eluting stents: a systematic review. *Catheter Cardiovasc Interv* 2013; **81**(3): 481–487.

82 Serruys PW, Ormiston JA, Onuma Y, *et al.* A bioabsorbable everolimus-eluting coronary stent system (ABSORB): 2-year outcomes and results from multiple imaging methods. *Lancet* 2009; **373**(9667): 897–910.

83 Serruys PW, Onuma Y, Dudek D, *et al.* Evaluation of the second generation of a bioresorbable everolimus-eluting vascular scaffold for the treatment of de novo coronary artery stenosis: 12-month clinical and imaging outcomes. *J Am Coll Cardiol* 2011; **58**(15): 1578–1588.

84 Alfonso F, Byrne RA, Rivero F, Kastrati A. Current treatment of in-stent restenosis. *J Am Coll Cardiol* 2014; **63**(24): 2659–2673.

85 Gutiérrez-Chico JL, Alegría-Barrero E, Teijeiro-Mestre R, *et al.* Optical coherence tomography: from research to practice. *Eur Heart J Cardiovasc Imaging* 2012; **13**(5): 370–384.

86 Gonzalo N, Serruys PW, Okamura T, *et al.* Optical coherence tomography patterns of stent restenosis. *Am Heart J* 2009; **158**(2): 284–293.

87 Takano M, Yamamoto M, Inami S, *et al.* Appearance of lipid-laden intima and neovascularization after implantation of bare-metal stents extended late-phase observation by intracoronary optical coherence tomography. *J Am Coll Cardiol* 2009; **55**(1): 26–32.

88 Kilickesmez K, Dall'Ara G, Rama-Merchan JC, *et al.* Optical coherence tomography characteristics of in-stent restenosis are different between first and second generation drug eluting stents. *IJC Heart Vessel* 2014; **3**: 68–74.

89 Kang S-J, Mintz GS, Akasaka T, *et al.* Optical coherence tomographic analysis of in-stent neoatherosclerosis after drug-eluting stent implantation. *Circulation* 2011; **123**(25): 2954–2963.

90 Miyazaki S, Hiasa Y, Takahashi T, *et al.* In vivo optical coherence tomography of very late drug-eluting stent thrombosis compared with late in-stent restenosis. *Circ J* 2012; **76**(2): 390–398.

91 Onuma Y, Serruys PW, Perkins LEL, *et al.* Intracoronary optical coherence tomography and histology at 1 month and 2, 3, and 4 years after implantation of everolimus-eluting bioresorbable vascular scaffolds in a porcine coronary artery model: an attempt to decipher the human optical coherence tomography. *Circulation* 2010; **122**(22): 2288–2300.

92 Mattesini A, Secco GG, Dall'Ara G, *et al.* ABSORB biodegradable stents versus second-generation metal stents: a comparison study of 100 complex lesions treated under OCT guidance. *JACC Cardiovasc Interv* 2014; **7**(7): 741–750.

93 Dempsey RJ, Davis DG, Buice RG, Lodder RA. Biological and medical applications of near-infrared spectrometry. *Appl Spectrosc OSA* 1996; **50**(2): 18A–34A.

94 Gardner CM, Tan H, Hull EL, *et al.* Detection of lipid core coronary plaques in autopsy specimens with a novel catheter-based near-infrared spectroscopy system. *JACC Cardiovasc Imaging* 2008; **1**(5): 638–648.

95 Waxman S, Dixon SR, L'Allier P, *et al.* In vivo validation of a catheter-based near-infrared spectroscopy system for detection of lipid core coronary plaques: initial results of the SPECTACL study. *JACC Cardiovasc Imaging* 2009; **2**(7): 858–868.

96 Davies MJ, Richardson PD, Woolf N, Katz DR, Mann J. Risk of thrombosis in human atherosclerotic plaques: role of extracellular lipid, macrophage, and smooth muscle cell content. *Br Heart J* 1993; **69**(5): 377–381.

97 Madder RD, Smith JL, Dixon SR, Goldstein JA. Composition of target lesions by near-infrared spectroscopy in patients with acute coronary syndrome versus stable angina. *Circ Cardiovasc Interv* 2012; **5**(1): 55–61.

98 Madder RD, Goldstein JA, Madden SP, *et al.* Detection by near-infrared spectroscopy of large lipid core plaques at culprit sites in patients with acute ST-segment elevation myocardial infarction. *JACC Cardiovasc Interv* 2013; **6**(8): 838–846.

99 Oemrawsingh RM, Cheng JM, García-García HM, *et al.* Near-infrared spectroscopy predicts cardiovascular outcome in patients with coronary artery disease. *J Am Coll Cardiol* 2014; **64**(23): 2510–2518.

100 Goldstein JA, Maini B, Dixon SR, *et al.* Detection of lipid-core plaques by intracoronary near-infrared spectroscopy identifies high risk of periprocedural myocardial infarction. *Circ Cardiovasc Interv* 2011; **4**(5): 429–437.

101 Raghunathan D, Abdel-Karim A-RR, Papayannis AC, *et al.* Relation between the presence and extent of coronary lipid core plaques detected by near-infrared spectroscopy with postpercutaneous coronary intervention myocardial infarction. *Am J Cardiol* 2011; **107**(11): 1613–1618.

102 Stone G. TCT Congress 2014. Washington DC, USA. CANARY: Evaluation of the relationship between intravascular ultrasound and near infrared spectroscopy lipid parameters with periprocedural myonecrosis, with an integrated randomized trial of distal protection to prevent PCI-related myocardial infarction. Washington DC; 2014.

103 Brilakis ES, Abdel-Karim A-RR, Papayannis AC, *et al.* Embolic protection device utilization during stenting of native coronary artery lesions with large lipid core plaques as detected by near-infrared spectroscopy. *Catheter Cardiovasc Interv* 2012; **80**(7): 1157–1162.

104 Dixon SR, Grines CL, Munir A, *et al.* Analysis of target lesion length before coronary artery stenting using angiography and near-infrared spectroscopy versus angiography alone. *Am J Cardiol* 2012; **109**(1): 60–66.

105 Kini AS, Baber U, Kovacic JC, *et al.* Changes in plaque lipid content after short-term intensive versus standard statin therapy: the YELLOW trial (reduction in yellow plaque by aggressive lipid-lowering therapy). *J Am Coll Cardiol* 2013; **62**(1): 21–29.

106 Osborn EA, Jaffer FA. The advancing clinical impact of molecular imaging in CVD. *JACC Cardiovasc Imaging* 2013; **6**(12): 1327–1341.

107 Jaffer FA, Verjans JW. Molecular imaging of atherosclerosis: clinical state-of-the-art. *Heart* 2014; **100**(18): 1469–1477.

108 Jaffer FA, Vinegoni C, John MC, *et al.* Real-time catheter molecular sensing of inflammation in proteolytically active atherosclerosis. *Circulation* 2008; **118**(18): 1802–1809.

109 Jaffer FA, Calfon MA, Rosenthal A, *et al.* Two-dimensional intravascular near-infrared fluorescence molecular imaging of inflammation in atherosclerosis and stent-induced vascular injury. *J Am Coll Cardiol* 2011; **57**(25): 2516–2526.

110 Yoo H, Kim JW, Shishkov M, *et al.* Intra-arterial catheter for simultaneous microstructural and molecular imaging in vivo. *Nat Med* 2011; **17**(12): 1680–1684.

111 Dixon AJ, Hossack JA. Intravascular near-infrared fluorescence catheter with ultrasound guidance and blood attenuation correction. *J Biomed Opt* 2013; **18**(5): 56009.

112 Ughi GJ. Abstract Presentation in TCT Congress 2014. Washington DC, USA. Next-Generation Intravascular Imaging: Dual-Modality OCT and Near-Infrared Auto-Fluorescence (NIRAF) for the Simultaneous Acquisition of Microstructural and Molecular/Chemical Information Within the Coronary Vasculature: Early Human Clinical Experience. Washington DC: 2014.

113 Vinegoni C, Botnaru I, Aikawa E, *et al.* Indocyanine green enables near-infrared fluorescence imaging of lipid-rich, inflamed atherosclerotic plaques. *Sci Transl Med* 2011; **3**(84): 84ra45.

114 Lee S, Lee MW, Cho HS, *et al.* Fully integrated high-speed intravascular optical coherence tomography/near-infrared fluorescence structural/molecular imaging in vivo using a clinically available near-infrared fluorescence-emitting indocyanine green to detect inflamed lipid-rich atherom. *Circ Cardiovasc Interv* 2014; **7**(4): 560–569.

115 Verjans JW, Osborn EA, Ughi GJ, *et al.* Targeted near-infrared fluorescence imaging of atherosclerosis: clinical and intracoronary evaluation of indocyanine green. *J Am Coll Cardiol Img.* Published online August 17, 2016. doi:10.1016/j.jcmg.2016.01.034.

116 Van Dam GM, Themelis G, Crane LMA, *et al.* Intraoperative tumor-specific fluorescence imaging in ovarian cancer by folate receptor-α targeting: first in-human results. *Nat Med* 2011; **17**(10): 1315–1319.

CHAPTER 9

Complementary Imaging Techniques: Multislice Computed Tomography of Coronary Arteries

Omosalewa O. Lalude[1], Francesca Pugliese[2], Pim J. de Feyter[2], and Stamatios Lerakis[3]

[1] Memorial Healthcare System, Hollywood, FL, USA

[2] Erasmus MC University Medical Center, Rotterdam, The Netherlands

[3] Emory University School of Medicine and Georgia Institute of Technology, Atlanta, GA, USA

The introduction of 4-slice computed tomography (CT) in 2000 was followed by rapid and revolutionary advances in multislice computed tomography (MSCT) technology. Currently, 64-MSCT and dual-source computed tomography (DSCT) are considered state-of-the-art for cardiac MSCT imaging with 320-slice systems also emerging in clinical practice.

Non contrast-enhanced MSCT scans allow visualization of cardiac and coronary artery calcification. After intravenous injection of iodinated contrast agent, MSCT can delineate cardiac chambers, great cardiac vessels, and coronary arteries (Figure 9.1).

The evaluation of general cardiac morphology is usually performed by echocardiography and/or magnetic resonance imaging (MRI) without the need for contrast injection or radiation exposure. Nevertheless, MSCT can be clinically helpful in a variety of situations, including the need for cross-sectional imaging in the event of inconclusive findings at echocardiography or in patients with pacemakers or other devices precluding MRI. Importantly, the main clinical focus of MSCT in cardiac imaging is the evaluation of the coronary arteries.

Coronary MSCT angiography—technique
Basic principles
In MSCT scanners, the X-rays are generated by an X-ray tube mounted on a rotating gantry. The patient is centered within the bore of the gantry such that the array of detectors is positioned to record incident photons after they have traversed the patient. MSCT differs from single detector CT principally by the design of the detector array, which allows the acquisition of multiple adjacent sections simultaneously.

MSCT systems have two principal modes of scanning (Figure 9.2). The first mode is *sequential* scanning, also known as "step-and-shoot," in which the table is advanced in a step-wise fashion. In this mode, the X-rays are generated during an imaging window positioned at a predetermined offset from the R wave (prospective ECG triggering; Figure 9.2a) while the table is stationary. The diastolic phase of the cardiac cycle is usually chosen because cardiac motion is reduced in diastole. Sequential scanning is the current mode for measuring coronary calcium at most centers using MSCT.

The second mode is *spiral* or helical scanning, in which the table moves continuously at a fixed speed relative to the gantry rotation.

The ECG trace of the patient is recorded during the scan. After data acquisition, the optimal reconstruction window is chosen among all available time positions to minimize motion artifacts (retrospective ECG gating; Figure 9.2b). Spiral scanning is the current mode for performing coronary MSCT angiography because it allows flexibility in the position of reconstruction windows, which is helpful to ensure the least motion artifacts. However, spiral scanning is associated with a higher X-ray radiation exposure than sequential scanning.

In order to reduce radiation exposure in spiral scanning, the X-ray tube current can be modulated prospectively: guided by the ECG, the full output occurs only during an interval of the cardiac cycle which will be used for image reconstruction (e.g. diastole), whereas the X-ray output will be reduced during the remaining cardiac cycle (Figure 9.2b).

Temporal resolution is the time for acquiring the data needed for the reconstruction of one image. Temporal resolution depends primarily on gantry rotation time. In particular, because reconstruction of MSCT images requires data acquired over half gantry rotation (180°), temporal resolution equals half of the gantry rotation time (Figure 9.3a). The latest development to improve temporal resolution and omit the need to lower patients' heart rates by pre-medication has been the introduction of MSCT scanners with two X-ray sources acquiring different projections simultaneously [1]. In DSCT, the two X-ray sources are mounted at an angle of 90°, therefore temporal resolution is equal to a quarter of the gantry rotation time (i.e., 330/4 = 83 ms) (Figures 9.3b and 9.4).

Coronary arteries have a diameter of 2–4 mm in their proximal tract and taper distally, therefore high *spatial resolution* is another prerequisite for MSCT coronary imaging. Spatial resolution of MSCT on the transverse plane (x, y) is 0.4×0.4 mm^2. Spatial resolution along patient's longitudinal axis (z-axis) is determined mainly by the individual detector width, which varies between 0.5 and 0.625 mm depending on the manufacturer. These features permit reconstruction of high quality images with similar sub-millimeter resolution along the x, y, and z axes. Although catheter angiography has a bi-dimensional spatial resolution of 0.2×0.2 mm^2, a major advantage of MSCT over catheter angiography is the ability to perform multi-planar reconstructed images. An overview of major image parameters, patient preparation, and contrast administration in catheter angiography, 64-MSCT, and DSCT is given in Table 9.1.

Interventional Cardiology: Principles and Practice, Second Edition. Edited by George D. Dangas, Carlo Di Mario, and Nicholas N. Kipshidze.
© 2017 John Wiley & Sons, Ltd. Published 2017 by John Wiley & Sons, Ltd.

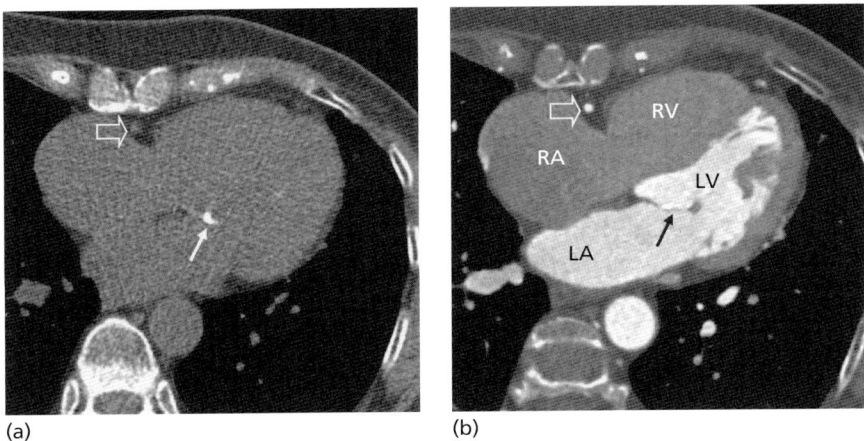

Figure 9.1 Axial images provide four-chamber views of the heart without (a) and with (b) injection of contrast agent. LA, left atrium; LV, left ventricle; RA, right atrium; RV, right ventricle; void arrow, right coronary artery; arrow, mild calcification of the mitral valve.

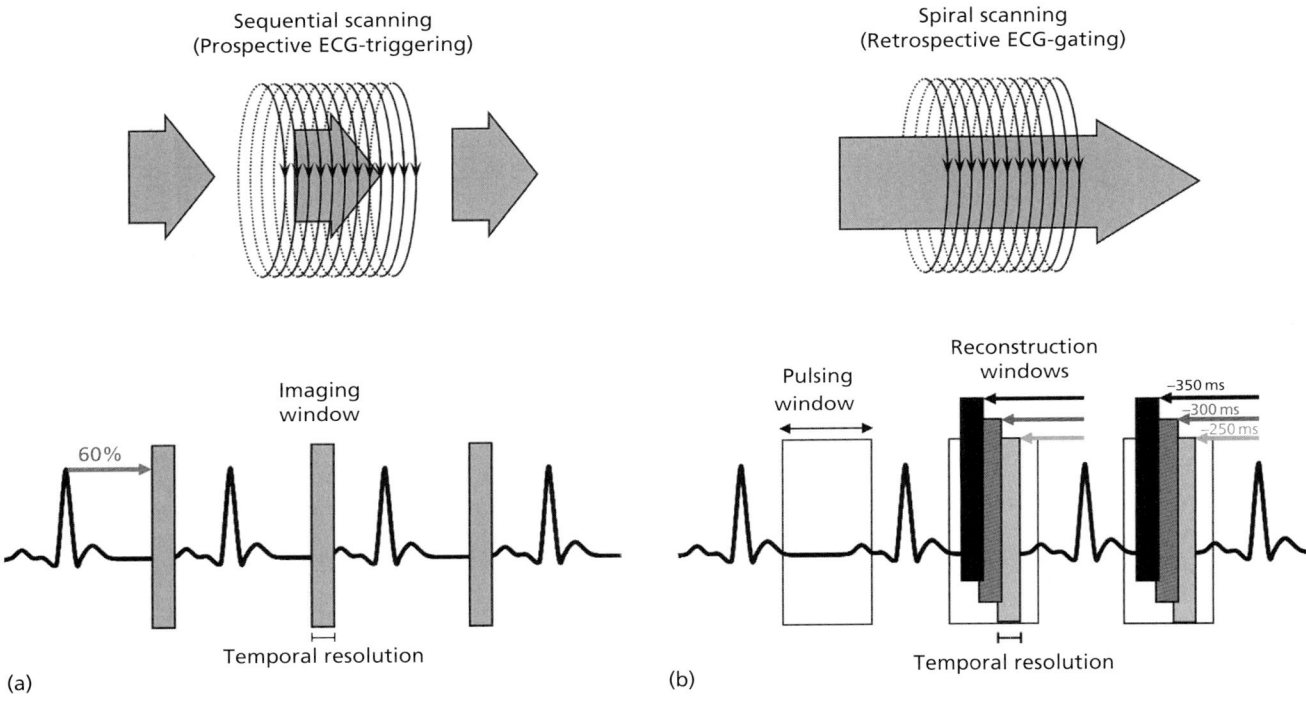

Figure 9.2 In sequential scanning, data for one axial slice are acquired, after which the table is advanced to the next position (a). Sequential scan protocols use prospective ECG-triggering to synchronize the data acquisition to cardiac motion. Based on the measured duration of previous heart cycles, the scan of one slice is initiated at a pre-specified moment after the R-wave. Diastole is commonly chosen to ensure the least motion artifacts (e.g., 60% of the previous R-R interval). Spiral scanners acquire data continuously and record the patient's ECG while the table moves at a constant speed (b). Images are reconstructed using retrospective ECG-gating. This mode is more flexible to minimize motion artifacts because reconstruction window can be positioned arbitrarily within the R-R interval. If X-ray tube modulation is used, the full output occurs only during an interval of the cardiac cycle (pulsing window) which can eventually be used for image reconstruction.

Contrast enhancement

Good contrast enhancement in coronary arteries is essential for the detection of atherosclerotic changes and luminal stenosis. An iodine flow in the range of 1.2–2 g/s is recommended [2]. This can be achieved by either injecting low concentration contrast material at high flow rates or by injection of high concentration contrast material at lower flow rates. However, it is standard practice to inject contrast agent at rates of at least 5 mL/s. Total contrast volume is determined by contrast injection rate multiplied by the scan time required to cover the heart. Typical injection volumes are in the range 60–100 mL. Dual injection (i.e., iodinated contrast followed by saline, 30–50 mL) is recommended for MSCT of the heart. Saline is helpful to avoid dense opacification of the right cardiac chambers and consequent artifacts which might limit the interpretation of the right coronary artery.

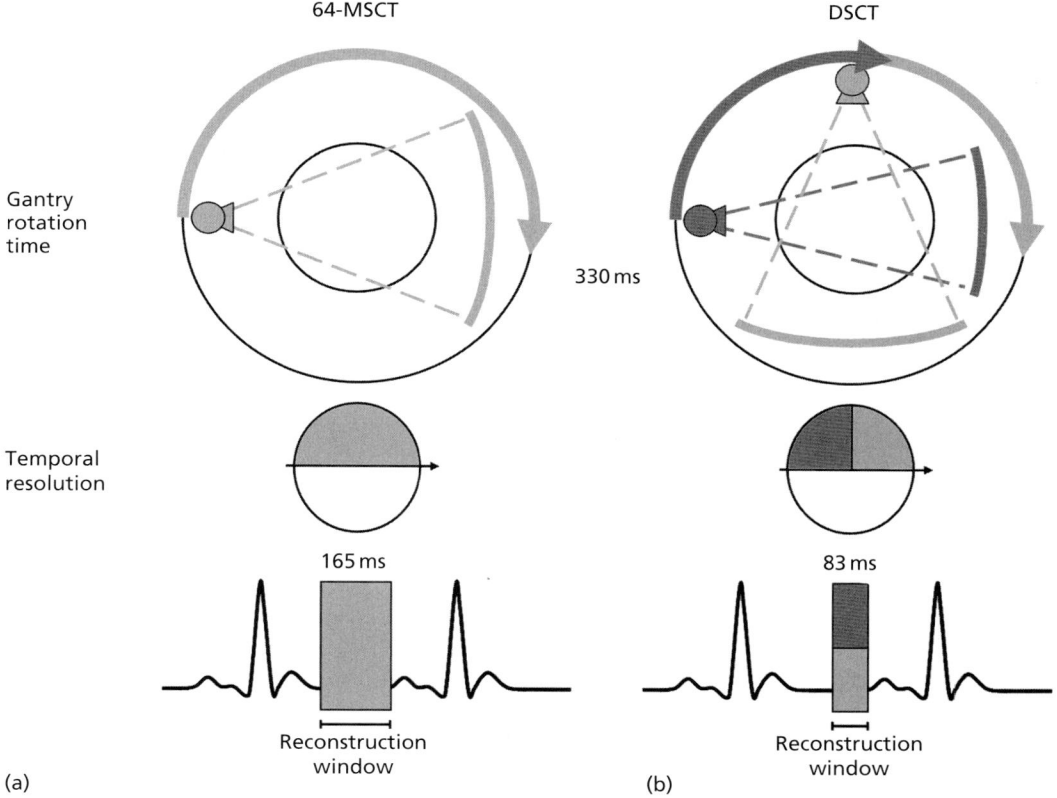

Figure 9.3 Reconstruction of multislice computed tomography (MSCT) images (a) uses data acquired over 180°, thus temporal resolution equals half of the gantry rotation time. Because the shortest gantry rotation time currently achievable by a 64-MSCT scanner is 330 ms, the corresponding temporal resolution is 165 ms. Temporal resolution corresponds to the width of reconstruction window. In dual-source computed tomography (DSCT) (b), two X-ray sources and two corresponding detector arrays are mounted at an angle of 90°, therefore only 90° rotation is needed to provide data from 180°. In DSCT, temporal resolution is equal to a quarter of the gantry rotation time (i.e., 330/4 = 83 ms).

Image post-processing

With image post-processing, the source axial images are modified and made useful for the observer [3] (Figure 9.5). With isotropic resolution, multiplanar reformats (MPR) and maximum intensity projections (MIP) along the course of the coronary arteries are the routinely methods for assessment of coronaries from MSCT datasets. Three-dimensional volume rendering technique (VRT) provides a helpful overview, for example in cases of complex anatomy such as coronary artery bypass grafts (CABG) or anomalous coronary arteries [4]. However, axial images may be best for the detection of coronary stenoses.

Typical artifacts

It is important to recognize a few typical MSCT artifacts that may lead to image misinterpretation. Motion artifacts typically blur the contours of the heart and coronary arteries (Figure 9.6). Inconsistent triggering or arrhythmias will lead to misalignment of adjacent image stacks. Partial voluming occurs when a pixel (i.e., smallest portion of an image) contains more than one type of tissue. In this setting, the attenuation value assigned to the pixel is the weighted average of the different attenuation values. Thus, when a pixel is only partially filled by a structure of very high attenuation (e.g., metal or bone), a high CT number is assigned to the complete pixel, which will thus appear bright on the image. This may lead

to overestimation of the size of high-attenuation objects (e.g., coronary calcifications and stents) (Figure 9.7).

Coronary MSCT angiography—clinical applications

Stenosis detection

Although conventional coronary angiography is still regarded as the reference standard for the detection and quantification of coronary artery stenosis, there are situations where sufficient information can be acquired by a non-invasive technique with benefits in terms of cost, patient risk, and discomfort.

Since 1999, when the first studies on MSCT coronary angiography were published, the development of MSCT technology has been tremendous. Numerous studies [5–21] have compared the accuracy of MSCT in the detection of coronary artery stenosis with invasive coronary angiography (Table 9.2). While sensitivity and specificity remained similar comparing 16-MSCT and 64-MSCT, 64-MSCT and DSCT became more robust for imaging the coronaries: in the segmental analysis, a decrease was shown for the number of coronary segments that had to be excluded due to insufficient image quality (Figure 9.8; Table 9.2) [22]. Importantly, in the per-patient analysis, which is clinically relevant because it explores the ability of MSCT to identify patients with or without

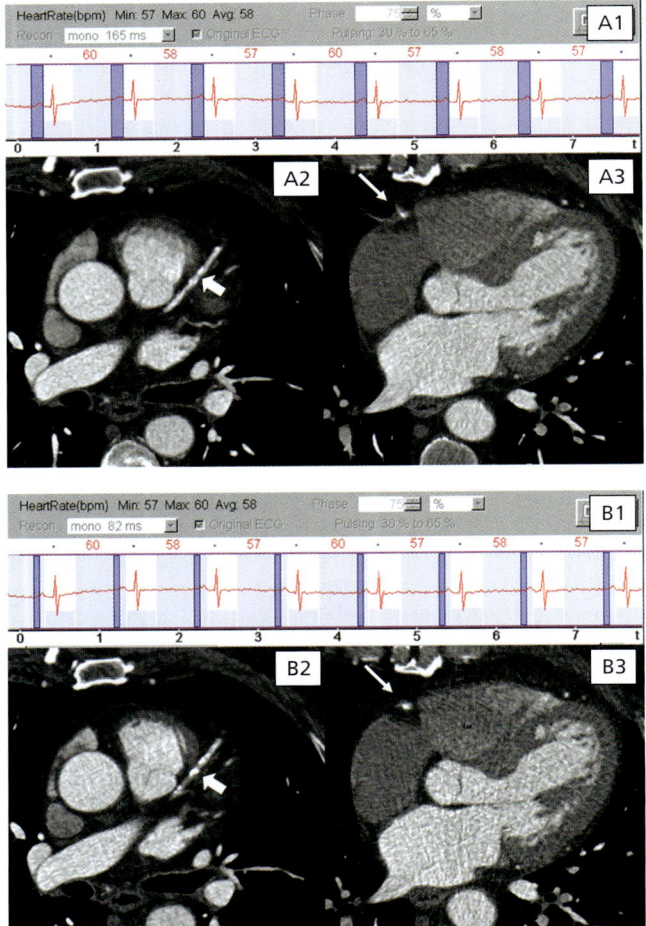

Figure 9.4 MSCT images display the average cardiac motion over the reconstruction window. A 165 mm-wide reconstruction window (A1–A3) averages MSCT views obtained during 180° gantry rotation. This is the reconstruction algorithm employed in 64-MSCT. An 83 mm-wide reconstruction window (B1–B3) averages MSCT views obtained (by two detector arrays) during 90° gantry rotation. This is the reconstruction algorithm employed in DSCT. Reconstruction using 180° data (A2) might improve image contrast when compared to reconstruction using 90° data (B2) because more MSCT views are averaged for the reconstruction of the same image (gross arrow = LAD). However, a wider reconstruction window worsens temporal resolution and can cause more blurring (A3) than the use of the narrowest reconstruction window (B3) (thin arrow = RCA).

significant coronary artery disease (CAD), the negative predictive value was consistently found to be high, in the range 92–100% (Table 9.2). These findings led to the hypothesis that a normal MSCT obviates the need for invasive angiography in properly selected clinical circumstances. The reported positive predictive values were lower, indicating the tendency of MSCT to overestimate the severity of disease in comparison to invasive coronary angiography. Especially in the presence of coronary calcifications and residual motion in the dataset, MSCT is presently limited to accurately grade lesion severity (percentage of stenosis). However,

Table 9.1 Overview of image parameters, patient preparation, and contrast administration.

	Catheter angiography	64-MSCT	DSCT
Spatial resolution	0.2 × 0.2 mm²	0.4 × 0.4 × 0.4 mm³	0.4 × 0.4 × 0.4 mm³
Temporal resolution (ms)	8	16	83
Preparation			
Beta-blockers	No	If heart rate ≥65 beats/min, metoprolol 100 mg orally 1 hr before scan or/and 5–15 mg i.v. in patients with aortic valve stenosis, severe hypotension, Mobitz heart block consider calcium channel blockers	(Optional)
Nitroglycerine	Intracoronary	(Optional— sublingual)	(Optional— sublingual)
Contrast	80–100 mL intracoronary	100 mL intravenous	60–100 mL intravenous

DSCT, dual-source computed tomography; MSCT, multislice computed tomography.

MSCT has a notably high sensitivity and negative predictive value for the detection of significant CAD, thus it may be well suited to clinical situations in which exclusion of CAD is of paramount concern (e.g., in patients with low to intermediate pretest likelihood of disease) [23]. The evolving indications of MSCT of the heart, with emphasis on the evaluation of coronary arteries, are shown in Table 9.3.

Bifurcations and ostial lesions

The angiographic evaluation of bifurcation lesions can be hindered by projectional foreshortening, vessel overlap, and insufficient vessel opacification; for these reasons, the assessment of the side branch ostium can be particularly challenging. Errors in diagnosis can lead to consequences for patient management: when CABG surgery is the treatment of choice, underestimation of a side branch lesion can result in the side branch not being grafted; when percutaneous coronary intervention (PCI) is preferred, detailed anatomic information permits selection of the optimal intervention strategy. Moreover, conventional angiography does not provide sufficient information on the plaque burden at the level of the bifurcation. In the presence of a high plaque burden, initial treatment of both the main and side branches (e.g., crush or culottes techniques) should be preferred over main branch stenting first followed by provisional balloon angioplasty (with or without stenting) of the side branch.

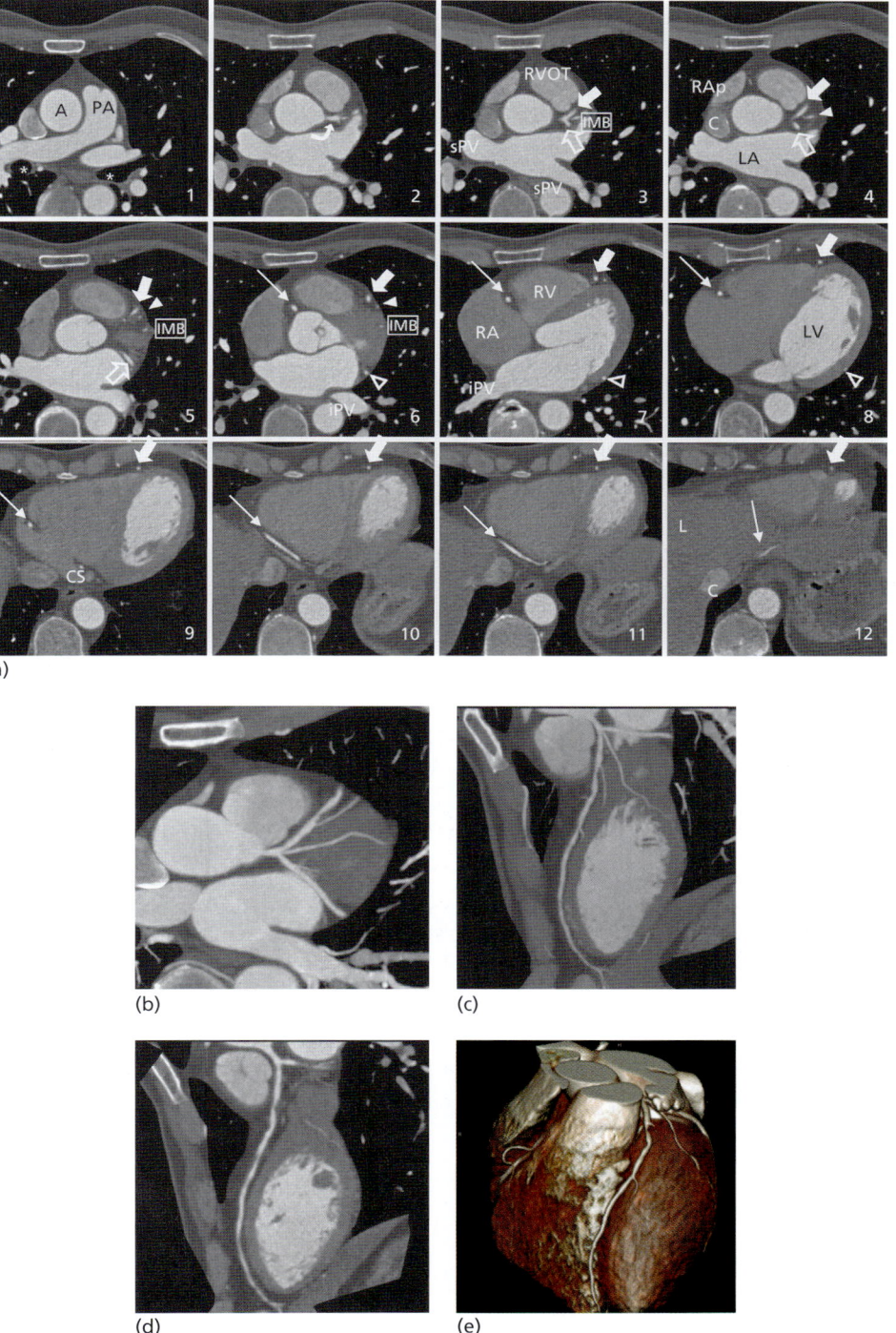

(a)

(b)

(c)

(d)

(e)

Figure 9.5 (a) (1–12): The basic information of MSCT is the axial images (a1–a12). Scrolling through them in the cranial to caudal direction shows any structure in the axial plane. The scan starts at the level of the tracheal bifurcation (a1) therefore the main bronchi (asterisks), the ascending aorta (A) and pulmonary artery (PA) are shown. As we scroll caudally, the origin of the left main coronary artery (a2, curved arrow) and its trifurcation (a3) into left anterior descending artery (gross arrow), circumflex artery (open arrow), and intermediate branch (IMB) are seen. The left anterior descending artery (a3–a12, gross arrow) courses along the superior interventricular groove and can be followed down to the apex of the heart. A diagonal branch is also seen (a4–a6, gross arrowhead). The left circumflex artery (a3–a5, open arrow) courses in the left atrioventricular groove and gives an obtuse marginal branch (a6–a8, open arrowhead). The proximal right coronary artery (a6, thin arrow) has a short horizontal course. Then the vessel courses caudally (a7–a9, thin arrow) in the right atrio-ventricular groove. The inferior inter-ventricular groove contains the posterior descending artery (a12, thin arrow). (A, aorta; asterisks, main bronchi; C, cava; CS, coronary sinus; IMB, intermediate branch; iPV, inferior pulmonary veins; L, liver; LA, left atrium; LV, left ventricle; PA, pulmonary artery; RA, right atrium; Rap, right appendage; RV, right ventricle; RVOT, right ventricular outflow tract; sPV, superior pulmonary veins.) (b–e) Axial images are reconstructed to form a volume. Post-processing is performed on this volume dataset. Multiplanar reconstructions (b) cut this volume according to planes arbitrarily tilted in any orientation. When the cut plane is not flat but curved, the result is a curved multiplanar reconstruction (c, d). This image is a flattened representation of the curved plane (d). Maximum intensity projection is an algorithm that visualizes only the structures with the highest attenuation along the observation line (c). Volume rendering (e) displays the volume based on the density of the structures. Color attribution is arbitrary; therefore the appearance will change when the operator changes the colors of the algorithm.

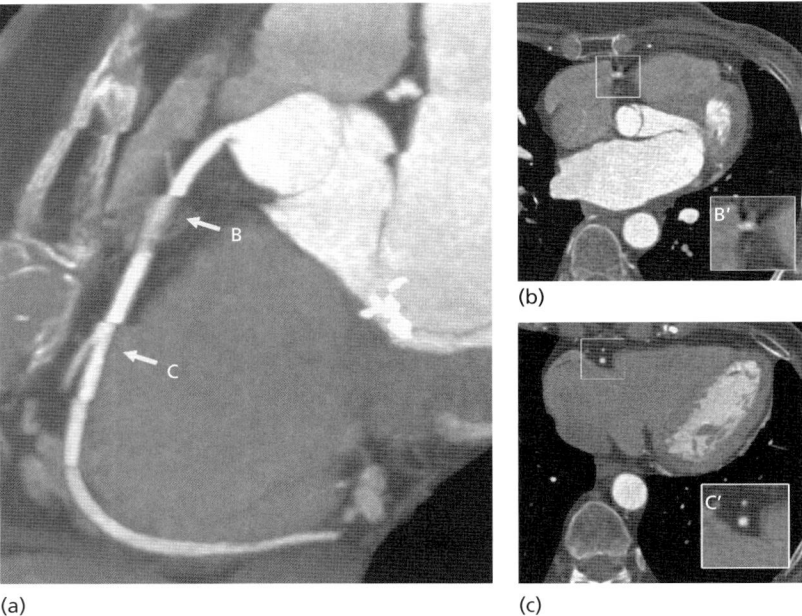

Figure 9.6 Typical artifacts in cardiac MSCT (a) include motion artifacts (b) and stack misalignment resulting from heart rate variations or slight arrhythmia (c). Whereas motion artifacts cause blurring (B), images within a misaligned stack are not blurred (C).

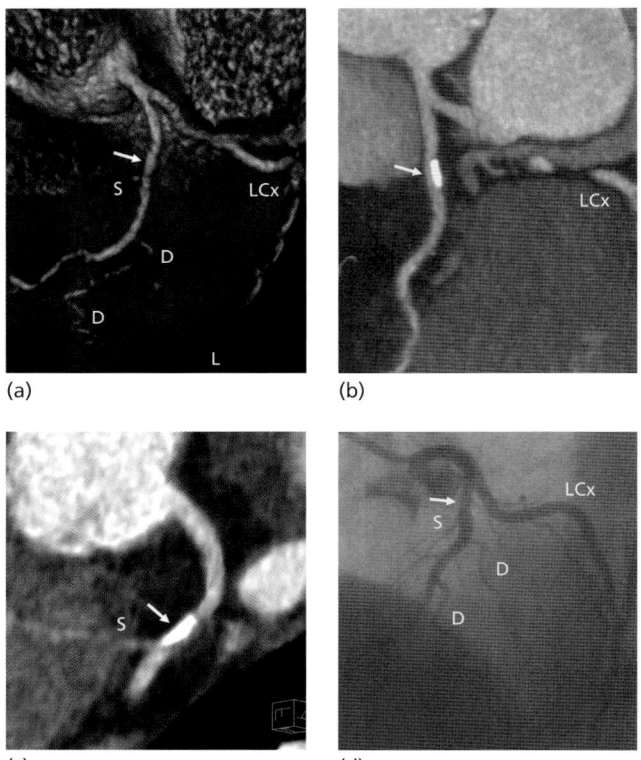

Figure 9.7 Volume rendered image (a), curved maximum intensity projection (b), and multiplanar reconstruction (c) show a calcified plaque (arrow) located in the left anterior descending (LAD) just proximal to the origin of a septal branch (S). The size of structures with high X-ray attenuation such as calcifications is overestimated in MSCT due to partial voluming. This calcification superimposes most of the coronary artery lumen. The conventional angiogram (d) shows a normal LAD. LCx, left circumflex.

Van Mieghem *et al.* [24] compared MSCT with conventional angiography for the detection and classification of coronary bifurcation lesions. In keeping with the available literature on non-bifurcation lesions, they reported 96% sensitivity, 97% specificity, 63% positive predictive value, and 99% negative predictive value for the detection of bifurcation lesions (Figure 9.9). MSCT was found to be accurate also in classifying bifurcation lesions according to the Medina classification system [25]. Furthermore, thanks to the three-dimensional nature of MSCT data, the bifurcation angle between the main vessel and the side branch could be measured accurately. In situations where both branches needed to be stented, information regarding the bifurcation angle was used to support the choice of the stenting technique.

The visualization of ostial lesions (Figure 9.10) can be affected by projectional limitations in conventional angiography. Occasionally, ostial lesions can be masked by the engagement of the catheter tip beyond the lesion. At a pre-interventional stage, MSCT can provide information on three-dimensional anatomy of ostial lesions and vessel take-off angle [26].

Chronic total occlusion

In the diagnostic work-up of patients with chronically occluded coronary arteries, MSCT can add important information to conventional angiography. Measurement of the length of the occluded segment, which has long been identified as a predictor of failed PCI, can be limited in conventional angiography by foreshortening, calibration limitations, and lack of collateral filling (Figure 9.11). Conversely, MSCT is a three-dimensional technique that allows reliable length measurement of coronary segments. Likewise, MSCT permits the evaluation of the proximal entry port, the severity of calcification (Figure 9.12), and the delineation of occlusion trajectory. Therefore, MSCT improves the ability to predict the success rate of PCI. Mollet *et al.* [27] found that a blunt entry point, an occlusion length >15 mm, and severe calcification, all determined by MSCT, were independent predictors of procedural failure.

Table 9.2 Detection of coronary stenosis—diagnostic performance of MSCT vs. conventional angiography.

	No. patients	Per segment					Per patient			
		Unevaluable segments (%)	Sensitivity (%)	Specificity (%)	PPV (%)	NPV (%)	Sensitivity (%)	Specificity (%)	PPV (%)	NPV (%)
16-MSCT										
Mollet [13]	128	7	92	95	79	98	100	86	97	100
Hoffman [9]	103	6	95	98	87	99	97	87	90	95
Achenbach [5]	50	4	94	96	69	99	100	83	100	86
Mollet [12]	51	0	95	98	87	99	97	84	89	95
Garcia [7]	187	29	85	91	36	99	98	55	50	99
Dewey [6]	129	9	83	86	90	95	93	74	93	92
Hausleiter [8]	129	11	93	87	46	99	–	–	–	–
64-MSCT										
Leschka [11]	53	0	94	97	87	99	100	100	100	100
Raff [18]	70	12	86	95	66	98	95	90	93	93
Leber [10]	59	0	88	97	–	99	94	–	–	–
Pugliese [17]	35	0	99	96	78	99	100	90	96	100
Mollet [14]	52	2	99	95	76	99	100	92	97	100
Ropers [19]	82	4	95	93	56	99	96	91	83	98
Nikolaou [15]	72	10	86	95	72	97	97	72	83	95
Hausleiter [8]	114	8	92	92	54	99	99	75	74	99
320-MSCT										
Dewey [46]	30	0	78	98	75	99	100	94	92	100
DSCT										
Nikolaou [16]	20	4	95	93	79	98	–	–	–	–
Scheffel [20]	30	1	96	98	86	99	–	–	–	–
Weustink [21]	100	0	95	95	75	99	99	87	96	95

Stents

Coronary stents are notoriously difficult to assess by MSCT. Partial voluming artifacts enlarge the apparent size of the stent; this is particularly disturbing in smaller stents, where the in-stent lumen might be completely obscured, and in overlapping and bifurcation stents due to an excess of metal. As demonstrated *in vitro*, types of metal and strut thickness also have an important role for in-stent lumen assessibility [28]; generally, stents with thinner struts (e.g., 0.14 mm) are less problematic than stents with thicker struts (e.g., 0.15 mm and above).

In the evaluation of coronary stents, the finding of contrast-enhancement distal to the stent is not foolproof for stent patency, because collateral pathways may fill the vessel retrograde; if the stent is being evaluated for the presence of non-occlusive in-stent restenosis, direct visualization of the in-stent lumen becomes the mandatory criterion.

Technical requirements for coronary stent imaging are 64-slice MSCT scanners with thin detectors in order to optimize spatial resolution and decrease partial voluming. High temporal resolution is also important because high density artifacts are exacerbated by the presence of residual motion in the MSCT dataset [29].

Clinical studies compared different generations of MSCT scanners with conventional angiography for the detection of in-stent restenosis, defined as ≥50% luminal narrowing (Table 9.4). Studies performed using 16-MSCT [30], 40-MSCT [31], and 64-MSCT [32–34] reported promising results with variable percentages of non-assessable stents. Using DSCT [35], the percentage of non-assessable stents was found to be low; whereas the diagnostic performance did not vary significantly between different stent configurations (i.e., single stents vs. overlapping/bifurcation stenting), the results were influenced importantly by the stent diameter. In particular, the ability of DSCT to exclude with certainty in-stent

Table 9.3 Evolving indications of MSCT of the heart with emphasis on the evaluation of coronary arteries [23].

Detection of CAD in symptomatic patients

1. Intermediate pre-test probability of CAD + equivocal ECG/unable to exercise

2. Equivocal exercise tests, perfusion imaging, stress echo

3. Evaluation of coronary arteries in patients with heart failure of new onset to assess etiology

Coronary anomalies

Exclusion of CAD prior to cardiac valve surgery/major non-cardiac surgery

Patients with recurrent chest pain after PCI with low probability of in-stent restenosis and large stents (≥3 mm)

Coronary artery bypass grafts

Acute chest pain

1. Non-ST segment elevation and initial troponin negative

2. Intermediate probability of aortic dissection/aneurysm, pulmonary emboli, obstructive CAD (triple rule out)

---

restenosis in stents with diameters ≤2.75 mm was significantly lower than that observed in larger stents.

Ideally, the stent type and diameter are known prior to the scan, therefore in-stent lumen assessability in a particular patient could be predicted from the available *in vitro* and *in vivo* data. However, MSCT was shown to have a constantly high negative predictive value, therefore it may be useful in patients with clinical symptoms but low pre-test probability for in-stent restenosis.

Stent implantation in the left main (LM) and proximal left anterior descending/circumflex (LAD/Cx) provides a suitable scenario for the use of MSCT in the detection of in-stent restenosis. This is mainly because of the relatively large size of stents implanted in the LM and proximal LAD/CX; moreover, this part of the coronary tree is relatively protected from motion artifacts. Although CABG surgery is still recommended in patients with LM disease, PCI is increasingly performed on the unprotected LM coronary artery in the drug-eluting stent (DES) era. However, in-stent restenosis still occurs with DES and can cause fatal myocardial infarction or sudden death [36], therefore surveillance with routinely angiography 6 months after PCI for LM stem is highly recommended [37]. A study by Van Mieghem *et al.* [38] showed that MSCT was safe and reliable in excluding in-stent restenosis in patients with LM and proximal LAD/CX stents; this study suggested that MSCT might be an acceptable first-line alternative to conventional angiography for the follow-up of patients after unprotected LM stenting.

MSCT also visualizes the configuration of bifurcation/overlapping stents (Figure 9.13) and the position of stents implanted in ostial lesions. Tissue prolapses, stent malapposition, and underexpansion are generally not clearly visualized by MSCT. It is conceivable that stents with thinner struts, absorbable and non-metallic stents (Figure 9.14) will be less affected by high density artifacts; the introduction of these new devices might increase the utility of MSCT in patients after PCI.

Coronary artery bypass grafts
General issues
Patients with prior CABG surgery usually present with comorbidity and have a higher prevalence of valve disease and ventricular dysfunction than non-CABG patients. They have a higher incidence of complications during invasive procedures, including

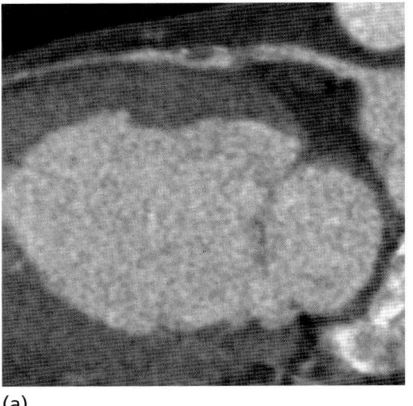 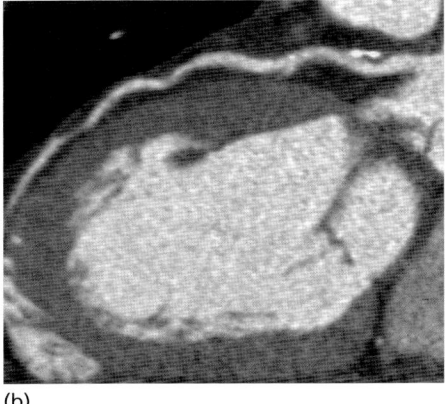 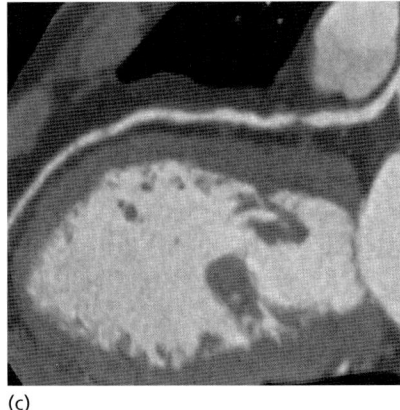

(a)   (b)   (c)

Figure 9.8 Curved multiplanar reconstructions of the left main (LM) and LAD arteries obtained in three different patients with 16-MSCT (a), 64-MSCT (b), and DSCT (c) show progressive improvement in image quality. All the patients had heart rates during the scan of 62–65 bpm.

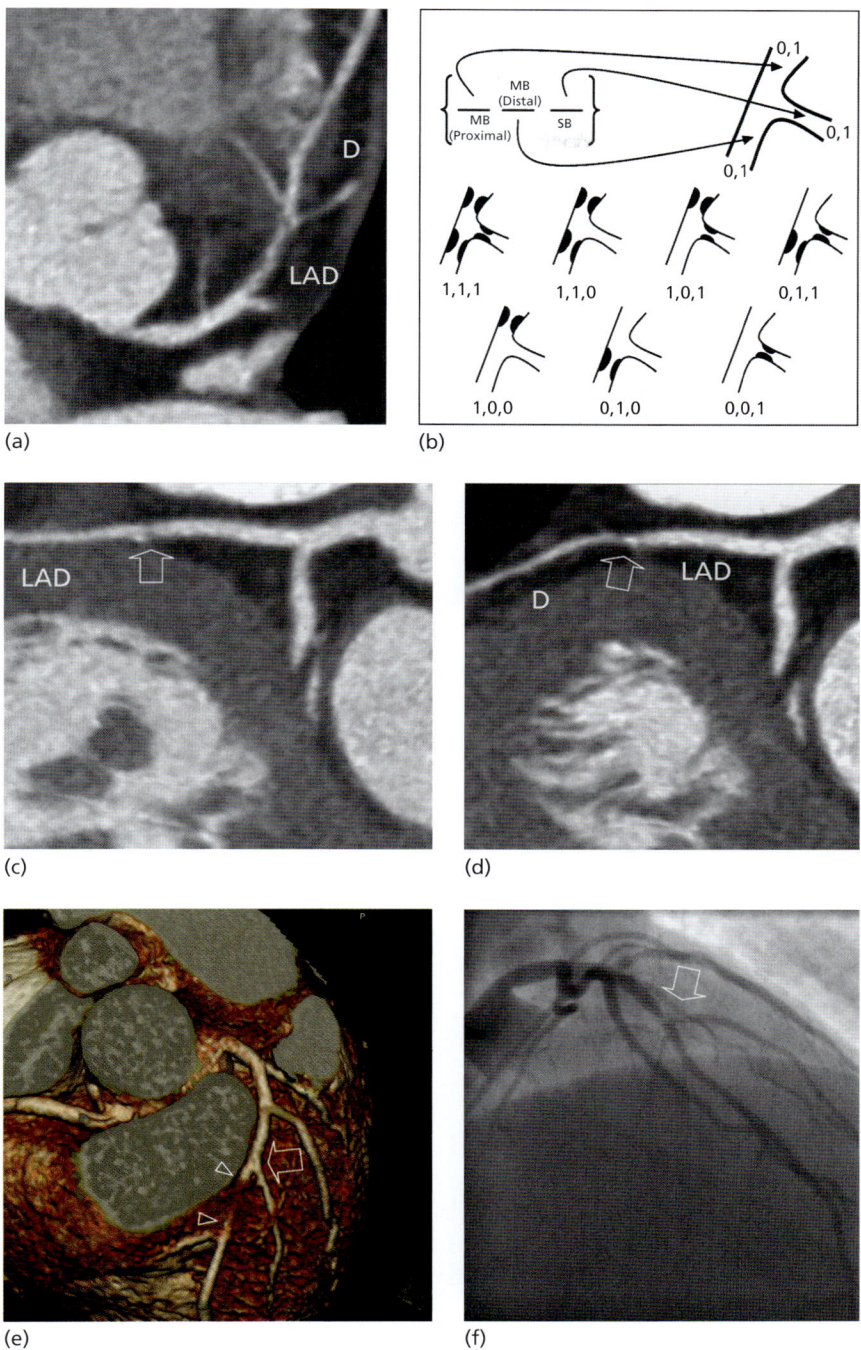

Figure 9.9 The DSCT multiplanar reconstruction (a) shows a proximal bifurcation lesion (arrows) in the left anterior descending (LAD) artery, also seen on the curved multiplanar reconstructions of the LAD (c) and diagonal branch (e). The lesion is confirmed by the conventional angiogram (f). According to the Medina classification system (b), the lesion involves proximal main branch and side branch whereas the distal main branch is unremarkable (1,0,1). The lesion is not clearly detectable in the volume rendered image (e); distally to the bifurcation, the LAD has intramyocardial course (d) (arrowheads).

cardiac catheterization, and can therefore benefit from non-invasive coronary angiography performed by MSCT.

Generally, bypass grafts are well visualized by MSCT because of their large diameter, limited calcification, and relative immobility. However, surgical opaque material, such as vascular clips, sternal wires, and graft orifice indicators, hinder the evaluability of coronary grafts (Figure 9.15).

Clinical performance and limitations

64-MSCT permits the evaluation of graft patency with a sensitivity approaching 100% in both arterial and venous grafts and without exclusion of grafts because of insufficient image quality (Table 9.5) [39–42]. However, ischemic symptoms in patients after CABG surgery can be caused by obstruction of bypass grafts or by disease progression in native coronary arteries. Comprehensive evaluation

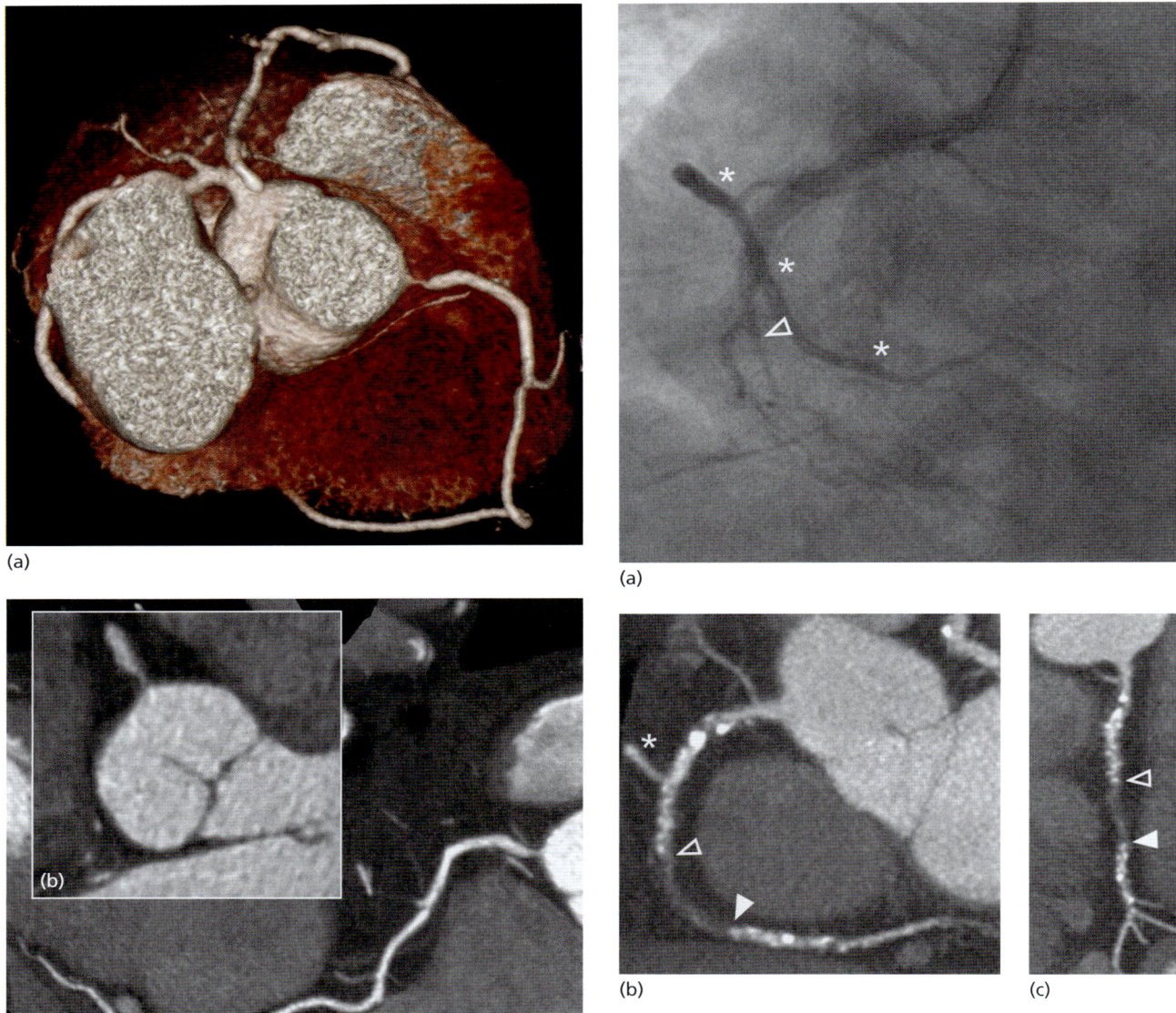

(a)

(b)

(c)

(a)

(b)   (c)

Figure 9.10 The volume rendered view after removal of the right atrium (a), axial image (b), and curved multiplanar reconstruction (c) demonstrate an ostial lesion of the right coronary artery (RCA).

Figure 9.11 Occlusion of the RCA (open arrowheads) is demonstrated by the conventional angiogram (a), DSCT multiplanar reconstruction (b), and curved multiplanar reconstruction (c) of the vessel. The distal patent RCA is not sharply visualized on the angiogram (a). The multiplanar reconstruction (b) and curved multiplanar reconstruction (c) of the RCA permit better visualization of the distal patent vessel (solid arrowheads) and thus of the actual occlusion length. Asterisks: right ventricular branch.

post-CABG surgery should also include the native coronary tree; assessment of the native coronary arteries can be difficult in these patients owing to the diffuse nature of the disease and the presence of severe calcifications [39].

Valve disease

Whereas the visualization of the tricuspid and pulmonary valves is generally inconsistent, the mitral and aortic valves can reliably be depicted in contrast-enhanced MSCT scans. While MSCT cannot provide measurements of transvalvular flow and pressure gradients, dynamic imaging of the open and closed valve is possible (Figure 9.16). For the normal and stenotic aortic valve, recent studies have demonstrated the ability of MSCT to measure the orifice area with close correlation to transesophageal echocardiography and invasive assessment of the aortic orifice area [43,44]. However, in the setting of severely calcified stenosis, measurements of the opening area by CT may become unreliable. Non-enhanced CT scans can be used to quantify aortic valve calcium [45].

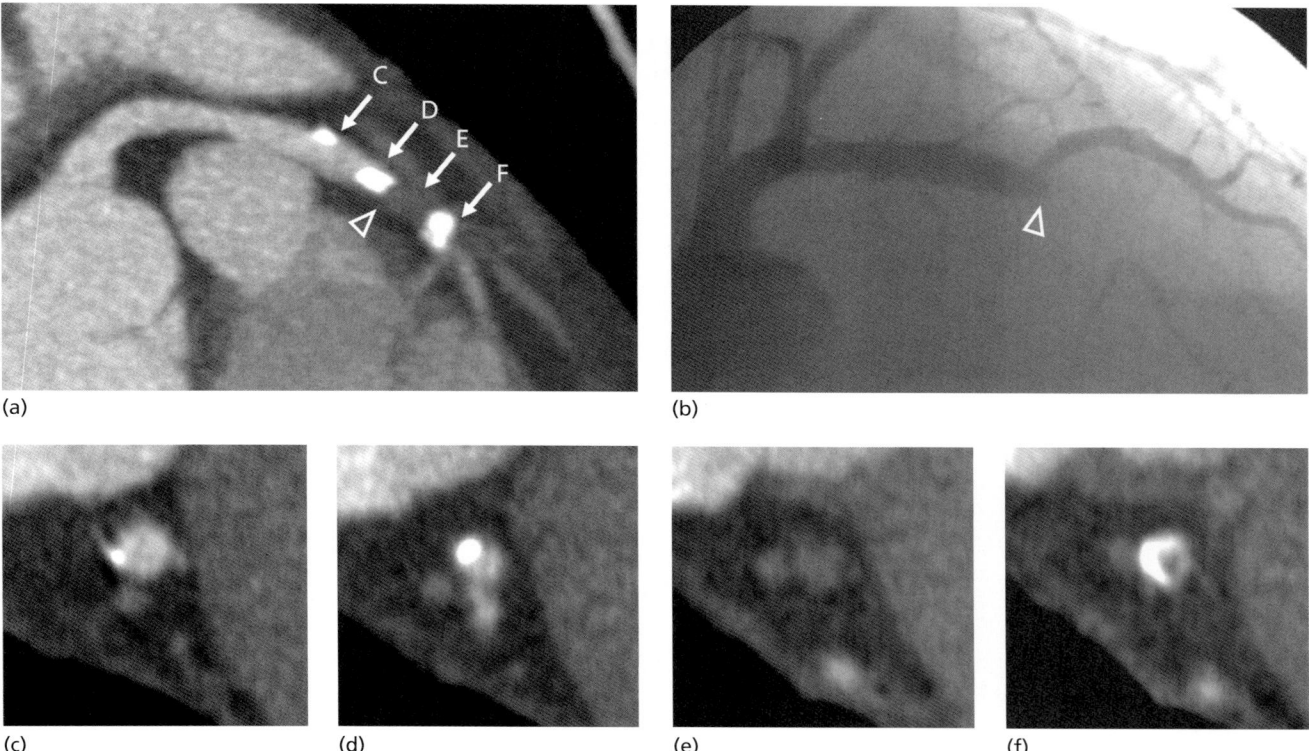

Figure 9.12 Occlusion of the proximal LAD (arrowheads) is demonstrated by the DSCT maximum intensity projection image (a) and conventional angiogram (b). The DSCT cross sections (c-f), obtained as indicated in (a), provide information on the severity of lesion calcification. Bulky calcifications are present proximally to the occlusion (c), at the level of the stump (d) and more distally (f).

Coronary anomalies

It can sometimes be difficult during invasive coronary angiography to define the origin and course of anomalous coronary arteries. MSCT is extremely reliable for visualizing the origin and course of anomalous coronary vessels and is well suited for investigating patients with known or suspected congenital coronary artery anomalies. MSCT permits morphologic analysis with very high resolution; moreover, this technique is not restricted by "echo windows" or by implanted devices such as pacemakers or implantable cardioverter defibrillators, which are frequently encountered in patients with congenital heart disease. The introduction of whole-heart 320-row CT, which reduces radiation exposure from intensive overscanning and overranging, makes this technique particularly attractive in women and younger age groups [46].

Recent clinical trials of CT coronary angiography
SCOT-HEART trial

CT coronary angiography in patients with suspected angina due to coronary heart disease (SCOT-HEART): an open-label, parallel-group, multicenter trial, is the first trial to assess the clinical impact of the addition of CT angiography (CTA) in patients presenting with suspected angina due to coronary heart disease (CHD) in the outpatient setting [47]. Previous trials have focused on assessing the accuracy and comparability of CTA for the identification of CHD [48–50] and the evaluation of low–intermediate risk patients with chest pain in emergency departments [51–53]. This prospective, parallel group trial included patients aged 18–75 years referred for the assessment of suspected angina due to CHD from 12 centers across Scotland. The final analysis included 4146 patents randomized to standard care plus CTA or standard care alone. Some 47% of subjects had a baseline diagnosis of CHD and 36% a diagnosis of angina due to coronary heart disease. AT 6 weeks, CTA reclassified the diagnosis of CHD in 558 (27%) of subjects assigned to CTA compared with 1% assigned to standard care and the diagnosis of angina due to CHD in 481 (23%) of subjects assigned to CTA compared with 1% to standard care ($p < 0.001$ for both).

The certainty (relative risk [RR] 2.56, 95% CI 2.33–2.79; $p < 0.0001$) and frequency (RR 1.09, CI 1.02–1.17; $p = 0.0172$) of the diagnosis of CHD increased with CTA compared with standard care. However, the certainty increased (RR 1.79, CI 1.62–1.96; $p < 0.0001$) and frequency appeared to decrease (RR 0.93, CI 0.85–1.02; $p = 0.1289$) for the diagnosis of angina due to CHD. This changed planned investigations (12% vs. 1%; $p < 0.0001$) and treatments (27% vs. 5%; $p < 0.0001$) but did not affect 6-week symptom severity or subsequent admittances to hospital for chest pain. After 1.7 years, CTA was associated with a 38% reduction in fatal and non-fatal myocardial infarction (26% vs. 42%, HR 0.62, 95% CI 0.38–1·01; $p = 0.0527$), but this was not significant.

Table 9.4 Detection of in-stent restenosis—diagnostic performance of MSCT vs. conventional angiography.

	Unevaluable stents (%)	Sensitivity (%)	Specificity (%)	PPV (%)	NPV (%)
16-MSCT Gilard [30]					
All diameters	36	–	–	–	–
>3 mm	19	86	100	100	99
≤3 mm	49	54	100	100	94
40-MSCT Gaspar [31]					
All diameters	5	89	81	47	97
64-MSCT Rixe [34]					
All diameters	42	86	98	86	98
>3 mm	22	100	100	100	100
3 mm	42	83	96	83	96
<3 mm*	92	–	100	–	100
Ehara [33]					
All diameters	12	92	81	54	98
Cademartiri [32]					
All diameters	7	90	86	44	98
DSCT Pugliese [35]					
All diameters	5	94	92	77	98
≥3.5 mm	0	100	100	100	100
3 mm	0	100	97	91	100
≤2.75 mm	22	84	64	52	90

NPV, negative predictive value; PPV, positive predictive value.
*Only one stent available, without in-stent restenosis.

In summary, CTA helped clarify the diagnosis and target interventions with a trend toward lower risk of myocardial infarction in this outpatient cohort with suspected angina due to CHD.

PROMISE trial

Outcomes of anatomic versus functional testing for coronary artery disease: the prospective multicenter imaging study for evaluation of chest pain (PROMISE) trial is the largest outcome study in cardiovascular imaging to date [54]. The trial randomized 10,003 symptomatic mostly intermediate-risk outpatients (mean age 60.8 years, 52.7% women, 87.7% with chest pain or dyspnea on exertion) without CAD to a strategy of initial anatomic testing with CTA or to functional testing (exercise electrocardiography, nuclear stress testing, or stress echocardiography). Additional inclusion criteria were an age of more than 54 years (in men) or more than 64 years (in women) or an age of 45–54 years (in men) or 50–64 years (in women) with at least one cardiac risk factor (diabetes, peripheral arterial

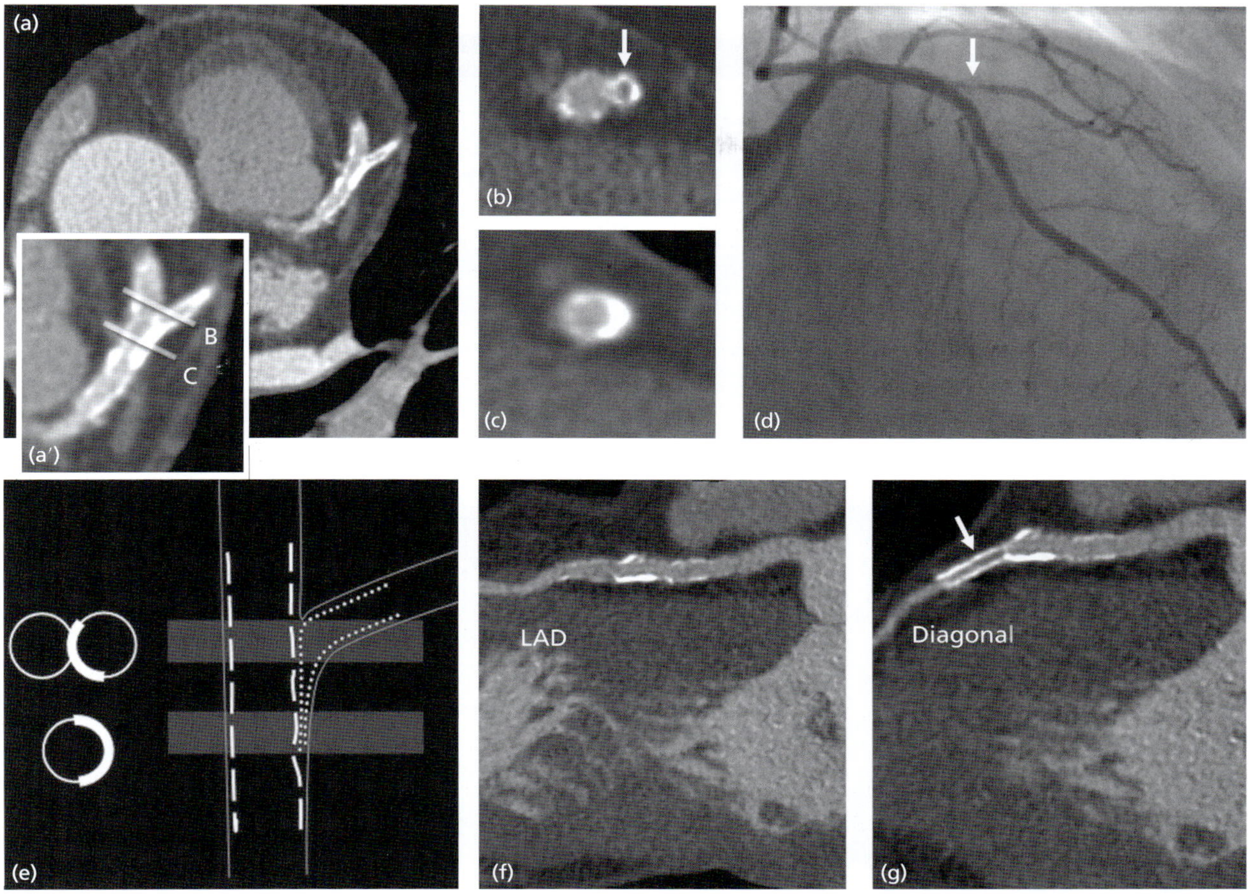

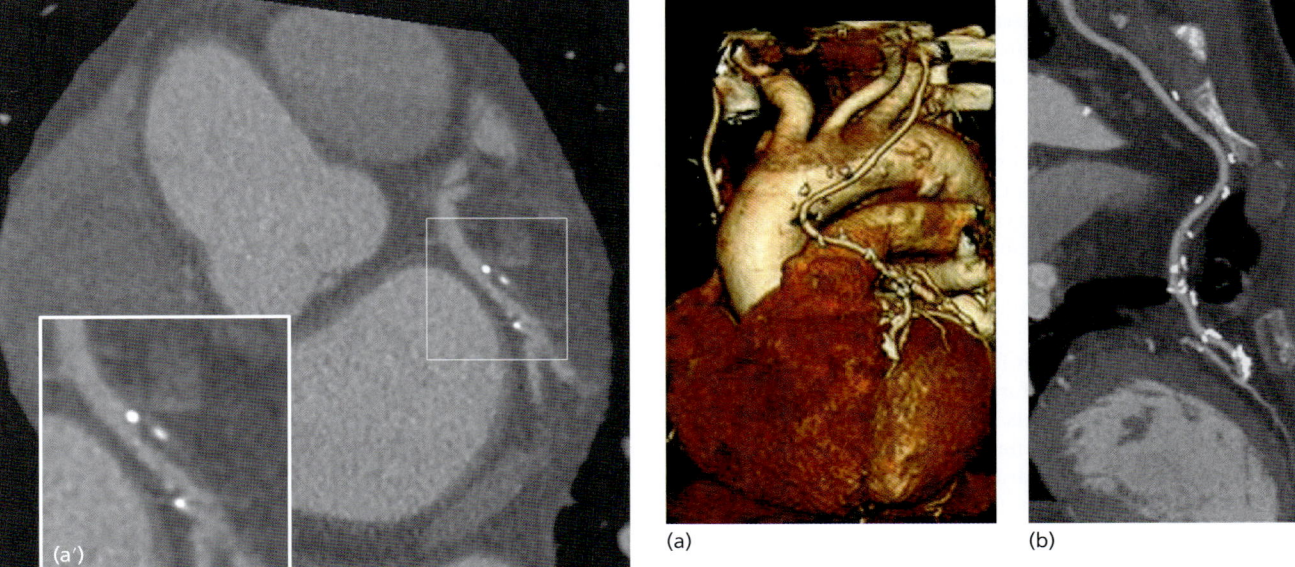

Figure 9.13 The DSCT axial image (a), its magnification (a'), the cross-sectional views (b, c) and the diagram (e) show the typical appearance of the crush stenting technique, characterized by three layers of metal crushed against the ostium of the side branch. The DSCT cross-section obtained at the level of the carina (B) and the curved multiplanar reconstruction of the diagonal branch (g) demonstrate in-stent restenosis in the diagonal branch stent (arrow). The LAD (main branch) is patent (f). The conventional angiogram (d) confirms the findings.

Figure 9.14 The DSCT multiplanar reconstruction (a) and its magnification (a') show a bioabsorbable stent placed in the LCx artery. The stent is radiolucent with radiopaque markers at the stent edges.

Figure 9.15 In a patient after coronary artery bypass graft surgery, the DSCT volume rendered image (a) and the curved multiplanar reconstruction (b) show patency of the left internal mammary artery graft and of the anastomosis of the graft onto the LAD. Notice the hyper-dense appearance of the surgical clips.

Table 9.5 Detection of coronary graft and native vessel stenosis—diagnostic performance of 64-MSCT vs. conventional angiography.

	Unevaluable (%)	Sensitivity (%)	Specificity (%)	PPV (%)	NPV (%)
Malagutti [39]					
All grafts	0	100	98	98	100
Arterial	–	100	100	100	100
Venous	–	100	96	98	100
Distal run-offs	0	89	93	50	99
Non-grafted natives	0	97	86	66	99
Ropers [42]					
All grafts	0	100	94	92	100
Distal run-offs	7	86	90	50	98
Non-grafted natives	9	86	76	44	96
Meyer [40]					
All grafts	2	97	97	93	99
Arterial	–	93	97	86	98
Venous	–	99	98	96	99
Pache [41]					
All grafts	3	98	89	90	98
Arterial	–	–	–	–	92
Venous	–	–	–	–	100

disease, cerebrovascular disease, current or past tobacco use, hypertension, or dyslipidemia).

Over a median follow-up period of 25 months, a primary endpoint event (death from any cause, myocardial infarction, hospitalization for unstable angina, and major complication of cardiovascular procedures or tests) occurred in 164 of 4996 patients in the CTA group (3.3%) and in 151 of 5007 (3.0%) in the functional testing group (adjusted hazard ratio 1.04; 95% CI 0.83–1.29; p = 0.75). At 12 months, the risk of death or non-fatal myocardial infarction was marginally lower in the CTA group than in the functional testing group (hazard ratio 0.66; 95% CI 0.44–1.00; p = 0.049).

CTA was associated with fewer catheterizations showing no obstructive CAD than was functional testing (3.4% vs. 4.3%; p = 0.02), although more patients in the CTA group underwent catheterization within 90 days after randomization (12.2% vs. 8.1%). Revascularization was performed within 90 days after randomization in 311 of 4996 patients (6.2%) in the CTA group compared with 158 of 5007 (3.2%) in the functional testing group (p < 0.001), including 72 and 38 patients, respectively, who underwent CABG. The median cumulative radiation exposure per patient was lower in the CTA group than in the functional testing group (10.0 vs. 11.3 mSv), but 32.6% of the patients in the

functional testing group had no exposure, so the overall exposure was higher in the CTA group (mean 12.0 vs. 10.1 mSv; p < 0.001).

In an economic sub-analysis there were no significant differences between the strategies in costs in that patient population over 3 years [55]. The costs per person for CTA were slightly more than costs for functional testing: $279 at 3 months, $358 at 12 months $388 at 24 months and $694 at 36 months. The jump in cost between 24 and 36 months was attributed to some outlier costs for non-cardiovascular care and increased revascularization in the CTA group.

In summary, in symptomatic patients with suspected CAD who required non-invasive testing, a strategy of initial CTA, as compared with functional testing, did not improve clinical outcomes over a median follow-up of 2 years. CTA remains a good initial testing option given the similarity in outcomes and costs to functional testing.

PLATFORM trial

A prospective trial recently evaluated the role of CTA with incorporation of CTA-based calculation of fractional flow reserve (CTA/FFR) of possibly significant lesions [56]. This prospective, randomized multicenter trial found significantly lower rate of

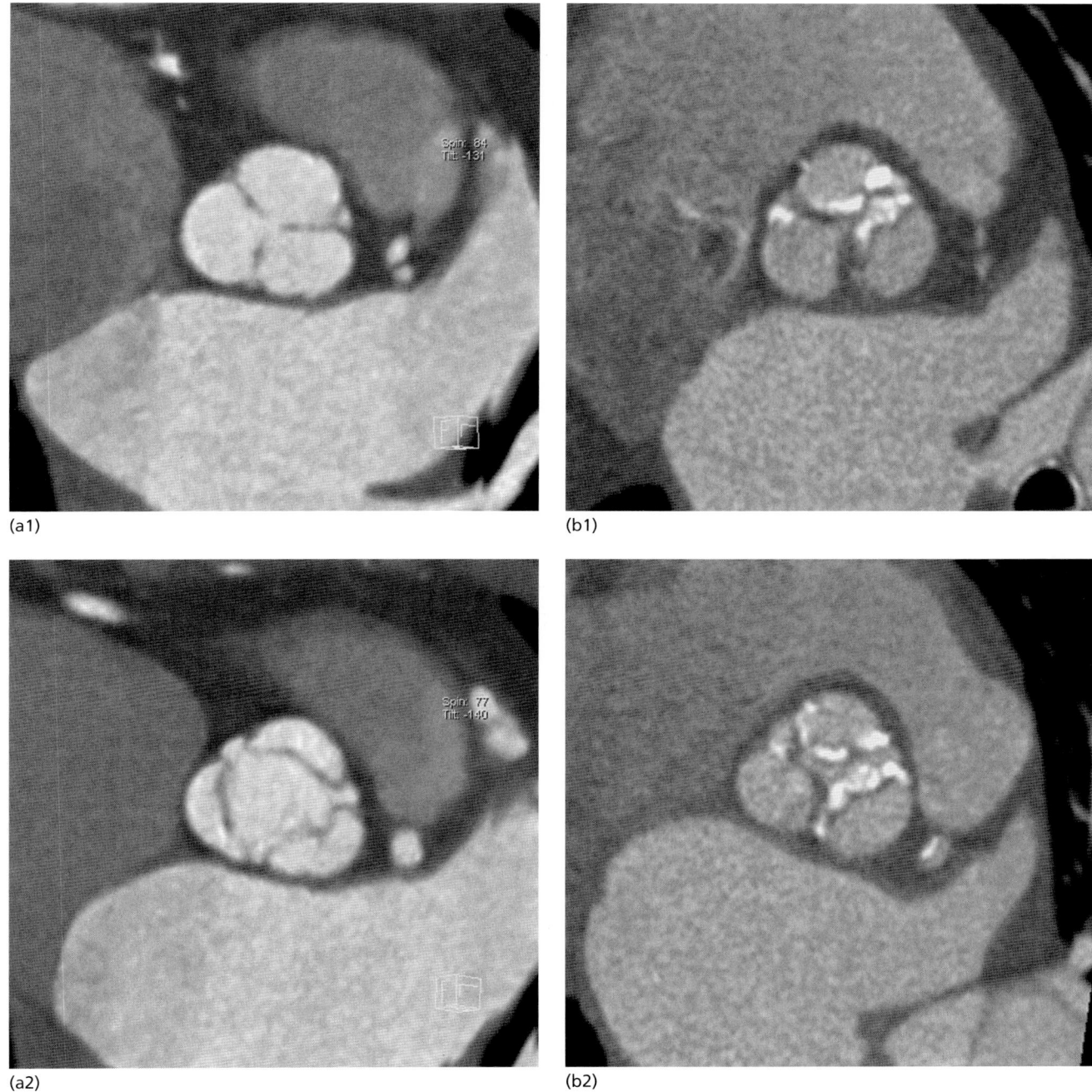

Figure 9.16 The MSCT multiplanar images were obtained in two different patients (A and B) parallel to the aortic valve. Images in the upper row (a1, b1) were obtained during diastole. Images in the lower row (a2, b2) were obtained in systole. In patient A, the cusps adapt during diastole (a1) and open during systole (a2); the aortic valve is normal. In patient B, aortic cusps are thickened and calcified (b1, b2). Opening is incomplete during systole (b2); the patient has aortic valve stenosis.

(futile) invasive coronary angiography in the group randomized to CTA/FFR imaging compared with control. However, this trial did not evaluate whether imaging with CTA alone versus CTA/FFR might have produced similar results.

The last three recent trials provide supporting evidence that coronary CTA should be incorporated in the testing armamentarium for evaluating patients with chest pain and possible coronary artery disease. The trials confirm the high clinical value of CTA in identifying high risk plaque and determining the existence and severity of coronary stenosis which can lead to alteration of treatment strategies with the potential to improve clinical outcomes of symptomatic patients. Notably, both confirmation but also exclusion of anatomic coronary disease can be of clinical importance in patient care because initiation of proper therapy (in the former case) or the avoidance of futile and potentially dangerous approaches (in the latter case). There is no doubt that

📖 Case study

A 44-year-old woman was seen in the outpatient cardiology clinic for vague left-sided chest pain sometimes aggravated by exertion. She has a history of mixed hyperlipidemia, depression, and morbid obesity (weight 264 lb, BMI 46.8) with a 40 lb weight gain in the last 5 years. Her baseline ECG was normal (Figure 9.17a).

An exercise echocardiogram was performed. She exercised for 6 minutes achieving a workload of 6 METs and 92% of the maximum predicted heart rate. The blood pressure response was hypertensive and there were equivocal ST changes with runs of ventricular bigeminy and symptoms of chest pain/shortness of breath during stress. There was augmentation of the left ventricular ejection fraction (LVEF) from 60% to 80% and no stress-induced wall motion abnormalities. Single vessel or distal vessel coronary artery disease could not be excluded.

A positron-emission tomography (PET) scan was planned. However, a pharmacologic single-photon emission CT (SPECT) study was performed with regadenoson. A moderate sized reversible anterior/anterolateral defect of moderate intensity was noted (Figure 9.17b). The LVEF was 60% at rest and >60% post-stress.

Cardiac catheterization was performed for possible ischemia on the SPECT study. Coronary angiography was performed which revealed an anomalous single coronary artery arising from the right coronary cusp giving rise to the left anterior descending (LAD) and left circumflex (LCx) arteries. There was no apparent angiographic stenosis of any other arteries although the LAD appeared small and could not be selectively engaged. A left ventriculogram revealed normal LV systolic function with an estimated LVEF of 60%. A coronary CTA was recommended for assessment of the course of the LAD and LCx arteries.

A multidetector CT coronary angiogram was obtained using retrospective ECG-gating after coronary vasodilatation with 0.4 mg of sublingual nitroglycerin. A single coronary artery arising from the right coronary cusp was seen (Figure 9.17c). The single coronary artery gives rise to the LAD, LCx, and right coronary (RCA) arteries and there was no stenosis of any of the arteries. The LAD follows a pre-pulmonic course and the left circumflex a retroaortic course (Figure 9.17d). The calcium score was zero. The LVEF was 81%.

This case illustrates the utility of coronary CTA in the assessment of chest pain in low to intermediate risk patients and for

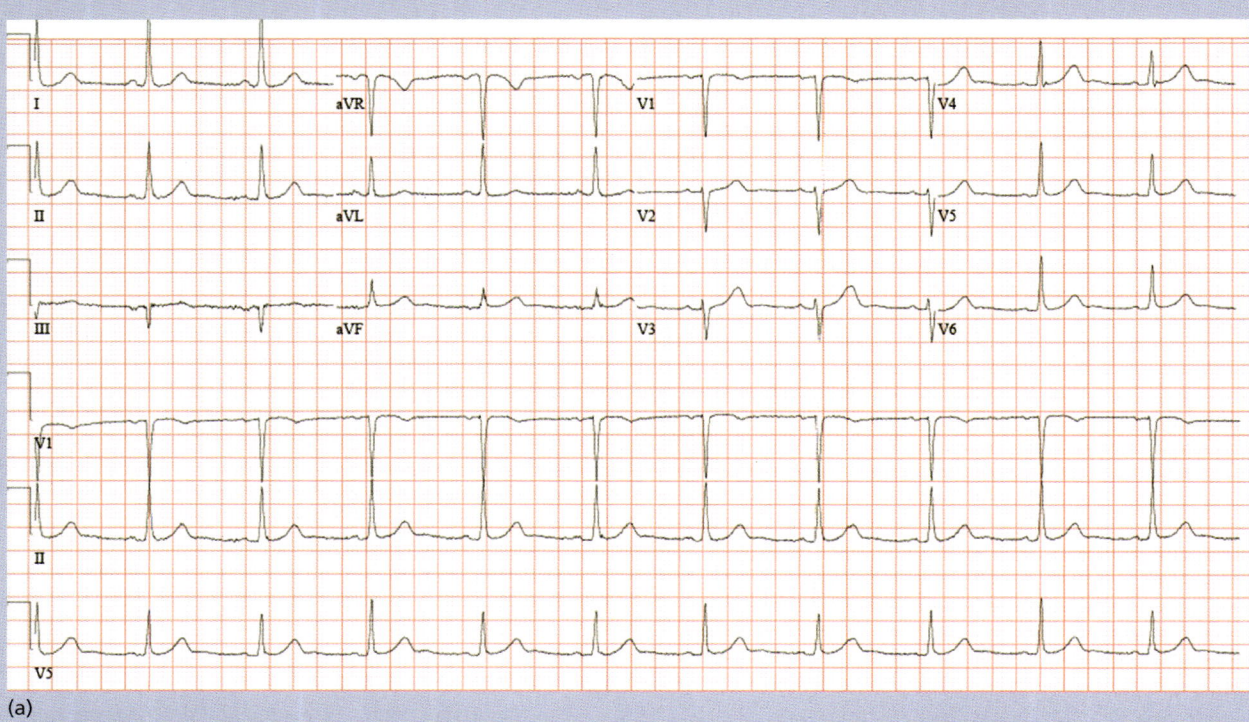

(a)

Figure 9.17 (a) Baseline normal ECG. (b) SPECT images with alternating rows of stress and rest images showing a basal anterior / anterolateral reversible defect (white arrows). (c) Axial projection showing anomalous large single coronary artery arising from the right coronary cusp (black arrow). (d) Sagittal projection showing all three coronary artery origins from the single coronary artery. The LAD has a course anterior to the pulmonary artery while the LCx runs retroaortic. AO, aorta; LAD, left anterior descending; LCx, left circumflex; PA, pulmonary artery; RCA, right coronary artery.

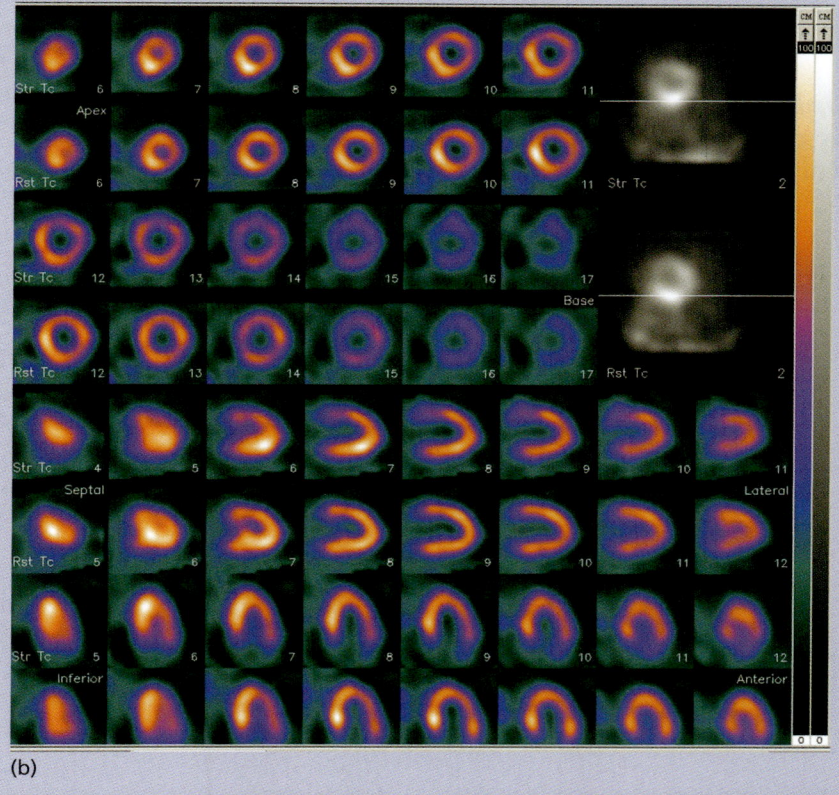

(b)

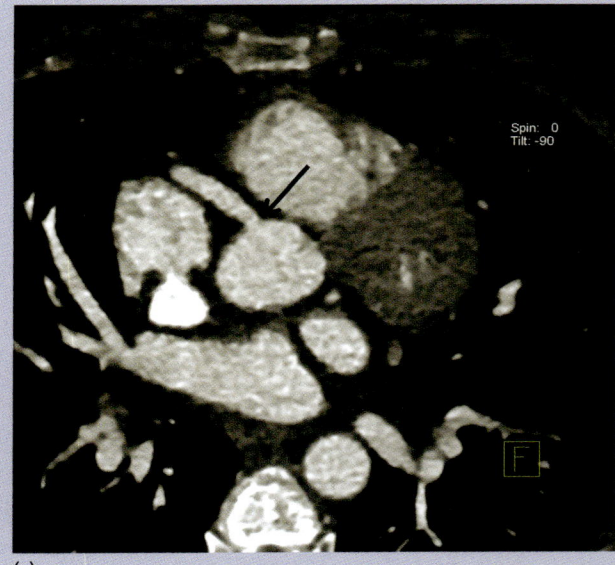

(c)

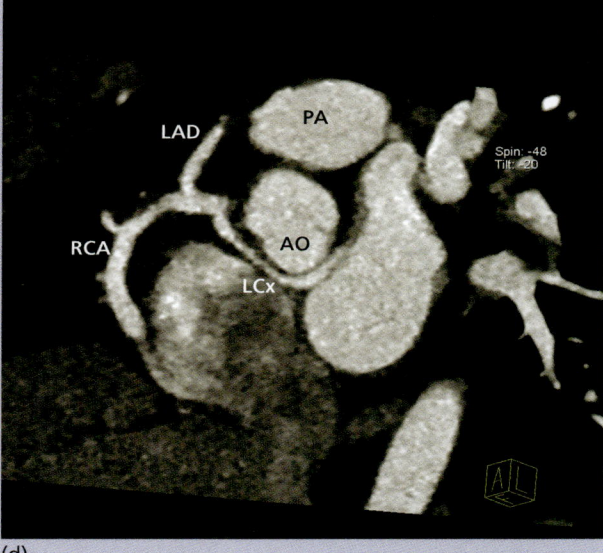

(d)

Figure 9.17 (Continued)

the evaluation of the origin, course, and patency of suspected anomalous coronary arteries. It would have been reasonable to proceed directly to coronary CTA after the equivocal stress echocardiogram instead of performing another functional stress test and the invasive coronary angiogram could also have been avoided. The basal anterior/anterolateral reversible defect was likely related to breast attenuation which was also seen on the raw projection images. Breast attenuation artifacts are common in obese women on SPECT studies and a PET study would have been a better choice as previously planned.

CTA imaging with and without functional lesion assessment should be the subject of future clinical trials.

 Interactive multiple choice questions are available for this chapter on www.wiley. com/go/dangas/cardiology

References

1 Flohr TG, McCollough CH, Bruder H, *et al*. First performance evaluation of a dual-source CT (DSCT) system. *Eur Radiol* 2006; **16**: 256–268.

2 Cademartiri F, Mollet NR, van der Lugt A, *et al*. Intravenous contrast material administration at helical 16-detector row CT coronary angiography: effect of iodine concentration on vascular attenuation. *Radiology* 2005; **236**: 661–665.

3 Fishman EK, Magid D, Ney DR, *et al*. Three-dimensional imaging. *Radiology* 1991; **181**: 321–337.

4 Vogl TJ, Abolmaali ND, Diebold T, *et al*. Techniques for the detection of coronary atherosclerosis: multi-detector row CT coronary angiography. *Radiology* 2002; **223**: 212–220.

5 Achenbach S, Ropers D, Pohle FK, *et al*. Detection of coronary artery stenoses using multi-detector CT with 16 × 0.75 collimation and 375 ms rotation. *Eur Heart J* 2005; **26**: 1978–1986.

6 Dewey M, Teige F, Schnapauff D, *et al*. Noninvasive detection of coronary artery stenoses with multislice computed tomography or magnetic resonance imaging. *Ann Intern Med* 2006; **145**: 407–415.

7 Garcia MJ, Lessick J, Hoffmann MH. Accuracy of 16-row multidetector computed tomography for the assessment of coronary artery stenosis. *JAMA* 2006; **296**: 403–411.

8 Hausleiter J, Meyer T, Hadamitzky M, *et al*. Non-invasive coronary computed tomographic angiography for patients with suspected coronary artery disease: the Coronary Angiography by Computed Tomography with the Use of a Submillimeter resolution (CACTUS) trial. *Eur Heart J* 2007; **28**: 3034–3041. doi:10.1093/eurheartj/ehm150. Available online http://eurheartj.oxfordjournals.org/cgi/content/full/ehm150v1 (accessed April 13, 2016).

9 Hoffmann MH, Shi H, Schmitz BL, *et al*. Noninvasive coronary angiography with multislice computed tomography. *JAMA* 2005; **293**: 2471–2478.

10 Leber AW, Knez A, von Ziegler F, *et al*. Quantification of obstructive and nonobstructive coronary lesions by 64-slice computed tomography: a comparative study with quantitative coronary angiography and intravascular ultrasound. *J Am Coll Cardiol* 2005; **46**: 147–154.

11 Leschka S, Alkadhi H, Plass A, *et al*. Accuracy of MSCT coronary angiography with 64-slice technology: first experience. *Eur Heart J* 2005; **26**: 1482–1487.

12 Mollet NR, Cademartiri F, Krestin GP, *et al*. Improved diagnostic accuracy with 16-row multi-slice computed tomography coronary angiography. *J Am Coll Cardiol* 2005; **45**: 128–132.

13 Mollet NR, Cademartiri F, Nieman K, *et al*. Multislice spiral computed tomography coronary angiography in patients with stable angina pectoris. *J Am Coll Cardiol* 2004; **43**: 2265–2270.

14 Mollet NR, Cademartiri F, van Mieghem CA, *et al*. High-resolution spiral computed tomography coronary angiography in patients referred for diagnostic conventional coronary angiography. *Circulation* 2005; **112**: 2318–2323.

15 Nikolaou K, Knez A, Rist C, *et al*. Accuracy of 64-MDCT in the diagnosis of ischemic heart disease. *AJR Am J Roentgenol* 2006; **187**: 111–117.

16 Nikolaou K, Saam T, Rist C, *et al*. Pre- and postsurgical diagnostics with dual-source computed tomography in cardiac surgery. *Radiologe* 2007; **47**: 310–318.

17 Pugliese F, Mollet NR, Runza G, *et al*. Diagnostic accuracy of non-invasive 64-slice CT coronary angiography in patients with stable angina pectoris. *Eur Radiol* 2006; **16**: 575–582.

18 Raff GL, Gallagher MJ, O'Neill WW, *et al*. Diagnostic accuracy of noninvasive coronary angiography using 64-slice spiral computed tomography. *J Am Coll Cardiol* 2005; **46**: 552–557.

19 Ropers D, Rixe J, Anders K, *et al*. Usefulness of multidetector row spiral computed tomography with 64- × 0.6-mm collimation and 330-ms rotation for the noninvasive detection of significant coronary artery stenoses. *Am J Cardiol* 2006; **97**: 343–348.

20 Scheffel H, Alkadhi H, Plass A, *et al*. Accuracy of dual-source CT coronary angiography: first experience in a high pre-test probability population without heart rate control. *Eur Radiol* 2006; **16**: 2739–2747.

21 Weustink AC, Meijboom WB, Mollet NR, *et al*. Reliable high-speed coronary computed tomography in symptomatic patients. *J Am Coll Cardiol* 2007; **50**: 786–794.

22 Pugliese F, Mollet NR, Hunink MG, *et al*. Diagnostic performance of computed tomography coronary angiography using different generations of multisection scanners: single-centre experience. *Radiology* 2008; **246**: 384–393.

23 Hendel RC, Patel MR, Kramer CM, *et al*. ACCF/ACR/SCCT/SCMR/ASNC/NASCI/SCAI/SIR 2006 appropriateness criteria for cardiac computed tomography and cardiac magnetic resonance imaging: a report of the American College of Cardiology Foundation Quality Strategic Directions Committee Appropriateness Criteria Working Group, American College of Radiology, Society of Cardiovascular Computed Tomography, Society for Cardiovascular Magnetic Resonance, American Society of Nuclear Cardiology, North American Society for Cardiac Imaging, Society for Cardiovascular Angiography and Interventions, and Society of Interventional Radiology. *J Am Coll Cardiol* 2006; **48**: 1475–1497.

24 Van Mieghem CA, Thury A, Meijboom WB, *et al*. Detection and characterization of coronary bifurcation lesions with 64-slice computed tomography coronary angiography. *Eur Heart J* 2007; **28**: 1968–1976.

25 Medina A, Suarez de Lezo J, Pan M. A new classification of coronary bifurcation lesions. *Rev Esp Cardiol* 2006; **59**: 183.

26 Aviram G, Shmilovich H, Finkelstein A, *et al*. Coronary ostium-straight tube or funnel-shaped? A computerized tomographic coronary angiography study. *Acute Card Care* 2006; **8**: 224–248.

27 Mollet NR, Hoye A, Lemos PA, *et al*. Value of preprocedure multislice computed tomographic coronary angiography to predict the outcome of percutaneous recanalization of chronic total occlusions. *Am J Cardiol* 2005; **95**: 240–243.

28 Maintz D, Seifarth H, Raupach R, *et al*. 64-slice multidetector coronary CT angiography: in vitro evaluation of 68 different stents. *Eur Radiol* 2006; **16**: 818–826.

29 Pugliese F, Cademartiri F, van Mieghem C, *et al*. Multidetector CT for visualization of coronary stents. *Radiographics* 2006; **26**: 887–904.

30 Gilard M, Cornily JC, Pennec PY, *et al*. Assessment of coronary artery stents by 16 slice computed tomography. *Heart* 2006; **92**: 58–61.

31 Gaspar T, Halon DA, Lewis BS, *et al*. Diagnosis of coronary in-stent restenosis with multidetector row spiral computed tomography. *J Am Coll Cardiol* 2005; **46**: 1573–1579.

32 Cademartiri F, Schuijf JD, Pugliese F, *et al*. Usefulness of 64-slice multislice computed tomography coronary angiography to assess in-stent restenosis. *J Am Coll Cardiol* 2007; **49**: 2204–2210.

33 Ehara M, Kawai M, Surmely JF, *et al*. Diagnostic accuracy of coronary in-stent restenosis using 64-slice computed tomography: comparison with invasive coronary angiography. *J Am Coll Cardiol* 2007; **49**: 951–959.

34 Rixe J, Achenbach S, Ropers D, *et al*. Assessment of coronary artery stent restenosis by 64-slice multi-detector computed tomography. *Eur Heart J* 2006; **27**: 2567–2572.

35 Pugliese F, Weustink AC, Van Mieghem C, *et al*. Dual-source coronary computed tomography angiography for detecting in-stent restenosis. *Heart* 2007; **94**: 848–854. doi:10.1136/hrt.2007.126474. Available online http://heart.bmj.com/cgi/content/abstract/hrt.2007.126474v1?papetoc (accessed 13 April 2016).

36 Takagi T, Stankovic G, Finci L, *et al*. Results and long-term predictors of adverse clinical events after elective percutaneous interventions on unprotected left main coronary artery. *Circulation* 2002; **106**: 698–702.

37 Smith SC Jr, Feldman TE, Hirshfeld JW Jr, *et al*. ACC/AHA/SCAI 2005 Guideline Update for Percutaneous Coronary Intervention—summary article: a report of the American College of Cardiology/American Heart Association Task Force on Practice Guidelines (ACC/AHA/SCAI Writing Committee to Update the 2001 Guidelines for Percutaneous Coronary Intervention). *Circulation* 2006; **113**: 156–175.

38 Van Mieghem CA, Cademartiri F, Mollet NR, *et al*. Multislice spiral computed tomography for the evaluation of stent patency after left main coronary artery stenting: a comparison with conventional coronary angiography and intravascular ultrasound. *Circulation* 2006; **114**: 645–653.

39 Malagutti P, Nieman K, Meijboom WB, *et al*. Use of 64-slice CT in symptomatic patients after coronary bypass surgery: evaluation of grafts and coronary arteries. *Eur Heart J* 2007; **28**: 1879–1885.

40 Meyer TS, Martinoff S, Hadamitzky M, *et al*. Improved noninvasive assessment of coronary artery bypass grafts with 64-slice computed tomographic angiography in an unselected patient population. *J Am Coll Cardiol* 2007; **49**: 946–950.

41 Pache G, Saueressig U, Frydrychowicz A, *et al*. Initial experience with 64-slice cardiac CT: non-invasive visualization of coronary artery bypass grafts. *Eur Heart J* 2006; **27**: 976–980.

42 Ropers D, Fohle FK, Kuettner A, Pflederer T, *et al*. Diagnostic accuracy of non-invasive coronary angiography in patients after bypass surgery using 64-slice spiral computed tomography with 330-ms gantry rotation. *Circulation* 2006; **114**: 2334–2341; quiz 2334.

43 Alkadhi H, Wildermuth S, Plass A, *et al*. Aortic stenosis: comparative evaluation of 16-detector row CT and echocardiography. *Radiology* 2006; **240**: 47–55.

44 Feuchtner GM, Dichtl W, Friedrich GJ, *et al.* Multislice computed tomography for detection of patients with aortic valve stenosis and quantification of severity. *J Am Coll Cardiol* 2006; **47**: 1410–1417.

45 Willmann JK, Weishaupt D, Lachat M, *et al.* Electrocardiographically gated multi-detector row CT for assessment of valvular morphology and calcification in aortic stenosis. *Radiology* 2002; **225**: 120–128.

46 Dewey M, Zimmermann E, Deissenrieder F, *et al.* Noninvasive coronary angiography by 320-row computed tomography with lower radiation exposure and maintained diagnostic accuracy: comparison of results with cardiac catheterization in a head-to-head pilot investigation. *Circulation* 2009; **120**: 867–875.

47 SCOT-HEART investigators. CT coronary angiography in patients with suspected angina due to coronary heart disease (SCOT-HEART): an open-label, parallel-group, multicentre trial. *Lancet* 2015; **385**: 2383–2391. Available from: http://linkinghub.elsevier.com/retrieve/pii/S0140673615602914 (accessed April 13, 2016).

48 Budoff MJ, Dowe D, Jollis JG, *et al.* Diagnostic performance of 64-multidetector row coronary computed tomographic angiography for evaluation of coronary artery stenosis in individuals without known coronary artery disease. *J Am Coll Cardiol* 2008; **52**(21): 1724–1732.

49 Dewey M, Zimmermann E, Deissenrieder F, *et al.* Noninvasive coronary angiography by 320-row computed tomography with lower radiation exposure and maintained diagnostic accuracy: comparison of results with cardiac catheterization in a head-to-head pilot investigation. *Circulation* 2009; **120**(10): 867–875.

50 Schroeder S, Achenbach S, Bengel F, *et al.* Cardiac computed tomography: indications, applications, limitations, and training requirements: Report of a Writing Group deployed by the Working Group Nuclear Cardiology and Cardiac CT of the European Society of Cardiology and the European Council of Nuclear Cardiology. *Eur Heart J* 2008; **29**(4): 531–556.

51 Goldstein JA, Chinnaiyan KM, Abidov A, *et al.* The CT-STAT (Coronary Computed Tomographic Angiography for Systematic Triage of Acute Chest Pain Patients to Treatment) Trial. *J Am Coll Cardiol* 2011; **58**(14): 1414–1422.

52 Hoffmann U, Truong QA, Schoenfeld DA, *et al.* Coronary CT angiography versus standard evaluation in acute chest pain. *N Engl J Med* 2012; **367**(4): 299–308.

53 Litt HI, Gatsonis C, Snyder B, *et al.* CT angiography for safe discharge of patients with possible acute coronary syndromes. *N Engl J Med* 2012; **366**(15): 1393–1403.

54 Douglas PS, Hoffmann U, Patel MR, *et al.* Outcomes of anatomical versus functional testing for coronary artery disease. *N Engl J Med* 2015; **372**(14): 1291–1300.

55 PROMISE Investigators. CTA, functional testing associated with similar outcomes in patients with suspected CAD. Available from: http://www.healio.com/cardiology/imaging/news/online/%7B3d4851fe-14bd-4679-91f2-7635497ecd07%7D/promise-cta-functional-testing-associated-with-similar-outcomes-in-patients-with-suspected-cad?utm_source=maestro&utm_medium=email&utm_campaign=cardiology+news#perspective (accessed April 13, 2016).

56 Douglas PS, Pontone G, Hlatky MA, *et al*; PLATFORM Investigators. Clinical outcomes of fractional flow reserve by computed tomographic angiography-guided diagnostic strategies vs. usual care in patients with suspected coronary artery disease: the prospective longitudinal trial of FFR(CT): outcome and resource impacts study. *Eur Heart J* 2015; **36**: 3359–3367.

CHAPTER 10
Cardiovascular Magnetic Resonance Imaging

Omosalewa O. Lalude[1] and Stamatios Lerakis[2]

[1] Memorial Healthcare System, Hollywood, FL, USA
[2] Emory University School of Medicine and Georgia Institute of Technology, Atlanta, GA, USA

In the last 15–20 years, cardiac magnetic resonance (CMR) has emerged as a useful non-invasive tool for the complete assessment of cardiovascular morphology and function in the absence of ionizing radiation. Although other imaging modalities such as echocardiography, nuclear imaging, and computed tomography (CT) are available for the assessment of cardiovascular pathology, CMR has imaging sequences that can be manipulated to generate varying degrees of soft-tissue contrast for cardiac tissue characterization. Coupled with this, is the excellent spatial (1–2 mm in-plane resolution), temporal (50 ms or better), and contrast resolutions which allow for routine assessment of cardiac function and blood flow [1,2]. Sequences involving the administration of gadolinium-based contrast agents (GBCAs) also allow for the assessment of myocardial perfusion, viability, and various myopericardial diseases.

The main limitations of CMR are inability to image very large or claustrophobic patients, the long scan time of 20–45 minutes and the risk of nephrogenic systemic fibrosis from gadolinium contrast in patients with impaired renal function (GFR <30 mL/min). The limitations notwithstanding, the ability of CMR to provide comprehensive evaluations of cardiovascular morphology, function, and pathology makes it an attractive tool for the assessment of patients undergoing cardiac interventional procedures and for the planning of such interventions. It is therefore imperative that the interventional cardiologist be familiar with the applications of CMR in this regard. This chapter provides a concise overview of the techniques for the CMR imaging, the applications of these techniques, and the use of CMR in the planning of interventional procedures.

CMR technical concepts
Image generation
CMR is based on the detection of the magnetic spin direction of protons from water and fat in the body. The human body is composed of ~70% water and water is formed from two hydrogen atoms and one oxygen atom. The hydrogen atom has a single proton in its nucleus and each proton functions as a molecular magnet within the magnetic field of the MRI scanner [3]. The intrinsic angular momentum of each proton results in rotation (or precession) around the longitudinal axis of the scanner's magnetic field. This is referred to as "spin." Application of radiofrequency (RF) energy at a flip angle to this axis with the precessing (Lamor) frequency tips the

proton spins toward the transverse plane generating a magnetization that emits a coherent oscillating signal that decays in amplitude and coherence with time. The decay of amplitude (T1 relaxation) and coherence (T2 relaxation) is unique to each tissue and generates energy which is measured by properly oriented receiver coils [1,4]. Using spatial modulation of the magnetic field strength, the received MR signal is spatially encoded for image generation. Parameters such as the flip angle, the time between the applications of successive RF pulses to generate a transverse magnetization (repetition time, TR), and the time at which the signal is measured after the excitation (TE) can be altered to generate images that highlight a specific type of soft-tissue contrast (i.e., T-1 weighted, T-2 weighted, or proton-density weighted) [1].

CMR techniques
There are multiple CMR sequences that can provide morphologic, cine, perfusion, viability, and velocity-encoded flow images. Morphologic black blood images for excellent depiction of myocardial structure and the relationship of the great vessels are typically performed with single-shot (i.e., static) double inversion recovery fast spin-echo techniques (Double–IR FSE) and half-Fourier acquisition turbo spin-echo (HASTE). A fat saturation prepulse can be applied if necessary and the images are obtained from fast acquisitions every other heartbeat and do not require a breath hold. Segmented (i.e., from several heart beats) FSE images are acquired when higher spatial resolution and improved T1 or T2-weighting are required for the characterization of cardiac masses [5].

Bright blood morphologic imaging was previously performed with gradient-recalled echo (GRE) pulse sequences but steady state free precession (SSFP) sequences have resulted in improved imaging. SSFP sequences are not dependent on the inflow effects of blood but on the T2/T1 ratio of the tissue being imaged and provide high intrinsic contrast between the blood and myocardium [6]. They are similar to HASTE sequences in that they do not require a breath hold and are a form of single-shot imaging. They are useful for the evaluation of intraluminal abnormalities as in aortic dissection or for the localization of pulmonary veins [5]. The SSFP technique can be used to produce cine images in which multiple images are obtained in the same slice location in rapid succession during different phases of the cardiac cycle and displayed as a continuous movie loop. The standard acquisition is a segmented retrospectively

Interventional Cardiology: Principles and Practice, Second Edition. Edited by George D. Dangas, Carlo Di Mario, and Nicholas N. Kipshidze.
© 2017 John Wiley & Sons, Ltd. Published 2017 by John Wiley & Sons, Ltd.

gated acquisition in which data are acquired throughout the cardiac cycle and "time stamped" to allow assignment to the proper cardiac phase. Cine imaging allows evaluation of ventricular wall motion, wall thickening, measurement of chamber sizes, and assessment of valvular morphology and function.

Cardiac tagging is a widely available technique that produces a deformable reference grid that allows visualization and quantification of regional heterogeneity in myocardial contraction in the setting of coronary artery disease (CAD) and non-ischemic cardiomyopathy [7–10]. It is also very useful for assessing the motion of the myocardium relative to the pericardium. Displacement encoding with stimulated echo (DENSE) is a tissue tracking variant that overcomes some of the limitations of tagging by allowing direct visualization of myocardial displacement and tracking of myocardial displacement on a pixel basis [3].

Tissue characterization is a unique feature of CMR. It uses the characteristics of proton relaxation (i.e., the relaxation times T1, T2, and T2*) to characterize myocardial or vascular tissue. T1 images are often used for contrast-enhanced studies while T2 and T2* imaging have mostly been used in non-contrast approaches. For example, within the myocardium, T2-weighted CMR imaging is sensitive to regional or global increases of myocardial water content as with acute transplant rejection, acute myocarditis, and acute myocardial infarction. T2* relaxation times are significantly altered by the myocardial iron content and their quantification provides an excellent marker for iron overload [2]. Pixelwise T1 and T2 maps whereby an estimate of T1/T2 is encoded in the intensity of each pixel allows for quantification of the parameter of interest. This permits establishment of normal ranges and the assignment of colors for simplification of visual interpretation [11–13].

Perfusion imaging for the assessment of myocardial blood flow and ischemia is performed at rest and with a pharmacologic vasodilator stress agent such as adenosine or regadenoson. T1-weighted GRE images are acquired every heart beat in diastole to study the first pass kinetics of GBCAs. Usually, 3–4 myocardial slices (depending on heart rate) are obtained to ensure adequate ventricular coverage and temporal resolution. T1-weighting is accentuated for accurate depiction of GBCAs which substantially shorten the T1 of the myocardium causing an increase in signal intensity. Signal intensity (SI) correlates with contrast concentration and analysis can be performed in a qualitatively or quantitatively. Most frequently, a trained observer qualitatively examines the myocardium for low signal or hypoperfusion relative to normally perfused segments. In delayed enhancement (DE) or late gadolinium enhancement (LGE) CMR, the differential distribution volume of GBCAs and T1 difference between necrotic or fibrotic and normal myocardium is exploited to generate contrast on an inversion recovery (IR) T1-weighted GRE sequence. The inversion delay is chosen such that normal myocardium is "nulled" (zero SI) and appears very dark while necrotic or fibrotic myocardium appears bright (Figure 10.1). This is a consequence of the loss of cell membrane integrity and interstitial edema associated with infarction that increases the volume of distribution of GBCAs in the extracellular space [14,15]. In addition, reduction in functional capillary density alters the contrast kinetics of GBCAs such that washout from infarcted myocardium occurs at a much slower rate than from normal myocardium [15]. Areas of prior infarction will have higher concentrations of contrast on DE images 5–10 minutes after intravenous administration of GBCAs. LGE due to ischemic heart disease is typically subendocardial but may be extensive and transmural. Left ventricular (LV) epicardial and midwall patterns of LGE are associated with

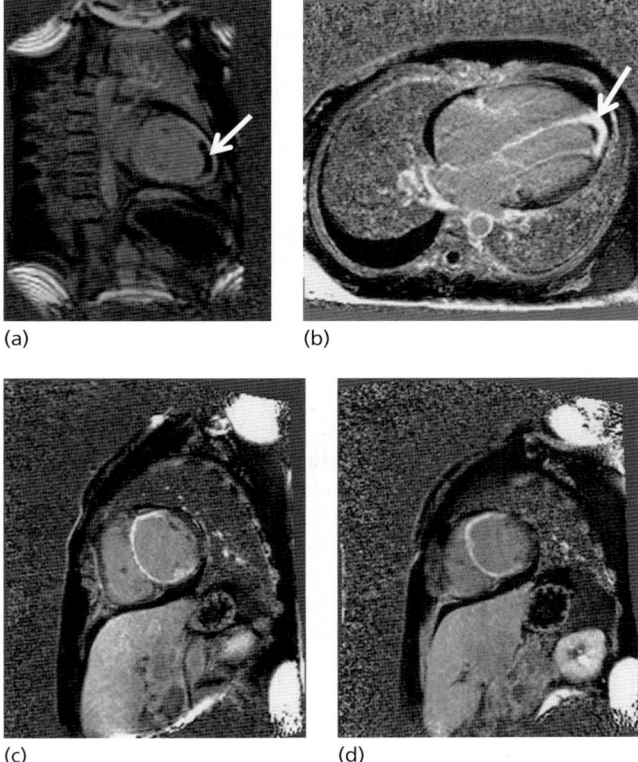

Figure 10.1 (a) Two-chamber view showing high signal intensity (SI) transmural late gadolinium enhancement (LGE) of the entire anterior wall, apex, and inferior wall with an apical thrombus (white arrow). (b) Four-chamber view showing high SI transmural delayed enhancement (DE) of the septum, apex and apical lateral walls with underlying thombus (white arrow). (c, d) Mid and distal short axis slices of the left ventricle showing delayed transmural enhancement of the anterior, septal, and inferior walls. Patient was a 37-year-old man who had an ST-segment elevation MI and received percutaneous intervention (PCI) to the let anterior descending (LAD) artery. He had a previous PCI to the obtuse marginal branch of the circumflex and the right coronary artery (RCA) is found to be occluded at that time. The study was performed for heart failure evaluation. Also note the four chamber dilatation and surrounding pericardial effusion. The circumflex artery territory is viable but there is no viable myocardium in the LAD and RCA territories.

infectious and inflammatory conditions such as myocarditis and sarcoidosis. In cardiac amyloidosis, molecular binding to amyloid protein and very rapid washout of GBCAs from blood results in extensive uptake in myocardial tissue. Single-shot LGE imaging using a long inversion time (~600 ms) is useful for detecting thrombi and can be obtained 2–5 minutes post contrast [5,16,17].

Blood flow can be quantified by phase contrast velocity mapping (PCVM) using velocity-encoded sequences. Velocity-encoding phase shifts result from the sequential application of bipolar magnetic field gradients of opposite polarity. The first gradient produces a phase shift that is reversed by the second pulse such that stationary spins will have no net phase at the end of the sequence. However, flowing spins will acquire a net phase change dependent on velocity in the direction of the flow-encoding gradients [18]. The maximum velocity encoded by the sequence is termed the Venc and should be set at a value just above the anticipated velocities to be measured to avoid aliasing. Aliasing results in artifactual reduction of measured flow while a Venc setting that is too high leads to increased noise or inaccuracy of flow or velocity measurement [5]. Two sets of data are obtained. The magnitude data provide the map of protons within the slice, giving the conventional cross-sectional image. The other set of data obtained is the phase data. This dataset provides a map of the velocity of the protons within the slice. The intensity of a pixel in a phase image reflects the velocity of the protons within that pixel. Evaluation of the intensity of a region of pixels provides quantitative data reflecting the flow of blood through a portion of the heart or artery [18].

Contrast enhanced MR angiography (CE-MRA) is most often performed using thin-section T1-weighted spoiled GRE image acquisitions during the arterial passage of intravenously administered contrast [5,19]. Mutiple thin slices are obtained in a 3D volumetric technique and then assembled into maximum intensity projection (MIP) and volume rendered images. Multiplanar review, which allows visualization of the vessel in cross-section and evaluation of vessel walls, can also be performed. The thoracic aorta is usually imaged in the axial or sagittal plane. An oblique sagittal "candy cane" view which reduces the thickness of the imaging slab can be used to minimize breath hold time. Sequences can be performed with electrocardiographic (ECG) gating and imaging in diastole to avoid image degradation in the aortic root from cardiac motion. Abdominal, pelvic, and lower extremity runoff studies are usually obtained in the coronal plane and are well accepted for comprehensive evaluation of the vasculature in patients likely to require revascularization [20,21]. MRA for the evaluation of renal artery stenosis in comparison with digital subtraction angiography has also been well validated [22].

The visualization of coronary arteries on MR has been a longstanding challenge because of the complexities of imaging small, tortuous vessels at high spatial resolution. This is further compounded by the fact that coronary arteries are only stationary for brief periods of the cardiac cycle. The most successful techniques for imaging coronary arteries utilize navigator echo-based cardiacgated techniques to minimize respiratory motion [23,24]. A high spatial resolution 3D GRE volume covering the proximal and mid coronary arteries is acquired in mid-diastole when coronary blood flow is maximized. The sequence is time consuming and the distal coronary segments are not well visualized. Thus, the major utility of this technique is for assessing the origins and to a limited degree the course of the coronary arteries.

Patient preparation and MRI safety

Although CMR is generally considered safe, there are three main categories of safety concerns: potential projectiles in the MR scanner room, implanted cardiovascular devices, and issues related to contrast administration.

The first step in the preparation of a patient is screening to ensure that there are no major contraindications such as implanted cerebrovascular clips, cochlear implants, ocular metallic fragments, neural stimulators, or insulin pumps. At most institutions, MRIs are not performed in patients with cardiac pacemakers or implantable cardioverter defibrillator (ICD) because of the potential risk and of device malfunction, excessive device or lead heating, or induction of currents within the leads. In addition, the wires and generator can sometimes be associated with significant artifact and other imaging modalities have to be considered. Recent reports, however,

suggest that CMR can be performed safely in patients with pacemakers and ICDs manufactured after 2000 if the benefits are deemed to outweigh the risks [25,26]. Consultation with a Pacemaker/ICD expert or electrophysiologist is recommended prior to CMR imaging [26]. Most coronary and peripheral stents are safe for CMR, even immediately after implantation, as are many nitinol-based devices, such as septal/left atrial appendage occluders and prosthetic valves [2]. If there is any doubt as to the safety of a device, further enquiry should be made, a CMR safety or physics expert may be consulted or an alternative procedure can be performed. GBCAs should not be administered patients with acute or chronic severe renal insufficiency (i.e., GFR <30 mL/min) who are at increased risk for nephrogenic systemic fibrosis or nephrogenic fibrosing dermopathy (NSF/NFD) [27] and pregnant patients.

The patient is then briefed on what to expect throughout the study and instructed on breath holding as most sequences are performed on end-expiration and require 5–10 second breath-holds. Informed consent is usually obtained for contrast and stress CMR studies. A 20-gauge intravenous catheter is placed in an arm vein for the administration of the contrast agent. A second intravenous line is placed in the contralateral arm if a pharmacologic stress agent is to be administered. Vector cardiographic chest leads are placed for ECG gating and respiratory monitoring can be achieved by attaching a bellows-type belt around the patient's waist. The phased array cardiac receiver coil is then placed on the precordium. Brachial cuff pressure and digital pulse oximetry is periodically measured for stress CMR or studies requiring sedation for claustrophobia. Patients undergoing CMR stress imaging with adenosine or regadenoson should avoid caffeine-containing substances for 12–24 hours before the test. Although anaphylactic reactions to GBCAs are rare [2], patients with prior documented reactions should be premedicated with steroids and antihistamines 12–24 hours prior to the scan.

Applications of CMR
Heart failure

Rest CMR is useful for the initial evaluation of cardiac structure and function for newly suspected or potential heart failure (HF): patients with new symptoms or signs of HF, prior to or during the use of cardiotoxic chemotherapy in patients without prior LV function assessment, in patients with familial or genetic dilated cardiomyopathies, in adult congenital heart disease, and in patients with acute myocardial infarction (AUC imaging in HF 2013). In the evaluation of ischemic etiology, stress/rest CMR can be performed in patients with or without angina or ischemic equivalent. After ischemic etiology is determined, in patients with mild–severe LV dysfunction, LV ejection fraction 30–49% and suitable coronary anatomy for revascularization, viability evaluation can be performed using stress/rest or rest CMR. CMR can also be use to determine candidacy for ICD or cardiac resynchronization therapy (CRT) and for pre-procedure planning (i.e., assessment of fibrosis, intracoronary thrombus, and coronary vein variations) [28].

CMR offers more accurate assessment of function and morphology than most other imaging modalities, providing reliable volumetric data with high diagnostic image quality in nearly all patients. High precision and avoidance of ionizing radiation allows CMR to be used in serial evaluations of patients with heart failure to assess response to medical therapy to follow disease progression. Cine SSFP sequences are used to visualize and quantify global left and right atrial and ventricular systolic function relative to reference datasets for normal subjects. Regional biventricular function can be assessed qualitatively and quantitatively by myocardial tagging. LV diastolic function parameters such as the mitral inflow and pulmonary vein flow patterns as well as tissue velocity and strain and strain rates can be obtained similar to echocardiography. The distribution of scarring on LGE allows for accurate discrimination of ischemic from non-ischemic cardiomyopathies [29]. Non-ischemic etiologies of heart failure either do not have detectable scars or have a non-subendocardial distribution that is very distinct from ischemic subendocardial to transmural patterns. In hypertrophic cardiomyopathy (HCM), the LGE is typically found in hypertrophied regions and in the interventricular septum close to the right ventricular (RV) insertion areas [30,31]. In dilated cardiomyopathy, a mid-myocardial stripe of septal fibrosis is more typical and is of strong prognostic value [32]. In patients with acute heart failure, T2-weighted CMR may be useful to detect myocardial inflammation due to acute myocarditis [33,34]. In cardiac iron overload, quantification of $T2^*$ relaxation times have proven useful for estimating intramyocardial iron content [35].

Coronary artery evaluation

CMR has evolved over the past 10–15 years as an important diagnostic modality for coronary anomalies and coronary artery aneurysms despite the limitations previously highlighted in the section on imaging techniques [23,36]. Coronary anomalies are rare (~1% of the general population [37]) and usually benign. Congenital coronary anomalies in which the anomalous segment courses between the aorta and pulmonary artery are a well-recognized cause of myocardial ischemia and sudden cardiac death, especially among young adults [38,39]. CMR is also very helpful for visualizing the course of coronaries especially when intramural segments are present [2]. Most acquired coronary aneurysms arise as sequelae of mucocutaneous lymph node syndrome (Kawasaki's disease) and are associated with short and long-term morbidity and mortality [40]. These aneurysms have been accurately identified and characterized on CMR [41,42].

In specialized academic centers, CMR has proven useful for the discrimination of multivessel CAD which is helpful in patients with a dilated cardiomyopathy and no clinical history of myocardial infarction. Focal stenosis usually appears as signal attenuation. An international multicenter, free-breathing, 3D volume targeted CMR study of patients without prior angiography showed a high sensitivity (100%) and specificity (85%) with high negative predictive value (100%) for the identification of left main and multivessel CAD (≥50% diameter stenosis) by quantitative angiography [24]. The study was not as predictive for single vessel CAD. Whole heart SSFP coronary CMR methods appear to be as accurate as free breathing methods and can be useful for heavily calcified vessels which cause blooming artifacts on CT [43]. However, the evaluation of coronary stents is limited by local signal void/image artifacts that are dependent on stent material and CMR sequence. In comparison with the native coronary arteries, reverse saphenous vein and internal mammary artery grafts are relatively easy to image because of their minimal motion during the cardiac and respiratory cycles and the larger lumen of reverse saphenous vein grafts. Coronary CMR bypass graft assessment is limited by local signal loss/artifact caused by implanted metallic objects (hemostatic clips, stainless steel graft markers, sternal wires, prosthetic valves or rings, and graft stents). The assessment of grafts has shown good correlation with quantitative X-ray angiography for both graft occlusion and stenosis. This resulted in a sensitivity and specificity of 61% (25/41 grafts) and 91% (114/125 grafts), respectively, for conventional gradient-echo CMR in detecting occlusions in grafts or recipient vessels. A sensitivity of 75% and specificity of 91% was found for grafts alone. The sensitivity and specificity for graft stenosis (≥50%; sensitivity) were 82–91% and 60–62%, respectively [44]. Saphenous vein and internal mammary bypass graft CMR has also been combined with rest and adenosine stress graft flow assessment with good results [44].

Ischemic heart disease

The combination of CMR stress perfusion, function, and LGE allows the use of CMR as a primary form of testing for: (i) identifying ischemic heart disease (IHD) in patients who have resting ECG abnormalities or are unable to exercise; or (ii) determining patients who are appropriate candidates for interventional procedures; and (iii) defining the distribution of large vessel CAD in candidates for interventional procedures [2].

Myocardial ischemia and perfusion Dobutamine stress (DS) CMR is useful for the assessment of inducible ischemia by the qualitative or quantitative (CMR tagging) evaluation of wall motion with increasing doses of dobutamine similar to DS echocardiography. Assessment of LV wall motion after low-dose dobutamine in patients with resting akinetic LV wall segments is useful for identifying patients who will develop improvement in LV systolic function after coronary arterial revascularization [2]. GRE DS CMR has high accuracy for detecting ischemia mainly because of the excellent LV endocardial visualization throughout the studies even at high heart rates and can be very useful for patients with poor echocardiographic windows [45,46]. On a meta-analysis of stress-functional CMR studies, stress-induced wall motion abnormality imaging demonstrated a sensitivity of 83% and specificity of 86% and perfusion imaging demonstrated a sensitivity of 91% and specificity of 81% on a patient level [47]. Abnormalities observed during DS or perfusion CMR have been shown to be independent predictors of adverse cardiac events [48]. Three-year event-free survival was been reported at 99.2% for patients with normal DS or stress perfusion CMR and 83.5% for those with abnormal studies. Ischemia on DS or stress perfusion CMR was predictive of cardiac events over the 3-year period with hazard ratios of 5.4 and 12.5, respectively, on univariate analysis and 10.6 and 4.72, respectively, on multivariate analysis [48].

Myocardial infarction and viability The spatial extent of LGE correlates with the distribution of myocyte necrosis in the early period following infarction and that of collagenous scar seen at 8 weeks [49–51], whereas in regions of the heart subjected to reversible injury, the retention of contrast does not occur. When compared with SPECT, LGE is more reliable in detecting subendocardial scar [52,53] in a study of patients evaluated for ischemic heart disease. Border zones of infarcts which contain healthy and necrotic myocytes have intermediate intensity LGE between normal and infarcted tissue and have been associated with the development of ventricular arrhythmias [54]. Areas of microvascular obstruction or "no-reflow" are areas of hyoenhancement surrounded by areas of scar with LGE and represent areas of severe capillary damage that do not allow penetration of contrast even after 10 minutes after contrast injection. These areas of non-viable tissue are usually seen in the 7–10 days post myocardial infarction (MI) and portend a worse prognosis (i.e., marker for post-MI complications and greater predictor of MACE than LGE infarct size) [55].

Myocarditis and non-ischemic cardiomyopathies

Acute viral myocarditis

CMR is considered to be the most versatile and powerful tool in the diagnosis of myocarditis. CMR should be performed when there are new or persisting symptoms (dyspnea, palpitations, effort intolerance, malaise or chest pain) suggestive of myocarditis; plus evidence of recent or ongoing myocardial injury (ventricular dysfunction, new or persisting ECG abnormalities or elevated troponin); plus suspected viral etiology (history of recent systemic viral illness or previous myocarditis, absence of risk factors for CAD/age <35 years, symptoms not explained by coronary stenosis on angiogram or recent negative stress test) [34]. The Lake Louise CMR diagnostic criteria developed by an expert consensus group is as follows. In the appropriate clinical setting, CMR findings are consistent with myocardial inflammation if at least two of the following criteria are present: regional or global myocardial SI increase in T2-weighted images; increased global myocardial early gadolinium enhancement (EGE) ratio between myocardium and skeletal muscle in gadolinium-enhanced T1-weighted images; and at least one focal lesion with non-ischemic regional distribution in inversion recovery LGE T1-weighted images [34]. Studies using combined (any two of three) criteria demonstrate high specificity (89–96%), accuracy (73–85%), and positive predictive value (88–95%) for the CMR diagnosis of myocarditis [56,57]. New native and post-contrast T1 mapping techniques with extracellular volume quantification improve the diagnostic criteria of CMR compared with the Lake Louise criteria [58,59].

CMR is useful for the diagnosis of various cardiomyopathies allowing for appropriate therapy and prognostication. CMR is considered to identify the etiology of cardiac dysfunction and heart failure including: (i) evaluation of dilated cardiomyopathy in the setting of normal coronary arteries; (ii) patients with positive cardiac enzymes without obstructive atherosclerosis on angiography; (iii) patients suspected of amyloidosis or other infiltrative diseases; (iv) HCM; (v) arrhythmogenic RV cardiomyopathy (ARVC); or (vi) syncope or ventricular arrhythmia [2].

Dilated cardiomyopathy

Progressive LV dilatation, LV systolic dysfunction, and regional mid-wall myocardial fibrosis associated with dilated cardiomyopathy can be evaluated by CMR. Fibrosis on LGE has been associated with adverse cardiac events [32] and focal interventricular mid-wall septal fibrosis has been linked to ventricular arrhythmias [60].

Stress (Takotsubo) cardiomyopathy

Stress cardiomyopathy (SC) is acute reversible LV dysfunction following a stressful event with a classic appearance of apical ballooning and hypercontractile basal segments. Other variants with mid or basal LV hypocontraction or RV involvement have also been described. This condition has typically been diagnosed on the basis of history, the ECG, cardiac enzyme profile, contraction pattern on echocardiography or ventriculography, and the absence of significant CAD on coronary angiography. CMR is uniquely suited for the evaluation of patients with SC because it allows for accurate visualization of regional wall motion abnormalities, precise quantification of LV and RV function, and assessment of concomitant abnormalities (e.g., pericardial and pleural effusion, LV and RV thrombi). CMR imaging also provides markers for reversible (inflammation, ischemic edema) and irreversible (necrosis/fibrosis) injury, which may be particularly important to verify SC and exclude similar diseases such as acute MI or myocarditis. On a retrospective study of

SC, myocardial edema with a distinct transmural, midventricular to apical distribution matching the distribution of LV dysfunction was observed. [61]. In the same study, there was no LGE at the threshold normally set for myocardial infarction of five standard deviations above remote myocardium. Also, of the patients who underwent the three CMR protocol requirements for the Lake Louise consensus criteria for myocarditis, 67% were positive for acute myocardial inflammation, with increased values for the T2 SI ratio and the EGE ratio during the acute phase [61].

Non-compaction cardiomyopathy

Non-compaction cardiomyopathy is characterized by a thin compacted myocardium in the mid and apical segments of the LV associated with regional dilatation, dysfunction, and hypertrabeculation. On CMR, an end-diastolic ratio of the non-compacted to compacted LV myocardium of ≥2.3 is considered diagnostic [62].

Arrhythmogenic RV cardiomyopathy

ARVC is characterized by global or regional dilatation of the RV (and in some cases the LV). Fatty and or fibrous replacement of the myocardium may be found on histology but this is not considered to be specific for the disease. As a result, the identification of myocardial fat on CMR is no longer considered a diagnostic criterion. Instead, RV dilatation with RV volumes indexed to body surface area with specific cut-offs for men and women and reduced RVEF as well as global and regional RV and LV myocardial dysfunction are the criteria released by the task force [63]. LGE of RV fibrosis has also been reported as a useful marker [64].

Hypertrophic cardiomyopathy

HCM is characterized by excessive myocardial hypertrophy, myocardial fibrosis, diastolic function abnormalities, and dynamic LV outflow tract obstruction. Cine images are useful for assessment of LV morphology, quantification of LV volumes and mass, and for visualization of the turbulent jet associated with systolic anterior motion of the mitral valve. Scattered areas of focal LGE are seen in the myocardium in areas of hypertrophy and are associated with decreased systolic thickening and perfusion deficits. In a recent study, LGE involving ≥15% of LV mass was identified as a novel risk marker for sudden cardiac death (SCD) which can be used as an arbiter when conventional risk stratification is ambiguous [65]. CMR is very sensitive for detecting HCM in first-degree relatives of those with clinical HCM [66] and can identify the effects of alcohol septal ablation [67].

Sarcoidosis

Up to 50% of patients with pulmonary sarcoidosis have cardiac involvement which is the leading cause of death in these patients. Early contrast enhancement is useful for demonstrating areas of inflammation while LGE shows areas of irreversible injury [68]. Myocardial involvement could be subendocardial to transmural and does not follow a coronary distribution.

Amyloidosis

Myocardial amyloid accumulation is often a consequence of systemic amyloidosis with resultant increase in ventricular wall thickness. The amyloid protein has increased affinity for GBCAs resulting in a much faster clearance of the contrast from the blood than in other patients. The classic appearance is of a low signal "dark" blood pool and a very high SI myocardium that is difficult to "null" on LGE images. The T1 and T2 relaxation times of the myocardium are shortened from the increased accumulation of GBCAs and this allows for detection with high accuracy [69].

Hemochromatosis

Cardiac iron overload in diseases such as thalassemia and hereditary hemochromatosis can lead to dilatation, hypertrophy, and dysfunction. The prognosis in this condition is based on the degree of cardiac involvement. Myocardial T2* quantification, which can be accurately determined, has been shown to be a more efficacious marker of cardiac iron involvement and guidance of chelation therapy than serial liver biopsies [35,70].

Pericardial disease

Pericardial disease represents a spectrum of diseases from congenital absence, pericardial effusion, and effusive constrictive pericarditis to constrictive pericarditis (CP) (Figure 10.2). CMR can provide information on the extent of pericardial disease (regardless of body habitus or prior surgical procedures), abnormalities in surrounding structures, and allows an accurate measurement of pericardial and related structures. It also provides superior tissue characterization including an estimate of inflammation [2,71]. Black blood T1-weighted SE CMR is used for morphologic assessment of the pericardium, intrathoracic and mediastinal structures. Black blood T2-weighted SE CMR highlights fluid-rich structures such as pericardial effusion or myocardial edema with concomitant myocarditis. SSFP cine allows visualization of effusion, the often tubular

configuration of the ventricles, and flattening/paradoxical motion of the interventricular septum in CP. It also allows for quantification of chamber size/function including RV/right atrial (RA) collapse. Ventricular interdependence, which is the sine qua non of diagnosis of CP differentiating it from restrictive cardiomyopathy, can be evaluated on real-time cine CMR. Other physiologic consequences of CP such as distension of the inferior vena cava/hepatic veins can be observed on various sequences. Tagged cine can be used to demonstrate tethering or adhesion of the pericardial layers which impairs the normal sliding motion of the pericardium across the myocardium. This is particularly helpful in the subset of patients with organized pericardial effusions or pericardial adhesions and normal pericardial thickness [2]. Perfusion CMR imaging is recommended to assess the blood supply of pericardial mass lesions and high SI on LGE suggests pericarditis.

Congenital heart disease

CMR may be used for assessing cardiac structure and function and blood flow through the heart, great vessels, cardiac shunts, and extracardiac conduits in individuals with simple and complex congenital heart disease (CHD) before and after surgical repair [72]. The ability of CMR to delineate complex anatomy and the lack of ionizing radiation is particularly attractive in the pediatric age group as serial follow-up studies are usually required [73]. CMR has high accuracy and reproducibility for assessment of ventricular cavity size and systolic function in CHD [74]. This is important as patients

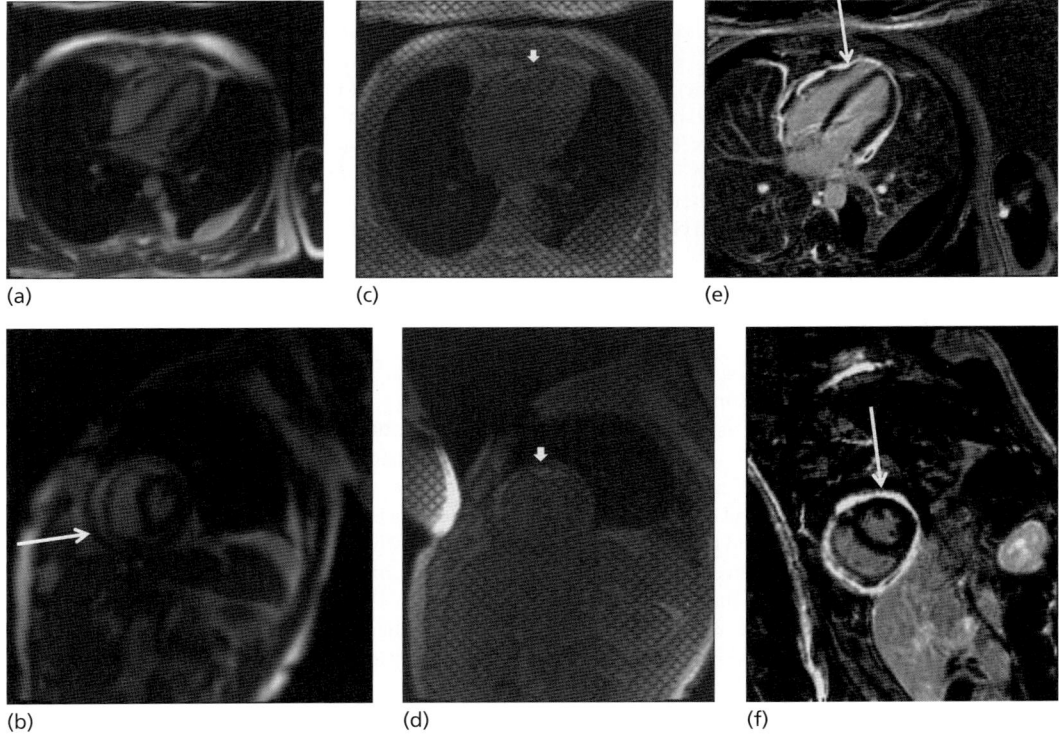

Figure 10.2 Free breathing cine sequences on inspiration. (a) Four-chamber view showing flattening of the septum and tubular elongation of the ventricles with a small left pleural effusion. (b) Mid-short axis showing thick pericardium of ~ 8 mm (white arrow), septal flattening, and circumferential pericardial effusion. Myocardial tagging in diastole. (c, d) Four-chamber and mid-short axis showing adherent pericardium (arrowheads). LGE imaging. (e, f) Four-chamber and mid-short axis showing marked circumferential pericardial thickening and enhancement (white arrows) consistent with pericarditis. Patient was a 56-year-old man who developed cough and fever after a vacation. He presented 1 month after the onset of symptoms with shortness of breath and CMR was consistent with constrictive pericarditis.

with CHD tend to have unusual cardiac chamber shapes and sizes as a consequence of the baseline altered physiology or the numerous corrective procedures with concomitant exposure to cardiopulmonary bypass or deep hypothermic circulatory arrest.

CMR with PCVM for quantification of the pulmonary to systemic flow ratio (Qp/Qs) (shunt fraction) is useful in patients with simple CHD such as atrial and ventricular septal defects [75,76]. In tetralogy of Fallot (TOF), the regurgitant fraction of the often disrupted pulmonic valve can be quantified. The caval contributions of blood flow to each lung in patients with single ventricle physiology who have undergone Glenn and Fontan procedures can be determined [77]. CMR, often with CE-MRA, is also helpful for the assessment of abnormalities of the great vessels such as transposition and obstructive aortic anomalies such as aortic coarctation and interruption. CMR (SE, cine, dynamic PCVM) with CE-MRA is superior to other imaging modalities including echocardiography for combined anatomic (location and severity of narrowing) and physiologic (trans-coarctation pressures gradient and collateral flow assessment) of coarctation [2]. CMR and CE-MRA are useful for distinguishing true from pseudocaoarctation and for assessing complications of repair such as restenosis or pseudoaneurysm formation [2]. Aortic arch anomalies and vascular rings (i.e., double aortic arch, right aortic arch with aberrant left subclavian artery, or mirror-image right aortic arch with left-sided ligamentum arteriosum) can cause varying degrees of compression of the trachea and/or esophagus, without or with symptoms stridor, dyspnea, cyanosis, or dysphagia. These anomalies and their potentially life-threatening complications can be imaged with CMR and/or CE-MRA [2].

Valvular heart disease

CMR may be used in the assessment of valvular stenosis, valvular and regurgitation, para- or perivalvular masses, perivalvular complications of infectious processes, or prosthetic valve disease. CMR is a particularly useful for identifying serial changes in LV volumes or mass that occurs with valvular dysfunction. Although cine SSFP is usually preferred for functional imaging, standard GRE sequences are preferred for jet visualization and qualitative assessment of valve disease because of their longer echo time [78]. Valve disease on GRE sequences is usually seen as a signal void or turbulent jet just above or below the valve. CMR planimetry of the aortic and mitral valves correlates with planimetry on echocardiography. CMR planimetry of the mitral valve often results in overestimation of the valve area relative pressure half-time secondary to translational motion of the heart [79,80]. Isolated mitral or tricuspid valve regurgitation can be estimated from the difference of the LV and RV stroke volumes. A more direct method for the outflow valves is to use PCVM to obtain the peak/mean velocities of the jet and the flow through a stenotic valve [81]. The pressure gradient is then calculated by plugging the velocities into the Bernoulli equation. Forward and reverse volume across a valve for the quantification of regurgitant fraction is also possible with PCVM. In-plane PCVM is helpful for assessing the direction of eccentric jets as is often the case with mitral or bicuspid aortic valve regurgitation.

Vascular disease

Aortic disease

CMR imaging techniques (e.g., spin echo, GRE, and cine PCVM; and 3D CE-MRA) permit the assessment of the anatomic abnormalities and the predisposing or resulting pathophysiologic changes associated with diseases of the aorta [2]. These techniques are used in the following conditions:

1 Aneurysm: to elucidate etiology and identify associated aortic valve abnormalities for pre-surgical planning
2 Atherosclerosis and penetrating ulcer: to identify aortic pseudoaneurysms, non-communicating dissection
3 Traumatic injury: to identify aortic wall hemorrhage and differentiate between partial and circumferential tears
4 Dissection: to identify acute versus chronic states, delineate the extent and locate antry and exit flaps, measure flow in the true and false lumen, differentiate from intramural hematoma and assess associated aortic valve involvement
5 Aortitis: detection of wall inflammation and measurement of wall thickness in response to treatment.

Post-surgical repair, CE-MRA can be used to assess disease progression or regression and postoperative complications [82,83].

Peripheral arterial disease

CMR is appropriate for patients with lower extremity claudication and for the evaluation of location and degree of stenosis for selection of patients for revascularization. 2D times of flight (TOF) techniques were used in the past but 3D CE-MRA has been shown to be more accurate for detecting and grading stenosis. For extended (up to 1 m) coverage, a multistation ("bolus chase") CE-MRA with a single contrast injection is preferred. A hybrid technique with a supplemental dedicated CE-MRA of the lower extremities improves visualization of the infrapopliteal arteries especially in diabetic patients in whom arterial enhancement can be variable or fast. Prospective studies have shown CE-MRA to be more sensitive and specific for the detection of arterial stenosis of greater than 50% compared with duplex ultrasound [84]. In a randomized study of consecutive patients [85] randomized to either peripheral CE-MRA or 16-slice cardiac CT angiography (CTA), CTA was found to be less expensive with no statistically significant differences in patient outcomes (i.e., quality of life). Mean therapeutic confidence for CE-MRA and CTA were similar and comparable to that for digital subtraction angiography. CTA exposed participants to ionizing radiation and ionic contrast. Compared with CTA and ultrasound, CMR has the additional advantage of being able to characterize atherosclerotic plaque components.

Carotid disease

Carotid endarterectomy (CEA) or carotid artery stenting (CAS) is recommended in appropriate patients with severe symptomatic stenosis (70–99%). Various techniques including 2D and 3D TOF with or without CE-MRA have been utilized for the assessment of the carotid arteries. Availability of 3.0-T CMR units and recent developments in parallel imaging have greatly improved the performance of CE-MRA such that it rivals CTA and conventional angiography for the assessment of coronary stenosis and aneurysms [86–88]. PCVM has been found useful for the evaluation of peak velocity and flow of stenotic carotid segments and vertebral artery flow in subclavian steal syndrome.

Renal artery disease

CMR can be used to assess renal artery stenosis, dissection, aneurysmal dilatation, and quantify renal blood flow. Multiple renal arteries are common and CMR is useful for detecting the number and location of the arteries as well as the configuration of renal blood supply in horseshoe kidneys. Renal and adrenal parenchymal mass lesions can also be detected on CMR. MRA for the assessment of renal artery stenosis including fibromuscular dysplasia has been well validated against digital subtraction angiography [16]. Some studies have estimated the sensitivity and specificity of 3.0-T MRA in the detection of intra-abdominal arterial stenosis as 100% and greater than 92%, respectively [89,90].

CMR for interventional cardiac procedures

Transcatheter aortic valve implantation

Transcatheter aortic valve implantation (TAVI) recently emerged as an alternative treatment option for patients considered high risk for surgical aortic valve replacement (SAVR). While CTA and echocardiography are more commonly applied in the evaluation of patients for TAVI, there are some specific situations in which CMR may be useful. Cine CMR can provide a detailed anatomic assessment of the AV that can be used to (i) identify the presence of congenital valvular abnormalities such as bicuspid aortic valve that may preclude TAVI, and (ii) obtain a directly planimetered aortic valve area [91] which is useful for assessing the severity of AS if there is a

discrepancy between clinical and echocardiographic findings. Direct comparison of CMR imaging and MDCT measurements of the aortic root and aortic annulus has shown close agreement [92,93]. In patients with renal insufficiency, gated non-enhanced MRA can be an alternative to CT for accurate measurements of the proximal aorta and evaluation of the aorto-iliofemoral system[94,95]. The major limitation of CMR for TAVI planning is inadequate visualization of calcified cardiac structures.

PCVM is useful for obtaining peak velocity of the aortic valve in patients with technically limited echocardiographic studies [96]. Significant mitral regurgitation is considered a relative contraindication to TAVI (primer) and concomitant aortic or mitral regurgitation can be quantified on PCVM. CMR is the ideal modality for assessing LV volumes, mass, and function to determine the optimal timing of intervention and identify patients in whom TAVI is contraindicated (i.e., LVEF <20%) [91]. LGE imaging can provide information about the extent of scarring related to CAD or help identify previously undiagnosed conditions such as cardiac amyloidosis which can alter prognosis [97].

CMR is beginning to show promise in the evaluation of post-TAVI complications (Figure 10.3). In general, GRE images with short echo times yield fewer artifacts from the implanted core valve than SSFP images [97]. The severity of perivalvular regurgitation

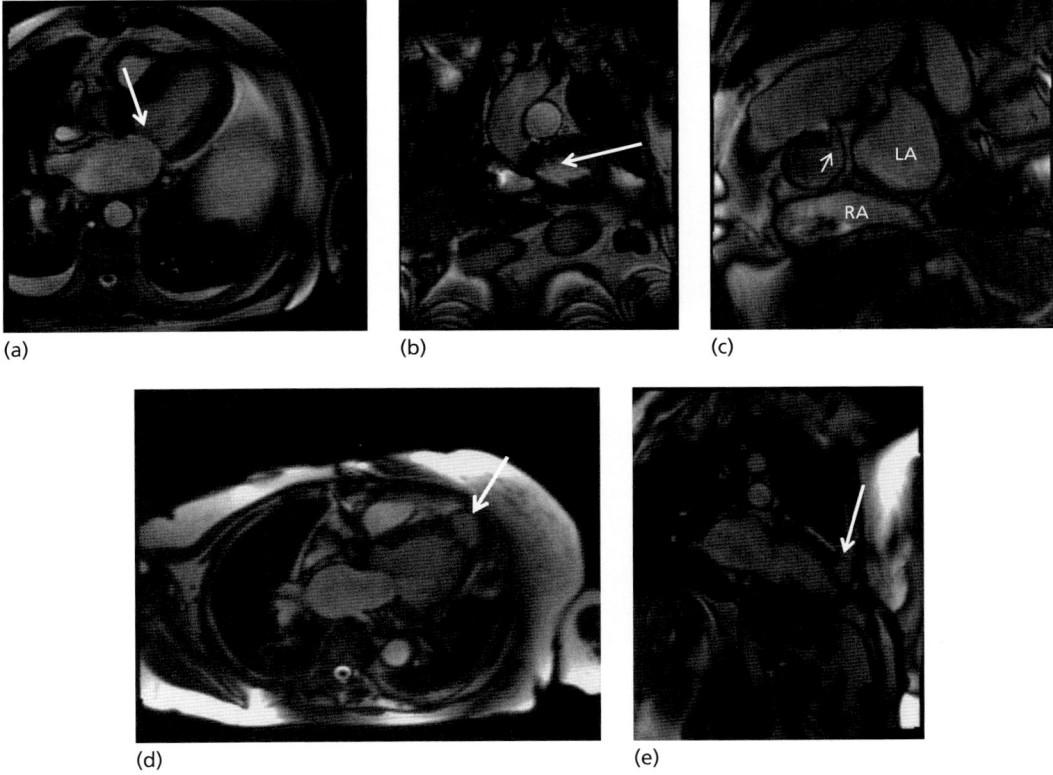

Figure 10.3 Post transcatheter aortic valve implantation (TAVI) complications: steady state free precession (SSFP) images showing a perivalvular aortic regurgitation 13 days post TAVI in a 90-year-old man. (a) Three-chamber view (white arrow). (b) Left ventricular outflow tract view showing the posterior jet (white arrow). (c) The jet (short white arrow) is located adjacent to the left atrium (LA) on the short-axis view. RA, right atrium. (d) SSFP images showing four-chamber view. (e) Two-chamber view of a pseudoaneurysm (white arrow) post-apical puncture for TAVI in an 86-year-old woman.

(PVR) was associated with increasing annulus diameter on both CMR imaging and MDCT [92]. The location and number of perivalvular regurgitation (PVR) jets can be determined and PCVM allows for quantification of aortic regurgitation which helps in the pre-procedural planning for closure devices when indicated. CMR is also useful for the assessment of PVR associated with longstanding surgically placed aortic and mitral valves.

Aortic coarctation

CMR has become the preferred non-invasive tool for selection for percutaneous intervention (PI) and surveillance after surgery or PI in patients with aortic coarctation. CMR is increasing being used due to its ability to generate both 3D anatomic and hemodynamic information without radiation exposure [98–101]. CE-MRA provides 3D visualization of arch geometry, aneurysmal formation, and collateral vessels. Aortic stents placed during intervention interfere with assessment of the coarctation post-intervention but collateral flow estimation is unaffected.

Right ventricular outflow tract dysfunction

Dysfunction of the right ventricular outflow tract (RVOT) post repair of TOF often leads to varying degrees of stenosis and regurgitation. CMR derived parameters of RV size and function are important for determining timing of intervention. CMR provides accurate information on anatomy, size, and geometry of the RVOT and pulmonary arteries. This is crucial in pre-procedural assessment for percutaneous pulmonary valve implantation, as certain anatomic criteria are to be met for the safe anchoring of the valve [98,102,103].

Emerging uses for CMR
Interventional CMR

Clinical cardiovascular interventional CMR (ICMR) has been demonstrated in specialized academic centers to be feasible and initial results are promising [104]. Using combined X-ray fluoroscopy (XRF) and MR (XMR), cardiac catheterizations have been performed in children for the last 10 years [105]. Invasive receiver coil imaging of peripheral arterial atheromata has been reported [106,107]. MRI datasets and real-time XRF have been combined for therapeutic procedures such as aortic stenting and high quality intra-arterial MRA with passive device placement in the iliofemoral arteries has also been reported [108–110].

Conclusions

CMR is a non-invasive radiation-free versatile imaging modality that allows high resolution visualization and functional assessment of cardiac structures; including wall motion analysis, quantification of cardiac function/blood flow, and myocardial tissue characterization. CMR also allows 3D anatomic depiction of cardiovascular structures but, unlike CT, does not require iodinated contrast. Although there are a few limitations of CMR, it has found wide application in the assessment of cardiovascular conditions and is also important in the multimodality planning of cardiac interventional procedures. Clinical ICMR is feasible and has the potential to revolutionize the field of interventional cardiology.

 Case Study

A 59-year-old man with a history of hypertension, hyperlipidemia, and cocaine abuse was admitted to a local hospital with a 3-day history of substernal chest pain, dyspnea, and diaphoresis. His EKG was consistent with inferior ST elevation myocardial infarction. Coronary angiography showed right coronary artery thrombosis and PCI with thrombectomy and stenting to the right coronary artery was performed. He had an uneventful hospital course and was discharged home on guideline directed medical therapy (GDMT).

One month after discharge, he presented in congestive heart failure with shortness of breath, a new murmur, and an enlarged cardiac silhouette on chest X-ray. He was transferred to a tertiary care institution for further management. A transthoracic echocardiogram showed a small pericardial effusion, moderate to severe mitral regurgitation, and severe left ventricular dysfunction, LVEF 25%, with a basal inferolateral pseudoaneurysm and an inferoseptal ventricular septal defect with left to right flow. A CMR was performed for better assessment of the extent of pathology as well as calculation of the shunt fraction. The CMR confirmed the presence of mitral regurgitation (Figure 10.4a), the extent of the large inferobasal pseudoaneurysm (Figure 10.4b, c), a true inferobasal aneurysm (Figure 10.4d), and communication between the left and right ventricles consistent with a rupture of the interventricular septum (Figure 10.4e). The calculated LVEF was 25%, RVEF 47% and the Qp/Qs was 1.9, consistent with a significant shunt.

He underwent surgical repair of the ventricular septal rupture and LV pseudoaneurysm/aneurysm. Six days post-surgery he had an episode of sustained monomorphic ventricular tachycardia. The electrophysiology team was consulted and an implantable cardiac defibrillator was placed. He was discharged home on the seventh postoperative day on GDMT. A pre-discharge echocardiogram showed slight improvement in LV systolic function, LVEF 30–35%, mild mitral regurgitation and a restrictive residual ventricular septal defect with a peak gradient of 102 mmHg.

This case illustrates the utility of CMR in the evaluation of complications post-MI/PCI in the stabilized patient. In this case, valuable information on the extent of ventricular damage was obtained for surgical planning.

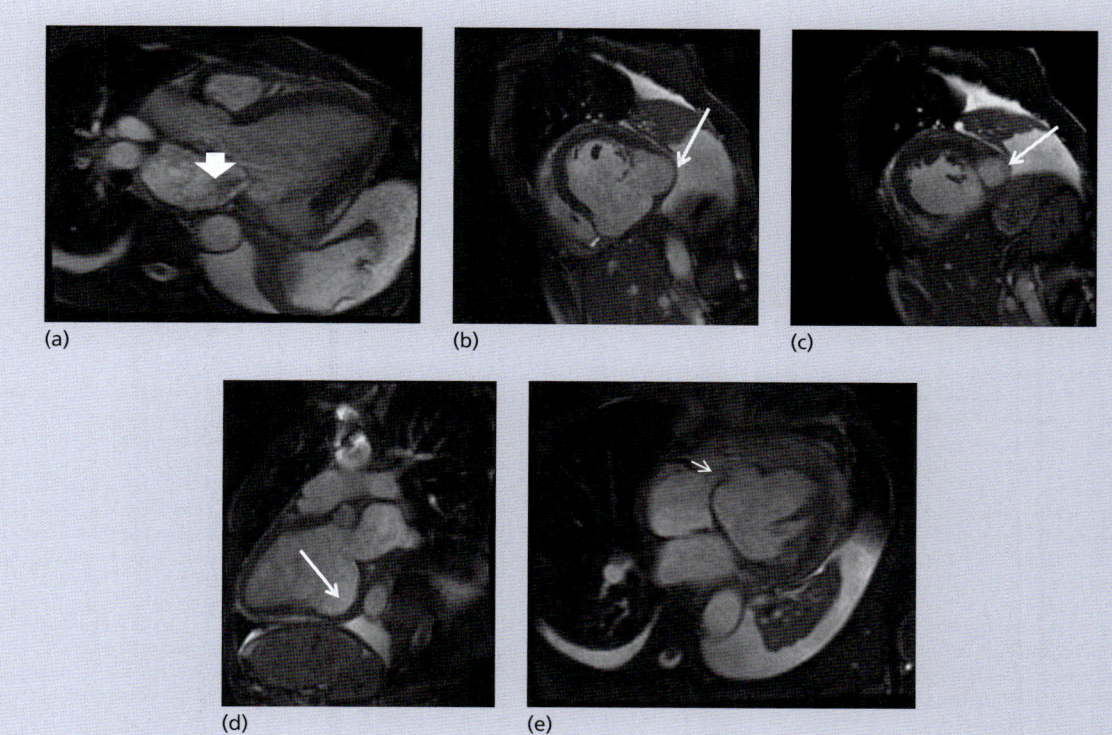

Figure 10.4 SSFP images. (a) Three-chamber, (b, c) short-axis views showing a posteriorly directed mitral regurgitation jet (arrowhead) and the inferobasal pseudoaneurysm (white arrows). (d) Two-chamber view showing the true LV aneurysm (white arrows). (e) Four-chamber view showing the ventricular septal rupture in the inferobasal septum (small white arrow).

Interactive multiple choice questions are available for this chapter on www.wiley. com/go/dangas/cardiology

References

1 Krishnamurthy R, Cheong B, Muthupillai R. Tools for cardiovascular magnetic resonance imaging. *Cardiovasc Diagn Ther* 2014; **4**(2): 104.

2 Hundley WG, Bluemke DA, Finn JP, *et al.* ACCF/ACR/AHA/NASCI/SCMR 2010 Expert Consensus Document on Cardiovascular Magnetic Resonance. *J Am Coll Cardiol* 2010; **55**(23): 2614–2662.

3 Biederman RWW, Doyle M, Yamrozik J. *Cardiovascular MRI Tutorial: Lectures and Learning.* Lippincott Williams & Wilkins, Philadelphia: 2007.

4 Ridgway JP. Cardiovascular magnetic resonance physics for clinicians: part I. *J Cardiovasc Magn Reson* 2010; **12**(1): 71.

5 Grizzard J, Judd R, Kim R. *Cardiovascular MRI in Practice: A Teaching File Approach.* Springer, London: 2008.

6 Reeder SB, Herzka DA, McVeigh ER. Signal-to-noise ratio behavior of steady-state free precession. *Magn Reson Med* 2004; **52**(1): 123–130.

7 Marcus JT, Götte MJ, Van Rossum AC, *et al.* Myocardial function in infarcted and remote regions early after infarction in man: assessment by magnetic resonance tagging and strain analysis. *Magn Reson Med* 1997; **38**(5): 803–810.

8 Fernandes VRS, Polak JF, Edvardsen T, *et al.* Subclinical atherosclerosis and incipient regional myocardial dysfunction in asymptomatic individuals. *J Am Coll Cardiol* 2006; **47**(12): 2420–2428.

9 Gerber BL, Belge B, Legros GJ, *et al.* Characterization of acute and chronic myocardial infarcts by multidetector computed tomography comparison with contrast-enhanced magnetic resonance. *Circulation* 2006; **113**(6): 823–833.

10 Young AA, Dokos S, Powell KA, *et al.* Regional heterogeneity of function in nonischemic dilated cardiomyopathy. *Cardiovasc Res* 2001; **49**(2): 308–318.

11 Messroghli DR, Niendorf T, Schulz-Menger J, Dietz R, Friedrich MG. T1 mapping in patients with acute myocardial infarction. *J Cardiovasc Magn Reson* 2003; **5**(2): 353–359.

12 Messroghli DR, Radjenovic A, Kozerke S, Higgins DM, Sivananthan MU, Ridgway JP. Modified Look-Locker inversion recovery (MOLLI) for high-resolution T1 mapping of the heart. *Magn Reson Med* 2004; **52**(1): 141–146.

13 Moon JC, Messroghli DR, Kellman P, *et al.* Myocardial T1 mapping and extracellular volume quantification: a Society for Cardiovascular Magnetic Resonance (SCMR) and CMR Working Group of the European Society of Cardiology consensus statement. *J Cardiovasc Magn Reson* 2013; **15**(1): 92.

14 Lima JAC, Judd RM, Bazille A, Schulman SP, Atalar E, Zerhouni EA. Regional heterogeneity of human myocardial infarcts demonstrated by contrast-enhanced mri potential mechanisms. *Circulation* 1995; **92**(5): 1117–1125.

15 Kim RJ, Chen E-L, Lima JAC, Judd RM. Myocardial Gd-DTPA kinetics determine MRI contrast enhancement and reflect the extent and severity of myocardial injury after acute reperfused infarction. *Circulation* 1996; **94**(12): 3318–3326.

16 Grizzard JD, Ang GB. Magnetic resonance imaging of pericardial disease and cardiac masses. *Magn Reson Imaging Clin N Am* 2007; **15**(4): 579–607, vi.

17 Barkhausen J, Hunold P, Eggebrecht H, *et al.* Detection and characterization of intracardiac thrombi on MR imaging. *Am J Roentgenol* 2002; **179**(6): 1539–1544.

18 Lotz J, Meier C, Leppert A, Galanski M. Cardiovascular Flow measurement with phase-contrast mr imaging: basic facts and implementation 1. *Radiographics* 2002; **22**(3): 651–671.

19 Edelman RR. MR angiography: present and future. *AJR Am J Roentgenol* 1993; **161**(1): 1–11.

20 Ruehm SG, Hany TF, Pfammatter T, Schneider E, Ladd M, Debatin JF. Pelvic and lower extremity arterial imaging: diagnostic performance of three-dimensional contrast-enhanced MR angiography. *Am J Roentgenol* 2000; **174**(4): 1127–1135.

21 Kreitner K-F, Kalden P, Neufang A, *et al.* Diabetes and peripheral arterial occlusive disease: prospective comparison of contrast-enhanced three-dimensional MR angiography with conventional digital subtraction. *Am J Roentgenol* 2000; **174**(1): 171–179.

22 Zhang H, Prince MR. Renal MR angiography. *Magn Reson Imaging Clin N Am* 2004; **12**(3): 487–503, vi.

23 Taylor AM, Thorne SA, Rubens MB, *et al.* Coronary artery imaging in grown up congenital heart disease complementary role of magnetic resonance and X-ray coronary angiography. *Circulation* 2000; **101**(14): 1670–1678.

24 Kim WY, Danias PG, Stuber M, et al. Coronary magnetic resonance angiography for the detection of coronary stenoses. N Engl J Med 2001; 345(26): 1863–1869.

25 Roguin A, Zviman MM, Meininger GR, et al. Modern pacemaker and implantable cardioverter/defibrillator systems can be magnetic resonance imaging safe: in vitro and in vivo assessment of safety and function at 1.5 T. Circulation 2004; 110: 475–482.

26 Levine GN, Gomes AS, Arai AE, et al. Safety of magnetic resonance imaging in patients with cardiovascular devices. Circulation 2007; 116: 2878-2891.

27 Food and Drug Administration. FDA Drug Safety Communication: new warnings for using gadolinium-based contrast agents in patients with kidney dysfunction. Available from: http://www.fda.gov/Drugs/DrugSafety/ucm223966.htm (accessed April 15, 2016).

28 Patel MR, White RD, Abbara S, et al. 2013 ACCF/ACR/ASE/ASNC/SCCT/SCMR appropriate utilization of cardiovascular imaging in heart failure. J Am Coll Cardiol 2013; 61(21): 2207–2231.

29 McCrohon JA, Moon JCC, Prasad SK, et al. Differentiation of heart failure related to dilated cardiomyopathy and coronary artery disease using gadolinium-enhanced cardiovascular magnetic resonance. Circulation 2003; 108(1): 54–59.

30 Choudhury L, Mahrholdt H, Wagner A, et al. Myocardial scarring in asymptomatic or mildly symptomatic patients with hypertrophic cardiomyopathy. J Am Coll Cardiol 2002; 40(12): 2156–2164.

31 Moon JC, McKenna WJ, McCrohon JA, Elliott PM, Smith GC, Pennell DJ. Toward clinical risk assessment inhypertrophic cardiomyopathy withgadolinium cardiovascular magnetic resonance. J Am Coll Cardiol 2003; 41(9): 1561–1567.

32 Assomull RG, Prasad SK, Lyne J, et al. Cardiovascular Magnetic resonance, fibrosis, and prognosis in dilated cardiomyopathy. J Am Coll Cardiol 2006; 48(10): 1977–1985.

33 Skouri HN, Dec GW, Friedrich MG, Cooper LT. Noninvasive imaging in myocarditis. J Am Coll Cardiol 2006; 48(10): 2085–2093.

34 Friedrich MG, Sechtem U, Schulz-Menger J, et al. Cardiovascular magnetic resonance in myocarditis: a JACC White Paper. J Am Coll Cardiol 2009; 53(17): 1475–1487.

35 Anderson LJ, Westwood MA, Prescott E, Walker JM, Pennell DJ, Wonke B. Development of thalassaemic iron overload cardiomyopathy despite low liver iron levels and meticulous compliance to desferrioxamine. Acta Haematol 2006; 115(1-2): 106–108.

36 McConnell MV, Ganz P, Selwyn AP, Li W, Edelman RR, Manning WJ. Identification of anomalous coronary arteries and their anatomic course by magnetic resonance coronary angiography. Circulation 1995; 92(11): 3158–3162.

37 Engel HJ, Torres C, Page HL. Major variations in anatomical origin of the coronary arteries: angiographic observations in 4,250 patients without associated congenital heart disease. Cathet Cardiovasc Diagn 1975; 1(2): 157–169.

38 Cheitlin MD, Castro CMD, Mcallister HA. Sudden death as a complication of anomalous left coronary origin from the anterior sinus of valsalva a not-so-minor congenital anomaly. Circulation 1974; 50(4): 780–787.

39 Levin DC, Fellows KE, Abrams HL. Hemodynamically significant primary anomalies of the coronary arteries: angiographic aspects. Circulation 1978; 58(1): 25–34.

40 Akagi T, Rose V, Benson LN, Newman A, Freedom RM. Outcome of coronary artery aneurysms after Kawasaki disease. J Pediatr 1992; 121(5 Pt 1): 689–694.

41 Mavrogeni S, Papadopoulos G, Douskou M, et al. Magnetic resonance angiography isequivalent to X-ray coronary angiography for the evaluation of coronary arteries in kawasaki disease. J Am Coll Cardiol 2004; 43(4): 649–652.

42 Mavrogeni S, Papadopoulos G, Douskou M, et al. Magnetic resonance angiography, function and viability evaluation in patients with Kawasaki disease. J Cardiovasc Magn Reson 2006; 8(3): 493–498.

43 Liu X, Zhao X, Huang J, et al. Comparison of 3D free-breathing coronary MR angiography and 64-MDCT angiography for detection of coronary stenosis in patients with high calcium scores. Am J Roentgenol 2007; 189(6): 1326–1332.

44 Langerak SE. Value of magnetic resonance imaging for the noninvasive detection of stenosis in coronary artery bypass grafts and recipient coronary arteries. Circulation 2003; 107(11): 1502–1508.

45 Nagel E, Lehmkuhl HB, Bocksch W, et al. Noninvasive diagnosis of ischemia-induced wall motion abnormalities with the use of high-dose dobutamine stress MRI comparison with dobutamine stress echocardiography. Circulation 1999; 99(6): 763–770.

46 Hundley WG, Hamilton CA, Thomas MS, et al. Utility of fast cine magnetic resonance imaging and display for the detection of myocardial ischemia in patients not well suited for second harmonic stress echocardiography. Circulation 1999; 100(16): 1697–1702.

47 Nandalur KR, Dwamena BA, Choudhri AF, Nandalur MR, Carlos RC. Diagnostic performance of stress cardiac magnetic resonance imaging in the detection of coronary artery disease. J Am Coll Cardiol 2007; 50(14): 1343–1353.

48 Jahnke C, Nagel E, Gebker R, et al. Prognostic value of cardiac magnetic resonance stress tests adenosine stress perfusion and dobutamine stress wall motion imaging. Circulation 2007; 115(13): 1769–1776.

49 Kim RJ, Lima JAC, Chen E-L, et al. Fast 23Na magnetic resonance imaging of acute reperfused myocardial infarction potential to assess myocardial viability. Circulation 1997; 95(7): 1877–1885.

50 Kim RJ, Fieno DS, Parrish TB, et al. Relationship of MRI delayed contrast enhancement to irreversible injury, infarct age, and contractile function. Circulation 1999; 100(19): 1992–2002.

51 Wu E, Judd RM, Vargas JD, Klocke FJ, Bonow RO, Kim RJ. Visualisation of presence, location, and transmural extent of healed Q-wave and non-Q-wave myocardial infarction. Lancet 2001; 357(9249): 21–28.

52 Wagner A, Mahrholdt H, Holly TA, et al. Contrast-enhanced MRI and routine single photon emission computed tomography (SPECT) perfusion imaging for detection of subendocardial myocardial infarcts: an imaging study. Lancet 2003; 361(9355): 374–379.

53 Ibrahim T, Bülow HP, Hackl T, et al. Diagnostic value of contrast-enhanced magnetic resonance imaging and single-photon emission computed tomography for detection of myocardial necrosis early after acute myocardial infarction. J Am Coll Cardiol 2007; 49(2): 208–216.

54 Yan AT, Shayne AJ, Brown KA, et al. Characterization of the peri-infarct zone by contrast-enhanced cardiac magnetic resonance imaging is a powerful predictor of post-myocardial infarction mortality. Circulation 2006; 114(1): 32–39.

55 Hombach V, Grebe O, Merkle N, et al. Sequelae of acute myocardial infarction regarding cardiac structure and function and their prognostic significance as assessed by magnetic resonance imaging. Eur Heart J 2005; 26(6): 549–557.

56 Abdel-Aty H, Boyé P, Zagrosek A, et al. Diagnostic performance of cardiovascular magnetic resonance in patients with suspected acute myocarditis: comparison of different approaches. J Am Coll Cardiol 2005; 45(11): 1815–1822.

57 Gutberlet M, Spors B, Thoma T, et al. Suspected chronic myocarditis at cardiac MR: diagnostic accuracy and association with immunohistologically detected inflammation and viral persistence. Radiology 2008; 246(2): 401–409.

58 Ferreira VM, Piechnik SK, Dall'Armellina E, et al. Native T1-mapping displays the extent and non-ischemic patterns of injury in acute myocarditis without the need for contrast agents. J Cardiovasc Magn Reson 2014; 16(Suppl 1): O6.

59 Radunski UK, Lund GK, Stehning C, et al. CMR in patients with severe myocarditis. JACC Cardiovasc Imaging 2014; 7(7): 667–675.

60 Nazarian S, Bluemke DA, Lardo AC, et al. Magnetic resonance assessment of the substrate for inducible ventricular tachycardia in nonischemic cardiomyopathy. Circulation 2005; 112(18): 2821–2825.

61 Eitel I, von Knobelsdorff-Brenkenhoff F, Bernhardt P, et al. Clinical characteristics and cardiovascular magnetic resonance findings in stress (takotsubo) cardiomyopathy. JAMA 2011; 306(3): 277–286.

62 Petersen SE, Selvanayagam JB, Wiesmann F, et al. Left ventricular non-compaction: insights from cardiovascular magnetic resonance imaging. J Am Coll Cardiol 2005; 46(1): 101–105.

63 Marcus FI, McKenna WJ, Sherrill D, et al. Diagnosis of arrhythmogenic right ventricular cardiomyopathy/dysplasia proposed modification of the task force criteria. Circulation 2010; 121(13): 1533–1541.

64 Tandri H, Saranathan M, Rodriguez ER, et al. Noninvasive detection of myocardial fibrosis in arrhythmogenic right ventricular cardiomyopathy using delayed-enhancement magnetic resonance imaging. J Am Coll Cardiol 2005; 45(1): 98–103.

65 Chan RH, Maron BJ, Olivotto I, et al. Prognostic value of quantitative contrast-enhanced cardiovascular magnetic resonance for the evaluation of sudden death risk in patients with hypertrophic cardiomyopathy. Circulation 2014; 130(6): 484–495.

66 Maron MS, Maron BJ, Harrigan C, et al. Hypertrophic cardiomyopathy phenotype revisited after 50 years with cardiovascular magnetic resonance. J Am Coll Cardiol 2009; 54(3): 220–228.

67 Valeti US, Nishimura RA, Holmes DR, et al. Comparison of surgical septal myectomy and alcohol septal ablation with cardiac magnetic resonance imaging in patients with hypertrophic obstructive cardiomyopathy. J Am Coll Cardiol 2007; 49(3): 350–357.

68 Schulz-Menger J, Wassmuth R, Abdel-Aty H, Siegel I, Franke A, Dietz R. Patterns of myocardial inflammation and scarring in sarcoidosis as assessed by cardiovascular magnetic resonance. Heart 2006; 92(3): 399–400.

69 Maceira AM, Joshi J, Prasad SK, et al. Cardiovascular magnetic resonance in cardiac amyloidosis. Circulation 2005; 111(2): 186–193.

70 Pennell DJ. T2* Magnetic resonance and myocardial iron in thalassemia. Ann N Y Acad Sci 2005; 1054(1): 373–378.

71 Cosyns B, Plein S, Nihoyanopoulos P, et al. European Association of Cardiovascular Imaging (EACVI) position paper: multimodality imaging in pericardial disease. Eur Heart J Cardiovasc Imaging 2015; 16(1): 12–31.

72 Warnes CA, Williams RG, Bashore TM, et al. ACC/AHA 2008 Guidelines for the management of adults with congenital heart disease: executive summary a report of the American College of Cardiology/American Heart Association Task Force on Practice Guidelines (Writing Committee to Develop Guidelines for the Management of Adults With Congenital Heart Disease): Developed in

Collaboration With the American Society of Echocardiography, Heart Rhythm Society, International Society for Adult Congenital Heart Disease, Society for Cardiovascular Angiography and Interventions, and Society of Thoracic Surgeons. *Circulation* 2008; **118**(23): 2395–2451.

73 Partington SL, Valente AM. Cardiac magnetic resonance in adults with congenital heart disease. *Methodist DeBakey Cardiovasc J* 2013; **9**(3): 156–162.

74 Mooij CF, de Wit CJ, Graham DA, Powell AJ, Geva T. Reproducibility of MRI measurements of right ventricular size and function in patients with normal and dilated ventricles. *J Magn Reson Imaging* 2008; **28**(1): 67–73.

75 Hundley WG, Li HF, Lange RA, et al. Assessment of left-to-right intracardiac shunting by velocity-encoded, phase-difference magnetic resonance imaging a comparison with oximetric and indicator dilution techniques. *Circulation* 1995; **91**(12): 2955–2960.

76 Beerbaum P, Körperich H, Barth P, Esdorn H, Gieseke J, Meyer H. Noninvasive quantification of left-to-right shunt in pediatric patients phase-contrast cine magnetic resonance imaging compared with invasive oximetry. *Circulation* 2001; **103**(20): 2476–2482.

77 Prakash A, Powell AJ, Geva T. Multimodality noninvasive imaging for assessment of congenital heart disease. *Circ Cardiovasc Imaging* 2010; **3**(1): 112–125.

78 Suzuki J, Caputo GR, Kondo C, Higgins CB. Cine MR imaging of valvular heart disease: display and imaging parameters affect the size of the signal void caused by valvular regurgitation. *AJR Am J Roentgenol* 1990; **155**(4): 723–727.

79 Djavidani B, Debl K, Lenhart M, et al. Planimetry of mitral valve stenosis by magnetic resonance imaging. *J Am Coll Cardiol* 2005; **45**(12): 2048–2053.

80 Debl K, Djavidani B, Seitz J, et al. Planimetry of aortic valve area in aortic stenosis by magnetic resonance imaging. *Invest Radiol* 2005; **40**(10): 631–636.

81 Kilner PJ, Manzara CC, Mohiaddin RH, et al. Magnetic resonance jet velocity mapping in mitral and aortic valve stenosis. *Circulation* 1993; **87**(4): 1239–1248.

82 Loubeyre P, Delignette A, Bonefoy L, Douek P, Amiel M, Revel D. Magnetic resonance imaging evaluation of the ascending aorta after graft-inclusion surgery: comparison between an ultrafast contrast-enhanced MR sequence and conventional cine-MRI. *J Magn Reson Imaging* 1996; **6**(3): 478–483.

83 Fattori R, Nienaber CA. MRI of acute and chronic aortic pathology: pre-operative and postoperative evaluation. *J Magn Reson Imaging* 1999; **10**(5): 741–750.

84 Leiner T, Kessels AGH, Nelemans PJ, et al. Peripheral Arterial disease: comparison of color duplex us and contrast-enhanced MR angiography for diagnosis. *Radiology* 2005; **235**(2): 699–708.

85 Ouwendijk R, de Vries M, Pattynama PMT, et al. Imaging peripheral arterial disease: a randomized controlled trial comparing contrast-enhanced MR angiography and multi-detector row CT angiography. *Radiology* 2005; **236**(3): 1094–1103.

86 Nael K, Villablanca JP, Saleh R, et al. Contrast-enhanced MR angiography at 3 T in the evaluation of intracranial aneurysms: a comparison with time-of-flight MR angiography. *Am J Neuroradiol* 2006; **27**(10): 2118–2121.

87 Villablanca JP, Nael K, Habibi R, Nael A, Laub G, Finn JP. 3 T contrast-enhanced magnetic resonance angiography for evaluation of the intracranial arteries: comparison with time-of-flight magnetic resonance angiography and multislice computed tomography angiography. *Invest Radiol* 2006; **41**(11): 799–805.

88 Nael K, Villablanca JP, Pope WB, McNamara TO, Laub G, Finn JP. Supraaortic arteries: contrast-enhanced MR angiography at 3.0 T—highly accelerated parallel acquisition for improved spatial resolution over an extended field of view. *Radiology* 2007; **242**(2): 600–609.

89 Kramer U, Nael K, Laub G, et al. High-resolution magnetic resonance angiography of the renal arteries using parallel imaging acquisition techniques at 3.0 T: initial experience. *Invest Radiol* 2006; **41**(2): 125–132.

90 Nael K, Saleh R, Lee M, et al. High-spatial-resolution contrast-enhanced MR angiography of abdominal arteries with parallel acquisition at 3.0 T: initial experience in 32 patients. *Am J Roentgenol* 2006; **187**(1): W77–85.

91 Hendel RC, Patel MR, Kramer CM, et al. ACCF/ACR/SCCT/SCMR/ASNC/NASCI/SCAI/SIR 2006 Appropriateness Criteria for Cardiac Computed Tomography and Cardiac Magnetic Resonance Imaging: A Report of the American College of Cardiology Foundation Quality Strategic Directions

Committee Appropriateness Criteria Working Group, American College of Radiology, Society of Cardiovascular Computed Tomography, Society for Cardiovascular Magnetic Resonance, American Society of Nuclear Cardiology, North American Society for Cardiac Imaging, Society for Cardiovascular Angiography and Interventions, and Society of Interventional Radiology. *J Am Coll Cardiol* 2006; **48**(7): 1475–1497.

92 Jabbour A, Ismail TF, Moat N, et al. Multimodality imaging in transcatheter aortic valve implantation and post-procedural aortic regurgitation: comparison among cardiovascular magnetic resonance, cardiac computed tomography, and echocardiography. *J Am Coll Cardiol* 2011; **58**(21): 2165–2173.

93 Koos R, Altiok E, Mahnken AH, et al. Evaluation of aortic root for definition of prosthesis size by magnetic resonance imaging and cardiac computed tomography: Implications for transcatheter aortic valve implantation. *Int J Cardiol* 2012; **158**(3): 353–358.

94 Miyazaki M, Lee VS. Nonenhanced MR angiography. *Radiology* 2008; **248**(1): 20–43.

95 Cavalcante JL, Schoenhagen P. Role of cross-sectional imaging for structural heart disease interventions. *Cardiol Clin* 2013; **31**(3): 467–478.

96 Cawley PJ, Maki JH, Otto CM. Cardiovascular magnetic resonance imaging for valvular heart disease technique and validation. *Circulation* 2009; **119**(3): 468–478.

97 Little SH, Shah DJ, Mahmarian JJ. Multimodality noninvasive imaging for transcatheter aortic valve implantation: a primer. *Methodist DeBakey Cardiovasc J* 2012; **8**(2): 29–37.

98 Carminati M, Agnifili M, Arcidiacono C, et al. Role of imaging in interventions on structural heart disease. *Expert Rev Cardiovasc Ther* 2013; **11**(12): 1659–1676.

99 Nielsen JC, Powell AJ, Gauvreau K, Marcus EN, Prakash A, Geva T. Magnetic resonance imaging predictors of coarctation severity. *Circulation* 2005; **111**(5): 622–628.

100 Didier D, Saint-Martin C, Lapierre C, et al. Coarctation of the aorta: pre and postoperative evaluation with MRI and MR angiography; comparison with echocardiography and surgery. *Int J Cardiovasc Imaging* 2006; **22**(3-4): 457–475.

101 Muzzarelli S, Meadows AK, Ordovas KG, Higgins CB, Meadows JJ. Usefulness of cardiovascular magnetic resonance imaging to predict the need for intervention in patients with coarctation of the aorta. *Am J Cardiol* 2012; **109**(6): 861–865.

102 Zahn EM, Hellenbrand WE, Lock JE, McElhinney DB. Implantation of the melody transcatheter pulmonary valve in patients with a dysfunctional right ventricular outflow tract conduit: early results from the U.S. clinical trial. *J Am Coll Cardiol* 2009; **54**(18): 1722–1729.

103 Eicken A, Ewert P, Hager A, et al. Percutaneous pulmonary valve implantation: two-centre experience with more than 100 patients. *Eur Heart J* 2011; **32**(10): 1260–1265.

104 Lederman RJ. Cardiovascular interventional magnetic resonance imaging. *Circulation* 2005; **112**(19): 3009–3017.

105 Pushparajah K, Tzifa A, Razavi R. Cardiac MRI catheterization: a 10-year single institution experience and review. *Interv Cardiol* 2014; **6**(3): 335–346.

106 Dick AJ, Raman VK, Raval AN, et al. Invasive human magnetic resonance imaging: feasibility during revascularization in a combined XMR suite. *Catheter Cardiovasc Interv* 2005; **64**(3): 265–274.

107 Hofmann LV, Liddell RP, Eng J, et al. Human peripheral arteries: feasibility of transvenous intravascular mr imaging of the arterial wall. *Radiology* 2005; **235**(2): 617–622.

108 Manke C, Nitz WR, Djavidani B, et al. MR imaging-guided Stent placement in iliac arterial stenoses: a feasibility study. *Radiology* 2001; **219**(2): 527–534.

109 Paetzel C, Zorger N, Seitz J, et al. Intraarterial contrast material-enhanced magnetic resonance angiography of the aortoiliac system. *J Vasc Interv Radiol* 2004; **15**(9): 981–984.

110 Paetzel C, Zorger N, Bachthaler M, et al. Magnetic resonance-guided percutaneous angioplasty of femoral and popliteal artery stenoses using real-time imaging and intra-arterial contrast-enhanced magnetic resonance angiography. *Invest Radiol* 2005; **40**(5): 257–262.

CHAPTER 11

Stable Coronary Artery Disease

Abhiram Prasad[1] and Bernard J. Gersh[2]
[1] St George's, University of London, London, UK
[2] Mayo Clinic and Mayo Clinic College of Medicine, Rochester, MN, USA

The main objectives of treatment for stable angina are the relief of symptoms related to myocardial ischemia and improvement in prognosis. Significant progress has been made over the past three decades in drug therapy, percutaneous coronary intervention (PCI), and coronary artery bypasses grafting (CABG). While this chapter focuses on percutaneous revascularization, it is important to remember that medical therapy and secondary prevention have a central role in the management of coronary atherosclerosis. Secondary prevention via lifestyle modification, treatment of conventional risk factors (Table 11.1), and drug therapy (Figure 11.1) [1–3] reduces cardiovascular mortality, myocardial infarction, unstable angina, onset of heart failure, and the need for revascularization, likely by plaque stabilization and limiting the progression of atherosclerosis.

Guidelines on the management of stable angina

The most recent guidelines on the management of stable angina have been published by the European Society of Cardiology in 2013 [4] as well as by the American College of Cardiology (ACC) and the American Heart Association (AHA) in 2012 [5]. Additional relevant guidelines include the 2014 ESC/EACTS Guidelines on myocardial revascularization (Tables 11.2 and 11.3) [6], and the ACCF/AHA/SCAI 2011 Guideline for Percutaneous Coronary Intervention [7]. These guidelines are evidence based and should be the basis for clinical practice. However, there are several fundamental limitations of the trial data available on the management of stable angina. First, as with many clinical trials, the rigorous inclusion and exclusion criteria have resulted in a relatively small number of the screened patients being enrolled into the studies. This significantly limits the ability to generalize the findings to the larger population in daily practice. Moreover, clinical trials have generally excluded high risk patients with severe angina, severe atherosclerosis, severely reduced left ventricular (LV) systolic function, or multiple comorbid conditions. Second, the findings of clinical trials comparing treatment strategies often become outdated quickly because of the rapid evolution in clinical practice.

Indications for coronary angiography

The decision regarding whether to treat a patient with medical therapy or revascularization is based on the fundamental principal of risk stratification. The spectrum of risk for myocardial infarction and cardiovascular death is wide even in "stable" coronary artery disease (CAD). Initial risk stratification and thereby the decision to perform coronary angiography can be determined by a combination of clinical evaluation, and in most cases stress testing and an assessment of left LV function (Figure 11.2). Those with high risk features on clinical evaluation such as severe angina, unstable angina, and severe heart failure should proceed directly to coronary angiography without being subjected to a stress test. Coronary angiography is not indicated in low risk patients (Figure 11.3). The decision in intermediate risk patients should be based on severity of symptoms, response to initial medical therapy, functional status, lifestyle, and occupation. Moreover, a detailed discussion with the patient regarding the risks, benefits, alternatives, and goals of invasive assessment is required prior to proceeding with coronary angiography. Coronary angiography is indicated in patients with high risk features on non-invasive assessment irrespective of symptoms, severe angina (Class 3 of Canadian Cardiovascular Society Classification; CCS), diagnostic uncertainty after non-invasive evaluation, and patients with the possibility of restenosis following PCI in a coronary distribution supplying a moderate to large amount of myocardium.

Percutaneous coronary intervention for stable angina

Several randomized trials have compared the outcomes following PCI with medical management for stable angina [8–11]. These include the studies from the balloon angioplasty era such as the second Randomized Intervention Treatment of Angina (RITA-2) [9] and the Angioplasty Compared to Medicine (ACME) trials [10]. The studies and meta-analyses of the randomized trials [12,13] have consistently demonstrates that PCI does not reduce the likelihood of death or myocardial infarction, but is more effective in

Interventional Cardiology: Principles and Practice, Second Edition. Edited by George D. Dangas, Carlo Di Mario, and Nicholas N. Kipshidze.
© 2017 John Wiley & Sons, Ltd. Published 2017 by John Wiley & Sons, Ltd.

Table 11.1 Optimal secondary prevention in stable coronary artery disease.

Risk factor	Goal/recommended intervention
Lipid management	LDL-C <1.8 mmol/L (<70 mg/dL) or >50% LDL-C reduction when target level cannot be reached
	Lifestyle modification including low fat-low cholesterol diet; and a moderate or high dose of a statin therapy should be prescribed, in the absence of contraindications or documented adverse effects
	Secondary goal is non-HDL cholesterol <130 mg/dL (<3.2 mmol/L) in pts with triglycerides >200 mg/dL (>2.2 mmol/L)
Blood pressure control	<140/90 mmHg (lowering to 130–139/80–85 mmHg may be better)
	Lifestyle modification and drug therapy (beta-blockers and ACE-inhibitors preferred)
Diabetes management	Hemoglobin A_{1c} <7.0%
	Lifestyle modification ± drug therapy
Smoking	Complete cessation. No environmental exposure
Weight management	Body mass index 18.5–24.9 kg/m², waist circumference: men <40 inches (<100 cm), and women <35 inches (88 cm)
	Regular physical exercise and restrict caloric intake
Physical activity	30–60 minutes of moderate-intensity aerobic activity, such as brisk walking, at least 5 days and preferably 7 days per week

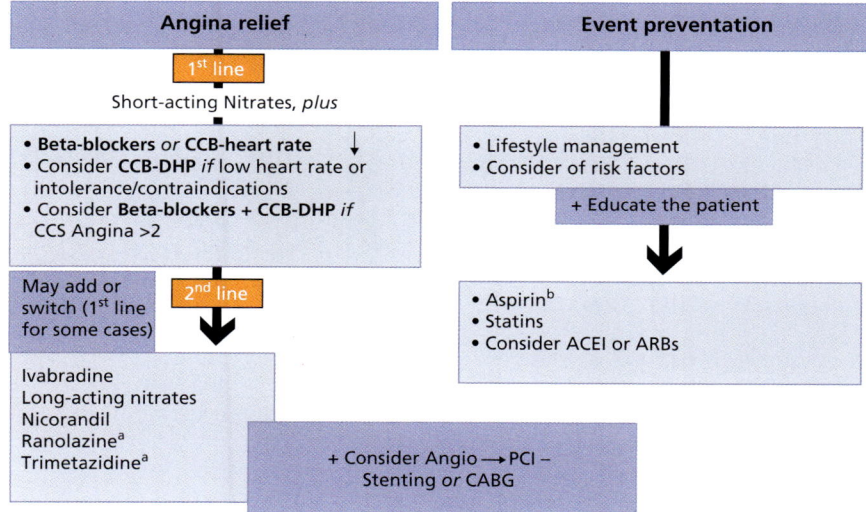

Figure 11.1 Medical management of stable angina (ESC guidelines). ACEI, angiotensin-converting enzyme inhibitor; CABG, coronary artery bypass graft; CCB, calcium channel blocker; CCS, Canadian Cardiovascular Society; DHP, dihydropyridine; PCI, percutaneous coronary intervention. [a]Data for diabetics. [b]If intolerance, consider clopidogrel. Source: Montalescot et al. 2013 [4]. Reproduced by permission of Oxford University Press.

relieving angina in patients with single and multivessel disease. Notably, there was an early hazard associated with PCI in the RITA-2 trial in which there was a greater likelihood of myocardial infarction related to the procedure, but the rates of death and myocardial infarction at 7 years was similar in both arms of the trial. In addition, studies conducted in the balloon angioplasty era had shown that there was an increased risk for emergency CABG in the PCI treated group, but this was not reported in the recent Clinical Outcomes Utilizing Revascularization and Aggressive Drug Evaluation (COURAGE) trial, presumably because of the routine use of stent [14].

The COURAGE trial is the largest study to compare medical therapy with PCI and its findings are consistent with previous studies. The trial enrolled 2287 patients (approximately two-thirds with

Table 11.2 ESC Guideline indications for revascularization in patients with stable angina or silent ischemia.

Extent of CAD (anatomical and/or functional)		Class[b]	Level[c]
For prognosis	Left main disease with stenosis >50%[a]	I	A
	Any proximal LAD stenosis >50%[a]	I	A
	Two-vessel or three-vessel disease with stenosis >50%[a] with impaired LV function (LVEF <40%)[a]	I	A
	Large area of ischemia (>10% of LV)	I	B
	Single remaining patent with coronary artery stenosis >50%[a]	I	C
For symptoms	Any coronary stenosis >50%[a] in the presence of limiting angina or angina equivalent, unresponsive to medical therapy	I	A

CAD, coronary artery disease; LAD, left anterior descending; LV, left ventricular; LVEF, left ventricular ejection fraction;
[a] With documented ischemia or FFR 0.80 for diameter stenosis <90%.
[b] Class of recommendation.
[c] Level of evidence.
Source: Windecker *et al.* 2014 [6]. Reproduced by permission of Oxford University Press.

Table 11.3 ESC guidelines for the type of revascularization (CABG or PCI) in patients with stable angina with suitable coronary anatomy for both procedures and low predicted surgical mortality.

Recommendations according to the extent of CAD	CABG		PCI	
	Class[a]	Level[b]	Class[a]	Level[b]
One- or two-vessel disease without proximal LAD stenosis	IIb	C	I	C
One-vessel disease with proximal LAD stenosis	I	A	I	A
Two-vessel disease with proximal LAD stenosis	I	B	I	C
Left main disease with a SYNTAX score ≤22	I	B	I	B
Left main disease with a SYNTAX score 23–32	I	B	IIa	B
Left main disease with a SYNTAX score >32	I	B	III	B
Three-vessel disease with a SYNTAX score ≤22	I	A	I	B
Three-vessel disease with a SYNTAX score 23–32	I	A	III	B
Three-vessel disease with a SYNTAX score >32	I	A	III	B

[a] Class of recommendation.
[b] Level of evidence.
Source: Windecker *et al.* 2014 [6]. Reproduced by permission of Oxford University Press.

two or three vessel disease) with stable CAD. The inclusion criteria were either a coronary stenosis ≥80% and classic angina without provocative stress testing, or a stenosis ≥70% in at least one proximal epicardial coronary artery and objective evidence of myocardial ischemia. A large number of patients were excluded from the trial because of high risk features such as a strongly positive stress test, persistent CCS class IV angina, an ejection fraction of <30%, refractory heart failure or cardiogenic shock, revascularization within the previous 6 months, and those with coronary anatomy unsuitable for PCI. The randomization was to either optimal medical therapy alone or PCI with optimal medical therapy. During a median follow-up duration of 4.6 years, there was no difference in the primary composite endpoint of death and nonfatal myocardial infarction (19.0% vs. 18.5%; p = 0.62). These findings must be to be interpreted in light of the facts that less than 10% of the patients screened met eligibility criteria for enrolment (as is the case in virtually all revascularization trials), 85% of patients were male, and that randomization was performed in the cardiac catheterization laboratory following angiography, which may have contributed to selection bias. The percentage of those requiring revascularization during follow-up were 21.1% of patients in the PCI arm, compared with 32.6% in the medical arm. The repeat revascularization rates in the PCI group would likely have been lower had drug-eluting stents (DES) been used. PCI was associated with a small reduction in the requirement for anti-anginal therapy and greater likelihood of freedom from angina; however, this benefit diminished over

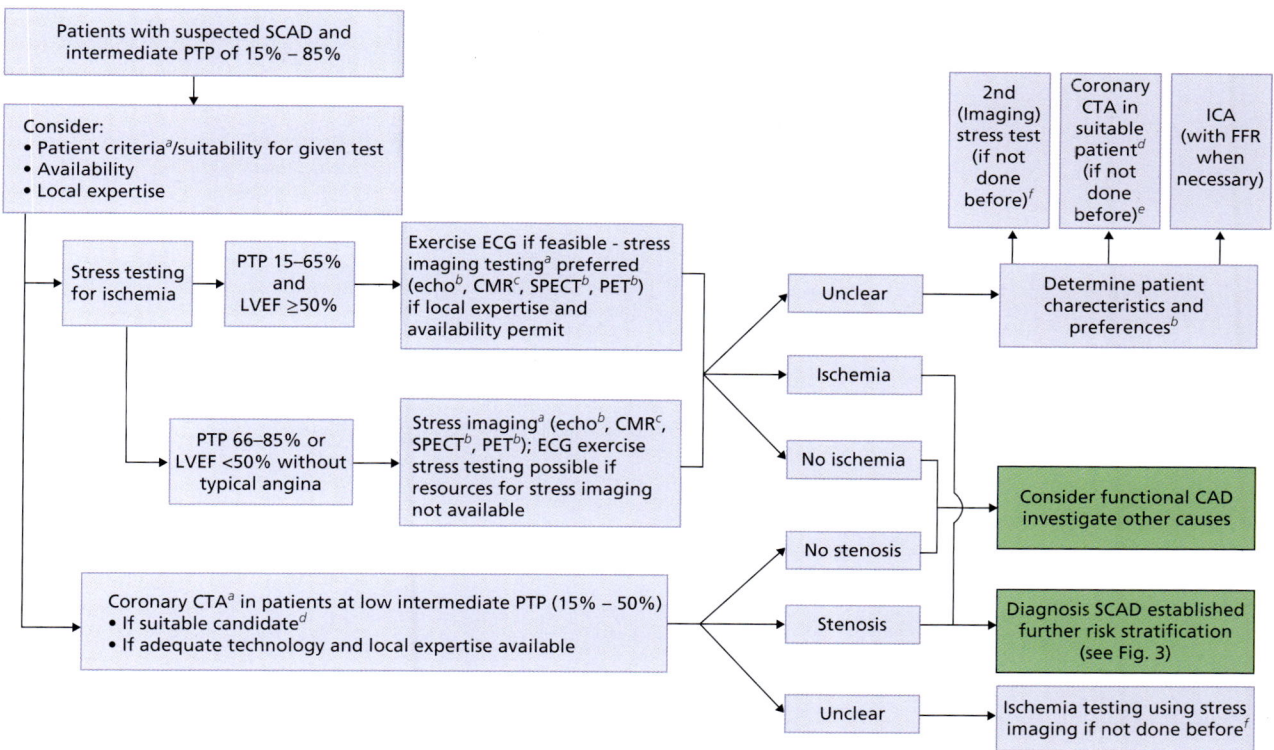

Figure 11.2 Non-invasive testing in patients with suspected stable coronary artery disease (SCAD) and intermediate pre-test probability (PTP) (ESC guidelines). CAD, coronary artery disease; CTA, computed tomography angiography; CMR, cardiac magnetic resonance; ECG, electrocardiogram; ICA, invasive coronary angiography; LVEF, left ventricular ejection fraction; PET, positron emission tomography; PTP, pre-test probability; SCAD, stable coronary artery disease; SPECT, single photon emission computed tomography.
[a] Consider age of patient versus radiation exposure.
[b] In patients unable to exercise use echo or SPECT/PET with pharmacologic stress instead.
[c] CMR is only performed using pharmacologic stress.
[d] Patient characteristics should make a fully diagnostic coronary CTA scan highly probable consider result to be unclear in patients with severe diffuse or focal calcification.
[e] Proceed as in lower left coronary CTA box.
[f] Proceed as in stress testing for ischemia box.
Source: Montalescot *et al.* 2013 [4]. Reproduced by permission of Oxford University Press.

time. Of note, approximately one-third of the patients in the medical arm had to cross over to PCI as a result of inadequate control of symptoms with optimal medical therapy. Finally, it is important to recognize that the findings of the COURAGE trial are also in keeping with earlier studies comparing CABG with medical therapy in which surgical revascularization did not improve survival or prevent myocardial infarction in patients with stable disease who had mild to moderate symptoms and good LV function.

Despite the overall conclusion of the COURAGE trial, the importance of risk stratification based on the magnitude of ischemic burden was highlighted by the results of the nuclear perfusion stress test substudy. The findings indicated that medical therapy alone was associated with a higher risk of mortality and infarction in patients who had a reversible perfusion defect involving more than 10% of the myocardium. These data suggest that a more sophisticated approach than subjective visual estimation of coronary stenoses and their ischemic potential is required in the management of stable CAD [15]. Measurement of fractional flow reserve (FFR) appears to be beneficial in the triage of patients with an intermediate stenosis who have not had a stress test prior to the angiogram. In the DEFER trial, patients with single vessel disease and an intermediate stenosis, an FFR ≥0.75 identified a low risk group of patients

who did not benefit from angioplasty at a follow-up of 5 years. In the more recent Fractional Flow Reserve versus Angiography for Multivessel Evaluation 2 (FAME 2) trial, the clinical utility of FFR measurement in patients with stable coronary artery disease being angiographically evaluated for PCI was assessed [16]. FFR was measured across all lesions with a ≥50% diameter reduction in a major native epicardial coronary artery with a diameter of at least 2.5 mm and supplying viable myocardium. Patients with at least one stenosis with an FFR of ≤0.80 were randomized to FFR-guided PCI of all stenoses with FFR ≤0.80 with DES plus best medical therapy, or best medical therapy alone. The primary endpoint was a composite of death, myocardial infarction, or unplanned hospitalization leading to urgent revascularization at 24 months. The study was stopped prematurely by the data and safety monitoring board. After a mean duration of follow-up of 213 days, after randomization of 888 of the planned 1632 patients, the primary endpoint occurred in 4.3% who had PCI compared to 12.7% who were managed medically (hazard ratio [HR] 0.32, 95% CI 0.19–0.53). The difference persisted at 2-year follow-up. The reduction was driven by a lower rate of urgent revascularization in the PCI group. Though "urgent revascularization" is considered a "soft" endpoint, the definition used to define the events met criteria for an acute coronary syndrome

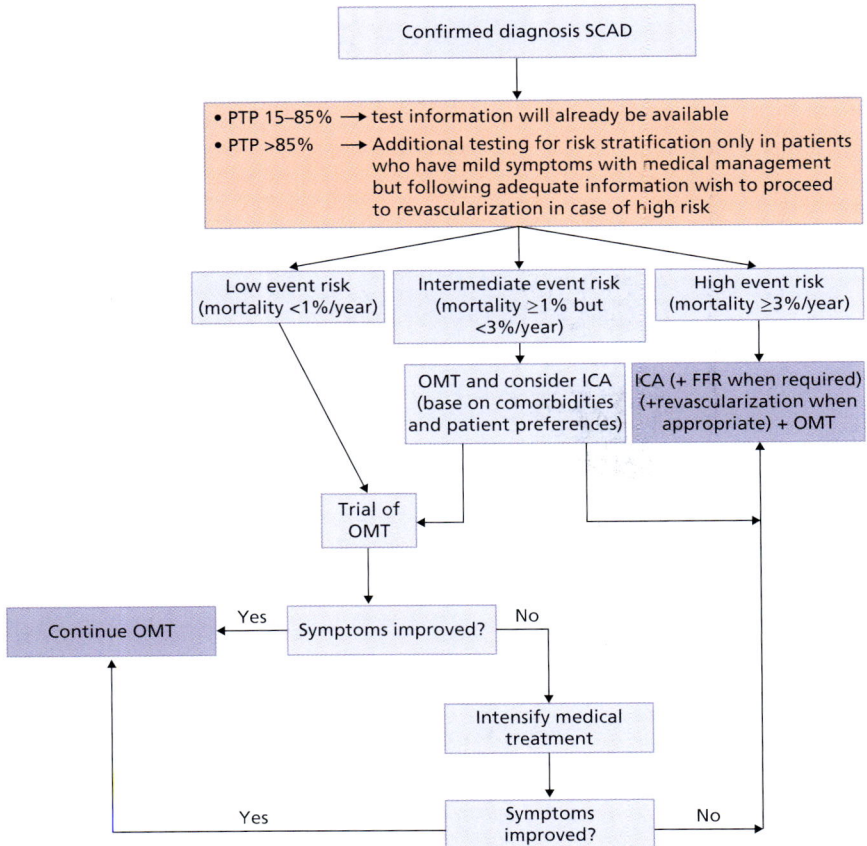

Figure 11.3 Management based on risk determination for prognosis in patients with chest pain and suspected stable coronary artery disease (SCAD) (ESC Guidelines). ICA, invasive coronary angiography; OMT, optimal medical therapy; PTP, pre-test probability; SCAD, stable coronary artery disease. Source: Montalescot *et al.* 2013 [4]. Reproduced by permission of Oxford University Press.

and 50% of the patients had objective evidence of ischemia. Limitations of FAME 2 include the premature termination of the trial, lack of non-invasive stress test documentation of ischemia prior to angiography, and the absence of double blinding of the assigned strategy such that the results of FFR measurement in the medical arm may have biased the patient's and/or physician's decision for preceding with crossover to PCI. Nevertheless, the findings of FAME 2 suggest that PCI is appropriate in patients with functionally significant stenosis involving a moderate or greater myocardial territory, and this is reflected in current guidelines (Table 11.2). Most interventionist use a FFR-guided strategy for intermediate (50–70% diameter stenosis) lesions in the absence of objective documentation of at least moderate ischemic burden in the coronary territory of interest or unclear results from stress testing.

The Medicine, Angioplasty, or Surgery Study (MASS) and MASS II trials have compared medical therapy with PCI and CABG in stable angina. The MASS trial enrolled patients with single vessel disease (>80% proximal left anterior descending artery stenosis) [17]. While balloon angioplasty and medical therapy were associated with greater need for revascularization, there was no difference in rate of death or myocardial infarction in the three groups during follow-up. The trial was conducted in the pre-stent era without modern medical therapy which limits the applicability of the findings to contemporary practice. The MASS II trial, however, was conducted in patients with multivessel disease, and had a similar design except that PCI was performed with bare metal stents in

most patients, and more contemporary medical therapy was implemented. At 5 years, the results were similar to the MASS trial in that there was no difference in death or myocardial infarction between the three treatment strategies, but the need for revascularization for refractory angina during follow-up was much higher with medical therapy and PCI [18].

A unique study in elderly patients with stable angina was the Trial of Invasive vs. Medical therapy in Elderly patients (TIME). At 1 year, the primary endpoint of quality of life was equally improved with both strategies. The invasive approach was associated with an early hazard, but there was no difference with regards to reduction in symptoms, death, or non-fatal infarction at 1 year. PCI did reduce the likelihood of subsequent hospitalization for uncontrolled symptoms [19].

A significant number of patients with CAD have asymptomatic or "silent" ischemia which is associated with an increased risk of cardiovascular events. The Asymptomatic Cardiac Ischemia Pilot (ACIP) study investigated the efficacy of three treatment strategies among patients with stable disease who had angina or silent ischemia from single or multivessel disease. Patients were randomized to angina-guided medical therapy, angina plus ischemia-guided medical therapy, or revascularization by either balloon angioplasty or CABG. At 2 years following randomization, revascularization was associated with a lower mortality and a reduction in the composite endpoint of death, myocardial infarction, and recurrent hospitalization [20]. An important study that evaluated treatment of silent ischemia is the Swiss Interventional Study on Silent Ischemia Type II (SWISSI II) trial which compared medical therapy with balloon angioplasty among patients who had suffered a myocardial infarction, and had one or two vessel disease [21]. A surprising finding was that cardiac death and myocardial infarction were significantly lower in the group randomized to balloon angioplasty. While the findings of the ACIP and SWISSI II trials are significant, they need to be interpreted with the knowledge that both enrolled relatively small number of patients and that optimal medical therapy, as defined in the COURAGE trial, was not implemented.

The studies to date have had significant crossover to revascularization in those originally randomized to medical therapy and hence have been trials of "initial treatment strategies" rather than specific treatments. Thus, based on the evidence from the COURAGE trial and the preceding randomized clinical trials, it is reasonable to conclude that medical therapy is an appropriate *initial strategy* for a substantial proportion of patients with mild to moderately severe stable angina. PCI is suitable for those patients who are significantly symptomatic despite optimal medical therapy, or as *initial strategy* for those with a positive stress test at low workload, or have a moderate to large ischemic territory. Aggressive secondary prevention is essential regardless of the treatment strategy utilized. The findings of the Atorvastatin versus Revascularization Treatment (AVERT) trial showed that PCI in combination with inadequate lipid lowering therapy is associated with worse outcomes in patients with angina when compared with a strategy of optimal lipid management and medical therapy alone [11].

In BARI 2D, 2368 patients with type 2 diabetes mellitus and stable coronary artery disease (defined as either a ≥50% stenosis of a major epicardial artery with a positive stress test or ≥70% stenosis and classic angina) were randomized to either revascularization (CABG or PCI) within 4 weeks together with intensive medical therapy or to intensive medical therapy alone [22]. The decision regarding CABG versus PCI was based on clinical judgment, and made prior to randomization. At 5 years, there was no difference in the primary endpoints of the rates of survival (88.3% vs. 87.8%) or freedom from the composite of death, myocardial infarction, and stroke (77.2% vs. 77.7%). In the PCI stratum, there was no significant difference in primary endpoints between the revascularization group compared to the medical-therapy only group. However, in the CABG stratum, the rate of major cardiovascular events was significantly lower in the revascularization group. Patients selected for CABG had higher angiographic and clinical risk scores than those selected for PCI, and it was those with the highest clinical and angiographic risk profile who seemed to derive a benefit from CABG.

A recent meta-analysis from 12 randomized clinical trials with 37,548 patient-years of follow-up demonstrated that PCI compared with medical therapy alone was associated with a statistically significant 24% relative reduction in the risk of spontaneous non-procedural myocardial infraction (MI), at the cost of a 317% relative increase in the risk of procedural MI, with no overall difference in the risk of all MI. The point estimate for PCI versus medical therapy for the outcome of all-cause mortality and cardiovascular mortality paralleled that of spontaneous non-procedural MI (incident rate ratio = 0.70; 95% CI 0.44–1.09), but was not statistically significant [23]. In a network meta-analysis from 100 trials in 93,553 patients with 262,090 patient years of follow-up, new generation drug eluting stents (everolimus: rate ratio 0.75, 95% CI 0.59–0.96; zotarolimus (Resolute): 0.65, 95% CI 0.42–1.00) were associated with improved survival compared with medical treatment. However, balloon angioplasty (0.85, 95% CI 0.68–1.04), bare metal stents (0.92, 95% CI 0.79–1.05), or early generation drug eluting stents (paclitaxel: 0.92,

95% CI 0.75–1.12; sirolimus: 0.91, 95% CI 0.75–1.10; zotarolimus (Endeavor): 0.88, 95% CI 0.69–1.10) were not associated with improved survival compared with medical treatment. The findings suggest that there may be improved survival with new (second) generation DES but not with other PCI technology, compared with medical treatment. These reports are provocative and challenge the general dogma that PCI has no impact on mortality. The findings are especially notable because the randomized trials have generally limited the enrolment to patients with single vessel disease and have excluded high risk patients with left main disease or chronic total occlusion for whom revascularization can offer greater benefit. Thus, until further data are available and strategies for risk stratification are improved, therapeutic decisions ought to be based on guidelines, but tailored according to a combined assessment of the patient's clinical presentation, severity of ischemia, and coronary anatomy [24].

Comparison of percutaneous and surgical revascularization

The available evidence suggests that PCI and CABG are equivalent for the treatment of single vessel disease. This was specifically investigated in the MASS trial at a single center in which patients with significant (>80%) proximal LAD stenosis were randomized to balloon angioplasty, CABG, or medical therapy. The data demonstrated that there was similar relief of symptoms with both forms of revascularization. However, revascularization resulted in a lower incidence of inducible ischemia compared to medical therapy alone, and all three strategies resulted in the effective treatment of limiting angina [17]. Similar findings have been reported from another small study of 134 patients with isolated proximal LAD stenosis in which angioplasty and CABG produced comparable results [25] also when the follow-up is prolonged to 10 years [26]. Importantly, the need for repeat revascularization during follow-up was greater with percutaneous revascularization using balloon angioplasty in both trials.

In the assessment of trials comparing surgery with PCI, an important premise is that none of these studies have specifically addressed the functional significance of the lesions treated. With respect to PCI in multivessel disease, the Fractional Flow Reserve vs. Angiography for Multivessel Evaluation (FAME) trial demonstrated that a targeted strategy guided by measurement of FFR provides superior outcomes at 1 year compared with treatment of all vessels with visually estimated significant stenoses [27]. Several randomized clinical trials [28–33] and meta-analyses of the data [34] have compared PCI directly with CABG for the treatment of single and multivessel disease. The studies, predominantly from the pre-stent era, were among relatively low risk patients with multivessel disease and preserved LV function. By design, the inclusion criteria for these trials had mandated that the coronary anatomy was suitable for both forms of revascularization, thereby excluding most patients with very complex coronary anatomy or chronic total occlusions. These older trials provided important lessons, but are not directly relevant to current practice because they predated stents and the widespread use of internal mammary artery graft in CABG.

The largest of these studies is the Bypass Angioplasty Revascularization Investigation (BARI) trial in which 1829 patients were enrolled. PCI was performed with balloon angioplasty which was associated with similar frequency of death, myocardial infarction, and recurrent angina when compared with CABG during 10 years of follow-up in the overall study population [35]. Not surprisingly, repeat revascularization was significantly less common in patients randomized to surgery. One notable finding that has influenced current practice is that cardiac mortality was significantly lower (19.4% vs. 34.5%; p = 0.003) amongst diabetics requiring glucose lowering therapy who were randomized to CABG and received at least one mammary graft. Potential explanations for this observation are that CABG offers complete revascularization and hence mitigates some of the adverse impact of the greater atherosclerotic burden and "future culprit" lesions, as well as the greater likelihood of restenosis and disease progression in diabetic patients. This finding has been confirmed in a more recent study [36] but the clinical relevance and applicability of the BARI study results have been questioned by the findings from the BARI registry, which highlighted the importance of clinical judgment. The patients in the registry had clinical characteristics that were similar to those in the randomized trial, but the survival among diabetic patients was similar regardless of whether angioplasty or CABG was performed. It has been speculated that the conflicting results between the registry and the trial may have been because the treatment assignment in the registry was at the discretion of the physicians who might have selected the most appropriate form of revascularization for each patient [37].

The Arterial Revascularization Therapy Study Part I (ARTS I) and the Stent or Surgery (SoS) trials have compared bare metal stent based PCI with CABG [38,39]. In the ARTS I trial, death and myocardial infarction were similar with both treatment strategies, but, as one might expect, complete revascularization was less often achieved and repeat revascularization was more frequent with percutaneous revascularization. The results of the SoS trial were similar but, for reasons that are unclear, there was an unexpected higher mortality associated with PCI (5% vs. 2%; p = 0.01), likely unrelated to treatment selection as the difference was entirely a result of non-cardiac deaths. The long-term results (5–6 years) of the ARTS, ERACI II, and SoS trials, and a large (7812 patients) meta-analysis including 10 randomized trials of balloon angioplasty or stenting vs. surgery with a median follow-up of 5.9 years has been published [40–43]. In the meta-analysis, long-term mortality was similar after CABG and PCI in patients with multivessel CAD (hazard ratio 0.91, 95% CI 0.82–1.02; p = 0.12). CABG was associated with a significantly lower mortality in patients with diabetes (HR 0.70, 0.56–0.87; p = 0.014 for interaction) and patients aged 65 years or older (0.82, 95% CI 0.70–0.97; p = 0.002 for interaction).

DES account for approximately 70–80% of stents used for contemporary PCI around the world but there are limited data comparing the outcomes between PCI using DES and CABG. There are three randomized clinical trials (SYNTAX, CARDia, and FREEDOM) to date [44–46]. Multicenter registry data from Arterial Revascularization Therapies Study II (ARTS II) has compared PCI using sirolimus DES with historical controls from the ARTS I trial [47]. The incidence of the composite primary endpoint of all-cause death, any cerebrovascular event, non-fatal myocardial infarction, or any repeat revascularization at 1 year in the DES group was similar to the CABG treatment arm of ARTS I. The rate of repeat revascularization was 8.5% in the DES group compared to 4.1% and 21.3% in CABG and PCI arms, respectively, of ARTS I. The 3-year results were consistent and confirmed, in patients with and without diabetes, the absence of significant differences in the combined endpoint when compared with the historical control of ARTS I surgical arm. While the data have inherent limitations of using historical controls, it had been suggested that PCI using DES might result in comparable outcomes to CABG, predominantly by decreasing repeat revascularization.

The Synergy Between PCI with TAXUS and Cardiac Surgery (SYNTAX) trial randomized 1800 patients with three vessel and/or left main disease to either CABG or PCI after a local interventional cardiologist and cardiac surgeon at each site prospectively evaluated eligible patients and determined that equivalent anatomic revascularization could be achieved with either strategy [44]. A score of anatomic complexity (SYNTAX score: www.syntaxscore.com) was prospectively calculated. Unlike most previous trials where a small minority of patients who were screened were ultimately enrolled, almost half of the 4337 screened were randomized, with the majority of those excluded were unsuitable for PCI. The rates of death and myocardial infarction at 12 months were similar in the two groups. Stroke was significantly more frequent in the CABG group (2.2% vs. 0.6%; p = 0.003) while the incidence of stent thrombosis and symptomatic graft occlusion at 12 months were similar in the two groups (3.3 and 3.4%, respectively). An increased rate of repeat revascularization in the PCI group (13.5% vs. 5.9%; p < 0.001) led to an excess of major cardiac and cardiovascular events in the PCI group, with the endpoint of the trial (non-inferiority of PCI using DES) not being met. Subgroup analysis based on the predetermined SYNTAX score showed that the negative outcome was confined to patients with high scores (>33, 10.9% in the surgical arm vs. 23.4% in the PCI arm). The patients with left main disease had similar incidence of 12 month MACE in the surgical and PCI groups (13.7 vs. 15.8%; p = 0.44). At 5-year follow-up, the composite primary endpoint (death from any cause, stroke, MI, or repeat revascularization) remained significantly higher (37.3% vs. 26.9%) in the PCI group due primarily to the higher rates of repeat revascularization and myocardial infarction. The rates of all-cause death and stroke were not different [48]. When analyzed by SYNTAX score, those with a score of <23, inclusive of left main patients, there was no difference in the composite primary endpoint (32.1% vs. 28.6%; p = 0.43). In those with a SYNTAX score of 23–32 with unprotected left main disease, the outcomes were similar (32.7% vs. 32.3%; p = 0.88); but not in patients with three vessel disease in whom PCI had higher event rates for the primary composite endpoint (37.9% vs. 22.6%; p = 0.0008). For patients with a SYNTAX score ≥33, the rates were higher in patients with left main disease (46.5% vs. 29.7%; p = 0.003) and those with three vessel disease without (41.9% vs. 24.1%; p = 0.0005) unprotected left main disease. The results of the SYNTAX trial indicate that CABG remains the standard for patients with complex three vessel disease. However, in patients with less complex disease (i.e., left main coronary disease with low or intermediate SYNTAX scores, or three vessel disease with low SYNTAX scores), PCI is a reasonable alternative treatment to CABG. In patients with a high SYNTAX score, the potential advantages of surgery should be stressed, but PCI should not be denied to patients who have a strong preference or a very high surgical risk. However, these conclusions must be interpreted in the context of the trial's limitations, such as the use of a first generation (paclitaxel-eluting) stent, which has a higher rate of restenosis than current second generation drug-eluting stents. Also, the analyses of subgroups by SYNTAX score was not pre-specified or adequately powered, and therefore the findings should be considered hypothesis generating.

In the Coronary Artery Revascularization in Diabetes (CARDia) trial, 510 diabetic patients with multivessel or complex single vessel coronary disease were randomized to PCI using a stent (and routine abciximab) or CABG. The trial was underpowered for the primary endpoint (composite of all-cause mortality, myocardial infarction, and stroke), and at 1 year there was no difference between CABG and the 69% of patients who received a DES (12.4% and 11.6%; p = 0.82) [45]. In the Future Revascularization Evaluation in Patients with Diabetes Mellitus: Optimal Management of Multivessel Disease (FREEDOM) trial, 1900 patients with diabetes and multivessel (83% with three vessel) disease (median SYNTAX score of 26) were randomized to either PCI with a first generation (paclitaxel or sirolimus-eluting) stent or CABG. Both groups received optimal medical therapy [46]. At a median follow-up of 3.8 years, the primary composite endpoint death from any cause, non-fatal myocardial infarction, or non-fatal stroke was more frequent in the PCI group (26.6% vs. 18.7%; p = 0.005). The benefit of CABG was predominantly because of lower rates of myocardial infarction and death from any cause while stroke was more frequent in the CABG group (2.4% vs. 5.2%; p = 0.03 at 5 years). The findings of FREEDOM suggest that in patients with diabetes and advanced CAD, CABG is superior to PCI using first generation stents.

Comparison of coronary artery bypass surgery with medical therapy for stable angina

The European Coronary Surgery Study (ECSS), Coronary Artery Surgery Study (CASS), and Veterans Administration Cooperative Study (VA Study) are large randomized trials that have compared CABG with medical therapy among patients with mild to moderate angina [49–51]. The consistent finding from these studies was that surgical revascularization provides better symptomatic relief from angina but the benefit is lost over time, most likely because of vein graft failure and subsequent crossover to CABG in the medical treatment arm. The randomized trials and a meta-analysis [52] indicate that an initial strategy of surgical revascularization does not improve survival in the general population of CAD, but that there are specific subsets that either have a large amount of ischemic myocardium or significant LV dysfunction. Thus, patients with three vessel disease (especially in those with abnormal LV function), two or three vessels disease with >75% stenosis of the LAD or a markedly positive stress test derive prognostic benefit from CABG. In general, patients with severe symptoms have been excluded from the trials, but an analysis from registry data of the CASS study indicates that surgical revascularization probably improves prognosis in patients with severe angina who have multivessel disease, even in the absence of LV function or proximal LAD stenosis [53]. It is important to be aware that this evidence, which has been used to craft current guidelines, is limited by the fact that the randomized trials were all conducted in the early years of bypass surgery, and are not representative of the contemporary surgical techniques such as the routine use of internal mammary grafts or minimally invasive and off-pump surgery [54]. Conversely, the medical group did not benefit from the aggressive preventive measures which are now routine nor did they consistently receive beta-blockers or angiotensin-converting enzyme (ACE) inhibitors. Furthermore, the general applicability of these trials is limited by the fact that they did not enrol many women or patients over 65 years old.

Recommendations for revascularization in stable angina

Broadly speaking, revascularization is appropriate for patients with limiting symptoms despite optimal medical therapy, strongly positive stress tests, proximal multivessel disease, and those who prefer an interventional approach over medical therapy. The choice between PCI and CABG in any one patient is determined by the risks of the procedure, likelihood of success, and ability to achieve complete revascularization with the two strategies as well as diabetic status and patient preference. While medical therapy is the cornerstone of treatment of stable angina, it is important to remember that there is no evidence that medical therapy alone improves prognosis in high risk patients, as defined in the clinical trials of medical treatment vs. CABG.

Patients with significant proximal LAD artery disease have a survival advantage with CABG over medical therapy, even in the absence of severe symptoms, LV dysfunction, or other lesions. PCI provides similar results among patients who have suitable anatomy for PCI of the proximal LAD and normal LV function (Tables 11.2 and 11.3).

CABG offers a survival advantage over medical therapy in patients with severe symptoms and three vessel disease, even in the absence of proximal LAD involvement or LV dysfunction. Patients with three vessel disease and LV dysfunction should have CABG. PCI is an alternative to CABG in those with angiographically suitable targets and normal LV function (e.g., SYNTAX score ≤22; Tables 11.2 and 11.3). Surgical revascularization is recommended for significant left main disease though PCI is an alternative in patients with SYNTAX score of ≤22, and should be considered for those with a SYNTAX score of 23–32 (Tables 11.2 and 11.3).

In patients with diabetes mellitus, particularly in the setting of multivessel or diffuse disease, there is a survival advantage with CABG over PCI. PCI is reasonable for diabetics with discrete two vessel disease (e.g., SYNTAX score ≤22) and preserved LV function.

For the majority of patients with stable CAD who do not fall into the subgroups described, there is no documented survival advantage with revascularization. PCI and CABG should be offered for the treatment of symptoms refractory to medical therapy. The guidelines state that both forms of revascularization are suitable for two vessel disease, but in current practice the majority of these patients and those with single vessel disease are treated with PCI unless the lesions are angiographically unsuitable, or involve the proximal LAD [55].

Revascularization in asymptomatic patients should only be considered with the goal of improving prognosis. The guidelines for the treatment of asymptomatic patients are similar to those for symptomatic patients. However, the level of evidence for asymptomatic patients is weaker as the clinical trials have mainly included symptomatic patients. However, ischemia is an important therapeutic target in contemporary practice over and above the treatment of symptoms.

Conclusions

Unlike PCI for acute coronary syndromes, percutaneous revascularization does not prevent death or myocardial infarction in patients with stable angina. There remains the possibility that PCI can reduce hard endpoints in high risk patients, but clinical trials in these patient subsets have not been conducted. For patients in low risk subgroups, the main advantage of PCI is the ability to effectively and more rapidly relieve symptoms. In general, therefore, PCI is indicated for the treatment of symptomatic coronary atherosclerosis, particularly in patients who remain symptomatic limited despite optimal medical therapy. PCI is the preferred revascularization strategy for single vessel disease, younger patients (age <50 years), elderly patients with significant comorbid conditions, and those who are not surgical candidates. There is no clear indication for PCI in the treatment of asymptomatic disease.

CABG is also highly effective in relieving symptoms, but importantly it reduces mortality in high risk patients. This benefit is proportional to baseline risk profile of the patient. Complete revascularization is more likely to be achieved with CABG. Thus, CABG is preferred for high risk patients such as those with multivessel disease where complete revascularization is an important goal, particularly in three vessel disease, and in the presence of significant LV systolic dysfunction. Subgroups that should be considered for surgery include significant unprotected left main disease, three vessel disease, especially if there is impaired LV function, diffuse atherosclerosis, or one or more chronic total occlusion. Another important group of patients who may benefit with CABG are diabetics with three vessel disease. However, as with PCI, CABG does not reduce the incidence of non-fatal myocardial infarction. PCI for multivessel disease, even with the use if DES, is associated with higher rates of repeat revascularization than CABG.

Developments in medical therapy for secondary prevention, PCI and CABG result in limited data being available from clinical trials that reflect contemporary practice, especially in high risk patients. With regards to PCI, the initial optimism for the current generation of DES has been tempered by the concerns of late stent thrombosis and the potential need for long-term dual antiplatelet therapy.

Interactive multiple choice questions are available for this chapter on www.wiley.com/go/dangas/cardiology

References

1   Perk J, De Backer G, Gohlke H, *et al.* European Guidelines on cardiovascular disease prevention in clinical practice (version 2012). *Eur Heart J* 2012; **33**: 1635–1701.

2   Stone NJ, Robinson JG, Lichtenstein AH, *et al.* 2013 ACC/AHA guideline on the treatment of blood cholesterol to reduce atherosclerotic cardiovascular risk in adults: a report of the American College of Cardiology/American Heart Association Task Force on Practice Guidelines. *Circulation* 2014; **129**(Suppl 2): 1–45.

3   Smith SC Jr, Benjamin EJ, Bonow RO, *et al.* AHA/ACCF secondary prevention and risk reduction therapy for patients with coronary and other atherosclerotic vascular disease: 2011update: a guideline from the American Heart Association and American College of Cardiology Foundation. *Circulation* 2011; **124**: 2458–2473.

4   Montalescot G, Sechtem U, Achenbach S, *et al.* 2013 ESC guidelines on the management of stable coronary artery disease: The Task Force on the management of stable coronary artery disease of the European Society of Cardiology. *Eur Heart J* 2013; **34**: 2949–3003.

5   Fihn SD, Gardin JM, Abrams J, *et al.* 2012 ACCF/AHA/ACP/AATS/PCNA/SCAI/STS guideline for the diagnosis and management of patients with stable ischemic heart disease: a report of the American College of Cardiology Foundation/American Heart Association Task Force on, American Association for Thoracic Surgery, Preventive Cardiovascular Nurses Association, Society for Cardiovascular Angiography and Interventions, and Society of Thoracic Surgeons. *J Am Coll Cardiol* 2012; **60**: e44–164.

6   Windecker S, Kolh P, Alfonso F, *et al.* 2014 ESC/EACTS Guidelines on myocardial Revascularization. The Task Force on Myocardial Revascularization of the European Society of Cardiology (ESC) and the European Association for Cardio-Thoracic Surgery (EACTS). *Eur Heart J* 2014; **35**(37): 2541–2619. doi:10.1093/eurheartj/ehu278.

7   Levine GN, Bates ER, Blankenship JC, *et al.* 2011 ACCF/AHA/SCAI guideline for percutaneous coronary intervention: a report of the American Collegeof Cardiology Foundation/American Heart Association Task Force on Practice Guidelinesand the Society for Cardiovascular Angiography and Interventions. *J Am CollCardiol* 2011; **58**: e44–122.

8   Parisi AF, Folland ED, Hartigan P. A comparison of angioplasty with medical therapy in the treatment of single-vessel coronary artery disease. *N Engl J Med* 1992; **326**: 10–16.

9   Anonymous. Coronary angioplasty versus medical therapy for angina: the second Randomised Intervention Treatment of Angina (RITA-2) trial. RITA-2 trial participants. *Lancet* 1997; **350**: 461–468.

10 Folland ED, Hartigan PM, Parisi AF. Percutaneous transluminal coronary angioplasty versus medical therapy for stable angina pectoris: outcomes for patients with double-vessel versus single-vessel coronary artery disease in a Veterans Affairs Cooperative randomized trial. Veterans Affairs ACME InvestigatorS. *J Am Coll Cardiol* 1997; **29**: 1505–1511.

11 Pitt B, Waters D, Brown WV, *et al.* Aggressive lipid-lowering therapy compared with angioplasty in stable coronary artery disease. Atorvastatin versus Revascularization Treatment Investigators. *N Engl J Med* 1999; **341**: 70–76.

12 Bucher HC, Hengstler P, Schindler C, *et al.* Percutaneous transluminal coronary angioplasty versus medical treatment for non-acute coronary heart disease: meta-analysis of randomised controlled trials. *BMJ* 2000; **321**: 73–77.

13 Katritsis DG, Ioannidis JP. Percutaneous coronary intervention versus conservative therapy in nonacute coronary artery disease: a meta-analysis. *Circulation* 2005; **111**: 2906–2912.

14 Boden WE, O'Rourke RA, Teo KK, *et al.* Optimal medical therapy with or without PCI for stable coronary disease. *N Engl J Med* 2007; **356**: 1503–1516.

15 Shaw LJ, Berman DS, Maron DJ, *et al.* COURAGE Investigators. Optimal medical therapy with or without percutaneous coronary intervention to reduce ischemic burden: results from the Clinical Outcomes Utilizing Revascularization and Aggressive Drug Evaluation (COURAGE) trial nuclear substudy. *Circulation* 2008; **117**(10): 1283–1291.

16 De Bruyne B, Fearon WF, Pijls NH, *et al.* Fractional flow reserve-guided PCI for stable coronary artery disease. *N Engl J Med* 2014; **371**: 1208–1217.

17 Hueb WA, Soares PR, Almeida De Oliveira S, *et al.* Five-year follow-up of the medicine, angioplasty or surgery study (MASS): a prospective, randomized trial of medical therapy, balloon angioplasty, or bypass surgery for single proximal left anterior descending coronary artery stenosis. *Circulation* 1999; **100**(Suppl II): 107–113.

18 Hueb W, Lopes NH, Gersh BJ, *et al.* Five-year follow-up of the Medicine, Angioplasty, or Surgery Study (MASS II): A randomized controlled clinical trial of 3 therapeutic strategies for multivessel coronary artery disease. *Circulation* 2007; **115**: 1082–1089.

19 Pfisterer M, Buser P, Osswald S, *et al.* Outcome of elderly patients with chronic symptomatic coronary artery disease with an invasive versus optimized medical treatment strategy: one-year results of the randomized TIME trial. *JAMA* 2003; **289**: 1117–1123.

20 Davies RF, Goldberg AD, Forman S, *et al.* Asymptomatic Cardiac Ischemia Pilot (ACIP) study two-year follow-up: outcomes of patients randomized to initial strategies of medical therapy versus revascularization. *Circulation* 1997; **95**: 2037–2043.

21 Erne P, Schoenenberger AW, Burckhardt D, *et al.* Effects of percutaneous coronary interventions in silent ischemia after myocardial infarction: the SWISSI II randomized controlled trial. *JAMA* 2007; **297**: 1985–1991.

22 Frye RL, August P, Brooks MM, *et al.* BARI 2D Study Group. A randomized trial of therapies for type 2 diabetes and coronary artery disease. *N Engl J Med* 2009; **360**: 2503–2511.

23 Bangalore S, Pursnani S, Kumar S, Bagos PG. Percutaneous coronary intervention versus optimal medical therapy for prevention of spontaneous myocardial infarction in subjects with stable ischemic heart disease. *Circulation* 2013; **127**: 769–781.

24 Epstein SE, Waksmar R, Pichard AD, Kent KM, Panza JA. Percutaneous coronary intervention versus medical therapy in stable coronary artery disease: the unresolved conundrum. *JACC Cardiovasc Interv* 2013; **10**: 993–998.

25 Goy JJ, Eeckhout E, Burnand B, *et al.* Coronary angioplasty versus left internal mammary artery grafting for isolated proximal left anterior descending artery stenosis. *Lancet* 1994; **343**: 1449–1453.

26 Goy JJ, Kaufmann U, Hurni M, *et al.* SIMA Investigators 10-year follow-up of a prospective randomized trial comparing bare-metal stenting with internal mammary artery grafting for proximal, isolated de novo left anterior coronary artery stenosis the SIMA (Stenting versus Internal Mammary Artery grafting) trial. *J Am Coll Cardiol* 2008; **52**(10): 815–817.

27 Tonino PA, De Bruyne B, Pijls NH, *et al.* FAME Study Investigators. Fractional flow reserve versus angiography for guiding percutaneous coronary intervention. *N Engl J Med*. 2009; **360**(3): 213–224.

28 Bypass Angioplasty Revascularization Investigation (BARI) Investigators. Comparison of coronary bypass surgery with angioplasty in patients with multi-vessel disease. *N Engl J Med* 1996; **335**: 217–225.

29 Anonymous. Coronary angioplasty versus coronary artery bypass surgery: the Randomized Intervention Treatment of Angina (RITA) trial. *Lancet* 1993; **341**: 573–580.

30 Hamm CW, Reimers J, Ischinger T, *et al.* A randomized study of coronary angioplasty versus bypass-surgery in patients with symptomatic multivessel coronary disease. *N Engl J Med* 1994; **331**: 1037–1043.

31 King SB III, Lembo, NJ, Weintraub WS, *et al.* A randomized trial comparing coronary angioplasty with coronary bypass surgery. *N Engl J Med* 1994; **331**: 1044–1050.

32 Anonymous. First-year results of CABRI (Coronary Angioplasty versus Bypass Revascularisation Investigation). CABRI Trial Participants. *Lancet* 1995; **346**: 1179–1184.

33 Rodriguez A, Boullon F, Perez-Balino N, *et al.* Argentine randomized trial of percutaneous transluminal coronary angioplasty versus coronary artery bypass surgery in multivessel disease (ERACI): in-hospital results and 1-year follow-up. *ERACI Group. J Am Coll Cardiol* 1993; **22**: 1060–1067.

34 Hoffman SN, TenBrook JA, Wolf MP, *et al.* A meta-analysis of randomized controlled trials comparing coronary artery bypass graft with percutaneous transluminal coronary angioplasty: one- to eight-year outcomes. *J Am Coll Cardiol* 2003; **41**: 1293–1304.

35 BARI Investigators. The final 10-year follow-up results from the BARI randomized trial. *J Am Coll Cardiol* 2007; **49**: 1600–1606.

36 Niles NW, McGrath PD, Malenka D, *et al.* Survival of patients with diabetes and multivessel coronary artery disease after surgical or percutaneous coronary revascularization: results of a large regional prospective study. Northern New England Cardiovascular Disease Study Group. *J Am Coll Cardiol* 2001; **37**: 1008–1015.

37 Gersh BJ, Frye RL. Methods of coronary revascularization: things may not be as they seem. *N Engl J Med* 2005; **352**: 2235–2237.

38 Serruys PW, Unger F, Sousa JE, *et al.* Comparison of coronary-artery bypass surgery and stenting for the treatment of multivessel disease. *N Engl J Med* 2001; **344**: 1117–1124.

39 Legrand VM, Serruys PW, Unger F, *et al.* Three-year outcome after coronary stenting versus bypass surgery for the treatment of multivessel disease. *Circulation* 2004; **109**: 1114–1120.

40 Serruys PW, Ong ATL, van Herwerden LA, *et al.* Five-year outcomes after coronary stenting versus bypass surgery for the treatment of multivessel disease: the final analysis of the Arterial Revascularization Therapies (ARTS) randomized trial. *J Am Coll Cardiol* 2005; **46**: 575–581.

41 Rodriguez AE, Baldi J, Pereira CF, *et al.* Five-year follow-up of the Argentine randomized trial of coronary angioplasty with stenting versus coronary bypass surgery in patients with multiple vessel disease (ERACI II). *J Am Coll Cardiol* 2005; **46**: 582–588.

42 Booth J, Clayton T, Pepper J, *et al.* Randomized, controlled trial of coronary artery bypass surgery versus percutaneous coronary intervention in patients with multivessel coronary artery disease: six-year follow-up from the Stent or Surgery trial (SoS). *Circulation* 2008; **118**: 381–388.

43 Hlatky MA, Boothroyd DB, Bravata DM, *et al.* Percutaneous coronary interventions for multivessel disease: a collaborative analysis of individual patient data from ten randomised trials. *Lancet* 2009; **373**: 1190–1197.

44 Serruys PW, Morice MC, Kappetein AP, *et al.* Percutaneous coronary intervention versus coronary-artery bypass grafting for severe coronary artery disease. *N Engl J Med* 2009; **360**: 961–972.

45 Kapur A, Hall RJ, Malik IS, *et al.* Randomized comparison of percutaneous coronary intervention with coronary artery bypass grafting in diabetic patients: 1-year results of the CARDia (Coronary Artery Revascularization in Diabetes) trial. *J Am Coll Cardiol.* 2010; **55**: 432–440.

46 Farkouh ME, Domanski M, Sleeper LA, *et al.* FREEDOM Trial Investigators. Strategies for multivessel revascularization in patients with diabetes. *N Engl J Med* 2012; **367**: 2375.

47 Valgimigli M, Dawkins K, Macaya C, *et al.* Impact of stable versus unstable coronary artery disease on 1-year outcome in elective patients undergoing multivessel revascularization with sirolimus-eluting stents: a subanalysis of the ARTS II trial. *J Am Coll Cardiol* 2007; **49**: 431–441.

48 Mohr FW, Morice MC, Kappetein AP, *et al.* Coronary artery bypass graft surgery versus percutaneous coronary intervention in patients with three-vessel disease and left main coronary disease: 5-year follow-up of the randomised, clinical SYNTAX trial. *Lancet* 2013; **381**: 629–638.

49 VA Coronary Artery Bypass Surgery Cooperative Study Group. Eighteen-year follow-up in the Veterans Affairs Cooperative Study of Coronary Artery Bypass Surgery for stable angina. *Circulation* 1992; **86**: 121–130.

50 Varnauskas E. Twelve-year follow-up of survival in the randomized European Coronary Surgery Study. *N Engl J Med* 1988; **319**: 332–337.

51 Passamani E, Davis KB, Gillespie MJ, Killip T. A randomized trial of coronary artery bypass surgery. Survival of patients with a low ejection fraction. *N Engl J Med* 1985; **312**: 1665–1671.

52 Yusuf S, Zucker D, Peduzzi P, *et al.* Effect of coronary artery bypass graft surgery on survival: overview of 10-year results from randomised trials by the Coronary Artery Bypass Graft Surgery Trialists Collaboration. *Lancet* 1994; **344**: 563–570.

53 Myers WO, Schaff HV, Gersh BJ, *et al.* Improved survival of surgically treated patients with triple vessel coronary artery disease and severe angina pectoris: a report from the Coronary Artery Surgery Study (CASS) registry. *J Thorac Cardiovasc Surg* 1989; **97**: 487–495.

54 Rihal CS, Raco DL, Gersh BJ, Yusuf S. Indications for coronary artery bypass surgery and percutaneous coronary intervention in chronic stable angina: review of the evidence and methodological considerations. *Circulation* 2003; **108**: 2439–2445.

55 Hannan EL, Racz MJ, Walford G, *et al.* Long-term outcomes of coronary-artery bypass grafting versus stent implantation. *N Engl J Med* 2005; **352**: 2174–2183.

CHAPTER 12

PCI Strategies in Acute Coronary Syndromes without ST Segment Elevation (NSTEACS)

Georgios E. Christakopoulos[1], Subhash Banerjee[1], and Emmanouil S. Brilakis[1,2]

[1]VA North Texas Health Care System and University of Texas Southwestern Medical Center, Dallas, TX, USA

[2]Minneapolis Heart Institute, Minneapolis, MN, USA

Coronary angiography and percutaneous coronary intervention (PCI) is key for the effective management of patients presenting with non-ST segment elevation acute coronary syndromes (NSTEACS), as reflected in both the European Society of Cardiology (ESC) [1] and the American Heart Association/American College of Cardiology (AHA/ACC) guidelines [2]. This chapter reviews risk stratification, patient selection for cardiac catheterization, the role of PCI for revascularizing these patients, and the recommended adjunctive pharmacologic therapy.

Risk stratification

Risk stratification is critical for selecting treatment strategy (invasive vs. ischemia-driven) and timing (urgent, early, or delayed). High risk patients derive more benefit from more aggressive management strategies. Risk stratification is based on clinical, electrocardiographic, and laboratory findings (Box 12.1) and is often facilitated by use of risk scores that synthesize the impact of various parameters on patient outcomes (Table 12.1).

High risk manifests as myocardial injury and ischemia (e.g., ongoing chest pain, electrocardiographic changes, and cardiac biomarker increase), decrease in left ventricular function (cardiogenic shock and heart failure symptoms), and arrhythmias (such as ventricular tachycardia or fibrillation). Moreover, patients with prior coronary artery bypass graft surgery (CABG) are at increased risk for complications, as are patients with recent PCI, and those with comorbidities, such as chronic kidney disease and diabetes.

Two risk scores that are commonly used currently for risk stratification of NSTEACS patients are the Global Registry of Acute Coronary Events (GRACE) score and the Thrombolysis in Myocardial Infarction (TIMI) score.

The GRACE risk score can be used in patients with both NSTEACS and ST-segment elevation acute myocardial infarction. It is often considered more applicable to everyday clinical practice compared with other scores, as it was derived from a multinational registry of unselected patients from several hospitals around the world (Europe, Asia, North America, South America, Australia, and New Zealand). Eight parameters are used for calculating GRACE score:

1 Patient's age
2 Heart rate
3 Systolic blood pressure
4 Killip class [3]
5 Serum creatinine level
6 Cardiac arrest at hospital admission
7 ST-segment deviation in ECG
8 Elevated cardiac biomarkers.

The TIMI risk score for NSTEACS is simpler than the GRACE score and is also widely used. It can be rapidly determined as the sum of seven variables (age ≥65, at least 3 risk factors for coronary artery disease, prior coronary stenosis of 50% or more, ST-segment deviation on electrocardiogram at presentation, at least two anginal events in the past 24 hours, use of aspirin in the prior 7 days, and elevated serum cardiac markers) and can predict the composite of all-cause mortality, new or recurrent myocardial infarction and severe recurrent ischemia requiring urgent revascularization within 14 days from presentation, as follows:

Score of 0–1 = 4.7%
Score of 2 = 8.3%
Score of 3 = 13.2%
Score of 4 = 19.9%
Score of 5 = 26.2%
Score of 6–7 = at least 40.9%.

Invasive versus ischemia-guided approach

Patients presenting with NSTEACS can be treated with a routine invasive strategy or with an initial ischemia-guided strategy. In general, the higher the baseline patient risk, the higher the likelihood of improving outcomes with aggressive treatment strategies, including cardiac catheterization and revascularization.

Patients with signs and symptoms of ongoing ischemia, such as refractory angina and hemodynamic or electrical instability, should undergo urgent/immediate angiography (within 2 hours).

Among stabilized NSTEACS patients, a routine invasive management (Table 12.1) is recommended in patients who present with high risk features (such as dynamic electrocardiographic changes suggestive of ischemia, increased levels of cardiac biomarkers, or high risk scores) unless they have serious comorbidities or contraindications to coronary angiography and revascularization.

Patients treated with an ischemia-guided strategy are treated with medical therapy alone unless they develop refractory angina, have myocardial ischemia in non-invasive evaluation, or are

Interventional Cardiology: Principles and Practice, Second Edition. Edited by George D. Dangas, Carlo Di Mario, and Nicholas N. Kipshidze.
© 2017 John Wiley & Sons, Ltd. Published 2017 by John Wiley & Sons, Ltd.

considered to have risk of adverse events (such as patients with high TIMI or GRACE risk score).

Several studies and meta-analyses have reported that a routine invasive approach is superior to a conservative approach in NSTEACS [4,5]. A meta-analysis of eight trials including >10,000 patients revealed significant reduction in the risk of death, myocardial infarction, or rehospitalization with an acute coronary syndrome with an invasive strategy (odds ratio 0.78, 95% confidence interval 0.61–0.98) [5]. The benefit was observed in both men and high risk women, but not in low risk women, supporting a conservative approach for the latter group [5].

The optimal timing of coronary angiography for NSTEACS patients undergoing invasive management remains controversial (Table 12.2); however, immediate coronary angiography (similar to primary PCI for ST-segment elevation acute myocardial infarction) is not warranted in NSTEACS patients, except for those with hemodynamic or electrical instability or medically refractory angina [6]. Early angiography (within 24 hours from presentation) provides rapid assessment of coronary anatomy and triage for revascularization, potentially preventing subsequent ischemic complications and expediting discharge from the hospital. Delayed angiography allows for stabilization of the patient and potential decrease of the intracoronary thrombus burden through antithrombotic therapy.

Some studies have suggested that delaying angiography for several days may be detrimental [7]. In the largest trial performed to date, the Timing of Intervention in Acute Coronary Syndromes (TIMACS) trial, routine early intervention (coronary angiography ≤24 hours after randomization) did not reduce the primary study endpoint (death, myocardial infarction, or stroke) compared with delayed intervention (coronary angiography ≥36 hours after randomization) in the overall study population [8]. However, early intervention was beneficial in the subgroup of patients with GRACE score >140 (13.9% vs. 21.0%; hazard ratio 0.65, 95% CI 0.48–0.89; p = 0.006) [8].

A delayed (25–72 hours) invasive strategy may be acceptable for intermediate risk patients with a GRACE score <140 who have one or more of the following clinical features: history of diabetes mellitus, renal insufficiency (GFR <60 mL/min/1.73 m^2), reduced systolic left ventricular function with an ejection fraction (EF) <40%, history of recent PCI or prior CABG. In patients at low risk without recurrent symptoms or signs of ongoing ischemia, a non-invasive assessment of inducible ischemia should be performed before discharge, followed by angiography if the findings suggest high risk.

Box 12.1 High-risk criteria for patients with non-ST segment elevation acute coronary syndromes (NSTEACS)

Primary criteria
- Relevant rise or fall in troponin
- Dynamic ST- or T-wave changes (symptomatic or silent)
- GRACE score >140

Secondary criteria
- Diabetes mellitus
- Renal insufficiency (GFR <60 mL/min/1.73 m^2)
- Reduced left ventricular function (ejection fraction <40%)
- Early post-infarction angina
- Recent PCI
- Prior CABG
- Intermediate to high GRACE risk score

CABG, coronary artery bypass graft surgery; GFR, glomerular filtration rate; GRACE, Global Registry of Acute Coronary Events; PCI, percutaneous coronary intervention.

Coronary revascularization in NSTEACS

In NSTEACS patients with single-vessel coronary artery disease, ad hoc PCI is most frequently performed. In patients with multivessel disease (who represent more than 50% of NSTEACS patients) the decision between culprit-lesion PCI, multivessel PCI, and CABG is more complex. In patients with hemodynamic instability, pulmonary edema, recurrent ventricular arrhythmias, or total occlusion of the culprit coronary artery, culprit lesion PCI is usually preferred. In contrast, CABG is preferred in stabilized patients with complex multivessel disease and a high SYNTAX score. In the Acute

---

Table 12.1 Comparison of three risk scores used for risk stratification in patients with non-ST segment elevation acute coronary syndromes (NSTEACS).

	PURSUIT	TIMI	GRACE
History	Age Gender Worst CCS class in last 6 weeks	Age ≥3 CAD risk factors Known CAD (stenosis ≥50%) Aspirin within 7 days Recent (<24 h) severe angina	Age Cardiac arrest during presentation
Examination	1. SBP 2. HR 3. Rales		1. SBP 2. HR 3. Killip class
ECG	ST-segment depression	ST-segment depression >0.5 mm	ST segment deviation
Laboratory tests		↑ Cardiac markers	↑ Cardiac markers Creatinine

CAD, coronary artery disease; CCS, Canadian Cardiovascular Society; GRACE, Global Registry of Acute Coronary Events; HR, heart rate; PURSUIT, Platelet glycoprotein IIb/IIIa in Unstable angina: Receptor Suppression Using Integrilin; SBP, systolic blood pressure; TIMI, Thrombolysis In Myocardial Infarction.

Table 12.2 Selection of an early invasive vs. ischemia-guided strategy in patients with non-ST segment elevation acute coronary syndromes (NSTEACS).

	ACC/AHA guidelines	ESC guidelines
Immediate invasive (<2 h)	Refractory angina	Refractory angina with associated heart failure
	Signs or symptoms of new or worsening mitral regurgitation	
	Hemodynamic instability	Hemodynamic instability
	Sustained VT or VF	Life-threatening ventricular arrhythmias
	Recurrent angina or ischemia at rest or with low level activities despite intensive medical therapy	
Early invasive (within 24 h)	None of the above, but GRACE risk score >140	Grace score >140
	Temporal change in troponin	Relevant rise or fall in troponin
	New or presumably new ST depression	Dynamic ST- or T-wave changes (symptomatic or silent)
Delayed invasive (within 25–72 h)	None of the above but diabetes mellitus	Diabetes mellitus
	Renal insufficiency (GFR <60 mL/min/1.73 m^2)	Renal insufficiency (GFR <60 mL/min/1.73 m^2)
	Reduced LV systolic function (EF <0.40)	Reduced LV systolic function (EF <0.40)
	Early post-infarction angina	Early post-infarction angina
	PCI within 6 months	Recent PCI
	Prior CABG	Prior CABG
	GRACE risk score 109–140; TIMI score ≥ 2	Intermediate to high GRACE risk score (<140)

ACC, American College of Cardiology; AHA, American Heart Association; CABG, coronary artery bypass graft; ESC, European Society of Cardiology; EF, ejection fraction; GFR, glomerular filtration rate; GRACE, Global Registry of Acute Coronary Events; LV, left ventricular; PCI, percutaneous coronary intervention; VF, ventricular fibrillation; VT, ventricular tachycardia.

Catheterization and Urgent Intervention Triage Strategy (ACUITY) trial compared with CABG, PCI for multivessel disease was associated with a lower risk of stroke, myocardial infarction, bleeding, and renal injury but significantly higher rates of subsequent revascularization at both 1 month and 1 year [9].

In a NSTEACS patient with multivessel coronary artery disease undergoing PCI there is no consensus about whether the culprit lesion only or all obstructive lesions should be treated concurrently [10]; both approaches are acceptable and decisions should be made on a case-by-case basis taking into account the potential risks and benefits of the procedure [2,11,12]. In general, complete revascularization is associated with improved clinical outcomes [13,14], and should be pursued regardless of whether revascularization is with PCI or with CABG. Occasionally, identification of the culprit lesion can be challenging and could be facilitated by use of intravascular imaging with optical coherence tomography, which can identify plaque rupture and thrombus formation [15]. In some cases no plaque rupture can be found, suggesting plaque erosion, which can often be successfully managed with medical therapy alone without stenting [16].

PCI: adjunctive pharmacologic treatment

Adjunctive pharmacologic therapy is critical for the success of PCI, but is also beneficial for patients treated with a conservative approach [17]. Table 12.3 summarizes the recommended antithrombotic therapy according to the ACC and ESC guidelines. Both guidelines recommend anticoagulation and dual antiplatelet therapy with aspirin (ASA) and a P2Y$_{12}$-receptor antagonist (prasugrel, clopidogrel, or ticagrelor) for NSTEACS patients undergoing PCI.

Table 12.3 Summary of the guideline recommendations for antiplatelet and anticoagulant therapy among patients with non-ST segment elevation acute coronary syndromes (NSTEACS).

ACC/AHA Guidelines	ESC Guidelines
Antiplatelet therapy	
1. Aspirin is recommended for all patients at an initial dose of 81–325 mg (325 mg for all patients if not already on aspirin prior to PCI) Maintenance dose: 81–325 mg (indefinitely) (class I)	**1. Aspirin** is recommended for all patients without contraindications at an initial oral loading dose of 150–300 mg (or 80–150 mg IV) Maintenance dose of 75–100 mg/day long term, regardless of treatment strategy (class I)
2. A P2Y12 inhibitor is recommended in addition to ASA, and maintained over 12 months unless there are contraindications such as excessive risk of bleeding (class I). Options include: • Prasugrel 60 mg loading dose, then 10 mg/day • Clopidogrel 600 mg loading dose, then 75 mg/day • Ticagrelor 180 mg loading dose, then 90 mg twice daily Ticagrelor is preferred to clopidogrel in patients treated with an early invasive strategy and/or stenting (class IIA) Prasugrel is preferred over clopidogrel in patients not at high risk of bleeding (class IIA), and without a history of stroke or TIA (prasugrel is class III in such patients) DAPT beyond 12 months may be considered in patients undergoing stent implantation (class IIb)	**2. A P2Y12 inhibitor** is recommended in addition to ASA, and maintained over 12 months unless there are contraindications such as excessive risk of bleeds (class IA): • Clopidogrel (300–600 mg loading dose, 75 mg/day dose), is recommended for patients who cannot receive ticagrelor or prasugrel or who require oral anticoagulation (class IB) • Ticagrelor (180 mg loading dose, 90 mg twice daily) is recommended, in the absence of contraindications, for all patients at moderate-to-high risk of ischemic events (e.g., elevated cardiac troponins), regardless of initial treatment strategy and including those pretreated with clopidogrel (which should be discontinued when ticagrelor is started) (class IB) • Prasugrel (60 mg loading dose, 10 mg daily dose) is recommended in patients who are proceeding to PCI if no contraindication (class IB) Pre-treatment with prasugrel in patients in whom coronary anatomy not known, is not recommended (class III)
3. GP IIb/IIIa inhibitors GP IIb/IIIa inhibitor at the time of PCI is recommended in patients with NSTEACS and high risk features (e.g., high troponin) not adequately pretreated with clopidogrel or ticagrelor (class I) or with high risk patients treated with UFH and adequately pretreated with clopidogrel (class IIa). Options include: abciximab, double-bolus eptifibatide or high dose tirofiban	**3. GP IIb/IIIa antagonists** should be considered for bail-out situations or thrombotic complications (class IIa) Pre-treatment with GP IIb/IIIa antagonists in patients in whom coronary artery anatomy is not known, is not recommended (class III)
Anticoagulation therapy	
Performance of PCI with enoxaparin may be reasonable in patients treated with upstream subcutaneous enoxaparin for NSTEACS (class IIb)	Fondaparinux (2.5 mg s.c. daily) is recommended as having the most favorable efficacy– safety profile regardless of the management strategy (class I)
Intravenous UFH is useful in patients with NSTEACS undergoing PCI (class I)	
Bivalirudin is useful as an anticoagulant with or without prior treatment with UFH in patients with NSTEACS undergoing PCI (class I) • For patients who have received UFH, wait 30 min, then give 0.75 mg/kg IV loading dose, then 1.75 mg/kg/h IV infusion • For patients already receiving bivalirudin infusion, give additional loading dose 0.5 mg/kg and increase infusion to 1.75 mg/kg/h during PCI In patients with NSTEACS undergoing PCI who are at high risk of bleeding, bivalirudin monotherapy is preferred to the combination of UFH and a GP IIb/IIIa receptor antagonist (class IIa)	Bivalirudin (0.75 mg/kg bolus, followed by 1.75 mg/kg/h for up to 4 h after the procedure) is recommended as alternative to UFH plus GP IIb/IIIa receptor inhibitor during PCI (class I) UFH 70–100 IU/kg i.v. (50–70 IU/kg if concomitant with GPIIb/IIIa inhibitors) is recommended in patients undergoing PCI who did not receive any anticoagulant (class I) Enoxaparin (1 mg/kg s.c. twice daily) or UFH are recommended when fondaparinux is not available (class I) Enoxaparin should be considered as an anticoagulant for PCI in patients pretreated with s.c. enoxaparin (class IIa)
Fondaparinux: If PCI is performed while the patient is on fondaparinux, an additional 85 IU/kg UFH should be given intravenously immediately before PCI because of the risk of catheter thrombosis (60 IU/kg IV if a GP IIb/IIIa inhibitor used with UFH dosing based on the target-activated clotting time) (class I) Fondaparinux should not be used as the sole anticoagulant to support PCI in patients with NSTEACS due to an increased risk of catheter thrombosis (class III)	Fondaparinux should not be used as the sole anticoagulant to support PCI in patients with NSTEACS due to an increased risk of catheter thrombosis In patients on fondaparinux (2.5 mg/day s.c.), a single bolus UFH (85 IU/kg, or 60 IU/kg in the case of concomitant use of GP IIb/IIIa receptor inhibitors) is indicated during PCI (class I)
Anticoagulation should be discontinued after invasive procedure unless otherwise indicated (class I)	Crossover of UFH and LMWH is not recommended (class III) Discontinuation of anticoagulation should be considered after PCI, unless otherwise indicated

ASA, aspirin; DAPT; dual antiplatelet therapy; GP, glycoprotein; LMWH, low-molecular weight heparin; PCI, percutaneous coronary intervention; IV, intravenous; s.c., subcutaneous; UFH, unfractionated heparin.

Aspirin

Aspirin irreversibly inhibits the platelet cyclo-oxygenase-1 (COX-1). In view of its efficacy, low cost, and widespread availability, all NSTEACS patients should receive it, unless they have a contraindication [18]. According to the AHA/ACC guidelines patients that are on aspirin before PCI, should take 81–325 mg non-enteric coated aspirin before PCI, whereas patients not on aspirin should be given non-enteric coated aspirin (325 mg dose) as soon as possible before PCI. After PCI, aspirin should be continued at a dose of 81–325 mg/day indefinitely, unless contraindicated [2]. The ESC guidelines differ on dosing, recommending ASA for all patients without contraindications at an initial oral loading dose of 150–300 mg (or 80–150 mg intravenously); after PCI patients should be kept on aspirin at a maintenance dose of 75–100 mg/day, regardless of treatment strategy [1].

P2Y$_{12}$ receptor inhibitor

An oral P2Y$_{12}$ inhibitor should be administered in addition to aspirin to all NSTEACS patients undergoing PCI. Three oral P2Y$_{12}$ receptor Inhibitors are currently used: clopidogrel, prasugrel, and ticagrelor (ticlopidine is seldom used currently because of potential for serious hematologic side effects).

In the Clopidogrel in Unstable Angina to Prevent Recurrent Events (CURE) trial, NSTEACS patients were randomized to clopidogrel or placebo. During a mean follow-up of 9 months, clopidogrel reduced the incidence of the cardiovascular death, MI, or stroke by 20% (9.3% vs. 11.4%; p < 0.001) [19]. In the Clopidogrel and Aspirin Optimal Dose Usage to Reduce Recurrent Events – Seventh Organization to Assess Strategies in Ischemic Syndromes (CURRENT–OASIS 7) trial, compared with standard dose clopidogrel (300-mg loading dose and 75 mg/day thereafter) double dose clopidogrel (600 mg loading dose on the first day, followed by 150 mg/day for 6 days and 75 mg/day thereafter) did not reduce the 30-day incidence of cardiovascular death, MI, or stroke (4.2% vs. 4.4%; p = 0.30), although it did reduce the risk of stent thrombosis among patients who underwent PCI [20].

Clopidogrel is a pro-drug that requires multistep activation and its efficacy is markedly affected by genetic factors, such as CYP 2C19 polymorphisms. In contrast, prasugrel and ticagrelor are more potent platelet inhibitors with consistent metabolism [21,22].

In the Trial to Assess Improvement in Therapeutic Outcomes by Optimizing Platelet Inhibition with Prasugrel–Thrombolysis in Myocardial Infarction 38 (TRITON–TIMI 38) 13,608 patients (74% of whom had NSTEACS) were randomized to prasugrel or clopidogrel (300 mg loading dose) [21]. Prasugrel was given after coronary angiography once the decision for PCI was made. During a median follow-up of 14.5 months, compared with clopidogrel prasugrel reduced the incidence of cardiovascular death, MI, or stroke (9.9% vs. 12.1%; p <0.001), and the risk for stent thrombosis (of both bare metal and drug-eluting stents) [23], but also increased the risk for TIMI major and fatal bleeding [21]. Prasugrel was harmful in patients with prior transient ischemic attack or stroke and did not provide clinical benefit among patients ≥75 years old or with <60 kg body weight [21]. In the Comparison of Prasugrel at the Time of Percutaneous Coronary Intervention (PCI) or as Pretreatment at the Time of Diagnosis in Patients with Non-ST Elevation Myocardial Infarction (ACCOAST) trial, pretreatment with prasugrel did not decrease ischemic complications when compared with administration at the time of PCI and was associated with higher risk for major bleeding [24]. In the Targeted Platelet

Inhibition to Clarify the Optimal Strategy to Medically Manage Acute Coronary Syndromes (TRILOGY ACS) study, prasugrel administration was not beneficial among NSTEACS patients treated with medical therapy without PCI [25].

The Study of Platelet Inhibition and Patient Outcomes (PLATO), randomized 18,624 patients (62% of whom had NSTEACS) to ticagrelor or clopidogrel [22,26]. Compared with clopidogrel, ticagrelor reduced the 12-month incidence of vascular death, MI, or stroke (9.8% vs. 11.7%; p <0.001) and also reduced all-cause mortality (4.5% vs. 5.9%; p <0.001). However, ticagrelor-treated patients had higher rate of non CABG-related major bleeding, dyspnea, and ventricular pauses lasting ≥3 s (but not requiring specific treatment). North American patients did not derive benefit from ticagrelor administration, likely because of co-administration of ≥100 mg/day aspirin [27].

Based on the benefits observed with prasugrel and ticagrelor in the above studies, the AHA/ACC guidelines favor them over clopidogrel (class IIa indication) [2]. The ESC guidelines go even further in recommending prasugrel and ticagrelor over clopidogrel, stating that clopidogrel should be used when prasugrel or ticagrelor are not available or are contraindicated in patients who cannot receive ticagrelor or prasugrel or who require oral anticoagulation (class I indication) [1].

The optimal duration of dual antiplatelet therapy after PCI for NSTEACS remains controversial. The currently guideline-recommended duration is 12 months unless there are contraindications or an excessive risk of bleeding [1,2]. Some studies have suggested that shorter duration of P2Y12 inhibitor administration could be equivalent or superior to longer duration [28]. However, the largest study performed to date, the Dual Antiplatelet Therapy (DAPT) study, reported that compared with 12 months, 30 months of dual antiplatelet therapy were associated with lower risk of stent thrombosis (0.4% vs. 1.4%; hazard ratio 0.29, 95% confidence interval 0.17–0.48; p <0.001), and myocardial infarction (2.1% vs. 4.1%; hazard ratio 0.47; p < 0.001), at the cost of increased risk for moderate to severe bleeding (2.5% vs. 1.6%, p = 0.001), and a nominal increase in all-cause mortality (2.0% vs. 1.5%; p = 0.05), although cardiac mortality was similar in both groups [29].

Glycoprotein IIb/IIIa inhibitors

Much of the evidence that supports use of glycoprotein (GP) IIb/IIIa inhibitors (abciximab, eptifibatide, or tirofiban) in NSTEACS patients was obtained in the era before the routine use of dual antiplatelet therapy. In a meta-analysis by Boersma et al. [30], GP IIa/IIIa inhibitors were only beneficial in patients with elevated troponin and in those who underwent revascularization within 30 days.

In the Early Glycoprotein IIb/IIIa Inhibition in Non-ST-Segment Elevation Acute Coronary Syndrome (EARLY-ACS) trial, routine upstream administration of eptifibatide did not benefit NSTEACS patients, except patients at the highest risk for ischemic complications (such as those with troponin elevation, ST deviation, diabetes, recurrent ischemia) and low risk for bleeding (age <75 years) [31]. In patients pre-treated with P2Y12 inhibitors, outcomes have been favorable with use of bivalirudin alone vs. UFH and GPI [9], leading to a significant reduction in GPI use in contemporary practice.

In summary, GP IIb/IIIa are infrequently used as pretreatment in NSTEACS patients who receive dual antiplatelet therapy and have intermediate/high risk features (class IIb indication in the AHA/ACC guidelines). They are indicated at the time of PCI in high-risk patients undergoing PCI, whether they have been pretreated with a P2Y12 inhibitor (class IIa indication if unfractionated heparin is used as anticoagulant) or not (class I indication) [2].

Anticoagulation

Anticoagulation is recommended for all NSTEACS patients undergoing PCI to reduce the risk of intracoronary and catheter thrombus formation. The type of anticoagulation is selected according to ischemic and bleeding risks as well as the efficacy–safety profile of the chosen agent for each patient individually. Parenteral anticoagulants used in patients with NSTEACS undergoing PCI include unfractionated heparin (UFH), low molecular weight heparin (LMWH, usully enoxaparin), bivalirudin, and fondaparinux.

Unfractionated heparin has been used for many years for PCI. It has low cost; however, response to unfractionated heparin is variable, requiring measurement of its antithrombotic effect. In the largest study of enoxaparin in NSTEACS, the Superior Yield of the New Strategy of Enoxaparin, Revascularization and Glycoprotein IIb/IIIa Inhibitors (SYNERGY) trial, 10,027 high-risk NSTEACS patients treated with an early invasive strategy were randomized to enoxaparin or UFH [32]. Enoxaparin-treated patients had similar incidence of death or MI compared with those treated with UFH, but higher incidence of major bleeding [32]. As a result enoxaparin is infrequently used during PCI for NSTEACS.

Bivalirudin is a direct thrombin inhibitor [9,33–35]. In the ACUITY trial, bivalirudin monotherapy was associated with a non-inferior rate of the composite ischemia endpoint (death, MI, or unplanned revascularization) (7.8% and 7.3%, respectively; p = 0.32) and significantly reduced the rates of major bleeding (3.0% vs. 5.7%; p < 0.001) as compared with bivalirudin + GP IIb/IIIa inhibitor and UFH + GP IIb/IIIa inhibitor [9,35]. However, among patients not pretreated with clopidogrel before PCI, the incidence of ischemic events was higher in the bivalirudin group (9.1% vs. 7.1%, RR 1.29; p = 0.054 for interaction) [9].

Fondaparinux is a factor Xa inhibitor. In the Fifth Organization to Assess Strategies in Acute Ischemic Syndromes (OASIS 5) trial, patients receiving fondaparinux had lower 30-day mortality compared with those receiving enoxaparin (2.9% vs. 3.5%, HR 0.83, 95% CI 0.71–0.97; p = 0.02), likely related to the lower risk for major bleeding (2.2% vs. 4.1% at 9 days; p < 0.001) [36]. Patients undergoing PCI on fondaparinux had a threefold higher rate of guide catheter thrombus (0.9% vs. 0.3%), hence UFH (85 IU/kg without or 60 IU/kg with a GP IIb/IIIa inhibitor) should be administered to patients on fondaparinux who require PCI [37].

The European and American guideline recommendations for anticoagulation in NSTEACS patients are summarized in Table 12.3 [1,2].

Conclusion

In summary, NSTEACS are commonly encountered in daily clinical practice. Risk stratification is key for determining optimal treatment strategies, with higher risk patients deriving more benefit from more aggressive strategies. An early invasive approach is preferred for most high risk patients. Clinical outcomes can be improved by optimal selection of anticoagulation and antiplatelet treatments.

*Interactive multiple choice questions are available for this chapter on **www.wiley. com/go/dangas/cardiology**.*

References

1 Roffi M, Patrono C, Collet JP, et al. 2015 ESC Guidelines for the management of acute coronary syndromes in patients presenting without persistent ST-segment elevation: Task Force for the Management of Acute Coronary Syndromes in Patients Presenting without Persistent ST-Segment Elevation of the European Society of Cardiology (ESC). *Eur Heart J* 2016; **37**: 267–315.

2 Amsterdam EA, Wenger NK, Brindis RG, et al. 2014 AHA/ACC Guideline for the management of patients with non-st-elevation acute coronary syndromes: a report of the American College of Cardiology/American Heart Association Task Force on Practice Guidelines. *J Am Coll Cardiol* 2014; **64**(24): e139–228. PubMed PMID: 25260718.

3 Killip T 3rd, Kimball JT. Treatment of myocardial infarction in a coronary care unit: a two year experience with 250 patients. *Am J Cardiol* 1967; **20**(4): 457–464.

4 Fox KA, Clayton TC, Damman P, et al. Long-term outcome of a routine versus selective invasive strategy in patients with non-ST-segment elevation acute coronary syndrome a meta-analysis of individual patient data. *J Am Coll Cardiol* 2010; **55**(22): 2435–2445. PubMed PMID: 20359842.

5 O'Donoghue M, Boden WE, Braunwald E, et al. Early invasive vs conservative treatment strategies in women and men with unstable angina and non-ST-segment elevation myocardial infarction: a meta-analysis. *JAMA* 2008; **300**(1): 71–80. PubMed PMID: 18594042.

6 Montalescot G, Cayla G, Collet JP, et al. Immediate vs delayed intervention for acute coronary syndromes: a randomized clinical trial. *JAMA* 2009; **302**(9): 947–954. PubMed PMID: 19724041.

7 Neumann FJ, Kastrati A, Pogatsa-Murray G, et al. Evaluation of prolonged antithrombotic pretreatment ("cooling-off" strategy) before intervention in patients with unstable coronary syndromes: a randomized controlled trial. *JAMA* 2003; **290**(12): 1593–1599. PubMed PMID: 14506118.

8 Mehta SR, Granger CB, Boden WE, et al. Early versus delayed invasive intervention in acute coronary syndromes. *N Engl J Med* 2009; **360**(21): 2165–2175. PubMed PMID: 19458363.

9 Stone GW, McLaurin BT, Cox DA, et al. Bivalirudin for patients with acute coronary syndromes. *N Engl J Med* 2006; **355**(21): 2203–2216. PubMed PMID: 17124018.

10 Blankenship JC, Moussa ID, Chambers CC, et al. Staging of multivessel percutaneous coronary interventions: an expert consensus statement from the Society for Cardiovascular Angiography and Interventions. *Catheter Cardiovasc Interv* 2012; **79**(7): 1138–1152. PubMed PMID: 22072562.

11 Shishehbor MH, Lauer MS, Singh IM, et al. In unstable angina or non-ST-segment acute coronary syndrome, should patients with multivessel coronary artery disease undergo multivessel or culprit-only stenting? *J Am Coll Cardiol* 2007; **49**(8): 849–854. PubMed PMID: 17320742.

12 Brener SJ, Milford-Beland S, Roe MT, et al. Culprit-only or multivessel revascularization in patients with acute coronary syndromes: an American College of Cardiology National Cardiovascular Database Registry report. *Am Heart J* 2008; **155**(1): 140–146. PubMed PMID: 18082505.

13 Garcia S, Sandoval Y, Roukoz H, et al. Outcomes after complete versus incomplete revascularization of patients with multivessel coronary artery disease: a meta-analysis of 89,883 patients enrolled in randomized clinical trials and observational studies. *J Am Coll Cardiol.* 2013; **62**(16): 1421–1431. PubMed PMID: 23747787.

14 Rosner GF, Kirtane AJ, Genereux P, et al. Impact of the presence and extent of incomplete angiographic revascularization after percutaneous coronary intervention in acute coronary syndromes: the Acute Catheterization and Urgent Intervention Triage Strategy (ACUITY) trial. *Circulation* 2012; **125**(21): 2613–2620. PubMed PMID: 22550156.

15 Kubo T, Imanishi T, Takarada S, et al. Assessment of culprit lesion morphology in acute myocardial infarction: ability of optical coherence tomography compared with intravascular ultrasound and coronary angioscopy. *J Am Coll Cardiol* 2007; **50**(10): 933–939. PubMed PMID: 17765119.

16 Prati F, Uemura S, Souteyrand G, et al. OCT-based diagnosis and management of STEMI associated with intact fibrous cap. *JACC Cardiovasc Imaging* 2013; **6**(3): 283–287.

17 Lindholm D, Varenhorst C, Cannon CP, et al. Ticagrelor vs. clopidogrel in patients with non-ST-elevation acute coronary syndrome with or without revascularization: results from the PLATO trial. *Eur Heart J* 2014; **35**(31): 2083–2093. PubMed PMID: 24727884. Pubmed Central PMCID: 4132637.

18 Brilakis ES, Patel VG, Banerjee S. Medical management after coronary stent implantation: a review. *JAMA* 2013; **310**(2): 189–198. PubMed PMID: 23839753. Epub 2013/07/11. eng.

19 Yusuf S, Zhao F, Mehta SR, Chrolavicius S, Tognoni G, Fox KK. Effects of clopidogrel in addition to aspirin in patients with acute coronary syndromes without ST-segment elevation. *N Engl J Med* 2001; **345**(7) :494-502. PubMed PMID: 11519503.

20 Mehta SR, Bassand JP, Chrolavicius S, *et al*. Dose comparisons of clopidogrel and aspirin in acute coronary syndromes. *N Engl J Med* 2010; **363**(10): 930–942. PubMed PMID: 20818903.

21 Wiviott SD, Braunwald E, McCabe CH, *et al*. Prasugrel versus clopidogrel in patients with acute coronary syndromes. *N Engl J Med* 2007; **357**(20): 2001–2015. PubMed PMID: 17982182.

22 Wallentin L, Becker RC, Budaj A, *et al*. Ticagrelor versus clopidogrel in patients with acute coronary syndromes. *N Engl J Med* 2009; **361**(11): 1045–1057. PubMed PMID: 19717846.

23 Wiviott SD, Braunwald E, McCabe CH, *et al*. Intensive oral antiplatelet therapy for reduction of ischaemic events including stent thrombosis in patients with acute coronary syndromes treated with percutaneous coronary intervention and stenting in the TRITON-TIMI 38 trial: a subanalysis of a randomised trial. *Lancet* 2008; **371**(9621): 1353–1363. PubMed PMID: 18377975.

24 Montalescot G, Bolognese L, Dudek D, *et al*. Pretreatment with prasugrel in non-ST-segment elevation acute coronary syndromes. *N Engl J Med* 2013; **369**(11): 999–1010. PubMed PMID: 23991622.

25 Roe MT, Armstrong PW, Fox KA, *et al*. Prasugrel versus clopidogrel for acute coronary syndromes without revascularization. *N Engl J Med* 2012; **367**(14): 1297–1309. PubMed PMID: 22920930.

26 Cannon CP, Harrington RA, James S, *et al*. Comparison of ticagrelor with clopidogrel in patients with a planned invasive strategy for acute coronary syndromes (PLATO): a randomised double-blind study. *Lancet* 2010; **375**(9711): 283–293. PubMed PMID: 20079528.

27 Mahaffey KW, Wojdyla DM, Carroll K, *et al*. Ticagrelor compared with clopidogrel by geographic region in the platelet inhibition and patient outcomes (PLATO) trial. *Circulation* 2011; **124**(5): 544–554. PubMed PMID: 21709065.

28 Stefanini GG, Siontis GC, Cao D, Heg D, Juni P, Windecker S. Short versus long duration of dapt after des implantation: a meta-analysis. *J Am Coll Cardiol* 2014; **64**(9): 953–954. PubMed PMID: 25169183.

29 Mauri L, Kereiakes DJ, Yeh RW, *et al*. Twelve or 30 months of dual antiplatelet therapy after drug-eluting stents. *N Engl J Med* 2014; **371**(23): 2155–2166. PubMed PMID: 25399658.

30 Boersma E, Harrington RA, Moliterno DJ, *et al*. Platelet glycoprotein IIb/IIIa inhibitors in acute coronary syndromes: a meta-analysis of all major randomised clinical trials. *Lancet* 2002; **359**(9302): 189–198. PubMed PMID: 11812552.

31 Giugliano RP, White JA, Bode C, *et al*. Early versus delayed, provisional eptifibatide in acute coronary syndromes. *N Engl J Med*. 2009; **360**(21): 2176–2190. PubMed PMID: 19332455.

32 Enoxaparin vs unfractionated heparin in high-risk patients with non–ST-segment elevation acute coronary syndromes managed with an intended early invasive strategy: primary results of the synergy randomized trial. *JAMA* 2004; **292**(1): 45–54.

33 Lincoff AM, Bittl JA, Harrington RA, *et al*. Bivalirudin and provisional glycoprotein IIb/IIIa blockade compared with heparin and planned glycoprotein IIb/IIIa blockade during percutaneous coronary intervention: REPLACE-2 randomized trial. *JAMA* 2003; **289**(7): 853–863. PubMed PMID: 12588269.

34 Lincoff AM, Kleiman NS, Kereiakes DJ, *et al*. Long-term efficacy of bivalirudin and provisional glycoprotein IIb/IIIa blockade vs heparin and planned glycoprotein IIb/IIIa blockade during percutaneous coronary revascularization: REPLACE-2 randomized trial. *JAMA* 2004; **292**(6): 696–703. PubMed PMID: 15304466.

35 Stone GW, White HD, Ohman EM, *et al*. Bivalirudin in patients with acute coronary syndromes undergoing percutaneous coronary intervention: a subgroup analysis from the Acute Catheterization and Urgent Intervention Triage strategy (ACUITY) trial. *Lancet* 2007; **369**(9565): 907–919. PubMed PMID: 17368152.

36 Fifth Organization to Assess Strategies in Acute Ischemic Syndromes I, Yusuf S, Mehta SR, Chrolavicius S, *et al*. Comparison of fondaparinux and enoxaparin in acute coronary syndromes. *N Engl J Med* 2006; **354**(14): 1464–1476. PubMed PMID: 16537663.

37 Levine GN, Bates ER, Blankenship JC, *et al*. 2011 ACCF/AHA/SCAI Guideline for percutaneous coronary intervention: a report of the American College of Cardiology Foundation/American Heart Association Task Force on Practice Guidelines and the Society for Cardiovascular Angiography and Interventions. *J Am Coll Cardiol* 2011; **58**(24): e44–122. PubMed PMID: 22070834.

CHAPTER 13

Primary and Rescue PCI in Acute Myocardial Infarction and Elements of Myocardial Conditioning

Tayo Addo[1], Neil Swanson[2], and Anthony Gershlick[2]

[1] University of Texas Southwestern Medical Center, Dallas, TX, USA
[2] University of Leicester, Leicester, UK

Acute myocardial infarction results when abrupt thrombotic occlusion of a major epicardial coronary occurs. Following extensive pathologic investigation, it is now quite clear that the underlying etiologic mechanism involves acute disruption of an atherosclerotic plaque generally previously moderate in severity. The resultant exposure of circulating blood to underlying plaque material results in platelet aggregation, thrombin generation, and thrombosis [1]. The severity of injury, often detected on the ECG as ST-segment elevation, indicates extensive and transmural myocardial ischemia owing to such abrupt termination of blood flow and lack of prior adaptation. A large region of myocardium undoubtedly suffers necrosis if not immediately addressed. Soon after the appreciation of thrombus and aggregated platelets at the occlusion site, substantial advances in care were made with the rapid administration of fibrinolytics, antiplatelets, and antithrombins aimed at re-establishing vessel patency. Collectively regarded as reperfusion therapy, these agents were studied extensively, in combination and with high efficiency, and resulted in improved survival [2–10]. Along with these reperfusion studies conducted in the late 1980s and throughout the 1990s, coronary angiography was employed to assess the efficacy of therapy and the following observations were made.

1 Reperfusion therapy, even with the most potent agents, did not always result in restoring optimal vessel patency.
2 Vessel patency and coronary myocardial blood flow were highly important determinants of survival.
3 Time to treatment was a powerful determinant of effectiveness.
4 The emerging technique of percutaneous transluminal coronary balloon angioplasty could be used effectively to establish blood flow either as the primary treatment or as salvage after unsuccessful medical reperfusion therapy [11].

Primary PCI

Initial experience and comparisons with thrombolytic therapy

The very early experience led by Hartzler and others indicated that percutaneous coronary intervention (PCI) was not only feasible in acute myocardial infarction, but the recanalization rate was very high, typically exceeding 90% [12]. However, others expressed caution, reporting high complication rates including major bleeding and recurrent infarction, particularly when performed shortly after thrombolytic therapy [13]. Several trials were subsequently conducted comparing thrombolytic therapy with primary PCI spanning over 10 years and ultimately summarized in a meta-analysis by Keeley et al. [14]. Comprising 7739 patients, short-term mortality was reduced from 9% to 7%. Even when patients with cardiogenic shock were excluded, mortality was still reduced from 7% to 5%, with benefits sustained at longer term follow-up. Recurrent myocardial infarction was reduced from 6.8% to 2.5% and stroke reduced from 2% to 1% (Figure 13.1). In these initial trials primary PCI was delivered efficiently and at institutions with experience in the procedure, so there were concerns if this could be duplicated in real-world practice. Nonetheless, the results were widely embraced as angiography and intervention was safer and more predictable than fibronolytic therapy. Efficacy was also confirmed in subsequent large non-randomized registries. In the Swedish Heart Intensive Care Admissions Registry [15], 16,034 patients receiving reperfusion with fibrinolytic therapy were compared with 7084 receiving primary PCI. Mortality at 1 year was reduced from 15.6% to 7.6% in favor of primary PCI. Given the limited number of hospitals capable of PCI and the resources required, it was initially unclear if this therapy could become the dominant strategy in reperfusion therapy. Over the past 15 years, however, access to primary PCI has risen substantially and it is now the treatment of choice in 80% of cases of acute myocardial infarction [16,17]. A number of small trials have compared thrombolytic therapy with primary PCI in patients presenting to non-PCI-capable hospitals where an efficient transfer could be accomplished. In a meta-analysis, these studies similarly confirmed the superiority of primary PCI in reducing ischemic outcomes [18]. The benefits of primary PCI have been noted despite a treatment-related delay of 60–120 minutes, and in subgroups such as the elderly, those with cardiogenic shock, and late presentation, where fibrinolytic therapy was much less effective.

Current delivery standards

The benefits of reperfusion therapy via primary angioplasty is similarly time dependent [19–21]. In the first few hours there is significant opportunity for myocardial salvage with demonstrable

Interventional Cardiology: Principles and Practice, Second Edition. Edited by George D. Dangas, Carlo Di Mario, and Nicholas N. Kipshidze.
© 2017 John Wiley & Sons, Ltd. Published 2017 by John Wiley & Sons, Ltd.

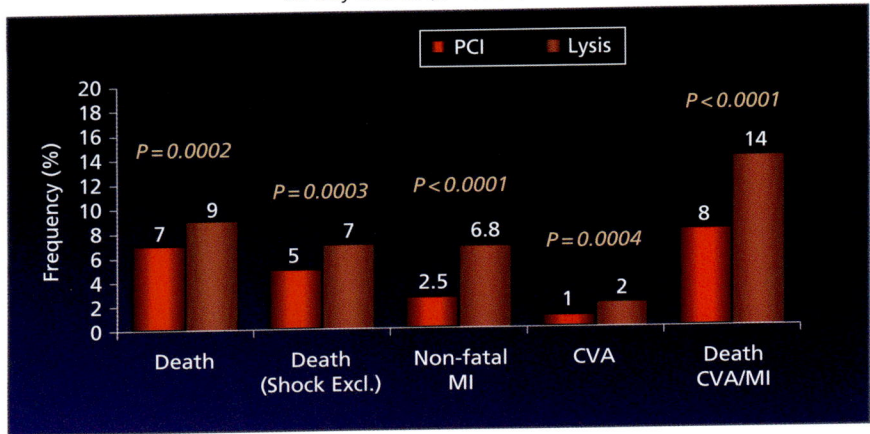

Figure 13.1 Results of 23 randomized trials of percutaneous coronary intervention (PCI) versus lysis. CVA, cerebrovascular accident. Source: Adapted from Keeley *et al*. 2003 [14].

reductions in infarct size and the greatest reductions in mortality. These benefits decline with time although outcomes with reperfusion remain better for 24 hours as long as there is evidence of ongoing ischemia. When compared with fibrinolytic therapy, primary PCI is more efficacious in patients presenting later in the course of myocardial infarction. PCI establishes better vessel patency, coronary blood flow, and tissue reperfusion, all determinants of improved outcomes [22]. The infarct-related vessel is also revascularized by stent implantation nowadays, almost eliminating the risk of recurrent ischemia and infarction [23]. However, primary PCI is associated with an inherent delay because of the logistics of performing PCI versus the ease of administering thrombolytics. PCI must be accomplished expeditiously as delay in delivery of this therapy is associated with increased mortality. The best results are seen when a door-2-reperfusion time of <90 minutes is achieved. Figure 13.2 shows the current American College of Cardiology Foundation guidelines for effective delivery of primary PCI. When arriving at a primary PCI-capable facility, a door-2-reperfusion time of <90 minutes is the treatment goal. When arriving at a non-primary PCI facility, a rapid transfer program should be in place such that total initial contact to reperfusion time does not exceed 120 minutes. Otherwise thrombolytic therapy should be first offered, if appropriate, followed by transfer for possible salvage PCI. The maximum PCI-related delay has been deduced from large registries of acute myocardial infarction and it is generally accepted that a delay of >120 minutes abolishes the advantage of primary PCI [24]. Nonetheless, in subgroups where thrombolytics perform poorly such as delayed presentation, advanced age, and cardiogenic shock, primary PCI remains preferable [22]. Substantial gains have been made in recent years at reducing door-2-reperfusion time in primary PCI through education and hospital system-wide efforts [25,26]. Unfortunately, further reductions in overall mortality have not been realized despite reductions to well below 90 minutes in recent years. Changes in demographics and patient risk could account for some of this attrition [27,28].

Technical approach and enhancements

The infarct-related vessel is occluded in most patients at the time of initial angiography. In others, a high grade stenosis is present with varying degrees of flow beyond the occlusion [22]. Thrombus accounts for most of the obstruction present and it is often easily traversed with a standard guidewire, although figuring the course of the occluded vessel can be difficult without experience. The obstruction is also easily dilatable given the contents are thrombus and soft plaque. Once dilatation has been performed, normal flow (TIMI 3) is often restored. Repeated angioplasty or stent implantation can then be performed to achieve definitive revascularization. In a few patients, angioplasty and even stent implantation does not establish normal flow. This is typically because of severe myocardial damage, tissue edema, or embolization of thrombotic debris to the distal microvasculature. In the most severe cases, referred to as no-reflow, there is no flow from the vessel into the myocardial tissue. Reperfusion in such cases is unsuccessful and the prognosis is poorer [29]. Most of the challenge that occurs in primary PCI is related to clinical and hemodynamic stability. For example, ventricular fibrillation is an ongoing risk given active severe ischemia, and acute heart failure and pulmonary edema can develop suddenly. Profound left ventricular failure and bradyarrythmias can also result in severe hypotension, shock, and cardiac arrest. The patient's clinical distress can also complicate the delicate measures required for vascular access and safe PCI, and the use of potent anticoagulants increases acute bleeding risk. The procedure must therefore be accomplished expeditiously to terminate ongoing ischemia but attention to safety and rapid management of ischemic complications cannot be understated.

The technique has evolved in much the same way as PCI for coronary disease. Optimal balloon angioplasty was the initial method of revascularization and often carried the risks of abrupt vessel closure and restenosis. Stent implantation was introduced to overcome these limitations and proved successful. In the Controlled Abciximab and Device Investigation to Lower Late Angioplasty Complication (CADILLAC) trial, stent implantation was associated with reduced risk of abrupt vessel closure, and restenosis as well as repeat revascularization at longer term follow-up were significantly reduced [30].

Drug-eluting stents These were introduced to further reduce restenosis in PCI and although there were initial concerns about increased risk of stent thrombosis, several trials have shown efficacy and safety in primary PCI. The Harmonizing Outcomes with Revascularization and Stents in AMI (HORIZONS) trial randomly

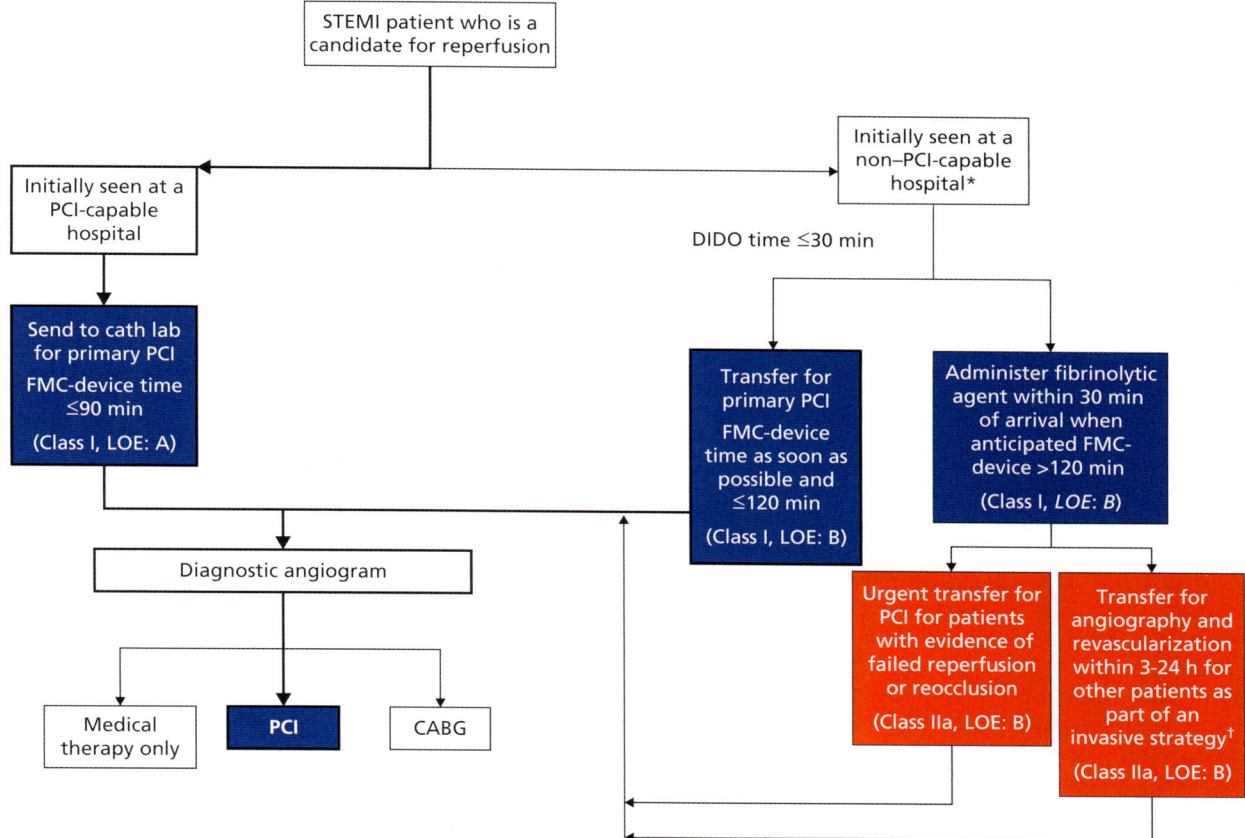

*Patients with cardiogenic shock or severe heart failure initially seen at a non–PCI-capable hospital should be transferred for cardiac catheterization and revascularization as soon as possible, irrespective of time delay from MI onset (*Class I, LOE: B*). †Angiography and revascularization should not be performed within the first 2 to 3 hours after administration of fibrinolytic therapy.

Figure 13.2 Reperfusion therapy for patients with ST-elevated myocardial infarction (STEMI). CAGB, coronary artery bypass graft; FMC, first medical contact. Source: O'Gara *et al.* 2013 [48].

assigned 3006 patients undergoing primary PCI to receive a pacli-taxel-eluting stent or a bare metal stent in 3 : 1 ratio. Ischemia-driven target lesion revascularization was reduced from 7.5% to 4.5% with no increase in stent thrombosis [31]. In a meta-analysis comparing first generation drug-eluting stents with bare metal stents, target vessel revascularization was significantly reduced and there was no increase in stent thrombosis [32]. Newer generation drug-eluting stents have further improved outcomes [33,34]. In the Clinical Evaluation of the Xience-V Stent in Acute Myocardial Infarction (EXAMINATION) trial comparing current generation everolimus-eluting stents with bare metal stents, both restenosis and stent thrombosis were reduced. Current generation drug-eluting stents are now preferred in primary PCI for better short- and longer term outcomes provided that the recommendations of dual antiplatelet therapy are feasible.

Thrombectomy The infarct vessel in primary PCI by definition contains thrombus; occasionally thrombus is extensive and compli-cates revascularization by causing distal embolization and micro-vascular occlusions. This results in failure to establish normal coronary blood flow or tissue perfusion. Both of these events have been repeatedly shown to be associated with worse outcomes including higher mortality. Thrombus burden within the coronary artery can be reduced by aspiration thrombectomy, accomplished

either by manual aspiration through a catheter or aided by a mechanical device. The technique can be applied expeditiously during primary PCI and in most trials applying thrombectomy, coronary perfusion is improved as measured by either ST-segment resolution, thrombolysis in myocardial infarction 3 (TIMI 3) flow achieved or myocardial blush score. Early data were very persuasive and the technique was widely used [35]. In two recently completed definitive large trials, however, the efficacy and safety of aspiration thrombectomy has been seriously questioned [36,37]. In the Thrombus Aspiration during ST-segment Elevation myocardial infarction (TASTE) trial, 7244 patients were randomized to receive either manual aspiration along with primary PCI or to standard primary PCI. There was no difference in primary endpoint of mor-tality at 30 days, and no difference in mortality or other major adverse cardiac events at 1 year. In the TOTAL trial, 10,732 patients were similarly randomized to adjunct manual aspiration or routine primary PCI. The primary endpoint of cardiovascular death, recur-rent myocardial infarction, cardiogenic shock, or severe heart fail-ure at 6 months was no different in the two groups. Moreover, a pre-specified safety endpoint of stroke at 30 days was increased in the aspiration group. Routine aspiration thrombectomy in primary PCI therefore can no longer be recommended based on these trials, although in special instances for severe persistent angiographic thrombus, aspiration can help enhance vessel patency.

Radial access An advance in angiography and PCI came with the use of the radial artery rather than the femoral artery for vascular access. This technique—now embraced by a substantial number of operators—is associated with reductions in major bleeding and other vascular complications. On the hand, the procedure is technically more challenging and ultimately unsuccessful in 5–10% of cases. A number of trials have evaluated radial versus femoral artery access in managing patients with acute coronary syndromes including primary PCI for STEMI. In the Radial Vs Femoral Access for Coronary Intervention (RIVAL) trial, 7021 patients with acute coronary syndromes were randomized to undergo angiography and PCI via the radial versus the femoral artery. Ischemic outcomes were comparable between the two groups; however, vascular complications were reduced from 3.8% to 1.4% in the radial arm. In a pre-specified subgroup of 1958 with STEMI, ischemic outcomes, driven by mortality, were unexpectedly reduced from 5.2% to 3.1% [38]. In the RIFLE-STEACS, 1001 patients undergoing primary PCI were similarly randomized to radial or femoral access. Outcomes with radial access were significantly better, driven by reductions in major bleeding and cardiac mortality [39]. In these as well as other trials, reperfusion time was not compromised with the radial approach. In a meta-analysis involving more than 5000 patients, mortality was reduced from 4.7% to 2.7% and major bleeding from 2.9% to 1.4% [40].

In summary, radial access in primary PCI is an attractive technique when it can be performed without compromising reperfusion times. Major vascular complications and bleeding can be reduced and there are now strong suggestions of reduced mortality. However, confirmation in more definitive trials is needed.

Mechanical support Cardiogenic shock complicates 5–7% of acute myocardial infarction and is primarily the result of left ventricular failure caused by extensive infarction or multivessel coronary disease [41,42]. Prompt revascularization is considered the most effective intervention [43] and is highly recommended; however, in many patients shock persists and results in progressive circulatory failure and multi-organ failure with a high mortality rate. Rapid support using intra-aortic balloon pump (IABP) counter pulsation was long thought to be highly effective by augmenting coronary perfusion and reducing systemic afterload. The IABP Shock II trial was designed to study the effectiveness of this intervention [44]. Six hundred patients with myocardial infarction complicated by cardiogenic shock were randomized to receive IABP support after successful primary PCI or to receive routine post-intervention care. The primary outcome of 30-day all-cause mortality was no different in both groups and at 1 year follow-up, there remained no differences in mortality or other major adverse cardiac events. It remains unclear at this point if there is a benefit of mechanical support for shock in STEMI following successful primary PCI. It is possible that a greater level of support beyond what is capable with IABP is needed and investigation is currently underway to test whether more robust support as provided with the Impella® left ventricular assist will be effective [45].

Multivessel intervention: Multivessel coronary disease is frequently noted in primary PCI and associated with a worse prognosis [46]. To date, however, guidelines have advocated focus of the infarct (culprit) vessel with additional intervention reserved for a later date or driven by ischemia,[47,48]. Part of the rationale behind this is to avoid inducing ischemia or complication in other vessel territories at the time of acute myocardial infarction. Randomized

trials to address this issue had been lacking until recently. In the Preventive Angioplasty in Myocardial Infarction (PRAMI) trial, 465 patients with multivessel disease, having undergone successful primary PCI, were randomized to undergo additional revascularization of non-culprit severe stenoses or to undergo standard care with additional intervention driven by refractory angina. Patients assigned to additional revascularization experienced significantly lower major adverse events of cardiac death, recurrent myocardial infarction, or refractory ischemia [49]. In the Complete versus Lesion-only Primary PCI (CvLPRIT) trial, 296 patients were similarly randomized and patients undergoing complete revascularization demonstrated reductions in major adverse cardiac events including cardiac death, myocardial infarction, heart failure, and ischemia-driven revascularization at 12 months [50]. These data, though preliminary, suggest more complete revascularization appears safe and beneficial in patients undergoing primary PCI. Larger, more definitive, randomized trials are needed to confirm these findings.

Salvage and rescue PCI

Despite the remarkable availability of primary PCI in many communities, this therapy cannot be delivered to all in an efficient manner with target goals described. Many patients therefore continue to receive thrombolytic therapy as their primary reperfusion strategy and outcomes are generally very good. Several studies have evolved to define how patients should be managed after thrombolytic therapy, whether successful or not. When thrombolytic therapy is considered unsuccessful, as characterized by persistent or recurrent angina and/or ST elevation, it is generally agreed that rapid PCI is effective at providing successful reperfusion [51]. The Rapid Early Action for Coronary Treatment (REACT) study showed that compared with conservative care salvage primary PCI resulted in improved major cardiovascular events for 6 months [52]. Such salvage/rescue PCI can be expected in 15–25% of patient receiving thrombolytics and so a mechanism to transfer to a PCI center should be in place.

Beyond rescue PCI, there appear to be benefits of ultimately performing urgent PCI in most patients who have received successful reperfusion with thrombolytics. Thrombolytics simply restore coronary blood flow in the infarct vessel. A high grade stenosis remains with a disrupted plaque and is a source for recurrent thrombosis or persistent ischemia. Such recurrent ischemia can be seen in up to 25% of patients and is associated with increased mortality. Several trials tested the hypothesis that routine early angiography and intervention would be superior to strategy of invasive management guided by recurrent or inducible ischemia. In the largest trial, the Trial of Routine Angioplasty and Stenting after Fibrinolysis to Enhance Reperfusion in Acute Myocardial Infarction (TRANSFER-AMI) randomized 1059 patients and found that routine PCI performed a median of 4 hours after successful fibrinolysis was associated with reductions in major adverse cardiac events [53]. In a meta-analysis of similar trials with routine PCI performed within the first 24 hours, reductions in death and myocardial infarction were demonstrated at 1 year follow-up [54].

When primary PCI cannot be delivered rapidly as in a 90-minute reperfusion time, a strategy of thrombolytic therapy with subsequent transfer for routine PCI appears to be a reasonable alternative. This is especially relevant when a patient first arrives at a hospital not capable of performing primary PCI and rapid transfer would be difficult. Rapid transfer is logistically difficult for many centers as delays eliminate the advantage of PCI over thrombolytics [55,56]. The Strategic Reperfusion Early after Myocardial Infarction (STREAM) trial randomized 1832 patients who could not receive primary PCI within expected guidelines to undergo pre-hospital fibrinolytics followed by salvage/routine PCI versus a strategy to proceed directly to primary PCI. Direct primary PCI was performed at a median of 178 minutes and >30% of the pre-hospital fibrinolytic therapy group required rescue PCI. Both arms ultimately had highly successful reperfusion and vessel patency. There was no difference in the primary endpoint of major adverse cardiac events; however, stroke was more common with the fibrinolytic arm [57].

Pharmacologic support before and during primary PCI

Pharmacologic therapy in primary PCI has evolved along with advances in supportive therapy for PCI in general, designed to enhance coronary patency, tissue level perfusion, and procedural safety. Numerous investigations of antiplatelets and antithrombins have been conducted since the initial procedural efficacy was shown utilizing standard intravenous heparin and oral aspirin.

Intra-procedural therapy investigations

To enhance thrombus management as was demonstrated with fibrinolytic therapy and in medical therapy for acute coronary syndromes, glycoprotein (GP) IIb/IIIa inhibitors were added to heparin in a series of primary PCI trials. The largest, the CADILLAC trial [58], randomized over 2000 patients to abciximab or placebo and found reductions in acute thrombotic complications including recurrent myocardial infarction. A meta-analysis of trials using abciximab showed clear reductions in recurrent myocardial infarction and trends toward lower mortality [59] but major bleeding was increased. Small molecule GP IIb/IIIa inhibitors, specifically high dose tirofiban and double bolus eptifibatide, were similarly investigated primarily in comparison with abciximab in multiple trials [60–62]. These generally showed comparable outcomes, particularly when viewed in aggregate, but no advantage in bleeding complications [63]. GP IIb/IIIa inhibitors are therefore a reasonable supportive therapy during primary PCI although they have been associated with an increase in major bleeding complications.

Bivalirudin, a potent and specific thrombin inhibitor, was introduced as an alternative to intravenous heparin in PCI and subsequently compared with strategies involving intravenous heparin with routine and then selective use of GP IIb/IIIa inhibitors. The largest trial to date was the HORIZONS trial, which randomly assigned 3602 patients to receive bivalirudin or heparin with a GP IIb/IIIa inhibitor [64]. Overall, major adverse cardiac events were not different, but major bleeding complication was reduced leading to a superior net clinical outcome. The EUROMAX trial randomized 2218 patients scheduled for primary PCI to receive bivalirudin or heparin with optional GP IIb/IIIa inhibitor [65]. Outcomes were similarly improved with the primary benefit coming from reduced bleeding complications. In both trials, an increase in acute stent thrombosis was noted but this did not affect long-term outcomes. In HEAT PPCI, 1829 patients were randomized to bivalirudin versus heparin and GP IIb/IIIa inhibitors used selectively in each group [66]. In this trial, adverse cardiovascular events including stent thrombosis were higher with bivalirudin and there was no bleeding advantage. Finally, in the recently published BRIGHT trial involving 2194 patients, bivalirudin utilizing a longer infusion

strategy was compared with a heparin alone and heparin plus GP IIb/IIIa infusion regimen [67]. There were no differences in acute ischemic outcomes; however, bleeding was lowest with the bivalirudin alone therapy. In summary, bivalirudin can be used as alternative to heparin or heparin with a GP IIb/IIIa inhibitor in primary PCI. Lower bleeding complications can be expected but there is a small risk of acute thrombotic events which can be mitigated by longer anticoagulant therapy. In a recent trial, Stone *et al.* [67] demonstrated a reduction in infarct size with intracoronary delivery of abciximab on a background of bivalirudin therapy in patients with large anterior myocardial infarction. GP IIb/IIIa inhibitors should therefore remain a consideration in selected patients even when on a background of bivalirudin.

Pre-procedural therapy investigations

To enhance early vessel patency, several drugs have been proposed to improve primary PCI efficacy, a strategy referred to as facilitated primary PCI. Among these, fibrinolytics and antiplatelets have received the most rigorous study. Early evaluations of this strategy were fraught with adverse outcomes and in a meta-analysis of these early trials Keeley and Grimes [68] found significantly higher bleeding and ischemic complications with no ischemic advantage. These studies were conducted before significant improvements in PCI technique including the use of thienopyridine oral antiplatelets and coronary stents. More contemporary evaluations began with the Facilitated Intervention with Enhanced Reperfusion Speed to Stop Events (FINESSE) trial where 2452 patients were randomly assigned to facilitated PCI using either abciximab or combined abciximab and retaplase, initiated before primary PCI, or to standard primary PCI with abciximab initiated during the procedure [69]. Facilitated PCI was associated with higher early ST-segment elevation resolution and higher baseline TIMI 3 flow rate but PCI was ultimately equally successful in both groups. There was no difference in major cardiovascular endpoints that included death, late ventricular fibrillation, cardiogenic shock, or heart failure. Major bleeding was increased with facilitated PCI. Similarly, in the Ongoing Tirofiban in Myocardial Infarction Evaluation 2 (ON-TIME 2) trial, tirofiban was randomly administered pre-hospitalization in a facilitated fashion among 936 patients undergoing primary PCI [70]. ST-segment resolution was improved as well as early stent thrombosis but overall clinical outcomes were comparable. The oral antiplatelet ticagrelor was similarly investigated as a facilitating therapy in the Administration of Ticagrelor in the Ambulance or in the Catheterization laboratory (ATLANTIC) trial [71]. A total of 1862 patients were randomly assigned to receive ticagrelor initiated in the ambulance well before primary PCI or to standard primary PCI with ticagrelor initiated in the catheterization laboratory. In this study, unlike FINESSE and ON-TIME 2, there was no improvement in ST-segment elevation resolution. There was also no difference in major clinical outcomes, although acute stent thrombosis—which occurred rarely—was further reduced with early ticagrelor.

Post-procedural therapy investigations

Recurrent thrombotic event rates are higher in patients following STEMI and contribute to late mortality and recurrent myocardial infarction. These may be the result of recurrent thrombosis of the infarct-related vessel, including stent thrombosis, or new plaque disruption and acute coronary syndrome elsewhere. As platelets have an important role in atherothrombosis, long-term oral antiplatelets have been extensively investigated. The CLARITY TIMI-28 trial first suggested the effectiveness of oral P2Y12 antagonists after myocardial infarction in patients who received thrombolytics along with aspirin [72]. In this trial, clopidogrel initiated soon after thrombolytics enhanced vessel patency at angiography days later and resulted in reduced risk for recurrent myocardial infarction at 30 days. In the Clopidogrel and Metoprolol in Myocardial Infarction Trial (COMMIT) trial, clopidogrel when added early to a large unselected population of patients with acute myocardial infarction resulted in reduced risk of overall death at as early as 4 weeks [73]. The CURRENT OASIS-7 trial investigated whether a short course of double dose clopidogrel soon after acute coronary syndrome would improve outcomes [74]. Among patients undergoing PCI, the higher dosing regimen resulted in reduced risk of recurrent myocardial infarction and stent thrombosis at 30 days. In this trial, over 6000 patients had STEMI and benefits were consistent in this group. The TRITON TIMI-38 trial tested the more potent oral thienopyridine prasugrel in patients with acute coronary syndrome including over 3500 patients with STEMI [75]. Prasugrel therapy was associated with significantly lower major adverse cardiac events, particularly recurrent myocardial infarction and stent thrombosis, over the 15-month period of study. The PLATO trial studied ticagrelor, a non-thienopyridine P2Y12 inhibitor high risk patients with acute coronary syndromes. The rate of cardiovascular death and recurrent myocardial infarction was reduced, as was stent thrombosis. There were also over 7000 patients enrolled with STEMI and outcomes were comparable [76].

In summary, dual oral antiplatelet therapies improve outcomes in acute myocardial infarction managed with PCI. More potent agents appear to further reduce the risk of recurrent thrombotic events including recurrent myocardial infarction and stent thrombosis compared with standard dose clopidogrel. These agents should therefore be initiated as early as feasible and continued long term as suggested by guidelines.

Myocardial conditioning

The prospect of protecting the myocardium from irreversible damage during acute myocardial infarction has long been considered the holy grail in this line of therapy. To date only early reperfusion therapy has been proven to terminate and minimize extent of injury. Nonetheless, several investigations have explored pathways such as reducing cardiac mechanical work, enhancing ischemic adaptation, enhancing tissue level perfusion, delivering supplemental oxygen, manipulating metabolism, and reducing free radical damage. In the CRISP-AMI trial, the use of IABP counter-pulsation aimed at reducing cardiac work did not reduce infarct size among 337 patients with anterior myocardial infarction [77]. The IABP SHOCK II trial also found no benefit of this therapy in patients with cardiogenic shock following successful primary PCI. Remote ischemic preconditioning to enhance ischemic adaptation has been applied successfully in transplantation organ harvest and minimizes injury during cardiac surgery. Botker et al. [78] tested intermittent forearm ischemia using blood pressure inflation in 333 patients with acute ST-elevation myocardial infarction (STEMI). A reduction in infarct size was noted; however, given the limited study size, a larger clinical is needed. Vasodilatation of the microvasculature during acute ischemic injury was proposed to be protective and initially appeared promising with adenosine. However, the Acute Myocardial Infarction Study of Adenosine-II (AMISTAD-II) trial tested this hypothesis in 2118 patients and found no significant improvement in infarct size or clinical

outcomes [79]. In the AMIHOT trials, the effect of supersaturated oxygen therapy was tested in patients with acute myocardial infarction [80,81]. A reduction in infarct size was noted in patients with anterior myocardial infarction treated. However, given the small sample size, a larger trial powered for clinical endpoints is needed. To minimize energy consumption by switching from fatty acid metabolism to glucose metabolism, the CREATE-ECLA trial evaluated the effect of a glucose insulin potassium infusion in 20,201 patients with acute STEMI [82]. Despite prior positive preliminary data, there was no effect on mortality or other major adverse events including cardiogenic shock, cardiac arrest, or reinfarction. To combat inflammation and cell death via the complement pathway, the APEX-AMI investigators tested the monoclonal antibody pexelizumab in over 5700 patients with acute myocardial infarction undergoing primary PCI [83]. There was no effect on mortality or endpoints such as cardiogenic shock at 30 or 90 days.

In summary, the ability to limit myocardial damage from prolonged ischemia in acute myocardial infarction has remained unproven. While more investigation is needed, the most effective intervention to date remains early recognition of STEMI and rapid mechanical reperfusion via primary PCI.

Interactive multiple choice questions are available for this chapter on www.wiley. com/go/dangas/cardiology.

References

1 Falk E, Nakano M, Bentzon JF, Finn AV, Virmani R. Update on acute coronary syndromes: the pathologists' view. *Eur Heart J* 2013; **34**: 719–728.

2 Gruppo Italiano per lo Studio della Streptochinasi nell'nfarctio Miocardico (GISSI). Effectiveness of intravenous thrombolytic treatment in acute myocardial infarction. *Lancet* 1986; **1**: 397–402.

3 Second International Study of Infarct Survival (ISIS-2) Collaborative Group. Randomized trial of intravenous streptokinase, oral aspirin, both, or neither among 17,187 cases of suspected acute myocardial infarction: ISIS-2. *Lancet* 1988; **2**: 349–360.

4 Third International Study of Infarct Survival (ISIS-3) Collaborative Group. ISIS-3: a randomized comparison of streptokinase vs tissue plasminogen activator vs anistreplase and of aspirin plus heparin vs aspirin alone in 41,299 cases of suspected acute myocardial infarction. *Lancet* 1992; **339**: 753–770.

5 The GUSTO Investigators. An international randomized trial comparing four thrombolytic strategies for acute myocardial infarction. *N Engl J Med* 1993; **329**: 673–682.

6 The GUSTO III Investigators. An International, multicenter, randomized comparison of reteplase with alteplase for acute myocardial infarction. *N Engl J Med* 1997; **337**: 1118–1123.

7 The GUSTO V Investigators. Reperfusion therapy for acute myocardial infarction with fibrinolytic therapy or combination low dose fibrinolytic therapy and platelet glycoprotein IIb/IIa inhibition: The GUSTO 5 Trial. *Lancet* 2001; **357**: 1905–1914.

8 HERO-2 Trial Investigators. Thrombin-specific anticoagulation with bivalirudin versus heparin in patients receiving fibrinolytic therapy for acute myocardial infarction: the HERO-2 Trial. *Lancet* 2002; **358**: 1855–1863.

9 OASIS-6 Trial Group. Effects of fondaparinux on mortality and reinfarction in patients with acute ST-segment elevation myocardial infarction. *JAMA* 2006; **295**: 1519–1530.

10 ExTRACT-TIMI 25 Investigators. Enoxaparin versus unfractionated heparin with fibrinolysis for acute myocardial infarction. *N Eng J Med* 2006; **354**: 1477–1488.

11 GUSTO Angiographic Investigators. The effects of tissue plasminogen activator, streptokinase or both on coronary artery patency, ventricular function, and survival after acute myocardial infarction. *N Engl J Med* 1993; **329**: 1615–1622.

12 O'Keefe J Jr, Bailey WL, Rutherford BD, Hartzler GO. Primary angioplasty for acute myocardial infarction in 1,000 consecutive patients: results in an unselected population and high-risk subgroups. *Am J Cardiol* 1993; **72**: 107G.

13 Every NR, Parsons LS, Hlatky M, Martin JS, Weaver WD. A comparison of thrombolytic therapy with primary coronary angioplasty for acute myocardial infarction. Myocardial Infarction Triage and Intervention Investigators. *N Engl J Med* 1996; **335**: 1253–1260.

14 Keeley E, Boura JA, Grines CL. Primary angioplasty versus intravenous thrombolytic therapy for acute myocardial infarction: a quantitative review of 23 randomized trials. *Lancet* 2003; **361**: 13–20.

15 Stenestrand U, Lindbäck J, Wallentin L; RIKS-HIA Registry. Long-term outcome of primary percutaneous coronary intervention vs prehospital and in-hospital thrombolysis for patients with ST-segment elevation myocardial infarction. *JAMA* 2006; **296**: 1749–1756.

16 Sugiyama T, Hasegawa K, Kobayashi Y, Takahashi O, Fukui T, Tsugawa Y. Differential time trends of outcomes and costs of care for acute myocardial infarction hospitalizations by ST elevation and type of intervention in the United States, 2001–2011. *J Am Heart Assoc* 2015; **4**: e001445.

17 Kristensen S, Laut KG, Fajadet J, et al. Reperfusion therapy for ST elevation myocardial Infarction 2010/2011: current status in 37 ESC countries. *Eur Heart J* 2014; **35**: 1957–1970.

18 Dalby M, Bouzamondo A, Lechat P, Montalescot G. Transfer for primary angioplasty versus immediate thrombolysis in acute myocardial infarction: a meta-analysis. *Circulation* 2003; **108**: 1809–1814.

19 De Luca G, Suryapranata H, Zijlstra F, et al. Symptom onset-to-balloon time and mortality in patients with acute myocardial infarction treated with primary angioplasty. *J Am Coll Cardiol* 2003; **42**: 991–997.

20 Brodie B, Hansen C, Stuckey TD, et al. Door-to-balloon time with primary percutaneous coronary intervention for acute myocardial infarction impacts late mortality in high-risk patients and patients presenting early after the onset of symptoms. *J Am Coll Cardiol* 2006; **47**: 289–295.

21 McNamara R, Wang Y, Herrin J, et al. Effect of door-to-balloon time on mortality in patients with ST-segment elevation myocardial infarction. *J Am Coll Cardiol* 2006; **47**: 2180–2186.

22 GUSTO IIb Angioplasty Substudy Investigators. A clinical trial comparing primary angioplasty with tissue plasminogen activator for acute myocardial infarction. *N Engl J Med* 1997; **336**: 1621–1628.

23 Armstrong PW, Fu Y, Chang WC, et al. GUSTO-IIb Investigators. Acute coronary syndromes in the GUSTO-IIb trial: prognostic insights and the impact of recurrent ischemia. *Circulation* 1998; **98**: 1860–1868.

24 Pinto D, Kirtane AJ, Nallamothu BK, et al. Hospital delays in reperfusion therapy for ST-segment elevation myocardial infarction: implications when selecting a reperfusion strategy. *Circulation* 2006; **114**: 2019–2025.

25 Jacobs AK, Antman EM, Ellrodt G, et al. Recommendation to develop strategies to increase the number of ST-segment elevation myocardial infarction patients with timely access to primary percutaneous coronary intervention. *Circulation* 2006; **113**: 2152–2163.

26 Krumholtz HM, Herrin J, Miller LE, et al. Improvements in door-to-balloon time in the United States, 2005 to 2010. *Circulation* 2011; **124**: 1038–1045.

27 Menees DS, Peterson ED, Wang Y, et al. Door-to-balloon time and mortality among patients undergoing primary PCI. *N Engl J Med* 2013; **369**: 901–909.

28 Nallamothu BK, NormandSL, Wang Y, et al. Relation between door-to-balloon times and mortality after primary percutaneous intervention over time: a retrospectively study. *Lancet* 2015; **385**: 1114–1122.

29 Rezkalla S, Kloner R. No-reflow phenomenon. *Circulation* 2002; **105**: 656–662.

30 Stone GW, Grines CL, Cox DA, et al. CADILLAC Investigators. Comparison of angioplasty or stenting, with or without abciximab in acute myocardial infarction. *N Engl J Med* 2002; **369**: 957–966.

31 Stone GW, Lansky AJ, Pocock SJ, et al. HORIZONS AMI trial investigators. Paclitaxel-eluting stents versus bare metal stents in acute myocardial infarction. *N Engl J Med* 2009; **360**: 1946–1959.

32 Kastrati A, Dibra A, Spaulding C, et al. Meta-analysis of randomized trials on drug eluting stents versus bare metal stents in acute myocardial infarction. *Eur Heart J* 2007; **28**: 2706–2713.

33 Sabate M, Cequier A, Iñiguez A, et al. Everolimus-eluting stent versus bare-metal stent in ST-segment elevation myocardial infarction (EXAMINATION): 1 year results of a randomized trial. *Lancet* 2012; **380**: 1482–1490.

34 Sabate M, Räber L, Heg D, et al. Comparison of newer-generation drug-eluting with bare-metal stents in patients with acute ST-elevation myocardial infarction: a pooled analysis of EXAMINATION and COMFORTABLE-AMI trials. *JACC Cardiovasc Interv* 2014; **7**: 55–63.

35 Svilaas T, Vlaar PJ, van der Horst IC, et al. TAPAS trial investigators. Thrombus aspiration during primary percutaneous coronary intervention. *N Engl J Med* 2008; **358**: 557–567.

36 Lagergvist B, Fröbert O, Olivecrona GK, et al. TASTE Trial investigators. Thrombus aspiration during ST segment elevation myocardial infarction. *N Engl J Med* 2014; **371**: 1111–1120.

37 Jolly S, Cairns JA, Yusuf S, et al. TOTAL Investigators. Randomized trial of manual aspiration with or without routine manual thrombectomy. *N Engl J Med* 2015; **372**: 1389–1398.

38 Mehta SR, Jolly S, Cairns J, et al. RIVAL investigators. Effects or radial versus femoral access in patients with acute coronary syndromes with or without ST-segment elevation. *J Am Coll Cardiol* 2012; **60**: 2490–2499.

39 Ramagnoli E, Bioni-Zoccai G, Sciahbasi A, et al. Radial versus femoral intervention in ST-segment elevation acute coronary syndrome: the RIFLE-STEACS study. *J Am Coll Cardiol* 2012; **60**: 2481–2489.

40 Karrowni W, Vyas A, Giacomino B, et al. Radial versus femoral access for primary percutaneous interventions in ST-segment elevation myocardial infarction: a meta-analysis of randomized trials. *JACC Cardiovasc Interv* 2013; **6**: 814–823.

41 Goldberg R, Spencer FA, Gore JM, et al. Thirty-year trends (1975 to 2005) in the magnitude of, management of, and hospital death rates associated with cardiogenic shock in patients with acute myocardial infarction: a population-based perspective. *Circulation* 2009; **119**: 1211–1219.

42 Babaev A, Frederick PD, Pasta DJ, et al. Trends in the management and outcomes of patients with acute myocardial infarction complicated by cardiogenic shock. *JAMA* 2005; **294**: 448–454.

43 Hochman JS, Sleeper LA, White HD, et al. One-year survival following early revascularization for cardiogenic shock. *JAMA* 2001; **285**: 190–192.

44 Thiele H, Schuler G, Neumann FJ, et al. Intra-aortic balloon pump counterpulsation in acute myocardial infarction complicated by cardiogenic shock (IABP-SHOCK II trial). *Lancet* 2013; **382**: 1638–1645.

45 O'Neill W, Kleiman NS, Moses J, et al. A prospective, randomized clinical trial of hemodynamic support with Impella 2.5 versus intra-aortic balloon pump in patients undergoing high risk percutaneous coronary intervention: the PROTECT II trial. *Circulation* 2012; **126**: 1717–1726.

46 Park DW, Clare RM, Schulte PJ, et al. Extent, location, and clinical significance of non-infarct-related coronary artery disease among patients with ST-elevation myocardial infarction. *JAMA* 2014; **312**: 2019–2027.

47 ESC guidelines for the management of acute myocardial infarction in patients presenting with ST-segment elevation. *Eur Heart J* 2012; **33**: 2569–2619.

48 O'Gara P, Kushner FG, Ascheim DD, et al. 2013 ACCF/AHA guideline for the management of ST-elevation myocardial infarction. a report of the ACCF/AHA task force on practice guidelines. *J Am Coll Cardiol* 2013; **61**: e78–140.

49 Wald D, Morris JK, Wald NJ, et al. Randomized trial of preventive angioplasty in myocardial infarction. *N Engl J Med* 2013; **369**: 1115–1123.

50 Gershlick A, Khan JN, Kelly DJ, et al. Randomized trial of complete versus lesion-only revascularization in patients undergoing primary PCI for STEMI and multivessel disease: the CvLPRIT trial. *J Am Coll Cardiol* 2015; **65**: 963–972.

51 Wijeysundera H, Vijayaraghavan R, Nallamothu BK, et al. Rescue angioplasty or repeat fibrinolysis after failed fibrinolytic therapy for ST-segment elevation myocardial infarction: a meta-analysis of randomized trials. *J Am Coll Cardiol* 2007; **49**: 422–430.

52 Gershlick A, Stephens-Lloyd A, Hughes S, et al. Rescue angioplasty after failed thrombolytic therapy for acute myocardial infarction. *N Engl J Med* 2005; **353**: 2758–2768.

53 TRANSFER-AMI trial investigators. Routine early angioplasty after fibrinolysis for acute myocardial infarction. *N Engl J Med* 2009; **360**: 2075–2018.

54 D'Souza SP, Mamas MA, Fraser DG, et al. Routine early coronary angioplasty versus ischaemia-guided angioplasty after thrombolysis in ST-elevation myocardial infarction: a meta-analysis. *Eur Heart J* 2011; **32**: 972–982.

55 Nallamothu BK, Bates ER, herrin J, et al. Times to treatment in transfer patients undergoing primary percutaneous coronary intervention in the United States: National Registry of Myocardial Infarction (NRMI)-3/4 analysis. *Circulation* 2005; **111**: 761–767.

56 Pinto D, Frederick PD, Chakrabarti AK, et al. Benefit of transferring ST-segment elevation myocardial infarction patients for percutaneous coronary intervention compared with onsite fibrinolytic declines as delay increases. *Circulation* 2011; **124**: 2512.

57 STREAM Investigative team. Fibrinolysis or primary PCI in ST elevation myocardial infarction. *N Engl J Med* 2013; **368**: 1379–1387.

58 Stone G, Grines CL, Cox DA, et al. Comparison of angioplasty or stenting, with or without abciximab in acute myocardial infarction. *N Engl J Med* 2002; **369**: 957–966.

59 De Luca G, Suryapranata H, Stone GW, et al. Abciximab as adjunct to reperfusion in ST-segment elevation myocardial infarction: a meta-analysis of randomized trials. *JAMA* 2005; **293**: 1759–1765.

60 Valgimigli M, Campo G, Gambetti S, et al. Tirofiban and sirolimus-eluting stent vs abciximab and bare-metal stent for acute myocardial infarction: a randomized trial. *JAMA* 2005; **293**: 2109–2117.

61 Akerblom A, James SK, Koutouzis M, et al. Eptifibatide is noninferior to abciximab in primary percuta neous coronary intervention: results from the SCAAR (Swedish Coronary Angiography and Angioplasty Registry). *J Am Coll Cardiol* 2010; **56**: 470–475.

62 De Luca G, Ucci G, Cassetti E, Marino P. Benefits of small molecule administration as compared with abciximab among patients with ST-segment myocardial infarction treated with primary angioplasty: a meta-analysis. *J Am Coll Cardiol* 2009; **53**: 1668–1673.

63 Stone G, Witzenbichler B, Guagliumi G, *et al;* HORIZONS AMI trial investigators. Bivalirudin during primary PCI in acute myocardial infarction. *N Engl J Med* 2008; **358**: 2218–2230.

64 Steg PG, van't Hof A, Hamm CW, *et al;* EUROMAX investigators. Bivalirudin started during emergency transport for primary PCI. *N Engl J Med* 2013; **369**: 2207–2217.

65 Shahzad A, Kemp I, Mars C, *et al.* HEAT-PPCI investigators: Unfractionated heparin versus bivalirudin in primary percutaneous coronary intervention. *Lancet* 2014; **384**: 1849–1858.

66 BRIGHT investigators. Bivalirudin versus heparin with or without tirofiban during primary percutaneous intervention in acute myocardial infarction. *JAMA* 2015; **313**: 1336–1346.

67 Stone GW, Maehara A, Witzenbichler B, *et al.* Intracoronary abciximab and aspiration thrombectomy in patients with large anterior myocardial infarction: the INFUSE-AMI randomized trial. *JAMA* 2012; **307**: 1817–1826.

68 Keeley EC, Boura JA, Grines CL. Comparison of primary and facilitated percutaneous coronary intervention for ST-segment elevation infarction: quantitative review of randomized trials. *Lancet* 2006; **367**: 578–586.

69 FINESSE investigators. Facilitated PCI in patients with ST-segment elevation myocardial infarction. *N Engl J Med* 2008; **358**: 2205–2217.

70 ON-TIME 2 study group. Prehospitalization of Tirofiban in patients with acute myocardial infarction undergoing primary angioplasty. *Lancet* 2008; **372**: 537–546.

71 ATLANTIC investigators. Prehospital ticagrelor in ST segment elevation myocardial infarction. *N Engl J Med* 2014; **371**: 1016–1027.

72 Sabatine MS, Cannon CP, Gibson CM, *et al.* Addition of clopidogrel to aspirin and fibrinolytic therapy after myocardial infarction with ST-segment elevation. *N Engl J Med* 2005; **352**: 1179–1189.

73 Chen Z, Jiang LX, Chen YP, *et al.* Addition of clopidogrel to aspirin in 45,852 patients with acute myocardial infarction. *Lancet* 2005; **366**: 1607–1621.

74 Mehta S, Tanquay JF, Eikelboom JW, *et al.* Double-dose versus standard dose clopidogrel and high-dose versus low-dose aspirin in individuals undergoing percutaneous coronary for acute coronary syndromes. (CURRENT-OASIS 7): a randomized factorial trial. *Lancet* 2010; **376**: 1233–1243.

75 Montalescot G, Wiviott SD, Braunwald E, *et al.* Prasugrel compared with clopidogrel in patients undergoing percutaneous revascularization for ST segment elevation myocardial infarction. *Lancet* 2009; **373**: 723–731.

76 Steg PG, James S, Harrington RA, *et al.* Ticagrelor versus clopidogrel in patients with ST-segment elevation acute coronary syndromes intended for reperfusion with primary percutaneous coronary intervention: PLATO trial subgroup analysis. *Circulation* 1210; **122**: 2131.

77 Patel M, Smalling RW, Thiele H, *et al.* Intra-aortic balloon counterpulsation and infarct size in patients with acute myocardial infarction and without shock: the CRISP-AMI randomized trial. *JAMA* 2011; **306**: 1329–1337.

78 Botker H, Kharbanda R, Schmidt MR, *et al.* Remote ischemic conditioning before hospital admission, as a complement to angioplasty, and effect on myocardial salvage in patients with acute myocardial infarction. *Lancet* 2010; **375**: 727–734.

79 Ross A, Gibbons RJ, Stone GW, *et al.* A randomized, double-blinded, placebo-controlled multi-center trial of adenosine as an adjunct to reperfusion in the treatment of acute myocardial infarction (AMISTAD-II). *J Am Coll Cardiol* 2005; **45**: 1775–1780.

80 Stone G, Martin JL, de Boer MJ, *et al.* Effect of supersaturated oxygen delivery on infarct size after percutaneous coronary intervention in acute myocardial infarction. *Circ Cardiovasc Interv* 2009; **2**: 366–375.

81 O'Neill, Martin JL, Dixon SR, *et al.* Acute myocardial infarction with hyperoxemic therapy: a prospective randomized trial of intracoronary hyperoxemic reperfusion after percutaneous coronary intervention. *J Am Coll Cardiol* 2007; **50**: 397–405.

82 Mehta S, Yusuf S, Diaz R, *et al.* Effect of glucose-insulin-potassium infusion on mortality in patients with acute ST-segment elevation myocardial infarction: the CREATE-ECLA randomized trial. *JAMA* 2005; **293**: 437–446.

83 Armstrong P, Granger CB, Adams PX, *et al;* APEX-AMI Investigators. Pexelizumab for ST-elevation acute myocardial infarction in patients undergoing primary percutaneous coronary intervention. *JAMA* 2007; **297**: 43–51.

CHAPTER 14

The Management of Cardiogenic Shock and Hemodynamic Support Devices and Techniques

Bimmer E.P.M. Claessen, Dagmar Ouweneel, and José P.S. Henriques

Department of Cardiology, Academic Medical Center—University of Amsterdam, Amsterdam, The Netherlands

Even in the current era of primary percutaneous intervention (PCI), cardiogenic shock remains a dramatic and lethal condition. The incidence of cardiogenic shock after myocardial infarction (MI) appears to be lowering from about 10% in the 1970s and 1980s to about 5–6% currently, potentially as a result of improvement in time-to-reperfusion and as a result of better techniques for reperfusion (primary PCI compared with thrombolysis) [1–5]. However, mortality after MI remains very high with recent studies reporting mortality rates of 40–65% [5,6]. This chapter reviews evidence on medical and mechanical management of cardiogenic shock.

Definition of shock

Shock is defined as a clinical condition where there is inadequate end-organ perfusion caused by failure of the heart to pump blood in adequate quantities. There is currently no uniform definition of cardiogenic shock in clinical practice or for research purposes. A couple of influential randomized clinical trials use definitions that are similar, but not identical.

In the SHOCK (should we emergently revascularize occluded coronaries for cardiogenic shock) trial, cardiogenic shock was defined by a combination of clinical and hemodynamic criteria [7,8]. Clinical criteria in SHOCK were hypotension (a systolic blood pressure of <90 mmHg for at least 30 minutes or the need for supportive measures to maintain a systolic blood pressure of ≥90 mmHg) and end-organ hypoperfusion (cool extremities or a urine output of <30 mL/hour, and a heart rate of ≥60 bpm). The hemodynamic criteria were a cardiac index of no more than 2.2 L/minute/m^2 of body-surface area and a pulmonary capillary wedge pressure of at least 15 mmHg [7,8].

In the IABP-SHOCK II (intra-aortic balloon pump in cardiogenic shock) trial, the following definition was used:
1 A systolic blood pressure of less than 90 mmHg for more than 30 minutes or needing infusion of catecholamines to maintain a systolic pressure above 90 mmHg;
2 Clinical signs of pulmonary congestion; and
3 Impaired end-organ perfusion.
The diagnosis of impaired end-organ perfusion required at least one of the following: altered mental status; cold, clammy skin and extremities; oliguria with urine output of less than 30 mL/hour; or serum lactate level higher than 2.0 mmol/L [9].

Epidemiology

Cardiogenic shock after MI occurs in about 5–6% of cases in the current era of primary PCI, and occurred in about 10% of cases in the era before rapid mechanical reperfusion [1–5]. The incidence of cardiogenic shock may have declined, but mortality after cardiogenic shock remains very high, even in contemporary cohorts, with mortality rates of 40–60% [10,11].

An early study of 845 patients presenting with acute MI, not treated with thrombolysis or mechanical reperfusion, investigated risk factors for the occurrence of cardiogenic shock [1]. In this study, cardiogenic shock occurred in 60 patients (7.1%). Predictors of cardiogenic shock included age >65 years, left ventricular ejection fraction at hospital admission <35%, large infarct size (peak creatine kinase-MB isoenzyme >160 IU/L), diabetes mellitus, and previous MI. Risk factors in the GUSTO (Global Utilization of Streptokinase and Tissue-plasminogen activator for Occluded coronary arteries) trial, conducted in the era of thrombolysis, included: age, systolic blood pressure, heart rate, and Killip class upon presentation [12].

In the large (n = 5745) APEX-AMI (assessment of pexelizumab in acute MI) trial, the incidence of shock was only 3.4% (n = 196), most likely because this randomized controlled trial enrolled a relatively low-risk patient population [11]. In APEX-AMI the following risk factors for developing cardiogenic shock were identified: older age, female sex, hypertension, diabetes mellitus, and being a non-smoker.

Management of cardiogenic shock
Impact of coronary revascularization

Since the shock trial, early revascularization has been recognized as the primary treatment modality for cardiogenic shock. Current American College of Cardiology/American Heart Association (ACC/AHA) guidelines state a class I, level of evidence B indication for emergency revascularization with either PCI or coronary artery bypass graft (CABG) in suitable patients with cardiogenic shock from pump failure after ST-elevation myocardial infarction (STEMI) irrespective of the time delay from MI onset [13].

Interventional Cardiology: Principles and Practice, Second Edition. Edited by George D. Dangas, Carlo Di Mario, and Nicholas N. Kipshidze.
© 2017 John Wiley & Sons, Ltd. Published 2017 by John Wiley & Sons, Ltd.

The landmark SHOCK trial randomized 302 patients with cardiogenic shock complicating MI in a 1 : 1 fashion to treatment with emergency revascularization (n = 152) or initial medical stabilization (n = 150). Revascularization incorporated emergency coronary angiography followed by either CABG or PCI. In the SHOCK trial, 30-day mortality rates were numerically lower in the early revascularization arm (46.7% vs. 56.0%; p = 0.11). However, at 6 months mortality rates were significantly lower with early revascularization (50.3% vs. 63.1%; p = 0.027) [7]. Furthermore, emergency revascularization was not only associated with improved survival, but also with improved quality of life, assessed by the multidimensional index of life quality and New York Heart Association (NYHA) heart failure class [14].

An important substudy investigated the clinical outcome in patients assigned to emergency revascularization in the SHOCK trial undergoing PCI compared with CABG [15]. Out of 128 patients undergoing emergency revascularization, 81 underwent PCI (63.3%) and 47 underwent CABG (36.7%). Patients undergoing CABG were at higher risk at baseline with a greater extent of coronary artery disease and a greater prevalence of diabetes mellitus. In the CABG group, 87.2% of patients were considered completely revascularized whereas only 23.1% of patients in the PCI group were considered completely revascularized. Despite the higher baseline risk profile of patients undergoing CABG, 1-year survival was similar in both treatment arms, suggesting a potential benefit of complete revascularization. Partly because of this substudy, current guidelines recommend complete revascularization during PCI for cardiogenic shock, as compared with culprit-vessel only PCI for MI without cardiogenic shock [13,16].

Left-ventricular assist devices and the intra-aortic balloon pump

Mechanical support devices aim to overcome the inability of the heart to pump adequate amounts of blood by supporting the circulation and increasing cardiac output. Moreover, support devices aim to unload the damaged left ventricle by afterload (pressure unloading) or pre-load reduction (volume unloading). Currently available devices include the intra-aortic balloon pump (IABP), the Impella axial flow pump, the TandemHeart device, and extracorporeal membrane oxygenation (ECMO) [17]. An overview of various characteristics of these devices is provided in Table 14.1.

IABP The IABP was introduced 1968. It is inserted percutaneously in the femoral artery and positioned in the descending thoracic aorta distal to the left subclavian artery and proximal to the renal artery branches. The IABP aims to augment coronary blood flow and systemic blood flow during diastole. The balloon is synchronized to the cardiac cycle and is rapidly inflated with helium gas during diastole and rapidly deflated immediately before systole. In a small study that randomized 40 patients in cardiogenic shock to optimal medical therapy alone or to optimal medical therapy and an IABP, no significant differences were observed in hemodynamic parameters such as cardiac output and systemic vascular resistance between the groups [18]. The IABP SHOCK II trial randomized 600 patients with cardiogenic shock complicating MI to treatment with an IABP or no IABP. Early revascularization and optimal medical therapy was provided in both study arms. The use of the IABP did not reduce 30-day or 1-year mortality [6,10]. Moreover, there were no differences in time to hemodynamic stabilization, the length of intensive care unit stay, serum lactate levels, dose and duration of catecholamine administration, or renal function [6].

Impella The Impella consists of a pigtail catheter at the tip functioning as the inlet for blood which is positioned in the left ventricle and uses a micro-axial rotary pump which is placed across the aortic valve to continuously expel blood into the aorta. There are three versions of the impella system: the Impella 2.5 which delivers up to 2.5 L/min of flow; the Impella CP delivering up to 3.5–4.0 L/min of flow which are both inserted percutaneously; and the Impella 5.0 which delivers up to 5.0 L/min but requires a surgical cutdown for insertion [17]. Currently available evidence on the use of the Impella device in cardiogenic shock is limited to observational studies and a small randomized trial [19–21]. In the ISAR-SHOCK (efficacy study of LV assist device to treat patients with cardiogenic shock) trial, 26 patients with cardiogenic shock were randomized to IABP or Impella [19]. In this small study the cardiac index after 30 minutes of support was significantly higher in the Impella group compared with the IABP group (delta 0.49 ± 0.46 L/min/m^2 vs. 0.11 ± 0.31 L/min/m^2; p = 0.02). Overall 30-day mortality was similar in both groups.

TandemHeart The TandemHeart uses a continuous flow centrifugal pump which can deliver up to 4 L/min of blood flow. It can be inserted using fluoroscopy guidance in the catheterization laboratory. The inflow cannula is inserted through the femoral vein and guided to the left atrium via an atrial septal puncture. The outflow cannula is inserted through the femoral artery and positioned at the level of the aortic bifurcation. In two small randomized clinical trials enrolling about 40 patients each, the TandemHeart was associated with significant improvements in hemodynamic parameters when compared with the IABP [22,23]. However, without direct left ventricular unloading the TandemHeart increases left ventricular afterload which partially offsets the potential cardiac workload benefits. Other concerns with the TandemHeart are the complications (bleeding and limb ischemia) and the complex insertion procedure.

ECMO Venoarterial ECMO consists of a centrifugal pump, a heat exchanger, and a membrane oxygenator. Venous blood is aspirated from the right atrium via the femoral vein, it is then guided to a pump which directs it to a membrane oxygenator, and is then guided via the outflow cannula into the descending aorta via the femoral artery. As this is quite a complex machine, it is associated with complications such as systemic inflammatory response, renal failure limb ischemia, and bleeding. Moreover, it increases both the afterload and the pre-load of the left ventricle resulting in increased oxygen demand which impedes myocardial protection [24].

Guideline recommendations for the IABP and left ventricular assist devices The 2014 European Society of Cardiology and the European Association for Cardio-Thoracic Surgery (ESC/EACTS) guidelines for myocardial revascularization no longer recommend the use of IABP in patients with cardiogenic shock (class III recommendation, level of eveidence A) [16]. These guidelines state a class IIb, level of evidence C recommendation for the use of left ventricular assist devices "short-term mechanical circulatory support in ACS patients with cardiogenic shock may be considered." The 2013 ACC/AHA guidelines state a class IIa level of evidence B recommendation for the use of the IABP. "The use of intra-aortic balloon pump (IABP) counterpulsation can be useful for patients with cardiogenic shock after STEMI who do not quickly stabilize with pharmacological therapy" [13]. The ACC/AHA recommendation for left ventricular assist devices is class IIb, level of evidence C "Alternative LV assist devices for circulatory support may be considered in patients with refractory cardiogenic shock."

Table 14.1 Overview of mechanical support devices.

	IABP	ECMO	TandemHeart	Impella 2.5	Impella CP	Impella 5.0
Pump mechanism	Pneumatic	Centrifugal	Centrifugal	Axial flow	Axial flow	Axial flow
Cannula size	7–9 Fr	18–21 Fr inflow; 15–22 Fr outflow	21 Fr inflow; 15–17 Fr outflow	13 Fr	14 Fr	22 Fr; Surgical cut-down
Insertion technique	Descending aorta via the femoral artery	Inflow cannula into the right atrium via the femoral vein, outflow cannula into descending aorta via femoral artery	21 Fr inflow cannula into left atrium via femoral vein and trans-septal puncture and 15–17 Fr outflow cannula into femoral artery	12 Fr catheter placed retrograde across the aortic valve via the femoral artery	14 Fr catheter placed retrograde across the aortic valve via the femoral artery	21 Fr catheter placed retrograde across the aortic valve via a surgical cut-down of the femoral artery
Hemodynamic support (L/min)	0.5–1.0	>4.5	4	2.5	3.5–4.0	5.0
Implantation time	+	++	++++	++	++	++++
Risk of limb ischemia	+	+++	+++	++	++	++
Anticoagulation	+	+++	+++	+	+	+
Hemolysis	+	++	++	++	++	++
Requires stable heart rhythm	Yes	No	No	No	No	No
Post-implantation management complexity	+	+++	++++	++	++	++

Source: Adapted from Ouweneel and Henriques 2012 [17]. Reproduced with permission of BMJ Publishing and the British Cardiovascular Society.

Vasopressors and inotropes

Rapid treatment of hypoperfusion and hypotension is essential when dealing with cardiogenic shock. Inotropes can be used to increase cardiac output and vasopressors to increase blood pressure. However, inotropes and vasopressors increase myocardial oxygen consumption and current guidelines suggest their use should be assessed on an individual patient basis [13]. Sympathomimetic agents are most commonly used in the setting of cardiogenic shock, but phosphodiesterase inhibitors and calcium sensitizers are also sometimes used.

Sympathomimetic agents Norephinephrine has a high affinity for the alpha-adrenergic receptor and has minor beta-agonistic effects. Therefore, norepinephrine is a potent vasopressor with limited inotropic effects. Dopamine has a variety of effects depending on the dosage. At low doses (1–2 µg/kg/min) it increases urine output by augmenting renal blood flow and natriuresis [25,26]. At intermediate doses (5–10 µg/kg/min) dopamine stimulates beta-1 adrenergic receptors, allowing for an increased stroke volume and an increased heart rate, increasing cardiac output. At high doses (>10 µg/kg/min) dopamine predominantly stimulates alpha-adrenergic receptors, causing vasoconstriction. A randomized study of 1679 patients with shock (septic, hypovolemic, and cardiogenic) assigned to dopamine or norepinephrine as the first line vasopressor showed more arrhythmic events in the dopamine group (24.1% vs. 12.4%; p <0.001). A subgroup analysis of patients with cardiogenic shock showed that dopamine was associated with increased 28-day mortality compared with norepinephrine [27]. An alternative is dobutamine, which is a synthethic catecholamine with strong beta-1 and beta-2 receptor affinity. The beta-2 affinity of dobutamine may cause vasodilatation and can cause hypotension.

Phosphodiesterase inhibitors and calcium sensitizers Agents such as milrinone and enoximone increase the intracellular concentration of cyclic adenosine monophosphate (cAMP) by inhibiting the action of phosphodiesterase 3 [28]. Phosphodiesterase 3 is an enzyme found in the sarcoplasmic reticulum of cardiac myocytes and vascular smooth muscle cells that breaks down cAMP into AMP. The increased intracellular concentration of cAMP causes increased myocardial contractility, improved diastolic relaxation, and vasodilatation. Milrinone, the most widely used phophodiesterase inhibitor, has a relatively long half-life of 2–4 hours. The calcium-sensitizer levosimendan sensitizes troponin C to calcium, thereby increasing the effects of calcium on cardiac myofilaments which increases cardiac contractility at low energy costs. Levosimendan also causes vasodilatation by opening ATP-dependent potassium channels [29,30]. Neither milrinone nor levosimendan have been tested in the setting of cardiogenic shock complicating MI and so experience with these agents in this setting is limited.

Conclusions

In conclusion, the incidence of cardiogenic shock is declining, but its clinical impact remains as significant as ever. Vasopressors and inotropes can be used to improve blood pressure and cardiac output, but they cause an increase in systemic vascular resistance and in pulmonary capillary wedge pressure and increase cardiac work and cardiac oxygen consumption. Therefore, the use of left ventricular assist devices is a promising treatment modality that is currently being investigated in larger randomized controlled trials.

Interactive multiple choice questions are available for this chapter on **www.wiley.com/go/dangas/cardiology**

References

1 Hands ME, Rutherford JD, Muller JE, *et al*. The in-hospital development of cardiogenic shock after myocardial infarction: incidence, predictors of occurrence, outcome and prognostic factors: the MILIS Study Group. *J Am Coll Cardiol* 1989; **14**(1): 40–46; discussion 7–8.

2 Goldberg RJ, Samad NA, Yarzebski J, Gurwitz J, Bigelow C, Gore JM. Temporal trends in cardiogenic shock complicating acute myocardial infarction. *N Engl J Med* 1999; **340**(15): 1162–1168.

3 Babaev A, Frederick PD, Pasta DJ, *et al*. Trends in management and outcomes of patients with acute myocardial infarction complicated by cardiogenic shock. *JAMA* 2005; **294**(4): 448–454.

4 Jeger RV, Radovanovic D, Hunziker PR, *et al*. Ten-year trends in the incidence and treatment of cardiogenic shock. *Ann Intern Med* 2008; **149**(9): 618–626.

5 Goldberg RJ, Spencer FA, Gore JM, Lessard D, Yarzebski J. Thirty-year trends (1975 to 2005) in the magnitude of, management of, and hospital death rates associated with cardiogenic shock in patients with acute myocardial infarction: a population-based perspective. *Circulation* 2009; **119**(9): 1211–1219.

6 Thiele H, Zeymer U, Neumann FJ, *et al*. Intraaortic balloon support for myocardial infarction with cardiogenic shock. *N Engl J Med* 2012; **367**(14): 1287–1296.

7 Hochman JS, Sleeper LA, Webb JG, *et al*. Early revascularization in acute myocardial infarction complicated by cardiogenic shock. SHOCK Investigators. Should we emergently revascularize occluded coronaries for cardiogenic shock. *N Engl J Med* 1999; **341**(9): 625–634.

8 Hochman JS, Sleeper LA, Godfrey E, *et al*. SHould we emergently revascularize occluded coronaries for cardiogenic shocK: an international randomized trial of emergency PTCA/CABG-trial design. The SHOCK Trial Study Group. *Am Heart J* 1999; **137**(2): 313–321.

9 Thiele H, Schuler G, Neumann FJ, *et al*. Intraaortic balloon counterpulsation in acute myocardial infarction complicated by cardiogenic shock: design and rationale of the Intraaortic Balloon Pump in Cardiogenic Shock II (IABP-SHOCK II) trial. *Am Heart J* 2012; **163**(6): 938–945.

10 Thiele H, Zeymer U, Neumann FJ, *et al*. Intra-aortic balloon counterpulsation in acute myocardial infarction complicated by cardiogenic shock (IABP-SHOCK II): final 12 month results of a randomised, open-label trial. *Lancet* 2013; **382**: 1638–1645.

11 French JK, Armstrong PW, Cohen E, *et al*. Cardiogenic shock and heart failure post-percutaneous coronary intervention in ST-elevation myocardial infarction: observations from "Assessment of Pexelizumab in Acute Myocardial Infarction". *Am Heart J* 2011; **162**(1): 89–97.

12 Hasdai D, Califf RM, Thompson TD, *et al*. Predictors of cardiogenic shock after thrombolytic therapy for acute myocardial infarction. *J Am Coll Cardiol* 2000; **35**(1): 136–143.

13 American College of Emergency Physicians, Society for Cardiovascular Angiography and Interventions, O'Gara PT, Kushner FG, Ascheim DD, *et al*. 2013 ACCF/AHA guideline for the management of ST-elevation myocardial infarction: a report of the American College of Cardiology Foundation/American Heart Association Task Force on Practice Guidelines. *J Am Coll Cardiol* 2013; **61**(4): e78–140.

14 Sleeper LA, Ramanathan K, Picard MH, *et al*. Functional status and quality of life after emergency revascularization for cardiogenic shock complicating acute myocardial infarction. *J Am Coll Cardiol* 2005; **46**(2): 266–273.

15 White HD, Assmann SF, Sanborn TA, *et al*. Comparison of percutaneous coronary intervention and coronary artery bypass grafting after acute myocardial infarction complicated by cardiogenic shock: results from the Should We Emergently Revascularize Occluded Coronaries for Cardiogenic Shock (SHOCK) trial. *Circulation* 2005; **112**(13): 1992–2001.

16 Authors/Task Force members, Windecker S, Kolh P, Alfonso F, *et al*. 2014 ESC/EACTS Guidelines on myocardial revascularization: the Task Force on Myocardial Revascularization of the European Society of Cardiology (ESC) and the European Association for Cardio-Thoracic Surgery (EACTS) Developed with the special contribution of the European Association of Percutaneous Cardiovascular Interventions (EAPCI). *Eur Heart J* 2014; **35**(37): 2541–2619.

17 Ouweneel DM, Henriques JP. Percutaneous cardiac support devices for cardiogenic shock: current indications and recommendations. *Heart* 2012; **98**(16): 1246–1254.

18 Prondzinsky R, Unverzagt S, Russ M, *et al*. Hemodynamic effects of intra-aortic balloon counterpulsation in patients with acute myocardial infarction complicated by cardiogenic shock: the prospective, randomized IABP shock trial. *Shock* 2012; **37**(4): 378–384.

19 Seyfarth M, Sibbing D, Bauer I, *et al*. A randomized clinical trial to evaluate the safety and efficacy of a percutaneous left ventricular assist device versus intra-aortic balloon pumping for treatment of cardiogenic shock caused by myocardial infarction. *J Am Coll Cardiol* 2008; **52**(19): 1584–1588.

20 Engstrom AE, Cocchieri R, Driessen AH, *et al*. The Impella 2.5 and 5.0 devices for ST-elevation myocardial infarction patients presenting with severe and profound cardiogenic shock: the Academic Medical Center intensive care unit experience. *Crit Care Med* 2011; **39**(9): 2072–2079.

21 O'Neill WW, Schreiber T, Wohns DH, *et al*. The current use of Impella 2.5 in acute myocardial infarction complicated by cardiogenic shock: results from the USpella Registry. *J Interv Cardiol* 2014; **27**(1): 1–11.

22 Burkhoff D, Cohen H, Brunckhorst C, O'Neill WW, TandemHeart Investigators G. A randomized multicenter clinical study to evaluate the safety and efficacy of the TandemHeart percutaneous ventricular assist device versus conventional therapy with intraaortic balloon pumping for treatment of cardiogenic shock. *Am Heart J* 2006; **152**(3): 469 e1–8.

23 Thiele H, Sick P, Boudriot E, *et al*. Randomized comparison of intra-aortic balloon support with a percutaneous left ventricular assist device in patients with revascularized acute myocardial infarction complicated by cardiogenic shock. *Eur Heart J* 2005; **26**(13): 1276–1283.

24 Kawashima D, Gojo S, Nishimura T, *et al*. Left ventricular mechanical support with Impella provides more ventricular unloading in heart failure than extracorporeal membrane oxygenation. *ASAIO J* 2011; **57**(3): 169–176.

25 Horwitz D, Fox Sm D, Goldberg LI. Effects of dopamine in man. *Circ Res* 1962; **10**: 237–243.

26 Dasta JF, Kirby MG. Pharmacology and therapeutic use of low-dose dopamine. *Pharmacotherapy* 1986; **6**(6): 304–310.

27 De Backer D, Biston P, Devriendt J, *et al*. Comparison of dopamine and norepinephrine in the treatment of shock. *N Engl J Med* 2010; **362**(9): 779–789.

28 Baim DS, McDowell AV, Cherniles J, *et al*. Evaluation of a new bipyridine inotropic agent—milrinone—in patients with severe congestive heart failure. *N Engl J Med* 1983; **309**(13): 748–756.

29 Yokoshiki H, Katsube Y, Sunagawa M, Sperelakis N. Levosimendan, a novel Ca2+ sensitizer, activates the glibenclamide-sensitive K+ channel in rat arterial myocytes. *Eur J Pharmacol* 1997; **333**(2-3): 249–259.

30 Pollesello P, Ovaska M, Kaivola J, *et al*. Binding of a new Ca2+ sensitizer, levosimendan, to recombinant human cardiac troponin C: A molecular modelling, fluorescence probe, and proton nuclear magnetic resonance study. *J Biol Chem* 1994; **269**(46): 28584–28590.

CHAPTER 15

Percutaneous Coronary Intervention in Unprotected Left Main

Gill Louise Buchanan[1], Alaide Chieffo[2], and Antonio Colombo[2]

[1]Department of Cardiology, North Cumbria University NHS Trust Carlisle, United Kingdom

[2]Interventional Cardiology Unit, San Raffaele Scientific Hospital, Milan, Italy

The presence of unprotected left main coronary artery (ULMCA) disease is a common finding in patients undergoing coronary angiography, typically observed in approximately 5–7% [1] and generally associated with concurrent triple vessel disease. Such patients receiving only medical therapy have increased mortality rates; indeed, data from the Coronary Artery Surgery Study (CASS) shows only 57% of those treated medically survive 5 years [2]. This is likely because the ULMCA subtends a large area [3] and significant disease can lead to left ventricular dysfunction and arrhythmias.

Until relatively recently the conventional form of treatment for the stenosed ULMCA has been coronary artery bypass grafting (CABG). The introduction of drug-eluting stents (DES) resulted in a significant reduction in restenosis and target lesion revascularization (TLR) following percutaneous coronary intervention (PCI) [4–18]. Due to such advances in coronary stent technology, in addition to antiplatelet pharmacology and adjunctive imaging techniques, the option of PCI has become more widely accepted. This has resulted in a change in the guidelines for myocardial revascularization, reducing the indication for CABG in this complex disease subset from Class I (level of evidence A) to Class I (level of evidence B) [19]. Indeed, the results of a number of clinical trials are awaited with anticipation, which may lead to further changes in the guidelines for ULMCA intervention in the future. This chapter discusses the available evidence for ULMCA PCI and practical issues that the operator encounters.

Current evidence for ULMCA revascularization

Numerous non-randomized, observational registries have demonstrated no significant differences between CABG and PCI in patients with ULMCA lesions with regards to major adverse cardiovascular and cerebrovascular events (MACCE), up to 5 years' follow-up (Table 15.1) [8,20–35].

Randomized trial data comparing PCI with CABG for the treatment of the ULMCA are shown in Table 15.2. The landmark Synergy between Percutaneous Coronary Intervention with TAXUS and Cardiac Surgery (SYNTAX) study was the first major randomized trial comparing CABG versus PCI with DES. The study included a pre-specified subgroup of patients with ULMCA (PCI n = 357; CABG n = 348). At 12 months in this group, there was non-inferiority in MACCE (PCI 15.8% vs. CABG 13.7%; p = 0.44), although there were higher rates of repeat revascularization amongst those undergoing PCI (PCI 11.8% vs. CABG 6.5%; p = 0.02). Conversely, in the CABG group there were significantly higher rates of cerebrovascular events (PCI 0.3% vs. CABG 2.7%; p = 0.01) [36].

The results of this study have now been published at 5 years' follow-up, confirming no differences in MACCE overall (PCI 36.9% vs. CABG 31.0%; p = 0.12) [37]. However, although the results were similar between those patients with low (0–22; 30.4% vs. 31.5%; p = 0.74) and intermediate (23–32; 32.7% vs. 32.3%; p = 0.88) SYNTAX scores, in the high SYNTAX score group, CABG did appear to be a superior treatment option (≥33; 46.5% in PCI vs. 29.7% in CABG; p = 0.003) [38]. It must be taken into account that these observations must be considered hypothesis-generating only, as non-inferiority was not achieved in the overall trial. Nonetheless, the results are encouraging for ULMCA PCI in those with low anatomic risk (<33 SYNTAX score). Of note, the SYNTAX study utilized first-generation DES which have consequently been shown to be inferior to the contemporary new generation DES in the incidence of repeat revascularization and, very importantly, stent thrombosis (ST).

There is growing evidence for the use of the new generation DES for ULMCA disease, with a number of registry studies reporting encouraging results. The Unprotected Left Main Stenting with a Second Generation Drug-Eluting Stent: One Year Outcomes of the LEft Main Xience V (LEMAX) Pilot Study was the first to publish the results assessing outcomes of 173 patients undergoing ULMCA PCI with the Xience V (Abbott Vascular, Santa Clara, CA, USA) everolimus-eluting stent (EES) [39]. Despite a relatively high risk group (mean SYNTAX score was 25.2 ± 9.5% and 81.0% of lesions affecting the distal bifurcation), the overall MACCE at 1 year was 15.1%, with all-cause mortality only being 2.9%. The occurrence of TLR and target vessel revascularization (TVR) were low overall (2.9% and 7.0%, respectively) and, moreover, the rate of probable or definite ST was low at only 0.6%. This study once more demonstrated higher MACCE in those with a high SYNTAX score (≥33) (25.0% vs. 12.0%, respectively; p = 0.05).

Interventional Cardiology: Principles and Practice, Second Edition. Edited by George D. Dangas, Carlo Di Mario, and Nicholas N. Kipshidze.
© 2017 John Wiley & Sons, Ltd. Published 2017 by John Wiley & Sons, Ltd.

Table 15.1 Observational registry studies comparing coronary artery bypass grafting versus percutaneous coronary intervention in the treatment of the unprotected left main coronary artery.

Study	Year	Patients (n)	Follow-up (months)	Cardiac death (%)	MACCE (%)
Palmerini et al. [21]	2006	311	12	NA	NA
Lee et al. [8]	2006	173	12	1.6 vs. 2.0	25.0 vs. 17.0
Sanmartin et al. [27]	2007	335	12	NA	11.4 vs. 10.4
Chieffo et al. [32]	2010	249	60	11.9 vs. 7.5	38.3 vs. 32.4
Park et al. [33]	2010	2240	60	9.9*	NA

MACCE, major adverse cardiovascular and cerebrovacular event; NA, not available.
*Cumulative for overall.

Table 15.2 Randomized controlled trials comparing coronary artery bypass grafting versus percutaneous coronary intervention in the treatment of the unprotected left main coronary artery. The table demonstrates results at 12 months.

	Le Mans [23]	SYNTAX Left Main [70]	Boudriot et al. [71]	PRECOMBAT [72]
Year	2008	2009	2010	2011
Patients (n)	105	705	201	600
Age (years)	61	65	68	62
SYNTAX Score	25	30	24	25
Death (%)	7.5 vs. 1.9; p=0.37	4.4 vs. 4.2; p=0.88	5.0 vs. 2.0; p<0.001	2.7 vs. 2.0; p=0.45
MACCE (%)	24.5 vs. 28.8; p=0.29	13.7 vs. 15.8; p=0.44	13.9 vs. 19.0; p=0.19	6.7 vs. 8.7; p=0.12

Le Mans, Study of Unprotected Left Main Stenting Versus Bypass Surgery; MACCE, major cardiovascular or cerebrovascular event; PRECOMBAT, Premier of Randomized Comparison of Bypass Surgery versus Angioplasty Using Sirolimus Eluting Stent in Patients with Left Main Coronary Artery Disease; SYNTAX, Synergy between Percutaneous Coronary Intervention with TAXUS and Cardiac Surgery.

There are a number of new generation DES, which have been demonstrated to have comparable outcomes in the treatment of the ULMCA. A total of 650 patients were randomized in the Drug Eluting Stent for Left Main Stem Disease (ISAR LEFT MAIN) 2 to EES versus zotarolimus-eluting stents (ZES), with a primary endpoint of death, myocardial infarction (MI), and TLR at 1 year. There were no differences between groups (ZES 17.5% vs. EES 14.3%; relative risk [RR] 1.26; 95% confidence interval [CI] 0.85–1.85; p=0.25) or in the risk of ST (0.9% vs. 0.6%; p>0.99) [40]. The currently available data are promising for the use of new generation DES for ULMCA PCI and the results of long-term follow-up are eagerly awaited.

There are a number of ongoing multicenter trials comparing new generation DES with CABG, such as the Premier of Randomized Comparison of Bypass Surgery versus Angioplasty Using Sirolimus-Eluting Stent in Patients with Left Main Coronary Artery Disease 2 (PRECOMBAT 2) which aims to evaluate the outcomes of 401 patients undergoing ULMCA PCI with EES with historical controls from the PRECOMBAT trial (randomized PCI with the first generation sirolimus-eluting stents [SES] versus CABG). The results of the landmark trial Evaluation of Xience Prime versus Coronary Artery Bypass Surgery for Effectiveness of Left Main Revascularization trial (EXCEL) are also expected. In this study, 2634 patients with ULMCA and a SYNTAX score ≤32 have been randomized to either CABG or EES (Xience Prime, Abbott Vascular,

Redwood City, CA, USA). The primary endpoint is the composite incidence of death, MI, or cerebrovascular events at a median follow-up duration of 3 years.

Current guidelines for ULMCA revascularization

As a result of the growing amount of positive data for the use of PCI in this high risk patient subset, current European practice guidelines have now accepted the role of ULMCA PCI [19]. Indeed, although CABG is a Class I indication (now level of evidence B), PCI in those patients with a SYNTAX score of ≤22 now has an equivalent Class I (level of evidence B) indication. Those patients with an intermediate SYNTAX score (22–32) have a Class IIa (level of evidence B) indication; however, CABG is still advocated in those with a SYNTAX score of ≥32. With regards to the American Heart Association/American College of Cardiology/Society for Cardiovascular and Angiographic Interventions (AHA/ACC/SCAI) guidelines, PCI has a Class IIa (level of evidence B) in those with favorable anatomy for PCI (SYNTAX ≤22) and clinical conditions that present a greater risk of adverse events with CABG. In certain scenarios (e.g., in patients presenting with acute coronary syndromes and ST-elevation MI), ULMCA PCI is a Class IIa (level of evidence B) indication [41].

Multidisciplinary assessment and the use of risk scores

Each individual with ULMCA disease differs, both with regards to their clinical condition and comorbidities as well as their coronary anatomy. As such, it is advisable that every patient is discussed by the "heart team" to determine the most appropriate revascularization strategy to produce the best long-term outcomes for the patient. Indeed, assessment by the heart team in complex pathologies now has a Class I (level of evidence C) indication in recent guidelines [19].

A number of scoring systems have been devised to help with risk stratification prior to undergoing intervention. The traditional scores used by cardiothoracic surgeons are the Society of Thoracic Surgeons (STS) score and the Logistic European System for Cardiac Operative Risk Evaluation (EuroSCORE). Newer scores have been devised and validated by the interventional cardiologists and include the SYNTAX score, a prospective angiographic tool that grades the anatomic complexity of coronary artery disease (an online calculator can be found at www.syntaxscore.com). The use of the STS score and SYNTAX score are commented upon in both the European and in the AHA/ACC/SCAI guidelines as reasonable to calculate in patients with ULMCA disease [19,41].

More recently, other scoring systems have been developed which do not rely solely on anatomic factors, but also take into account other clinical issues relevant to the patient. Potentially, this leads to an improved means of risk stratification for the individual patient. The SYNTAX Score II considers coronary anatomy in addition to the factors assessed in the more traditional surgical scoring systems, which were associated with mortality at 4 years in the SYNTAX study (including age, creatinine clearance, left ventricular ejection fraction, peripheral vascular disease, female sex, and chronic obstructive pulmonary disease) [42]. A further risk model is the Global Risk Classification (GRC), which combines the SYNTAX score with the EuroSCORE [43] and has been demonstrated in patients undergoing ULMCA PCI to be a superior predictor of cardiac mortality. The New Risk Stratification Score (NERS) has been shown to more reliably predict major adverse cardiac events (MACE) than the SYNTAX score in high risk patients requiring ULMCA PCI [44]. Regardless, it is essential that each individual patient undergoes a thorough assessment of clinical and anatomic factors to enable effectual risk stratification and allow guidance in treatment strategy decision making.

Imaging and lesion assessment

The identification of the ULMCA generally arises following conventional diagnostic coronary angiography. This common tool allows basic assessment of the severity of disease, disease location (including involvement of the distal bifurcation), and lesion length. However, there is a large variability in intra- and inter-observer of the ULMCA [45,46] due to the short length of the vessel, with the absence of a normal segment for comparison. In addition, because of positive remodeling it can be difficult to form an accurate assessment and hence the use of adjunctive imaging modalities can have a crucial role prior to consideration of ULMCA revascularization.

Tools such as intravascular ultrasound (IVUS) and optical coherence tomography (OCT) allow more accurate assessment of the morphology of the disease and the significance in often complex coronary angiograms. The size of the vessel and the length of the lesion can be accurately determined by IVUS, to enable precise stent sizing in patients undergoing PCI. Furthermore, IVUS is vital to guarantee adequate stent expansion and apposition following stent implantation, to potentially reduce the risk of events such as ST. The use of IVUS guidance over angiography guidance alone has been shown to reduce 3-year mortality in a subgroup analysis of patients treated with DES from the MAIN-COMPARE registry (IVUS 4.7% vs. no IVUS 16.0%; p = 0.049) [47]. A more recent patient level pooled analysis of four registry studies demonstrated the use of IVUS to be associated with less cardiac death, MI, and TLR at 3 years (IVUS 11.3% vs. no IVUS 16.4%; p = 0.04) and a lower incidence of definite and probable ST (0.6% vs. 2.2%; p = 0.04) [48].

More recently, the use of OCT has come to the fore in the assessment and treatment of complex patient subsets undergoing PCI and due to the 10-fold higher axial resolution compared with IVUS, it has been demonstrated to be more sensitive in detecting malapposition and edge dissections in the assessment of the ULMCA [49]. This modality may gain an increasing role in the future in determining factors that may predispose an individual to ST (e.g., delayed or incomplete stent endothelialization or stent malapposition).

As an alternative to an anatomic assessment, it is possible to obtain an invasive functional assessment of the significance of an ULMCA "angiographically" intermediate lesion with the use of fractional flow reserve (FFR). A reading following achievement of maximal hyperemia of ≤0.75 is known to be an indicator of significant stenosis. Indeed, in patients with an equivocal ULMCA stenosis on coronary angiography, a strategy of revascularization based on the FFR measurement was associated with excellent survival and freedom from events at up to 3 years' follow-up [50]. Another study of 213 patients with angiographically equivocal ULMCA lesions underwent FFR assessment and were referred for CABG if FFR <0.80 (surgical group) or remained on medical management or underwent PCI to another target if FFR to ULMCA was ≥0.80 (non-surgical group). At 5 years, there was no difference in survival (surgical group 85.4% vs. non-surgical group 89.8%; p = 0.48) [51]. These data support the notion that we should consider revascularization when ULMCA disease is functionally significant and not driven by the angiographic appearance alone.

Interventional approach

The ULMCA is as unique as each coronary artery and is made up of three diverse segments: the ostium, the main shaft, and the distal bifurcation. The bifurcation is more likely to form atherosclerotic plaque from shear stresses and subsequent flow disturbances, with the carina typically free of disease [52]. However, when the distal bifurcation is involved, this not only adds to the technical difficulties for the operator, but also leads to less favorable clinical outcomes and increased need for repeat revascularization than disease affecting only the ostium or the mid shaft [10,12]. Indeed, a large registry study comparing outcomes following ostial or shaft versus distal bifurcation disease in 1612 patients demonstrated the latter to have a higher MACE (propensity-score adjusted HR 1.48, 95% CI 1.16–1.89; p = 0.001), at a median follow-up period of 1250 (inter-quartile range 987–1564) days. This again was largely because of the higher rate of TLR in this group [53]. Moreover, a recent study has shown that a true bifurcation lesion is a significant predictor of restenosis (23.0% vs 14.0%; p = 0.008) [54].

Clinical outcomes when treating the ostium of the ULMCA alone are favorable with either revascularization strategy and a registry study has demonstrated comparable outcomes [55]. In this lesion subset, a number of studies have shown low event rates following PCI [5–7,55,56] and such a procedure is less technically

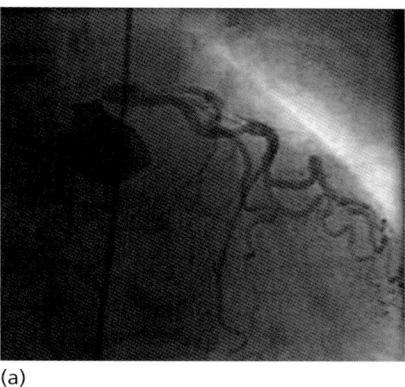
(a)

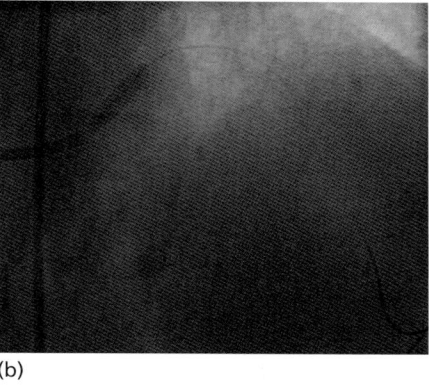
(b)

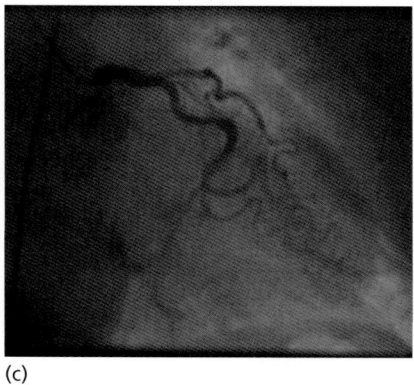
(c)

Figure 15.1 The treatment of an ostial left main stem lesion in an 84-year-old female patient with a SYNTAX score of 11. (a) shows the lesion at baseline; (b) demonstrates the implantation of a 3.5 × 8 mm drug-eluting stent; (c) the final angiographic end result.

challenging. Figure 15.1 illustrates a successful case of PCI to an ostial lesion.

Ideally, DES should be utilized in all ULMCA PCI, unless there are strong reasons not to use such a stent. A multicenter study of 147 patients undergoing PCI with DES ULMCA disease not involving the bifurcation, demonstrated a TLR rate of 0.7%, cardiac death rate of 2.7%, and MACE rate of 7.4% at long-term clinical follow-up (886 ± 308 days) [10]. The ULMCA ostium is typically large in diameter and, ideally, the stent should protrude back into the aorta by 1–2 mm and avoid the distal bifurcation. Several cine projections should be used to ensure accurate positioning of the stent, with the use of the left anterior oblique cranial view of particular value in clearly visualizing the ostium. In a similar fashion, ULMCA lesions involving the shaft alone should be treated, again avoiding the distal bifurcation if possible.

However, it is not surprising that the distal bifurcation is involved in 60–90% [57] and because of the marked variation in anatomy, no solo PCI strategy can be applied. Factors that need to be considered in determining the best form of intervention include the bifurcation angulation, distribution of the disease, the side branch size, and presence of disease. Conventionally, the main branch is the left anterior descending coronary artery, with the side branch the circumflex or intermediate artery. However, it must be remembered that the side branch can be just as important in terms of size and territory of distribution.

The important thing is to keep it simple if at all possible and if the disease affects the main branch alone (Medina classification 1,1,0 or 1,0,0), a provisional one-stent strategy with stent implantation from the ULMCA into the main branch would be the preferred option. Following optimization with post-dilatation and final kissing balloon inflation, a second stent should only be considered if dissection with reduced TIMI flow is apparent or if there is a significant residual stenosis (which could be assessed for functional significance with FFR). It is well known that a single stent approach for PCI of the ULMCA distal bifurcation has been demonstrated to have better outcomes [58,59] including a TLR rate almost equivalent to that for PCI of the ostium or body when DES are used [5,60].

In certain circumstances, two stents should be the strategy from the outset: if there is significant disease affecting both branches which are of favorable size with a large area of distribution and if the side branch disease is longer than 3–5 mm in length. Restenosis is typically confined to the side branch ostium [59,61]; however, TLR

rates can be up to 26%. A study has randomized 419 patients with distal bifurcation ULMCA disease to either the double kiss crush versus the culotte technique. The latter group sustained more MACE (16.3% vs. 6.2%; p < 0.05) largely because of higher TVR (11.0% vs. 4.3%; p < 0.05) [62]. Figure 15.2 illustrates the results following treatment of the distal bifurcation with the mini-crush technique. However, it must be emphasized that whichever technique is used, the operator should be confident and final kissing balloon inflation is essential to obtain the optimal result.

More recently, dedicated bifurcation stents have become a novel topic for consideration by interventional cardiologists. The Tryton® (Tryton Medical, Inc., Durham, NC, USA) can be used alongside a conventional DES in a "reverse culotte" technique, facilitating stenting and potentially improving angiographic results and clinical outcomes. The feasibility of this stent with EES was demonstrated in a prospective single arm study, including 52 patients with stable ULMCA disease. There was angiographic success in 100% and at 6 months' follow-up TLR occurred in 12%, MI in 10%, and MACE in 22%, with importantly no ST [63]. In the future, with improvements in technology, there may be a greater usage of similar stents if procedural ease and outcomes become favorable.

Pharmacotherapy in ULMCA intervention

There are a number of different adjunctive pharmacologic agents available currently for use during PCI, including unfractionated heparin, bivalirudin, and the glycoprotein IIb/IIIa antagonists, the choice of which generally lies with the operator. However, a recent pooled dataset from three large randomized trials comparing bivalirudin with heparin has suggested that in the ULMCA group (177 patients) bivalirudin was associated with significantly less non-CABG-related bleeding (4.5% vs. 14.6%; RR 0.27; 95% CI 0.09–0.83; p = 0.013) despite a similar composite endpoint of death, MI, and TVR at 30 days (11.4% vs. 12.4%; p = 0.513) [64].

The stent type of choice is the DES and the typical accepted duration of treatment following elective DES implantation is at least 12 months of dual antiplatelet therapy (DAPT), with aspirin therapy continued indefinitely thereafter [41,65]. However, despite the fact that some current DES have CE mark for only 3 months DAPT, many interventionalists may actually recommend more prolonged DAPT because of the potentially catastrophic consequences should ST occur in the ULMCA. Indeed, the recent Dual Antiplatelet

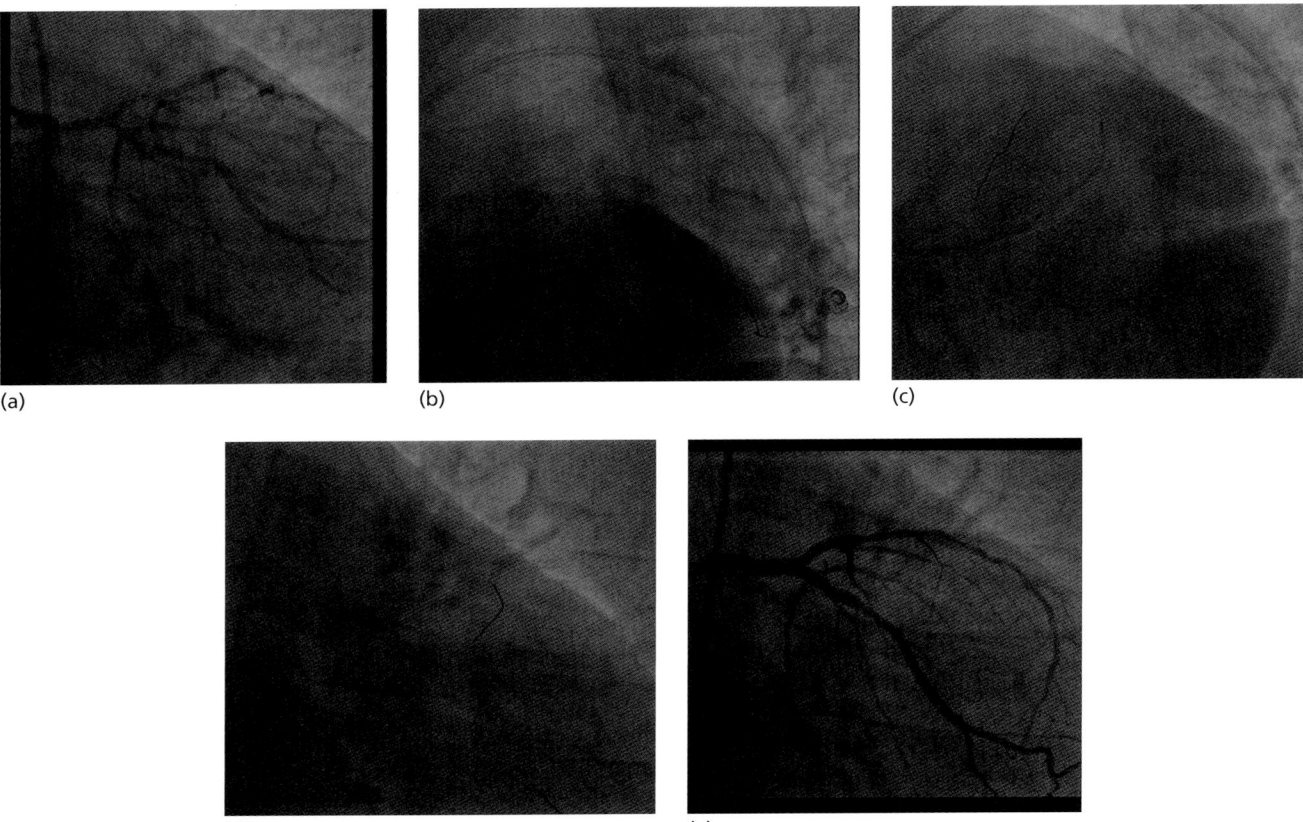

Figure 15.2 The use of a two stent mini-crush strategy for the treatment of a 69-year-old male patient with a SYNTAX score of 24. (a) shows the disease affecting the distal bifurcation. (b) and (c) show positioning of the circumflex (3.0 × 18 mm) and left anterior descending coronary artery (3.5 × 23 mm) stents respectively. (d) demonstrates final kissing balloon inflation and (e) the final angiographic end result.

Therapy Study randomized 9961 patients to 12 months versus 30 months of DAPT. Prolonged treatment with DAPT reduced the rate of ST (0.4% vs. 1.4%; HR 0.29; 95% CI 0.17–0.48; p < 0.001) and MACCE (4.3% vs. 5.9%; HR 0.71; 95% CI 0.59–0.85; p < 0.001), with conversely more bleeding in the prolonged treatment group (2.5% vs. 1.6%; p = 0.001) [66]. Further studies are necessary to clarify the optimum regimen and duration of DAPT following the treatment of ULMCA with DES.

Hemodynamic support

Generally with good left ventricular function, patients can tolerate ULMCA PCI well with no requirement for hemodynamic support electively. Indeed, the risk of acute instability requiring intra-aortic balloon pump (IABP) support is only 8% [67]. However, if there is severe left ventricular dysfunction, systolic blood pressure <90 mmHg, or acute coronary syndrome, a prophylactic IABP can be considered prior to the procedure. In addition, certain anatomic subsets, such as an occluded right coronary artery, dominant circumflex artery, or a heavy calcium burden that requires rotational atherectomy may undergo such support.

Currently the Impella 2.5 system (Abiomed Inc., Danvers, MA, USA), a minimally invasive left ventricular assist device, is available as an alternative means of hemodynamic support [68]. This device has been compared with the IABP in a randomized study of 452

patients requiring non-emergent PCI with complex triple vessel coronary artery disease or ULMCA with severely depressed left ventricular function. There was no difference in 30-day MACE between groups (IABP 40.1% vs. Impella 35.1%; p = 0.227); however, a trend for improved MACE at 90 days with the Impella 2.5 (IABP 49.3% vs. Impella 40.6%; p = 0.066) suggested there may be a benefit of this novel device in such situations if hemodynamic support is deemed necessary [69].

Conclusions

The treatment of the ULMCA remains a challenge for the interventional cardiologist, not only in procedural complexity but also the concurrent disease affecting many of the patients undergoing such a procedure. There has been increased enthusiasm in recent years because of a number of improvements within the field, including stent technology, adjunctive imaging, and pharmacotherapy which has resulted in the emergence of encouraging outcomes.

It must be remembered that each patient is an individual and should be risk stratified as such with the heart team involvement and careful consideration should be given to the strategy and pharmacotherapy regime. The results of randomized trials are eagerly awaited, which in time may lead to further changes in the guidelines for ULMCA PCI.

Interactive multiple choice questions are available for this chapter on www.wiley. com/go/dangas/cardiology

References

1 DeMots H, Rösch J, McAnulty JH, Rahimtoola SH. Left main coronary artery disease. *Cardiovasc Clin* 1977; **8**(2): 201–211.

2 Taylor HA, Deumite NJ, Chaitman BR, Davis KB, Killip T, Rogers WJ. Asymptomatic left main coronary artery disease in the Coronary Artery Surgery Study (CASS) registry. *Circulation* 1989; **79**(6): 1171–1179.

3 Kalbfleisch H, Hort W. Quantitative study on the size of coronary artery supplying areas postmortem. *Am Heart J* 1977; **94**(2): 183–188.

4 de Lezo JS, Medina A, Pan M, et al. Rapamycin-eluting stents for the treatment of unprotected left main coronary disease. *Am Heart J* 2004; **148**(3): 481–415.

5 Chieffo A, Stankovic G, Bonizzoni E, et al. Early and mid-term results of drug-eluting stent implantation in unprotected left main. *Circulation* 2005; **111**(6): 791–795.

6 Park SJ, Kim YH, Lee BK, et al. Sirolimus-eluting stent implantation for unprotected left main coronary artery stenosis: comparison with bare metal stent implantation. *J Am Coll Cardiol* 2005; **45**(3): 351–356.

7 Valgimigli M, van Mieghem CA, Ong AT, et al. Short- and long-term clinical outcome after drug-eluting stent implantation for the percutaneous treatment of left main coronary artery disease: insights from the Rapamycin-Eluting and Taxus Stent Evaluated At Rotterdam Cardiology Hospital registries (RESEARCH and T-SEARCH). *Circulation* 2005; **111**(11): 1383–1389.

8 Lee MS, Kapoor N, Jamal F, et al. Comparison of coronary artery bypass surgery with percutaneous coronary intervention with drug-eluting stents for unprotected left main coronary artery disease. *J Am Coll Cardiol* 2006; **47**(4): 864–870.

9 Valgimigli M, Malagutti P, Aoki J, et al. Sirolimus-eluting versus paclitaxel-eluting stent implantation for the percutaneous treatment of left main coronary artery disease: a combined RESEARCH and T-SEARCH long-term analysis. *J Am Coll Cardiol* 2006; **47**(3): 507–514.

10 Chieffo A, Park SJ, Valgimigli M, et al. Favorable long-term outcome after drug-eluting stent implantation in nonbifurcation lesions that involve unprotected left main coronary artery: a multicenter registry. *Circulation* 2007; **116**(2): 158–162.

11 Sheiban I, Meliga E, Moretti C, et al. Long-term clinical and angiographic outcomes of treatment of unprotected left main coronary artery stenosis with sirolimus-eluting stents. *Am J Cardiol* 2007; **100**(3): 431–435.

12 Biondi-Zoccai GG, Lotrionte M, Moretti C, et al. A collaborative systematic review and meta-analysis on 1278 patients undergoing percutaneous drug-eluting stenting for unprotected left main coronary artery disease. *Am Heart J* 2008; **155**(2): 274–283.

13 Chieffo A, Part SJ, Meliga E, et al. Late and very late stent thrombosis following drug-eluting stent implantation in unprotected left main coronary artery: a multicentre registry. *Eur Heart J* 2008; **29**(17): 2108–2115.

14 Kim YH, Dangas GD, Solinas E, et al. Effectiveness of drug-eluting stent implantation for patients with unprotected left main coronary artery stenosis. *Am J Cardiol* 2008; **101**(6): 801–806.

15 Tamburino C, Di Salvo ME, Capodanno D, et al. Are drug-eluting stents superior to bare-metal stents in patients with unprotected non-bifurcational left main disease? Insights from a multicentre registry. *Eur Heart J* 2009; **30**(10): 1171–1179.

16 Tamburino C, Di Salvo ME, Capodanno D, et al. Comparison of drug-eluting stents and bare-metal stents for the treatment of unprotected left main coronary artery disease in acute coronary syndromes. *Am J Cardiol* 2009; **103**(2): 187–193.

17 Kim YH, Park DW, Lee SW, et al. Long-term safety and effectiveness of unprotected left main coronary stenting with drug-eluting stents compared with bare-metal stents. *Circulation* 2009; **120**(5): 400–407.

18 Meliga E, Garcia-Garcia HM, Valgimigli M, et al. Longest available clinical outcomes after drug-eluting stent implantation for unprotected left main coronary artery disease: the DELFT (Drug Eluting stent for LeFT main) Registry. *J Am Coll Cardiol* 2008; **51**(23): 2212–2219.

19 Authors/Task Force members, Windecker S, Kolh P, Alfonso F, et al. 2014 ESC/EACTS Guidelines on myocardial revascularization: The Task Force on Myocardial Revascularization of the European Society of Cardiology (ESC) and the European Association for Cardio-Thoracic Surgery (EACTS)Developed with the special contribution of the European Association of Percutaneous Cardiovascular Interventions (EAPCI). *Eur Heart J* 2014; **35**(37): 2541–2619.

20 Chieffo A, Morici N, Maisano F, et al. Percutaneous treatment with drug-eluting stent implantation versus bypass surgery for unprotected left main stenosis: a single-center experience. *Circulation* 2006; **113**(21): 2542–2547.

21 Palmerini T, Marzocchi A, Marrozzini C, et al. Comparison between coronary angioplasty and coronary artery bypass surgery for the treatment of unprotected left main coronary artery stenosis (the Bologna Registry). *Am J Cardiol* 2006; **98**(1): 54–59.

22 Palmerini T, Barlocco F, Santarelli A, et al. A comparison between coronary artery bypass grafting surgery and drug eluting stent for the treatment of unprotected left main coronary artery disease in elderly patients (aged > or =75 years). *Eur Heart J* 2007; **28**(22): 2714–2719.

23 Buszman PE, Kiesz SR, Bochenek A, et al. Acute and late outcomes of unprotected left main stenting in comparison with surgical revascularization. *J Am Coll Cardiol* 2008; **51**(5): 538–545.

24 Seung KB, Park DW, Kim YH, et al. Stents versus coronary-artery bypass grafting for left main coronary artery disease. *N Engl J Med* 2008; **358**(17): 1781–1792.

25 Park DW, Kim YH, Yun SC, et al. Long-term outcomes after stenting versus coronary artery bypass grafting for unprotected left main coronary artery disease: 10-year results of bare-metal stents and 5-year results of drug-eluting stents from the ASAN-MAIN (ASAN Medical Center-Left MAIN Revascularization) Registry. *J Am Coll Cardiol* 2010; **56**(17): 1366–1375.

26 Brener SJ, Galla JM, Bryant R 3rd, Sabik JF 3rd, Ellis SG. Comparison of percutaneous versus surgical revascularization of severe unprotected left main stenosis in matched patients. *Am J Cardiol* 2008; **101**(2): 169–172.

27 Sanmartin M, Baz JA, Claro R, et al. Comparison of drug-eluting stents versus surgery for unprotected left main coronary artery disease. *Am J Cardiol* 2007; **100**(6): 970–973.

28 Hsu JT, Chu CM, Chang ST, Kao CL, Chung CM. Percutaneous coronary intervention versus coronary artery bypass graft surgery for the treatment of unprotected left main coronary artery stenosis: in-hospital and one year outcome after emergent and elective treatments. *Int Heart J* 2008; **49**(3): 355–370.

29 Makikallio TH, Niemelä M, Kervinen K, et al. Coronary angioplasty in drug eluting stent era for the treatment of unprotected left main stenosis compared to coronary artery bypass grafting. *Ann Med* 2008; **40**(6): 437–443.

30 Rodes-Cabau J, Deblois J, Bertrand OF, et al. Nonrandomized comparison of coronary artery bypass surgery and percutaneous coronary intervention for the treatment of unprotected left main coronary artery disease in octogenarians. *Circulation* 2008; **118**(23): 2374–2381.

31 Wu C, Hannan EL, Walford G, Faxon DP. Utilization and outcomes of unprotected left main coronary artery stenting and coronary artery bypass graft surgery. *Ann Thorac Surg* 2008; **86**(4): 1153–1159.

32 Chieffo A, Magni V, Latib A, et al. 5-year outcomes following percutaneous coronary intervention with drug-eluting stent implantation versus coronary artery bypass graft for unprotected left main coronary artery lesions the milan experience. *JACC Cardiovasc Interv* 2010; **3**(6): 595–601.

33 Park DW, Seung KB, Kim YH, et al. Long-term safety and efficacy of stenting versus coronary artery bypass grafting for unprotected left main coronary artery disease: 5-year results from the MAIN-COMPARE (Revascularization for Unprotected Left Main Coronary Artery Stenosis: Comparison of Percutaneous Coronary Angioplasty Versus Surgical Revascularization) registry. *J Am Coll Cardiol* 2010; **56**(2): 117–124.

34 Park IS, Cho AH, Lee SJ, Kim JS, Lee KS, Kim YI. Life-threatening anaphylactoid reaction in an acute ischemic stroke patient with intravenous rt-PA thrombolysis, followed by successful intra-arterial thrombolysis. *J Clin Neurol* 2008; **4**(1): 29–32.

35 Cho S, Park TS, Yoon DH, et al. Identification of genetic polymorphisms in FABP3 and FABP4 and putative association with back fat thickness in Korean native cattle. *BMB Rep* 2008; **41**(1): 29–34.

36 Serruys PW, Morice MC, Kappetein AP, et al. Percutaneous coronary intervention versus coronary-artery bypass grafting for severe coronary artery disease. *N Engl J Med* 2009; **360**(10): 961–972.

37 Morice MC, Serruys PW, Kappetein AP, et al. Five-year outcomes in patients with left main disease treated with either percutaneous coronary intervention or coronary artery bypass grafting in the synergy between percutaneous coronary intervention with taxus and cardiac surgery trial. *Circulation* 2014; **129**(23): 2388–2394.

38 Mohr FW, Morice MC, Kappetein AP, et al. Coronary artery bypass graft surgery versus percutaneous coronary intervention in patients with three-vessel disease and left main coronary disease: 5-year follow-up of the randomised, clinical SYNTAX trial. *Lancet* 2013; **381**(9867): 629–638.

39 Salvatella N, Morice MC, Darremont O, et al. Unprotected left main stenting with a second-generation drug-eluting stent: one-year outcomes of the LEMAX Pilot study. *EuroIntervention* 2011; **7**(6): 689–696.

40 Mehilli J, Richardt G, Valgimigli M, et al. Zotarolimus- versus everolimus-eluting stents for unprotected left main coronary artery disease. *J Am Coll Cardiol* 2013; **62**(22): 2075–2082.

41 Levine GN, Bates ER, Blankenship JC, et al. 2011 ACCF/AHA/SCAI Guideline for Percutaneous Coronary Intervention. *J Am Coll Cardiol* 2011; **58**(24): e44–122.

42 Farooq V, van Klaveren D, Steyerberg EW, et al. Anatomical and clinical characteristics to guide decision making between coronary artery bypass surgery and

percutaneous coronary intervention for individual patients: development and validation of SYNTAX score II. *Lancet* 2013; 381(9867): 639–650.

43 Capodanno D, Miano M, Cincotta G, et al. EuroSCORE refines the predictive ability of SYNTAX score in patients undergoing left main percutaneous coronary intervention. *Am Heart J* 2010; 159(1): 103–109.

44 Chen SL, Chen JP, Mintz G, et al. Comparison between the NERS (New Risk Stratification) score and the SYNTAX (Synergy between Percutaneous Coronary Intervention with Taxus and Cardiac Surgery) score in outcome prediction for unprotected left main stenting. *JACC Cardiovasc Interv* 2010; 3(6): 632–641.

45 Fisher LD, Judkins MP, Lesperance J, et al. Reproducibility of coronary arteriographic reading in the coronary artery surgery study (CASS). *Catheter Cardiovasc Diagn* 1982; 8(6): 565–575.

46 Isner JM, Kishel J, Kent KM, Ronan JA Jr, Ross AM, Roberts WC. Accuracy of angiographic determination of left main coronary arterial narrowing: angiographic–histologic correlative analysis in 28 patients. *Circulation* 1981; 63(5): 1056–1064.

47 Park SJ, Kim YH, Park DW, et al. Impact of intravascular ultrasound guidance on long-term mortality in stenting for unprotected left main coronary artery stenosis. *Circ Cardiovasc Interv* 2009; 2(3): 167–177.

48 de la Torre Hernandez JM, Baz Alonso JA, Gómez Hospital JA, et al. IVUS-TRONCO-ICP Spanish study., Clinical impact of intravascular ultrasound guidance in drug-eluting stent implantation for unprotected left main coronary disease: pooled analysis at the patient-level of 4 registries. *JACC Cardiovasc Interv* 2014; 7: 244–254.

49 Fujino Y, Bezerra HG, Attizzani GF, et al. Frequency-domain optical coherence tomography assessment of unprotected left main coronary artery disease: a comparison with intravascular ultrasound. *Catheter Cardiovasc Interv* 2013; 82(3): E173–183.

50 Jasti V, Ivan E, Yalamanchili V, Wongpraparut N, Leesar MA. Correlations between fractional flow reserve and intravascular ultrasound in patients with an ambiguous left main coronary artery stenosis. *Circulation* 2004; 110(18): 2831–2836.

51 Hamilos M, Muller O, Cuisset T, et al. Long-term clinical outcome after fractional flow reserve-guided treatment in patients with angiographically equivocal left main coronary artery stenosis. *Circulation* 2009; 120(15): 1505–1512.

52 Prosi M, Perktold K, Ding Z, Friedman MH. Influence of curvature dynamics on pulsatile coronary artery flow in a realistic bifurcation model. *J Biomech* 2004; 37(11): 1767–1775.

53 Naganuma T, Chieffo A, Meliga E, et al. Long-term clinical outcomes after percutaneous coronary intervention for ostial/mid-shaft lesions versus distal bifurcation lesions in unprotected left main coronary artery. The DELTA Registry (drug-eluting stent for left main coronary artery disease): a multicenter registry evaluating percutaneous coronary intervention versus coronary artery bypass grafting for left main treatment. *JACC Cardiovasc Interv* 2013; 6(12): 1242–1249.

54 Tiroch K, Mehilli J, Byrne RA, et al. Impact of coronary anatomy and stenting technique on long-term outcome after drug-eluting stent implantation for unprotected left main coronary artery. *JACC Cardiovasc Interv* 2014; 7(1): 29–36.

55 Naganuma T, Chieffo A, Meliga E, et al. Long-term clinical outcomes after percutaneous coronary intervention versus coronary artery bypass grafting for ostial/ midshaft lesions in unprotected left main coronary artery from the DELTA registry: a multicenter registry evaluating percutaneous coronary intervention versus coronary artery bypass grafting for left main treatment. *JACC Cardiovasc Interv* 2014; 7(4): 354–361.

56 Valgimigli M, Malagutti P, Rodriguez-Granillo GA, et al. Distal left main coronary disease is a major predictor of outcome in patients undergoing percutaneous intervention in the drug-eluting stent era: an integrated clinical and angiographic analysis based on the Rapamycin-Eluting Stent Evaluated At Rotterdam Cardiology Hospital (RESEARCH) and Taxus-Stent Evaluated At Rotterdam Cardiology Hospital (T-SEARCH) registries. *J Am Coll Cardiol* 2006; 47(8): 1530–1537.

57 Park SJ, Park DW. Percutaneous coronary intervention with stent implantation versus coronary artery bypass surgery for treatment of left main coronary artery disease: is it time to change guidelines? *Circ Cardiovasc Interv* 2009; 2(1): 59–68.

58 Kim YH, Park SW, Hong MK, et al. Comparison of simple and complex stenting techniques in the treatment of unprotected left main coronary artery bifurcation stenosis. *Am J Cardiol* 2006; 97(11): 1597–1601.

59 Palmerini T, Marzocchi A, Tamburino C, et al. Impact of bifurcation technique on 2-year clinical outcomes in 773 patients with distal unprotected left main coronary artery stenosis treated with drug-eluting stents. *Circ Cardiovasc Interv* 2008; 1(3): 185–192.

60 Agostoni P, Valgimigli M, Van Mieghem CA, et al. Comparison of early outcome of percutaneous coronary intervention for unprotected left main coronary artery disease in the drug-eluting stent era with versus without intravascular ultrasonic guidance. *Am J Cardiol* 2005; 95(5): 644–647.

61 Mehilli J, Kastrati A, Byrne RA, et al. Paclitaxel- versus sirolimus-eluting stents for unprotected left main coronary artery disease. *J Am Coll Cardiol* 2009; 53(19): 1760–1768.

62 Chen SL, Xu B, Han YL, et al. Comparison of double kissing crush versus Culotte stenting for unprotected distal left main bifurcation lesions: results from a multicenter, randomized, prospective DKCRUSH-III study. *J Am Coll Cardiol* 2013; 61(14): 1482–1488.

63 Magro M, Girasis C, Bartorelli AL, et al. Acute procedural and six-month clinical outcome in patients treated with a dedicated bifurcation stent for left main stem disease: the TRYTON LM multicentre registry. *EuroIntervention* 2013; 8(11): 1259–1269.

64 Geisler T, Müller K, Karathanos A, et al. Impact of antithrombotic treatment on short-term outcomes after percutaneous coronary intervention for left main disease: a pooled analysis from REPLACE-2, ACUITY, and HORIZONS-AMI trials. *EuroIntervention* 2014; 10(1): 97–104.

65 Wijns W, Kolh P, Danchin N, et al. Guidelines on myocardial revascularization: The Task Force on Myocardial Revascularization of the European Society of Cardiology (ESC) and the European Association for Cardio-Thoracic Surgery (EACTS). *Eur Heart J* 2010; 31(20): 2501–2555.

66 Mauri L, Kereiakes DJ, Yeh RW, et al. Twelve or 30 months of dual antiplatelet therapy after drug-eluting stents. *N Engl J Med* 2014; 371(23): 2155–2166.

67 Briguori C, Airoldi F, Chieffo A, et al. Elective versus provisional intraaortic balloon pumping in unprotected left main stenting. *Am Heart J* 2006; 152(3): 565–572.

68 Dixon SR, Henriques JP, Mauri L, et al. A prospective feasibility trial investigating the use of the Impella 2.5 system in patients undergoing high-risk percutaneous coronary intervention (The PROTECT I Trial): initial US experience. *JACC Cardiovasc Interv* 2009; 2(2): 91–96.

69 O'Neill WW, Kleiman NS, Moses J, et al. A prospective, randomized clinical trial of hemodynamic support with Impella 2.5 versus intra-aortic balloon pump in patients undergoing high-risk percutaneous coronary intervention: the PROTECT II study. *Circulation* 2012; 126(14): 1717–1727.

70 Morice MC, Serruys PW, Kappetein AP, et al. Outcomes in patients with de novo left main disease treated with either percutaneous coronary intervention using paclitaxel-eluting stents or coronary artery bypass graft treatment in the Synergy Between Percutaneous Coronary Intervention with TAXUS and Cardiac Surgery (SYNTAX) trial. *Circulation* 2010; 121(24): 2645–2653.

71 Boudriot E, Thiele H, Walther T, et al. Randomized comparison of percutaneous coronary intervention with sirolimus-eluting stents versus coronary artery bypass grafting in unprotected left main stem stenosis. *J Am Coll Cardiol* 2011; 57(5): 538–545.

72 Park SJ, Kim YH, Park DW, et al. Randomized trial of stents versus bypass surgery for left main coronary artery disease. *N Engl J Med* 2011; 364(18): 1718–1727.

CHAPTER 16

Bifurcation Lesion Stenting

Yves Louvard, Thierry Lefevre, Bernard Chevalier, and Philippe Garot

Institut Cardiovasculaire Paris Sud, Hôpital Privé Jacques Cartier, Massy and Hôpital Privé Claude Galien, Quincy, France

The history of coronary bifurcation treatment is superimposed with that of coronary angioplasty as illustrated in the early 1980s by the description of the kissing balloon technique [1]. Many technical strategies have been proposed under various names since the advent of stenting but they have not always been adequately assessed.

Results achieved in coronary bifurcations with bare metal stents were clearly not as good as those achieved in non-bifurcated lesions, especially with respect to restenosis and repeat interventions (TLR). These poor results fueled the development of dedicated stents while drug-eluting stents (DES) paved the way for enhanced techniques aiming at optimal angiographic results [2].

In order to compare the various techniques, a substantial number of randomized trials were carried out, the majority of which supported the provisional side branch (SB) stenting strategy (2013 ACC/AHA and 2014 ESC recommendations). The strategies recommended for the most complex lesions are still the subject of heated debate. Angioplasty of the distal left main is similar to bifurcation percutaneous coronary intervention (PCI) without any specific difficulties, but with a higher procedural risk. Indeed, as the angle between the two distal branches is wider and the vessel diameters are larger, many stents are unsuitable for treating such cases. Although provisional stenting is regarded as superior on the basis of findings from registries and sub-group analyses, no randomized trial has yet been performed.

Anatomy and function of a coronary bifurcation

As is the case for trees in nature or in other parts of the human body, coronary trees have a pseudo-fractal geometry consisting of self-similar repetition of the same modules which are asymmetrical and increasingly smaller coronary bifurcations (Figure 16.1). Each bifurcation is a single anatomic and functional entity with diameters defined by Murray's law as follows: D^3 proximal = D3 main distal + D^3 side branch. For Huo and Kassab the exponent is 2.3. Finet's formula is simpler: D proximal = (D main distal + D side branch) 0.678 [3]. When two diameters of a bifurcation are known, the third can be calculated [4].

A coronary bifurcation is not only an anatomic entity, it is also a functional entity. There are, indeed, linear relationships between diameter, length, flow, and the myocardial mass supplied by a vessel [3]. The bifurcation carena or flow divider plays an important part in the distribution of flow required to supply the myocardium.

The anatomic configuration of coronary bifurcations has multiple implications for treatment strategies and also for quantitative angiography (QCA). From the origin of the vessel down to its distal extremity, the diameter decreases unevenly at each bifurcation and does not follow a linear pattern as in standard QCA software [5]. With this type of software in the main vessel segment proximal (PM) to the SB, the reference diameter is underestimated and the degree of stenosis is overestimated. In the segment distal to the SB (DM), the reference is overestimated as is the degree of stenosis compared to the actual dimensions of the vessel segments. By conventional QCA, the SB can be measured using two methods. Measurement from the ostium underestimates the degree of an ostial lesion as well as the reference diameter. The most commonly used method includes the proximal main branch in the analysis and overestimates the diameter, the degree of stenosis, and the frequency of ostial lesions. There is currently a variety of dedicated software products which have become indispensable for coronary bifurcation QCA [6].

Coronary bifurcation: a pro-atherogenic anatomy

In a linear coronary vessel, blood flow velocity is high during diastole (with a symmetric profile) generating high wall shear stress (WSS). In a vessel loop, the profile becomes asymmetric with high WSS on the outside and lower WSS on the inside of the loop.

In a bifurcation, the velocity is high at the level of the carena, generating high WSS on both sides of the carena, whereas flow is turbulent and even recirculating on the opposite walls resulting in low WSS [7]. High velocity persists in the coronary tree beyond the epicardial segments where the vascular area does not vary.

Low WSS is a documented pro-atherogenic factor whereas high WSS has a protective effect. In areas of high WSS, the endothelial

Interventional Cardiology: Principles and Practice, Second Edition. Edited by George D. Dangas, Carlo Di Mario, and Nicholas N. Kipshidze.
© 2017 John Wiley & Sons, Ltd. Published 2017 by John Wiley & Sons, Ltd.

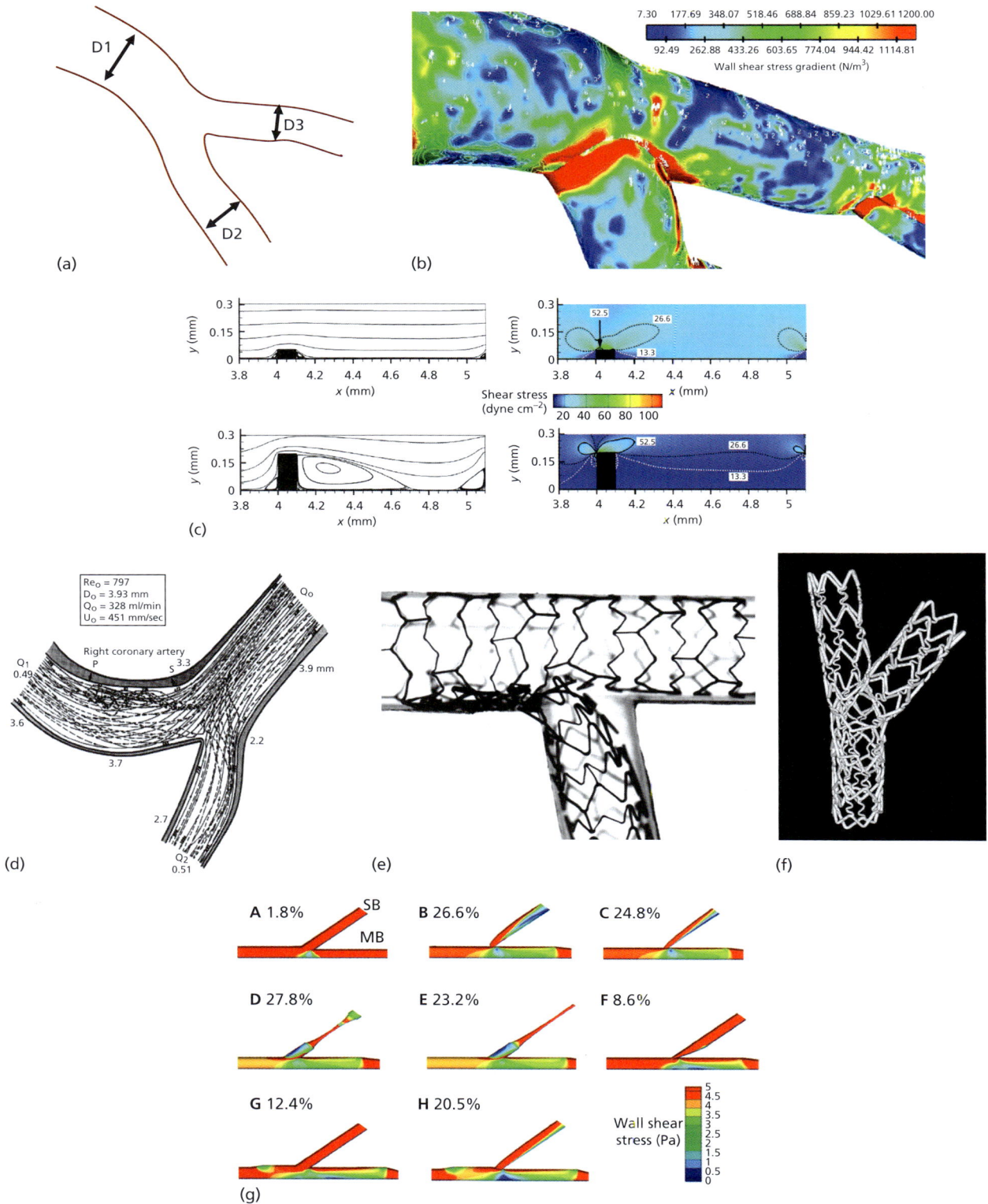

Figure 16.1 Coronary bifurcation fundamental aspects. (a): asymmetric branching, the modulus of the pseudo-fractal coronary tree. (b): Map of wall shear stress (WSS) derived from patient anatomy. Dark blue color corresponds to low WSS (Source: Soulis J, *et al. Hippokratia* 2014; **18**(1): 12–16). (c): Turbulences generated by stent struts, more important for thick stents, responsible for low WSS distal to a thick strut, as there is high WSS on the top of the strut (Source: Chestnutt and Han 2015 [18]). (d): flow in coronary bifurcation, linear with high velocity outside the curve and on both sides of the carena, turbulent (low WSS) opposite the carena (Source: reproduced from Asakura and Karino 1990 [7], Fig. 13, with permission of Wolters Kluwer). (e): Classic crush in an open angle bench bifurcation. The side branch (SB) stent is not apposed on the carena, there is an excess of metal in the proximal (PM) segment, if a kissing balloon (KB) is attempted there is a risk of crossing to the SB outside the stent (Source: Ormiston JA, *et al. Catheter Cardiovasc Interv* 2004; **63**(3): 332–336). (f): example of micro CT-scan of a bench stent deployment (Source: Ormiston JA, *et al. Catheter Cardiovasc Interv* 2004; **63**(3): 332–6). (g): WSS in various post-treatment scenarios in bifurcation models. In models with significant SB stenosis (B–E), low WSS areas were observed in the SB and lateral side of main branch (MB). Low WSS areas in the lateral side of MB were also more exaggerated in the post-kissing balloon angioplasty models (G and H) and carina shift model (F). Percentages of low WSS are indicated in each scenario. A is the original normal model and has the lowest surface of low WSS (Source: Na and Koo. *Korean Circ J* 2011; **41**: 91–96. Published under Creative Commons License 3.0).

cells are aligned along the flow with no intercellular space, whereas low WSS is associated with cellular disorientation, presence of intercellular space, and various other modifications [8].

Maps of WSS in a coronary vessel can be produced in models derived from real patients, confirming the relationship between low WSS and presence of atheroma. In a bifurcation, atheroma initially develops opposite the carena, as shown by anatomo-pathologic examination. Development of atheroma affects the pattern of intra-coronary flow, which may in turn lead to circular progression of the plaque toward the carena [9].

Stent behavior in bifurcations

The deployment of stents in bench models reproducing more or less accurately "real" coronary bifurcations has considerably helped operators to identify difficulties and implement successful strategies. These models have been designed to match the technical conditions of "real" interventions as closely as possible.

The opening of a stent strut toward the SB in bifurcations with an acute angle results in the protrusion of struts in the SB ostium as well as stent distortion on the side opposite the SB. This double phenomenon is even more marked when opening a distal strut next to the carena and can be corrected by performing kissing balloon inflation. This is the basis of the provisional stenting strategy [10].

By systematically assessing techniques and dedicated stents in basic models of both bifurcations and non-bifurcations, Ormiston *et al.* [11] demonstrated the inadequacy of the Crush and Culotte technical strategies in bifurcations with an open B angle, which was further confirmed in clinical settings. Similarly, the Simultaneous Kissing Stent (SKS) technique is less attractive than initially thought, because it generates a neocarena, two semi-cylindrical channels wrapped up around each other, as well as malapposition areas.

Bench testing images using micro CT scan have become very useful investigation and teaching tools. The use of electron microscopes has made possible the analysis of polymer damage in certain settings. The most elaborate benches allow the analysis of bioresorbable stent deployment at 37° [12]. They are even sometimes derived from the anatomy of real patients with pulsatile perfusion or cyclic angle modification in order to test stent resistance to fracture. Modern DES are almost exclusively based on an open-cell design. Strut dimensions (thickness, but here more importantly width) and strut shape (rectangular, round, elliptical, and so on) influence the impact on SB origin and can affect re-crossing. The main differences between design are related to the number of connectors (two or three) and their types as they can connect to peak or to valleys in a straight or an oblique way; some designs include variations in strut connector width. The range of diameters are usually covered by two or three designs, with different cut-off according to the brand, which can impact the capability of overexpansion and maximal cell size opening as they have a different number of crowns [11]. A good knowledge of these data when selecting stents to treat bifurcation is the key to success. Bench tests have been carried out to evaluate the impact of different types of stent at the different steps of bifurcation stenting particularly in terms of residual ostial SB obstruction and malapposition [11]. However, differences are usually limited and the most important factor of variability is not the stent design but the relation of crowns and connectors with the SB ostium due to the absence of possible control at the time of implantation *in vivo*, when using non-dedicated stents. The result could be a V, W, T, or H shape of struts obstructing the SB, which explains the variability of final results in terms of strut apposition at the SB ostium after SB inflation and/or kissing balloon technique.

Digital simulation bench tests have recently been developed using more or less realistic bifurcation models and virtual stents with the same characteristics as commercially available stents. The most sophisticated models are derived from digital reconstruction based on angiographic, CT scan, or intraluminal (IVUS or OCT) patient data [13,14]. These simulation models have allowed the evaluation of technical strategies whose clinical outcome was uncertain: selection of the crossover stent diameter in provisional stenting and effect of proximal optimization technique (POT). Digital simulation provides data that cannot be obtained in real patients such as flow geometry before and after stenting, circumferential stress generated by stenting (overdilatation) with documented clinical impact [15], mapping and significance of low WSS areas in bifurcations with neointimal hyperplasia (NIH) opposite the carena [16].

Variations in flows can be analyzed according to strut thickness as there is recirculation behind the struts (known factor of restenosis) [17]. Analysis of flow behind the stent struts enables the identification of the triggering factors of thrombosis [18]. These data can be used to develop enhanced technical strategies as well as for teaching purposes or even for future pre-treatment

Coronary bifurcation stenosis

Definitions of coronary bifurcation lesions are generally based on the SB ostium diameter with relation to the potential myocardial complications associated with SB occlusion. This diameter is often similar to that of the smallest available stent (2.25 mm) which can be used to stent a 2-mm artery (1.1 : 1 ratio).

In order to include factors such as myocardial viability in the SB territory or its collateralizing role, the European Bifurcation Club (EBC), a coronary bifurcation treatment think tank founded in 2004, proposed the following definition: "a coronary artery narrowing occurring adjacent to, and/or involving the origin of a significant SB." A significant SB is a branch that the operator does not want to lose [19].

Many classifications of bifurcation lesions based on angiography have been proposed, all of which are difficult to memorize. Some of these classifications are associated with arbitrary treatment strategies for each bifurcation type [20]. Medina's is the simplest classification (Figure 16.2) [21] but does not provide complete lesion characterization and must be combined with dedicated QCA and other imaging methods which are now indexed as new Medina intravenous ultrasound (IVUS) or fractional flow reserve (FFR) classifications. The important characteristics to be taken into account before performing coronary angioplasty are the presence of calcifications, the length and degree of the SB ostium stenosis, the angle between the PM segment and the SB (A for access), or the angle between the two distal segments (B for between) [19]. Medina's classification should be associated with precise delineation of the SB (before treatment for comparative studies) preferably based on the diameter and length of the distal artery. This description could follow Medina's classification and be expressed as LAD1, LAD2, Dg2 [19].

Stenting techniques

Describing the techniques of coronary bifurcation stenting has become a difficult task owing to the creativity deployed by interventional cardiologists. Certain very similar technical strategies are known under different names, whereas very dissimilar techniques can be designated by the same name. Very few classifications of

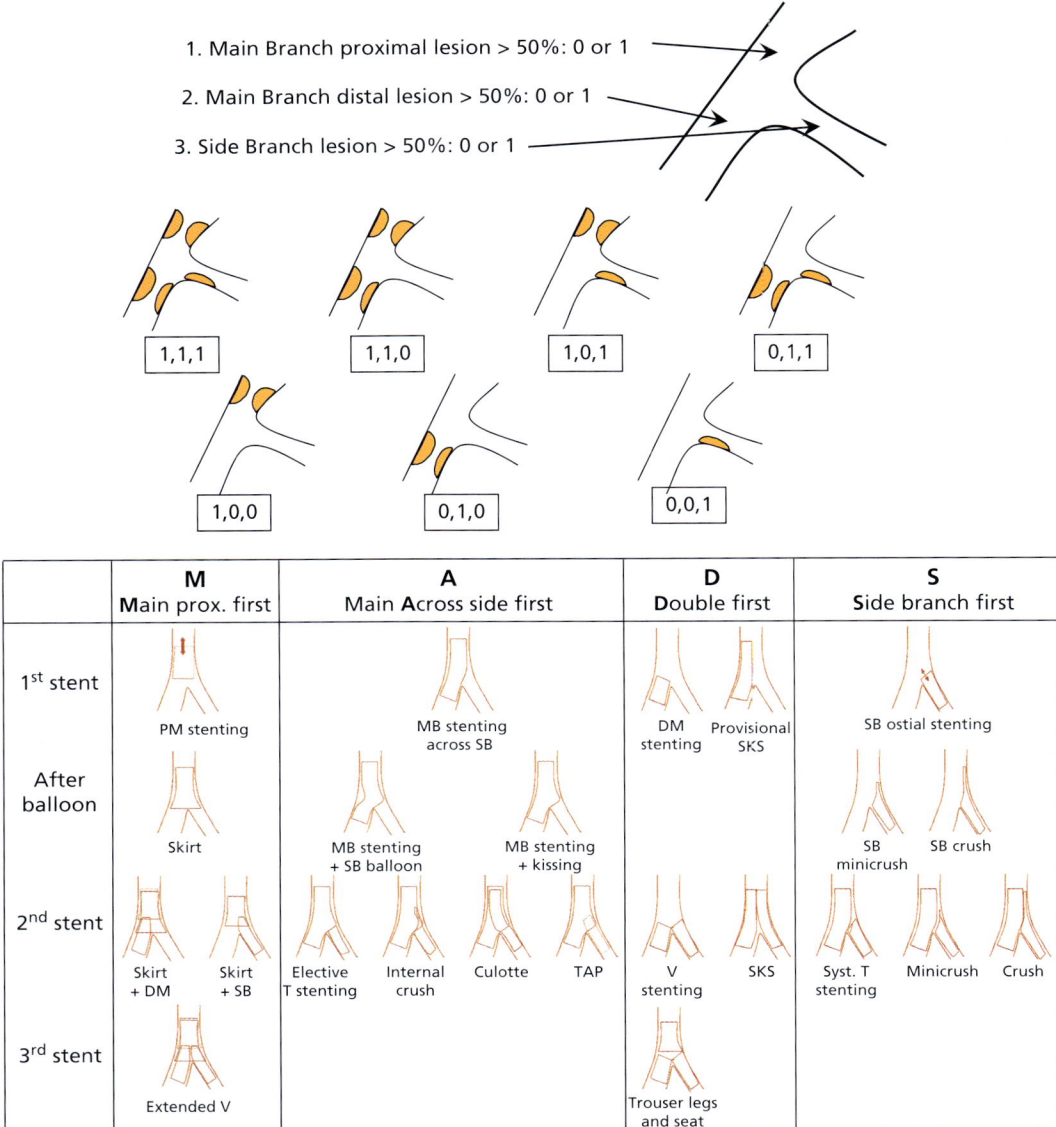

Figure 16.2 Top: the Medina classification: It consists in giving a binary value (1, 0) according to whether each of the segments (PM, DM, SB) previously defined is compromised or not (Source: Medina *et al.* 2006 [21]). Bottom: the MADS classification of bifurcation stenting techniques. Stenting strategies are indexed according to final stent placement. There are classified into strategies according to the position of the first implanted stent: M, proximal main; A, across; D, double; S, side branch.

stenting techniques have been published. The EBC has tried to find a method of classification that is both simple and open. The MADS classification is based exclusively on the final position of stents and on the order in which they are implanted (Figure 16.2) [19], thus allowing a simplified description according to the strategy implemented, namely, the position of the first stent. All strategies share common technical issues.

All the various strategies of stent placement in the MADS classification have been carried out in patients and have been published or reported. However, most of the recent techniques have not been specifically listed in the classification because their main variations from the standard techniques only involve balloon or wire maneuvers. Inverted strategies have been included in the classification to describe stent implantation techniques from the main artery to the smallest distal branch (i.e., "straight" Culotte described first

by Chevalier [22], A for "Across" strategy and the inverted Culotte stenting from PM to SB) all with their own technical problems.

The only way to perfectly describe and classify the various technical strategies implemented in patients would be an e-reporting sytem including all the preparation techniques, wire and balloon maneuvers.

Non-left main and left main stenosis clinical trials

One versus two stents?

Many trials, non-randomized in the era of bare metal stents (BMS), randomized or not in the era of DES, have compared the use of one vs. two stents in non-left main bifurcations.

In the era of BMS, the meta-analysis by Zamani and Kinlay [23] clearly underlined the benefit of single stent placement with respect to the occurrence of clinical events. Six randomized trials comparing single- versus double-stenting were carried out in Europe and were included in several meta-analyses which confirmed the absence of any differences in terms of mortality or repeat intervention [24–29]. The single-stent strategy was associated with a lower rate of myocardial infarction (MI) and a trend toward a reduced incidence of stent thrombosis. A meta-analysis of both randomized and non-randomized studies comparing QCA results showed a better acute gain in the SB ostium associated with the dual-stent technique, but also a higher late loss, which translated into an absence of mid-term differences in minimal luminal diameter (MLD) [30].

European studies comparing one- or two-stent strategies were discussed in reports of Asian trials in the DES era. The DK-Crush II trial [31], in particular, compared the provisional stenting strategy in patients with true bifurcation lesions (Medina 1,1,1 or 0,1,1) with the double kissing crush technique whereby two kissing balloon inflations are performed, the first inflation after placement of the first stent in the SB with minimal proximal crush using a balloon, and the second inflation at the end of the procedure. This randomized trial, which included 185 patients in each study group, observed no significant clinical differences at 6 months, but significant differences in the rates of death, MI, and TVR at 12 months after systematic follow-up angiography at 8 months. This study was included in a meta-analysis which highlighted a trend toward a potential benefit associated with a double stenting strategy in bifurcations with a large-diameter SB (sub-group analysis).

In the Korean randomized trial, PERFECT, no differences were observed between the Crush and the Provisional strategies in bifurcations with SB stenosis: MACE at 12 months: 17.8 vs. 18.5 for Crush and single stenting, respectively [32].

The patient-level meta-analysis of the Nordic I and BBC 1 trials generated particularly interesting findings [33]. Indeed, at 9 months a difference emerged with respect to the rates of death, MI, and TVR in favor of the single-stent strategy. This difference was consistent across all subgroups, especially in patients with a large SB and long lesions. Procedural time, X-ray exposure, and volume of contrast used were also lower in recipients of a single stent. The 5-year overall mortality rate was inferior in the single-stent strategy group (3.8% vs. 7.0%; p = 0.04) [Behan, personal communication, EBC meeting 2014].

Final kissing balloon or not?

The potential benefits of final kissing balloon (FKB) are considered irrefutable when both branches of the bifurcation are stented [34]. The benefits of final kissing in provisional stenting procedures are still controversial. The Nordic III randomized study [35] did not show any clinical difference at 6 months, but demonstrated a difference in favor of kissing with respect to SB restenosis at 8 months. The COBIS I registry [36] pointed to a higher risk of TLR and MACE associated with FKB in contrast to COBIS II [37] which showed a reduction in target vessel revascularization in the main vessel or in both branches.

Two recent Korean randomized studies confirmed that systematic final kissing is not superior to the simple crossover strategy in bifurcations with a lesion-free SB. A higher restenosis rate was observed in the main vessel (3.8% vs. 7.0%; p = 0.018) in the CROSS study [32]. In this study, systematic angiographic follow-up examination was performed at 8 months before clinical endpoint analysis (MACE: death, MI, TVR). The SMART-STRATEGY trial [38]

compared a conventional with an aggressive strategy after crossover stenting. In the "aggressive" strategy group the SB was treated in the presence of< TIMI 3 flow or >75% stenosis, in non-LM bifurcations, and with >50% SB stenosis in LM bifurcations. The conservative strategy was associated with a lower incidence of procedure-related myocardial necrosis (5.5% vs. 17.7%; p = 0.002) and at 12 months the incidence of target vessel failure was similar in both groups (9.2–9.4%).

The efficiency of kissing and prevention of its potentially negative effects depend on the manner in which it is carried out [35]: use of non-compliant balloons at least in unstented SB in order to prevent the occurrence of dissection, short balloons to avoid oval distortion in the PM segment, stent diameters adapted to the distal diameters of the bifurcation, inflations in the SB in preparation for kissing, prolonged inflations, inflation in the SB first.

Which double stent technique?

Like the provisional stenting strategy, double stenting techniques have evolved. Crush has now become mini-crush whereby a stent strut is opened toward the SB following each stent implantation, with kissing inflation in most cases (Mini-DK-Crush) [39], which improves the success rate of final kissing. With respect to the Culotte technique, the proximal overlapping area has been reduced to a minimum (mini-Culotte) and POT is carried out at each stage of the procedure.

Two randomized trials compared two bifurcation stenting techniques: the NORDIC II trial found no significant differences between Crush and Culotte techniques at 6 months. However, there was a lower use of FKB in the Crush group (failure) as well as a trend toward more frequent biomarker elevation [40,41]. Opposite findings in the left main were reported in the DK-Crush III study [42].

The Simultaneous Kissing Stent (SKS) technique described by Sharma et al. [43] consists of the simultaneous deployment of two stents from the PM segment toward each of the two branches. This technique has not been compared with other strategies. It has inherent technical difficulties which are not easy to overcome. For instance, in cases of proximal dissection, a neocarena of variable length is generated, making any repeat intervention difficult. The advocates of this technique recommend the implementation of a life-long dual antiplatelet treatment.

Double stenting: a pro-thrombotic situation

The meta-analysis by Zimarino et al. [44] clearly demonstrated the excess rate of stent thrombosis in cases of double stenting (OR 2.31) associated with an increase in MI (OR 1.86). It also showed the relation between infarction and thrombosis. Peri-procedural biomarker elevation associated with double stenting techniques has no impact on patient outcome.

Are results applicable to distal left main stenting?

There are no randomized studies comparing the single and double stenting strategies in distal left main lesions. The findings of many registries suggest that the provisional SB stenting strategy should also be recommended in distal left main segments in the majority of cases.

Several important registries pointed to the superiority of the provisional strategy: improved TLR-free survival in a population of 773 patients with left main lesions undergoing single stent implantation, no differences between the double stenting, T, V, or Crush techniques in the Italian multicenter study by Palmerini et al. [45], lower rate of cardiac death at 3 years in the study by Toyofuku *et al.* [46], a lower 1-year MACE rate in a sub-group of the Syntax trial.

Workhorse versus dedicated stents

Very few randomized studies comparing the provisional strategy with the use of a dedicated stent have been carried out. Recently, the Tryton dedicated stent was compared with the provisional strategy in bifurcations with a large SB. The TRYTON trial did not meet its non-inferiority primary endpoint as a result of an increased rate of peri-procedural MI [47]. However, bifurcations included in the study had an SB diameter often lower than specified in the inclusion criteria. A sub-group analysis of SBs with a diameter >2.25 mm demonstrated the non-inferiority of the TRYTON stent [48].

Bifurcation stenting general principles

Based on fundamental clinical data pertaining to non-left main and left main bifurcation stenting, three recommendations can be made:

1 The number of implanted stents should be limited, which may lead to implementation of the provisional SB stenting strategy. Alternatively, an SB stenting predictive score [49] or SB occlusion predictive score can be used in order to weigh up the advantages of stenting the SB first. A comparison between the two strategies in the same population would show that using the score used in the DEFINITON study, 30% of double stenting starting with the SB would be performed and 70% of provisional SB stenting strategies. If the provisional strategy were to be used, the percentage of double stenting after final kissing balloon would be probably lower than 30% even in left main lesions.

2 Full deployment and apposition of a single stent layer is needed.

3 Compliance with the branching law of bifurcation should be respected.

Provisional side branch stenting strategy

Step-by-step provisional SB stenting is described in Figures 16.3 and 16.4. A jailed wire in the SB, hydrophilic or not, is a safe technique if the crossover stent is not deployed on the radiopaque segment of the wire.

Many predictors of SB occlusion have been described. They involve the presence of ostial lesions of the SB, lesion length, stenosis or homolateral plaque at the SB of the PM segment, calcified plaque opposite the SB, an acute coronary syndrome, lesions outside the left main. An acute B angle has been considered a predictive factor of occlusion resulting from carena shift when a stent larger than the diameter of the DM segment is implanted [50]. However, Zhang *et al.* [51] states that an open angle is a predictor of occlusion whereas Hahn *et al.* [52] concludes that the angle has no impact.

This recent study also questions the efficacy of a jailed wire in preserving SB patency. However, the jailed wire strategy can be considered as a predictor of patency restoration because of its use as a "landmark," the change in the angle of SB access or in the setting of a salvage maneuver (reopening of the SB with a very small balloon inflated outside the stent). The size of the stent is selected on the basis of the DM segment diameter. The purpose of the POT is to give

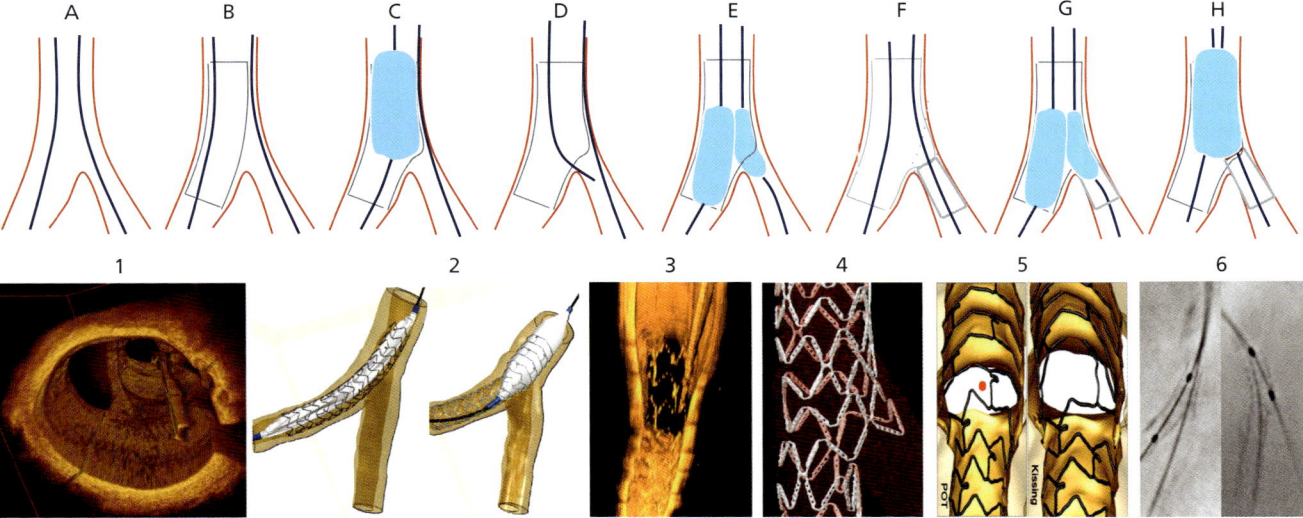

Figure 16.3 Provisional stenting strategy. A: 2 wires beginning with the most difficult branch 1: Axial OCT view showing the position of the carena (flow divider). B: Stenting of the main branch across the SB protected by a jailed wire, diameter chosen from the DM segment. C: Proximal optimization technique (POT) proposed by Darremont, to give a second diameter, the one of the PM segment (matching that of the PM segment), to the stent. 2: Crossover stent deployment in a specific patient model, proximal malapposition. After POT the proximal segment of the stent is apposed, the cells are more opened in front of the SB if the big and short POT balloon is inflated with the distal marker in front of the carena. D: Main vessel wire, prepared with a long shape, is pulled slowly in front of the SB to enter the most distal cell facilitated by POT. 3: Online 3D OCT reconstruction showing the wire in the most distal cell. E: after dejailing of the SB wire pushed in the distal main vessel, kissing balloon using short balloons, non-compliant for the SB, chosen from the two distal segments. Begin the inflation with the SB balloon. 4: When the most distal cell is entered toward the SB, there is metal projection in the ostium of the SB. 5. Ostium of the SB after POT only (left) and after kissing balloon (right). F: SB stenting when necessary performed as a T stenting or a TAP (T and Protrusion). 6: Stent enhancement showing on the left projection of metal in the SB ostium, ideal for T stenting, absence of projection after proximal cell crossing on the right leading to TAP stenting. G: Mandatory FKB after any double stenting implantation. H: Final POT to correct potential elliptical distortion created by kissing.

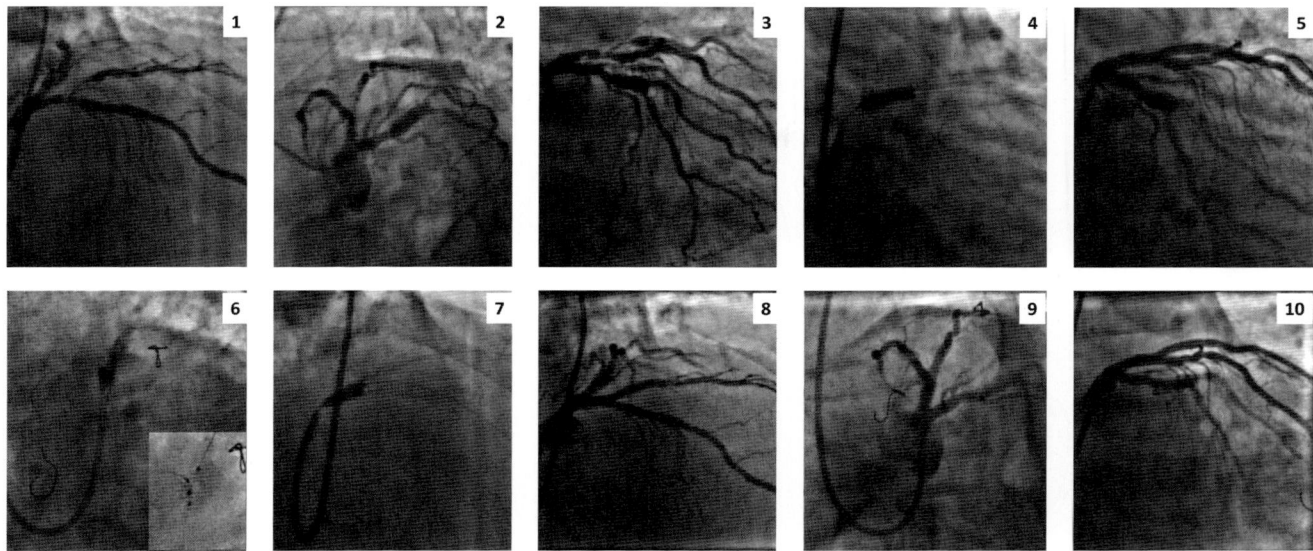

Figure 16.4 Inverted provisional stenting. 1–3: Bifurcation stenosis 1,0,1; LAD1,LAD1,Dg1. 4: After stenting from left anterior descending (LAD) to diagonal with a stent diameter adapted to diagonal, a POT is performed with a short balloon adapted to LAD diameter. 5: Result after POT. 6: Kissing balloon with short balloons adapted to the two distal diameters, non-compliant for LAD. 7: Second POT with the same balloon to correct the proximal oval distortion. 8–10: Result in three initial projections.

the crossover stent two distinct diameters corresponding to those of the two covered segments. This technique allows the reconstruction of the initial anatomy of the bifurcation and facilitates wire exchange when SB treatment is implemented by avoiding wire exchange outside the proximal part of the main branch (MB) [53].

The "crossover" stent should be implanted sufficiently proximal to the SB to accommodate a short, large-diameter balloon. Guidewire exchange is normally carried out by pulling back the main vessel wire (in the absence of any untreated dissection) in order to insert it in the SB through the most distal cell, thus allowing the projection of struts in the ostial segment of the SB opposite the carena. The jailed wire is subsequently removed from the SB and inserted into the DM segment. Though relatively safe, this maneuver can be associated with a risk of guiding-catheter penetration resulting in dissection or longitudinal stent distortion particularly in the setting of left main PCI.

Guide-wire exchange generally aims at treating the origin of the SB which is often stenosed as a consequence of the carena shift phenomenon. The resulting stenosis is non-significant in most instances as shown by FFR assessment of angiographically tight lesions [54]. This can be explained by the oval configuration of the SB ostium as visualized using the least optimal angiographic view, even though the actual reduction of the vascular area is minimal.

Kissing balloon inflation was the first specific technique applied to bifurcations and is still the subject of controversy. Alternatives to kissing balloon have been proposed on the basis of *in vitro* tests that need clinical validation. These include successive inflations in the side and main branches (Side, Main, Side: SMS) and above all POT-side-POT. It is sometimes recommended that a second stent should be implanted in the SB ostium in the presence of a dissection or residual stenosis, or even systematically in long lesions located in large vessels. In such cases, T or TAP (T and Protrusion) [55] placement can be performed depending on the coverage of the ostium by a crossover stent as visualized using

the stent enhancement technique (when the SB wire has been inserted in the most distal strut). Though a more complex technique, the straight Culotte stenting technique can also be used to treat the SB. In all cases, final kissing balloon with short non-compliant balloons after double stenting is indispensable and final POT useful to correct oval distortion.

The major advantage of provisional SB stenting lies in the fact that each step of the procedure can be adapted according to the results of the previous step. In small-diameter SBs, simple protection (use of a protection wire) during crossover stenting is sufficient. In large-diameter SBs, when flow in the SB is < TIMI 3, associated with chest pain and/or ST segment changes, reopening of the branch (SMS, POT-side-POT, or kissing balloon inflation) is necessary. If there is a significant difference between the PM and the DM diameters, POT should be performed and a cell should be opened toward the SB by means of kissing balloon or POT-side-POT, in order to ensure SB access in case further treatment should be required or to put the carena in its place.

Beginning with SB stenting

The initial stenting techniques starting with the SB were conventional T stenting with the frequent disadvantage of a gap at the SB ostium in Y-shaped bifurcations (Figure 16.5) [2]. This led to the modified T stenting whereby the SB stent protrudes into the MB in which a balloon has been inflated [2]. In the conventional Crush technique strategy, the SB stent is implanted far into the PM segment, then crushed with the crossover stent in the MB. Subsequently wiring the SB to perform the indispensable final kissing balloon inflation can prove difficult.

The most elaborate version of the Crush technique is currently the mini DK-Crush described by Chen *et al.* (Figure 16.3) [39]. This specific strategy does not use POT and, consequently, the size of the selected stent must match the PM diameter. Performing

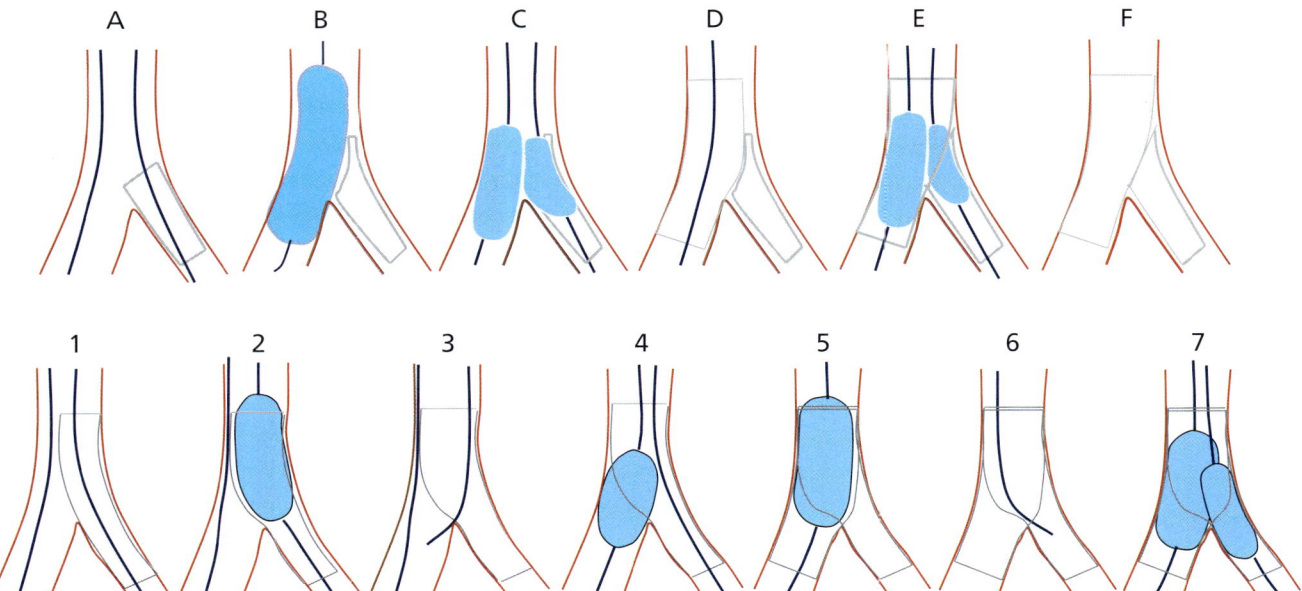

Figure 16.5 Mini-DK-Crush technique. A: Two wires, implantation of a stent in the ostium of the SB with a small protrusion. B: Crush of the protrusion with balloon inflation in the main branch after SB wire removal. C: After recrossing toward the SB with a wire, first KB. D: Crossover stent implantation in the main vessel after SB wire removal. E: After rewiring the SB, second KB. F: final result. 1–7: Inverted Culotte. 1: Two wires, implantation of a stent chosen from SB diameter from PM to SB. 2: POT with a balloon adapted to PM diameter to avoid unintentional crush. 3: Use of the SB wire to re-enter the distal (DM) close to the carena. 4: After dejailing the main vessel wire, insertion in the SB and pre-dilatation toward the DM to prepare stenting. 5: Stent from PM (short protrusion) to DM, followed by POT after SB wire removal. 6: Wire recrossing th SB, close to the carena (distal cell). 7: Final KB.

kissing balloon inflation after Crush in the SB facilitates both the passage of the wire through the struts of the stent which is subsequently implanted in the MB and final kissing inflation.

There are two distinct Culotte techniques. The first was initially described as part of the provisional strategy. The second begins with stent implantation in the PM segment toward the SB, in order to avoid losing the SB. As the difference between the PM and SB diameters is sometimes significant, the second technique (Figure 16.3) requires POT in the PM on the SB wire immediately after implantation of the first stent in order to prevent the occurrence of wire exchange outside the stent toward the DM, which would result in unintended Crush.

Dedicated stent implantation

Bifurcation-dedicated stents represent the holy grail for the interventional cardiologist. Although many dedicated stents have been evaluated in the past 10 years, their superiority over the provisional strategy has not been demonstrated. There are currently four dedicated stents commercially available worldwide.

The BIOSS stent is the most recent dedicated device. Data pertaining to this stent have been collected in small registry studies. It is a balloon-expandable DES with large struts at the bifurcation level facilitating access to the SB. There is currently a sirolimus-eluting version of this stent.

The Stentys device was also evaluated in registry studies. It is a balloon-expandable stent, initially eluting TAXUS. The new generation is a sirolimus-eluting stent allowing accurate placement (inflation of the balloon results in the rupture of the sheath covering the stent). The design of this stent enables easy access to the bifurcation branches with the possibility of "breaking" a strut during SB dilatation in order to achieve optimal SB coverage in cases of distal access.

The Axxess stent was broadly evaluated and compared with the provisional strategy in non-randomized studies. It is a balloon-expandable Biolimus A9-eluting stent. The stent design enables treatment of the MB segment proximal to the bifurcation with partial coverage of the SB ostium and distal MB segment. It is often necessary to implant one or even two additional stents for adequate coverage of the lesion. A version of this stent was specifically designed for left main lesions.

The Tryton stent is a balloon-expandable bare stent designed to facilitate bifurcation treatment using the Culotte technique. This stent is intended for "true" bifurcation lesions requiring a double stent technique. The stent design allows optimal coverage of the SB as well as loose coverage of the proximal MB facilitating access to the MB and placement of a DES in the MB. This is the only dedicated stent that has been assessed in comparison with the provisional strategy in a randomized trial in patients with "true" bifurcation lesions. The study failed to demonstrate the non-inferiority of the dedicated stent compared with the provisional strategy. However, the inclusion criteria, and especially the SB size >2.5 mm, were not adequately fulfilled in this study.

When taking into account patients meeting the inclusion criteria, the Tryton stent appears to be non-inferior to the provisional strategy. A study evaluating the Tryton stent specifically designed for left main lesions is currently underway. The new stent iteration will be a DES.

Bifurcation stenting with bioresorbable stents

The potential advantages of BRS in the treatment of bifurcations are the conformability of the scaffold, the absence of fracture at the level of the carena when two stents are implanted, and the possibility of restoring patency in the SB. However, given the long resorption time, especially with bioresorbable vascular scaffolds (BVS), the risk of thrombosis at 1–4 years cannot be eliminated.

Bench testing data pertaining to BVS [11] have evidenced some limitations for the treatment of bifurcations. Although BVS are compatible with a conventional provisional strategy with appropriate sizing, conventional kissing should not be performed as it can result in BVS fracture. According to the recommendations issued by the EBC, POT-side-POT should be performed if the SB needs attention or alternatively, "mini kissing" using short, non-compliant balloons which do not extend beyond the polygone of confluence, inflated at low pressures (≤5 atm).

Given the thickness of BVS (150 μm), dual-stent techniques may increase the risk of thrombosis. The only technique that we can currently recommend is T stenting with two BVS or one BVS in the MB and a DES in the SB. There are few data regarding the other BRS, but some seem to have a broader expansion potential, which could allow stenting with 2 BRS. The new BVS generation with 100-μm thickness provides interesting treatment possibilities.

Role of imaging in bifurcation stenting

The role of imaging (IVUS or OCT) in the treatment of bifurcations is still the subject of controversy. Although IVUS and OCT provide interesting information (apposition, stent positioning, access to the distal strut, technical mistakes) likely to improve the final result, only a few retrospective studies have shown potential benefits for left main stenting in particular.

In routine practice, we recommend that imaging techniques should be used when in doubt or during the learning phase, especially for left main treatment or when BRS are used.

Conclusions

The safe and efficient treatment of coronary bifurcation lesions requires appropriate knowledge of the anatomy and function of this specific entity. Remembering the lessons learned from bench testing during the procedure can help the operator overcome inherent difficulties. Simulation models are more associated with strategy and can be instrumental in achieving a reduction in the number of stents used, in avoiding stent overlap, and enabling appropriate stent apposition in order to restore an optimal anatomic configuration.

Several strategies have been accurately delineated. The Mini-DK-Crush and mini-Culotte techniques are recommended for complex lesions, whereas the provisional strategy can be implemented in practically all lesions.

One might have been justified in thinking that the advent of BRS would solve the issues related to bifurcation stenting. However, early experience has shown that these stents generate new technical and clinical problems such as thrombosis.

Acknowledgment

The authors would like to thank Catherine Dupic for her assistance in the preparation of this chapter.

Interactive multiple choice questions are available for this chapter on www.wiley. com/go/dangas/cardiology

References

1 Meier B. Kissing balloon coronary angioplasty. *Am J Cardiol* 1984; **54**(7): 918–920.

2 Louvard Y, Lefèvre T, Morice MC. Percutaneous coronary intervention for bifurcation coronary disease. *Heart* 2004; **90**(6): 713–722. Review.

3 Kassab GS, Finet G. Anatomy and function relation in the coronary tree: from bifurcations to myocardial flow and mass. *EuroIntervention* 2015; **11**(Suppl V): 13–17.

4 Kassab GS. Mathematical modeling of coronary arterial tree. Available at: http://www.bifurc.net/files/medtool/webmedtool/icpstool01/stud0714/pdf00001.pdf (accessed April 18, 2016).

5 Lansky A, Tuinenburg J, Costa M, *et al*; European Bifurcation Angiographic Sub-Committee. Quantitative angiographic methods for bifurcation lesions: a consensus statement from the European Bifurcation Group. *Catheter Cardiovasc Interv* 2009; **73**(2): 258–266.

6 Grundeken MJ, Ishibashi Y, Ramcharitar S, *et al*. The need for dedicated bifurcation quantitative coronary angiography (QCA) software algorithms to evaluate bifurcation lesions. *EuroIntervention* 2015; **11**(Suppl V): 44–49.

7 Asakura T, Karino T. Flow patterns and spatial distribution of atherosclerotic lesions in human coronary arteries. *Circ Res* 1990; **66**(4): 1045–1066.

8 Chatzizisis YS, Coskun AU, Jonas M, *et al*. Role of endothelial shear stress in the natural history of coronary atherosclerosis and vascular remodeling: molecular, cellular, and vascular behavior. *J Am Coll Cardiol* 2007; **49**(25): 2379–2393. Review.

9 van der Giessen AG, Wentzel JJ, Meijboom WB, *et al*. Plaque and shear stress distribution in human coronary bifurcations: a multislice computed tomography study. *EuroIntervention* 2009; **4**(5): 654–661.

10 Lefèvre T, Louvard Y, Morice MC, *et al*. Stenting of bifurcation lesions: classification, treatments, and results. *Catheter Cardiovasc Interv* 2000; **49**(3): 274–283.

11 Ormiston J, Darremont O, Iwasaki K, *et al*. Lessons from the real bench: non-BRS. *EuroIntervention* 2015; **11**(Suppl V): 27–30.

12 Ormiston J, Motreff P, Darremont O, Webber B, Guerin P, Webster M. Bioresorbable scaffolds on the bench. *EuroIntervention* 2015; **11**(Suppl V): 166–169.

13 Antoniadis AP, Mortier P, Kassab G, *et al*. Biomechanical modeling to improve coronary artery bifurcation stenting: expert review document on techniques and clinical implementation. *JACC Cardiovasc Interv* 2015; **8**(10): 1281–1296. Review.

14 Migliavacca F, Chiastra C, Chatzizisis YS, *et al*. Virtual bench testing to study coronary bifurcation stenting. *EuroIntervention* 2015; **11**(Suppl V): 31–34.

15 Costa MA, Angiolillo DJ, Tannenbaum M, *et al*; STLLR Investigators. Impact of stent deployment procedural factors on long-term effectiveness and safety of sirolimus-eluting stents (final results of the multicenter prospective STLLR trial). *Am J Cardiol* 2008; **101**(12): 1704–1711.

16 Nakazawa G, Yazdani SK, Finn AV, *et al*. Pathological findings at bifurcation lesions: the impact of flow distribution on atherosclerosis and arterial healing after stent implantation. *J Am Coll Cardiol* 2010; **55**(16): 1679–1687.

17 Kastrati A, Mehilli J, Dirschinger J, *et al*. Intracoronary Stenting and Angiographic Results Strut Thickness Effect on Restenosis Outcome (ISAR-STEREO) Trial. *Vestn Rentgenol Radiol* 2012; **2**: 52–60.

18 Chesnutt JK, Han HC. Simulation of the microscopic process during initiation of stent thrombosis. *Comput Biol Med* 2015; **56**: 182–191.

19 Louvard Y, Thomas M, Dzavik V, *et al*. Classification of coronary artery bifurcation lesions and treatments: time for a consensus! *Catheter Cardiovasc Interv* 2008; **71**(2): 175–183.

20 Movahed MR. Major limitations of randomized clinical trials involving coronary artery bifurcation interventions: time for redesigning clinical trials by involving only true bifurcation lesions and using appropriate bifurcation classification. *J Interv Cardiol* 2011; **24**(4): 295–301.

21 Medina A, Suárez de Lezo J, Pan M. A new classification of coronary bifurcation lesions. *Rev Esp Cardiol* 2006; **59**(2): 183.

22 Chevalier B, Glatt B, Royer T, *et al*. Placement of coronary stents in bifurcation lesions by the "culotte" technique. *Am J Cardiol* 1998; **82**(8): 943–949.

23 Zamani P, Kinlay S. Long-term risk of clinical events from stenting side branches of coronary bifurcation lesions with drug-eluting and bare-metal stents: an observational meta-analysis. *Catheter Cardiovasc Interv* 2011; **77**(2): 202–212.

24 Colombo A, Moses JW, Morice MC, *et al*. Randomized study to evaluate sirolimus-eluting stents implanted at coronary bifurcation lesions. *Circulation* 2004; **109**(10): 1244–1249.

25 Pan M, de Lezo JS, Medina A, *et al*. Rapamycin-eluting stents for the treatment of bifurcated coronary lesions: a randomized comparison of a simple versus complex strategy. *Am Heart J* 2004; **148**(5): 857–864.

26 Steigen TK, Maeng M, Wiseth R, et al; Nordic PCI Study Group. Randomized study on simple versus complex stenting of coronary artery bifurcation lesions: the Nordic bifurcation study. *Circulation* 2006; **114**(18): 1955–1961.

27 Ferenc M, Gick M, Kienzle RP, et al. Randomized trial on routine vs. provisional T-stenting in the treatment of de novo coronary bifurcation lesions. *Eur Heart J* 2008; **29**(23): 2859–2867.

28 Colombo A, Bramucci E, Saccà S, et al. Randomized study of the crush technique versus provisional side-branch stenting in true coronary bifurcations: the CACTUS (Coronary Bifurcations: Application of the Crushing Technique Using Sirolimus-Eluting Stents) Study. *Circulation* 2009; **119**(1): 71–78.

29 Hildick-Smith D, de Belder AJ, Cooter N, et al. Randomized trial of simple versus complex drug-eluting stenting for bifurcation lesions: the British Bifurcation Coronary Study: old, new, and evolving strategies. *Circulation* 2010; **121**(10): 1235–1243.

30 Athappan G, Ponniah T, Jeyaseelan L. True coronary bifurcation lesions: meta-analysis and review of literature. *J Cardiovasc Med (Hagerstown)* 2010; **11**(2): 103–110.

31 Chen SL, Santoso T, Zhang JJ, et al. A randomized clinical study comparing double kissing crush with provisional stenting for treatment of coronary bifurcation lesions: results from the DKCRUSH-II (Double Kissing Crush versus Provisional Stenting Technique for Treatment of Coronary Bifurcation Lesions) trial. *J Am Coll Cardiol* 2011; **57**(8): 914–920.

32 Kim YH, Lee JH, Roh JH, et al. Randomized comparisons between different stenting approaches for bifurcation coronary lesions with or without side branch stenosis. *JACC Cardiovasc Interv* 2015; **8**(4): 550–560.

33 Behan MW, Holm NR, Curzen NP, et al. Simple or complex stenting for bifurcation coronary lesions: a patient-level pooled-analysis of the Nordic Bifurcation Study and the British Bifurcation Coronary Study. *Circ Cardiovasc Interv* 2011; **4**(1): 57–64.

34 Murasato Y, Finet G, Foin N. Final kissing balloon inflation: the whole story. *EuroIntervention* 2015; **11**(Suppl V): 81–85.

35 Niemelä M, Kervinen K, Erglis A, et al.; Nordic-Baltic PCI Study Group. Randomized comparison of final kissing balloon dilatation versus no final kissing balloon dilatation in patients with coronary bifurcation lesions treated with main vessel stenting: the Nordic-Baltic Bifurcation Study III. *Circulation* 2011; **123**(1): 79–86.

36 Gwon HC, Hahn JY, Koo BK, et al. Final kissing ballooning and long-term clinical outcomes in coronary bifurcation lesions treated with1-stent technique: results from the COBIS registry. *Heart* 2012; **98**(3): 225–231.

37 Yu CW, Yang JH, Song YB, et al. Long-term clinical outcomes of final kissing ballooning in coronary bifurcation lesions treated with the 1-stent technique: results from the COBIS II Registry (Korean Coronary Bifurcation Stenting Registry). *JACC Cardiovasc Interv* 2015; **8**(10): 1297–1307.

38 Song YB, Hahn JY, Song PS, et al. Randomized comparison of conservative versus aggressive strategy for provisional side branch intervention in coronary bifurcation lesions: results from the SMART-STRATEGY (SmartAngioplasty Research Team-Optimal Strategy for Side Branch Intervention in Coronary BifurcationLesions) randomized trial. *JACC Cardiovasc Interv* 2012; **5**(11): 1133–1140.

39 Chen SL, Zhang JJ, Ye F, et al. Comparison of DK crush with classical crush technique with drug-eluting stents for the treatment of coronary bifurcation lesions from DKCRUSH-1 study. *Zhonghua Xin Xue Guan Bing Za Zhi* 2008; **36**(2): 100–107.

40 Erglis A, Kumsars I, Niemelä M, et al; Nordic PCI Study Group. Randomized comparison of coronary bifurcation stenting with the crush versus the culotte technique using sirolimus eluting stents: the Nordic stent technique study. *Circ Cardiovasc Interv* 2009; **2**(1): 27–34.

41 Kervinen K, Niemelä M, Romppanen H, et al; Nordic PCI Study Group. Clinical outcome after crush versus culotte stenting of coronary artery bifurcation lesions: the Nordic Stent Technique Study 36-month follow-up results. *JACC Cardiovasc Interv* 2013; **6**(11): 1160–1165.

42 Chen SL, Xu B, Han YL, et al. Comparison of double kissing crush versus Culotte stenting for unprotected distal left main bifurcation lesions: results from a multi-center, randomized, prospective DKCRUSH-III study. *J Am Coll Cardiol* 2013; **61**(14): 1482–1488.

43 Sharma SK, Choudhury A, Lee J, et al. Simultaneous kissing stents (SKS) technique for treating bifurcation lesions in medium-to-large size coronary arteries. *Am J Cardiol* 2004; **94**(7): 913–917.

44 Zimarino M, Corazzini A, Ricci F, et al. Late thrombosis after double versus single drug-eluting stent in the treatment of coronary bifurcations: a meta-analysis of randomized and observational Studies. *JACC Cardiovasc Interv* 2013; **6**(7): 687–695.

45 Palmerini T, Marzocchi A, Tamburino C, et al. Impact of bifurcation technique on 2-year clinical outcomes in 773 patients with distal unprotected left main coronary artery stenosis treated with drug-eluting stents. *Circ Cardiovasc Interv* 2008; **1**(3): 185–192.

46 Toyofuku M, Kimura T, Morimoto T, et al; j-Cypher Registry Investigators. Comparison of 5-year outcomes in patients with and without unprotected left main coronary artery disease after treatment with sirolimus-eluting stents: insights from the j-Cypher registry. *JACC Cardiovasc Interv* 2013; **6**(7): 654–663.

47 Généreux P, Kumsars I, Lesiak M, et al. A randomized trial of a dedicated bifurcation stent versus provisional stenting in the treatment of coronary bifurcation lesions. *J Am Coll Cardiol* 2015; **65**(6): 533–543.

48 Généreux P, Kini A, Lesiak M, et al. Outcomes of a dedicated stent in coronary bifurcations with large side branches: a subanalysis of the randomized TRYTON bifurcation study. *Catheter Cardiovasc Interv* 2015 Sep 23. doi: 10.1002/ccd.26240.

49 Chen SL, Sheiban I, Xu B, et al. Impact of the complexity of bifurcation lesions treated with drug-eluting stents: the DEFINITION study (Definitions and impact of complex bifurcation lesions on clinical outcomes after percutaneous coronary intervention using drug-eluting stents). *JACC Cardiovasc Interv* 2014; **7**(11): 1266–1276.

50 Vassilev D, Gil R. Clinical verification of a theory for predicting side branch stenosis after main vessel stenting in coronary bifurcation lesions. *J Interv Cardiol* 2008; **21**(6): 493–503.

51 Zhang D, Xu B, Yin D, et al. How bifurcation angle impacts the fate of side branch after main vessel stenting: a retrospective analysis of 1,200 consecutive bifurcation lesions in a single center. *Catheter Cardiovasc Interv* 2015; **85**(Suppl 1): 706–715.

52 Hahn JY, Chun WJ, Kim JH, et al. Predictors and outcomes of side branch occlusion after main vessel stenting in coronary bifurcation lesions: results from the COBIS II Registry (COronary BIfurcation Stenting). *J Am Coll Cardiol* 2013; **62**(18): 1654–1659.

53 Darremont O, Leymarie JL, Lefèvre T, et al. Technical aspects of the provisional side branch stenting strategy. *EuroIntervention* 2015; **11**(Suppl V): 86–90.

54 Koo BK, Kang HJ, Youn TJ, et al. Physiologic assessment of jailed side branch lesions using fractional flow reserve. *J Am Coll Cardiol* 2005; **46**(4): 633–637.

55 Burzotta F, Gwon HC, Hahn JY, et al. Modified T-stenting with intentional protrusion of the side-branch stent within the main vessel stent to ensure ostial coverage and facilitate final kissing balloon: the T-stenting and small protrusion technique (TAP-stenting). Report of bench testing and first clinical Italian-Korean two-centre experience. *Catheter Cardiovasc Interv* 2007; **70**(1): 75–82.

CHAPTER 17

Risk Stratification Approach to Multivessel Coronary Artery Disease

Davide Capodanno and Corrado Tamburino
Ferrarotto Hospital, University of Catania, Catania, Italy

Myocardial revascularization in patients with multivessel coronary artery disease (MVD) can be accomplished by percutaneous coronary interventions (PCI) or coronary artery bypass grafting (CABG). Approximately two-thirds of patients who require revascularization have MVD and two-thirds of these have anatomy that is amenable to treatment by PCI or surgery. Today, more complex lesions and sicker patients are being taken for multivessel PCI than in the past. This has been brought about by increasing operator experience, technological advances such as the availability of drug-eluting stents (DES), and more potent antiplatelet therapy with glycoprotein IIb/IIIa receptor antagonists and clopidogrel. Other contemporary procedural improvements, such as the availability of newer generation DES and more potent antiplatelet drugs than clopidogrel for patients with acute coronary syndromes (ACS) (i.e., prasugrel or ticagrelor), are anticipated to improve further the outcomes of patients with MVD undergoing PCI. As a result, the frequency of multivessel PCI is expected to increase in the future.

Many factors must be considered when approaching a patient with MVD. First, these patients have a less favorable long-term outcome. They are more likely to have adverse clinical features including diabetes mellitus, prior myocardial infarction (MI), and reduced left ventricular function. Second, the functional significance and complexity of each lesion need to be assessed to determine the appropriate percutaneous strategy. Procedural complexity and the risk of multivessel intervention is increased when unfavorable anatomy such as chronic total occlusions (CTO), calcified bifurcation lesions, and diffusely diseased small vessels are present (Box 17.1). Third, the impact of restenosis needs to be considered. The decision to choose PCI as a revascularization strategy should be based not only on whether it can be done safely and successfully, but also on its short- and long-term benefits when compared with the alternative of medical or surgical treatment. A risk stratification approach in decision-making for revascularization of MVD is currently endorsed by clinical practice guidelines.

Revascularization strategy

The extent of planned revascularization, on all diseased lesions or directed to selectively targeted coronary segments, is a major determinant of treatment strategy.

Complete revascularization

The concept of complete revascularization was initiated from early studies on CABG which demonstrated that patients who were completely revascularized derived symptomatic and survival benefits over those who were incompletely revascularized. Patients with diabetes mellitus, extensive coronary artery disease, large ischemic burden, and left ventricular dysfunction required the most complete revascularization to achieve long-term event-free survival.

There is large variability in the definition of completeness of myocardial revascularization adopted by different studies. We propose a simple definition that takes into account the size of the vessel, the severity of the lesion, and the viability of the myocardial territory (Table 17.1). An anatomically complete revascularization is accomplished when all vessels with clinically significant stenosis (≥50% stenosis in vessel >1.5 mm diameter) are treated irrespective of the underlying myocardial function. A functionally complete revascularization refers to cases in which only lesions supplying viable myocardium are treated. Therefore, revascularization may be anatomically incomplete but functionally adequate.

Although complete revascularization is the goal in most patients undergoing multivessel intervention, incomplete revascularization is common in clinical practice. The ability to achieve complete revascularization depends on the selection of patients. Reasons for not attempting to treat all diseased vessels include the presence of CTO, the presence of serious medical conditions such as severe left ventricular dysfunction, or the decision to treat only the "culprit lesion" that is thought to be responsible for the patient's symptoms. Functionally adequate revascularization aims to treat all significant stenoses in vessels that supply viable myocardium. Lesions in small or diffusely diseased vessels and lesions serving infarcted territories can be safely left alone. Recently, some evidence has emerged that the prognosis of patients with MVD remains acceptable when the amount of incomplete revascularization does not exceed specific thresholds measured by adaptations of the anatomic SYNTAX score (i.e., residual SYNTAX score) [1].

Culprit lesion strategy

Culprit lesion refers to the lesion responsible for the acute coronary syndrome or the stenosis most likely responsible for the patient's symptoms. The decision of whether to perform culprit vessel or

Interventional Cardiology: Principles and Practice, Second Edition. Edited by George D. Dangas, Carlo Di Mario, and Nicholas N. Kipshidze.
© 2017 John Wiley & Sons, Ltd. Published 2017 by John Wiley & Sons, Ltd.

Box 17.1 High-risk multivessel coronary artery disease patient subsets

Diabetes mellitus
Renal failure
Impaired left ventricular function
Inability to achieve complete revascularization with percutaneous coronary intervention
Multiple chronic total occlusions
Left main disease
Three vessel disease
Diffuse disease

Table 17.1 Revascularization strategies in patients with multivessel coronary artery disease.

Complete numerical revascularization	The number of stenotic vessels must equal the number of distal anastomoses applied
Complete anatomic revascularization	Unconditional: all stenotic vessels are revascularized, irrespective of size and territory supplied Conditional: all stenotic vessels >1.5 mm in diameter and ≥50% diameter stenosis are revascularized
Complete functional revascularization	All ischemic myocardial territories are reperfused; areas of old infarction with no viable myocardium are not required to be reperfused
Complete revascularization by a predetermined scoring cut-off value	Scoring of stenoses in different vessels at different locations (weightings may be used). The overall extent of disease is a continuous variable, the treatment is another variable, and the post-treatment score determines completeness of revascularization Anatomic: irrespective of viable myocardium Functional: the post-revascularization score is calculated on the basis of the amount of remaining myocardium at risk (Jeopardy score)

complete revascularization needs to be individualized. In most cases of MVD, target or culprit lesion can be identified by a combination of historical data, electrocardiographic findings, angiography supplemented by radionuclide studies or intravascular imaging. Morphologic characteristics that are associated with an unstable or culprit lesion include scalloped edges, irregular borders, and the presence of thrombus. In patients in whom a culprit lesion or lesions can be determined, PCI can be directed to treat that lesion alone without exposing the patient to the risks of dilating other lesions not responsible for the patient's symptoms. If the patient continues to have angina or a subsequent stress test shows ischemia in that territory, a second procedure can be performed to revascularize the vessel that was previously not attempted.

Staged PCI

The decision to perform multivessel PCI in the same procedure or planned staged procedures include the desire to diminish procedural risk, avoid excessive contrast use, lessen patient discomfort,

and reduce physician fatigue. Whereas it is reasonable to attempt two simple lesions during the same procedure, the presence of complex lesion should deter the operator from attempting more than one lesion at a time. Staging potentially limits the amount of myocardium at risk in the event of acute closure. However, the incidence of acute closure is rare with the advent of stents and dual-antiplatelet therapy. In case of staging, the time interval for planning the second procedure varies from days to few months according to the operator's discretion. One approach is to stage at an interval of 4–8 weeks to allow the first lesion to stabilize.

On the other hand, multivessel PCI in a single procedure can be associated with several inherent advantages. It expedites patient care, avoids a second invasive procedure with its associated morbidity, and reduces total radiation exposure and potentially cost. However, multivessel intervention is associated with a higher procedural contrast use and should be avoided in situations where the risk of contrast-induced nephropathy is high.

Regardless of the strategy (staged or multivessel PCI), the order in which diseased vessels are treated needs to planned. In ACS, the culprit lesion is treated first. In elective PCI for stable angina, the artery either supplying the largest amount of myocardium or involving the technically most difficult lesion is usually approached first. CTO are often the most technically demanding lesions to treat and are usually approached first in multivessel PCI. In the event of failed PCI to the CTO, the patient could be referred for CABG. Before attempting to open a CTO, it is important to determine the viability of the myocardium supplied by the occluded artery. The hypothesis that late mechanical reperfusion in patients with asymptomatic occluded infarct-related artery will improve long-term clinical outcomes remains to be proved.

Assessment of non-culprit or intermediate lesion

Assessment of a coronary lesion of intermediate severity continues to be a challenge. There can be significant observer variability in interpretation of the severity of an intermediate coronary lesion defined as luminal stenosis >40% but <70%. Intravascular imaging with intravascular ultrasound (IVUS) or optical coherence tomography (OCT) has become a more accurate standard for defining the severity of atherosclerosis and luminal dimensions compared to angiography. In the cardiac catheterization laboratory, coronary pressure wire-derived fractional flow reserve (FFR) can be used to determine the physiologic significance of a coronary stenosis that is distinct from the anatomic visualization provided by IVUS or OCT. This method relies on the decrease in intra-arterial pressure induced by a functionally significant stenosis to determine whether an intermediate lesion is producing ischemia.

High risk patients and risk stratification

The risk–benefit ratio must be assessed carefully for each patient with MVD. The risks of complications from PCI depend on several factors, including specific anatomic features of the artery and lesion, the overall cardiac and non-cardiac condition of the patient, and the clinical setting.

Risk models can be used to help predict the likelihood of procedural complication. For example, the Mayo Clinic risk score using seven variables (age, MI less than or equal to 24 hours, pre-procedural shock, serum creatinine level, left ventricular ejection

Table 17.2 SYNTAX score and SYNTAX-based model for risk stratification in MVD

Score	Components	Objective
SYNTAX score	Anatomic (angiographic)	Assessment of the location, extent, and complexity of coronary artery disease
Functional SYNTAX score	Anatomic + FFR	Similar to the SYNTAX score but calculated only on hemodynamically significant lesions
Residual SYNTAX score	SYNTAX score after PCI	A marker of completeness of revascularization by PCI
CABG SYNTAX score	Residual SYNTAX score after CABG	A marker of completeness of revascularization by CABG
SYNTAX Revascularization Index	1-[rSS/bSS]) × 100	A marker of the proportion of CAD burden treated by PCI
Global Risk Score	SYNTAX score + EuroSCORE	Developed to improve the predictive power of the SYNTAX score by inclusion of clinical variables
Clinical SYNTAX score	SYNTAX score * ACEF score	Developed to improve the predictive power of the SYNTAX score by inclusion of clinical variables
Logistic Clinical SYNTAX score	SYNTAX score + ACEF Score	Developed to improve the predictive power of the SYNTAX score by inclusion of clinical variables
SYNTAX score II	SYNTAX score + clinical variables	Decision making for PCI vs. CABG

fraction, congestive heart failure, and peripheral artery disease) has been validated to predict MACE and procedural death with excellent discrimination [2]. The model was robust across many subgroups, including those undergoing elective PCI, those with diabetes mellitus, and in elderly patients.

Recently, novel scores have been developed to assess the long-term impact of PCI. Many of them originate from the pivotal SYNTAX score, an anatomic risk model created by merging of different existing angiographic classifications (Table 17.2). The SYNTAX score was originally conceived as an instrument to facilitate the discussion of interventional cardiologists and surgeons about revascularization options for a given left main or MVD patient during the so-called heart team meetings [3]. However, limitations of this score have been highlighted over time, which include the lack of clinical variables in the score algorithm [4]. The recently introduced SYNTAX score II tries to address this limitation (Table 17.2), but no validation of this score in patients with MVD is available so far.

Acute coronary syndrome

Patients with ACS frequently present with multiple complex coronary plaques. About 40–60% of patients who presented with acute MI have evidence of ulcerated plaques or thrombus in other than the infarct-related artery. Patients with intermediate to high risk non-ST elevation ACS, based on clinical, biomarker, and angiographic assessment, should undergo early revascularization. In this scenario, initial incomplete revascularization with PCI of the culprit lesion(s) is frequently preferred with subsequent staged PCI to non-culprit lesions if required. Whether the patient will ultimately need surgical bypass or staged PCI should be determined at time of initial angiography. If the patient is a surgical candidate, balloon

angioplasty alone or stents with a early coverage pattern (i.e., bare metal stents or certain second-generation DES) should be used to avoid delay to surgery caused by the need for prolonged dual-antiplatelet therapy.

In patients with MVD and ST-elevation MI (STEMI), the conventional strategy for primary PCI is recanalization of the infarct-related artery with decisions about PCI of non-culprit lesions at later follow-up guided by objective evidence of residual ischemia. The decision to defer non-culprit lesion PCI is supported by evidence of possible overestimation of non-culprit lesion severity in the setting of MI due to enhanced vascular tone often resistant to nitrate administration. However, with the improvement of PCI outcomes, recent studies have shown multivessel PCI during STEMI to be safe in selected patients compared with treating only the infarct-related artery [5]. Multivessel PCI during STEMI should be always considered when the patient remains hemodynamically unstable after PCI of the infarct-related artery. This can occur if there is more than one culprit vessel or critical stenoses in non-culprit vessels that supply a significant amount of myocardium not collateralized by the infarct-related artery. Potential advantages of multivessel PCI during STEMI include decrease in ischemic burden and improvement of left ventricular function.

Diabetes mellitus

Diabetic patients with MVD typically have smaller vessel size, longer lesion length, and greater plaque burden than non-diabetic patients. These adverse characteristics are associated with accelerated atherosclerosis, high restenosis rates, and less favorable long-term survival following PCI than non-diabetic patients. Most trials comparing CABG with PCI in diabetic patients have shown increased long-term survival with CABG. Based on a recent large meta-analysis, CABG remains the preferred treatment for diabetic patients with MVD [6]. Whether the advent of second-generation DES can narrow the gap between PCI and CABG in MVD in terms of the need for repeat revascularization remains to be demonstrated.

The elderly

Elderly patients have a higher risk profile than younger patients and mandate thorough clinical evaluation before acceptance for PCI or CABG. The long-term benefit of PCI in the elderly remains controversial. Culprit lesion PCI for symptom relief may be adequate in most patients rather than aiming for complete revascularization despite more extensive coronary disease than younger patients.

Left ventricular dysfunction

Left ventricular dysfunction is a major determinant of peri-procedural risk. Complete revascularization of viable myocardium in patients with MVD and left ventricular dysfunction is associated with improved survival, although this relationship was not significant after adjustment for other baseline variables in the post-hoc analysis of a randomized trial [7]. Currently available non-invasive techniques to assess myocardial viability include thallium single photon emission computed tomography, dobutamine echocardiography, positron emission tomography with ^{18}F-fluoro-deoxyglucose, and contrast-enhanced magnetic resonance imaging.

Renal dysfunction

Patients with renal dysfunction are at increased risk of developing contrast-induced nephropathy (CIN) and long-term mortality after PCI. The cornerstone of CIN prevention is adequate pre-hydration. In patient at increased risk for CIN, nephrotoxic medications should be withheld, renal protective strategies be considered for prophylaxis, and low or iso-osmolar contrast agents should be utilized. A strategy of staging the PCI initially targeting the culprit lesion is preferable to minimize contrast volume.

Three vessel disease

Triple vessel PCI is more likely to result in incomplete revascularization and less favorable outcomes than CABG. However, triple vessel disease can be highly heterogeneous. Patients with multifocal discrete stenoses are generally amendable to PCI whereas CABG is preferable for those with diffuse disease and multiple CTO. The SYNTAX score can help to identify those patients with three-vessel disease at lower risk of adverse long-term prognosis with PCI (i.e., those with SYNTAX score <22).

Revascularization in the era of drug-eluting stents

Three randomized trials (CARDIA, SYNTAX, and FREEDOM) have compared the outcomes of DES with CABG in patients with MVD. The Coronary Artery Revascularization in Diabetes (CARDIA) trial was designed to demonstrate non-inferiority of PCI to CABG in diabetic patients with MVD. The trial fell short of its planned recruitment, enrolling only 510 patients out of the intended 600, meaning that the non-inferiority parameters set for the trial were not reached because of insufficient power [8]. Twelve-month results showed no apparent difference between CABG and PCI in terms of the composite endpoints of death, non-fatal MI, and non-fatal stroke (10.5% vs. 13.0%; p = 0.39). Comparing CABG

with a small subgroup of PCI patients who received DES rather than bare metal stents, the composite endpoint of death, non-fatal MI, and non-fatal stroke was 12.4% vs. 11.6% (p = 0.82) again showing no difference in this composite endpoint.

The SYNergy between percutaneous coronary intervention with TAXus and cardiac surgery (SYNTAX) trial was the first randomized controlled trial to compare PCI using a first-generation DES with CABG in patients with left main disease and three-vessel disease. A total of 1800 patients were randomized in a 1 : 1 fashion to PCI or CABG. At 5 years, MACCE were 26.9% in the CABG group and 37.3% in the PCI group (p <0.0001), driven by significant increases in MI and repeat revascularization in the PCI group [9]. In the analysis of the cohort of patients with three-vessel disease, MACCE at 5 years were significantly higher with PCI than CABG (37.5% vs. 24.2%; p <0.001) [10]. PCI was also associated with higher rates of all-cause death, repeat revascularization, and the composite of death, stroke or MI, whereas the incidence of stroke was similar in the two groups. The risk of MACCE with PCI was significantly higher in patients with intermediate and high SYNTAX scores, but not in those with low SYNTAX score. The differences in MACCE between PCI and CABG were larger in diabetic patients. Overall, the SYNTAX trial suggests that CABG should remain the standard of care for patients with MVD when compared with first-generation DES, with the possible exception of those with less complex anatomy (i.e., low SYNTAX score), where PCI may be an acceptable revascularization strategy.

The Future Revascularization Evaluation in Patients with Diabetes Mellitus: Optimal Management of Multivessel Disease (FREEDOM) study compared PCI and CABG in 1900 diabetic patients with MVD. The primary outcome, a composite of death from any cause, non-fatal MI, or non-fatal stroke, occurred more frequently in the PCI group (p = 0.005), with 5-year rates of 26.6% in the PCI group and 18.7% in the CABG group [11]. The benefit of CABG was driven by differences in rates of both MI and death from any cause, while stroke was more frequent with CABG.

Medical therapy

Patients with MVD have diffuse disease and progression of untreated plaques. Multiple stents only treat focal areas of most significant stenosis. Untreated vulnerable plaques could potentially develop into culprit lesions over time. Aggressive medical therapy with risk factor modification and lipid lowering is essential.

Conclusions

Patients with MVD comprise the majority of those undergoing PCI today and will likely remain so. With improved techniques, stents, and adjunctive drugs, short- and medium-term outcomes after PCI have improved significantly. However, based on the results of contemporary trials, CABG remains the standard of care for most of the patients with MVD and those with diabetes in particular.

If long-term outcomes after second-generation DES prove to be comparable with CABG, PCI may become the preferred revascularization strategy for many patients. The role of PCI in patients with multivessel disease will depend both on the patient's anatomy and the clinical setting in which the revascularization is planned. For each patient, the risk–benefit ratio should be examined, and risk scores can be helpful for decision-making. A PCI procedure should be performed only after considering all therapeutic options and their short- and long-term outcomes.

(⊞) ***Interactive multiple choice questions are available for this chapter on www.wiley. com/go/dangas/cardiology***

References

1 Farooq V, Serruys PW, Bourantas CV, *et al.* Quantification of incomplete revascularization and its association with five-year mortality in the synergy between percutaneous coronary intervention with taxus and cardiac surgery (SYNTAX) trial validation of the residual SYNTAX score. *Circulation* 2013; **128**: 141–151.

2 Singh M, Rihal CS, Lennon RJ, Spertus J, Rumsfeld JS, Holmes DR Jr. Bedside estimation of risk from percutaneous coronary intervention: the new Mayo Clinic risk scores. *Mayo Clin Proc* 2007; **82**: 701–708.

3 Sianos G, Morel MA, Kappetein AP, *et al.* The SYNTAX Score: an angiographic tool grading the complexity of coronary artery disease. *EuroIntervention* 2005; **1**: 219–227.

4 Capodanno D, Tamburino C. Integrating the Synergy between percutaneous coronary intervention with Taxus and Cardiac Surgery (SYNTAX) score into practice: use, pitfalls, and new directions. *Am Heart J* 2011; **161**: 462–470.

5 Wald DS, Morris JK, Wald NJ, *et al.* Randomized trial of preventive angioplasty in myocardial infarction. *N Engl J Med* 2013; **369**: 1115–1123.

6 Verma S, Farkouh ME, Yanagawa B, *et al.* Comparison of coronary artery bypass surgery and percutaneous coronary intervention in patients with diabetes: a meta-analysis of randomised controlled trials. *Lancet Diabetes* 2013; **1**: 317–328.

7 Bonow RO, Maurer G, Lee KL, *et al.* Myocardial viability and survival in ischemic left ventricular dysfunction. *N Engl J Med* 2011; **364**: 1617–1625.

8 Kapur A, Hall RJ, Malik IS, *et al.* Randomized comparison of percutaneous coronary intervention with coronary artery bypass grafting in diabetic patients. 1-year results of the CARDia (Coronary Artery Revascularization in Diabetes) trial. *J Am Coll Cardiol* 2010; **55**: 432–440.

9 Mohr FW, Morice MC, Kappetein AP, *et al.* Coronary artery bypass graft surgery versus percutaneous coronary intervention in patients with three-vessel disease and left main coronary disease: 5-year follow-up of the randomised, clinical SYNTAX trial. *Lancet* 2013; **381**: 629–638.

10 Head SJ, Davierwala PM, Serruys PW, *et al.* Coronary artery bypass grafting vs. percutaneous coronary intervention for patients with three-vessel disease: final five-year follow-up of the SYNTAX trial. *Eur Heart J* 2014; **35**: 2821–2830.

11 Farkouh ME, Domanski M, Sleeper LA, *et al.* Strategies for multivessel revascularization in patients with diabetes. *N Engl J Med* 2012; **367**: 2375–2384.

CHAPTER 18

Chronic Total Coronary Occlusion

Gerald S. Werner[1] and Emmanouil S. Brilakis[2,3]

[1] Klinikum Darmstadt GmbH, Darmstadt, Germany

[2] Cardiac Catheterization Laboratories, VA North Texas Health Care System, Dallas, TX, USA

[3] Minneapolis Heart Institute, Minneapolis, MN, USA

Coronary chronic total occlusions (CTO) make up 18% of all significant coronary lesions observed during diagnostic angiography, as demonstrated recently in a cohort study of 14,400 angiographies from three Canadian centers [1]. The term "chronic coronary occlusion" had not been rigidly defined in recent years regarding the duration of the occlusion, and whether the inclusion was complete (TIMI 0 flow) or functional (TIMI I).

In order to find common ground for future development and discussion of technique and patient outcome, a consensus was reached by an European experts group which has now been accepted as the uniform definition of chronic total coronary occlusions as those with a documented duration of occlusion of at least 3 months, with absolutely no flow through the lesion itself (TIMI 0 flow) [2]. Occlusions within 1–3 months' duration should be addressed as recent occlusions, and within a period of 4 weeks after an acute myocardial infarction, as subacute occlusions (e.g., lesions that were included in the Occluded Artery Trial [3].

Morphology of the occlusion

Another important characteristic of a CTO is the length of the actually occluded segment. This can only be assessed through simultaneous visualization of the proximal (ipsilateral) segment and the distal segment through collateral filling. As the majority of collaterals originate from the contralateral artery, this requires double injection with the contrast injection started first in the contralateral donor artery, then followed by the injection into the occluded artery.

For the interventional strategy of entering, passing, and leaving the occluded segment, the basic pathoanatomic features of a CTO have to be kept in mind (Figure 18.1). We discriminate a proximal cap of the occlusion, which is often fibrotic or calcified and can provide considerable resistance to the wire advancement. Then along the occlusion length follows a segment of loose fibrous tissue or organized thrombus. Especially in long-standing occlusions, it may include islets of calcifications, which provide an obstacle to the advancement of the wire through this part of the occlusion until the distal cap is encountered. The resistance of the distal cap is usually lower than the proximal cap, presumably because of the lower pressure of about 30–40 mmHg existing in this collateralized segment of the occluded

artery [4]. The segment distal to the occlusion is often tapered and constricted and provides a small target for the distal wire entry.

A few pathologic studies carried out more than 15 years ago in small number of patients, often with functional occlusions, reported a considerable number of residual channels and also so called microchannels (diameter <200 μm) within the occlusion [5,6]. However, a recent pathohistologic study in a larger number of patients provided evidence that microchannels are not a typical feature of CTOs; instead negative remodeling is frequently observed [7].

Indications for treatment

The CTO is a unique set of lesions with regard to the complexity of the required interventional technique, but also with regard to the discordant view on the indication to treat these lesions. The latter is reflected by the low representation of CTOs among lesions treated by percutaneous coronary intervention (PCI) [1], while on the other hand, the presence of a CTO appears to bear a specific additional prognostic risk if left untreated [8–10]. Patients with a CTO sometimes present with stable angina pectoris, but especially exercise limitation and dyspnea are more prevalent than in non-occlusive lesions [11].

Sometimes, CTOs are detected when other coronary lesions progress and lead to unstable angina. Patients with acute coronary syndrome and ST-elevation infarct are at particularly high risk if the collateral supplying artery is involved in an acute myocardial infarction as the territory at risk is larger than with a single acute occlusion [12].

A limitation to accept CTOs as a unanimous target for PCI is the lack of a randomized study to answer this issue. However, the wealth of data from prospective registries and meta-analyses already provide considerable evidence to treat CTOs [13,14]. The indication is based on three basic goals:

1 To relieve exercise limiting symptoms of angina or dyspnea, especially in patients with preserved left ventricular (LV) function, or to resolve ischemia caused by the CTO, similar to the indication in stable angina caused by non-occlusive lesions;
2 To improve regional LV dysfunction in the territory of the occluded artery, provided there is residual viability; the latter can nowadays be readily assessed by magnetic resonance imaging with late contrast enhancement [15,16];

Interventional Cardiology: Principles and Practice, Second Edition. Edited by George D. Dangas, Carlo Di Mario, and Nicholas N. Kipshidze.
© 2017 John Wiley & Sons, Ltd. Published 2017 by John Wiley & Sons, Ltd.

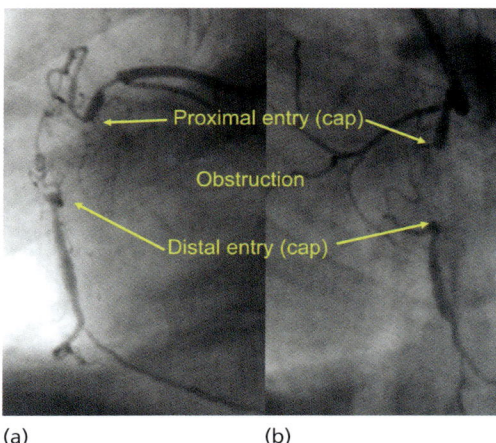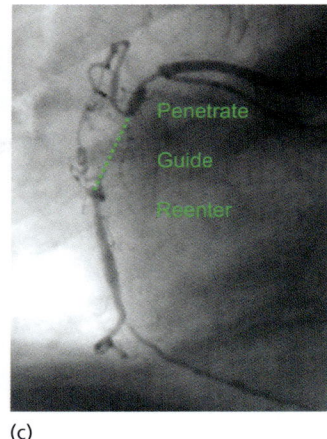

Figure 18.1 The basic features of a chronic total coronary occlusion (a and b) and the technical steps of recanalization (c).

3 To achieve complete revascularization in patients with multivessel coronary artery disease, as leaving a CTO untreated affects the outcome in these patients, as demonstrated by the post hoc analysis of the SYNTAX trial and other subanalysis [10].

An indispensable prerequisite to opening a CTO is the presence of collaterals to supply the distal occluded segment. In the absence of collaterals, no viable myocardium would have survived. On the other hand, physiologic assessment of collateral function demonstrated that even angiographically well-developed collaterals are not sufficient to prevent ischemia and cannot be an excuse for not revascularizing a CTO [17,18]. The fractional flow reserve measured distal to an occlusion before actually opening it is about 0.4, which is well below the level of 0.8 uniformly accepted as threshold for interventional treatment in non-occlusive lesions (see Chapter 6).

Patients with a concomitant CTO and an acute coronary syndrome caused by a non-occlusive lesion should be treated for this culprit lesion first, before considering the recanalization of a CTO. In stable patients, however, complete revascularization should be the ultimate goal. Therefore, a staged PCI approach should start with the CTO first, especially as lesions in the collateral supplying artery would be treated at increased risk if the CTO were not treated [19]. If the CTO procedure fails, the patient can still be referred for coronary artery bypass graft (CABG) surgery for complete revascularization [10].

Basic rules of engagement

To cross a CTO we need to visualize the distal segment in order to direct our guidewire progress, and we often need to resort to more rigid wires than in non-occlusive lesions. The latter go along with a potential damage of the arterial wall, deviation into the subintimal vascular space, or even perforation toward the pericardium, which requires special emphasis on control of the wire position during each and every step of wire advancement (Figure 18.2).

The absolute prerequisite for a CTO procedure is to reduce risk and avoid complications. The indication is a mere symptomatic one, as prognostic considerations are not backed by randomized trials. Therefore the CTO procedure should not harm the patient in any way, and the first rule of engagement is to always be absolutely sure where the tip of the wire is positioned. A second sheath for injection of contrast to visualize the collateral filling from the

contralateral artery is therefore always mandatory except in those cases where a coronary occlusion is approached, and there is collateral filling from ipsilateral branches. However, the most frequent occlusion, the right coronary and the left anterior descending (LAD) artery, usually require such a double injection. For a regular antegrade recanalization approach it is often sufficient to use a small diagnostic sheath (4 or 5 Fr) for the contralateral visualization to save on contrast volume, but if visualization is poor, larger catheter sizes should be chosen.

The second rule of engagement is to provide optimum backup for the procedure. Even if a wire can be passed rather effortlessly, the passage of balloons and stents can fail because of lack of backup. Especially for the right coronary artery, the regular JR guide may not provide adequate support, and an AL1 is generally preferred. However, there is a balance to be made between catheter size and shape, and this requires careful planning right at the start of the procedure. A large diameter such as 8 Fr (preferred by Japanese operators) will provide enforced support even with less aggressive shapes, and it provides ample working space for complex techniques using double wires with microcatheters, double balloons, and so on. The large diameter is also recommended when a subintimal re-entry approach might be necessary using special devices (Stingray re-entry balloon and wire). A large diameter with less aggressive shape is especially important for proximal or ostial occlusions, where deep guide engagement is not possible or counterproductive. In non-ostial lesions, a smaller guide size of 6 Fr will require deeper engagement for adequate support. The predominantly used catheter size in Europe is 7 Fr, which provides proper support and working lumen. It is important to always use catheters with side holes, especially for the right coronary artery, to avoid local dissections during contrast injection into the occluded proximal artery, and to avoid hypoperfusion of proximal side branches.

For the left coronary artery (LCA), the guide catheter has to be selected according to the length of the left main artery, and the angle of take off of the occluded artery. For LAD occlusions an extra backup shape provides the ideal support, while occasionally the classic AL2 or 3 may be ideal for proximal circumflex occlusions.

The third rule of engagement is to advance guidewires with the support of a microcatheter, to start with soft wires in order not to damage the proximal arterial segments with aggressive rigid wires. For example, a sharp-angled take off from the LCA may require

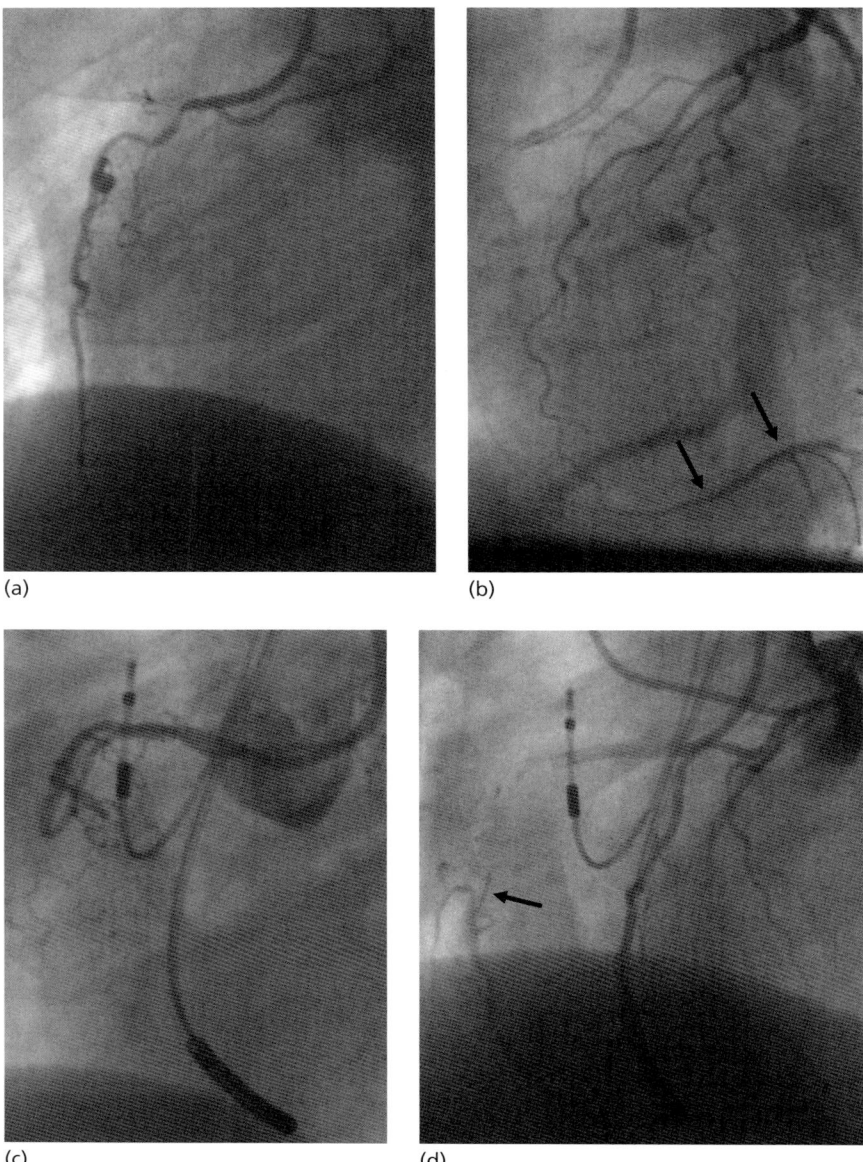

Figure 18.2 Bilateral contrast injection is essential for control of the wire position and advancement and direction. Proximal right coronary artery (RCA) occlusion (a) with recanalization wire in a posterolateral side branch (b, arrows). Proximal RCA occlusion (c) with recanalization wire outside of the distal vessel lumen (d, arrow).

soft hydrophilic wires to negotiate it, whereas the required angle and the wire stiffness will be inadequate for the actual occlusion. The advancement of a microcatheter through the difficult proximal angulation will be almost always possible, and once positioned at the proximal end of the CTO, the soft wire can be exchanged for a dedicated recanalization wire (Figure 18.3).

Guidewire selection and handling

Guidewire selection incorporates a great deal of personal preference and operator experience [20,21]. In general, however, one can discriminate and advise on the use of the two basic guidewire features—hydrophilic PTFE wires and metal wires—which have hydrophilic coating to various extents.

There is not a single wire that serves all lesions and all circumstances, and a familiarity with several wires from each family is mandatory. For CTO procedures, two features of a guidewire are of utmost importance: tip stiffness and torque control. Wires can be used in incremental fashion with increasing tip stiffness when the previous wire encounters resistance. Torque control is a major feature of dedicated CTO wires in order to facilitate maneuvering of the wire in long resistive lesions.

While wire development was a gradual and slow process for many years, now an ever-wider and improved variety of guidewires have become available which have led to changes in wire selection and preference over the past 5 years. Wire selection depends on the planned approach to the occlusion, which is determined by the angiographic features of the lesion. Basically, three technical approaches

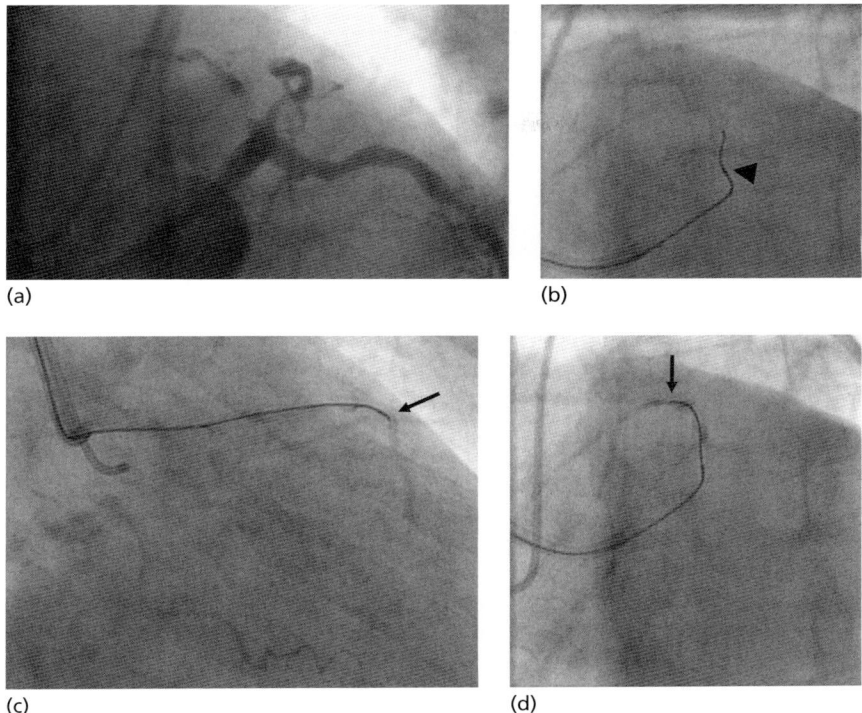

Figure 18.3 Proximal left anterior descending (LAD) occlusion with tapered entry (a). The tip shape for entering the LAD is different from what is required for navigation within the occlusion. After advancing a soft wire into the LAD, a microcatheter (b, arrow tip) is advanced, and the wire exchanged with a different tip shape. Further advancement is controlled by bilateral contrast injection in two planes (c and d).

are discriminated; drilling, penetrating, and sliding techniques. Some wires suit one of these categories best, but basically, each wire can be manipulated to work in one of these basic modes. A wire can be selected to "test" the proximal cap, but often needs to be changed during the procedure. Flexibility in wire selection is required throughout the whole procedure.

The tip shape is the first and basic step of wire manipulation, and often requires modification during the progress of the procedure. In non-occlusive lesions a basic rule of thumb is to adapt the radius of the tip angle to the size of the artery in which the wire is to be advanced. A major difference with tip shapes in CTOs is that the vessel diameter at the lesion site is practically zero, because it is occluded. Therefore the length of the proximal tip angle should be as short as possible with a moderate 30–45° angle. Within the occlusion, no secondary angle is added. Most recent wires are even shipped with preformed tiny preshaped tips of less than 1 mm length.

A detailed description of how to select wires would go beyond the scope of this chapter, and, most importantly, would be outdated before its publication given the current speed of wire development, but the following remarks give a brief idea of the criteria and sequence of wire selection.

Occlusions with a distinct entry point

Depending on the resistance of the proximal cap, which may be deduced from information on the duration of the occlusion or visible calcification, the wire can be selected accordingly (Figure 18.3). For presumably soft plaques (CTO <1 year) a Fielder XT could be selected, or a Gaia 1. For more resistant occlusions, a Gaia 2 might work as primary wire, or an Ultimate 3. The Fielder XT (more recently XT-A) is a tapered low tip force wire, the tapered Gaia

wires have higher tip force with high torque control, and the Ultimate has a tip diameter like normal workhorse wires of 0.014 inch. Wire manipulation is improved by advancing the microcatheter about 1 cm close to the wire tip. The wire is carefully rotated and advanced mainly by observing the fluoroscopic image, less so according to tactile feedback.

Occlusions without any discernible entry point

These occur typically at the site of side branches (Figure 18.4). Penetration requires tapered tip wires such as the Confianza Pro 9 and 12 g wire with 0.009 inch tip diameter, or the Progress 140 T or 200 T. The recently available Gaia 2 and 3 are also ideal wires for penetrating the proximal cap; however, with calcified caps the Confianza wires are preferable. Penetration into the subintimal vessel space can occur and therefore requires careful monitoring and control of the wire approach.

Occlusions with suspected residual lumen

The sliding technique rests on the low friction advancement of PTFE wires and is ideal for occlusions with suspected residual lumen (Figure 18.5). These wires are widely (over)used, as they promise a fast approach because of the low friction, but they are poorly steerable and will easily leave the vessel lumen. Typical wires of this type are the Pilot family wires. Recently, low tip force wires became available like the Fielder XTR, which is ideal for atraumatic probing of residual channels. The Pilot wire, if used gently and carefully, will also be successful in crossing even difficult-looking occlusions (Figure 18.6). High tip force Pilot wires can also be used in in-stent CTOs.

No single technique serves all lesions, and all approaches should be utilized and combined as required.

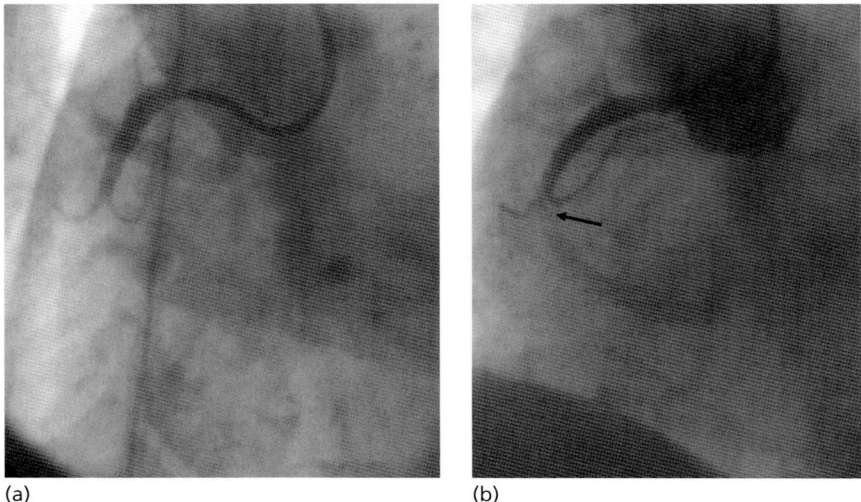

Figure 18.4 Proximal RCA occlusion with two side branches (a). Perforation of the proximal cap is required with a Confianza wire (b arrow).

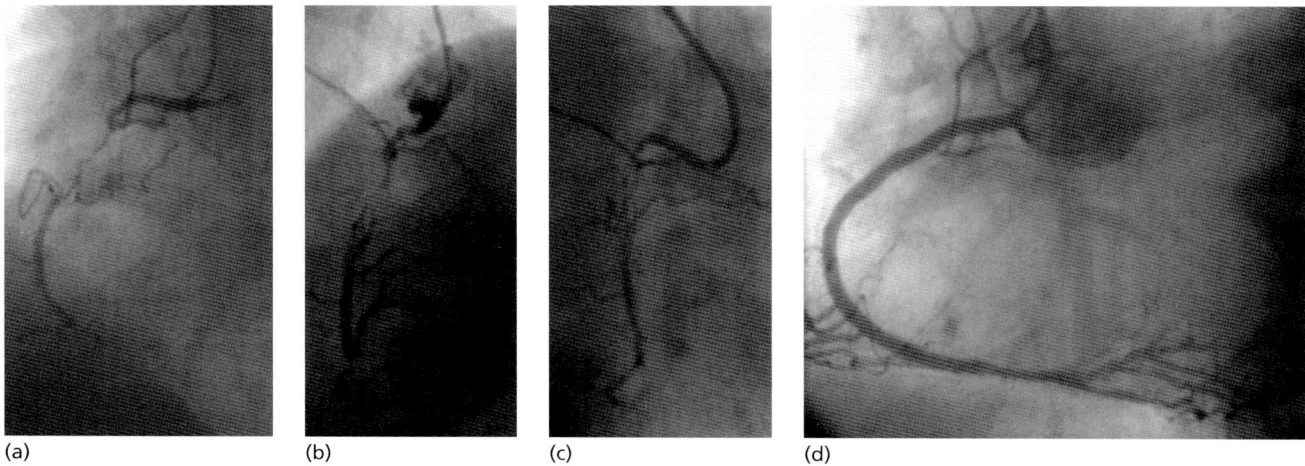

Figure 18.5 (a) Proximal RCA occlusion with a long intracoronary channel (spontaneous secondary recanalization). A Whisper LS wire is gently advanced and successfully reaches the distal vessel lumen (b and c), and the procedure is concluded successfully (d).

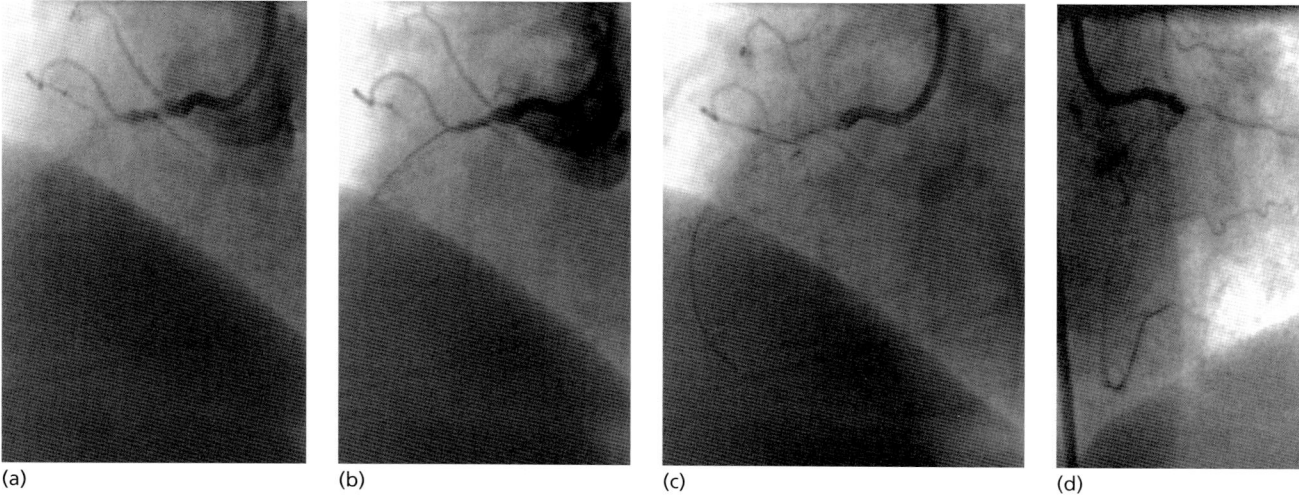

Figure 18.6 A proximal RCA occlusion with sidebranch and no visible entry (a). Still, a Pilot 50 wire can be successfully advanced gently (b) and reaches the distal vessel (c and d) as confirmed by contrast staining around the wire.

Advanced antegrade recanalization techniques

The basic approach is to advance a single wire gently with just enough force for slow advancement. The tip of the wire gives tactile feedback to the experienced operator about the intravascular position; however, this is not always reliable. Wire advancement requires fluoroscopic checking by monitoring in at least two orthogonal projections and occasional contralateral contrast injections. Not infrequently, the first wire enters the subintimal space, which is recognized by missing the distal entry of the occlusion outside of the contrast-filled lumen. A decision then needs to be made either to proceed with wire manipulation or switch to a subintimal re-entry approach. This decision is based on familiarity with the technique, and anatomic features of the distal cap.

If a wire-based approach is used, then the first wire can be used as a helpful guide to the general direction of the vessel course and can enable the manipulation of a second parallel wire slightly deviating from the initial course to successfully enter the distal lumen. This is the parallel wire technique (Figure 18.7). Often, the first wire is a moderately stiff wire and the second wire is of increased stiffness, but a tapered wire (e.g., Gaia 2 or Confianza Pro). This technique can be accommodated by modern 6 Fr guide catheters. However, if both wires are supported by a microcatheter or over-the-wire balloon (the see-saw technique), a larger diameter of 7 or 8 Fr is required [22]. If necessary a third wire can even be introduced.

The main issue with the multiple wire approach is not to advance the primary wire within the false lumen far beyond the distal entry point in order to avoid a subintimal hematoma that might obstruct the distal entry and make the manipulation of a second wire difficult or even impossible because of loss of contrast filling of the compressed distal lumen.

The deviation of the primary wire from the true vessel lumen can occur at any point during advancement, but it often happens at the entry into the proximal cap. A refined technique to control this and modify the entry point is by use of intravascular ultrasound (IVUS). An IVUS probe is advanced, after purposeful dilatation of the wrong channel, into this false lumen, and under IVUS imaging and orientation of the relative wire positions and the IVUS catheter on fluoroscopy, a wire can be redirected into the true lumen [23].

Sometimes, when an occlusion includes several side branches, the wire can be directed only in one of the secondary branches. If this cannot be controlled after some effort, it may be prudent to dilate the occlusion toward this side branch with a small-sized balloon. Not infrequently, this maneuver then provides easy access to the other occluded branches: termed the sesame open approach. In these situations, where the operator wants to access another branch at often acute angles, the use of a dual-lumen microcatheter (TwinPass, Crusade) is helpful, with an over-the-wire lumen ending at a distal side port [24].

In situations where the direction of the guidewire advancement is defined, but the wire will simply not penetrate the intended segment, the support of the wire needs enhancement. This can be achieved by inflating an over-the-wire balloon proximal to the occlusion, or by using other enhancements of guide support such as the anchoring balloon technique or the Guideliner or Guidezilla guide extension catheters.

Antegrade dissection and re-entry

A frequent situation during the course of antegrade wire manipulation is the subintimal wire position. Antegrade dissection and re-entry techniques aim to cross the occluded vessel segment through the more compliant subintimal space, followed by re-entry into the distal true lumen. Antegrade dissection can be achieved using a "knuckled" guidewire (usually a polymer-jacketed guidewire) (STAR [25], mini-STAR [26]), but the reliability of the wire re-entry

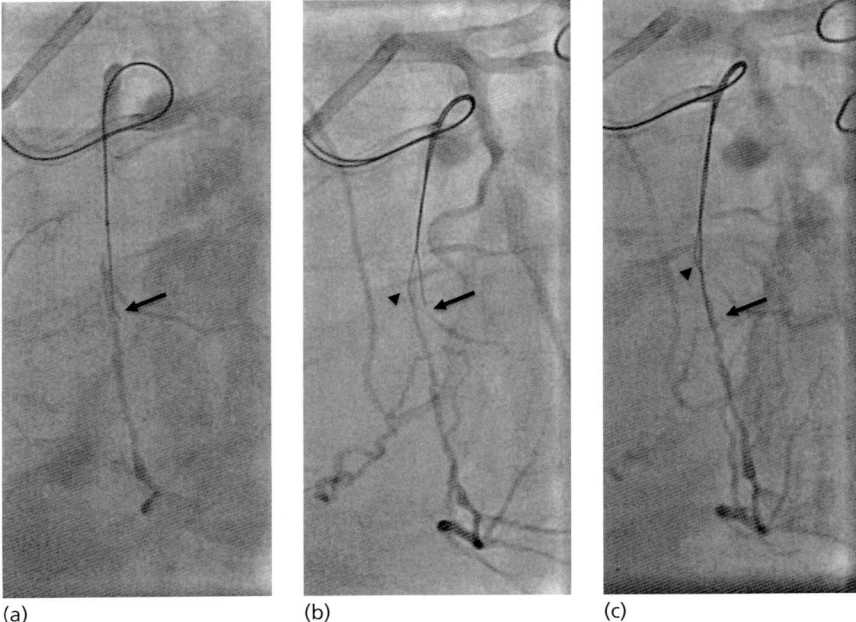

(a)   (b)   (c)

Figure 18.7 Typical example of the advantage of parallel wiring: the first wire Gaia 2 misses the distal target to the right (a, arrow), and a second Gaia 2 in parallel misses the target initially to the left (b, arrow tip); finally the first wire is redirected to enter the distal lumen (c, arrow), which was confirmed in a second plane.

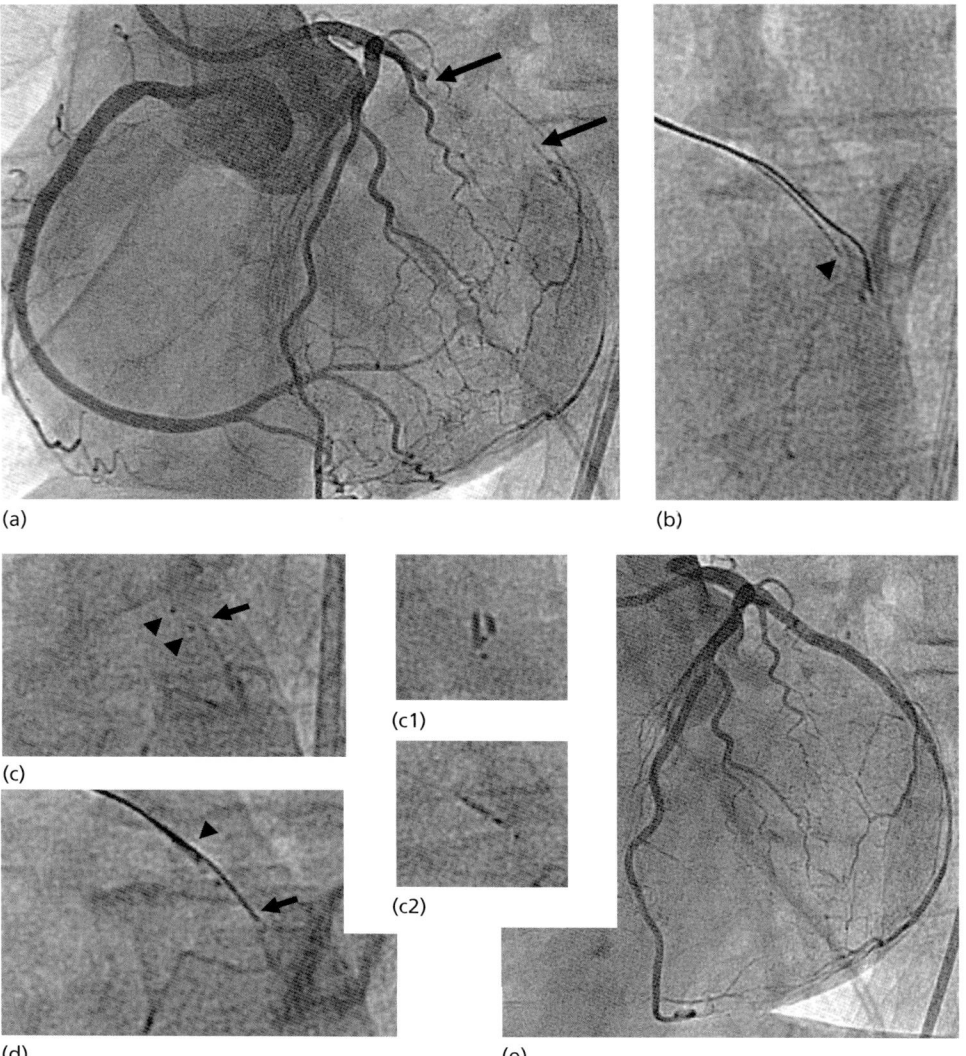

Figure 18.8 Long occlusion of the left circumflex artery (a; between arrows) with collateral supply from the contralateral right artery, and also from epicardial diagonal branches. Initial attempt with parallel wire technique, both wires below or above the distal target (arrow head) in LAO projection (b). The StingRay catheter with two radiopaque dot markers (arrow heads) is advanced into the subintimal space below the distal collateral-filled target (c; arrow). The StingRay balloon is inflated and appears as parallel lines in the RAO projection (c1) and single line in LAO projection (c2). The single line indicates, that we look from the side on the catheter, with one side port exiting on top, one below. The StingRay wire is then directed toward the side port, that points toward the target (d; arrow), and exits in this example at the proximal side port before the two markers (arrow). The catheter is then exchanged for a microcatheter, then advanced into the true distal lumen, and a soft wire exchanged for the StingRay wire. The final result after stenting of this limited subintimal re-entry (e).

is not controllable. With the advent of the dedicated BridgePoint re-entry device (Boston Scientific; Natick, MA, USA), a more reliable re-entry can be achieved. It consists of the CrossBoss catheter, a metal catheter with a 1-mm distal atraumatic tip that is advanced with a rapid-spin technique to provide either a passage through the occlusion or a passage into the subintimal space. In the latter case, re-entry can then be achieved with the Stingray system. The Stingray balloon has a flat shape with two side exit ports, and self-orients so that one exit port faces the true lumen and the other faces the adventitia upon low-pressure inflation (2–4 atm) [27]. The Stingray guidewire is a stiff (12 g) guidewire with a 0.009 inch tapered tip which is advanced through the side port of the Stingray balloon facing the distal true lumen under fluoroscopic guidance

until it re-enters the true lumen (Figure 18.8) [28,29]. The length of the dissection should be minimized [30], as extensive dissection–re-entry techniques have been associated with high restenosis and re-occlusion rates [31,32].

Retrograde approach

The success rate of conventional and advanced wire techniques has been increased by wires with improved torque control. However, there remain limitations in long and calcified occlusions, and in those with inadequate guide catheter support. Often it is difficult to determine the entry into the occlusion, and therefore alternative approaches are desirable. The retrograde approach provides such

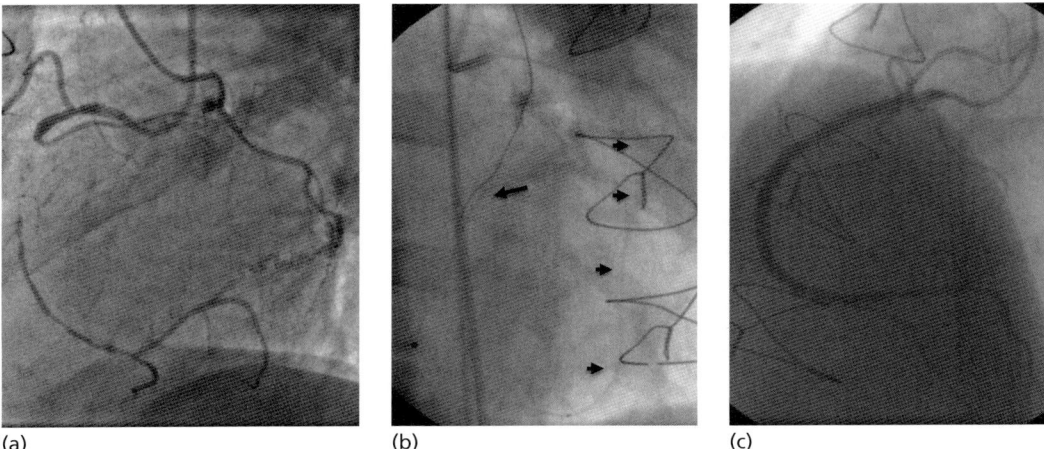

(a)   (b)   (c)

Figure 18.9 A proximal RCA occlusion in a post coronary artery bypass graft (CABG) patient, which was tried twice before antegradely (a), but could not be crossed with successful distal re-entry. A retrograde approach is chosen (b) and a wire passed through a septal perforator into the posterior descending artery (b; arrow heads) and then advanced toward the distal cap of the occlusion. The recanalization was completed with the reverse CART technique at the point where the wire overlap (b; arrow), and then followed by stent placement (c).

an enhancement of technical means by taking the reverse route of occlusion passage from the distal to the proximal cap. As the distal cap is often softer than the proximal cap, the advancement of the wire may be easier than from the antegrade approach. This can be achieved via a patent bypass graft, but as this is a rare coincidence, the retrograde approach via collateral connections is the most frequent means of access as developed by Dr. Osamu Katoh [33–35]. In principle, several pathways can be used, but the septal connections are those best approached causing the least danger to the patient in case of collateral damage. Ideally, small trans-septal thread-like collateral connections (CC1 collateral connections [36]) should be used for the approach to either the occluded right coronary artery or LAD. This approach should be used only after extensive experience with the antegrade approach and so is only briefly mentioned and described here (Figure 18.9).

The rapid development of wires to cross the collaterals and devices to support this approach (microcatheters) have made it more easily applicable than 5 years ago. In principle, either the retrograde wire is used as a marker for the antegrade approach, or the retrograde wire is advanced through the occlusion into the proximal artery and into the antegrade guiding catheter. The first approach is still valid, especially to save contrast medium, but the latter retrograde passage is the most frequently applied technique. Depending on whether the wire passes through the lumen (true lumen crossing) or deviates into the plaque wall, passage needs to be facilitated by inflating a balloon over an antegrade wire (reverse CART technique) [37].

The retrograde approach proceeds by means of very structured steps, but it requires in all cases, except for an ostial occlusion, the positioning of an antegrade wire into the body of the occlusion. This can be done as a first step, or needs to be done after collateral passage. The steps are as follows:

1 Selection and passage of the collateral, now achieved in the majority of cases with a soft and atraumatic Sion wire; even epicardial collateral connections can now be successfully passed. The main obstacle remains the tortuosity of the collateral path.
2 After reaching the vessel distal to the occlusion a microcatheter is advanced through the collateral (Corsair) which dilates the

collaterals and serves as an extension of the guide catheter. In epicardial tortuous connections, a Finecross or similar microcatheter is preferred.
3 Exchange the microcatheter for a wire to pass the occlusion. Here often softer wires than for the antegrade approach can be used, but basically wires are used as required. The goal is to achieve either a passage through the occlusion or at least a long zone of overlap with the antegrade wire. If no passage is possible, then the CART maneuver is applied with antegrade balloon inflations to open the space for passing the retrograde wire into the proximal true lumen.
4 The wire then is advanced into the guiding catheter or an extension of the guiding catheter (GuideLiner, Guidezilla [38]), followed by the microcatheter. The retrograde wire is then exchanged for a >300 cm wire to enable externalization of this wire from the antegrade Y-connector.

Thus, a wire is provided that extends via the collateral through the occlusion and provides ideal support to perform the final steps of dilatation and stent placement. The collaterals need to remain protected from this wire by the microcatheter, which is retracted into the artery distal to the occlusion. Before finally removing the collateral "gear," a contrast injection ensures the integrity of the passed collateral.

Hybrid approach for intervention of chronic total occlusions

In the USA, the "hybrid" approach had been promoted as a means to structure the approach to CTOs as an algorithm based on four CTO angiographic features obtained using dual injection: (i) proximal cap ambiguity; (ii) lesion length; (iii) quality of the distal vessel; and (iv) presence of collateral vessels that are appropriate for the retrograde approach [39]. When the proximal cap is ambiguous or the distal target vessel is diffusely diseased, a primary retrograde approach is favored. Otherwise, an antegrade approach is initially pursued using guidewire escalation for short (<20 mm in length) lesions, and a primary antegrade dissection strategy for longer (≥20 mm) lesions. Early change in crossing strategy is recommended if the initially selected approach fails to achieve progress.

Balloon dilatation

After the guidewire is successfully advanced across the occlusion, and most importantly, its correct intravascular position checked in at least two orthogonal views with a contralateral injection, a balloon needs to be advanced. This is facilitated by modern low-profile balloons with diameters down to 1–1.25 mm to be followed by an adequately sized balloon [21].

There are several techniques available to increase support if even a small balloon cannot be advanced [40,41]. They are intended to improve and stabilize the guide catheter position in the ostium. In some instances with heavily calcified lesions a rotablator is required; however, it can be extremely difficult to exchange the recanalization wire for the delicate 0.010 inch rotablator guidewire. This can be achieved with the aid of a support catheter, which is advanced as far as possible into the occlusion. If this can be achieved, a small rotablator burr is used. Another device useful in this situation is a laser catheter, but because of high hardware costs and limited applications these devices are rarely found in catheterization laboratories [42]. A device that can help in achieving the initial headway through the occlusion is the Tornus support catheter (ASAHI Intec Inc.) which can be screwed across the occlusion once a guidewire is in position [43].

Deciding the appropriate balloon size for the subsequent full lesion dilatation can be difficult. Therefore, nitroglycerine is frequently given intracoronary to increase the distal vessel size which is always constricted after the recanalization [44,45].

Stent placement

The advent of the drug-eluting stent reduced the target vessel failure rate considerably into ranges that are comparable with non-occlusive lesions [46,47]. The need for long and multiple stents no longer appears to have a considerable impact on vessel patency, although the issue of long-term freedom from very late stent thrombosis is not yet established in this specific lesion subset. When comparing previous and present results of stents in CTOs it needs to be kept in mind that parallel to the introduction of DES the complexity of CTOs successfully recanalized tended to increase in dedicated centers with improved techniques.

When planning stent coverage after balloon dilatation of a CTO, liberal coverage and maximizing stent expansion is advantageous to avoid focal restenosis at the edges of the stent when they are implanted within severely atherosclerotic segments, and to reduce flow turbulence to avoid stent thrombosis. However, extensive stenting can lead to stent fractures, which was observed in first generation DES, but is still a problem in more recent DES [48]. All available data show that the frequently diffuse and often occlusive restenosis in bare metal stents changed with DES to predominantly focal restenosis at the edge or within the stent, which can be treated by focal stenting.

The future perhaps lies with bioabsorbable scaffolds, and initial experience appears promising, but it remains to be established whether a full-metal jacket can and should be replaced with a full-plastic jacket after complex recanalization procedures especially of the right coronary artery.

Intravascular ultrasound in CTOs

IVUS can be of use during several steps of the interventional process. As an advanced adjunctive technique requiring considerable expertise and experience, it can be used to locate the entry into an occlusion if a side branch takes off right at the proximal cap and the IVUS can be positioned at the take off of this side branch. If the guidewire is advanced into the subintimal space, an IVUS catheter advanced into this false space can help with re-entering the true lumen [20].

With increasing use of the retrograde approach, IVUS is used to identify the wire position of the antegrade and retrograde wire with respect to lumen and subintimal space, and to assist in decision making as to the most appropriate technique [20,49]. Where IVUS is of general advantage, even with less experience in the abovementioned fields, is the assessment of stent placement and optimal stent expansion [50,51]. Diffuse atherosclerosis makes it difficult to place the proximal and distal stent borders within a less diseased segment to avoid edge stenosis, and to expand the stent fully because of underestimation of the actual media to media vessel diameter. Full lesion coverage and expansion are key factors to obtain long-term success in these lesions.

When to stop a procedure

The important question arises, if a procedure appears not to be achieving success, as to when to stop, either to opt for a subsequent second attempt, which is sometimes a feasible choice, or to opt for alternative methods like surgical revascularization. There may be technical reasons to stop the procedure, and also safety aspects. From the outset it must be clear that a recanalization requires considerable laboratory time, typically 90–120 minutes, but can extend well beyond these limits. Therefore, a sufficient time slot must be reserved to avoid the abortion of a potentially successful procedure because of logistic reasons.

There are three main reasons to stop the procedure.

1 To avoid radiation damage [52,53]. Fluoroscopy time will run typically into 40–60 minutes, sometimes even longer. To avoid radiation damage to the patient's skin low radiation dose protocols should be applied, the fluoro pulse rate reduced, and fluoro image storage preferred to filming whenever possible. From the start of the procedure, radiation should be at a minimum. Angulation must be changed and adjusted frequently to avoid a single spot high radiation load [54].

2 To avoid contrast-induced nephropathy [55,56]. The maximum amount of contrast for each individual patient should be set before the start of the procedure with reference to the patient's age and kidney function. Contrast use can be reduced by using the retrograde marker wire technique to avoid repetitive contrast injections during wire manipulation, and by using IVUS to assess the vessel instead of contrast agent. Additional technical devices are also available and can be used in critical patients (see Chapter 27).

3 The procedure should be stopped if complications occur that cannot be easily managed, or the strategy fails, with no alternative plan. In general, a second attempt after 4–6 weeks can be attempted if there are viable alternative options for a successful conclusion [21].

Complications

The published data show no difference in complication rates between occlusive and non-occlusive lesions, but these comparisons were not made with advanced techniques and new dedicated guidewires [57,58]. A recent meta-analysis gives an estimate of typical CTO complications such as perforation and tamponade, but other complications seem to be underestimated, as radiation damage and contrast-induced nephropathy especially were not regularly reported in previous studies [59]. More recent data show that the retrograde approach seems to be safe with only moderately higher risk regarding perforations [60,61]. In view of the often disputed indication for CTO PCI, and the viable option of surgical revascularization, the interventional procedure must be undertaken safely.

To avoid the complication of vessel perforation every care has to be taken to recognize and correct false wire positions, and never following these wires with balloons without absolute certainty of the correct intraluminal wire position. Dissections and perforations can lead to contrast staining of the myocardium, which is not necessarily a reason to stop the procedure so long as it does not compromise the collateral vessel supply.

The wire can also leave the lumen once it has passed the occlusion and is positioned distally. The stiff wires can easily damage the distal vessel lumen when they are left in place during the balloon and stent procedure. Therefore, the distal wire tip should be always kept in view, and very stiff wires should be exchanged for regular guidewires with soft tips as soon as possible, for example after the first balloon dilatation.

However, as vessel damage and pericardial effusion is an intrinsic risk, a basic rule is to avoid any other anticoagulant than heparin during the procedure, which can be readily reversed by protamine sulfate. There are also no data to support the use of gycoprotein IIb/IIIa antagonists in CTOs.

The operator needs to be experienced in placing a pericardial drain if needed, but often this can be avoided by rapidly obstructing the leakage with a balloon inflated for several (more than 10) minutes to seal the damage. If this does not work, negative pressure suction on a microcatheter advanced far into the distal vessel helps, or thrombus injection through this microcatheter. The problem will be difficult to control if the leakage is fed not only by the antegrade course, but also via collaterals. If the sources of the leakage cannot be sealed, for example by the use of coils, removal of the coronary gear and then reversal of heparin anticoagulation with protamine sulfate and a pericardial drainage for some time is the only option, and in case of continuing effusion a surgical repair.

Other complications observed are inflicted on neighboring vessels during the approach toward the occlusion. Here particular care is required as damage with partial vessel occlusion can put the patient at severe risk as one artery is already chronically occluded. Stiff wires should not be advanced through the left main artery across angles to avoid such damage, and should rather be advanced through over-the-wire catheters, which are put into position with the help of regular floppy guidewires.

New types of complications occur through the application of the retrograde wire technique. Particular care and foresight is required not to use the singular principal supplying collateral as any damage would immediately lead to severe ischemia. Furthermore, epicardial and specifically apical collateral connections are prone to damage and may even be ruptured, leading to a life-threatening acute tamponade. On the other hand, damage inflicted within the transseptal pathway is rarely severe and resolves without sequelae. These advanced techniques should only be carried out by the most experienced operators after extensive experience in safe application of conventional and advanced antegrade wire techniques.

Interactive multiple choice questions are available for this chapter on www.wiley.com/go/dangas/cardiology

References

1 Fefer P, Knudtson ML, Cheema AN, *et al.* Current perspectives on coronary chronic total occlusions: the Canadian Multicenter Chronic Total Occlusions Registry. *J Am Coll Cardiol* 2012; **59**: 991–997.

2 Di Mario C, Werner GS, Sianos G, *et al.* European perspective in the recanalisation of Chronic Total Occlusions (CTO): consensus document from the EuroCTO Club. *EuroIntervention* 2007; **3**: 30–43.

3 Hochman JS, Lamas GA, Buller CE, *et al.* Coronary intervention for persistent occlusion after myocardial infarction. *N Engl J Med* 2006; **355**: 2395–407.

4 Werner GS, Ferrari M, Betge S, Gastmann O, Richartz BM, Figulla HR. Collateral function in chronic total coronary occlusions is related to regional myocardial function and duration of occlusion. *Circulation* 2001; **104**: 2784–2790.

5 Katsuragawa M, Fujiwara H, Miyamae M, Sasayama S. Histologic studies in percutaneous transluminal coronary angioplasty for chronic total occlusion: comparison of tapering and abrupt types of occlusion and short and long occluded segments. *J Am Coll Cardiol* 1993; **21**: 604–11.

6 Srivatsa SS, Edwards WD, Boos CM, *et al.* Histologic correlates of angiographic chronic total coronary artery occlusions: influence of occlusion duration on neovascular channel patterns and intimal plaque composition. *J Am Coll Cardiol* 1997; **29**: 955–963.

7 Sakakura K, Nakano M, Otsuka F, *et al.* Comparison of pathology of chronic total occlusion with and without coronary artery bypass graft. *Eur Heart J* 2014; **35**: 1683–1693.

8 Hannan EL, Racz M, Holmes DR, *et al.* Impact of completeness of percutaneous coronary intervention revascularization on long-term outcomes in the stent era. *Circulation* 2006; **113**: 2406–2412.

9 Valenti R, Migliorini A, Signorini U, *et al.* Impact of complete revascularization with percutaneous coronary intervention on survival in patients with at least one chronic total occlusion. *Eur Heart J* 2008; **29**: 2336–2342.

10 Farooq V, Serruys PW, Garcia-Garcia HM, *et al.* The negative impact of incomplete angiographic revascularization on clinical outcomes and its association with total occlusions: the SYNTAX (Synergy Between Percutaneous Coronary Intervention with Taxus and Cardiac Surgery) trial. *J Am Coll Cardiol* 2013; **61**: 282–294.

11 Safley DM, Grantham JA, Hatch J, Jones PG, Spertus JA. Quality of life benefits of percutaneous coronary intervention for chronic occlusions. *Catheter Cardiovasc Interv* 2014; **84**: 629–634.

12 Claessen BE, van der Schaaf RJ, Verouden NJ, *et al.* Evaluation of the effect of a concurrent chronic total occlusion on long-term mortality and left ventricular function in patients after primary percutaneous coronary intervention. *JACC Cardiovasc Interv* 2009; **2**: 1128–1134.

13 Joyal D, Afilalo J, Rinfret S. Effectiveness of recanalization of chronic total occlusions: a systematic review and meta-analysis. *Am Heart J* 2010; **160**: 179–187.

14 Pancholy SB, Boruah P, Ahmed I, Kwan T, Patel TM, Saito S. Meta-analysis of effect on mortality of percutaneous recanalization of coronary chronic total occlusions using a stent-based strategy. *Am J Cardiol* 2013; **111**: 521–525.

15 Werner GS, Surber R, Kuethe F, *et al.* Collaterals and the recovery of left ventricular function after recanalization of a chronic total coronary occlusion. *Am Heart J* 2005; **149**: 129–137.

16 Kirschbaum SW, Baks T, van den Ent M, *et al.* Evaluation of left ventricular function three years after percutaneous recanalization of chronic total occlusions. *Am J Cardiol* 2008; **101**: 179–185.

17 Werner GS, Fritzenwanger M, Prochnau D, *et al.* Determinants of coronary steal in chronic total coronary occlusions donor artery, collateral, and microvascular resistance. *J Am Coll Cardiol* 2006; **48**: 51–58.

18 Werner GS, Surber R, Ferrari M, Fritzenwanger M, Figulla HR. The functional reserve of collaterals supplying long-term chronic total coronary occlusions in patients without prior myocardial infarction. *Eur Heart J* 2006; **27**: 2406–2412.

19 Migliorini A, Valenti R, Parodi G, *et al.* The impact of right coronary artery chronic total occlusion on clinical outcome of patients undergoing percutaneous coronary intervention for unprotected left main disease. *J Am Coll Cardiol* 2011; **58**: 125–130.

20 Sumitsuji S, Inoue K, Ochiai M, Tsuchikane E, Ikeno F. Fundamental wire technique and current standard strategy of percutaneous intervention for chronic total occlusion with histopathological insights. *JACC Cardiovasc Interv* 2011; **4**: 941–951.

21 Sianos G, Werner GS, Galassi AR, *et al.* Recanalisation of chronic total coronary occlusions: 2012 consensus document from the EuroCTO club. *EuroIntervention* 2012; **8**: 139–145.

22 Mitsudo K, Yamashita T, Asakura Y, *et al.* Recanalization strategy for chronic total occlusions with tapered and stiff-tip guidewire: the results of CTO new techniQUE for STandard procedure (CONQUEST) trial. *J Invasive Cardiol* 2008; **20**: 571–577.

23 Ito S, Suzuki T, Ito T, *et al.* Novel technique using intravascular ultrasound-guided guidewire cross in coronary intervention for uncrossable chronic total occlusions. *Circ J* 2004; **68**: 1088–1092.

24 Arif I, Callihan R, Helmy T. Novel use of twin-pass catheter in successful recanalization of a chronic coronary total occlusion. *J Invasive Cardiol* 2008; **20**: 309–311.

25 Colombo A, Mikhail GW, Michev I, *et al.* Treating chronic total occlusions using subintimal tracking and reentry: the STAR technique. *Catheter Cardiovasc Interv* 2005; **64**: 407–411; discussion 412.

26 Galassi AR, Tomasello SD, Costanzo L, *et al.* Mini-STAR as bail-out strategy for percutaneous coronary intervention of chronic total occlusion. *Catheter Cardiovasc Interv* 2012; **79**: 30–40.

27 Werner GS. The BridgePoint devices to facilitate recanalization of chronic total coronary occlusions through controlled subintimal reentry. *Expert Rev Med Devices* 2011; **8**: 23–29.

28 Werner GS, Schofer J, Sievert H, Kugler C, Reifart NJ. Multicentre experience with the BridgePoint devices to facilitate recanalisation of chronic total coronary occlusions through controlled subintimal re-entry. *EuroIntervention* 2011; **7**: 192–200.

29 Whitlow PL, Burke MN, Lombardi WL, *et al*; Investigators FA-CT. Use of a novel crossing and re-entry system in coronary chronic total occlusions that have failed standard crossing techniques: results of the FAST-CTOs (Facilitated Antegrade Steering Technique in Chronic Total Occlusions) trial. *JACC Cardiovasc Interv* 2012; **5**: 393–401.

30 Mogabgab O, Patel VG, Michael TT, *et al.* Long-term outcomes with use of the CrossBoss and stingray coronary CTO crossing and re-entry devices. *J Invasive Cardiol* 2013; **25**: 579–585.

31 Godino C, Latib A, Economou FI, *et al.* Coronary chronic total occlusions: mid-term comparison of clinical outcome following the use of the guided-STAR technique and conventional anterograde approaches. *Catheter Cardiovasc Interv* 2012; **79**: 20–27.

32 Valenti R, Vergara R, Migliorini A, *et al.* Predictors of reocclusion after successful drug-eluting stent-supported percutaneous coronary intervention of chronic total occlusion. *J Am Coll Cardiol* 2013; **61**: 545–550.

33 Surmely JF, Tsuchikane E, Katoh O, *et al.* New concept for CTO recanalization using controlled antegrade and retrograde subintimal tracking: the CART technique. *J Invasive Card* 2006; **18**: 334–338.

34 Sianos G, Barlis P, Di Mario C, *et al.* European experience with the retrograde approach for the recanalisation of coronary artery chronic total occlusions: a report on behalf of the euroCTO club. *EuroIntervention* 2008; **4**: 84–92.

35 Brilakis ES, Grantham JA, Thompson CA, *et al.* The retrograde approach to coronary artery chronic total occlusions: a practical approach. *Catheter Cardiovasc Interv* 2012; **79**: 3–19.

36 Werner GS, Ferrari M, Heinke S, *et al.* Angiographic assessment of collateral connections in comparison with invasively determined collateral function in chronic coronary occlusions. *Circulation* 2003; **107**: 1972–1977.

37 Rathore S, Katoh O, Tuschikane E, Oida A, Suzuki T, Takase S. A novel modification of the retrograde approach for the recanalization of chronic total occlusion of the coronary arteries intravascular ultrasound-guided reverse controlled antegrade and retrograde tracking. *JACC Cardiovasc Interv* 2010; **3**: 155–164.

38 Mozid AM, Davies JR, Spratt JC. The utility of a guideliner catheter in retrograde percutaneous coronary intervention of a chronic total occlusion with reverse cart-the "capture" technique. *Catheter Cardiovasc Interv* 2014; **83**: 929–932.

39 Brilakis ES, Grantham JA, Rinfret S, *et al.* A percutaneous treatment algorithm for crossing coronary chronic total occlusions. *JACC Cardiovasc Interv* 2012; **5**: 367–379.

40 Hirokami M, Saito S, Muto H. Anchoring technique to improve guiding catheter support in coronary angioplasty of chronic total occlusions. *Catheter Cardiovasc Interv* 2006; **67**: 366–371.

41 Kovacic JC, Sharma AB, Roy S, *et al.* GuideLiner mother-and-child guide catheter extension: a simple adjunctive tool in pci for balloon uncrossable chronic total occlusions. *J Interv Cardiol* 2013; **26**: 343–350.

42 Azzalini L, Ly HQ. Laser atherectomy for balloon failure in chronic total occlusion. *Int Heart J* 2014; **55**: 546–549.

43 Tsuchikane E, Katoh O, Shimogami M, *et al.* First clinical experience of a novel penetration catheter for patients with severe coronary artery stenosis. *Catheter Cardiovasc Interv* 2005; **65**: 368–373.

44 Galassi AR, Tomasello SD, Crea F, *et al.* Transient impairment of vasomotion function after successful chronic total occlusion recanalization. *J Am Coll Cardiol* 2012; **59**: 711–718.

45 Brugaletta S, Martin-Yuste V, Padro T, *et al.* Endothelial and smooth muscle cells dysfunction distal to recanalized chronic total coronary occlusions and the relationship with the collateral connection grade. *JACC Cardiovasc Interv* 2012; **5**: 170–178.

46 Colmenarez HJ, Escaned J, Fernandez C, *et al.* Efficacy and safety of drug-eluting stents in chronic total coronary occlusion recanalization: a systematic review and meta-analysis. *J Am Coll Cardiol* 2010; **55**: 1854–1866.

47 Saeed B, Kandzari DE, Agostoni P, *et al.* Use of drug-eluting stents for chronic total occlusions: a systematic review and meta-analysis. *Catheter Cardiovasc Interv* 2011; **77**: 315–332.

48 Imai M, Kadota K, Goto T, *et al.* Incidence, risk factors, and clinical sequelae of angiographic peri-stent contrast staining after sirolimus-eluting stent implantation. *Circulation* 2011; **123**: 2382–2391.

49 Tsujita K, Maehara A, Mintz GS, *et al.* Intravascular ultrasound comparison of the retrograde versus antegrade approach to percutaneous intervention for chronic total coronary occlusions. *JACC Cardiovasc Interv* 2009; **2**: 846–854.

50 Hong SJ, Kim BK, Shin DH, *et al.* Usefulness of intravascular ultrasound guidance in percutaneous coronary intervention with second-generation drug-eluting stents for chronic total occlusions (from the Multicenter Korean-Chronic Total Occlusion Registry). *Am J Cardiol* 2014; **114**: 534–540.

51 Estevez-Loureiro R, Ghione M, Kilickesmez K, Agudo P, Lindsay A, Di Mario C. The role for adjunctive image in pre-procedural assessment and peri-procedural management in chronic total occlusion recanalisation. *Curr Cardiol Rev* 2014; **10**: 120–126.

52 Kato M, Chida K, Sato T, *et al.* The necessity of follow-up for radiation skin injuries in patients after percutaneous coronary interventions: radiation skin injuries will often be overlooked clinically. *Acta Radiol* 2012; **53**: 1040–1044.

53 Vano E, Escaned J, Vano-Galvan S, Galvan C. Importance of a patient dosimetry and clinical follow-up program in the detection of radiodermatitis after long percutaneous coronary interventions. *Cardiovasc Intervent Radiol* 2013; **36**: 330–337.

54 Suzuki S, Furui S, Isshiki T, *et al.* Patients' skin dose during percutaneous coronary intervention for chronic total occlusion. *Catheter Cardiovasc Interv* 2008; **71**: 160–164.

55 Pucelikova T, Dangas G, Mehran R. Contrast-induced nephropathy. *Catheter Cardiovasc Interv* 2008; **71**: 62–72.

56 Morino Y, Kimura T, Hayashi Y, *et al.* In-hospital outcomes of contemporary percutaneous coronary intervention in patients with chronic total occlusion insights from the J-CTO Registry (Multicenter CTO Registry in Japan). *JACC Cardiovasc Interv* 2010; **3**: 143–151.

57 Stone GW, Kandzari DE, Mehran R, *et al.* Percutaneous recanalization of chronically occluded coronary arteries: a consensus document: Part I. *Circulation* 2005; **112**: 2364–2372.

58 Stone GW, Reifart NJ, Moussa I, *et al.* Percutaneous recanalization of chronically occluded coronary arteries: a consensus document: Part II. *Circulation* 2005; **112**: 2530–2537.

59 Patel VG, Brayton KM, Tamayo A, *et al.* Angiographic success and procedural complications in patients undergoing percutaneous coronary chronic total occlusion interventions: a weighted meta-analysis of 18,061 patients from 65 studies. *JACC Cardiovasc Interv* 2013; **6**: 128–136.

60 Rathore S, Matsuo H, Terashima M, *et al.* Procedural and in-hospital outcomes after percutaneous coronary intervention for chronic total occlusions of coronary arteries 2002 to 2008: impact of novel guidewire techniques. *JACC Cardiovasc Interv* 2009; **2**: 489–497.

61 Galassi AR, Tomasello SD, Reifart N, *et al.* In-hospital outcomes of percutaneous coronary intervention in patients with chronic total occlusion: insights from the ERCTO (European Registry of Chronic Total Occlusion) registry. *EuroIntervention* 2011; **7**: 472–479.

CHAPTER 19

Percutaneous Coronary Intervention of Arterial and Vein Grafts

Bimmer E.P.M. Claessen[1], José P.S. Henriques[1], and George D. Dangas[2]

[1]Department of Cardiology, Academic Medical Center—University of Amsterdam, Amsterdam, The Netherlands

[2]Department of Cardiology, Mount Sinai Medical Center, New York, NY, USA

Coronary artery bypass graft (CABG) surgery was introduced in the 1960s and is an effective technique to treat coronary artery disease [1]. In CABG, coronary stenoses or occlusions are bypassed using arterial (most commonly the left internal mammary artery; LIMA) or venous conduits (most commonly the greater saphenous vein). In recent years, the number of CABG surgeries has been in decline as a result of technical advances in percutaneous coronary intervention (PCI) which is now the most commonly used coronary revascularization technique [2]. However, even in the era of PCI with drug-eluting stents (DES) and dual antiplatelet therapy (DAPT), CABG surgery is associated with improved 5-year clinical outcomes, with the most outspoken benefit in patients with diabetes mellitus and complex coronary artery disease [3–5]. Nonetheless, long-term results of CABG surgery are limited by gradual progression of coronary artery disease in the native vessels but also by gradual failure of bypass conduits [6]. Therefore, patients who underwent CABG surgery may require secondary revascularization. This chapter provides an overview of the challenges of PCI in patients with failing arterial or venous bypass grafts.

Scope of the problem

Secondary revascularization after previous bypass surgery is not uncommon. For example, in the contemporary Synergy Between Percutaneous Coronary Intervention with Taxus and Cardiac Surgery (SYNTAX) trial, repeat revascularization had occurred in 13.7% of patients undergoing CABG surgery afer 5 years' follow-up [5]. In the SYNTAX trial, 1800 patients with multivessel coronary artery disease were randomized to treatment with CABG surgery using state-of-the-art techniques using arterial grafts where possible, or PCI with TAXUS paclitaxel-eluting stents (Boston Scientific, Natick, MA, USA) [7]. An analysis from the US National Cardiovascular Data Registry (NCDR) reported that between 2004 and 2009 17.5% of all PCI procedures (300,902 of 1,721,046) were performed with patients who had previously undergone CABG surgery [8].

The etiology of graft failure after CABG surgery is different depending on its timing. Graft occlusion of venous conduits within the first year after CABG surgery occurs in approximately 3–10% of patients in contemporary trials and registries and aspirin has been useful in diminishing this problem [7,9,10]. This is mostly caused by surgical problems such as kinking due to excessive graft length, pre-existing pathology in the vein graft, poor flow distal to the anastomosis resulting in acute postoperative failure, or as a response to vascular injury analogous to vascular injury after PCI. Late failure of bypass graft conduits results from attrition of saphenous vein grafts (SVGs) and/or progression of atherosclerotic disease in the native coronary arteries.

Arterial conduits are superior to venous conduits in terms of long-term graft patency. A study in 1254 patients who underwent CABG surgery reported 10-year patency rates of 61% for SVGs and 85% for internal mammary artery (IMA) grafts. Recent evidence from a meta-analysis comparing bilateral IMA and single IMA grafting showed a survival benefit with bilateral IMA grafting after a mean follow-up period of 9 years [11]. A secondary analysis in a cohort of 1419 patients undergoing CABG with an arterial graft to the left anterior descending artery (LAD) from the SYNTAX trial and registry showed that 5-year clinical outcomes in the CABG cohort were comparable in patients who received venous conduits or arterial conduits as a second graft [12]. Therefore, the follow-up duration in the SYNTAX subanalysis may be too short to detect an advantage with arterial conduits which is likely to arise between 5 and 20 years of follow-up.

Secondary revascularization after CABG surgery: PCI or repeat surgery?

As of 2015, only one randomized trial has compared PCI with CABG in post-CABG patients. The Angina with Extremely Serious Operative Mortality Evaluation (AWESOME) trial included 142 patients in a randomized trial comparing CABG with PCI in post-CABG patients [13]. Additionally, 719 patients were enrolled in a physician-directed registry. In this small randomized trial, there were no differences in terms of survival between the CABG and PCI arms at 3-year follow-up (73% vs. 76%, respectively).

Current US and European guidelines recommend a heart team approach in order to decide on the optimal revascularization technique in patients undergoing secondary revascularization

Interventional Cardiology: Principles and Practice, Second Edition. Edited by George D. Dangas, Carlo Di Mario, and Nicholas N. Kipshidze.
© 2017 John Wiley & Sons, Ltd. Published 2017 by John Wiley & Sons, Ltd.

after previous CABG surgery for ischemia refractory to medical therapy [14,15]. The 2011 American College of Cardiology/ American Heart Association (ACC/AHA) guideline on coronary artery bypass surgery states that a number of factors favoring repeat CABG include "vessels unsuitable for PCI, the number of diseased bypass grafts, availability of the LIMA for grafting, chronically occluded arteries and good distal targets for bypass graft placement. Factors favoring PCI over CABG include limited areas of ischemia causing symptoms, suitable PCI targets, a patent graft to the LAD artery, poor CABG targets, and comorbid conditions" [16].

PCI for acute postoperative graft failure

Occlusion of SVGs has been reported to occur in approximately 10% of grafts within 30 days of CABG surgery [10]. Acute graft failure after CABG surgery can be suspected by changes in the electrocardiogram (ECG) such as ST segment elevation or the development of new Q waves, by elevated biomarkers, by new wall motion abnormalities on echocardiography, hemodynamic instability, or a combination of these findings. Emergency angiography followed by PCI is the preferred strategy to manage acute postoperative graft failure [17]. However, redo CABG surgery is performed if multiple grafts are occluded or if the anatomy is not suited for PCI. Even with rapid emergency angiography and PCI, acute graft failure is associated with high in-hospital mortality, analogous to mortality after acute stent thrombosis after PCI [18]. For example, a recently published observational study of 54 patients undergoing emergency coronary angiography within 30 days after CABG surgery between 2004 and 2008 reported a 30-day mortality rate of 26% [17]. In the context of PCI within hours to days after CABG surgery there is an increased risk of perforation at the site of the freshly made anastomosis [17]. Current guidelines recommend that the target for PCI should be the body of the native vessel or the IMA graft, while the acutely occluded SVG should be avoided because of the risk of embolization and/or perforation [15].

PCI in degenerated saphenous vein grafts

The majority of PCIs after CABG surgery are performed in the native coronary system as reported by an analysis in 300,902 procedures from the NCDR comprising patients with previous CABG [8]; 62.5% of patients in this study underwent PCI in native vessels only and 37.5% underwent PCI in at least one bypass graft with the vast majority of these grafts being SVGs (SVG 34.9%, arterial graft 2.5%, both arterial and SVGs 0.2%).

Treatment of SVGs with PCI is associated with high rates of major adverse cardiac events (MACE). A patient-pooled meta-analysis of 3958 patients included in five randomized controlled trials and one registry investigating embolic protection devices in SVGs reported a 30-day MACE (defined as death, myocardial infarction, or target vessel revascularization) rate of 13.8% in patients treated with conventional guidewires and 9.6% in patients with embolic protection devices [19]. The strongest predictors of 30-day MACE were a larger estimated plaque volume and a high degree of SVG degeneration. Analyses from a registry of approximately 1000 patients undergoing PCI with bare metal stents (BMS) in SVGs have shown that female gender and diabetes mellitus are both associated with an increased risk of adverse events after SVG PCI [20,21].

Another prognostically unfavorable characteristic of patients undergoing SVG or arterial graft PCI, particularly in the presence of extensive occlusions in the native coronary circulation, is that they typically have a low left ventricular ejection fraction. In these patients, the use of a hemodynamic support device can be indicated to optimize the extent of complete revascularization and minimize peri-procedural complications [22,23].

Guiding catheter selection

Guiding catheter selection depends on the insertion site of aorto-coronary bypass grafts in the aorta. Usually, grafts to the distal right coronary artery (RCA) or distal left circumflex coronary artery (CX) are located cranially above the ostium of the RCA; these grafts can be engaged by a Multipurpose, Judkins Right, or Amplatz Right or Left guiding catheter [24]. Grafts to the left coronary artery (LCA) are usually inserted in the aorta cranially to the ostium of the LCA; these grafts can be engaged by a Judkin Right, Hockey Stick, Left Coronary Bypass, or Amplatz Left guiding catheter.

Bare metal or drug-eluting stents in SVG interventions

In *de novo* coronary artery lesions the use of current-generation DES is associated with improved outcomes in terms of safety (death, myocardial infarction, stent thrombosis) and efficacy (target lesion and target vessel revascularization) compared with first-generation DES and BMS [25,26]. A large number of studies have also shown that DES implantation reduces the risk of repeat revascularization compared with BMS in SVG PCI [27]. Moreover, an analysis from 3063 patients undergoing SVG PCI in the Swedish Coronary Angiography and Angioplasty Registry (SCAAR) reported lower mortality rates in patients who received DES compared with BMS [28]. Current guidelines support the use of DES in SVGs (Class I, level of evidence A) [15]. A significant vessel mismatch occurs (particularly in SVG to diagonal or distal marginal branches) at the distal anastomosis level, which occasionally precludes the use of any stent at these locations. A particularly challenging situation is SVG disease in association with significant stenosis in the native coronary artery distal to the SVG anastomosis: typically, those distal vessels are of small caliber and present with diffuse disease and calcification. It is not unusual that no revascularization option is possible and cell or gene therapy protocols have been employed in such cases. Interestingly, this type of unfavorable anatomy is not necessarily related to low global regional systolic function.

Embolic protection devices in SVG interventions

Because of the high atheromatous load of degenerated vein grafts, PCI of SVGs is associated with an increased risk for distal embolization resulting in peri-procedural myocardial infarction [19]. A number of individual clinical trials and meta-analyses of clinical trials support the use of embolic protection devices in SVG intervention to reduce the occurrence of distal embolization [19,29–31].

Three distinct types of embolic protection devices have been developed. Distal occlusion aspiration devices comprise the first class; these devices contain an inflatable occlusion balloon which is passed distal to the lesion and inflated to prevent antegrade blood flow. The balloon is mounted on a hypotube which is used as the guidewire for stenting or balloon angioplasty. The PCI is performed while the blood in the SVG is stagnant, and any debris is subsequently removed by an aspiration catheter. Examples of this type of embolic protection device include the PercuSurge GuardWire (Medtronic, Minneapolis, MN, USA) and the TriActiv System (Kensey Nash Corp, Exton, PA, USA).

Distal embolic filters are the second class of embolic protection devices and the most commonly used type. These devices have a shrunken filter mounted on the distal part of a guidewire. The filter with a pore size of 100–110 μm is positioned distal to the lesion and subsequently deployed. Distal embolic filters allow for antegrade blood flow while capturing debris of similar size to the aforementioned distal occlusion system [32]. After stenting or balloon angioplasty, accumulated plaque debris is retrieved using a retrieval catheter. Examples of this type of embolic protection device include the Spider (Abbott Vascular, Abbott Park, IL), the FilterWire (Boston Scientific, Natick, MA, USA), and the Interceptor Plus (Medtronic Vascular, Santa Rosa, CA, USA).

Finally, a proximal occlusion aspiration device (Proxis, St. Jude Medical, Minneapolis, MN, USA) was found to be effective in SVG PCI, but its manufacture was discontinued and it is no longer commercially available [33].

Currently, the use of embolic protection devices is listed as a Class I, level of evidence B recommendation by both the ESC and ACC/AHA guidelines [15,34].

Use of glycoprotein IIb/IIIa inhibitors in vein graft PCI

Because of the high thrombotic burden of degenerated vein grafts, the glycoprotein IIb/IIIa inhibitors (GPIs) which inhibit platelet aggregation have been investigated in SVG PCI. However, use of GPIs in SVG PCI was not found to result in a reduction of adverse ischemic events. A pooled analysis of individual patient data ($n = 627$) from five randomized controlled trials investigating GPIs in SVG PCI reported a numerically higher rate of adverse events (death, myocardial infarction, or revascularization) at 6-month follow-up in SVG PCI when GPIs where used compared with placebo (39.4% vs. 32.7%; $p = 0.07$) [35].

Radial approach in vein graft PCI

A recent randomized controlled trial investigated 128 consecutive patients who had previously undergone CABG surgery and who were referred for cardiac catheterization to radial or femoral vascular access [36]. In this small study, radial access was associated with longer procedural time (34.2 ± 14.7 vs. 21.9 ± 6.8 minutes; $p < 0.01$), longer fluoroscopy time (12.7 ± 6.6 vs. 8.5 ± 4.7 minutes; $p < 0.01$), and increased contrast use (171 ± 72 mL vs. 142 ± 39 mL; $p < 0.01$). Moreover, access site crossover occurred in 17.2% of patients in the radial group. However, outcomes were similar in patients who underwent PCI. This study suggests that the radial approach in vein graft PCI should preferably be used by operators who have extensive experience with radial PCI and angiography. In our opinion, the exact location of the graft and the distance of its proximal anastomosis from the innominate artery, and its relation to the great vessel and arch tortuosity are very important factors in determining the feasibility of a radial approach and the access site laterality (left versus right radial).

PCI in arterial conduits

If arterial grafts require intervention, this need most commonly arises during the first year after CABG surgery as the most common mechanism of arterial graft narrowing is a response to injury (analogous to the mechanism of restenosis after PCI) [8]. Arterial grafts using the radial artery are known to have a tendency to develop coronary spasm, which complicates PCI of these types of grafts [37]. Calcium channel blockers have been used empirically by many surgeons after arterial graft conduit implantation (particularly radial grafts). Arterial grafts are notably resistant to atherosclerotic deterioration particularly within their shafts; therefore anastomotic lesions are the most common. There is limited clinical evidence on the subject of PCI of arterial grafts. A different behavior of anastomotic and shaft lesions has been suggested with use of BMS and balloons, respectively, as first line of treatment; DES implantation has changed this practice. A small retrospective study suggests that DES implantation in arterial grafts results in a reduction in target lesion revascularization compared with BMS [38].

Guiding catheter selection for LIMA and RIMA grafts

A LIMA graft can be engaged via the left radial artery or via the femoral route. The most commonly used catheter shapes or the Judkins Right 4 or the IMA. For successful wiring of a tortuous LIMA a soft hydrophilic wire, perhaps supported by a 1.5 mm balloon may be required. In patients where the LIMA takes off from the proximal ascending part of the left subclavian artery, the use of a guiding catheter with a 0.035 inch glidewire inside can allow nonselective injection and advancement of a 0.014 inch wire into the IMA, then the glidewire can be retracted and the catheter directed toward the IMA with help from the 0.014 inch wire.

The right IMA (RIMA) can be engaged by IMA or Judkins Right 4 shaped catheters using the right radial artery or the femoral approach. When using the femoral approach, engaging the RIMA may prove challenging, and an approach using a glidewire as described above can be helpful.

Conclusions

PCI in patients who have undergone CABG surgery is a frequently encountered clinical problem. These are typically patients with high rates of risk factors for coronary sclerosis in addition to numerous extracardiac comorbidities. In patients with medically refractory anginal complaints after previous CABG surgery, a tailored approach to secondary revascularization should be devised by the heart team. If PCI is deemed the most appropriate revascularization technique, guidelines recommend treatment of the native coronary artery system. If this is contraindicated and PCI of degenerated vein grafts is performed, the use of embolic protection devices and placement of DES rather than BMS is recommended. We have to also keep in mind that the achievement of the most optimal final luminal diameter in graft lesions has been associated with a greater post-procedure myocardial injury and operators should take account of this trade-off [39].

Interactive multiple choice questions are available for this chapter on www.wiley. com/go/dangas/cardiology

References

1 Cheng TO. History of coronary artery bypass surgery: half of a century of progress. *Int J Cardiol* 2012; **157**(1): 1–2.

2 Epstein AJ, Polsky D, Yang F, Yang L, Groeneveld PW. Coronary revascularization trends in the United States, 2001–2008. *JAMA* 2011; **305**(17): 1769–1776.

3 Farkouh ME, Domanski M, Sleeper LA, *et al.* Strategies for multivessel revascularization in patients with diabetes. *N Engl J Med* 2012; **367**(25): 2375–2384.

4 Group BDS, Frye RL, August P, *et al.* A randomized trial of therapies for type 2 diabetes and coronary artery disease. *N Engl J Med* 2009; **360**(24): 2503–2515.

5 Mohr FW, Morice MC, Kappetein AP, *et al.* Coronary artery bypass graft surgery versus percutaneous coronary intervention in patients with three-vessel disease and left main coronary disease: 5-year follow-up of the randomised, clinical SYNTAX trial. *Lancet* 2013; **381**(9867): 629–638.

6 Sabik JF 3rd, Blackstone EH, Gillinov AM, Smedira NG, Lytle BW. Occurrence and risk factors for reintervention after coronary artery bypass grafting. *Circulation* 2006; **114**(1 Suppl): I454–460.

7 Serruys PW, Morice MC, Kappetein AP, *et al.* Percutaneous coronary intervention versus coronary-artery bypass grafting for severe coronary artery disease. *N Engl J Med* 2009; **360**(10): 961–972.

8 Brilakis ES, Rao SV, Banerjee S, *et al.* Percutaneous coronary intervention in native arteries versus bypass grafts in prior coronary artery bypass grafting patients: a report from the National Cardiovascular Data Registry. *JACC Cardiovasc Interv* 2011; **4**(8): 844–850.

9 Thielmann M, Massoudy P, Jaeger BR, *et al.* Emergency re-revascularization with percutaneous coronary intervention, reoperation, or conservative treatment in patients with acute perioperative graft failure following coronary artery bypass surgery. *Eur J Cardiothorac Surg* 2006; **30**(1): 117–125.

10 Harskamp RE, Lopes RD, Baisden CE, de Winter RJ, Alexander JH. Saphenous vein graft failure after coronary artery bypass surgery: pathophysiology, management, and future directions. *Ann Surg* 2013; **257**(5): 824–833.

11 Yi G, Shine B, Rehman SM, Altman DG, Taggart DP. Effect of bilateral internal mammary artery grafts on long-term survival: a meta-analysis approach. *Circulation* 2014; **130**(7): 539–545.

12 Parasca CA, Head SJ, Mohr FW, *et al.* The impact of a second arterial graft on 5-year outcomes after coronary artery bypass grafting in the Synergy Between Percutaneous Coronary Intervention With TAXUS and Cardiac Surgery Trial and Registry. *J Thorac Cardiovasc Surg* 2015; **150**(3): 597–606.

13 Morrison DA, Sethi G, Sacks J, *et al.* Percutaneous coronary intervention versus repeat bypass surgery for patients with medically refractory myocardial ischemia: AWESOME randomized trial and registry experience with post-CABG patients. *J Am Coll Cardiol* 2002; **40**(11): 1951–1954.

14 Fihn SD, Blankenship JC, Alexander KP, *et al.* 2014 ACC/AHA/AATS/PCNA/SCAI/STS focused update of the guideline for the diagnosis and management of patients with stable ischemic heart disease: a report of the American College of Cardiology/American Heart Association Task Force on Practice Guidelines, and the American Association for Thoracic Surgery, Preventive Cardiovascular Nurses Association, Society for Cardiovascular Angiography and Interventions, and Society of Thoracic Surgeons. *J Am Coll Cardiol* 2014; **64**(18): 1929–1949.

15 Authors/Task Force members, Windecker S, Kolh P, Alfonso F, *et al.* 2014 ESC/EACTS Guidelines on myocardial revascularization: The Task Force on Myocardial Revascularization of the European Society of Cardiology (ESC) and the European Association for Cardio-Thoracic Surgery (EACTS) Developed with the special contribution of the European Association of Percutaneous Cardiovascular Interventions (EAPCI). *Eur Heart J* 2014; **35**(37): 2541–2619.

16 Hillis LD, Smith PK, Anderson JL, *et al.* 2011 ACCF/AHA Guideline for Coronary Artery Bypass Graft Surgery. A report of the American College of Cardiology Foundation/American Heart Association Task Force on Practice Guidelines. Developed in collaboration with the American Association for Thoracic Surgery, Society of Cardiovascular Anesthesiologists, and Society of Thoracic Surgeons. *J Am Coll Cardiol* 2011; **58**(24): e123–210.

17 Babiker A, Del Angel JG, Perez-Vizcayno MJ, *et al.* Rescue percutaneous intervention for acute complications of coronary artery surgery. *EuroIntervention* 2009; **5**(Suppl D): 64–69.

18 Claessen BE, Henriques JP, Jaffer FA, Mehran R, Piek JJ, Dangas GD. Stent thrombosis: a clinical perspective. *JACC Cardiovasc Interv* 2014; **7**(10): 1081–1092.

19 Coolong A, Baim DS, Kuntz RE, *et al.* Saphenous vein graft stenting and major adverse cardiac events: a predictive model derived from a pooled analysis of 3958 patients. *Circulation* 2008; **117**(6): 790–797.

20 Ahmed JM, Dangas G, Lansky AJ, *et al.* Influence of gender on early and one-year clinical outcomes after saphenous vein graft stenting. *Am J Cardiol* 2001; **87**(4): 401–405.

21 Ahmed JM, Hong MK, Mehran R, *et al.* Influence of diabetes mellitus on early and late clinical outcomes in saphenous vein graft stenting. *J Am Coll Cardiol* 2000; **36**(4): 1186–1193.

22 Dangas GD, Kini AS, Sharma SK, *et al.* Impact of hemodynamic support with Impella 2.5 versus intra-aortic balloon pump on prognostically important clinical outcomes in patients undergoing high-risk percutaneous coronary intervention (from the PROTECT II randomized trial). *Am J Cardiol* 2014; **113**(2): 222–228.

23 O'Neill WW, Kleiman NS, Moses J, *et al.* A prospective, randomized clinical trial of hemodynamic support with Impella 2.5 versus intra-aortic balloon pump in patients undergoing high-risk percutaneous coronary intervention: the PROTECT II study. *Circulation* 2012; **126**(14): 1717–1727.

24 Hindnavis V, Cho SH, Goldberg S. Saphenous vein graft intervention: a review. *J Invasive Cardiol* 2012; **24**(2): 64–71.

25 Navarese EP, Tandjung K, Claessen B, *et al.* Safety and efficacy outcomes of first and second generation durable polymer drug eluting stents and biodegradable polymer biolimus eluting stents in clinical practice: comprehensive network meta-analysis. *BMJ* 2013; **347**: f6530.

26 Palmerini T, Biondi-Zoccai G, Della Riva D, *et al.* Stent thrombosis with drug-eluting and bare-metal stents: evidence from a comprehensive network meta-analysis. *Lancet* 2012; **379**(9824): 1393–1402.

27 Paradis JM, Belisle P, Joseph L, *et al.* Drug-eluting or bare metal stents for the treatment of saphenous vein graft disease: a Bayesian meta-analysis. *Circ Cardiovasc Interv* 2010; **3**(6): 565–576.

28 Frobert O, Schersten F, James SK, Carlsson J, Lagerqvist B. Long-term safety and efficacy of drug-eluting and bare metal stents in saphenous vein grafts. *Am Heart J* 2012; **164**(1): 87–93.

29 Baim DS, Wahr D, George B, *et al.* Randomized trial of a distal embolic protection device during percutaneous intervention of saphenous vein aorto-coronary bypass grafts. *Circulation* 2002; **105**(11): 1285–1290.

30 Carrozza JP Jr, Mumma M, Breall JA, *et al.* Randomized evaluation of the TriActiv balloon-protection flush and extraction system for the treatment of saphenous vein graft disease. *J Am Coll Cardiol* 2005; **46**(9): 1677–1683.

31 Stone GW, Rogers C, Hermiller J, *et al.* Randomized comparison of distal protection with a filter-based catheter and a balloon occlusion and aspiration system during percutaneous intervention of diseased saphenous vein aorto-coronary bypass grafts. *Circulation* 2003; **108**(5): 548–553.

32 Quan VH, Huynh R, Seifert PA, *et al.* Morphometric analysis of particulate debris extracted by four different embolic protection devices from coronary arteries, aortocoronary saphenous vein conduits, and carotid arteries. *Am J Cardiol* 2005; **95**(12): 1415–1419.

33 Mauri L, Cox D, Hermiller J, *et al.* The PROXIMAL trial: proximal protection during saphenous vein graft intervention using the Proxis Embolic Protection System: a randomized, prospective, multicenter clinical trial. *J Am Coll Cardiol* 2007; **50**(15): 1442–1449.

34 Levine GN, Bates ER, Blankenship JC, *et al.* 2011 ACCF/AHA/SCAI Guideline for Percutaneous Coronary Intervention: a report of the American College of Cardiology Foundation/American Heart Association Task Force on Practice Guidelines and the Society for Cardiovascular Angiography and Interventions. *J Am Coll Cardiol* 2011; **58**(24): e44–122.

35 Roffi M, Mukherjee D, Chew DP, *et al.* Lack of benefit from intravenous platelet glycoprotein IIb/IIIa receptor inhibition as adjunctive treatment for percutaneous interventions of aortocoronary bypass grafts: a pooled analysis of five randomized clinical trials. *Circulation* 2002; **106**(24): 3063–3067.

36 Michael TT, Alomar M, Papayannis A, *et al.* A randomized comparison of the transradial and transfemoral approaches for coronary artery bypass graft angiography and intervention: the RADIAL-CABG Trial (RADIAL Versus Femoral Access for Coronary Artery Bypass Graft Angiography and Intervention). *JACC Cardiovasc Interv* 2013; **6**(11): 1138–1144.

37 Sharma AK, Ajani AE, Garg N, *et al.* Percutaneous interventions in radial artery grafts: clinical and angiographic outcomes. *Catheter Cardiovasc Interv* 2003; **59**(2): 172–175.

38 Buch AN, Xue Z, Gevorkian N, *et al.* Comparison of outcomes between bare metal stents and drug-eluting stents for percutaneous revascularization of internal mammary grafts. *Am J Cardiol* 2006; **98**(6): 722–724.

39 Iakovou I, Mintz GS, Dangas G, *et al.* Increased CK-MB release is a "trade-off" for optimal stent implantation: an intravascular ultrasound study. *J Am Coll Cardiol* 2003; **42**: 1900–1905.

CHAPTER 20

Interventional Approach in Small Vessel, Diffuse, and Tortuous Coronary Artery Disease

Robert Pyo

Montefiore Medical Center, Albert Einstein College of Medicine, New York, NY, USA

Unfavorable factors for percutaneous coronary intervention (PCI) include small caliber of coronary vessels, diffuse lesion length, and significant coronary artery tortuosity. Small caliber of coronary arteries is associated with increased restenosis. Diffuse or long lesions are associated with decreased procedural success and are associated with higher rates of restenosis. PCI of tortuous lesions are also associated with decreased procedural success rates which stem chiefly from difficulty in delivering devices. Difficulty in device delivery not only makes intervention challenging, but also makes anatomic and physiologic assessment of lesions difficult. However, with thoughtful application of technique and use of supportive equipment, PCI of these difficult lesion subsets can be accomplished with a high degree of success and safety.

Small vessel disease

Definition and prevalence

A small coronary artery is defined as a vessel with a reference vessel diameter of less than 2.5–2.75 mm [1,2]. Usually, the caliber of the vessel is determined by angiographic evaluation. However, if there is diffuse coronary artery disease, the reference vessel diameter may not be easily discernable and the true vessel diameter can easily be underestimated by using angiography-based estimates. In these cases, imaging with intravascular ultrasound (IVUS) or optical coherence tomography (OCT) is sometimes needed to confirm true vessel size.

Percutaneous interventions of small vessels are relatively common and compromise approximately 25–30% of coronary procedures [3,4]. Patients with small diameter coronary arteries tend to be older and are more likely to be female. They also tend to have higher frequencies of concomitant disease such as heart failure and diabetes [5].

Anatomic and physiologic assessment

Physiologic assessment of small vessel coronary artery disease is important. Because of the relatively poorer outcomes after PCI, intervention should be entertained only for clinically significant lesions. Lesions with angiographic diameter stenosis of greater than 70% when compared to reference vessel diameter are generally considered physiologically important and are thought to potentially cause ischemia [6,7]. However, visual estimation of stenosis severity by angiography alone can be difficult if the reference vessel diameter is small. IVUS, OCT, and fractional flow reserve (FFR) can be employed to aid in the evaluation of the clinical significance of small vessel disease.

Intravascular ultrasound

Evaluation of small vessel coronary arteries with IVUS can be performed effectively. Availability of smaller 5 Fr IVUS catheters makes delivery easier. Images are assessed in a similar fashion to larger arteries and the principal analysis is assessment of minimal lumen cross-sectional area (CSA). For larger vessels with reference diameters of greater than 3.0 mm, a CSA of less than 4.0 mm^2 is generally correlated with ischemia which is proven by nuclear imaging [8]. For smaller vessels, the cut-off CSA below which ischemia is thought to occur is smaller. In the Fractional Flow Reserve and Intravascular Ultrasound Relationship Study (FIRST), coronary artery lesions in vessels with varying reference vessel diameters were evaluated with FFR. The best cut-off CSA for lesions in vessels with reference vessel diameters less than 3.0 mm was 2.4 mm^2. Lesions with CSA below this cut-off were likely to have an "ischemic" FFR value of less than 0.8 [9].

Fractional flow reserve

Measurement of FFR can be useful in assessing the physiologic significance of lesions in small coronary arteries. FFR has been validated as an important tool for identifying lesions that when treated with PCI lead to improved clinical outcome. Although most of the data supporting the use of FFR have been derived from studies that evaluated larger coronary arteries, evidence supports the use of this modality in smaller coronary arteries as well [10]. In the FAME study, 20–30% of the coronary arteries that were studied were less than 3.0 mm in diameter and the average reference vessel diameter was 2.5 mm [11]. In the Phantom study, evaluation of patients with FFR could identify those patients with small coronary artery disease in whom PCI could be safely be deferred [12]. The FFR cut-off for physiologic significance in small coronary arteries appears to be in the range 0.75–0.80, and values less than this cut-off range correlate with ischemia.

Interventional Cardiology: Principles and Practice, Second Edition. Edited by George D. Dangas, Carlo Di Mario, and Nicholas N. Kipshidze.
© 2017 John Wiley & Sons, Ltd. Published 2017 by John Wiley & Sons, Ltd.

Optical coherence tomography

OCT is a relatively new imaging modality compared to IVUS. Rather than using ultrasound, it uses infrared light to obtain cross-sectional images of coronary arteries. Compared with IVUS, it has the distinct advantage of having superior resolution. In order to image optimally, the blood in the coronary artery must be washed out with dye. In smaller vessels, this washout may not be optimal because of the distal location of the vessels. The correlation between ischemia and OCT-derived CSA has not been rigorously validated.

Technical aspects

PCI of small vessel disease can be challenging. Delivery of devices is often difficult because of the distal location of the small vessels. Small vessels can also be at bifurcations and all the challenges of bifurcation PCI are compounded by the small size of the vessel. Stent sizing can be difficult because of tapering of a small vessel to even smaller dimensions. However, the application of a well-executed plan can make intervention easier.

Device delivery

Delivery of devices to the distal portion of the coronary bed is difficult but can be accomplished safely with application of the correct technique and equipment. A "buddy wire" is often used [13,14]. In this technique, two wires are delivered into the target vessel. One of the wires is a stiff support wire that enhances delivery. Commonly used wires in this category are the Mailman™ (Boston Scientific, Marlborough, MA, USA) and the Grand Slam (Abbott, Abbott Park, IL, USA). These wires enhance delivery by "straightening" bends proximal to the lesion and provide a "rail" over which device delivery is facilitated. Furthermore, in cases where guide support is suboptimal, the use of a stiff support wire will help to support the guide in a coaxial position for optimal device delivery. The second wire is the delivery wire or the wire over which the balloon or stent will be delivered. This wire is a softer wire which allows passage of devices, even through tortuous vessel segments, without significant biasing effect (for more on wire bias see the section on diffuse vessel disease).

In cases where equipment delivery is particularly difficult even with the use of the buddy wire technique, mother-and-child guide extenders facilitate delivery. Two commonly used varieties are the Guideliner (Vascular Solutions, Minneapolis, MN, USA) and Guidezilla (Boston Scientific, Marlborough, MA, USA). These devices provide additional support for device passage by allowing deep intubation of coronary arteries. Additionally, in cases of unusual take off angle of the coronary ostium or anomalous coronary ostium take off, these devices can provide coaxial support. In particularly challenging cases, these devices can be advanced over the shaft of an inflated balloon to "super" deep seat the device into the coronary vasculature (for details of this technique see the section on tortuous vessel disease). The balloon can then be deflated, withdrawn, and the stent can be delivered through the deep-seated guide extender. Care must be taken when using these devices for deep intubation because coronary dissections can occur as these devices are advanced into the coronary vasculature.

Bifurcation lesions

Treatment of bifurcation lesions in small vessels should employ a one-stent strategy. The stent should be placed into the larger branch after ballooning the smaller branch pre-emptively to prevent abrupt closure. Re-crossing into the jailed side branch routinely to treat an angiographically "pinched" side branch with balloon dilatation should not be performed because of the possibility of causing stent deformation [15]. If ischemic symptoms develop or angiographically suboptimal flow is observed in the unstented side branch, the stent strut should be re-crossed into the smaller unstented side branch with a guidewire and the jailing stent strut opened with a small non-compliant balloon inflated to high pressure. The segment of the vessel before the bifurcation is small and therefore may not allow simultaneous kissing balloon inflation. A final high pressure inflation of a non-compliant balloon in the stented main branch will in most cases be sufficient to re-align the stent struts without re-closure of the unstented side branch. Use of sequential balloon inflation rather than simultaneous kissing balloon inflation does not appear to make a difference in clinical outcome [16]. In fact, sequential balloon dilatation rather than simultaneous kissing balloon dilatation was associated with a more favorable anatomic outcome in the main branch [17]. The small caliber of the parent portion of the vessel can preclude any meaningful two-stent strategy and even if such a strategy is employed the in-stent restenosis rate is high. In general, a one-stent strategy should be used to treat bifurcation lesions in small coronary arteries.

Device size

The availability of smaller balloons and stents has made PCI of small vessel disease easier and safer. Balloons as small as 1.2 mm allow crossing and dilatation of distal lesions in small vessels feasible [18]. Some of these smaller balloons are mounted on relatively stiff shafts that promote efficient delivery of forward force. Plain old balloon angioplasty (POBA) has produced acceptable results [3]. However, if vessel size allows, treatment with drug-eluting stents (DES) is preferred to balloon angioplasty alone. DES are now available in diameters as small as 2.25 mm.

Clinical outcomes

Clinical outcomes of percutaneous intervention of small vessel disease are poor compared to similar procedures of larger caliber vessels [19]. Poor outcomes are primarily brought about by the increased rates of in-stent restenosis (ISR) and target vessel revascularization (TVR). POBA was often used as a treatment for small vessels and, at least when compared to bare metal stents (BMS), appeared to yield equal results. The TVR rate at 6 months was approximately 20% at 6 months' follow-up [3]. This rate is much higher than the 6 month TVR rate of approximately 10% following placement of BMS in large vessels [20]. The advent of DES substantially improved ISR and TVR rates after stenting in small coronary arteries. The rate of revascularization was 4% at 9 months' follow-up [21,22]. With the advent of second generation DES, patency rates after stenting small coronary arteries have improved even more [23].

Key points and summary

- Intervention of small vessel coronary arteries is relatively common and comprises 20–30% of all percutaneous interventions in some series.
- Angiography is the most commonly employed method of assessing small vessel disease severity. However, other modalities including IVUS and FFR have been validated in studies and are reasonable adjunctive modalities to assess physiologic importance of small vessel coronary artery disease.
- PCI of small vessel disease can be challenging. Factors that contribute to difficulty include potential distal location of small vessels, proximal tortuosity, and location at bifurcation points. However, with use of proper equipment and technique, percutaneous intervention can be performed safely.

- A small diameter makes matching vessel to equipment size potentially challenging. However, recent introduction of smaller balloons and DES have made PCI more effective. Second generation DES as small as 2.25 mm in diameter are available and the use of these stents is associated with good clinical outcomes which are superior to simple balloon angioplasty and use of BMS.

Diffuse vessel disease
Definition and prevalence
Diffuse coronary artery disease is characterized by atherosclerotic plaques greater than 20 mm in length [24]. Certain subsets of patients are more likely to have diffuse coronary artery disease. Diabetic patients tend to have diffuse, multivessel coronary artery disease and are more likely to undergo surgical revascularization. South Asian patients as a whole tend to have severe diffuse coronary artery disease that may not be amenable to either surgical or percutaneous revascularization [25]. Patients who have undergone cardiac transplantation sometimes present with diffuse occlusive coronary artery disease. In this group of patients, the disease is often caused by transplant vasculopathy which is a result of a diffuse proliferation of smooth muscle cells [26]. Less commonly, atherosclerotic lesions can occur in coronary arteries of transplanted hearts, but these lesions tend to occur in a more focal pattern [27]. Uncommonly, diffuse coronary artery disease develops in response to a general inflammatory process in patients with vasculopathies [28].

Anatomic and physiologic assessment
Coronary angiography is most often used to identify diffuse coronary artery disease. However, because of diffuse involvement of the coronary artery, it is often difficult to determine the disease-free reference diameter of the vessel and thus makes estimation of percent stenosis problematic. Indeed, in some cases an estimation of the reference vessel size is impossible and the vessel as a whole is described as "moderately diffusely" or "severely diffusely" diseased. Therefore, modalities other than angiography are needed in some cases to quantify the extent of diffuse coronary artery disease.

Intravascular ultrasound and optical coherence tomography
IVUS is useful in characterizing diffuse coronary artery disease. In cases where assessment of percent stenosis is difficult because of lack of a clear reference vessel diameter, measurement with IVUS is an alternate method to assess severity of disease and implications for physiologic importance. A plaque with a CSA of less than 4.0 mm^2 measured by IVUS in a vessel with a reference vessel diameter of at least 3.0 mm is generally thought to cause ischemia [8]. Lower CSA thresholds for ischemia have been identified in vessels with reference diameters of less than 3.0 mm [9]. In addition, imaging with IVUS identifies more severe segments of diffuse disease which can be selectively stented. IVUS-guided spot stenting of the most severely diseased areas spares the need for implantation of long stents and can be associated with better outcomes [29].

OCT yields similar information to IVUS. Additionally, it has the advantage of superior resolution and can yield important qualitative data about the lesion such as degree of calcification [30]. Furthermore, its superior resolution facilitates identification of stent malapposition which occurs relatively more frequently when diffuse lesions are stented. OCT can then be used to guide corrective measures with high pressure balloon dilatation.

Fractional flow reserve
Because it is often difficult to ascertain an accurate percent stenosis of a diffuse lesion, FFR is a valuable tool to gauge its physiologic importance. Particularly in cases where there are severe lesions in tandem that are separated by less severely diseased segments, pullback of the FFR wire can isolate lesions that are hemodynamically significant. In this technique, the FFR wire is placed across a diffuse lesion and under maximal hyperemia a hemodynamic assessment of the entire lesion is made. If the FFR value is significant ($\leq$0.8) under maximal hyperemia, the wire is pulled back proximally from the most distal portion of a diffuse lesion. If there is a significant pressure drop across a lesion (approximately 10 mmHg), that lesion is treated with PCI. It is important to perform a FFR measurement of the entire diffuse lesion again after stenting, because the physiologic interaction between serial lesions is accounted for by more than a hemodynamic drop which is simply the additive effect of the serial lesions [31]. For example, an initially hemodynamically insignificant proximal lesion can become significant by FFR after the more distal lesion is treated with a stent. This more proximal lesion should be treated in order to render the entire diffuse lesion hemodynamically insignificant. This concept is illustrated in Figure 20.1. In cases where there is no significant drop across a particular area of a diffuse lesion, either the entire lesion has to be stented to obtain hemodynamic benefit or the patient is not a good candidate for PCI and should be considered for surgical revascularization.

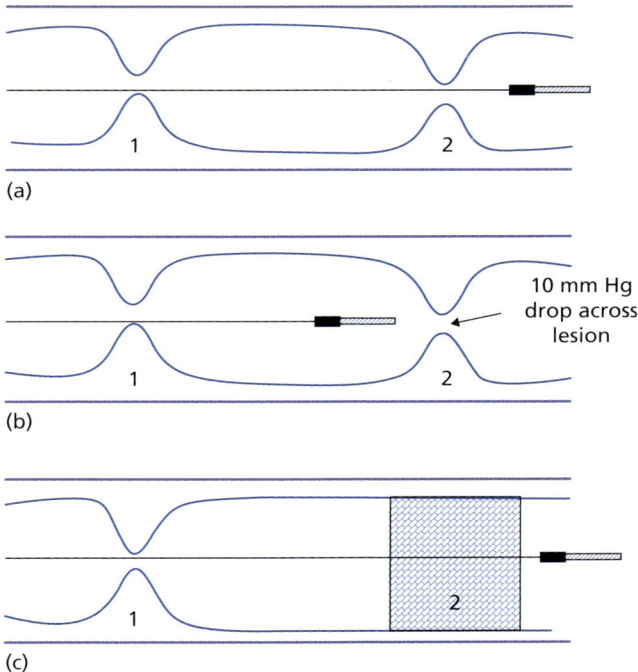

Figure 20.1 (a) A fractional flow reserve (FFR) wire advanced beyond two sequential lesions (1 and 2) registers a clinically significant value. (b) During pullback, a 10 mmHg drop is registered across the distal lesion (2) but a significant pressure drop is not registered across the proximal lesion (1). (c) Once the distal lesion is treated with a stent (2) the FFR wire is placed distal to the stent and pulled back again. No pressure drop is registered across the stented segment (2), but a significant pressure drop is recorded across the proximal lesion (1) – the proximal lesion should be stented.

Technical aspects

Percutaneous intervention of diffuse coronary artery disease is challenging. Deciding how much of the vessel to stent may not be straightforward and therefore adjunctive diagnostic modalities to coronary angiography, such as IVUS or FFR, may have to be employed to determine the extent of stenting. Even after deciding which segment to treat, delivery of devices across areas of diffuse disease can be difficult. In particular, lesions that are calcified and or occupy bends in the vessel can be particularly challenging.

Device delivery

Stent delivery into diffuse coronary artery lesions can be difficult because of increased mechanical resistance, location of disease around vessel bends, and in certain subsets of patients such as those with chronic kidney disease associated with calcification. Therefore it is important to pre-treat these lesions adequately prior to making an attempt to deliver a stent. There should be a low threshold for preparing a lesion with rotational atherectomy in diffusely calcified lesions (see Chapter 22 for details of this technique). Use of rotational atherectomy will significantly increase the likelihood that all portions of the diffuse lesion will be uniformly and adequately dilatable with a balloon. After rotational atherectomy, a high pressure balloon sized 0.5 mm smaller than the reference vessel diameter should be inflated to high pressures at the areas to be stented. The use of a balloon sized slightly smaller than the vessel, inflated to high pressures ensures adequate expansion of the lesion without undue barotrauma.

Even after adequate balloon dilatation and expansion, delivery of a stent can be difficult. The same techniques to enhance stent delivery in small vessels can be used. The use of a stiff support wire enhances delivery by providing a more stable platform to advance devices such as a balloon or stent. If a "buddy wire" system is used and the lesion occurs at a bend in the vessel, it is helpful to advance the stent over the softer non-support wire, because there will be less biasing against the vessel wall. This concept is illustrated in Figure 20.2. In straight lesions, delivery of the stent can be tried over the support wire if it fails to deliver on the softer wire. Guide extenders provide further support. Care should be used when "deep seating" these devices into coronary arteries with diffuse disease, because the risk of dissection is higher than when it is advanced into relatively disease-free segments of coronary arteries. In general, these devices should not be advanced into a segment of the artery that for whatever reason cannot be stented.

Plain old balloon angioplasty

In some cases diffuse coronary artery disease is not amenable for therapy with stents: the stents is undeliverable or the vessel size too small. If surgical revascularization is not feasible, stand-alone balloon angioplasty may be the only treatment option. When treating a lesion with only angioplasty or POBA, a long non-compliant balloon sized 1 : 1 to the vessel should be inflated to nominal pressure. Contemporary non-compliant balloons come in lengths of up to 30 mm. After the lesion is sufficiently dilated, the balloon should be kept inflated for about 1 minute at 50% of nominal pressure. This prolonged ballooning at less than nominal pressure will "tack up" potential dissection flaps without causing excessive barotrauma to the vessel. It is important to utilize a non-compliant balloon. Inflation of a long compliant balloon in a diffuse lesion at the high pressures that are required to adequately dilate a lesion can result in severe local barotrauma and flow-limiting dissection as a result of uneven inflation. The results from balloon-only treatment

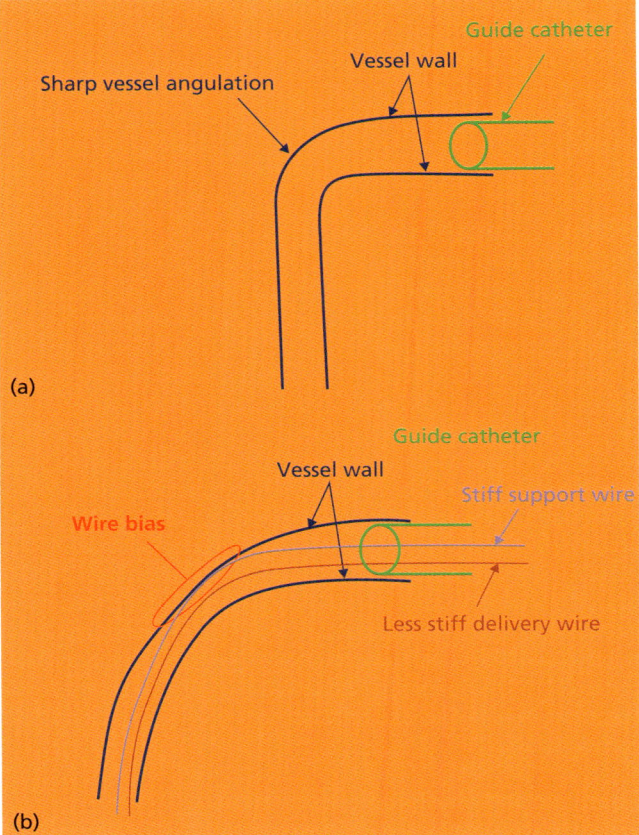

Figure 20.2 (a) 90° angulation in the vessel has set up a condition for wire bias. (b) The stiff support wire has "straightened" the vessel at the expense of causing wire bias against the vessel. Delivery of a device over this wire may be problematic because it may be "biased" against the vessel wall. Delivery over the device over the less stiff delivery wire is associated with less bias.

of diffuse coronary artery disease when compared to stenting are poor. Restenosis rates and target lesion revascularization rates can be as high as 42% and 21%, respectively [32]. Furthermore, balloon angioplasty of diffuse lesions can result in flow-limiting dissections demanding bailout stenting, which is associated with a high rate of peri-procedure myocardial infarction [32,33]. POBA should be used as a last option for treatment of diffuse coronary artery disease.

Stent

The use of BMS in the treatment of diffuse coronary artery disease improved procedural success when compared to balloon angioplasty only, but TVR rates remained high [32,33]. The use of DES significantly improved patency rates over the use of BMS and decreased revascularization rates to single digits [21,22]. Long second generation DES are available: both everolimus- and zotarolimus-eluting stents are available in 38 mm lengths. Revascularization rates after 9–12 months' follow-up after treatment of lesions longer than 30 mm with these stents are under 10% [34–36]. For lesions longer than 38 mm, placement of sequential stents with overlap is required. First generation DES overlap has been associated with increased in-stent restenosis rates [37]. Second generation

DES have been associated with better outcomes when placed in an overlapping configuration [38,39]. When more than two stents are used, overlap length should be minimized. The newer generation stents have thin strut architecture and therefore can be hard to visualize with fluoroscopy. Use of enhanced stent visualization imaging techniques ("stent boost") can improve visualization to minimize overlap length [40].

Clinical outcomes

Percutaneous treatment of diffuse coronary artery disease is associated with less favorable outcome than treatment of more focal disease. Stand-alone balloon angioplasty is associated with poor outcome and should be avoided. Stenting diffuse coronary artery disease has been associated with poorer outcome than stenting focal disease. In fact, stent length has been identified as an independent predictor of in-stent restenosis [41]. Diffuse disease is prevalent in diabetics and presents a therapeutic dilemma. These patients are often not ideal candidates for surgical bypass because of poor targets for distal anastomosis [25]. Use of second generation DES have produced acceptable outcome in patients with diffuse coronary artery disease and should be used when possible.

Key points and summary

- The prevalence of diffuse coronary artery disease is high in patient subsets such as diabetics. The diffuse nature of disease can make them poor targets for bypass surgery and clinically significant disease must be treated percutaneously in selected cases.
- Angiography is the most common way to assess the severity of diffuse coronary artery disease. However, in some cases identifying a non-diseased part of the vessel to measure a reference vessel diameter can be challenging, and imaging modalities such as IVUS or OCT have to be employed. Additionally, the use of FFR is especially useful in evaluating severe sequential lesions in diffuse coronary artery disease.
- Delivery of equipment can be difficult in diffuse coronary artery disease, especially if the lesion is calcified or occupies a bend. Adequate vessel preparation prior to stent delivery is essential. Treatment with rotational atherectomy, followed by high-pressure balloon angioplasty, is essential prior to stent delivery if calcification is present. Use of buddy wire technique and guide extenders can help overcome resistance caused by biasing effects and long lesion length.

Tortuous vessel disease
Definition and prevalence

Coronary artery tortuosity is simply the presence of significant bends in the coronary vasculature. In the setting of PCI, vessel tortuosity is assessed in the portion of the vessel prior to the lesion. Various schemes have been proposed for quantifying the severity of coronary tortuosity [24,42]. Excessive tortuosity is defined by at least one bend >90° or >2 bends >60°. Therefore, in general, the more acute the angle and the more bends prior to the lesion characterize increasingly tortuous coronary arteries. Excessive tortuosity is associated with decreased chance of PCI success and is associated with a greater likelihood of adverse outcome.

Coronary tortuosity is not infrequent. In some series, the prevalence of this anatomic finding is as high as 39% [43]. Although coronary tortuosity can occur in any vessel, the prevalence is higher in the left circumflex artery simply because the first bend of this artery as it comes off the left main artery can occur at a steep angle.

Additionally, the obtuse marginal branches of the left circumflex coronary artery often arise at close to 90° angles and contribute to general vessel tortuosity. The left anterior descending coronary artery has the second highest incidence of coronary tortuosity followed by the right coronary artery [43]. Fortunately, there is an inverse relationship of coronary tortuosity and presence of atherosclerotic coronary artery disease. However, in some cases, tortuosity itself can lead to ischemia because of changes in blood flow through the tortuous segments [42,44].

Anatomic and physiologic assessment

Coronary angiography is the mainstay of assessing lesions in tortuous coronary arteries and analysis of multiple views is required to assess lesions. If significant tortuosity is present in more than one coronary artery, overlap of the vessels results in an illusion of stenosis because of the Mach effect [45]. Every effort should be made to "open up" bifurcation points where this effect can be especially misleading. Lesion assessment should be undertaken before wiring tortuous coronary arteries because pseudo-lesions can appear [46]. Other modalities can be used to supplement data obtained from the coronary angiogram, but vessel tortuosity makes any method prone to producing artifactual data.

Intravascular ultrasound

Use of IVUS can be challenging in imaging tortuous vessels because it can be difficult to deliver in tortuous coronary arteries. The use of smaller 5 Fr imaging systems can make delivery easier. In particularly challenging cases, the IVUS catheter can be delivered using the buddy wire technique. Even after successful delivery of an IVUS catheter, care must be used in interpreting the data. Images obtained from tortuous segments of a coronary artery are difficult to analyze because wire bias can make acquisition of coaxial images difficult. Sudden decrease in CSA without corresponding increase in plaque burden, abrupt change in vessel geometry from a circular shape to an oval shape, or inexplicable changes in the relative areas of the vessel structures are clues that point to potential introduction of artifacts by vessel tortuosity.

Fractional flow reserve

FFR data can be difficult to obtain because of the challenges of negotiating vessel tortuosity with the wire. FFR wires can be difficult to maneuver. One way to overcome this is to use a more maneuverable wire to "straighten" the coronary artery prior to advancing the FFR wire. When using this technique, it is important to remove the non-FFR wire prior to obtaining hemodynamic data. Failure to do so can introduce artifact. Alternatively, the Acist Rxi™ (Eden Prairie, MN, USA) system allows delivery of the FFR device over any wire the interventional cardiologist chooses. Once an FFR device is delivered, care must be taken in analyzing the data as the accordion effect of the FFR device in a tortuous vessel can yield false positive results [47].

Technical aspects
Device delivery

Device delivery can be difficult in tortuous coronary artery disease. Use of the buddy wire system is a commonly used technique to overcome vessel tortuosity. Often, a stiff "support wire" is paired with a softer wire. Examples of support wires include the Mailman™ (Boston Scientific, Marlborough, MA, USA) and the Grand Slam (Abbott, Abbott Park, IL, USA). It is easier to wire with the non-support wire first and then wire with the less maneuverable support

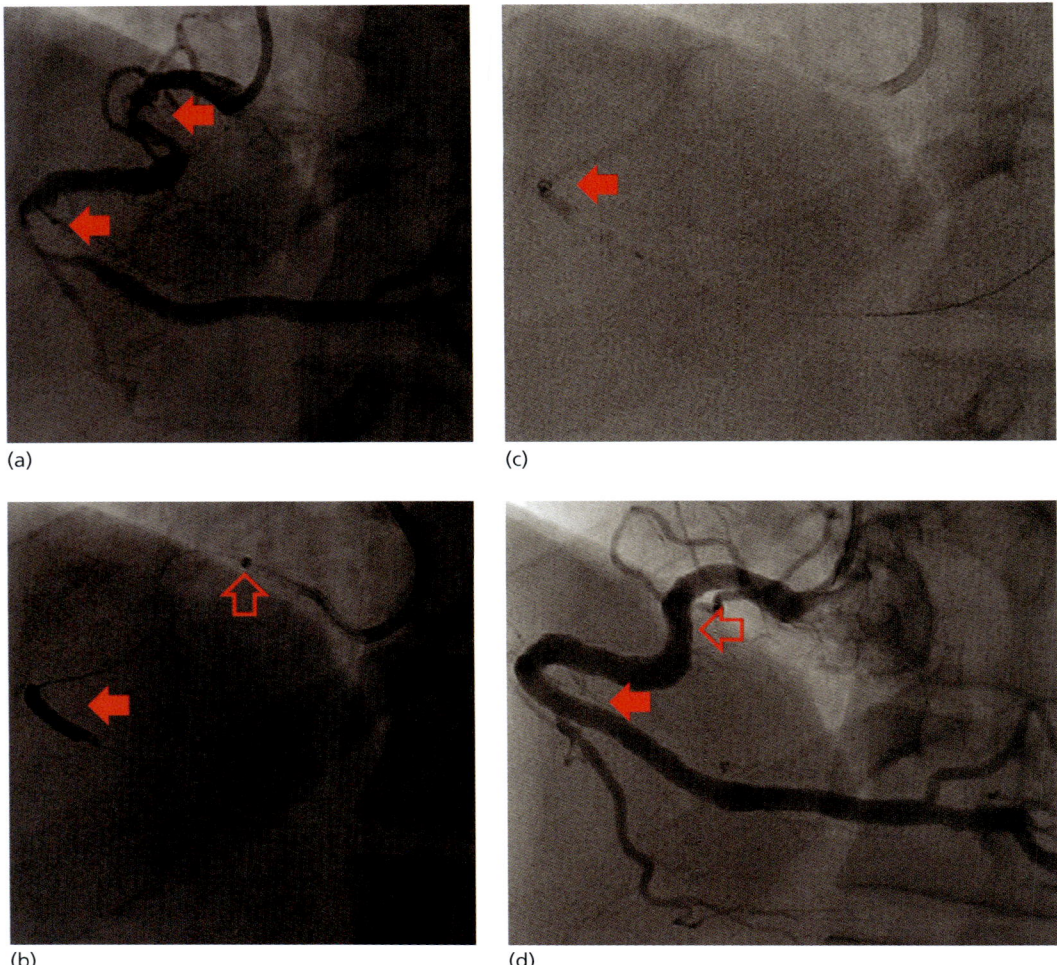

Figure 20.3 (a) A severely tortuous right coronary artery with severe lesions in the proximal and distal portions (red arrows). (b) A 2.5 mm non-compliant balloon inflated in the distal right coronary artery to serve as anchor (red arrow). A Guideliner™(Vascular Solutions, Minneapolis, MN, USA) is introduced into the proximal right coronary artery over the shaft of the inflated balloon (open arrow). (c) A Guideliner™ is advanced over the inflated balloon anchor to the distal right coronary artery (red arrow). (d) A stent was delivered through the Guideliner™ and successfully deployed in the distal lesion (red arrow). A similar approach was used to successfully treat the proximal right coronary artery lesion (open arrow).

wire. Initially, devices should be advanced on the softer non-support wire. Often, the support wire will be so biased against the tortuosity that device delivery over this wire is difficult (Figure 20.2). If delivery over the softer wire is unsuccessful, an attempt to deliver the device over the support wire is sometimes successful.

Use of guide extenders can be crucial in successful completion of a tortuous coronary artery percutaneous intervention. These devices provide added support and allow a coaxial configuration of the guide–guidewire system to enhance delivery. The guide extenders can be "delivered" or deep-seated into the coronary artery over a wire. Deep seating is enhanced by advancing the guide extenders over two wires or over a support wire. In particularly tough cases, a balloon can be advanced into the distal portion of the target coronary artery and the guide liner can be advanced over the uninflated balloon. If the guide extender cannot be advanced over the uninflated balloon, further support can be obtained by inflating the balloon to serve as an anchor. The guide extender can then be advanced over the shaft of the inflated balloon. The anchoring balloon should be sized 0.5 mm smaller than the reference vessel diameter so that barotrauma to the vessel is minimized. This concept is illustrated in Figure 20.3. In some cases the guide extender can be advanced over the inflated balloon shaft past the coronary artery lesion. If this is accomplished, the stent can then be advanced within the guide extender to the desired location and then unsheathed. Using this technique long stents can be delivered in extremely tortuous vessels.

When using deep seating techniques with the guide extenders, one should be aware of pitfalls. Significant decrease in coronary perfusion can occur due to the physical presence of the guide extender and straightening of the vessel. As a result the arterial pressure from the guide system may be damped and frequent non-invasive blood pressure monitoring has to be performed to assess for true systemic pressure. Frequent and repeated checks for ischemia should be performed and if detected the guide extender should be withdrawn immediately. Contrast dye injection through a deep-seated guide extender should be avoided as much as possible. When it is absolutely necessary, cautious injections of small volumes of dye should be utilized. Large volume dye injection through a damped guide system can result in ventricular fibrillation. Additionally, hydrostatic trauma from an aggressive dye injection causes dissection. Significant dissection can also occur when advancing the guide extenders. This complication can be mitigated by advancing the guide extender over the shaft of the balloon.

Rotational atherectomy

Percutaneous intervention of tortuous coronary arteries with concomitant calcification can be particularly challenging. The key challenge is to deliver stents past a calcified tortuous bend. The use of rotational atherectomy can make delivery of devices much easier, but care must be taken because the risks of causing serious flow-limiting dissection and life-threatening coronary perforation are much higher when used in this subset of coronary artery disease. Often, the floppy RotaWire™ (Boston Scientific, Marlborough, MA, USA) is used, because this causes less bias than the extra support variety. In particularly challenging vessels, a transit catheter such as the Finecross™ (Terumo Cardiovascular Systems, Ann Arbor, MI, USA) is used to facilitate wiring of the lesion with a guidewire. Wires without a spring coil configuration at the tip such as the Fielder™ (Abott Laboratories, Abbott Park, IL, USA) or the Kinetix™ (Boston Scientific, Natik, MA, USA) can negotiate a tortuous coronary artery effectively and efficiently. Once the lesion is wired, the transit catheter is advanced past the lesion, the initial guidewire withdrawn, and the RotaWire™ advanced past the lesion through the transit catheter. The transit catheter is then withdrawn over the RotaWire™. A 1.25 mm burr is recommended to treat tortuous vessels, particularly if the lesion encompasses a bend. As a result of the bias caused by the wire, the 1.25 mm burr will make contact with the vessel wall and adequate vessel modification can be accomplished. Use of a larger burr greatly increases the probability of complications.

In tortuous vessels, the treatment of complications can be challenging. For example, it can be impossible to deliver a covered stent in cases of perforation. In cases of flow-limiting dissections, an unplanned quick delivery of a stent into a suboptimally prepared lesion is challenging. If the dissection is in the proximal portion of a major vessel, prolonged slow flow or no flow can result in catastrophic hemodynamic or arrhythmogenic consequences. Therefore, deliberate, carefully conducted, rotational atherectomy with a small burr is essential. In this very challenging subset of vessels, "less" may truly be "more."

Clinical outcomes

Percutaneous coronary intervention of tortuous coronary artery disease can be difficult and fraught with potential complications. Significantly tortuous coronary arteries, designated AHA vessel classification types B and C, are associated with low success rates for successful intervention. Tortuous coronary arteries that are calcified are particularly difficult to address with percutaneous intervention. Potentially life-threatening complications can occur and prove difficult to treat.

Key points and summary

- Coronary tortuosity is not an infrequent finding. Tortuous coronary arteries with associated calcification represent one of the most challenging subset of vessels to perform percutaneous interventions.
- Assessment of coronary artery disease is performed primarily with angiography. Use of adjunctive imaging modalities such as

IVUS can be problematic because vessel tortuosity may not yield coaxial views. FFR should be used with caution because significant accordion effects yield false positive results.

- Adequately preparing the vessel prior to attempting stent delivery is crucial. Rotational atherectomy is very useful to prepare calcified vessels, but should be used cautiously because significant complications can occur and often these complications cannot be addressed quickly because of the difficulty in delivering corrective devices. Use of small burr size (1.25 mm) is mandatory and atherectomy runs should be deliberately slow and cautious.
- Device delivery can be enhanced by using buddy wire techniques and by using guide extenders. Guide extenders can be associated with significant complications such as vessel dissection. Guide extenders should never be traversed over a vessel segment that for whatever reason cannot or should not be stented.

Interactive multiple choice questions are available for this chapter on www.wiley.com/go/dangas/cardiology

References

1 Biondi-Zoccai G, Moretti C, Abbate A, Sheiban I. Percutaneous coronary intervention for small vessel coronary artery disease. *Cardiovasc Revasc Med* 2010; **11**(3): 189–198.

2 Ardissino D, Cavallini C, Bramucci E, et al. Sirolimus-eluting vs uncoated stents for prevention of restenosis in small coronary arteries: a randomized trial. *JAMA* 2004; **292**(22): 2727–2734.

3 Kastrati A, Schömig A, Dirschinger J, et al. A randomized trial comparing stenting with balloon angioplasty in small vessels in patients with symptomatic coronary artery disease. ISAR-SMART Study Investigators. Intracoronary Stenting or Angioplasty for Restenosis Reduction in Small Arteries. *Circulation* 2000; **102**(21): 2593–2598.

4 Chamie D, Costa JR Jr, Abizaid A, et al. Serial angiography and intravascular ultrasound: results of the SISC Registry (Stents In Small Coronaries). *JACC Cardiovasc Interv* 2010; **3**(2): 191–202.

5 Schunkert HL, Harrell L, Palacios IF. Implications of small reference vessel diameter in patients undergoing percutaneous coronary revascularization. *J Am Coll Cardiol* 1999; **34**(1): 40–48.

6 Uren NG, Melin JA, De Bruyne B, et al. Relation between myocardial blood flow and the severity of coronary-artery stenosis. *N Engl J Med* 1994; **330**(25): 1782–1788.

7 Gould KL, Lipscomb K, Hamilton GW. Physiologic basis for assessing critical coronary stenosis. Instantaneous flow response and regional distribution during coronary hyperemia as measures of coronary flow reserve. *Am J Cardiol* 1974; **33**(1): 87–94.

8 Nishioka T, Amanullah AM, Luo H, et al. Clinical validation of intravascular ultrasound imaging for assessment of coronary stenosis severity: comparison with stress myocardial perfusion imaging. *J Am Coll Cardiol* 1999; **33**(7): 1870–1878.

9 Waksman R, Legutko J, Singh J, et al. FIRST: Fractional Flow Reserve and Intravascular Ultrasound Relationship Study. *J Am Coll Cardiol* 2013; **61**(9): 917–923.

10 Puymirat E, Peace A, Mangiacapra F, et al. Long-term clinical outcome after fractional flow reserve-guided percutaneous coronary revascularization in patients with small-vessel disease. *Circ Cardiovasc Interv* 2012; **5**(1): 62–68.

11 Tonino PA, De Bruyne B, Pijls NH, et al. Fractional flow reserve versus angiography for guiding percutaneous coronary intervention. *N Engl J Med* 2009; **360**(3): 213–224.

12 Costa MA, Sabate M, Staico R, et al. Anatomical and physiologic assessments in patients with small coronary artery disease: final results of the Physiologic and Anatomical Evaluation Prior to and After Stent Implantation in Small Coronary Vessels (PHANTOM) trial. *Am Heart J* 2007; **153**(2): 296 e1–7.

13 Burzotta F, Trani C, Mazzari MA, et al. Use of a second buddy wire during percutaneous coronary interventions: a simple solution for some challenging situations. *J Invasive Cardiol* 2005; **17**(3): 171–174.

14 Jafary FH. When one won't do it, use two-double "buddy" wiring to facilitate stent advancement across a highly calcified artery. *Catheter Cardiovasc Interv* 2006; **67**(5): 721–723.

15 Niemela M, Kervinen K, Erglis A, *et al.* Randomized comparison of final kissing balloon dilatation versus no final kissing balloon dilatation in patients with coronary bifurcation lesions treated with main vessel stenting: the Nordic-Baltic Bifurcation Study III. *Circulation* 2011; **123**(1): 79–86.

16 Brueck M, Scheinert D, Flachskampf FA, Daniel WG, Ludwig J. Sequential vs. kissing balloon angioplasty for stenting of bifurcation coronary lesions. *Catheter Cardiovasc Interv* 2002; **55**(4): 461–466.

17 Foin N, Torii R, Mortier P, *et al.* Kissing balloon or sequential dilation of the side branch and main vessel for provisional stenting of bifurcations: lessons from micro-computed tomography and computational simulations. *JACC Cardiovasc Interv* 2012; **5**(1): 47–56.

18 Cardiac Interventions Today. 2013 *Buyer's Guide.* November/December **6**(6).

19 Togni M, Eber S, Widmer J, *et al.* Impact of vessel size on outcome after implantation of sirolimus-eluting and paclitaxel-eluting stents: a subgroup analysis of the SIRTAX trial. *J Am Coll Cardiol* 2007; **50**(12): 1123–1131.

20 Kaiser C, Galatius S, Erne P, *et al.* Drug-eluting versus bare-metal stents in large coronary arteries. *N Engl J Med* 2010; **363**(24): 2310–2319.

21 Schampaert E, Cohen EA, Schlüter M, *et al.* The Canadian study of the sirolimus-eluting stent in the treatment of patients with long de novo lesions in small native coronary arteries (C-SIRIUS). *J Am Coll Cardiol* 2004; **43**(6): 1110–1115.

22 Schofer J, Schlüter M, Gershlick AH, *et al.* Sirolimus-eluting stents for treatment of patients with long atherosclerotic lesions in small coronary arteries: double-blind, randomised controlled trial (E-SIRIUS). *Lancet* 2003; **362**(9390): 1093–1099.

23 Bartorelli AL, Serruys PW, Miquel-Hébert K, Yu S, Pierson W, Stone GW; SPIRIT II SPIRIT III Investigators. An everolimus-eluting stent versus a paclitaxel-eluting stent in small vessel coronary artery disease: a pooled analysis from the SPIRIT II and SPIRIT III trials. *Catheter Cardiovasc Interv* 2010; **76**(1): 60–66.

24 Smith SC Jr, Dove JT, Jacobs AK, *et al.* ACC/AHA guidelines for percutaneous coronary intervention (revision of the 1993 PTCA guidelines)-executive summary: a report of the American College of Cardiology/American Heart Association task force on practice guidelines (Committee to revise the 1993 guidelines for percutaneous transluminal coronary angioplasty) endorsed by the Society for Cardiac Angiography and Interventions. *Circulation* 2001; **103**(24): 3019–3041.

25 Jolicoeur EM, Cartier R, Henry TD, *et al.* Patients with coronary artery disease unsuitable for revascularization: definition, general principles, and a classification. *Can J Cardiol* 2012; **28**(2 Suppl): S50–59.

26 Schmauss D, Weis M. Cardiac allograft vasculopathy: recent developments. *Circulation* 2008; **117**(16): 2131–2141.

27 Weisz G. NIRS Imaging of Cardiac allograft vasculopathy. *J Invas Cardiol* 2013; **25**(Suppl A): 35–36.

28 Waller BF, Fry ET, Hermiller JB, Peters T, Slack JD. Nonatherosclerotic causes of coronary artery narrowing: Part III. *Clin Cardiol* 1996; **19**(8): 656–661.

29 Colombo A, De Gregorio J, Moussa I, *et al.* Intravascular ultrasound-guided percutaneous transluminal coronary angioplasty with provisional spot stenting for treatment of long coronary lesions. *J Am Coll Cardiol* 2001; **38**(5): 1427–1433.

30 Prati F, Regar E, Mintz GS, *et al.* Expert review document on methodology, terminology, and clinical applications of optical coherence tomography: physical principles, methodology of image acquisition, and clinical application for assessment of coronary arteries and atherosclerosis. *Eur Heart J* 2010; **31**(4): 401–415.

31 Pijls NH, De Bruyne B, Bech GJ, *et al.* Coronary pressure measurement to assess the hemodynamic significance of serial stenoses within one coronary artery: validation in humans. *Circulation* 2000; **102**(19): 2371–2377.

32 Serruys PW, Foley DP, Suttorp MJ, *et al.* A randomized comparison of the value of additional stenting after optimal balloon angioplasty for long coronary lesions: final results of the additional value of NIR stents for treatment of long coronary lesions (ADVANCE) study. *J Am Coll Cardiol* 2002; **39**(3): 393–399.

33 Tenaglia AN, Zidar JP, Jackman JD Jr, *et al.* Treatment of long coronary artery narrowings with long angioplasty balloon catheters. *Am J Cardiol* 1993; **71**(15): 1274–1277.

34 Ahn JM, Park DW, Kim YH, *et al.* Comparison of resolute zotarolimus-eluting stents and sirolimus-eluting stents in patients with de novo long coronary artery lesions: a randomized LONG-DES IV trial. *Circ Cardiovasc Interv* 2012; **5**(5): 633–640.

35 Hermiller JJ. Clinical outcomes after PCI treatment of very long coronary lesions with the XIENCE V everolimus eluting stent (EES): pooled analysis from the SPIRIT and XIENCE V USA Prospective Multi-Center Trials. *J Am Coll Cardiol* 2013; **62**(18 Suppl B): B56.

36 Teirstein P, Stone GW, Meredith IT, *et al.* Three-year results of the PLATINUM small vessel and long lesion trials evaluating the platinum chromium everolimus-eluting stent in de novo coronary artery lesions. *J Am Coll Cardiol* 2013; **62**(18 Suppl B): B57.

37 Raber L, Jüni P, Löffel L, *et al.* Impact of stent overlap on angiographic and long-term clinical outcome in patients undergoing drug-eluting stent implantation. *J Am Coll Cardiol* 2010; **55**(12): 1178–1188.

38 Farooq V, Vranckx P, Mauri L, *et al.* Impact of overlapping newer generation drug-eluting stents on clinical and angiographic outcomes: pooled analysis of five trials from the international Global RESOLUTE Program. *Heart* 2013; **99**(9): 626–633.

39 Kitabata H, Loh JP, Pendyala LK, *et al.* Safety and efficacy outcomes of overlapping second-generation everolimus-eluting stents versus first-generation drug-eluting stents. *Am J Cardiol* 2013; **112**(8): 1093–1098.

40 Mutha V, Asrar Ul, Haq M, *et al.* Usefulness of enhanced stent visualization imaging technique in simple and complex PCI cases. *J Invasive Cardiol* 2014; **26**(10): 552–557.

41 Kobayashi Y, De Gregorio J, Kobayashi N, *et al.* Stented segment length as an independent predictor of restenosis. *J Am Coll Cardiol* 1999; **34**(3): 651–659.

42 Groves SS, Jain AC, Warden BE, Gharib W, Beto RJ 2nd. Severe coronary tortuosity and the relationship to significant coronary artery disease. *W V Med J* 2009; **105**(4): 14–17.

43 Li Y, Shen C, Ji Y, Feng Y, Ma G, Liu N. Clinical implication of coronary tortuosity in patients with coronary artery disease. *PLoS One* 2011; **6**(8): e24232.

44 Li Y, Liu NF, Gu ZZ, *et al.* Coronary tortuosity is associated with reversible myocardial perfusion defects in patients without coronary artery disease. *Chin Med J (Engl)* 2012; **125**(19): 3581–3583.

45 Randall PA. Mach bands in cine coronary arteriography. *Radiology* 1978; **129**(1): 65–66.

46 Koh TW, Kelly P, Timmis AD. Images in cardiology: artefactual coronary artery lesions caused by effect of guidewire on tortuous coronary arteries: angiographic appearances during right coronary angioplasty. *Heart* 2001; **86**(6): 655.

47 Muller O, Hamilos M, Ntalianis A, Sarno G, De Bruyne B. Images in cardiovascular medicine. The accordion phenomenon: lesson from a movie. *Circulation* 2008; **118**(18): e677–678.

CHAPTER 21

In-Stent Restenosis in New Generation DES Era

Marco G. Mennuni and Patrizia Presbitero

Department of Cardiology, Humanitas Research Hospital, Rozzano, Milan, Italy

In-stent restenosis (ISR) represents the key limitation of bare metal stent (BMS) implantation as a result of excessive neointimal hyperplasia within the implanted stent. Drug-eluting stents (DES) were developed to address this limitation [1]. At the beginning of the DES era, the rate of restenosis reported was around zero [2]. Since then, interventionists have progressively employed DES in the treatment of patients with increasingly complex disease. As a consequence, DES restenosis rates have risen [3]. During the last decade, early generation DES were replaced by new generation devices releasing limus analogues, through more biocompatible polymer coatings, applied on thinner stent platforms. The favorable biocompatibility of new generation DES translated into an improved safety and efficacy profile, rendering these devices the standard of care for percutaneous coronary intervention (PCI) in current clinical practice. Nevertheless, ISR with the subsequent need for repeat revascularization is still observed in up to 10% of patients treated with new generation DES during long-term follow-up [4].

Definition

Angiographic restenosis, or "binary restenosis" after PCI, is defined as ≥50% luminal narrowing at follow-up angiography. The most widely accepted definition of clinical restenosis, assessed as a requirement for ischemia-driven repeat revascularization, was proposed by the Academic Research Consortium, and it requires both an assessment of luminal narrowing and the patient's clinical context [5].

Incidence

ISR was observed in around 20–30% of patients treated in BMS pivotal trials. The antiproliferative effectiveness of early generation DES reduced this incidence by approximately 70% [3]. A further significant improvement was obtained with new generation DES. It is noteworthy that antiproliferative effectiveness of DES was shown to be consistent across a wide spectrum of patient populations, including those traditionally considered at higher risk of ISR such as patients with acute myocardial infarction and with diabetes mellitus (Table 21.1). Clinical registries, which include patients with more complex coronary lesions, are probably more accurate in revealing the true incidence of ISR in the real world, but could underestimate the restenosis rate because of underreporting of clinical events and low rates of angiographic follow-up. Restenosis rates from registries are 30%, 15%, and 12% at 6–8 months with BMS, first generation, and new generation DES, respectively [4].

The last technical evolution of DES is the bioresorbable vascular scaffold (BVS) system. This platform has a bioabsorbable polylactic acid scaffold with a bioabsorbable polylactic acid coating that elutes everolimus. At the beginning of BVS use, they had similar problems to BMS, which were mainly a result of the inadequacy of preimplant lesion preparation and stent deployment issues, such as lack of good expansion, geographic missing, and overlapping of thick struts, leading to a high incidence of restenosis. Nowadays, following the improvement in BVS technology and deployment technique, the rate of restenosis is around 3–5%; however, data are limited [6].

Clinical presentation

Although some cases of ISR are silent, the majority lead to ischemic symptoms. Reports on the presentation of both BMS and DES restenosis have shown that unstable angina is a frequent manifestation (20–60%). Moreover, depending on the definitions applied, both BMS and DES restenosis presented as myocardial infarction in 1–20% of patients [3]. During the last decade, among patients treated with DES, clinical presentation seems to be similar irrespective of DES generation [7].

Pathophysiologic mechanisms

Possible mechanisms of ISR after DES implantation have been thoroughly studied in the last decade. According to the available evidence, specific mechanisms have a different role according to timing of ISR presentation. The majority of data is derived from studies on ISR occurring within the first 12 months after DES implantation (early ISR) when excessive neointimal formation appears to be the dominant mechanism [8,9]. Conversely, late ISR—occurring beyond the first 12 months after DES implantation—appears to be triggered by different biologic mechanisms.

Interventional Cardiology: Principles and Practice, Second Edition. Edited by George D. Dangas, Carlo Di Mario, and Nicholas N. Kipshidze.
© 2017 John Wiley & Sons, Ltd. Published 2017 by John Wiley & Sons, Ltd.

Table 21.1 Incidence of restenosis after first and new generation DES implantation in the randomized trial, grouped by selected population, all-comers, diabetic, and acute myocardial infarction patients.

Selected population [reference]	DES type	Patients (n)	Angiography rate at follow-up (%)	Follow-up period (months)	In-stent restenosis (%)	In-segment restenosis (%)	TLR (%)	Long-term follow-up (months)	Long-term TLR (%)
TAXUS II SR [80]	PES	131	98	6	2.3	5.5	–	60	10.3
TAXUS VI [81]	PES	219	96	9	9.1	12.4	–	60	14.6
TAXUS IV [51]	PES	662	44	6	5.5	7.9	–	60	9.1
REALITY [82]	PES	669	91	8	8.3	11.1	–		
ISAR-SMART 3 [83]	PES	100	92	6–8	18.5	21.7	–		
ISAR-DESIRE 2 [84]	PES	225	85	6–8	–	20.6	–		
ISAR-DESIRE [85]	PES	125	82	6–8	13.6	16.5	–		
ENDEAVOR IV [86]	PES	772	17.5	8	6.7	10.4	–	60	8.6
SPIRIT II [87]	PES	77	92	6	3.5	5.8	–	4	12.7
SPIRIT III [88]	PES	332	50	8	5.7	8.9	–	36	8.9
SPIRIT IV [89]	PES	1229	Not routinely performed	12	–	–	4.6	24	9.9
NOBORI [90]	PES	90	78	9	6.2	6.2	–		
RAVEL [91]	SES	120	89	6	0	0	–	60	10.3
SIRIUS [92]	SES	533	66	8	3.2	8.9	–	60	9.4
C-SIRIUS [39]	SES	50	88	8	0	2.3	–		
E-SIRIUS [40]	SES	175	92	8	3.9	5.9	–		
SES SMART71 [93]	SES	129	95	8	4.9	9.8	–	24	7.9
REALITY [82]	SES	648	93	8	7.0	9.6	–		

ISAR-SMART 3 [83]	SES	100	91	6–8	11.0	14.3	–		
ISAR-DESIRE 2 [84]	SES	225	84.9	6–8	–	19.0	–		
ISAR-DESIRE [85]	SES	125	82	6–8	4.9	6.9	–		
ENDEAVOR III [94]	SES	113	83.2	8	2.1	4.3	–	60	6.5
EXCELLENT [95]	SES	364	65	9	1.4	2.8	–		
ENDEAVOR II [96]	ZES	598	88.5	8	9.4	13.2	–	60	7.5
ENDEAVOR III [94]	ZES	323	87.3	8	9.2	11.7	–	60	8.1
ENDEAVOR IV [86]	ZES	770	18.7	8	13.3	15.3	–	60	7.7
SPIRIT II [87]	EES	223	92	6	1.3	3.4	–	48	5.9
SPIRIT III [88]	EES	669	51	8	2.3	4.7	–	36	5.4
SPIRIT IV [89]	EES	2458	Not routinely performed	12	–	–	2.5	24	6.9
EXCELLENT [95]	EES	1079	67	9	2.0	3.4	–		
EVOLVE [97]	EES	98	97	6	3.2	5.3	–	24	10.2
EVOLVE II [98]	EES	838	Not routinely performed	12	–	–	1.7		
NOBORI 180	Bp-BES	153	93	9	0.7	0.7	–		
EVOLVE [97]	Bp-EES	94	96	6	0.0	2.3	–	24	3.3
EVOLVE [97]	Bp-EES	89	89	6	0.0	1.1	–	24	4.2
EVOLVE II [98]	Bp-EES	846	Not routinely performed	12	–	–	2.6		
ABSORB [85]	BVS	30	86	6	7.7	7.7	–		

(Continued)

Table 21.1 (Continued)

	DES type	Patients (n)	Angiography rate at follow-up (%)	Follow-up period (months)	In-stent restenosis (%)	In-segment restenosis (%)	TLR (%)	Long-term follow-up (months)	Long-term TLR (%)
All-comers									
COMPARE [99]	PES	903	70	12	–	–	5.3	24	6.4
SIRTAX [100]	PES	569	54	8	7.5	11.7	–	60	17.9
LEADERS [101]	PES	850	Not routinely performed	12	–	–	5.7	48	13
SIRTAX [100]	SES	503	53	8	3.2	6.6	–	60	14.9
NEXT [102]	EES	1618	14	9	–	–	7.5		
EVERBIO II [103]	EES	80	90	9	3.8	8.7	–		
COMPARE77	EES	897	70	12	–	–	2.0	24	2.9
COMPARE II [104]	EES	912	Not routinely performed	12	–	–	3.7		
EVERBIO II [103]	BES	80	94	9	4.7	9.4	–		
LEADERS [101]	Bp-BES	857	Not routinely performed	12	–	–	5.1	48	11
COMPARE II [104]	Bp-BES	1795	Not routinely performed	12	–	–	4.2		
NEXT [102]	Bp-BES	1617	14	9	–	–	7.1		
EVERBIO II [103]	BVS	78	88	9	5.3	10.6	–		
Diabetic									
DES-DIABETES [105]	PES	200	77	6	18.2	20.8	–	48	12.0
TAXUS IV diabetes [106]	PES	78	72	9	5.1	6.4	–		
ISAR-DIABETIC [107]	PES	180	88	6–8	14.9	19.0	–		

	Stent type	N	%						
ENDEAVOR IV diabetes [108]	PES	236	18	8	23.8	16.7	–		–
SPIRIT IV diabetes [109]	PES	399	Not routinely performed	12	–	–	4.7		–
ISAR-DIABETIC [107]	SES	180	86	6–8	8.0	11.4	–		–
DECODE [110]	SES	54	96	6	9.0	12.8	–		–
DES-DIABETES [105]	SES	200	88	6	3.4	4.0	–	48	7.5
DIABETES [111]	SES	80	93	9	3.9	7.8	–	24	7.7
ENDEAVOR IV diabetes [108]	ZES	241	18	8	25.0	27.3	–		–
SPIRIT IV diabetes [109]	EES	786	Not routinely performed	12	–	–	4.2		–
STEMI									
HORIZONS-AMI [112]	PES	2257	40	13	8.2	9.6	–	36	10.2
TYPHOON [113]	SES	335	82	8	3.5	7.1	–	48	7.6
DEDICATION [114]	SES/ PES/ ZES	313	Not routinely performed	8	–	–	13.1	36	16.3
EXAMINATION [115]	EES	751	Not routinely performed	12	–	–	2.1	24	2.9
COMFORTABLE [116]	Bp-BES	575	Not routinely performed	12	–	–	1.6	12	1.6

Bp, bioabsorbable polymer-coated; BES, biolimus-eluting stent; BVS, bioresorbable vascular scaffold; EES, everolimus-eluting stent; PES, paclitaxel-eluting stent; SES, sirolimus-eluting stent; TLR, target lesion revascularization; ZES, zotarolimus-eluting stent.

Early restenosis
Biologic factors
Drug resistance Excessive neointimal hyperplasia is characterized by proliferation and migration of vascular smooth muscle cells and extracellular matrix formation as a response to local injury after stent deployment. Antiproliferative agents released by DES aim to suppress this process by inhibiting the cell cycle. Two classes of agents have been applied to DES for this purpose: paclitaxel and rapamycin analogues (i.e., "limus").

Paclitaxel binds to the β-tubulin subunit of microtubules and interferes with microtubule dynamics during mitosis [10]. Resistance to paclitaxel has been described and appears to be associated with increased expression of the *mdr-1* gene and its product P-glyxoprotein, β-tubulin mutation, changes in apoptotic regulatory and mitosis checkpoint proteins, and potentially the overexpression of interleukin-6 [11,12]. Currently, the relevance of paclitaxel resistance in the context of ISR remains unknown.

Limus agents inhibit the function of the mammalian target of rapamycin (mTOR), blocking protein synthesis, cell cycle progression, and cell migration [13]. Genetic mutations and defects of mTOR or mTOR-related proteins (FKB12P, p27-Kip1, etc.) can influence the sensitivity to limus agents, and confer drug resistance [14]. Moreover, it has been suggested that the presence of diabetes with hyperinsulinemia can determine mTOR-inhibition resistance of vascular smooth muscle cells proliferation [15–17]. This evidence could explain the strong association between insulin resistance and ISR [18,19]. Nevertheless, this hypothesis has not been confirmed by prospective clinical investigations.

Hypersensitivity In the BMS era, allergic reactions to nickel and molybdenum released from stainless steel stents were potential triggering mechanisms for ISR. The platform material used in many novel DES are alloys (e.g., cobalt chromium), which have a lower nickel content than stainless steel, and do not appear to trigger the adverse proliferative response and hypersensitivity [3].

Mechanical factors
The efficacy of DES is based on delivering therapeutic concentrations of drug to the underlying tissue. Hemodynamic environments surrounding the stent modulate the drug distribution pattern to the arterial wall. *In vitro* and *in vivo* studies have shown that drug release appears to be sensitive to flow alteration secondary to wall displacement and stent malapposition [20,21]. Therefore, a number of mechanical factors could determine the occurrence of ISR.

Incomplete stent apposition Incomplete stent apposition, defined as the lack of contact between at least one stent strut and the underlying intimal surface of the vessel, increases the risk of ISR. Typical causes of incomplete stent apposition:
1 Inadequate stent implantation because of stent–vessel size mismatch; stent under-expansion despite adequate stent–vessel ratio because of low implantation pressure or complex plaque;
2 Acute or chronic stent recoil;
3 Resolution over time of thrombus located between the stent struts and the vessel wall; and
4 Positive vessel remodeling.
A further classification has been created according to the timing of incomplete stent apposition diagnosis: acute (i.e., diagnosed post-stent deployment) or acquired (i.e., not present post-procedure, but identified at follow-up assessment). Early detection of incomplete stent apposition remains crucial, because acute incomplete stent apposition affects the overall vascular response, leading to delayed stent strut coverage [22].

Stent fractures Stent fractures have been associated with ISR, because of its potential decrease in local drug delivery at the fracture point and/or mechanical injury. Stent fracture after both first generation DES have been reported, with an incidence rate of 2–3% [23,24], with a restenosis rate ranging from 15% to 65% [25–28]. Predictors of stent fracture:
1 Use of long stent
2 Use of large high-pressure balloon post-dilatation
3 Use of sirolimus-eluting stent (SES)
4 Stenting on a bend >75°, and
5 Stenting in a right coronary artery or in a saphenous vein graft [29–32].
The observed rate of stent fracture and the association with major adverse pathologic events were comparable across first and new generation devices, indicating that careful long-term follow-up remains important even after everolimus-eluting stent (EES) implantation [33].

Technical factors
Stent gap and incomplete plaque coverage represents a theoretical mechanism of stent restenosis. Stent gap has been demonstrated to be associated with ISR [34]. Theoretically, the amount of local drug deposition to the vessel wall decreases at the gap site. Considering that the safety and efficacy of overlapping DES have been reported, stent gaps should be avoided [35]. When treating ostial, bifurcation, and/or long lesions, it is sometimes difficult to avoid incomplete lesion coverage [36]. The presence of geographic miss during the procedure (injured or diseased segment not covered by stent or balloon-artery size ratio <0.9 or >1.3) is associated with increased risk of total vascular reocclusion (TVR) and myocardial infarction at 1 year [37]. Today, the availability of new generation DES with better mechanical performance characteristics and greater stent length allow them to cover very long lesions, avoiding multiple stents [38]. The recommended technique includes predilatation with shorter balloons, using a longer single stent to cover the entire area of balloon injury, and post-dilatation within the stented regions using short high-pressure balloons. Following these recommendations, the proximal margin restenosis rates have decreased [39,40]. However, recent data studying angiographic patterns of restenosis demonstrate the persistence of a high rate of edge restenosis among those with a focal presentation [7].

Late restenosis
In addition to early restenosis factors, a late restenosis might be secondary to hypersentivity reactions or new atherosclerotic processes. Early generation DES are associated with delayed arterial healing and hypersensitivity reactions resulting in chronic inflammation. A hypersensitivity reaction to polymer, drug, or scaffold leads to restenosis [41]. Second-generation DES have been developed to overcome these issues. In a pathologic study, use of new generation cobalt chromium EES (CoCr-EES) resulted in greater strut coverage with less inflammation than SES or

paclitaxel-eluting stent (PES) [33]. Nevertheless, a hypersensitivity reaction has been reported in second generation DES in both CoCr-EES stent and zotarolimus-eluting stent (ZES) [42].

The presence of chronic hypersensitivity phenomena can also trigger a neoatherosclerotic process. Late and impaired healing of the endothelium, after DES, facilitates lipid deposition within neointima [43]. In this setting, neointima is more prone to develop neoatherosclerosis and unstable plaque either behind the stent or within the intraluminal neointima [44–46]. In light of the fact that late DES failure is more likely to progress to acute myocardial infarction, and worse outcomes [47], early detection of subcritical in-stent neoatherosclerotic plaques can be used as a marker of high risk lesions and patients.

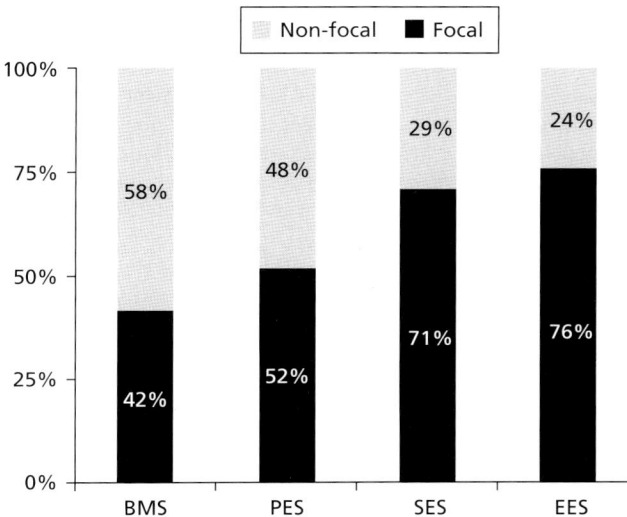

Figure 21.1 Morphologic pattern of restenosis across different stent generation. BMS, bare metal stent; EES, everolimus-eluting stent; PES, paclitaxel-eluting stent; SES, sirolimus-eluting stent. Source: Adapted from Mehran *et al.* [48], Cosgrave *et al.* [57], and Lee *et al.* [8].

Morphologic pattern of DES restenosis

The classification of angiographic patterns of ISR has been shown to be of crucial prognostic significance [48–50]. The incidence and pattern of restenosis were different between BMS and DES, and among different type of DES. In particular, BMS resulted in a diffuse pattern in 60% of restenosis cases. The rate of diffuse restenosis decreased to 40–50% with use of first generation PES [51], and further lowered with SES (about 20%) in both randomized trial and registry (Figure 21.1) [52,53]. A comparison study between PES and SES confirmed higher incidence of diffuse and occlusive restenosis with PES when compared with SES use [54]. Restenosis presenting as total occlusion is rare, but remains associated with worse outcome at follow-up [55]. Recently, a restrospective study on new generation DES (everolimus and zotarolimus) reported diffuse restenosis rate similar to SES, around 15–20% of ISR cases [56].

Prognostic implications for morphologic patterns of ISR

Mehran *et al.* [48] reported that target lesion revascularization (TLR) at 1 year after repeat intervention for ISR increased progressively with ISR classification (focal 19%, intra-stent 35%, proliferative 50%, total occlusion 83%; p < 0.001). Similar to BMS, first generation DES ISR studies demonstrated that diffuse patterns were associated with worse clinical outcomes [3,49,57]. The diffuse pattern even in new generation DES is theoretically associated with adverse events, but no evidence has yet been reported.

Predictors of DES restenosis

Unfavorable demographic, clinical, and angiographic characteristics confer an increased risk for ISR after DES implantation. These data are mainly based on first generation DES experience and are summarized in Table 21.2. The predictive factors for first generation DES restenosis identified from real-world data seem to be similar to those for BMS, such as small vessels, longer stents, and stent underexpansion [58–61]. Currently, with use of newer generation DES, lesion length might not be associated with higher risk of restenosis, because of better healing properties, thinner profile, and availability of longer sizes that lead to a theoretical reduction of stent overlapping. On the other hand, thinner struts might result in a higher rate of stent fractures, which is strongly

Table 21.2 Predictors of restenosis.

Demographics characteristics	Clinical characteristics	Lesion characteristics	Procedural characteristics
Age Female gender	Diabetes mellitus Multivessel CAD	Multivessel coronary disease ISR Bypass graft LAD Ostial lesion Chronic total occlusion Small vessel Length Severe calcification	Multiple lesion treatment Type of DES Final MLD

CAD, coronary artery disease; DES, drug-eluting stent; ISR, in-stent restenosis; LAD, left anterior descending; MLD, minimum lumen diameter.

associated with restenosis [61]. Recent studies confirmed older age, multivessel treatment, small vessel size, increased stented length, complex lesion morphology, diabetes mellitus, and prior bypass surgery as predictors of restenosis after new generation DES implantation [4,62,63]. Considering that post-minimal lumen diameter is a major factor in restenosis, optimal acute angiographic result remains crucial even after new generation DES implantation.

Role of intravascular imaging

Intravascular ultrasound (IVUS) and optical coherence tomography (OCT) permit detailed cross-sectional imaging of the deployed stents. Factors associated with DES restenosis can be detected through IVUS and or OCT information. IVUS and OCT complement each other for the study and diagnosis of incomplete stent apposition. IVUS has higher tissue penetration power (4–8 mm) compared with OCT (1–3 mm), but it has lower axial resolution (150 vs. 15 μm). With these characteristics IVUS enables the visualization of the external elastic membrane, to quantify the vessel size and to assess positive vascular remodeling [64], while OCT allows a sharper picture of the stent–lumen interface [65]. IVUS is important in evaluation of the mechanical factors that contribute to stent restenosis:

1 Stent underexpansion
2 Edge problems and stent gaps in multiple stenting
3 Stent fracture
4 New atherosclerosis vs. neointimal hyperplasia.

Furthermore, intravascular imaging is very important in the optimization of restenosis to guide the choice between new balloon and stent size.

Approach to DES restenosis

Despite the many studies analyzing the best treatments for stent restenosis that have been published, the optimal strategy for DES restenosis remains poorly defined. Evidence from meta-analyses seems to suggest a similar efficacy of drug-eluting balloons (DEB) and DES [66].

Drug-eluting balloon

The local application of antiproliferative drugs with a balloon for treatment of ISR emerged from the limitations of current techniques: the high occurrence of restenosis with conventional balloon angioplasty or with the debulking technique, and the shortfalls of implanting an additional metal layer, particularly in small vessels and in bifurcations. The available DEB deliver paclitaxel, eluted at 3 μg/mm². DEB are coated with a matrix composed of paclitaxel and a hydrophilic spacer (matrix carrier). This coating method allows the best solubility of paclitaxel and its transfer to the vessel wall [67]. The hydrophilic character of the matrix carrier and the lipophilic properties of paclitaxel support the release of the drug from the balloon to the vascular wall, and the drug elution lasts 1 week. However, matrix represents a key limitation of this technology; it makes DEBs rigid and thick compared to the conventional balloon, so it is more difficult to navigate them through tortuous and narrow vessels. Nevertheless, DEB has some theoretical advantages over DES:

1 Avoiding stent-polymer inflammation trigger
2 Delivery of antiproliferative drug exactly where the barotrauma has been induced by balloon, and
3 Avoiding multiple layers of stents.

Several studies on DEB either vs. conventional balloon angioplasty (BA), DES, or both showed a better performance of DEB compared with BA, and an equivalent or only mildly worse performance in comparison with PES in term of clinical and angiographic outcomes [68–75]. As a matter of fact, although binary restenosis and late lumen loss were similar between DEB and PES, target lesion revascularization was only mildly higher in DEB than PES. These findings suggest that in big vessels, use of new DES for treatment of restenosis might offer better results in term of further revascularization [72]. Theoretically, the extent of restenosis burden, such as in case of diffuse ISR or total occlusion, may be responsible for a suboptimal performance of DEB. The persistence of large amount of intimal hyperplasia or neoatherosclerotic plaque not properly squeezed after preliminary ballooning is well detectable by angiography; it is important to carefully evaluate the angiographic result after a balloon pre-dilatation, before deciding to proceed with DEB or to shift to DES implantation.

Drug-eluting stent

As the clinical and angiographic results of DES use for BMS restenosis were superior to those with conventional therapy in several randomized trials, DES are also used as a re-treatment modality for DES restenosis. Almost all the studies comparing clinical and angiographic effects of re-DES treatment with conventional therapy for DES restenosis showed a superiority of DES. As a result, guidelines recommend DES to treat patients with ISR irrespective of the type of the initial stent (BMS or DES) [76]. The longer follow-up at 4 years after treatment of BMS restenosis with SES reported an incidence of further restenosis of 25% [77]. The incidence of new restenosis after DES re-treatment varies greatly between 4% and 20% in the various series within 1 year; for these reasons the long-term efficacy of further DES deployment remains uncertain. As drug resistance may be the mechanism of DES restenosis, it was conceived that the placement of a different DES could be more effective in treating DES restenosis compared with the same DES. However, (i) almost all the studies available compared SES vs. PES and few data are available with different "limus" stent, and (ii) the studies showed contradictory results [78]. More recently, use of new generation DES for treatment of BMS restenosis was tested in the RIBS-V trial [74]. This study showed that both EES and PEB provided very low clinical and angiographic recurrence of restenosis, but with EES showing superior angiographic results. Likewise, the RIBS-IV trial analyzed the treatment of DES restenosis and it resulted in similar findings to RIBS-V [79]. From these data it seems that the new generation DESs represent a good approach even in patients with focal pattern to treat DES ISR.

As far as BVS is concerned in treatment of ISR, anecdotal reports show that its use is feasible and theoretically attractive because it avoids multiple metal layers deployed on the vessel wall. However, many concerns regard strut thickness, lack of flexibility, radial strength, and recoil, to contraindicate BVS use for restenosis treatment.

Proposed treatment strategies of DES restenosis

As the etiologies of DES restenosis are diverse, it is recommended to use IVUS or OCT in order to understand the mechanism of restenosis, and to drive therapeutic strategy. Figure 21.2 proposes an algorithm for the current approach to new generation DES restenosis. If restenosis is focal within the stent body or secondary to stent underexpansion, DEB use is recommended; while if the focal edge is involved, which probably means uncovered atherosclerotic plaque or plaque shift, a new generation DES is recommended, and

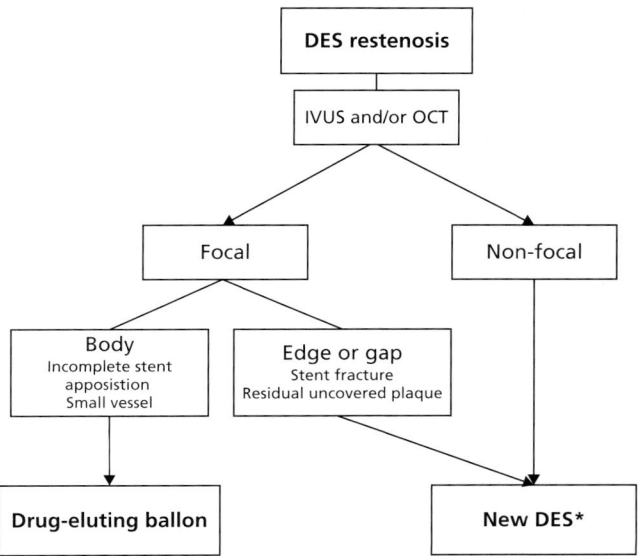

Figure 21.2 Algorithm for the treatment of drug-eluting stent (DES) restenosis. CABG, coronary artery bypass graft; IVUS, intravenous ultrasound; OCT, optical coherence tomography.

different drug elution use might be considered. In small vessels (diameter less than 2.5 mm) use of DEB is preferable in order to avoid a further metallic layer. In diffuse disease, which is currently rare, DEB could be a good choice, because of lack of long-term follow-up after second generation DES used in this setting. However, in case of suboptimal angiographic results, after high-pressure balloon angioplasty resulting in persistence of a high amount of material unable to be squeezed by the balloon, DES in DES is the best option.

Interactive multiple choice questions are available for this chapter on www.wiley. com/go/dangas/cardiology

References

1 Stettler C, Wandel S, Allemann S, *et al.* Outcomes associated with drug-eluting and bare-metal stents: a collaborative network meta-analysis. *Lancet* 2007; **370**: 937–948.

2 Morice MC, Serruys PW, Sousa JE, *et al.* A randomized comparison of a sirolimus-eluting stent with a standard stent for coronary revascularization. *N Engl J Med* 2002; **346**: 1773–1780.

3 Dangas GD, Claessen BE, Caixeta A, Sanidas EA, Mintz GS, Mehran R. In-stent restenosis in the drug-eluting stent era. *J Am Coll Cardiol* 2010; **56**: 1897–1907.

4 Cassese S, Byrne RA, Tada T, *et al.* Incidence and predictors of restenosis after coronary stenting in 10 004 patients with surveillance angiography. *Heart* 2014; **100**: 153–159.

5 Cutlip DE, Windecker S, Mehran R, *et al.* Clinical end points in coronary stent trials: a case for standardized definitions. *Circulation* 2007; **115**: 2344–2351.

6 Patel N, Banning AP. Bioabsorbable scaffolds for the treatment of obstructive coronary artery disease: the next revolution in coronary intervention? *Heart* 2013; **99**: 1236–1243.

7 Magalhaes MA, Minha S, Chen F, *et al.* Clinical presentation and outcomes of coronary in-stent restenosis across 3-stent generations. *Circ Cardiovasc Interv* 2014; **7**: 768–776.

8 Lee MS, Pessegueiro A, Zimmer R, Jurewitz D, Tobis J. Clinical presentation of patients with in-stent restenosis in the drug-eluting stent era. *J Invasive Cardiol* 2008; **20**: 401–403.

9 Kang SJ, Mintz GS, Park DW, *et al.* Mechanisms of in-stent restenosis after drug-eluting stent implantation: intravascular ultrasound analysis. *Circ Cardiovasc Interv* 2011; **4**: 9–14.

10 Costa MA, Simon DI. Molecular basis of restenosis and drug-eluting stents. *Circulation* 2005; **111**: 2257–2273.

11 Yusuf RZ, Duan Z, Lamendola DE, Penson RT, Seiden MV. Paclitaxel resistance: molecular mechanisms and pharmacologic manipulation. *Curr Cancer Drug Targets* 2003; **3**: 1–19.

12 Orr GA, Verdier-Pinard P, McDaid H, Horwitz SB. Mechanisms of Taxol resistance related to microtubules. *Oncogene* 2003; **22**: 7280–7295.

13 Fattori R, Piva T. Drug-eluting stents in vascular intervention. *Lancet* 2003; **361**: 247–249.

14 Inoue T, Node K. Molecular basis of restenosis and novel issues of drug-eluting stents. *Circ J* 2009; **73**: 615–621.

15 Lightell DJ Jr, Woods TC. Relative resistance to mammalian target of rapamycin inhibition in vascular smooth muscle cells of diabetic donors. *Ochsner J* 2013; **13**: 56–60.

16 Stout RW, Bierman EL, Ross R. Effect of insulin on the proliferation of cultured primate arterial smooth muscle cells. *Circ Res* 1975; **36**: 319–327.

17 Zhang Y, Wang Q, Yang D, *et al.* Expression of mammalian target of rapamycin in atherosclerotic plaques is decreased under diabetic conditions: a mechanism for rapamycin resistance. *Mol Med Rep* 2014; **9**: 2388–2392.

18 Zhao LP, Xu WT, Wang L, *et al.* Influence of insulin resistance on in-stent restenosis in patients undergoing coronary drug-eluting stent implantation after long-term angiographic follow-up. *Coron Artery Dis* 2015; **26**: 5–10.

19 Virmani R, Liistro F, Stankovic G, *et al.* Mechanism of late in-stent restenosis after implantation of a paclitaxel derivate-eluting polymer stent system in humans. *Circulation* 2002; **106**: 2649–2651.

20 Balakrishnan B, Tzafriri AR, Seifert P, Groothuis A, Rogers C, Edelman ER. Strut position, blood flow, and drug deposition: implications for single and overlapping drug-eluting stents. *Circulation* 2005; **111**: 2958–2965.

21 O'Brien CC, Kolachalama VB, Barber TJ, Simmons A, Edelman ER. Impact of flow pulsatility on arterial drug distribution in stent-based therapy. *J Control Release* 2013; **168**: 115–124.

22 Attizzani GF, Capodanno D, Ohno Y, Tamburino C. Mechanisms, pathophysiology, and clinical aspects of incomplete stent apposition. *J Am Coll Cardiol* 2014; **63**: 1355–1367.

23 Hoye A, Iakovou I, Ge L, *et al.* Long-term outcomes after stenting of bifurcation lesions with the "crush" technique: predictors of an adverse outcome. *J Am Coll Cardiol* 2006; **47**: 1949–1958.

24 Hamilos MI, Papafaklis MI, Ligthart JM, Serruys PW, Sianos G. Stent fracture and restenosis of a paclitaxel-eluting stent. *Hellenic J Cardiol* 2005; **46**: 439–442.

25 Aoki J, Nakazawa G, Tanabe K, *et al.* Incidence and clinical impact of coronary stent fracture after sirolimus-eluting stent implantation. *Catheter Cardiovasc Interv* 2007; **69**: 380–386.

26 Lee SH, Park JS, Shin DG, *et al.* Frequency of stent fracture as a cause of coronary restenosis after sirolimus-eluting stent implantation. *Am J Cardiol* 2007; **100**: 627–630.

27 Okumura M, Ozaki Y, Ishii J, *et al.* Restenosis and stent fracture following sirolimus-eluting stent (SES) implantation. *Circ J* 2007; **71**: 1669–1677.

28 Popma JJ, Tiroch K, Almonacid A, Cohen S, Kandzari DE, Leon MB. A qualitative and quantitative angiographic analysis of stent fracture late following sirolimus-eluting stent implantation. *Am J Cardiol* 2009; **103**: 923–929.

29 Sianos G, Hofma S, Ligthart JM, *et al.* Stent fracture and restenosis in the drug-eluting stent era. *Catheter Cardiovasc Interv* 2004; **61**: 111–116.

30 Umeda H, Gochi T, Iwase M, *et al.* Frequency, predictors and outcome of stent fracture after sirolimus-eluting stent implantation. *Int J Cardiol* 2009; **133**: 321–326.

31 Halkin A, Carlier S, Leon MB. Late incomplete lesion coverage following Cypher stent deployment for diffuse right coronary artery stenosis. *Heart* 2004; **90**: e45.

32 Shaikh F, Maddikunta R, Djelmami-Hani M, Solis J, Allaqaband S, Bajwa T. Stent fracture, an incidental finding or a significant marker of clinical in-stent restenosis? *Catheter Cardiovasc Interv* 2008; **71**: 614–618.

33 Otsuka F, Vorpahl M, Nakano M, *et al.* Pathology of second-generation everolimus-eluting stents versus first-generation sirolimus- and paclitaxel-eluting stents in humans. *Circulation* 2014; **129**: 211–223.

34 Hecht HS, Polena S, Jelnin V, *et al.* Stent gap by 64-detector computed tomographic angiography relationship to in-stent restenosis, fracture, and overlap failure. *J Am Coll Cardiol* 2009; **54**: 1949–1959.

35 Kereiakes DJ, Wang H, Popma JJ, *et al.* Periprocedural and late consequences of overlapping Cypher sirolimus-eluting stents: pooled analysis of five clinical trials. *J Am Coll Cardiol* 2006; **48**: 21–31.

36 Costa MA, Angiolillo DJ, Tannenbaum M, *et al.* Impact of stent deployment procedural factors on long-term effectiveness and safety of sirolimus-eluting stents (final results of the multicenter prospective STLLR trial). *Am J Cardiol* 2008; **101**: 1704–1711.

37 Colombo A, Moses JW, Morice MC, et al. Randomized study to evaluate sirolimus-eluting stents implanted at coronary bifurcation lesions. Circulation 2004; **109**: 1244–1249.

38 Schmidt W, Lanzer P, Behrens P, Topoleski LD, Schmitz KP. A comparison of the mechanical performance characteristics of seven drug-eluting stent systems. Catheter Cardiovasc Interv 2009; **73**: 350–360.

39 Schampaert E, Cohen EA, Schluter M, et al. The Canadian study of the sirolimus-eluting stent in the treatment of patients with long de novo lesions in small native coronary arteries (C-SIRIUS). J Am Coll Cardiol 2004; **43**: 1110–1115.

40 Schofer J, Schluter M, Gershlick AH, et al. Sirolimus-eluting stents for treatment of patients with long atherosclerotic lesions in small coronary arteries: double-blind, randomised controlled trial (E-SIRIUS). Lancet 2003; **362**: 1093–1099.

41 Nebeker JR, Virmani R, Bennett CL, et al. Hypersensitivity cases associated with drug-eluting coronary stents: a review of available cases from the Research on Adverse Drug Events and Reports (RADAR) project. J Am Coll Cardiol 2006; **47**: 175–181.

42 Otsuka F, Yahagi K, Ladich E, et al. Hypersensitivity reaction in the US Food and Drug Administration-approved second-generation drug-eluting stents: histopathological assessment with ex vivo optical coherence tomography. Circulation 2015; **131**: 322–324.

43 Finn AV, Joner M, Nakazawa G, et al. Pathological correlates of late drug-eluting stent thrombosis: strut coverage as a marker of endothelialization. Circulation 2007; **115**: 2435–2441.

44 Nakazawa G, Otsuka F, Nakano M, et al. The pathology of neoatherosclerosis in human coronary implants bare-metal and drug-eluting stents. J Am Coll Cardiol 2011; **57**: 1314–1322.

45 Otsuka F, Nakano M, Ladich E, Kolodgie FD, Virmani R. Pathologic etiologies of late and very late stent thrombosis following first-generation drug-eluting stent placement. Thrombosis 2012; **2012**: 608593.

46 Ino Y, Kubo T, Kitabata H, et al. Difference in neointimal appearance between early and late restenosis after sirolimus-eluting stent implantation assessed by optical coherence tomography. Coron Artery Dis 2013; **24**: 95–101.

47 Lee CW, Ahn JM, Yoon SH, et al. Temporal patterns of drug-eluting stent failure and its relationship with clinical outcomes. Catheter Cardiovasc Interv 2015; **85**: 515–521.

48 Mehran R, Dangas G, Abizaid AS, et al. Angiographic patterns of in-stent restenosis: classification and implications for long-term outcome. Circulation 1999; **100**: 1872–1878.

49 Rathore S, Kinoshita Y, Terashima M, et al. A comparison of clinical presentations, angiographic patterns and outcomes of in-stent restenosis between bare metal stents and drug eluting stents. EuroIntervention 2010; **5**: 841–846.

50 Corbett SJ, Cosgrave J, Melzi G, et al. Patterns of restenosis after drug-eluting stent implantation: insights from a contemporary and comparative analysis of sirolimus- and paclitaxel-eluting stents. Eur Heart J 2006; **27**: 2330–2337.

51 Stone GW, Ellis SG, Cox DA, et al. A polymer-based, paclitaxel-eluting stent in patients with coronary artery disease. N Engl J Med 2004; **350**: 221–231.

52 Popma JJ, Leon MB, Moses JW, et al. Quantitative assessment of angiographic restenosis after sirolimus-eluting stent implantation in native coronary arteries. Circulation 2004; **110**: 3773–3780.

53 Colombo A, Orlic D, Stankovic G, et al. Preliminary observations regarding angiographic pattern of restenosis after rapamycin-eluting stent implantation. Circulation 2003; **107**: 2178–2180.

54 Solinas E, Dangas G, Kirtane AJ, et al. Angiographic patterns of drug-eluting stent restenosis and one-year outcomes after treatment with repeated percutaneous coronary intervention. Am J Cardiol 2008; **102**: 311–315.

55 Nikolsky E, Gruberg L, Rosenblatt E, et al. Chronic total occlusion due to diffuse in-stent restenosis: is brachytherapy the solution? Int J Cardiovasc Intervent 2004; **6**: 33–38.

56 Lee S, Yoon CH, Oh IY, et al. Angiographic patterns of restenosis with second generation drug-eluting stent: comparative analysis from a 10-year single-center experience. Int Heart J 2015; **56**: 6–12.

57 Cosgrave J, Melzi G, Biondi-Zoccai GG, et al. Drug-eluting stent restenosis the pattern predicts the outcome. J Am Coll Cardiol 2006; **47**: 2399–2404.

58 Kastrati A, Schomig A, Elezi S, et al. Predictive factors of restenosis after coronary stent placement. J Am Coll Cardiol 1997; **30**: 1428–1436.

59 Cutlip DE, Chhabra AG, Baim DS, et al. Beyond restenosis: five-year clinical outcomes from second-generation coronary stent trials. Circulation 2004; **110**: 1226–1230.

60 Stone GW, Ellis SG, Cannon L, et al. Comparison of a polymer-based paclitaxel-eluting stent with a bare metal stent in patients with complex coronary artery disease: a randomized controlled trial. JAMA 2005; **294**: 1215–1223.

61 Kuramitsu S, Iwabuchi M, Yokoi H, et al. Incidence and clinical impact of stent fracture after the Nobori biolimus-eluting stent implantation. J Am Heart Assoc 2014; **3**: e000703.

62 Niccoli G, Stuteville M, Sudhir K, et al. Incidence, time course and predictors of early vs. late target lesion revascularisation after everolimus-eluting stent implantation: a SPIRIT V substudy. EuroIntervention 2013; **9**: 353–359.

63 Grube E, Chevalier B, Smits P, et al. The SPIRIT V study: a clinical evaluation of the XIENCE V everolimus-eluting coronary stent system in the treatment of patients with de novo coronary artery lesions. JACC Cardiovasc Interv 2011; **4**: 168–175.

64 Maehara A, Mintz GS, Weissman NJ. Advances in intravascular imaging. Circ Cardiovasc Interv 2009; **2**: 482–490.

65 Bezerra HG, Costa MA, Guagliumi G, Rollins AM, Simon DI. Intracoronary optical coherence tomography: a comprehensive review clinical and research applications. JACC Cardiovasc Interv 2009; **2**: 1035–1046.

66 Piccolo R, Galasso G, Piscione F, et al. Meta-analysis of randomized trials comparing the effectiveness of different strategies for the treatment of drug-eluting stent restenosis. Am J Cardiol 2014; **114**: 1339–1346.

67 Scheller B, Speck U, Abramjuk C, Bernhardt U, Bohm M, Nickenig G. Paclitaxel balloon coating, a nove. method for prevention and therapy of restenosis. Circulation 2004; **110**: 810–814.

68 Scheller B, Hehrlein C, Bocksch W, et al. Treatment of coronary in-stent restenosis with a paclitaxel-coated balloon catheter. N Engl J Med 2006; **355**: 2113–2124.

69 Unverdorben M, Vallbracht C, Cremers B, et al. Paclitaxel-coated balloon catheter versus paclitaxel-coated stent for the treatment of coronary in-stent restenosis. Circulation 2009; **119**: 2986–2994.

70 Habara S, Mitsudo K, Kadota K, et al. Effectiveness of paclitaxel-eluting balloon catheter in patients with sirolimus-eluting stent restenosis. JACC Cardiovasc Interv 2011; **4**: 149–154.

71 Rittger H, Brachmann J, Sinha AM, et al. A randomized, multicenter, single-blinded trial comparing paclitaxel-coated balloon angioplasty with plain balloon angioplasty in drug-eluting stent restenosis: the PEPCAD-DES study. J Am Coll Cardiol 2012; **59**: 1377–1382.

72 Byrne RA, Neumann FJ, Mehilli J, et al. Paclitaxel-eluting balloons, paclitaxel-eluting stents, and balloon angioplasty in patients with restenosis after implantation of a drug-eluting stent (ISAR-DESIRE 3): a randomised, open-label trial. Lancet 2013; **381**: 461–467.

73 Habara S, Iwabuchi M, Inoue N, et al. A multicenter randomized comparison of paclitaxel-coated balloon catheter with conventional balloon angioplasty in patients with bare-metal stent restenosis and drug-eluting stent restenosis. Am Heart J 2013; **166**: 527–533.

74 Alfonso F, Perez-Vizcayno MJ, Cardenas A, et al. A randomized comparison of drug-eluting balloon versus everolimus-eluting stent in patients with bare-metal stent-in-stent restenosis: the RIBS V Clinical Trial (Restenosis Intra-stent of Bare Metal Stents: paclitaxel-eluting balloon vs. everolimus-eluting stent). J Am Coll Cardiol 2014; **63**: 1378–1386.

75 Xu B, Gao R, Wang J, et al. A prospective, multicenter, randomized trial of paclitaxel-coated balloon versus paclitaxel-eluting stent for the treatment of drug-eluting stent in-stent restenosis: results from the PEPCAD China ISR trial. JACC Cardiovasc Interv 2014; **7**: 204–211.

76 Authors/Task Force members, Windecker S, Kolh P, Alfonso F, et al. 2014 ESC/EACTS Guidelines on myocardial revascularization: The Task Force on Myocardial Revascularization of the European Society of Cardiology (ESC) and the European Association for Cardio-Thoracic Surgery (EACTS)Developed with the special contribution of the European Association of Percutaneous Cardiovascular Interventions (EAPCI). Eur Heart J 2014; **35**: 2541–2619.

77 Alfonso F, Perez-Vizcayno MJ, Hernandez R, et al. Long-term clinical benefit of sirolimus-eluting stents in patients with in-stent restenosis results of the RIBS-II (Restenosis Intra-stent: Balloon angioplasty vs. elective sirolimus-eluting Stenting) study. J Am Coll Cardiol 2008; **52**: 1621–1627.

78 Vyas A, Schweizer M, Malhotra A, Karrowni W. Meta-analysis of same versus different stent for drug-eluting stent restenosis. Am J Cardiol 2014; **113**: 601–606.

79 Alfonso F. A prospective, randomized trial of paclitaxel-eluting balloons versus everolimus-eluting stents in patients with coronary in-stent restenosis of drug-eluting stents: the RIBS IV Clinical Trial TCT. Washington, DC, 2014.

80 Colombo A, Drzewiecki J, Banning A, et al. Randomized study to assess the effectiveness of slow- and moderate-release polymer-based paclitaxel-eluting stents for coronary artery lesions. Circulation 2003; **108**: 788–794.

81 Dawkins KD, Grube E, Guagliumi G, et al. Clinical efficacy of polymer-based paclitaxel-eluting stents in the treatment of complex, long coronary artery lesions from a multicenter, randomized trial: support for the use of drug-eluting stents in contemporary clinical practice. Circulation 2005; **112**: 3306–3313.

82 Morice MC, Colombo A, Meier B, et al. Sirolimus- vs paclitaxel-eluting stents in de novo coronary artery lesions: the REALITY trial: a randomized controlled trial. JAMA 2006; **295**: 895–904.

83 Mehilli J, Dibra A, Kastrati A, Pache J, Dirschinger J, Schomig A. Intracoronary drug-eluting stenting to abrogate restenosis in small arteries study I: randomized trial of paclitaxel- and sirolimus-eluting stents in small coronary vessels. *Eur Heart J* 2006; **27**: 260–266.

84 Mehilli J, Byrne RA, Tiroch K, *et al.* Randomized trial of paclitaxel- versus sirolimus-eluting stents for treatment of coronary restenosis in sirolimus-eluting stents: the ISAR-DESIRE 2 (Intracoronary Stenting and Angiographic Results: Drug Eluting Stents for In-Stent Restenosis 2) study. *J Am Coll Cardiol* 2010; **55**: 2710–2716.

85 Kastrati A, Mehilli J, von Beckerath N, *et al.* Sirolimus-eluting stent or paclitaxel-eluting stent vs balloon angioplasty for prevention of recurrences in patients with coronary in-stent restenosis: a randomized controlled trial. *JAMA* 2005; **293**: 165–171.

86 Kirtane AJ, Leon MB, Ball MW, *et al.* The "final" 5-year follow-up from the ENDEAVOR IV trial comparing a zotarolimus-eluting stent with a paclitaxel-eluting stent. *JACC Cardiovasc Interv* 2013; **6**: 325–333.

87 Garg S, Serruys PW, Miquel-Hebert K. Four-year clinical follow-up of the XIENCE V everolimus-eluting coronary stent system in the treatment of patients with de novo coronary artery lesions: the SPIRIT II trial. *Catheter Cardiovasc Interv* 2011; **77**: 1012–1017.

88 Applegate RJ, Yaqub M, Hermiller JB, *et al.* Long-term (three-year) safety and efficacy of everolimus-eluting stents compared to paclitaxel-eluting stents (from the SPIRIT III Trial). *Am J Cardiol* 2011; **107**: 833–840.

89 Stone GW, Rizvi A, Sudhir K, *et al.* Randomized comparison of everolimus- and paclitaxel-eluting stents. 2-year follow-up from the SPIRIT (Clinical Evaluation of the XIENCE V Everolimus Eluting Coronary Stent System) IV trial. *J Am Coll Cardiol* 2011; **58**: 19–25.

90 Chevalier B, Silber S, Park SJ, *et al.* Randomized comparison of the Nobori Biolimus A9-eluting coronary stent with the Taxus Liberte paclitaxel-eluting coronary stent in patients with stenosis in native coronary arteries: the NOBORI 1 trial--Phase 2. *Circ Cardiovasc Interv* 2009; **2**: 188–195.

91 Morice MC, Serruys PW, Barragan P, *et al.* Long-term clinical outcomes with sirolimus-eluting coronary stents: five-year results of the RAVEL trial. *J Am Coll Cardiol* 2007; **50**: 1299–1304.

92 Weisz G, Leon MB, Holmes DR Jr, *et al.* Five-year follow-up after sirolimus-eluting stent implantation results of the SIRIUS (Sirolimus-Eluting Stent in De-Novo Native Coronary Lesions) Trial. *J Am Coll Cardiol* 2009; **53**: 1488–1497.

93 Menozzi A, Solinas E, Ortolani P, *et al.* Twenty-four months clinical outcomes of sirolimus-eluting stents for the treatment of small coronary arteries: the long-term SES-SMART clinical study. *Eur Heart J* 2009; **30**: 2095–2101.

94 Kandzari DE, Mauri L, Popma JJ, *et al.* Late-term clinical outcomes with zotarolimus- and sirolimus-eluting stents. 5-year follow-up of the ENDEAVOR III (A Randomized Controlled Trial of the Medtronic Endeavor Drug [ABT-578] Eluting Coronary Stent System Versus the Cypher Sirolimus-Eluting Coronary Stent System in De Novo Native Coronary Artery Lesions). *JACC Cardiovasc Interv* 2011; **4**: 543–550.

95 Park KW, Chae IH, Lim DS, *et al.* Everolimus-eluting versus sirolimus-eluting stents in patients undergoing percutaneous coronary intervention: the EXCELLENT (Efficacy of Xience/Promus Versus Cypher to Reduce Late Loss After Stenting) randomized trial. *J Am Coll Cardiol* 2011; **58**: 1844–1854.

96 Fajadet J, Wijns W, Laarman GJ, *et al.* Long-term follow-up of the randomised controlled trial to evaluate the safety and efficacy of the zotarolimus-eluting driver coronary stent in de novo native coronary artery lesions: five year outcomes in the ENDEAVOR II study. *EuroIntervention* 2010; **6**: 562–567.

97 Meredith IT, Verheye S, Dubois CL, *et al.* Primary endpoint results of the EVOLVE trial: a randomized evaluation of a novel bioabsorbable polymer-coated, everolimus-eluting coronary stent. *J Am Coll Cardiol* 2012; **59**: 1362–1370.

98 Kereiakes DJ. *Primary outcome of the EVOLVE II trial: a prospective randomized investigation of a novel bioabsorbable polymer-coated, everolimus-eluted coronary stent American Heart Association Scientific Session.* Chicago, IL: 2014.

99 Kedhi E, Joesoef KS, McFadden E, *et al.* Second-generation everolimus-eluting and paclitaxel-eluting stents in real-life practice (COMPARE): a randomised trial. *Lancet* 2010; **375**: 201–209.

100 Raber L, Wohlwend L, Wigger M, *et al.* Five-year clinical and angiographic outcomes of a randomized comparison of sirolimus-eluting and paclitaxel-eluting stents: results of the Sirolimus-Eluting Versus Paclitaxel-Eluting Stents for Coronary Revascularization LATE trial. *Circulation* 2011; **123**: 2819–2828.

101 Stefanini GG, Kalesan B, Serruys PW, *et al.* Long-term clinical outcomes of biodegradable polymer biolimus-eluting stents versus durable polymer sirolimus-eluting stents in patients with coronary artery disease (LEADERS): 4 year follow-up of a randomised non-inferiority trial. *Lancet* 2011; **378**: 1940–1948.

102 Natsuaki M, Kozuma K, Morimoto T, *et al.* Biodegradable polymer biolimus-eluting stent versus durable polymer everolimus-eluting stent: a randomized, controlled, noninferiority trial. *J Am Coll Cardiol* 2013; **62**: 181–190.

103 Puricel S, Arroyo D, Corpataux N, *et al.* Comparison of everolimus- and biolimus-eluting coronary stents with everolimus-eluting bioresorbable vascular scaffolds. *J Am Coll Cardiol* 2015; **65**: 791–801.

104 Smits PC, Hofma S, Togni M, *et al.* Abluminal biodegradable polymer biolimus-eluting stent versus durable polymer everolimus-eluting stent (COMPARE II): a randomised, controlled, non-inferiority trial. *Lancet* 2013; **381**: 651–660.

105 Lee SW, Park SW, Kim YH, *et al.* A randomized comparison of sirolimus- versus paclitaxel-eluting stent implantation in patients with diabetes mellitus: 4-year clinical outcomes of DES-DIABETES (drug-eluting stent in patients with DIABETES mellitus) trial. *JACC Cardiovasc Interv* 2011; **4**: 310–316.

106 Hermiller JB, Raizner A, Cannon L, *et al.* Outcomes with the polymer-based paclitaxel-eluting TAXUS stent in patients with diabetes mellitus: the TAXUS-IV trial. *J Am Coll Cardiol* 2005; **45**: 1172–1179.

107 Dibra A, Kastrati A, Mehilli J, *et al.* Paclitaxel-eluting or sirolimus-eluting stents to prevent restenosis in diabetic patients. *N Engl J Med* 2005; **353**: 663–670.

108 Kirtane AJ, Patel R, O'Shaughnessy C, *et al.* Clinical and angiographic outcomes in diabetics from the ENDEAVOR IV trial: randomized comparison of zotarolimus- and paclitaxel-eluting stents in patients with coronary artery disease. *JACC Cardiovasc Interv* 2009; **2**: 967–976.

109 Kereiakes DJ, Cutlip DE, Applegate RJ, *et al.* Outcomes in diabetic and nondiabetic patients treated with everolimus- or paclitaxel-eluting stents: results from the SPIRIT IV clinical trial (Clinical Evaluation of the XIENCE V Everolimus Eluting Coronary Stent System). *J Am Coll Cardiol* 2010; **56**: 2084–2089.

110 Chan C, Zambahari R, Kaul U, *et al.* A randomized comparison of sirolimus-eluting versus bare metal stents in the treatment of diabetic patients with native coronary artery lesions: the DECODE study. *Catheter Cardiovasc Interv* 2008; **72**: 591–600.

111 Sabate M, Jimenez-Quevedo P, Angiolillo DJ, *et al.* Randomized comparison of sirolimus-eluting stent versus standard stent for percutaneous coronary revascularization in diabetic patients: the diabetes and sirolimus-eluting stent (DIABETES) trial. *Circulation* 2005; **112**: 2175–2183.

112 Stone GW, Witzenbichler B, Guagliumi G, *et al.* Heparin plus a glycoprotein IIb/IIIa inhibitor versus bivalirudin monotherapy and paclitaxel-eluting stents versus bare-metal stents in acute myocardial infarction (HORIZONS-AMI): final 3-year results from a multicentre, randomised controlled trial. *Lancet* 2011; **377**: 2193–2204.

113 Spaulding C, Teiger E, Commeau P, *et al.* Four-year follow-up of TYPHOON (trial to assess the use of the CYPHer sirolimus-eluting coronary stent in acute myocardial infarction treated with BallOON angioplasty). *JACC Cardiovasc Interv* 2011; **4**: 14–23.

114 Holmvang L, Kelbaek H, Kaltoft A, *et al.* Long-term outcome after drug-eluting versus bare-metal stent implantation in patients with ST-segment elevation myocardial infarction: 5 years follow-up from the randomized DEDICATION trial (Drug Elution and Distal Protection in Acute Myocardial Infarction). *JACC Cardiovasc Interv* 2013; **6**: 548–553.

115 Sabate M, Brugaletta S, Cequier A, *et al.* The EXAMINATION trial (Everolimus-Eluting Stents Versus Bare-Metal Stents in ST-Segment Elevation Myocardial Infarction): 2-year results from a multicenter randomized controlled trial. *JACC Cardiovasc Interv* 2014; **7**: 64–71.

116 Raber L, Kelbaek H, Ostojic M, *et al.* Effect of biolimus-eluting stents with biodegradable polymer vs bare-metal stents on cardiovascular events among patients with acute myocardial infarction: the COMFORTABLE AMI randomized trial. *JAMA* 2012; **308**: 777–787.

CHAPTER 22

Laser, Rotational, and Orbital Coronary Atherectomy

Kaleab N. Asrress[1], Peter O'Kane[2], Robert Pyo[3], and Simon R. Redwood[1]

[1] Department of Cardiology, St Thomas' Hospital, and King's College London British Heart Foundation Centre of Excellence, The Rayne Institute, St. Thomas' Hospital, London, UK
[2] Dorset Heart Centre, Royal Bournemouth Hospital, Bournemouth, UK
[3] Montefiore Medical Center, Albert Einstein College of Medicine, New York, NY, USA

Despite advances in percutaneous coronary intervention (PCI) technology, difficulty in crossing or dilating calcified coronary lesions remains one of the greatest challenges in contemporary practice. Given that the aging population, increased rates of renal failure, and diabetes mellitus all contribute to the burden of coronary calcification, it is likely that this will be a growing problem. Compared with non-calcified lesions, increased intracoronary calcium deposition leads to a higher incidence of major adverse cardiovascular events, particularly myocardial infarction [1]. They are also associated with a higher frequency of restenosis, target lesion revascularization (TLR), vessel dissection during PCI, failure to deliver a stent, balloon ruptures, and undilatable lesions [2–7]. Furthermore, up to 50% of stents deployed in calcified lesions have been shown to have asymmetric expansion, potentially increasing the likelihood of restenosis and stent thrombosis [8,9].

Many of these challenges can be overcome by adequate lesion preparation. This chapter summarizes three atherectomy techniques (AT) that are employed as treatment strategies for calcific coronary lesions:

1 Rotational atherectomy (RA) – the oldest and perhaps most widely used
2 Orbital atherectomy (OA) – a relatively newly developed modality, and
3 Excimer laser coronary atherectomy (ELCA).

Background
Rotational atherectomy
Arterial dissection, early vessel elastic recoil, and later restenosis because of cell proliferation lead to a failure to maintain vessel patency after plain old balloon angioplasty (POBA). Long and calcified lesions are particularly non-compliant and high balloon inflation pressures may be needed. Shearing forces, persistence of the shifted atheromatous mass (containing cells capable of proliferation), and a stimulus to proliferation resulting from balloon injury are important features in determining POBA failures. An ablative technique that can restore vessel patency by selectively removing atheromatous bulk without injuring more normal vessel components has the potential to overcome some of the shortcomings of POBA. In this context, RA was developed in the late 1980s as an alternative

percutaneous method for lumen enlargement [10,11]. Randomized trials demonstrated some advantages of RA over POBA in procedural success but not in reducing rates of restenosis [12,13]. Additionally, the subsequent development of routine stenting very effectively solved the POBA problems of vessel dissection and elastic recoil thereby discouraging more widespread adoption of RA.

However, problems with cell proliferation and in-stent restenosis (ISR) remained major determinants of TLR, affecting as many as one-third of stented lesions. Balloon treatment of ISR was frequently complicated by recurrent restenosis, particularly when restenosis was diffuse along the length of the stent. The persistence and elastic recoil of the proliferating cell mass were thought to be responsible for balloon failure and recurrent restenosis. Therefore a benefit for lesion ablation with RA was postulated. However, the success of RA in this situation remained equivocal after the publication of two randomized trials with contrary findings [12,14,15]. Stent development, with the introduction of drug-eluting stents (DES), has significantly reduced rates of ISR as a reason for TLR. However, a major challenge to contemporary PCI is the accessibility of some lesions, particularly calcified lesions, to balloon or stent placement, or to balloon dilatation. In complex lesions, even high inflation pressures may not achieve satisfactory stent expansion in as many as half of the cases. Restenosis and acute stent thrombosis occur more frequently following such procedures.

RA alters the physical characteristics of the obstructing lesion, reducing its physical bulk and rigidity, and increasing the accessibility of the debulked coronary segment to balloon and stent devices. As such, RA improves lesion access and can optimize minimum lumen diameter (MLD) gains as an adjunctive technique to enable and/or optimize stenting. RA offers more predictable lesion preparation and consequently avoids the risk of vessel perforation from very high balloon dilatation inflation pressures.

Excimer coronary laser atherectomy
Excimer lasers are pulsed gas lasers that use a mixture of a rare gas and halogen as an active medium to generate pulses of short wavelength, high-energy ultraviolet light. After application of an electrical discharge, energy absorbed by the individual atoms results in their being in a higher energy state. Electronic excitation of one of the atoms (halogen) initiates bonding with the other atomic species

Interventional Cardiology: Principles and Practice, Second Edition. Edited by George D. Dangas, Carlo Di Mario, and Nicholas N. Kipshidze.
© 2017 John Wiley & Sons, Ltd. Published 2017 by John Wiley & Sons, Ltd.

(argon, krypton, or xenon), resulting in the formation of an electronically "excited dimer" molecule or "excimer." As the molecule returns toward the ground state, short wavelength (and corresponding high photon energy) ultraviolet radiation is emitted. Work in the 1980s demonstrated that the ultraviolet radiation emitted by an excimer laser could be used to inscribe exceptionally clean and precise etching cuts in cardiovascular tissue including atherosclerotic coronary artery segments [16], and subsequently in vein grafts [17] and native coronary artery disease [18–20]. Early clinical results in the era of POBA were mixed [21,22]. Randomized studies comparing ELCA, RA, and POBA showed that procedural success was better with RA than ELCA and POBA but high rates of TLR were seen with all three modalities at 6 months' follow-up [23].

The development of coronary stents, with adjunctive RA, resulted in reduced use of ELCA as a routine technique. However, it still has a key role as an adjunct in specific clinical situations: the treatment of non-crossable or non-expandable coronary lesions; under-expanded stents [24,25]; and in aortocoronary saphenous vein grafts where there is a preponderance of fibro-calcific as well as thrombotic material [26–28]. It has also shown utility in the setting of acute myocardial infarction and large thrombus burden [29,30].

Orbital atherectomy

The Orbital Atherectomy System (Diamondback 360° OAS, Cardiovascular Systems, CSI, St. Paul, MN, USA) is a technique that has recently become available as an adjunctive tool for coronary lesion preparation. This has become an established technique in the treatment of calcific peripheral vascular disease and has recently shown utility in the coronary arena. Although relatively new, with the first study showing safety and efficacy only being published in 2014 [31], it will add to the catheter laboratory armamentarium in the treatment of severe coronary calcification.

Rotational atherectomy
Technical considerations

The business end of rotational atherectomy (Rotablator, Boston Scientific, MA, USA) is a nickel-plated brass elliptical burr coated with diamond microchips on the front or crossing surface of the burr, with the rear half of the burr having no diamond chips and therefore no ablating surface (Figure 22.1). Rotational speeds up to 190,000 rpm are transmitted via a flexible drive shaft enclosed within a Teflon sheath (4.3 Fr) connected to a gas-driven turbine. Burr sizes

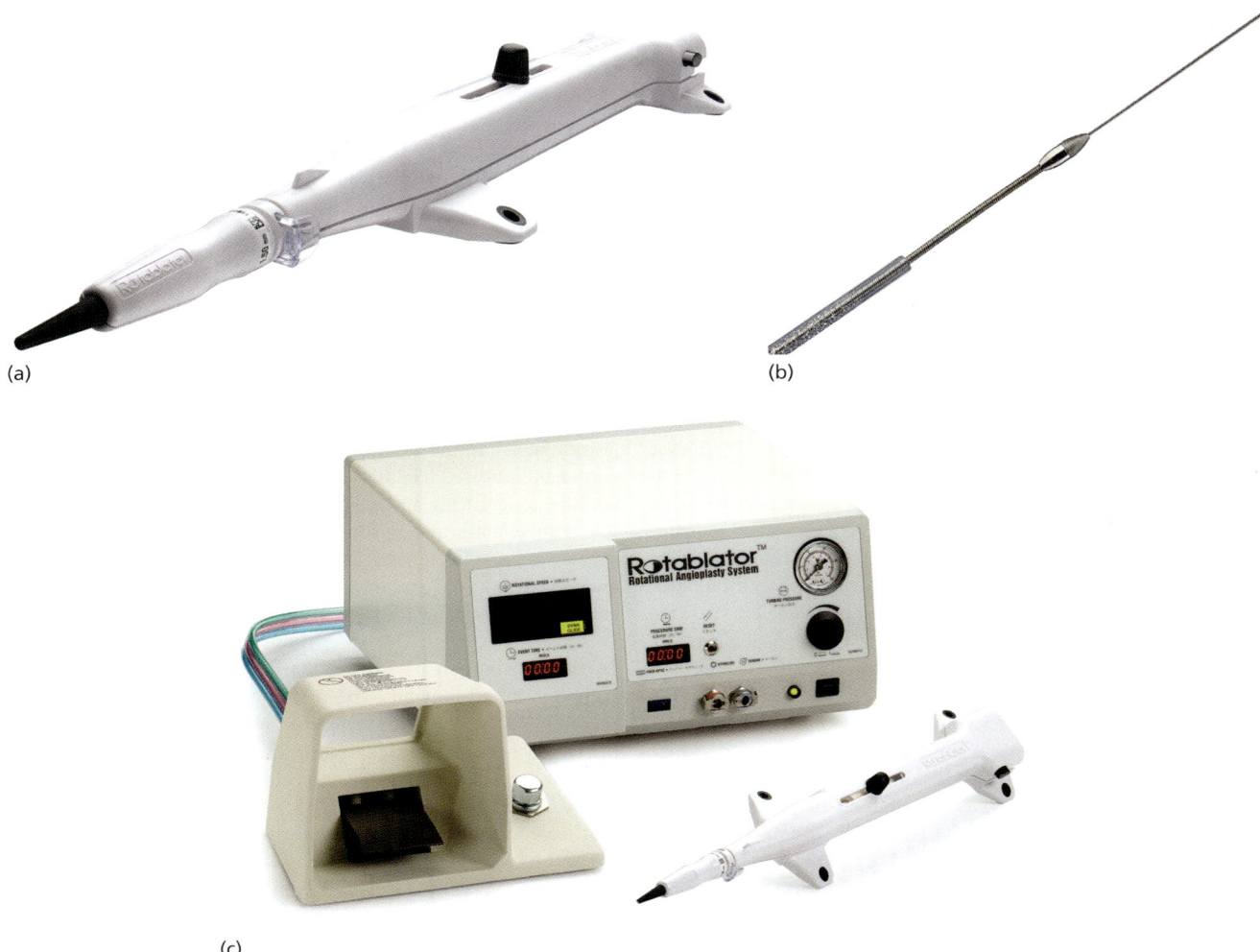

(a)

(b)

(c)

Figure 22.1 Rotablator system with burrs, console, Rotalink system. (a) A single advancer can be used for multiple burr exchanges. (b) The diamond-coated burr is advanced on the guidewire and torque transmitted via the Teflon-coated 4.3 Fr sheath. (c) Control console and foot pedal. Images courtesy of Boston Scientific.

of 1.25, 1.5, and 1.75 mm can be accommodated by most 6 Fr guiding catheters. Notably, the use of a 1.75 mm burr with the 6 Fr guide will cause pressure dampening. The minimum guide size for a 2.0 mm burr is 7 Fr. Burr sizes of 2.15 and 2.25 mm can be accommodated by most 8 and 9 Fr guiding catheters. Burr sizes of 2.38 and 2.50 mm require alternative guides with 9 and 10 Fr lumen diameters, respectively. Following passage of a proprietary spring-tipped steel guide-wire (Boston Scientific, RotaWire, 0.009 inches) into the distal vessel beyond the target lesion, the shaft-mounted burr is advanced into position proximal to the lesion over the RotaWire.

In some of the early RA studies, inability to pass the RotaWire into the distal vessel accounted for most procedural failures. A variety of RotaWires with different characteristics is now available. Many operators believe that these wires are less torque responsive than other coronary guidewires, and therefore it can be difficult to wire a complex lesion primarily with a RotaWire. In this instance, a regular .014 inch guidewire can be used to cross the lesion and an over-the-wire balloon or microcatheter tracked through the lesion after which the crossing wire is exchanged for a RotaWire. This technique can be used to traverse particularly challenging lesions such as chronic total occlusions (CTO).

A saline-based infusion cocktail delivered through the Teflon-coated sheath provides lubrication for the drive shaft. Heparin anti-coagulation (typically 70 IU/kg 5000 IU in 500 mL normal saline) and vasodilators (verapamil 5 mg and isosorbide dinitrate 5 mg) are frequently added to the cocktail and are delivered directly into the coronary artery. Systemic anticoagulation aims for an activated clotting time of about 300 seconds. Historically, a temporary trans-venous pacemaker was often positioned when rotablating right coronary artery disease or dominant left circumflex lesions to manage the transient atrioventricular block that often occurred. However, with contemporary practice using smaller burrs, shorter runs, and atropine pre-treatment, bradyarrhythmic complications are rare and pacing is unnecessary.

Once an appropriately sized burr is in position proximal to the lesion and it is confirmed that cocktail is reliably being delivered, the drive is switched on and engaged. Rotational speeds are typically between 130,000 and 150,000 rpm [7,13]. More rapid rotational speeds generate excessive heat and also result in greater platelet activation [32]. Lower speeds can result in ablative behavior less selective for atheroma, but in general is associated with fewer complications. The burr is advanced slowly into and beyond the target lesion and with care taken to maintain rotational speed as the burr encounters friction; if rotational speed drops, retreat from the target lesion may be necessary. Significant decrements in rotational speed (>5000 rpm) must be avoided as these are associated with excessive heat production through friction and are associated with poorer immediate and long-term outcomes [33,34]. Sudden drop in burr speed is also associated with burr trapping in the lesion, hence the cautious advancement and attention to burr speed.

Burr advancement is best accomplished in a piecemeal "pecking" fashion rather than through steady constant movement. The recommended movement comprises short (about 10–20 second) runs of slow, smooth advances of the burr into the lesion followed by retreat. The burr should not be forced through the lesion. Because the rear of the burr does not have an abrading surface, the device can become trapped beyond the lesion and it can be difficult to pull back. The operator should retreat from the lesion between "pecks" in order to maintain rotational speed and enable coronary blood flow to flush ablative debris beyond the lesion.

After the lesion is crossed, the spinning burr is passed back and forth across the lesion until the operator feels no further significant resistance to the burr. Larger burrs can then be selected and the procedure repeated, typically until a maximum burr size of 60–80% of the reference vessel diameter has successfully crossed the lesion. More modest degrees of ablation can be associated with fewer short and long-term complications [34,35], and in any case may be considered satisfactory if the principal indication for RA has been to debulk rather than abolish the lesion (as an adjunct to stenting) or to facilitate tracking of balloons or stents across the target lesion. A strategy using a single 1.5 or 1.75 mm burr is satisfactory for the majority of cases.

The rotating burr abrades atherosclerotic material, selectively removing non-compliant tissue to improve vessel patency. Intravascular ultrasound (IVUS) examination following RA typically demonstrates a circular lumen with a smooth distinct luminal–vessel wall interface distinct from that seen following balloon barotrauma [36]. The diameter of the newly created lumen usually tends to exceed that of the largest burr used, perhaps because of non-axial movement of the burr about its long axis, or as a consequence of vessel spasm during ablation [11,36].

In vitro studies suggest that normal (compliant, soft) vascular tissue is relatively unharmed and therefore not easily abraded, but that more rigid, calcified structures are more amenable to abrasion [11,36]. Burr abrasion generates minute particles (5–10 μm) which are propagated distally into and through the coronary microcirculation. Consequences of distal microembolization of these atheromatous particles and of platelet activation by the rotating burr are believed to contribute to vessel spasm and no-reflow complications observed during RA. *In vitro*, glycoprotein (GP) IIb/IIIa inhibitors attenuate platelet activation resulting from RA, and are associated with fewer ischemic complications although in practice with good technique and appropriate burr sizing, no-reflow is a rare complication. A small randomized study showed that use of GP IIb/IIIa inhibitors results in lower increases in serum cardiac enzyme concentrations during RA [37], although larger studies are required to support routine use.

Indications for RA
Calcific lesions
The principal indication for RA is in the treatment of calcific lesions, which in the absence of lesion preparation or modification confer an increased likelihood of procedural failure, stent underdeployment, restenosis, and major complications [38]. In such lesions, RA both enables and optimizes stenting, facilitating procedural success in complex lesions, chronic total occlusions, ostial lesions, and bifurcation lesions associated with bulky plaque and vessel geometry unfavorable for stent deployment [8,23,39–44].

In-stent restenosis
Although it had previously been established as a promising treatment option for ISR with favorable outcomes, in the DES era RA has largely been superseded in this situation by balloon angioplasty, drug-eluting balloons, cutting or scoring balloons, DES, or coronary artery bypass grafting (CABG) [45]. The two randomized studies that have addressed this issue have reported apparently discrepant results. The single-center US Rotational Atherectomy versus Balloon Angioplasty for Diffuse In-Stent Restenosis (ROSTER) study [15] reports that RA was associated with a much lower rate of repeat stenting than POBA (10% vs. 31%%; p <0.001) and a lower TLR incidence (32% vs. 45%; p = 0.042). Importantly, one-third of patients evaluated for inclusion in ROSTER were excluded from the study if prior IVUS demonstrated evidence of inadequate stent expansion.

The multicenter European Angioplasty versus Rotational Atherectomy for Treatment of Diffuse In-Stent Resenosis Trial (ARTIST) [14] did not evaluate adequacy of stent expansion with IVUS prior to randomization. Balloon treatment was associated with better outcome; 6-month event-free survival was significantly better after POBA than with RA (91% vs. 80%; p < 0.01). IVUS results at follow-up are consistent with the interpretation that a factor favoring POBA was the resulting stent overexpansion. As registry data suggest that as many as 50% of stents are incompletely deployed [8], and ROSTER detected this in one-third of their ISR patients, ARTIST results may be heavily biased by results of balloon treatment of inadequate stent expansion. ARTIST should therefore not be considered to have evaluated the efficacy of RA for treating ISR occurring in optimally deployed bare metal stents (BMS). It is intuitive that RA is most beneficial for removal of intimal hyperplasia but less effective for radial expansion of an underexpanded stent. If RA is contemplated for use in DES ISR, pre-treatment imaging with IVUS or optical coherence tomography (OCT) may be warranted to first elucidate the mechanism of restenosis.

Contraindications to RA

Contraindications to RA include saphenous vein graft lesions, thrombus, dissection, and occlusions through which a guidewire will not pass, although there are reports in the literature of successful use of RA despite contraindications.

Avoiding complications

The complications of RA are similar to those of PCI, and include vascular access complications, stroke, myocardial infarction, urgent CABG, death, dissection, perforation, acute vessel closure, side branch loss, and slow-flow and/or no-reflow. Additional complications of RA includes burr entrapment, estimated at 0.5–1%. Smaller burr sizes (burr–artery ratio <0.7) reduces angiographic complications and peri-procedural enzyme release with similar procedural success [34,35]. Smaller burrs permit use of smaller guide catheters and therefore sheaths, permitting safe and effective transradial RA in the majority of cases, and resulting in fewer vascular complications. Smaller guide catheter use also limits RA-associated stroke [46].

Slow-flow and no-reflow during RA are likely related to microvascular embolization of atherosclerotic debris and thrombus. Strategies to prevent this include antiplatelet therapy, vasodilators, and meticulous technique. Vasodilators used for the purpose of reducing slow-flow and no-reflow include adenosine, calcium antagonists, nitroglycerine, and nicorandil.

Techniques to avoid burr entrapment have been described earlier. If this does occur, timely action is required to remove the entrapped burr. The most common solution in the literature is surgical removal with CABG; however, interventional approaches can be divided into two techniques: dilation of the lesion with balloon angioplasty, and burr removal facilitated by deep catheter intubation. These are described in detail elsewhere [47].

Excimer laser coronary atherectomy
Technical considerations

Background technical considerations to ELCA have already been described. The CVX-300 cardiovascular laser excimer system (Spectranetics, Colorado Springs, CO, USA) uses xenon chloride (XeCl) as the active medium. Consequently, the light emitted is pulsed and lies in the ultraviolet B (UVB) region of the spectrum with a wavelength of 308 nm and a tissue penetration depth of 30–50 μm. This shallow absorption depth limits medial and adventitial tissue damage in standard PCI. Significant thermal ablation is avoided because of the pulsed delivery of high-energy pulses that last only a fraction of a second. The number of pulses emitted during a 1 second period is known as the pulse repetition rate. The duration of each pulse is termed a pulse width, which can be modified according to the nature of the treated lesion.

Tissue breakdown via photo-ablation occurs in three steps. First, rapid UV light absorption occurs resulting in severing of carbon–carbon bonds, with subsequent dissipation of energy. This energy dissipation leads to evaporation of intracellular water to produce a steam bubble that advances ahead of the laser catheter. Tissue breakdown occurs as a result of rapid expansion and contraction of these steam bubbles. The threshold energy required for the penetration of UV light into the surrounding tissue and the subsequent creation of a steam bubble is called fluence (range: 30–80 mJ/mm²). High pulse energy delivery is more efficacious in managing calcified lesions. The resultant debris particles are <10 μm in diameter with minimal risk of distal embolization [48].

ELCA catheters are compatible with a standard 0.014 inch guidewire and are available in four diameters for use in the coronary artery (0.9, 1.4, 1.7, and 2.0 mm). The catheters most commonly used have a concentric array at the tip, but eccentric laser catheters are also available which are potentially better for debulking in ISR (Figure 22.2a). The larger diameter devices (1.7 and 2.0 mm catheters) are primarily used in straight sections of large diameter vessels, for example saphenous vein grafts. They require 7 and 8 Fr guide catheters, respectively. Both the 0.9 and 1.4 mm are 6 Fr compatible catheters but only the 0.9 mm X-80 ELCA catheter is routinely used in balloon failure and CTO cases because of its excellent deliverability, high power, and repetition rate settings. The 0.9 mm catheter contains 65 fibers of 50 μm diameter each and the radiopaque marker on this catheter is set back from the tip, making the device extremely deliverable.

In cases where the balloon has failed to cross a lesion, this rapid-exchange ELCA catheter is advanced to the lesion and, during continuous saline flush, lasing commences with gentle slow forward traction of the catheter. As the pulsed UV light emitted has a shallow penetration depth there is a low risk of dissection and vessel perforation. However, it is imperative to advance the catheter slowly and cautiously when dealing with very resistant lesions. In these cases there is often a tendency for even a supportive guide catheter to "back out" of the coronary artery, which would prevent saline from reaching the point of laser–plaque interaction, and increase the risk of complications.

Saline infusion technique

It is critically important to note that both blood and iodinated contrast media, in comparison to water or saline, almost completely absorb the excimer laser energy. This results in the formation of cavity microbubbles at the site of energy delivery (Figure 22.2c, d) which subsequently potentiates the effects of pressure waves increasing the likelihood of vessel wall dissection [49]. Therefore the removal of contrast media and blood at the laser tip or energy delivery site has become mandatory; this is achieved with saline flushing [50]. This results in direct delivery of the energy to the atherosclerotic material and leads to lower dissection rates [51].

This is achieved in practical terms by attaching a 1 L bag of 0.9% saline to the manifold via a three-way tap allowing saline to be injected with a 20 mL Leur-lock syringe when required. It is

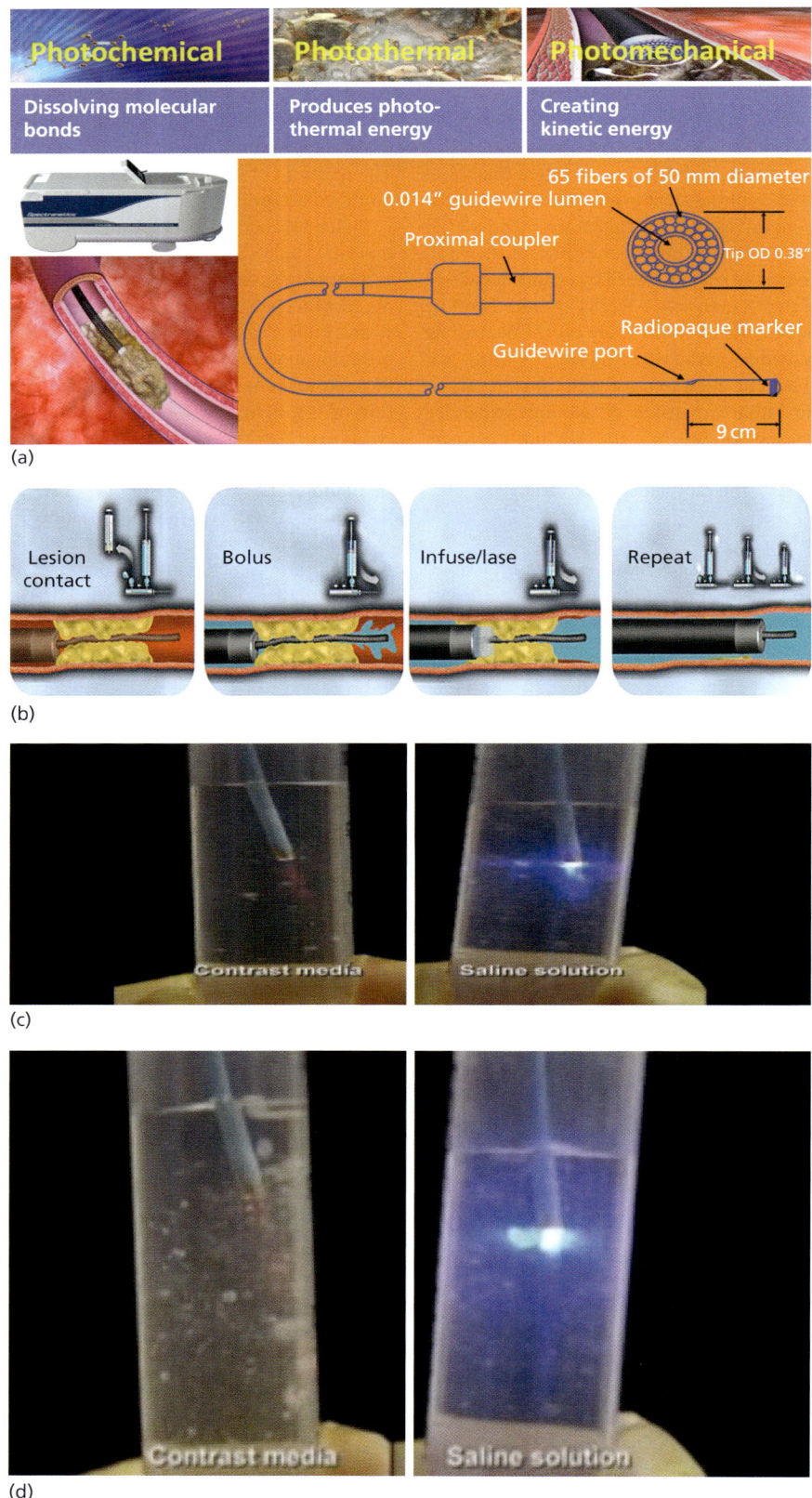

Figure 22.2 Excimer coronary laser atherectomy (ECLA). (a) Mechanism of action of ECLA. (b) Process of preforming a saline bolus and infusion in the ECLA process. (c, d) Demonstration of the importance of saline infusion to prevent the formation of microbubbles that are evident when the laser is activated in contrast medium. Images courtesy of Cardiovascular Systems, Inc.

important to visualize directly under fluoroscopy that all contrast is flushed from the guide catheter in the selected starting position for lasing, and that the saline does not get mixed with contrast. Some 5 mL of saline should be infused prior to laser activation followed by a slow injection continued at a rate of 2–3 mL/s throughout the lasing process (usually 5–10 seconds; Figure 22.2b). It is important to ensure that the guide catheter is well intubated into the coronary artery to ensure saline delivery to the laser catheter tip.

When dealing with CTO lesions, it is advisable not to use the saline technique. When crossing the CTO with a guidewire, a section of the guidewire passage can be outside the true lumen of the vessel. Any anterograde injection can result in propagation of a dissection plane and ultimately result in a longer length of stenting if not immediate no-reflow phenomena. Furthermore, the saline infusion is unlikely to reach the intended target given the lack of runoff from the lesion and will therefore be ineffective. It is also likely that using ELCA without saline in this setting will permit greater energy at the proximal or distal cap of the occlusion, ultimately facilitating the ELCA effect.

It should be noted that ELCA is not recommended when the operator is aware that there is a long length of subintimal guidewire positioning as can occur during typical anterograde dissection re-entry. ELCA catheters are relatively indiscriminate in performing tissue ablation and will essentially "modify" any tissue in their field of delivery. Within the subintimal space the catheter would lie in closer proximity to the media and adventitia of the vessel and could cause perforation. For non-crossable and non-dilatable lesions, whether or not in the context of CTO, the highly deliverable 0.9 mm X-80 catheter is favored with a maximum fluence (energy) of 80 mJ/mm² and a repetition rate of 80 Hz. Activation for 10 seconds is followed by a mandatory rest of 5 seconds between each lasing period, which is continued until either the catheter has traversed the lesion or sufficient lesion modification has occurred to permit balloon crossing or expansion.

The major advantage of ELCA is that the catheter is utilized on the standard 0.014 inch guidewire and so, unlike RA, it can be used more easily without the need to exchange wires. This is of particular importance during CTO because it prevents any loss of distal wire position once the lesion has been crossed. Once ELCA has successfully traversed the lesion the procedure can be completed with balloon angioplasty and stenting.

We have previously reported the combined use of ELCA and RA as the "RASER" technique and have utilized this in many procedures [52]. Lesions that cannot be treated with RA initially, because of inability to advance a RotaWire, can first be treated with ELCA with the understanding that the device will not fully debulk the lesion to permit stenting. However, the "pilot hole" created by ELCA can then be used to pass a RotaWire, either independently or via a microcatheter exchange technique, to permit subsequent RA and achieve procedural success.

Indications for ELCA
Chronic total occlusions
ELCA has additional beneficial properties other than simply being able to cross or adequately debulk the resistant lesion. The ablative effect is transmitted across the atherosclerotic plaque, any organized thrombus, fibrosis, and calcification, which comprise the main architecture of a CTO. During recanalization attempts, the friable thrombus can induce platelet aggregation and promote the release of vasoconstrictor agents. This leads to a pro-thrombotic milieu that presents an additional challenge to an already technically demanding procedure. ELCA has a suppressive effect on platelet

aggregation and can sever links within the fibrin mesh leading to clot dissolution [52,53]. ELCA is unlikely to have any significant effect on the calcification within a lesion but the ablation of material supporting the calcified plaque weakens the overall lesion to permit successful balloon traversing and expansion.

Non-dilatable lesions
ELCA was first approved for use in cases of balloon failure during PCI in the USA in 1992 by the US Food and Drug Administration. However, there are few data on its use, particularly in contemporary practice. There are several reports of its use for balloon failure in the balloon angioplasty era [54–56]. The technology available at that time was limited to 1.4, 1.7, and 2.0 mm laser catheters and the laser energy delivered was much lower than in current practice with a maximum of 60 fluence and 25 Hz. It was also prior to the practice of continuous saline flushing during lasing, which has been shown to decrease complications [51]. Complication rates in these patients were high (8% significant dissection, 3% perforation, 3% acute stent thrombosis, and 3% emergency bypass surgery) and laser success rates were only 37%, although clinical success was obtained in 89%. Advances in PCI (with improved wire and balloon technology, the near universal use of coronary stents and the introduction of various drug-eluting stents) have increased the range of indications for PCI and improved outcomes since the 1990s.

Underexpanded stents
The ablative capabilities of ELCA are based on absorption of its energy in the atheroma, leading to photomechanical and photothermal processes. Using high power energy, the 0.9 X-80 catheter has been shown to cross even heavily calcified lesions. Even if the target lesions are not directly in the focus of laser beam, the specific interaction of ELCA energy in blood vessels induces acoustic shock waves propagating on to the surrounding structures. This effect becomes even more desirable when treating underexpanded coronary stents. Underexpanded coronary stents pose a significant risk for stent thrombosis and subsequent adverse clinical outcomes. There are very few reports on the use successful use of ELCA to treat under expanded stents [57,58]. In our experience, this is a very good indication, in the presence of calcific coronary stenosis, for the use of ELCA. The laser catheter ablates tissue on the abluminal surface of the stent allowing lesion modification and subsequent expansion of an originally underexpanded stent.

Avoiding complications
ELCA complications are on the whole similar to those encountered during routine PCI as described earlier with RA. Specific issues arise from interruption of the continuous saline flush or contamination with contrast which can generate excessive heat and bubbles. Dissection re-entry techniques for CTO also require specific attention if the catheter is subintimal. Scrupulous technique and a procedure volume to maintain operator skills are essential to utilizing this technology safely.

Orbital atherectomy
Despite the mature nature of RA, which has been in clinical use since the 1980s, the persistence of angiographic and clinical complications highlights the potential for further progress in technology and technique. OA is a technique that has recently become available for coronary intervention (Diamondback 360° OAS, Cardiovascular Systems, CSI, St. Paul, MN, USA). Distinct from

52 McKenzie DB, Talwar S, Jokhi PP, *et al.* How should I treat severe coronary artery calcification when it is not possible to dilate a balloon or deliver a Rotawire™? *EuroIntervention* 2011; **6**: 779–783.

53 Topaz O. On the hostile massive thrombus and the means to eradicate it. *Catheter Cardiovasc Interv* 2005; **65**: 280–281.

54 Ahmed WH, al-Anazi MM, Bittl JA. Excimer laser-facilitated angioplasty for undilatable coronary narrowings. *Am J Cardiol* 1996; **78**: 1045–1046.

55 Shen ZJ, García-García HM, Schultz C, van der Ent M, Serruys PW. Crossing of a calcified "balloon uncrossable" coronary chronic total occlusion facilitated by a laser catheter: a case report and review recent four years' experience at the thoraxcenter. *Int J Cardiol* 2010; **145**: 251–254.

56 Bittl JA, Ryan TJ, Keaney JF, *et al.* Coronary artery perforation during excimer laser coronary angioplasty: the percutaneous excimer laser coronary angioplasty registry. *J Am Coll Cardiol* 1993; **21**: 1158–1165.

57 Fernandez JP, Hobson AR, McKenzie DB, Talwar S, O'Kane PD. How should I treat severe calcific coronary artery disease? *EuroIntervention* 2011; **7**: 400–407.

58 Lam SC, Bertog S, Sievert H. Excimer laser in management of underexpansion of a newly deployed coronary stent. *Catheter Cardiovasc Interv* 2014; **83**: E64–68.

59 Parikh K, Chandra P, Choksi N, Khanna P, Chambers J. Safety and feasibility of orbital atherectomy for the treatment of calcified coronary lesions: the ORBIT I trial. *Catheter Cardiovasc Interv* 2013; **81**: 1134–1139.

60 Kini A, Marmur JD, Duvvuri S, Dangas G, Choudhary S, Sharma SK. Rotational atherectomy: improved procedural outcome with evolution of technique and equipment. Single-center results of first 1,000 patients. *Catheter Cardiovasc Interv* 1999; **46**: 305–311.

61 Adams GL, Khanna PK, Staniloae CS, Abraham JP, Sparrow EM. Optimal techniques with the diamondback 360° system achieve effective results for the treatment of peripheral arterial disease. *J Cardiovasc Transl Res* 2011; **4**: 220–229.

CHAPTER 23

Thrombus-Containing Lesions

Giovanni Luigi De Maria and Adrian P. Banning

Oxford Heart Centre, Oxford University Hospitals, John Radcliffe Hospital, Oxford, UK

Atherosclerotic plaque disruption is a key event in the pathophysiology of acute coronary syndromes (ACS). Plaque erosion and rupture are identified as potential mechanisms associated with atherosclerotic plaque instability [1] and result in the exposure to the bloodstream of plaque components and procoagulant molecules. Subsequent intraluminal activation of the coagulative cascade results in platelet activation and formation of blood clot and thrombus [2].

Intraluminal thrombus is probably a universal feature of ACS as it is predominantly responsible for the accelerated process of vessel occlusion or subocclusion that characterizes the spectrum of ACS, from ST elevation ACS to non-ST-elevation ACS. However, the prevalence of thrombus-containing lesions identifiable on angiography varies across the spectrum of coronary syndromes from 5–17 % in patients with stable angina [3–5], to 75–90% [3–5] in patients with unstable angina or non-ST-elevation ACS [5,6], and almost 100% patients with ST-elevation myocardial infarction (STEMI).

Understanding the potential hazards that can be encountered when treating thrombotic lesions is crucial and being familiar with the strategies to deal with thrombus-containing lesion is mandatory for an interventional cardiologist.

Initial management requires:

1 Recognition of the presence of thrombus and its quantification.
2 Understanding that a thrombus-containing lesion is unpredictable and prone to sudden evolution; during the course of the procedure an apparent type A lesion with TIMI flow 3 can rapidly evolve into a blocked vessel with TIMI flow 0 and consequent hemodynamic deterioration.
3 Understanding that thrombus and debris deriving from the disrupted unstable plaque can embolize distally downstream of the coronary microcirculation, blunting the benefit of revascularization.
4 Being aware that thrombotic lesions are usually associated with high vascular tone and this, together with the presence of thrombotic debris, presents challenges to optimal stent sizing, with consequent increased risks of stent underexpansion and/or malapposition.

Consequently, the approach to achieving a successful interventional outcome for a patient with thrombus-containing lesion requires "recognition and a cautious respect to minimize distal embolization and optimize flow." This chapter describes an interventional approach to managing thrombus-containing coronary lesions. Advice on the adjunctive pharmacologic management of thrombotic lesions is detailed in Chapters 41–42.

How to deal with thrombus-containing lesions

Access site

When dealing with thrombus-containing lesions, selection of vascular access site is critical, especially in the setting of STEMI. There is no doubt that the radial approach is the preferred strategy for any interventional procedure and this has been confirmed recently by demonstration of a mortality benefit associated with a lower risk of bleeding with a radial than a femoral approach [7–9]. This benefit is especially evident in the acute setting with the potential requirement for potent antiplatelet agents (e.g., GP IIb/IIIa inhibitors).

When faced with the potential restrictions of the radial route, especially in smaller female patients, patients with arterial spasm, or complex tortuous anatomies with radial loops or remnants [10], options include sheathless guiding catheters [11], or balloon-assisted tracking to deal with radial artery spasm. This allows access to the aortic root with a 6 Fr guiding catheter without needing to downsize to 5 Fr [12]. Starting the procedure with a 5 Fr guiding catheter precludes the possibility of performing thrombus aspiration in most left coronary cases (occasionally a 5 Fr guide can be used in the right coronary as a thrombus aspiration device). Switching to a femoral approach should be undertaken when the balance of risk favors this approach.

Identification of thrombus

Identification and quantification of thrombus are extremely important as they tailor the appropriate management in terms of adjunctive pharmacotherapy and adjunctive mechanical devices to minimize the occurrence of distal embolization. Recognizing that we are dealing with a thrombus-containing lesion is usually straightforward based on the clinical presentation and angiography. Sometimes, however, distinguishing thrombus and calcium on angiography alone can be challenging. Troponin elevation prior to arrival in the catheter laboratory, suggesting ongoing myocardial damage, can be considered to be a marker of possible thrombotic burden but there are situations in which troponin negative patients

Interventional Cardiology: Principles and Practice, Second Edition. Edited by George D. Dangas, Carlo Di Mario, and Nicholas N. Kipshidze.
© 2017 John Wiley & Sons, Ltd. Published 2017 by John Wiley & Sons, Ltd.

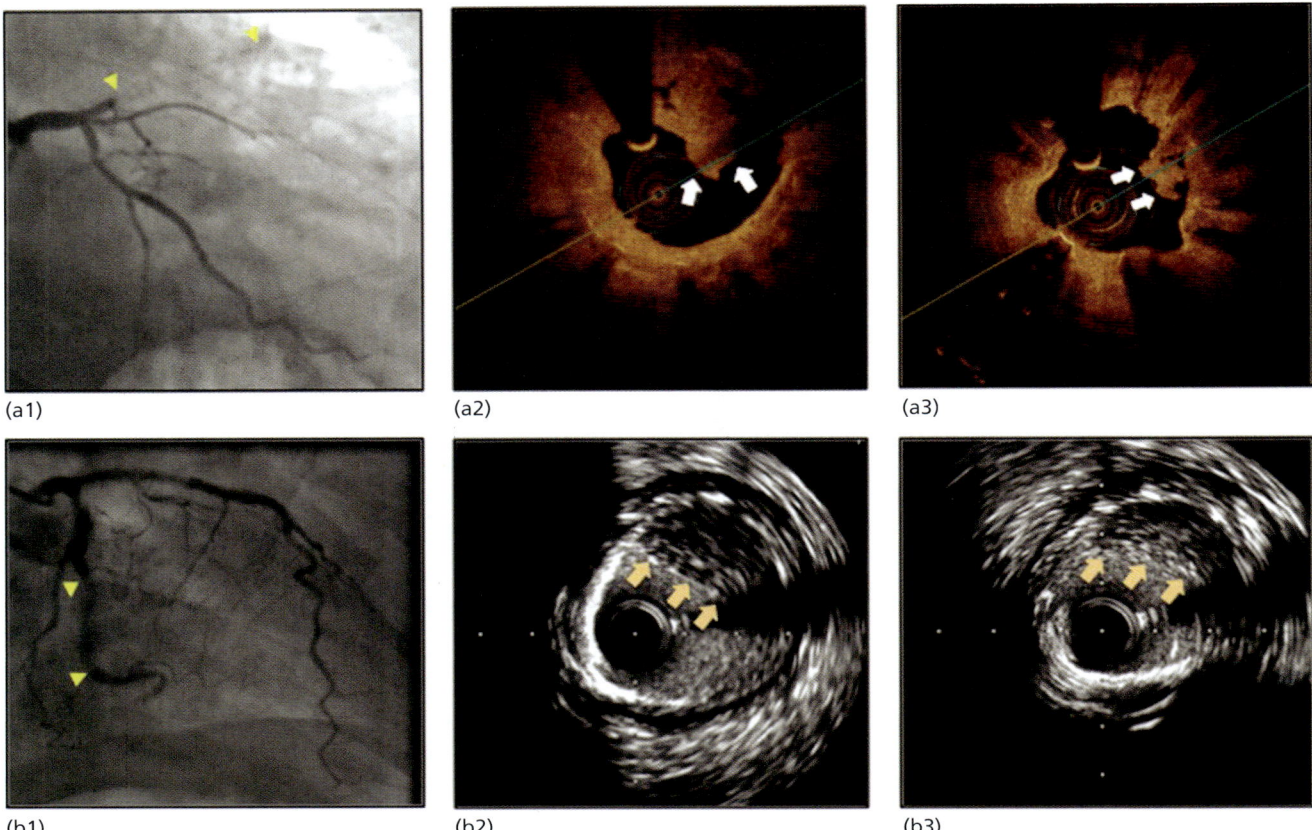

Figure 23.1 Two examples of stent thrombosis. Panels a1, b1 show the variable appearance of thrombus at coronary angiogram. In panel a1 the vessel is completely occluded at the site of the old stent (edges highlighted by yellow arrowheads) with TIMI 0 flow. In panel b1 blood flow is maintained but there is a clear area of haziness at the site of the stent (yellow arrowheads). Panels a2, a3 provide the OCT appearance of the thrombotic lesion with clear and well detailed identification of the thrombotic material protruding toward the lumen (white arrows). The lack of shadowing confirms the possible "young" age of the thrombus, which looks like a white thrombus. Panels b2, b3 provide the intravenous ultrasound (IVUS) appearance of the thrombotic lesion. The lower spatial resolution of IVUS accounts for a less detailed definition of the thrombotic material, appearing as a low echogenic (black) area (pale yellow arrows). Compared with optical coherence tomography (OCT), the highest penetration of the ultrasound accounts for the better visualization of the whole vessel wall behind the thrombotic material.

can have considerable thrombus demonstrable by angiography, as for example in patients with degenerate vein grafts.

Thrombus identification on angiography is considered routine but operators should remember that angiography has only 26% sensitivity in predicting the presence of thrombus [5,13]. Thrombotic lesions are usually identified on angiography as an area of vessel filling defect or vessel haziness during contrast injection. Thrombus can cause different degrees of vessel stenosis and blood flow impairment, and it is possible to find vessel occlusion with TIMI flow 0 or alternatively a normal flow in a non-diseased vessel and an imposed area of haziness corresponding to adherent thrombotic material. When this type of angiographic appearance occurs in the absence of atherosclerosis a potential embolic pathogenesis associated with atrial fibrillation or paradoxical embolism should be considered.

A useful method to quantify coronary thrombus on angiography is represented by the Thrombus Score, proposed by Sianos *et al.* [14]. Five classes are described with progressively increasing gravity: grade 0 corresponds to no angiographic evidence of thrombotic material; grade 1 is possible thrombus, appearing as a convex hazy lesion with irregular contours; grade 2 is definite thrombus ≤1/2 the vessel diameter; grade 3 is definite thrombus >1/2 but <2 vessel diameters; grade 4 is definite thrombus ≥2 vessel diameters; grade 5

is inability of thrombus burden assessment, also after guidewire passage, for persistence of TIMI flow 0.

Intracoronary intravascular ultrasound (IVUS) and optical coherence tomography (OCT) have higher sensitivity and specificity than angiography and allow better thrombus definition, quantification, and characterization. Historically, care was needed when using intracoronary imaging for thrombotic lesions but this is now usually safe. However, in cases of massive thrombus, high quality interpretable images are not possible unless anterograde coronary flow is established.

The high spatial resolution of OCT (Figure 23.1) allows the most detailed definition of thrombus, appearing as a mass attached to luminal surface or floating within the lumen, and even makes possible the discrimination between red and white thrombus [15]. Red thrombus has high backscatter and high attenuation while white (platelet-rich) thrombus has less backscatter, is homogeneous, and has low attenuation. Besides qualitative assessment, OCT offers the possibility for an accurate quantitative assessment of thrombotic burden; a number of classification criteria have been proposed [16–19]. Additionally, OCT can detect mechanical issues associated with stent thrombosis [20]. Both case series and studies have showed the high sensitivity and specificity of OCT in detecting stent malapposition, stent underexpansion, incomplete strut coverage, and new atherosclerosis, thus providing information about the pathophysiology of early and late stent thrombosis. This is especially useful when excluding pharmacologic issues, such as non-response or early interruption of antiplatelet drugs [21,22]. Consequently, OCT should currently be considered the imaging modality of choice when investigating the mechanisms of stent thrombosis.

Although OCT has the best spatial resolution, IVUS has the advantage of providing detail about the vessel wall behind the thrombus. However, identifying fresh thrombus on IVUS can be challenging especially when flow is slow and thus careful examination of images is recommended. Compared to infrared light, ultrasound can penetrate thrombus, which appears as a non-homogenous hypoechogenic (dark) intraluminal area, overlying the vessel wall inner surface which can be completely assessed [23]. It must be noted that organized thrombus usually appears more echogenic (gray–white) and can be difficult to differentiate from intimal hyperplasia or fibrous plaque. According to its collagen content it can produce an acoustic shadow making the thrombus hard to distinguish from fibrous plaque.

Routine intravascular imaging techniques are not recommended when dealing with thrombotic lesions but can be useful in the following situations:

1 Mismatch between clinical presentation and the angiographic appearance. Is this thrombus or calcium?
2 Uncertain non-obstructive or partially obstructive angiographic plaque appearance.
3 Exact thrombotic burden quantification for research purposes.
4 Optimizing difficult stent sizing.

Wiring

Conventional workhorse guidewires are usually considered as first choice for wiring the vast majority of thrombus-containing lesions, especially in situations in which coronary anatomy downstream to the culprit lesion is unknown because of vessel occlusion.

A first attempt to pass a wire is useful to "feel" the lesion typology, facilitating the initial discrimination of fresh thrombus from old thrombus and/or a thrombus-containing lesion from a chronic total occlusion. Particular care must be taken when approaching the thrombotic lesions with the guidewire. The wire might (i) be occlusive to flow; (ii) disrupt the unstable plaque with possible dissection; or (iii) dislodge the overlying thrombus downstream with possible vessel occlusion from distal embolization. The general rule "never let the guidewire come back from a safe position distally to the target lesion" is especially valid when dealing with thrombotic lesions.

When a first attempt at wiring using a workhorse guidewire has failed it is usual to step up to a hydrophilic guidewire. The hydrophilic coating reduces friction significantly increasing the trackability, making such guidewires helpful tools in localizing channels through the thrombus or to negotiate the true lumen in cases of dissection. Recommendations in handling this type of guidewire are no different from those applied in the context of non-thrombotic lesions. The low tactile sense associated with this typology of guidewires favours subintimal passage, coronary dissection, or perforation. For these reasons, (i) these wires should be handled by experienced operators; (ii) tip wire position should always be tested with contrast injection before moving to the next step of the procedure, and (iii) ideally, whenever it is possible and safe, these guidewires should be exchanged with a workhorse guidewire before moving to the next stage of the procedure.

To confirm wire position when TIMI flow is still 0 or becomes 0 after guidewire passage, an easy approach is to gently advance a low profile deflated balloon and to reassess. Subsequently, if there is persistent uncertainty, a second approach with a microcatheter (FinecrossMG, Terumo, Japan; or Corasir, Asahi Intecc Co., Japan) can be used to visualize the distal portion of the coronary tree, thus confirming the position of the guidewire which can then be replaced with a workhorse wire.

Lesion preparation

The most serious complication during treatment of thrombus-containing lesions is the occurrence of distal embolization of athero-thrombotic material with consequent microvascular obstruction and no-reflow phenomenon. Consequently, despite evolution in practice, thrombus-containing lesions continue to be associated with poor procedural results and higher rates of death, myocardial infarction, arrhythmic complications, and the need for urgent revascularization [24].

It has been demonstrated that thrombus manipulation during balloon angioplasty and stenting is associated with the "cheese grater" effect, leading to thrombus detachment and downstream washout of athero-thrombotic debris [25].

Thrombus debulking can be achieved by two approaches: pharmacologic and mechanic. These strategies are not mutually exclusive, but can have an additive effect, especially in the setting of large myocardial infarction [26,27]. The first approach relies mainly on GP IIb/IIIa inhibitors and is dealt in detail in Chapter 42. The second strategy consists of mechanical prevention of distal embolization by either: (i) balloon and/or filter protection devices aiming to trap debris liberated during predilation/stenting; or (ii) thrombectomy, aiming to directly remove the thrombotic material from the lesion site.

Proximal and distal protection devices

There are currently three main types of balloon and filter protection devices [28]:

1 Distal occlusion devices (Percusurge, Medtronic, Santa Rosa, CA, USA; TriActiv system, Kensey Nash, Exton, PA, USA).
2 Distal filters (FilterWire EX, Boston Scientific, Natick, MA, USA; SpiderRX and SpiderFX, ev3 Inc., Plymouth, MN, USA).
3 Proximal occlusion devices (Proxis (St. Jude Medical, St. Paul, MN, USA).

Distal occlusion devices mainly consist of a balloon inflated distally to the thrombotic lesion soon after the passage of the guidewire. In this way debris dislodged during predilation and stenting phases will be prevented from reaching the coronary microcirculation by the inflated balloon. The debris is then aspirated before the distal balloon is deflated. The main advantages of these devices are their relatively smaller profile (usually 0.026–0.033 inch) and their theoretical ability to trap most debris including small particles and even soluble matter. Conversely, the main drawbacks are (i) the prolonged ischemia associated to distal occlusion during their application; (ii) the risk of proximal side branch embolization; (iii) inability to visualize the target vessel distally to the occlusive device; and (iv) potential inability to aspirate debris located at the fornices of the inflated balloon [28].

Distal filters consist of baskets placed distally to the lesion with the intention to trap debris liberated during predilation and stenting. At the end of the procedure, the filter packed with athero-thrombotic debris is retrieved by means of a "filter retriever." The main advantages offered by filter devices are their ease of use, the possibility of preserving distal perfusion during the adoption, and the possibility of keeping visualization of the target vessel distally to the filter device during the procedure. The main limitations of filter devices consist in the larger profile of the sheath (0.040–0.050 inch) needed to keep the filter folded during the crossing of the target lesion with consequent risk of dislodgement of athero-thrombotic debris. The larger profile may eventually require a gentle predilation before the deployment of the device with increased risk of distal embolization. Compared with distal occlusive devices, filter devices are prone to the passage of distal emboli (especially if small in size, e.g., <100 µm) through filter pores or between the filter and the vessel wall if the filter is not completely apposed to the vessel wall [28].

Finally, proximal occlusion devices consist of a balloon inflated proximally to the lesion, thus blocking blood flow and thus the driving force washing athero-thrombotic debris toward the coronary microvasculature. Proximal protection offers theoretical advantages over distal protection including the ability to protect the distal vascular bed without first crossing the lesion with a bulky device, which may itself cause distal embolization. Additionally, some vessels are not suitable for distal protection systems because of the lack of an appropriate "landing zone" for the device, because of tortuosity, plaque disease, or both.

Of all these protection devices, only distal filters are regularly used in clinical practice. Their adoption has been established in percutaneous coronary intervention (PCI) on saphenous vein grafts [29,30], because randomized trials failed to show a clinical benefit in PCI on native vessels [31,32]. Embolization during device deployment, a delay to PCI due to device deployment, and "filter no-reflow" occurrence have been claimed as possible mechanisms explaining the failure of filters in PCI on native vessels [28,33].

Thrombectomy

Theoretically, reduction of thrombus burden by thrombectomy should (i) prevent the risk of distal embolization; (ii) improve a better visualization of the atherosclerotic lesion; (iii) improve the evaluation of vessel size; (iv) favor direct stenting; (v) prevent stent malapposition, after disappearance of the thrombus initially located between the stent struts and the vessel wall [34].

Two main kinds of thrombectomy devices are available: manual (or aspiration) and mechanical. In manual thrombectomy devices, thrombus aspiration is obtained by application of a suction force exerted by the operator. In mechanical devices, aspirating force is produced by specific device-related mechanisms.

Manual thrombectomy

Manual thrombus aspiration devices consist of 6 Fr compatible dual lumen catheters. The smaller lumen is used to deliver the device over a conventional 0.014 inch guidewire over a short monorail rapid exchange system. The larger lumen presents one or more distal apertures and is connected to a Luer lock syringe. By creating a vacuum in the Luer lock syringe a negative pressure is produced leading to aspiration of thrombotic material while crossing the lesion site. Figure 23.2 summarizes the main steps for the preparation of the thrombus aspiration catheter.

A successful manual thrombectomy is performed by: (i) aspirating while crossing the thrombus; (ii) performing multiple passes across the target thrombus; and (iii) aspirating while withdrawing the aspiration catheter back into the guiding catheter. Aspirating while crossing the thrombus reduces the risk of distal embolization, conversely aspirating during withdrawal prevents the risk that the

aspirated thrombus is lost downstream in the coronary artery or, even worse, in the aorta (Figure 23.3). For this reason a deep intubation of the guiding catheter during thrombus aspiration catheter withdrawal, and complete clearance of the guiding catheter (by blood aspiration and/or by blood back-spilling through the open valve of the Y connector) before proceeding to contrast injection are recommended. The optimal number of aspiration passes is debated but theoretically at least three passes are recommended. It is possible that the amount of residual thrombus detected by intravascular imaging could be a guide in the decision to make additional catheter passes [35].

Two parameters determine the efficacy of a manual thrombectomy: deliverability and aspiration rate. The main technical characteristics of manual thrombus aspiration catheters available on the market are summarized in Figure 23.4. The catheter deliverability depends on catheter pushability and trackability and on coronary anatomy (tortuosity, calcifications, and vessel size). Hydrophilic coating, metallic braided shaft, or metallic stylet have been applied to the most recent generation of thrombectomy catheters to improve their trackability and pushability.

Aspiration rate is expressed by the formula: $\Delta P\pi r4/8\,\mu L$ [36,37]. The aspiration rate is thus affected positively by the depression created by the Luer lock syringe (ΔP) and by the minimum radius of the aspiration catheter (r). Conversely, high thrombus viscosity (μ) and aspiration catheter length (L) negatively affect the aspiration rate. It is thus clear that larger lumen aspiration catheters are more effective at the expense of difficult application in thrombotic lesions located in small vessels. Similarly, thrombus aspiration performance can be hampered in very old, organized, and high viscous thrombi. It possible to hypothesize that modification of thrombus viscosity might improve the efficacy of thrombus aspiration, for example by local injection of GP IIb/IIIa inhibitors through dedicated a delivery device (Clearway RX, Atrium Medical, Hudson, NH, USA; Amicath, IHT, Spain) or through the thrombectomy catheter itself [17].

A drawback of aspiration catheters is the ability to extract thrombotic material from the region of the vessel closer to the tip of the device. It is logical to think that the aspiration performance is affected by the distance of the thrombotic material from the tip of the device itself. The position of the catheter within the lumen is definitely affected by the position of the guidewire and thus the "bias wire" strategy can help to improve aspiration efficacy. This technique consists of changing the position of the guidewire toward a side branch [38], thus changing the position of the thrombus aspiration catheter itself, eventually facilitating closer position of its tip toward the thrombotic lesion. Intravascular imaging helps to guide this maneuver by showing very high residual thrombotic burden after the first thrombus aspiration pass and thus favoring a further thrombectomy pass after the guidewire position has been changed.

Although they are user-friendly devices, manual thrombus aspiration catheters are associated with several complications: (i) coronary spasm; (ii) distal embolization during crossing; (iii) dissection; (iv) perforation; and (v) proximal displacement of thrombus with potential embolization down to previously unaffected arteries [39].

After the first studies ascertaining the benefit of manual thrombectomy in terms of myocardial reperfusion (assessed by ST resolution, myocardial blush grade (MBG) [40–45], contrast echocardiography [46,47], and cardiac magnetic resonance [48]), it was the TAPAS trial that suggested a potential benefit in terms

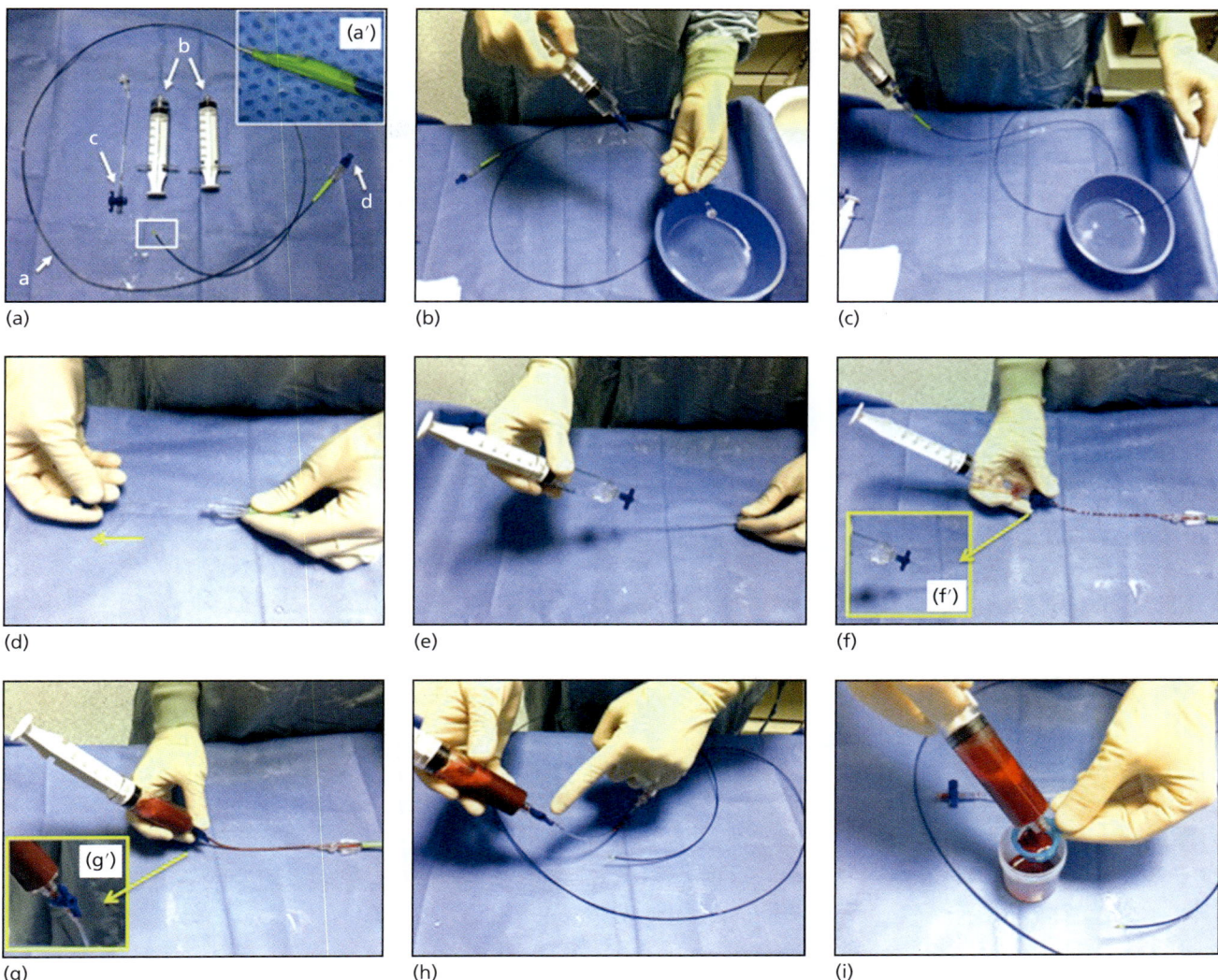

Figure 23.2 The preparation of a thrombus aspiration catheter (Export Advance, Medtronic in the example). (a) Elements of the manual thrombus aspiration system (a, thrombus aspiration catheter; b, Luer lock syringes; c, extension tube with one-way-tap; d, stylet [specifically of the Export Advance system]). (a'). Detail of thrombus aspiration catheter tip. (b, c) Flushing tube extension and aspiration catheter. (d) Once the aspiration catheter is placed at the site of the target lesion the stylet is removed (this step is to be considered only for aspiration catheter with stylet). (e, f) Luer lock syringe is connected and vacuum is made. (f'): Detail of the one-way-tap orientation in this stage. (g) By opening the one-way tap aspiration is started. (g'): Detail of the one-way-tap orientation during aspiration. (h) At the end of the aspiration the catheter is retrieved keeping the one-way tap open in order to maintain aspiration during the withdrawal. (i) The syringe is emptied into the filter and debris collection can be assessed.

of long-term mortality leading to a change in the guidelines. More recently, the TASTE trial failed to show a clear benefit from *routine* manual thrombectomy in a larger population of 7244 patients with STEMI [49]. Notably, 40% of potential patients were excluded and up to two-thirds of patients presented with a low thrombotic burden and all-cause mortality was the primary endpoint. The recently published results of the larger TOTAL study conducted on 10,063 patients confirmed a lack of benefit from routine manual thrombus aspiration [50]. In line with the previous smaller trial, the TOTAL trial detected a benefit of thrombectomy in terms of soft endpoints like ST resolution and occurrence of distal embolization; however, the trial showed no difference in major adverse cardiac event (MACE) rate at 180 days in patients

treated with thrombectomy compared with those receiving PCI alone [50]. Even if a longer follow-up is needed before drawing definite conclusions, it is evident that both the TASTE and TOTAL studies highlight the need for a more accurate use of thrombectomy. Accordingly, the recent European guidelines recommend manual thrombectomy only in selected patients: those with clear evidence of high thrombotic burden and feasible coronary anatomy [51].

Mechanical thrombectomy

With mechanical thrombectomy devices the thrombus is first lysed before extraction. Thrombus lysis is achieved through different mechanisms according to the device adopted.

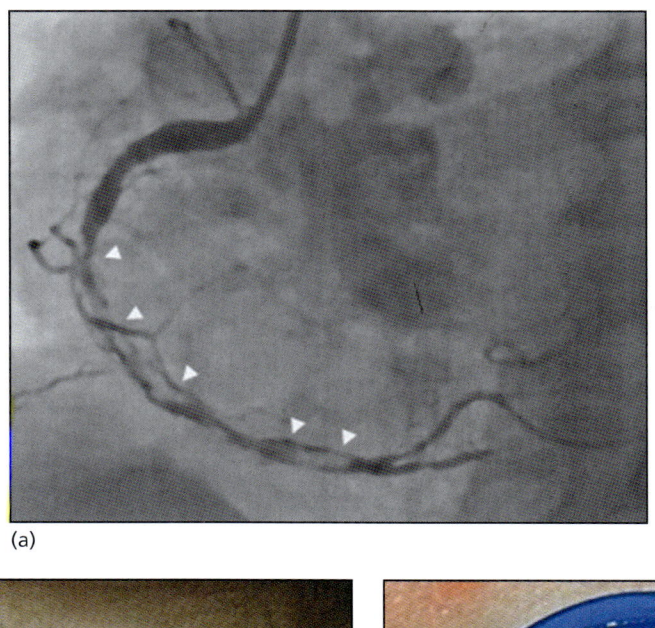

(a)

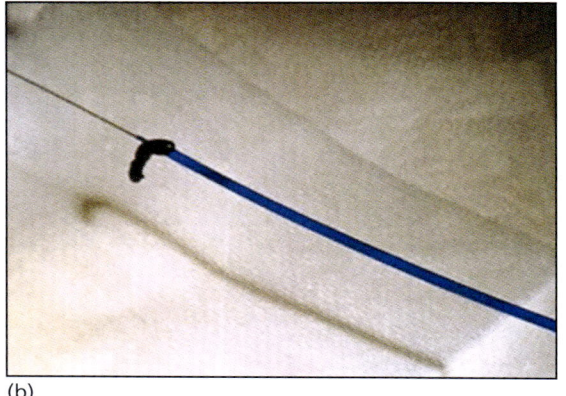

(b)

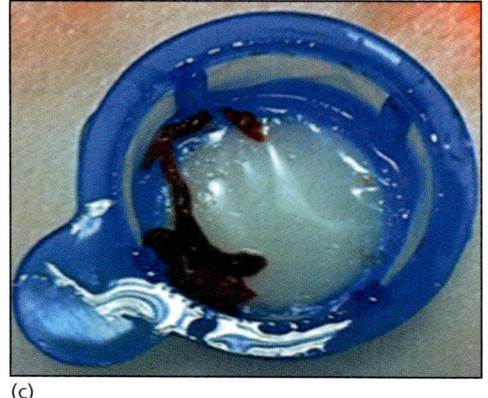

(c)

Figure 23.3 Keeping aspiration maintaining a negative pressure in the Luer lock syringe is essential during withdrawal of the aspiration catheter. In this case, manual thrombus aspiration was performed in a very highly thrombotic lesion of the right coronary artery (a). During the first pass with the thrombus aspiration catheter, blood back-spilling in the syringe stopped relatively soon. The thrombus aspiration catheter was then withdrawn and a large amount of thrombotic debris attached to the tip of the aspiration catheter was observed (b). Withdrawing the aspiration catheter maintaining aspiration was crucial in this case, preventing the embolization of thrombotic debris. For safety reasons the guiding catheter was replaced with a new one and further passes with a new thrombus aspiration catheter were performed retrieving a very large amount of thrombotic material (c).

The X-Sizer (ev3 Inc., Plymouth, MN, USA) is an over-the-wire dual-channeled catheter with a spinning helical tip in the first channel, which fragments the thrombus. At the same time, a miniature vacuum system in the second channel removes the debris created.

The AngioJet rheolytic thrombectomy System (Possis Medical, Inc. Minneapolis, MN, USA) makes use of the Venturi effect to remove thrombus. Saline is injected at high pressure through small steel tubing by an external pump, creating an area of low pressure around the jet, which pulls surrounding blood, including thrombus, into the catheter.

The ThromCat XT (Kensey Nash, Exton, PA, USA) combines flushing via three ports at the distal tip, with powerful suction from five ports, with a helix spinning at 95,000 rpm macerating the thrombus retrieved.

The Rinspiration System (Kerberos Proximal Solutions Inc., Sunnyvale, CA, USA) employs simultaneous irrigation and aspiration of the vessel to remove thrombus by three lumens: a 25 cm monorail wire lumen allows passage over a standard 0.014 inch coronary guidewire, a second lumen for aspiration, and a third lumen for injection of saline through perforations located proximal to the aspiration lumen.

Mechanical thrombectomy devices have a theoretical advantage of better thrombus extraction and greater profiles, but lower flexibility and steeper learning curve are their main weak points. Furthermore, the high risk of device stent-entrapment observed for the X-Sizer has led to the withdraw of this device from the market. Randomized trials directly comparing manual with mechanical aspiration have reported no differences between the two approaches in terms of MACE, but highlighting a higher

		Aspiration rate		Trackability/pushability			
	Guide-catheter compatibility	Distal extraction area	Proximal extraction area	Hydrophilic coating	Braided coiled shaft	Stylet	Buddy-wire compatibility
Export AP *Medtronic*	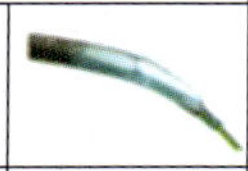 6F	0.87 mm^2	0.85 mm^2	Yes	Yes	No	No
Export advanced *Medtronic*	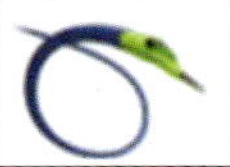 6F	0.93 mm^2	0.98 mm^2	Yes	Yes	Yes	Yes
Hunter *IHT Cordynamic*	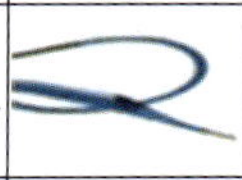 6F	0.95 mm^2	1.04 mm^2	Yes	Yes	No	No
Vmax *Stron Medical*	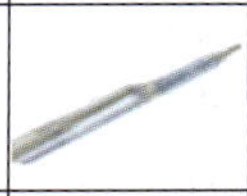 6F (available 5F compatible)	0.95 mm^2	0.95 mm^2	Yes	No	Yes	No
Drive CE *Invatec Medtronic*	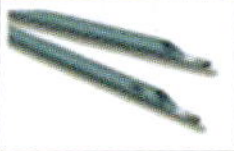 6F	1.12 mm^2	0.77 mm^2	Yes	No	No	No
Eliminate *Terumo*	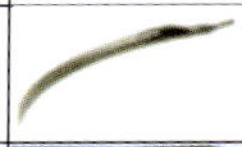 6F	0.79 mm^2	0.95 mm^2	Yes	Yes	Yes	Yes
ProntoV3 *Vascular Solutions*	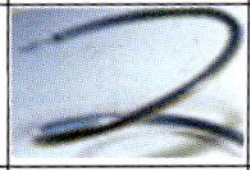 6F	0.90 mm^2	0.90 mm^2	Yes	Yes	No	No
Quick cat *Spectranetics*	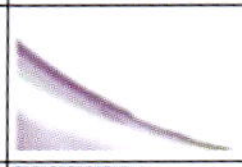 6F	0.87 mm^2	0.75 mm^2	Yes	No	No	No
ThrombusterII *Kaneka Medics*	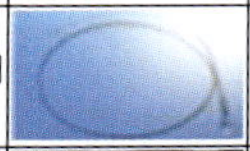 6F	0.78 mm^2	0.95 mm^2	Yes	No	Yes	No
Fetch2 *Boston Scientific*	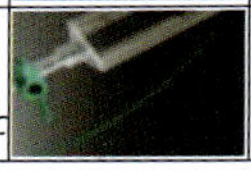 6F	---- mm^2	---- mm^2	Yes	Yes	No	No

Figure 23.4 Summary of the main technical characteristics of the manual thrombus aspiration catheters available on the market. The technical characteristics are grouped according their influence on aspiration rate and trackability/pushability, which are the two main parameters determining the performance of a manual thrombus aspiration device.

rate of successful deployment with the manual thrombectomy devices [52,53].

Consequently, mechanical thrombus aspiration has a niche role in very thrombotic lesions; for example, in patients with large thrombus burden located at the site of very ectatic segments where, for obvious "geographic" reasons, the performance of conventional manual aspiration catheters is expected to be limited (Figure 23.5).

Excimer laser

Excimer laser coronary angioplasty (ELCA) is used to reduce thrombotic burden. The system consists of an excimer laser generator (CVX-300, Spectranetics, CO, USA) and a pulsed xenon-chlorine laser catheter (available diameters 0.9, 1.4, 1.7, and 2.0 mm). The laser catheter delivers excimer energy (wavelength 308 nm, pulse length 185 ns) with a fluence (energy per surface unit) ranging from 30 to 80 mJ/mm^2 and a pulse repetition rate ranging 25–80 Hz. Fluence and pulse repetition rate are parameters that the operator can modify to improve the performance according to the characteristics of the target lesion.

A safe and effective laser photo-ablation strategy requires attention to the three "S's": size, slow, and saline. In other words, (i) it is crucial to choose a laser catheter correctly sized to the target vessel diameter; (ii) the catheter must be advanced slowly; and (iii) constant saline flushing at the tip of the catheter during its advancement is required. Saline infusion guarantees that blood and contrast dye are cleared from the tip of the catheter. Blood and contrast dye can absorb the energy delivered by the catheter and favor the development of microbubbles with increased risk of vessel dissection.

The excimer laser produces vaporization of the thrombus through three mechanisms: photochemical, photothermal, and photomechanical [54]. The photochemical action is the result of UV light hitting the tissue at a rate of up to 125 billions per second, with a 50 μm penetration, and leading to billions of molecular bonds fractured per second. The photothermal effect derives from absorption of energy by the thrombus, with consequent molecular vibration and heating and vaporization of intracellular water, ultimately ending in cellular rupture and thrombus disruption by vapor bubbles. Finally, the photomechanical effect derives from

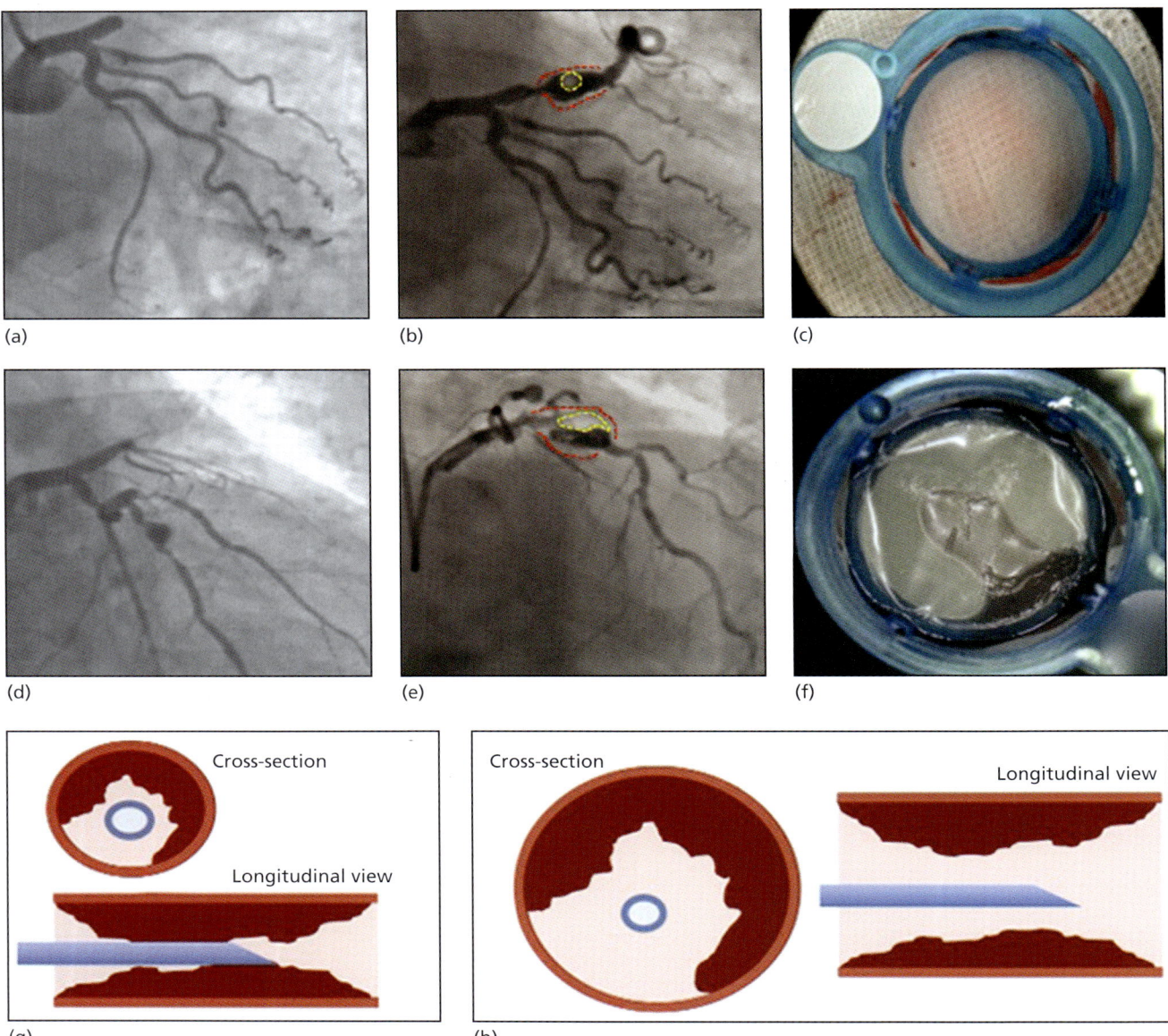

Figure 23.5 Ectatic and aneurismatic coronary segments represent an anatomic scenario in which performance of manual thrombus aspiration can be suboptimal for evident "geographic" reason. (a, b) and (d, e) show two examples of patients with anterior ST-elevation myocardial infarction (STEMI), with culprit lesion located at the site of a large aneurimatic segment containing a large amount of thrombus. The dotted red lines detect the contours of the aneurism, while the dotted yellow lines detect the contours of the thrombotic material. Manual thrombus aspiration was performed in both cases with retrieve of no thrombus in the filter (c, f). In normal vessels (g) the manual aspiration catheter is able to get in touch with the thrombus, with higher probability of removing both thrombus hanging in the lumen as "parietal" thrombus adherent to vessel wall. In large ectatic/aneurismatic segments a geographic miss because of the large dimension of the vessel accounts for the lower ability of the manual aspiration catheter to reach thrombotic debris, especially when adherent to the vessel wall (h). For this reason thrombus-containing lesions at the site of ectatic/aneurimatic segments could be a scenario for a possible application of mechanical thrombus aspiration devices, known to have a theoretically higher thrombus aspiration capacity.

the vibration and collapse of vapor bubbles mechanically breaking down the target tissue. Excimer laser adopts light in the UV range and spectroscopy analysis on thrombus reveals how excimer wavelength is ideally suited for absorption by the fresh thrombus [55], to the point that a "platelet stunning" action has been described,

resulting in a local, direct, and inhibitory effect on platelet aggregation kinetics [56].

In the CARMEL study, the excimer laser has been tested in a population of 151 patients with myocardial infarction resulting in an improvement of both residual stenosis and flow rate. Interestingly, the greater benefit from laser application was observed in patients with larger thrombotic burden [57]. Encouraging results have also been described in terms of improved reperfusion assessed by TIMI flow and MBG in patients with myocardial infarction treated with excimer laser [58].

Stenting

Stenting, with or without post-dilatation, is usually the final step of the revascularization procedure. It has a recommendation IA according to the current guidelines for the treatment of patients with both non-ST-segment elevation ACS and STEMI and thus also with thrombotic lesions [51].

Considerations during stent deployment include: (i) stent sizing, as undersizing with consequent malapposition is possible in the acute vasospastic environment; and (ii) the process of stent expansion is associated with increased risk of distal embolization. In order to minimize the risk of distal embolization associated with stenting, two modifications are currently under consideration. The first is deferring stenting in the acute phase, especially in the setting of STEMI and the second is the use of dedicated mesh stents.

Some studies have reported the feasibility and safety of a deferring stent strategy with restoration of TIMI flow by balloon dilatation or thrombectomy alone [59], which demonstrated a lower final infarct size in some patients with STEMI [60]. This approach needs to be tested in larger randomized clinical trials, but should be considered when thrombosis is evident on chronic or severe calcific lesions. In these cases, deferring stenting for a staged rotablation-assisted PCI or excimer laser should be considered.

Beside the deferring stent approach, evidence is also growing in favour of stents designed to reduce the occurrence of distal embolization. The MGuard (InspireMD, Tel Aviv, Israel) is a newly developed metal stent designed to trap the athero-thrombotic debris behind a polyethylene-terephthalate mesh anchored to the external surface of the struts. So far the stent has shown positive results for soft endpoints such as final TIMI flow and MBG, while no differences have observed in terms of mortality or MACE rate compared to conventional bare metal stents [61].

Conclusions

In the treatment of thrombus-containing lesions, each step of the procedure, from access selection to stenting, is of crucial importance and requires clear planning and understanding of the underlying coronary anatomy and lesion characteristics. A large armamentarium of drugs and devices is available for the interventional cardiologist; however, as the TASTE trial demonstrates, indiscriminate adoption of every technique in every patient is not to be recommended. Consequently, identification of the subset of patients at higher risk of suboptimal final result that might benefit from additional or alternative strategies is desirable and this represents the new challenge in the treatment of thrombus-containing lesions.

📖 Case study

A 50-year-old man with no previous past cardiologic history presented with anterior STEMI. Coronary angiogram confirmed acute occlusion of large left anterior descending (LAD) (Figure 23.6a). After wiring, thrombus aspiration was performed and TIMI 3 flow was restored (b). Predilatation was then performed with 2.0×15 mm (c), 2.5×15 mm (d) semi-compliant balloons and even 3.0×15 (e) and 3.5×15 mm non-compliant balloons inflated at high pressure (up to 20 atmospheres). In all cases, however, a complete inflation of the balloon (highlighted by yellow arrows in c, d, and e) was impossible to achieve because of possible high calcific burden. After a failed attempt to cross the lesion with a cutting balloon, the patient's clinical condition was reviewed (patient was symptom-free and TIMI 3 flow) and the procedure was stopped. The patient was transferred to the coronary care unit to complete the bivalarudin infusion and continue double antiplatelet therapy with 75 mg aspirin and 90 mg ticagrelor twice daily. A rotablation-assisted PCI to LAD was scheduled within 48 hours from the index procedure.

After 48 hours the patient had a second angiogram as scheduled (f). Before proceeding to rotablation an intravascular imaging with optical coherence tomography (OCT) was performed. OCT was useful because it excluded the presence of high residual thrombotic burden and confirmed the presence of a high calcific burden (g, white arrowheads). Rotablation with a 1.75 mm burr was then performed. Balloon expansion was still limited so rotablation with a 2.00 mm burr was performed allowing a successful predilation with a full expansion of a 3.0×15 mm non-compliant balloon (h). The procedure was then completed with stenting with a 3.5×38 mm drug-eluting stent post-dilated with a 4.0×15 mm non-compliant balloon, achieving a good final angiographic result (i).

The case shows how deferring stenting in the setting of a thrombus-containing lesion is safe and should be considered when even an aggressive predilatation resulted in a suboptimal outcome. In such a scenario, deferring a hemodynamically stable patient with good TIMI flow to a rotablation-assisted PCI after 24–48 hours is a reasonable option. In this case, intravascular imaging not only confirmed the large calcific component of the plaque, but it was also useful in excluding large residual thrombus, thus allowing rotablation to be performed with fewer concerns about the risk of distal embolization.

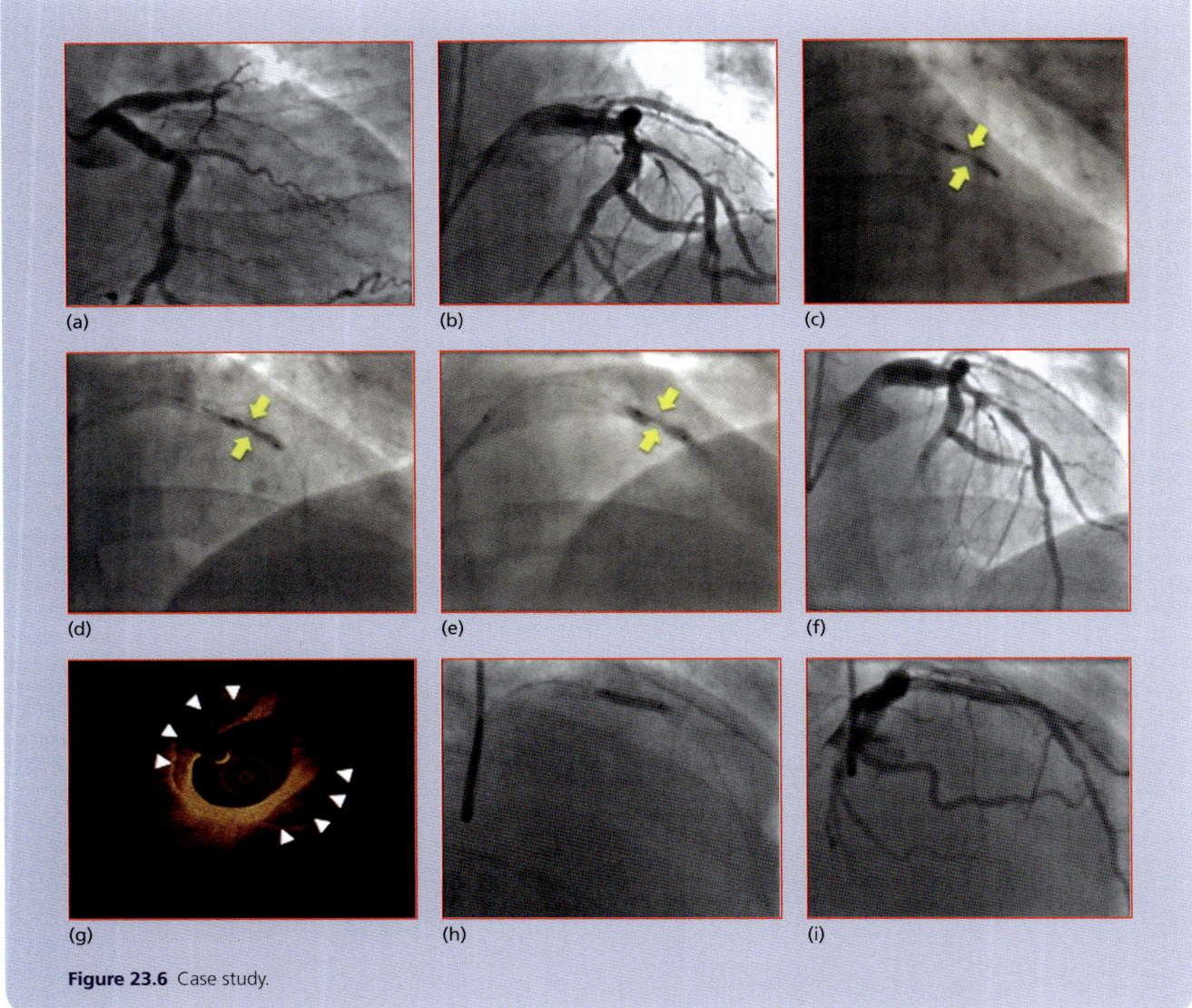

Figure 23.6 Case study.

Interactive multiple choice questions are available for this chapter on www.wiley.com/go/dangas/cardiology

References

1 Arbab-Zadeh A, Nakano M, Virmani R, Fuster V. Acute coronary events. *Circulation* 2012; **125**: 1147–1156.

2 Srikanth S, Ambrose JA. Pathophysiology of coronary thrombus formation and adverse consequences of thrombus during PCI. *Curr Cardiol Rev* 2012; **8**: 169–176.

3 de Feyter PJ, Ozaki Y, Baptista J, *et al.* Ischemia-related lesion characteristics in patients with stable or unstable angina: a study with intracoronary angioscopy and ultrasound. *Circulation* 1995; **92**: 1408–1413.

4 Hussain KM, Gould L, Bharathan T, *et al.* Arteriographic morphology and intracoronary thrombus in patients with unstable angina, non-Q wave myocardial infarction and stable angina pectoris. *Angiology* 1995; **46**: 181–189.

5 White CJ, Ramee SR, Collins TJ, *et al.* Coronary thrombi increase PTCA risk: angioscopy as a clinical tool. *Circulation* 1996; **93**: 253–258.

6 Mizuno K, Miyamoto A, Satomura K, *et al.* Angioscopic coronary macromorphology in patients with acute coronary disorders. *Lancet* 1991; **337**: 809–812.

7 Jolly SS, Yusuf S, Cairns J, *et al.* Radial versus femoral access for coronary angiography and intervention in patients with acute coronary syndromes (RIVAL): a randomised, parallel group, multicentre trial. *Lancet* 2011; **377**: 1409–1420.

8 Romagnoli E, Biondi-Zoccai G, Sciahbasi A, *et al.* Radial versus femoral randomized investigation in ST-segment elevation acute coronary syndrome: the RIFLE-STEACS (Radial Versus Femoral Randomized Investigation in ST-Elevation Acute Coronary Syndrome) study. *J Am Coll Cardiol* 2012; **60**: 2481–2489.

9 Valgimigli M, Gagnor A, Calabro P, *et al.* Radial versus femoral access in patients with acute coronary syndromes undergoing invasive management: a randomised multicentre trial. *Lancet* 2015; **385**: 2465–2476.

10 Burzotta F, Trani C, De Vita M, Crea F. A new operative classification of both anatomic vascular variants and physiopathologic conditions affecting transradial cardiovascular procedures. *Int J Cardiol* 2010; **145**: 120–122.

11 Cheaito R, Benamer H, Hovasse T, *et al.* Feasibility and safety of transradial coronary interventions using a 6.5-F sheathless guiding catheter in patients with small radial arteries: a multicenter registry. *Catheter Cardiovasc Interv* 2015; **86**: 51–58.

12 Pavlidis AN, Karamasis GV, Rees P. Balloon-assisted tracking during primary percutaneous coronary intervention. *Acute Cardiac Care* 2015; **17**: 26–28.

13 Zhao XQ, Théroux P, Snapinn SM, Sax FL. Intracoronary thrombus and platelet glycoprotein IIb/IIIa receptor blockade with tirofiban in unstable angina or non-Q-wave myocardial infarction: angiographic results from the PRISM-PLUS trial (Platelet receptor inhibition for ischemic syndrome management in patients limited by unstable signs and symptoms). *Circulation* 1999; **100**: 1609–1615.

14 Sianos G, Papafaklis MI, Serruys PW. Angiographic thrombus burden classification in patients with ST-segment elevation myocardial infarction treated with percutaneous coronary intervention. *J Invasive Cardiol* 2010; **22**(10 Suppl B): 6B–14B.

15 International Working Group for Intravascular Optical Coherence Tomography (IWG-IVOCT). Consensus standards for acquisition, measurement, and reporting

of intravascular optical coherence tomography studies: a report from the International Working Group for Intravascular Optical Coherence Tomography Standardization and Validation. *J Am Coll Cardiol* 2012; **59**: 1058–1072.

16 Porto I, Mattesini A, Valente S, Prati F, Crea F, Bolognese L. Optical coherence tomography assessment and quantification of intracoronary thrombus: Status and perspectives. *Cardiovasc Revasc Med* 2015; **16**: 172–178.

17 Prati F, Capodanno D, Pawlowski T, et al. Local delivery versus intracoronary infusion of abciximab in patients with acute coronary syndromes. *JACC Cardiovasc Interv* 2010; **3**: 928–934.

18 Onuma Y, Thuesen L, van Geuns RJ, et al. Randomized study to assess the effect of thrombus aspiration on flow area in patients with ST-elevation myocardial infarction: an optical frequency domain imaging study—TROFI trial. *Eur Heart J* 2013; **34**: 1050–1060.

19 Magro M, Regar E, Gutiérrez-Chico JL, et al. Residual atherothrombotic material after stenting in acute myocardial infarction: an optical coherence tomographic evaluation. *Int J Cardiol* 2013; **167**: 656–663.

20 Kang SJ, Lee CW, Song H, et al. OCT analysis in patients with very late stent thrombosis. *JACC Cardiovasc Imaging* 2013; **6**: 695–703.

21 Parodi G, La Manna A, Di Vito L, et al. Stent-related defects in patients presenting with stent thrombosis: differences at optical coherence tomography between subacute and late/very late thrombosis in the Mechanism Of Stent Thrombosis (MOST) study. *EuroIntervention* 2013; **9**: 936–944.

22 Prati F, Kodama T, Romagnoli E, et al. Suboptimal stent deployment is associated with subacute stent thrombosis: optical coherence tomography insights from a multicenter matched study. From the CLI Foundation investigators: the CLI-THRO study. *Am Heart J* 2015; **169**: 249–256.

23 Mintz GS, Nissen SE, Anderson WD, et al. American College of Cardiology Clinical Expert Consensus Document on Standards for Acquisition, Measurement and Reporting of Intravascular Ultrasound Studies (IVUS). A report of the American College of Cardiology Task Force on Clinical Expert Consensus Documents. *J Am Coll Cardiol* 2001; **37**: 1478–1492.

24 Freeman MR, Williams AE, Chisholm RJ, Armstrong PW. Intracoronary thrombus and complex morphology in unstable angina. Relation to timing of angiography and in-hospital cardiac events. *Circulation* 1989; **80**: 17–23.

25 Okamura A, Ito H, Iwakura K, et al. Detection of embolic particles with the Doppler guide wire during coronary intervention in patients with acute myocardial infarction: efficacy of distal protection device. *J Am Coll Cardiol* 2005; **45**: 212–215.

26 Stone GW, Witzenbichler B, Godlewski J, et al. Intralesional abciximab and thrombus aspiration in patients with large anterior myocardial infarction: one-year results from the INFUSE-AMI trial. *Circ Cardiovasc Interv* 2013; **6**: 527–534.

27 Pyxaras SA, Mangiacapra F, Verhamme K, et al. Synergistic effect of thrombus aspiration and abciximab in primary percutaneous coronary intervention. *Catheter Cardiovasc Interv* 2013; **82**: 604–611.

28 Mauri L, Rogers C, Baim DS. Devices for distal protection during percutaneous coronary revascularization. *Circulation* 2006; **113**: 2651–2656.

29 Baim DS, Wahr D, George B, et al. Randomized trial of a distal embolic protection device during percutaneous intervention of saphenous vein aorto-coronary bypass grafts. *Circulation* 2002; **105**: 1285–1290.

30 Stone GW, Rogers C, Hermiller J, et al. Randomized comparison of distal protection with a filter-based catheter and a balloon occlusion and aspiration system during percutaneous intervention of diseased saphenous vein aorto-coronary bypass grafts. *Circulation* 2003; **108**: 548–553.

31 Kelbaek H, Terkelsen CJ, Helqvist S, et al. Randomized comparison of distal protection versus conventional treatment in primary percutaneous coronary intervention: the drug elution and distal protection in ST-elevation myocardial infarction (DEDICATION) trial. *J Am Coll Cardiol* 2008; **51**: 899–905.

32 Haeck JD, Kuijt WJ, Koch KT, et al. Infarct size and left ventricular function in the PRoximal Embolic Protection in Acute myocardial infarction and Resolution of ST-segment Elevation (PREPARE) trial: ancillary cardiovascular magnetic resonance study. *Heart* 2010; **96**: 190–195.

33 Porto I, Belloni F, Niccoli G, et al. Filter no-reflow during percutaneous coronary intervention of saphenous vein grafts: incidence, predictors and effect of the type of protection device. *EuroIntervention* 2011; **7**: 955–961.

34 De Luca G, Verdoia M, Cassetti E. Thrombectomy during primary angioplasty: methods, devices, and clinical trial data. *Curr Cardiol Rep* 2010; **12**: 422–428.

35 Wieringa WG, Lexis CP, Diercks GF, et al. The feasibility of optical coherence tomography guided thrombus aspiration in patients with non-ST-elevation myocardial infarction after initial conservative therapy: a pilot study. *Int J Cardiol* 2013; **168**: 4981–4982.

36 Hara H, Nakamura M, Komatsu H, et al. Comparison of the in vitro performance of 6 and 7 French aspiration catheters. *EuroIntervention* 2007; **2**: 487–492.

37 Rioufol G, Collin B, Vincent-Martin M, et al. Large tube section is the key to successful coronary thrombus aspiration: findings of a standardized bench test. *Catheter Cardiovasc Interv* 2006; **67**: 254–257.

38 Yan W, Ward MR, Nelson G, Figtree GA, Bhindi R. Overcoming limited depth penetration of optical coherence tomography with wire bias. *JACC Cardiovasc Interv* 2012; **5**: e1–e2.

39 Serdoz R, Pighi M, Konstantinidis NV, Kilic ID, Abou-Sherif S, Di Mario C. Thrombus aspiration in primary angioplasty for ST-segment elevation myocardial infarction. *Curr Atheroscler Rep* 2014; **16**: 431.

40 Svilaas T, Vlaar PJ, van der Horst IC, et al. Thrombus aspiration during primary percutaneous coronary intervention. *N Engl J Med* 2008; **358**: 557–567.

41 Dudek D, Mielecki W, Burzotta F, et al. Thrombus aspiration followed by direct stenting: a novel strategy of primary percutaneous coronary intervention in ST-segment elevation myocardial infarction: results of the Polish-Italian-Hungarian RAndomized ThrombEctomy Trial (PIHRATE Trial). *Am Heart J* 2010; **160**: 966–972.

42 Silva-Orrego P, Colombo P, Bigi R, et al. Thrombus aspiration before primary angioplasty improves myocardial reperfusion in acute myocardial infarction: the DEAR-MI (Dethrombosis to Enhance Acute Reperfusion in Myocardial Infarction) study. *J Am Coll Cardiol* 2006; **48**: 1552–1559.

43 Burzotta F, Trani C, Romagnoli E, et al. Manual thrombus-aspiration improves myocardial reperfusion: the randomized evaluation of the effect of mechanical reduction of distal embolization by thrombus-aspiration in primary and rescue angioplasty (REMEDIA) trial. *J Am Coll Cardiol* 2005; **46**(2): 371–376.

44 De Luca L, Sardella G, Davidson CJ, et al. Impact of intracoronary aspiration thrombectomy during primary angioplasty on left ventricular remodelling in patients with anterior ST elevation myocardial infarction. *Heart* 2006; **92**: 951–957.

45 Lipiecki J, Monzy S, Durel N, et al. Effect of thrombus aspiration on infarct size and left ventricular function in high-risk patients with acute myocardial infarction treated by percutaneous coronary intervention: results of a prospective controlled pilot study. *Am Heart J* 2009; **157**: 583.e1–7.

46 Galiuto L, Garramone B, Burzotta F, et al. Thrombus aspiration reduces microvascular obstruction after primary coronary intervention: a myocardial contrast echocardiography substudy of the REMEDIA Trial. *J Am Coll Cardiol* 2006; **48**: 1355–1360.

47 Liistro F, Grotti S, Angioli P, et al. Impact of thrombus aspiration on myocardial tissue reperfusion and left ventricular functional recovery and remodeling after primary angioplasty. *Circ Cardiovasc Interv* 2009; **2**: 376–383.

48 Sardella G, Mancone M, Bucciarelli-Ducci C, et al. Thrombus aspiration during primary percutaneous coronary intervention improves myocardial reperfusion and reduces infarct size: the EXPIRA (thrombectomy with export catheter in infarct-related artery during primary percutaneous coronary intervention) prospective, randomized trial. *J Am Coll Cardiol* 2009; **53**: 309–315.

49 Lagerqvist B, Fröbert O, Olivecrona GK, et al. Outcomes 1 year after thrombus aspiration for myocardial infarction. *N Engl J Med* 2014; **371**: 1111–1120.

50 Jolly SS, Cairns JA, Yusuf S, et al. Randomized trial of primary PCI with or without routine manual thrombectomy. *N Engl J Med* 2015; **372**: 1389–1398.

51 Authors/Task Force members. 2014 ESC/EACTS Guidelines on myocardial revascularization: The Task Force on Myocardial Revascularization of the European Society of Cardiology (ESC) and the European Association for Cardio-Thoracic Surgery (EACTS) Developed with the special contribution of the European Association of Percutaneous Cardiovascular Interventions (EAPCI). *Eur Heart J* 2014; **35**: 2541–2619.

52 Vink MA, Patterson MS, van Etten J, et al. A randomized comparison of manual versus mechanical thrombus removal in primary percutaneous coronary intervention in the treatment of ST-segment elevation myocardial infarction (TREAT-MI). *Catheter Cardiovasc Interv* 2011; **78**: 14–19.

53 Parodi G, Valenti R, Migliorini A, et al. Comparison of manual thrombus aspiration with rheolytic thrombectomy in acute myocardial infarction. *Circ Cardiovasc Interv.* 2013; **6**: 224–230.

54 Fracassi F, Roberto M, Niccoli G. Current interventional coronary applications of excimer laser. *Expert Rev Med Devices* 2013; **10**: 541–549.

55 Lee G, Ikeda RM, Stobbe D, et al. Effects of laser irradiation on human thrombus: demonstration of a linear dissolution–dose relation between clot length and energy density. *Am J Cardiol* 1983; **52**: 876–877.

56 Topaz O, Minisi AJ, Bernardo NL, et al. Alterations of platelet aggregation kinetics with ultraviolet laser emission: the "stunned platelet" phenomenon. *Thromb Haemost* 2001; **86**: 1087–1093.

57 Topaz O, Ebersole D, Das T, et al. Excimer laser angioplasty in acute myocardial infarction (the CARMEL multicenter trial). *Am J Cardiol* 2004; **93**: 694–701.

58 Dahm JB, Ebersole D, Das T, et al. Prevention of distal embolization and no-reflow in patients with acute myocardial infarction and total occlusion in the infarct-related vessel: a subgroup analysis of the cohort of acute revascularization in myocardial infarction with excimer laser-CARMEL multicenter study. *Catheter Cardiovasc Interv* 2005; **64**: 67–74.

59 Escaned J, Echavarría-Pinto M, Gorgadze T, et al. Safety of lone thrombus aspiration without concomitant coronary stenting in selected patients with acute myocardial infarction. *EuroIntervention* 2013; **8**: 1149–1156.

60 Carrick D, Oldroyd KG, McEntegart M, et al. A randomized trial of deferred stenting versus immediate stenting to prevent no- or slow-reflow in acute ST-segment elevation myocardial infarction (DEFER-STEMI). *J Am Coll Cardiol* 2014; **63**: 2088–2098.

61 Stone GW, Abizaid A, Silber S, et al. Prospective, Randomized, Multicenter Evaluation of a Polyethylene Terephthalate Micronet Mesh-Covered Stent (MGuard) in ST-Segment Elevation Myocardial Infarction: The MASTER Trial. *J Am Coll Cardiol* 2012; **60**: 1975–1984.

CHAPTER 24

Specialized Balloons in Percutaneous Coronary Intervention: Cutting, Scoring, Gliding, and Drug-Eluting Balloons

Bimmer E.P.M. Claessen[1], José P.S. Henriques[1], and George D. Dangas[2]

[1]Department of Cardiology, Academic Medical Center—University of Amsterdam, Amsterdam, The Netherlands
[2]Department of Cardiology, Mount Sinai Medical Center, New York, NY, USA

Balloon angioplasty was the only available treatment in the early days of percutaneous coronary intervention (PCI). Major drawbacks of balloon angioplasty alone were elastic recoil, acute vessel closure, and restenosis [1]. The development of coronary artery stents subsequently revolutionized the field of interventional cardiology, virtually eliminating elastic recoil and acute vessel closure [1,2], but they also introduced the new problem of stent thrombosis and were still limited by relatively high rates of in-stent restenosis [3,4]. Bare metal stents (BMS) were succeeded by drug-eluting stents (DES) which currently are the standard of care for treating most coronary artery lesions [5]. Nonetheless, balloon angioplasty is still an integral part of interventional cardiology in the current era. Lesion preparation by predilation is vital for allowing stent delivery to severely narrowed and calcified lesions. This is particularly important in the current era of bioresorbable vascular scaffolds (BVS) which require meticulous lesion preparation before implantation [6]. A number of specialized balloons such as cutting balloons and scoring balloons have been developed to facilitate lesion preparation. Moreover, several specialized balloons have been developed specifically for a dedicated purpose, for example a short gliding balloon which can be employed for side branch ostial dilatation in bifurcation lesions, or the clearway catheter which is designed for intracoronary delivery of pharmaceutical agents [7–11]. Finally, a new class of drug-coated balloons have been developed which show great potential in treating in-stent restenosis lesions and *de novo* lesions [12]. This chapter provides an overview of specialty balloons currently used in the field of interventional cardiology.

Cutting and scoring balloons

Cutting balloons were introduced in the early 1990s in an attempt to limit vascular injury and elastic recoil [13]. On a cutting balloon a number of cutting edges of small metal blades are mounted on the surface of the balloon along the longitudinal axis. As compared with regular angioplasty balloons, cutting balloons were hypothesized to have an advantage by cutting into the media with a sharp incision, inducing less medial smooth muscle cell stretch leading to fewer stimuli for intimal proliferation. Although the initial clinical experience with the cutting balloon was favorable [14], the introduction of coronary artery stents proved more effective at reducing restenosis and reducing acute vessel closure [1,2], thus reducing the indications for using a cutting balloon. Current European Society of Cardiology (ESC) guidelines mention that preparation and debulking with a cutting balloon may be useful in highly calcified, rigid, ostial lesions [15]. The American College of Cardiology/American Heart Association (ACC/AHA) guidelines include a class III recommendation (level of evidence A) stating that cutting balloon angioplasty should not be performed routinely during PCI [16]. There is also a class IIb recommendation (level of evidence C) stating that cutting balloon angioplasty might be considered to avoid slippage-induced coronary artery trauma during PCI for in-stent restenosis or ostial lesions in side branches.

Scoring balloons are composed of a minimally compliant balloon encircled by a scoring element (typically a wire) which creates focal concentrations of dilating force, minimizing balloon slippage and assisting in the expansion of stenotic coronary arteries. Essentially this recreates the local environment of a regular balloon inflation alongside a "buddy wire" which is embedded into the lesion and also acts as an anti-slippage element. Starting with the FX-minirail (Abbott Vascular, no longer manufactured), several different types of scoring balloons are currently commercially available, the most common being the AngioSculpt Scoring Balloon Catheter (AngioScore, Fremont, CA, USA), which is a conventional nylon-blend balloon encircled with spiral nitinol scoring wires, and the Scoreflex scoring catheter (OrbusNeich, Hong Kong, China), which has only one protruding element on the surface of the balloon; it has an extremely short tip which wraps the guidewire used to deliver the device longitudinally along the balloon as a second scoring element. Their use has evolved in similar indications as the cutting balloon. The AngioScore balloon has been tested in a small cohort (n = 93) of patients undergoing PCI of bifurcation lesions with a provisional side branch stenting approach and DES in the main branch [17]. At 9-month follow-up this simple provisional strategy for complex true bifurcation PCI resulted in low rates of target lesion revascularization (3.3%).

Interventional Cardiology: Principles and Practice, Second Edition. Edited by George D. Dangas, Carlo Di Mario, and Nicholas N. Kipshidze.
© 2017 John Wiley & Sons, Ltd. Published 2017 by John Wiley & Sons, Ltd.

The Glider balloon in coronary bifurcation lesions

The Glider balloon (TriReme Medical, Pleasanton, CA, USA) is a short balloon (4 mm) that is specifically designed for use in bifurcation lesions. In the most commonly used technique for bifurcation lesion PCI, provisional side branch stenting, final kissing balloons to correct carina shift after deployment of the main vessel stent is frequently performed. However, final kissing balloons can be technically challenging because of challenges in crossing the main vessel stent struts with a balloon. The Glider balloon is designed with an oblique cut at the distal tip to facilitate crossing into the side branch: once the shorter aspect of the oblique tip has stopped at the difficult to cross side branch ostium, the balloon is rotated and the longer aspect of the balloon is then expected to emerge beyond the ostium allowing opening of the strut with inflation. In theory, because of its short length (4 mm) it also minimizes the risk of side branch dissection [18].

An observational study in 236 consecutive bifurcation lesions where final kissing balloon dilatation was attempted reported successful kissing balloons with conventional angioplasty balloons in 221 lesions (93.5%) [11]. In the 15 lesions where conventional balloons did not pass, the Glider balloon crossed in 12 patients (80%). Similar results were reported in another registry study comprising 125 patients with 131 bifurcation lesions [19]. These data suggest that the Glider balloon is a useful bail-out device for recrossing stent struts in bifurcation stenting if conventional angioplasty balloons fails.

Clearway catheter for intracoronary drug delivery

The Clearway catheter (Atrium Medical, Hudson, NH, USA) is a microporous PTFE balloon mounted on a 2.7 Fr rapid exchange catheter which has been investigated in patients undergoing primary PCI for ST-segment elevation myocardial infarction (STEMI). This balloon occludes coronary blood flow, contains the thrombus, and allows for local infusion of a pharmaceutical agent [20]. It was investigated in the INFUSE-AMI trial (intracoronary abciximab infusion and aspiration thrombectomy in patients undergoing percutaneous coronary intervention for anterior ST-segment elevation myocardial infarction) which randomized 452 patients with an anterior STEMI and an occluded proximal or mid left anterior descending coronary artery (LAD) [10]. All patients underwent primary PCI using bivalirudin and were randomized in a 2 × 2 factorial design to one of four arms:

1 Local infusion of the glycoprotein IIb/IIIa platelet inhibitor abciximab using the Clearway catheter and thrombus aspiration using a manual thrombus aspiration device
2 Local infusion of abciximab but no thrombus aspiration
3 Thrombus aspiration but no abciximab infusion, or
4 No abciximab infusion and no thrombus aspiration.

In this relatively small study, infarct size at 30-day follow-up was significantly smaller in patients treated with local infusion of abciximab, but not in patients undergoing manual thrombus aspiration.

Flash Ostial dual balloon angioplasty catheter

This specialized balloon catheter (Cardinal Health, CA, USA) is designed to address the protrusion of stent struts to the aorta when a stent is placed in an aorto-ostial lesion. It is designed to use as the final step of angioplasty/stent implantation. It consists of a balloon-in-balloon technology and is delivered as a monorail over a 0.014 inch wire. The inner balloon is inflated first (nominal diameter to the stent implanted) and anchors at the ostium; then the outer (soft) balloon is inflated which dilates up to 20 mm within the aorta, thereby pushing the protruding struts toward the aortic wall. Ideally, this facilitates strut apposition and allows easier re-engagement of catheters at future procedures. The current sizes allow its use in left and right coronary as well as renal and subclavian procedures.

Drug-eluting balloons

Drug-eluting balloons, also often referred to as drug-coated balloons, were designed to facilitate local delivery of anti-restenotic drugs. By using highly lipophilic drugs, short contact times of a few minutes are sufficient for adequate drug delivery. The majority of drug-eluting balloons currently used in clinical practice elute the cytotoxic drug paclitaxel, which is also sometimes used on drug-eluting stents (DES). However, most current DES types elute an analogue of the anti-inflammatory and cytostatic drug sirolimus. Paclitaxel is excellently suited for use on drug-eluting balloons because of its rapid uptake and prolonged retention into the coronary vessel wall [21]. Given the paclitaxel-eluting DES have not fared as well as the DES eluting limus-type drugs, reservations remain on whether the paclitaxel-eluting balloons indeed represent the maximum capacity this technology offers. Recent developments in drug delivery have led to sirolimus (analogue) -eluting balloons using nanomicrospheres. By using lipophilic nanospheres to encapsulate the drug, the uptake of the drug can be enhanced by the increased lipophilicity and the duration of drug elution can be lengthened by regulating drug release from the nanosphere–drug complexes. Studies using these novel nanotechnology-based sirolimus (analogue)-eluting balloons are currently being performed and are anticipated over the next years. In the following section, the drug-eluting balloons discussed are all paclitaxel-eluting balloons.

DEB in in-stent restenosis lesions

The widespread use of second-generation DES has drastically reduced the incidence of in-stent restenosis (ISR), a common problem with BMS [22]. Nonetheless, ISR still occurs in 2–10% of lesions treated with DES, depending on stent type and lesion characteristics, and is notoriously hard to treat [4]. DES ISR can be treated by repeat placement of a DES, but concern exists about negative consequences of having multiple layers of stent [23]. Therefore, a drug-eluting balloon may be well suited for treatment of ISR lesions, allowing for acute lumen gain and local delivery of antiproliferative pharmaceutical agents.

The safety and efficacy of the drug-eluting balloon for treatment of BMS ISR was established in the small PEPCAD II (paclitaxel-eluting PTCA-balloon catheter in coronary artery disease) randomized trial which enrolled 131 patients with BMS ISR who were randomly allocated to treatment with a TAXUS paclitaxel-eluting stent or a drug-eluting balloon [24]. At 6 month-angiographic follow-up, in-segment lumen loss was significantly lower in the drug-eluting balloon group (0.17 ± 0.42 vs. 0.38 ± 0.61 mm; p = 0.03), with binary restenosis rates (defined as >50% stenosis) of 20% in the TAXUS group and 9% in the drug-eluting balloon group (p = 0.08). At 3-year clinical follow-up, rates of target lesion revascularization (TLR) were 9.1% in the drug-eluting balloon group and 18.5% in the TAXUS group (p = 0.14) [25].

The performance of drug-eluting balloons in the treatment of DES ISR was evaluated in the ISAR-DESIRE 3 (intracoronary stenting and angiographic results: drug-eluting stent in-stent restenosis: 3 treatment approached), PEPCAD China ISR, and RIBS IV (restenosis intra-stent of drug-eluting stents: drug-eluting balloon versus everolimus-eluting stent) randomized controlled trials [26–28]. These studies showed that using a paclitaxel-eluting balloon results in comparable or superior outcomes compared with using paclitaxel-eluting DES in ISR lesions. However, the RIBS IV trial, which compared the paclitaxel-eluting balloon with the second generation everolimus-eluting stent, reported superior outcomes in terms of angiographic (late loss) and clinical (TLR) endpoints with the everolimus-eluting stent [27]. Another recent observational study raised concerns about the durability of the efficacy of the drug-eluting balloon in 468 patients with 550 ISR lesions (of which 436 lesions were DES ISR; 79.3%) [29]. Patients underwent quantitative coronary angiography analysis at 6 and 18 months after the index procedure. At 18 months, late lumen loss was significantly greater in patients with DES ISR compared with BMS ISR. Moreover, in the DES ISR group, approximately 25% of patients underwent TLR after 18 months. These results underscore the complexity of the problem of DES ISR and suggest that DES ISR treatment with drug-eluting balloons could benefit from more aggressive lesion preparation, for example with scoring or cutting balloons before deployment of the drug-eluting balloon.

DEB in de novo lesions

Drug-eluting balloons have also been used for treatment of de novo coronary artery lesions, either by themselves, or combined with BMS implantation. A small study randomized 30 patients with a single de novo coronary artery lesion to treatment with BMS alone, predilatation with a drug-eluting balloon followed by BMS implantation, or BMS implantation followed by postdilatation with a drug-eluting balloon. In this small study, angiographic outcomes were better when drug-eluting balloons were used, with no difference between use before or after BMS implantation [30].

This potential clinical application of drug-eluting balloons was coined as a potentially safe alternative to first-generation drug-eluting stents, which were hampered by high rates of very late stent thrombosis [31]. However, the introduction of second-generation DES with biocompatible or bioresorbable polymers eluting sirolimus or its analogues has since been proven to be a safer and more effective alternative to first generation DES with better angiographic results compared with drug-eluting balloons for de novo coronary artery lesions [5,32].

Nonetheless, drug-eluting balloons could be an attractive treatment option for small coronary vessels which was first studied in the small (n = 182) randomized BELLO (balloon elution and late loss optimization) trial [33]. Patients undergoing PCI of a lesion with a reference vessel diameter <2.8 mm by visual estimation were randomized to treatment with a drug-eluting balloon and provisional BMS (which was used in 20% of patients) or a TAXUS paclitaxel-eluting stent. At 2-year clinical follow-up, TLR rates were numerically lower in the drug-eluting balloon group (6.8% vs. 12.1%; p = 0.25). A major shortcoming of this study is the fact that paclitaxel-eluting DES were used, whereas next generation everolimus-eluting DES have been shown to yield superior outcomes in terms of repeat revascularization and death/myocardial infarction compared with paclitaxel-eluting DES [34].

The drug-eluting balloon has also been investigated in bifurcation lesions, where they may form an attractive option to minimize side branch restenosis. The BABILON trial (paclitaxel-coated balloon catheter in bifurcated coronary lesions) enrolled 108 patients with de novo bifurcation lesions which were randomized to treatment with provisional T-stenting with BMS or everolimus-eluting DES. In this study, all patients underwent sequential main branch and side branch dilatation with a drug-eluting balloon [35]. At 2-year clinical follow-up, angiographic outcomes were similar for the side branches. However, in the main branches, everolimus-eluting DES implantation led to reduced TLR rates compared with BMS implantation (3.6% vs. 15.4%; p = 0.045). Therefore, the role for drug-eluting balloons in de novo coronary artery lesions seems limited to treatment of side branches in bifurcation lesions or vessels with small reference diameters that do not allow for stent implantation.

DEB in acute myocardial infarction

The use of drug-eluting balloons in acute myocardial infarction has been investigated because it theoretically eliminates the risk of stent thrombosis after primary PCI. To date, a total of two non-randomized observational studies have reported on the use of drug-eluting balloons in the setting of acute myocardial infarction. A 100-patient registry from a large tertiary referral center in the Netherlands showed that a drug-eluting balloon-only strategy was feasible in 41 patients, while 59 patients required additional stenting [36]. At 1-year clinical follow-up, two patients had died, while three patients had undergone TLR. Another non-randomized study of 40 patients with STEMI undergoing primary PCI with drug-eluting balloons showed less favorable results with the drug-eluting balloon [37]. At 6-month clinical follow-up, seven major adverse cardiovascular events occurred (17.5%); one non-cardiac death, five TLRs, and one target vessel revascularization. Given the conflicting results of these two studies, the role of the drug-eluting balloon in primary PCI is currently not clear, and more research is needed to provide additional data on safety and efficacy of this treatment strategy.

Conclusions

Specialized balloons of several types have been developed, each with their own clinical applications. In most day-to-day PCI cases, "standard" compliant and non-compliant balloons are sufficient. Nonetheless, specialized balloons are of particular value in select situations, and can be used to optimize lesion preparation (cutting balloon, scoring balloon), to treat ISR (cutting balloon, scoring balloon, and drug-eluting balloon), intracoronary drug delivery (clearway catheter), or treatment of side branches in bifurcation lesions (Glider balloon, drug-eluting balloon). Further research is needed to establish the applicability of novel sirolimus (analogue) -eluting balloons, and the use of drug-eluting balloons in de novo coronary artery disease and acute myocardial infarction.

Interactive multiple choice questions are available for this chapter on www.wiley. com/go/dangas/cardiology

References

1 Serruys PW, de Jaegere P, Kiemeneij F, *et al.* A comparison of balloon-expandable-stent implantation with balloon angioplasty in patients with coronary artery disease. Benestent Study Group. *N Engl J Med* 1994; **331**(8): 489–495.

2 Fischman DL, Leon MB, Baim DS, *et al.* A randomized comparison of coronary-stent placement and balloon angioplasty in the treatment of coronary artery disease. Stent Restenosis Study Investigators. *N Engl J Med* 1994; **331**(8): 496–501.

3 Claessen BE, Henriques JP, Jaffer FA, Mehran R, Piek JJ, Dangas GD. Stent thrombosis: a clinical perspective. *JACC Cardiovasc Interv* 2014; 7(10): 1081–1092.

4 Dangas GD, Claessen BE, Caixeta A, Sanidas EA, Mintz GS, Mehran R. In-stent restenosis in the drug-eluting stent era. *J Am Coll Cardiol* 2010; 56(23): 1897–907.

5 Navarese EP, Tandjung K, Claessen B, et al. Safety and efficacy outcomes of first and second generation durable polymer drug eluting stents and biodegradable polymer biolimus eluting stents in clinical practice: comprehensive network meta-analysis. *BMJ* 2013; 347: f6530.

6 Serruys PW, Chevalier B, Dudek D, et al. A bioresorbable everolimus-eluting scaffold versus a metallic everolimus-eluting stent for ischaemic heart disease caused by de-novo native coronary artery lesions (ABSORB II): an interim 1-year analysis of clinical and procedural secondary outcomes from a randomised controlled trial. *Lancet* 2015; 385(9962): 43–54.

7 Kawase Y, Saito N, Watanabe S, et al. Utility of a scoring balloon for a severely calcified lesions: bench test and finite element analysis. *Cardiovasc Interv Ther* 2014; 29(2): 134–139.

8 Schmidt T, Hansen S, Meincke F, Frerker C, Kuck KH, Bergmann MW. Safety and efficacy of lesion preparation with the AngioSculpt Scoring Balloon in left main interventions: the ALSTER Left Main registry. *EuroIntervention* 2016; 11: 1346–1354.

9 Moses JW, Carlier S, Moussa I. Lesion preparation prior to stenting. *Rev Cardiovasc Med* 2004; 5(Suppl 2): S16–21.

10 Stone GW, Maehara A, Witzenbichler B, et al. Intracoronary abciximab and aspiration thrombectomy in patients with large anterior myocardial infarction: the INFUSE-AMI randomized trial. *JAMA* 2012; 307(17): 1817–1826.

11 Briguori C, Visconti G, Donahue M, Chiariello GA, Focaccio A. The glider balloon: a useful device for the treatment of bifurcation lesions. *Int J Cardiol* 2013; 168(4): 3208–3211.

12 Indermuehle A, Bahl R, Lansky AJ, et al. Drug-eluting balloon angioplasty for in-stent restenosis: a systematic review and meta-analysis of randomised controlled trials. *Heart* 2013; 99(5): 327–333.

13 Barath P, Fishbein MC, Vari S, Forrester JS. Cutting balloon: a novel approach to percutaneous angioplasty. *Am J Cardiol* 1991; 68(11): 1249–1252.

14 Popma JJ, Lansky AJ, Purkayastha DD, Hall LR, Bonan R. Angiographic and clinical outcome after cutting balloon angioplasty. *J Invasive Cardiol* 1996; 8(Suppl A): 12A–19A.

15 Authors/Task Force m, Windecker S, Kolh P, Alfonso F, et al. 2014 ESC/EACTS Guidelines on myocardial revascularization: The Task Force on Myocardial Revascularization of the European Society of Cardiology (ESC) and the European Association for Cardio-Thoracic Surgery (EACTS). Developed with the special contribution of the European Association of Percutaneous Cardiovascular Interventions (EAPCI). *Eur Heart J* 2014; 35(37): 2541–2619.

16 Levine GN, Bates ER, Blankenship JC, et al. 2011 ACCF/AHA/SCAI Guideline for Percutaneous Coronary Intervention. A report of the American College of Cardiology Foundation/American Heart Association Task Force on Practice Guidelines and the Society for Cardiovascular Angiography and Interventions. *J Am Coll Cardiol* 2011; 58(24): e44–122.

17 Weisz G, Metzger DC, Liberman HA, et al. A provisional strategy for treating true bifurcation lesions employing a scoring balloon for the side branch: final results of the AGILITY trial. *Catheter Cardiovasc Interv* 2013; 82(3): 352–359.

18 Secco GG, Di Mario C. A new dedicated ultrashort steerable balloon for side branch ostial dilatation. *Catheter Cardiovasc Interv* 2011; 77(3): 363–366.

19 Secco GG, Rittger H, Hoffmann S, et al. The glider registry: a prospective multicentre registry of a new ultrashort dedicated balloon for side-branch ostial dilatation. *Catheter Cardiovasc Interv* 2013.

20 Saraf S, Ong PJ, Gorog DA. ClearWay RX: rapid exchange therapeutic perfusion catheter. *EuroIntervention* 2008; 3(5): 639–642.

21 Axel DI, Kunert W, Goggelmann C, et al. Paclitaxel inhibits arterial smooth muscle cell proliferation and migration in vitro and in vivo using local drug delivery. *Circulation* 1997; 96(2): 636–645.

22 Bangalore S, Toklu B, Amoroso N, et al. Bare metal stents, durable polymer drug eluting stents, and biodegradable polymer drug eluting stents for coronary artery disease: mixed treatment comparison meta-analysis. *BMJ* 2013; 347: f6625.

23 Tagliareni F, La Manna A, Saia F, Marzocchi A, Tamburino C. Long-term clinical follow-up of drug-eluting stent restenosis treatment: retrospective analysis from two high volume catheterisation laboratories. *EuroIntervention* 2010; 5(6): 703–708.

24 Unverdorben M, Vallbracht C, Cremers B, et al. Paclitaxel-coated balloon catheter versus paclitaxel-coated stent for the treatment of coronary in-stent restenosis. *Circulation* 2009; 119(23): 2986–2994.

25 Unverdorben M, Vallbracht C, Cremers B, et al. Paclitaxel-coated balloon catheter versus paclitaxel-coated stent for the treatment of coronary in-stent restenosis: the three-year results of the PEPCAD II ISR study. *EuroIntervention* 2015; 11: 926–934.

26 Kufner S, Cassese S, Valeskini M, et al. Long-term efficacy and safety of paclitaxel-eluting balloon for the treatment of drug-eluting stent restenosis: 3-year results of a randomized controlled trial. *JACC Cardiovasc Interv* 2015; 8(7): 877–884.

27 Alfonso F, Perez-Vizcayno MJ, Cardenas A, et al. A prospective randomized trial of drug-eluting balloons versus everolimus-eluting stents in patients with in-stent restenosis of drug-eluting stents: The RIBS IV Randomized Clinical Trial. *J Am Coll Cardiol* 2015; 66(1): 23–33.

28 Xu B, Gao R, Wang J, et al. A prospective, multicenter, randomized trial of paclitaxel-coated balloon versus paclitaxel-eluting stent for the treatment of drug-eluting stent in-stent restenosis: results from the PEPCAD China ISR trial. *JACC Cardiovasc Interv* 2014; 7(2): 204–211.

29 Habara S, Kadota K, Shimada T, et al. Late restenosis after paclitaxel-coated balloon angioplasty occurs in patients with drug-eluting stent restenosis. *J Am Coll Cardiol* 2015; 66(1): 14–22.

30 Burzotta F, Brancati MF, Trani C, et al. Impact of drug-eluting balloon (pre- or post-) dilation on neointima formation in de novo lesions treated by bare-metal stent: the IN-PACT CORO trial. *Heart Vessels* 2015.

31 Stone GW, Moses JW, Ellis SG, et al. Safety and efficacy of sirolimus- and paclitaxel-eluting coronary stents. *N Engl J Med* 2007; 356(10): 998–1008.

32 Fischer D, Scheller B, Schafer A, et al. Paclitaxcel-coated balloon plus bare metal stent vs. sirolimus-eluting stent in de novo lesions: an IVUS study. *EuroIntervention* 2012; 8(4): 450–455.

33 Naganuma T, Latib A, Sgueglia GA, et al. A 2-year follow-up of a randomized multicenter study comparing a paclitaxel drug-eluting balloon with a paclitaxel-eluting stent in small coronary vessels the BELLO study. *Int J Cardiol* 2015; 184: 17–21.

34 Baber U, Mehran R, Sharma SK, et al. Impact of the everolimus-eluting stent on stent thrombosis: a meta-analysis of 13 randomized trials. *J Am Coll Cardiol* 2011; 58(15): 1569–1577.

35 Lopez Minguez JR, Nogales Asensio JM, Doncel Vecino LJ, et al. A prospective randomised study of the paclitaxel-coated balloon catheter in bifurcated coronary lesions (BABILON trial): 24-month clinical and angiographic results. *EuroIntervention* 2014; 10(1): 50–57.

36 Vos NS, Dirksen MT, Vink MA, et al. Safety and feasibility of a PAclitaxel-eluting balloon angioplasty in Primary Percutaneous coronary intervention in Amsterdam (PAPPA): one-year clinical outcome of a pilot study. *EuroIntervention* 2014; 10(5): 584–590.

37 Nijhoff F, Agostoni P, Belkacemi A, et al. Primary percutaneous coronary intervention by drug-eluting balloon angioplasty: the nonrandomized fourth arm of the DEB-AMI (drug-eluting balloon in ST-segment elevation myocardial infarction) trial. *Catheter Cardiovasc Interv* 2015; 86(Suppl 1): 34–44.

CHAPTER 25

Coronary Artery Dissections, Perforations, and the No-Reflow Phenomenon

Adriano Caixeta[1], Luiz Fernando Ybarra[1], Azeem Latib[2], Flavio Airoldi[3], Roxana Mehran[4], and George D. Dangas[4]

[1] Hospital Israelita Albert Einstein; Universidade Federal de São Paulo, São Paulo, Brazil
[2] San Raffaele Scientific Institute, Milan, Italy
[3] IRCCS Multimedica, Sesto San Giovanni, Italy
[4] Department of Cardiology, Mount Sinai Medical Center, New York, NY, USA

Coronary dissection, perforation, and the no-reflow phenomenon are some of the most dreaded complications occurring in the catheterization laboratory and have been associated with a high rate of major adverse outcomes [1–14]. Although operator experience, equipment, drugs, and device technology continually improve, major dissection, abrupt closure, arterial perforation, and no-reflow remain the primary reasons for failure of percutaneous coronary intervention (PCI). While some instances of these complications are subtle, others are dramatic and can result in abrupt vessel closure, myocardial infarction, need for urgent coronary artery bypass surgery, pericardial tamponade, heart failure, cardiogenic shock, and even death. As a result, interventional cardiologists need to be vigilant for these complications and initiate therapy without delay. Improvements in PCI technique and equipment, primarily with the widespread use of coronary stents, has significantly decreased the incidence of acute closure and the need for emergency revascularization. Furthermore, innovative percutaneous approaches to the management of coronary perforation have included the use of covered stents and microcoil vessel occlusion. This chapter discusses the risk factors, recognition, and contemporary approach to managing peri-procedural complications related to PCI.

Coronary artery dissection
Dissection following PCI

By definition, separation of the media by hemorrhage with or without an associated intimal tear is termed coronary artery dissection. PCI depends upon mechanical dilatation of the artery or ablation of atherosclerotic plaque and is therefore essentially associated with plaque fracture, intimal splitting, and localized medial dissection; these tears can extend into the media for varying distances and degrees, and even extend through the adventitia resulting in frank perforation. Historically, acute vessel closure is the most feared complication of coronary artery dissection, and in the pre-stent era occurred in 2–14% of patients [15–19]. Subsequently, because of improvements in PCI technique and equipment, primarily the widespread use of coronary stents—compared to balloon angioplasty—acute closure and the need for emergency coronary artery bypass surgery (CABG) have decreased significantly, despite the increasing complexity of cases. In contemporary interventional

practice, including the use of stents in patients with moderate to high risk acute coronary syndromes, the incidence of abrupt vessel closure is less than 1% [20], and most laboratories report emergency CABG rates below 0.5% [21].

Dissections have been classified by the National Heart, Lung, and Blood Institute (NHLBI) according to their angiographic appearance [22,23]. The modified NHLBI criteria defined dissection as angiographically detectable intimal or medial damage manifesting as a radiolucent area within the vessel or as an extravasation of contrast medium after an interventional procedure. These criteria were refined into a more detailed classification system and are graded based upon their angiographic appearances as types A–F (Table 25.1). Type A dissections represent minor radiolucent areas within the coronary lumen during contrast injection, with little or no persistence of contrast after the dye has cleared. Type B dissections are parallel tracts or a double lumen separated by a radiolucent area during contrast injection, with minimal or no persistence after dye clearance (Figure 25.1). Type C dissections appear as contrast outside the coronary lumen ("extraluminal cap"), with persistence of contrast after dye has cleared from the lumen (Figure 25.2). Type D dissections represent spiral ("barber shop pole") luminal filling defects, frequently with excessive contrast staining of the dissected false lumen (Figure 25.3). Type E dissections appear as new, persistent filling defects within the coronary lumen (Figure 25.4). Type F dissections represent those that lead to total occlusion of the coronary lumen without distal antegrade flow (Figure 25.5) [24].

During the balloon angioplasty era, some studies have attempted to distinguish minor dissections from detrimental major ones. In general, type A and B dissections are clinically benign and do not adversely affect procedural outcome. Conversely, types C–F are considered major dissections and carry a significant increase in morbidity and mortality. Major dissections are characterized by numerous morphologic features: (i) a linear intraluminal filling defect or luminal staining evident in two projections; (ii) a linear filling defect extending greater than 20 mm; and (iii) dissection types C–F according to NHLBI criteria [25]. Major dissections also create intraluminal filling defects of sufficient size to produce a reduction in luminal diameter of at least 50% and/or a reduction in distal coronary flow. Huber *et al.* [25] demonstrated that abrupt closure, myocardial infarction, and bypass grafting occurred in fewer

Interventional Cardiology: Principles and Practice, Second Edition. Edited by George D. Dangas, Carlo Di Mario, and Nicholas N. Kipshidze.
© 2017 John Wiley & Sons, Ltd. Published 2017 by John Wiley & Sons, Ltd.

than 3% of patients with NHLBI type B dissections. Conversely, dissection types C–F were associated with complication rates of 12–37%. Persistent extraluminal contrast, new persistent filling defects, and spiral dissections portend adverse clinical outcomes.

Previous studies in the pre-stent era identified risk factors for the development of coronary artery dissection. Angiographic predictors include calcified lesions, eccentric lesions, long lesions, complex lesion morphology (ACC/AHA type B or C), and vessel tortuosity. A balloon to artery ratio >1.2 also predisposes to dissection [26,27].

The dissection can occur after overly vigorous attempts at guidewire passage, following balloon predilatation before the planned stent implantation, or even after stenting.

Stent edge dissections are common as the junction between stent metal—and more recently between bioresorbable vascular scaffold (BVS) strut—and reference segment tissue is a site of compliance mismatch (Figure 25.6). Intracoronary ultrasound (IVUS) or optical coherence tomography (OCT) does not seem to predict coronary dissection on preintervention analysis of lesion morphology or plaque composition [28]. A recent study evaluated the frequency, predictors, and detailed assessment of OCT detected stent edge dissections in 230 patients. The overall incidence of OCT-detected edge

Table 25.1 National Heart, Lung and Blood Institute (NHLBI) classification system for coronary artery dissection types. Types A and B are generally clinically benign, whereas types C–F portend significant morbidity and mortality.

Type A	Coronary dissection with only minor radiolucent areas within the coronary lumen without a reduction in coronary flow
Type B	Minimal or no dye persistence in the presence of parallel track or a double lumen separated by a radiolucent area during contrast injection
Type C	Dissection with persistent extraluminal dye after contrast injection
Type D	Spiral dissection
Type E	Dissection with new and filling defects
Type F	This dissection does not fit any of the above types A–E and is associated with impaired flow or total occlusion of the vessel

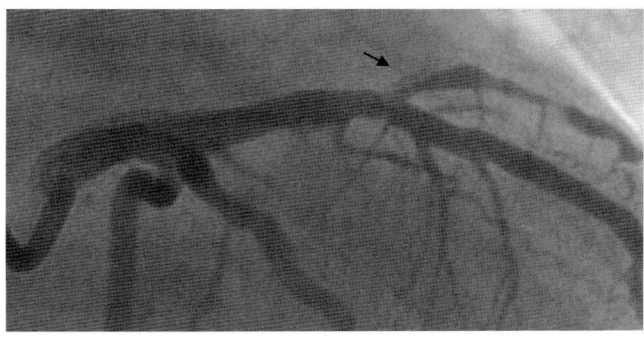

Figure 25.2 Type C dissection at diagonal branch after balloon dilatation. The arrow shows a focal and persistent extraluminal dye contrast.

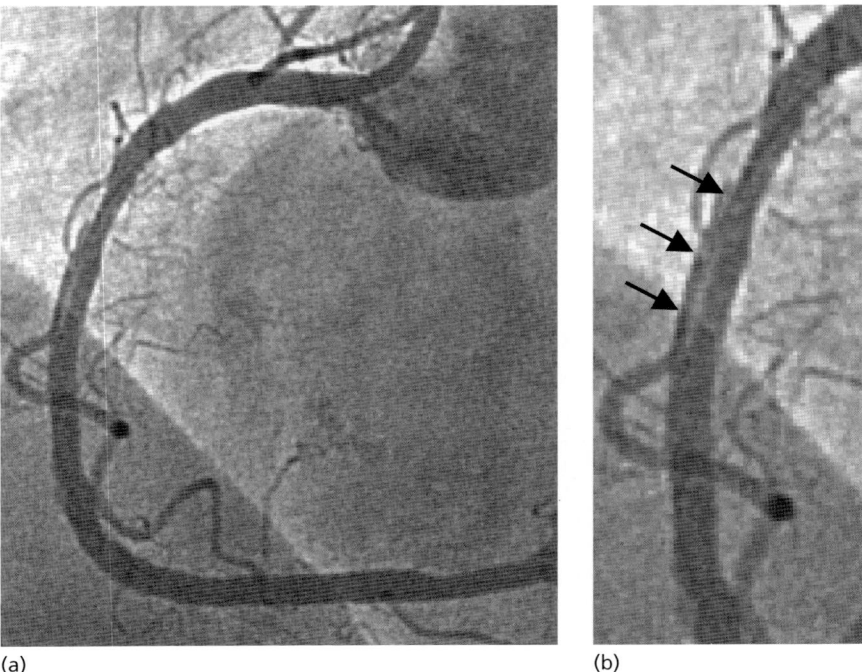

(a)   (b)

Figure 25.1 Type B dissection after balloon dilatation at right coronary artery (a). Notice the radiolucent parallel track at proximal and mid segments of the vessel (arrows) (b).

dissection was 37.8%, and most (84%) of them were not apparent on angiography. Additional stenting was performed in one-fourth of all dissections, which were longer, had bigger dimensions, and promoted deeper vascular injury. Of note, non-flow-limiting, small, and superficial dissections left untreated proved benign over time [29].

Ischemic complications in the current era usually occur as manifestations of edge dissections after metallic stent or BVS implantation, which can predispose to device thrombosis. The treatment of coronary edge dissection with stent implantation depends on the combination of angiographic assessment, flow assessment, and signs or symptoms of ischemia. Minor dissections should not be treated unless they result in lumen compromise; the vast majority have sealed when imaged at follow-up. In contrast, larger dissections are associated with an increased risk of progression to total occlusion (abrupt closure) of the treated arterial segment [16,25]. The potential strategies of treatment include: (i) stent implantation; (ii) bypass surgery; or (iii) medical treatment alone. The choice of stenting vs. conservative management or surgery is therefore made on a case-by-case basis. In general, in the vast majority of dissections necessitating treatment, stent implantation is the first choice [29].

Intramural hematoma is a variant of dissection. By IVUS or OCT, intramural hematomas are typically crescent-shaped, with straightening of the internal elastic membrane (Figure 25.7). In general, unless focal, superficial, and small, an intramural hematoma should be treated because of the propensity for propagation and lumen compromise.

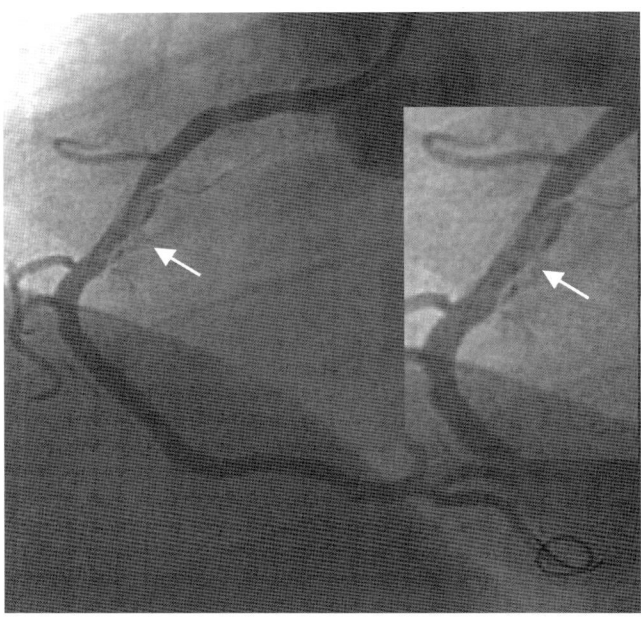

Figure 25.3 Type D dissection at right coronary artery after balloon dilatation for planned stent implantation. Despite the spiral dissection, there is no flow impairment.

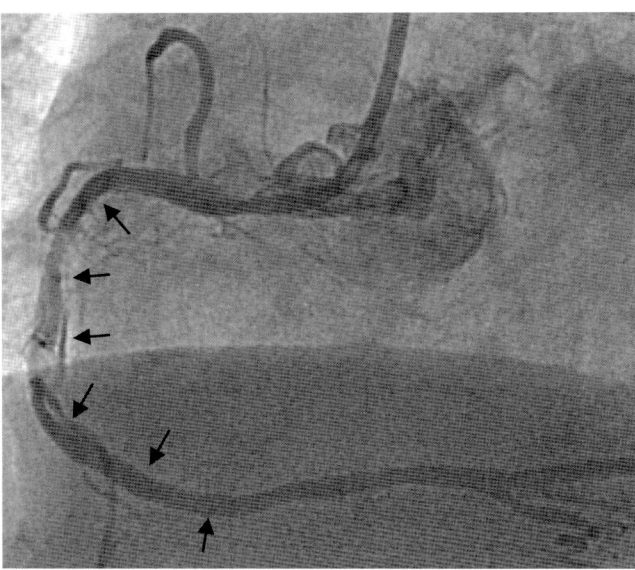

Figure 25.4 Type E dissection. A spiral dissection at the right coronary artery after balloon angioplasty dilatation for stenting. Notice the extensive filling defects (arrows) with lumen narrowing at the mid portion of the artery.

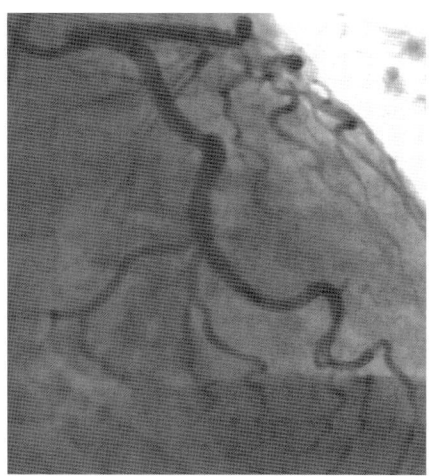
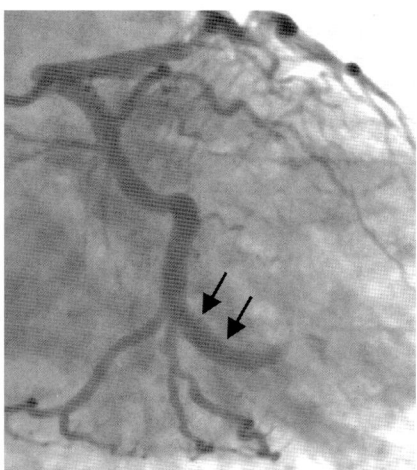

Figure 25.5 Mild disease at circumflex artery by angiogram. Diagnostic IVUS was performed to interrogate the plaque stenosis. During the procedure a type F dissection has been observed; notice the spiral dissection (arrows) associated with total occlusion of the vessel.

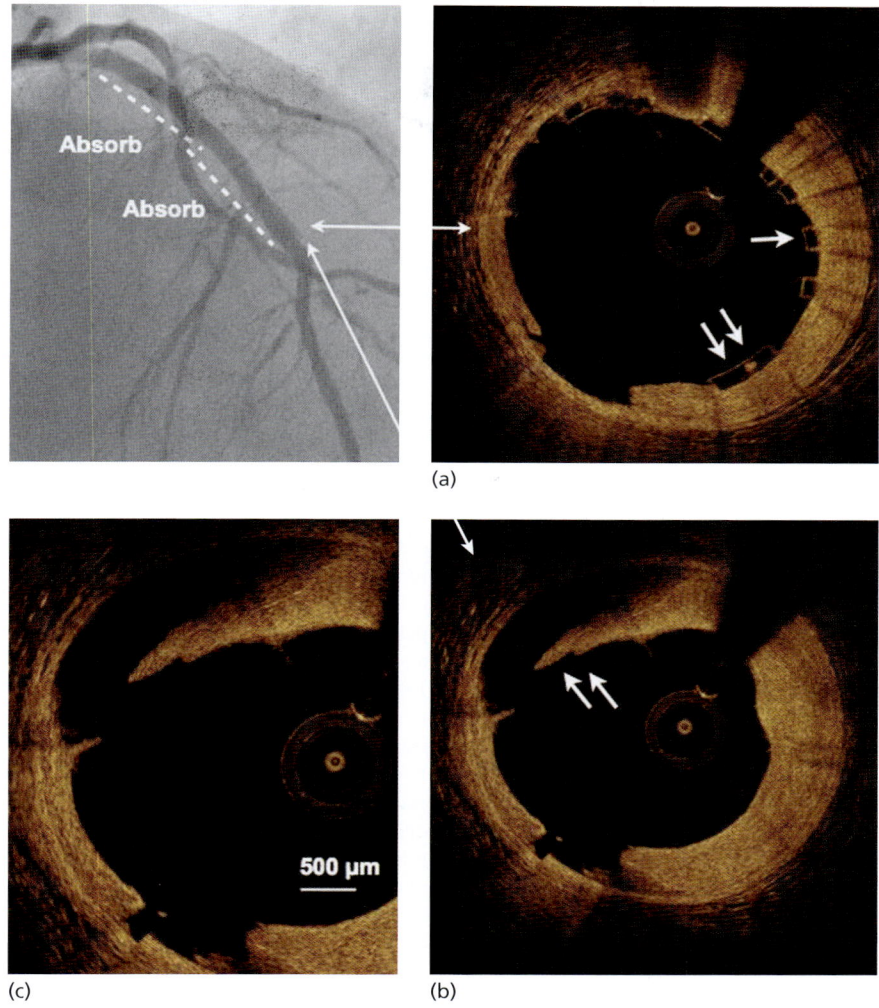

Figure 25.6 Distal edge dissection by angiography and optical coherence tomography (OCT). Left anterior descending artery in the anterior–posterior cranial view after two Absorb bioresorbable vascular scaffold (BRS) implantations. Note a subtle distal edge dissection by angiography (arrows). OCT shows that the BRS struts are well apposed and expanded (a, arrows); note a deep edge dissection just beyond the BRS struts involving the intima and media with a flap (b, arrows). (c) is a magnified image.

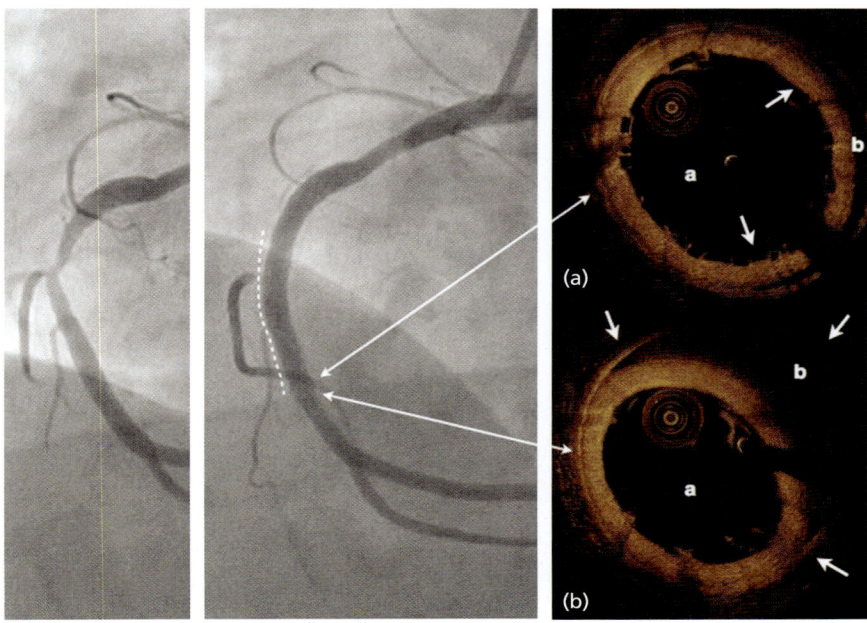

Figure 25.7 Edge coronary hematoma with true (a) and false (b) lumen by Optical coherence tomography (OCT). Right coronary artery in LAO view pre (left) and post (middle) after Absorb bioresorbable vascular scaffold (BRS) implantation. There is no sign of distal edge dissection by angiography. OCT (right) shows that BRS struts are well apposed and expanded (**a**, arrows); there is also a small hematoma/dissection behind the struts (**a** in panel a); note an edge hematoma from 11 to 5 o'clock (**a** in panel b) with crescent shape, but with no lumen compromise **b**.

Guide catheter-induced dissection

The incidence of iatrogenic coronary artery dissection at the time of cardiac catheterization or PCI is not known. Catheter-induced dissection with retrograde extension to the aortic root is rare and has been estimated to occur in approximately 0.008–0.02% of diagnostic catheterizations and 0.06–0.07% of PCIs (Figure 25.8) [30,31]. The natural history of catheter-induced coronary artery dissections is varied. In some cases, dissections lead to acute closure of the vessel with myocardial infarction [32]. In other circumstances, retrograde extension of the dissection back to involve the aorta can occur [33,34], and in other cases, dissections of the coronary artery have been associated with persistently normal (TIMI-3) flow without ischemia, and have healed without any intervention [35]. Several factors are associated with increased risk for catheter-induced artery dissection:

1 Left main disease
2 Use of Amplatz-shaped catheters
3 Catheterization for acute myocardial infarction
4 Catheter manipulations
5 Vigorous contrast media injection
6 Deep intubations of the catheter within the coronary artery
7 Variant anatomy of the coronary ostia, and
8 Vigorous, deep inspiration [36], and the recanalization of chronic total occlusion (CTO) [37].

The management of catheter-induced coronary dissection depends on the patency of the distal vessel and the extent of propagation of the dissection. In general, in the presence of myocardial ischemia or acute closure, PCI or CABG is mandated to prevent acute myocardial infarction or even death. There have been reports of successful outcomes with coronary artery stenting [38] and CABG [32,39]. Nevertheless, in the absence of ischemia the therapeutic options are less clear. Conservative management of guide catheter-induced coronary artery dissection has met with successful outcomes in selected patients [32,35]. The choice of stenting vs. conservative management is therefore made on a case-by-case basis.

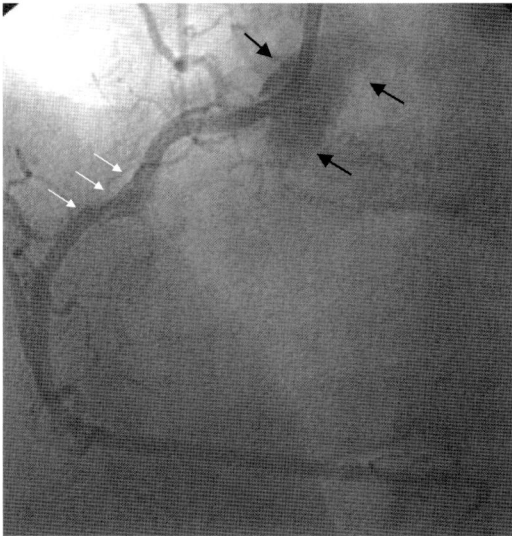

Figure 25.8 Catheter-induced dissection with retrograde extension of the dissection back to involve the aorta root (black arrows). Notice the spiral dissection with narrowing at the right coronary artery (white arrows).

Coronary artery perforation

Incidence

Coronary artery perforation represents a disruption of the vessel wall through the intima, media, and adventitia. Coronary perforation can engender localized pseudoaneurysm, perivascular hematoma, arterioventricular fistula, or hemopericardium. Angiographically, a perforation is defined as evidence of extravasation of contrast medium or blood from the coronary artery, during or following PCI. Few data are available on the true incidence of coronary perforation with balloon angioplasty alone. Various case series, many of which include the use of atherectomy devices, report an incidence ranging from 0.1% to 0.9% [2,25,40–43]. Some studies have described the incidence of coronary perforation to be 2–10 times higher in all published series using atheroablative techniques (directional atherectomy, excimer laser, rotablator, and transluminal extraction catheter) than with balloon angioplasty with or without stenting [44,45]. Ellis *et al.* [1] have reported the first large-scale series reflecting practice in 1990 and 1991. Of 12,900 procedures, 0.5% were complicated by coronary perforation. The incidence of perforations with balloon angioplasty alone was 0.1%, while that associated with rotablation was 1.3% and with excimer laser was 1.9%. The excimer laser probably carries the highest risk of coronary perforation (up to 3%) [1,46]. However, the device-related learning curve can also explain the higher rates of complications. For example, in a series, coronary perforation in conjunction with excimer laser use occurred in 1.2% of 3000 consecutive patients, but decreased to 0.3% in the last 1000 patients [46]. Other important information emerged from the Ellis *et al.* report. First, over-sizing of the angioplasty balloon was one of the key causes of perforation. Second, and most importantly, the development of cardiac tamponade was associated with high mortality (20%).

The actual incidence of guidewire-related coronary perforation is most likely higher than reported because it remains unrecognized and self-limited in several cases. The incidence of coronary perforation by the guidewire was 0.21% in the series by Dippel *et al.* [41] and 0.36% in the series by Fukutomi *et al.* [42]. In the later series, perforation occurred at the treatment site in 12 cases, in a distal vessel in 10 cases, and could not be localized in 5 cases [42]. In the series by Witzke *et al.* [47], coronary perforation by guidewire use was observed in 20 of 39 cases (51%). Of these cases, perforations occurred while trying to cross the lesion with a guidewire in 11 patients (55%). Based on these data, the authors emphasized that the distal migration of the guidewire is an important factor contributing to coronary perforation, and that meticulous care of the guidewire should be taken, especially in patients treated with glycoprotein platelet (GP) IIb/IIIa receptor inhibitors. The use of hydrophilic-coated guidewires, especially in complex cases, can be associated with higher rates of distal perforation than non-hydrophilic wires because of wire migration.

In the largest experience thus far assessing the incidence and outcomes of coronary perforation, our group analyzed of 12,921 patients treated with PCI in three randomized trials: REPLACE-2, ACUITY, and HORIZONS-AMI [48]. We found that coronary perforation occurred in 0.27% of cases. Noteworthy, at 30 days, patients with versus those without coronary perforation had significantly (all p values <0.001) higher rates of 30-day mortality (11.4% vs. 1.0%), myocardial infarction (MI) (Q-wave, 22.9% vs. 5.7%; non-Q wave, 17.1% vs. 4.9%), target vessel revascularization (TVR) (20.1% vs. 1.8%), and composite endpoint of death/MI/TVR (31.4% vs. 7.8%). The proportion of perforation that progress on to tamponade ranges between 10% and 50%. In Fejka *et al.*'s series [44], almost 50% of those developing tamponade died. Of note, of 31 cases of tamponade, 14 presented more than 4 h after the procedure. The mortality of these later presenters was lower than those who had a more precipitous course within the catheterization laboratory (21% vs. 59%), but it was still considerable. In addition, according to the authors it was not possible to identify by angiography the bleeding point leading to tamponade in 10 of the 14 late presenters, suggesting that the most likely mechanism was guidewire distal branch perforation. In our study [48], mortality of the patients who developed hemopericardium and tamponade following perforation was 80%.

In cases involving CTOs, perforations from the use of stiff guidewires are the most commonly observed type, mainly divided into: (i) perforation of the false lumen while advancing a stiff wire into the false lumen; and (ii) distal small branch perforation after crossing a CTO lesion. The most important recommendation during CTO angioplasty is to not advance any device over the guidewire unless the operator is sure of where the distal end of the guidewire lies. In general, special treatment is not required for false lumen perforation because it usually disappears after dilatation of another false lumen. However, if a device is advanced over the guidewire through the perforation, this usual self-limited complication can become a life-threatening situation. In distal small branch perforations, the most important consideration is performing careful observation via angiography. These perforations can cause late tamponade because the operator is often not able to detect them. At the end of the procedure, even in successful cases, a final angiography should be carefully performed.

Classification

A classification system for coronary perforations related to the angiographic appearance of blood extravasation (Table 25.2) was created based on the analysis of prospectively recorded data from a total of 12,900 PCI procedures from 11 US sites during a 2-year period [1]. Coronary perforation occurred in 62 patients (0.5%). Type II perforation was the most frequent perforation type in this series (50%), followed by type III (25.8%), and type I (21%); the minority of cases were characterized by cavity spilling (3.2%) [1]. Of note, the NHLBI classification system for coronary dissections overlaps with the Ellis classification model, with NHLBI type C coronary dissections corresponding angiographically with Ellis type I perforations (Figures 25.9, 25.10, and 25.11) [25].

In addition, other studies have evaluated the proposed classification system as a tool to predict outcome and to serve as the basis of management [1,49–51]. Analysis showed that:

- Type I perforations rarely result in tamponade or in myocardial ischemia.
- Type II perforations have high treatment success rates when managed with prolonged balloon inflation, and commonly have

Table 25.2 Classification of coronary perforations.

Type I	Extraluminal crater without extravasation
Type II	Pericardial or myocardial blush without contrast jet extravasation
Type III	Extravasation through frank (≥1 mm) perforation
Cavity spilling	Perforation into anatomic cavity chamber, coronary sinus, etc.

low occurrence of persistent contrast extravasation, consequently resulting in a low incidence of adverse sequelae [49].

- Type III perforations are associated with the rapid development of hemodynamic compromise and life-threatening complications, including abrupt tamponade, need for emergent bypass surgery, and very high mortality. Notably, type III perforations with contrast spilling into either the left or right coronary ventricle or coronary sinus do not have catastrophic consequences and are commonly benign [50,51].

Risk factors for coronary perforation

Risk factors for coronary perforation during standard PCI can be classified as: (i) patient-related; (ii) procedure-related; or (iii) device-related risk factors (Table 25.3).

Patient-related factors

Patient characteristics that have been associated with a risk of perforation include age, female gender, renal insufficiency, and history of prior CABG [1,40,48,52,53]. In a multicenter study by Ellis et al. [1], patients who developed perforation were almost 10 years older than those who had no perforation. In addition, women represented 46% of patients with perforation but only 16% of patients without this complication. Calcification presents a technical challenge for the interventionist. It often requires very high-pressure balloon inflation—either for predilatation or for post-dilatation—in order to achieve success [40]. The study found that 93% were complex, ACC/AHA class B2 or C, and 58% exhibited heavy calcification. Recently, Généraux et al. [54] evaluated data from 6855 patients presenting with acute coronary syndromes in whom PCI was performed from two large-scale randomized controlled trials: ACUITY and HORIZONS-AMI. By multivariable analysis, the presence of moderate or severe target lesion calcification was an independent predictor of 1-year definite stent thrombosis and ischemic target lesion revascularization (TLR).

Procedure-related factors

The use of oversized compliant balloons coupled with relatively high deployment or post-dilatation inflation pressures to achieve full stent expansion and minimize residual stenosis after stent implantation can cause vessel wall perforation [1,40,55]. Several mechanisms are involved, including overstretching of the most compliant coronary artery segment, a high-pressure jet caused by balloon rupture, and outward pushing of a stent strut through the vessel wall. Procedural success and complication rates as a function of balloon-to-vessel ratio and high inflation pressure have been reported in numerous studies. In a study by Colombo et al. [55], the use of a high balloon-to-vessel ratio (1.2 : 1) with a mean pressure of 12 atm for the treatment of coronary stenosis in 60 patients was associated with a mean final percent stenosis of −8% with one case of a coronary rupture. Conversely, usage of a similar balloon-to-vessel ratio with a higher inflation pressure (mean of 15 atm), applied in the next 300 patients yielded a slight improvement in the final percent stenosis (mean −10%), but at the expense of an increase in the incidence of vessel rupture and major dissection (3.4%). Finally, in a different subgroup, usage of a smaller balloon-to-vessel ratio of only 1.0 but with a higher mean pressure (16 atm), applied in 162 patients, yielded a percent residual stenosis of 1% with a rate of coronary rupture reduced to 0.7%. Similarly, in a series by Ellis et al. [1] the mean balloon-to-artery ratio in patients treated with plain balloon angioplasty was significantly higher in those who developed coronary perforation compared with those

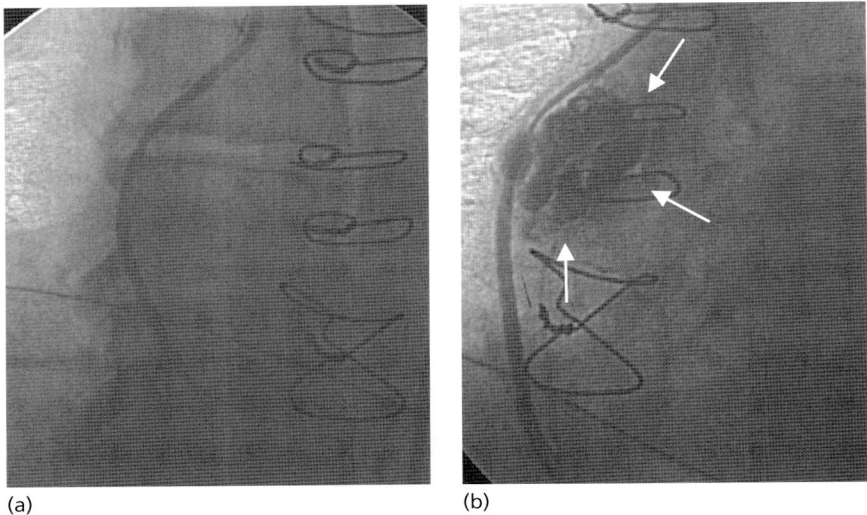

Figure 25.9 (a) An example of type III perforation; arrows (b) show post-balloon dilatation of a small saphenous vein graft to right coronary artery.

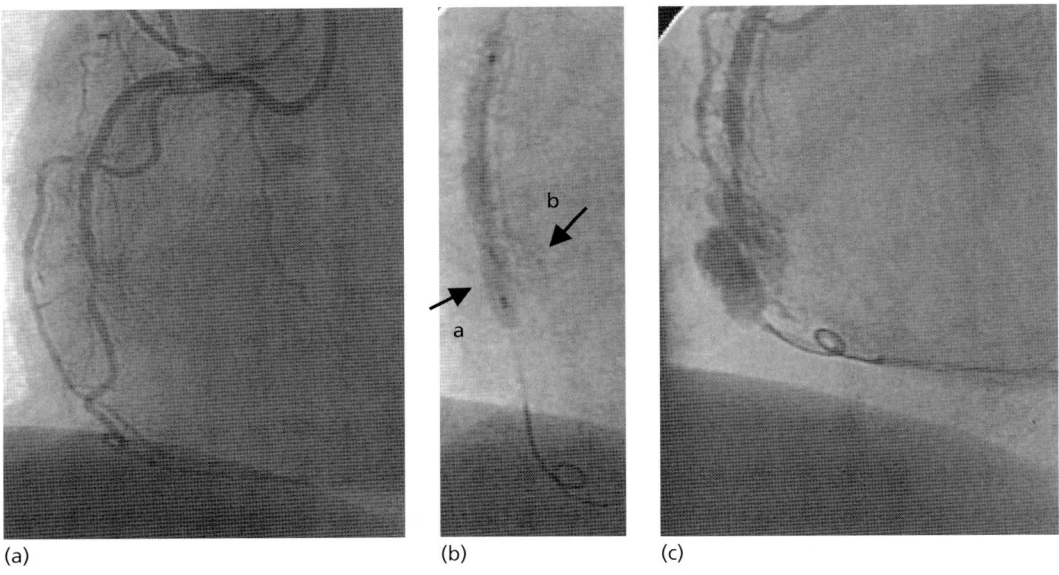

Figure 25.10 Type III perforation. This patient underwent a previous stent implantation in the mid right coronary artery. Follow-up catheterization showed restenosis with chronic total occlusion (a). (b) shows that the guidewire has been crossed and the balloon has been inflated at the origin of the acute marginal branch **a**; the distal portion of the stent is shown in (b), arrow **b**. Notice the perforation with contrast extravasation in (c).

who did not (1.19 ± 0.17 vs. 0.92 ± 0.16; $p = 0.03$). The same findings were reported by Stankovic *et al.* [56], where a high balloon-to-artery ratio was associated with a 7.6-fold increase in the odds of coronary perforation.

Vessel determinants associated with coronary rupture include lesion severity with American College of Cardiology/American Heart Association (ACC/AHA) type B or C lesions, and the presence of a more highly calcified lesion has also been associated with coronary rupture [52,57,58]. Of note, PCI for CTO is also associated with an increased risk [40].

Device-related factors

Coronary perforation can be caused by the guiding catheter, balloon rupture, guidewire, IVUS/OCT catheter, embolic protection device, and atheroablative and CTO devices [56,59,60]. Dippel *et al.* [41] reported that, of more than 6000 interventions, ablative procedures were accorded a 6.8-fold risk of perforation. In addition, the perforations with these technologies were often Ellis type III. Recently, stiffer wires for CTO procedures have been developed to dramatically enhance the ability to cross the lesions. Vessel perforation has become particularly important with the introduction of stiff wires

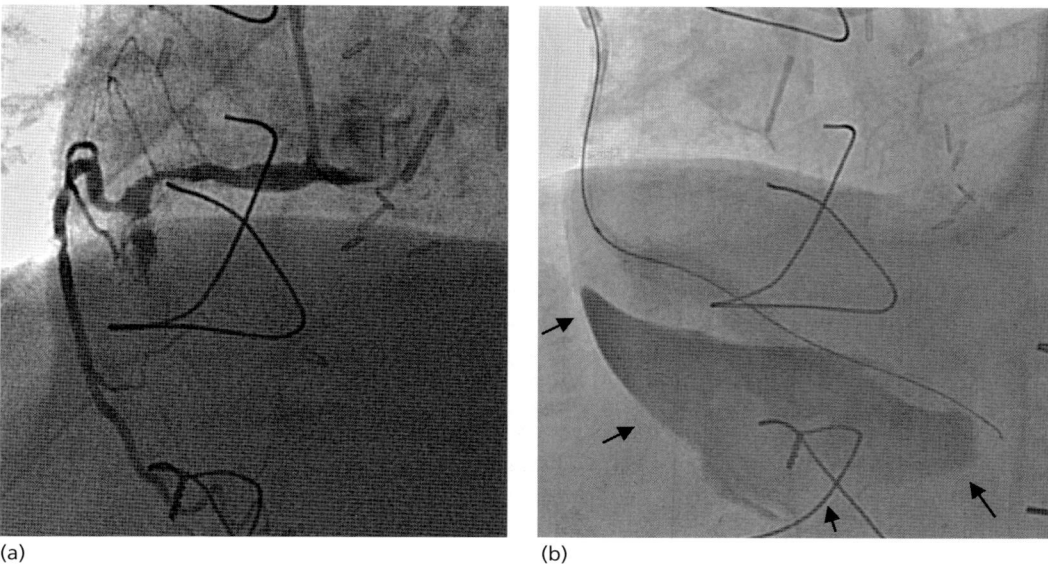

(a)   (b)

Figure 25.11 Chronic total occlusion at mid right coronary artery (a). Failed attempts leads to vessel dissection and perforation type III with pericardial effusion (b).

Table 25.3 Risk factors for coronary perforation.

Patient-related	Procedure-related	Device-related
Female gender	High balloon/stent-to-artery ratio	Stiff wire
Older age Renal insufficiency	High inflation or post-dilatation pressure	Hydrophilic-coated wire
	Extremely distal location of the guidewires Treatment of chronic total occlusion	Cutting balloon
		Atheroablative devices
		IVUS/OCT in the false lumen

IVUS, intravenous ultrasound; OCT, optical coherence tomography.

for penetrating the proximal and distal caps of CTO. However, dilating a subintimal channel can not only result in vessel occlusion or perforation, but also prohibit future surgical grafting of the coronary artery. Special attention must also be taken when hydrophilic wires are used because of their propensity for subintimal passage and perforation of end capillaries. These wires easily enter thin-walled vasa vasorum, which are prone to perforation either directly from the wire or from the subsequent dilatations. Recently, Stathopoulos *et al.* [61] analyzed 23,399 PCI and identified 73 patients complicated by coronary perforation, of which 31 were guidewire induced. In-hospital mortality was similar for patients with guidewire-induced and non-guidewire-induced perforations. Tamponade conferred a threefold increase in the long-term probability of death and guidewire-induced coronary perforation during elective PCI had the best survival.

Cardiac tamponade as well as requirement for emergency surgery are important risk factors for overall mortality with coronary perforation [1,57].

Management and treatment of perforation
Coronary perforation carries a significant mortality risk. Therefore, management and treatment are important and should be initiated very rapidly. The strategy for treating coronary perforation is best determined by specific angiographic type and clinical circumstances. Based on angiographic classification, a treatment algorithm for coronary perforations was proposed by Dippel *et al.* [41]. In general, type I perforations usually respond to conservative measurements. Stenting over the blemish often successfully deals with the problem site. In many of these conditions, prolonged proximal balloon inflation helps solve the problem. When limited pericardial effusion occurs, as in type I or II perforations, serial echocardiography can suggest clues to ongoing leakage, as evidenced by changes in the effusion size. Early diastolic right ventricular collapse and late diastolic right atrial collapse are early signs of cardiac tamponade and precede the onset of hypotension.

In limited perforations (types I and II) not caused by guidewire use, maintaining guidewire position across the perforation site is crucial, and careful balloon compression of the perforation site is usually recommended to limit further extravasation. In patients receiving heparin, reversal of the anticoagulant effects should be considered. In an analysis of the Mayo Clinic PCI database, administration of protamine sulfate and prolonged balloon inflation were the most common treatments performed after identification of a coronary perforation [52]. In those patients receiving unfractionated heparin (UFH), IV protamine sulfate should be given, with subsequent dose titration guided by anticoagulation status, to rapidly and easily reverse the anticoagulation effects [42,62]. Reversal of heparin anticoagulation should target an activated clotting time (ACT) of 150 seconds. Protamine partially neutralizes the anti-IIa activity, but not the anti-Xa activity of low-molecular-weight heparin [63,64]. Importantly, protamine has been safely administered to facilitate hemostasis following coronary stent deployment without adverse ischemic sequelae [65]. However, this safety has not been well demonstrated following drug-eluting stent (DES) implantation [66]. GP IIb/IIIa inhibitor infusion should be stopped whenever perforation occurs, regardless of the severity. The effects of abciximab can be reversed by platelet transfusion; eptifibatide and tirofiban have no antidote but have a relatively short half-life lasting several hours. Direct antithrombin agents (e.g., bivalirudin) are more problematic, as there is no antidote for this class of agents. However, we have shown treatment of patients experiencing coronary perforation with adjunctive antithrombotic therapy of bivalirudin monotherapy was not associated with worse outcomes compared than treatment with UFH plus GP IIb/IIIa inhibitors [48].

Pericardiocentesis should be performed only in the presence of cardiac tamponade with hemodynamic or echocardiographic cardiac compromise [41].

In type I perforation, management is commonly limited to careful observation for 15–30 minutes with repeated injections of contrast media, associated with the measures described above. In type II perforation, the first step in management is placement of a standard balloon catheter (2–3 atm pressure) to seal the perforation [41,67]. Then, heparin reversal and GP IIb/IIIa inhibitor discontinuation should be promptly instituted. Echocardiographic assessment should be performed without delay. Emergent cardiac surgery is reserved for those patients who do not achieve hemostasis with these conservative measures. In type III perforation, an immediate aggressive treatment strategy is required, including adequate volume resuscitation, administration of catecholamines, and, frequently, urgent pericardiocentesis. Immediate reversal of anticoagulation with IV protamine sulfate and platelet transfusion in abciximab-treated patients is critical. According to the algorithm proposed by Dippel et al. [41], treatment of type III perforation should start with standard balloon catheter inflation at the site of perforation for at least 5–10 minutes to provide time to perform pericardiocentesis. Subsequent prolonged balloon inflation can successfully seal a type III perforation or provide time to place an additional device to assist the treatment. The site of coronary perforation must be completely sealed and confirmed by an angiogram performed at least 10 minutes following treatment. Intermittent or continuous pericardial catheter aspiration should be employed overnight. Furthermore, the authors recommend in-hospital observation for an additional 24 hours with repeat echocardiography prior to discharge or on the day following pericardial catheter removal [41].

Devices and materials for coronary perforation

Several devices and materials have been used for sealing the perforation site, such as plugs, coils, glues, beads, and covered-stents. Plugs, coils, glues, and beads are usually used for small (types I or II) or distal perforations caused by the guidewire. These perforations cannot be sealed with covered stents, which are more useful for pinhole perforations. Coil embolization of coronary perforations, especially of the distal vessel, has also been used as a percutaneous bailout treatment [68,69]. In general, most studies report microcoil embolization with platinum or stainless steel coils ranging from 0.014 to 0.025 inches in diameter [70,71]. These are delivered through dedicated microcatheters and are ideal suited to this purpose (Figure 25.12). However, larger coils have been used in coronary artery ruptures or in large segment perforations [72,73]. Other, rather innovative methods of sealing distal vessel perforation have been reported: injection of thrombin [70,74]; autologous clotted blood [75]; tris-acrylgelatin microspheres [76]; fibrin glue [77]; subcutaneous adipose tissue [78]; polyvinyl alcohol foam [79]; and ethylene-vinyl-alcohol-copolymer (Onix) [80]. Any material that includes clotting and plugging the small perforation will suffice. Autologous vein-covered stents have also been described as an effective treatment option for successful percutaneous sealing of perforations [81,82]. However, isolating the graft (typically a cephalic vein) by cutdown and mounting and suturing it onto a metallic stent is time-consuming and an improbable emergency treatment for free-flowing perforation and pericardial tamponade [83].

If cardiac tamponade develops and low blood pressure ensues, pericardiocentesis and drainage with a pigtail catheter are required. An important point to consider is the need to use two guiding catheters in order to be able to control the perforation with the inflated balloon while being ready to advance a covered stent if needed. When extravascular flow is observed on angiography despite prolonged balloon inflation, a covered stent should be used to stop the leakage. If a life-threatening perforation occurs while working with a smaller guide requiring the covered stent for sealing, a balloon angioplasty catheter (or stent delivery balloon) should immediately be inflated across the tear in the coronary vessel to provide temporary hemostasis. Another guide catheter should then be introduced via contralateral femoral artery access and used to cannulate the coronary ostium after gently disengaging the other guide. The covered stent should be introduced into the new guide over a second guidewire and passed just proximal to the occluding balloon, which is then deflated and retracted, allowing passage of the new guidewire and the covered stent for definite closure of the perforation [84].

A bare metal stent covered by an ultrathin polymer (polyethylene terephthalate) mesh sleeve on its external surface, the MGuard® stent (InspireMD, Tel Aviv, Israel), has been described as an option for sealing coronary perforations (Figure 25.13) [85,86]. The protective net is composed of micron-level fibers with pore size of ≤200 μm. It was developed to block the plaque and thrombus detachment from the arterial wall during and after the intervention to reduce embolization. The MGuard® stent is a combination of a bare metal stent and an embolic protection device, intended to represent a feasible and safe treatment option in patients with STEMI and saphenous vein graft (SVG) intervention.

Covered stent device description

The most widely used device is the polytetrafluoroethylene (PTFE) covered stent which can reduce the mortality related to coronary perforation to 10% [56]. The currently available coronary stent graft is a balloon expandable, slotted-tube stent. The Jostent/Graftmaster RX® coronary stent graft device (AbbottVascular Devices, Abbott Park, IL, USA) consists of an ultrathin (75 μm), biocompatible, and expandable PTFE layer sandwiched in between two coaxial 316 L stainless steel, slotted-tube, balloon-expandable stents. Available lengths of the stent are 16, 19, and 26 mm, with diameters of 2.8–4.8 mm. The main limitations of the stent are an enhanced propensity for stent thrombosis, which can be diminished by high-pressure prolonged balloon inflation (for optimal expansion, the recommended inflation pressure is 15–16 atm for at least 30 seconds to allow for complete stent expansion), IVUS/OCT evaluation for proper implantation, and prolonged antiplatelet therapy that includes aspirin and thienopyridines. Several reports have described the use of the PTFE-covered stent in treating coronary perforations, with favorable results [1,81,84,87–89].

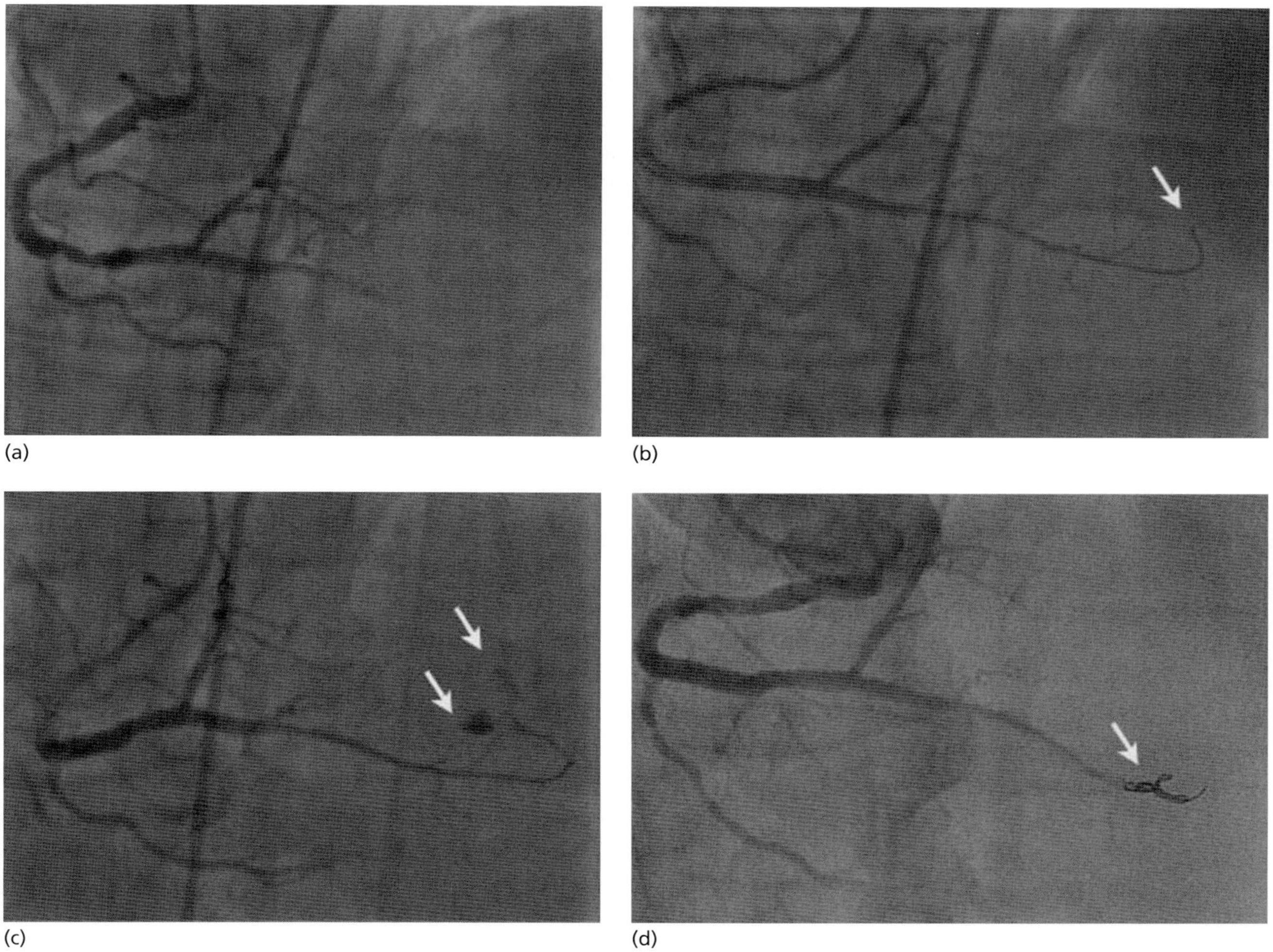

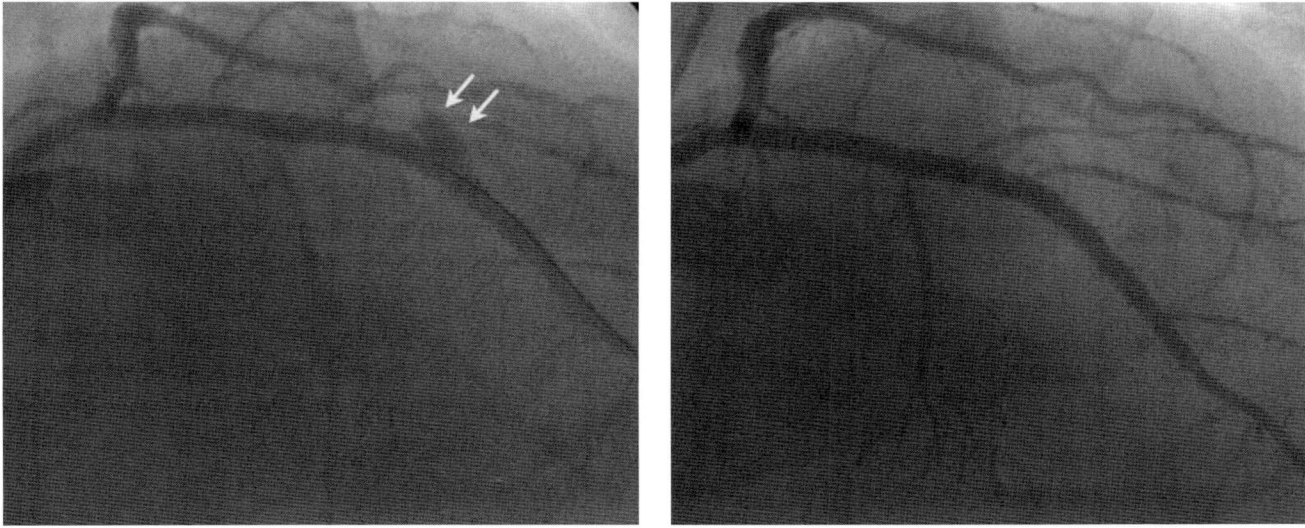

Figure 25.12 Right coronary artery in the RAO cranial view pre PCI in a patient with non-ST elevation myocardial infarction. The target vessel was the posterior descending artery, which is occluded. (a) After vessel recanalization using Whisper hidrophilic coated wire (Abbott Vascular, USA), the tip of the wire went inadvertently through in the very distal part of the vessel (b) causing perforation with contrast jet extravasation to the left ventricule (c). The perforation was sucessfully sealed using Azur platinum coil with expandable hydrogel polymer (d) (Terumo, Japan).

Figure 25.13 Left anterior descending artery in the RAO cranial view after multiple DES implantation (left). After post-dilatation with non-compliant balloon a type I perforation with extraluminal crater without extravasation is noted (arrows). Protamine was administered for heparin reversal following Mguard stent implantation. The site of the perforation is completely sealed after stenting (right).

In a multicenter, retrospective, international registry, Lansky et al. [84] reported the use of Jostent® coronary stent grafts in 41 cases of coronary perforations. Perforations were relatively severe: 16.7% Ellis type I, 54.2% type II, and 29.1% type III. Of the 41 patients, >1/3 (n = 14) experienced life-threatening complications before stent graft implantation, including pericardial tamponade (12.2%), cardiogenic shock (9.8%), and cardiac arrest (2.4%). A total of 52 coronary stent grafts were used to treat the 41 perforations (mean 1.3 per lesion). All coronary stent grafts were placed successfully, with 92.9% of the perforations sealed completely and 7.1% partially. One patient developed abrupt vessel closure after coronary stent graft deployment, resulting in an overall procedure success rate of 96.4%.

Based on a comparison of outcomes of coronary perforations in two Milan centers before and after 1998, Stankovic et al. [56] showed that the use of the covered stent was associated with a significant reduction of in-hospital major adverse cardiac events (MACE) (death, any MI, and TVR) in type III perforations (91–33%), but had no impact on the clinical course of type II perforations. A two-center study in Europe reported 49 cases of coronary perforation complicating a total of 10,945 PCI procedures (0.45%) [87]. Adequate sealing of the perforation was not achieved by conventional methods (perfusion balloon, reversal of anticoagulation, platelet transfusion with/without pericardiocentesis) in 29 of 49 patients (59%). The first 17 of 29 patients in this series were treated with Palmaz-Schatz™ stents (attempted in five but successful in only two patients) and/or with emergent cardiac surgery (15 patients). In the subsequent 12 of 29 patients, perforations were treated with PTFE-covered stents. In this series, PTFE-covered stents successfully sealed 91% of coronary perforations after other conservative approaches failed. In the same series, pericardial effusion without hemodynamic impairment was identified less frequently in patients receiving another stent and/or undergoing urgent cardiac surgery. Although PTFE-covered stents are considered to be the device of choice in the treatment of coronary perforations, in some situations the use of this stent is technically difficult or even impossible because of its limitations, including limited flexibility and tractability, especially in diffusely diseased vessels. Furthermore, the use of covered stents in native coronary arteries must be undertaken with caution, given the potential for side branch coverage with subsequent myonecrosis. Another recently available covered stent outside the USA is the Direct-Stent® Stent-Graft (InSitu Technologies InC. MN, USA), which consists of a single layer of ePTFE polymer with proprietary micro-porous technology. Available lengths of the stent are 10 and 38 mm, with diameters of 2.25–60 mm.

Early and late clinical outcome

For the patient with major perforation in hospital, careful observation with frequent hemodynamic monitoring is required after the procedure, and follow-up angiographic examination should be performed the next day. After making sure there are no adverse findings, the patient can be discharged.

Sequelae of coronary perforations range in severity from none to devastating, and are fraught with early (often instant) and/or late complications. Based on the series by Ellis et al. [1], a clear correlation exists between the angiographic type of coronary perforation and early complications. In this series, mortality and Q-wave MI were entirely limited to type III perforations. The majority of cases of emergent CABG and tamponade were also associated with type III perforations (63% for both complications), while emergent CABG and tamponade were remarkably lower in type I and II

coronary perforations. Interestingly, a recent study showed that despite treatment of more complex disease, the incidence of coronary perforation has not increased, which has been confirmed by a meta-analysis performed by Shimony et al. [90,91].

In the series described by Dippel et al. [41], clinical outcomes were quite favorable in patients with type II perforations: there were no cases of death or emergency CABG, with only one patient (5.3%) requiring pericardiocentesis. Importantly, these outcomes were achieved despite fairly infrequent reversals of procedural anticoagulation (21.1%), platelet transfusion (15.8%), or the use of prolonged perfusion balloon catheter inflation (26.3%), although the majority of patients (73.7%) received abciximab during PCI. In contrast, patients with type III perforations had a higher rate of mortality (21.4%), pericardial tamponade (42.9%), and emergent CABG (50.0%), despite more aggressive therapies including the use of protamine (64.3%), platelet transfusions (50.0%), and prolonged perfusion balloon catheter inflations (87.7%). Similarly, in a series by Stankovic et al. [56], all cases of in-hospital death and/or emergency CABG were associated exclusively with type III coronary perforations. Al-Lamee et al. [92] confirmed those findings, showing a high acute mortality (during the procedure and in-hospital mortality of 3.6% and 14.8%, respectively) and high long-term mortality and MACE rates (15.2% and 41.3%, respectively) after grade III coronary perforation.

A number of reports have emphasized that pericardial tamponade can develop several hours after coronary perforation. In a series by Ellis et al. [1], there was a 5–10% incidence of delayed (24 hours or more post-PCI) tamponade, arguing for careful patient monitoring, especially during that time period. Delayed pericardial tamponade typically results from a guidewire-related perforation and occurs not infrequently in patients undergoing recanalization of a CTO. Fukutomi et al. [42] reported five cardiac tamponades occurring in a total of 25 patients; in 12 patients, signs of tamponade emerged immediately after coronary perforation, while a delayed presentation (after a mean time of 4.9 ± 3.4 hours) occurred in 13 patients who were all treated for CTO lesions. In the same series, a guidewire caused coronary perforations in 8 of 13 patients (61.5%), with a delayed development of pericardial tamponade. Finally, in a series by Fejka et al. [44] analyzing 31 cases of cardiac tamponade occurring in a total of 25,697 procedures (0.12%) during a 7-year period, tamponade was diagnosed during the procedure in 17 patients (55%) at a mean time of 18 minutes from the start of PCI; in 14 patients (45%), tamponade presented later (mean time 4.4 hours post-PCI, range 2–15 hours). The same study clearly demonstrated that cardiac tamponade related to coronary perforation was associated with high rates of mortality; 13 of 31 patients (42%) in this series died. Mortality was especially high for those patients who developed cardiac tamponade during PCI compared with those who developed delayed tamponade (59% vs. 21% of patients).

The no-reflow phenomenon

No-reflow (or slow-flow or slow-reflow) phenomenon during PCI refers to a condition of decreased or absent antegrade coronary blood flow without angiographic evidence of a persistent mechanical obstruction [93,94]. By definition, no-reflow can be diagnosed only after excluding other causes of reduced antegrade flow such as dissection, spasm, thrombus, or a residual high-grade stenosis. It occurs rarely in elective PCI, but far more frequently in patients who present with acute MI. Persistent no-reflow has important prognostic implications and has been associated with unfavorable clinical outcomes [8–10,95]. Patients who develop no-reflow during PCI have a significantly higher incidence of in-hospital and long-term complications such as MI, stent thrombosis, heart failure, negative ventricular remodeling, ventricular tachycardia, and death [8–14,96].

Incidence

The overall incidence of angiographic no-reflow phenomenon during PCI ranges from 0.2% to 2%. Higher rates have been reported for primary PCI (5–23%), SVG (9%), and rotational atherectomy (12%) [8,13,96–98]. It has been observed more commonly in diabetics, in lesions with a large thrombotic burden, and in patients without pre-infarction angina, suggesting a protective effect from ischemic preconditioning [6,7,12,14,93]. Also, it is more pronounced with longer periods of coronary occlusions [94]. Of note, except for thrombus-containing long lesions and degenerative SVGs, it can be difficult to predict the risk of no-reflow based on the angiographic appearance of a lesion. Furthermore, other causes of impaired coronary flow can simulate no-reflow including dissection, intracoronary thrombus formation, intracoronary bubble injection, epicardial coronary spasm, or remaining high-grade stenosis.

Pathophysiology

The pathophysiology of no-reflow is complex and not entirely understood, but appears to be multifactorial. Potential mechanisms differ depending on the clinical setting and lesion type undergoing PCI. In humans, it appears to be a combination of distal embolization, inflammation, and microvascular spasm [12,14,93,99–101]. Substantial capillary damage can also be seen with intraluminal obstruction resulting from endothelial swelling, capillary plugging, and microthombi. An observed relationship between plaque volume, necrotic core, and distal coronary perfusion after PCI suggests that the release of material from the plaque is related to, if not causal, in distal microvascular obstruction. In fact, aspiration of coronary arteries in patients with thrombotic lesions and no-reflow has shown embolic debris (containing both thrombi and atheromatous gruel) in the majority of cases [100]. Vasospasm appears to have a central role in the pathogenesis of no-reflow irrespective of the clinical scenario in which it occurs. Experimental data suggest that microvascular vasospasm is caused by the release of serotonin, angiotensin II, thromboxane, and α-adrenergic agonists [8,102–104]. The local release of these vasoconstrictor substances impairs capillary autoregulation and increases reflex sympathetic activity.

Other mechanisms that have been implicated include oxygen free radical-mediated injury, reperfusion injury with loss of microvascular integrity [100,101], endothelial dysfunction, neutrophil infiltration, platelet aggregation, plasminogen activator inhibitor-1, tissue factor, and inflammatory factors (sCD40L, soluble E-selectin) [93,100,101,105]. The triggers of no-reflow during PCI appear to be distal embolization of plaque and/or thrombus with subsequent microcirculatory spasm. Thus, no-reflow is a major problem in the treatment of acute MI, thrombus-containing lesions, large plaque burden, rotational atherectomy, and SVG (Figure 25.14) [106].

Prevention

Possible approaches to prevent the no-reflow phenomenon include the use of mechanical aspiration, distal embolic protection, direct stenting, systemic infusion of GP IIb/IIIa inhibitors, and intracoronary infusion of vasodilating or antithrombotic/thrombolytic agents. Apart from antiplatelet agent, all pharmacological drugs should be injected superselectively into the target vessel in order to reach effectively areas of myocardium.

Thrombectomy and aspiration

Occlusive thrombosis from an unstable atherosclerotic plaque is the substrate of most acute MIs. Therefore, macro- and micro-embolization during PCI in acute MI results in obstruction of the microvascular network and subsequently in reduced efficacy of reperfusion and myocardial salvage [107]. Use of adjunctive thrombectomy during primary PCI has been associated with significant improvement in coronary flow before stent implantation as well as post-procedural epicardial and myocardial perfusion with less distal embolization. However, its benefit for long-term survival is controversial [108–110]. For instance, in the INFUSE-AMI trial [109], patients randomized to aspiration thrombectomy vs. no aspiration had no significant difference in infarct size at 30 days, absolute infarct mass, or abnormal wall motion score. The multicenter, prospective, randomized TASTE trial [110], enrolled 7244 patients from the national comprehensive Swedish Coronary Angiography and Angioplasty Registry (SCAAR). Patients with STEMI undergoing PCI were randomly assigned to manual thrombus aspiration followed by PCI or to PCI only. Disappointingly, routine thrombus aspiration before PCI compared with PCI alone did not reduce 30-day mortality among patients with STEMI (2.8% vs. 3.0%). Finally, with regard to mechanical thrombectomy, the results of randomized trials do not show benefit [111,112].

Distal protection devices

The use of distal protection devices during SVG PCI has decreased the incidence of no-reflow during PCI in several studies, and confirmed the role of distal embolization in the development of this complication. As a result of their proven effectiveness in preventing distal embolization, no-reflow and MACE, the AHA/ACC/SCAI recommend the use of distal embolic protection devices when technically feasible in patients undergoing PCI to SVGs [113,114]. The SAFER trial established that the routine use of a distal protection device is associated with a reduced incidence of no-reflow in the treatment of degenerated SVGs [115].

The efficacy of a distal embolic protective device in acute STEMI was addressed in the multicenter EMERALD trial. Despite the removal of debris, there was no difference between the two groups in terms of ST segment resolution at 30 minutes (63% vs. 62%) and left ventricular infarct size (12.0% vs. 9.5%). In addition, MACE at 6 months were similar in the two groups (10% vs. 11%). The lack of benefit persisted when only patients undergoing primary PCI were evaluated [116]. Other subgroup analysis did not identify any subset of patients in whom an advantage of distal protection occurred [116,117].

Several explanations can be proposed regarding these negative findings. First of all, we should consider that in the setting of acute MI distal embolization can induce an additional, although limited, myocardial necrosis. This increase plays a minor part against the large background of necrosis resulting from ischemia and/or reperfusion. This condition differs from embolization that may occur in SVGs, in which the myocardial area distal to the graft is viable. Also, the type of device used and its crossing profile, operator experience, and technique of usage may have a relevant role. Whatever part embolic protection devices might play, they cannot be employed in all patients, but only in a minority of them with particular clinical or anatomic features and the problem is how to select patients who

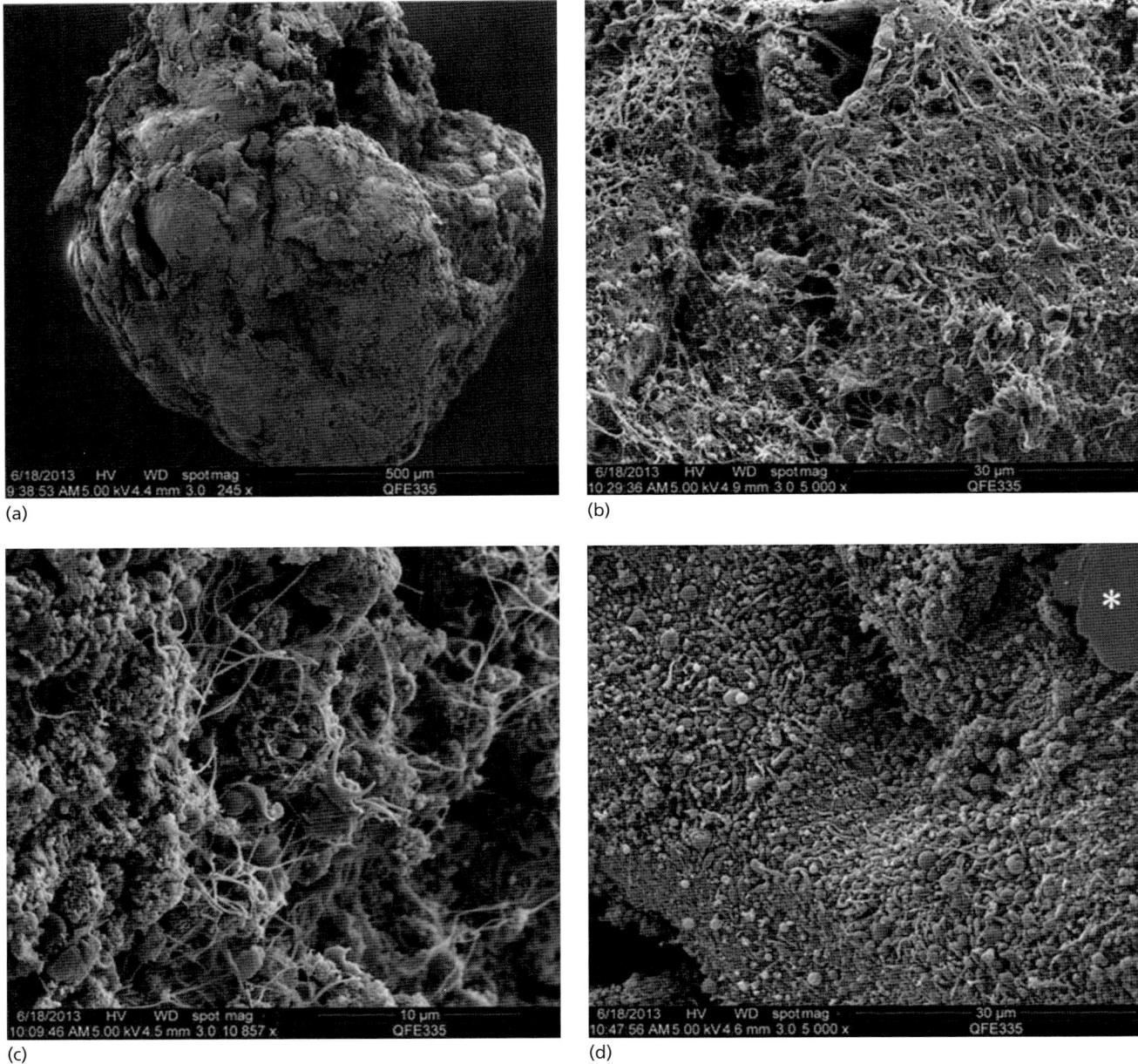

Figure 25.14 Scanning electron microscopy (SEM) of the aspirated material from saphenous vein graft in an 80-year-old patient with a history of prior coronary artery bypass graft surgery. Coronary angiography showed a severe lesion in the saphenous vein graft to obtuse marginal (a). Slow-phenomenon was observed even after thrombus aspiration (b) and distal protection distal. SEM showing fibrin network, entrapped erythrocytes, activated platelets, and cholesterol crystals (*) (c, d).

may benefit from dedicated devices. The indiscriminate utilization of this resource to all patients not only represents an unjustified adjunctive cost, but is also associated with increased procedural time and reperfusion delay.

Direct stenting

In patients with an acute STEMI undergoing primary PCI, direct stenting can reduce embolization of plaque constituents, lowering the incidence of the no-reflow phenomenon, thereby increasing myocardial perfusion and salvage. Direct stenting can also

improve myocardial perfusion and the incidence of death, MI, or heart failure compared with conventional stenting in patients who undergo PCI after fibrinolysis [118–121].

Systemic glycoprotein IIb/IIIa inhibitors

It is unclear whether GP IIb/IIIa inhibitors when infused peripherally reduce the incidence of no-reflow, because data addressing this issue are limited and inconsistent.

The effect of GP IIb/IIIa receptor inhibitors in preventing no-reflow during SVG intervention has been disappointing [122].

Roffi *et al.* [123] performed a pooled analysis of five randomized intravenous GP IIb/IIIa inhibitor trials (EPIC, EPILOG, EPISTENT, IMPACT II, and PURSUIT) showing that prophylactic administration of these agents does not improve outcomes during PCI of SVG.

Intracoronary infusions

An intracoronary infusion of adenosine, verapamil, streptokinase, or abciximab has been evaluated studies for its ability to improve myocardial reperfusion, prevent reperfusion injury, and salvage ischemic myocardium at the time of primary PCI. In the INFUSE-AMI trial [109], patients with large anterior STEMI presenting early after symptom onset and undergoing primary PCI with bivalirudin anticoagulation, infarct size at 30 days was significantly reduced by bolus intracoronary abciximab (6.8% vs. 17.9%) delivered to the infarct lesion site but not by manual aspiration thrombectomy. Patients randomized to intracoronary abciximab also had a significant reduction in absolute infarct mass (18.7 vs. 24.0 g). The routine use of abciximab during primary PCI has yet to be adopted after the results of larger clinical trials.

Verapamil pre-treatment has been shown to be effective in reducing no-reflow during SVG intervention in a small (n = 32) randomized trial [124]. However, the intragraft verapamil failed to reduce the mortality or MI in patients with no-reflow and has not been incorporated into clinical practice.

Chronic statin therapy

It has been suggested that statin therapy reduces myocardial injury after PCI. Plaque stabilization and other pleiotropic effects of statin therapy could lower rate of no-reflow, improve wall motion, and left ventricular ejection fraction [125].

Treatment

Once no-reflow occurs, every attempt must be made to reverse it in order to reduce the risk of adverse outcome [126]. During PCI procedures, no-reflow can manifest as acute ischemia and be associated with chest pain, ECG changes, bradycardia, conduction disturbances, and hypotension leading to marked hemodynamic instability and cardiogenic shock. However, there are also rare cases of no-reflow that occur without any clinical sequelae. The initial evaluation and treatment of no-reflow consists of maintaining hemodynamic and electrophysiological stability. Box 25.1 provides a guide to the evaluation and management of no-reflow.

As the predominant abnormality during no-reflow appears to be microvascular constriction, different vasoactive drugs have been employed for the treatment of this phenomenon and their efficacy depends on coronary artery vasodilatation and hyperemia induction especially at the microvascular level [7,93,99,122].

Nitroglycerin

In fact, nitroglycerin (NTG) is not effective in reversing no-reflow and is given at the onset of no-reflow in order to exclude epicardial coronary spasm. It has been shown that NTG administration results in an increase in minimum lumen diameter that is not further increased by nitroprusside [127]. NTG also did not change any of the examined angiographic parameters (TIMI grade, corrected TIMI frame count, and TIMI myocardial blush) compared with baseline values (after stent deployment). This lack of effect on no-reflow has been confirmed in a number of studies [8,11].

> **Box 25.1** Strategy for evaluating and management of no-reflow
>
> 1 Exclude dissection, epicardial spasm, thrombus at lesion site, distal macro-embolism or air embolism
> 2 Check ACT levels (250–300 s)
> 3 Ensure oxygenation, hemodynamic stability, and maintain adequate coronary perfusion pressures
> 4 Intracoronary nitrates to exclude epicardial coronary artery spasm
> 5 Administer pharmacologic agents super-selectively into distal arterial bed by infusion catheter/microcatheter or over-the-wire balloon
>   a. Nitroprusside 80–200 µg bolus (up to 1000 µg total dose). Consider alternating with boluses of epinephrine 50–200 µg
>   b. Adenosine 10–20 µg high velocity boluses repeated as needed (10–30 doses)
>   c. Verapamil 50–200 µg bolus (up to 1000 µg total dose with temporary pacemaker standby)
>   d. Second-line agents for which evidence is less strong: epinephrine 50–200 µg, nicorandil 2 µg, papaverine 10–20 µg, nicardipine 200 µg, diltiazem 0.5–2.5 mg over 1 min up to 5 mg
> 6 Consider administering a glycoprotein IIb/IIIa receptor inhibitor intracoronary/intragraft or intravenous

Nitroprusside

NTG and nitroprusside (NTP) are both donors of nitric oxide, an endothelium-derived compound that has multiple vascular functions, including vasodilatation, inhibition of platelet adhesion, and anti-inflammatory activity [128]. Nitric oxide is a potent vasodilator in the resistance arteriolar circulation [129] and plays a significant part in the control of coronary blood flow through the microcirculation [130]. However, there is an important distinction between NTG and NTP. Resistance vessels, which primarily determine coronary blood flow, have a decreased capacity for enzymatic conversion of NTG into nitric oxide. Unlike NTG, NTP is a direct donor of nitric oxide and is reported to require no intracellular metabolism to derive nitric oxide; thus making nitric oxide available to the microcirculation and effectively dilating these distal vessels.

NTP has gained favor with many operators for its rapid and marked vasodilating effect with limited systemic hypotension. However, its dosage and efficacy in different clinical settings are not yet clearly established, because available information is derived from retrospective analysis of angiographic findings in different clinical conditions with different doses, routes of administration, and efficacy assessments [99,127,128]. A standardized NTP protocol has been suggested [127]:

1 Insert a multifunction catheter or over-the-wire balloon into the culprit vessel

2 Initial 80-µg bolus of NTP is selectively administered distal to the site of stent implantation or balloon dilatation via the multifunction catheter.

3 If no response, boluses of NTP with an increment of 40 µg each time is repeated every 2 minutes.

4 NTP boluses are continued until TIMI 3 flow is achieved or systolic blood pressure decreases to <80 mm Hg.

It was observed that the initial 80-µg bolus restored normal TIMI flow normal in 58% of patients (7 of 12) with acute MI and in 44% of patients (4 of 9) with SVG stenosis. The maximal dose (120–160 µg) restored normal TIMI flow in all remaining patients with acute MI but in only one additional patient with SVG stenosis. This standardized protocol for intracoronary NTP administration succeeded in normalizing coronary flow in all patients with acute MI but in only 55% of patients with slow flow in SVG.

Two important factors why NTP has not been shown to be effective in some of the previous studies:

1 *Local drug delivery:* we believe that selectively delivering the drug distal in the coronary bed via a microcatheter is essential and superior to injection via guiding catheter or systemically. This exploits its maximal effect at the target site and allowing, when necessary, the use of higher doses of NTP without detrimental systemic effects on blood pressure. Agents administered via the guiding catheter will preferentially distribute to areas with normal flow.

2 *Incremental doses:* in a large proportion of patients only large doses of NTP were effective. Because of its relatively short half-life (50–70 s), a greater effect of NTP cannot be obtained by repeated cumulative small boluses but only by single large boluses.

Verapamil

Intracoronary calcium-channel blockers such as verapamil have been administered for no-reflow during PCI for acute MI and have been shown to improve microvascular perfusion and myocardial salvage [104]. Although microvascular and macrovascular spasm may be calcium mediated [131], their mechanism of action may go beyond the fact that they act directly on the vascular smooth muscle rather than nitric oxide. In the setting of acute ischemia invoked by balloon inflations during PTCA, verapamil has been shown to increase the ischemic tolerance significantly. Its cardioprotective effects are ascribed to the reduction of calcium influx into the ischemic myocardial cell, restitution of the calcium homeostasis, and improved myocardial blood flow by relief of microvascular spasm [132,133]. Verapamil can also affect platelet aggregation in the setting of acute MI by reducing the effects of catecholamines [132–134].

Verapamil is the most studied drug for the treatment of no-reflow. It has been shown that verapamil only improves TIMI flow grade in 67–89% and up to 88% when administered with NTG [6,8,11,104,135].

A major limitation of verapamil and the main reason why many interventionalists are reluctant to use it are because of its adverse effects such as hypotension, prolonged heart block, and a negative inotropic effect. In a patient who is already hypotensive or having conduction disturbances from no-reflow, we would strongly advise not using verapamil. Similarly, in patients with severe left ventricular dysfunction, this negative inotropic agent should not be used.

Adenosine

Adenosine has a very short half-life (usually a few seconds) and is well tolerated without significant side effects. It is capable of dilating the coronary resistance vessels and appears to be more potent than verapamil for relieving microvascular spasm. The vasodilator effect of this drug is mediated by specific adenosine A2A and A2B receptors and related to the opening of ATP-sensitive K+ channels. Furthermore, adenosine has been suggested to have a role in the preservation of endothelium integrity [136–138]. In experimental studies, adenosine has also been shown to inhibit neutrophil accumulation, superoxide generation, and adherence of coronary endothelium as well as cardiac release of endothelin [136]. Although the preventive effect of adenosine against no-reflow may be due to both the vasodilator and anti-inflammatory actions of the drug, the beneficial effect observed after no-reflow is more likely a result of its vasodilator action. Unlike verapamil, adenosine has little potential to cause prolonged detrimental effects upon atrioventricular conduction or myocardial contractility.

Prior studies [138,139] have shown that adenosine has a beneficial effect in treating no-reflow during SVG intervention. One of the novel aspects of the study by Fischell *et al.* [139] was the use of repetitive forceful injections of adenosine and saline flushes using a small-volume (3 mL) syringe. In an *ex vivo* model intended to simulate the conditions of no-reflow, the authors demonstrated the potentially beneficial effects of this approach in generating greater velocity and pressure during saline administration. It is likely that the mechanical advantage afforded by a small syringe allows more effective delivery of the active vasodilator to the target vascular bed, without the need for a drug infusion catheter. It is also possible that these forceful injections help to mechanically drive debris and/or aggregating platelets through the microvascular bed and into the coronary and then systemic venous circulation. Two studies have compared the combination of adenosine and NTP, at doses of 50–200 μg, with adenosine alone. Both agents mediate vasodilatation in the coronary microcirculation in different but potentially additive mechanisms and the combination has been shown to be superior to adenosine alone [136,140].

Other agents

Several other approaches to the treatment of no-reflow have been published such as intracoronary or intragraft injections of abciximab, nicorandil, epinephrine, nicardipine, diltiazem, urokinase, abciximab, intra-aortic balloon pumps, and papaverine [6,141–144].

Intravenous platelet GP IIb/IIIa receptor inhibitors are usually administered in cases of no-reflow when distal embolization is considered to be the predominant underlying cause. They resolve any platelet-rich thrombi that has occurred and prevent platelet plugs from developing. However, only a single case report suggests utility in this setting [142]. There are also anecdotal reports regarding the use of antiplatelet agents (abciximab) to treat no-reflow after failed treatment with intracoronary verapamil in native coronary arteries. In addition, a report by Heitzer *et al.* [145] has found that the GP IIb/IIIa inhibitors (tirofiban and eptifibatide) improve the bioavailability of vascular nitric oxide in patients with coronary artery disease, by blocking platelet–endothelial interactions, which potentially adds vasodilator properties to these agents.

Nicorandil is a direct ATP K+ channel opener and as the vasodilatory action of adenosine is mediated by these channels, nicorandil has been attempted in treating no-reflow, either alone or in combination with adenosine. However, data are still limited [146]. Finally, intracoronary epinephrine has been shown to improve flow in 69% of PCI patients with refractory no-reflow [147]. However, data on all the above agents are still limited to small case series or anecdotal reports and thus these agents have not been incorporated into daily practice.

Prognosis of no-reflow

No-reflow has been associated with an increase in MI of up to 32% and a 5–15% higher incidence of death [6–8]. The reversibility of no-flow is an important prognostic factor in that it has been associated with a lower 30-day mortality rate [126]. Although restoration of epicardial flow does not always imply complete reperfusion at the myocardial level, achievement of TIMI 3 flow is extremely important for improvement of myocardial function and outcome [6,9]. No-reflow has also been associated with long-term detrimental effects, including an increased risk for cardiac death, congestive heart failure, malignant arrhythmias, and a decrease in ejection fraction. The predictors of death with no-reflow include cardiogenic shock, large amount of jeopardized myocardium, history of congestive heart failure or left ventricular ejection fraction < 30%, age ≥ 65–70 years, multivessel disease (especially with collaterals from the index vessel to another location), female gender, and prolonged time needed to restore flow [6–8]. We have recently shown in a large-scale HORIZONS-AMI trial that failure to restore normal TIMI flow after PCI in STEMI occurred in 12.9% of patients, and was associated with a twofold higher mortality at 3-year follow-up [96].

Conclusions

Coronary dissection with vessel occlusion, coronary perforation following coronary angiography or PCI, and the no-reflow phenomenon are dreaded complications occurring in the catheterization laboratory. These complications can result in acute MI, need for urgent coronary artery bypass surgery, pericardial tamponade, heart failure, and death.

The management of coronary dissection depends on the patency of the distal vessel and the extent of propagation of the dissection. In general, in the presence of MI or acute closure, coronary stenting is mandated.

For coronary perforation, the treatment strategy depends on the type of vessel and the location of the injury. Principles include prompt recognition of perforation, immediate balloon tamponade of the injured vessel, rapid reversal of anticoagulation or antiplatelet therapy, addressing hemodynamic instability, involvement of surgeons if appropriate, and specific treatment of the vessel perforation or rupture with a bailout device such as embolization coils or covered stents.

The no-reflow phenomenon is a diagnosis of exclusion and needs to be treated promptly with superselective distal intracoronary injection of nitroprusside (associated or not to adenosine) using an over-the-wire angioplasty balloon or intracoronary infusion microcatheter. During SVG intervention, an embolic protection device should always be used if technically feasible to prevent no-reflow.

Interactive multiple choice questions are available for this chapter on www.wiley.com/go/dangas/cardiology

References

1 Ellis SG, Ajluni S, Arnold AZ, et al. Increased coronary perforation in the new device era. Incidence, classification, management, and outcome. *Circulation* 1994; **90**(6): 2725–2730.

2 Ajluni SC, Glazier S, Blankenship L, O'Neill WW, Safian RD. Perforations after percutaneous coronary interventions: clinical, angiographic, and therapeutic observations. *Catheter Cardiovasc Diagn* 1994; **32**(3): 206–212.

3 Elsner M, Zeiher AM. [Perforation and rupture of coronary arteries]. *Herz* 1998; **23**(5): 311–8.

4 Holmes DR Jr, Reeder GS, Ghazzal ZM, et al. Coronary perforation after excimer laser coronary angioplasty: the Excimer Laser Coronary Angioplasty Registry experience. *J Am Coll Cardiol* 1994; **23**(2): 330–335.

5 Kini A, Marmur JD, Duvvuri S, Dangas G, Choudhary S, Sharma SK. Rotational atherectomy: improved procedural outcome with evolution of technique and equipment. Single-center results of first 1,000 patients. *Catheter Cardiovasc Interv* 1999; **46**(3): 305–311.

6 Abbo KM, Dooris M, Glazier S, et al. Features and outcome of no-reflow after percutaneous coronary intervention. *Am J Cardiol* 1995; **75**(12): 778–782.

7 Klein LW, Kern MJ, Berger P, et al. Society of cardiac angiography and interventions: suggested management of the no-reflow phenomenon in the cardiac catheterization laboratory. *Catheter Cardiovasc Interv* 2003; **60**(2): 194–201.

8 Piana RN, Paik GY, Moscucci M, et al. Incidence and treatment of "no-reflow" after percutaneous coronary intervention. *Circulation* 1994; **89**(6): 2514–2518.

9 Ito H, Maruyama A, Iwakura K, et al. Clinical implications of the "no reflow" phenomenon: a predictor of complications and left ventricular remodeling in reperfused anterior wall myocardial infarction. *Circulation* 1996; **93**(2): 223–228.

10 Resnic FS, Wainstein M, Lee MK, et al. No-reflow is an independent predictor of death and myocardial infarction after percutaneous coronary intervention. *Am Heart J* 2003; **145**(1): 42–46.

11 Kaplan BM, Benzuly KH, Kinn JW, et al. Treatment of no-reflow in degenerated saphenous vein graft interventions: comparison of intracoronary verapamil and nitroglycerin. *Catheter Cardiovasc Diagn* 1996; **39**(2): 113–118.

12 Kaul S, Ito H. Microvasculature in acute myocardial ischemia: part II: evolving concepts in pathophysiology, diagnosis, and treatment. *Circulation* 2004; **109**(3): 310–315.

13 Morishima I, Sone T, Okumura K, et al. Angiographic no-reflow phenomenon as a predictor of adverse long-term outcome in patients treated with percutaneous transluminal coronary angioplasty for first acute myocardial infarction. *J Am Coll Cardiol* 2000; **36**(4): 1202–1209.

14 Kaul S, Ito H. Microvasculature in acute myocardial ischemia: part I: evolving concepts in pathophysiology, diagnosis, and treatment. *Circulation* 2004; **109**(2): 146–149.

15 Detre K, Holubkov R, Kelsey S, et al. Percutaneous transluminal coronary angioplasty in 1985–1986 and 1977–1981. The National Heart, Lung, and Blood Institute Registry. *N Engl J Med* 1988; **318**(5): 265–270.

16 Ellis SG, Roubin GS, King SB 3rd, et al. Angiographic and clinical predictors of acute closure after native vessel coronary angioplasty. *Circulation* 1988; **77**(2): 372–379.

17 Detre KM, Holmes DR Jr, Holubkov R, et al. Incidence and consequences of periprocedural occlusion. The 1985–1986 National Heart, Lung, and Blood Institute Percutaneous Transluminal Coronary Angioplasty Registry. *Circulation* 1990; **82**(3): 739–750.

18 de Feyter PJ, van den Brand M, Laarman GJ, van Domburg R, Serruys PW, Suryapranata H. Acute coronary artery occlusion during and after percutaneous transluminal coronary angioplasty: frequency, prediction, clinical course, management, and follow-up. *Circulation* 1991; **83**(3): 927–936.

19 de Feyter PJ, de Jaegere PP, Serruys PW. Incidence, predictors, and management of acute coronary occlusion after coronary angioplasty. *Am Heart J* 1994; **127**(3): 643–651.

20 Stone GW, Ware JH, Bertrand ME, et al. Antithrombotic strategies in patients with acute coronary syndromes undergoing early invasive management: one-year results from the ACUITY trial. *JAMA* 2007; **298**(21): 2497–2506.

21 Seshadri N, Whitlow PL, Acharya N, Houghtaling P, Blackstone EH, Ellis SG. Emergency coronary artery bypass surgery in the contemporary percutaneous coronary intervention era. *Circulation* 2002; **106**(18): 2346–2350.

22 Dorros G, Cowley MJ, Simpson J, et al. Percutaneous transluminal coronary angioplasty: report of complications from the National Heart, Lung, and Blood Institute PTCA Registry. *Circulation* 1983; **67**(4): 723–730.

23 Holmes DR Jr, Holubkov R, Vlietstra RE, et al. Comparison of complications during percutaneous transluminal coronary angioplasty from 1977 to 1981 and from 1985 to 1986: the National Heart, Lung, and Blood Institute Percutaneous Transluminal Coronary Angioplasty Registry. *J Am Coll Cardiol* 1988; **12**(5): 1149–1155.

24 Rogers JH, Lasala JM. Coronary artery dissection and perforation complicating percutaneous coronary intervention. *J Invasive Cardiol* 2004; **16**(9): 493–499.

25 Huber MS, Mooney JF, Madison J, Mooney MR. Use of a morphologic classification to predict clinical outcome after dissection from coronary angioplasty. *Am J Cardiol* 1991; **68**(5): 467–471.

26 Sharma SK, Israel DH, Kamean JL, Bodian CA, Ambrose JA. Clinical, angiographic, and procedural determinants of major and minor coronary dissection during angioplasty. *Am Heart J* 1993; **126**(1): 39–47.

27 Bansal A CN, Levine, AB, et al. *Determinants of arterial dissection during PTCA: lesion type versus inflation rate. J Am Coll Cardiol* 1989; **12**: 229A.

28 Athanasiadis A, Haase KK, Wullen B, et al. Lesion morphology assessed by pre-interventional intravascular ultrasound does not predict the incidence of severe coronary artery dissections. *Eur Heart J* 1998; **19**(6): 870–878.

29 Chamie D, Bezerra HG, Attizzani GF, et al. Incidence, predictors, morphological characteristics, and clinical outcomes of stent edge dissections detected by optical coherence tomography. *JACC Cardiovasc Interv* 2013; **6**(8): 800–813.

30 Perez-Castellano N, Garcia-Fernandez MA, Garcia EJ, Delcan JL. Dissection of the aortic sinus of Valsalva complicating coronary catheterization: cause, mechanism, evolution, and management. *Catheter Cardiovasc Diagn* 1998; **43**(3): 273–279.

31 Carter AJ, Brinker JA. Dissection of the ascending aorta associated with coronary angiography. *Am J Cardiol* 1994; **73**(12): 922–923.

32 Awadalla H, Sabet S, El Sebaie A, Rosales O, Smalling R. Catheter-induced left main dissection incidence, predisposition and therapeutic strategies experience from two sides of the hemisphere. *J Invasive Cardiol* 2005; **17**(4): 233–236.

33 Goldstein JA, Casserly IP, Katsiyiannis WT, Lasala JM, Taniuchi M. Aortocoronary dissection complicating a percutaneous coronary intervention. *J Invasive Cardiol* 2003; **15**(2): 89–92.

34 Dunning DW, Kahn JK, Hawkins ET, O'Neill WW. Iatrogenic coronary artery dissections extending into and involving the aortic root. *Catheter Cardiovasc Interv* 2000; **51**(4): 387–393.

35 Nikolsky E, Boulos M, Amikam S. Spontaneous healing of long, catheter-induced right coronary artery dissection. *Int J Cardiovasc Interv* 2003; **5**(4): 211.

36 Boyle AJ, Chan M, Dib J, Resar J. Catheter-induced coronary artery dissection: risk factors, prevention and management. *J Invasive Cardiol* 2006; **18**(10): 500–503.

37 Boukhris M, Tomasello SD, Marza F, Azzarelli S, Galassi AR. Iatrogenic aortic dissection complicating percutaneous coronary intervention for chronic total occlusion. *Can J Cardiol* 2015; **31**(3): 320–327.

38 Kim JY, Yoon J, Jung HS, Yoo BS, Lee SH. Percutaneous coronary stenting in guide-induced aortocoronary dissection: angiographic and CT findings. *Int J Cardiovasc Imaging* 2005; **21**(4): 375–378.

39 Gur M, Yilmaz R, Demirbag R, Kunt AS. Large atherosclerotic plaque related severe right coronary artery dissection during coronary angiography. *Int J Cardiovasc Imaging* 2006; **22**(3–4): 321–325.

40 Javaid A, Buch AN, Satler LF, et al. Management and outcomes of coronary artery perforation during percutaneous coronary intervention. *Am J Cardiol* 2006; **98**(7): 911–914.

41 Dippel EJ, Kereiakes DJ, Tramuta DA, et al. Coronary perforation during percutaneous coronary intervention in the era of abciximab platelet glycoprotein IIb/IIIa blockade: an algorithm for percutaneous management. *Catheter Cardiovasc Interv* 2001; **52**(3): 279–286.

42 Fukutomi T, Suzuki T, Popma JJ, et al. Early and late clinical outcomes following coronary perforation in patients undergoing percutaneous coronary intervention. *Circulation J* 2002; **66**(4): 349–356.

43 Gunning MG, Williams IL, Jewitt DE, Shah AM, Wainwright RJ, Thomas MR. Coronary artery perforation during percutaneous intervention: incidence and outcome. *Heart* 2002; **88**(5): 495–498.

44 Fejka M, Dixon SR, Safian RD, et al. Diagnosis, management, and clinical outcome of cardiac tamponade complicating percutaneous coronary intervention. *Am J Cardiol* 2002; **90**(11): 1183–1186.

45 Cohen BM, Weber VJ, Relsman M, Casale A, Dorros G. Coronary perforation complicating rotational ablation: the U.S. multicenter experience. *Catheter Cardiovasc Diagn* 1996; **Suppl 3**: 55–59.

46 Litvack F, Eigler N, Margolis J, et al. Percutaneous excimer laser coronary angioplasty: results in the first consecutive 3,000 patients. The ELCA Investigators. *J Am Coll Cardiol* 1994; **23**(2): 323–329.

47 Witzke CF, Martin-Herrero F, Clarke SC, Pomerantzev E, Palacios IF. The changing pattern of coronary perforation during percutaneous coronary intervention in the new device era. *J Invasive Cardiol* 2004; **16**(6): 257–301.

48 Doll JA, Nikolsky E, Stone GW, et al. Outcomes of patients with coronary artery perforation complicating percutaneous coronary intervention and correlations with the type of adjunctive antithrombotic therapy: pooled analysis from REPLACE-2, ACUITY, and HORIZONS-AMI trials. *J Invasive Cardiol* 2009; **22**(5): 453–459.

49 Del Campo C, Zelman R. Successful non-operative management of right coronary artery perforation during percutaneous coronary intervention in a patient receiving abciximab and aspirin. *J Invasive Cardiol* 2000; **12**(1): 41–43.

50 Korpas D, Acevedo C, Lindsey RL, Gradman AH. Left anterior descending coronary artery to right ventricular fistula complicating coronary stenting. *J Invasive Cardiol* 2002; **14**(1): 41–43.

51 Hering D, Horstkotte D, Schwimmbeck P, Piper C, Bilger J, Schultheiss HP. [Acute myocardial infarct caused by a muscle bridge of the anterior interventricular ramus: complicated course with vascular perforation after stent implantation]. *Z Kardiol* 1997; **86**(8): 630–638.

52 Fasseas P, Orford JL, Panetta CJ, et al. Incidence, correlates, management, and clinical outcome of coronary perforation: analysis of 16,298 procedures. *Am Heart J* 2004; **147**(1): 140–145.

53 Colombo A, Mikhail GW, Michev I, et al. Treating chronic total occlusions using subintimal tracking and reentry: the STAR technique. *Catheter Cardiovasc Interv* 2005; **64**(4): 407–411; discussion 412.

54 Genereux P, Madhavan MV, Mintz GS, et al. Ischemic outcomes after coronary intervention of calcified vessels in acute coronary syndromes: pooled analysis from the HORIZONS-AMI (Harmonizing Outcomes With Revascularization and Stents in Acute Myocardial Infarction) and ACUITY (Acute Catheterization and Urgent Intervention Triage Strategy) TRIALS. *J Am Coll Cardiol* 2014; **63**(18): 1845–1854.

55 Colombo ATJ. *Techniques in Coronary Artery Stenting*. London: 2000.

56 Stankovic G, Orlic D, Corvaja N, et al. Incidence, predictors, in-hospital, and late outcomes of coronary artery perforations. *Am J Cardiol* 2004; **93**(2): 213–216.

57 Gruberg L, Pinnow E, Flood R, et al. Incidence, management, and outcome of coronary artery perforation during percutaneous coronary intervention. *Am J Cardiol* 2000; **86**(6): 680–682, A8.

58 Reimers B, von Birgelen C, van der Giessen WJ, Serruys PW. A word of caution on optimizing stent deployment in calcified lesions: acute coronary rupture with cardiac tamponade. *Am Heart J* 1996; **131**(1): 192–194.

59 Pasquetto G, Reimers B, Favero L, et al. Distal filter protection during percutaneous coronary intervention in native coronary arteries and saphenous vein grafts in patients with acute coronary syndromes. *Italian Heart J* 2003; **4**(9): 614–619.

60 Mauser M, Ennker J, Fleischmann D. [Dissection of the sinus valsalvae aortae as a complication of coronary angioplasty]. *Z Kardiol* 1999; **88**(12): 1023–1027.

61 Stathopoulos I, Panagopoulos G, Kossidas K, Jimenez M, Garratt K. Guidewire-induced coronary artery perforation and tamponade during PCI: in-hospital outcomes and impact on long-term survival. *J Invasive Cardiol* 2014; **26**(8): 371–376.

62 Stoelting RK. Allergic reactions during anesthesia. *Anesth Analg* 1983; **62**(3): 341–356.

63 Van Ryn-McKenna J, Cai L, Ofosu FA, Hirsh J, Buchanan MR. Neutralization of enoxaparine-induced bleeding by protamine sulfate. *Thromb Haemost* 1990; **63**(2): 271–274.

64 Massonnet-Castel S, Pelissier E, Bara L, et al. Partial reversal of low molecular weight heparin (PK 10169) anti-Xa activity by protamine sulfate: in vitro and in vivo study during cardiac surgery with extracorporeal circulation. *Haemostasis* 1986; **16**(2): 139–146.

65 Briguori C, Di Mario C, De Gregorio J, Sheiban I, Vaghetti M, Colombo A. Administration of protamine after coronary stent deployment. *Am Heart J* 1999; **138**(1 Pt 1): 64–68.

66 Cosgrave J, Qasim A, Latib A, Aranzulla TC, Colombo A. Protamine usage following implantation of drug-eluting stents: a word of caution. *Catheter Cardiovasc Interv* 2008; **71**(7): 913–914.

67 Maruo T, Yasuda S, Miyazaki S. Delayed appearance of coronary artery perforation following cutting balloon angioplasty. *Catheter Cardiovasc Interv* 2002; **57**(4): 529–531.

68 Assali AR, Moustapha A, Sdringola S, Rihner M, Smalling RW. Successful treatment of coronary artery perforation in an abciximab-treated patient by microcoil embolization. *Catheter Cardiovasc Interv* 2000; **51**(4): 487–489.

69 Gaxiola E, Browne KF. Coronary artery perforation repair using microcoil embolization. *Catheter Cardiovasc Diagn* 1998; **43**(4): 474–476.

70 Fischell TA, Korban EH, Lauer MA. Successful treatment of distal coronary guidewire-induced perforation with balloon catheter delivery of intracoronary thrombin. *Catheter Cardiovasc Interv* 2003; **58**(3): 370–374.

71 Aslam MS, Messersmith RN, Gilbert J, Lakier JB. Successful management of coronary artery perforation with helical platinum microcoil embolization. *Catheter Cardiovasc Interv* 2000; **51**(3): 320–322.

72 Dorros G, Jain A, Kumar K. Management of coronary artery rupture: covered stent or microcoil embolization. *Catheter Cardiovasc Diagn* 1995; **36**(2): 148–154; discussion 155.

73 Mahmud E, Douglas JS Jr. Coil embolization for successful treatment of perforation of chronically occluded proximal coronary artery. *Catheter Cardiovasc Interv* 2001; **53**(4): 549–552.

74 Jamali AH, Lee MS, Makkar RR. Coronary perforation after percutaneous coronary intervention successfully treated with local thrombin injection. *J Invasive Cardiol* 2006; **18**(4): E143–145.

75 Hadjimiltiades S, Paraskevaides S, Kazinakis G, Louridas G. Coronary vessel perforation during balloon angioplasty: a case report. *Catheter Cardiovasc Diagn* 1998; **45**(4): 417–420.

76 To AC, El-Jack SS, Webster MW, Stewart JT. Coronary artery perforation successfully treated with tris-acryl gelatin microsphere embolisation. *Heart Lung Circ* 2008; **17**(5): 423–426.

77 Storger H, Ruef J. Closure of guide wire-induced coronary artery perforation with a two-component fibrin glue. *Catheter Cardiovasc Interv* 2007; **70**(2): 237–240.

78 Oda H, Oda M, Makiyama Y, et al. Guidewire-induced coronary artery perforation treated with transcatheter delivery of subcutaneous tissue. *Catheter Cardiovasc Interv* 2005; **66**(3): 369–374.

79 Iakovou I, Colombo A. Management of right coronary artery perforation during percutaneous coronary intervention with polyvinyl alcohol foam embolization particles. *J Invasive Cardiol* 2004; **16**(12): 727–728.

80 Asouhidou I, Katsaridis V. Successful embolization of iatrogenic ruptured coronary artery using Onyx: a new technique. *Acute Cardiac Care* 2014; **16**(4): 123–126.

81 Colombo A, Itoh A, Di Mario C, et al. Successful closure of a coronary vessel rupture with a vein graft stent: case report. *Catheter Cardiovasc Diagn* 1996; **38**(2): 172–174.

82 Colon PJ 3rd, Ramee SR, Mulingtapang R, Pridjian A, Bhatia D, Collins TJ. Percutaneous bailout therapy of a perforated vein graft using a stent-autologous vein patch. *Catheter Cardiovasc Diagn* 1996; **38**(2): 175–178.

83 Satler LF. A revised algorithm for coronary perforation. *Catheter Cardiovasc Interv* 2002; **57**(2): 215–216.

84 Lansky AJ, Yang YM, Khan Y, et al. Treatment of coronary artery perforations complicating percutaneous coronary intervention with a polytetrafluoroethylene-covered stent graft. *Am J Cardiol* 2006; **98**(3): 370–374.

85 Romaguera R, Gomez-Hospital JA, Cequier A. Novel use of the Mguard mesh-covered stent to treat coronary arterial perforations. *Catheter Cardiovasc Interv* 2012; **80**(1): 75–78.

86 Fogarassy G, Apro D, Veress G. Successful sealing of a coronary artery perforation with a mesh-covered stent. *J Invasive Cardiol* 2012; **24**(4): E80–83.

87 Briguori C, Nishida T, Anzuini A, Di Mario C, Grube E, Colombo A. Emergency polytetrafluoroethylene-covered stent implantation to treat coronary ruptures. *Circulation* 2000; **102**(25): 3028–3031.

88 Ramsdale DR, Mushahwar SS, Morris JL. Repair of coronary artery perforation after rotastenting by implantation of the JoStent covered stent. *Catheter Cardiovasc Diagn* 1998; **45**(3): 310–313.

89 von Birgelen C, Haude M, Herrmann J, et al. Early clinical experience with the implantation of a novel synthetic coronary stent graft. *Catheter Cardiovasc Interv* 1999; **47**(4): 496–503.

90 Hendry C, Fraser D, Eichhofer J, et al. Coronary perforation in the drug-eluting stent era: incidence, risk factors, management and outcome: the UK experience. *EuroIntervention* 2012; **8**(1): 79–86.

91 Shimony A, Joseph L, Mottillo S, Eisenberg MJ. Coronary artery perforation during percutaneous coronary intervention: a systematic review and meta-analysis. *Can J Cardiol* 2011; **27**(6): 843–850.

92 Al-Lamee R, Ielasi A, Latib A, et al. Incidence, predictors, management, immediate and long-term outcomes following grade III coronary perforation. *JACC Cardiovas Interv* 2011; **4**(1): 87–95.

93 Eeckhout E, Kern MJ. The coronary no-reflow phenomenon: a review of mechanisms and therapies. *Eur Heart J* 2001; **22**(9): 729–739.

94 Kloner RA, Ganote CE, Jennings RB. The "no-reflow" phenomenon after temporary coronary occlusion in the dog. *J Clin Invest* 1974; **54**(6): 1496–1508.

95 Ito H, Tomooka T, Sakai N, et al. Lack of myocardial perfusion immediately after successful thrombolysis: a predictor of poor recovery of left ventricular function in anterior myocardial infarction. *Circulation* 1992; **85**(5): 1699–1705.

96 Caixeta A, Lansky AJ, Mehran R, et al. Predictors of suboptimal TIMI flow after primary angioplasty for acute myocardial infarction: results from the HORIZONS-AMI trial. *EuroIntervention* 2013; **9**(2): 220–227.

97 Mehta RH, Harjai KJ, Cox D, et al. Clinical and angiographic correlates and outcomes of suboptimal coronary flow inpatients with acute myocardial infarction undergoing primary percutaneous coronary intervention. *J Am Coll Cardiol* 2003; **42**(10): 1739–1746.

98 Stone GW, Grines CL, Cox DA, et al. Comparison of angioplasty with stenting, with or without abciximab, in acute myocardial infarction. *N Engl J Med* 2002; **346**(13): 957–966.

99 Silva JA WC. Large thrombus burden, slow flow, no-reflow, and distal embolization. In: Martinez EE LP, Ong ATL, Serruys PW (eds) *Common Clinical Dilemmas in Percutaneous Coronary Interventions*. Informa Healthcare: 2007; 261–282.

100 Kotani J, Nanto S, Mintz GS, et al. Plaque gruel of atheromatous coronary lesion may contribute to the no-reflow phenomenon in patients with acute coronary syndrome. *Circulation* 2002; **106**(13): 1672–1677.

101 Rezkalla SH, Kloner RA. No-reflow phenomenon. *Circulation* 2002; **105**(5): 656–662.

102 Leosco D, Fineschi M, Pierli C, et al. Intracoronary serotonin release after high-pressure coronary stenting. *Am J Cardiol* 1999; **84**(11): 1317–1322.

103 Wilson RF, Laxson DD, Lesser JR, White CW. Intense microvascular constriction after angioplasty of acute thrombotic coronary arterial lesions. *Lancet* 1989; **1**(8642): 807–811.

104 Taniyama Y, Ito H, Iwakura K, et al. Beneficial effect of intracoronary verapamil on microvascular and myocardial salvage in patients with acute myocardial infarction. *J Am Coll Cardiol* 1997; **30**(5): 1193–1199.

105 Salloum J, Tharpe C, Vaughan D, Zhao DX. Release and elimination of soluble vasoactive factors during percutaneous coronary intervention of saphenous vein grafts: analysis using the PercuSurge GuardWire distal protection device. *J Invasive Cardiol* 2005; **17**(11): 575–579.

106 Borges MD, Aguillera AH, Brilhante JJ, Caixeta A. Saphenous vein graft thrombus findings by scanning electron microscopy in a patient with acute myocardial infarction. *Einstein* 2013; **11**(3): 398–399.

107 Antoniucci D, Valenti R, Migliorini A. Thrombectomy during PCI for acute myocardial infarction: are the randomized controlled trial data relevant to the patients who really need this technique? *Catheter Cardiovasc Interv* 2008; **71**(7): 863–869.

108 Svilaas T, Vlaar PJ, van der Horst IC, et al. Thrombus aspiration during primary percutaneous coronary intervention. *N Engl J Med* 2008; **358**(6): 557–567.

109 Stone GW, Maehara A, Witzenbichler B, et al. Intracoronary abciximab and aspiration thrombectomy in patients with large anterior myocardial infarction: the INFUSE-AMI randomized trial. *JAMA* 2012; **307**(17): 1817–1826.

110 Frobert O, Lagerqvist B, Olivecrona GK, et al. Thrombus aspiration during ST-segment elevation myocardial infarction. *N Engl J Med* 2013; **369**(17): 1587–1597.

111 Burzotta F, Trani C, Romagnoli E, et al. Manual thrombus-aspiration improves myocardial reperfusion: the randomized evaluation of the effect of mechanical reduction of distal embolization by thrombus-aspiration in primary and rescue angioplasty (REMEDIA) trial. *J Am Coll Cardiol* 2005; **46**(2): 371–376.

112 Ali A, Cox D, Dib N, et al. Rheolytic thrombectomy with percutaneous coronary intervention for infarct size reduction in acute myocardial infarction: 30-day results from a multicenter randomized study. *J Am Coll Cardiol* 2006; **48**(2): 244–252.

113 King SB 3rd, Smith SC Jr, Hirshfeld JW Jr, et al. 2007 focused update of the ACC/AHA/SCAI 2005 guideline update for percutaneous coronary intervention: a report of the American College of Cardiology/American Heart Association Task Force on Practice guidelines. *J Am Coll Cardiol* 2008; **51**(2): 172–209.

114 Smith SC Jr, Feldman TE, Hirshfeld JW Jr, et al. ACC/AHA/SCAI 2005 Guideline Update for Percutaneous Coronary Intervention—summary article: a report of the American College of Cardiology/American Heart Association Task Force on Practice Guidelines (ACC/AHA/SCAI Writing Committee to Update the 2001 Guidelines for Percutaneous Coronary Intervention). *Circulation* 2006; **113**(1): 156–175.

115 Baim DS, Wahr D, George B, et al. Randomized trial of a distal embolic protection device during percutaneous intervention of saphenous vein aorto-coronary bypass grafts. *Circulation* 2002; **105**(11): 1285–1290.

116 Stone GW, Webb J, Cox DA, et al. Distal microcirculatory protection during percutaneous coronary intervention in acute ST-segment elevation myocardial infarction: a randomized controlled trial. *JAMA* 2005; **293**(9): 1063–1072.

117 Gick M, Jander N, Bestehorn HP, et al. Randomized evaluation of the effects of filter-based distal protection on myocardial perfusion and infarct size after primary percutaneous catheter intervention in myocardial infarction with and without ST-segment elevation. *Circulation* 2005; **112**(10): 1462–1469.

118 Loubeyre C, Morice MC, Lefevre T, Piechaud JF, Louvard Y, Dumas P. A randomized comparison of direct stenting with conventional stent implantation in selected patients with acute myocardial infarction. *J Am Coll Cardiol* 2002; **39**(1): 15–21.

119 Ly HQ, Kirtane AJ, Buros J, et al. Angiographic and clinical outcomes associated with direct versus conventional stenting among patients treated with fibrinolytic therapy for ST-elevation acute myocardial infarction. *Am J Cardiol* 2005; **95**(3): 383–386.

120 Antoniucci D, Valenti R, Migliorini A, et al. Direct infarct artery stenting without predilation and no-reflow in patients with acute myocardial infarction. *Am Heart J* 2001; **142**(4): 684–690.

121 Mockel M, Vollert J, Lansky AJ, et al. Comparison of direct stenting with conventional stent implantation in acute myocardial infarction. *Am J Cardiol* 2011; **108**(12): 1697–1703.

122 Movahed MR, Butman SM. The pathogenesis and treatment of no-reflow occurring during percutaneous coronary intervention. *Cardiovasc Revasc Med* 2008; **9**(1): 56–61.

123 Roffi M, Mukherjee D, Chew DP, et al. Lack of benefit from intravenous platelet glycoprotein IIb/IIIa receptor inhibition as adjunctive treatment for percutaneous interventions of aortocoronary bypass grafts: a pooled analysis of five randomized clinical trials. *Circulation* 2002; **106**(24): 3063–3067.

124 Michaels AD, Appleby M, Otten MH, et al. Pretreatment with intragraft verapamil prior to percutaneous coronary intervention of saphenous vein graft lesions: results of the randomized, controlled vasodilator prevention on no-reflow (VAPOR) trial. *J Invasive Cardiol* 2002; **14**(6): 299–302.

125 Iwakura K, Ito H, Kawano S, et al. Chronic pre-treatment of statins is associated with the reduction of the no-reflow phenomenon in the patients with reperfused acute myocardial infarction. *Eur Heart J* 2006; **27**(5): 534–539.

126 Lee CH, Wong HB, Tan HC, et al. Impact of reversibility of no reflow phenomenon on 30-day mortality following percutaneous revascularization for acute myocardial infarction-insights from a 1,328 patient registry. *J Intervent Cardiol* 2005; **18**(4): 261–266.

127 Airoldi F, Briguori C, Cianflone D, et al. Frequency of slow coronary flow following successful stent implantation and effect of nitroprusside. *Am J Cardiol* 2007; **99**(7): 916–920.

128 Hillegass WB, Dean NA, Liao L, Rinehart RG, Myers PR. Treatment of no-reflow and impaired flow with the nitric oxide donor nitroprusside following percutaneous coronary interventions: initial human clinical experience. *J Am Coll Cardiol* 2001; **37**(5): 1335–1343.

129 Myers PR, Banitt PF, Guerra R Jr, Harrison DG. Characteristics of canine coronary resistance arteries: importance of endothelium. *Am J Physiol* 1989; **257**(2 Pt 2): H603–610.

130 Kuo L, Chilian WM, Davis MJ. Interaction of pressure- and flow-induced responses in porcine coronary resistance vessels. *Am J Physiol* 1991; **261**(6 Pt 2): H1706–1715.

131 Villari B, Ambrosio G, Golino P, *et al.* The effects of calcium channel antagonist treatment and oxygen radical scavenging on infarct size and the no-reflow phenomenon in reperfused hearts. *Am Heart J* 1993; **125**(1): 11–23.

132 Brogden RN, Benfield P. Verapamil: a review of its pharmacological properties and therapeutic use in coronary artery disease. *Drugs* 1996; **51**(5): 792–819.

133 Campbell CA, Kloner RA, Alker KJ, Braunwald E. Effect of verapamil on infarct size in dogs subjected to coronary artery occlusion with transient reperfusion. *J Am Coll Cardiol* 1986; **8**(5): 1169–1174.

134 Werner GS, Lang K, Kuehnert H, Figulla HR. Intracoronary verapamil for reversal of no-reflow during coronary angioplasty for acute myocardial infarction. *Catheter Cardiovasc Interv* 2002; **57**(4): 444–451.

135 Pomerantz RM, Kuntz RE, Diver DJ, Safian RD, Baim DS. Intracoronary verapamil for the treatment of distal microvascular coronary artery spasm following PTCA. *Catheter Cardiovasc Diagn* 1991; **24**(4): 283–285.

136 Barcin C, Denktas AE, Lennon RJ, *et al.* Comparison of combination therapy of adenosine and nitroprusside with adenosine alone in the treatment of angiographic no-reflow phenomenon. *Catheter Cardiovasc Interv* 2004; **61**(4): 484–491.

137 Hein TW, Kuo L. cAMP-independent dilation of coronary arterioles to adenosine: role of nitric oxide, G proteins, and K(ATP) channels. *Circ Res* 1999; **85**(7): 634–642.

138 Sdringola S, Assali A, Ghani M, *et al.* Adenosine use during aortocoronary vein graft interventions reverses but does not prevent the slow-no reflow phenomenon. *Catheter Cardiovasc Interv* 2000; **51**(4): 394–399.

139 Fischell TA, Carter AJ, Foster MT, *et al.* Reversal of "no reflow" during vein graft stenting using high velocity boluses of intracoronary adenosine. *Catheter Cardiovasc Diagn* 1998; **45**(4): 360–365.

140 Parikh KH, Chag MC, Shah KJ, *et al.* Intracoronary boluses of adenosine and sodium nitroprusside in combination reverses slow/no-reflow during angioplasty: a clinical scenario of ischemic preconditioning. *Can J Physiol Pharmacol* 2007; **85**(3-4): 476–482.

141 Ishihara M, Sato H, Tateishi H, *et al.* Attenuation of the no-reflow phenomenon after coronary angioplasty for acute myocardial infarction with intracoronary papaverine. *Am Heart J* 1996; **132**(5): 959–963.

142 Rawitscher D, Levin TN, Cohen I, Feldman T. Rapid reversal of no-reflow using Abciximab after coronary device intervention. *Catheter Cardiovasc Diagn* 1997; **42**(2): 187–190.

143 Huang RI, Patel P, Walinsky P, *et al.* Efficacy of intracoronary nicardipine in the treatment of no-reflow during percutaneous coronary intervention. *Catheter Cardiovasc Interv* 2006; **68**(5): 671–676.

144 Fugit MD, Rubal BJ, Donovan DJ. Effects of intracoronary nicardipine, diltiazem and verapamil on coronary blood flow. *J Invasive Cardiol* 2000; **12**(2): 80–85.

145 Heitzer T, Ollmann I, Koke K, Meinertz T, Munzel T. Platelet glycoprotein IIb/IIIa receptor blockade improves vascular nitric oxide bioavailability in patients with coronary artery disease. *Circulation* 2003; **108**(5): 536–541.

146 Lim SY, Bae EH, Jeong MH, *et al.* Effect of combined intracoronary adenosine and nicorandil on no-reflow phenomenon during percutaneous coronary intervention. *Circ J* 2004; **68**(10): 928–932.

147 Skelding KA, Goldstein JA, Mehta L, Pica MC, O'Neill WW. Resolution of refractory no-reflow with intracoronary epinephrine. *Catheter Cardiovasc Interv* 2002; **57**(3): 305–309.

CHAPTER 26

Access Site Complications

Jose M. Wiley[1], Fernando Pastor[2], and Cristina Sanina[3]

[1] Albert Einstein College of Medicine, and Montefiore Einstein Center for Heart & Vascular Care, Bronx, NY, USA
[2] Instituto Cardiovascular Cuyo, Sanatorio La Merced, Villa Mercedes, Argentina
[3] University of Miami Miller School of Medicine, Miami, FL, USA

Technologic advances in the design of catheters and devices have allowed a more aggressive approach to percutaneous coronary intervention (PCI), which has resulted in an increase in the volume and complexity of procedures. As a result, the frequency of non-cardiac complications has also risen. The most common complications following percutaneous interventions are related to vascular access and are linked to the complexity of the coronary intervention. Muller *et al.* [1] reported a 2.6% incidence of vascular access complications following routine PCI, which increased to 6% (p < 0.0001) after complex interventions. The purpose of this chapter is to describe the incidence, predisposing factors, and treatment options for some of the most common non-cardiac complications following PCI.

Femoral vascular access complications
Bleeding

Access site bleeding is the most frequent complication following femoral arterial access. Transfusion of red blood cells after PCI has been reported in 1.8–6.5% of cases [2–4]. Risk factors associated with bleeding complications are shown in Box 26.1.

Fewer femoral complications have been noted in patients undergoing elective PCI using 6 Fr compared to 7 or 8 Fr guiding catheters (13.8% vs. 23.5%; p < 0.01) [5,6]. However, other studies have not shown sheath size to be an important risk factor [7,8]. Bleeding complications are reduced when heparin is discontinued after the procedure without any adverse impact on cardiac outcomes [9,10]. Likewise, sheath removal as early as possible after the procedure can also decrease bleeding [7,11,12]. Bleeding complications associated with glycoprotein IIb/IIIa platelet receptor inhibitor use have been reduced by reducing the heparin dosage (70 IU/kg) [4,12].

A mass or fullness at the access site suggests the presence of a hematoma. However, this finding can be difficult to appreciate in obese patients in whom significant blood loss can occur without obvious physical signs. The management of access site bleeding depends on the severity and hemodynamic consequences of bleeding.

In general, access site bleeding is controlled by manual or mechanical compression and reversal of anticoagulation. If bleeding continues despite these steps, more aggressive therapies including percutaneous intervention or surgical therapy are considered.

If patients with bleeding complications have received abciximab (Reopro, Eli Lilly, Indianapolis, IN, USA), normally functioning platelets can be transfused without interference from the tightly bound drug. The same does not apply to the small molecule platelet glycoprotein IIb/IIIa inhibitors, eptifibatide (Integrilin, Cor Therapeutics, South San Francisco, CA, USA) and tirofiban (Aggrastat, Merck, West Point, PA, USA). These small molecules are competitive inhibitors, not tightly bound to the receptor, leaving excess-free drug available to inhibit the transfused platelets. However, their shorter half-life allows the antiplatelet effects to wear off after several hours.

Retroperitoneal bleeding

The incidence of retroperitoneal hematoma formation has been reported in 0.12–0.44% of patients after an interventional procedure [13–15]. The risk of bleeding into the retroperitoneal space is increased with a high femoral puncture (above the inguinal ligament) and with a back wall puncture of the vessel [15]. Knowledge of the femoral vascular and inguinal anatomy is helpful in minimizing this risk. The goal is to access the common femoral artery corresponding to the vascular segment overlying the medial third of the femoral head.

The signs and symptoms of retroperitoneal bleeding include hypotension, abdominal distension or fullness, and pain [15,16]. The diagnosis of retroperitoneal bleeding are confirmed by computed tomography (CT) or abdominal/pelvic ultrasound [17,18]. If retroperitoneal bleeding is suspected, anticoagulation should be reversed and discontinued. Volume resuscitation with crystalloid solutions and/or blood products should be administered if volume depletion is clinically evident. Alternatively, if bleeding causes hemodynamic embarrassment, emergency angiography from the contralateral femoral access site can be considered to localize the bleeding site. Once the bleeding site has been identified, tamponade of the bleeding with an angioplasty balloon will stabilize the patient. If prolonged balloon inflation is not effective in stopping the blood loss, consideration is given to placing a covered stent (Wallgraft, BSC, Watertown, MA, USA) to seal the leak. Open surgical repair may also be considered [19].

Pseudoaneurysm

A pseudoaneurysm occurs when a hematoma continues to communicate with the arterial lumen. Following PCI, routine ultrasound screening will reveal pseudoaneurysms in up to 6% of

Interventional Cardiology: Principles and Practice, Second Edition. Edited by George D. Dangas, Carlo Di Mario, and Nicholas N. Kipshidze.
© 2017 John Wiley & Sons, Ltd. Published 2017 by John Wiley & Sons, Ltd.

Box 26.1 Risk factors for femoral access bleeding [2–4]

Female gender
Elevated blood pressure
Prolonged in-dwelling sheath time
Larger diameter sheath
Older age
Low body weight
Obesity
Larger heparin dose
Thrombolytic agents

---

patients compared to a 3% incidence if symptoms initiate the ultrasound investigation [20]. Low arterial access (superficial femoral artery or profunda femoris artery entry) has been associated with pseudoaneurysm formation [21]. Other risk factors include female sex, age greater than 70 years, diabetes mellitus, and obesity [8].

Patients with pseudoaneurysms often present with pain at the access site several days following the intervention. On physical examination, a pulsatile hematoma can be present with a systolic bruit. Management of a femoral pseudoaneurysm is dependent on its size, severity of symptoms, and need for continued anticoagulation. A small pseudoaneurysm (≤2 cm) will often resolve spontaneously. Larger pseudoaneurysms should be treated with ultrasound-guided compression, percutaneous thrombin/collagen injection, endovascular coil insertion, or by placement of covered stents. Surgical repair of pseudoaneurysms is usually reserved for the failure of less invasive approaches.

Ultrasound-guided compression

In 1991, Fellmeth et al. [22] described ultrasound-guided compression repair (UGCR) of femoral artery pseudoaneurysms. This method causes thrombosis of the pseudoaneurysm by compressing the neck of the pseudoaneurysm with the ultrasound probe and causing stasis. Variable success rates, ranging from 55% to 90%, have been reported [22–26].

Although many pseudoaneurysms can be successfully treated by this technique, UGCR does have limitations. It is time-consuming and labor-intensive. Compression times vary from 10 minutes to as long as 300 minutes, with 30 minutes being the average [27]. Intravenous sedation and analgesia are often required because this procedure can be uncomfortable for the patient. If the patient must continue anticoagulation after successful compression, close follow-up is necessary as the risk of recurrence or rupture of the pseudoaneurysm is increased [25]. Predictors of failure of UGCR to treat pseudoaneurysms include obesity, large pseudoaneurysm size, concomitant anticoagulation therapy, and groin discomfort [25–27]. Ultrasound-guided compression is unattractive or contraindicated in the presence of infection, a tense hematoma, or limb-threatening ischemia.

Ultrasound-guided thrombin injection

Percutaneous thrombin injection into the pseudoaneurysm with ultrasound guidance is another technique to treat pseudoaneurysms [28–34]. Despite its introduction in 1986, this technique has only recently gained wide acceptance. Multiple series have reported success rates of 86–97% for treatment of femoral artery

pseudoaneurysms using bovine thrombin (500–10,000 IU) with sonographic guidance [29,30,32,34].

A risk associated with thrombin injection is that the injected thrombin can exit the pseudoaneurysm, enter the native circulation, and cause distal extremity thrombosis. Pezzullo et al. [34] described distal thrombin embolization in 1 of 23 patients, and Cope and Zeit [35] reported distal thrombin embolization in 2 of 4 (50%) patients. The risk of distal embolization can be minimized by directing the needle away from the neck of the pseudoaneurysm, thereby minimizing the risk of injecting thrombin into the native circulation.

Another technique to prevent distal thrombin embolization is the use of angioplasty balloon occlusion of the femoral artery at the site of the pseudoaneurysm neck during thrombin injection to prevent embolization. We have reported the successful closure of four femoral pseudoaneurysms using percutaneous thrombin injection with balloon occlusion (Figure 26.1) [36]. Briefly, the technique requires contralateral femoral artery access and inflation of a peripheral angioplasty balloon, sized 1 : 1 to the diameter of the reference vessel, across the origin of the pseudoaneurysm. This occludes flow in the common femoral artery and completely obstructs any flow into or out of the pseudoaneurysm. Thrombin is then percutaneously injected into the pseudoaneurysm sac without risk of distal embolization. The stasis induced by balloon occlusion facilitates thrombosis of the pseudoaneurysm with very small amounts of thrombin.

Patients who have had previous exposure to thrombin or bovine proteins are at risk of immunologic cross-reactivity. Reported side effects include the development of hypotension, bradycardia, and the formation of inhibitors of coagulation factors, all presumed secondary to the immunologic cross-reactivity of bovine thrombin [37–39]. One report described an anaphylactic reaction after thrombin injection of a femoral pseudoaneurysm in a patient who had had repeated exposures to bovine thrombin [33]. Patients who have had prior exposure to bovine thrombin should undergo skin testing to detect possible allergy.

Biodegradable collagen injection

Percutaneous closure of femoral pseudoaneurysm by biodegradable collagen injection is an innovative approach. Hamraoui et al. [40] described this technique by injecting bovine collagen guided by angiography from the contralateral site. The overall success rate for this procedure was 108/110 (98%).

The advantages of this treatment include reduction in the risk of migration of the collagen plug through the neck of the pseudoaneurysm, and no reported cross-reaction to human factor V [40]. However, its disadvantages include the need for contralateral femoral arterial access, and utilization of a large introducer sheath [41].

Covered stents

Covered stents have been used successfully to exclude femoral artery pseudoaneurysms [41,42]. Waigand et al. [41] described the successful treatment of 32 pseudoaneurysms with a covered stent. Thalhammer et al. [42] reported the successful treatment of 16 pseudoaneurysms with covered stents. The use of covered stents is not ideal if the pseudoaneurysm involves the bifurcation of the common femoral artery into the superficial femoral artery and the profunda femoris artery, as it will cause occlusion of the branch vessels. Placement of a self-expanding covered stent into the common femoral artery may preclude future vascular access at this site. Covered stents can also be associated with an increased risk of

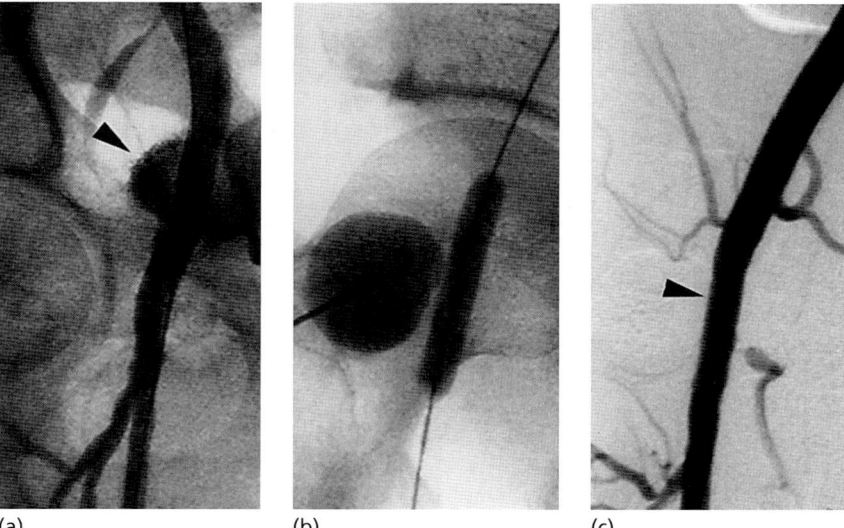

(a)   (b)   (c)

Figure 26.1 (a) Arrowhead points to the pseudoaneurysm in the common femoral artery. (b) Isolation of the pseudoaneurysm with an inflated peripheral balloon catheter; pseudoaneurysm is filled by direct contrast injection. (c) Arrowhead points to the site of the resolved pseudoaneurysm after thrombin injection into aneurysm sac.

subacute stent thrombosis and late stent occlusion, especially when deployed in a common femoral artery with poor run-off [41,42].

Coil embolization
Successful closure of pseudoaneurysms has been reported with coil embolization [41,43]. Waigand *et al.* [41] reported closure of the channel between the artery and the pseudoaneurysm by placing coils in 12 patients. In smaller channels, 0.014 inch coils (3 × 40 mm) were delivered through a 3 Fr Tracker (Target Therapeutics) catheter, while larger coils (0.35 inch, 6 × 30 mm) were delivered in larger channels through a 5 Fr angiographic catheter.

Coil embolization of femoral pseudoaneurysms appears to be effective, but can be time-consuming [41]. Other disadvantages include the potential for persistent flow between loosely packed coils. If the coils are placed superficially, local discomfort and pressure necrosis of the overlying skin can occur [43].

Surgical repair
Surgical repair, the conventional treatment of femoral artery pseudoaneurysms, has largely been replaced with non-surgical techniques. While surgery is effective, it is associated with significant morbidity, including postoperative discomfort, wound infection, increased costs, and prolonged hospital stay. The current strategy in most centers is to reserve surgical repair of a femoral pseudoaneurysm for those instances in which percutaneous therapies fail.

Arteriovenous fistulae
Arteriovenous fistulae (AVF) occur during vascular access when the percutaneous needle punctures the femoral artery and the overlying vein, creating a fistulous communication when the sheath is removed. The incidence of post-catheterization AVF is approximately 0.4% [14]. The risk of creating an AVF is increased by either a high or low femoral puncture, multiple puncture attempts, and prolonged clotting times [8]. Fistulae may not be clinically evident for several days following the procedure. Clinically, AVF is characterized by a continuous to-and-fro murmur over the access site. In some cases, there may be a swollen and tender extremity as a result of venous dilatation, and in severe circumstances arterial insufficiency (steal syndrome) occurs [41]. The diagnosis of a suspected AVF can be confirmed by color flow Doppler ultrasound.

Most AVF following PCI are small, not hemodynamically significant, and close spontaneously [42]. Symptomatic AVF require closure to prevent increased shunting and distal swelling and tenderness. Ultrasound-guided compression and the use of covered stents on the arterial side of the fistula have been successful in small numbers of patients [44]. In 1994, Uhlich *et al.* [44] successfully closed a large AVF with a covered stent. Waigand *et al.* [42] reported successfully closing 21 AVF using covered stents. Thalhammer *et al.* [42] reported the use of covered stents in nine AVF. A significant disadvantage related to the use of covered stents for closure of an AVF is the increased incidence (12–17%) of stent thrombosis [44].

Percutaneous coil embolization has also been described in a small number of patients for the treatment of AVF. However, experience with this technique remains limited [45]. Surgical repair, the traditional therapy for closure of catheterization-related AVF, when necessary, has been displaced by percutaneous methods. Once again, surgical correction is reserved for those patients who fail a less invasive approach.

Lower extremity ischemia
Local thrombosis of the femoral artery or lower extremity vessel related to the access site is unusual, reported to occur in less than 1% [46,47]. Risk factors include larger catheters or sheaths in relatively small arteries (catheter–artery mismatch), the presence of peripheral vascular disease, advanced age, cardiomyopathy, and the presence of hypercoagulable states (e.g., protein C or protein S deficiency, the lupus anticoagulant). In the absence of predisposing factors, vessel dissection or spasm can contribute to arterial thrombosis.

Signs and symptoms are those typically found with acute extremity ischemia (the five Ps): pain, pallor, paresthesia, pulseless, and polar (cold). The diagnosis of ischemia is suggested by physical examination and can be confirmed by duplex ultrasound. Patients with symptomatic, acute limb ischemia following vascular access should undergo angiography to characterize the anatomic basis for the ischemia. Treatment options include balloon angioplasty to restore flow with or without a selective infusion of thrombolytic therapy, stents, or catheter thrombectomy. If percutaneous methods fail, surgical thrombectomy and repair are required [47].

Dissection

Iatrogenic dissection of the femoral or iliac artery from PCI ranges from 0.01% to 0.4% [48,49]. Vascular access dissection contributes to the development of distal extremity ischemia, pseudoaneurysm, or thrombus formation. The recognition of a vascular dissection should be followed by angiography to characterize the extent of the dissection. Treatment includes balloon angioplasty, endovascular stent placement, or surgical repair to stabilize a flow-limiting dissection.

Infection

Local infection at the site of arterial access occurs in less than 1% of patients following coronary interventional procedures [50]. The most common organisms isolated are *Staphylococcus aureus* and *S. epidermidis* [33]. Pyrogenic reactions following cardiac catheterization generally occur within 1 hour of the procedure and manifest as fever, chills, and lethargy.

Upper extremity vascular access complications

Radial artery access

Transradial access for interventional coronary catheterization is being performed with increasing frequency because hemostasis can be obtained easily by local compression of the superficial course of the radial artery. Patients ambulate immediately after the procedure. A normal Allen's test prior to the radial artery access ensures that radial arterial occlusion does not endanger the viability of the hand.

Kiemeneij *et al.* [51] reported successful coronary cannulation in 93%, 95.7%, and 99.7% of patients randomized to undergo percutaneous transluminal coronary angioplasty (PTCA) by the radial, brachial, and femoral approaches, respectively. A randomized comparative study of PTCA using the radial, brachial, and femoral approaches reported that major access site complications were similar for brachial (2.3%) and femoral artery access (2.0%) but that no major complications occurred with radial artery access [51,52]. In a series of 563 patients who underwent transradial angioplasty with 6 Fr guiding catheters, asymptomatic radial artery occlusion was found in only 2.8% of patients.

Although the radial artery is small in size, the availability of low profile catheters and devices makes it possible to perform PCI using 6 or 7 Fr sheaths via the radial artery. In a study comparing PTCA with abciximab using either transradial or transfemoral approaches, no major access site bleeding complications occurred in the radial artery group, compared to 7.4% in the femoral artery group (p = 0.04) [53]. The transradial approach allows immediate postprocedural ambulation resulting in increased patient comfort. The disadvantages of the transradial approach include more frequent access failure than for the femoral approach, and the inability to perform procedures requiring larger sized sheaths.

Brachial artery access

Percutaneous brachial access has largely replaced the surgical cutdown (Sones technique) method for obtaining brachial artery access. The Society for Cardiac Angiography and Intervention registry data suggested that the risk of access site-related thrombosis increases fourfold with the brachial approach (0.96% vs. 0.22%; p < 0.001) compared with the femoral approach [47]. The most common complications associated with brachial artery access are bleeding, thrombosis, pseudoaneurysm formation, and brachial nerve compression. Thrombotic complications are more common than bleeding complications for brachial access compared to the femoral approach [54]. If a pulse deficit or other ischemic symptom suggests thrombosis after cannulation of the brachial artery, local thrombolysis or catheter thrombectomy are performed. If the problem is an intimal flap or dissection, angioplasty or stent placement can be required to restore antegrade flow. If these less invasive measures are not successful, surgical repair is required.

Complications related to vascular closure devices

Vascular access closure devices are designed to facilitate hemostasis after percutaneous interventions and have been used to reduce the time to ambulation and to decrease hospital length of stay. In these regards, all currently available devices in the USA have shown favorable results [55–60]. However, these devices are prone to specific complications and have not been demonstrated to reduce access site complications.

A retrospective single-center experience of 425 patients treated with a collagen plug closure device (Angioseal, Daig, St. Paul, MN, USA) reported device failure (8%), bleeding (0.2%), pseudoaneurysm formation (0.5%), femoral artery stenosis (1.4%) as shown in Figure 26.2, infection (0.2%), and the need for surgical repair in 1.6% [56].

In another trial of 1001 patients, two collagen plug devices, Vasoseal (Datascope, Montvale, NJ, USA) and Angioseal, and a suture-mediated device (Techstar, Perclose, Redwood City, CA, USA) were compared to manual compression for hemostasis. Both collagen plug devices were found to have higher complication rates (1.5%; p = 0.02, and 2.6%; p = 0.0002, respectively) than manual compression (0.5%). The complications associated with the suture-mediated device, Techstar, were not different from those of manual compression [56]. In a series including 1200 consecutive suture closure (Techstar) patients, complications included the development of a hematoma (2.1%), the need for vascular surgery (0.6%), retroperitoneal hemorrhage (0.3%), blood transfusion (0.7%), local infection (0.5%), and pseudoaneurysm formation (0.1%) [57].

In the initial US Feasibility Trial using the Duett vascular closure device (Vascular Solutions, Minneapolis, MN, USA), a vascular sealing device comprised of a balloon delivery catheter and a flowable procoagulant consisting of thrombin and collagen, Mooney *et al.* [58] reported 4.7% of patients developed hematomas larger than 6 cm in diameter, and 2.3% of patients developed pseudoaneurysms.

A few centers around the country have developed endovascular rescue procedures for acute vessel closure related to abrupt femoral access closure devises, particularly for Angioseal (Daig, St. Paul, MN, USA) (Figure 26.2) and Perclose (Redwood City, CA, USA) (Figure 26.3), with anecdotal encouraging results. This involves obtaining contralateral femoral access, crossing over to the affected

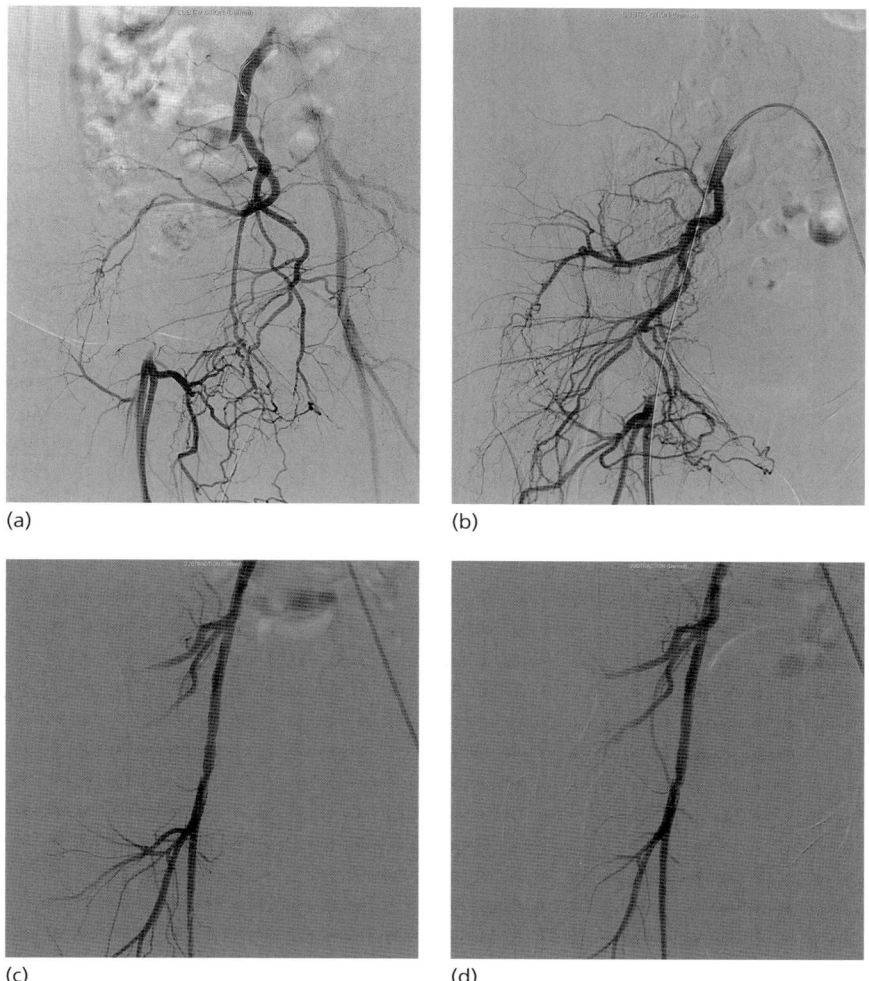

Figure 26.2 Angioseal common femoral artery injury. (a) demonstrates Angioseal closure injury of the common femoral artery with thrombus. (b) shows the lesion crossed with a 0.14 inch wire, distal embolic protection, and a balloon in place for dilatation. (c) shows the lesion after balloon dilatation and embolic debris in the filter. (d) shows the final result with wire and embolic protection removed.

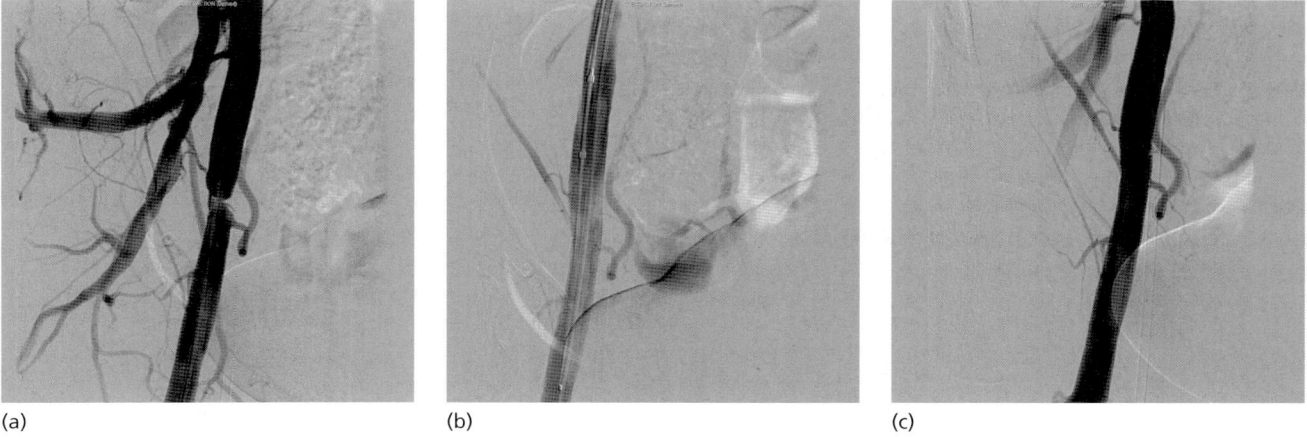

Figure 26.3 Perclose common femoral artery injury. (a) demonstrates Perclose closure injury of the common femoral artery. (b) shows balloon dilatation of the injury site. (c) shows final result with wire and balloon removed.

Table 26.1 Comparison of femoral artery hemostasis techniques.

	Pneumatic (%)	Manual (%)	C-clamp (%)	p
Prolonged time	35	13	20	<0.0001
Bleeding	16	3	4	<0.0001
Crossover	27	1	1	<0.001
Discomfort	3.1	2.2	1.9	<0.001

Prolonged time = greater than 13 min. Bleeding = in-laboratory bleeding. Crossover occurred when an alternative method was required to achieve hemostasis. Discomfort was measured on a 1 (min) to 10 (max) point scale. Source: Lehmann KG, *et al.* 1999 [59].

limb, advancing a 0.035 inch hydrophilic wire, traversing the closure device lesion, and exchanging the wire with a 0.035 inch exchange catheter. A 0.014 inch filter is then advanced into the superficial femoral artery and a 0.014–0.035 inch balloon is advanced into the lesion and inflated; progressively larger balloons are used until the lesion is expanded and closure device is released. The filter is then retrieved with the remnants of the closure device and antegrade flow is usually re-established. Directional atherectomy can be used in cases of endovascular deployment of plug-based devices (e.g., Angioseal collagen plug) after wire crossing and distal filter deployment. A stent is rarely advisable in the common femoral artery location. Referral for surgical repair of the femoral arterial access should also be considered because the exposure is rather superficial, often under local anesthesia and sedation.

Complications related to compression devices

Manual femoral artery compression has been compared with device compression with either a C-clamp or a pneumatic compression device (Femostop, RADI Medical Systems, Uppsala, Sweden) in 400 patients [59]. The pneumatic compression device required longer compression time, and patients experienced an increased frequency of bleeding, more frequent crossover to an alternate technique, and an increase in patient discomfort (Table 26.1) [59]. In another study of 185 PCI patients in whom abciximab was given, Chamberlain *et al.* [60] compared three different methods of femoral artery closure: Vasoseal (collagen plug), Perclose (suture closure), and Femostop (pneumatic compression). Vasoseal and Perclose had significantly lower rates of successful hemostasis than Femostop (78.8%, 85.7%, 100%, respectively; p < 0.001). Vasoseal was the only device with infection reported as a complication (1.9%; p = NS) [60].

Interactive multiple choice questions are available for this chapter on www.wiley. com/go/dangas/cardiology

References

1 Muller DW, Shamir KJ, Ellis SG, Topol EJ. Peripheral vascular complications after conventional and complex percutaneous coronary interventional procedures. *Am J Cardiol* 1992; **69**(1): 63–68.

2 Schomig A, Neumann FJ, Kastrati A, *et al.* A randomized comparison of antiplatelet and anticoagulant therapy after the placement of coronary-artery stents. *N Engl J Med* 1996; **334**(17): 1084–1089.

3 Leon MB, Baim DS, Popma JJ, *et al.* A clinical trial comparing three antithrombotic-drug regimens after coronary-artery stenting. Stent Anticoagulation Restenosis Study Investigators. *N Engl J Med* 1998; **339**(23): 1665–1671.

4 Investigators E. Platelet glycoprotein IIb/IIIa receptor blockade and low-dose heparin during percutaneous coronary revascularization. *N Engl J Med* 1997; **336**(24): 1689–1696.

5 Metz D, Meyer P, Touati C, *et al.* Comparison of 6 F with 7 F and 8 F guiding catheters for elective coronary angioplasty: results of a prospective, multicenter, randomized trial. *Am Heart J* 1997; **134**(1): 131–137.

6 Aguirre FV, Topol EJ, Ferguson JJ, *et al.* Bleeding complications with the chimeric antibody to platelet glycoprotein IIb/IIIa integrin in patients undergoing percutaneous coronary intervention. EPIC Investigators. *Circulation* 1995; **91**(12): 2882–2890.

7 Popma JJ, Satler LF, Pichard AD, *et al.* Vascular complications after balloon and new device angioplasty. *Circulation* 1993; **88**(4 Pt 1): 1569–1578.

8 Waksman R, King SB 3rd, Douglas JS, *et al.* Predictors of groin complications after balloon and new-device coronary intervention. *Am J Cardiol* 1995; **75**(14): 886–889.

9 Friedman HZ, Cragg DR, Glazier SM, *et al.* Randomized prospective evaluation of prolonged versus abbreviated intravenous heparin therapy after coronary angioplasty. *J Am Coll Cardiol* 1994; **24**(5): 1214–1219.

10 Rabah M, Mason D, Muller DW, *et al.* Heparin after percutaneous intervention (HAPI): a prospective multicenter randomized trial of three heparin regimens after successful coronary intervention. *J Am Coll Cardiol* 1999; **34**(2): 461–467.

11 Mandak JS, Blankenship JC, Gardner LH, *et al.* Modifiable risk factors for vascular access site complications in the IMPACT II Trial of angioplasty with versus without eptifibatide. Integrilin to Minimize Platelet Aggregation and Coronary Thrombosis. *J Am Coll Cardiol* 1998; **31**(7): 1518–1524.

12 Lincoff AM, Tcheng JE, Califf RM, *et al.* Standard versus low-dose weight-adjusted heparin in patients treated with the platelet glycoprotein IIb/IIIa receptor antibody fragment abciximab (c7E3 Fab) during percutaneous coronary revascularization. PROLOG Investigators. *Am J Cardiol* 1997; **79**(3): 286–291.

13 Omoigui NA, Califf RM, Pieper K, *et al.* Peripheral vascular complications in the Coronary Angioplasty Versus Excisional Atherectomy Trial (CAVEAT-I). *J Am Coll Cardiol* 1995; **26**(4): 922–930.

14 Johnson LW, Esente P, Giambartolomei A, *et al.* Peripheral vascular complications of coronary angioplasty by the femoral and brachial techniques. *Catheter Cardiovasc Diagn* 1994; **31**(3): 165–172. Epub 1994/03/01.

15 Sreeram S, Lumsden AB, Miller JS, Salam AA, Dodson TF, Smith RB. Retroperitoneal hematoma following femoral arterial catheterization: a serious and often fatal complication. *Am Surg* 1993; **59**(2): 94–98.

16 Kent KC, Moscucci M, Mansour KA, *et al.* Retroperitoneal hematoma after cardiac catheterization: prevalence, risk factors, and optimal management. *J Vasc Surg* 1994; **20**(6): 905–910; discussion 910–913.

17 Shih HC WY, Ko TJ, Wu JK, Su CH, Lee CH. Noninvasive evaluation of blunt abdominal trauma: prospective study using diagnostic algorithms to minimize nontherapeutic laparotomy. *World J Surg* 1999; **23**: 265–270.

18 Rothlin MA, Naf R, Amgwerd M, Candinas D, Frick T, Trentz O. Ultrasound in blunt abdominal and thoracic trauma. *J Trauma* 1993; **34**(4): 488–495.

19 Kazmers A, Meeker C, Nofz K, *et al.* Nonoperative therapy for postcatheterization femoral artery pseudoaneurysms. *Am Surg* 1997; **63**(2): 199–204.

20 Moote DJ, Hilborn MD, Harris KA, Elliott JA, MacDonald AC, Foley JB. Postarteriographic femoral pseudoaneurysms: treatment with ultrasound-guided compression. *Ann Vasc Surg* 1994; **8**(4): 325–331.

21 Kim D, Orron DE, Skillman JJ, *et al.* Role of superficial femoral artery puncture in the development of pseudoaneurysm and arteriovenous fistula complicating percutaneous transfemoral cardiac catheterization. *Catheter Cardiovasc Diagn* 1992; **25**(2): 91–97.

22 Fellmeth BD, Baron SB, Brown PR, *et al.* Repair of postcatheterization femoral pseudoaneurysms by color flow ultrasound guided compression. *Am Heart J* 1992; **123**(2): 547–551.

23 Feld R, Patton GM, Carabasi RA, Alexander A, Merton D, Needleman L. Treatment of iatrogenic femoral artery injuries with ultrasound-guided compression. *J Vasc Surg* 1992; **16**(6): 832–840.

24 Hajarizadeh H, LaRosa CR, Cardullo P, Rohrer MJ, Cutler BS. Ultrasound-guided compression of iatrogenic femoral pseudoaneurysm failure, recurrence, and long-term results. *J Vasc Surg* 1995; **22**(4): 425–430; discussion 430–433.

25 Dean SM, Olin JW, Piedmonte M, Grubb M, Young JR. Ultrasound-guided compression closure of postcatheterization pseudoaneurysms during concurrent anticoagulation: a review of seventy-seven patients. *J Vasc Surg* 1996; **23**(1): 28–34, discussion 35.

26 Chatterjee T, Do DD, Kaufmann U, Mahler F, Meier B. Ultrasound-guided compression repair for treatment of femoral artery pseudoaneurysm: acute and follow-up results. *Catheter Cardiovasc Diagn* 1996; **38**(4): 335–340.

27 Schaub F, Theiss W, Busch R, Heinz M, Paschalidis M, Schomig A. Management of 219 consecutive cases of postcatheterization pseudoaneurysm. *J Am Coll Cardiol* 1997; **30**(3): 670–675. Epub 1997/09/01.

28 Liau CS, Ho FM, Chen MF, Lee YT. Treatment of iatrogenic femoral artery pseudoaneurysm with percutaneous thrombin injection. *J Vasc Surg* 1997; **26**(1): 18–23. Epub 1997/07/01.

29 Kang SS, Labropoulos N, Mansour MA, et al. Expanded indications for ultrasound-guided thrombin injection of pseudoaneurysms. *J Vasc Surg* 2000; **31**(2): 289–298. Epub 2000/02/09.

30 Brophy DP, Sheiman RG, Amatulle P, Akbari CM. Iatrogenic femoral pseudoaneurysms: thrombin injection after failed US-guided compression. *Radiology* 2000; **214**(1): 278–282. Epub 2000/01/22.

31 Paulson EK, Sheafor DH, Kliewer MA, *et al.* Treatment of iatrogenic femoral arterial pseudoaneurysms: comparison of US-guided thrombin injection with compression repair. *Radiology* 2000; **215**(2): 403–408. Epub 2000/05/05.

32 La Perna L, Olin JW, Goines D, Childs MB, Ouriel K. Ultrasound-guided thrombin injection for the treatment of postcatheterization pseudoaneurysms. *Circulation* 2000; **102**(19): 2391–2395. Epub 2000/11/09.

33 McNeil NL, Clark TW. Sonographically guided percutaneous thrombin injection versus sonographically guided compression for femoral artery pseudoaneurysms. *AJR Am J Roentgenol* 2001; **176**(2): 459–462. Epub 2001/02/13.

34 Pezzullo JA, Dupuy DE, Cronan JJ. Percutaneous injection of thrombin for the treatment of pseudoaneurysms after catheterization: an alternative to sonographically guided compression. *AJR Am J Roentgenol* 2000; **175**(4): 1035–1040. Epub 2000/09/23.

35 Cope C, Zeit R. Coagulation of aneurysms by direct percutaneous thrombin injection. *AJR Am J Roentgenol* 1986; **147**(2): 383–387. Epub 1986/08/01.

36 Samal AK, White CJ, Collins TJ, Ramee SR, Jenkins JS. Treatment of femoral artery pseudoaneurysm with percutaneous thrombin injection. *Catheter Cardiovasc Interv* 2001; **53**(2): 259–263. Epub 2001/06/02.

37 Information Ad. *Hemostatics* 1997; **20**: 12–16.

38 Dorion RP, Hamati HF, Landis B, Frey C, Heydt D, Carey D. Risk and clinical significance of developing antibodies induced by topical thrombin preparations. *Arch Path Lab Med* 1998; **122**(10): 887–894. Epub 1998/10/24.

39 Pope M, Johnston KW. Anaphylaxis after thrombin injection of a femoral pseudoaneurysm: recommendations for prevention. *J Vasc Surg* 2000; **32**(1): 190–191. Epub 2000/07/06.

40 Hamraoui K, Ernst SM, van Dessel PF, *et al.* Efficacy and safety of percutaneous treatment of iatrogenic femoral artery pseudoaneurysm by biodegradable collagen injection. *J Am Coll Cardiol* 2002; **39**(8): 1297–1304. Epub 2002/04/17.

41 Waigand J, Uhlich F, Gross CM, Thalhammer C, Dietz R. Percutaneous treatment of pseudoaneurysms and arteriovenous fistulas after invasive vascular procedures. *Catheter Cardiovasc Interv* 1999; **47**(2): 157–164. Epub 1999/06/22.

42 Thalhammer C, Kirchherr AS, Uhlich F, Waigand J, Gross CM. Postcatheterization pseudoaneurysms and arteriovenous fistulas: repair with percutaneous implanta-

tion of endovascular covered stents. *Radiology* 2000; **214**(1): 127–131. Epub 2000/01/22.

43 Murray A BT, Belli AM. Direct puncture coil embolization of iatrogenic pseudoaneurysms. *J Intervent Radiol* 1994; **9**: 183–186.

44 Uhlich FGM, Willenbrock R, Dietz R. Successful percutaneous closure of an arteriovenous fistula with a covered stent. *J Invasive Cardiol* 1995; **7**: 28A.

45 Lemaire JM, Dondelinger RF. Percutaneous coil embolization of iatrogenic femoral arteriovenous fistula or pseudo-aneurysm. *Eur J Radiol* 1994; **18**(2): 96–100. Epub 1994/05/01.

46 Matsi PJ, Manninen HI. Complications of lower-limb percutaneous transluminal angioplasty: a prospective analysis of 410 procedures on 295 consecutive patients. *Cardiovasc Interv Radiol* 1998; **21**(5): 361–366. Epub 1998/12/16.

47 Dacie JE, Goldin J. The value of interventional techniques in the management of symptomatic leg ischaemia complicating transfemoral cardiac procedures. *Clin Radiol* 1994; **49**(11): 779–783. Epub 1994/11/01.

48 Manke C, Geissler A, Seitz J, *et al.* Temporary Strecker stent for management of acute dissection in popliteal and crural arteries. *Cardiovasc Interv Radiol* 1999; **22**(2): 141–143. Epub 1999/03/30.

49 Jahnke T, Voshage G, Muller-Hulsbeck S, Grimm J, Heller M, Brossmann J. Endovascular placement of self-expanding nitinol coil stents for the treatment of femoropopliteal obstructive disease. *J Vasc Interv Radiol* 2002; **13**(3): 257–266. Epub 2002/03/05.

50 Samore MH, Wessolossky MA, Lewis SM, Shubrooks SJ Jr, Karchmer AW. Frequency, risk factors, and outcome for bacteremia after percutaneous transluminal coronary angioplasty. *Am J Cardiol* 1997; **79**(7): 873–877. Epub 1997/04/01.

51 Kiemeneij F, Laarman GJ, Odekerken D, Slagboom T, van der Wieken R. A randomized comparison of percutaneous transluminal coronary angioplasty by the radial, brachial and femoral approaches: the access study. *J Am Coll Cardiol* 1997; **29**(6): 1269–1275. Epub 1997/05/01.

52 Stella PR, Kiemeneij F, Laarman GJ, Odekerken D, Slagboom T, van der Wieken R. Incidence and outcome of radial artery occlusion following transradial artery coronary angioplasty. *Catheter Cardiovasc Diagn* 1997; **40**(2): 156–158. Epub 1997/02/01.

53 Choussat R, Black A, Bossi I, Fajadet J, Marco J. Vascular complications and clinical outcome after coronary angioplasty with platelet IIb/IIIa receptor blockade: comparison of transradial vs transfemoral arterial access. *Eur Heart J* 2000; **21**(8): 662–667. Epub 2000/03/25.

54 Jevnikar AM, Finnie KJ, Dennis B, Plummer DT, Avila A, Linton AL. Nephrotoxicity of high- and low-osmolality contrast media. *Nephron* 1988; **48**(4): 300–305. Epub 1988/01/01.

55 Eidt JF, Habibipour S, Saucedo JF, et al. Surgical complications from hemostatic puncture closure devices. *Am J Surg* 1999; **178**(6): 511–516. Epub 2000/02/12.

56 Carey D, Martin JR, Moore CA, Valentine MC, Nygaard TW. Complications of femoral artery closure devices. *Catheter Cardiovasc Interv* 2001; **52**(1): 3–7; discussion 8. Epub 2001/01/09.

57 Fram DB, Giri S, Jamil G, *et al.* Suture closure of the femoral arteriotomy following invasive cardiac procedures: a detailed analysis of efficacy, complications, and the impact of early ambulation in 1,200 consecutive, unselected cases. *Catheter Cardiovasc Interv* 2001; **53**(2): 163–173. Epub 2001/06/02.

58 Mooney MR, Ellis SG, Gershony G, Yehyawi KJ, Kummer B, Lowrie M. Immediate sealing of arterial puncture sites after cardiac catheterization and coronary interventions: initial US feasibility trial using the Duett vascular closure device. *Catheter Cardiovasc Interv* 2000; **50**(1): 96–102. Epub 2000/05/18.

59 Lehmann KG, Heath-Lange SJ, Ferris ST. Randomized comparison of hemostasis techniques after invasive cardiovascular procedures. *Am Heart J* 1999; **138**(6 Pt 1): 1118–1125. Epub 1999/11/30.

60 Chamberlin JR, Lardi AB, McKeever LS, *et al.* Use of vascular sealing devices (VasoSeal and Perclose) versus assisted manual compression (Femostop) in transcatheter coronary interventions requiring abciximab (ReoPro). *Catheter Cardiovasc Interv* 1999; **47**(2): 143–147; discussion 8. Epub 1999/06/22.

CHAPTER 27

Renal Insufficiency and the Impact of Contrast Agents

Michael Donahue and Carlo Briguori

Laboratory of Interventional Cardiology and Department of Cardiology, Clinica Mediterranea, Naples, Italy

Chronic kidney disease (CKD) is recognized as a major global public health problem affecting 8–16% of the adult population worldwide [1]. The Kidney Disease: Improving Global Outcomes (KDIGO) study defines CKD as abnormalities of kidney structure or function, present for 3 months or longer, with implications for health. Glomerular filtration rate (GFR) is generally accepted as the best overall index of kidney function while albuminuria is the best marker of kidney damage. The preferred equation to calculate estimated glomerular filtration rate is that of the Chronic Kidney Disease Epidemiology Collaboration (commonly known as the CKD-EPI) [2]. CKD is classified into six stages of estimated GFR (1, 2, 3A, 3B, 4, and 5) and three albuminuria stages (1, 2, and 3), with stage 1 representing normal values and the higher stages reflecting more severe disease [3]. A GFR <60 mL/min/1.73 m^2 is referred as decreased GFR and a GFR <15 mL/min/1.73 m^2 as kidney failure [3].

The prevalence of coronary artery disease (CAD) in patients with CKD is high and is a major cause of morbidity and mortality [4]. A meta-analysis by the CKD Prognosis Consortium demonstrated associations of GFR <60 mL/min/1.73 m^2 with subsequent risk of all-cause and cardiovascular mortality, kidney failure, acute kidney injury (AKI), and CKD progression in the general population and in populations with increased risk for cardiovascular disease [4,5].

Myocardial revascularization in patients with CKD by either percutaneous or surgical approaches is aggravated by a higher rate of complications than in patients without CKD [6–12]. Contrast-induced acute kidney injury (CIAKI) represents one of the most common complications in this subset of patients.

Contrast-induced acute kidney injury

CIAKI is defined as the acute kidney damage occurring following iodinated contrast media (CM) exposure in the absence of other causes.

CIAKI is the third most common cause of hospital-acquired AKI after impaired renal perfusion and use of nephrotoxic medications, and accounts for 10% of all causes of hospital-acquired renal failure [13–15]. CIAKI is also associated with increased health resource utilization, prolongation of hospital stay, increased long-term mortality, and accelerated progression of CKD and represents a powerful predictor of poor early and late outcome [16].

Risk factors and scores

Various cut-off criteria have been proposed to identify a clinically relevant renal function deterioration following contrast agent exposure. Currently, an increase in serum creatinine (sCr) ≥25% and/or ≥0.5 mg/dL (44 mmol/L) from baseline assessed within 48 hours after CM exposure is generally accepted as the recommended threshold [17,18].

Several risk scores have been proposed to assess the individual risk of developing CIAKI. They represent an effective tool to identify patients at high risk for CIAKI who would benefit from prophylactic therapy. Risk factors for CIAKI are: age ≥75 years, pre-existing CKD, diabetes mellitus, high volume of CM, multiple myeloma, heart failure, hemodynamic instability, or other cause of reduced renal perfusion. CKD (defined as a eGFR < 60 mL/min/1.73 m^2) represents the most important predictor, therefore it is recommended to estimate in each patient exposed to CM the baseline renal function by estimating the glomerular filtration rate (eGFR) using the CKD-EPI or the Modification of Diet on Renal Disease (MDRD) equations to estimate GFR (eGFR), instead of focusing solely on sCr. The risk score proposed by Mehran et al. [19] is simple to calculate and very useful for individual patient risk assessment. An increased score is strongly associated with CIAKI, from 7.5% (low risk score) to 57.3% (high risk score). A new score has been recently elaborated by Gurm et al. [20] which requires a computer for calculation and, unlike the previous score, has the benefit of being composed solely of preprocedural variables. The prediction model stratifies patients into low risk (<1%), intermediate risk (1–7%), and high-risk (>7%) categories based on the risk of CIAKI and has a higher discrimination than previously reported models. These scores are very useful in clinical practice for two reasons: (i) because they allow better definition of the risk in individual patients before contrast exposure, and (ii) consequently, help clinicians to target the most appropriate prophylactic strategy in each patient.

Pathophysiology

The mechanisms by which CIAKI occurs are complex and not well understood. However, it is widely held that a combination of mechanisms (hemodynamic, toxic, and osmotic) need to act in concert to cause CIAKI (Figure 27.1) [21].

Interventional Cardiology: Principles and Practice, Second Edition. Edited by George D. Dangas, Carlo Di Mario, and Nicholas N. Kipshidze.
© 2017 John Wiley & Sons, Ltd. Published 2017 by John Wiley & Sons, Ltd.

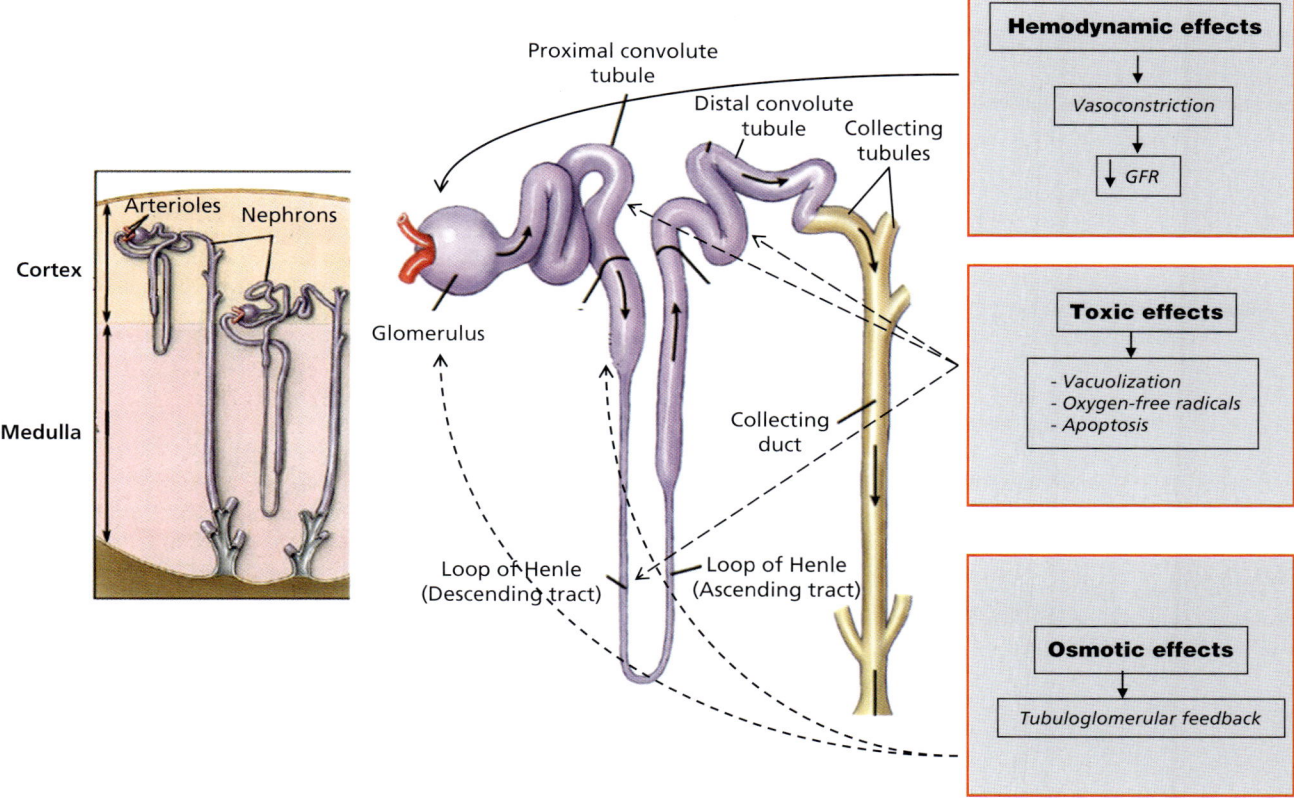

Figure 27.1 Pathogenesis of contrast-induced acute kidney injury (CIAKI): the combination of mechanisms that acting in concert lead to CIAKI.

Medullary hypoxia

The deeper portion of the outer medulla, which is particularly exposed to hypoxic damage, is the kidney region where contrast nephrotoxicity take place. Hypoxia derives mainly from decrease in renal medullary perfusion. CM augments fluid viscosity and the resistance to flow in renal tubules; the increase of renal interstitial pressure reduces both renal medullary flow and glomerular filtration rate and can lead to diminished renal perfusion (tubuloglomerular feedback). Contrast osmolarity seems to have a role, but only if it is high (>1000 mOsm/kg of H_2O).

Renal tubular damage

CM promote reactive oxygen species (ROS) generation. Oxygen radicals are highly reactive and can directly damage renal endothelial–epithelial cells or induce renal microvessel constriction (e.g., via endothelin-A receptor activation). In addition to the ischemic changes to the renal tubules, CM has a cytotoxic effect on the tubular epithelial cells by activating apoptosis via three mechanisms: (i) ROS, (ii) JNK and p38 kinases, and (iii) the intrinsic (or mitochondrial) pathway of apoptosis [22,23]. This effect seems to be time- and dosage-dependent.

Diagnosis and novel biomarkers

The classifications of CIAKI proposed are based on the variation of two parameters: sCr or GFR, and urinary flow. The diagnostic criteria for kidney damage are summarized in Table 27.1 [24,25]. Levels of sCr usually begin to rise within 24–48 hours of CM exposure, peaking at 2–3 days and returning to baseline values within 2 weeks. This is mainly caused by two significant limitations of

dosing sCr. First, creatinine excreted in the urine is not solely a result of glomerular filtration, but also of renal tubular secretion. This means that changes in sCr will underestimate the true fall in GFR. Second, following an acute fall in GFR, less creatinine is excreted. The retained creatinine is distributed in total body water and, although the injury induced by CM impairs GFR almost immediately, it requires 24–48 h for the fall in GFR to be reflected in an elevated level of sCr. This implies an intrinsic delay of treatment of patients who will develop CIAKI and, on the contrary, a prolonged hospital stay in patients who will not develop CIAKI. Serum creatinine levels are still considered the major marker of CIAKI, but for these limitations other biomarkers that allow an earlier diagnosis of AKI have been proposed [26].

The cystatin C (CyC) is produced at a relatively constant rate by nucleated cells and is not affected by renal tubular secretion or pharmacologic treatments [27]. In a study on 410 patients with CKD undergoing percutaneous procedures, an increase in serum CyC ≥10% in 24 hours after the procedure showed a sensitivity of 100% and a specificity of 86% in predicting CIAKI [28]. In addition, the CyC demonstrated to be an independent predictor of adverse events at follow-up [28,29].

The neutrophil gelatinase associated lipocalin (NGAL) is a protein whose production is induced by an acute injury to the renal tubular epithelium. The NGAL has been shown to be one of the most promising biomarkers of AKI, an increase both in the serum and urinary NGAL within 2–4 hours after administration of CM is a strong predictor of CIAKI [30–32]. A recent meta-analysis found that NGAL levels between 100 and 270 ng/mL have a high sensitivity and specificity for AKI [33].

Table 27.1 RIFLE and AKIN criteria [24,25].

RIFLE criteria (7 days)		
Class	**Criteria: GFR**	**Criteria: urine output**
R–Risk	Increase sCr × 1.5 or GFR decrease >25%	<0.5 mL/kg/hr for 6 hr
I–Injury	Increase sCr × 2 or GFR decrease >25%	<0.5 mL/kg/hr for 12 hr
F–Failure	Increase sCr × 3 or GFR decrease >75% or SCr ≥4 mg/dL	<0.3 mL/kg/hr for 24 hr or anuria for 12 hr
L–Loss	Persistent kidney failure >4 weeks	
E–ESKD	Terminal kidney injury >3 months	

AKIN criteria (48 hour)		
Stage	**Criteria: serum creatinine**	**Criteria: urine output**
1	Increase of sCr × 1.5 or >0.3 mg/dL	< 0.5 mL/kg/hr for 6 hr
2	Increase of sCr × 2	< 0.5 mL/kg/hr for 6 hr
3	Increase of sCr × 3 or >4 mg/dL	< 0.3 mL/kg/hr for >24 hr or anuria for 12 hr

eGFR, estimated glomerular filtration rate; sCr, serum creatinine.

The kidney injury molecule-1 (KIM-1) is a transmembrane adhesion protein of type 1, the expression of which increases in the proximal tubule cells in response to ischemic injury. A soluble form can be detected in the urine of animal models and in patients with acute renal failure due to CIAKI [34].

Prevention of CIAKI

The optimal strategy to prevent CIAKI remains uncertain. At present, the best approach to prevent CIAKI is to identify patients at risk using risk scores, to minimize the amount of administered CM (low or iso-osmolality contrast) and provide adequate peri-procedural hydration [35]. The use of antioxidant compounds like *N*-acetylcysteine (NAC) or statins, although not part of the official recommendations, also seems to have a role in preventing CIAKI [36–39], while the use of nephrotoxic drugs should be suspended for at least 2 days prior to CM exposure. The role of prophylactic renal replacement therapies (RRT), such as hemofiltration, is still debated and limited to patients at very high risk.

Volume supplementation

Hydration is considered one of the major beneficial measures for prevention of CIAKI [35]. Volume supplementation prevents CIAKI mostly via two mechanisms:

1 The inhibition of arginine-vasopressine (via vagal inputs from the mechanoreceptors located at the atrial–venous junctions and by a direct effect of osmolality on the supra-aortic nuclei), and

2 The increase in medullary perfusion and regional pO_2 by inducing an increase of urine flow rates, that reduces the concentration of CM in the tubule and expedites CM excretion [21,40].

This implies a reduction of the exposure time of tubular cells to the toxic effects of CM. Hydration with isotonic saline (0.9% NaCl) should be started intravenously 12 hours prior to the procedure at a rate of 1 mL/kg/h and should be continued for 12 hours following the procedure. In patients with unstable hemodynamic conditions, where there is a particular concern regarding volume overload, at least 0.5 mL/kg/h intravenous saline infusion should be received before contrast exposure. The post-procedure hydration target can be adjusted according to urine output which should remain above 150 mL/h. The optimal hydration regimen should be defined according to a pre-defined clinical marker. Two markers have been identified: (i) urine flow rate [41], and (ii) left ventricular end-diastolic pressure (LVEDP) [42].

Urine flow rate High urine flow rate reduces the incidence of CIAKI via several effects. Data from the PRINCE study indicated that the increase in urine flow rate (≥150 mL/h) reduces the toxic effect of CM [43]. The RenalGuard system (PLC Medical System, Inc. Franklin, MA, USA) has been developed to facilitate optimal hydration therapy [44]. This device allows high urine output to be achieved while simultaneously balancing urine output and venous fluid infusion to prevent hypovolemia. Randomized trials [45,46] have demonstrated the effectiveness of this system in significantly reducing the incidence of CIAKI compared with standard hydration in patients at high risk.

Left ventricular end diastolic pressure The POSEIDON trial [42] sought to determine the efficacy of a novel fluid protocol based upon the LVEDP. This single center study included 396 patients undergoing cardiac catheterization with an estimated GFR ≤60 mL/min/1.73 m² and one or more of diabetes mellitus, history of congestive heart failure, hypertension, or age >75 years and who were randomly allocated to LVEDP guided volume expansion or standard hydration (control group). Both groups received intravenous 0.9% sodium chloride at 3 mL/kg for 1 hour prior to cardiac catheterization. In the LVEDP group, the fluid rate was adjusted according to the LVEDP as follows: 5 mL/kg/hr for LVEDP <13 mmHg; 3 mL/kg/hr for 13–18 mmHg, and 1.5 mL/kg/hr for >18 mmHg. The control group hydration rate was 1.5 mL/kg/hr. For both groups, the fluid rate was set at the start of the procedure, continued during the procedure, and for 4 hours post-procedure. CIAKI occurred less frequently among patients randomized to the LVEDP-guided group than the control group (6.7% vs. 16.3%; p = 0.005).

It is still controversial whether some solutions are superior to others. Evidence suggests that hydration with sodium bicarbonate, compared with isotonic saline, represents an effective strategy to prevent CIAKI [47–51]. However, the recent randomized trial for the prevention of contrast induced nephropathy in patients with chronic kidney disease, the Bicarbonate or Saline Study (BOSS) trial, enrolling 376 patients who underwent either coronary or peripheral angiogram, failed to demonstrate a superiority of sodium bicarbonate over sodium chloride solution in preventing CIAKI, although a reduction in the the death rate was seen [52]. The use of sodium bicarbonate infusion allows volume supplementation for shorter periods and can also further reduce the generation of injurious oxygen-free radicals. The higher amount of bicarbonate in the proximal convoluted tubule can buffer the higher amount of

H+ due to cellular hypoxia and facilitate Na+ reabsorption through the electrogenic co-transposer [53]. Free-radical formation is promoted by an acidic environment typical of tubular urine but is inhibited by the higher pH of normal extracellular fluid [54]. It has been hypothesized that alkalinizing renal tubular fluid with bicarbonate reduces injury [47]. Patients undergoing volume supplementation with the abovementioned protocol should receive 154 mEq/L NaHCO3, as a bolus of 3 mL/kg/hour for 1 hour prior to CM administration, followed by an infusion of 1 mL/kg/hour for 6 hours after the procedure.

Contrast media
Type of contrast agents
Osmolality has an important role in the pathophysiology of CIAKI [21]. It has been reported that low osmolality (LOCM) and iso-osmolality contrast agent (IOCM) are less nephrotoxic than high osmolar contrast agents (HOCM) [55]. HOCM is highly charged and highly osmolar ($\approx$1500 mOsm/kg H_2O). It is still controversial whether IOCM ($\approx$290 mOsm/kg H_2O) is less nephrotoxic than LOCM ($\approx$700–800 mOsm/kg H_2O). While early studies suggested a role for osmolality in the pathogenesis of CIAKI at high osmolalities (>1000 mOsm/kg H_2O), for CM with an osmolality in the range of 290 to approximately 800 mOsm/kg H_2O, other physicochemical characteristics, such as viscosity, perhaps have a greater role in the development of CIAKI blocking the protective benefit of lower osmolality [56]. To date, no consensus has been reached on the relative importance of osmolality and viscosity and the current guidelines recommend the use of either IOCM or LOCM (other than iohexol and ioxaglate) in patients with CKD undergoing angiography [57].

In the NEPHRIC trial [58], enrolling 126 patients with diabetes mellitus and CKD, CIAKI occurred in 3% of patients in the IOCM group and 25% in the LOCM group (p = 0.003). However, this result has not been confirmed in other observational [59] and randomized trials [60]. In the CARE trial [60], 414 patients with an eGFR of 20–59 mL/min scheduled for a percutaneous coronary procedure were randomized to LOCM iopamidol (796 mOsm/kg of H_2O) or IOCM iodixanol (290 mOsm/kg H_2O). No significant differences overall and in the subgroup of diabetic patients existed in the primary CIAKI endpoint (a post-procedural sCr increase of $\geq$0.5 mg/dL) or in the secondary CIAKI endpoints (a post-procedural sCr increase of $\geq$25% over baseline, a post-dose eGFR decrease of $\geq$25% and the mean peak change in serum creatinine of >0.50 mg/dL). Finally, in a meta-analysis comparing the iso-osmolar iodixanol with LOCM, the pooled relative rate (RR) was 0.68 (95% CI 0.46–1.01; p = 0.06), while in the studies that included only patients with decreased kidney function after CM administration the RR was 0.59 (95% CI 0.33–1.07; p = 0.08). However, when iohexol was the LOCM used, the risk of CIAKI was significantly lower than with iodixanol (RR 0.38; 95% CI 0.21–0.68; p <0.01) [61].

Volume of contrast agents
The use of a small volume of contrast dye and the avoidance of closely spaced repetitive studies represents one of the most important recommendations to prevent CIAKI [18]. Low volume has been variably defined as a total absolute volume <100 mL, <125 mL, <140 mL, or a volume adjusted for body weight of <5 mL/kg (to a maximum of 300 mL) divided by the plasma creatinine concentration [62]. It has been suggested that use of the iodine dose : glomerular filtration rate (I/GFR) ratio may be a more expedient way of

improving risk assessment of CIAKI than the most common practice of estimating CM dose from body weight alone [63]. Chapters 4, 7, and 18 illustrate some of the principles used to minimize contrast use. General recommendations include limitations in the diagnostic angiogram pre-PCI to few essential views especially for urgent unstable patients for whom treatment should be limited to the culprit artery, injections limited to the minimum required to assess proper positioning of devices and final result, filming the balloon during expansion or using fluoroscopic optimization of the stent visualization (stent "boost" modality), or using automated contrast injectors and catheters without side holes.

Pharmacologic therapy
The generation of ROS subsequent to CM exposure of vasa recta and tubule cells and the consequent apoptosis activation have been considered an important pathophysiologic cause of CIAKI [21]. In recent years many clinical studies have been conducted to test the use of antioxidant compounds in an attempt to prevent CIAKI. The most investigated drugs are NAC, ascorbic acid, and statins.

N-acetylcysteine
NAC is a thiol compound classically known as a mucolytic agent, which is used to thin mucus especially in patients with respiratory disease. NAC is a potent antioxidant that scavenges a wide variety of oxygen-derived free-radicals. It may be capable of preventing CIAKI by stopping direct oxidative tissue damage and also by improving renal hemodynamics [64–66]. The antioxidant effect of NAC seems to be dose-dependent [67,68]. The molecular mechanisms of NAC on CIAKI prevention have been clearly elucidated in in vitro experiments. Recent studies demonstrate that NAC exerts its antioxidant properties preventing kidney cell death by inhibiting oxygen-free radical production and thus stress kinases and apoptosis activation upon CM exposure [69,70]. However, the results on the use of NAC are conflicting. While initial studies by Tepel et al. [64] showed that NAC (600 mg orally twice daily) plus hydration was more effective than hydration alone in preventing CIAKI in patients with CKD undergoing computed tomography, a recent large randomized trial [71] failed to demonstrate the superiority of NAC versus placebo in reducing the incidence of CIAKI in patients undergoing coronary angiography. Although a recent meta-analysis of 30 trials showed a renoprotective benefit with NAC [72], the most recent guidelines do not recommend NAC for CIAKI prevention [35].

Ascorbic acid
Additional evidence of the effectiveness of an antioxidant strategy comes from the observation by Spargias et al. [73], who investigated the impact of ascorbic acid in preventing CIAKI. In vitro and in vivo studies have also demonstrated a role for ascorbic acid in the prevention of CIAKI [74,75]. A combination of different antioxidant compounds was tested by Briguori et al. [76]. Consecutive patients with CKD were randomly assigned to prophylactic administration of 0.9% saline infusion plus NAC, sodium bicarbonate infusion plus NAC, or 0.9% saline plus ascorbic acid plus NAC. The combined prophylactic strategy of sodium bicarbonate plus NAC was superior in preventing CIAKI in patients at medium-to-high risk undergoing contrast exposure. The lack of favorable protective effect of the combination of ascorbic acid plus NAC compared to NAC alone suggests additional and/or alternative mechanism(s) (other than antioxidant effect) which require further investigation. We

hypothesize that NAC and ascorbic acid work through similar pathways while the protective action of bicarbonate may be different in comparison to NAC and therefore additive.

Statins

Besides the common use of the 3-hydroxy-3-methylglutaryl coenzyme A (HMG-CoA) reductase inhibitors to decrease cholesterol levels, they have several "pleiotropic" effects through their non-lipid-related mechanisms acting on inflammation responses, endothelial function, plaque stability, thrombus formation, and apoptotic pathway [77]. *In vitro* models indicate that pre-treatment with atorvastatin prevents CM-induced renal cell apoptosis by reducing stress kinase activation and restored the survival signals mediated by Akt and Erks signal transduction pathways [78]. Many studies have investigated the effectiveness of statins pre-treatment in reducing the incidence of CIAKI [78–83] and demonstrated that preprocedural high dose statin treatment reduces the risk of CIAKI and the need for RRT in patients undergoing coronary angiography and/or percutaneous interventions. Moreover, most recent investigations confirmed that rosuvastatin in statin-naïve patients with both stable and acute coronary syndrome scheduled for early invasive procedure could prevent CIAKI [82,83]. The most recent guidelines recommend high doses of statin for CIAKI prevention [35].

Other medications

Because of the potential role of focal renal vasoconstriction induced by contrast agents, numerous vasodilator drugs have been tested for prevention of CIAKI. Theophylline [84], nifedipine [85], adenosine [86], endothelin receptor antagonists [87], atrial natriuretic peptide [88], dopamine, and fenoldopam [89–91] do not seem to be effective. A randomized double-blind placebo-controlled trial showed that prophylactic administration of iloprost in patients with CKD, undergoing coronary angiography and/or intervention, may protect against CIAKI [92].

Compelling data support that neither mannitol nor furosemide offer additional protection against radiocontrast-induced nephrotoxicity as compared with saline hydration alone in either diabetic or non-diabetic patients [93,94].

Ischemic remote preconditioning

In addition to the effects of local ischemia, remote ischemia can protect distant organs or tissue during subsequent ischemia [95]. This has been termed remote ischemic preconditioning (RIPC) [96]. RIPC is a method by which the deliberate induction of transient non-lethal ischemia of an organ protects against subsequent ischemic injury of another organ. The potential use of RIPC has been mostly evaluated in the setting of myocardial protection. There are also preliminary data suggesting that RIPC prior to both cardiac surgery and CM administration protects against AKI [97]. In a randomized double-blind trial, 100 patients with CKD were subjected to RIPC or to a sham procedure prior to elective coronary angiography [98]. RIPC was induced by intermittent arm ischemia generated by four cycles of 5-minute inflation of a blood pressure (BP) cuff to 50 mmHg above individual systolic pressure within 45 minutes before angiography. The sham procedure consisted of inflation of a BP cuff to individual diastolic pressure, followed by deflation to 10 mmHg. All patients received also acetylcysteine and a continuous saline infusion. The incidence of CIAKI was 6% in the RIPC group versus 20% in the sham group (OR 0.21, 95% CI 0.07–0.57). In a second trial, 225 patients with a

non-ST-segment elevation myocardial infarction were randomly assigned to receive RIPC or a sham procedure prior to the coronary intervention [99]. RIPC consisted of four cycles of 30 second inflation, followed by 30 seconds deflation of the stent balloon during the PCI procedure; the sham procedure consisted of four cycles of 30-second inflation to only 3 atm pressure, followed by deflation. Even in this study, CIAKI occurred less frequently in the RIPC group than in the sham group (12.4% vs. 29.5%, respectively, OR 0.34, 95% CI 0.16–0.71). These results, although compelling (particularly because RIPC is conferred using different modalities and at different time points prior to contrast exposure), require confirmation in larger randomized trials to determine the underlying mechanism of protection and before RIPC can be recommended as a preventive measure for CIAKI [100]. In addition, the safety of repetitive balloon inflations in a coronary artery poststenting remains unclear.

Renal replacement therapy

Hemofiltration is expensive, time consuming, logistically cumbersome, and associated with significant risks. Its effectivess compared with other less expensive strategies is not well established so this treatment modality should be reserved for patients who already have fairly advanced renal insufficiency [101]. Marenzi *et al.* [102] found that, compared with intravenous saline, hemofiltration administered as prophylactic therapy in high-risk patients was associated with: (i) a lesser likelihood of the serum creatinine rising >25% (5% vs. 50%); (ii) a lesser likelihood of requiring dialysis (3% vs. 25%), and (iii) a lower in-house (2% vs. 14%) and 1-year mortality (10% vs. 30%). However, it has been pointed out that creatinine removal by the hemofiltration procedure can be sufficient to explain the decreased frequency of elevation in the serum creatinine. Moreover, the control group had an unusually high incidence of acute renal failure, attributable to the excessive volume of contrast media used and, possibly, to the absence of optimal pharmacologic prophylaxis. Patients in the hemofiltration group were cared for in an intensive care unit; their greater intensity of care relative to the control group may explain why hemofiltration was associated with improved short- and long-term survival. In contrast, the same authors found that hemofiltration performed only post-contrast exposure is not effective [103]. Recently, data from Spini *et al.* [104] confirmed that continuous renal replacement therapy (CRRT) performed before and after PCI is more effective for CIAKI prevention in patients with severe CKD in comparison to CRRT performed only after, is capable of significantly reducing sCr levels and increasing eGFR values, and is associated with a lower mortality rate during follow-up. Given the aforementioned limitations, the applicability of these findings to current clinical practice remains unclear. Table 27.2 depicts the approach proposed to prevent CIAKI based on current evidence.

Conclusions

The optimal strategy to prevent CIAKI remains uncertain. The most recent guidelines [35,105] recommend: (i) a peri-procedural intravenous volume expansion with isotonic sodium chloride, (ii) the use of a low or iso-osmolality contrast agents, and (iii) to limit the volume of the administered contrast agent. Adequate hydration should be guided according to LVEDP and/or urine flow rate. The RenalGuard system seems to be helpful in preventing CIAKI by allowing a high urine flow rate and optimal fluid balance. Statins can be effective in reducing oxidative stress and therefore preventing

Table 27.2 Checklist for estimating the risk of CIAKI and prevention strategies in patients undergoing percutaneous procedures.

Risk assessment

1 eGFR calculation
2 Risk score assessment (Mehran, Gurm)
3 Nephrologic consulation (eGFR <15 mL/min/1.73 m²). Indication for elective RRT

Prophylaxis

1 Intravenous hydration 2 Drugs	Normal saline	0.5–1 mL/kg/hr 12 hr before and 12 hr after Maintain urine flow rate >150 mL/hr *or* LVEDP-guided: <13 mmHg = 5 mL/kg/hr 13–18 mmHg = 3 mL/kg/hr >18 mmHg = 1.5 mL/kg/hr
	Sodium bicarbonate	154 mEq/L 3 mL/kg/hr ≥1 hr before and 1 mL/kg/hr for 6 hr after
	Renalguard system (eGFR < 30 mL/min/1.73 m² and/or Mehran risk score >11) Statins	Maintain urine flow rate ≥300 mL/hr Atorvastatin 80 mg Rosuvastatin 40 mg
	N-acetylcysteine	1200 mg b.i.d. before and after
Iodinated contrast media	Iso- and low osmolar (beside ioxalate and ioexol) Limited volume (mL)	• Prolong the time-interval between CM-enhanced studies • Staged procedures for complex multivessel disease • Alternative CM (CO₂ for peripheral procedures • Automated contrast injectors
Serial control of serum creatinine	At 48–72 hr: additional controls if clinically indicated	

CM, contrast media; eGFR, estimated glomerular filtration rate; LVEDP, left ventricular end-diastolic pressure; RRT, renal replacement therapy.

renal cell apoptosis. Additional data are necessary to clarify the role of RIPC in routine clinical practice.

Interactive multiple choice questions are available for this chapter on www.wiley. com/go/dangas/cardiology

References

1 Jha V, Garcia-Garcia G, Iseki K, *et al.* Chronic kidney disease: global dimension and perspectives. *Lancet* 2013; **382**(9888): 260–272.

2 Gansevoort RT, Correa-Rotter R, Hemmelgarn BR, *et al.* Chronic kidney disease and cardiovascular risk: epidemiology, mechanisms, and prevention. *Lancet* 2013; **382**(9889): 339–352.

3 Kidney Disease: Improving Global Outcomes (KDIGO) CKD Work Group. KDIGO 2012 clinical practice guideline for the evaluation and management of chronic kidney disease. *Kidney Int Suppl* 2013; **3**: 1–150.

4 Levey AS, Beto JA, Coronado BE, *et al.* Controlling the epidemic of cardiovascular disease in chronic renal disease: What do we know? What do we need to learn? Where do we go from here? National Kidney Foundation Task Force on Cardiovascular Disease. *Am J Kidney Dis* 1998; **32**: 853–906.

5 Matsushita K, van der Velde M, Astor BC, *et al.* Association of estimated glomerular filtration rate and albuminuria with all-cause and cardiovascular mortality in general population cohorts: a collaborative meta-analysis. *Lancet* 2010; **375**: 2073–2081.

6 Hillis GS, Croal BL, Buchan KG, *et al.* Renal function and outcome from coronary artery bypass grafting: impact on mortality after a 2.3-year follow-up. *Circulation* 2006; **113**: 1056–1062.

7 Cooper WA, O'Brien SM, Thourani VH, *et al.* Impact of renal dysfunction on outcomes of coronary artery bypass surgery: results from the Society of Thoracic Surgeons National Adult Cardiac Database. *Circulation* 2006; **113**: 1063–1070.

8 Hassani SE, Chu WW, Wolfram RM, *et al.* Clinical outcomes after percutaneous coronary intervention with drug-eluting stents in dialysis patients. *J Invasive Cardiol* 2006; **18**(6): 273–277.

9 Hemmelgarn BR, Southern D, Culleton BF, *et al.* Survival after coronary revascularization among patients with kidney disease. *Circulation* 2004; **110**: 1890–1895.

10 Aoki J, Ong AT, Hoye A, *et al.* Five year clinical effect of coronary stenting and coronary artery bypass grafting in renal insufficient patients with multivessel coronary artery disease: insights from ARTS trial. *Eur Heart J* 2005; **26**: 1488–1493.

11 Briguori C, Airoldi F, Chieffo A, Carlino M, Montorfano M, Colombo A. Renal function and drug-eluting stent. *Int J Cardiol* 2010; **142**(1): 92–94.

12 Iakovou I, Schmidt T, Bonizzoni E, *et al.* Incidence, predictors, and outcome of thrombosis after successful implantation of drug-eluting stents. *JAMA* 2005; **293**(17): 2126–2130.

13 Nash K, Hafeez A, Hou S. Hospital-acquired renal insufficiency. *Am J Kidney Dis* 2002; **39**: 930–936.

14 Tepel M, Aspelin P, Lameire N. Contrast-induced nephropathy: a clinical and evidence-based approach. *Circulation* 2006; **113**: 1799–1806.

15 Gruberg L, Mehran R, Dangas G, *et al.* Acute renal failure requiring dialysis after percutaneous coronary interventions. *Catheter Cardiovasc Interv* 2001; **52**: 409–416.

16 Subramanian S, Tumlin J, Bapat B, Zyczynski T. Economic burden of contrast-induced nephropathy: implications for prevention strategies. *J Med Econ* 2007; **10**: 119–134.

17 Mehran R, Nikolsky E. Contrast-induced nephropathy: definition, epidemiology, and patients at risk. *Kidney Int* 2006; **100**: 11–15.

18 Solomon R, Deray G. How to prevent contrast-induced nephropathy and manage risk patients: practical recommendations. *Kidney Int Suppl* 2006; **100**: S51–53.

19 Mehran R, Aymong ED, Nikolsky E, *et al.* A simple risk score for prediction of contrast-induced nephropathy after percutaneous coronary intervention: development and initial validation. *J Am Coll Cardiol* 2004; **44**: 1393–1399.

20 Gurm HS, Seth M, Kooiman J, Share D.A. Novel tool for reliable and accurate prediction of renal complications in patients undergoing percutaneous coronary intervention. *J Am Coll Cardiol* 2013; **61**(22): 2242–2428.

21 Persson PB, Hansell P, Liss P. Pathophysiology of contrast medium-induced nephropathy. *Kidney Int* 2005; **68**: 14–22.

22 Quintavalle C, Brenca M, De Micco F, et al. In vivo and in vitro assessment of pathways involved in contrast media-induced renal cells apoptosis. *Cell Death Dis* 2011; **2**: e155.

23 Romano G, Briguori C, Quintavalle C, et al. Contrast agents and renal cell apoptosis. *Eur Hearth J* 2008; **29**: 2569–2576.

24 Bellomo R, Ronco C, Kellum JA, et al. Acute renal failure: definition, outcome measures, animal models, fluid therapy and information technology needs. The Second International Consensus Conference of the Acute Dialysis Quality Initiative (ADQI) Group. *Crit Care* 2004; **8**(4): R204–R212.

25 Mehta RL, Kellum JA, Shah SV, et al. Acute Kidney Injury Network: report of an initiative to improve outcomes in acute kidney injury. *Crit Care* 2007; **11**: R31.

26 Guitterez NV, Diaz A, Timmis GC, et al. Determinants of serum creatinine trajectory in acute contrast nephropathy. *J Interv Cardiol* 2002; **15**: 349–354.

27 Tenstad O, Roald AB, Grubb A, Aukland K. Renal handling of radio labelled human cystatin C in the rat. *Scand J Clin Lab Invest* 1996; **56**(5): 409–414.

28 Briguori C, Visconti G, Rivera NV, et al. Cystatin C and contrast-induced acute kidney injury. *Circulation* 2010; **121**(19): 2117–2122.

29 Solomon RJ, Mehran R, Natarajan MK, et al. Contrast-induced nephropathy and long-term adverse events: cause and effect? *Clin J Am Soc Nephrol* 2009; **4**(7): 1162–1169.

30 Mishra J, Ma Q, Kelly C, et al. Kidney NGAL is a novel early marker of acute injury following transplantation. *Pediatr Nephrol* 2006; **21**(6): 856–863.

31 McCullough PA, Williams FJ, Stivers DN, et al. Neutrophil gelatinase-associated lipocalin: a novel marker of contrast nephropathy risk. *Am J Nephrol* 2012; **35**(6): 509–514.

32 Tasanarong A, Hutayanon P, Piyayotai P. Urinary neutrophil gelatinase-associated lipocalin predicts the severity of contrast-induced acute kidney injury in chronic kidney disease patients undergoing elective coronary procedures. *BMC Nephrol* 2013; **14**(1): 270.

33 Haase M, Devarajan P, Haase-Fielitz A, et al. The outcome of neutrophil gelatinase-associated lipocalin-positive subclinical acute kidney injury: a multicenter pooled analysis of prospective studies. *J Am Coll Cardiol* 2011; **57**(17): 1752–1761.

34 Han WK, Bailly V, Abichandani R, Thadhani R, Bonventre JV. Kidney Injury Molecule-1 (KIM-1): a novel biomarker for human renal proximal tubule injury. *Kidney Int* 2002; **62**(1): 237–244.

35 Windecker S, Kolh P, Alfonso F. 2014 ESC/EACTS Guidelines on myocardial revascularization: The Task Force on Myocardial Revascularization of the European Society of Cardiology (ESC) and the European Association for Cardio-Thoracic Surgery (EACTS) Developed with the special contribution of the European Association of Percutaneous Cardiovascular Interventions (EAPCI). *Eur Heart J* 2014; **35**(37): 2541–2619.

36 Kelly AM, Dwamena B, Cronin P, et al. Meta-analysis: effectiveness of drugs for preventing contrast-induced nephropathy. *Ann Intern Med* 2008; **148**: 284–294.

37 Briguori C, Quintavalle C, De Micco F, Condorelli G. Nephrotoxicity of contrast media and protective effects of acetylcysteine. *Arch Toxicol* 2011; **85**: 165–173.

38 Toso A, Maioli M, LeonCIAKIi M, et al. Usefulness of atorvastatin (80 mg) in prevention of contrast-induced nephropathy in patients with chronic renal disease. *Am J Cardiol* 2010; **105**: 288–292.

39 Patti G, Ricottini E, Nusca A, et al. Short-term, high-dose atorvastatin pretreatment to prevent contrast-induced nephropathy in patients with acute coronary syndromes undergoing percutaneous coronary intervention (from the ARMYDA-CIAKI [Atorvastatin for Reduction of MYocardial Damage during Angioplasty—Contrast-Induced Nephropathy] Trial. *Am J Cardiol* 2011; **108**: 1–7.

40 Seeliger E, Becker K, Ladwig M, et al. Up to 50-fold increase in urine viscosity with iso-osmolar contrast media in the rat1. *Radiology* 2010; **256**: 406–414.

41 Brown JR, Thompson CA. Contrast-induced acute kidney injury: the at-risk patient and protective measures. *Curr Cardiol Rep* 2010; **12**: 440–445.

42 Brar SS, Aharonian V, Mansukhani P, et al. Haemodynamic-guided fluid administration for the prevention of contrast-induced acute kidney injury: the POSEIDON randomised controlled trial. *Lancet* 2014; **383**(9931): 1814–1823.

43 Stevens MA, McCullough PA, Tobin KJ, et al. A prospective randomized trial of prevention measures in patients at high risk for contrast nephropathy: Results of the PRINCE study. *J Am Coll Cardiol* 1999; **33**: 403–411.

44 Dorval J-F, Dixon SR, Zelman RB, et al. Feasibility study of the RenalGuard balanced hydration system: a novel strategy for the prevention of contrast-induced nephropathy in high risk patients. *Int J Cardiol* 2013; **166**: 482–486.

45 Briguori C, Visconti G, Focaccio F, et al. Renal Insufficiency After Contrast Media Administration Trial II (REMEDIAL II): RenalGuard System in high-risk patients for contrast-induced acute kidney injury. *Circulation* 2011; **124**: 1260–1269.

46 Marenzi G, Ferrari C, Marana I, et al. Prevention of contrast nephropathy by furosemide with matched hydration: the MYTHOS (Induced Diuresis With Matched Hydration Compared to Standard Hydration for Contrast Induced Nephropathy Prevention) trial. *JACC Cardiovasc Interv* 2012; **5**: 90–97.

47 Merten GJ, Burgess WP, Gray LV, et al. Prevention of contrast-induced nephropathy with sodium bicarbonate: a randomized controlled trial. *JAMA* 2004; **291**: 2328–2334.

48 Briguori C, Airoldi F, D'Andrea D, et al. Renal Insufficiency Following Contrast Media Administration Trial (REMEDIAL): a randomized comparison of 3 preventive strategies. *Circulation* 2007; **115**(10): 1211–1217.

49 Trivedi H, Nadella R, Szabo A. Hydration with sodium bicarbonate for the prevention of contrast-induced nephropathy: a meta-analysis of randomized controlled trials. *Clin Nephrol* 2010; **74**: 288–296.

50 Kunadian V, Zaman A, Spyridopoulos I, Qiu W. Sodium bicarbonate for the prevention of contrast induced nephropathy: a meta-analysis of published clinical trials. *Eur J Radiol* 2011; **79**: 48–55.

51 Tamai N, Ito S, Nakasuka K, et al. Sodium bicarbonate for the prevention of contrast-induced nephropathy: the efficacy of high concentration solution. *J Invasive Cardiol* 2012; **24**: 439–442.

52 Solomon R. Randomized trial for the prevention of contrast induced nephropathy in patients with chronic kidney disease: The Bicarbonate or Saline Study (BOSS), TCT 2013 meeting. San Francisco. Available at http://www.tctmd.com/show. aspx?id=121633 (accessed April 23, 2016).

53 Boron WF. Acid–base transport by the renal proximal tubule. *J Am Soc Nephrol* 2006; **17**: 2368–2382.

54 Alpem R. Renal acidification mechanisms. In: Barry M. Brenner, ed. *The Kidney*. WB Saunders, Philadelphia, PA: 2000; 455–469.

55 Barrett BJ, Carlisle EJ. Meta-analysis of the relative nephrotoxicity of high and low-osmolality iodinated contrast media. *Radiology* 1993; **188**: 171–178.

56 Solomon R. The role of osmolality in the incidence of contrast-induced nephropathy: a systematic review of angiographic contrast media in high risk patients. *Kidney Int* 2005; **68**: 2256–2263.

57 Kushner FG, Hand M, Smith Jr SC, et al. 2009 focused updates: ACC/AHA guidelines for the management of patients with ST-elevation myocardial infarction (updating the 2004 guideline and 2007 focused update) and ACC/AHA/SCAI guidelines on percutaneous coronary intervention (updating the 2005 guideline and 2007 focused update) a report of the American College of Cardiology Foundation/American Heart Association Task Force on Practice Guidelines. *J Am Coll Cardiol* 2009; **54**: 2205–2241.

58 Aspelin P, Aubry P, Fransson SG, et al. Nephrotoxic effects in high-risk patients undergoing angiography. *N Engl J Med* 2003; **348**: 491–499.

59 Briguori C, Colombo A, Airoldi F, et al. Nephrotoxicity of low-osmolality versus iso-osmolality contrast agents: impact of N-acetylcysteine. *Kidney Int* 2005; **68**: 2250–2255.

60 Solomon RJ, Natarajan MK, Doucet S, et al. Cardiac Angiography in Renally Impaired Patients (CARE) study: a randomized double-blind trial of contrast-induced nephropathy in patients with chronic kidney disease. *Circulation* 2007; **115**: 3189–3196.

61 Heinrich MC, Haberle L, Muller V, et al. Nephrotoxicity of iso-osmolar iodixanol compared with nonionic low-osmolar contrast media: metaanalysis of randomized controlled trials. *Radiology* 2009; **250**: 68–86.

62 Cigarroa RG, Lange RA, Williams RH, et al. Dosing of contrast material to prevent contrast nephropathy in patients with renal disease. *Am J Med* 1989; **86**: 649–652.

63 Nyman U, Almen T, Aspelin P, et al. Contrast-medium-induced nephropathy correlated to the ratio between dose in gram iodine and estimated GFR in ml/min. *Acta Radiol* 2005; **46**: 830–842.

64 Tepel M, van der Giet M, Schwarzfeld C, et al. Prevention of radiographic-contrast-agent-induced reductions in renal function by acetylcysteine. *N Engl J Med* 2000; **343**: 180–184.

65 DiMari J, Megyesi J, Udvarhelyi N, et al. N-acetylcysteine ameliorates ischemic renal failure. *Am J Physiol* 1997; **272**: F292–298.

66 Heyman SN, Goldfarb M, Shina A, et al. N-acetylcysteine ameliorates renal microcirculation: studies in rats. *Kidney Int* 2003; **63**: 634–641.

67 Briguori C, Colombo A, Violante A, et al. Standard vs. double dose of N-acetylcysteine to prevent contrast agent associated nephrotoxicity. *Eur Heart J* 2004; **25**: 206–211.

68 Marenzi G, Assanelli E, Marana I, et al. N-acetylcysteine and contrast-induced nephropathy in primary angioplasty. *N Engl J Med* 2006; **354**: 2773–2782.

69 Quintavalle C, Brenca M, De Micco F, et al. In vivo and in vitro assessment of pathways involved in contrast media-induced renal cells apoptosis. *Cell Death Dis* 2011; **2**: e155.

70 Briguori C, Quintavalle C, De Micco F, Condorelli G. Nephrotoxicity of contrast media and protective effects of acetylcysteine. *Arch Toxicol* 2011; **85**: 165–173.

71 Investigators ACT. Acetylcysteine for prevention of renal outcomes in patients undergoing coronary and peripheral vascular angiography: main results from the

randomized acetylcysteine for contrast-induced nephropathy trial (ACT). *Circulation* 2011; **124**: 1250–1259.

72 Kelly AM, Dwamena B, Cronin P, *et al.* Meta-analysis: effectiveness of drugs for preventing contrast-induced nephropathy. *Ann Intern Med* 2008; **148**: 284–294.

73 Spargias K, Alexopoulos E, Kyrzopoulos S, *et al.* Ascorbic acid prevents contrast-mediated nephropathy in patients with renal dysfunction undergoing coronary angiography or intervention. *Circulation* 2004; **110**: 2837–2842.

74 Dillioglugil MO, Maral Kir H, Gulkac MD, *et al.* Protective effects of increasing vitamin E and A doses on cisplatin-induced oxidative damage to kidney tissue in rats. *Urol Int* 2005; **75**: 340–344.

75 Shimizu MHM, Araujo M, Borges SMM, de Tolosa EMeC, Seguro AC. Influence of age and vitamin E on post-ischemic acute renal failure. *Exp Gerontol* 2004; **39**: 825–830.

76 Briguori C, Airoldi F, D'Andrea D, *et al.* Renal Insufficiency Following Contrast Media Administration Trial (REMEDIAL): a randomized comparison of 3 preventive strategies. *Circulation* 2007; **115**: 1211–1217.

77 Lev EI, Kornowski R, Vaknin-Assa H, *et al.* Effect of previous treatment with statins on outcome of patients with ST-segment elevation myocardial infarction treated with primary percutaneous coronary intervention. *Am J Cardiol* 2009; **103**: 165–169.

78 Quintavalle C, Fiore D, De Micco F, *et al.* Impact of a high loading dose of atorvastatin on contrast-induced acute kidney injury. *Circulation* 2012; **126**: 3008–3016.

79 Toso A, Maioli M, Leoncini M, *et al.* Usefulness of atorvastatin (80 mg) in prevention of contrast-induced nephropathy in patients with chronic renal disease. *Am J Cardiol* 2010; **105**: 288–292.

80 Patti G, Ricottini E, Nusca A, *et al.* Short-term, high-dose atorvastatin pretreatment to prevent contrast-induced nephropathy in patients with acute coronary syndromes undergoing percutaneous coronary intervention (from the ARMYDA-CIN [Atorvastatin for Reduction of MYocardial Damage during Angioplasty--Contrast-Induced Nephropathy] Trial. *Am J Cardiol* 2011; **108**: 1–7.

81 Xinwei J, Xianghua F, Jing Z, *et al.* Comparison of usefulness of simvastatin 20 mg versus 80 mg in preventing contrast-induced nephropathy in patients with acute coronary syndrome undergoing percutaneous coronary intervention. *Am J Cardiol* 2009; **104**: 519–524.

82 Han Y, Zhu G, Han L, *et al.* Short-term rosuvastatin therapy for prevention of contrast-induced acute kidney injury in patients with diabetes and chronic kidney disease. *J Am Coll Cardiol* 2014; **63**(1): 62–70.

83 Toso A, Leoncini M, Maioli M, *et al.* Early high dose rosuvastatin for contrast induced nephropathy prevention in acute coronary syndrome: results from the PRATO-ACS Study (Protective Effect of Rosuvastatin and Antiplatelet Therapy On contrast induced acute kidney injury and myocardial damage in patients with Acute Coronary Syndrome). *J Am Coll Cardiol* 2014; **63**(1): 71–79.

84 Katholi RE, Taylor GJ, McCann WP, *et al.* Nephrotoxicity from contrast media: attenuation with theophylline. *Radiology* 1995; **195**: 17–22.

85 Bakris GL, Burnett JC Jr. A role for calcium in radiocontrast-induced reductions in renal hemodynamics. *Kidney Int* 1985; **27**: 465–468.

86 Pflueger A, Larson TS, Nath KA, *et al.* Role of adenosine in contrast media-induced acute renal failure in diabetes mellitus. *Mayo Clin Proc* 2000; **75**: 1275–1283.

87 Wang A, Holcslaw T, Bashore TM, *et al.* Exacerbation of radiocontrast nephrotoxicity by endothelin receptor antagonism. *Kidney Int* 2000; **57**: 1675–1680.

88 Kurnik BR, Allgren RL, Genter FC, *et al.* Prospective study of atrial natriuretic peptide for the prevention of radiocontrast-induced nephropathy. *Am J Kidney Dis* 1998; **31**: 674–680.

89 Stone GW, McCullough PA, Tumlin JA, *et al.* Fenoldopam mesylate for the prevention of contrast-induced nephropathy: a randomized controlled trial. *JAMA* 2003; **290**: 2284–2291.

90 Briguori C, Colombo A, Airoldi F, *et al.* N-Acetylcysteine versus fenoldopam mesylate to prevent contrast agent-associated nephrotoxicity. *J Am Coll Cardiol* 2004; **44**: 762–765.

91 Bakris GL, Lass NA, Glock D. Renal hemodynamics in radiocontrast medium-induced renal dysfunction: a role for dopamine-1 receptors. *Kidney Int* 1999; **56**: 206–210.

92 Spargias K, Adreanides E, Demerouti E, *et al.* Iloprost prevents contrast-induced nephropathy in patients with renal dysfunction undergoing coronary angiography or intervention. *Circulation* 2009; **120**: 1793–1799.

93 Solomon R, Werner C, Mann D, *et al.* Effects of saline, mannitol, and furosemide to prevent acute decreases in renal function induced by radiocontrast agents. *N Engl J Med* 1994; **331**: 1416–1420.

94 Weinstein JM, Heyman S, Brezis M. Potential deleterious effect of furosemide in radiocontrast nephropathy. *Nephron* 1992; **62**(4): 413–415.

95 Przyklenk K, Bauer B, Ovize M, Kloner RA, Whittaker P. Regional ischemic "preconditioning" protects remote virgin myocardium from subsequent sustained coronary occlusion. *Circulation* 1993; **87**(3): 893.

96 Hausenloy DJ, Yellon DM. Remote ischaemic preconditioning: underlying mechanisms and clinical application. *Cardiovasc Res* 2008; **79**(3): 377.

97 Igarashi G, Iino K, Watanabe H, Ito H. Remote ischemic pre-conditioning alleviates contrast-induced acute kidney injury in patients with moderate chronic kidney disease. *Circ J* 2013; **77**(12): 3037–3044.

98 Er F, Nia AM, Dopp H, *et al.* Ischemic preconditioning for prevention of contrast medium-induced nephropathy: randomized pilot RenPro Trial (Renal Protection Trial). *Circulation* 2012; **126**: 296–303.

99 Deftereos S, Giannopoulos G, Tzalamouras V, *et al.* Renoprotective effect of remote ischemic post-conditioning by intermittent balloon inflations in patients undergoing percutaneous coronary intervention. *J Am Coll Cardiol* 2013; **61**(19): 1949–1955.

100 Bonventre JV. Limb ischemia protects against contrast-induced nephropathy. *Circulation* 2012; **126**(4): 384–387.

101 Klarenbach SW, Pannu N, Tonelli MA, *et al.* Cost-effectiveness of hemofiltration to prevent contrast nephropathy in patients with chronic kidney disease. *Crit Care Med* 2006; **34**: 1044–1051.

102 Marenzi G, Marana I, Lauri G, *et al.* The prevention of radiocontrast-agent-induced nephropathy by hemofiltration. *N Engl J Med* 2003; **349**: 1333–1340.

103 Marenzi G, Lauri G, Campodonico J, *et al.* Comparison of two hemofiltration protocols for prevention of contrast-induced nephropathy in high-risk patients. *Am J Med* 2006; **119**: 155–162.

104 Spini V, Cecchi E, Chiostri M, *et al.* Effects of two different treatments with continuous renal replacement therapy in patients with chronic renal dysfunction submitted to coronary invasive procedures. *J Invasive Cardiol* 2013; **25**(2): 80–84.

105 Kidney Disease: Improving Global Outcomes (KDIGO) Work Group. KDIGO Clinical Practice Guideline for Acute Kidney Injury. *Kidney Int Suppl* 2012; **2**: 1–141.

CHAPTER 28

Radiation Management in Interventional Cardiology

Stephen Balter[1] and Charles E. Chambers[2]

[1] Columbia University Medical Center, New York, NY, USA
[2] Penn State Hershey Medical Center, Hershey, PA, USA

Optimal clinical outcomes, the minimum of clinical complications, and the avoidance of harm to staff are among the pillars supporting any successful interventional cardiac laboratory. Achieving such results requires continuing diligence and commitment from the host institution, all physician operators, and laboratory staff. Space constraints limit this chapter to selected topics but additional reviews are available in the literature [1–4].

Fluoroscopically guided interventions (FGI) can be unnecessarily radiologically hazardous to the patient [5] unless a knowledgeable operator [3] takes appropriate precautions. High level factors that should be considered include the following:

- The total "dose" delivered to the patient is influenced by equipment configuration, individual patient factors, and the operator's skill. Caution: dose in a radiologic sense has several different connotations beyond, the usual meaning found in pharmacology; this difference is discussed later. Operators are expected to be mindful of radiation use during each procedure and continuously justify continuing with the procedure based on the current risk–benefit balance.
- Technology can only serve to define dose rates. The total dose delivered by a FGI procedure is dependent upon both dose rates and the time that the beam is on.
- Fluoroscopes are general purpose instruments. Appropriate configuration to accommodate the current clinical task is an essential part of continuous optimization of the procedure. Unacceptable patient irradiation and/or image quality will occur if the equipment is not appropriately configured.

Measurements of radiation

X-rays are classified as a form of ionizing radiation because each X-ray photon contains enough energy to ionize atoms and disrupt molecular bonds. The biologic effects of ionizing radiation are different from the essentially thermal effects of non-ionizing radiation (e.g., microwaves) on tissue. The detection and management of X-ray injury is substantially different from conventional burn management.

The common pharmacologic usage of *dose* is the entire aspirin tablet administered to a patient. The concentration of aspirin in the patient's blood (e.g., ng/100 mL) can be measured when necessary. Radiologic *dose* is the local concentration of energy extracted from a radiation field when it interacts with matter. Because the radiation field in a patient is never uniform, different regions of the patient receive different *doses* from a fluoroscopic procedure. Figure 28.1 schematically illustrates these concepts.

No single number can describe either the total physical distribution of radiologic dose in a patient from a FGI or the overall biologic risk of that irradiation. Nevertheless, multiple "dose" indicators have been developed and are used for patient radiation management and risk evaluation.

The five fluoroscopic "dose" indicators commonly used in interventional cardiology are shown in Table 28.1. Peak skin dose (PSD) and reference point air kerma ($K_{a,r}$) provide indices of tissue reaction risk in individual patients. Kerma area product (KAP) relates to the total amount of radiation experienced by patients and staff. Effective dose (E) is used to estimate cancer risk (for populations, not for individuals). Although commonly reported, fluoroscopic time is of little value for estimating patient risk.

Interventional fluoroscopes are flexible instruments that are configurable on a case-by-case basis to meet the requirements of that procedure. Figure 28.2 is a block diagram of the key components of an interventional fluoroscope. System operation is determined by the combination of operator selectable parameters and feedback elements designed to stabilize system performance and imaging. The operator is a crucial element in many of these control loops.

Radiobiology

Although radiation exposure associated with isolated episodes of care is typically limited, all radiation exposure confers risk, and these risks are well established. Deterministic effects are dose dependent direct health effects of radiation, for which a threshold is believed to exist. Deterministic effects of fluoroscopy typically present within weeks of exposure as skin injury. For the operator and staff, eye injury in the form of a specific fluoroscopic related cataract, posterior subscapular, is seen in individuals with high dose exposure over time [6–8].

Patient-related factors associated with skin injury include smoking, poor nutrition, compromised skin integrity, obesity, overlapping skin folds, and skin location [9]. Ethnic differences are seen, with those individuals with light-colored hair or skin being more susceptible. An autosomal recessive ATM gene present

Interventional Cardiology: Principles and Practice, Second Edition. Edited by George D. Dangas, Carlo Di Mario, and Nicholas N. Kipshidze.
© 2017 John Wiley & Sons, Ltd. Published 2017 by John Wiley & Sons, Ltd.

in 1% of the population predisposes an individual to increased radio sensitivity. Certain diseases states, hyperthyroidism, diabetes, and autoimmune and connective tissue disorders, as well as chemotherapeutic agents, place an individual at increased risk for

tissue injury. Individuals who have had recent radiation exposure or any previous high dose radiation tissue injury are more susceptible to subsequent tissue injury.

Stochastic effects are biologic effects of radiation that occur by chance in a population of exposed persons, for which no clear threshold exists; whereas probability is proportional to radiation dose, severity is dose-independent. A stochastic injury occurs when there is injury to the DNA backbone that does not properly heal itself. The result is not cell death but a mutation leading to either a cancer or a genetic abnormality. A single X-ray photon can cause this change; it is not directly dose related, even though the risk of acquiring such injury increases with dose. Because of the time required for one transformed cell to multiply into an observable tumor, the latent period for cancer induction is years to decades after the irradiation.

Patient radiation management

Managing patient radiation is generally divided into actions that are required before, during, and after a procedure [4,10,11]. Additional considerations are needed for pregnant and pediatric patients. Box 28.1 is a sample check-list covering key points. A few of these points are also essential for staff safety. Each facility should develop its own check-list.

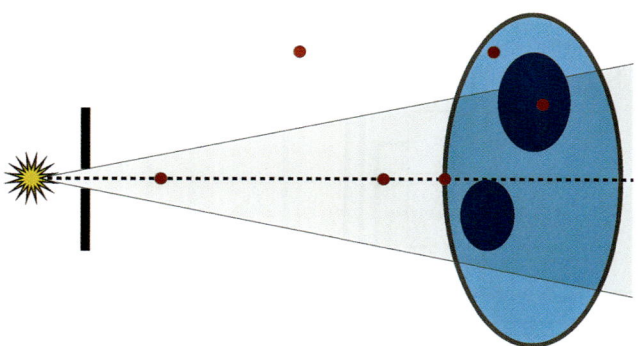

Figure 28.1 Radiologic dose is the concentration of energy received by a small mass of matter (1 Gy = 1 joule/kG) at a specific point. None of the (red) points in this figure received the same dose from the irradiation. Factors include distance from the source, tissue attenuation, and scatter.

Table 28.1 Radiologic dose indicators.

Indicator	Unit	Definition	Comments
Peak skin dose (PSD)	gray	Maximum dose delivered to any portion of the patient's skin during a procedure (includes backscatter from the patient's tissues)	Severity of injury is related to the PSD Real-time PSD displays on interventional fluoroscopes are available on some newer fluoroscopes PSD can be evaluated after the procedure if direct measurement film is used during the case or by calculations in newer systems
Reference point air kerma ($K_{a,r}$)	gray	Total air kerma delivered to a defined point relative to the X-ray gantry from a procedure (excludes scatter)	Usable to estimate the risk of a skin reaction $K_{a,r}$ displays are currently available on essentially all interventional fluoroscopes The relationship between PSD and $K_{a,r}$ is highly dependent on beam motion and geometry
Kerma area product (KAP)	$Gycm^2$	Total amount of radiation emitted from an X-ray tube during a procedure (excludes scatter)	Used to estimate staff irradiation and patient effective dose, KAP displays are currently available on essentially all interventional fluoroscopes KAP can be calculated by multiplying $K_{a,r}$ by the field size at the reference point
Effective dose (E)	mSv	Calculated value representing a risk weighted whole-body irradiation	Used to estimate the cancer risk to a hypothetical person, E can be estimated from KAP and other factors E cannot be measured; it is always a calculated quantity
Fluoroscopic time (FT) *Should NOT be used as the only radiation metric for interventional procedures*	min	Time that the X-ray beam is on in a fluoroscopic mode. *(Obsolete as a quantity for estimating radiation risk)*	FT does not account for variations in X-ray output with changes in patient size and ignores the much higher dose rate contribution from cine

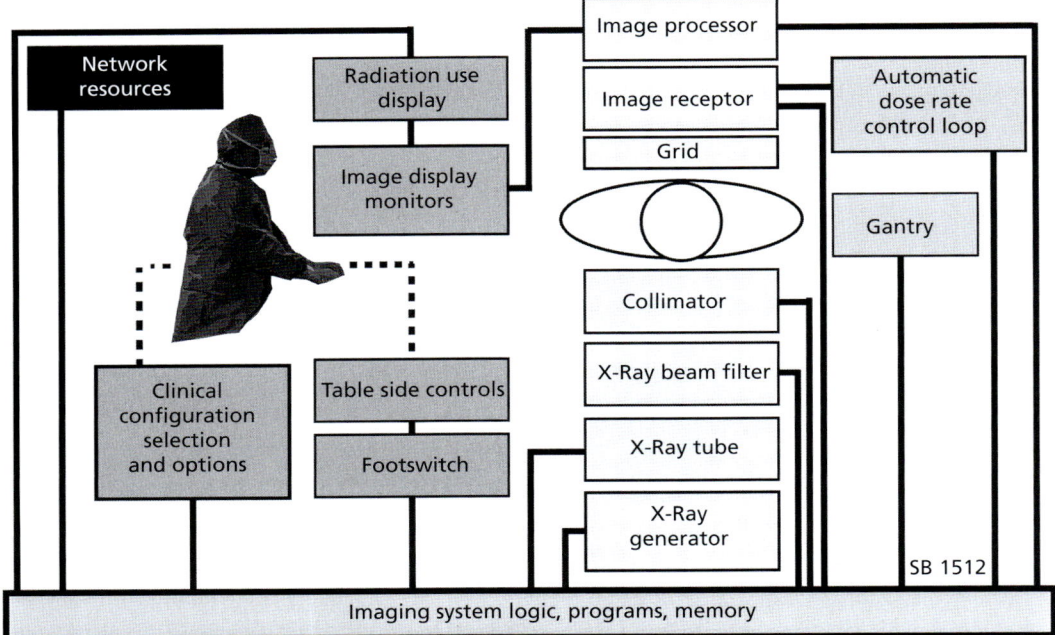

Figure 28.2 Block diagram of an interventional fluoroscope showing key components and control loops. Note that the operator functions as an important control element by selecting technique factors, FOV, geometry, etc.

Box 28.1 Example of a radiologic check-list

Pre-procedure:
- Obtain patient's radiation history; check patient's skin if positive for prior recent exposure
- Extend radiation aspects of informed consent when appropriate for high risk cases
- Plan alternative beam orientations for forthcoming case when necessary

Time out:
- Verify that fluoroscopic system settings are correct for the planned procedure
- All staff should be wearing their personal radiation monitors (staff safety item)
- All staff wearing their radiation and non-radiation personal protective equipment (staff safety item)
- Ancillary radiation shielding devices present in laboratory (staff safety item)

During procedure (reminders to be reviewed during time out):
- Use lowest dose rate settings consistent with immediate clinical goal
- Operator (and staff) aware of radiation use during procedure
- Operator aware of beam angles used during procedure
- Operator assess risk–benefit at each dose notification

Post-procedure:
- Complete patient dosimetry recorded in medical record and case report
- Substantial dose of radiation justified in medical record when appropriate
- Patient notified if substantial dose of radiation was used; and given their initial follow-up processes
- Patents receiving substantial doses are followed as appropriate

---

Pre-procedure aspect of radiation dose management

Assess the risk–benefit ratio of performing the procedure. Radiation should be one element of this assessment particularly in heavy patients, patients who have undergone multiple procedures, and in patients who have had a major interventional procedure within a few months prior to the planned procedure.

Informed consent should appropriately include radiation issues. In most cases, the focus should be on potential skin reactions. This is especially important for complex procedures and for patients who are at increased risk because of their body size or radiation history. Fetal risk and its management must be discussed with pregnant patients. A discussion of cancer risks should be included for patients below the age of 60 and might be offered to all patients.

Time out

The physician should personally verify that the patient identification has been entered into the fluoroscope and that it is properly configured for the planned procedure. One of the standard protocols installed on the machine may be appropriate; however, adjusted protocols can be used to meet specific clinical requirements. The time-out process should also include verification that all staff are wearing appropriate radioprotective equipment and radiation monitors. Available radioprotective shielding (table, face, and mobile) should be properly deployed.

Procedural aspects of radiation management

The physician must continuously manage radiation from the onset to the completion of the procedure. Conceptually, radiation management is similar to contrast agent or other drug management during the procedure. The dose needed from moment to moment, and for the entire procedure, is titrated in the patient's best interest.

Table 28.2 summarizes physician radiation management during a procedure. Some items are focused on minimizing staff irradiation. Most serve to avoid unnecessary patient irradiation. Steps taken to

Table 28.2 Procedural physician radiation management items.

	Management	Effect
General		
A	The system should be configured to the lowest dose-rate modes consistent with immediate clinical activities. Reconfiguration is needed either when images are clinically inadequate or when a lower dose rate mode will comfortably suffice for present activities. (Check during time out)	Incorrect technique selection might increase patient dose by a factor of 10 without contributing to the needs of the procedure
B	Never produce radiation unless the operator's eyes are on the primary image monitor	This might save 10% or more of the entire radiation dose
C	The use of retrospectively stored fluoroscopy instead of cine documentation will always save radiation and also can save contrast media	Saves several 10s of % when stored fluoro replaces cine for documenting inflations, etc.
Specific		
1	The low dose rate mode (for both fluoro and cine) should be initially tried in every case. Escalate the dose rate only when images are inadequate for procedural requirements. The goal is sufficient image quality to perform the procedure without spending radiation and other resources on unnecessarily high quality image	Typically each higher step doubles the dose rate for that mode
2	Fluoroscopic and cine frame rates should be set to the minimum required for adequate temporal resolution and image noise	Dose rate decreases with decreasing frame rate. % change differs between manufacturers
3	The primary operator should control beam on time. The beam should only be on when needed by this person to observe motion	Irradiating the patient without observing the monitor is a total waste of radiation
4	Where possible, change the imaging beam angle during long procedures. This will help minimize peak skin dose	Dose is always local. Sufficient beam motion irradiates different tissue and minimizes reactions
5	Minimize beam orientations that place a great thickness of tissue between the patient and image receptor	Every 4–5 cm additional tissue in the beam doubles the skin dose rate
6	The X-ray tube should be as far from the patient as possible. Spacing reduces skin dose by increasing the Source to Image receptor distance	Increasing the spacing from 38 cm (minimum defined by spacer) to 45 cm decreases skin dose rate by approximately a factor of 2 (All else constant)
7	Examination table height should to facilitate the primary operator's comfort. This often contributes to quicker device manipulation and therefore less beam on time	Total dose = dose-rate × time. Reduced time may be a greater benefit than maximizing spacing
8	The image receptor should always be as close to the patient as practicable. This minimizes input dose rates	Reducing spacing as much as possible can save 25% of dose-rate in thick patients
9	Cine should only be used only when necessary. Most interventional fluoroscopes have the capability of retrospectively storing the most recent 10–30 seconds of fluoroscopy. The judicious use of this mode avoids the higher dose rates required for cine and can reduce the total contrast volume	Typical cine dose rates are 10 times as high as fluoro dose rates for the same view
10	Higher magnification factors usually require higher levels of patient irradiation. They should be avoided where possible	Dose rates for image intensifiers usually increase by a factor of 4 when the magnification is doubled. For flat-panel detectors the increase is usually a factor of 2

Table 28.3 Notification and substantial radiation dose level (SRDL) levels [4].

Dose metric	First notification	Subsequent notifications (increments)	SRDL
$D_{skin,max}$[a]	2 Gy	0.5 Gy	3 Gy
$K_{a,r}$[b]	3 Gy	1 Gy	5 Gy[b]
KAP (P_{KA}[c])	300 Gy cm²[d]	100 Gy cm²[d]	500 Gy cm²[d]
Fluoroscopy time	30 min	15 min	60 min

[a] $D_{skin,max}$ is peak skin dose, requiring calculations by physicist.
[b] $K_{a,r}$ is total air kerma at the reference point.
[c] P_{KA} is air kerma-area product. Caution: different fluoroscopes use different display units.
[d] Assuming a 100 cm² field at the patient's skin. For other field sizes, the P_{KA} values should be adjusted proportionally to the actual procedural field size (e.g., for a field size of 50 cm², the SRDL value for P_{KA} would be 250 Gy cm²). Source: NCRP 2010 [4], Fig. 4.7. Reprinted with permission of the National Council on Radiation Protection and Measurements, http://NCRPpublications.org.

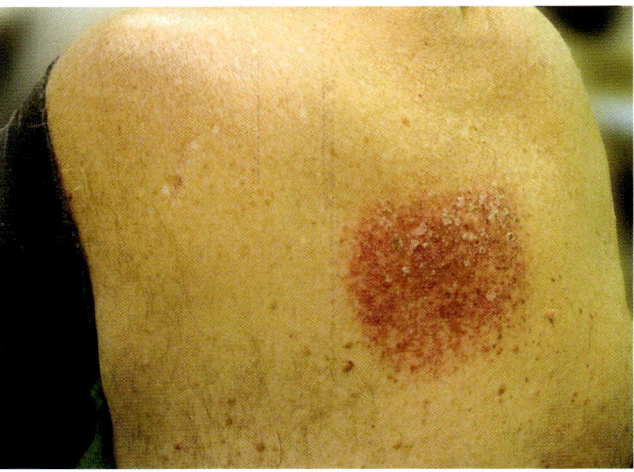

Figure 28.3 Dry desquamation (poikiloderma) at 1 month in a patient receiving approximately 11 Gy calculated peak skin dose. Source: Chambers CE, *et al.* 2011 [1].

avoid wasting patient irradiation will often simultaneously reduce irradiation to staff.

Integrating other imaging modalities during catheterization (trans-esophageal and intracardiac echocardiography) reduces radiation exposure. CT three-dimensional reconstruction can be used for intra-procedural real-time overlays during complex transcatheter interventions, such as closure of para-valvular leaks. Rotational angiography might be used as well [12]. The information obtained through 3D reconstructions eliminates the need for several biplane cine acquisitions and is particularly useful in patients requiring complex pulmonary artery rehabilitation, where it allows the operator to exactly determine the best angles that profile individual lesions requiring transcatheter interventions.

Staff should periodically remind operators of radiation use [4]. Table 28.3 summarizes dose metrics that are available on a specific fluoroscope and can be used for this purpose.

Post-procedural aspects of radiation management

Actual radiation use for every procedure should be documented in the patient's medical record and procedure report [13]. Fluoroscopic time is a totally inadequate measure of either potential skin injury or of cancer risk. Data must include all of the available dose metrics shown in Table 28.3 which are reported by the interventional fluoroscope.

Exceeding the predefined substantial radiation dose level (SRDL) triggers additional clinical documentation and patient communication. Procedures performed below this the SRDL are unlikely to result in clinically important tissue reactions. Injuries are rare below twice the SRDL but become more frequent at higher doses (Figure 28.3). The default SRDL for interventional cardiology is a $K_{a,r}$ of 5 Gy at the reference point.

The operator should explicitly report the medical necessity for the documented radiation level in the procedure report using enough detail to be understandable for case review purposes. These events, as with all essential aspects of laboratory radiation safety,

should be a regular component of the catheterization laboratory quality improvement program.

The patient (and family) should receive pre-discharge radiation instructions when an SRDL is exceeded. (Fluoroscopic time should only be used as the trigger if none of the other metrics in Table 28.3 are available for a specific procedure.) The key points relevant to this process are shown in Table 28.4.

Staff radiation safety

"X-rays" are essential for both diagnosis and therapy. Though the benefits are quantifiable with decreased morbidity and mortality, the risks of radiation are less clear. In interventional cardiology, the importance of a radiation-conscious environment is stressed where protection for the patient protects the staff and vice versa. Methods for measuring patient dose, monitoring staff dose, implementing appropriate training, and managing radiation dose from the outset of the procedure are important components of a catheterization laboratory radiation safety program.

Personal dose monitoring

Staff radiation levels are known [4,14] and generally well below regulatory dose limits provided that best practices are followed. However, there is no way to detect radiologic safety failures unless all individuals in the laboratory always wear and return their radiation monitors as specified by the institution's radiation safety officer (RSO) (different institutions use different protocols). The RSO will contact individuals when radiation levels are of concern (generally between 10% and 30% of the regulatory limits). Nevertheless, all users should periodically review their records with the RSO.

Shielding

Protective garments must be worn by all persons who are in the procedure room when the X-ray beam is on. These garments are designed to protect the gonads and 80% of the active bone marrow. The standard is a 0.25–0.5 mm lead apron, which stops approximately 90% of the scattered radiation [15]. Separate thyroid shielding (also approximately 90% reduction) is recommended for younger workers as well as all individuals whose externally worn dosimeter at collar level exceeds 4 mSv in a month [16]. Long-term deleterious

Table 28.4 Post-procedure patient notification and follow-up.

Patient-centric: pre-discharge	
This should always be done as a personal communication. it should be supplemented by a written reminder	
1	Your procedure required a substantial amount of radiation for its completion
1a	(Less than twice a SRDL): Because of this, it is possible that you might have some skin reddening from this. In many cases, it will fade in time and not reoccur. In some cases you will have some cosmetic skin discoloration
1b	(More than twice a SRDL): You are at increased risk for a clinically significant skin reaction from the procedure. (Escalate the warning for higher values)
2	Avoid damaging your skin. Do not scratch or scrub the area where we worked
3	For the next year, please tell all of your healthcare providers that you had a procedure that used radiation and may have caused a skin reaction
4	In a month, have a family member examine your back for a red area about the size of a hand. If anything is seen please contact the catheterization laboratory for further instructions. (Figure 28.3 illustrates a fluoroscopic radiation injury)
Physicians and laboratory staff	
A	Patient should be called proactively at 1.5 × SRDL
	If the patient cannot be directly contacted, consider informing the referring physician
B	The laboratory must be prepared to handle such calls. The discussion should be with a physician or radiation trained mid-level provider
C	If the individual taking the call cannot absolutely rule out a radiation etiology, the patient should be scheduled for an examination by the physician performing the procedure. If a physician visit is needed, the patient should be reminded to avoid further skin injury
D	Based on the physician's examination of the patient's skin, appropriate follow-up visits, referrals, or treatments should be recommended

SRDL, substantial radiation dose level.

effects from protective garments are well documented with methods for potential improvement currently being addressed by the multispecialty occupational health group in the interventional laboratory [17]. Proper protective garment care, including hanging aprons on designated racks with adequate hangers and periodic inspection for damage, is an essential part of radiation safety.

Recent epidemiologic studies give reason for concern regarding potential eye injury, presenting as posterior subcapsular cataract formation [6,7,18–20]. Radiation-specific eye protection works if properly selected and used [21,22]. The glasses must fit properly for both protection and comfort, provide 0.25 mm lead equivalent protection, and have additional side shielding. Well-designed eye shielding reduces dose to the lens of the eye by approximately two-thirds.

Radiation shielding of the operator's hands is generally counterproductive when the hands are in the useful beam because the shielding drives the system to greater output, increasing patient and often staff dose. Protective hand equipment is often labeled with warnings against placing the hands in or near the beam. The best rule is to avoid seeing your hands on the monitor. Labeling on "protective" gloves often warns users not to put their hands in the beam while wearing the gloves (Figure 28.4).

Current shielding provides substantial reduction in operator dose and should be used routinely [23–25]. Transparent ceiling-mounted shielding with a patient contour cutout protects the operator's upper body. When positioning this shield, the origin of scatter X-rays is from the patient, to block this scatter directed toward the operator's head and arms. The operator should only see the area being imaged by looking through the shield. In-laboratory moveable barriers provide protection for staff required to be in the procedure room, while individuals not required in the fluoroscopic suite should remain in the control room. Disposable radiation-absorbing non-lead patient sterile drapes also help to reduce staff dose but do not always provide a substantial benefit [26].

Specific radiation safety considerations
Women and fluoroscopic guided procedures

The fetus of a pregnant patient can be at risk for potential stochastic injury and, at high (fetal) dose, the induction of a deterministic effect [27,28]. Deterministic effects in the embryo-fetus for absorbed doses below 50 mGy are seldom detectable, while doses in excess of 100 mGy can cause gestation time and dose-dependent developmental effects. The safest policy is to avoid elective procedures during pregnancy. The benefits and risks to both mother and fetus of performing a planned procedure need to be carefully considered with informed consent essential. Even in the absence of known risk factors, approximately 5% of live births possess some form of congenital malformation. With proper procedure planning to exclude abdomen or pelvis exposure (consider radial access) and, if available, consultation with a qualified medical physicist, embryo-fetus exposure can be limited to scatter radiation with very low and usually acceptable risk.

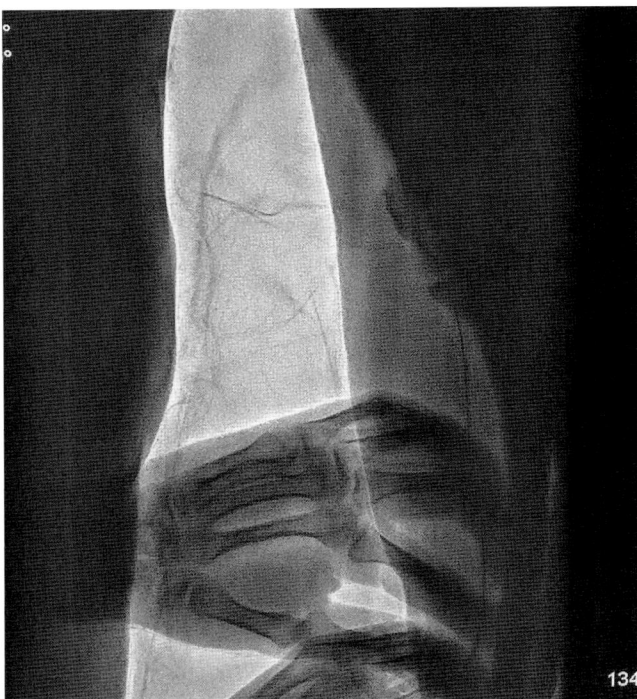

Figure 28.4 Worst practice: an example of unnecessary irradiation of an operator's hands during the insertion of a transradial device. A radiation shield is seen on the left and the patient's arm on the right. The majority of the operator's hands are irradiated by the unattenuated beam passing between the shield and patient. Safety rule: operators should not see their hands on the monitor.

Whether it is staff or physician, the pregnant worker is best protected in a laboratory that utilizes best practices for radiation safety. Each hospital should have a radiation safety policy for pregnant workers that addresses occupational exposure, dosimeter use and readings, duties including call, and risk–benefit of additional shielding. It is unlawful to prevent pregnant employees from working in occupations that may expose them to radiation. All pregnant workers should have a specific dosimeter, to be worn at the waist under the protective garment, issued and read monthly. The work-related restriction limit for the embryo-fetus radiation exposure equivalent dose is 0.5 mSv/month. Once a pregnancy is identified, the expectant mother should not receive more than 1 mSv according to the International Commission on Radiation Protection (ICRP) and 5 mSv according to the National Commission on Radiation Protection (INCRP) for the remainder of the pregnancy [28,29]. It should be noted that reference values of 1 mSv are seldom recorded *for an entire year* in this location [30].

Pediatric patients

Equipment routinely used for pediatric procedures of any kind should be appropriately designed, equipped, and configured for this purpose. Appropriate modifications should be made to accommodate the variable procedural requirements as well as the wide age and weight range of these patients [31,32]. The use of unmodified adult settings for small patients (<40 kG) can result in both unnecessary patient irradiation and substandard image quality.

Children born with congenital heart disease frequently undergo numerous diagnostic and therapeutic catheterizations, with potential harmful cumulative long-term effects of radiation exposure [33,34]. This raises significant concern when children survive to potentially manifest these late effects of radiation exposure. The importance of radiation dose reduction in the pediatric patient has been emphasized through the Image Gently and Step Lightly campaigns [31,32].

Training and education

The potential benefits for all operators, no matter what skill level (achieved or perceived), to be thoroughly trained in radiation safety with regularly updates should not be understated. Fetterly and colleagues at the Mayo Clinic succeeded in a 40% radiation dose reduction (CAK) over a 3-year period by implementing a culture and philosophy of radiation safety in the catheterization laboratory [1,35,36]. The interventional cardiologists' goal is to do the best for their patients, and in so doing, protect the staff and themselves. In the multi-task environment of the cardiac catheterization laboratory, mandatory radiation safety training, with annual updates, will allow all operators, new and experienced, to achieve this goal throughout their career.

Radiation quality processes

The American College of Cardiology Foundation/American Heart Association/Society for Cardiovascular Angiography and Interventions (ACC/AHA/SCAI) 2011 PCI Guidelines [37] reconfirmed the requirements for all cardiac catheterization laboratories with interventional programs have a quality improvement program specific for the laboratory. This requires more than just outcomes review; it necessitates appropriate processes for best patient care be implemented. Radiation safety, including patient radiation dose review [38], must be among these processes. Compliance with local regulatory requirements only assures a basic level of safety anywhere in an institution. The catheterization laboratory is a much more demanding environment [35,39,40] and should accept the financial and administrative responsibilities of maintaining greater safety margins for both patients and staff [41].

Key topics include the following: design of the laboratory and adjacent spaces; equipment selection, configuration, quality control, and service; staff radiation protection; and patient radiation management. Degrees of assistance with these topics can be provided by experts, such as medical and health physicists. The laboratory medical director should accept the responsibility of keeping these experts engaged in laboratory operations on a routine basis instead of relying on "strangers" when an emergency occurs.

Both the physician and support staffs need enough usable current knowledge to recognize problems and ask for help when necessary. Ultimately, operator training and experience are essential to maintaining radiation safety on a case-by-case basis.

Conclusions

Radiation safety is one of several priorities that must be attended to in the cardiac catheterization laboratory. The interventional cardiologist is required to take the leadership role. Establish a radiation safety program for the laboratory, incorporating the physicist for radiation training, equipment purchase, and safe maintenance. Require and document the appropriate radiation safety training both upon employment and with annual updates. Purchase and properly operate imaging equipment with dose limiting capabilities and appropriate dose notification. Utilize all available above and below table shielding as well as personal protective garments and glasses. Mandate the wearing of the dosimetry badge(s) by incorporating badge use as a component of the pre-procedure "time out." Manage radiation dose throughout the case, not just upon high dose notification. Establish follow-up parameters with policies for those patients receiving high radiation doses. When a radiation conscious environment has been established in the cardiac catheterization laboratory, the patients, staff, and physicians will all benefit.

Interactive multiple choice questions are available for this chapter on www.wiley.com/go/dangas/cardiology

References

1 Chambers CE, Fetterly KA, Holzer R, *et al.* Radiation safety program for the cardiac catheterization laboratory. *Catheter Cardiovasc Interv* 2011; **77**(4): 546–556.

2 Cousins C, Miller DL, Bernardi G, *et al.* ICRP Publication 120: Radiological protection in cardiology. *Ann ICRP* 2013; **42**(1): 1–125.

3 Hirshfeld JW Jr, Balter S, Brinker JA, *et al.* ACCF/AHA/HRS/SCAI clinical competence statement on physician knowledge to optimize patient safety and image quality in fluoroscopically guided invasive cardiovascular procedures: a report of the American College of Cardiology Foundation/American Heart Association/American College of Physicians Task Force on Clinical Competence and Training. *J Am Coll Cardiol* 2004; **44**(11): 2259–2282.

4 National Council on Radiation Protection and Measurements (NCRP). Report 168: Radiation Dose Management for Fluoroscopically Guided Interventional Medical Procedures. NRCP: 2010.

5 Balter S, Miller DL. Patient skin reactions from interventional fluoroscopy procedures. *AJR Am J Roentgenol* 2014; **202**(4): W335–342.

6 Vano E, Kleiman NJ, Duran A, Romano-Miller M, Rehani MM. Radiation-associated lens opacities in catheterization personnel: results of a survey and direct assessments. *J Vasc Interv Radiol* 2013; **24**(2): 197–204.

7 Jacob S, Boveda S, Bar O, *et al.* Interventional cardiologists and risk of radiation-induced cataract: results of a French multicenter observational study. *Int J Cardiol* 2013; **167**(5): 1843–1847.

8 Jacob S, Michel M, Spaulding C, *et al.* Occupational cataracts and lens opacities in interventional cardiology (O'CLOC study): are X-rays involved? *Radiation-induced cataracts and lens opacities. BMC Public Health* 2010; **10**: 537.

9 Balter S, Hopewell JW, Miller DL, Wagner LK, Zelefsky MJ. Fluoroscopically guided interventional procedures: a review of radiation effects on patients' skin and hair. *Radiology* 2010; **254**(2): 326–341.

10 Bartal G, Vano E, Paulo G, Miller DL. Management of patient and staff radiation dose in interventional radiology: current concepts. *Cardiovasc Intervent Radiol* 2014; **37**: 289–298.

11 Stecker MS. Patient radiation management and preprocedure planning and consent. *Tech Vasc Interv Radiol* 2010; **13**(3): 176–182.

12 Sawdy JM, Gocha MD, Olshove V, *et al.* Radiation protection during hybrid procedures: innovation creates new challenges. *J Invasive Cardiol* 2009; **21**(9): 437–440.

13 Miller DL, Balter S, Dixon RG, *et al.* Quality improvement guidelines for recording patient radiation dose in the medical record for fluoroscopically guided procedures. *J Vasc Interv Radiol* 2012; **23**(1): 11–18.

14 Kim KP, Miller DL, Berrington de Gonzalez A, *et al.* Occupational radiation doses to operators performing fluoroscopically-guided procedures. *Health Phys* 2012; **103**(1): 80–99.

15 Balter S, Sones FM Jr, Brancato R. Radiation exposure to the operator performing cardiac angiography with U-arm systems. *Circulation* 1978; **58**(5): 925–932.

16 Schueler BA. Operator shielding: how and why. *Tech Vasc Interv Radiol* 2010; **13**(3): 167–171.

17 Miller DL, Klein LW, Balter S, *et al.* Occupational health hazards in the interventional laboratory: progress report of the Multispecialty Occupational Health Group. *J Vasc Interv Radiol* 2010; **21**(9): 1338–1341.

18 Kleiman NJ. Radiation cataract. *Ann ICRP* 2012; **41**(3–4): 80–97.

19 Authors on behalf of ICRP. IRCP Publication 118: ICRP statement on tissue reactions and early and late effects of radiation in normal tissues and organs: threshold doses for tissue reactions in a radiation protection context. *Ann ICRP* 2012; **41**(1-2): 1–322.

20 Hall EJ, Giaccia AJ. *Radiobiology for the Radiologist*, 7th edn. Philadelphia: Wolters Kluwer Health/Lippincott Williams & Wilkins: 2012.

21 Sturchio GM, Newcomb RD, Molella R, Varkey P, Hagen PT, Schueler BA. Protective eyewear selection for interventional fluoroscopy. *Health Phys* 2013; **104**(2 Suppl 1): S11–16.

22 McVey S, Sandison A, Sutton DG. An assessment of lead eyewear in interventional radiology. *J Radiol Prot* 2013; **33**(3): 647–659.

23 Duran A, Hian SK, Miller DL, Le Heron J, Padovani R, Vano E. A summary of recommendations for occupational radiation protection in interventional cardiology. *Catheter Cardiovasc Interv* 2013; **81**(3): 562–567.

24 Thornton RH, Dauer LT, Altamirano JP, Alvarado KJ, St Germain J, Solomon SB. Comparing strategies for operator eye protection in the interventional radiology suite. *J Vasc Interv Radiol* 2010; **21**(11): 1703–1707.

25 Kim KP, Miller DL. Minimising radiation exposure to physicians performing fluoroscopically guided cardiac catheterisation procedures: a review. *Radiat Prot Dosimetry* 2009; **133**(4): 227–233.

26 Politi L, Biondi-Zoccai G, Nocetti L, *et al.* Reduction of scatter radiation during transradial percutaneous coronary angiography: a randomized trial using a lead-free radiation shield. *Catheter Cardiovasc Interv* 2012; **79**(1): 97–102.

27 Hall EJ. Radiation biology for pediatric radiologists. *Pediatr Radiol* 2009; **39**(Suppl 1): S57–64.

28 International Commission on Radiation Protection (ICRP). ICRP Report 84: Pregnancy and Medical Radiation. ICRP: 2000.

29 Martins BI. NRC, NCRP, ICRP and recommendations on prenatal radiation exposure. *Health Phys* 1989; **56**(4): 572–523.

30 Chandra V, Dorsey C, Reed AB, Shaw P, Banghart D, Zhou W. Monitoring of fetal radiation exposure during pregnancy. *J Vasc Surg* 2013; **58**(3): 710–714.

31 Hernanz-Schulman M, Goske MJ, Bercha IH, Strauss KJ. Pause and pulse: ten steps that help manage radiation dose during pediatric fluoroscopy. *AJR Am J Roentgenol* 2011; **197**(2): 475–481.

32 Sidhu M. Radiation safety in pediatric interventional radiology: step lightly. *Pediatr Radiol* 2010; **40**(4): 511–513.

33 Mettler FA Jr, Constine LS, Nosske D, Shore RE. Ninth Annual Warren K. Sinclair Keynote Address: effects of childhood radiation exposure: an issue from computed tomography scans to Fukushima. *Health Phys* 2013; **105**(5): 424–429.

34 International Commission on Radiation Protection (ICRP). ICRP Publication 121: radiological protection in paediatric diagnostic and interventional radiology. *Ann ICRP* 2013; **42**(2): 1–63.

35 Fetterly KA, Mathew V, Lennon R, Bell MR, Holmes DR Jr, Rihal CS. Radiation dose reduction in the invasive cardiovascular laboratory: implementing a culture and philosophy of radiation safety. *JACC Cardiovasc Interv* 2012; **5**(8): 866–873.

36 Fetterly KA, Lennon RJ, Bell MR, Holmes DR Jr, Rihal CS. Clinical determinants of radiation dose in percutaneous coronary interventional procedures: influence of patient size, procedure complexity, and performing physician. *JACC Cardiovasc Interv* 2011; **4**(3): 336–343.

37 Levine GN, Bates ER, Blankenship JC, *et al.* 2011 ACCF/AHA/SCAI Guideline for Percutaneous Coronary Intervention: executive summary: a report of the American College of Cardiology Foundation/American Heart Association Task Force on Practice Guidelines and the Society for Cardiovascular Angiography and Interventions. *Catheter Cardiovasc Interv* 2012; **79**(3): 453–495.

38 Miller DL, Hilohi CM, Spelic DC. Patient radiation doses in interventional cardiology in the US: advisory data sets and possible initial values for US reference levels. *Med Phys* 2012; **39**(10): 6276–6286.

39 Klein LW, Miller DL, Goldstein J, *et al.* The catheterization laboratory and interventional vascular suite of the future: anticipating innovations in design and function. *Catheter Cardiovasc Interv* 2011; **77**(3): 447–455.

40 Fazel R, Gerber TC, Balter S, *et al.* Approaches to enhancing radiation safety in cardiovascular imaging: a scientific statement from the American Heart Association. *Circulation* 2014; **130**(19): 1730–1748.

41 Balter S, Rosenstein M, Miller DL, Schueler B, Spelic D. Patient radiation dose audits for fluoroscopically guided interventional procedures. *Med Phys* 2011; **38**(3): 1611.

CHAPTER 29

Concepts of Cell Therapy and Myocardial Regeneration

Kevin O'Gallagher[1], Zoë Astroulakis[2], Alex Sirker[3], and Jonathan M. Hill[1]

[1]Department of Cardiology, King's College Hospital NHS Foundation Trust, London, UK
[2]Department of Cardiology, St George's Hospital, London, UK
[3]Department of Cardiology, UCLH and St Bartholomew's Hospital, London, UK

Over the past 15 years, stem cell therapy has emerged as a potential therapeutic intervention in ischemic heart disease, engaging the interests of basic scientists and cardiologists alike. Despite recent advances in pharmacologic and catheter-based interventions for coronary heart disease, myocardial salvage is often incomplete resulting in a process of adverse left ventricular (LV) remodeling leading to symptomatic heart failure. This chapter discusses the relevance of cell therapy to interventional cardiology, outlining the progress of over a decade of clinical trials, and looks to future directions for clinical research.

Origin of concept

The concept of the adult stem cell was born over 30 years ago, following the identification of a bone marrow cell capable of reconstituting hematopoiesis in irradiated mice [1]. However, it is only in the last 15 years that the relevance of this work to cardiology was realized with the description, from the late Jeffrey Isner's laboratory, of bone marrow derived stem/progenitor cells that could regenerate cells constituting the cardiovascular system [2]. This challenged the previously held belief that the vascularization of adult ischemic tissue was restricted to the proliferation and migration of mature endothelial cells. Indeed, Isner's group went on to provide evidence that these cells could home to sites of ischemia and participate in new blood vessel formation, a process previously thought to be restricted to embryonic development. Furthermore, work involving animal models of ischemia demonstrated that bone marrow mononuclear cells (BMNCs) and endothelial progenitor cells (EPC) could participate in myocardial neovascularization with evidence of functional improvement [3–7].

The next key development, and now widely recognized as the landmark paper within the field of cardiovascular cell therapy, was the description by Orlic et al. [8] working in Piero Anversa's group, that a bone marrow derived population of cells from one mouse could be transplanted into recipient mice with myocardial infarction and become incorporated into the area of myocardial injury, exhibiting immunohistochemical evidence of transdifferentiation as well as leading to demonstrable changes in LV function. Further work has shown that stem cells are able to transdifferentiate into multiple different cardiovascular cell types including endothelial cells, vascular smooth muscle cells, and cardiac myocytes [9–12].

Subsequent controversies notwithstanding, the papers from the Isner and Anversa groups heralded the beginning of intense activity in cardiovascular therapy which continues to this day. However, many key questions remain regarding the putative mechanisms of action.

Myocardial regeneration

Within cardiology, stem cell therapy has generated huge interest by challenging the long-held paradigm of developmental biology that the heart is a terminally differentiated organ, and as such cannot be repaired. Previously, the extent of myocardial necrosis had been shown to be intimately linked to the duration of coronary artery occlusion [13,14]. Such studies were critical in creating the drive forward in reperfusion therapy, but also led clinicians and scientists alike to think of myocardial injury as an irreversible event. Indeed, any improvement in LV function post-myocardial infarction (MI) was thought to result from a combination of hypertrophy and fibrosis. Such ideas were called into question with the observation that adult hearts contained large numbers of mitotic figures [15–17]. However, the proportion of mitotic cardiomyocytes was extremely small, suggesting they could not function alone as an effective repair system. The possibility that these dividing cells might have arisen from an extra-cardiac source, such as the bone marrow, was postulated by studies performed in sex-mismatched cardiac transplant patients. In males receiving female hearts, cardiac biopsies revealed Y-chromosome-carrying cardiomyocytes [17–19], intimating that cells from an extra-cardiac source could potentially engraft and differentiate into cardiac tissue. This marked the first recognition that the heart could receive cells from an extra-cardiac source. To explain this phenomenon, it was suggested that these cells might have arisen from the bone marrow, being released and engrafting either as a low-level process of continual renewal or in direct response to injury [8,11]. Alternative suggestions included the possibility of a locally resident population of cardiac stem cells, with self-renewing, multipotent, and clonogenic potential [20].

Interventional Cardiology: Principles and Practice, Second Edition. Edited by George D. Dangas, Carlo Di Mario, and Nicholas N. Kipshidze.
© 2017 John Wiley & Sons, Ltd. Published 2017 by John Wiley & Sons, Ltd.

Mobilization of stem/progenitor cells

Studies in humans have confirmed that BMNCs and EPCs are indeed mobilized from the bone marrow to sites of ischemia at the time of myocardial infarction [21]. This occurs in response to the release of cytokines leading to the chemotactic migration of stem and progenitor cells to the area of injury. Such cytokines include vascular endothelial growth factor (VEGF) and stromal derived factor-1 (SDF-1) [22]. Reduced oxygen tension in ischemic tissue leads to an increase in SDF-1 levels in response to the upregulation of hypoxia-inducible factor-1 (HIF-1) in endothelial cells [23,24]. This hypoxic gradient directs the migration and homing, and increases the adhesion of, CXCR4-expressing progenitor cells to ischemic tissue [25]. It has been shown that impaired CXCR4-mediated cell signaling contributes to the reduced neovascularization capacity seen in patients with coronary artery disease [26], and modifications of this pathway appear to offer promise for the enhancement of cell homing and retention. In addition, the capture of cells at the site of ischemia has been shown to be aided by the upregulation of integrins and intercellular adhesion molecules [27–30], and by the mediation of platelets [31].

Mechanism of action

However, it is still unclear as to the exact mechanism by which transplanted cells exert their beneficial effects on cardiac function. Proposed mechanisms include endothelial differentiation (thereby aiding vascular regeneration and improving blood supply to the infarct border zone and so improving regional/global systolic LV function), cellular fusion, transdifferentiation to cardiomyocytes and/or via paracrine effects on the local cellular milieu, and the issue remains controversial.

Several studies have suggested that BMNCs co-localize with non-myocardial cells such as fibroblasts [32]. However, these observations are so far anecdotal and could be explained by methodologic issues such as the release of dye from apoptotic cells in the area of fibrosis or by the use of unfractionated bone marrow, which includes other cell precursor populations. Nonetheless, they are consistent with the basic postulate that stem cells differentiate along milieu-dependent pathways. Damaged adult myocardium is devoid of key embryonic growth factors, meaning an inability to recreate the necessary environment to stimulate myocyte growth or regeneration. This presents a challenge, and accordingly stimulates the search for novel strategies to encourage transplanted cells down the cardiac differentiation pathway prior to transplantation, if not *in situ*.

Choice of cell type for cardiac cell therapy

Although the majority of work has been performed using BMNCs (either selected or unselected), other cell types can be used, including mesenchymal stem cells, skeletal muscle myoblasts, and cardiac stem cells. Mesenchymal stem cells (MSC) are stromal cells, found both in the bone marrow and adipose tissue. The "immune-privileged" status [33] of MSC allows both autologous and allogenic use: this, combined with the ability to deliver the treatment intravenously, represents an attractive "off-the-shelf" aspect to this therapy. Skeletal myoblasts (SMs) can be easily and conveniently harvested via muscle biopsy. However, there is debate surrounding the safety of this technique, particularly on the issue of their potential for arrhythmogenesis [34–36]. Cardiac stem cells (CSC), either as ckit+ cells or cardiosphere-derived cells, are resident undifferentiated cells with the ability to differentiate into beating myocytes.

Cell therapy following acute myocardial infarction

The first wave of trials examining bone marrow (BM) cell therapy in the setting of acute MI indicated that autologous unselected BM cell therapy was indeed both safe and feasible, and the noted improvements in LV function paved the way for larger scale randomized clinical trials which unfortunately sometimes generated conflicting and controversial results. This has largely arisen as a result of key differences in the cell population used, the time and mode of delivery, and the different methodologies used to assess changes in LV function. For many clinicians, the demonstration of safety alone is insufficient grounds on which to proceed to larger clinical studies. Indeed, many cite that the statistically significant changes in LV function are clinically insignificant, and further studies are not currently justified.

Cell type

The transfer of autologous BMNCs is attractive as a form of cell therapy because of the relative ease by which it can be obtained, the lack of requirement for *ex vivo* expansion, and of course the lack of risk of rejection by the recipient. It also supports the idea that no particular cell type should be omitted, and that functional recovery is dependent upon a balance between the various sub-populations present in the mononuclear fraction. As such, the majority of clinical trials so far have used unfractionated BMNCs [37–40].

The problem with using unfractionated BMNCs, however, is that any functionally superior subgroup of cells would have to compete for engraftment along with all the other "non-stem" cells. CD34+ cells have been shown to mediate cardiac repair by inducing angiogenesis, inhibiting apoptosis and by promoting myocyte recovery in experimental models of myocardial infarction [41]. Indeed, it has been shown that CD34+ enriched BM cells are up to seven times more efficient at engrafting in ischemic myocardium [42]. In addition to the CD34+ marker expressed by stem/progenitor cells, CD133 (a prominin 5 transmembrane glycoprotein 1 marker) is co-expressed in a substantial number of hematopoietic cells with potent angiogenic capacity [43–45]. The intracoronary injection of CD133+ enriched BM cells has been shown to be feasible, and to be associated with the promotion of cardiac recovery in a small study, albeit with a slightly increased incidence of in-stent restenosis and re-occlusion [46]. CD133+ cells have been shown to enhance functional response in patients following an acute MI [47].

Timing of cell delivery

The timing of cell delivery is an obvious design difference between trials. The course of the normal healing processes at the time of MI seems to coincide with the expression of putative homing signals favoring cell engraftment via transendothelial passage during the early days post-reperfusion. However, when cells were transplanted within 24 hours of optimal reperfusion therapy no benefit was seen in global left ventricular ejection fraction (LVEF) [39]. This has led to the suggestion that the early pro-inflammatory environment required for healing in MI is toxic to stem/progenitor cells either in terms of survival or function or both, given that initial ischemia and reperfusion injury are characterized by the rapid rise of reactive oxygen radicals and inflammatory cytokines, and that this explains the lack of benefit seen when therapy is delivered within the first 24 hours. Consistent with this theory are the findings of the sub-analysis of the REPAIR-AMI trial [40] indicating that the greatest benefit is seen when delivery occurs more than 4 days post-reperfusion. However, this suggestion was not borne out in the Timing in Myocardial infarction Evaluation (TIME) trial, which found that, following acute MI, timing of cell therapy (3 vs. 7 days) had no significant effect on either global or regional parameters of LV function [48]. Similar, negative results were also reported from the SWISS-AMI (no significant different in early (5–7 days) or late (3–4 weeks) administration of BMNC versus control) [49] and LateTIME (BMNC 2–3 weeks post acute MI) [50] trials. Furthermore, collaborative meta-analysis suggests that timing of cell therapy has no significant effect on markers of LV remodeling [51].

Homing and engraftment

Even the positive reports from randomized clinical trials using autologous BMNC transplantation have shown at best a 6–9% increase in measures of LV function, and it is difficult to understand how such a small increase in global LVEF could be translated into significant clinical improvement. Countering the idea that stem cells transdifferentiate into functioning cardiomyocytes, Hofmann et al. [42] used 2-[^{18}F]-fluoro-2-deoxy-D-glucose (18F-FDG) labeling to follow the fate of intracoronary delivered unselected and CD34$^+$ enriched autologous BMNCs in patients following acute MI. They noted that only 1.3–2.6% of unselected BMNCs could be detected in the myocardium following intracoronary delivery, with the majority of detected activity in the liver and spleen. However, when they delivered CD34$^+$ enriched BMNCs they found increased engraftment in the infarct border zone to 14–39% of the total detectable activity. Furthermore, a study examining the 1 day kinetics of transplanted cells indicated that engraftment is a temporary phenomenon, with myocardial activity dropping off between 2 and 20 hours post-intracoronary delivery from ~5% to ~1% [52–54]. Additionally, in patients with a history of MI more than 6 months prior, myocardial activity disappeared altogether. This would suggest any positive effects are likely to occur by means other than by direct tissue incorporation. Factors accounting for the transiency of cell retention could be related to a reduced adhesive status of the myocardial microcirculation, and/or the functional performance of delivered cells. Studies are required to investigate this further, and to examine whether pharmacologic manipulation of the microcirculation either at the time of, or prior to, cell delivery makes any difference. Further important differences between trials include whether they were randomized/blinded and/or placebo-controlled, the methods used in assessing LV function and duration of follow-up.

Non-BMNC cell therapy

Although the majority of trials have been performed using BMNC, other sources have been used. The CArdiosphere-Derived aUtologous stem CElls to reverse ventricUlar dySfunction (CADUCEUS) prospective, randomized, controlled study studied the effect of intracoronary administration of cardiosphere-derived stem cells (CDC) post-MI. Both 6-month and 1-year follow-up suggest significant improvement in scar size, mass, and viable mass, but no improvement in LVEF compared with controls [55,56].

Trials and meta-analyses

The majority of trials utilizing cell therapy in the context of acute MI have utilized BMNC as the therapy of choice. REPAIR-AMI, REGENT, and SWISS-AMI are the largest studies to date. REPAIR-AMI was a multicenter double-blinded randomized placebo-controlled trial of patients with ST-elevation MI (STEMI) and impaired LV function, with the treatment arm receiving unfractionated BMNC. In the treatment arm there was a significant improvement in LV function (as measured by quantitative LV angiography) compared with placebo [40]. One-year follow-up for a combined endpoint of death, recurrence of MI, or revascularization was significantly reduced in the treatment arm [57]. The REGENT randomized placebo-controlled trial compared the use of selected (CD34$^+$, CXCR4$^+$) with unfractionated BMNC in patients with revascularized acute MI and reduced LVEF [58]. No significant difference in ΔLVEF, quantified by MRI, was seen between treatment groups and control; however, there was a trend for benefit in those with lower baseline LVEF.

Several meta-analyses, utilizing data from published studies, have been produced in recent years. Unfortunately, the results of these are in many ways as disparate as the results of individual studies themselves.

Delewi et al. [51] report in a collaborative meta-analysis of clinical trials that intracoronary injection of BMNC in patients with acute MI is associated with a significant improvement in LVEF (2.55%, with a reduction in left ventricular end-systolic volume index (LVESI) and end-diastolic volume index (LVEDI)) compared with placebo. Subgroup analysis suggested that the largest benefit is seen in those <55 years old and those with baseline LEVF <40%. However, de Jong et al. [59] found that the significant improvement in LVEF seen in cell therapy is abolished when only MRI-derived (rather than other modalities) data is used. The Francis group have raised concerns regarding discrepancies in reporting of cell therapy trials [60]. A meta-analysis from the same group found that in the minority of studies where no discrepancies could be identified, the mean change in LVEF from cell therapy was –0.4% [61]. Most recently in the ACCRUE study, Gyöngyösi et al. [62] reported the results of a prospective Individual Patient Data meta-analysis of 1252 patients from 12 trials utilizing intracoronary cell therapy in patients with recent MI. No clinical benefit, either from avoidance of major adverse cerebrovascular and cardiac events (MACCE) or improvement in LV function, was identified.

Current trials

The Effect of Intracoronary Reinfusion of Bone-Marrow-derived Mononuclear Cells on All Cause Mortality in Acute Myocardial Infarction (BAMI) study, currently recruiting, promises to be the largest randomized controlled trial investigating cell therapy following acute MI (n = 3000) [63]. Given the large number of intended participants compared to previously published studies (both trials and meta-analyses) and the use of mortality as primary endpoint, its results are eagerly awaited.

Cell therapy in chronic ischemic heart disease

While the majority of trials have examined the effects of cell therapy in acute MI, only a limited number of trials have focused their attention on its use in chronic ischemic heart disease. One of the first studies looked at a small group of patients undergoing elective coronary artery bypass graft surgery (CABG), in whom they found improved myocardial perfusion and metabolism after enriched CD133$^+$ cells were injected into the infarct border zone [64]. Similar observations were noted in an open-label randomized study where patients with LV dysfunction undergoing CABG surgery together with direct intramyocardial injection of BMNCs showed better functional improvement than with CABG alone [65].

Perin *et al.* [66] went on to study the electromechanically mapped guidance of transendomyocardially injected BMNCs in patients with refractory angina and myocardial ischemia. They demonstrated not only that it was procedurally safe, but that it was associated with clinical improvement detectable at 3 months and maintained to 12 months. However, when the Perin group carried out the FOCUS-CCTRN study, a phase 2 randomized double-blind, placebo-controlled trial utilizing endomyocardial injection of BMNC in symptomatic patients with ischemic cardiomyopathy (BMNC arm n = 61, control n = 31), no significant improvement in left ventricular end-systolic volume (LVESV), maximal oxygen consumption, or reversibility (assessed by SPECT) was demonstrated [67].

A randomized, blinded placebo-controlled trial of 26 patients with chronic total arterial occlusions was conducted, where autologous granulocyte colony-stimulating factor (G-CSF) mobilized circulating progenitor cells were injected down percutaneously revascularized coronary arteries. Assessment of LV function by magnetic resonance imaging showed that LVEF in treated patients had increased by 14% while infarct size had been reduced by 16%. Notably, there was a demonstrable improvement in regional wall motion at the target site [68].

The controlled crossover Transplantation of Progenitor Cells and Regeneration Enhancement–Chronic Heart Disease (TOPCARE-CHD) trial enrolled 75 patients with stable chronic ischemic heart disease who had previously sustained an MI [69]. Here, patients were randomly assigned to receive BMNCs, circulating progenitor cells, or no cells into the (patent) coronary artery supplying the most dyskinetic LV region. The increase in mean LVEF seen in the BMNC group was modest (2.9%), but significantly greater than in the circulating progenitor and control groups. The crossover phase of the study indicated that BMNC therapy was indeed associated with a greater increase in both global and regional LV function.

Poglajen *et al.* [70] published the results of a prospective crossover trial (n = 33) in which the effect of endomyocardial implantation of selected CD34+ cells in patients with ischemic cardiomyopathy. The 6-month treatment phase was associated with significant improvements in LVEF, NT-proBNP, and 6 minute walk test.

The CAuSMIC Study, a phase I randomized, open-label, controlled trial studying endomyocardial implantation of skeletal myoblasts in patients with ischemic cardiomyopathy, with improved New York Heart Association (NYHA) functional status and a trend toward reduction in LV dimensions [71].

The Scipio trial, a randomized phase 1 trial assessing cardiac stem cells (SCS) in patients with chronic ischemic cardiomyopathy undergoing CABG, produced early reports indicating feasibility and safety in addition to significant improvement in LVEF and reduction in infarct size [72]. It should be noted, however, that "concerns about the integrity of certain data" in the published study have been raised and are being investigated at the time of writing [73].

The POSEIDON trial (a comparison of allogenic vs. autologous MSC in chronic ischemic cardiomyopathy), while lacking a control group, met its primary endpoint in demonstrating the safety of allogenic MSC [74].

National and international task forces

The European Society of Cardiology has established a task force for the future of stem cell therapy in cardiology [75]. A similar task force has been established by the National Heart, Lung and Blood Institute, which has provided a framework to coordinate the resources and funding of cardiovascular cell-based therapy in the USA [76]. Both of these groups offer clear advice, and warn against research proceeding without international consensus, aiming to avoid further small, underpowered studies.

Conclusions

Despite recent technological and pharmacologic advances made within the field of interventional cardiology reducing mortality from coronary artery disease, it continues to cause significant morbidity and efforts have been directed to developing ways of improving endothelial and myocardial function in patients in order to prevent future coronary events. The last two decades have seen an explosion of interest in the use of autologous stem cell therapy to improve the outcome for patients living with coronary heart disease. Unfortunately, the results of published randomized controlled trials and indeed meta-analyses have been conflicting, particularly in the post-acute MI population. Although the delivery of autologous stem cells to the heart appears to be safe, many unanswered questions remain regarding their mechanism of action, the optimum cell type, method, and timing of delivery. It is anticipated that future larger scale randomized controlled trials, particularly the BAMI trial, will provide us with the answers to some of these in due course.

Interactive multiple choice questions are available for this chapter on www.wiley.com/go/dangas/cardiology

References

1 McCulloch EA, Till JE. The radiation sensitivity of normal mouse bone marrow cells, determined by quantitative marrow transplantation into irradiated mice. *Radiat Res* 1960; **13**: 115–125.

2 Asahara T, Murohara T, Sullivan A, *et al.* Isolation of putative progenitor endothelial cells for angiogenesis. *Science* 1997; **275**(5302): 964–967.

3 Shi Q, Rafii S, Wu MH, *et al.* Evidence for circulating bone marrow-derived endothelial cells. *Blood* 1998; **92**(2): 362–367.

4 Takahashi T, Kalka C, Masuda H, *et al.* Ischemia- and cytokine-induced mobilization of bone marrow-derived endothelial progenitor cells for neovascularization. *Nat Med* 1999; **5**(4): 434–438.

5 Kawamoto A, Gwon HC, Iwaguro H, *et al.* Therapeutic potential of ex vivo expanded endothelial progenitor cells for myocardial ischemia. *Circulation* 2001; **103**(5): 634–637.

6 Kocher AA, Schuster MD, Szabolcs MJ, *et al.* Neovascularization of ischemic myocardium by human bone-marrow-derived angioblasts prevents cardiomyocyte apoptosis, reduces remodeling and improves cardiac function. *Nat Med* 2001; **7**(4): 430–436.

7 Tateishi-Yuyama E, Matsubara H, Murohara T, *et al.* Therapeutic angiogenesis for patients with limb ischaemia by autologous transplantation of bone-marrow cells: a pilot study and a randomised controlled trial. *Lancet* 2002; **360**(9331): 427–435.

8 Orlic D, Kajstura J, Chimenti S, *et al.* Mobilized bone marrow cells repair the infarcted heart, improving function and survival. *Proc Natl Acad Sci U S A* 2001; **98**(18): 10344–10349.

9 Forbes SJ, Vig P, Poulsom R, *et al.* Adult stem cell plasticity: new pathways of tissue regeneration become visible. *Clin Sci (Lond)* 2002; **103**(4): 355–369.

10 Eisenberg LM, Burns L, Eisenberg, CA. Hematopoietic cells from bone marrow have the potential to differentiate into cardiomyocytes in vitro. *Anat Rec A Discov Mol Cell Evol Biol* 2003; **274**(1): 870–882.

11 Jackson KA, Majka SM, Wang H, *et al.* Regeneration of ischemic cardiac muscle and vascular endothelium by adult stem cells. *J Clin Invest* 2001; **107**(11): 1395–1402.

12 Kajstura J, Rota M, Wang B, *et al.* Bone marrow cells differentiate in cardiac cell lineages after infarction independently of cell fusion. *Circ Res* 2005; **96**(1): 127–137.

13 Maroko PR, Libby P, Ginks WR, *et al*. Coronary artery reperfusion. I. Early effects on local myocardial function and the extent of myocardial necrosis. *J Clin Invest* 1972; **51**(10): 2710–2716.

14 Ginks WR, Sybers HD, Maroko PR, *et al*. Coronary artery reperfusion. II. Reduction of myocardial infarct size at 1 week after the coronary occlusion. *J Clin Invest* 1972; **51**(10): 2717–2723.

15 Kajstura J, Leri A, Finato N, *et al*. Myocyte proliferation in end-stage cardiac failure in humans. *Proc Natl Acad Sci U S A* 1998; **95**(15): 8801–8805.

16 Beltrami AP, Urbanek K, Kajstura J, *et al*. Evidence that human cardiac myocytes divide after myocardial infarction. *N Engl J Med* 2001; **344**(23): 1750–1757.

17 Quaini F, Urbanek K, Beltrami AP, *et al*. Chimerism of the transplanted heart. *N Engl J Med* 2002; **346**(1): 5–15.

18 Laflamme MA, Myerson D, Saffitz JE, *et al*. Evidence for cardiomyocyte repopulation by extracardiac progenitors in transplanted human hearts. *Circ Res* 2002; **90**(6): 634–640.

19 Muller P, Pfeiffer P, Koglin J, *et al*. Cardiomyocytes of noncardiac origin in myocardial biopsies of human transplanted hearts. *Circulation* 2002; **106**(1): 31–35.

20 Oh H, Bradfute SB, Gallardo TD, *et al*. Cardiac progenitor cells from adult myocardium: homing, differentiation, and fusion after infarction. *Proc Natl Acad Sci U S A* 2003; **100**(21): 12313–12318.

21 Shintani S, Murohara T, Ikeda H, *et al*. Mobilization of endothelial progenitor cells in patients with acute myocardial infarction. *Circulation* 2001; **103**(23): 2776–2779.

22 Yamaguchi J, Kusano KF, Masuo O, *et al*. Stromal cell-derived factor-1 effects on ex vivo expanded endothelial progenitor cell recruitment for ischemic neovascularization. *Circulation* 2003; **107**(9): 1322–1328.

23 Ceradini DJ, Kulkarni AR, Callagham MJ, *et al*. Progenitor cell trafficking is regulated by hypoxic gradients through HIF-1 induction of SDF-1. *Nat Med* 2004; **10**(8): 858–864.

24 De Falco, E, Porcelli D, Torella AR, *et al*. SDF-1 involvement in endothelial phenotype and ischemia-induced recruitment of bone marrow progenitor cells. *Blood* 2004; **104**(12): 3472–3482.

25 Peled A, Petit I, Collet O, *et al*. Dependence of human stem cell engraftment and repopulation of NOD/SCID mice on CXCR4. *Science* 1999; **283**(5403): 845–848.

26 Walter DH, Haendeler J, Reinhold J, *et al*. Impaired CXCR4 signaling contributes to the reduced neovascularization capacity of endothelial progenitor cells from patients with coronary artery disease. *Circ Res* 2005; **97**(11): 1142–1151.

27 Yoon CH, Hur J, Oh IY, *et al*. Intercellular adhesion molecule-1 is upregulated in ischemic muscle, which mediates trafficking of endothelial progenitor cells. *Arterioscler Thromb Vasc Biol* 2006; **26**(5): 1066–1072.

28 Vajkoczy P, Blum S, Lamparter M, *et al*. Multistep nature of microvascular recruitment of ex vivo-expanded embryonic endothelial progenitor cells during tumor angiogenesis. *J Exp Med* 2003; **197**(12): 1755–1765.

29 Chavakis E, Aicher A, Heeschen C, *et al*. Role of beta2-integrins for homing and neovascularization capacity of endothelial progenitor cells. *J Exp Med* 2005; **201**(1): 63–72.

30 Jin H, Aiyer A, Su J, *et al*. A homing mechanism for bone marrow-derived progenitor cell recruitment to the neovasculature. *J Clin Invest* 2006; **116**(3): 652–662.

31 Massberg S, Konrad I, Schurzinger K, *et al*. Platelets secrete stromal cell-derived factor 1alpha and recruit bone marrow-derived progenitor cells to arterial thrombi in vivo. *J Exp Med* 2006; **203**(5): 1221–1233.

32 Wang JS, Shum-Tim D, Galipeau J, *et al*. Marrow stromal cells for cellular cardiomyoplasty: feasibility and potential clinical advantages. *J Thorac Cardiovasc Surg* 2000; **120**(5): 999–1005.

33 Pittinger MF, Martin BJ. Mesenchymal stem cells and their potential as cardiac therapeutics. *Circ Res* 2004; **95**: 9–20.

34 Menache P, Hagege AA, Vilquin JT *et al*. Autologous skeletal myoblast transplantation for severe postinfarction left ventricular dysfunction. *J Am Coll Cardiol* 2003; **41**(7): 1078–1083.

35 Dib N, Michler RE, Pagani FD *et al*. Safety and feasibility of autologous myoblast transplantation in patients with ischaemic cardiomyopathy: four-year follow-up. *Circulation* 2005; **112**: 1748–1755.

36 Menasche P, Alfieri O, Janssens S *et al*. The Myoblast Autologous Grafting in Ischemic Cardio-myopathy (MAGIC) trial: first randomized placebo-controlled study of myoblast transplantation. *Circulation* 2008; **117**: 1189–1200.

37 Wollert KC, Meyer GP, Lotz J, *et al*. Intracoronary autologous bone-marrow cell transfer after myocardial infarction: the BOOST randomised controlled clinical trial. *Lancet* 2004; **364**(9429): 141–148.

38 Lunde K, Solheim S, Aakhus S, *et al*. Intracoronary injection of mononuclear bone marrow cells in acute myocardial infarction. *N Engl J Med* 2006; **355**(12): 1199–1209.

39 Janssens S, Dubois C, Bogaert J, *et al*. Autologous bone marrow-derived stem-cell transfer in patients with ST-segment elevation myocardial infarction: double-blind, randomised controlled trial. *Lancet* 2006; **367**(9505): 113–121.

40 Schachinger V, Erbs S, Elsasser A, *et al*. Intracoronary bone marrow-derived progenitor cells in acute myocardial infarction. *N Engl J Med* 2006; **355**(12): 1210–1221.

41 Katritsis DG, Sotiropoulou A, Karvouni E, *et al*. Transcoronary transplantation of autologous mesenchymal stem cells and endothelial progenitors into infarcted human myocardium. *Catheter Cardiovasc Interv* 2005; **65**(3): 321–329.

42 Hofmann M, Wollert KC, Meyer GP, *et al*. Monitoring of bone marrow cell homing into the infarcted human myocardium. *Circulation* 2005; **111**(17): 2198–2202.

43 Bhatia M. AC133 expression in human stem cells. *Leukemia* 2001; **15**(11): 1685–1688.

44 Quirici N, Soligo D, Caneva L, *et al*. Differentiation and expansion of endothelial cells from human bone marrow CD133(+) cells. *Br J Haematol* 2001; **115**(1): 186–194.

45 Kuci S, Wessels JT, Buhring HJ, *et al*. Identification of a novel class of human adherent CD34– stem cells that give rise to SCID-repopulating cells. *Blood* 2003; **101**(3): 869–876.

46 Bartunek J, Vanderheyden M, Vandekerckhove B, *et al*. Intracoronary injection of CD133-positive enriched bone marrow progenitor cells promotes cardiac recovery after recent myocardial infarction: feasibility and safety. *Circulation* 2005; **112**(9 Suppl): I178–183.

47 Voo S, Eggermann J, Dunaeva M, *et al*. Enhanced functional response of CD133+ circulating progenitor cells in patients early after acute myocardial infarction. *Eur Heart J* 2008; **29**(2): 241–250.

48 Traverse JH, Henry TD, Pepine CJ, *et al*. Effect of the use and timing of bone marrow mononuclear cell delivery on left ventricular function after acute myocardial infarction: the TIME randomized trial. *JAMA* 2012; **308**(22): 2380–2389.

49 Surder D, Manka R, Lo Cicero V, *et al*. Intracoronary injection of bone marrow-derived mononuclear cells early or late after myocardial infarction: effects on global left ventricular function. *Circulation* 2013; **127**(19): 1968–1979.

50 Traverse JH, Henry TD, Ellis SG, *et al*. Effect of intracoronary delivery of autologous bone marrow mononuclear cells 2 to 3 weeks following myocardial infarction on left ventricular function: the LateTIME randomized trial. *JAMA* 2011; **306**(19): 2110–2119.

51 Delewi R, Hirsch A, Tijssen JG, *et al*. Impact of intracoronary bone marrow cell therapy on left ventricular function in the setting of ST-segment elevation myocardial infarction: a collaborative meta-analysis. *Eur Heart J* 2014; **35**(15): 989–998.

52 Nyolczas N, Gyongyosi M, Beran G, *et al*. Design and rationale for the Myocardial Stem Cell Administration After Acute Myocardial Infarction (MYSTAR) Study: a multicenter, prospective, randomized, single-blind trial comparing early and late intracoronary or combined (percutaneous intramyocardial and intracoronary) administration of nonselected autologous bone marrow cells to patients after acute myocardial infarction. *Am Heart J* 2007; **153**(2): 212 e1–7.

53 Bartunek J, Vanderheyden M, Wijns W, *et al*. Bone-marrow-derived cells for cardiac stem cell therapy: safe or still under scrutiny? *Nat Clin Pract Cardiovasc Med* 2007; **4**(Suppl 1): S100–105.

54 Penicka M, Lang O, Widimsky P, *et al*. One-day kinetics of myocardial engraftment after intracoronary injection of bone marrow mononuclear cells in patients with acute and chronic myocardial infarction. *Heart* 2007; **93**(7): 837–841.

55 Makkar RR, Smith RR, Cheng K, *et al*. Intracoronary cardiosphere-derived cells for heart regeneration after myocardial infarction (CADUCEUS): a prospective, randomised phase 1 trial. *Lancet* 2012; **379**(9819): 895–904.

56 Malliaras K, Makkar RR, Smith RR, *et al*. Intracoronary cardiosphere-derived cells after myocardial infarction: evidence of therapeutic regeneration in the final 1-year results of the CADUCEUS trial (CArdiosphere-Derived aUtologous stem CElls to reverse ventricUlar dySfunction. *J Am Coll Cardiol* 2014; **63**(2): 110–122.

57 Schachinger V, Erbs S, Elsasser A, *et al*. Improved clinical outcome after intracoronary administration of bone-marrow-derived progenitor cells in acute myocardial infarction: final 1-year results of the REPAIR-AMI trial. *Eur Heart J* 2006; **27**(23): 2775–2783.

58 Tendera M, Wojakowski W, Ruzyllo W, *et al*. Intracoronary infusion of bone marrow-derived selected CD34+ CXCR4+ cells and non-selected mononuclear cells in patients with acute STEMI and reduced left ventricular ejection fraction: results of randomized, multicentre Myocardial Regeneration by Intracoronary Infusion of Selected Population of Stem Cells in Acute Myocardial Infarction (REGENT) Trial. *Eur Heart J* 2009; **30**(11): 1313–1321.

59 de Jong R, Houtgraaf JH, Samiei S, *et al*. Intracoronary stem cell infusion after myocardial infarction: a meta-analysis and update on clinical trials. *Circ Cardiovasc Interv* 2014; **7**(2): 156–167.

60 Francis DP, Mielewczik M, Zargaran D, *et al*. Autologous bone marrow-derived stem cell therapy in heart disease: discrepancies and contradictions. *Int J Cardiol* 2013; **168**: 3381–3403.

61 Nowbar AN, Mielewczik M, Karavassilis M, *et al*. Discrepancies in autologous bone marrow stem cell trials and enhancement of ejection fraction (DAMASCENE): weighted regression and meta-analysis. *BMJ* 2014; **348**: g2688.

62 Gyöngyösi M, Wojakowski, Lemarchand P, *et al*. Meta-Analysis of Cell-based CarDiac studies (ACCRUE) in patients with acute myocardial infarction based on individual patient data. *Circ Res* 2015; **116**(8): 1346–1360.

63 BAMI. The effect of intracoronary reinfusion of bone marrow-derived mononuclear cells (BM-MNC) on all cause mortality in acute myocardial infarction (BAMI). Available at: https://clinicaltrials.gov/ct2/show/nct01569178 (accessed April 24, 2016).

64 Stamm C, Kleine HD, Choi YH, *et al*. Intramyocardial delivery of CD133+ bone marrow cells and coronary artery bypass grafting for chronic ischemic heart disease: safety and efficacy studies. *J Thorac Cardiovasc Surg* 2007; **133**(3): 717–725.

65 Patel AN, Geffner L, Vina RF, *et al*. Surgical treatment for congestive heart failure with autologous adult stem cell transplantation: a prospective randomized study. *J Thorac Cardiovasc Surg* 2005; **130**(6): 1631–1638.

66 Perin EC, Dohmann HF, Borojevic, *et al*. Transendocardial, autologous bone marrow cell transplantation for severe, chronic ischemic heart failure. *Circulation* 2003; **107**(18): 2294–2302.

67 Perin EC, Willerson JT, Pepine CJ, *et al*. Effect of transendocardial delivery of autologous bone marrow mononuclear cells on functional capacity, left ventricular function, and perfusion in chronic heart failure: the FOCUS-CCTRN trial. *JAMA* 2012; **307**(16): 1717–1726.

68 Erbs S, Linke A, Adams V, *et al*. Transplantation of blood-derived progenitor cells after recanalization of chronic coronary artery occlusion: first randomized and placebo-controlled study. *Circ Res* 2005; **97**(8): 756–762.

69 Assmus B, Fischer-Rasokat U, Honold J, *et al*. Transcoronary transplantation of functionally competent BMCs is associated with a decrease in natriuretic peptide serum levels and improved survival of patients with chronic postinfarction heart failure: results of the TOPCARE-CHD Registry. *Circ Res* 2007; **100**(8): 1234–1241.

70 Poglajen G, Sever M, Cukjati M, *et al*. Effects of transendocardial CD34+ cell transplantation in patients with ischemic cardiomyopathy. *Circ Cardiovasc Interv* 2014; **4**: 552–559.

71 Dib N, Dinsmore J, Lababidi Z, *et al*. One-year follow-up of feasibility and safety of the first U.S., randomized, controlled study using 3-dimensional guided catheter-based delivery of autologous skeletal myoblasts for ischemic cardiomyopathy (CAuSMIC study). *JACC Cardiovasc Interv* 2009; **2**: 9–16.

72 Bolli R, Chugh AR, D'Amario D, *et al*. Cardiac stem cells in patients with ischaemic cardiomyopathy (SCIPIO): initial results of a randomised phase 1 trial. *Lancet* 2011; **378**(9806): 1847–1857.

73 The Lancet Editors. Expression of concern: the SCIPIO trial. *Lancet* 2014; **383**(9925): 1279.

74 Hare JM, Fishman JE, Gerstenblith G, *et al*. Comparison of allogenic vs autologous bone marrow-derived mesenchymal stem cells delivered by transendocardial injection in patients with ischemic cardiomyopathy: the POSEIDON randomized tial. *JAMA* 2012; **308**(22): 2369–2379.

75 Bartunek J, Dimmeler S, Drexler H, *et al*. The consensus of the task force of the European Society of Cardiology concerning the clinical investigation of the use of autologous adult stem cells for repair of the heart. *Eur Heart J* 2006; **27**(11): 1338–1340.

76 Thomas JW. National Heart, Lung and Blood Institute resources and programs for cell-based therapies. *Circ Res* 2007; **101**(1): 1–6.

CHAPTER 30

Statistical Essentials in the Design and Analysis of Clinical Trials

Usman Baber[1] and Stuart J. Pocock[2]
[1] Icahn School of Medicine at Mount Sinai, New, NY, USA
[2] London School of Hygiene and Tropical Medicine, University of London, London, UK

The rapidly changing landscape of cardiology has been driven by an increasing wealth of clinical data within the scientific literature. Clinical decisions are therefore strongly influenced by the appropriate implementation of evidence-based medicine, requiring the clinician to have an understanding of clinical trial design, and commonly utilized biostatistical analyses. The chapter begins with succinct descriptions of fundamental statistical principles. Significance testing, the estimation of the magnitude of effect, and the interpretation of p-values are discussed, before the discussion of advanced techniques, such as the analysis of time to event data. This is followed by brief explanations of the basic principles of clinical trial design and planning, addressing issues of bias, sample size and power, and commonly used trial designs. Each topic is coupled with examples from published clinical trials.

The fundamentals

Significance tests and p-values

In a well-conducted clinical trial, particularly with double-blind randomized trials, the possibility of bias is minimal and therefore the observed outcome difference between treatment groups is either a genuine effect or due to chance variation. Significance tests enable one to assess the strength of evidence that a real effect is present rather than a chance finding. There are three main types of outcome data analyzed in contemporary studies with different measures and tests of association as shown in Table 30.1.

While the calculations differ, the underlying principle is the same for all significance tests. For example, in the Strategies for Multivessel Revascularization in Patients with Diabetes (FREEDOM) trial, 1900 patients with diabetes mellitus (DM) were randomly allocated to either percutaneous coronary intervention (PCI) (n = 953) or coronary artery bypass graft (CABG) (n = 947) and followed for at least 2 years with a primary composite outcome of death, non-fatal myocardial infarction, or non-fatal stroke. At 5 years, the number (%) of patients with a primary outcome event in the PCI and CABG groups was 205 (26.6%) and 147 (18.7%), respectively, with a log-rank p-value of 0.005.

The interpretation of the p-value is predicated on the formulation of the null hypothesis, which in the case of the FREEDOM trial assumed that both PCI and CABG were equally effective revascularization approaches in patients with DM and multivessel coronary artery disease (CAD). Then the p-value is defined as the probability p of detecting a difference of 26.6% vs. 18.7% or larger under the assumption that no true difference exists (i.e., the null hypothesis is true).

The answer from the log-rank test is p = 0.005.

The smaller the probability p, the more convincing the evidence to contradict the null hypothesis. In the case of the FREEDOM trial, we have strong evidence that CABG reduces the risk of the primary endpoint compared to PCI.

Estimating the magnitude of effect

Conventional metrics to quantify the magnitude of a treatment effect (i.e., measure of association) include the risk ratio or relative risk; relative risk reduction, odds ratio, and number needed to treat. Examples of calculating each are provided in Table 30.2 with corresponding examples from the FREEDOM trial.

There is no "correct" singular metric to quantify a treatment effect. Often, it is recommended to incorporate several of these to appreciate both relative and absolute effects.

Ninety-five percent confidence interval to express uncertainty

Any estimate of treatment effect in a clinical trial contains some random error, and calculating a confidence interval (CI) enables one to see within what range it is plausible that the true effect lies. For instance, the observed relative risk in the TYPHOON trial is 0.51 while the 95% CI is 0.33–0.80. This means that one is 95% sure that the true relative risk is in this interval. To be precise, there is a 2.5% chance that the true RR lies below 0.33 and 2.5% that the true RR is greater than 0.80. The larger the trial, the tighter the CI becomes. Specifically, to halve the CI width one needs a trial four times the size.

Interventional Cardiology: Principles and Practice, Second Edition. Edited by George D. Dangas, Carlo Di Mario, and Nicholas N. Kipshidze.
© 2017 John Wiley & Sons, Ltd. Published 2017 by John Wiley & Sons, Ltd.

Table 30.1 Three main types of outcome data are analyzed in contemporary studies with different measures and tests of association.

Type of data	Example	Measure of association	Test of association
Binary	In-stent restenosis	Odds ratio	Chi-square test
Time to event	Time to death	Hazard ratio	Log-rank test
Quantitative	Late loss (mm)	Mean	t-test

Table 30.2 Common measures of association and calculations.

Measure of association	Calculation	FREEDOM example
Relative risk (RR)	Event rate in group 1 Event rate in group 2	0.187/0.266 = 0.70
Relative risk reduction (RRR)	1–RR	1–0.70 = 0.3
Odds ratio (OR)	(Prob of event in group 1/Probability of no event in group 1) / (Prob of event in group 2/Probability of no event in group 2)	(0.187/0.813) / (0.266/0.734) =0.63
Number needed to treat (NNT)	1/Absolute risk reduction	1/(0.266–0.187) ~ 13

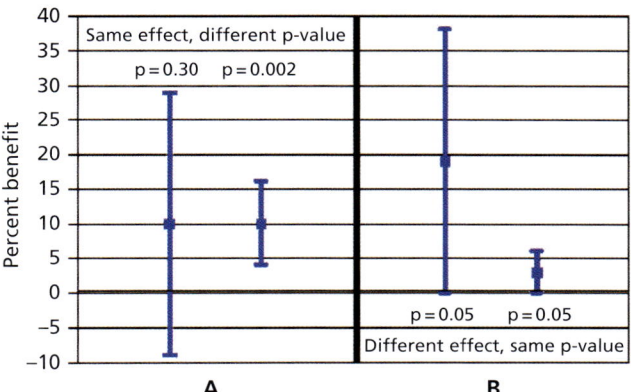

Figure 30.1 Interpreting p-values.

Interpreting p-values

Use of significance tests is often misleadingly oversimplified by putting too much emphasis on whether p is above or below 0.05. A p < 0.05 means the result is statistically significant at the 5% level, but is an arbitrary guideline. It does not mean one has firm proof of an effect. By definition, even if two treatments are truly identical there is a 1 in 20 chance of reaching p < 0.05. Also, p > 0.05, not statistically significant (or n.s.), does not necessarily mean no true difference exists.

This concept is illustrated graphically in Figure 30.1. In the left-hand panel of this figure, similar treatment effects are obtained from two different studies, one of which is significant and one is not. The lack of significance alone should not be the sole metric on which to interpret the findings, particularly as the effect size appears to be large, albeit imprecise. In contrast, in the right-hand panel, a p-value of 0.05 is obtained with two very different effect sizes, one which is large and another that is much smaller. Again, focusing on the p-value alone as the sole discriminator of importance in treatment effect would ignore the very large and perhaps clinically relevant gradient of effect between the treatments.

Link between p-values and confidence intervals

If we have p < 0.05 then the 95% CI for the risk ratio (or odds ratio) will exclude 1, while if p > 0.05 is observed then the 95% CI will include 1. Thus, by looking at the CI alone one can infer whether the treatment difference is significant at the 5% level.

Time to event data

Many major trials study time to a primary event outcome. For instance, the ACUITY trial studied composite ischemia: death, myocardial infarction, or unplanned revascularization over 1 year follow-up.

A Kaplan–Meier life-table plot is the main method of displaying such data by treatment group (Figure 30.2). It displays the cumulative percentage of patients experiencing the event over time for each group. This method takes account of patients having different lengths of follow-up (e.g., any lost to follow-up before the intended 1 year).

Such a plot is a useful descriptive tool, but one needs to use a log-rank test to see if there is evidence of a treatment difference in the incidence of events. For instance, the heparin + IIb/IIIa (n = 4603) and bivalirudin alone (n = 4612) groups had composite ischemia in 15.4% and 16.0% of patients, respectively. The log-rank test uses the total data by group displayed to obtain p = 0.29 (i.e., the data are consistent with the null hypothesis of no treatment difference). The log-rank test can be thought of as an extension, indeed improvement, to the simpler chi-squared test comparing two percentages because it takes into account the fact that patients have been followed for, and deaths occur at, differing times from randomization.

With time to event data, the *hazard ratio* is used to estimate any relative treatment differences in risk. It is similar to, but more complicated to calculate, than the simple relative risk already mentioned. It effectively averages the instantaneous relative risk occurring at different follow-up times, using what is commonly called a Cox proportional hazards model. In this case the hazard ratio comparing bivalirudin with heparin + IIa/IIIa is 1.06 with 95% CI 0.95–1.17. Thus, there is an observed 6% increase in hazard but the 95% CI includes 1 reflecting the lack of statistical significance.

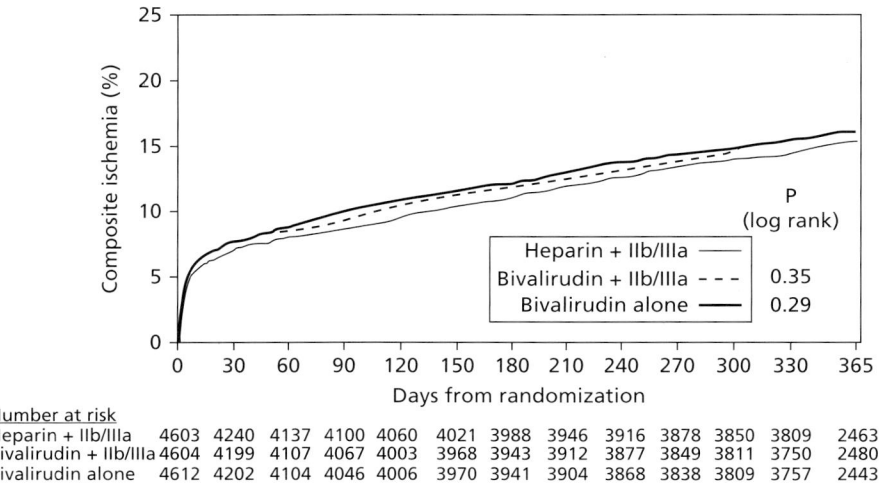

Figure 30.2 Kaplan–Meier life-table plot showing pattern of treatment difference over time (e.g., ACUITY 1-year follow-up).

Quantitative data

For a quantitative measure of patient outcome it is common to compare the mean outcomes in each treatment group. For example, in the SYMPLICITY HTN-3 study, 535 patients with resistant hypertension were randomized in a blinded fashion to either renal denervation or sham control with a primary efficacy endpoint of change in office systolic blood pressure (SBP) at 6 months. The mean change from baseline in the renal denervation and sham groups was -14.1 ± 23.9 mmHg and -11.7 ± 25.9 mmHg, respectively. The mean change between groups was -2.39 mmHg (95% CI -6.89 to 2.12; $p = 0.26$).

The standard deviation (SD) summarizes the extent of individual patient variation around each mean. If the data are normally distributed then appropriately 95% of individuals will have a value within two standard deviations either side of the mean. This is sometimes called the *reference range*. However, for a clinical trial outcome measure it is more useful to calculate the *standard error of the mean* (SEM) which is $SD / \sqrt{N}$. That is, precision in the estimated mean increases proportionately with the square root of the number of patients. The 95% confidence for the mean is mean $\pm 1.96 \times$ SEM.

Trial design: the fundamentals

When planning a clinical trial much energy is devoted to defining exactly what is the *new treatment*, who are the eligible *patients*, and what are the primary and secondary *outcomes*. Then the following statistical design issues need to be considered.

Control group

One essential is that the trial is *comparative* (i.e., one needs a *control group* of patients receiving a standard treatment who will be compared with patients receiving the new treatment). Such standard treatment can either be an established active treatment or no treatment (possibly a placebo). Of course, all patients in both groups have good medical care in all other respects.

Randomization

One needs a fair (unbiased) comparison between new treatment and control, and *randomization* is the key requirement in this regard. That is, each patient has an equal chance of being randomly assigned to new or standard treatment. Furthermore, the method of handling random assignments is such that no one can predict in advance what each next patient will be assigned to. Thus, randomization ensures there is no selection bias in deciding which patients get new or standard treatment. Such selection bias is a serious problem in any observational (non-randomized) studies comparing treatments, making them notoriously unreliable in their conclusions.

As a consequence, randomization minimizes the possibility that treatment groups will significantly differ in baseline characteristics. The possibility for chance variation can never be completely eliminated, however, even in a randomized study design. To further guarantee that key baseline features will not influence the treatment effect, randomization can also be stratified, a common approach in multicenter studies.

In addition, randomization helps to ensure that all other aspects of patient care, and also the evaluation of patient outcome, is identical in both treatment groups. In this respect it is often important to make the trial *double blind* whereby neither patients nor those treating them and evaluating their response know which treatment each individual patient is receiving.

If a trial cannot be made double blind one can nevertheless require *blinded evaluation* of outcome by people not aware of which treatment each patient is on.

Trial size and power calculations

For a trial to provide a reliably precise answer as to the relative merits of the randomized treatments one needs a sufficiently large number of patients. *Power calculations* are the most commonly used statistical method for determining the required trial size.

Each power calculation entails the following five steps, itemized in Table 30.3:

1 Choose a *primary outcome* for the trial.
2 Decide on a *level of statistical significance* required for declaring a "positive" trial. Five percent significance is usually chosen.
3 Declare what you expect the *control groups results* to be.
4 Declare the *smallest true treatment difference* that is important to detect. Large treatment effects, if present, can be detected in relatively small trials so it is relevant to focus on what reasonably modest effect one would not wish to miss.

Table 30.3 Key components of sample size/power calculations.

Component	Comments
Outcome type	Proportion; time to event; mean
Type I error (alpha)	Level of significance to declare a "significant" result. Typically 0.05
Control group rate	Risk for events in non-experimental arm
Meaningful difference	Smallest true difference with clinical impact
Type II error (beta)	Probability of declaring no difference when in fact one exists. Typically 0.1 or 0.2. Power = 1 – Beta

Table 30.4 Impact of incorrect sample size assumptions on study power.

Component of power calculation	Assumption compared to actual	Effect on power	Example
Sample size	Lower than expected	Reduced	VA CARDS
Detectable difference	Higher than expected	Increased	FAME 2
Event rate	Lower than expected	Reduced	GRAVITAS

5 Declare with what *degree of certainty* (statistical power) one wishes to detect such a difference as statistically significant. From such information there are statistical formulae that provide the required number of patients.

It is important to note that sample size is estimated in the design phase of a study using a priori assumptions that may or may not end up being correct. The implications of incorrect assumptions are not trivial. Poor design can result in an underpowered study that is unable to demonstrate reductions with a treatment effect that is in fact beneficial, thereby depriving patients of a therapeutic option. Alternatively, poor enrolment or event rate assumptions that are not realistic can result in significant expenditure of both human and financial resources in the execution of a study that is ultimately futile. Appreciating the nuances of sample size calculations is critical to the interpretation of clinical trial results, both positive and negative. Table 30.4 provides several examples of trials that were either under- or overpowered based on initial assumptions.

In the VA CARDS trial, investigators designed a multicenter randomized trial comparing CABG with PCI in patients with DM and CAD. The trial required 790 patients to yield 90% power to detect a 40% reduction in the primary endpoint. However, the trial was stopped early because of slow enrolment, after enrolling only 198 patients. The CI for the treatment effect was very wide, 0.47–1.71, and although this included the detectable difference for which the study was powered (RR 0.6), the small sample size rendered the results imprecise and non-significant. In contrast, in FAME 2, De Bruyne *et al.* compared revascularization versus medical therapy in patients with stable CAD and fractional flow reserve (FFR) values

≤0.8. The study assumed an event rate of 18.0% in the control arm, relative risk reduction of 30%, and 816 patients per group to provide 84% power. Although the event rate assumption in the control arm was close to actual (19.5%), the study was halted after only 54% of projected enrolment because of a much larger than expected relative risk reduction of 61%. Finally, Price *et al.* designed the GRAVITAS trial to examine the impact of standard vs. high-dose clopidogrel on reducing 6-month outcomes in patients with high on-treatment platelet reactivity. The investigators assumed a 6-month event rate of 5.0%, risk reduction of 50%, and a sample size of 2200 to provide 80% power. Although the trial enrolled the required sample size, event rates were only 2.3% in each group, yielding a non-significant and imprecise treatment effect of 1.01 (0.58–1.76).

Often, a single clinical trial is neither large nor representative enough to evaluate a particular therapeutic issue. Then, *meta-analyses* can be of value in combining evidence from several related trial to reach an overall conclusion.

Additional topics in clinical design and analysis
Superiority and non-inferiority designs
This chapter so far has discussed the fundamentals of trial design and statistical analysis. Clearly there are many other important issues that need to be tackled in the design, conduct, analysis, and interpretation of clinical trials. All we can do here is briefly alert the reader to these topics and encourage them to pursue further from other courses, textbooks, publications, and so on.

In *trial design* we have concentrated on parallel group trial with just two treatments. In this context the most common trial types include superiority and non-inferiority designs. The key difference between these trial types relates to the expression of the null and alternative hypotheses for each respective design. In a classic superiority trial the null hypothesis states that there are no differences between the experimental and control treatments whereas in a non-inferiority trial the null hypothesis is formulated as the experimental treatment is worse than control by a pre-specified margin. Similarly, the alternative hypothesis for a superiority trial assumes that the experimental and control treatments are different (i.e., experimental is "superior") while in a non-inferiority framework the alternative hypothesis states that the experimental arm is no worse than the control by a pre-specified margin. The possible interpretation of trial results is predicated on the study design, as shown in Figure 30.3. The choice of superiority as compared to a non-inferiority design is influenced by a number of factors including cost, existing therapies, and side effect profiles of different treatments. Novel oral anticoagulants (NOACs), for example, require less monitoring than conventional anticoagulation with oral vitamin K antagonists. Demonstration of non-inferiority, therefore, may be sufficient evidence to choose a NOAC as was shown in the large randomized ROCKET-AF trial comparing rivoraxaban to warfarin. In addition, the great efficacy of certain treatments can require prohibitively large and expensive trials designed to show superiority.

Intention to treat and per-protocol analyses
Most major trials use *analysis by intention to treat* whereby all patients are included in their randomized groups even though they did not all fully comply with the intended treatments. Such an analysis gives an unbiased comparison of the treatment policies as they were delivered in practice, a so-called *pragmatic trial*. *Per protocol analyses,* which exclude any patient follow-up when not on

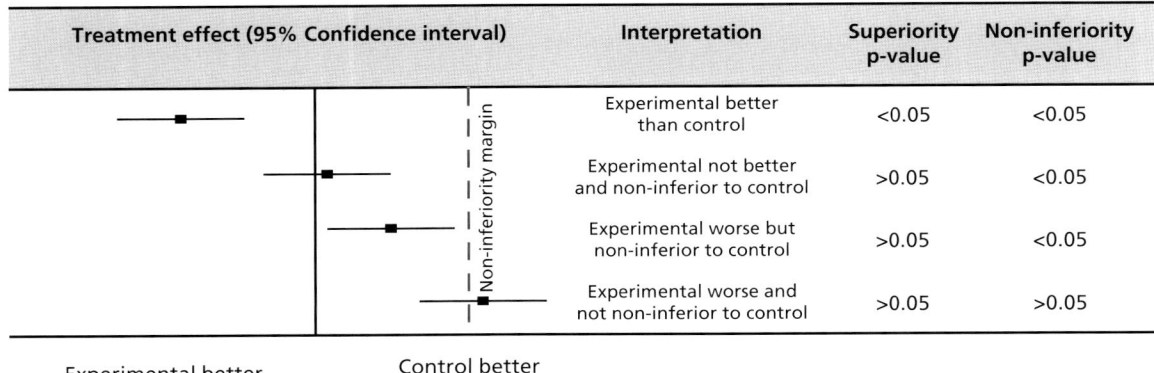

Figure 30.3 Example of the most common trial type, including superiority and non-inferiority designs. The possible interpretation of trial results is predicated on the study design.

randomized treatment, are potentially biased as it could be the sicker patients who opt out.

Reporting of trial findings in medical journals, at conference presentations, and to regulatory authorities need to be of the highest standards whereby an unbiased and detailed report of all relevant findings is presented.

The objectives, methods, discussion, and conclusions need to be clearly presented in a balanced report. In particular, results and interpretations should include any safety issues (adverse events) as well as efficacy findings. For publications in medical journals, the CONSORT guidelines are helpful to authors, editors, referees, and readers in enhancing the quality assessment of any trial report.

Interactive multiple choice questions are available for this chapter on www.wiley.com/go/dangas/cardiology

Historical Perspective of Sirolimus and Paclitaxel-Eluting Stent Clinical Studies

Adriano Caixeta[1], Leonardo Guimarães[1], Philippe Généreux[2], and George D. Dangas[3]

[1] Hospital Israelita Albert Einstein; Universidade Federal de São Paulo, São Paulo, Brazil
[2] Columbia University Medical Center, New York, NY, USA
[3] Department of Cardiology, Mount Sinai Medical Center, New York, NY, USA

Over the past decades, the field of percutaneous coronary intervention (PCI) has been rapidly evolving since the first balloon angioplasty in 1977. Bare metal stents (BMS) were developed and significantly improved the acute success and reproducibility of PCI results compared to balloon angioplasty [1,2]. However, stent-mediated arterial injury elicited neointimal hyperplasia, leading to restenosis and the need for repeat revascularization in about one-third of patients [3–6]. Drug-eluting stents (DES) with antiproliferative drugs attached via polymer on the stent surface were developed as a logical next step in the evolution of PCI. These devices were designed to maintain the mechanical advantages of BMS over stand-alone balloon angioplasty, while releasing antiproliferative agents directly to the arterial wall to combat the neointimal hyperplasia occurring after conventional BMS placement. First-generation DES including sirolimus and paclitaxel have shown clear evidence of clinical success with the application of the right dose and release kinetics. This chapter discusses the clinical data on sirolimus and paclitaxel-eluting stents from pivotal trial to multivessel disease treatment, focusing on their historical contribution to interventional cardiology.

Initial studies of first-generation DES

In 2003, the Food and Drug Administration (FDA) approved the use of the two first-generation DES: the CYPHER sirolimus-eluting stent (SES; Cordis Corporation, Johnson & Johnson, Miami Lakes, FL), and the TAXUS paclitaxel-eluting stent (PES; Boston Scientific Corporation, Maple Grove, MN). The FDA decision was based on the results of pivotal randomized clinical trials comparing a given DES with a comparator BMS in relatively non-complex lesions that constitute the "on-label" indications for DES use. In these early trials, the use of DES was demonstrated to reduce restenosis and repeat revascularization rates by 50–90% compared to BMS across all lesion and patients subsets [7].

In addition, DES has shown benefits with respect to reduced repeat revascularization and other restenosis-related endpoints in more complex lesions, including acute myocardial infarction (MI), chronic total occlusions, in-stent restenosis, diffuse disease, saphenous vein grafts, and bifurcation lesions [8–13]. In fact, given the observed relative reductions in restenosis-related endpoints with DES, it follows that as the overall (absolute) risk of restenosis rises—as is observed with more complex lesion subsets—the absolute benefit of DES over BMS should increase. Thus, confidence in DES subsequently swelled, and as positive results from subsequent trials for a variety of expanded indications surfaced, physicians rapidly expanded the patient populations treated with DES to include other "off-label" indications. In the years immediately after DES approval, "off-label" use of these devices was estimated to occur in up to 65% of cases [14,15].

Paclitaxel-eluting stent

Paclitaxel was approved by the FDA in 1992 as an antineoplastic agent to treat metastatic ovarian malignancies. Paclitaxel is a natural diterpenoid extracted from the bark, roots, and leaves of several Taxus species, including *Taxus brevifolia* and *Taxus media*. Its effect has been mainly explained by its ability to stabilize microtubules and thereby inhibit cell division in the G0/G1 and G2/M phases [16]. Several studies have shown that paclitaxel inhibits the development of neointimal hyperplasia in different *in vitro* and in animal models of restenosis [17–20].

Overview of the TAXUS clinical trials

The safety and efficacy of the polymer-based paclitaxel-eluting TAXUS stent system have been investigated in six studies: TAXUS I [21], TAXUS II [22], TAXUS III [23], TAXUS IV [24,25], TAXUS V *de novo* [8], and TAXUS VI [26]. All studies, with the exception of TAXUS III, were randomized, double-blind, multicenter investigations that compared the paclitaxel-eluting Taxus™ stent with BMS. TAXUS III was an open-label investigation. Primary endpoints varied by study and included one or more of the following: 30-day major adverse cardiac events (MACE) (TAXUS I and TAXUS III), 6-month in-stent volume obstruction caused by neointimal proliferation (TAXUS II), and 9-month ischemia driven target vessel revascularization (TVR) (TAXUS IV, TAXUS V *de novo*, and TAXUS VI).

TAXUS I enrolled 61 patients and was a feasibility study designed to assess the safety of Taxus™ slow-release vs. BMS. At 12 months, the MACE rates were 10% and 3% in the control and Taxus™ groups, respectively, demonstrating excellent long-term safety. These results

Interventional Cardiology: Principles and Practice, Second Edition. Edited by George D. Dangas, Carlo Di Mario, and Nicholas N. Kipshidze.
© 2017 John Wiley & Sons, Ltd. Published 2017 by John Wiley & Sons, Ltd.

were maintained through the 4-year follow-up with no new MACE in any TAXUS patient between 1 and 4 years.

TAXUS II studied 536 patients in 38 sites in a randomized, double-blind, controlled study of the safety and efficacy of the Taxus stent system on the NIRx stent platform. In this study, two sequential cohorts (testing slow and moderate-release TAXUS formulations) enrolled patients with standard risk de novo coronary artery lesions. The 6-month results showed strong clinical performance as demonstrated by lower MACE and target lesion revascularization (TLR) rates in TAXUS patients compared with patients who received a BMS. The 6-month MACE rates were reduced from 19.8% in the control group to 8.5% for the slow-release formulation cohort (p = 0.0035) and 7.8% for the moderate-release formulation cohort (p = 0.0019). At 12 months, the MACE rate in the slow-release cohort remained low at 10.9% compared with the control rate of 21.7% (p = 0.0082) and the TLR rate was 4.7% compared with 14.4% for the control group (p = 0.0035). At 12 months, the moderate-release formulation cohort reported a 9.9% MACE rate (p = 0.0048 vs. control) with a 3.8% TLR rate (p = 0.0010 vs. control). The 3-year follow-up for TAXUS II results were maintained with no new TLR or stent thrombosis occurring in the TAXUS groups.

TAXUS III was a single-arm registry examining the feasibility of implanting Taxus stent for the treatment of in-stent restenosis. The trial enrolled 29 patients, of whom 28 were treated with the Taxus NIRx stent platform. The trial confirmed safety and reported no stent thrombosis, no deaths, and a binary restenosis rate of 16% at 6 months. From 6 months to 3 years, there was only one cardiac death and no stent thrombosis.

Similarly, in the large randomized TAXUS IV trial, randomizing 1314 patients with single de novo non-complex coronary lesions, the 9-month rate of ischemia-driven TVR was 4.7% with PES vs. 12.0% with BMS, again a highly significant difference with similar relative effects observed across all subgroups [25].

TAXUS V was a randomized, double-blind trial studying 1156 patients at 66 sites in the USA using the slow-release formulation (Express² stent platform). TAXUS V expanded on the TAXUS IV pivotal trial by studying a higher risk patient population, including patients with small vessels, and long lesions requiring multiple overlapping stents—the most challenging lesions and highest risk patients ever studied in a randomized controlled DES trial in the USA. The primary endpoint of the trial was 9-month TVR, which was significantly lower in the TAXUS group (12.1%) than in the control group (17.3%; p = 0.0184). At 9 months, the overall MACE rate in the TAXUS group was 15.0%, compared with 21.2% in the control group (p = 0.0084). The study also reported a TLR rate of 8.6% in the Taxus™ cohort compared with 15.7% in the control group (p = 0.0003). In addition, stent thrombosis rates were identical between Taxus™ and control group stents (0.7% each). These clinical benefits were maintained at 1 year with an overall MACE rate of 18.9% in the TAXUS group compared to 25.9% in the control group (p = 0.0052) and a TLR rate of 11.2% in the TAXUS group vs. 19.0% in the control group (p = 0.0003).

TAXUS VI, an international trial studying 446 patients with complex coronary artery disease at 44 sites, was designed to establish the safety and efficacy of the moderate-release formulation (on the Express² stent platform) in the treatment of longer lesions. The trial had a primary endpoint of 9-month TVR. The study's TVR rate was 9.1% in the TAXUS group vs. the control group rate of 19.4% at 9 months (p = 0.0027). Additionally, the Taxus™ group had a TLR rate of 6.8% (compared with 18.9% in the control group; p = 0.0001) and an in-segment binary restenosis rate of 12.4% (compared with 35.7% in the control group; p < 0.0001). The results sup-

ported safety as demonstrated by low MACE rates (16.4% MACE rate at 9 months in the TAXUS group compared with 22.5% in the control group; p = 0.1208). The 2-year follow-up data for TAXUS VI demonstrated that the safety and efficacy benefits associated with a moderate-release formulation of the Taxus™ were maintained at 2 years; a continued significant reduction in TLR rate (9.7% for the TAXUS group, as compared with 21.0% for the control group; p = 0.0013). Stent thromboses remained low and comparable to control rates (0.9% for both the Taxus™ group and the control group). The 2-year results for TAXUS VI support long-term safety with increased local exposure of the vessel to paclitaxel released from the moderate-release formulation compared to the levels released from the slow-release formulation. Even with an *in vitro* dosing rate 8–10 times greater than the commercialized slow-release formulation, no compromise in safety was observed.

Longer-term data from the five pivotal PES trials, including 3513 patients, has been reported; these data demonstrate durable reductions in clinical restenosis endpoints with similar overall safety for Taxus™ vs. BMS (Figure 31.1) [24]. The cumulative incidence of stent thrombosis was similar between Taxus™ and BMS (2.1% vs. 1.7%; p = 0.46). Subgroup analyses also demonstrated a similar relative benefit of Taxus™ vs. BMS for diabetics, and all vessel sizes (Figure 31.2). In brief, this patient-level meta-analysis

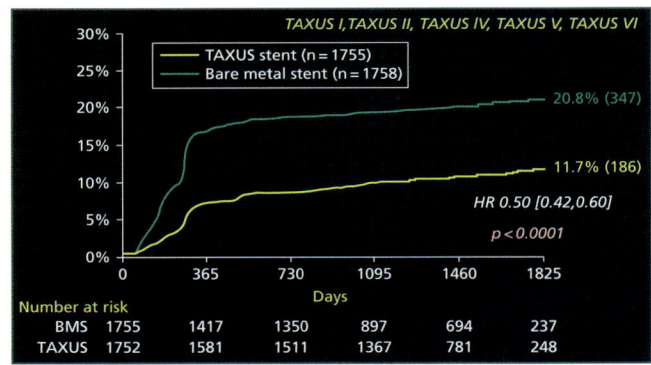

Figure 31.1 Pooled analysis from five TAXUS randomized clinical trials. Kaplan–Meier curves of cumulative rates of target vessel revascularization comparing Taxus™ stent with bare metal stent (BMS).

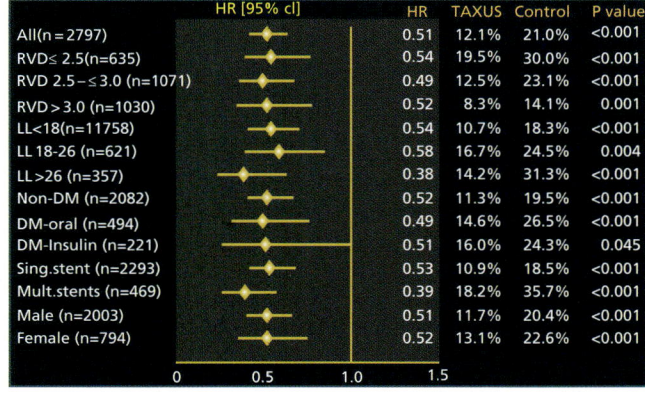

Figure 31.2 Target lesion revascularization up to 5-year follow-up. Subgroup analysis summary from 5 TAXUS pivotal randomized clinical trial. Subgroup analysis shows relative benefit of Taxus™ vs. BMS for diabetics, all vessel sizes and all lesion length.

from the five principal TAXUS trials concluded that at 3–5 year follow-up, polymer-based PES compared to BMS stents result in:

1 No significant differences in death or MI;
2 No significant increase in stent thrombosis;
3 No significant increase in late stent thrombosis by Academic Research Consortium (ARC) definitions; and
4 Sustained reduction in target lesion and TVR.

Sirolimus-eluting stent

First FDA approved in 1999 as prophylaxis for kidney transplant rejection, sirolimus is a macrolytic lactone produced by *Streptomyces hygroscopicus*. The primary mechanism of action of sirolimus's inhibition of neointimal hyperplasia is probably related to its ability to bind to FK binding protein-12 (FKBP-12) in cells; this complex binds to and inhibits activation of the mammalian target of rapamycin (mTOR), preventing progression in the cell cycle form the G1 phase to the S phase [27]. Its anti-inflammatory and antiproliferative properties reduce smooth muscle cell proliferation in the arterial wall following stent-induced injury [28,29]. With the low-release formulation of the Cypher™, 50% of the drug is released in the first 2 weeks and most of the sirolimus is released within 4 weeks after stent implantation.

Overview of the Cypher® clinical trials

Following the success of the first pilot study of the SES in 45 patients for suppressing intimal hyperplasia [30,31], the safety and efficacy of the polymer-based sirolimus-eluting Cypher® stent system have been investigated in four major studies: RAVEL [32], SIRIUS [33], E-SIRIUS [34], and C-SIRIUS [35].

The RAVEL trial, a randomized trial of 238 patients, compared SES with a standard BMS in patients with angina pectoris. At 6-month angiographic follow-up, the in-stent late luminal loss was significantly lower in the SES group (−0.01 ± 0.33 mm) than in the standard stent group (0.80 ± 0.53 mm; p <0.001), with a remarkable reduction in the rate of restenosis (0% vs. 26.6%; p <0.001). The rate of MACE, a composite of death, MI, coronary artery bypass grafting (CABG), or TVR at 1 year was 5.8% for SES-treated patients vs. 28.8% for BMS-treated patients (p <0.001), mostly driven by a higher rate of revascularization of the target vessel in the standard stent group. At 3-year follow-up, these results were maintained, demonstrating a persistent reduction in MACE with SES compared to BMS (15.5% vs. 33.1%; p = 0.002) [36].

The SIRIUS trial, a 1058-patient randomized trial comparing the Cypher® DES to its uncoated BMS, has led to FDA approval of SES in 2003. More complex than in the RAVEL trial, lesion length was 15–30 mm with vessel diameters of 2.5–3.5 mm. Both the primary endpoint, the rate of target vessel failure (a composite of cardiac death, MI, or revascularization of the target vessel) and the rate of MACE at 9 months was markedly lower among SES-treated patients (8.6% vs. 21.0%; p <0.001 and 7.1% vs. 18.9%; p <0.001, respectively). The benefit of SES was observed in all tested subgroups in the trial, including diabetic patients, and irrespective of vessel size. Additionally, longer term follow-up from SIRIUS has also demonstrated a persistently maintained benefit of SES over BMS, with 5-year rates of target vessel failure of 22.5% vs. 34.7% (p <0.0001) and MACE of 20.3% vs. 33.5% (p <0.0001), respectively [37].

Performed in Canada and Europe, C-SIRIUS and E-SIRIUS have shown similar results to the SIRIUS study. In these trials, the overall rate of angiographic restenosis was markedly lower with SES than BMS (in-stent: 3.1% vs. 42.7%; p <0.001; in-segment: 5.1% vs. 44.2%;

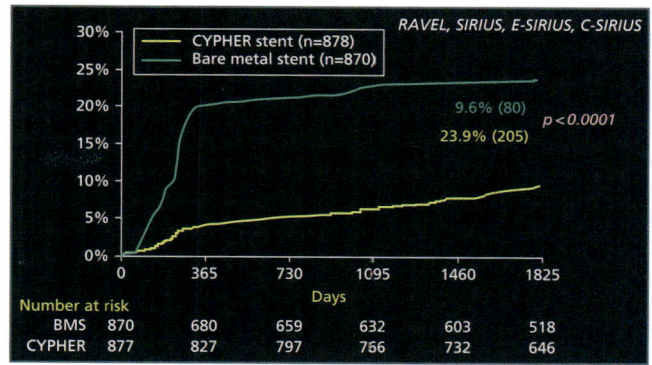

Figure 31.3 Pooled analysis from four Cypher® randomized clinical trials. Kaplan–Meier curves of cumulative rates of target vessel revascularization comparing Cypher® stent with BMS.

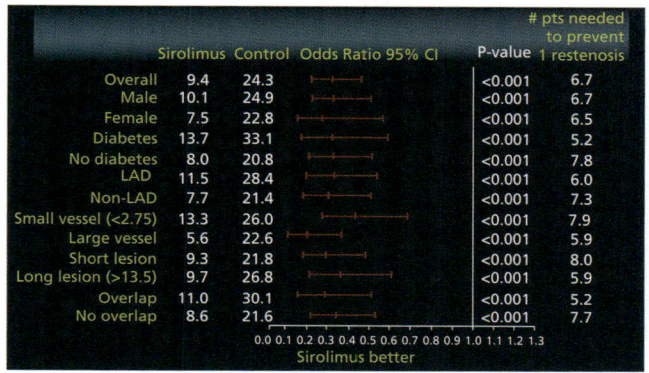

Figure 31.4 Target lesion revascularization up to 5-year follow-up. Subgroup analysis from four Cypher® randomized clinical trials. Subgroup analysis shows relative benefit of Cypher® vs. BMS for diabetics and vessel sizes, and all lesion length.

p < 0.001). Reductions in MACE with the use of SES compared to BMS were also observed. A pooled analysis at 2-year follow-up of the three SIRIUS studies has shown significant reductions in MACE (10.6% vs. 26.3%; p < 0.001) with SES compared to BMS [38].

Longer term data from the four pivotal SES trials, including 1748 patients, has been reported; these data demonstrate durable reductions in clinical restenosis endpoints with similar overall safety for Cypher® vs. BMS (Figure 31.3) [39]. The cumulative incidence of stent thrombosis was similar with Cypher® and BMS (2.1% vs. 2.0%; p = 0.99). Subgroup analyses from the 5-year follow-up of the SIRIUS study also demonstrated a similar relative benefit of Cypher® vs. BMS for diabetics and all vessel sizes (Figure 31.4). From this independent, patient-level meta-analysis from the four principal Cypher® trials it may be concluded that at 5-year follow-up of patients with single de novo native coronary lesions 2.5–3.5 mm in diameter and ≤30 mm in length, polymer-based SES compared to otherwise equivalent BMS result in:

1 No significant differences in death or MI;
2 No significant increase in stent thrombosis;
3 No significant increase in late stent thrombosis by ARC definitions; and
4 Sustained reduction in target lesion and TVR.

Acute myocardial infarction

The use of DES in acute MI has been studied in both observational registries as well as in randomized clinical trials. In a recent meta-analysis of eight randomized trials in 2786 patients with a follow-up of up to 24 months, the use of first-generation DES compared to BMS was associated with a significantly reduced risk of reintervention, without any difference in the rate of death, recurrent MI, and stent thrombosis [40]. First-generation DES have shown to decrease significantly the TLR and repeat revascularization at 2 years with a significant decrease of the 2-year risk-adjusted mortality rate [41]. These data are quite reassuring regarding the safety of use of DES in acute coronary syndrome.

The TYPHOON trial, a randomized trial of in 712 patients, compared SES with BMS in patients undergoing primary PCI. This study has shown a significant reduction in MACE in favor of the SES treatment (5.6% vs. 13.4% with BMS; p <0.001), largely driven by a lower rate of TVR [10]. At 8 months, angiographic follow-up demonstrated reductions in late loss and restenosis among patients treated with SES. No differences between the two groups were seen in term of rates of death, recurrent MI, and stent thrombosis.

In the SESAMI trial of 320 patients, treatment with SES was associated with a lower rate of restenosis (9.3% vs. 21.3%; p = 0.032) and with a reduction in TLV and MACE [42]. In the MISSION! trial, a randomized trial of SES vs. BMS in 310 patients undergoing primary PCI, treatment with SES was associated with a lower in-segment late luminal loss at 9 months (0.68 ± 0.57 mm vs. 0.12 ± 0.43 mm) and a lower TLV rate (3.2% vs. 11.3%; p = 0.006) [43]. Rates of death, MI, and stent thrombosis were not different. However, IVUS study shows that late stent malapposition at 9 months was present in 12.5% of BMS patients and in 37.5% of SES patients (p <0.001), raising concern about the long-term safety of SES in patients with ST-elevation MI (STEMI). However, the PASSION trial, a randomized trial of PES vs. BMS in 619 patients undergoing primary PCI, treatment with PES was associated with a non-significant trend in the rate of death from cardiac causes or recurrent MI (5.5% vs. 7.2%; p = 0.40) and in the rate of TLV (5.3% vs. 7.8%; p = 0.23) [9]. There was a trend toward a lower rate of serious adverse events in the PES group than in the uncoated-stent group (8.8% vs. 12.8%; p = 0.09).

The Harmonizing Outcomes with Revascularization and Stents in Acute Myocardial Infarction (HORIZONS AMI) trial [44] randomized 3602 patients from 123 centers in 11 countries. All patients had STEMI with a symptom onset of less than 12 hours. Patients were first randomized in a 1 : 1 fashion to unfractionated heparin plus a glycoprotein (GP) IIb/IIIa inhibitor (abciximab or eptifibatide) or to bivalirudin monotherapy plus provisional GP IIb/IIIa inhibitors. The implantation of the paclitaxel-eluting Taxus™ stent compared with the BMS Express™ stent resulted in a significant 41% reduction at 1 year in the primary efficacy endpoint of ischemia-driven TLR (4.5% vs. 7.5%, HR 0.59, 95% CI 0.43–0.83) and a significant 56% (10.0% vs. 22.9%, HR 0.44, 95% CI 0.33–0.57) reduction in the major secondary efficacy endpoint of binary restenosis. MACE, a composite of all-cause mortality, reinfarction, stroke, and stent thrombosis, were equivalent with the two stents (8.1% vs. 8.0%, HR 1.02, 95% CI 0.76–1.36). At 3 years, compared with 1802 patients allocated to receive heparin plus a GP inhibitor, 1800 patients allocated to bivalirudin monotherapy had lower rates of all-cause mortality (5.9% vs. 7.7%; p = 0.03), cardiac mortality (2.9% vs. 5.1%; p = 0.001), reinfarction (6.2% vs. 8.2%; p = 0.04), and major bleeding not related to bypass graft surgery (6.9% vs. 10.5%, p = 0.0001), with no significant differences in ischemia-driven TVR, stent thrombosis, or composite adverse events. Compared

with 749 patients who received BMS, 2257 patients who received a PES had lower rates of ischemia-driven TLR (9.4% vs. 15.1%; p <0.0001) after 3 years, with no significant differences in the rates of death, reinfarction, stroke, or stent thrombosis. Stent thrombosis was high (≥4.5%) in both groups [45,46]. Combining the HORIZONS study with other registries and randomized trials increases the number of patients with MI treated with DES and provides reassurances about efficacy and safety of DES in this clinical setting [47]. Currently, novel generation of DES implantation is the default therapy for patients with STEMI [48].

Multivessel disease

Patients with complex multivessel coronary disease represent a high risk subgroup of patients for PCI. Three randomized trials have compared first-generation DES with CABG, which comprises the main data in recent guidelines on myocardial revascularization [49,50].

The Coronary Artery Revascularization in Diabetes (CARDia) study [51] enrolled 510 patients in a randomized trial from 24 centers in the UK and Ireland, to compare the safety and efficacy of PCI with stenting against CABG in patients with diabetes and symptomatic multivessel coronary artery disease. This trial initially began using BMS, but when DES became available patients received Cypher™ stents. Cypher™ stents were used in 69% of patients and BMS in 31% patients undergoing PCI. A total of 254 patients were randomized for CABG and 256 for PCI, and at 1 year follow-up the composite rate of death, MI, and stroke was 10.5% in the CABG group and 13% in the PCI group (HR 1.25, 95% CI 0.752.09), and repeat revascularization rates of 2.0% and 11,8%, respectively. There was no difference in all-cause mortality rates. The CARDia study was the first trial of coronary ravascularization in diabetic patients but did not show that PCI was non-inferior to CABG for a period of up to 5 years.

The Future Revascularization Evaluation in Patients with Diabetes Mellitus: Optimal Management of Multivessel Disease (FREEDOM) trial [52] enrolled 1900 patients with multivessel coronary artery disease (mean SYNTAX score: 26.2 ± 8.6) and diabetes; these patients were randomized 1 : 1 to CABG or PCI and followed for a minimum of 2 years. In the PCI group, Cypher and Taxus stents were used in 51% and 43% of patients, respectively. At 30 days, the primary outcome (composite of death from any cause, non-fatal MI, or non-fatal stroke) occurred in fewer patients in the PCI group than in the CABG group. However, 5-year events rate were 26.6% in the PCI group and 18.7% in CABG group (95% CI 3.3–12.5). Five year rates of all-cause mortality were 16.3% in the PCI group versus 10.9% in the CABG group (p = 0.049), MI also statistically differed favoring CABG group with 13.9% in PCI group and 6.0% in the CABG group. There were fewer strokes in the PCI group (2.4% vs. 5.2%; p = 0.03). In summary, the FREEDOM trial found that CABG was superior to PCI in patients with diabetes and advanced coronary artery disease. CABG was associated with significantly reduced risks of death and MI but a higher risk of stroke during the 5-year study (Figure 31.5). The results in favor of CABG were consistent across all the prespecified subgroups, including severity of disease as assessed by the SYNTAX score (Figure 31.6).

Synergy between PCI with Taxus and Cardiac Surgery (SYNTAX) trial was a prospective multicenter study, which randomized 1800 patients with three-vessel or left main coronary artery disease to undergo CABG (897 patients) or PCI with Taxus stent (903 patients). At 1 year, the rate of primary endpoint was higher in the PCI group than the CABG group (17.8% vs. 12.4%; p = 0.002), mainly because of higher rates of repeat revascularization in the

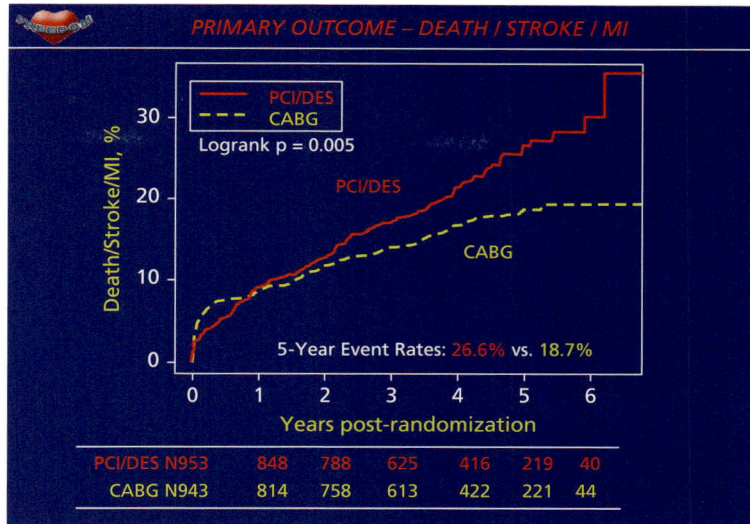

Figure 31.5 FREEDOM study. Kaplan–Meier estimates of the composite primary outcome of death, myocardial infarction (MI), or stroke truncated at 5 years after randomization.

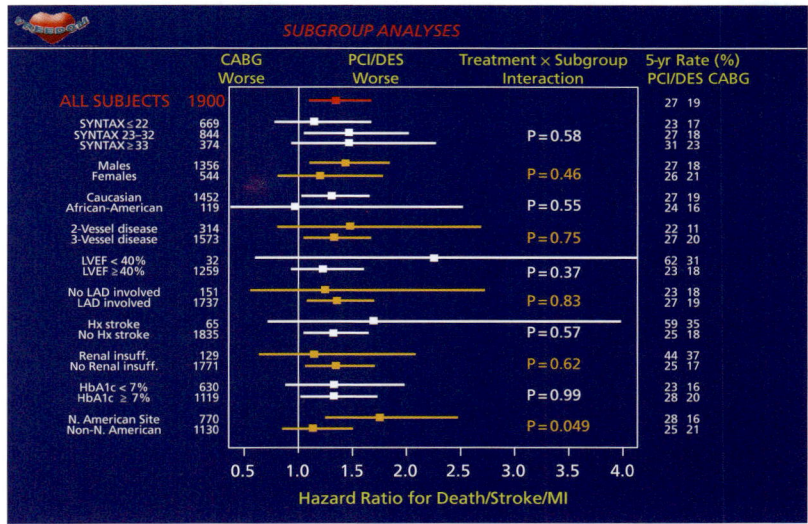

Figure 31.6 FREEDOM study. Primary composite outcome according to subgroup. Five-year composite event rates for death, myocardial infarction, or stroke are shown. LAD, left anterior descending artery; LVEF, left ventricular ejection fraction.

stent group (13.5% vs. 5.9%). Patients were stratified into three groups: low SYNTAX scores (0–22), intermediate scores (23–32), and high scores (≥32). The rate of primary endpoint in the stent group was similar to that in surgery group in patients with low complexity of disease (SYNTAX score ≤22; 32,1% vs. 28.6%, respectively; p = 0.43). The benefit of CABG emerged among patients with intermediate (SYNTAX score 23–32; 36% vs. 25.8%; p = 0.008) or high disease complexity (SYNTAX ≥33; 44% vs. 26.8%; p = 0.001) [53]. Based on these findings, CABG remains the standard treatment for patients with multivessel artery disease [54]. After 5 years' follow-up, Kaplan–Meier estimates of major adverse cardiac or cerebrovascular events (MACCE) were 26.9% in the CABG group and 37.3% in the PCI group (p <0.0001). Estimates of MI (3.8% in the CABG group vs. 9.7% in the PCI group; p <0.0001) and repeat revasculari-

zation (13.7% vs. 25.9%; p <0.0001) were significantly increased with PCI versus CABG. All-cause death (11.4% in the CABG group vs. 13.9% in the PCI group; p = 0.10) and stroke (3.7% vs. 2.4%; p = 0.09) were not significantly different between groups. In the CABG group, 28.6% of patients with low SYNTAX scores had MACCE versus 32.1% of patients in the PCI group (p = 0.43); however, in patients with intermediate or high SYNTAX scores MACCE was significantly increased with PCI (intermediate score, 25.8% of the CABG group vs. 36.0% of the PCI group; p = 0.008; high score, 26.8% vs. 44.0%; p <0.0001) (Figures 31.7, 31.8, 31.9 and 31.10).

From this independent large-scale trial it can be concluded that at 5-year follow-up of patients with multivessel disease that CABG should remain the standard of care for patients with complex lesions (high or intermediate SYNTAX scores). For patients with less complex disease

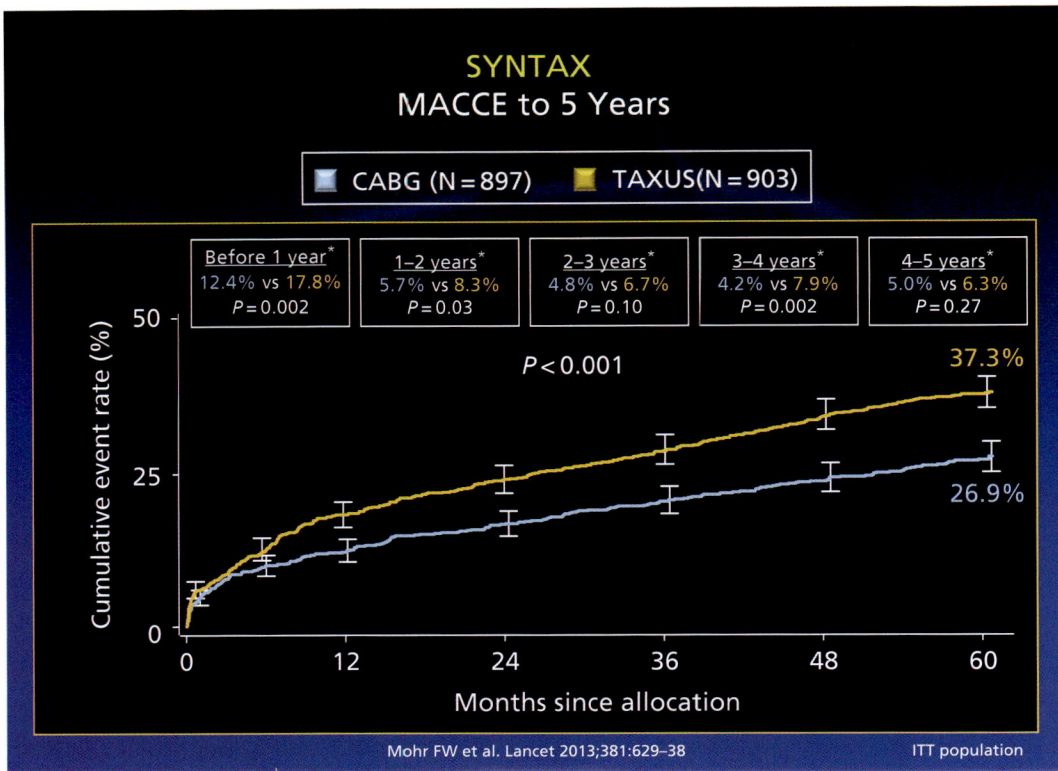

Figure 31.7 SYNTAX trial. Kaplan–Meier estimates of major adverse cardiac or cerebrovascular events (MACCE) at 5-year follow-up in the overall population.

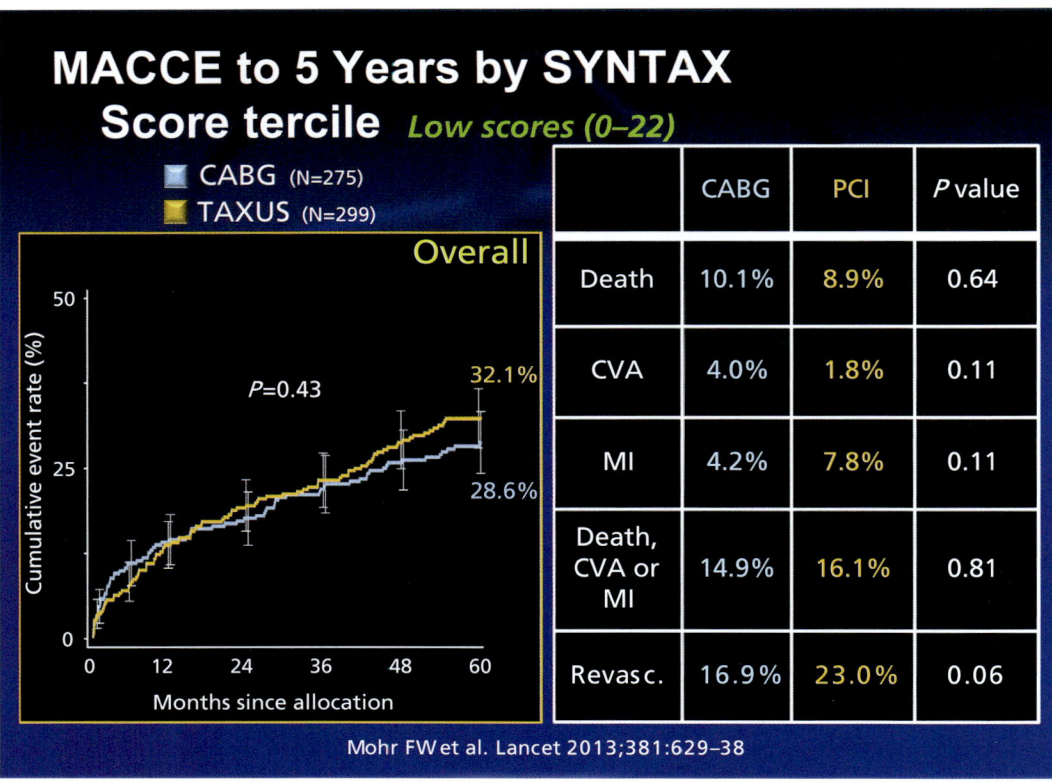

Figure 31.8 SYNTAX trial. Kaplan–Meier estimates of MACCE at 5-year follow-up in patients with lower SYNTAX score.

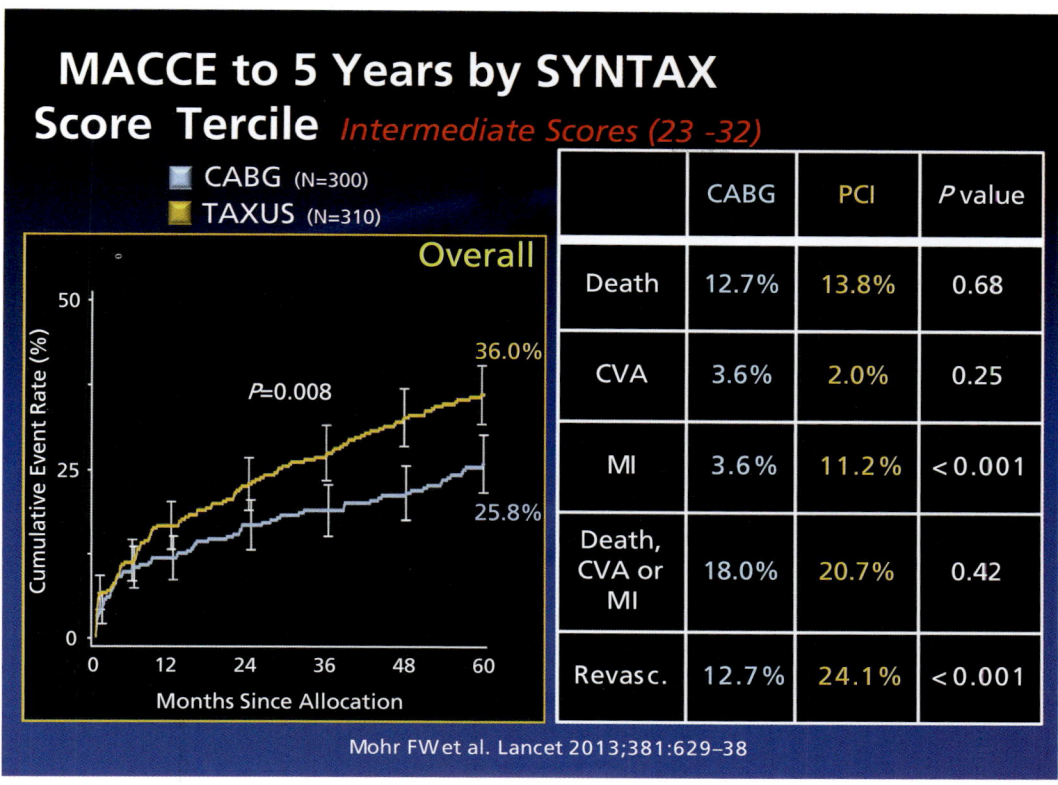

Figure 31.9 SYNTAX trial. Kaplan–Meier estimates of MACCE at 5-year follow-up in patients with intermediate SYNTAX score.

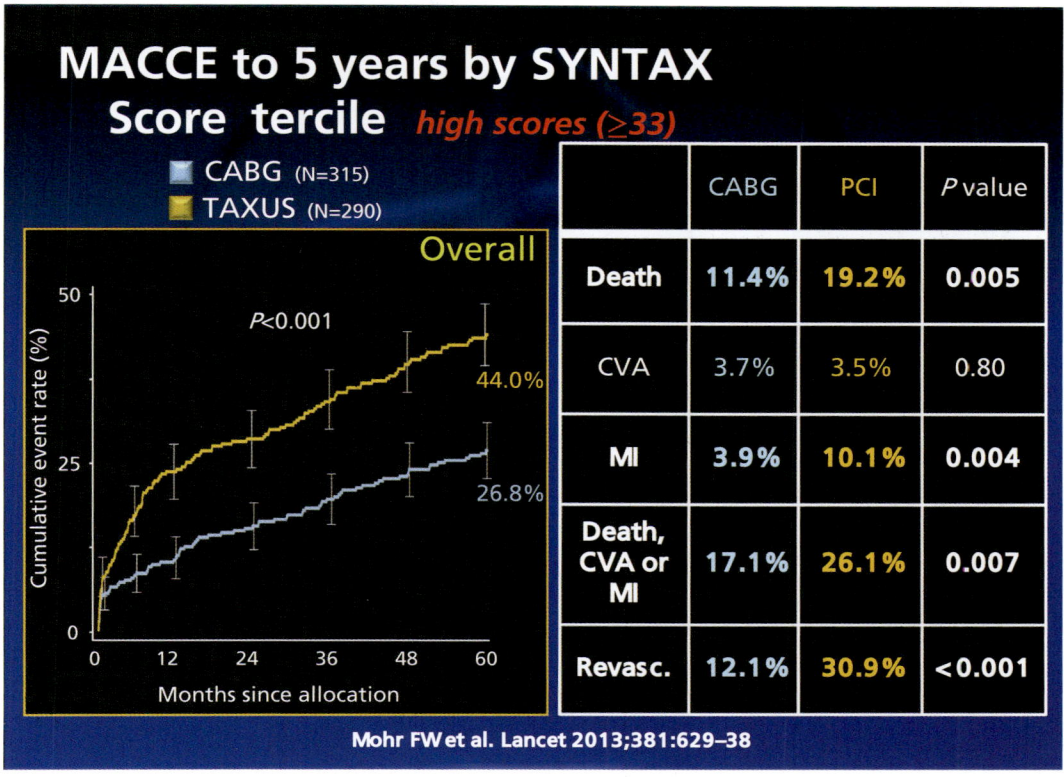

Figure 31.10 SYNTAX trial. Kaplan–Meier estimates of MACCE at 5-year follow-up in patients with higher SYNTAX score.

(low SYNTAX scores) or left main coronary disease (low or intermediate SYNTAX scores), PCI is an acceptable alternative. Notwithstanding, all patients with complex multivessel coronary artery disease should be reviewed by both a cardiac surgeon and an interventional cardiologist to reach consensus on optimum treatment [55].

Left main coronary artery disease

CABG is considered as the treatment of choice for unprotected left main coronary artery stenosis, although PCI can be an acceptable alternative in some patients with left main stenosis.

The Premier of Randomized Comparison of Bypass Surgery versus Angioplasty Using Sirolimus-Eluting Stent in Patients with Left Main Coronary Artery Disease (PRECOMBAT), a prospective, open-label trial, randomized 600 patients to PCI with SES (300 patients) or to CABG (300 patients). The primary endpoint of MACCE after 1 year occurred in 26 patients in the PCI group and 20 patients in the CABG group. In the PRECOMBAT trial, PCI with Cypher stents were shown to be non-inferior to CABG in patients with left main coronary artery disease with respect to the composite endpoint of death, MI, stroke or TVR at 1 year [56]. At 5 years, MACCE occurred in 52 patients in the PCI group and 42 patients in the CABG group (cumulative event rates of 17.5% and 14.3%; p=0.26). The two groups did not differ significantly in terms of death from any cause, MI, or stroke as well as their composite (8.4% and 9.6%; p=0.66). Ischemia-driven TVR occurred more frequently in the PCI group than in the CABG group (11.4% and 5.5%; p=0.012).

In the SYNTAX trial, unprotected left main cohort (n=705) was predefined and powered. The MACCE rate at 5 years was 36.9% in PCI patients and 31.0% in CABG patients (p=0.12). The mortality rate was 12.8% and 14.6% in PCI and CABG patients, respectively (p=0.53). Stroke was significantly increased in the CABG group (PCI 1.5% vs. CABG 4.3%; p=0.03) and repeat revascularization in the PCI arm (26.7% vs. 15.5%; p <0.01). MACCE events were similar between arms in patients with low–intermediate SYNTAX scores but significantly increased in PCI patients with high scores (≥33) [57].

Randomized trials, meta-analyses, and registries

Five-year follow-up data from the pivotal randomized trials has demonstrated durable and sustained reductions in TLR and TVR with both first-generation DES compared with BMS, with no significant differences in endpoints such as death, MI, or stent thrombosis [39]. These findings have been paralleled in meta-analyses of randomized trials comparing DES with BMS including not only the pivotal trials, but also trials for a variety of other indications, including acute MI [40,58].

One of the most extensive meta-analyses to date comparing BMS with DES included 38 trials, a total of 18,023 patients, at a follow-up of up to 4 years [59]. There was no significant difference in overall or cardiac mortality in this analysis between BMS, SES, or PES. Moreover, both SES and PES had significantly lower rates of repeat TLR than BMS. While SES was associated with lower rates of MI when compared with both BMS and PES, the number of patients needed to treat to prevent one MI event was about 100, which did not impact overall or cardiac mortality. With regard to stent thrombosis, there were no differences between BMS, SES, or PES with respect to overall stent thrombosis. Interestingly, there was trend of late temporal separation, suggesting that BMS had a lower incidence of definite stent thrombosis at 4 years. While the reported rate of late stent thrombosis was higher with PES than BMS and SES, wide confidence intervals preclude any definitive conclusions in this regard

(Figure 31.11). Although this large collaborative meta-analysis has clearly demonstrated no worse safety of both first-generation DES (SES and PES) compared to BMS with reductions in revascularization endpoints, head-to-head comparative data of SES with PES

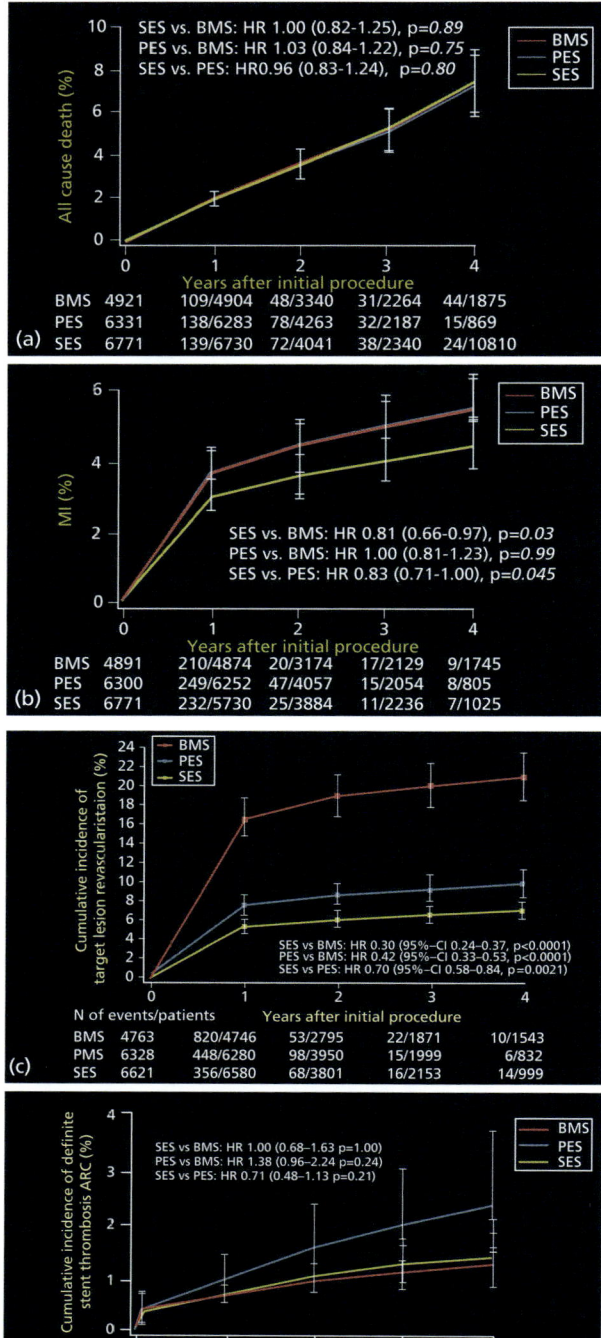

Figure 31.11 Network meta-analyses comparing BMS and drug-eluting stents (DES) included 38 trials, a total of 18,023 patients, at a follow-up of up to 4 years. Kaplan–Meier curve for death (a); myocardial infarction (b); target lesion revascularization (c); and ARC definite stent thrombosis (d).

have been mixed. In a meta-analysis of 16 randomized trials comparing SES with PES including 8695 patients, SES reduced the risk of target lesion and stent thrombosis compared to PES, without significant differences in risk of death or MI [60]. However, in the latest randomized trial comparing SES with PES in 2098 patients, there were no differences between SES and PES in the rate of MACE, defined as cardiac death, MI, TLR, or TVR.

In addition to data from randomized trials and meta-analyses of these trials, there has been a great deal of data presented and published recently from "real-world" registries of first-generation DES use. While a detailed summary of these data is beyond the scope of this review, a brief overview of the types of registry data currently available is instructive, and illustrates both the strengths and weaknesses of these types of analyses.

Most of these observational, non-randomized comparisons of BMS and first-generation DES fall into two types. The first type consists of a comparison between BMS and DES use occurring during two distinct time periods, a period with predominant use of BMS use (before or in the early stages of DES adoption) and a period with predominant DES use. The second type of analysis consists of a comparison between BMS and DES from a single period of concurrent BMS and DES use. Unlike randomized trials, these types of analyses evaluate both BMS and DES use in "real-world" patients, without restrictions of relatively strict patient and lesion inclusion and exclusion criteria. However, both types of analysis are of course observational, and are limited by differences between patients treated with BMS or DES. While the sequential type of comparison attempts to limit selection bias (or decision making swaying the choice of one type of stent over the other), this analysis is subject to bias relating to differences in case selection, adjunctive pharmacology, and procedural factors between two different time periods. Similarly, while the concurrent type of registry may be less subject to these latter biases, selection bias can have a major role in explaining differences between treatment groups. As a result, observational, non-randomized comparisons between treatment groups are extremely valuable, but must be interpreted with caution despite efforts to statistically adjust for baseline differences between comparator groups.

Historically, the majority of registry data comparing first-generation DES with BMS included follow-up of up to 4 years. Consistent with randomized trial data, these registries demonstrate significant reductions in TLV and other clinical endpoints related to restenosis. In addition, with the exception of the original presentation of the Swedish SCAAR registry that demonstrated increased mortality among DES-treated patients, no other registry (including the re-analysis of SCAAR) has demonstrated a statistically detectable increase in mortality or MI with DES compared to BMS [13,61–65]. In fact, the greater part of these registries have demonstrated up to 20% reductions in all-cause mortality with DES compared to BMS even in adjusted analyses.

Additionally, several registries have assessed the risks and benefits of first-generation DES use specifically in "off-label" patients, or patients who would have been excluded from the pivotal DES vs. BMS trials. In a single center registry of 1164 consecutive patients receiving BMS and 1285 consecutive patients receiving DES, the use of DES was associated with lower all-cause mortality (HR 0.72, 95% CI 0.54–0.94), and non-fatal MI or death (HR 0.78, 95% CI 0.62–0.98) compared to BMS in cases of "off-label" stenting. This study demonstrated an elevated risk associated with "off-label" use independent of stent type, but simultaneously demonstrated a greater relative benefit to DES vs. BMS when "off-label" stenting occurs [13]. Although late stent thrombosis occurred with first-generation DES in "off-label" settings, and did not happen with BMS, the relative

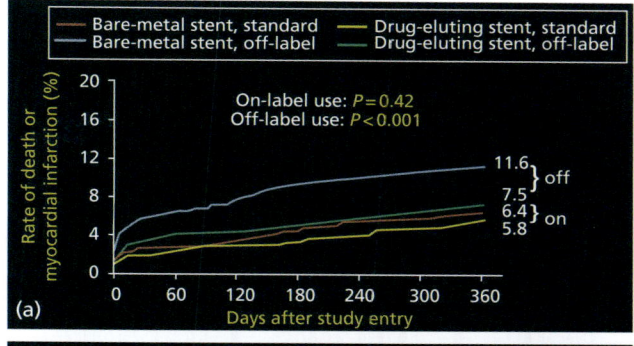

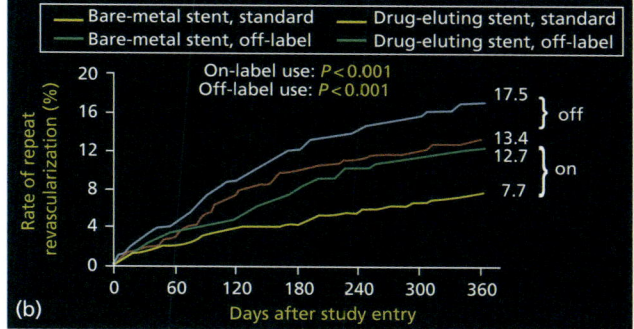

Figure 31.12 NHLBI Registry. Kaplan–Meier curves of death or myocardial infarction (a) and for target vessel revascularization (b) between "on-label" vs. "off-label" use.

benefit of reduced TLV, non-fatal MI, or death, and all-cause mortality would appear to outweigh this risk in "off-label" settings. Similarly, in the NHLBI Dynamic registry, there was no difference in the adjusted risk of death or MI at 1 year associated with "off-label" first-generation DES use compared to BMS use despite a greater prevalence of comorbid conditions among DES-treated patients. Consistent with other randomized trial and registry data, the risk of repeat revascularization was significantly lower with first-generation DES, regardless of the setting (Figure 31.12) [63].

In summary, the preponderance of both randomized and registry data including thousands of patients with follow-up in some cases of up to 5 years, supported the use of first-generation DES in reducing restenosis-related events with no untoward effects related to death or MI, and in fact a possible reduction in mortality observed in registry series.

Finally, in a recent head-to-head comparison of Cypher vs. Taxus, Zhang *et al.* [66] evaluated 76 studies including more than 15,000 patients in randomized controlled trials and over 70,000 patients in adjusted observational studies. At overall-term follow-up, SES significantly reduced TLR (RR 0.61, 95% CI 0.49–0.76), TVR (RR 0.67, 95% CI 0.54–0.83), MACE (RR 0.79, 95% CI 0.72–0.87), MI (RR 0.85, 95% CI 0.73–0.99), in-segment restenosis (RR 0.50. 95% CI 0.38–0.65) in randomized controlled trials compared with PES. In addition, lower rates of death (RR 0.91, 95% CI 0.83–1.00), any stent thrombosis (RR 0.62. 95% CI 0.45–0.86), definite stent thrombosis (RR 0.59; 95% CI 0.45–0.77) were found in patients receiving SES in adjusted observational studies (Figures 31.13 and 31.14). Largely similar results were found at short and long-term follow-up, and in patients with diabetes, acute MI, or long lesions. From this independent meta-analysis the authors concluded that SES significantly reduced the short, long, and overall-term risk of TLR/TVR, MACE, and restenosis, and overall-term risk of MI in randomized controlled trials, compared

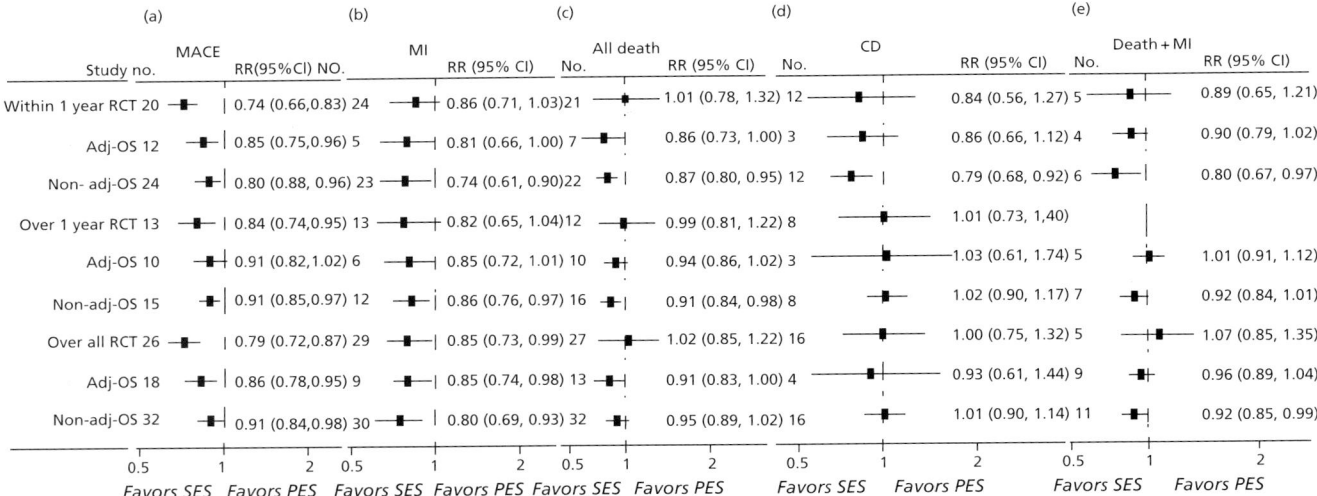

Figure 31.13 Relative risks and 95% confidence intervals of other clinical endpoints associated with SES versus PES. MACE (a), MI (b), all-cause death (c), cardiac death (d), death/MI (e) were evaluated in short-term (≤1 year), long-term (>1 year), and overall-term follow-up. Adj-OS, adjusted observational study; CD, cardiac death; CI, confidence interval; Death + MI, the composite of death and myocardial infarction; MACE, major adverse cardiac event; MI, myocardial infarction; No., number of the studies; Non-adj OS, non-adjusted observational study; PES, paclitaxel-eluting stents; RCT, randomized controlled trial; RR, relative risk; SES, sirolimus-eluting stent. Source: Zhang X, *et al.* 2014. Copyright PLoS One.

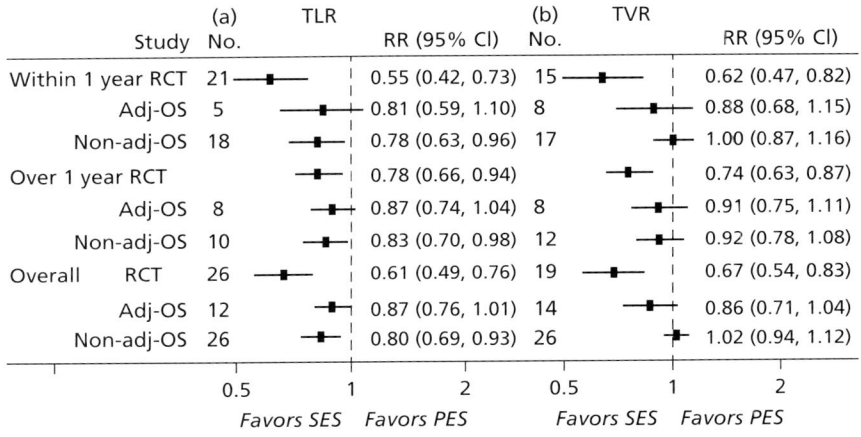

Figure 31.14 Relative rates and 95% confidence intervals of target lesion revascularization (TLR) (a) and target vessel revascularization (TVR) (b) associated with SES versus PES. Short-term (≤1 year), long-term (>1 year), and overall-term TLR and TVR in patients treated with SES versus PES were evaluated. Adj-OS, adjusted observational study; CI, confidence interval; No., number of the studies; Non-adj OS, non-adjusted observational study; PES, paclitaxel-eluting stents; RCT, randomized controlled trial; RR, relative risk; SES, sirolimus-eluting stent; TLR, target lesion revascularization; TVR, target vessel revascularization. Source: Zhang X, *et al.* 2014. Copyright PLoS One.

with PES. Lower rates of death and stent thrombosis were also observed in observational studies in SES-treated patients.

Nevertheless, issues such as incomplete delayed re-endothelialization and neointimal growth, enhanced platelet aggregation and inflammation, late-acquired incomplete stent apposition, and localized hypersensitivity reaction have been observed to occur with both first-generation DES. Novel DES systems have been introduced with the aim to improve outcomes while diminishing adverse events.

Safety concerns with DES and the introduction of novel generation DES

In late 2006, safety concerns were raised about these first-generation DES. Two meta-analyses and a large observational registry study individually suggested increases in adverse clinical endpoints with

DES largely emerging following the first year of stent implantation [67–69]. These initial data, combined with additional data demonstrating that first-generation DES are associated with a small but measurable risk of late stent thrombosis (stent thrombosis occurring beyond 30 days) [70,71], were widely reported in the media and lay press, and generated considerable controversy and concern for patients, physicians, device companies, and regulatory bodies alike.

Data from numerous trials and registries have shown that the overall rate of acute and subacute stent thrombosis appears to be no different for DES or BMS [25,33]. However, in analyses incorporating long-term follow-up, there is a small but finite risk of late stent thrombosis associated with DES use [70,72]. In theory, this occurrence of late stent thrombosis would be expected to increase mortality and non-fatal MI rates for DES-treated patients, but most studies, including meta-analyses inclusive of the early cautionary data, found no differences in death and MI at extended follow-up [58,72]. Moreover, subsequent re-analysis of the large Swedish registry study that initially raised concerns over DES safety with additional follow-up to 4 years and the addition of more patients has demonstrated no differences in hard clinical endpoints between DES and BMS.

As part of interventional cardiology history, there appears to be some consensus that while first-generation DES was likely associated with a slightly increased rate of late stent thrombosis compared to BMS, at least with "on-label" DES use, these risks appeared to be offset by reductions in restenosis-related outcomes, and thus there was no observed increases in hard safety endpoints such as death or MI with the use of first-generation DES compared to BMS. Finally, new generation DES and bioresorbable vascular scaffolds have been introduced in the armamentum of interventional cardiology in recent years; novel generation DES (including everolimus, zotarolimus, and biolimus-eluting stents) have been demonstrated to be safer and more efficacious than first-generation DES and are discussed in other chapters.

Conclusions

Historical approaches to SES and PES development and clinical data are reviewed in this chapter. The first-generation DES has overcome the obstacle of restenosis and consequent need for repeat revascularization over BMS. However, long-term safety issues have arisen. While there was a likely greater risk of late stent thrombosis with first-generation DES, the preponderance of data suggested that they were not associated with increases in death, MI, or other "hard clinical endpoints" compared to BMS, and were durably associated with reductions in restenosis-related endpoints, with potentially even greater absolute benefits (and risks) in "off-label" utilization.

As PCI continues to adapt and evolve, new developments in DES technology are currently in use. Aside from novel-generation stents, a whole host of new DES technologies are currently under active investigation. Bifurcation DES systems, DES with bioresorable polymers, non-polymer DES approaches with surface modification to obviate the use of a polymer, and even wholly bioresorbable vascular scaffolds are all currently in use in clinical practice or are being tested in clinical trials.

References

1 Leon MB, Baim DS, Popma JJ, et al. A clinical trial comparing three antithrombotic-drug regimens after coronary-artery stenting. Stent Anticoagulation Restenosis Study Investigators. *N Engl J Med* 1998; **339**(23): 1665–1671.

2 Serruys PW, de Jaegere P, Kiemeneij F, et al. A comparison of balloon-expandable-stent implantation with balloon angioplasty in patients with coronary artery disease. Benestent Study Group. *N Engl J Med* 1994; **331**(8): 489–495.

3 Serruys PW, Kutryk MJ, Ong AT. Coronary-artery stents. *N Engl J Med* 2006; **354**(5): 483–495.

4 Nayak AK, Kawamura A, Nesto RW, et al. Myocardial infarction as a presentation of clinical in-stent restenosis. *Circ J* 2006; **70**(8): 1026–1029.

5 Chen MS, John JM, Chew DP, et al. Bare metal stent restenosis is not a benign clinical entity. *Am Heart J* 2006; **151**(6): 1260–1264.

6 Schuhlen H, Kastrati A, Mehilli J, et al. Restenosis detected by routine angiographic follow-up and late mortality after coronary stent placement. *Am Heart J* 2004; **147**(2): 317–322.

7 Jeremias A, Kirtane A. Balancing efficacy and safety of drug-eluting stents in patients undergoing percutaneous coronary intervention. *Ann Intern Med* 2008; **148**(3): 234–238.

8 Stone GW, Ellis SG, Cannon L, et al. Comparison of a polymer-based paclitaxel-eluting stent with a bare metal stent in patients with complex coronary artery disease: a randomized controlled trial. *JAMA* 2005; **294**(10): 1215–1223.

9 Laarman GJ, Suttorp MJ, Dirksen MT, et al. Paclitaxeleluting versus uncoated stents in primary percutaneous coronary intervention. *N Engl J Med* 2006; **355**(11): 1105–1113.

10 Spaulding C, Henry P, Teiger E, et al. Sirolimus-eluting versus uncoated stents in acute myocardial infarction. *N Engl J Med* 2006; **355**(11): 1093–1104.

11 Lemos PA, Serruys PW, van Domburg RT, et al. Unrestricted utilization of sirolimus-eluting stents compared with conventional bare stent implantation in the "real world": The Rapamycin- Eluting Stent Evaluated At Rotterdam Cardiology Hospital (RESEARCH) registry. *Circulation* 2004; **109**(2): 190–195.

12 Urban P, Gershlick AH, Guagliumi G, et al. Safety of coronary sirolimus-eluting stents in daily clinical practice: one-year follow-up of the e-Cypher registry. *Circulation* 2006; **113**(11): 1434–1441.

13 Applegate RJ, Sacrinty MT, Kutcher MA, et al. "Off-label" stent therapy 2-year comparison of drug-eluting versus bare-metal stents. *J Am Coll Cardiol* 2008; **51**(6): 607–614.

14 Kip KE, Hollabaugh K, Marroquin OC, et al. The problem with composite end points in cardiovascular studies: the story of major adverse cardiac events and percutaneous coronary intervention. *J Am Coll Cardiol* 2008; **51**(7): 701–707.

15 Win HK, Caldera AE, Maresh K, et al. Clinical outcomes and stent thrombosis following off-label use of drug-eluting stents. *JAMA* 2007; **297**(18): 2001–2009.

16 Rowinsky EK, Donehower RC. Paclitaxel (taxol). *N Engl J Med* 1995; **332**(15): 1004–1014.

17 Axel DI, Kunert W, Göggelmann C, et al. Paclitaxel inhibits arterial smooth muscle cell proliferation and migration in vitro and in vivo using local drug delivery. *Circulation* 1997; **96**(2): 636–645.

18 Drachman DE, Edelman ER, Seifert P, et al. Neointimal thickening after stent delivery of paclitaxel: change in composition and arrest of growth over six months. *J Am Coll Cardiol* 2000; **36**(7): 2325–2332.

19 Heldman AW, Cheng L, Jenkins GM, et al. Paclitaxel stent coating inhibits neointimal hyperplasia at 4 weeks in a porcine model of coronary restenosis. *Circulation* 2001; **103**(18): 2289–2295.

20 Sollott SJ, Cheng L, Pauly RR, et al. Taxol inhibits neointimal smooth muscle cell accumulation after angioplasty in the rat. *J Clin Invest* 1995; **95**(4): 1869–1876.

21 Grube E, Silber S, Hauptmann KE, et al. TAXUS I: six-and twelve-month results from a randomized, double-blind trial on a slow-release paclitaxel-eluting stent for de novo coronary lesions. *Circulation* 2003; **107**(1): 38–42.

22 Colombo A, Drzewiecki J, Banning A, et al. Randomized study to assess the effectiveness of slow-and moderate-release polymer-based paclitaxel-eluting stents for coronary artery lesions. *Circulation* 2003; **108**(7): 788–794.

23 Tanabe K, Serruys PW, Grube E, et al. TAXUS III Trial: in-stent restenosis treated with stent-based delivery of paclitaxel incorporated in a slow-release polymer formulation. *Circulation* 2003; **107**(4): 559–564.

24 Stone GW, Ellis SG, Cox DA, et al. A polymer-based, paclitaxel-eluting stent in patients with coronary artery disease. *N Engl J Med* 2004; **350**(3): 221–231.

25 Stone GW, Ellis SG, Cox DA, et al. One-year clinical results with the slow-release, polymer-based, paclitaxel-eluting TAXUS stent: the TAXUS-IV trial. *Circulation* 2004; **109**(16): 1942–1947.

26 Dawkins KD, Grube E, Guagliumi G, et al. Clinical efficacy of polymer-based paclitaxel-eluting stents in the treatment of complex, long coronary artery lesions from a multicenter, randomized trial: support for the use of drug-eluting stents in contemporary clinical practice. *Circulation* 2005; **112**(21): 3306–3313.

27 Marx SO, Marks AR. Bench to bedside: the development of rapamycin and its application to stent restenosis. *Circulation* 2001; **104**(8): 852–855.

28 Marx SO, Jayaraman T, Go LO, et al. Rapamycin-FKBP inhibits cell cycle regulators of proliferation in vascular smooth muscle cells. *Circ Res* 1995; **76**(3): 412–417.

29 Poon M, Marx SO, Gallo R, et al. Rapamycin inhibits vascular smooth muscle cell migration. *J Clin Invest* 1996; **98**(10): 2277–2783.

30 Sousa JE, Costa MA, Abizaid A, et al. Lack of neointimal proliferation after implantation of sirolimus-coated stents in human coronary arteries: a quantitative coronary angiography and three-dimensional intravascular ultrasound study. *Circulation* 2001; **103**(2): 192–195.

31 Sousa JE, Costa MA, Abizaid AC, et al. Sustained suppression of neointimal proliferation by sirolimus-eluting stents: one-year angiographic and intravascular ultrasound follow-up. *Circulation* 2001; **104**(17): 2007–2011.

32 Morice MC, Serruys PW, Sousa JE, et al. A randomized comparison of a sirolimus-eluting stent with a standard stent for coronary revascularization. *N Engl J Med* 2002; **346**(23): 1773–1780.

33 Moses JW, Leon MB, Popma JJ, et al. Sirolimus-eluting stents versus standard stents in patients with stenosis in a native coronary artery. *N Engl J Med* 2003; **349**(14): 1315–1323.

34 Schofer J, Schluter M, Gershlick AH, et al. Sirolimus-eluting stents for treatment of patients with long atherosclerotic lesions in small coronary arteries: double-blind, randomised controlled trial (E-SIRIUS). *Lancet* 2003; **362**(9390): 1093–1099.

35 Schampaert E, Cohen EA, Schluter M, *et al.* The Canadian study of the sirolimus-eluting stent in the treatment of patients with long de novo lesions in small native coronary arteries (C-SIRIUS). *J Am Coll Cardiol* 2004; **43**(6): 1110–1115.

36 Fajadet, J., Morice MC, Bode C, *et al.* Maintenance of long-term clinical benefit with sirolimus-eluting coronary stents: three-year results of the RAVEL trial. *Circulation* 2005; **111**(8): 1040–1044.

37 Leon MB. Unpublished data. Paper presented at: American College of Cardiology Scientific Meeting, 2007.

38 Schampaert E, Moses JW, Schofer J, *et al.* Sirolimus-eluting stents at two years: a pooled analysis of SIRIUS, E-SIRIUS, and C-SIRIUS with emphasis on late revascularizations and stent thromboses. *Am J Cardiol* 2006; **98**(1): 36–41.

39 Caixeta A, Leon MB, Lansky MDA, *et al.* Five-year clinical outcomes after sirolimus-eluting stent implantation: insights from a patient-level pooled analysis of four randomized trials comparing sirolimus-eluting stents with bare-metal stents. *J Am Coll Cardiol* 2009; **54**(10): 894–902.

40 Kastrati A, Dibra A, Spaulding C, *et al.* Meta-analysis of randomized trials on drug-eluting stents vs. bare-metal stents in patients with acute myocardial infarction. *Eur Heart J* 2007; **28**(22): 2706–2713.

41 Mauri L, Silbaugh TS, Garg P, *et al.* Drug-eluting or bare-metal stents for acute myocardial infarction. *N Engl J Med* 2008; **359**(13): 1330–1342.

42 Menichelli M, Parma A, Pucci E, *et al.* Randomized trial of Sirolimus-Eluting Stent Versus Bare-Metal Stent in Acute Myocardial Infarction (SESAMI). *J Am Coll Cardiol* 2007; **49**(19): 1924–1930.

43 van der Hoeven BL, Liem SS, Jukema JW, *et al.* Sirolimus-eluting stents versus bare-metal stents in patients with ST-segment elevation myocardial infarction: 9-month angiographic and intravascular ultrasound results and 12-month clinical outcome results from the MISSION! Intervention Study. *J Am Coll Cardiol* 2008; **51**(6): 618–626.

44 Stone GW, HORIZONS AMI: a prospective randomized trial of paclitaxel-eluting stents vs baremetal stents in patients with acute ST-segment elevation myocardial infarction. Paper presented at: Transcatheter Cardiovascular Therapeutics (TCT) 20th Annual Scientific Symposium, 2008.

45 Dangas GD, Caixeta A, Mehran R, *et al.* Frequency and predictors of stent thrombosis after percutaneous coronary intervention in acute myocardial infarction. *Circulation* 2011; **123**(16): 1745–1756.

46 Stone GW, Witzenbichler B, Guagliumi G, *et al.* Heparin plus a glycoprotein IIb/IIIa inhibitor versus bivalirudin monotherapy and paclitaxel-eluting stents versus bare-metal stents in acute myocardial infarction (HORIZONS-AMI): final 3-year results from a multicentre, randomised controlled trial. *Lancet*, 2011. **377**(9784): 2193–2204.

47 Wallace EL, Abdel-Latif A, Charnigo R, *et al.* Meta-analysis of long-term outcomes for drug-eluting stents versus bare-metal stents in primary percutaneous coronary interventions for ST-segment elevation myocardial infarction. *Am J Cardiol* 2012; **109**(7): 932–940.

48 Sabate M, Räber L, Heg D, *et al.* Comparison of newer-generation drug-eluting with bare-metal stents in patients with acute ST-segment elevation myocardial infarction: a pooled analysis of the EXAMINATION (clinical Evaluation of the Xience-V stent in Acute Myocardial INfArcTION) and COMFORTABLE-AMI (Comparison of Biolimus Eluted From an Erodible Stent Coating With Bare Metal Stents in Acute ST-Elevation Myocardial Infarction) trials. *JACC Cardiovasc Interv* 2014; **7**(1): 55–63.

49 Kolh P, Windecker S, Alfonso F, *et al.* 2014 ESC/EACTS Guidelines on myocardial revascularization: the Task Force on Myocardial Revascularization of the European Society of Cardiology (ESC) and the European Association for Cardio-Thoracic Surgery (EACTS). Developed with the special contribution of the European Association of Percutaneous Cardiovascular Interventions (EAPCI). *Eur J Cardiothorac Surg* 2014; **46**(4): 517–592.

50 Fihn SD, Gardin JM, Abrams J, *et al.* 2012 ACCF/AHA/ACP/AATS/PCNA/SCAI/STS Guideline for the diagnosis and management of patients with stable ischemic heart disease: a report of the American College of Cardiology Foundation/American Heart Association Task Force on Practice Guidelines, and the American College of Physicians, American Association for Thoracic Surgery, Preventive Cardiovascular Nurses Association, Society for Cardiovascular Angiography and Interventions, and Society of Thoracic Surgeons. *J Am Coll Cardiol* 2012; **60**(24): e44–e164.

51 Kapur A, Hall RJ, Malik IS, *et al.* Randomized comparison of percutaneous coronary intervention with coronary artery bypass grafting in diabetic patients. 1-year results of the CARDia (Coronary Artery Revascularization in Diabetes) trial. *J Am Coll Cardiol* 2010; **55**(5): 432–440.

52 Farkouh ME, Domanski M, Sleeper LA, *et al.* Strategies for multivessel revascularization in patients with diabetes. *N Engl J Med* 2012; **367**(25): 2375–2384.

53 Head SJ, Davierwala PM, Serruys PW, *et al.* Coronary artery bypass grafting vs. percutaneous coronary intervention for patients with three-vessel disease: final five-year follow-up of the SYNTAX trial. *Eur Heart J* 2014; **35**(40): 2821–2830.

54 Levine GN, Bates ER, Blankenship JC, *et al.* 2011 ACCF/AHA/SCAI Guideline for Percutaneous Coronary Intervention. A report of the American College of Cardiology Foundation/American Heart Association Task Force on Practice Guidelines and the Society for Cardiovascular Angiography and Interventions. *J Am Coll Cardiol* 2011; **58**(24): e44–122.

55 Mohr FW, Morice MC, Kappetein AP, *et al.* Coronary artery bypass graft surgery versus percutaneous coronary intervention in patients with three-vessel disease and left main coronary disease: 5-year follow-up of the randomised, clinical SYNTAX trial. *Lancet* 2013; **381**(9867): 629–638.

56 Park SJ, Kim Yh, Park DW, *et al.* Randomized trial of stents versus bypass surgery for left main coronary artery disease. *N Engl J Med* 2011; **364**(18): 1718–1727.

57 Morice MC, Serruys PW, Kappetein AP, *et al.* Five-year outcomes in patients with left main disease treated with either percutaneous coronary intervention or coronary artery bypass grafting in the synergy between percutaneous coronary intervention with taxus and cardiac surgery trial. *Circulation* 2014; **129**(23): 2388–2394.

58 Kastrati A, Mehilli J, Pache J, *et al.* Analysis of 14 trials comparing sirolimus-eluting stents with bare-metal stents. *N Engl J Med* 2007; **356**(10): 1030–1039.

59 Stettler C, Wandel S, Allemann S, *et al.* Outcomes associated with drug-eluting and bare-metal stents: a collaborative network meta-analysis. *Lancet* 2007; **370**: 937–948.

60 Schomig A, Dibra A, Windecker S, *et al.* A meta-analysis of 16 randomized trials of sirolimus-eluting stents versus paclitaxel-eluting stents in patients with coronary artery disease. *J Am Coll Cardiol* 2007; **50**(14): 1373–1380.

61 Abbott JD, Dibra A, Windecker S, *et al.* Unrestricted use of drug-eluting stents compared with bare-metal stents in routine clinical practice: findings from the National Heart, Lung, and Blood Institute Dynamic Registry. *J Am Coll Cardiol* 2007; **50**(21): 2029–2036.

62 Jensen LO, Maeng M, Kaltoft A, *et al.* Stent thrombosis, myocardial infarction, and death after drug-eluting and bare-metal stent coronary interventions. *J Am Coll Cardiol* 2007; **50**(5): 463–470.

63 Marroquin OC, Selzer F, Mulukutla SR, *et al.* A comparison of bare-metal and drug-eluting stents for off-label indications. *N Engl J Med* 2008; **358**(4): 342–352.

64 Marzocchi A, Saia F, Piovaccari G, *et al.* Long-term safety and efficacy of drug-eluting stents: two-year results of the REAL (REgistro AngiopLastiche dell'Emilia Romagna) multicenter registry. *Circulation* 2007; **115**(25): 3181–3188.

65 Tu JV, Bowen J, Chiu M, *et al.* Effectiveness and safety of drug-eluting stents in Ontario. *N Engl J Med* 2007; **357**(14): 1393–1402.

66 Zhang X, Xie J, Li G, Chen Q, Xu B. Head-to-head comparison of sirolimus-eluting stents versus paclitaxel-eluting stents in patients undergoing percutaneous coronary intervention: a meta-analysis of 76 studies. *PLoS One* 2014; **9**(5): e97934.

67 Camenzind E, Steg PG, Wijns W. Stent thrombosis late after implantation of first-generation drug-eluting stents: a cause for concern. *Circulation* 2007; **115**(11): 1440–1455; discussion 1455.

68 Lagerqvist B, James SK, Stenestrand U, *et al.* Long-term outcomes with drug-eluting stents versus bare-metal stents in Sweden. *N Engl J Med* 2007; **356**(10): 1009–1019.

69 Nordmann AJ, Briel M, Bucher HC. Mortality in randomized controlled trials comparing drug-eluting vs. bare metal stents in coronary artery disease: a meta-analysis. *Eur Heart J* 2006; **27**(23): 2784–2814.

70 Daemen J, Wenaweser P, Tsuchida K, *et al.* Early and late coronary stent thrombosis of sirolimus-eluting and paclitaxel-eluting stents in routine clinical practice: data from a large two-institutional cohort study. *Lancet* 2007; **369**(9562): 667–678.

71 Pfisterer M, Brunner-La Rocca HP, Buser PT, *et al.* Late clinical events after clopidogrel discontinuation may limit the benefit of drug-eluting stents: an observational study of drug-eluting versus bare-metal stents. *J Am Coll Cardiol* 2006; **48**(12): 2584–2591.

72 Stone GW, Moses JW, Ellis SG, *et al.* Safety and efficacy of sirolimus- and paclitaxel-eluting coronary stents. *N Engl J Med* 2007; **356**(10): 998–1008.

CHAPTER 32

Cobalt-Chromium Everolimus-Eluting Stents

Vikas Thondapu[1], Yoshinobu Onuma[2], Bimmer E.P.M. Claessen[3], Patrick W. Serruys[4], and Peter Barlis[1]

[1] Melbourne Medical School, Faculty of Medicine, Dentistry and Health Sciences, The University of Melbourne, Australia
[2] Thoraxcenter, Erasmus Medical Center, Rotterdam, The Netherlands
[3] Department of Cardiology, Academic Medical Center—University of Amsterdam, Amsterdam, The Netherlands
[4] Faculty of Medicine, National Heart & Lung Institute, Imperial College London, London, UK

Compared to their bare metal predecessors, drug-eluting stents (DES) have undisputed efficacy in preventing in-stent restenosis. First-generation DES pushed the boundaries of percutaneous coronary intervention, permitting the application of minimally invasive techniques to clinical scenarios that once fell strictly in the surgical domain. Despite their efficacy and resulting enthusiastic use, however, concerns rapidly surfaced over their long-term safety. Evidence suggesting an increased risk of late stent thrombosis and restenosis resulted in a comprehensive reconsideration of the first-generation DES.

The countless studies that emerged from this reassessment provided new insights into the complex relationship between stent and vessel wall, and a renewed focus on the stent platform, polymer, and drug. Factors such as strut thickness, polymer biocompatibility, and drug release kinetics are now known to influence vascular endothelial healing, a major factor in long-term stent outcomes. Such insights have subsequently informed the design of the second-generation DES, resulting in the use of more biocompatible drug-eluting polymers, more effective drug formulations, and more resilient platform materials.

Cobalt-chromium (CoCr) stents were largely born out of the need for a new generation of coronary stents preserving or improving the safety, efficacy, and deliverability of earlier iterations. The superior biomechanics and biocompatibility of these alloys serve as the platform for increasingly varied and innovative approaches to stent design. Overall, it appears that the second-generation DES retain the anti-restenotic efficacy of first-generation DES while maintaining protection against late stent thrombosis [1–4]. While several second-generation DES are now in clinical use, this chapter focuses on the market-leading CoCr everolimus-eluting stents (EES), which have become the standard against which new stents and scaffolds are compared.

This chapter begins with a brief discussion of several material and chemical properties of CoCr alloys that contribute to these stents' superior biomechanics and biocompatibility. This discussion provides context for the subsequent technical description of the CoCr-EES and the clinical trials evaluating their safety and efficacy. Finally, it should be understood that the chemical and material properties discussed are not meant to be exhaustive nor meant to suggest that CoCr alloys are the single best material for coronary stents; other excellent materials exist and more are in development.

Rather, the goal is to illustrate that while CoCr alloys do have their limitations, they achieve a better balance than materials such as stainless steel. These concepts not only help explain the clinical success of CoCr-DES, but may also serve as a framework to better understand the performance of other important and commonly used stent materials such as the titanium and platinum alloys.

Material and chemical properties of cobalt-chromium alloys

The three overarching elements in the design of traditional DES are platform, polymer, and drug. Alteration in these features accounts for much of the variety seen in currently available stents (Figure 32.1). Although each element is critical, the platform's biomechanics and biocompatibility have key roles in a stent's overall performance. The CoCr alloys possess key material and chemical properties that improve their performance compared to stainless steel and many other materials used in coronary stents.

Platform biomechanics
Role of strut thickness

For more than a decade, stent design has prioritized thinner struts as a result of numerous studies demonstrating significantly improved outcomes compared to stents with thick struts [5,6]. While thick struts provide radial and longitudinal strength, they characteristically lack the flexibility and conformability critical in maintaining stent apposition without inducing vessel deformity and injury. Thinner struts demonstrate better apposition to the vessel wall and cause less disruption of local hemodynamics [7–11]. Stents with thinner struts also show less vascular inflammation [12,13] and thrombosis [7]. These findings may partially explain rapid and more complete endothelial healing seen with thin struts [14].

Strut thickness also impacts stent deliverability, the qualitative ease with which a stent is visualized, tracked to the target, and adequately deployed. Thinner struts increase flexibility to better negotiate complex vascular anatomy, reduce crossing profiles to navigate across lesions, and present less obstruction of side branch access. Thin struts, however, are less radio-opaque and thus decrease the operator's ability to visualize the stent under fluoroscopy to ensure safe and effective deployment.

Interventional Cardiology: Principles and Practice, Second Edition. Edited by George D. Dangas, Carlo Di Mario, and Nicholas N. Kipshidze.
© 2017 John Wiley & Sons, Ltd. Published 2017 by John Wiley & Sons, Ltd.

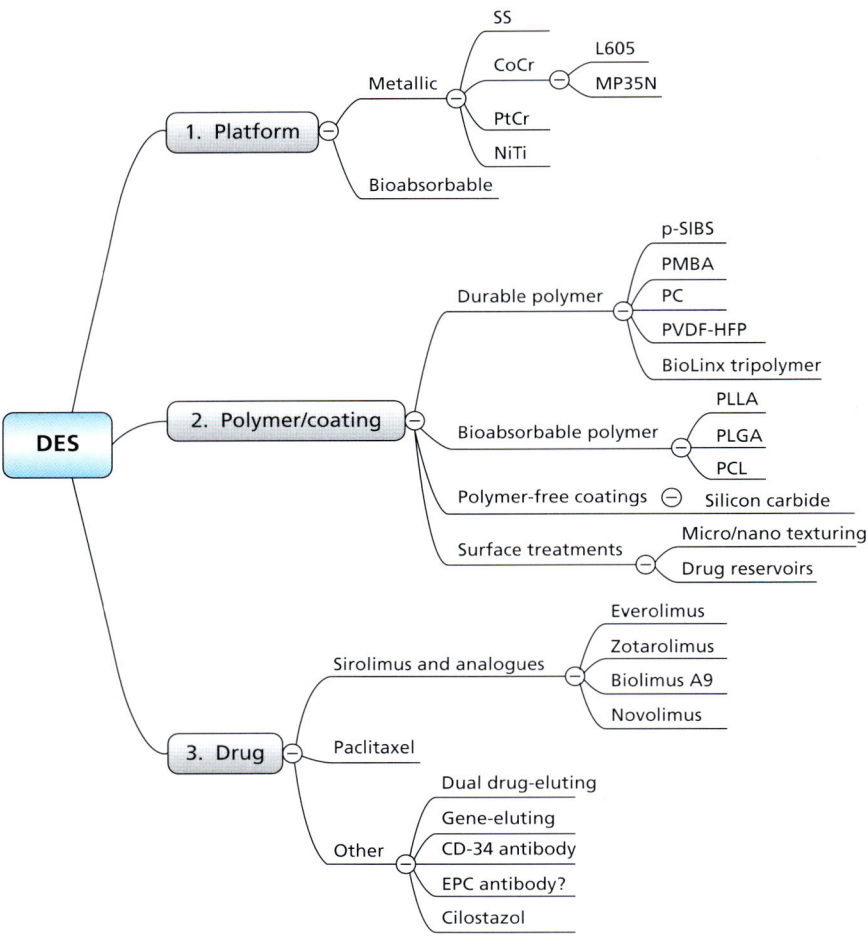

Figure 32.1 Components of drug-eluting stents (DES).

While these observations formed a strong driving force toward thinner struts, stainless steel was not strong or dense enough to fabricate thin struts while maintaining characteristics essential to coronary stents. In fact, the push toward thinner and thinner struts has led to concerns about recoil, longitudinal stent deformation, and stent fracture with newer stent platforms [15,16]. While these mechanical complications remain rare events overall, they have been associated with restenosis and thrombosis [17]. Some reports suggest, for instance, that longitudinal deformation occurs more frequently with platinum-chromium based stents [18] whereas others have found no correlation [19]. Ongoing studies suggest that in addition to certain clinical factors such as stent length and vessel diameter, the number and arrangement of longitudinal connectors between hoops are more significant determinants than strut thickness or material [15,16,20–22].

Ultimately, the material properties of the platform outline the fundamental limits of its design and deliverability. The tensile strength, yield strength, elasticity, and density of the platform material define the thinnest struts possible while maintaining strength, flexibility, and radio-opacity. While stainless steel has long been used in medical devices, it has several limitations in the context of coronary stents and the particular need for thinner stent struts. Relative to stainless steel, the CoCr alloys have struck a better balance. The most commonly used CoCr alloys, L605 and MP35N, vary in composition, but their biomechanical properties are similar

Table 32.1 Composition of stainless steel and cobalt-chromium alloys.

| Alloy | Element composition (%) | | | | | | | |
	C	Fe	Co	Cr	Ni	W	Mo	Mn
316L	0.03	64	—	18	14	—	2.6	2.0
MP35N	0.025	1.0	35	20	35	—	10	0.15
L605	0.1	3.0	52	20	10	15	—	1.5

(Table 32.1) [23]. Both L605 and MP35N have higher tensile strength, yield strength, elastic modulus, and density than 316 L stainless steel because of key differences in chemical composition.

Crystal structure of metals

The mechanical properties of alloys depend on their chemical composition and crystal structure of the metal (Table 32.2). Most metals have a crystalline structure in which atoms form repeating unit cells that can take various arrangements such as face-centered cubic, body-centered cubic, and hexagonal closely packed. Simplistically speaking, these arrangements determine how closely atoms are packed together, thereby determining properties such as strength, density, and magnetism. Further, unit cell arrangements can transform from one to another depending on factors such as temperature and the presence of impurities.

Many pure metals contain defects in the regular crystalline arrangement because of atoms missing from their expected position, interjection of atoms where they are not expected, or slight misalignment of bonds. Ultimately, these defects result in a polycrystalline material with countless crystal grains and planar facets (Figure 32.2a–c). Crystal defects partially account for the brittleness of pure metals and the deformability of metals in general, but defects can be removed or mitigated by various metallurgical techniques, thereby altering mechanical properties of the metal.

Alloying, or solid-solution strengthening, is one technique to stabilize crystal defects and strengthen pure metals. The addition of other elements effectively hinders deformation around defects due to differences in intermetallic bond strength and atom size (Figure 32.2d). Another technique is grain-boundary strengthening, which involves applying a force (such as with a hammer) to the metal or alloy to decrease grain size and reposition the defects to coalesce with the newly formed grain boundaries*. This is relevant because certain alloyed elements can also affect grain size; elements that reduce grain size can effectively increase the overall alloy strength. Finally, the temperature at which alloys are worked can induce transformations in the unit cell arrangement (such as

Table 32.2 Mechanical properties of stainless steel and cobalt-chromium alloys.

Material	Density (g/cm^3)	UTS (MPa)	Yield strength (MPa)	Elastic modulus (GPa)
316L	7.9	670	340	193
MP35N	8.4	930	414	233
L605	9.1	1000	500	243

UTS, ultimate tensile strength.

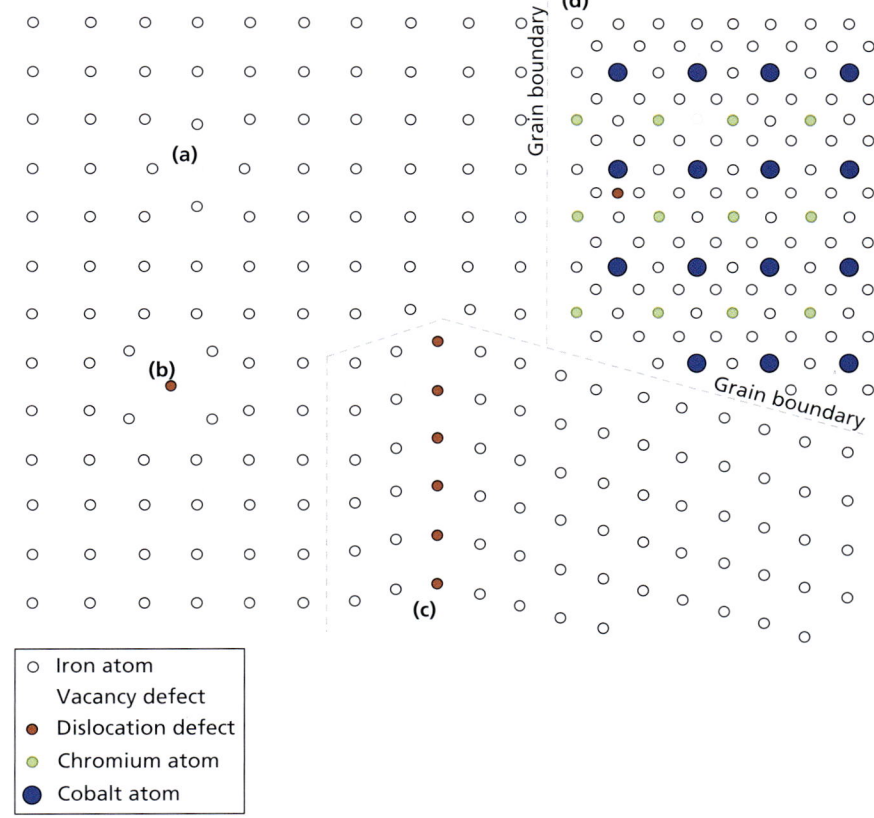

- ○ Iron atom
-   Vacancy defect
- ● Dislocation defect
- ● Chromium atom
- ● Cobalt atom

Figure 32.2 Schematic representation of metallic crystal structure, defects, and strengthening. (a) Vacancy defects in the crystal cause misalignment of bonds and a point susceptible to deformation. (b) Dislocation defects result in misalignment of bonds and susceptibility to deformation. (c) Linear or planar dislocation defects result in the formation of a new crystal grain and boundary. (d) Cobalt and chromium atoms stabilize defects and allow closer packing of atoms to strengthen alloys and increase wear resistance.

*As the surface of a crystal grain is generally formed by planes, planar boundaries define the interface where two crystal grains meet. Given a constant volume of polycrystalline metal, decreasing crystal grain size increases the number of grains and planar boundaries, akin to increasing surface area. Grain-boundary strengthening effectively ushers atomic crystal defects into planar boundaries, an inherently less unstable arrangement than randomly dispersed defects. In short, point and line defects are less stable than plane defects, although this mechanism breaks down with extreme reductions in grain size.

body-centered to face-centered cubic transformation), which again affects electromagnetic and mechanical behavior.

These concepts are introduced in order to demonstrate that the increased strength, elasticity, and density of CoCr alloys can be tied to the specific effects of cobalt, chromium, tungsten, and molybdenum on the crystal structure of the alloy. During CoCr alloy fabrication, the atomic structure of cobalt (more specifically, the number and arrangement of its electrons) facilitates a partial transformation of the unit cell arrangement from face-centered cubic to hexagonal closely packed structure. The resulting combination of closely packed but distinct unit cell configurations significantly increases the alloy's strength and wear resistance [24]. This type of unit cell rearrangement and strengthening does not occur in stainless steel.

In many alloys, chromium binds with carbon to form extremely strong chromium-carbides, which stabilize defects and grain boundaries. While carbides in CoCr alloys are generally chromium-based, cobalt, tungsten, and molybdenum can substitute for chromium and exert their own strengthening effects. Furthermore, tungsten promotes even distribution of carbides through the alloy; molybdenum decreases crystal grain size, reducing the destabilizing effect of crystal defects [24,25].

Thus, the specific chemical composition of CoCr alloys imbues the material with properties that allow the fabrication of thin-strut (<100 μm) stents while maintaining strength, flexibility, and radiopacity in addition to long-term resistance to wear, fatigue, and corrosion [25–28]. From a clinical standpoint, these biomechanical characteristics have contributed to reduced endothelial injury, thrombosis, and restenosis compared to stents with thicker struts [29,30]. These concepts help explain some of the limitations of stainless steel and some of the reasons cobalt, platinum, and titanium alloys perform so well in coronary stents.

Platform biocompatibility

Biocompatibility is an obvious requirement for any implanted device, but its definition has evolved over time and fluctuates considerably in accordance with the setting and desired outcomes [31]. For metallic coronary stents, biocompatibility requires resistance to thrombosis and low inflammatory potential. These characteristics are not inherent even to gold and turbostratic carbon, materials successfully used in other blood-contacting devices, but which have not worked well in coronary stents [32–35]. The CoCr alloys, however, continue to show their biocompatibility through low rates of restenosis and thrombosis [29,30] in addition to reduced need for revascularization historically compared to stainless steel BMS [36]. While likely related to thinner struts and improved biomechanics, several material and chemical properties of CoCr also contribute to improved resistance to thrombosis and inflammation.

Surface characteristics and resistance to thrombosis

Resistance to thrombosis is a vital characteristic of any coronary stent as metal is a potent trigger of fibrin deposition and platelet adhesion. While the detailed thermodynamic and electrochemical mechanisms of stent thrombosis are beyond the scope of this discussion, this process is again influenced by stent material properties and surface characteristics [12,37,38].

In brief, the energy differential between blood and metallic stent surface contributes not only to protein deposition on the stent, but also influences which proteins are deposited (fibrin, fibronectin, albumin, etc.) and the extent to which these proteins are denatured by contact with the metallic surface [38]. In fact, varying conformations of adherent fibronectin have been shown to have differential affinity for platelet, monocyte, and endothelial cell adhesion depending on which intermolecular binding domains are exposed upon adhering to metal [39]. This can influence propensity for thrombosis, restenosis, and endothelial coverage.

The energy differential between the stent surface and blood depends upon the material surface energy, a measure of the stability of molecular bonds at the surface relative to that of internal molecules; surface potential, a measure of electrical conductivity; and surface texture [38,40]. The empirical characterization of surfaces is extremely complex, and a clearly defined relationship between surface characteristics and thrombosis has remained elusive [41,42]. Simplistically speaking, however, CoCr alloys have low surface energy, low surface potential, and a surface readily electro-polished relative to other materials used in stents, all of which contribute to reduced thrombogenicity [37,43].

These observations are supported by the empirical measurement of fibrin and platelet adhesion *in vitro*, which can reasonably approximate the thrombo-resistance and inflammatory nature of various materials. For example, materials such as gold, manganese, and turbostatic carbon have high rates of *in vitro* fibrin, platelet, and monocyte adhesion [44], corresponding to high rates of restenosis seen with stents containing these materials [33,34]. In contrast, L605 CoCr shows a low rate of fibrin deposition, minimal monocyte adhesion, and good endothelial cell migration characteristics [44], again supported by clinical results demonstrating low thrombogenicity and restenosis [29,30].

Corrosion resistance and reduced inflammation

In addition to thick stent struts and early durable polymers, metal release from corroding stent platforms has been suggested as another source of vascular toxicity and chronic inflammation [45]. Corrosion has been postulated to explain the singular failure of gold-coated stents: surface irregularities imparted by the galvanization-coating technique may have caused cracks in the gold layer resulting in corrosion and leaching of toxic and inflammatory metal ions into surrounding tissues [33,42,46]. Refinement of the gold coating technique resulted in better surface texture and integrity, and eliminated excessive restenosis altogether [46].

Clearly, corrosion resistance depends on mechanical integrity of the platform. As seen with the gold-coated stents, cracks and fissures may have acted as a nidus for propagating corrosion (Figure 32.3). The high elasticity, wear, and fatigue resistance of the CoCr alloys reduce their propensity to fracture, and thus partially explain their superior corrosion resistance. However, compared with stainless steel and other commonly used device materials, CoCr alloys demonstrate superior corrosion resistance mainly because of *in vivo* oxidation of the metallic stent surface [25,47]. Surface oxidation creates a passive film that acts somewhat like a natural sealant and reduces metal release into surrounding tissues [48]. The importance of surface oxide formation cannot be overstated when considering that, as lone elements, cobalt, chromium, and nickel are highly toxic, yet once alloyed and oxidized they form a highly biocompatible, non-toxic material.

Interestingly, the stability of the formed oxide is more important in preventing metal release than quantitative metal content itself. Although both L605 and MP35N CoCr alloys contain a relatively high percentage by weight of nickel (10% and 35%, respectively), their superior oxide stability prevents nickel release seen in slightly more corrosion-prone alloys such as stainless steel. This superior

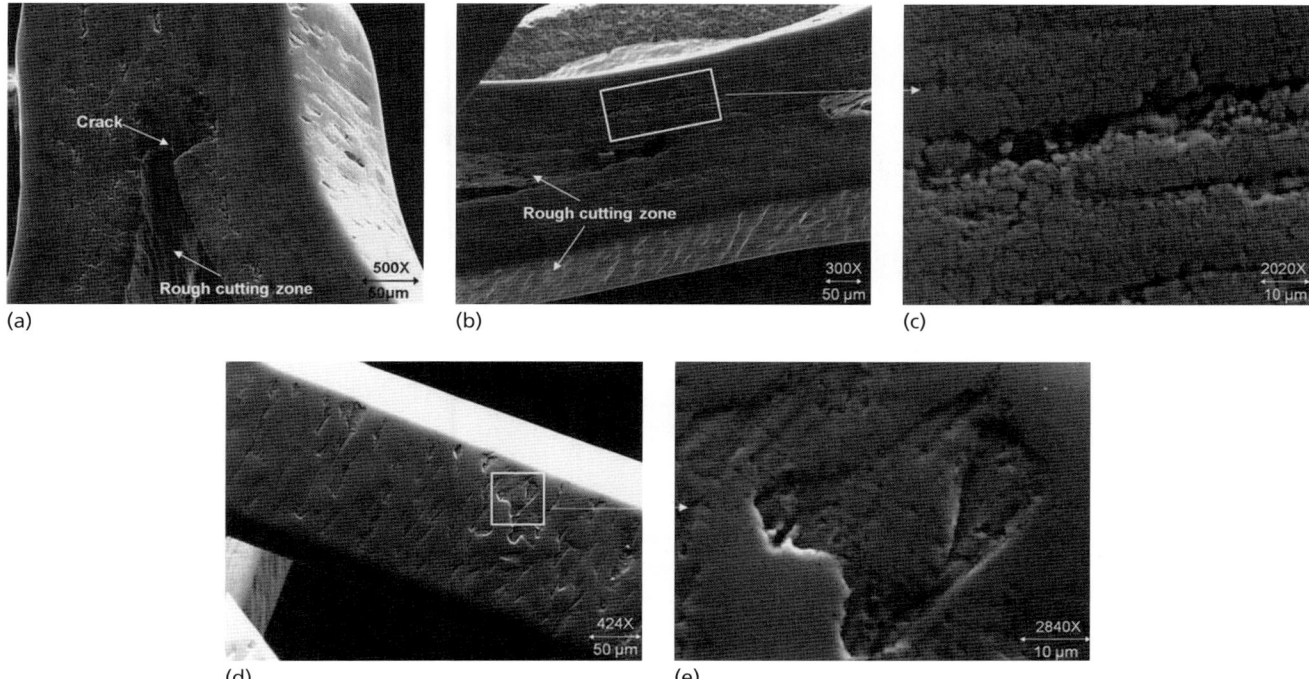

Figure 32.3 Stent corrosion. Scanning electron micrograph of the surface of a nickel-titanium stent with cracks (a, b, d) and corrosion pits upon closer examination (c, e). Source: Halwani DO, *et al.J Biomed Mater Res B* 2010; 95B: 225–238. Reproduced with permission. Copyright © 2010 Wiley Periodicals, Inc.

oxide stability is mainly because of high chromium content of CoCr alloys, although nickel and molybdenum also contribute. In a cobalt matrix, high chromium content in particular induces spontaneous surface oxidation to form a highly stable Cr_2O_3 oxide [24]. As a result, CoCr alloys have significantly greater corrosion resistance than stainless steel [47].

Lastly, it should be noted that the same element can have opposing effects on mechanical strength and corrosion resistance, hence the difficulty and importance of achieving balanced performance. Tungsten, for instance, improves strength and wear resistance of L605, but may also contribute to its slightly lower corrosion resistance than MP35N. On the other hand, MP35N lacks tungsten and can therefore be slightly more corrosion resistant at the expense of some mechanical strength. These are, of course, simplified explanations of highly complex phenomena, but still serve to illustrate how chemical and material properties relate to real-world clinical performance.

Cobalt-chromium everolimus-eluting stents: technical overview
Platform
The CoCr-EES are conscribed by the Xience V, Prime, Xpedition, and Alpine (Abbott Vascular, Santa Clara, CA, USA). Since the initial introduction of the Xience V in 2006, these stents have undergone only incremental changes marked by minor alterations in the platform design and delivery system.

The Xience V was based on the L605-CoCr Multi-Link Vision (Abbott Vascular) platform, which features 81 μm struts and an open-cell design characterized by in-phase sinusoidal hoops linked by three longitudinal connectors per hoop. Each longitudinal connector has a small C-shaped loop to enhance flexibility (Figure 32.4). The Xience V was subsequently replaced by the Xience Prime, and more recently by the Xpedition and Alpine.

The Xience Prime, Xpedition, and Alpine EES are based on the L605-CoCr Multi-Link 8 (Abbott Vascular), which features slightly longer cells and minor modifications to the proximal hoop, but is otherwise nearly identical to the Multi-Link Vision. Both of these platforms provide thin struts while maintaining excellent radial strength, longitudinal strength, flexibility, and radio-opacity [15,20,26].

Polymer
All of the Xience stents employ a biocompatible durable polymer coating consisting of a primer layer and a polymer-drug layer with a total thickness of 7.8 μm. The primer, poly n-butyl methylacrylate (PMBA), is synthesized from methylacrylate monomers and serves to adhere the drug-eluting polymer to the platform. The drug-eluting layer is a combination of polyvinylidene fluoride-hexafluoropropylene (PVDF-HFP) and everolimus mixed in a ratio of 83 : 17%, which is then applied to the entire PMBA-primed stent surface.

As the durable drug-eluting polymers are permanent, rapid endothelial healing and long-term resistance to thrombosis and chronic inflammation are essential to long-term safety. As with the CoCr alloys, the PVDF-HFP polymer possesses chemical and material properties that significantly enhance its clinical performance.

Polymer chemical structure
PVDF-HFP is a semi-crystalline polymer with an entirely saturated carbon-carbon backbone, which increases resistance to hydrolysis, oxidation, and enzymatic cleavage. This oxidative stability may

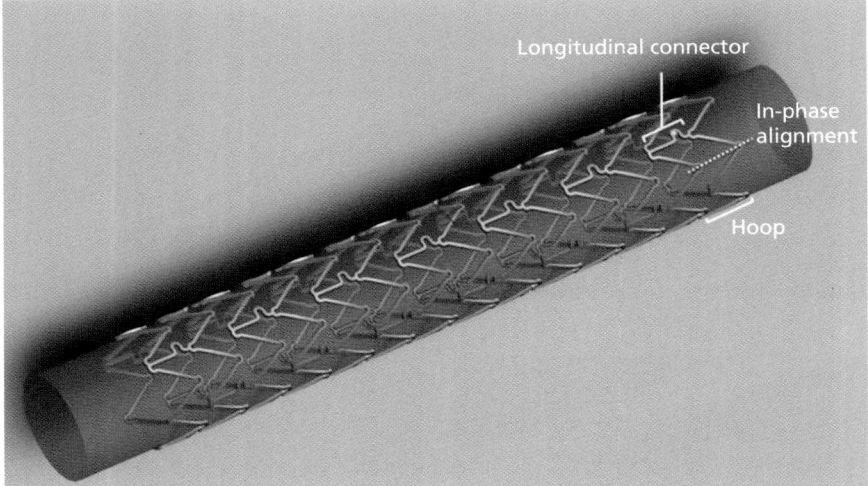

Figure 32.4 Xience stent. The Xience V/Multi-Link Vision has an open-cell, in-phase sinusoidal pattern with three longitudinal connectors between adjacent hoops. The longitudinal connectors feature a C-shaped loop (asterisk) to increase flexibility. The Xience Prime, Xpedition, and Alpine are based on the Multi-Link 8 platform, which features slightly longer connectors resulting in longer cells, but is otherwise identical to the Multi-Link 8.

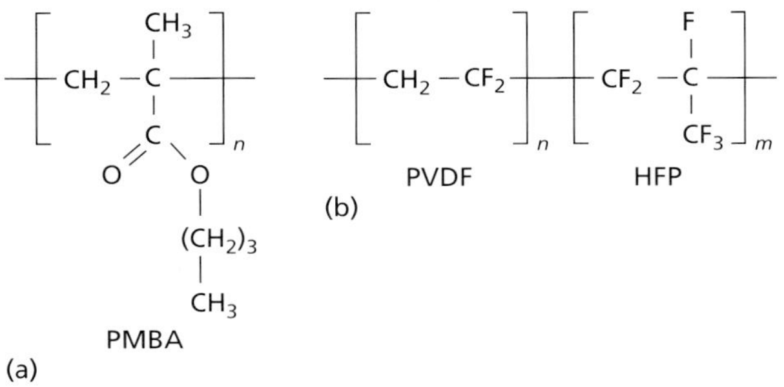

Figure 32.5 Chemical structure of poly n-butyl methylacrylate (PMBA) and polyvinylidene fluoride-hexafluoropropylene (PVDF-HFP). (a) Chemical structure of PMBA. (b) The completely saturated, partially fluorinated carbon-carbon backbone of PVDF-HFP increases its oxidative stability and resistance to thrombosis.

reduce the formation of inflammatory degradation products. Additionally, approximately 50% of the carbon backbone is saturated with fluorine to form a highly inert, hydrophobic stent surface resistant to thrombosis (Figure 32.5) [39]. Although hydrophobic surfaces are theoretically more prone to thrombosis, this has not been borne out by experiments comparing hydrophilic polymers to hydrophobic fluorinated polymers [49]. Instead, the high energy C-F bond's thermodynamic stability and relative non-polarity lower the surface energy and potential, respectively, of the CoCr platform [50]. These characteristics explain fluoropassivation, an empirically observed improvement in endothelial healing, resistance to thrombosis, and reduced inflammatory potential of fluorinated polymers [3,39,49–52].

Glass transition temperature for polymers

A brief word about glass transition temperature for polymers, T_g, the temperature below which polymers are brittle and prone to cracking, and above which they are pliable and elastic; it is the energy required to overcome intermolecular forces resisting fluid

motion of polymer chains. PVDF-HFP has a very low T_g of $-29\,°C$, resulting in inherently high elasticity and fatigue resistance at body temperature. This is particularly important in both the short and long term, as more brittle polymers can crack during balloon expansion or with constant cardiac motion and arterial pulsatility.

In summary, the semi-crystalline fluorinated structure and low T_g of PVDF-HFP contribute to high oxidative stability, resistance to fatigue and cracking, low thrombogenicity, and favorable drug release kinetics.

Drug

Everolimus is a partially synthetic analogue of sirolimus (rapamycin), a naturally occurring compound formed by *Streptomyces hygroscopicus*. Sirolimus and its analogues bind cytosolic FK-506 Binding Protein-12 (FKBP12) to form a complex inhibiting the mammalian target of rapamycin (MToR), resulting in cytostatic G1-phase cell cycle arrest. Everolimus may also selectively clear macrophages from atheromas, theoretically stabilizing vulnerable plaques, but the clinical significance remains to be elucidated [53].

Sirolimus analogues are synthesized by manipulating various carbon side-chain atoms. The sirolimus derivatives have similar *in vivo* potency and efficacy in their formulations for coronary DES but have highly varied lipophilicity. Everolimus is more lipophilic than sirolimus, resulting in increased local vascular uptake, particularly into lipid-rich atheroma, and lower systemic distribution. This has allowed the EES to contain a lower concentration of drug ($100\,\mu g/cm^2$).

The CoCr-EES has demonstrated excellent short- and long-term endothelial healing similar to bare metal stents and superior to the first-generation DES (Figure 32.6) [54]. This is partially caused by the kinetics of drug release, an important contributor to endothelial healing and clinical outcomes. The polymer-drug formulation of the CoCr-EES results in approximately 30% drug release within the first 24 hours after implantation, leading to 80% release by 30 days and complete elution by 120 days. The mechanisms of polymeric drug-elution are complex, but suffice it to say that the low T_g of

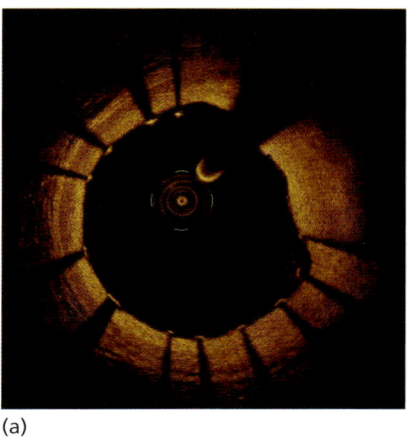
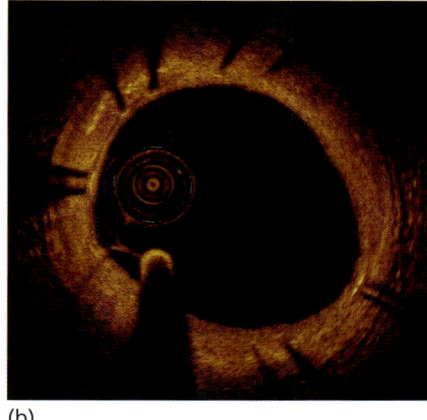

(a)   (b)

Figure 32.6 Cobalt-chromium everolimus-eluting stents (CoCr-EES) apposition and tissue coverage by optical coherence tomography (OCT). Intracoronary OCT provides high-resolution *in vivo* imaging of the coronary lumen, intimal-medial vessel structure, and stent struts. (a) Post-intervention OCT imaging shows good stent apposition to the vessel wall. (b) The same coronary segment imaged by OCT 6 months later shows even tissue coverage without hyperplastic response.

PVDF-HFP and the miscibility of polymer and drug (as both are hydrophobic) factor into controlled drug release.

Xience stents: clinical trials

A multitude of trials have proven the short- and long-term safety and efficacy of the CoCr-EES compared to first generation DES, and now these stents are considered the standard comparator for newer devices and scaffolds. As such, several landmark studies investigating the Xience EES are presented (Table 32.3).

SPIRIT I–IV

SPIRIT FIRST was a prospective trial randomizing 56 patients to the Xience V-EES or the Multi-Link Vision (Guidant/Abbott Vascular, Santa Clara, CA, USA) L605 CoCr BMS [55]. Early angiographic results from SPIRIT FIRST showed excellent performance of the Xience V-EES compared to the Multi-Link Vision CoCr BMS (6-month in-stent late lumen loss of 0.1 vs. 0.87 mm; p <0.001), along with a non-significantly lower rate of clinical events (7.7% vs. 21.4%; p =NS), as a result of low sample size resulting in lack of power to assess clinical outcomes. Long-term data confirmed that the early findings of superior safety and efficacy of the Xience V-EES over the Multi-Link Vision were consistently maintained over 5 years [56].

The SPIRIT II-IV trials compared the Xience V-EES with the Taxus paclitaxel-eluting stent (PES) (Boston Scientific, Natick, MA, USA). Early angiographic results from SPIRIT II demonstrated superior performance of the XV-EES compared to the Taxus PES, with a 6-month in-stent late lumen loss of 0.11 vs. 0.36 mm (p <0.0001) [57]. Although 2-year angiographic and intravascular ultrasound (IVUS) outcomes suggested a "late catch up" phenomenon with the XV-EES, there was no concomitant increase in adverse clinical events [58]. After 5 years, the XV-EES remained superior to the Taxus PES as evidenced by lower cardiac mortality, clinically driven TLR, and ischemia-driven MACE [59]. Interestingly, there was a lower incidence of definite or probable stent thrombosis in the EES group despite significantly lower dual antiplatelet therapy (DAPT) adherence at 5 years.

SPIRIT III showed a similar pattern of early angiographic superiority of the Xience V-EES over the Taxus PES in terms of 8-month in-stent late lumen loss (0.16 vs. 0.30 mm; p =0.002), along with significantly lower 1-year major adverse cardiac events (MACE) (6.0% vs. 10.3%; p =0.02) [60]. Superiority of the Xience V-EES was maintained at 5 years, with significantly lower rates of target vessel failure (TVF), target lesion failure (TLF), MACE, and all-cause death than the Taxus PES [2].

SPIRIT IV randomized 3690 patients with broad inclusion criteria to the Xience V-EES or the Taxus Express 2 PES (Boston Scientific). At 1 year, the EES showed significant reduction in ischemia-driven target lesion revascularization (TLR), TLF, target vessel revascularization (TVR), TVF, MACE, definite stent thrombosis, and any MI compared to the PES [61]. At 3 years, the Xience V-EES remained superior in terms of rates of death, target-vessel MI, TLF, and definite or probable stent thrombosis. Only ischemia-driven TLR became non-significant, though trended lower, for the EES. These results suggest that the main advantage of the Xience V-EES is its persistent and superior safety rather than efficacy over the Taxus PES [1].

A patient-pooled meta-analysis of 4989 patients (EES n =3350; PES n =1639) in the SPIRIT II, III, and IV randomized trials reaffirmed superior outcome with the EES compared with the TAXUS PES up to 3-years follow-up (as the final follow-up data for SPIRIT IV were collected at 3 years) [1]. This meta-analysis showed a reduction in all-cause mortality (3.2% vs. 5.1%; p =0.003) with the EES compared with the TAXUS PES. It has been hypothesized that reduced rates of repeat revascularization, myocardial infarction, and stent thrombosis with the EES have subsequently led to a significant reduction in this hard endpoint.

COMPARE I

The COMPARE I trial examined clinical outcomes in 1800 patients undergoing elective or emergent PCI randomized to the Xience V-EES or the TaxusLiberte PES (Boston Scientific). Of note, 74% of lesions were complex (Type B2/C) and the study population had a high acuity, with 27% of all participants presenting with ST-elevation myocardial infarction (STEMI). At 1 year, the Xience V-EES showed significantly lower clinical event rates [62]. After 2 years, the continued superiority of the Xience V-EES was driven mainly by decreased TVR, MI, and definite or probable stent thrombosis, as the difference between stents widened further for these measures [63].

Table 32.3 Selected trials

Trial	XV-EES versus:	Trial design	Selected inclusion/exclusion criteria	n	1° endpoint	Outcomes*	Conclusions
SPIRIT FIRST	MLV-BMS	Prospective, randomized, single-blind	I: One de novo lesion treatable with single 3.0 x 18 mm stent; silent, stable or unstable ischemia E: AMI; unprotected LM lesions, CTO, bifurcation lesions, heavy calcification, ISR; thrombus, LVEF <30%	60	In-stent LLL at 6 months	1°: 0.10 vs. 0.87 mm, p <0.001	XV-EES significantly reduced restenosis versus BMS; non-significantly lower rate of clinical events with EES
SPIRIT II	Taxus PES	Prospective, randomized, single-blind	I: up to 2 de novo lesions in different arteries; RVD 2.5–4.25 mm, length ≤28 mm E: AMI within 3 days; LVEF <30%; ostial, LM, bifurcation lesions; heavy calcification, thrombus	300	In-stent LLL at 6 months	1°: 0.11 vs. 0.36 mm, p <0.0001 for superiority	XV-EES superior to PES in reducing in-stent LLL; low rates of clinical events in both groups
SPIRIT III	Taxus PES	Prospective, randomized, single-blind	I: up to 2 de novo lesions in different coronary arteries; RVD 2.5–3.75 mm, length ≤28 mm; stable or unstable angina, or inducible ischemia E: Acute or recent MI, prior PCI in target vessel or planned within 9 months, non-target vessel intervention within 90 days prior or 9 months after	1002	In-segment LLL at 8 months	1°: 0.14 vs. 0.26 mm, p=0.003	XV-EES significantly reduced in-segment LLL compared to PES; lower rates of 12-month TVF and MACE
SPIRIT IV	Taxus Express 2 PES	Prospective, randomized, single-blind	I: Up to 3 de novo lesions in 1–2 epicardial arteries; RVD 2.5–3.75 mm, length ≤28 mm E: Left main trunk disease; recent MI, CTO, thrombus, or complex bifurcation	3687	Ischemia-driven TLF (CD, TV-MI, ID-TLR)	1°: 4.2% vs. 6.8%, p=0.001	XV-EES superior to PES for TLF; significantly lower rates of ID-TLR MI, and ST
XIENCE V USA	none	Prospective, observational, single-arm	I: treatment with only EES E: Limited exclusion criteria	5054	Definite and probable ST; Composite CD and MI at 12 months	1°: ST - 0.84% CD/MI - 6.5%	XV-EES shows excellent safety and efficacy in an unselected population
COMPARE I	TaxusLiberte PES	Prospective, randomized, single-blind	I: Elective or emergent PCI; complex lesions (type B2/C) E: limited exclusion criteria; non-compliance or contraindication to 12 months DAPT; planned major surgery within 30 days	1800	Composite of all death, non-fatal MI, TVR at 12 months	1°: 6.2% vs. 9.2%, p=0.02	XV-EES safe and effective in an all-comer population

	Design	Inclusion (I:) / Exclusion (E:) criteria	N	Primary endpoint	Result	Conclusion
EXAMINATION	Prospective, randomized	**I:** STEMI within 48 hours **E:** limited exclusion criteria; STEMI due to stent thrombosis	1498	Composite all death, any recurrent MI, any revascularization	1°: 11.9% vs. 14.2%, p = 0.19	XV-EES did not lower primary composite endpoint, but reduced TLR and ST
EXCELLENT	Prospective, randomized, open-label	**I:** Any number and location of lesions; silent ischemia, stable and unstable angina; RVD 2.25–4.25 mm **E:** STEMI within 72 hours, LVEF <25%, >50% stenosis of LM; CTO, in-stent restenosis, bifurcations requiring 2 stents	1443	In-segment LLL at 9 months	1°: 0.11 vs. 0.06 mm, p = 0.09 ($p_{non\text{-}inferiority}$ = 0.0382)	XV-EES non-inferior to SES for inhibition of LLL; similarly low rates of clinical events in both groups
EXECUTIVE: Prospective arm	Prospective, randomized	**I:** Multivessel disease; RVD 2.5–4.0 mm; length <28 mm; acceptable candidate for CABG **E:** AMI within 72 hours; LM, arterial or venous graft lesion; heavy calcification	200	In-stent LLL at 9 months	1°: –0.03 vs. 0.23 mm, p = 0.001	XV-EES significantly lowers LLL versus PES in patients with multivessel disease and low-to-intermediate SYNTAX score
EXECUTIVE: Retrospective arm	Single-arm	**I:** Multivessel disease; RVD 2.5–4.0 mm; length <28 mm; acceptable candidate for CABG **E:** AMI within 72 hours; LM, arterial or venous graft lesion; heavy calcification	400	Composite of all-cause death, MI, or ischemia-driven TVR at 12 months	1°: 9.2%	XV-EES shows low MACE rate in patients with multivessel disease
TWENTE	Prospective, randomized, single-blind	**I:** Stable or unstable ischemia; no limits on lesion length or RVD **E:** STEMI; limited exclusion criteria	1391	Composite of CD, MI, clinically-driven TVR at 12 months	1°: 8.1% vs. 8.2%, p = 0.94	XV-EES and R-ZES have similarly low clinical event rates in an unselected, complex population

AMI, acute myocardial infarction; CABG, coronary artery bypass graft; CD, cardiac death; C-SES, Cypher sirolimus-eluting stent; CTO, chronic total occlusion; DAPT, dual antiplatelet therapy; ISR, in-stent restenosis; LLL, late lumen loss; LM, left main; MLV-BMS, Multi-Link Vision bare metal stent; RVD, reference vessel diameter; R-ZES, Resolute zotarolimus-eluting stent; ST, stent thrombosis; STEMI, ST-elevation myocardial infarction; TLF, target lesion failure; T-PES, Taxus paclitaxel-eluting stent; TVR, target vessel revascularization; XV-EES, Xience V everolimus-eluting stent.

* All values are presented as XV-EES versus comparator stent.

EXAMINATION

The EXAMINATION trial studied 1498 patients presenting with STEMI, randomized to the Xience V-EES or the Multi-Link Vision (Abbott Vascular) CoCr BMS [64]. The primary endpoint was the composite of all-cause death, any MI, any revascularization at 1 year, and was specifically chosen to encompass the wide range of variables that may account for post-STEMI outcomes.

Ultimately, while the composite primary endpoint results did not show a significant difference between groups, the Xience V-EES significantly reduced TLR, TVR, and definite early stent thrombosis at 1 year [64]. These differences were maintained at 2 years: the Xience V-EES significantly reduced any repeat revascularization (TLR 2.9% vs. 5.6%; p = 0.009; TVR 4.8% vs. 7.9%; p = 0.014) and definite or probable stent thrombosis compared to BMS (1.3% vs. 2.8%; p = 0.04). However, overall rates of all cause death, cardiac death, and MI remained similar [65].

It is interesting to note that the Xience V's reduction in definite or probable stent thrombosis was driven mainly by lower early ST despite nearly 100% DAPT compliance in both groups. It remains unclear if this can be attributed to a polymer-mediated protective effect against thrombosis, but may be of particular significance in patients presenting with STEMI, where thrombus dissolution can lead to late acquired incomplete stent apposition (ISA), uncovered struts, and stent thrombosis.

EXCELLENT

The EXCELLENT trial compared clinical and angiographic outcomes of 1443 patients randomized to the Xience V/Promus EES or the Cypher sirolimus-eluting stent (SES) (Cordis, Miami, Florida) over 5 years. The primary endpoint, in-segment late lumen loss at 9 months, was similar for both stents (EES 0.11 vs. 0.06 mm, p = 0.09), as were all other angiographic and clinical outcome measures [66]. Long-term data will be critical in demonstrating any differences in the incidence of very late stent thrombosis and other measures of clinical safety and efficacy of the Xience V against the standard bearer Cypher SES.

EXECUTIVE

While the landmark SYNTAX study demonstrated the role of angiographically determined disease complexity in delineating surgical versus percutaneous management of patients with multivessel disease [67], these studies were based largely on first-generation DES data.

The EXECUTIVE trial prospectively and retrospectively evaluated outcomes in patients with multivessel disease and low-to-intermediate SYNTAX scores [68]. The prospective arm examined 200 patients randomly receiving either EES or PES, with a primary endpoint of 9-month in-stent late lumen loss and secondary endpoint of 12-month composite all-cause death, MI, or ischemia-driven TVR. The retrospective arm evaluated outcomes from a registry of 400 patients who received EES, with a primary endpoint of composite all-cause death, MI, or clinically driven TLR.

For the prospective arm, 9-month in-stent late lumen loss results showed superiority of the EES over PES (−0.03 vs. 0.23 mm; p = 0.001). Comparison of 12-month clinical outcomes for the prospective and retrospective arms showed that the composite endpoint was reached in 9.2% of the registry patients, 11.1% of EES, and 16.5% of PES (p = 0.30). The EXECUTIVE study showed that in patients with multivessel disease and low-to-intermediate SYNTAX scores treated with PCI, EES provides significantly better 9-month angiographic outcomes over PES, but clinical outcomes at 1 year are similar.

TWENTE

The TWENTE trial randomized 1391 patients to the Xience V-EES or the Resolute-ZES (Medtronic, Santa Rosa, CA, USA). Of note, the study protocol had limited exclusion criteria, mandated strict discontinuation of DAPT at 12 months, and encouraged stent post-dilatation. The primary endpoint of TVF at 1 year was similar between stents (ZES 8.2% vs. 8.1%; p = 0.94) [69].

At 2 years, the TWENTE trial showed overall similar clinical results between stents in patients with complex lesions and off-label indications [70]. Despite lower clinically driven TLR with the Xience V-EES, this did not translate to higher rates of TLF or cardiac death in the Resolute-ZES group (TLF: ZES 10.8% vs. 11.6%; p = 0.65; cardiac death: ZES 1.6% vs. 2.7%; p = 0.14). Similiarly, the incidence of late stent thrombosis was similar (ZES 1.2% vs. 1.4%; p = 0.65), as was the rate of very late stent thrombosis (VLST; ZES 0.3% vs. 0.3%; p = 1.00) after discontinuation of thienopyridine. Of the four patients with VLST, there was no clear temporal association between discontinuation of DAPT and thrombosis.

Most interesting is that while DAPT adherence at 2 years was extremely low as a result of protocol mandate (much lower than other comparable trials, such as Leaders, Resolute AC, Compare, Spirit IV), the rate of very late stent thrombosis was similar to these studies. These observations have raised significant questions regarding the optimal duration of DAPT.

Second-generation DES and dual-antiplatelet therapy

The excellent overall hemocompatibility of the CoCr stents has led to preliminary observations that early discontinuation of standard 12-month duration of DAPT may not increase the rate of late stent thrombosis in low-risk patients [71–74]. Several meta-analyses further suggest that longer durations of DAPT do not reduce adverse cardiovascular event rates but significantly increase the risk of bleeding [75,76].

A substudy of the EXCELLENT trial, which evaluated 1443 patients with EES or SES, further randomized these patients to 6 or 12 months of DAPT [71]. At 12 months, the primary endpoint of TVF was 4.8% for 6-month DAPT versus 4.3% for 12-month DAPT (p = 0.001 for non-inferiority). The risk of TVF was non-significantly higher in patients with SES in the 6-month group compared to 12 months, but there was no difference in the EES groups. Additionally, while there was a non-significantly increased rate of stent thrombosis in the 6-month group, five out of six events occurred while still on DAPT. Interestingly, subgroup analysis showed that diabetic patients in the 6-month group had higher TVF than the 12-month group, suggesting that a longer duration of DAPT could be beneficial in diabetic and other high-risk patients.

One-year results from the Xience V USA Registry of over 8000 real-world patients suggest that whereas DAPT discontinuation prior to 30 days post-PCI is a strong, independent predictor of stent thrombosis (HR 8.63; p = 0.008), discontinuation after 30 days is not a risk factor for late stent thrombosis at 1 year [77]. Pooled analysis of the RESOLUTE trials reported similar findings with the Resolute ZES, showing that the 1-year stent thrombosis rate in patients who interrupted DAPT prior to 30 days was 3.61%, compared to 0.11% in patients who interrupted DAPT after 30 days [78]. Both of these studies show that regardless of DAPT status, most stent thrombosis occurred within 30 days, suggesting that other factors likely contribute to early stent thrombosis.

While these results are not definitive and no conclusive recommendations have been made pending ongoing studies, they highlight the clinical relevance of hemocompatibility of all stent components.

CoCr-EES in specific lesion subsets
Bifurcation lesions

PCI of true bifurcation lesions is regarded as technically challenging and many studies have compared an initial one-stent or a dedicated two-stent strategy in this lesion subset. A single-center observational study of 319 patients undergoing true bifurcation PCI with CoCr-EES reported superior angiographic outcomes and comparable clinical outcomes with a two-stent strategy compared with a one-stent strategy [79]. Acute gain was improved with a two-stent strategy (0.65 ± 0.41 vs. 1.11 ± 0.47 mm; p >0.0001) and at 1-year clinical follow-up rates of target vessel revascularization (two-stent 5.8% vs. one-stent 7.4%; p = 0.31), myocardial infarction (two-stent 7.8% vs. one-stent 12.2%; p = 0.31), and major adverse cardiovascular events (two-stent 16.6% vs. one-stent 21.8%; p = 0.21) were non-significantly lower with a two-stent strategy. A similar study by the same investigators including only diabetic patients showed qualitatively similar results [80]. These studies suggest that the CoCr-EES may be well-suited for a dedicated two-stent approach in true bifurcation lesions.

In-stent restenosis

The performance of the CoCr-EES in in-stent restenosis lesions (ISR) was evaluated in the XIENCE V USA prospective multicenter registry [81]. A total of 383 out of 5215 patients underwent PCI of ISR lesions (7.4%). At 1 year, target lesion failure occurred in 10.9% of patients, MI in 2.2%, TLR in 10.3%, and cardiac death in 1.4% of patients. This study showed that the treatment of ISR with CoCr-EES is sage and efficacious at 1 year follow-up. However, rates of adverse events were significantly higher than patients who underwent PCI of non-ISR lesions. The use of CoCr-EES for ISR lesions was compared with paclitaxel-eluting balloons, balloon angioplasty, PES, and SES in a network meta-analysis of seven randomized trials [82]. This Bayesian meta-analysis showed that paclitaxel-eluting balloons and Co-Cr EES had the highest probabilities for being the best treatment option.

Small vessels and long lesions

A patient-pooled meta-analysis using data from 6283 patients included in the SPIRIT II, III, IV, and COMPARE randomized controlled trials (EES n = 3944; PES n = 2239) showed that patients with long lesions (>13.4 mm) in small vessels (<2.65 mm) have the lowest rates of adverse events [83]. This study showed that the CoCr-EES as compared with the PES resulted in significantly improved outcomes in patients with long lesions and/or small vessels, and non-significantly improved outcomes in patients with short lesions in large vessels.

Multivessel disease

The recently published Randomized Comparison of Coronary Artery Bypass Surgery and Everolimus-Eluting Stent Implantation in the Treatment of Patients with Multivessel Coronary Artery Disease (BEST) trial included a total of 880 patients with multivessel coronary artery disease who were randomly assigned to PCI with EES or CABG [84]. Patients with left main coronary artery disease were excluded. At a median follow-up of 4.6 years, there were no significant differences in terms of death or myocardial infarction between both groups. There was, however, an increased rate of repeat revascularization, because of a significantly higher rate of non-target lesion revascularization in the PCI group. This study suggests that PCI with CoCr EES may be an alternative to CABG surgery in anatomically complex multivessel disease.

Conclusions

The CoCr-EES have repeatedly and consistently demonstrated safety, efficacy, and deliverability compared to earlier stainless steel bare metal and first-generation DES. Their clinical success can be attributed to improvements in each of the three design elements of DES: the platform, polymer, and drug. The detailed mechanistic exploration of these improvements lends insight into factors that will continue to be important in stent design and optimizing clinical outcomes. In particular, what has emerged is the absolute importance of vascular endothelial integrity and function.

The CoCr-EES are now the standard comparator for new stents and scaffolds, but regardless of their excellent safety and efficacy, the permanent nature of these devices remains their lasting pitfall as persistent sources of endothelial injury. It is expected that ongoing advances in stent design will continue to shift the paradigm toward bioabsorbable materials that better maintain endothelial integrity and natural vasomotor function over time.

Interactive multiple choice questions are available for this chapter on www.wiley.com/go/dangas/cardiology

References

1 Dangas GD, Serruys PW, Kereiakes DJ, *et al*. Meta-analysis of everolimus-eluting versus paclitaxel-eluting stents in coronary artery disease: final 3-year results of the SPIRIT clinical trials program (Clinical Evaluation of the Xience V Everolimus Eluting Coronary Stent System in the Treatment of Patients With De Novo Native Coronary Artery Lesions). *JACC Cardiovasc Interv* 2013; **6**: 914–922.

2 Gada H, Kirtane AJ, Newman W, *et al*. 5-year results of a randomized comparison of XIENCE V everolimus-eluting and TAXUS paclitaxel-eluting stents: final results from the SPIRIT III trial (clinical evaluation of the XIENCE V everolimus eluting coronary stent system in the treatment of patients with de novo native coronary artery lesions). *JACC Cardiovasc Interv* 2013; **6**(12): 1263–1266.

3 Tada T, Byrne RA, Simunovic I, *et al*. Risk of stent thrombosis among bare-metal stents, first-generation drug-eluting stents, and second-generation drug-eluting stents: results from a registry of 18,334 patients. *JACC Cardiovasc Interv* 2013; **6**(12): 1267–1274.

4 Kirtane AJ, Leon MB, Ball MW, *et al*. The "final" 5-year follow-up from the ENDEAVOR IV trial comparing a zotarolimus-eluting stent with a paclitaxel-eluting stent. *JACC Cardiovasc Interv* 2013; **6**(4): 325–333.

5 Briguori C, Sarais C, Pagnotta P, *et al*. In-stent restenosis in small coronary arteries impact of strut thickness. *J Am Coll Cardiol* 2002; **40**: 403–409.

6 Kastrati A, Mehilli J, Dirschinger J, *et al*. Intracoronary Stenting and Angiographic Results: Strut Thickness Effect on Restenosis Outcome (ISAR-STEREO) Trial. *Circulation* 2001; **103**(23): 2816–2821.

7 Kolandaivelu K, Swaminathan R, Gibson WJ, *et al*. Stent thrombogenicity early in high-risk interventional settings is driven by stent design and deployment and protected by polymer-drug coatings. *Circulation* 2011; **123**(13): 1400–1409.

8 Foin N, Gutiérrez-Chico JL, Nakatani S, *et al*. Incomplete stent apposition causes high shear flow disturbances and delay in neointimal coverage as a function of strut to wall detachment distance: implications for the management of incomplete stent apposition. *Circ Cardiovasc Interv* 2014; **7**(2): 180–189.

9 LaDisa JF Jr, Olson LE, Douglas HA, Warltier DC, Kersten JR, Pagel PS. Alterations in regional vascular geometry produced by theoretical stent implantation influence distributions of wall shear stress: analysis of a curved coronary artery using 3D computational fluid dynamics modeling. *Biomed Eng Online* 2006; **5**: 40.

10 Tanigawa J, Barlis P, Dimopoulos K, Dalby M, Moore P, Di Mario C. The influence of strut thickness and cell design on immediate apposition of drug-eluting stents assessed by optical coherence tomography. *Int J Cardiol* 2009; **134**(2): 180–188.

11 Wentzel JJ, Whelan DM, van der Giessen WJ, *et al*. Coronary stent implantation changes 3-D vessel geometry and 3-D shear stress distribution. *J Biomechanics* 2000; **33**: 1287–1295.

12 Hara H, Nakamura M, Palmaz JC, Schwartz RS. Role of stent design and coatings on restenosis and thrombosis. *Adv Drug Deliv Rev* 2006; **58**(3): 377–386.

13 Sullivan TM, Ainsworth SD, Langan EM, et al. Effect of endovascular stent strut geometry on vascular injury, myointimal hyperplasia, and restenosis. *J Vasc Surg* 2002; **36**(1): 143–149.

14 Papayannis AC, Cipher D, Banerjee S, Brilakis ES. Optical coherence tomography evaluation of drug-eluting stents: a systematic review. *Catheter Cardiovasc Interv* 2013; **81**(3): 481–487.

15 Ormiston JA, Webber B, Webster MW. Stent longitudinal integrity bench insights into a clinical problem. *JACC Cardiovasc Interv* 2011; **4**(12): 1310–1317.

16 Pitney M, Pitney K, Jepson N, et al. Major stent deformation/pseudofracture of 7 Crown Endeavor/Micro Driver stent platform: incidence and causative factors. *EuroIntervention* 2011; **7**(2): 256–262.

17 Inaba S, Mintz GS, Yun KH, et al. Mechanical complications of everolimus-eluting stents associated with adverse events: an intravascular ultrasound study. *EuroIntervention* 2014; **9**: 1301–1308.

18 Abdel-Wahab M, Sulimov DS, Kassner G, Geist V, Toelg R, Richardt G. Longitudinal deformation of contemporary coronary stents: an integrated analysis of clinical experience and observations from the bench. *J Interv Cardiol* 2012; **25**(6): 576–585.

19 Kereiakes DJ, Popma JJ, Cannon LA, et al. Longitudinal stent deformation: quantitative coronary angiographic analysis from the PERSEUS and PLATINUM randomized controlled clinical trials. *EuroIntervention* 2012; **8**(2): 187–195.

20 Ormiston JA, Webber B, Ubod B, White J, Webster MW. Stent longitudinal strength assessed using point compression: insights from a second-generation, clinically related bench test. *Circ Cardiovasc Interv* 2014; **7**(1): 62–69.

21 Ota H, Kitabata H, Magalhaes MA, et al. Comparison of frequency and severity of longitudinal stent deformation among various drug-eluting stents: an intravascular ultrasound study. *Int J Cardiol* 2014; **175**(2): 261–267.

22 Romaguera R, Roura G, Gomez-Lara J, et al. Longitudinal deformation of drug-eluting stents: evaluation by multislice computed tomography. *J Invasive Cardiol* 2014; **26**(4): 161–166.

23 Poncin P, et al. *Comparing and Optimizing Co-Cr Tubing for Stent Applications. in Materials & Processes for Medical Devices.* Anaheim, CA, USA: 2004.

24 Chen Q, Thouas GA. Metallic implant biomaterials. *Materials Sci Eng R Rep* 2015; **87**: 1–57.

25 Hanawa T. Materials for metallic stents. *J Artif Organs* 2009; **12**(2): 73–79.

26 He Y, Maehara A, Mintz GS, et al. Intravascular ultrasound assessment of cobalt chromium versus stainless steel drug-eluting stent expansion. *Am J Cardiol* 2010; **105**(9): 1272–1275.

27 Kapnisis K, Constantinides G, Georgiou H, et al. Multi-scale mechanical investigation of stainless steel and cobalt-chromium stents. *J Mech Behav Biomed Mater* 2014; **40**: 240–251.

28 Lewis G. Materials, fluid dynamics, and solid mechanics aspects of coronary artery stents: a state-of-the-art review. *J Biomed Mater Res B Appl Biomater* 2008; **86**(2): 569–590.

29 Kereiakes DJ, Cox DA, Hermiller JB, et al. Usefulness of a cobalt chromium coronary stent alloy. *Am J Cardiol* 2003; **92**(4): 463–466.

30 Sketch MH Jr, Ball M, Rutherford B, et al. Evaluation of the Medtronic (Driver) cobalt-chromium alloy coronary stent system. *Am J Cardiol* 2005; **95**(1): 8–12.

31 Williams DF. On the mechanisms of biocompatibility. *Biomaterials* 2008; **29**(20): 2941–2953.

32 Kastrati A, Mehilli J, Dirschinger J, et al. Restenosis after coronary placement of various stent types. *Am J Cardiol* 2001; **87**: 34–39.

33 Kastrati A, Schömig A, Dirschinger J, et al. Increased risk of restenosis after placement of gold-coated stents. results of a randomized trial comparing gold-coated with uncoated steel stents in patients with coronary artery disease. *Circulation* 2000; **101**: 2478–2483.

34 Sick PB, Brosteanu O, Ulrich M, et al. Prospective randomized comparison of early and late results of a carbonized stent versus a high-grade stainless steel stent of identical design: the PREVENT Trial [corrected]. *Am Heart J* 2005; **149**(4): 681–688.

35 Sick PB, Gelbrich G, Kalnins U, et al. Comparison of early and late results of a Carbofilm-coated stent versus a pure high-grade stainless steel stent (the Carbostent-Trial). *Am J Cardiol* 2004; **93**(11): 1351–1356, A5.

36 Kastrati A, Dirschinger J, Boekstegers P, et al. Influence of stent design on 1-year outcome after coronary stent placement: a randomized comparison of five stent types in 1,147 unselected patients. *Catheter Cardiovasc Interv* 2000; **50**: 290–297.

37 Mani G, Feldman MD, Patel D, Agrawal CM. Coronary stents: a materials perspective. *Biomaterials* 2007; **28**(9): 1689–1710.

38 Ruckenstein E, Gourisankar SV. A surface energetic criterion of blood compatibility of foreign surfaces. *J Colloid Interface Science* 1984; **101**(2): 436–451.

39 Chin-Quee SL, Hsu SH, Nguyen-Ehrenreich KL, et al. Endothelial cell recovery, acute thrombogenicity, and monocyte adhesion and activation on fluorinated copolymer and phosphorylcholine polymer stent coatings. *Biomaterials* 2010; **31**(4): 648–657.

40 Palmaz JC. New advances in endovascular technology. *Texas Heart Inst J* 1997; **24**: 156–159.

41 DePalma VA, et al. Investigation of three-surface properties of several metals and their relation to blood compatibility. *J Biomed Mater Res Symp* 1972; **3**: 37–75.

42 Hehrlein C, Zimmermann M, Metz J, Ensinger W, Kübler W. Influence of surface texture and charge on the biocompatibility of endovascular stents. *Coron Artery Dis* 1995; **6**: 581–586.

43 Aihara H. Surface and biocompatibility study of electropolished L605, in General Engineering. 2009, San Jose State University.

44 Sprague EA, Palmaz JC. A model system to assess key vascular responses to biomaterials. *J Endovasc Ther* 2005; **12**: 594–604.

45 Koster R, Vieluf D, Kiehn M, et al. Nickel and molybdenum contact allergies in patients with coronary in-stent restenosis. *Lancet* 2000; **356**(9245): 1895–1897.

46 Edelman ER, Seifert P, Groothuis A, Morss A, Bornstein D, Rogers C. Gold-coated NIR stents in porcine coronary arteries. *Circulation* 2001; **103**: 429–434.

47 Yan Y, Neville A, Dowson D. Tribo-corrosion properties of cobalt-based medical implant alloys in simulated biological environments. *Wear* 2007; **263**(7-12): 1105–1111.

48 Okazaki Y, Gotoh E. Metal release from stainless steel, Co–Cr–Mo–Ni–Fe and Ni–Ti alloys in vascular implants. *Corrosion Sci* 2008; **50**(12): 3429–3438.

49 Gutierrez-Chico JL, van Geuns RJ, Regar E, et al. Tissue coverage of a hydrophilic polymer-coated zotarolimus-eluting stent vs. a fluoropolymer-coated everolimus-eluting stent at 13-month follow-up: an optical coherence tomography substudy from the RESOLUTE All Comers trial. *Eur Heart J* 2011; **32**(19): 2454–2463.

50 Xie X, Guidoin R, Nutley M, Zhang Z. Fluoropassivation and gelatin sealing of polyester arterial prostheses to skip preclotting and constrain the chronic inflammatory response. *J Biomed Mater Res B Appl Biomater* 2010; **93**(2): 497–509.

51 Guidoin R, Marois Y, Zhang Z, et al. The benefits of fluoropassivation of polyester arterial prostheses as observed in a canine model. *ASAIO J* 1994; **40**: M870–879.

52 Raber L, Magro M, Stefanini GG, et al. Very late coronary stent thrombosis of a newer-generation everolimus-eluting stent compared with early-generation drug-eluting stents: a prospective cohort study. *Circulation* 2012; **125**(9): 1110–1121.

53 Verheye S, Martinet W, Kockx MM, et al. Selective clearance of macrophages in atherosclerotic plaques by autophagy. *J Am Coll Cardiol* 2007; **49**(6): 706–715.

54 Joner M, Nakazawa G, Finn AV, et al. Endothelial cell recovery between comparator polymer-based drug-eluting stents. *J Am Coll Cardiol* 2008; **52**(5): 333–342.

55 Serruys PW, Ong AT, Piek JJ, et al. A randomized comparison of a durable polymer Everolimus-eluting stent with a bare metal coronary stent: The SPIRIT first trial. *EuroIntervention* 2005; **1**(1): 58–65.

56 Wiemer M, Serruys PW, Miquel-Hebert K, et al. Five-year long-term clinical follow-up of the XIENCE V everolimus eluting coronary stent system in the treatment of patients with de novo coronary artery lesions: the SPIRIT FIRST trial. *Catheter Cardiovasc Interv* 2010; **75**(7): 997–1003.

57 Serruys PW, Ruygrok P, Neuzner J, et al. A randomised comparison of an everolimus-eluting coronary stent with a paclitaxel-eluting coronary stent: the SPIRIT II trial. *EuroIntervention* 2006; **2**: 286–294.

58 Claessen BE, Beijk MA, Legrand V, et al. Two-year clinical, angiographic, and intravascular ultrasound follow-up of the XIENCE V everolimus-eluting stent in the treatment of patients with de novo native coronary artery lesions: the SPIRIT II trial. *Circ Cardiovasc Interv* 2009; **2**(4): 339–347.

59 Onuma Y, Miquel-Hebert K, Serruys PW. Five-year long-term clinical follow-up of the XIENCE V everolimus-eluting coronary stent system in the treatment of patients with de novo coronary artery disease: the SPIRIT II trial. *EuroIntervention* 2013; **8**: 1047–1051.

60 Stone GW, Midei M, Newman W, et al. Comparison of an everolimus-eluting stent and a paclitaxel-eluting stent in patients with coronary artery disease a randomized trial. *JAMA* 2008; **299**(16): 1903–1913.

61 Stone GW, Rizvi A, Newman W, et al. Everolimus-eluting versus paclitaxel-eluting stents in coronary artery disease. *N Engl J Med* 2010; **362**(18): 1663–1674.

62 Kedhi E, Joesoef KS, McFadden E, et al. Second-generation everolimus-eluting and paclitaxel-eluting stents in real-life practice (COMPARE): a randomised trial. *Lancet* 2010; **375**: 205–209.

63 Smits PC, Kedhi E, Royaards KJ, et al. 2-year follow-up of a randomized controlled trial of everolimus- and paclitaxel-eluting stents for coronary revascularization in daily practice. COMPARE (Comparison of the everolimus eluting XIENCE-V stent with the paclitaxel eluting TAXUS LIBERTE stent in all-comers: a randomized open label trial). *J Am Coll Cardiol* 2011; **58**(1): 11–18.

64 Sabate M, Cequier A, Iñiguez A, et al. Everolimus-eluting stent versus bare-metal stent in ST-segment elevation myocardial infarction (EXAMINATION): 1 year results of a randomised controlled trial. *Lancet* 2012; **380**(9852): 1482–1490.

65 Sabate M, Brugaletta S, Cequier A, et al. The EXAMINATION trial (Everolimus-Eluting Stents Versus Bare-Metal Stents in ST-Segment Elevation Myocardial Infarction): 2-year results from a multicenter randomized controlled trial. *JACC Cardiovasc Interv* 2014; **7**(1): 64–71.

66 Park KW, Chae IH, Lim DS, *et al.* Everolimus-eluting versus sirolimus-eluting stents in patients undergoing percutaneous coronary intervention: the EXCELLENT (Efficacy of Xience/Promus Versus Cypher to Reduce Late Loss After Stenting) randomized trial. *J Am Coll Cardiol* 2011; **58**(18): 1844–1854.

67 Serruys PW, Morice MC, Kappetein AP, *et al.* Percutaneous coronary intervention versus coronary-artery bypass grafting for severe coronary artery disease. *N Engl J Med* 2009; **360**(10): 961–972.

68 Ribichini F, Romano M, Rosiello R, *et al.* A clinical and angiographic study of the XIENCE V everolimus-eluting coronary stent system in the treatment of patients with multivessel coronary artery disease: the EXECUTIVE trial (EXecutive RCT: evaluating XIENCE V in a multi vessel disease). *JACC Cardiovasc Interv* 2013; **6**(10): 1012–1022.

69 von Birgelen C, Basalus MW, Tandjung K, *et al.* A randomized controlled trial in second-generation zotarolimus-eluting Resolute stents versus everolimus-eluting Xience V stents in real-world patients: the TWENTE trial. *J Am Coll Cardiol* 2012; **59**(15): 1350–1361.

70 Tandjung K, Sen H Lam MK, *et al.* Clinical outcome following stringent discontinuation of dual antiplatelet therapy after 12 months in real-world patients treated with second-generation zotarolimus-eluting resolute and everolimus-eluting Xience V stents: 2-year follow-up of the randomized TWENTE trial. *J Am Coll Cardiol* 2013; **61**(24): 2406–2416.

71 Gwon HC, Hahn JY, Park KW, *et al.* Six-month versus 12-month dual antiplatelet therapy after implantation of drug-eluting stents: the Efficacy of Xience/Promus Versus Cypher to Reduce Late Loss After Stenting (EXCELLENT) randomized, multicenter study. *Circulation* 2012; **125**(3): 505–513.

72 Kim BK, Hong MK, Shin DH, *et al.* A new strategy for discontinuation of dual antiplatelet therapy: the RESET Trial (REal Safety and Efficacy of 3-month dual antiplatelet Therapy following Endeavor zotarolimus-eluting stent implantation). *J Am Coll Cardiol* 2012; **60**(15): 1340–1348.

73 Park SJ, Park DW, Kim YH, *et al.* Duration of dual antiplatelet therapy after implantation of drug-eluting stents. *N Engl J Med* 2010; **362**: 1374–1382.

74 Valgimigli M, Campo G, Monti M, *et al.* Short- versus long-term duration of dual-antiplatelet therapy after coronary stenting: a randomized multicenter trial. *Circulation* 2012; **125**(16): 2015–2026.

75 Cassese S, Byrne RA, Tada T, King LA, Kastrati A. Clinical impact of extended dual antiplatelet therapy after percutaneous coronary interventions in the drug-eluting stent era: a meta-analysis of randomized trials. *Eur Heart J* 2012; **33**(24): 3078–3087.

76 Valgimigli M, Park SJ, Kim HS, *et al.* Benefits and risks of long-term duration of dual antiplatelet therapy after drug-eluting stenting: a meta-analysis of randomized trials. *Int J Cardiol* 2013; **168**(3): 2579–2587.

77 Naidu SS, Krucoff MW, Rutledge DR, *et al.* Contemporary incidence and predictors of stent thrombosis and other major adverse cardiac events in the year after XIENCE V implantation: results from the 8,061-patient XIENCE V United States study. *JACC Cardiovasc Interv* 2012; **5**(6): 626–635.

78 Silber S, Kirtane AJ, Belardi JA, *et al.* Lack of association between dual antiplatelet therapy use and stent thrombosis between 1 and 12 months following resolute zotarolimus-eluting stent implantation. *Eur Heart J* 2014; **35**(29): 1949–1956.

79 Kherada NI, Sartori S, Tomey MI, *et al.* Dedicated two-stent technique in complex bifurcation percutaneous coronary intervention with use of everolimus-eluting stents: the EES-bifurcation study. *Int J Cardiol* 2014; **174**(1): 13–17.

80 Meelu OA, Tomey MI, Sartori S, *et al.* Comparison of provisional 1-stent and 2-stent strategies in diabetic patients with true bifurcation lesions: the EES bifurcation study. *J Invasive Cardiol* 2014; **26**(12): 619–623.

81 Lee MS, Yang T, Mahmud E, *et al.* Clinical outcomes in the percutaneous coronary intervention of in-stent restenosis with everolimus-eluting stents. *J Invasive Cardiol* 2014; **26**(9): 420–426.

82 Piccolo R, Galasso G, Piscione F, *et al.* Meta-analysis of randomized trials comparing the effectiveness of different strategies for the treatment of drug-eluting stent restenosis. *Am J Cardiol* 2014; **114**(9): 1339–1346.

83 Claessen BE, Smits PC, Kereiakes DJ, *et al.* Impact of lesion length and vessel size on clinical outcomes after percutaneous coronary intervention with everolimus- versus paclitaxel-eluting stents pooled analysis from the SPIRIT (Clinical Evaluation of the XIENCE V Everolimus Eluting Coronary Stent System) and COMPARE (Second-generation everolimus-eluting and paclitaxel-eluting stents in real-life practice) Randomized Trials. *JACC Cardiovasc Interv* 2011; **4**(11): 1209–1215.

84 Park SJ, Ahn JM, Kim YH, *et al.* Trial of everolimus-eluting stents or bypass surgery for coronary disease. *N Engl J Med* 2015; **372**(13): 1204–1212.

CHAPTER 33

Platinum-Chromium Everolimus-Eluting Stents

Vikas Thondapu[1], Bimmer E.P.M. Claessen[2], George D. Dangas[3], Patrick W. Serruys[4], and Peter Barlis[1]

[1] Melbourne Medical School, Faculty of Medicine, Dentistry and Health Sciences, The University of Melbourne, Australia
[2] Department of Cardiology, Academic Medical Center—University of Amsterdam, Amsterdam, The Netherlands
[3] Department of Cardiology, Mount Sinai Medical Center, New York, NY, USA
[4] Faculty of Medicine, National Heart & Lung Institute, Imperial College London, London, UK

The critical role of intravascular injury in thrombosis has been well understood for over a century [1]. The advent of coronary intervention further underscored the potentially catastrophic consequences of vessel injury, namely stent thrombosis and restenosis. Interventional practice has evolved in the face of these clinical pressures and as a result, stent thrombosis and restenosis have become increasingly rare. Along with dual antiplatelet therapy and refined stent deployment technique, advances in stent design have revolutionized the treatment of ischemic heart disease.

With the goal of reducing vessel injury, the conventional approach to stent design has prioritized flexibility and conformability to the vessel wall. This strategy has contributed to several immensely successful devices, among them the platinum-chromium everolimus-eluting stents. From alloy composition to polymer and drug biocompatibility, the platinum-chromium stents have benefited from deeply considered design. These stents have capitalized upon the strengths of the platinum-chromium alloy along with the demonstrated safety and efficacy of the everolimus-fluorinated polymer combination. A more recent variant utilizing a fully biodegradable drug-eluting polymer has also shown promising results [2].

The second-generation drug-eluting stents have undoubtedly reduced vessel injury and resulted in excellent clinical outcomes [3,4]. There are concerns, however, that the design elements contributing to high flexibility have also increased risk for mechanical compromise [5,6]. While the clinical significance remains inconclusive, the observations of longitudinal stent deformation with newer platforms have renewed the understanding that stent design and performance are, in essence, a study of compromise and balance.

This chapter begins with a brief discussion of the platinum-chromium alloy and then examines the role of stent architecture in the risk for longitudinal deformation. We present technical aspects of the platinum-chromium everolimus-eluting stents and several landmark trials evaluating their clinical performance.

Material properties and biomechanics of the platinum-chromium alloy

As with cobalt-chromium (CoCr) alloys, development of the platinum-chromium (PtCr) alloy was driven by the clinical need for stronger and denser materials than stainless steel. These materials allow fabrication of thinner stent struts, which have repeatedly been shown to improve clinical restenosis outcomes [7].

In searching for new stent alloys, extensive analysis identified platinum as an ideal material partly because it is very soluble in stainless steel in the austenitic phase. That is, unlike many other materials, platinum stabilizes the iron-chromium matrix in a way that allows the further addition of platinum without development of brittle or magnetic phases [8]. Further testing of the PtCr alloy showed that 33% platinum content provided optimum characteristics for both ease of fabrication and stent biomechanics [9,10].

The success of the PtCr alloy derives, in part, from the fact that platinum largely replaces iron and nickel while maintaining adequate levels of chromium and molybdenum (Table 33.1). Certain elements such as chromium and molybdenum stabilize natural defects in the alloy's crystal structure through mechanisms such as solid-solution strengthening, grain refinement, and development of extremely strong metal carbides. Upon detailed analysis, PtCr alloy demonstrates a face centered cubic arrangement of atoms, fine grain crystals, and chromium carbides [8,10]. These characteristics contribute to high mechanical strength and fatigue resistance.

PtCr is significantly denser than stainless steel and the CoCr alloys, but its elastic modulus and tensile strength lie between the two. These properties have translated to the ability to fabricate thin struts (<100 μm) while maintaining necessary strength and radio-opacity. Additionally, compared with CoCr alloys, lower elastic modulus has contributed to less stent recoil [11,12]. In essence, materials with a high elastic modulus require a higher degree of deforming force to overcome the elastic limit in order to induce permanent deformation. Because CoCr alloys have a high elastic modulus, CoCr stents are theoretically at higher risk of recoil than PtCr and stainless steel stents given the same expanding force (Table 33.2). While this has been supported experimentally, however, the clinical relevance of this difference is unclear [12].

Biocompatibility: surface characteristics and resistance to corrosion

Stent corrosion and metal ion release into vascular tissues are increasingly viewed as contributors to vascular inflammation and perhaps even thrombosis [1,13,14]. In addition to mechanical

---

Interventional Cardiology: Principles and Practice, Second Edition. Edited by George D. Dangas, Carlo Di Mario, and Nicholas N. Kipshidze.
© 2017 John Wiley & Sons, Ltd. Published 2017 by John Wiley & Sons, Ltd.

Table 33.1 Composition of platinum-chromium (PtCr) compared with stainless steel and cobalt-chromium (CoCr) alloys.

Alloy	Element composition (%)							
	Pt	Fe	Co	Cr	Ni	W	Mo	Mn
PtCr	33	37	–	18	9	–	2.6	0.05
SS (316L)	–	64	–	18	14	–	2.6	2
CoCr (MP35N)	–	1	35	20	35	–	10	0.15
CoCr (L605)	–	3	52	20	10	15	–	1.5

Table 33.2 Mechanical properties of PtCr compared with stainless steel and CoCr alloys.

Material	Density (g/cm³)	UTS (MPa)	Yield strength (MPa)	Elastic modulus (GPa)
PtCr	9.9	834	480	203
316L	7.9	670	340	193
MP35N	8.4	930	414	233
L605	9.1	1000	500	243

UTS, ultimate tensile strength.

integrity of the stent platform, resistance to corrosion is primarily due to the formation of metal oxides at the stent surface. Certain surface oxides can act as a passive film reducing corrosion and metal ion release; chromium oxide is particularly resistant to corrosion [15]. Experimental data show that PtCr alloy preferentially forms chromium oxide over less effective iron and nickel oxides, likely because platinum has replaced these elements in the alloy [10,15].

In addition to corrosion resistance, biomaterial characteristics such as surface energy, potential, and texture are postulated to have a role in the propensity to induce thrombosis and inflammation. The precise molecular mechanisms of thrombosis and inflammation are outside the scope of the current discussion, but the process can be roughly conceptualized as a balance between thermodynamic, kinetic, and electrochemical factors that favor protein and cell deposition ultimately leading to coagulation and inflammation [16–26]. This balance is affected by the total energy of the system conscribed by the stent, vessel, and blood components [18,19].

Briefly, almost immediately upon device exposure to blood, a thin layer of protein and water are adsorbed onto the device surface. The deposited proteins undergo varying degrees of conformational change and denaturation depending on the surface characteristics of the device. The induced protein conformational changes expose different molecular binding domains that have varying affinity for other blood proteins. Protein adsorption and conformational changes that result in endothelial cell adhesion can protect against thrombosis and improve vascular healing. In contrast, protein adsorption and conformational changes that lead to

platelet activation and leukocyte adhesion ultimately predispose to thrombosis and inflammation [27].

Generally, blood-contacting materials with more stable surfaces tend to be less thrombogenic and inflammatory [24,28]. As a noble metal, the inert nature of platinum is also thought to contribute to the surface stability and biocompatibility of the PtCr stents [8,10]. Experimental observations show that platinum is present in relatively high quantities at the surface of PtCr stents [8,10]. Further biocompatibility studies demonstrate high rates of endothelial cell coverage and low rates of fibrin and platelet adhesion to PtCr stents [10,28–30]. Most recently, the OMEGA trial of the PtCr bare metal stent showed low rates of clinical restenosis and stent thrombosis (target lesion failure in 11.5% at 9 months, stent thrombosis in 0.6% at 12 months) [31], demonstrating *in vivo* biocompatibility comparable to or better than previous stainless steel and CoCr bare metal stents [32,33].

Longitudinal stent deformation and the role of stent architecture

Longitudinal stent deformation (LSD) refers to the elongation or shortening of a stent after deployment. Several mechanisms of LSD have been proposed, and most cases result from impingement of guidewires and secondary devices, or traction by deflated balloons caught on stent struts [34,35]. In other words, LSD is typically caused by the application of an external force resulting in mechanical distortion rather than spontaneous stent deformation. The majority occurs in the proximal region of stents [34]. Other risk factors associated with LSD include calcified and tortuous arteries, left main stenting, bifurcation stenting, small vessel diameter, longer lesions, and more stents, as these factors presumably increase the chance of guidewire impingement or balloon traction [36,37].

LSD appears to be extremely rare, having been discovered in less than 1% of deployed stents [35,37–41]. Given the rarity of LSD, the true incidence and clinical significance remain unclear. Whereas some studies have associated LSD with a higher risk of adverse events such as in-stent restenosis and stent thrombosis [34,42], other studies have found no correlation [35,40]. Similarly, some studies suggest that the PtCr stents are most commonly affected [35,38,40,41], but others show no particular susceptibility [39,43,44]. Several significant confounding biases have been proposed, most notably observer bias due to operators' heightened sensitivity to this complication, and detection bias due to the increased radio-opacity of platinum resulting in increased detection rates with these stents [34,38]. Nevertheless, a number of bench studies conducted thus far have elucidated factors in stent design that predispose the PtCr stents to longitudinal compromise [5,6,38,45].

In examining design factors contributing to LSD, it is worth considering the Promus Element (Boston Scientific, Natick, MA, USA), an early PtCr stent featuring 81 μm struts and an offset peak-to-valley serpentine ring design. Widened peaks were designed to redistribute intra-stent forces to improve radial strength and longitudinal flexibility [11]. Adjacent rings were joined by two short longitudinal connectors angled at approximately ~45° from the longitudinal axis. These connectors together formed a secondary double helix structure along the length of the stent, purported to add another element of longitudinal flexibility (Figure 33.1).

Susceptibility to LSD is primarily because of the number of connectors between rings and the arrangement of rings. Bench tests suggest that stents with three or more longitudinal connectors per

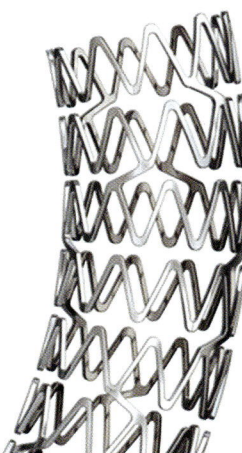

Figure 33.1 Promus Element stent. Image provided courtesy of Boston Scientific. © 2016 Boston Scientific Corporation or its affiliates. All rights reserved.

ring are less susceptible to deformation than those with two connectors [5,6,45]. This makes sense as the connectors help maintain a constant distance between adjacent rings. Additionally, the alignment of the Element's connectors have made these stents particularly susceptible to torque exerted by guidewire impingement. Because the connectors were angled at ~45° from the longitudinal axis, applied force is redirected to the joint between the connector and ring thereby increasing susceptibility to compression [5,37].

The arrangement of rings also contributes to longitudinal integrity. In-phase or offset ring patterns easily nest together upon bending or compression, clearly increasing flexibility but also the risk of deformation [45]. In stents with an out-of-phase ring pattern, the peak-to-peak arrangement of struts acts like surrogate longitudinal connectors or welded points; that is, with a longitudinal compressive force the rings do not nest together and instead, the peaks abut against each another, reducing susceptibility to both diffuse and point compression.

While bench testing has elucidated important stent design factors and potential mechanisms of LSD, the clinical applicability of these results is still debatable. Furthermore, it still remains unclear whether the early PtCr stent platforms were definitively prone to longitudinal deformation. Regardless, documented observations of mechanical compromise have underscored the role of stent architecture in biomechanical performance. Minor design changes to the Promus Element that followed seem to have improved the longitudinal integrity of the PtCr stents [5], and large-scale trials suggest that these stents are, at the very least, non-inferior to the cobalt-chromium based stents [3,4,35,40].

Promus Element and Premier EES
Platform
As previously described, the Promus Element (Boston Scientific, Natick, MA, USA) is based on the Omega bare metal PtCr platform, which features 81–86 μm struts (81 μm for 2.25–3.5 mm diameter and 86 μm for 4.0 mm diameter) and serpentine rings with two short longitudinal connectors per ring. These connectors are angled at approximately 45° relative to the longitudinal axis of the stent. The Element Plus is identical except for an updated balloon catheter delivery system.

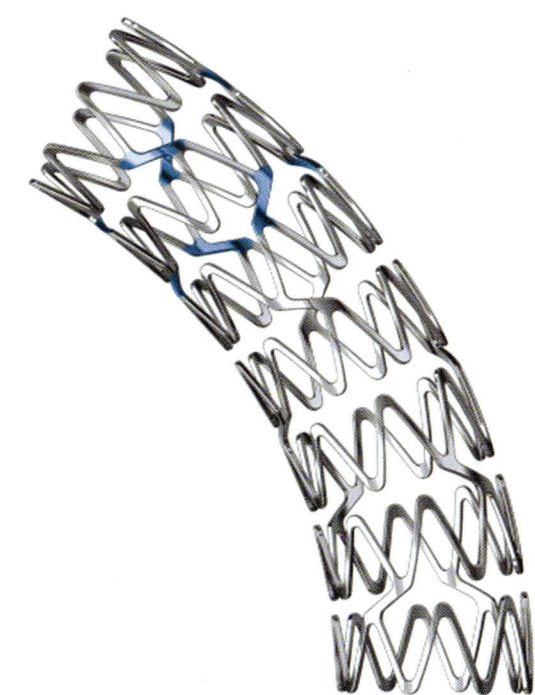

Figure 33.2 Promus Premier stent. Image provided courtesy of Boston Scientific. © 2016 Boston Scientific Corporation or its affiliates. All rights reserved.

In response to concerns about longitudinal stent deformation, the Omega platform was modified and renamed the Rebel. This updated platform now has four connectors between the first and last two rings (Figure 33.2) and serves as the basis for the Promus Premier (Boston Scientific).

Polymer
The Promus Element and Premier stents have a biocompatible, durable polymer consisting of a poly n-butyl methylacrylate (PMBA) primer and polyvinylidene fluoride-hexafluoropropylene (PVDF-HFP)-everolimus drug-eluting layer identical to the Xience V CoCr-EES (Abbott Vascular, Santa Clara, CA, USA). The total thickness of the polymer layer is approximately 7 μm. The biocompatibility and clinical performance of this drug-polymer combination has been demonstrated by numerous studies [46–50].

In brief, the excellent performance of this durable polymer lies in its completely saturated, partially fluorinated carbon-carbon backbone structure which results in a highly stable drug-eluting polymer resistant to oxidative breakdown and inflammatory response. The PVDF-HFP chemical structure also confers a high degree of surface stability, which may contribute to thromboresistance [24,51–53]. Lastly, the high flexibility of PVDF-HFP at body temperature (glass transition temperature for polymers) improves its resistance to peeling and cracking over the long term, further enhancing its durability and biocompatibility.

Drug
Everolimus is a partially synthetic analogue of sirolimus (rapamycin), a naturally occurring compound. These drugs function by binding FK-506 binding protein-12 (FKBP12) and inhibiting the mammalian target of rapamycin (MToR), causing cytostatic G1-phase cell cycle

arrest. Some evidence suggests that everolimus can also selectively clear macrophages from atheromas, theoretically stabilizing vulnerable plaques [54].

Everolimus is more lipophilic than sirolimus, which increases local vascular uptake particularly into lipid-rich atheroma, and lowers systemic distribution. This has allowed the EES to contain a lower concentration of drug ($100\,\mu g/cm^2$). The polymer-drug formulation of the PtCr-EES results in approximately 30% drug release within the first 24 hours after implantation, leading to 80% release by 30 days and complete elution by 120 days.

Clinical trials
PLATINUM QCA

In PLATINUM QCA, 100 patients with a single de novo lesion treated with a single PtCr-EES stent had 30-day follow-up for clinical events, and later underwent repeat angiography and intravascular ultrasound (IVUS) at 9 months to evaluate in-stent late lumen loss (Table 33.3) [55]. The primary endpoint, 30-day composite of cardiac death, myocardial infarction (MI), target lesion revascularization (TLR), or ARC-defined definite or probable stent thrombosis, was 1.0% due to a single case of peri-procedural stent thrombosis. Coronary angiography at 9 months demonstrated an overall in-stent late lumen loss of 0.20 ± 0.28 mm, comparable to historical data for the CoCr-EES from SPIRIT I, II, and III [50,56,57]. Post-procedure IVUS imaging further demonstrated a low rate of acute incomplete stent apposition (ISA; 5.7% for PtCr-EES vs. 34.4% for CoCr-EES in SPIRIT III) and no persistent or late acquired ISA at 9 months (vs. 25.6% for CoCr-EES in SPIRIT III at 8 months) [55,57].

PLATINUM

The PLATINUM trial randomized 1530 patients to either the PtCr-EES or CoCr-EES [58]. The primary endpoint, target lesion failure (TLF) at 12 months, demonstrated no significant difference between the stents (PtCr-EES 3.4% vs. CoCr-EES 2.9%; $p_{non-inferiority} = 0.001$, $p_{superiority} = 0.60$). Intention-to-treat analysis further demonstrated no significant differences in 12-month rates of TLF (3.5% vs. 3.2%; p = 0.72), cardiac death or MI (2.0% vs. 2.5%; p = 0.56), TLR (1.9% vs. 1.9%; p = 0.96), or ARC-defined definite or probable stent thrombosis (0.4% vs. 0.4%; p = 1.00) [58].

Three-year results of the PLATINUM study demonstrated comparable clinical outcomes between the PtCr-EES and CoCr-EES, with similar rates of all-cause death (PtCr-EES 3.7% vs. CoCr-EES 4.3%; p = 0.62), cardiac death (1.2% vs. 1.9%; p = 0.27), MI (2.3% vs. 2.5%; p = 0.81), ischemia-driven TLR (3.5% vs. 4.9%; p = 0.21), and ARC-defined definite or probable ST (0.7% vs. 0.5%; p = 0.76) [59].

As an early pivotal trial, the PLATINUM study necessarily excluded complex patients, which may explain the low overall rates of clinical events compared with earlier studies of the CoCr-EES [60–62]. Nonetheless, this trial has demonstrated the clinical safety and efficacy of the PtCr-EES through at least 3 years.

PLATINUM Small Vessel and Long Lesions

More complex lesions were evaluated in the PLATINUM Small Vessel and Long Lesion trial [63]. The small vessel arm included 94 patients receiving a single 2.25 mm-diameter Promus Element stent for lesions in vessels with a reference diameter of 2.25–2.5 mm. At 1 year, the rate of TLR was 2.4%, considerably lower than historical data for small caliber Taxus Element (7.3%), BioMatrix Flex (9.6%),

and Xience V (5.1%) stents [64–66]. The rate of TLR continues to remain low through at least 2 years (2.5%), and preliminary 4-year data show a TLR of 3.6% [63,67].

Similarly, the PLATINUM long lesion arm evaluated 102 patients receiving a 38 mm stent for lesions 24–34 mm in length [63]. In this group the 1-year rate of TLR was 3.1%, similar to historical data for the Cypher (Cordis/Johnson & Johnson, Warren, NJ, USA) sirolimus-eluting stent (2.4%) and lower than for the Taxus Express (7.2%) and BioMatrix Flex (12.4%) [68,69]. At 2 years, TLR is 5.2% and preliminary 3-year results show a TLR rate of 6.2% [63,67]. Collectively, these findings demonstrate the long-term clinical safety and efficacy of the PtCr-EES in patients with long lesions and small vessel disease.

DUTCH PEERS

The DUTCH PEERS trial evaluated 1811 patients randomized 1 : 1 to the Resolute Integrity (Medtronic) CoCr zotarolimus-eluting stent or the Promus Element [40]. This study was particularly noteworthy for its minimal exclusion criteria and complex patient population: 20% of subjects presented with ST-elevation MI, 25% presented with non-ST-elevation MI, and 66% of lesions were complex (type B2/C). The primary endpoint of target-vessel failure at 1 year demonstrated no significant difference between stents (ZES 6% vs. EES 5%; $p_{non-inferiority} = 0.006$). Similarly, there was no significant difference in the rate of definite ST (ZES 0.3% ves. EES 0.7%; p = 0.34), and no ST occurred beyond 3 months [40].

In DUTCH PEERS, operators reported suspicion for longitudinal deformation based on visualization during angiography. Further evaluation of these selected cases showed that while LSD occurred in none of the Resolute Integrity stents and in 0.6% (9/1591) of Promus Element stents (p = 0.002), none of these cases of LSD were associated with adverse clinical events [40]. A systematic analysis of LSD was not undertaken in DUTCH PEERS, and several biases such as the higher radio-opacity of platinum stents preclude any conclusions about the risk of LSD with the Promus Element in this study.

HOST-ASSURE

The HOST-ASSURE trial randomized 3755 South Korean patients 2 : 1 to the Promus Element PtCr-EES or the Resolute (Medtronic) CoCr-ZES, respectively, with minimal exclusion criteria [35]. The primary endpoint, TLF at 1 year, was reached in 2.9% of PtCr-EES and 2.9% of CoCr-ZES patients ($p_{non-inferiority} = 0.0247$). The rate of definite or probable stent thrombosis at 1 year was low and showed no significant difference between stents (PtCr-EES 0.36% vs. CoCr-ZES 0.67%; p = 0.229). A systematic study of angiograms demonstrated a 0.21% incidence of LSD with PtCr-EES (7/2491 studies) whereas no LSD was observed with CoCr-ZES. Similar to other studies, however, these cases of LSD were not associated with adverse events at 1 year [35].

SCAAR

Analysis of clinical outcomes from the Swedish Coronary Angiography and Angioplasty Registry (SCAAR) has demonstrated the clinical safety and efficacy of the Promus Element stent in a large and unselected population [70]. This study compared the rates of restenosis and definite stent thrombosis among 13,577 first and second-generation DES implanted in 8375 procedures. At 1 year, the rates of restenosis and definite stent thrombosis were not

Table 33.3 Summary of clinical trials of Promus Element.

Trial	Trial design	PtCr-EES versus:	Selected inclusion/ exclusion criteria	n	1° endpoint	Outcomes*	Conclusions
PLATINUM QCA	Prospective, single-arm	none	I: Single de novo lesion; silent, stable or unstable ischemia; RVD 2.25–4.0 mm E: MI within 72 hours; elevated cardiac enzymes at PCI; unprotected LM lesions, CTO, bifurcation lesions, heavy calcification, ISR; thrombus, LVEF <30%	100	Composite of cardiac death, MI, TLR, definite or probable ST at 30 days	1°: 1.0% 2°: In-stent LLL at 9 months; 0.17±0.25 mm	The PtCr-EES demonstrates acceptable safety and efficacy through 12 months
PLATINUM	Prospective, randomized, single-blind	CoCr-EES (XV)	I: Up to two de novo lesions; RVD 2.5–4.25 mm, length ≤24 mm E: AMI within 72 hours; LVEF <30%; ostial, LM, true bifurcation lesions; heavy calcification, thrombus, angulation, tortuosity	1530	TLF at 12 months	1°: 3.4% vs. 2.9%, $p_{superiority} = 0.60$, $p_{non-inferiority} = 0.001$	PtCr-EES non-inferior to CoCr-EES for TLF at 12 months; acceptable safety and efficacy with both stents
PLATINUM SV	Prospective, single-arm	none	I: Single de novo lesion; RVD 2.25–2.5 mm, length ≤28 mm E: Acute or recent MI, LVEF <30%, CTO, LM lesions, bifurcation lesions, thrombus	94	TLF at 12 months	1°: 2.4% 2°: TLF at 2 years 4.7%	PtCr-EES shows low rate of TLF in small vessels; acceptable safety and efficacy in small vessels
PLATINUM LL	Prospective, single-arm	none	I: Single de novo lesion; RVD 2.5–4.25 mm, length 24–34 mm E: Acute or recent MI, LVEF <30%, CTO, LM lesions, bifurcation lesions, thrombus	102	TLF at 12 months	1°: 3.2% 2°: TLF at 2 years 8.8%	PtCr-EES shows low rate of TLF in long lesions; acceptable safety and efficacy in long lesions
DUTCH PEERS	Prospective, randomized, single-blind	CoCr-ZES (RI)	I: Treatment with only EES E: Limited exclusion criteria	1811	TVF at 12 months	1°: 5% vs. 6%; p=0.42	Both stents are safe and effective in an all-comer population
HOST-ASSURE	Prospective, randomized, single-blind	CoCr-ZES (R)	I: Broad E: LVEF <25%	3755	TLF at 12 months	1°: 2.9 vs. 2.9%, $p_{superiority} = 0.98$; $p_{noninferiority} = 0.0247$	PtCr-EES non-inferior to CoCr-ZES for TLF at 1 year; LSD seen only in PtCr-EES but not associated with adverse clinical events
SCAAR	Observational	CoCr-EES (XP, XV), CoCr-ZES (E, R), SS-SES (C), SS-PES (TE, TL)	I: Treatment with DES E: None	13577 stents	Clinical restenosis and stent thrombosis at 12 months	Restenosis: 2.8% vs. 2.7% (all other DES) Stent thrombosis: 0.2% vs. 0.5% (all other DES)	PtCr-EES demonstrates similar rates of restenosis and stent thrombosis to all other DES combined

AMI, acute myocardial infarction; BMS, bare metal stent; C, Cypher; CD, cardiac death; CoCr, cobalt-chromium; CTO, chronic total occlusion; DAPT, dual antiplatelet therapy; E, Endeavor; EES, everolimus-eluting stent; ISR, in-stent restenosis; LLL, late lumen loss; MLV, Multi-Link Vision; PE, Promus Element/Premier; PES, paclitaxel-eluting stent; PtCr, platinum-chromium; R, Resolute; RI, Resolute Integrity; S, Synergy; SES, sirolimus-eluting stent; SS, stainless steel; ST, stent thrombosis; TE, Taxus Express; TL, Taxus Liberte ; TLF, target lesion failure; TLR, target lesion revascularization; XP, Xience Prime; XV, Xience V; ZES, zotarolimus-eluting stent.

* All values are presented as PE-EES versus comparator stent.

significantly different between the Promus Element and all other DES (restenosis, PtCr-EES 2.8% vs. 2.7%; stent thrombosis, PtCr-EES 0.2% vs. 0.5%). When compared with individual stents, however, the Promus Element showed significantly lower rates of restenosis and stent thrombosis than the Endeavor (Medtronic) ZES. Although LSD was not evaluated in this study, if it did occur with the Promus Element, it did not appear to significantly influence clinical events at 1 year [70].

Synergy EES
Platform
The platform of the Synergy (Boston Scientific) PtCr-EES has 74–81 μm struts (74 μm for 2.25–3.5 mm and 81 μm for 4.0 mm). The overall architecture of this stent is similar to the Rebel BMS, namely featuring an offset peak-to-valley ring arrangement, two short, angled longitudinal connectors in the body of the stent, and four connectors at the proximal and distal ends. Aside from thinner struts, the main alterations include reduced peak radius and less angled connectors, which collectively improve longitudinal strength.

Polymer
The Synergy employs a fully biodegradable poly-DL-lactide-coglycolide (PLGA) polymer applied to the abluminal surface of the stent with a maximum thickness of 4 μm. Compared with the Element and Premier stents, this formulation results in a greater than 50% reduction in the total weight of polymer used [11]. Spontaneous hydrolysis of the ester bonds of PLGA results in complete degradation to CO_2 and water by 4 months after implantation, leaving a bare metal stent in place.

Drug
Everolimus has demonstrated excellent safety and efficacy in its formulation for coronary stents. Combination with the PLGA polymer, however, results in a slightly different drug release profile than previous EES. The co-formulation of PLGA-everolimus used in the Synergy stent results in a burst of drug release in the first 7 days, leading to approximately 50% release in 30 days, 80% by 60 days, and nearly complete release by 90 days. Because of its lipophilic properties, everolimus is preferentially taken up by local vascular tissues and continues to be released from this tissue reservoir through 120 days post-implantation. *In vivo* porcine studies demonstrate that the Synergy-EES elicits vascular tissue responses similar to the Xience V and Promus Element, and is completely endothelialized by 30 days [30,71].

Clinical trials
EVOLVE I
The EVOLVE I first-in-human trial examined the early safety and efficacy of full-dose and half-dose Synergy EES compared to the benchmark durable polymer Promus Element (Table 33.4). In this trial 291 patients were randomised 1 : 1 : 1 to the Promus Element, Synergy, or Synergy reduced-dose stents and were subsequently followed for 30-day clinical events and 6-month angiographic measures [2]. The primary clinical endpoint was 30-day TLF, which occurred in 0, 1.1%, and 3.1% of patients in the Promus Element, Synergy, and Synergy half-dose, respectively; the rate of

TLF at 6 months was 3.1%, 2.2%, and 4.1%, respectively. The primary angiographic endpoint of 6-month in-stent late lumen loss demonstrated non-inferiority of both Synergy stents compared to the Promus Element (Promus Element: 0.15 ± 0.34 mm; Synergy: 0.10 ± 0.25 mm ($p_{noninferiority} < 0.001$), Synergy half-dose: 0.13 ± 0.26 mm ($p_{noninferiority} < 0.001$). These findings remained consistent even after adjustment for small but statistically significant differences in baseline reference vessel diameter. While the study was underpowered to detect significant differences in clinical outcomes, the overall the rate of clinical events remained low and similar between all three stents, with no cases of stent thrombosis over 6 months [2].

EVOLVE II
EVOLVE II randomized 1684 patients 1 : 1 to the Synergy or Promus Element Plus stents for treatment of stable CAD or NSTEMI [72]. Other inclusion criteria included ≤3 lesions in ≤2 vessels, lesions ≤34 mm in length and RVD 2.25–4 mm. Major exclusion criteria included STEMI, left main disease, chronic total occlusion, graft occlusion, and in-stent restenosis. The primary endpoint, 12-month TLF, was reached in 6.7% of Synergy patients versus 6.5% of the Promus Element Plus patients ($p = 0.83$, $p_{noninferiority} = 0.0005$). Similarly, no significant differences were observed for clinically indicated TLR (2.6% vs. 1.7%; $p = 0.21$) or definite or probable stent thrombosis (0.4% vs. 0.6%; $p = 0.50$) [72]. Overall, this study demonstrated that the Synergy stent is non-inferior to the Promus Element Plus for TLF at 1 year; other clinical measures show similar safety and efficacy between the stents in relatively uncomplicated disease. The EVOLVE II pharmacokinetic and diabetes substudies are ongoing.

BIO-RESORT TWENTE
BIORESORT TWENTE is an ongoing trial evaluating 3540 patients with minimal exclusion criteria. Patients are randomized 1 : 1 : 1 to the Synergy, Orsiro (Biotronik) thin-strut CoCr platform with degradable sirolimus-eluting PLLA polymer, and Resolute Integrity (Medtronic) CoCr platform with durable zotarolimus-eluting polymer [73].

Conclusions
Because of their deeply considered design, the platinum-chromium EES have demonstrated excellent overall safety and efficacy since their introduction. While the early Promus Element was hampered by concern over longitudinal deformation, larger studies suggest that this complication remains extremely rare and does not appear to be systematically associated with significant adverse clinical events. The subsequently redesigned Promus Premier has largely mitigated the risk for longitudinal compromise, and long-term clinical outcomes demonstrate continued safety and efficacy of these stents. Along with the CoCr-EES, these stents have taken their place as standard comparators against which new stents must be proven. Finally, the recent biodegradable polymer Synergy-EES has shown clinical outcomes comparable to the benchmark DES in early pivotal studies. Larger, longer-term studies in more complex patients are ongoing. Given the novelty and promise of fully biodegradable drug-eluting polymers, these results are awaited with anticipation.

Table 33.4 Summary of clinical trials of Synergy stent.

Trial	Synergy versus:	Trial design	Selected inclusion/exclusion criteria	n	1° endpoint	Outcomes*	Conclusions
EVOLVE I	Promus Element, Synergy ½-dose	Prospective, randomized, single-blind	**I:** Single de novo lesion; RVD 2.25–3.5 mm; length <28 mm **E:** Acute or recent MI; LM or bifurcation lesions; thrombus	291	Clinical: 30 day TLF Angiographic: 6 month in-stent LLL	30 day TLF: PE 0% vs. Sy 1.1% vs. Sy½ 3.1% 6-mo LLL: PE: 0.15±0.34 mm Sy: 0.10±0.25 mm, p_{noninf} <0.001 Sy½: 0.13±0.26 mm, p_{noninf} <0.001)	Synergy demonstrates noninferior angiographic efficacy to the Promus Element at 6 months; the rate of adverse clinical events was low
EVOLVE II	Promus Element Plus	Prospective, randomized, single-blind	**I:** ≤3 lesions in ≤2 vessels; RVD 2.5–4.0 mm; length <34 mm **E:** STEMI; LM or graft lesions; CTO; in-stent restenosis	1684	TLF at 12 months	6.7% v 6.5%; p=0.83, p_{noninf} =0.0005	Synergy noninferior to Promus Element Plus for TLF at 1 year; both stents demonstrate low rates of adverse clinical events at 1 year
BIO-RESORT TWENTE	Orsiro, Resolute Integrity	Prospective, randomized, single-blind	**I:** Broad **E:** Limited exclusion criteria	3540	TVF at 12 months	(Study ongoing)	(Study ongoing)

LLL, late lumen loss; PE, Promus Element stent; RVD, reference vessel diameter; STEMI, ST-elevation myocardial infarction; Sy, Synergy stent; Sy½, Synergy half-dose stent; TLF, target lesion failure; TVF, target vessel failure.
* All outcome data presented as Synergy stent versus comparator unless otherwise noted.

Interactive multiple choice questions are available for this chapter on www.wiley. com/go/dangas/cardiology

References

1 Ruygrok P, Serruys PW. Intracoronary stenting from concept to custom. *Circulation* 1996. **94**: 882–890.

2 Meredith IT, Verheye S, Dubois CL, *et al.* Primary endpoint results of the EVOLVE trial: a randomized evaluation of a novel bioabsorbable polymer-coated, everolimus-eluting coronary stent. *J Am Coll Cardiol* 2012; **59**(15): 1362–1370.

3 Sarno G, Lagerqvist B, Fröbert O, *et al.* Lower risk of stent thrombosis and restenosis with unrestricted use of "new-generation" drug-eluting stents: a report from the nationwide Swedish Coronary Angiography and Angioplasty Registry (SCAAR). *Eur Heart J* 2012; **33**(5): 606–613.

4 Sarno G, Lagerqvist B, Nilsson J, *et al.* Stent thrombosis in new-generation drug-eluting stents in patients with STEMI undergoing primary PCI: a report from SCAAR. *J Am Coll Cardiol* 2014; **64**(1): 16–24.

5 Ormiston JA, Webber B, Ubod B, White J, Webster MW. Stent longitudinal strength assessed using point compression: insights from a second-generation, clinically related bench test. *Circ Cardiovasc Interv* 2014; **7**(1): 62–69.

6 Ormiston JA, Webber B, Webster MW. Stent longitudinal integrity bench insights into a clinical problem. *JACC Cardiovasc Interv* 2011; **4**(12): 1310–1317.

7 Briguori C, Sarais C, Pagnotta P, *et al.* In-stent restenosis in small coronary arteries impact of strut thickness. *J Am Coll Cardiol* 2002; **40**: 403–409.

8 Craig CH, *et al.* Mechanical properties and microstructure of platinum enhanced radiopaque stainless steel (PERSS) alloys. *J Alloys Compounds* 2003; **361**(1-2): 187–199.

9 Menown IB, Noad R, Garcia EJ, Meredith I. The platinum chromium element stent platform: from alloy, to design, to clinical practice. *Adv Ther* 2010; **27**(3): 129–141.

10 O'Brien BJ, Stinson JS, Larsen SR, Eppihimer MJ, Carroll WM. A platinum-chromium steel for cardiovascular stents. *Biomaterials* 2010; **31**(14): 3755–3761.

11 Bennett J, Dubois C. A novel platinum chromium everolimus-eluting stent for the treatment of coronary artery disease. *Biologics* 2013; **7**: 149–159.

12 Ota T, Ishii H, Sumi T, *et al.* Impact of coronary stent designs on acute stent recoil. *J Cardiol* 2014; **64**(5): 347–352.

13 Gutensohn K, Beythien C, Bau J, *et al.* In vitro analyses of diamond-like carbon coated stents: reduction of metal ion release, platelet activation, and thrombogenicity. *Thromb Res* 2000; **99**: 577–585.

14 Koster R, Vieluf D, Kiehn M, *et al.* Nickel and molybdenum contact allergies in patients with coronary in-stent restenosis. *Lancet* 2000; **356**(9245): 1895–1897.

15 Chen Q, Thouas GA. Metallic implant biomaterials. *Mat Sci Eng: R Rep* 2015; **87**: 1–57.

16 Chiu TH, Nyilas E, Lederman DM. Thermodynamics of native protein/foreign surface interactions. *Trans Amer Soc Artif Int Organs* 1976; **22**: 498–512.

17 de Mel A, Cousins BG, Seifalian AM. Surface modification of biomaterials: a quest for blood compatibility. *Int J Biomater* 2012; **2012**: 707863.

18 Fang F, Satulovsky J, Szleifer I. Kinetics of protein adsorption and desorption on surfaces with grafted polymers. *Biophys J* 2005; **89**(3): 1516–1533.

19 Fang F, Szleifer I. Kinetics and thermodynamics of protein adsorption: a generalized molecular theoretical approach. *Biophys J* 2001; **80**: 2568–2589.

20 Hoffman AS. Modification of material surfaces to affect how they interact with blood. *Ann N Y Acad Sci* 1987; **516**: 96–101.

21 Huck V, Schneider MF, Gorzelanny C, Schneider SW. The various states of von Willebrand factor and their function in physiology and pathophysiology. *Thromb Haemost* 2014; **111**(4): 598–609.

22 Sawyer PN, Srinivasan S. The role of electrochemical surface properties in thrombosis as vascular interfaces: cumulative experience of studies in animals and man. In *Symposium on Problems in Evaluating the Blood Compatibility of Biomaterials.* New York, NY: 1972.

23 Tanaka M, Motomura T, Kawada M, *et al.* Blood compatible aspects of poly(2-methoxyethylacrylate)(PMEA): relationship between protein adsorption and platelet adhesion on PMEA surface. *Biomaterials* 2000; **21**: 1471–1481.

24 Tokuda K, *et al.* Simple method for lowering poly(methyl methacrylate) surface energy with fluorination. *Polymer J* 2014; **47**(1): 66–70.

25 Vroman L, Adams AL. Identification of rapid changes at plasma–solid interfaces. *J Biomed Mater Res* 1969; **3**: 43–67.

26 Srokowski EM, Woodhouse KA. Evaluation of the bulk platelet response and fibrinogen interaction to elastin-like polypeptide coatings. *J Biomed Mater Res A* 2014; **102A**: 540–551.

27 Gray JJ. The interaction of proteins with solid surfaces. *Curr Opin Struct Biol* 2004; **14**(1): 110–115.

28 Eppihimer MJ, Sushkova N, Grimsby JL, *et al.* Impact of stent surface on thrombogenicity and vascular healing: a comparative analysis of metallic and polymeric surfaces. *Circ Cardiovasc Interv* 2013; **6**(4): 370–377.

29 Soucy NV, Feygin JM, Tunstall R, *et al.* Strut tissue coverage and endothelial cell coverage: a comparison between bare metal stent platforms and platinum chromium stents with and without everolimus-eluting coating. *EuroIntervention* 2010; **6**: 630–637.

30 Wilson GJ, Huibregtse BA, Stejskal EA, *et al.* Vascular response to a third generation everolimus-eluting stent. *EuroIntervention* 2010; **6**: 512–519.

31 Wang JC, Carrié D, Masotti M, *et al.* Primary endpoint results of the OMEGA Study: one-year clinical outcomes after implantation of a novel platinum chromium bare metal stent. *Cardiovasc Revasc Med* 2015; **16**(2): 65–69.

32 Kastrati A, Mehilli J, Dirschinger J, *et al.* Restenosis after coronary placement of various stent types. *Am J Cardiol* 2001; **87**: 34–39.

33 Sketch MH Jr, Ball M, Rutherford B, *et al.* Evaluation of the Medtronic (Driver) cobalt-chromium alloy coronary stent system. *Am J Cardiol* 2005; **95**(1): 8–12.

34 Mamas MA, Williams PD. Longitudinal stent deformation: insights on mechanisms, treatments and outcomes from the Food and Drug Administration Manufacturer and User Facility Device Experience database. *EuroIntervention* 2012; **8**(2): 196–204.

35 Park KW, Kang SH, Kang HJ, *et al.* A randomized comparison of platinum chromium-based everolimus-eluting stents versus cobalt chromium-based Zotarolimus-Eluting stents in all-comers receiving percutaneous coronary intervention: HOST-ASSURE (harmonizing optimal strategy for treatment of coronary artery stenosis-safety and effectiveness of drug-eluting stents and anti-platelet regimen), a randomized, controlled, noninferiority trial. *J Am Coll Cardiol* 2014; **63**(25 Pt A): 2805–2816.

36 Hanratty CG, Walsh SJ. Longitudinal compression: a "new" complication with modern coronary stent platforms: time to think beyond deliverability? *EuroIntervention* 2011; **7**(7): 872–877.

37 Leibundgut G, Gick M, Toma A, *et al.* Longitudinal compression of the platinum-chromium everolimus-eluting stent during coronary implantation: predisposing mechanical properties, incidence, and predictors in a large patient cohort. *Catheter Cardiovasc Interv* 2013; **81**(5): E206–214.

38 Abdel-Wahab M, Sulimov DS, Kassner G, Geist V, Toelg R, Richardt G. Longitudinal deformation of contemporary coronary stents: an integrated analysis of clinical experience and observations from the bench. *J Interv Cardiol* 2012; **25**(6): 576–585.

39 Dvir D, Kitabata H, Barbash IM, *et al.* In vivo evaluation of axial integrity of coronary stents using intravascular ultrasound: Insights on longitudinal stent deformation. *Catheter Cardiovasc Interv* 2014; **84**(3): 397–405.

40 von Birgelen C, Sen H, Lam MK, *et al.* Third-generation zotarolimus-eluting and everolimus-eluting stents in all-comer patients requiring a percutaneous coronary intervention (DUTCH PEERS): a randomised, single-blind, multicentre, non-inferiority trial. *Lancet* 2014; **383**(9915): 413–423.

41 Williams PD, Mamas MA, Morgan KP, *et al.* Longitudinal stent deformation: a retrospective analysis of frequency and mechanisms. *EuroIntervention* 2012; **8**(2): 267–274.

42 Inaba S, Mintz GS, Yun KH, *et al.* Mechanical complications of everolimus-eluting stents associated with adverse events: an intravascular ultrasound study. *EuroIntervention* 2014; **9**: 1301–1308.

43 Kereiakes DJ, Popma JJ, Cannon LA, *et al.* Longitudinal stent deformation: quantitative coronary angiographic analysis from the PERSEUS and PLATINUM randomized controlled clinical trials. *J Am Coll Cardiol* 2012; **8**(2): 187–195.

44 Lupi A, Porto I, Rognoni A, *et al.* Clinical and biomechanical behavior of a platinum-chromium stent platform in a large all-comer single-center population: insights from the Novara-PROMETEUS Registry. *J Invasive Cardiol* 2014; **26**: 311–317.

45 Prabhu S, Schikorr T, Mahmoud T, Jacobs J, Potgieter A, Simonton C. Engineering assessment of the longitudinal compression behaviour of contemporary coronary stents. *EuroIntervention* 2012; **8**(2): 275–281.

46 Brener SJ, Kereiakes DJ, Simonton CA, *et al.* Everolimus-eluting stents in patients undergoing percutaneous coronary intervention: final 3-year results of the Clinical Evaluation of the XIENCE V Everolimus Eluting Coronary Stent System in the Treatment of Subjects With de Novo Native Coronary Artery Lesions trial. *Am Heart J* 2013; **166**(6): 1035–1042.

47 Gada H, Kirtane AJ, Newman W, *et al.* 5-year results of a randomized comparison of XIENCE V everolimus-eluting and TAXUS paclitaxel-eluting stents: final results from the SPIRIT III trial (clinical evaluation of the XIENCE V everolimus eluting coronary stent system in the treatment of patients with de novo native coronary artery lesions). *JACC Cardiovasc Interv* 2013; **6**(12): 1263–1266.

48 Gutierrez-Chico JL, van Geuns RJ, Regar E, *et al.* Tissue coverage of a hydrophilic polymer-coated zotarolimus-eluting stent vs. a fluoropolymer-coated everolimus-eluting stent at 13-month follow-up: an optical coherence tomography substudy from the RESOLUTE All Comers trial. *Eur Heart J* 2011; **32**(19): 2454–2463.

49 Onuma Y, Miquel-Hebert K, Serruys PW. Five-year long-term clinical follow-up of the XIENCE V everolimus-eluting coronary stent system in the treatment of patients with de novo coronary artery disease: the SPIRIT II trial. *EuroIntervention* 2013; **8**: 1047–1051.

50 Serruys PW, Ong AT, Piek JJ, *et al.* A randomized comparison of a durable polymer Everolimus-eluting stent with a bare metal coronary stent: the SPIRIT first trial. *EuroIntervention* 2005; **1**(1): 58–65.

51 Ai F, *et al.* Surface characteristics and blood compatibility of PVDF/PMMA membranes. *J Materials Sci* 2012; **47**(12): 5030–5040.

52 Kanno M, Kawakami H, Nagaoka S, Kubota S. Biocompatibility of fluorinated polyimide. *J Biomed Mater Res* 2002; **60**(1): 53–60.

53 Kawakami H, Kanno M, Nagaoka S, Kubota S. Competitive plasma protein adsorption onto fluorinated polyimide surfaces. *J Biomed Mater Res* 2003; **67A**: 1393–1400.

54 Verheye S, Martinet W, Kockx MM, *et al.* Selective clearance of macrophages in atherosclerotic plaques by autophagy. *J Am Coll Cardiol* 2007; **49**(6): 706–715.

55 Meredith I, Whitbourn R, Scott D, *et al.* PLATINUM QCA: a prospective, multicentre study assessing clinical, angiographic, and intravascular ultrasound outcomes with the novel platinum chromium thin-strut PROMUS Element everolimus-eluting stent in de novo coronary stenoses. *EuroIntervention* 2011; **7**: 84–90.

56 Serruys PW, Ruygrok P, Neuzner J, *et al.* A randomised comparison of an everolimus-eluting coronary stent with a paclitaxel-eluting coronary stent: the SPIRIT II trial. *EuroIntervention* 2006; **2**: 286–294.

57 Stone GW, Midei M, Newman W, *et al.* Comparison of an everolimus-eluting stent and a paclitaxel-eluting stent in patients with coronary artery disease a randomized trial. *JAMA* 2008; **299**(16): 1903–1913.

58 Stone GW, Teirstein PS, Meredith IT, *et al.* A prospective, randomized evaluation of a novel everolimus-eluting coronary stent: the PLATINUM (a Prospective, Randomized, Multicenter Trial to Assess an Everolimus-Eluting Coronary Stent System [PROMUS Element] for the Treatment of Up to Two de Novo Coronary Artery Lesions) trial. *J Am Coll Cardiol* 2011; **57**(16): 1700–1708.

59 Meredith IT, Teirstein PS, Bouchard A, *et al.* Three-year results comparing platinum-chromium PROMUS element and cobalt-chromium XIENCE V everolimus-eluting stents in de novo coronary artery narrowing (from the PLATINUM Trial). *Am J Cardiol* 2014; **113**(7): 1117–1123.

60 Ribichini F, Romano M, Rosiello R, *et al.* A clinical and angiographic study of the XIENCE V everolimus-eluting coronary stent system in the treatment of patients with multivessel coronary artery disease: the EXECUTIVE trial (EXecutive RCT: evaluating XIENCE V in a multi vessel disease). *JACC Cardiovasc Interv* 2013;. **6**(10): 1012–1022.

61 Serruys PW, Silber S, Garg S, *et al.* Comparison of zotarolimus-eluting and everolimus-eluting coronary stents. *N Engl J Med* 2010; **363**: 136–146.

62 von Birgelen C, Basalus MW, Tandjung K, *et al.* A randomized controlled trial in second-generation zotarolimus-eluting Resolute stents versus everolimus-eluting Xience V stents in real-world patients: the TWENTE trial. *J Am Coll Cardiol* 2012; **59**(15): 1350–1361.

63 Teirstein PS, Meredith IT, Feldman RL, *et al.* Two-year safety and effectiveness of the platinum chromium everolimus-eluting stent for the treatment of small vessels and longer lesions. *Catheter Cardiovasc Interv* 2015; **85**(2): 207–215.

64 Cannon LA, Kereiakes DJ, Mann T, *et al.* A prospective evaluation of the safety and efficacy of TAXUS Element paclitaxel-eluting coronary stent implantation for the treatment of de novo coronary artery lesions in small vessels: the PERSEUS Small Vessel trial. *EuroIntervention* 2011; **6**: 920–927.

65 Cannon LA, Simon DI, Kereiakes D, *et al.* The XIENCE nano everolimus eluting coronary stent system for the treatment of small coronary arteries: the SPIRIT Small Vessel trial. *Catheter Cardiovasc Interv* 2012; **80**(4): 546–553.

66 Wykrzykowska JJ, Serruys PW, Onuma Y, *et al.* Impact of vessel size on angiographic and clinical outcomes of revascularization with biolimus-eluting stent with biodegradable polymer and sirolimus-eluting stent with durable polymer the LEADERS trial substudy. *JACC Cardiovasc Interv* 2009; **2**(9): 861–870.

67 Teirstein P, *et al.* TCT-236 Four-year outcomes following implantation of the promus Element* platinum chromium everolimus-eluting stent in de novo coronary artery lesions in small vessels and long lesions: results of the platinum small vessel and long lesion trials. *J Am Coll Cardiol* 2014; **64**(11): B69.

68 Kim YH, Park SW, Lee SW, *et al.* Sirolimus-eluting stent versus paclitaxel-eluting stent for patients with long coronary artery disease. *Circulation* 2006; **114**(20): 2148–2153.

69 Wykrzykowska J, Räber L, de Vries T, *et al.* Biolimus-eluting biodegradable polymer versus sirolimus-eluting permanent polymer stent performance in long lesions: results from the LEADERS multicentre trial substudy. *EuroIntervention* 2009; **5**: 310–317.

70 Sarno G, Lagerqvist B, Carlsson J, *et al.* Initial clinical experience with an everolimus eluting platinum chromium stent (Promus Element) in unselected patients from the Swedish Coronary Angiography and Angioplasty Registry (SCAAR). *Int J Cardiol* 2013; **167**(1): 146–150.

71 Wilson GJ, Huibregtse BA, Pennington DE, Dawkins KD. Comparison of the SYNERGY with the PROMUS (XIENCE V) and bare metal and polymer-only Element control stents in porcine coronary arteries. *EuroIntervention* 2012; **8**: 250–257.

72 Kereiakes DJ, Meredith IT, Windecker S, *et al.* Efficacy and safety of a novel bioabsorbable polymer-coated, everolimus-eluting coronary stent: the EVOLVE II Randomized Trial. *Circ Cardiovasc Interv* 2015; **8**(4): pii.

73 Lam MK, Sen H, Tandjung K, *et al.* Comparison of 3 biodegradable polymer and durable polymer-based drug-eluting stents in all-comers (BIO-RESORT): rationale and study design of the randomized TWENTE III multicenter trial. *Am Heart J* 2014; **167**(4): 445–451.

CHAPTER 34
Bioresorbable Stents

Gianluca Caiazzo[1,2], Alessio Mattesini[3], Ciro Indolfi[1], and Carlo Di Mario[2,4]

[1]Division of Cardiology, Department of Medical and Surgical Sciences, Magna Graecia University, Catanzaro, Italy
[2]National Institute of Health Research (NIHR), Royal Brompton & Harefield NHS Foundation Trust, London, UK
[3]Department of Heart and Vessels, AOUC Careggi, Florence, Italy
[4]National Heart & Lung Institute, Imperial College London, London, UK

Metallic stents represent one of the most important steps for the treatment of coronary artery disease (CAD) and the second revolution in interventional cardiology after the introduction of plain old balloon angioplasty (POBA) by Gruntzig [1–3]. The long search for the ideal stent made some improvements along the way, sometimes by taking two steps forward and one step back, but today the question whether the ideal stent exists is still open.

The biodegradable vascular scaffold (BVS) technology represents one of the most interesting developments in the field of interventional cardiology in recent years, because in theory BVS yield the same results as metal stents but, by being completely resorbable in time, also carrying the exciting possibility of complete anatomic and functional "vascular restoration." This phenomenon is a continuous process with three main phases: revascularization, reabsorption of the device, and restoration of vessel integrity and function [4]. Key steps in the biodegradable stent revolution, including the first-in-man results of magnesium [5,6] and poly-L-lactide (PLLA) stents [7,8], have been reported and future clinical trials will test whether "vascular restoration therapy" could provide greater durability of results following percutaneous coronary intervention (PCI). A growing number of studies is being published on this topic, and a large number of devices are being tested on humans.

The ABSORB BVS (Abbott Vascular, Santa Clara, CA, USA) is the most used biodegradable stent on the market, with more than 100,000 devices implanted in patients all over the world. However, only one randomized trial is available, the ABSORB II randomized controlled trial, which compared the ABSORB BVS with the Xience drug-eluting stent (DES) at 1 year [9].

ABSORB bioresorbable vascular scaffold
The device
The ABSORB BVS is constituted by a PLLA backbone covered by a 1:1 mixture of an amorphous matrix of poly-D, L-lactide (PDLLA) and the antiproliferative drug everolimus ($100\,\mu L/cm^2$). PLLA is a semi-crystalline polymer consisting of crystal lamella (regions with high concentrations of polymer with crystalline structure) interconnected with random polymer chains forming an amorphous segment [10]. The first version of this scaffold (1.0), used in the ABSORB Cohort A study, had a crossing profile of 1.4 mm, strut thickness of $150\,\mu m$, and consisted of out-of-phase zigzag hoops

linked together by thin and straight bridges. This device had to be kept refrigerated at –20°C to ensure device integrity. The second generation (1.1), tested in Cohort B, can be stored at room temperature, has the same strut thickness but in-phase zigzag hoops linked by bridges (Figure 34.1) [11]. Also, the polymer has a lower hydrolysis (*in vivo* degradation) rate in order to improve the radial force of the device.

Several studies have reported similar performances with the Absorb 1.1 and the everolimus-eluting metallic stent in terms of acute gain and late lumen loss (LLL) [12]. Also, non-significant differences were recently found for acute absolute recoil when comparing Absorb BVS with Xience (0.20 ± 0.21 and 0.13 ± 0.21 mm, respectively; $p = 0.32$), implying that both devices have similar radial strength [13]. Importantly, the higher conformability and flexibility shown by Absorb BVS contribute to less change in vessel geometry and curvature; these properties could finally restore a healthy balance between the shear stress and cyclic strain interplay, possibly resulting in restoration of vasomotor tone, late luminal enlargement with late expansive remodeling, and vessel compliance restoration [14–16].

The reabsorption process
The main chemical process responsible for *in vivo* molecular weight degradation of BVS is hydrolysis. The amorphous regions binding the crystallites are less packed and therefore water can penetrate more easily and start the process. The whole process of hydrolysis has five stages: hydration, depolymerization by hydrolysis (reduction of molecular weight), loss of mass (with scission of amorphous tie chains and subsequent loss of radial strength), dissolution of the monomer, and formation of carbon dioxide and water into the Krebs cycle, excreted through the kidneys or lungs [17]. The timing of the whole process is of paramount importance for its performance. The mechanical integrity and the absence of recoil should continue over a period of 6 months, during which time the biologic process of restenosis decreases (according to this, a permanent device would be possibly unnecessary beyond this time) [18]. Over time, the polymer is replaced by a provisional matrix made of proteoglycan and then by de novo connective tissue (Figure 34.2) [19].

The whole reabsorption process has also been demonstrated with the use of optical coherence tomography (OCT) and

Interventional Cardiology: Principles and Practice, Second Edition. Edited by George D. Dangas, Carlo Di Mario, and Nicholas N. Kipshidze.
© 2017 John Wiley & Sons, Ltd. Published 2017 by John Wiley & Sons, Ltd.

qualitative assessment of BVS struts over time has been proposed as follows: preserved box, open box, dissolved bright box, and dissolved black box, in order of decreasing reflectivity (Figure 34.3) [20]. The OCT analysis performed within the ABSORB Cohort A study has shown that the complete absorption of the scaffold takes place up to 3 years from implantation [8]. After the reabsorption process, tissue adaptation seems to cause a cellular reorganization, which positively impacts on the key step of "vascular restoration" [20].

BVS implantation technique

The mechanical properties of the BVS substantially differ from metal stents and consequently the implantation technique differs slightly from the standard for metal stents. The Abbott Vascular elaborated a list of manufacturer's advice according to which some steps are of paramount importance in order to achieve a safe and effective scaffold deployment: pre-dilatation of the lesion in all cases; slow scaffold expansion (increasing of 2 atmospheres every 5 seconds); treatment of bifurcation lesions is discouraged as well as post-dilatation, which is suggested only in case of unsatisfactory angiographic results. If post-dilatation has to be performed, balloons should be ≤0.25 mm larger than the nominal diameter of the Absorb scaffold; inflation pressure should remain in accordance with the characteristic of the balloon expandability to avoid unacceptable dilatation of the scaffold, which is 0.5 mm over the nominal value. Atherectomy, cutting balloon, or brachytherapy are also discouraged. Given these recommendations, BVS deployment still represents a delicate procedure where each step, such as

accurate scaffold sizing, pre-dilatation, and post-deployment optimization, is extremely important.

The ABSORB program

The Absorb BVS has been supported by a robust, well-structured, international, investigator-sponsored (ABBOTT Vascular) program, designed to promote the clinical use of the Absorb BVS for the treatment of atherosclerotic vascular lesions (Table 34.1). The first-in-man study using BVS was the Absorb Cohort A study which enrolled 30 patients undergoing first generation (Absorb BVS 1.0) scaffold implantation for the treatment of single, not complex, lesions [9]. The 5-year clinical outcomes have been excellent, with 3.4% of major adverse cardiovascular events (MACE) mainly being myocardial infarction (MI) occurrence [21]. Subsequently, to enhance the mechanical strength of the struts and to reduce immediate and late recoil, the revised version BVS 1.1 was introduced and tested in the ABSORB Cohort B study [11]. It reported good clinical and imaging outcomes at 6 months on a larger population of patients (n = 101) for up to 3 years, with a MACE rate of 10.1% [22]. In order to build a body of evidence to support a broader utilization of the Absorb BVS, a prospective, single-arm, open-label clinical study (the ABSORB EXTEND) was designed [23]. The 1-year results were reassuring, with rates of 4.3% MACE, 2.9% MI, and 0.8% scaffold thrombosis (ST). To date, the 3-year follow-up data of 250 patients implanted with BVS in the ABSORB EXTEND study showed 9.3% cumulative MACE, with 6.0% TLR and 1.2% definite/probable ST rate [24]. Importantly, in the ABSORB EXTEND, as per study protocol (same for Cohorts A and B), left main and arterial or saphenous vein graft (SVG) lesions were excluded, as well as in-stent restenosis, totally occluded vessels, lesions treated with brachytherapy or Rotablator, lesions involving a bifurcation or ostial lesions. Also, lesions with excessive tortuosity, heavy calcification, or visible thrombus were not treated with the Absorb BVS. The same types of lesion have been treated in the first randomized study comparing metallic with fully biodegradable stents eluting the same drug (everolimus) [9]. The ABSORB II randomized controlled trial had a 2:1 single-blinded design with a sample population of 501 patients and a sophisticated quantitative computerized angiography (QCA) primary endpoint of nitrate-induced vasomotion and in-stent late loss at 3 years [9]. The 1-year clinical follow-up

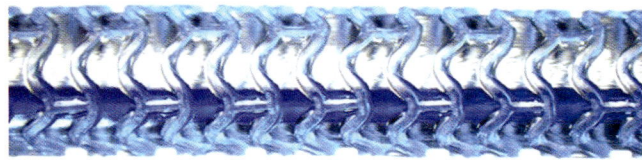

Figure 34.1 Absorb biodegradable vascular scaffold (BVS) structure and design (high-resolution microscope image).

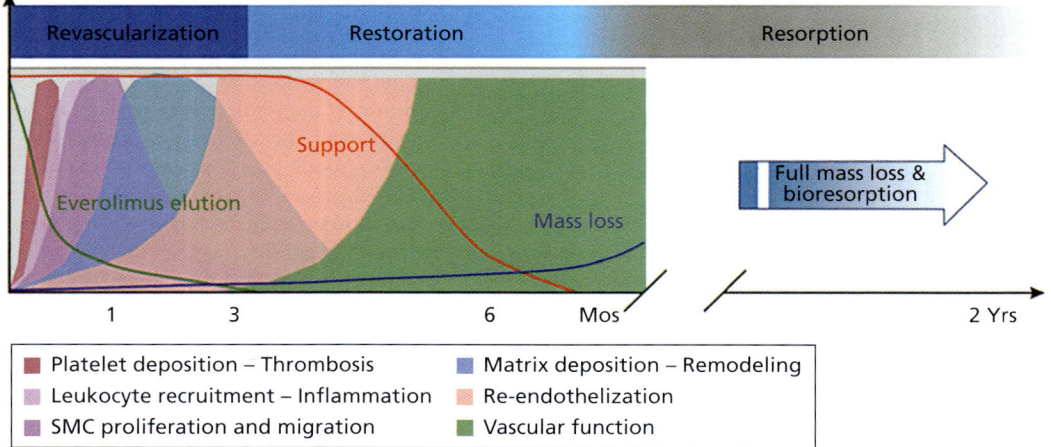

Figure 34.2 Conceptual representation of the three phases of bioresorbable scaffold functionality and the relationship to physiological following implantation. Source: Oberhauser *et al.* 2009 [66], p. F.18.

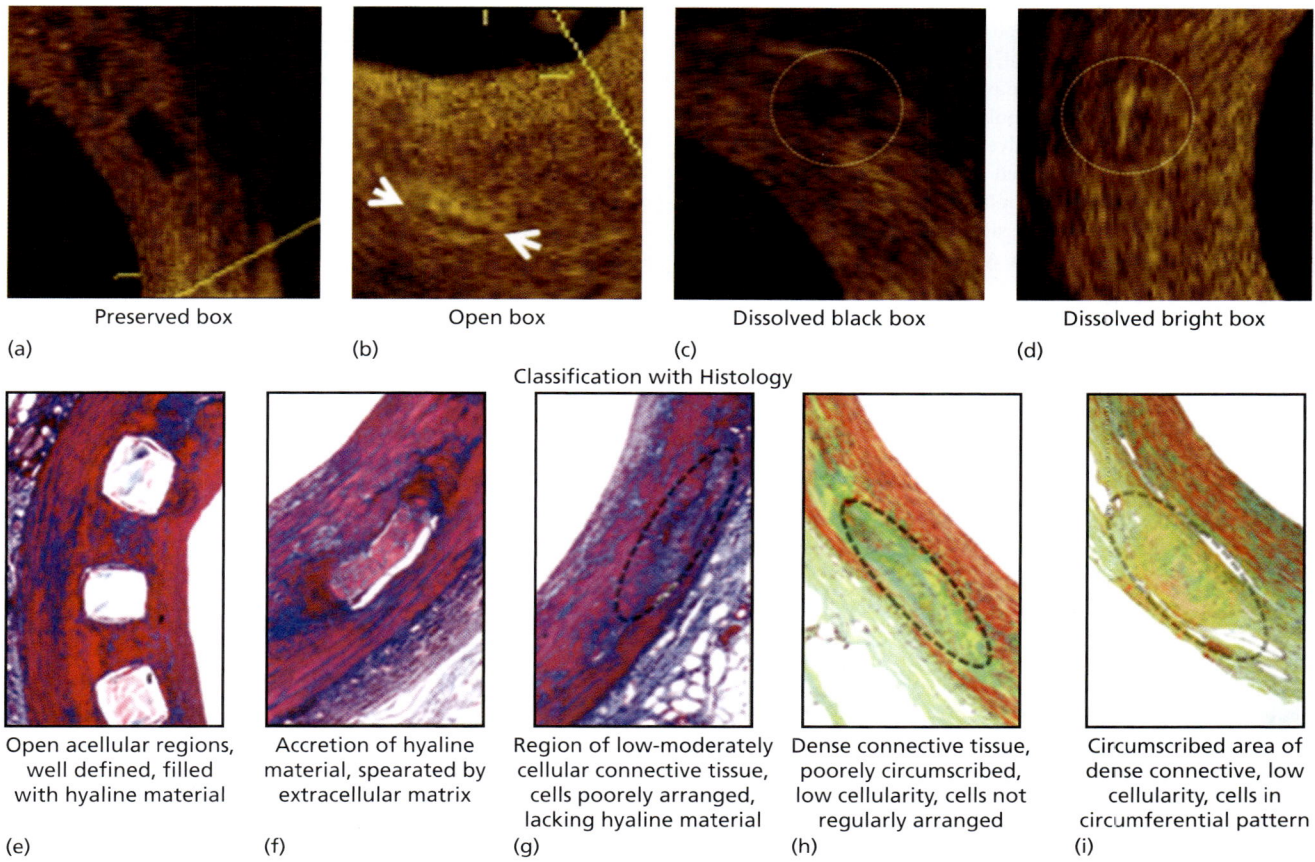

Classification with OCT

Preserved box (a)   Open box (b)   Dissolved black box (c)   Dissolved bright box (d)

Classification with Histology

Open acellular regions, well defined, filled with hyaline material (e)

Accretion of hyaline material, spearated by extracellular matrix (f)

Region of low-moderately cellular connective tissue, cells poorly arranged, lacking hyaline material (g)

Dense connective tissue, poorly circumscribed, low cellularity, cells not regularly arranged (h)

Circumscribed area of dense connective, low cellularity, cells in circumferential pattern (i)

Figure 34.3 Classification of Absorb BVS struts with OCT and histology over time (porcine coronary arteries). Progressive morphologic phases of struts degradation are shown: preserved box (a and e), open box (b, f, g), dissolved bright box (c and h), and dissolved black box (d and i) in order of decreasing reflectivity. Source: Adapted from Onuma et al. 2010 [20]. Reproduced with permission from Wolters Kluwer Health.

Table 34.1 The ABSORB Program (manufacturer-sponsored studies).

Study	Study design	Stage	n[a]	Follow-up
ABSORB cohort A	Observational, prospective	Completed	30	5 years
ABSORB cohort B	Non randomized, open label	Completed	101	5 years
ABSORB EXTEND	Observational, prospective	Active, not recruiting	=1000	3 years
ABSORB II	Randomized, single blind	Active, not recruiting	330	3 years
ABSORB PHYSIOLOGY*	Randomized, single blind	Terminated	35	2 years
ABSORB FIRST	Observational, perspective	Recruiting	1800	2 years
ABSORB III	Randomized, single blind	Recruiting	1502	3 years
ABSORB IV	Randomized, single blind	Recruiting	3000	3 years
ABSORB Japan	Randomized, single blind	Active, not recruiting	265	3 years
ABSORB China	Randomized, open label	Active, not recruiting	200	2 years
ABSORB UK	Observational, prospective registry	Recruiting	100	3 years

* 1 patient recruited
[a] n = number of patients.

included an elaborated analysis of immediate results including QCA and IVUS data. In this trial, the Absorb scaffold did not show any significant difference on the primary endpoint compared with the Xience at 1 year; a lower cumulative rate of recurrent or worsening angina reported through adverse event forms was reported in the Absorb arm when compared with the Xience arm. However, final in-stent minimum lumen diameter and IVUS minimum lumen cross-sectional area were significantly smaller in the Absorb group than in the Xience group. Also of interest, there was a trend toward higher MI and ST in the Absorb arm (4.5% vs. 1.2%; $p = 0.06$ for MI and 0.9% vs. 0.0%; $p = 0.55$ for ST) [9, 25]. The B-SEARCH Registry by Simsek et al. [26] has to be mentioned here because it enrolled patients (n = 88) from ABSORB Cohort A, Cohort B, and ABSORB EXTEND studies (thus, with same characteristics of lesion complexity); only one adverse event was recorded (non-target vessel revascularization) at 1-month follow-up. Of note, in order to test the performances of the Absorb BVS in more complex settings, some sub-studies involving ABSORB EXTEND population of patients were conducted, with interesting results [27–29]. Muramatsu et al. [27] analyzed 1209 side branches from 436 patients treated with BVS and found that scaffold implantation was associated with a higher incidence of post-procedural side branch occlusion compared with EES. Another study from Muramatsu et al. [28] evaluated the device-oriented composite endpoint (DoCE) at 1-year follow-up including cardiac death, target vessel MI, and target lesion revascularization, in a population of diabetic patients treated with BVS. They compared diabetic patients from ABSORB Cohort B and ABSORB EXTEND studies to diabetic patients treated with everolimus-eluting metal stents (EES) in pooled data from the SPIRIT trials, by applying propensity score matching. Diabetic patients treated with the BVS had a similar incidence of the DoCE compared with diabetic patients treated with EES in the matched study group (3.9% for the BVS vs. 6.4% for EES; $p = 0.38$), with no differences in the incidence of definite or probable ST (0.7% for both diabetic and non-diabetic patients with the BVS; 1.0% for diabetic patients with the BVS vs. 1.7% for diabetic patients with EES in the matched study group).

Also interesting results come from a recent study by Diletti et al. [29], aiming to assess the impact of vessel size on long-term outcomes after Absorb BVS implantation in the Cohort B population of patients. At 2 years' follow-up, similar clinical and angiographic outcomes were reported in small and large vessel groups. Notably, a significant late lumen enlargement and positive vessel remodeling were observed in small vessels.

In summary, in the ABSORB program, Absorb BVS has shown very good safety and efficacy results in not complex lesions, even when compared with its metallic counterpart, Xience. Several studies are ongoing within the same program and will further evaluate this device in different populations of patients with different endpoints.

Registries

To date, taking into account published and ongoing studies, there are almost 30 "real-world" studies or registries using the Absorb BVS worldwide. For this reason, a huge and still accumulating number of data are being reported, justifying the interest of the interventional cardiology community. The GHOST-EU Registry has recently been published and is the first large multicenter international registry assessing the early and mid-term clinical outcomes of PCI with everolimus-eluting Absorb BVS [30]. The study involved 10 European centers, enrolling 1189 patients with 1731 Absorb BVS implanted. The percentage of type B2 or C treated lesions (51%, according to the ACC/AHA classification) roughly represents a "real-world" scenario. The primary outcome, target lesion failure (TLF), defined as the combination of cardiac death, target vessel MI, or clinically driven target lesion revascularization (TLR), showed a cumulative incidence of 2.2% at 30 days and 4.4% at 6 months. Interestingly, the GHOST-EU Registry recorded a high 6-month ST of 1.5% and an annual ST of 2.1% (Table 34.1). Even higher ST rates were found in the "real-world" AMC Registry where 135 patients were included [31]. In this study, Kraak et al. [31] treated a real-world population of patients (62% of type B2 or C lesions) with both Absorb BVS and Xience DES, and reported a MI rate of 3.0% vs. 3.0%, respectively, while worse outcomes were observed for cardiac death (0.8% vs. 0%), TLR (6.3% vs. 3%), and ST (3.3% vs. 0%), the latter representing the higher 6-month rate of ST to date (3%). Interesting data come from two single-center studies evaluating the BVS performance in the highest setting of lesion complexity (both enrolling >80% type B2 + C lesions, according to the ACC/AHA classification) [32, 33]. The first study, by Costopoulos et al. [32], yielded 92 patient pairs (92 patients with 137 lesions treated with BVS and 92 patients with 124 lesions treated with EES), by propensity score matching. Clinical outcomes at 6 months were similar between the two groups with respect to TLR (3.3% vs. 5.4%; $p = 0.41$) and MACE (3.3% vs. 7.6%; $p = 0.19$). Importantly, the ST rate was 0% in both groups. Similarly, Mattesini et al. [33] performed the same comparison in 100 patients (50 treated with BVS and 50 with second-generation DES) presenting only with complex lesions (B2 or C in 100% of cases); they reported a low percentage of malapposed struts in both groups (BVS 2.1% vs. DES 2.4%), with 4% MACE and no ST.

A small number of "real-world" studies enrolling only patients with acute coronary syndrome (ACS) have been published to date, with interesting data from small populations of patients. The Prague 19 study by Kočka et al. [34], enrolling consecutive patients with ST-elevation MI (STEMI), compared 41 patients implanted with Absorb BVS with 57 patients who received a metal stent. Interestingly, in the BVS group, the study reported a lower percentage of diabetic patients (2.5% vs. 24.1%; $p = 0.003$) but a higher percentage of manual aspiration thrombectomy (37.5% vs. 12.3%; $p = 0.011$). The latter finding is of interest because the higher strut thickness of BVS should allow better entrapment of thrombotic material between the stent and the vessel, the "snow racket concept," which is the main feature of this novel device [35, 36]. The Prague 19 study reported only two adverse events in the BVS arm, with only one ST (subacute) also documented at OCT (which was available for 21 patients). Diletti et al. [35] recently published the results of the BVS STEMI study, a prospective single-arm study enrolling patients with STEMI (n = 49) undergoing BVS implantation. OCT imaging was also performed in 31 patients, revealing a low malapposition rate (seven scaffolds with >5% malapposed struts). The clinical outcomes at 1 month follow-up were excellent with only 2.6% MACE (one non-Q wave MI) and no ST. The largest study to date involving ACS patients by Gori et al. [37] reported results from 150 consecutive patients after BVS implantation, compared with 103 patients implanted with EES in the same time period. The 6-month MACE rate was similar between both groups (all $p > 0.5$), but a high definite/probable ST rate was reported (2.7%), mostly acute and subacute. In two out of the three ST cases, authors found an incomplete expansion of the BVS at OCT as a possible explanation.

Recently, the EVERBIO II study design has been published [38]. This is a single-center, randomized study comparing three typologies of drug-eluting stents (the Absorb™, the Promus Element™, and the Biomatrix Flex™) in a broader setting of lesions. The primary endpoint is in-stent LLL at 9 months as assessed by QCA; the secondary endpoints are divided into angiographic and clinical findings at up to 5 years' follow-up. A standard implantation technique was used for all devices and post-dilatation was performed in 36% of cases in the Absorb group. The 9-month results did not find any significant difference in LLL among devices, but in-segment LLL was significantly higher in the Absorb BVS than the EES/BES group (NCT01711931). The constrictive effect found by Gogas et al. [39] and the neointimal hyperproliferation at the scaffold proximal edge have been claimed as possible explanations [40]. The most recent published study enrolling patients with ACS, the RAI Registry, reported the 6-month outcomes from a population of 74 patients with STEMI, showing very high procedural success rate (97.3%) as well as low TLR and ST rates (4.1% and 1.3%, respectively). Of note, multiple overlapping BVS during primary PCI did not show any significant difference in clinical outcome when compared with single BVS implantation [41].

Intracoronary imaging guidance
IVUS
Several large studies have been published indicating that IVUS can be important for optimal DES stent expansion and lower malapposition rates in complex PCIs (multivessel disease and/or left main coronary artery stenting) [42], and its value has also been recognized in improving clinical outcomes after PCI [43–47]. A recent meta-analysis of more than 24,000 patients comparing IVUS with angiography-guided PCI outcomes showed lower rates of all-cause mortality, MI, target vessel revascularization, and ST in the IVUS-guided group [48]. Interestingly, OCT has been extensively used throughout most of the ABSORB program studies; however, given the wide availability of IVUS-guided PCI clinical data and the presence of standardized criteria for optimizing stent implantation, IVUS still represents a widely used tool for intracoronary imaging trials [49].

Optical coherence tomography
OCT is an established tool for the diagnosis and treatment of coronary lesions; its utility in improving clinical outcomes of patients undergoing PCI has been demonstrated [50]. This technology allows better visualization of both struts and the vessel wall, with an axial resolution 10-fold higher (14 μm) than IVUS, thus allowing better identification of stent failure (e.g., stent malapposition, dissection, tissue protrusion, and thrombus). However, OCT is not able to measure plaque burden because of its shallow penetration depth (1–2 mm) [51].

A recent study by Allahwalla et al. [52] reported that despite achieving angiographic success in all BVS implantations, further optimization was required in over one-quarter of patients on the basis of OCT findings. Although a comprehensive consensus document has been developed for acquisition, measurement, and reporting of intravascular optical coherence [53], whether IVUS criteria for optimal stent placement can be translated to OCT-guided stent implantation is still unknown. Notwithstanding these limitations, OCT is currently considered the "gold standard" imaging technique for the evaluation of biodegradable scaffolds; in fact, the BVS allows the assessment of the vessel wall behind the struts without the usual shadowing of metallic struts as seen in OCT analysis [54]. As a result, the use of OCT for BVS deployment has been widely accepted, and has contributed significantly to the

knowledge of the Absorb BVS characteristics and its interplay with the coronary wall [8,54]. OCT is especially recognized as an essential tool for the optimization of BVS in complex lesions such as bifurcations [55,56]. Looking at the most recent data, possible explanations of results from BVS "real-world" studies could also be reached for the use of intracoronary imaging guidance.

In conclusion, intracoronary imaging with IVUS and OCT is a useful tool in guiding BVS implantation, and the two modalities seem to be complementary. While IVUS could be more helpful for the evaluation of the plaque morphology and in the preparation phase, OCT allows better qualitative scaffold analysis and follow-up evaluation. Overall, both technologies ensure reliable lumen and scaffold measurements.

Clinically tested bioresorbable vascular scaffolds
During the long hunt for the ideal bioresorbable stent several attempts have been made. However, only a few of the proposed devices have been clinically tested on humans and an even smaller number have been clinically safe and effective enough to be commercialized. In this section we provide an overview of those BVS clinically tested in humans (Figure 34.4).

Igaki-Tamai Stent
The Igaki-Tamai PLLA coronary stent was the first fully bioresorbable stent to be implanted in humans, with complete degradation taking 18–24 months. The stent has a helical zigzag design, which differs from previous knitted formats. This results in less vessel wall injury during implantation and therefore less initial thrombus formation and reduced intimal hyperplasia [57]. The stent is mounted on a standard angioplasty balloon and is both self-expanding thermally and by balloon. Self-expansion occurs in response to heating the PLLA, which is achieved by the use of heated contrast (up to 70°C) to inflate the delivery balloon. Stent expansion is further optimized by inflating the delivery balloon to 6–14 atm for 30 seconds, and the nominal size of the stent is achieved by continued self-expansion at 37°C in the 20–30 minutes after stent deployment. The stent has a standard length of 12 mm and is available in diameters of 3, 3.5, and 4 mm; the stent strut thickness is 0.17 mm. An 8-Fr guiding catheter is required because the stent is initially constrained by a sheath that is removed once it crosses the lesion. At either end of the stent, to aid visualization, are two radio-opaque cylindrical gold markers.

The first-in-humans study of the Igaki-Tamai stent (15 patients, 19 lesions, 25 stents) demonstrated no MACEs or ST within 30 days and 1 repeat PCI at the 6-month follow-up. Encouragingly, the loss index (late loss/acute gain) was 0.48 mm, which was comparable to BMS, and demonstrated for the first time that BRS did not induce an excess of intimal hyperplasia. Furthermore, IVUS imaging demonstrated no significant stent recoil at day 1, and continued stent expansion was observed in the first 3 months of follow-up [58].

A second, larger study of 50 elective patients (63 lesions, 84 stents) also showed promising results. IVUS performed at the 3-year follow-up demonstrated the complete absence of stent struts, and angiographic analysis demonstrated a mean diameter stenosis of 25% compared with 38%, 29%, and 26% at 6, 12, and 24 months, respectively. Clinical outcomes at 4-year follow-up showed rates of overall and MACE-free survival of 97.7% and 82.0%, respectively [59].

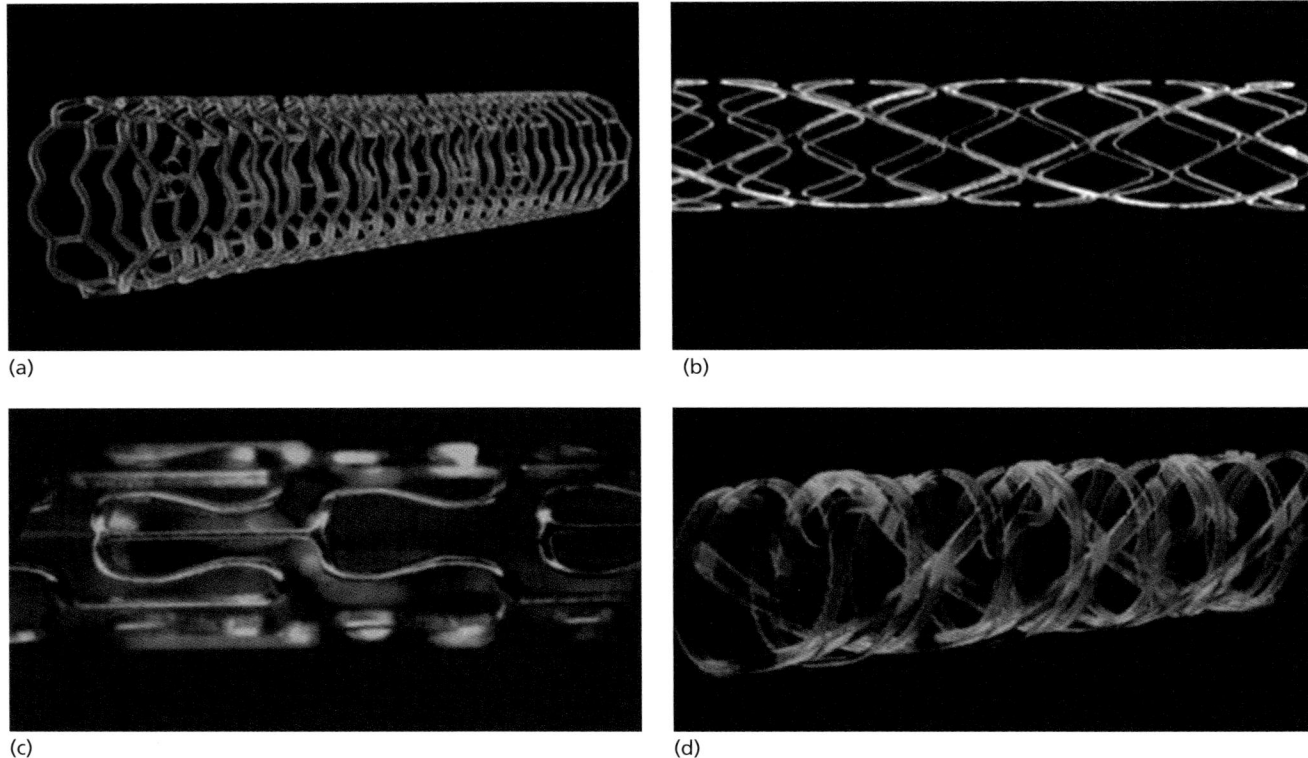

Figure 34.4 Structures and designs of clinically tested BVS: (a) DESolve, (b) Igaki Tamay, (c) AMS, (d) Rezolve.

Despite these impressive results, the failure of the stent to progress was related primarily to the use of heat to induce self-expansion. There were concerns that this could cause necrosis of the arterial wall, leading to excessive intimal hyperplasia or increased platelet adhesion, leading to ST [60]. None of these concerns were substantiated in the initial studies; however, only low-risk patients were enrolled. After completion of the Biodegradable peripheral Igaki-Tamai stents PERSEUS study [61], the stent became available in Europe for peripheral use, but so far it is not available for coronary use.

Tyrosine polycarbonate: REVA stent

The REVA stent (Boston Scientific, Natick, MA, USA) is a tyrosine poly (desaminotyrosyltyrosine ethyl ester) carbonate stent that is both resorbable and radio-opaque after the chemical modification of tyrosine to incorporate iodine molecules. The polymer degrades into water, carbon dioxide, and ethanol; in addition, tyrosine is metabolized by the Krebs cycle. The resorption time of the stent is dependent on the mass of the polymer, with reported times of 18 or 12 months for the high- and low-molecular weight polymers, respectively. In addition to its radio-opacity, the REVA stent also has a distinctive slide-and-lock design that provides both flexibility and strength. During the deployment of a standard deformable stent, significant strain is concentrated at hinge points; the consequence of straining a polymer beyond its yield point is a significant loss of mechanical strength. The slide-and-lock design eliminates hinge points and therefore minimizes polymer strain by 75% over a wide range of deployment diameters, thereby preventing deformation and weakening of the polymer during stent deployment. The locking mechanism maintains the acute lumen gain after stent deployment and provides additional support to the stent during vessel remodeling. Company data report negligible recoil and a radial force that is superior to the Multi-Link Vision BMS (Abbott Vascular, Santa Clara, CA, USA) [62].

The multicenter first-in-human clinical study of the REVA stent, the REVA Endovascular Study of a Bioresorbable Coronary Stent (RESORB) study, enrolled 30 patients from June 2007. The study was designed to evaluate the safety of the stent in de novo lesions 12 mm in length and 3.0–3.5 mm in diameter. The primary endpoint was MACE at 30 days; the secondary endpoint was IVUS and QCA-derived parameters at the 6-month follow-up. Follow-up at 6 months showed the absence of any significant vessel recoil as indicated by the external elastic lamina, which went from 15.5 ± 4.0 to $15.3 \pm 3.1\,\text{mm}^2$. Unfortunately, focal mechanical failures driven by polymer embrittlement led to a higher-than-anticipated rate of TLR (66.7%) at 4–6 months' follow-up [63].

Redesign of the stent has ensued, resulting in the second-generation ReZolve (Rezolve2) stent. This stent has a more robust polymer, a spiral slide-and-lock mechanism to improve clinical performance, and a coating of sirolimus. ReZolve2 is a lower profile and sheath-less version of the first-generation ReZolve scaffold and offers significantly improved deliverability and an approximate 30% increase in scaffold strength to provide increased support to significant coronary artery lesions before being resorbed by the body. REVA began implanting ReZolve2 in patients in March 2013. So far no results are available in literature.

Poly (anhydride ester) salicylic acid: IDEAL stent

The IDEAL biodegradable stent (Bioabsorbable Therapeutics Inc, Menlo Park, CA, USA) consists of a backbone of polyanhydride ester based on salicylic acid and adipic acid anhydride and an 8.3-μg/mm coating of sirolimus, potentially giving the stent both anti-inflammatory and antiproliferative properties. The vascular compatibility and efficacy of this biodegradable salicylate-based polymer have previously been demonstrated in the porcine model. Most notably, the polymer was associated with reduced inflammation compared with a standard BMS and Cypher stent [64]. This was very likely because of the anti-inflammatory properties of salicylic acid following absorption by the vessel wall after its release. Drug elution was found to be complete after 30 days, and complete stent degradation occurred over a 9- to 12-month period. The 8-Fr compatible, balloon-expandable stent is radio-opaque and does not require any special storage.

In July 2009, the 11 patients enrolled in the multicenter first-in-humans Whisper trial completed their 12-month follow-up. Primary results have shown stent safety and confirmed structural integrity of the stent with no evidence of acute or chronic recoil. Unfortunately, insufficient neointimal suppression has been demonstrated [65]. This is likely to be the consequence of inadequate drug dosing, particularly considering that the surface area dose of sirolimus is only one-quarter of that found on the Cypher stent. The rapid elution of sirolimus may also be a contributing factor.

A second-generation stent has been developed with a higher dose of sirolimus and a slower drug release pattern. Furthermore, the stent design has been optimized, which has resulted in a reduced crossing profile (6-Fr compatible) and thinner struts (175 μm). Although the program was on hold in early 2009, there are no results available in literature yet.

The DESolve scaffold

The DESolve Myolimus-Eluting Bioresorbable Coronary Scaffold System (Elixir Medical Corporation, Sunnyvale, CA, USA) is a PLLA-based polymer scaffold coated with the antiproliferative drug myolimus mounted on a rapid exchange balloon catheter delivery system. The DESolve scaffold is formed using proprietary techniques from a bioresorbable polylactide-based polymer with strut thickness of 150 mm and incorporates two platinum-based radio-opaque markers at either end to aid in placement. The scaffold is coated with a matrix of polylactide-based polymer and myolimus at a 3 mg/mm dose; more than 85% of the drug is released over 4 weeks. The system has a crossing profile of 1.47 mm and is 6-Fr catheter compatible. The scaffold is designed to resorb in about 1 year. The degradation process of PLLA-based polymers occurs primarily by hydrolysis and is metabolized *in vivo* via the Krebs cycle into carbon dioxide and water [66]. Important differentiating features of the DESolve scaffold include:

1 Its ability to self-correct to the vessel wall in cases of minor malapposition when expanded to the nominal diameter, which is accomplished using a proprietary processing technique;

2 The ability of the scaffold to maintain radial strength and vessel support for the critical 3- to 4-month period of vessel healing [67] while subsequently resorbing in about 1 year;

3 A wide safety margin for expansion where a 3.0-mm scaffold can be expanded to 4.5 mm in diameter without strut fracture.

Pre-clinical *in vivo* test results assessing the bioresorption profile of the DESolve scaffold using molecular weight measurements by gel permeation chromatography have demonstrated bioresorption of the DESolve scaffold with molecular weight reduction of >95% takes about 1 year.

The first-in-man trial assessing the safety of the DESolve scaffold has been recently published [68,69]. The study enrolled 16 patients with simple lesions (<12 mm). Acute procedural success was

achieved in 15 of 15 patients receiving a study scaffold. At 12 months, there was no scaffold thrombosis and no MACE directly attributable to the scaffold. At 6 months, in-scaffold LLL (by QCA) was 0.19 ± 0.19 mm; neointimal volume (by IVUS) was 7.19 ± 3.56%, with no evidence of scaffold recoil or late malapposition. Findings were confirmed with OCT and showed uniform, thin neointimal coverage (0.12 ± 0.04 mm). At 12 months, multislice computed tomography demonstrated excellent vessel patency.

The DESolve scaffold has been available in Europe since the beginning of 2014. To the best of our knowledge so far there are no data available from the aforementioned first-in-man trial.

Interactive multiple choice questions are available for this chapter on www.wiley. com/go/dangas/cardiology

References

1 Serruys PW, de Jaegere P, Kiemeneij F, *et al.* A comparison of balloonexpandable-stent implantation with balloon angioplasty in patients with coronary artery disease. Benestent Study Group. *N Engl J Med* 1994; **331**: 489–495.

2 Fischman DL, Leon MB, Baim DS, *et al.* A randomized comparison of coronary-stent placement and balloonangioplasty in the treatment of coronary artery disease. Stent Restenosis Study Investigators. *N Engl J Med* 1994; **331**: 496–501.

3 Gruntzig A. Transluminal dilatation of coronary-artery stenosis. *Lancet* 1978; **1**: 263.

4 Serruys PW, Garcia-Garcia HM, Onuma Y. From metallic cages to transient bioresorbable scaffolds: change in paradigm of coronary revascularization in the upcoming decade. *Eur Heart J* 2012; **33**(1): 16–25. doi: 10.1093/eurheartj/ehr384. Epub 2011 Oct 31.

5 Erbel R, Di Mario C, Bartunek J, *et al.* Temporary scaffolding of coronary arteries with bioabsorbable magnesium stents: a prospective, nonrandomised multicentre trial. *Lancet* 2007; **369**: 1869–1875.

6 Haude M, Erbel R, Erne P, *et al.* Safety and performance of the drug-eluting absorbable metal scaffold (DREAMS) in patients with de-novo coronary lesions: 12 month results of the prospective, multicentre, first-in-man BIOSOLVE-I trial. *Lancet* 2013; **381**: 836–844.

7 Ormiston JA, Serruys PW, Regar E, *et al.* A bioabsorbable everolimus-eluting coronary stent system for patients with single de-novo coronary artery lesions (ABSORB): a prospective open-label trial. *Lancet* 2008; **371**: 899–907.

8 Serruys PW, Ormiston JA, Onuma Y, *et al.* A bioabsorbable everolimuseluting coronary stent system (ABSORB): 2-year outcomes and results from multiple imaging methods. *Lancet* 2009; **373**: 897–910.

9 Serruys PW, Chevalier B, Dudek D, *et al.* A bioresorbable everolimus-eluting scaffold versus a metallic everolimus-eluting stent for ischaemic heart disease caused by de-novo native coronary artery lesions (ABSORB II): an interim 1-year analysis of clinical and procedural secondary outcomes from a randomised controlled trial. *Lancet* 2015; **385**: 43–54.

10 Ormiston JA, Serruys PW, Regar E, *et al.* A bioabsorbable everolimus-eluting coronary stent system for patients with single de-novo coronary artery lesions (ABSORB): a prospective open-label trial. *Lancet* 2008; **371**(9616): 899–907. doi: 10.1016/S0140-6736(08)60415-8.

11 Serruys PW, Onuma Y, Ormiston JA, *et al.* Evaluation of the second generation of a bioresorbable everolimus drug-eluting vascular scaffold for treatment of de novo coronary artery stenosis: six-month clinical and imaging outcomes. *Circulation* 2010; **122**(22): 2301–2312. doi: 10.1161/CIRCULATIONAHA.110.970772. Epub 2010 Nov 15.

12 Zhang YJ, Bourantas CV, Muramatsu T, *et al.* Comparison of acute gain and late lumen loss after PCI with bioresorbable vascular scaffolds versus everolimus-eluting stents: an exploratory observational study prior to a randomised trial. *EuroIntervention* 2014; **10**(6): 672–680.

13 Tanimoto S, Serruys PW, Thuesen L, *et al.* Comparison of in vivo acute stent recoil between the bioabsorbable everolimus-eluting coronary stent and the everolimus-eluting cobalt chromium coronary stent: insights from the ABSORB and SPIRIT trials. *Catheter Cardiovasc Interv* 2007; **70**(4): 515–523.

14 Gomez-Lara J, Garcia-Garcia HM, Onuma Y, *et al.* A comparison of the conformability of everolimus-eluting bioresorbable vascular scaffolds to metal platform coronary stents. *JACC Cardiovasc Interv* 2010; **3**(11): 1190–1198. doi: 10.1016/j.jcin.2010.07.016.

15 Gyongyosi M, Yang P, Khorsand A, Glogar D; Austrian Wiktor. Stent Study Group and European Paragon Stent Investigators. Longitudinal straightening effect of stents is an additional predictor for major adverse cardiac events. *J Am Coll Cardiol* 2000; **35**: 1580–1589.

16 Wentzel JJ, Whelan DM, van der Giessen WJ, *et al.* Coronary stent implantation changes 3-D vessel geometry and 3-D shear stress distribution. *J Biomech* 2000; **33**: 1287–1295.

17 Hollinger JO, Battistone GC. Biodegradable bone repair materials: synthetic polymers and ceramics. *Clin Orthop Relat Res* 1986; **(207)**: 290–305.

18 Serruys PW, Luijten HE, Beatt KJ, *et al.* Incidence of restenosis after successful coronary angioplasty: a time-related phenomenon: a quantitative angiographic study in 342 consecutive patients at 1, 2, 3, and 4 months. *Circulation* 1988; **77**(2): 361–371.

19 Ciccone WJ 2nd, Motz C, Bentley C, Tasto JP. Bioabsorbable implants in orthopaedics: new developments and clinical applications. *J Am Acad Orthop Surg* 2001; **9**(5): 280–208.

20 Onuma Y, Serruys PW, Perkins LE, *et al.* Intracoronary optical coherence tomography and histology at 1 month and 2, 3, and 4 years after implantation of everolimus-eluting bioresorbable vascular scaffolds in a porcine coronary artery model: an attempt to decipher the human optical coherence tomography images in the ABSORB trial. *Circulation* 2010; **122**(22): 2288–2300. doi: 10.1161/CIRCULATIONAHA.109.921528. Epub 2010 Oct 25.

21 Onuma Y, Dudek D, Thuesen L, *et al.* Five-year clinical and functional multislice computed tomography angiographic results after coronary implantation of the fully resorbable polymeric everolimus-eluting scaffold in patients with de novo coronary artery disease: the ABSORB Cohort A trial. *JACC Cardiovasc Interv* 2013; **6**(10): 999–1009. doi: 10.1016/j.jcin.2013.05.017.

22 Serruys PW, Onuma Y, Garcia-Garcia HM, *et al.* Dynamics of vessel wall changes following the implantation of the absorb everolimus-eluting bioresorbable vascular scaffold: a multi-imaging modality study at 6, 12, 24 and 36 months. *EuroIntervention* 2014; **9**(11): 1271–1284.

23 Abizaid A, Costa JR Jr, Bartorelli AL, *et al.* The ABSORB EXTEND study: preliminary report of the twelve-month clinical outcomes in the first 512 patients enrolled. *EuroIntervention* 2014 Apr 29. pii: 20130827-06. [Epub ahead of print].

24 Smits PC. TCT-615 ABSORB EXTEND: an interim report on the 36-month clinical outcomes from the first 250 patients enrolled. *J Am Coll Cardiol* 2014; **64**(11S). doi:10.1016/j.jacc.2014.07.681.

25 Di Mario C, Caiazzo G. Biodegradable stents: the golden future of angioplasty? *Lancet* 2014 Sep 12. pii: S0140-6736(14)61636-6. doi: 10.1016/S0140-6736(14)61636-6. [Epub ahead of print].

26 Simsek C, Magro M, Onuma Y, *et al.* Procedural and clinical outcomes of the Absorb everolimus-eluting bioresorbable vascular scaffold: one-month results of the Bioresorbable vascular Scaffold Evaluated At Rotterdam Cardiology Hospitals (B-SEARCH). *EuroIntervention* 2014; **10**(2): 236–240. doi: 10.4244/EIJV10I2A38.

27 Muramatsu T, Onuma Y, García-García HM, *et al.*; ABSORB-EXTEND Investigators. Incidence and short-term clinical outcomes of small side branch occlusion after implantation of an everolimus-eluting bioresorbable vascular scaffold: an interim report of 435 patients in the ABSORB-EXTEND single-arm trial in comparison with an everolimus-eluting metallic stent in the SPIRIT first and II trials. *JACC Cardiovasc Interv* 2013; **6**(3): 247–257. doi: 10.1016/j.jcin.2012.10.013.

28 Muramatsu T, Onuma Y, van Geuns RJ, *et al.*; ABSORB Cohort B Investigators; ABSORB EXTEND Investigators; SPIRIT FIRST Investigators; SPIRIT II Investigators; SPIRIT III Investigators; SPIRIT IV Investigators. 1-year clinical outcomes of diabetic patients treated with everolimus-eluting bioresorbable vascular scaffolds: a pooled analysis of the ABSORB and the SPIRIT trials. *JACC Cardiovasc Interv* 2014; **7**(5): 482–493. doi: 10.1016/j.jcin.2014.01.155. Epub 2014 Apr 16.

29 Diletti R, Farooq V, Girasis C, *et al.* Clinical and intravascular imaging outcomes at 1 and 2 years after implantation of absorb everolimus eluting bioresorbable vascular scaffolds in small vessels. Late lumen enlargement: does bioresorption matter with small vessel size? Insight from the ABSORB Cohort B trial. *Heart* 2013; **99**(2): 98–105. doi: 10.1136/heartjnl-2012-302598. Epub 2012 Oct 31.

30 Capodanno D, Gori T, Nef H, *et al.* Percutaneous coronary intervention with everolimus-eluting bioresorbable vascular scaffolds in routine clinical practice: early and midterm outcomes from the European multicentre GHOST-EU registry. *EuroIntervention* 2014; published online July 18. doi:10.4244/EIJY14M07_11.

31 Kraak RP, Hassell ME, Grundeken MJ, *et al.* Initial experience and clinical evaluation of the Absorb bioresorbable vascular scaffold (BVS) in real-world practice: the AMC Single Centre Real World PCI Registry. *EuroIntervention* 2014; published online Aug 20. doi:10.4244/EIJY14M08_08.

32 Costopoulos C, Latib A, Naganuma T, *et al.* Comparison of early clinical outcomes between absorb bioresorbable vascular scaffold and everolimus-eluting stent implantation in a real-world population. *Catheter Cardiovasc Interv* 2014 Jun 6. doi: 10.1002/ccd.25569. [Epub ahead of print].

33 Mattesini A, Secco GG, Dall'Ara G, *et al.* ABSORB biodegradable stents versus second-generation metal stents: a comparison study of 100 complex lesions treated

under OCT guidance. *JACC Cardiovasc Interv* 2014; **7**(7): 741–750. doi: 10.1016/j.jcin.2014.01.165.

34 Kočka V, Malý M, Toušek P, *et al.* Bioresorbable vascular scaffolds in acute ST-segment elevation myocardial infarction: a prospective multicentre study "Prague 19." *Eur Heart J* 2014; **35**: 787–794.

35 Diletti R, Karanasos A, Muramatsu T, *et al.* Everolimus-eluting bioresorbable vascular scaffolds for treatment of patients presenting with ST-segment elevation myocardial infarction: BVS STEMI first study. *Eur Heart J* 2014; **35**(12): 777–786. doi: 10.1093/eurheartj/eht546. Epub 2014 Jan 6.

36 Stone GW, Abizaid A, Silber S, *et al.* Prospective, randomized, multicenter evaluation of a polyethylene terephthalate micronet mesh-covered stent (MGuard) in ST-segment elevation myocardial infarction: the MASTER trial. *J Am Coll Cardiol* 2012; **60**: 1975–1984.

37 Gori T, Schulz E, Hink U, *et al.* Early outcome after implantation of Absorb bioresorbable drug-eluting scaffolds in patients with acute coronary syndromes. *EuroIntervention* 2014; **9**: 1036–1041.

38 Arroyo D, Togni M, Puricel S, *et al.* Comparison of everolimus-eluting and biolimus-eluting coronary stents with everolimus-eluting bioresorbable scaffold: study protocol of the randomized controlled EVERBIO II trial. *Trials* 2014; **15**: 9. doi: 10.1186/1745-6215-15-9.

39 Gogas BD, Serruys PW, Diletti R, *et al.* Vascular response of the segments adjacent to the proximal and distal edges of the ABSORB everolimus-eluting bioresorbable vascular scaffold: 6-month and 1-year follow-up assessment: a virtual histology intravascular ultrasound study from the first-in-man ABSORB Cohort B trial. *JACC Cardiovasc Interv* 2012; **5**(6): 656–665. doi: 10.1016/j.jcin.2012.02.017.

40 Indolfi C, Mongiardo A, Spaccarotella C, Caiazzo G, Torella D, De Rosa S. Neointimal proliferation is associated with clinical restenosis 2 years after fully bioresorbable vascular scaffold implantation. *Circ Cardiovasc Imaging* 2014; **7**(4): 755–757. doi: 10.1161/CIRCIMAGING.114.001727.

41 Ielasi A1, Cortese B, Varricchio A, *et al.* Immediate and midterm outcomes following primary PCI with bioresorbable vascular scaffold implantation in patients with ST-segment myocardial infarction: insights from the multicentre "Registro ABSORB Italiano" (RAI registry). *EuroIntervention* 2014 Oct 30 [Epub ahead of print], pii: 20140629-04. doi: 10.4244/EIJY14M10_11.

42 Chieffo A, Latib A, Caussin C, *et al.* A prospective, randomized trial of intravascular-ultrasound guided compared to angiography guided stent implantation in complex coronary lesions: the AVIO trial. *Am Heart J* 2013; **165**(1): 65–72. doi: 10.1016/j.ahj.2012.09.017. Epub 2012 Nov 20.

43 Roy P, Steinberg DH, Sushinsky SJ, *et al.* The potential clinical utility of intravascular ultrasound guidance in patients undergoing percutaneous coronary intervention with drug-eluting stents. *Eur Heart J* 2008; **29**(15): 1851–1857. doi: 10.1093/eurheartj/ehn249. Epub 2008 Jun 11.

44 Claessen BE, Mehran R, Mintz GS, *et al.* Impact of intravascular ultrasound imaging on early and late clinical outcomes following percutaneous coronary intervention with drug-eluting stents. *JACC Cardiovasc Interv* 2011; **4**(9): 974–981. doi: 10.1016/j.jcin.2011.07.005. Erratum in: JACC Cardiovasc Interv 2011; **4**(11): 1255.

45 Park SJ, Kim YH, Park DW, *et al.*; MAIN-COMPARE Investigators. Impact of intravascular ultrasound guidance on long-term mortality in stenting for unprotected left main coronary artery stenosis. *Circ Cardiovasc Interv* 2009; **2**(3): 167–177. doi: 10.1161/CIRCINTERVENTIONS.108.799494. Epub 2009 Apr 21.

46 Mudra H, di Mario C, de Jaegere P, *et al.*; OPTICUS (OPTimization with ICUS to reduce stent restenosis) Study Investigators. Randomized comparison of coronary stent implantation under ultrasound or angiographic guidance to reduce stent restenosis (OPTICUS Study). *Circulation* 2001; **104**(12): 1343–1349.

47 Oemrawsingh PV, Mintz GS, Schalij MJ, Zwinderman AH, Jukema JW, van der Wall EE; TULIP Study. Thrombocyte activity evaluation and effects of ultrasound guidance in long intracoronary stent placement. Intravascular ultrasound guidance improves angiographic and clinical outcome of stent implantation for long coronary artery stenoses: final results of a randomized comparison with angiographic guidance (TULIP Study). *Circulation* 2003; **107**(1): 62–67.

48 Jang JS, Song YJ, Kang W, *et al.* Intravascular ultrasound-guided implantation of drug-eluting stents to improve outcome: a meta-analysis. *JACC Cardiovasc Interv* 2014; **7**(3): 233–243. doi: 10.1016/j.jcin.2013.09.013. Epub 2014 Feb 13.

49 Waksman R, Kitabata H, Prati F, Albertucci M, Mintz GS. Intravascular ultrasound versus optical coherence tomography guidance. *J Am Coll Cardiol* 2013; **62**(17 Suppl): S32–40. doi: 10.1016/j.jacc.2013.08.709.

50 Prati F, Di Vito L, Biondi-Zoccai G, *et al.* Angiography alone versus angiography plus optical coherence tomography to guide decision-making during percutaneous coronary intervention: the Centro per la Lotta contro l'Infarto-Optimisation of Percutaneous Coronary Intervention (CLI-OPCI) study. *EuroIntervention* 2012; **8**(7): 823–829. doi: 10.4244/EIJV8I7A125.

51 Gomez-Lara J, Diletti R, Brugaletta S, *et al.* Angiographic maximal luminal diameter and appropriate deployment of the everolimus-eluting bioresorbable vascular scaffold as assessed by optical coherence tomography: an ABSORB Cohort B trial sub-study. *EuroIntervention* 2012; **8**(2): 214–224. doi: 10.4244/EIJV8I2A35.

52 Allahwala UK, Cockburn JA, Shaw E, Figtree GA, Hansen PS, Bhindi R. Clinical utility of optical coherence tomography (OCT) in the optimisation of Absorb bioresorbable vascular scaffold deployment during percutaneous coronary intervention. *EuroIntervention* 2014 Mar 20. pii: 20130415-05. [Epub ahead of print].

53 Tearney GJ, Regar E, Akasaka T, *et al.*; International Working Group for Intravascular Optical Coherence Tomography (IWG-IVOCT). Consensus standards for acquisition, measurement, and reporting of intravascular optical coherence tomography studies: a report from the International Working Group for Intravascular Optical Coherence Tomography Standardization and Validation. *J Am Coll Cardiol* 2012; **59**(12): 1058–1072. doi: 10.1016/j.jacc.2011.09.079.

54 Gutiérrez-Chico JL, Gijsen F, Regar E, *et al.* Differences in neointimal thickness between the adluminal and the abluminal sides of malapposed and side-branch struts in a polylactide bioresorbable scaffold: evidence in vivo about the abluminal healing process. *JACC Cardiovasc Interv* 2012; **5**(4): 428–435. doi: 10.1016/j.jcin.2011.12.015.

55 Foin N, Ghione M, Mattesini A, Davies JE, Di Mario C. Bioabsorbable scaffold optimization in provisional stenting: insight from optical coherence tomography. *Eur Heart J Cardiovasc Imaging* 2013; **14**(12): 1149. doi: 10.1093/ehjci/jet137. Epub 2013 Jul 24.

56 Alegría-Barrero E, Foin N, Chan PH, *et al.* Optical coherence tomography for guidance of distal cell recrossing in bifurcation stenting: choosing the right cell matters. *EuroIntervention* 2012; **8**(2): 205–213. doi: 10.4244/EIJV8I2A34

57 Pitt CG, Zhong-wei G. Modification of the rates of chain cleavage of poly(-caprolactone) and related polyesters in the solid state. *J Control Release* 1987; **4**: 283–292

58 Pitt CG, Chasalow FI, Hibionada YM, Klimas DM, Schindler A. Aliphatic polyesters, I: the degradation of poly(-caprolactone) in vivo. *J Appl Polym Sci* 1981; **26**: 3779–3787.

59 Tsuji T, Tamai H, Igaki K, *et al.* Four-year follow-up of the biodegradable stent (Igaki-Tamai stent). *Circ J* 2004; **68**: 135

60 Post MJ, de Graaf-Bos AN, van Zanten HG, de Groot PG, Sixma JJ, Borst C. Thrombogenicity of the human arterial wall after interventional thermal injury. *J Vasc Res* 1996; **33**: 156–163.

61 Biamino G, Schmidt A, Scheinert D. Treatment of SFA lesions with PLLA biodegradable stents: results of the PERSEUS Study. *J Endovasc Ther* 2005; **12**: 5.

62 Schulze R. REVA Medical, Inc. Bioresorbable stent. Presented at: Cardiovascular Revascularization Therapies Conference; March 7–9, 2007; Washington, DC.

63 Grube E. Bioabsorbable stent: the Boston Scientific and REVA technology. Presented at: EuroPCR; May 19–22, 2009; Barcelona, Spain.

64 Jabara R, Chronos N, Robinson K. Novel bioabsorbable salicylate-based polymer as a drug-eluting stent coating. *Catheter Cardiovasc Interv* 2008; **72**: 186–194.

65 Jabara R, Pendyala L, Geva S, Chen J, Chronos N, Robinson K. Novel fully bioabsorbable salicylate-based sirolimus-eluting stent. *EuroIntervention* 2009; **5**: F58–F64.

66 Oberhauser JP, Hossainy S, Rapoza RJ. Design principles and performance of bioresorbable polymeric vascular scaffolds. *EuroIntervention* 2009; **5**(Suppl F): 15–22.

67 Eglin D, Alini M. Degradable polymeric materials for osteosynthesis: tutorial. *Eur Cell Mater* 2008; **16**: 80–91.

68 Verheye S, Webster M, Stewart J, *et al.* TCT-563: Multicenter, first-in-man evaluation of the myolimus-eluting bioresorbable coronary scaffold: 6-month clinical and imaging results (abstr) *J Am Coll Cardiol* 2012; **60**(Suppl): B163.

69 Verheye S, Ormiston JA, Stewart J, *et al.* A next-generation bioresorbable coronary scaffold system: from bench to first clinical evaluation: 6- and 12-month clinical and multimodality imaging results. *JACC Cardiovasc Interv* 2014; **7**(1): 89–99. doi: 10.1016/j.jcin.2013.07.007. Epub 2013 Oct 16.

CHAPTER 35
The Biolimus Stent Family

Anna Franzone, Raffaele Piccolo, and Stephan Windecker
Department of Cardiology, Bern University Hospital, Bern, Switzerland

Biolimus
Chemical features and properties

The Biolimus peculiar chemical structure ($C_{55}H_{87}NO_{14}$, molecular weight 986.29 Da) consists of a 31-membered triene macrolide lactone that preserves the core sirolimus ring structure with a 2-ethoxyethyl group addition to the hydroxy group at position C(40) of the sirolimus molecule. The modification at position 40 of the rapamycin ring confers higher lipophilicity (approximately more than 10-fold) than sirolimus (Figure 35.1). As a consequence, it attaches more rapidly and enters the smooth muscle cell (SMCs) membranes in the coronary vessel wall and inhibits their proliferation. In the STent Eluting A9 BioLimus Trial in Humans (STEALTH PK) study, blood levels of Biolimus were measured through a liquid chromatography–tandem mass spectrometry assay in 27 moderate to high risk patients, 28 days and 6 months after receiving the BioMatrix stent. The highest measured blood concentration at any time point was 394 pg/mL. At 28 days following stent placement, 51.8% of patients had Biolimus concentrations less than the lower limit of quantitation (LLOQ; 10 pg/mL). Drug concentrations in the blood samples collected after 3 and 6 months were not detectable. At 9-month follow-up, no adverse events possibly, probably, or definitely related to Biolimus were reported [1].

The drug acts through the binding to an intracellular immunophilin, the FK506-binding protein 12 (FKBP12), which is upregulated in human neointimal SMCs [2]. The FKBP12–rapamycin complex, in turn, binds to a specific cell cycle-regulatory protein, the phosphoinositide 3-kinase mammalian target of rapamycin (mTOR), and inhibits its activation. mTOR is involved in crucial steps of cell proliferation, because it regulated the transition from the G_1 to S phase of the cell cycle [2]. It acts by phosphorylating a number of key proteins including those associated with protein synthesis (p70s6kinase) and initiation of translation (phas-1). The inhibition of mTOR is ultimately associated with a cytostatic effect with the arrest of the cell cycle in the late G_1 phase (Figure 35.2).

The Biosensor stent family

Biosensor International has pioneered the use of the Biolimus within a biodegradable-polymer coated device, the BioMatrix stent. Changes of the metal platform and/or the delivery system compared

with the first BioMatrix stent generated three new devices: BioMatrix Flex, BioMatrix NeoFlex, and Axxess (a bifurcation-dedicated stent). Moreover, a polymer-free Biolimus-eluting stent (BES; the BioFreedom) has also been launched (Figure 35.3).

In the BioMatrix, BioMatrix Flex, and BioMatrix NeoFlex, Biolimus is immersed at a dose of 15.6 µg/mm into the biodegradable L-polylactic acid (PLA) polymer. This is a synthetic polymer (aliphatic polyester) obtained from processing and polymerization of lactic acid monomers. Its degradation occurs within 6–9 months, primarily by hydrolysis and through two stages: (i) a non-enzymatic chain scission of the ester groups leads to a reduction in molecular weight; and (ii) the low molecular weight oligomers are metabolized by microorganisms in carbon dioxide and water through interaction with the Krebs cycle [3]. PLA acts by protecting the drug from contacts with body substances that could modify its chemistry before reaching the targeted area and by controlling the concentration of active ingredient release. The high drug-carrying capacity of PLA results in a significant reduction of the amount of carrier polymer used as compared with durable coatings of the first generation drug-eluting stent (DES; 225 vs. 1227 µg for the paclitaxel-eluting (PES) Taxus stent and 301 for the sirolimus-eluting (SES) Cypher stent).

PLA and Biolimus are mixed in a 1 : 1 ratio to create a 10-µm thick matrix that covers solely the abluminal surface of the stents. This asymmetrical coating allows a targeted drug release that attains directly in the surrounding coronary wall with limited systemic exposure. These stents differ in the specific metal platform and the delivery catheter.

The BioMatrix stent consists of the S-Stent™ Platform that is made of a 316 low carbon vacuum melt (LVM) stainless steel, laser-cut, tubular stent with 16.3–18.4% metal surface area, a strut thickness of 112 µm, and coated with a layer of parylene C that serves as primer for the adhesion of the matrix to the stent surface. The coating formulation is applied to the stent via an automatic micropipette coating process. The stent is pre-mounted on to a high pressure, semi-compliant rapid exchange balloon delivery system available in six and nine cell models. The delivery catheter has two radio-opaque markers, which fluoroscopically mark the ends of the stent to facilitate its proper placement. The typical platform with corrugated ring and Quadrature Link™ design combines high flexibility and deliverability with adequate support and scaffolding.

Interventional Cardiology: Principles and Practice, Second Edition. Edited by George D. Dangas, Carlo Di Mario, and Nicholas N. Kipshidze.
© 2017 John Wiley & Sons, Ltd. Published 2017 by John Wiley & Sons, Ltd.

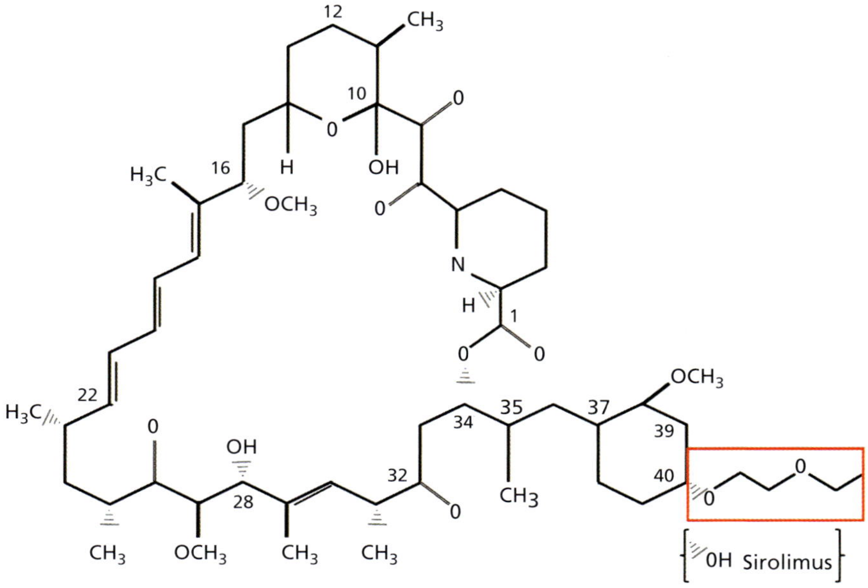

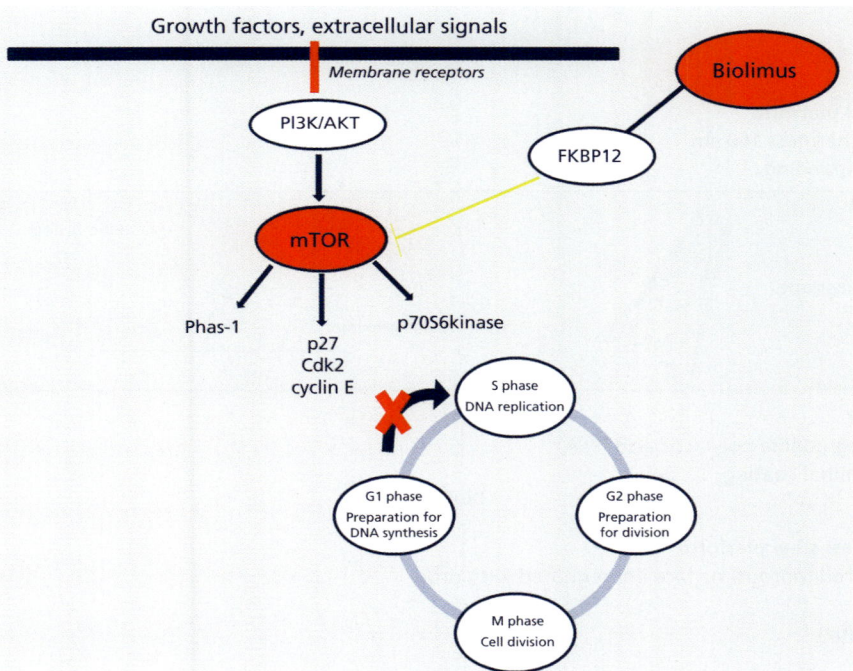

Figure 35.1 Chemical structure of Biolimus. The replacement of hydrogen by alkoxy-alkyl group at C(40) position of the sirolimus structure provides higher lipophilicity and peculiar pharmacokinetic properties.

Figure 35.2 Mechanism of action of Biolimus. The cytostatic effect (arrest of the cell cycle in the transition from phase G1 to phase S) is achieved through the FKBP12-mediated inhibition of mammalian target of rapamycin (mTOR).

The BioMatrix Flex (Conformité Européenne (CE) marked in 2010) has a modified platform design, the Juno™ Stent Platform, in which a curved strut connector (radius-shaped) substitutes the straight connector of the existing platform. Moreover, its additional features include a larger initial cell opening than the original (improving side branch accessibility), an increased between struts difference (1.47–1.56 mm), and the absence of a primer coating (parylene C) to adhere the polymer and drug to the stent.

The BioMatrix NeoFlex was launched in 2013 and presents superior trackability, crossability, and pushability as consequence of an additional improvement of the delivery system (lower lesion entry profile). It also features a further improvement of the Quadrature link design of the platform with a novel "S-shaped" connector link.

The AXXESS stent is a self-expanding, bifurcation dedicated device, CE marked in July 2010. It has a nitinol (nickel-titanium alloy) platform with a conical shape (flared distal diameter) and a

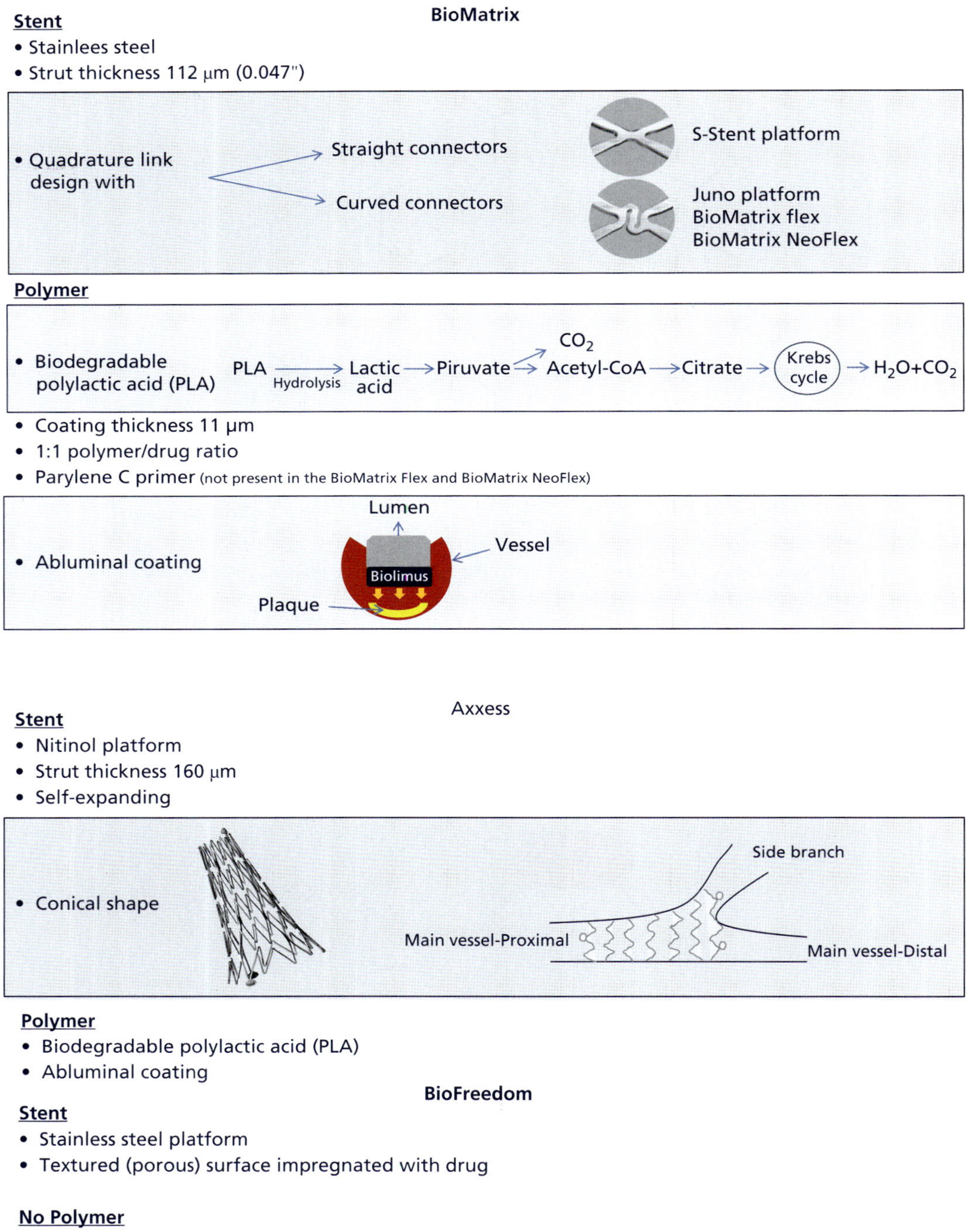

BioMatrix

Stent
- Stainlees steel
- Strut thickness 112 μm (0.047")

- Quadrature link design with → Straight connectors
- → Curved connectors

S-Stent platform

Juno platform
BioMatrix flex
BioMatrix NeoFlex

Polymer

- Biodegradable polylactic acid (PLA)

$PLA \xrightarrow{Hydrolysis} Lactic\ acid \rightarrow Piruvate \xrightarrow{} Acetyl\text{-}CoA \rightarrow Citrate \rightarrow \text{Krebs cycle} \rightarrow H_2O + CO_2$

with CO_2 produced at Acetyl-CoA

- Coating thickness 11 μm
- 1:1 polymer/drug ratio
- Parylene C primer (not present in the BioMatrix Flex and BioMatrix NeoFlex)

- Abluminal coating

Lumen
Vessel
Biolimus
Plaque

Axxess

Stent
- Nitinol platform
- Strut thickness 160 μm
- Self-expanding

- Conical shape

Side branch
Main vessel-Proximal
Main vessel-Distal

Polymer
- Biodegradable polylactic acid (PLA)
- Abluminal coating

BioFreedom

Stent
- Stainless steel platform
- Textured (porous) surface impregnated with drug

No Polymer

Figure 35.3 The main components of the Biosensor International Biolimus-eluting stents.

strut thickness of 0.16 mm and is specifically designed to conform to anatomy at the level of the bifurcation carina (up to an angle of 70°). Hereto, the device can accommodate vessels of 3.0–4.25 mm diameter, and is available in three different lengths (9, 11, and 14 mm). The stent elutes Biolimus at a concentration of 22 μg/mm of stent length.

The deployment requires a 7-Fr approach and is made easier through four highly visible radio-opaque markers, three located at the tip of the stent and the fourth pointing the proximal edge of the stent. The crimped stent is contained in a cover sheath. Before definite deployment, stent position can be further adjusted as long as the cover sheath contains more than half of the stent length and the radio-opaque markers can be used to control the retrieval of the stent by the sheath. Pre-dilatation of main vessel and side branch (using one of the standard bifurcation techniques) is highly recommended for tight lesions and calcified vessel segments as it can facilitate lesion crossing and optimal distal flaring at the carina site. After the AXXESS stent is implanted, additional stents can be placed through it in the distal main branch and/or distal side branch to achieve an acceptable angiographic result. Final high pressure and kissing balloon inflations are recommended in this overlap region, while avoiding vessel damage outside the stent edges.

A specific version of the AXXESS System has been designed for left main coronary artery (LMCA) bifurcation lesions, allowing for larger diameters (up to 4.75 mm) and distinct bifurcation angles (flare-end diameters of 8, 10, and 12 mm).

The BioFreedom drug-coated stent (DCS; CE approved in 2013) consists of a stainless platform with a micro-structured abluminal (outer) surface which allows the controlled release of Biolimus without the use of a polymer. The drug is harbored in crevices on the abluminal surface and almost completely (98%) transferred to the vessel wall within 28 days.

Clinical evidence

Table 35.1 provides an overview of the studies investigating the performance of the Biosensor International BES.

BioMatrix

Registries and non-randomized studies The STEALTH PK study was designed to specifically assess the pharmacokinetics of Biolimus after elution from the BioMatrix stent.

The Biolimus Eluting A-9 Coronary Stent Obviating Luminal Narrowing I (BEACON I) was a prospective registry compiled in multiple centers in Asia. It included 443 patients (602 lesions) with de novo or restenotic native coronary artery lesions treated with the BioMatrix stent. The primary endpoint was target vessel revascularization (TVR) at 6 months, and secondary endpoints included major adverse cardiac events (MACE; defined as composite of death, coronary artery bypass graft (CABG), Q-wave and non-Q-wave myocardial infarction (MI), and TVR) at 30 days, 6 months, and 12 months. The 30-day MACE was 3.5% with no events of new revascularization. At a median follow-up of 7.2 months, the MACE rate was 5.2% including 0.9% TVR and 0.2% target lesion revascularization (TLR) [4].

The BEACON II was a prospective, observational registry assessing clinical outcomes in real world, all-comers patients (n = 497) receiving the BioMatrix stent at the site of native coronary artery or saphenous vein graft (SVG) lesions (with the exception of protected or unprotected left main) in Asia-Pacific countries. The primary endpoint was the 12-month rate of MACE, defined as a composite of cardiac death, MI, and ischemia driven-TLR. Key secondary endpoints included ischemia-driven target lesion failure (TLF) and TLR at 12 months; rates of MACE and definite stent thrombosis (ST) up to 5 years. In a total number of 742 target lesions (mean target lesions per patient 1.49 ± 0.74), 31% were longer than 20 mm, 24% showed moderate–severe calcification, and 14% were bifurcation lesions (side branch >2 mm). Device success (defined as achievement of a final residual in-stent diameter stenosis of <30%) was 98.5%; lesion success (defined as attainment of <30% in-stent residual stenosis of the target lesion using any percutaneous method) was 98.7% and procedural success (defined as achievement of device success without the occurrence of in-hospital MACE) was 97.8%. MACE rate at 4-year follow-up was 9.4%. Definite very late stent thrombosis (VLST) events were rare (0.4%) and specifically none of these events occurred in patients receiving the BioMatrix stent in native coronary arteries [5,6].

The e-BioMatrix Registry was a prospective, multicenter, observational registry designed to assess outcomes in 5472 all-comers patients treated with either the BioMatrix or the BioMatrix Flex

stent across 57 European sites between April 2008 and August 2011. Criteria for inclusion were age >18 years and implantation of one of the BioMatrix family DES (any size, any vessel) without limitations of the number of treated lesions, vessels, or lesion length. Approximately 50% of patients presented with acute coronary syndrome (ACS). Patients were excluded if additional stents (different from the study stent) were used or if any lesions were treated with other techniques (e.g., stand-alone balloon angioplasty, atherectomy). The primary endpoint was the incidence of MACE at 12 months, defined as a composite of cardiac death, any MI, and clinically indicated TVR. Pre-defined secondary endpoints included the individual components of the primary endpoint, ST, major bleeding, and MACE at 24 months. The registry had two components: the e-BioMatrix PMS (Post-Marketing Surveillance) and the e-BioMatrix PMR (Post-Marketing Registry), which differ only with regard to the level of source data verification. The PMS registry collected all baseline data, all MACE, ST, and bleeding events through a monitoring system; the PMR registry monitors only cardiac-related events. The overall incidence of MACE was 4.5% (cardiac death 0.9%, MI 1.7%, clinically indicated TVR 2.8%) at 12 months and 6.8% at 24 months (cardiac death 1.5%, MI 2.4%, clinically indicated TVR 4.3%). Rate of definite or probable ST was 0.6% at 12 months and 0.2% between 12 and 24 months; the majority of such events occurred within the first 30 days (58.5%) and in patients still on dual antiplatelet therapy (DAPT). Despite its low incidence, ST was associated with high 24-month mortality (27.5%). Major bleeding occurred in 1.7% of patients at 12 months and 0.4% at 12–24 months with a mortality rate of 9.1%. Contrary to 12-month observations, comorbidities (as expressed by the Charlson index) were found independent predictors of MACE at 21 months by multivariate analysis [7,8].

The e-BioMatrix registry family also include arms enrolling patients treated with the BioMatrix in non-European countries. The e-BioMatrix India aims to evaluate the 2-year clinical safety and efficacy outcomes in 1189 patients (1418 lesions) prospectively enrolled between December 2008 and February 2012. An interim analysis involving 987 patients showed a 12-month incidence of MACE and ST of 0.45 and 0.2 per 100 person-years, respectively. No case of ST was reported among the 37% of patients who completed the 2-year follow-up [9]. A subgroup analysis showed comparable clinical outcomes among patients with diabetes mellitus (n = 485) with a MACE rate of 0.62% and a single case of probable ST reported [10].

Asia-Pacific registries also include single-center experiences from Thailand and Indonesia confirming satisfactory early angiographic performance of the BioMatrix stent and mid-term clinical outcomes in more than 400 patients [5].

Randomized studies (Figure 35.4)
BioMatrix vs. bare metal stent The STEALTH I trial was a first-in-man, multicenter, prospective study assessing the safety and efficacy of the BioMatrix stent. It randomly assigned, in a 2 : 1 ratio, 120 patients with single de novo lesions, undergoing percutaneous coronary intervention (PCI), to receive the BioMatrix Stent (n = 80, 82 lesions) or the control Gazelle S-Stent (n = 40, 40 lesions), a bare metal stent (BMS) with identical design. The angiographic primary endpoint, in-lesion late lumen loss (LLL) at 6-month follow-up, was significantly reduced in the BioMatrix group (0.14 ± 0.45 mm) compared to the control group (0.40 ± 0.41 mm; p = 0.004). A significant reduction of the in-stent LLL was also reported (0.26 ± 0.43 vs. 0.74 ± 0.45 mm; p <0.001). Binary restenosis rates were low in both

Table 35.1 Overview of clinical studies with the Biosensor International Biolimus-eluting stents.

Study name [ref], year (results available)	Design	Country	Patients	Setting	Planned follow-up	Primary endpoint	Status
BioMatrix							
STEALTH PK [1], 2011	Single Arm Registry	Europe	27	Stable CAD	1 year	Systemic concentrations of Biolimus at 28 days and 6-months	Completed
BEACON I [4], 2006	Single Arm Multicenter Registry	Asia	292	Stable CAD and UA	1 year	TVR at 6 months	Completed
BEACON II [5,6], 2012	Single Arm Multicenter Registry	Asia-Pacific	497	Stable CAD and UA	5 years	MACE* at 12 months	4-year FU completed
e-BioMatrix [7,8], 2015	Single Arm Multicenter Registry	Europe	5000	Stable CAD and ACS	5 years	MACE† at 12 months	2-year FU completed
STEALTH I [12,13], 2005	Randomized Multicenter BioMatrix vs. Gazelle BMS	Europe South America	120	Stable CAD	5 years	In-lesion LLL at 6 months	Completed
LEADERS [16,17], 2008	Randomized Multicenter BioMatrix vs. Cypher Select SES	Europe	1707	Stable CAD and ACS	5 years	CV death, MI, clinically indicated TVR at 9 months	Completed
COMFORTABLE AMI [14,15], 2012	Randomized Multicenter BioMatrix vs. Gazelle BMS	Europe Asia	1161	STEMI	2 years	Cardiac death, target vessel-related reinfarction, and ischemia-driven TLR at 1 year	Completed
EVERBIO II [23], 2015	Randomized Single Center BioMatrix vs. Promus Element EES and vs. Absorb BVS	Europe	240	Stable CAD	5 years	Angiographic LLL at 9 months	9-month FU completed
SORT OUT VI [21], 2015	Randomized Multicenter BioMatrix vs. Resolute Integrity ZES	Europe	1502	Stable CAD and ACS	5 years	Composite of safety (cardiac death and MI) and efficacy (TLR) at 12 months	1-year FU completed
Separham et al. [22], 2011	Randomized Single Center BioMatrix vs Xience EES	Asia	200	Stable CAD and ACS	1 year	Composite of cardiac death, MI, and clinically driven TVR at 1 year	Completed
STACCATO [24], 2014	Randomized Single Center BioMatrix vs Xience EES	Europe	64	Stable CAD and ACS	9 months	Percentage of uncovered struts assessed with OCT, at 9 months	Completed

AXXESS

Study	Design	Region	N	Population	Follow-up	Primary endpoint	Status
AXXESS Plus [25], 2007	Single Arm Multicenter Registry	Europe South America Oceania	139	Stable CAD and UA	5 years	In-stent LLL in parent vessel and side branch at 6 months	Completed
DIVERGE [26,27], 2009	Single Arm Multicenter Registry	Europe Australia Oceania	302	Stable CAD and UA	5 years	MACE rate at 9 months[‡]	Completed
AXXENT [28], 2009	Single Arm Multicenter Registry	Europe	33	Stable CAD	6 months	Percent neointimal volume obstruction (IVUS) at 6 months	Completed
COBRA [29], 2015	Randomized Multicenter AXXESS vs. Xience	Europe	40	Stable CAD and UA	9 months	Stent strut coverage as assessed with OCT at 9 months	Ongoing (preliminary results for 20 patients)

BioFreedom

Study	Design	Region	N	Population	Follow-up	Primary endpoint	Status
BioFreedom FIM [31,32], 2008	Randomized Single Center BioFreedom vs. Taxus Liberte	Europe	180	Stable CAD and UA	5 years	In-stent LLL at 12 months	4-year FU Completed
EGO-BIOFREEDOM [33], 2015	Single Arm Prospective Study	Europe	100	Stable CAD and UA	2 years	Strut coverage assessed with OCT at 9 months	Completed

ACS, acute coronary syndrome; BMS, bare metal stent; BVS, bioresorbable vascular scaffold; CAD, coronary artery disease; CV, cardiovascular; EES, everolimus-eluting stent; FU, follow-up; IVUS, intravascular ultrasound; LLL, late lumen loss; MACE, major adverse cardiac events; MI, myocardial infarction; OCT, optical coherence tomography; SES, sirolimus-eluting stent; TLR, target lesion revascularization; TVR, target vessel revascularization; UA, unstable angina; ZES,: zotarolimus-eluting stent.

* Cardiac death, clinically indicated MI (Q-wave and non-Q-wave) and clinically indicated TLR.

† Cardiac death, MI (Q-wave and non-Q-wave), or clinically indicated TVR.

‡ All-cause death, MI, and ischemia-driven TLR.

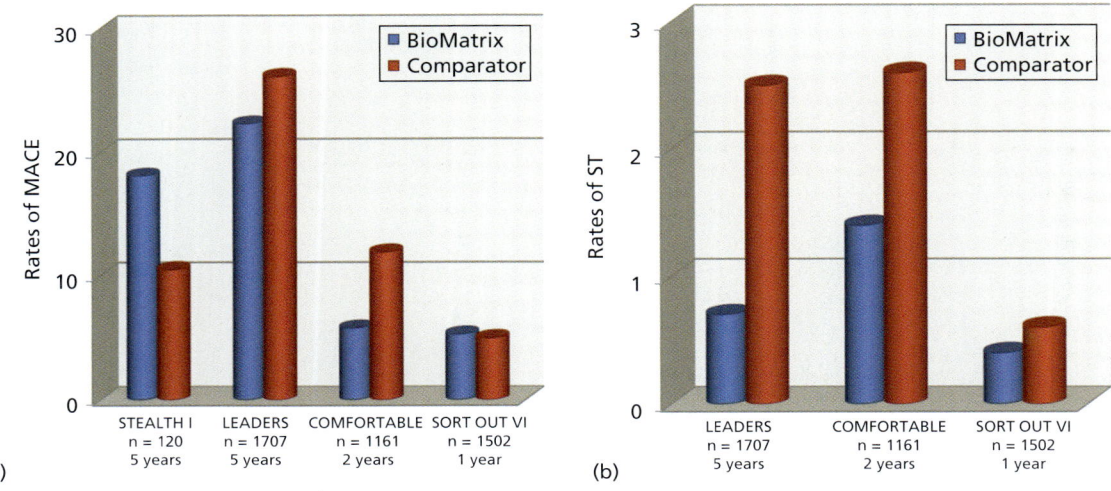

	STEALTH I (n = 120)		LEADERS (n = 335)		COMFORTABLE AMI (n = 103)		EVERBIO II (n = 238)			STACCATO (n = 58)	
	Biomatrix	Gazelle	Biomatrix	Cypher	Biomatrix	Gazelle	Biomatrix	Promus	Absorb	Biomatrix	Xience
Follow-up	6 months		9 months		13 months		9 months			9 months	
Late loss (mm)	0.14 ± 0.45	0.40 ± 0.41	0.13 ± 0.46	0.19 ± 0.50	0.11 ± 0.24	0.97 ± 0.75	0.25 ± 0.41	0.24 ± 0.32	0.28 ± 0.39	0.10 ± 0.31	0.15 ± 0.25
Diameter stenosis (mm)	22.0 ±12.1	30.9 ± 11.9	20.9 ±17.5	23.3 ± 19.6	12.02 ± 7.23	39.6 ±25.2	12.6 ± 14.9	11.3 ± 9.8	16.9 ± 11.6	14.9 ± 9.5	10.8 ± 7.9
Binary restenosis (%)	3.9	7.7	5.5	8.7	0	25.93	5	4	5	0	0
TLR (%)	1.3	0	6.5	7.4	3.5	9.5	5	14	10	-	-

(c)

Figure 35.4 Rates of major adverse cardiac events (MACE) (a) and stent thrombosis (ST) (b) and key angiographic findings (c) across the main randomized trials evaluating the performance of the BioMatrix stent.

groups (3.9% vs. 7.7%; p = NS) and lower than expected particularly in the control group [11]. Intravascular ultrasound (IVUS) analysis performed at the time of the angiographic follow-up revealed a comparable incidence of late incomplete apposition (3%) for both groups and a significantly lower percentage of neointimal volume (ratio between neointimal volume and stent volume) in patients receiving the BioMatrix stent (2.6% vs. 23.5%; p <0.001). Comparable clinical safety emerged with similar 6-month event-free survival (96.3% vs. 97.5%; p = 0.72) without significant difference in TLR rates [12]. The preserved safety profile persisted until 5-year follow-up with a MACE (death, MI, or TLR) rate of 18.1% in the BioMatrix group and 10.5% in the control group [13].

The Comparison of Biolimus Eluted From an Erodible Stent Coating With Bare Metal Stents in Acute ST-Elevation Myocardial Infarction (COMFORTABLE AMI) was a randomized, superiority trial comparing the efficacy and safety of the BioMatrix stent with the Gazelle BMS in 1161 patients presenting with STEMI undergoing primary PCI, at 11 sites in Europe and Israel, between September 2009 and January 2011. Patients were excluded in presence of

mechanical complications of acute MI, known allergy to any study medication, use of vitamin K antagonists, planned surgery unless DAPT could be maintained throughout the peri-surgical period, history of bleeding diathesis or known coagulopathy, pregnancy, participation in another trial, inability to provide informed consent, and life expectancy of less than 1 year. The pre-specified primary study endpoint was the device-oriented composite of cardiac death, target vessel-related reinfarction, and ischemia-driven TLR. Secondary endpoints included the patient-oriented composite of death, any reinfarction, and any revascularization, as well as target vessel-related reinfarction, and any revascularization (percutaneous and surgical procedures), cardiac death, all-cause mortality, Q-wave and non-Q-wave reinfarction, stroke, and ST. At 1 year, the primary endpoint occurred in 4.3% of patients receiving the BES and in 8.7% of patients receiving the BMS (HR 0.49, 95% CI 0.30–0.80; p = 0.004). The difference was driven by a lower risk of target vessel-related reinfarction (0.5% vs. 2.7%, HR 0.20, 95% CI 0.06–0.69; p = 0.01) and ischemia-driven TLR (1.6% vs. 5.7%, HR 0.28, 95% CI 0.13–0.59; p <0.001). Cardiac death was not significantly different (2.9% vs. 20 3.5%; p = 0.53). The rate of definite ST was 0.9% in patients treated with BES and 2.1% in patients treated with BMS (HR 0.42, 95% CI 0.15–1.19; p = 0.10) [14]. These differences were maintained at 2-year follow-up. The rate of the primary endpoint was 5.8% in patients assigned to receive the BioMatrix stent and 11.9% in control group (HR 0.48, 95% CI 0.31–0.72; p < 0.001). The angiographic control performed in 103 patients at 13 months showed a significant lower in-stent percent diameter stenosis in BES patients compared with patients treated with BMS (12.0 ± 7.2 vs. 39.6 ± 25; p < 0.001). No differences in DAPT compliance were observed between the study groups at any time point and approximately 18% of all patients continued thienopyridines throughout 2 years [15].

BioMatrix vs. first generation DES The Limus Eluted From A Durable Versus ERodable Stent Coating (LEADERS) was a prospective, multicenter, non-inferiority trial including 1707 patients, randomized, after coronary angiography, to receive the BioMatrix Flex or the durable polymer SES Cypher SELECT stent (Cordis, Miami Lakes, FL, USA). Patients with stable coronary artery disease (CAD) or ACS at presentation could be enrolled; other inclusion criteria were the presence of one or more, significant (>50%), coronary artery stenosis in a native vessel or SVG. Exclusion criteria included pregnancy; known intolerance to aspirin, clopidogrel, heparin, stainless steel, sirolimus, biolimus, or contrast material; inability to provide informed consent; participation in another trial; or planned surgery within 6 months of PCI unless DAPT was maintained throughout the peri-operative period. The primary endpoint of the trial was the rate of MACE, defined as the composite of cardiac death, MI, or clinically indicated TVR within 9 months. Secondary endpoints included MACE and its individual components, angiographic and clinical ST at 30 days, 6 months, 9 months and 1–5 years. BES proved to be non-inferior to SES for the primary endpoint at 9 months (9% vs. 11%, RR 0.88, 95% CI 0.64–1.19; p for non-inferiority = 0.003, p for superiority = 0.39) [16]. Optical coherence tomography (OCT) performed during angiographic follow-up at 9 months showed a more complete strut coverage in 20 patients treated with the BioMatrix stent (29 lesions with 4592 struts) compared with patients receiving SES (26 patients, 35 lesions with 6476 struts). Three lesions in the former group and 15 lesions in the latter had ≥5% of all struts uncovered (difference 233.1%, 95% CI 261.7–210.3; p <0.01) [17].

Early findings were confirmed up to 5-year follow-up: MACE rate 22.3% vs. 26.1%, RR 0.83 (95% CI 0.68–1.02; p for non-inferiority <0.0001, p for superiority = 0.069). Moreover, at this time point, the more comprehensive patient-oriented composite endpoint (including all-cause death, any MI, and all-cause revascularization) was significantly reduced with the BioMatrix stent (35.1% vs. 40.4%, RR 0.84, 95% CI 0.71–0.98; p for superiority = 0.023). Definite VLST from 1 to 5 years was also significantly reduced with the BioMatrix stent (0.7% vs. 2.5%, RR 0.26, 95% CI 0.10–0.68; p = 0.003) [18]. Several post hoc analyses explored the performance of the novel device in specific clinical and/or angiographic settings. The non-inferiority of the BioMatrix was confirmed in 429 patients with small vessel disease (defined as reference diameter <2.75 mm) as equivalent LLL (0.17 ± 0.47 vs. 0.22 ± 0.51 mm; p = NS), percent diameter stenosis (24.9% ± 20.7% vs. 23.8% ± 21.3%), and binary restenosis rates (12.8% vs. 9.7%) were reported, compared with 434 patients in the durable polymer SES arm. Moreover, rates of MACE and TLR at 1 year were similar (12.1% vs. 11.8%; p = 0.89 and 9.6% vs. 7.4%; p = 0.26, respectively) [19]. Patients with acute MI (ST-segment elevation MI (STEMI) and non-ST-segment elevation MI

(NSTEMI)) treated with the BioMatrix stent (n = 280) experienced lower rate of the patient-oriented composite endpoint compared with the SES at 5-year follow-up (28.9% vs. 42.3%, RR 0.61, 95% CI 0.47–0.82; p = 0.001). In patients with STEMI, specifically, the BioMatrix stent implantation significantly reduced the rate of the primary endpoint (24.4% vs. 39.3%, RR 0.55, 95% CI 0.36–0.85; p = 0.006), MACE (12.6% vs. 25.0%, RR 0.47, 95% CI 0.26–0.83; p = 0.008), and cardiac death (3.0% vs. 11.4%, RR 0.25, 95% CI 0.08–0.75; p = 0.007). Moreover, a trend toward reduction in definite ST was observed (3.7% vs. 8.6%, RR 0.41, 95% CI 0.15–1.18; p = 0.088) [20].

BioMatrix vs. second generation DES The Scandinavian Organization for Randomized Trials with Clinical Outcome VI (SORT OUT VI) was an open-label, randomized, multicenter, non-inferiority trial performed at three sites across Denmark including 1502 patients (1883 lesions) assigned to receive the durable-polymer zotarolimus-eluting stent (ZES) (Resolute Integrity, Medtronic CardioVascular, Santa Rosa, CA, USA) and 1497 patients (1791 lesions) to receive the BioMatrix Flex stent. Patients with stable CAD or ACS and at least one coronary lesion with more than 50% stenosis in a vessel with a diameter of 2.25–4.00 mm were included. The primary endpoint was a combination of safety (cardiac death or MI not clearly attributable to a non-target lesion) and efficacy (clinically indicated TLR) at 1 year. It occurred in 79 (5.3%) and 75 (5.0%) patients, respectively, proving the non-inferiority of the ZES compared with the BES (absolute risk difference 0.0025, upper limit of one-sided 95% CI 0.016%; p = 0.004) [21].

Separham et al. [22] randomly assigned 200 patients undergoing PCI of de novo coronary lesions to receive the BioMatrix or the Xience everolimus-eluting stent (EES; Abbott Vascular). At 1 year, the rates of cardiac death (0% in both groups), MI (2% vs. 0%; p = 0.49), and clinically driven TVR (0% in both groups) were similar for the study groups. No ST was reported in either group.

The performance of the BioMatrix Flex stent was tested in comparison with that of a durable polymer EES (Promus Element, Boston Scientific) and with the everolimus-eluting bioresorbable scaffold (Absorb BVS, Abbott Vascular) in the Comparison of Everolimus- and Biolimus-Eluting Stents With Everolimus-Eluting Bioresorbable Vascular Scaffold Stents II (EVERBIO II) trial. This was a single-center trial including 240 all-comers patients randomly assigned to receive one of the abovementioned devices in a 1 : 1 : 1 ratio. The only study exclusion criteria was a reference vessel diameter >4.0 mm which does not allow the Absorb implantation. The angiographic follow-up showed similar LLL among groups, at 9 months (primary endpoint). Clinical outcomes were also comparable: the rates of patient-oriented MACE (death, MI, and any revascularization) were 27% in patients treated with bioresorbable vascular scaffolds (BVS) and 26% in the EES/BES group (p = 0.83) and the device-oriented MACE (cardiac death, MI, and TLR) rates were 12% in BVS and 9% in the EES/BES group (p = 0.6) [23].

The Assessment of Stent sTrut Apposition and Coverage in Coronary ArTeries with Optical coherence tomography in patients with STEMI, NSTEMI and stable/unstable angina undergoing everolimus vs. biolimus A9-eluting stent implantation (STACCATO) study was a single-center, prospective, randomized trial comparing tissue coverage in coronary lesions stented with durable fluoropolymer-coated EES (Xience V/Xience PRIME) or with the BioMatrix stent. It included 64 patients (64 lesions) with stable CAD or ACS at presentation and de novo coronary lesions. The primary endpoint, percentage of uncovered struts as assessed with OCT 9 months after

PCI, was significantly lower with the use of the EES (4.3 ± 4.8% vs. 8.7 ± 7.8%; p = 0.019). No difference in the average percentage of malapposed struts at baseline (6.8 ± 6.9% vs. 6.9 ± 7.0%, respectively; p = 0.974) and at follow-up (0.1 ± 0.3% vs. 0.6 ± 1.3%; p = 0.143) was reported. Neointimal thickness at 9 months was 109 ± 43 μm in EES vs. 64 ± 18 μm in BES (p < 0.001), and angiographic LLL was 0.15 mm in EES vs. 0.10 mm in BES (p = 0.581). Comparable rates of MACE and ST were reported [24].

Ongoing studies Table 35.2 lists the ongoing studies evaluating the performance of the BioMatrix stent. Among these, the Comparative Effectiveness of 1 Month of Ticagrelor Plus Aspirin Followed by Ticagrelor Monotherapy Versus a Current-day Intensive Dual Antiplatelet Therapy in All-comers Patients Undergoing Percutaneous Coronary Intervention With Bivalirudin and BioMatrix Family Drug-eluting Stent Use (GLOBAL LEADERS, NCT01813435) is an investigator-sponsored trial aiming to enroll around 16,000 all-comer patients in approximately 132 centers (in Europe, North America, South America, and Asia-Pacific) to assess the potential benefits of new antiplatelet regimens. The randomization will occur at the time of the index procedure prior to PCI. Subjects will be stratified according to center and according to the clinical presentation (stable CAD or ACS). All the randomized patients will be treated with the BioMatrix Flex stent or the BioMatrix NeoFlex stent and will receive peri-procedural bivalirudin. After PCI, they will receive (1 : 1) either ticagrelor plus aspirin for 1 month followed by 23 months of ticagrelor monotherapy or standard DAPT for 12 months followed by aspirin monotherapy for 12–24 months. The primary study outcome will be the composite of all-cause mortality or non-fatal new Q-wave MI at 2 years.

AXXESS

The AXXESS Plus was a prospective, single-arm, multicenter, and non-randomized study evaluating the safety and efficacy of the AXXESS BES for the treatment of patients with de novo bifurcation lesions. A total of 139 patients from Europe, Brazil, and New Zealand, with history of stable or unstable angina, met the following inclusion criteria and were entered in the study: target lesion located within 5 mm of a bifurcation; main branch reference vessel diameter between 2.5–4.0 mm; side branch diameter >2.25 mm and lesion length <15 mm; total length of the lesion in the main branch <34 mm. The primary endpoint was in-stent LLL in parent vessel and side branch at 6-month follow-up, as measured by quantitative computerized angiographic analysis (QCA). The safety endpoint was a composite of MACE at 6 months after the procedure, defined as any death, Q-wave or non-Q-wave MI, or ischemia-driven TLR. Satisfactory levels of procedural and angiographic success were reported (94.9% and 100%, respectively). All patients were stented

Table 35.2 Ongoing BioMatrix stent studies.

Study name and/or identifier number	Sites	Design	Setting	Endpoints
NCT01947439	Asia	Randomized BES vs. ZES	Multivessel PCI	All-cause death, non-fatal MI, any revascularization at 2 years
SORT-OUT VIII NCT02093845	Europe	Randomized BES vs. EES (Synergy stent)	Non-selected patients with ischemic heart disease	Device-related TLF at 1 year
OCT SORT-OUT VIII NCT02253108	Europe	Randomized BES vs. EES (Synergy stent)	Non-selected patients with ischemic heart disease	Combined endpoint of vessel wall healing parameters assessed by OCT at 3 months
PONTINA NCT01060306	Europe	Observational BES vs. BMS	Patients with stable CAD or ACS undergoing LM PCI	Assessment of neointimal coverage by OCT at 6 months
CHOICE NCT01397175	Asia	Randomized BES vs. EES vs. ZES	All-comers patients	Device-oriented composite at 2 years
DETECT-OCT NCT01752894	Asia	Randomized BES vs. EES (angio- vs. OCT-guided PCI)	Stable CAD or unstable angina	Percentage of neointimal coverage by OCT at 3 months
DESTINY TRIAL NCT01856088	South America	Randomized BES vs. SES (Inspiron Stent)	Stable or unstable angina	LLL at 9 months
ROBUST NCT00888758	Europe	Randomized BES vs. EES	STEMI	MACE at 9 months

ACS, acute coronary syndrome; BES, Biolimus-eluting stent; CAD, coronary artery disease; EES, everolimus-eluting stent; LLL, late lumen loss; LM, left main; MACE, major adverse cardiac events; MI, myocardial infarction; OCT, optical coherence tomography; PCI, percutaneous coronary intervention; SES, sirolimus-eluting stent; TLF, target lesion failure; ZES, zotarolimus-eluting stent.

with the Axxess-Plus stent, with 80.9% having additional stents placed distally (42% having stents in both the distal main vessel and side branch, 29.4% having stents into the distal main vessel only, and 9.6% with a stent into only the side branch). In-stent late loss in the AXXESS group was 0.09 ± 0.56 mm. Late ST was observed in three cases, two of which were associated with confirmed premature DAPT discontinuation. In-stent restenosis in the main vessel was 7.1% and in the side branch was 13.7% (7.9% when a DES was implanted). The TLR rate at 6 months was 7.5%. Six-month IVUS analysis was performed in 49 cases (35.2%) and showed effective lesion coverage along with significant neointimal suppression: the neointimal volume obstruction percentage was $2.28 \pm 2.17\%$, with a minimum lumen area of 7.86 ± 2.63 mm^2 [25].

The Drug-Eluting Stent Intervention for Treating Side Branches Effectively (DIVERGE) study was a prospective, multicenter registry with the aim of expanding the results of the AXXESS Plus study to a broader population while keeping strict protocol indications such as the obligatory use of SES as additional stents for the parent vessel and the side branch if the residual diameter stenosis exceeded 30%. Lesion criteria for inclusion were any bifurcation with significant side branch (≥ 2.25 mm) and parental vessel-side branch angulation <70°. The primary endpoint was the rate of MACE, a composite of death, MI, and TLR at 9 months. Secondary endpoints included in-segment restenosis, late loss, and percent neointimal volume obstruction. Overall, 302 patients were included across 14 sites in Europe, Australia, and New Zealand. Of procedures, 12.3% involved AXXESS only; additional stenting of side branch involved 21.7 % patients (17.7% in the distal parent vessel and 4.0% in the side branch vessel); 64.7% received stents in both vessels. The 9-month MACE rate was 7.7% (0.7% death, 3.3% non-Q-wave MI, 1.0% Q-wave MI, 4.3% TLR) and 21.3% at 5 years (6.5% death, 8.6% MI, 12.4% TLR). Of patients originally enrolled in the study, 96.3% (291) were available for this long-term follow-up. Only five cases (1.7%) of definite VLST were reported, none of them resulting in death [26,27].

The AXXESS Stent in Left Main Coronary Artery Bifurcation Lesions (AXXENT) trial was a prospective, single-arm, multicenter study designed to evaluate the safety and efficacy of the AXXESS BES for the treatment of LMCA bifurcation lesions in 33 patients. Six-month IVUS analysis (performed in 26 subjects) showed 12.4% increase in volume and significant neointimal suppression (percent neointimal volume obstruction was $3.0\% \pm 4.1\%$ with a minimal lumen area of 10.3 ± 2.6 mm). Interestingly, lumen area was significantly smaller in the left circumflex coronary ostium compared with the left anterior descending ostium at follow-up, probably because of greater neointimal formation and inadequate stent expansion [28].

The multicenter Complex Coronary Bifurcation Lesions: Randomized Comparison Of a Strategy using a Dedicated Self-Expanding Biolimus A9-eluting Stent vs Culotte Strategy using Everolimus-eluting Stents (COBRA) trial aims to compare the dedicated AXXESS stent with a conventional Culotte strategy assessing vessel healing (through OCT and QCA at 9 months) and clinical outcomes. Patients with true bifurcation lesions will be randomized to receive the AXXESS stent plus two BioMatrix or two Xience EES implanted with the Culotte technique (encompassing minimized overlap and final kissing balloon). The primary endpoint is strut coverage at 9-month follow-up. Secondary endpoints will include OCT and QCA parameter at 9 months and clinical outcomes up to 5 years. Preliminary analysis performed on the first 40 patients enrolled (20 for each arm) showed no significant difference in the percentage of uncovered struts at 9 months. Furthermore, a delayed neointimal coverage was observed in the proximal main vessel

compared with more distal segments in patients receiving the Culotte technique whereas a trend toward a higher percentage of uncovered struts in all bifurcation segments was reported for subjects in the AXXESS arm. These findings have been related to differences in strut thickness, polymer, and antiproliferative drug between the study devices [29].

BioFreedom

Pre-clinical studies proved the long-term efficacy of the BioFreedom stent compared with SES in terms of late restenosis (reduced neointimal proliferation) and persistent inflammation (decreased fibrin, granuloma, and giant cells) [30].

The BioFreedom FIM included a total of 182 patients diagnosed with symptomatic ischemic heart disease and coronary lesions amenable to percutaneous treatment with DES. Inclusion criteria also were native vessels diameter ≥ 2.25 and ≤ 3 and lesion length ≤ 14 mm. Patients were divided in two cohorts on the basis of different time-point for angiographic and IVUS follow-up (after 4 or 9 months for cohort 1 and 2, respectively) and randomized to receive either the BioFreedom standard dose (15.6 μg/mm) or the BioFreedom low dose (7.8 μg/mm) or the PES Taxus Liberté (Boston Scientific). DAPT was recommended for at least 6 months after stent implantation. The primary endpoint was in-stent LLL at 12 months (cohort 2). Secondary endpoints included in-stent LLL at 4 months (cohort 1), MACE (composite of all death, MI, emergent CABG and TLR) and ST rate at 30 days, 4, 12 months and up to 5 years; clinically driven TLR, TVR, and TVF at 4, 12 months, and up to 5 years; in-stent/in-segment binary restenosis at 4 months; in-stent/in-segment Minimum Lumen Diameter (MLD) at 4 months; neointimal hyperplasia volume at 4 and 12 months measured by IVUS; biolimus concentrations pre/post procedure at discharge and 30 days. Both BioFreedom SD (0.08 mm) and LD (0.12 mm) groups demonstrated a significant reduction in late loss at 4 months compared to Taxus (0.37 mm) ($p < 0.0001$ and 0.002, respectively). The percentage of neointimal volume obstruction was significantly reduced in the BioFreedom Standard Dose arm, compared to both BioFreedom Low Dose and Taxus Liberté. In the second study cohort (including 107 patients), in-stent LLL in patients receiving BioFreedom SD was 0.17 mm, compared with an in-stent LLL of 0.35 mm in the Taxus Liberté group. When combining the cohorts, BioFreedom SD demonstrated sustained safety up to 12 months, including absence of ST [31]. After 4 years, similar rates of MACE in the BioFreedom SD and Taxus Liberté groups were reported (13.6% vs. 13.3%) with no evidence of ST [32].

The EGO-BIOFREEDOM trial was designed to assess the time frame, degree of endothelialization, and the subsequent neointimal proliferation through OCT evaluation in patients treated with the BioFreedom stent. This single center study included 100 "real-world" patients (with the exclusion of those with STEMI at presentation) who received baseline and 9-month OCT and were randomized to six groups according to timing of the blinded OCT follow-up. The primary outcome included OCT findings on coverage (degree of endothelialization/coverage) from 1 to 9 months. Secondary outcomes were OCT endpoints (neointimal area and neointimal thickness), QCA endpoints (LLL at 9 months), and clinical endpoints (MACE and ST at 9 and 12 months). Early strut coverage was classified into six categories (A, B, C: uncovered struts; D, E, F: covered struts); early coverage increased progressively from a minimum of 48.16% at 1 month to 97.14% (median) at 5 months. In each group of 20 patients, the range variations of percentage of coverage were much wider in the earlier (1–2 months) groups whereas nearly complete coverage was observed in the later months with more mature neointimal tissue (brighter intensity and more homogenous in appearance). Median strut coverage at 9 months reaches 99.55% (IQR 98.17–99.93%; min 85.41%, max 100%). Nine-month neointimal thickness remained very low at 0.10 mm (0.05–0.16 mm) in 55 patients. In-stent neointimal volume percentage increased from 4.3% (IQR 2.1–7.5%) in the first 5 months to 13% (9.4–15.9%) at 9 months. Four patients had in-stent restenosis requiring treatment (TLR rate 4%); no other target vessel-related infarct or cardiac death or definite or probable late ST were recorded [33].

The Leaders Free trial (NCT01623180) is an ongoing multicenter, randomized, double-blind trial comparing the BioFreedom stent with the Gazelle stent in approximately 2500 patients at high bleeding risk using a short (1 month) course of DAPT testing the non-inferiority for the primary safety endpoint (a composite of cardiac death, MI, and ST) and the superiority for the primary efficacy endpoint (clinically driven TLR) at 1 year.

The BioFreedom US IDE Feasibility Trial (NCT02131142) is a multicenter, prospective study started in August 2014, with the aim to collect additional safety (MACE, defined as the composite of cardiac death, MI, TLR, and definite ST) and effectiveness (LLL at 9 months) data for the use of the BioFreedom stent in patients with de novo, native coronary lesions.

The Nobori stent

The Nobori stent (Terumo, Tokyo, Japan) resembles the two main components of the BioMatrix stent: (i) the bare metal (stainless steel) platform with open cell, quadrature link design and strut thickness of 120 μm; (ii) the abluminal coating (toward vessel) with the biodegradable PLA as drug carrier, parylene C as primer coating and Biolimus at dose of 15.6 μg/mm stent length. The main difference is related to a different coating process: chemical vapor deposition is used for the Nobori whereas automated autopipette are used for the BioMatrix stent.

Preclinical and pharmacokinetic studies

Endothelial coverage proved to be complete 14 days after the implantation of the Nobori stent in porcine coronary arteries evaluated with the scanning electronic microscope without a significant vessel reaction up to 15 months compared with vessels treated with BMS [34]. Other reports showed a lower inflammatory profile compared with vessels implanted with the first generation SES or with the durable-polymer EES [35].

The NOBORI PK study evaluated the pharmacokinetics of Biolimus eluted from Nobori stent as well its tolerability and safety profile in 20 patients with de novo coronary lesions: the highest Biolimus blood concentration measured in blood samples obtained at different time points (before the procedure and 48 h, 7 and 28 days, 3, 6, and 9 months after stent implantation) was 32.2 pg/mL and was not associated with the occurrence of adverse events. The median time for the maximum concentration was 2 hours (0.05 hours to 3 months). After 6 months, only one patient had detectable Biolimus systemic levels whereas no measurable concentrations were found at 9 months [36].

Clinical evidence (Table 35.3)
Registries
The NOBORI CORE study compared the Nobori stent with first-generation Cypher SES in 107 patients with de novo coronary lesions (142, diameter 2.5–3.5 mm). Angiographic 9-month follow-up revealed a similar in-stent LLL (0.10±0.26 vs. 0.12±0.43; p=0.66) and binary restenosis (1.7 vs. 6.3%; p=0.32) whereas in-stent diameter stenosis was significantly lower in the Nobori group (13±10% vs. 20±12%; p=0.002) [37]. In a subgroup of patients (n=43), rapid atrial pacing was used to evaluate the endothelial function through the assessment of vasomotion: the use of the Nobori was associated with a preserved endothelial function and vasomotion [38]. Several factors contribute to this effect (polymer, asymmetric coating, drug); however, the clinical relevance of this effect needs further investigation.

The NOBORI 2 was a prospective, multicenter, single-arm registry evaluating the performance of the Nobori stent in a broad range of clinical settings. Indeed, it included 3067 patients across Europe and Asia between April 2008 and March 2009; approximately 73% of them had an off-label indication for the use of the Nobori stent. At 1 year, the overall rate of the device oriented endpoint or TLF (composite of cardiac death, MI, and TLR) was 3.9% (5.1% after 2 years). Patients in off-label group experienced significantly higher rates of the primary endpoint both after 1 and 2 years (TLF: 4.5% vs. 2.2% at 1 year and 5.9% vs. 2.8% at 2 years). The rates of ST were 0.68% and 0.80%, at 1 and 2 years, respectively [39].

The Italian Nobori Stent ProspectIve Registry (INSPIRE 1) included 1066 all-comers patients (1589 lesions) treated with the Nobori stent at seven Italian sites between February 2008 and July 2012. At 1 year, the primary endpoint (composite of cardiac death, MI, and clinically driven TVR) occurred in 4.0% of patients. TLF (secondary endpoint) occurred in 4.6% of patients. The rates of both primary and secondary endpoints were higher in patients with complex lesions. Definite and probable ST rate was 0.6% and was not significantly higher in the complex lesions group (0.9%) [40].

Randomized studies (Figure 35.5)

Nobori vs. first generation DES The NOBORI I trial compared the Nobori stent with the Taxus stent. The study was a randomized (2 : 1), prospective, controlled, non-inferiority trial with two arms: in the NOBORI I Phase I trial patients in the comparator group received the Taxus Express PES (Boston Scientific, Natick, MA, USA) whereas in the NOBORI I Phase II trial the Taxus Liberté PES was used. Overall, 362 patients with up to two de novo lesions in two epicardial vessels were included. The primary endpoint was angiographic in-stent LLL at 9 months, while secondary endpoints were MACE at 30 days, 4, 9, and 12 months, and yearly up to 5 years. In the NOBORI I Phase I, LLL was significantly lower in the Nobori group (0.15±0.27 vs. 0.32±0.33 mm; p=0.006). The NOBORI I Phase II proved both the non-inferiority and the superiority of the Nobori stent over the Taxus in terms of LLL (0.11±0.30 vs. 0.32±0.50 mm; p<0.001). Binary restenosis and neointimal volume obstruction were also significantly lower in the Nobori group. Regarding overall clinical outcomes after 5 years, no differences were reported in the composite of death and MI (10.9% vs. 11.2%) and the number of TLR was lower in patients treated with the Nobori stent (6.3% vs. 16%). The rates of ST were 0.0% and 3.2% in the Nobori and Taxus groups, respectively (p=0.014) [41].

In the SORT-OUT V trial 2468 patients were randomized (1 : 1) to the Nobori or the Cypher stent at three Danish sites. It was a non-inferiority trial and the primary endpoint was a composite of cardiac death, MI, definite ST, and TVR at 9 months. Clinical baseline features identified a moderate risk population with a considerable number of patients in both groups with diabetes, history of PCI and ACS at presentation. The primary endpoint occurred in 4.1% of

Table 35.3 Overview of clinical studies with the Nobori Biolimus-eluting stent.

Study name [ref], year (results available)	Design	Country	Patients	Setting	Planned follow-up	Primary endpoint	Status
NOBORI PK [36], 2008	Single Arm Registry	Europe	20	Stable CAD	1 year	Systemic concentrations of Biolimus A9 after 28 days and 6 months	Completed
NOBORI CORE [37,38], 2008	Prospective Multicenter Comparative	Europe	107	Stable CAD	1 year	In-stent LLL at 9 months	Completed
NOBORI 2 [39], 2012	Prospective Multicenter Single Arm Registry	Europe Asia	3067	All-comers	2 years	TLF* at 12 months	Completed
INSPIRE-1 [40], 2014	Multicenter Registry	Europe	1066	All-comers	NA	Composite of safety† and efficacy‡ at 12 months	1-year FU completed
NOBORI I [41], 2014	Randomized Multicenter Nobori vs. Taxus Express PES (Phase I or Taxus Liberté (Phase II)	Europe	362	Stable CAD and unstable angina	5 years	In-stent LLL at 9 months	Completed
COMPARE II [43], 2013	Randomized Multicenter Nobori vs. Xience	Europe	2707	Stable CAD and ACS	5 years	Composite of safety† and efficacy‡ at 12 months	1-year FU completed
NEXT [44,45], 2013	Randomized Multicenter Nobori vs. XIENCE/ Promus	Asia	3235	Stable CAD	10 years	TLR at 1 year	3-year FU completed
SORT OUT V [42], 2013	Randomized Multicenter Nobori vs. Cypher	Europe	2468	Stable CAD and ACS	1 year	Composite of cardiac death, MI, definite ST, TVR at 9 months	Completed
SORT OUT VII [46], 2015	Randomized Multicenter Nobori vs. Orsiro	Europe	2525	Stable CAD and ACS	1 year	Composite of cardiac death, MI, TLR at 12 months	Completed
LONG DES V [47], 2014	Randomized Multicenter Nobori vs. Promus Element	Asia	500	Stable CAD and unstable angina	1 year	In-segment LLL at 9 months	Completed
BASKET-PROVE II [48], 2015	Randomized Single center Nobori vs. Xience vs. PRO-kinetic	Europe	2291	Stable CAD and ACS	2 years	Cardiac death, MI and TVR at 9 months	Completed

ACS, acute coronary syndrome; CAD, coronary artery disease; FU, follow-up; LLL, late lumen loss; MI, myocardial infarction; ST, stent thrombosis; TLF, target lesion failure; TLR, target lesion revascularization; TVR, target vessel revascularization.

* Cardiac death, MI, and clinically indicated TLR.

† Cardiac death and non-fatal MI.

‡ Clinically indicated target vessel revascularization (TVR).

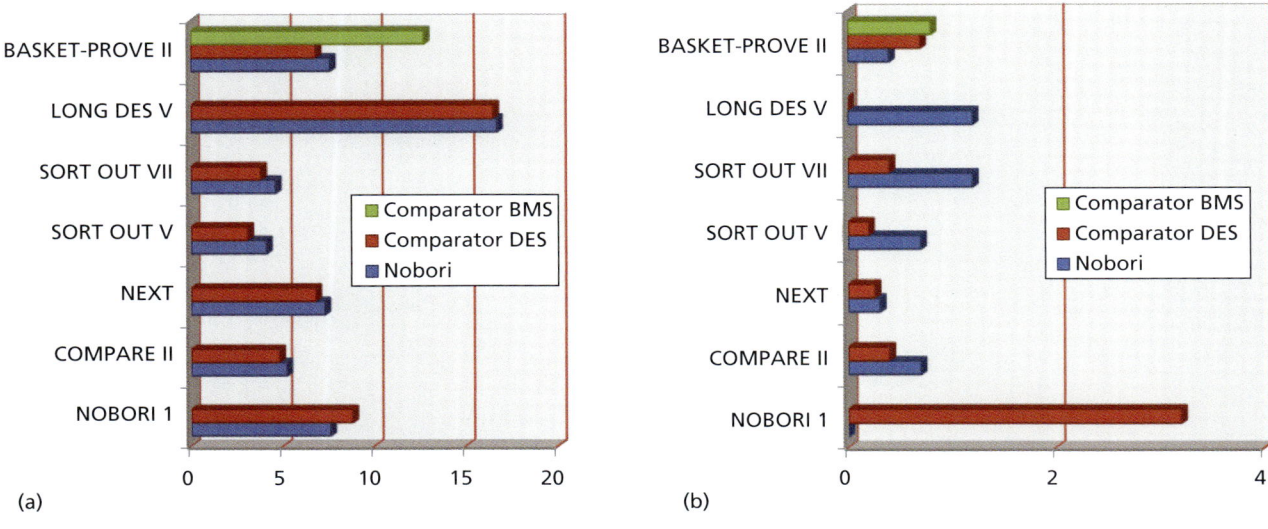

	NOBORI I Phase 1 (n = 120)		NOBORI I Phase 2 (n = 243)		NEXT (n = 457)		LONG DES V (n = 500)	
	Nobori	Taxus Express	Nobori	Taxus Liberté	Nobori	Xience	Nobori	Promus
Follow-up	9 months		9 months		8 months		8 months	
Late loss (mm)	0.15 ± 0.27	0.33 ± 0.34	0.11 ± 0.30	0.32 ± 0.50	0.17 ± 0.35	0.14 ± 0.36	0.20 ± 0.41	0.24 ± 0.38
Diameter stenosis (mm)	14.0 ± 8	19 ± 10	14 ± 8	21 ± 15	14.8 ± 13.8	14.1 ± 12	17.3 ± 15.6	20.5 ± 13.9
Binary restenosis (%)	0	0	0.7	6.2	7.1	7.5	3.7	4.9
TLR (%)	0	2.9	0	1.1	4.2	4.2	0.8	0.4

(c)

Figure 35.5 Rates of MACE (a) and ST (b) and key angiographic findings (c) across the main randomized trials evaluating the performance of the Nobori stent.

patients in the Nobori group and 3.1% of patient in the SES group (p for non-inferiority = 0.06, and p for superiority = 0.22). However, a significantly larger proportion of patients in the Nobori stent group had definite ST at 12 months than did those in the SES group (0.7% vs. 0.2%, risk difference 0.6%, 95% CI 0.0–1.1; p = 0.034) questioning the non-inferiority of the novel device [42].

Nobori vs. second generation DES The COMPARE II was an open-label, prospective, randomized (2 : 1), controlled, non-inferiority trial enrolling 2707 patients (4025 lesions) across 12 European sites between January 2009 and February 2011. Patients were randomized to receive the Nobori stent (n = 1795) or the thin strut Xience stent (n = 912). High-risk patients were largely represented in the study population: 58% presented with an ACS, 22% had diabetes, and 63.5% of lesions were classified as B2/C type according to

AHA/ACC classification. At 12 months, the primary endpoint, a composite of safety (cardiac death and non-fatal MI) and efficacy (clinically indicated TVR) occurred in 5.2% and 4.8% of patients treated with Nobori and Xience, respectively, proving the non-inferiority of the Nobori stent. Definite ST was 0.7% in the Nobori and 0.4% in Xience group [43].

The NOBORI Biolimus-Eluting Versus XIENCE/PROMUS Everolimus-Eluting Stent Trial (NEXT) was a prospective, multicenter, randomized, open-label trial evaluating the non-inferiority of the Nobori stent compared with a durable polymer EES (Xience or PROMUS) in terms of TLR at 1 year in 3235 patients mainly suffering from stable CAD (83% of patients). The study proved the non-inferiority of the Nobori stent with a TLR rate of 4.2% in both study arms (p for non-inferiority <0.0001, and p for superiority = 0.93). The cumulative rate of definite ST was also similar

Table 35.4 Ongoing Nobori stent studies.

Study name and/or identifier number	Sites	Design	Setting	Endpoints
e-NOBORI Registry NCT01261273	Europe Asia, Central and South America	Observational	All-comers	Freedom from TLF (cardiac death, target vessel MI and TLR) at 1 year
IRIS NOBORI NCT01348360	Asia	Observational Comparative (vs. first-generation DES)	Non-selected patients with ischemic heart disease	Composite of cardiac death, MI, and TVR at 1 year
NAUSICA NCT01401036	Asia	Randomized Nobori vs. uncoated stent	Acute MI	MACE at 1 year
BEGIN NCT01574586	Asia	Randomized Nobori vs. Xience	Patients with stable CAD undergoing bifurcation lesions PCI	Minimum lumen diameter of the side branch ostium in bifurcation at 8 months
ISAR-TEST 6 NCT01068106	Europe	Randomized Nobori vs. Xience	All-comers	Composite of cardiac death, MI, and TVR at 1 year

ACS, acute coronary syndrome; CAD, coronary artery disease; DES, drug-eluting stents; LLL, late lumen loss; MACE, major adverse cardiac events; MI, myocardial infarction; PCI, percutaneous coronary intervention; TLF, target lesion failure; TLR, target-lesion revascularization; TVR, target-vessel revascularization.

between the two study groups (0.25 vs. 0.06%; p = 0.18). The angiographic sub-study, including 528 patients, confirmed the non-inferiority by showing an in-segment LLL of 0.03 ± 0.39 vs. 0.06 ± 0.45 mm (p for non-inferiority <0.0001; p for superiority = 0.52) [44]. The safety and efficacy outcomes remained comparable through 3 year and beyond 1 year after stent implantation: TLR rates were 7.4% and 7.1%, p = 0.8; cardiac death 2.7% vs. 2.4%, p = 0.57; MI 4.0% vs. 3.7%, p = 0.72; TVR 11.3% vs. 9.9%, p = 0.21; ST 0.31% vs. 0.26%, p = 0.74 in the Nobori and in the EES groups, respectively [45].

The SORT OUT VII trial compared the efficacy and safety of the thin strut, cobalt-chromium biodegradable polymer sirolimus-eluting Orsiro stent (Biotronik, Switzerland) and the Nobori stent in 2525 all-comers patients. At 1 year, the primary endpoint (target lesion failure defined as a composite of cardiac death, MI not related to other than index lesion, and TLR) occurred in 3.8% of patients receiving the Orsiro stent and in 4.6% of patients receiving the Nobori stent (p for non-inferiority <0.0001). Moreover, patients treated with the Orsiro stent experienced a significantly lower rate of definite ST (0.4% vs. 1.2%, RR 0.33, 95% CI 0.12–0.92; p = 0.03) [46].

The randomized, multicenter, prospective LONG-DES V trial compared the Nobori stent with the Promus Element EES (Boston Scientific, USA) in 500 patients with long (≥25 mm) coronary lesions. In-segment LLL (primary endpoint) was comparable between the two groups at 9 months (0.14 ± 0.38 vs. 0.11 ± 0.37 mm; 95% CI −0.053 to 0.091; p for non-inferiority = 0.03, p for superiority = 0.45), as well as in-stent LLL (0.20 ± 0.41 vs. 0.24 ± 0.38 mm; p = 0.29). No significant differences in the rate of composite outcome of death, MI, and TVR were reported (41, 16.7% in Nobori arm vs. 42, 16.5% in Promus arm; p = 0.94) [47].

However, the performance of the Nobori stent in large vessels (≥3.0 mm in diameter) was evaluated in the BAsel Stent Kosten-Effektivitäts Trial–PROspective Validation Examination II (BASKET-PROVE II) study, a randomized, multicenter European

trial assigning, in a 1 : 1 : 1 ratio, 2291 patients to either the Nobori or the Xience or to the thin-strut silicon-carbide-coated BMS, PRO-Kinetic (Biotronik). The cumulative incidence of the primary endpoint (combined cardiac death, MI, and TVR) was 7.6% with the Nobori, 6.8% with Xience, and 12.7% with PRO-Kinetic. The Nobori stent proved non-inferiority to the Xience (absolute risk difference 0.78%; p for non-inferiority = 0.042) and superior to BMS (absolute risk difference, −5.16; −8.32 to −2.01; p = 0.0011). However, the use of the Nobori stent was not associated with an improved safety profile because no decrease in the occurrence of very late ST was reported [48].

Ongoing studies assessing the performance of the Nobori stents are reported in Table 35.4.

The Xtent

The XTENT Custom NX stent (Xtent, Menlo Park, CA, USA) was a customizable BES with a modular design made of multiple interdigitated 6-mm segments whose length could be customized according to the lesion length at the treatment site. This peculiar feature had the potential advantage to avoid overlapping stents when treating long lesions. Three studies proved the safety and effectiveness of this device (CUSTOM I, II, III) in 220 patients. However, because of industrial financial difficulties it has not been available since August 2009.

Evidence from pooled data

The considerable number of studies comparing biodegradable polymer BES with durable-polymer DES prompt the pooling of the available data in several meta-analyses. Biodegradable polymer BES did not significantly reduce the risk of MACE but demonstrated a significantly lower risk of very late ST when compared with durable polymer DES in a meta-analysis including eight randomized trials [49]. In a large-scale network meta-analysis, biodegradable polymer BES were associated with superior clinical outcomes compared with BMS and first-generation DES, similar rates of cardiac death, MI, and TVR when compared with second-generation durable-polymer DES, and higher rate of definite ST compared with cobalt-chromium EES [50].

Safety concerns were also issued by two other network meta-analyses assessing the safety and efficacy of durable polymer DES and biodegradable polymer BES: at 1 year, higher rates of ST and MI were reported for patients treated with BES compared with patients receiving new-generation, cobalt chromium EES [51,52].

Interactive multiple choice questions are available for this chapter on www.wiley.com/go/dangas/cardiology

References

1 Ostojic MC, Perisic Z, Sagic D, *et al.* The pharmacokinetics of Biolimus A9 after elution from the BioMatrix II stent in patients with coronary artery disease: the Stealth PK Study. *Eur J Clin Pharmacol* 2011; **67**(4): 389–398.

2 Sabatini DM, Erdjument-Bromage H, Lui M, Tempst P, Snyder SH. RAFT1: a mammalian protein that binds to FKBP12 in a rapamycin-dependent fashion and is homologous to yeast TORs. *Cell* 1994; **78**(1): 35–43.

3 Gunatillake PA, Adhikari R. Biodegradable synthetic polymers for tissue engineering. *Eur Cell Mater* 2003; **5**: 1–16.

4 Hai K. Initial results from the prospective, multicenter, observational, web-based BEACON Registry. *Cardiovasc Revasc Med* 2006; **7**: 81–126.

5 Santoso T. BEACON II: 3 year outcome. Asia PCR 2012.

6 D. W. The BEACON II registry: 4 year outcomes in an Asian Pacific patient population, oral presentation. Asia PCR 2013.

7 Urban P, Valdes M, Menown I, *et al.* Outcomes following implantation of the biolimus A9-eluting BioMatrix coronary stent: primary analysis of the e-BioMatrix registry. *Catheter Cardiovasc Interv* 2015; **86**(7): 1151–1160.

8 Eberli F. Comorbidities determine prognosis in patients undergoing coronary stenting: results from the e-BioMAtrix registry. Euro PCR 2013.

9 Mehta AB, Chandra P, Dalal J, *et al.* One-year clinical outcomes of BioMatrix-Biolimus A9 eluting stent: the e-BioMatrix multicenter post marketing surveillance registry in India. *Indian Heart J* 2013; **65**(5): 593–599.

10 Goyal BK, Metha A, Chandra P, *et al.* A two year analysis of diabetic subset "e-BioMatrix" prospective, multicenter, all-comers registry in India. *Indian Heart J* 2014; epub ahead of print.

11 Grube E, Hauptmann KE, Buellesfeld L, Lim V, Abizaid A. Six-month results of a randomized study to evaluate safety and efficacy of a Biolimus A9 eluting stent with a biodegradable polymer coating. *EuroIntervention* 2005; **1**(1):53–57.

12 Grube E. *Biolimus A9 Drug-Eluting Stents: The Biosensors STEALTH I Results.* Angioplasty Summit, Korea, 2005.

13 Grube E. STEALTH I: 5-year follow-up from a prospective randomized study of Biolimus A9-Eluting Stent with a biodegradable polymer coating vs. a bare metal stent. TCT 2011.

14 Raber L, Kelbaek H, Ostojic M, *et al.* Effect of biolimus-eluting stents with biodegradable polymer vs bare-metal stents on cardiovascular events among patients with acute myocardial infarction: the COMFORTABLE AMI randomized trial. *JAMA* 2012; **308**(8):777–787.

15 Raber L, Kelbaek H, Taniwaki M, *et al.* Biolimus-eluting stents with biodegradable polymer versus bare-metal stents in acute myocardial infarction: two-year clinical results of the COMFORTABLE AMI trial. *Circ Cardiovasc Interv* 2014; **7**(3): 355–364.

16 Windecker S, Serruys PW, Wandel S, *et al.* Biolimus-eluting stent with biodegradable polymer versus sirolimus-eluting stent with durable polymer for coronary revascularisation (LEADERS): a randomised non-inferiority trial. *Lancet* 2008; **372**(9644): 1163–1173.

17 Barlis P, Regar E, Serruys PW, *et al.* An optical coherence tomography study of a biodegradable vs. durable polymer-coated limus-eluting stent: a LEADERS trial sub-study. *Eur Heart J* 2010; **31**(2): 165–176.

18 Serruys PW, Farooq V, Kalesan B, *et al.* Improved safety and reduction in stent thrombosis associated with biodegradable polymer-based biolimus-eluting stents versus durable polymer-based sirolimus-eluting stents in patients with coronary artery disease: final 5-year report of the LEADERS (Limus Eluted From A Durable Versus ERodable Stent Coating) randomized, noninferiority trial. *JACC Cardiovasc Interv* 2013; **6**(8): 777–789.

19 Wykrzykowska JJ, Serruys PW, Onuma Y, *et al.* Impact of vessel size on angiographic and clinical outcomes of revascularization with biolimus-eluting stent with biodegradable polymer and sirolimus-eluting stent with durable polymer the LEADERS trial substudy. *JACC Cardiovasc Interv* 2009; **2**(9): 861–870.

20 Zhang YJ, Iqbal J, Windecker S, *et al.* Biolimus-eluting stent with biodegradable polymer improves clinical outcomes in patients with acute myocardial infarction. *Heart* 2015; **101**(4): 271–278.

21 Raungaard B, Jensen LO, Tilsted HH, *et al.* Zotarolimus-eluting durable-polymer-coated stent versus a biolimus-eluting biodegradable-polymer-coated stent in unselected patients undergoing percutaneous coronary intervention (SORT OUT VI): a randomised non-inferiority trial. *Lancet* 2015; **385**(9977): 1527–1535.

22 Separham A, Sohrabi B, Aslanabadi N, Ghaffari S. The twelve-month outcome of biolimus eluting stent with biodegradable polymer compared with an everolimus eluting stent with durable polymer. *J Cardiovasc Thorac Res* 2011; **3**(4): 113–116.

23 Puricel S, Arroyo D, Corpataux N, *et al.* Comparison of everolimus- and biolimus-eluting coronary stents with everolimus-eluting bioresorbable vascular scaffolds. *J Am Coll Cardiol* 2015; **65**(8): 791–801.

24 Adriaenssens T, Ughi GJ, Dubois C, *et al.* STACCATO (Assessment of Stent sTrut Apposition and Coverage in Coronary ArTeries with Optical coherence tomography in patients with STEMI, NSTEMI and stable/unstable angina undergoing everolimus vs. biolimus A9-eluting stent implantation): a randomised controlled trial. *EuroIntervention* 2014; **11**: e1619–1626.

25 Grube E, Buellesfeld L, Neumann FJ, *et al.* Six-month clinical and angiographic results of a dedicated drug-eluting stent for the treatment of coronary bifurcation narrowings. *Am J Cardiol* 2007; **99**(12): 1691–1697.

26 Verheye S, Agostoni P, Dubois CL, *et al.* 9-month clinical, angiographic, and intravascular ultrasound results of a prospective evaluation of the Axxess self-expanding biolimus A9-eluting stent in coronary bifurcation lesions: the DIVERGE (Drug-Eluting Stent Intervention for Treating Side Branches Effectively) study. *J Am Coll Cardiol* 2009; **53**(12): 1031–1039.

27 Chavarri V. *The AXXESS Plus and the DIVERGE studies results at 5 years.* Sao Paulo, July 24, 2013.

28 Hasegawa T, Ako J, Koo BK, *et al.* Analysis of left main coronary artery bifurcation lesions treated with biolimus-eluting DEVAX AXXESS plus nitinol self-expanding stent: intravascular ultrasound results of the AXXENT trial. *Catheter Cardiovasc Interv* 2009; **73**(1): 34–41.

29 Dubois C, Bennett J, Dens J, *et al.* COmplex coronary Bifurcation lesions: RAndomized comparison of a strategy using a dedicated self-expanding biolimus-eluting stent versus a culotte strategy using everolimus-eluting stents: primary results of the COBRA trial. *EuroIntervention* 2015; **11**(1): 1457–1467.

30 Tada N, Virmani R, Grant G, *et al.* Polymer-free biolimus a9-coated stent demonstrates more sustained intimal inhibition, improved healing, and reduced inflammation compared with a polymer-coated sirolimus-eluting cypher stent in a porcine model. *Circ Cardiovasc Interv* 2010; **3**(2): 174–183.

31 Grube E. BioFreedom First In Man Progress Report. TCT 2008.

32 Grube E. Very long-term results of biofreedom first-in-man, a randomized trial comparing polymer-free biofreedom stents with durable polymer Taxus Liberté Stent. TCT2013.

33 Lee WLS. The first establishment of early healing profile and 9-month outcomes of a new polymer-free Biolimus-A9 drug-coated-stent by longitudinal sequential OCT follow-ups: the EGO-BioFreedom study. Presented at EuroPCR, 2015.

34 Hagiwara H, Hiraishi Y, Terao H, *et al.* Vascular responses to a biodegradable polymer (polylactic acid) based biolimus A9-eluting stent in porcine models. *EuroIntervention* 2012; **8**(6):743–751.

35 Sumida AN, H. Gogas, B. *et al.* Comparison of coronary artery endothelial function after Nobori and Xience V stent implantation in swine model. *J Am Coll Cardiol* 2012; **59**: E58.

36 Ostojic M, Sagic D. Jung R, *et al.* The pharmacokinetics of Biolimus A9 after elution from the Nobori stent in patients with coronary artery disease: the NOBORI PK study. *Catheter Cardiovasc Interv* 2008; **72**(7): 901–908.

37 Ostojic M, Sagic D. Beleslin B, *et al.* First clinical comparison of Nobori -Biolimus A9 eluting stents with Cypher-Sirolimus eluting stents: Nobori Core nine months angiographic and one year clinical outcomes. *EuroIntervention* 2008; **3**(5): 574–579.

38 Hamilos MI, Ostojic M, Beleslin B, *et al.* Differential effects of drug-eluting stents on local endothelium-dependent coronary vasomotion. *J Am Coll Cardiol* 2008; **51**(22): 2123–2129.

39 Morice MC, Chevalier B, Tresukosol D, *et al.* Clinical outcomes of bifurcation stenting in NOBORI 2 study. *EuroIntervention* 2010; **6**: Suppl H.

40 Godino C, Parenti DZ, Regazzoli D, *et al.* One-year outcome of biolimus eluting stent with biodegradable polymer in all comers: the Italian Nobori Stent Prospective Registry. *Int J Cardiol* 2014; **177**(1): 11–16.

41 Chevalier B, Wijns W, Silber S, *et al.* Five-year clinical outcome of the Nobori drug-eluting coronary stent system in the treatment of patients with coronary artery disease: final results of the NOBORI 1 trial. *EuroIntervention* 2015; **11**(5): 549–554.

42 Christiansen EH, Jensen LO, Thayssen P, *et al.* Biolimus-eluting biodegradable polymer-coated stent versus durable polymer-coated sirolimus-eluting stent in unselected patients receiving percutaneous coronary intervention (SORT OUT V): a randomised non-inferiority trial. *Lancet* 2013; **381**(9867): 661–669.

43 Smits PC, Hofma S, Togni M, *et al.* Abluminal biodegradable polymer biolimus-eluting stent versus durable polymer everolimus-eluting stent (COMPARE II): a randomised, controlled, non-inferiority trial. *Lancet* 2013; **381**(9867): 651–660.

44 Natsuaki M, Kozuma K, Morimoto T, *et al.* Biodegradable polymer biolimus-eluting stent versus durable polymer everolimus-eluting stent: a randomized, controlled, noninferiority trial. *J Am Coll Cardiol* 2013; **62**(3):181–190.

45 Natsuaki M. Final 3-year outcome of a randomised trial comparing second-generation DES using either biodegradable polymer or durable polymer: the Norobi biolimus-eluting versus Xience/Promus everolimus-eluting stent trial (NEXT). Presented at EuroPCR 2015.

46 Jensen LO. Randomised comparison of a sirolimus-eluting stent with a biolimus-eluting stent in patients treated with PCI: the SORT OUT VII trial. EuroPCR 2015.

47 Lee JY, Park DW, Kim YH, *et al.* Comparison of biolimus A9-eluting (Nobori) and everolimus-eluting (Promus Element) stents in patients with de novo native long coronary artery lesions: a randomized long drug-eluting stent V trial. *Circ Cardiovasc Interv* 2014; **7**(3): 322–329.

48 Kaiser C, Galatius S, Jeger R, *et al.* Long-term efficacy and safety of biodegradable-polymer biolimus-eluting stents: main results of the Basel Stent Kosten-Effektivitats Trial-PROspective Validation Examination II (BASKET-PROVE II), a randomized, controlled noninferiority 2-year outcome trial. *Circulation* 2015; **131**(1): 74–81.

49 Ye Y, Xie H, Zeng Y, Zhao X, Tian Z, Zhang S. Efficacy and safety of biodegradable polymer biolimus-eluting stents versus durable polymer drug-eluting stents: a meta-analysis. *PLoS One* 2013; **8**(11): e78667.

50 Palmerini T, Biondi-Zoccai G, Della Riva D, *et al.* Clinical outcomes with bioabsorbable polymer- versus durable polymer-based drug-eluting and bare-metal stents: evidence from a comprehensive network meta-analysis. *J Am Coll Cardiol* 2014; **63**(4): 299–307.

51 Kang SH, Park KW, Kang DY, *et al.* Biodegradable-polymer drug-eluting stents vs. bare metal stents vs. durable-polymer drug-eluting stents: a systematic review and Bayesian approach network meta-analysis. *Eur Heart J* 2014; **35**(17): 1147–1158.

52 Navarese EP, Tandjung K, Claessen B, *et al.* Safety and efficacy outcomes of first and second generation durable polymer drug eluting stents and biodegradable polymer biolimus eluting stents in clinical practice: comprehensive network meta-analysis. *BMJ* 2013; **347**: f6530.

CHAPTER 36

The Biotronik Stent Family

Anna Franzone, Raffaele Piccolo, and Stephan Windecker

Department of Cardiology, Bern University Hospital, Bern, Switzerland

The Pro-Kinetic Energy and the Orsiro stent share two main components: the cobalt chromium platform and the unique passive coating (PROBIO).

Cobalt chromium platform

The introduction of cobalt chromium (CoCr) alloys in place of stainless steel as metallic platforms when manufacturing coronary stents aimed to improve the devices' properties and their final performance. Specifically, the CoCr alloy L605 is comprised of cobalt (52%), chromium (20%), nickel (10%), tungsten (15%), manganese (1.5%), and iron (3%). Its higher density than stainless steel (9.1 vs. 8 g/cm^3) ensures higher radio-opacity. Moreover, this platform features excellent radial strength as a consequence of higher tensile strength (1000 vs. 595 MPa) and elastic modulus (243 vs. 193 GPa); thinner struts (in the region of 80–90 μm compared to strut thicknesses of 130–140 μm for earlier 316 L devices); high toughness, corrosion resistance, and wear resistance [1,2].

Passive coating

PROBIO is a highly biocompatible, thin-layer (80 nm), amorphous silicon carbide (hydrogen-rich, phosphorous-doped modification a-SiC:H coating with two main functions: (i) to reduce the thrombogenic properties of metal stents and (ii) to promote regenerative endothelial coverage. It is deposited onto the surface of the stent through a plasma-enhanced chemical vapor deposition technique.

The coating acts mainly by inhibiting unwanted interactions between stent and surrounding tissue which promote platelet aggregation, leukocyte and complement activation, smooth muscle cell proliferation, and other reactions favoring thrombus formation and neointimal hyperplasia.

PROBIO is a "non-activating passive" biomaterial that blocks the electron transfer processes on the stent surface. The latter phenomenon results from the contact between the metal platform and blood cells and is ultimately responsible for the transformation of fibrinogen to fibrin. The unique PROBIO electronic structure inhibits the deposition and activation of cells and proteins on the stent surface. Moreover, this coating reduces metal ion (cobalt, tungsten, nickel, and chromium) diffusion from the stent platform by creating a diffusion barrier that seals the bare metal surface and prevents corrosion and the associated immune vessel reaction [3].

PROBIO has also been proved to facilitate endothelial coverage: endothelial cells (the best interface between blood and vessel) have shown a superior ability to form a continuous layer on the PROBIO-coated stent surface than on the 316 L stent surface [4].

Carrie et al. [5] evaluated the performance of the a-SiC:H coated stainless steel Tenax stent in 241 moderate-risk patients: successful deployment without procedural or clinical events were recorded in 95.4% of patients, with a 7.1% 1-year target lesion revascularization (TLR) rate and 15.8% 1-year incidence of major adverse cardiac events (MACE). The Tenax for the Prevention of Restenosis and Acute Thrombotic Complications, a Useful Stent Trial in Patients with ACS (TRUST) study randomly assigned 485 patients with unstable angina to percutaneous coronary intervention (PCI) with a Tenax stent or non-coated stent. In the subgroup of patients with Braunwald IIIB symptoms, those receiving a Tenax stent, compared to those receiving a non-coated stent, had a lower incidence of death, myocardial infarction (MI), or ischemia-driven target vessel revascularization (TVR) at 6 months (4.7% vs. 15.3%; p = 0.02) with a trend to reduced events at 9- and 18-month follow-up [6].

PRO-Kinetic Energy

The PRO-Kinetic coronary stent system is a cobalt chromium alloy tubular stent sculpted by laser from a single tube of L-605 CoCr alloy, pre-mounted on a semi-compliant, low profile balloon. The stent consists of circular segments at each end followed by a transition zone and helicoidally arranged struts in the middle. Each loop of the helix is connected to the next loop by three longitudinal struts. The three main stent components have a specific role: (i) helical meanders give flexibility to the stent and allow a smooth crimped profile; (ii) wedge-shaped transitions at the stent ends allow consistent scaffolding throughout the entire length of the stent; (iii) longitudinal connectors provide stability and support. The strut thickness is 60 μm/0.0024 inch per 2.0–3.0 mm stent, 80 μm/0.0031 inch per 3.5–4.0 mm stent, and 120 μm/0.0047 inch per 4.5–5.0 mm stent. The delivery system consists of a rapid exchange catheter (5 Fr compatible) with the PANTERA balloon (made of semi-crystalline co-polymer material); the enhanced force transmission (EFT) shaft improves kink resistance and pushability

Interventional Cardiology: Principles and Practice, Second Edition. Edited by George D. Dangas, Carlo Di Mario, and Nicholas N. Kipshidze.
© 2017 John Wiley & Sons, Ltd. Published 2017 by John Wiley & Sons, Ltd.

because of the gradual transition from the proximal to the distal part of the shaft. Device crimping is achieved through an advanced thermal technique ensuring secure stent retention forces as well as a smooth, low crossing profile (0.95 mm/0.037 inch).

Clinical evidence

The PRO-Heal registry included 145 patients with symptomatic coronary artery disease (CAD) treated with the PRO-Kinetic stent (161 lesions, 59% B2 and C lesions according to AHA/ACC classification) at a single German center, between February 2006 and June 2007. Procedural success was achieved for almost all patients (141/145, 97.2%). After 6 months, late lumen loss (LLL) was 0.75 ± 0.71 mm (in-stent) and 0.79 ± 0.72 mm (in-segment); TLR occurred in 4.9% of patients and the MACE rate was 5.6%. These results were considered encouraging and achieved through the beneficial effect of the passive coating on endothelial coverage [7].

Kornowski *et al.* [4] conducted a single-center, non-randomized, consecutive registry to evaluate the short and intermediate-term clinical performance of the PRO-Kinetic coronary stent in 515 all-comers patients (540 lesions) with moderate–high clinical and angiographic profile risk. At 6 months they reported a MACE rate of 8.7% (3.5% mortality, 1.9% cardiac mortality, 1.4% of any MI, TVR 6.4%).

The larger MULTIBENE study was a prospective, non-randomized study including 202 patients with single de novo lesions treated with the PRO-Kinetic stent at 10 European sites. At 6 months, the primary endpoint, target vessel failure (TVF), defined as a composite of cardiac death, MI, and TVR, occurred in 10.9% of patients while the rate of MACE (a composite of cardiac death, MI, TLR, and coronary artery bypass graft, CABG) was 11.4%. No cardiac death or stent thrombosis (ST) occurred. In-segment LLL was 0.66 ± 0.61 mm and binary restenosis was 20.8%, as determined in the angiographic subgroup including 72 subjects [8].

The ENERGY registry was a prospective, non-randomized, multi-center, observational registry evaluating the safety and effectiveness of the PRO-Kinetic stent in 1016 all-comers patients (1074 lesions, 61% A/B1). MACE (composite of cardiac death, MI, and clinically driven TLR) rates at 6, 12, and 24 months were 4.9%, 8.1%, and 9.4%; TLR rates were 2.8%, 4.9%, and 5.4%; and definite ST rates were 0.5%, 0.6%, and 0.6%, respectively [9].

The Efficacy and Safety of PRO-Kinetic Metal Alloy Stent in Hospitalized Patients with Acute ST-Elevation Myocardial Infarction (PROMETHEUS) was a prospective, open-label, single-arm cohort design involving multiple Korean sites. A total of 64 patients undergoing primary PCI were enrolled. Procedural success was achieved in 100% of the lesions. There was one case of in-hospital death resulting from cardiac tamponade. At 6 months' clinical follow-up, the rate of MACE (defined as all-cause death, new MI, and TLR) was 7.8% with TLR occurring in four patients (6.3%). Angiographic follow-up data were available for 42 patients (65.6%) and showed an in-stent LLL of 1.02 ± 0.62 mm and in-segment LLL of 0.99 ± 0.64 mm. Binary restenosis occurred in 53% of lesions with reference vessel diameters (RVDs) ≤ 3.0 mm, 25% of lesions with RVDs between 3.0 and 3.5 mm, and 0% of lesions with RVDs >3.5 mm ($p = 0.006$), suggesting a better performance of the stent in large vessels [10].

Similar results were reported for a retrospective study on a cohort of 117 patients presenting with acute coronary syndrome (32% unstable angina, 36% non-ST-segment elevation myocardial infarction (NSTEMI), 33% ST-segment elevation myocardial infarction (STEMI). MACE rates were 8.5% and 11.1% at 6 and 12 months' follow-up, respectively. The incidence of cardiac death, MI, and

TLR was 2.6%, 3.4%, and 2.6%, respectively, at 6 months, and 4.3%, 4.3%, 2.6%, respectively, at 12 months [11].

In the PRO-Vision Study, the PRO-Kinetic stent was compared with an uncoated stent with the same alloy (MULTI-LINK VISION; Abbott Vascular, Santa Clara, CA, USA) in terms of 1-year rate of TLR (defined as either reintervention in the stent, including 5-mm proximal and distal margins, or CABG because of restenosis). In the PRO-Kinetic group (n = 1353) TLR was significantly higher (9.0% vs. 5.6%; unadjusted OR 1.61, 95% CI 1.24–2.08; p <0.001) than the Vision group (n = 1378). Even after adjustment for multiple factors (post-intervention minimal luminal diameter, total implanted stent length, NSTEMI or unstable angina at presentation, triple vessel stenting), the use of PRO-Kinetic stents remained an independent predictor for revascularization (adjusted OR 1.57, 95% CI 1.18–2.10; p = 0.002) [12].

The BIOHELIX-I (NCT01612767) is a prospective, non-randomized, multicenter study to support the US Food and Drug Administration approval of the PRO-Kinetic stent. It has recently completed the enrolment of 329 patients in the USA, Europe, and South America. The primary endpoint for the study is the rate of TVF, encompassing cardiac death, MI, and ischemia-driven TVR, 9 months after stent implantation.

Orsiro

The Orsiro stent consists of an ultrathin (60 μm) CoCr alloy platform with a hybrid combination of passive and active coatings: the PROBIO (silicon carbide) and the high molecular poly-L lactic acid (PLLA) polymer. This polymer compound is used as a carrier for the supply and release of sirolimus and completely degrades during a period of 12–24 months (Figure 36.1). PLLA and the drug are mixed in a matrix (BIOlute) that completely coats the stent body surface; it has an asymmetric thickness (7.5 μm abluminal and

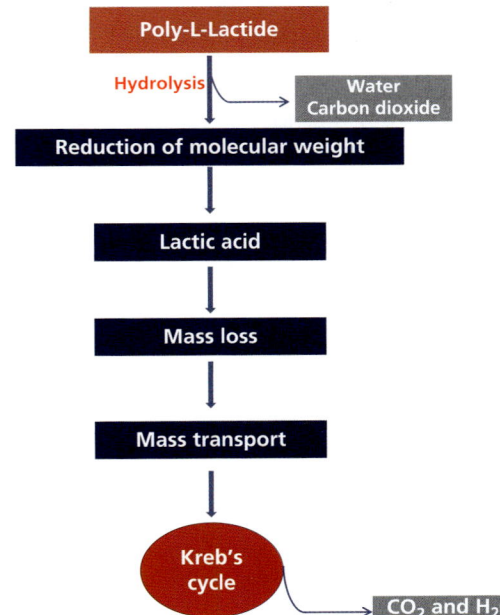

Figure 36.1 Metabolism of poly-L-lactic acid (PLLA). Hydrolysis of PLLA results in the loss of molecular weight, and reduction in strength and mass; ultimately the PLLA is metabolized into lactic acid, carbon dioxide (CO_2), and water (H_2O).

3.5 μm luminal) enabling a greater drug dose on the abluminal side. The drug load is 1.4 μg/mm^2 stent surface. The thickness of the coated stent struts is 60 μm for stents with a nominal diameter of 2.25–3.0 mm and 80 μm for the two larger sizes (3.50–4.00 mm).

Clinical evidence

Table 36.1 provides an overview of completed and ongoing studies evaluating the performance of the Orsiro stent.

The BIOFLOW-I was a prospective first-in-man trial including 30 patients with significant (diameter stenosis 50–90%) single de novo lesion in one coronary artery (with a reference vessel diameter between 2.5 and 3.5 mm and lesion length ≤22 mm) treated with the Orsiro stent at two sites in Romania. Patients were all followed up with angiography at 4 and 9 months and a small subgroup (15 patients) also had a concomitant intravascular ultrasound (IVUS) evaluation. Angiographic LLL was 0.12 ± 0.19 mm and 0.05 ± 0.22 mm at 4 and 9 months, respectively. At 1 year, the composite MACE (cardiac death, ischemia-driven TLR, and target vessel MI) was 10%. There was no report of ST. The IVUS analysis showed that the majority of patients did not develop any neointimal hyperplasia with a volume obstruction not measurable (0%) and extremely small (0.07%) at 4 and 9-month follow-up, respectively [13].

The multicenter, randomized BIOFLOW-II trial established the non-inferiority of the Orsiro stent compared to the durable polymer everolimus-eluting Xience stent (X-EES) in a total of 452 patients with stable or unstable CAD. The primary endpoint, LLL at 9 months, was 0.10 ± 0.32 mm in the Orsiro group vs. 0.11 ± 0.29 mm in the X-EES group (95% CI 0.06–0.07; p for non-inferiority <0.0001). At 1 year, similar rates of target lesion failure (TLF) were reported (6.5% vs. 8.0%, HR 0.82, 95% CI 0.40–1.68, log rank test; p = 0.58) without cases of ST. This trend was confirmed at 2 years in the overall population (10.0% vs. 8.4%; p = 0.5648) as well as in the diabetic subgroup (n = 128, 9.7% vs. 9.1%; p = 0.8975) and in patients with small vessels disease (n = 259, 9.4% vs. 13.3%; p = 0.3153).

At 9 months, two subgroups of patients were followed up with serial optical coherence tomography (OCT) and IVUS (n = 55 and 56, respectively). OCT showed similar neointimal thickness among lesions allocated to Orsiro and X-EES (0.10 ± 0.04 mm^2 vs. 0.11 ± 0.04 mm^2; p = 0.37) whereas a potential difference in neointimal area at follow-up was argued by IVUS (Orsiro: 0.16 ± 0.33 mm^2 vs. X-EES: 0.43 ± 0.56 mm^2; p = 0.04) [14,15].

The multicenter randomized BIOSCIENCE trial proved the non-inferiority of the Orsiro stent to the X-EES in a broad population including 2119 patients with stable CAD or acute coronary syndromes (ACS). There was no significant difference in the rate of the primary endpoint, TLF (composite of cardiac death, target vessel MI, and clinically indicated TLR) at 12 months: 6.5% in patients assigned to the Orsiro group (n = 1063) and 6.6% in patients assigned to the X-EES group (n = 1056) (p for non-inferiority <0.0004). Similarly, no significant differences were reported for definite ST (0.9% vs. 0.4%; p = 0.16) (Figure 36.2). This trend was preserved up to 2-year follow-up (TLF 10.5% vs. 10.4%, RR 1.00, 95% CI 0.77–1.31; p = 0.979). Two pre-specified subgroup analyses were performed to assess the outcomes in patients with STEMI at presentation (n = 407) and in patients with diabetes mellitus (n = 486). Improved clinical outcomes were reported for STEMI patients treated with the Orsiro as compared with the X-EES (TLF 3.3% vs. 8.7%, RR 0.38, 95% CI 0.16–0.91; p = 0.014) whereas the non-inferiority to the X-EES was confirmed among the high-risk diabetic patients (TLF 10.9% vs. 9.3%, RR 1.19, 95% CI 0.67–2.10; p = 0.56) [16,17].

In order to monitor the performance of the Orsiro in the real-world practice, the BIOFLOW-III was initiated as an international, prospective, multicenter, open-label study. It included 1356 all-comers patients between August 2011 and March 2012. At 1 year, the primary endpoint (TLF defined as composite of cardiac death, target vessel Q-wave or non-Q wave MI, emergent CABG, clinically driven TLR) occurred in 5.1% of patients. A comparable performance was reported in subgroups of patients with multivessel disease and acute MI [18].

In the prospective multicenter HATTRICK-OCT study, 44 patients presenting with ACS were randomly assigned (1 : 1) to be implanted with the Orsiro stent or with the Resolute zotarolimus-eluting stent (R-ZES) with the aim of comparing tissue coverage and apposition by OCT after 3 months. The percentages of uncovered and malapposed struts were significantly lower in patients treated with the Orsiro (3.9% and 2.6% vs. 8.9% and 5.3%, respectively). To test the effect of stent composition on coronary vasodilator function, coronary flow reserve (CFR) was also measured at the procedure. However, no significant differences were found [19].

The SORT OUT VII compared the efficacy and safety of the Orsiro stent and the Nobori stent in 2525 all-comers patients. At 1 year, the primary endpoint (TLF defined as a composite of cardiac death, MI not related to other than index lesion, and TLR) occurred in 3.8% of patients receiving the Orsiro stent and in 4.6% of patients receiving the Nobori stent (p for non-inferiority <0.0001). Moreover, patients treated with the Orsiro experienced a significantly lower rate of definite ST (0.4% vs. 1.2%, RR 0.33, 95% CI 0.12–0.92; p = 0.03) [20].

Absorbable metal scaffolds

The evolution of the Biotronik Absorbable Magnesium Scaffolds is depicted in Table 36.2.

Magnesium in bioresorbable devices

Magnesium is a mineral with an essential role for human physiology: it is responsible for bone metabolism, supports the immune functions, helps to maintain normal muscle and nerve function, and has a role in maintaining a normal heart rhythm. It is also a biocompatible metal whose two major limitations are low corrosion resistance and insufficient mechanical strength. As consequence, alloys with other metals such as calcium, zinc, manganese, and other rare earth elements have been developed for specific use into bioresorbable and biocompatible implant materials. These alloys have a strength-to-weight ratio comparable with that of strong aluminum alloys and alloy steels [21]. Because of its unique electrochemical properties, magnesium is more electronegative than other metals used for implants and has shown antithrombogenic properties *in vivo* [22,23]. Heublein *et al.* [24] were the first to investigate magnesium alloys for cardiovascular stents. They implanted an AE21 alloy stent in the coronary artery of experimental animals and observed a negligible inflammatory response up to 56 days. The Lekton Magic coronary stent (made of the WE43 magnesium alloy) was then produced by Biotronik and tested in porcine coronary arteries. Despite not being associated with larger lumen, at 28 days and 3 months neointimal area was significantly lower in magnesium alloy stent vessel segments than stainless steel vessel segments [25].

The first successful implantation of a biodegradable metal stent in human was performed by Zartner *et al.* [26] in the left pulmonary artery of a preterm baby with a congenital heart disease.

Table 36.1 The Orsiro Clinical Program.

Study name (identifier number). [ref]	Design	Country	Patients	Setting	Primary endpoint	Status
BIOFLOW-I (NCT 01214148), [13]	Prospective Multicenter FIM	Europe	30	Stable CAD	LLL at 9 months	Completed
BIOFLOW-II (NCT 01356888), [14,15]	Multicenter Randomized Orsiro vs. Xience	Europe	452	Stable CAD or unstable angina	In-stent LLL at 9 months	Completed
BIOFLOW-III (NCT01553526)	Prospective Multicenter Registry	Europe	1356	Stable CAD and ACS	TLF* at 12 months	Completed
BIOFLOW-IV (NCT01939249)	Multicenter Randomized Orsiro vs. Xience	Asia	~500	Stable CAD and ACS	TVF† at 12 months	Enrollment completed
BIOFLOW-INDIA (NCT01426139)	Prospective Multicenter Observational	India	120	Stable CAD	In-stent LLL at 9 months	Completed
BIOSCIENCE (NCT01443104), [16]	Randomized Multicenter Orsiro vs. Xience	Europe	2119	Stable CAD and ACS	TLF† at 12 months	Completed
HATTRICK-OCT (NCT01391871), [19]	Randomized Multicenter Orsiro vs. Resolute Integrity	Europe	44	Stable CAD	Stent strut coverage at 3 months	Completed
PRISON IV (NCT01516723)	Randomized Multicenter Orsiro vs. Xience	Europe	330	Stable CAD and ACS	In-stent LLL at 9 months	Ongoing
ORSIRO OCT (NCT01594736)	Randomized Multicenter Orsiro vs. Xience	Europe	30	Stable CAD	Stent strut coverage at 6 months	Ongoing
ORIENT (NCT01826552)	Randomized Multicenter Orsiro vs. Resolute Integrity	Asia	375	Stable CAD and ACS	In-segment LLL at 9 months	Ongoing

(Continued)

Table 36.1 (Continued)

Study name (identifier number). [ref]	Design	Country	Patients	Setting	Primary endpoint	Status
BIO-RESORT (NCT01674803)	Randomized Multicenter Orsiro vs. Sinergy vs. Resolute Integrity	Europe	3540	Stable CAD and ACS	TVF[†]at 12 months	Ongoing
SORT OUT VII (NCT01826552), [20]	Randomized Multicenter Orsiro vs. Nobori	Europe	2525	Stable CAD and ACS	Composite of cardiac death, MI, TLR at 12 months	Completed
BIODEGRADE (NCT02299011)	Randomized Multicenter Orsiro vs. BioMatrix	Asia	3850	Stable CAD and ACS	TLF[§] at 18 months	Ongoing
IRIS ORSIRO (NCT02039739)	Prospective Multicenter Observational	Asia	1000	All-comers	Composite event rate at 12 months	Ongoing

ACS, acute coronary syndrome; BMS, bare metal stent; BVS, bioresorbable vascular scaffold; CABG, coronary artery bypass graft; CAD, coronary artery disease; CV, cardiovascular; EES, everolimus-eluting stent; FU, follow-up; IVUS, intravascular ultrasound; LLL, late lumen loss; MACE, major adverse cardiac events; MI, myocardial infarction; OCT, optical coherence tomography; SES, sirolimus-eluting stent; TLR, target lesion revascularization; TVR, target vessel revascularization; UA, unstable angina; ZES, zotarolimus-eluting stent.

* Cardiac death, clinically indicated MI (Q-wave and NQ-wave), or clinically indicated TLR.

[†] Cardiac death, MI (Q-wave and NQ-wave), emergent CABG, and clinically indicated TLR.

[‡] Cardiac death, MI (Q-wave and NQ-wave), or clinically indicated TVR.

[§] Cardiac death, MI (Q-wave and NQ-wave), or clinically indicated TLR.

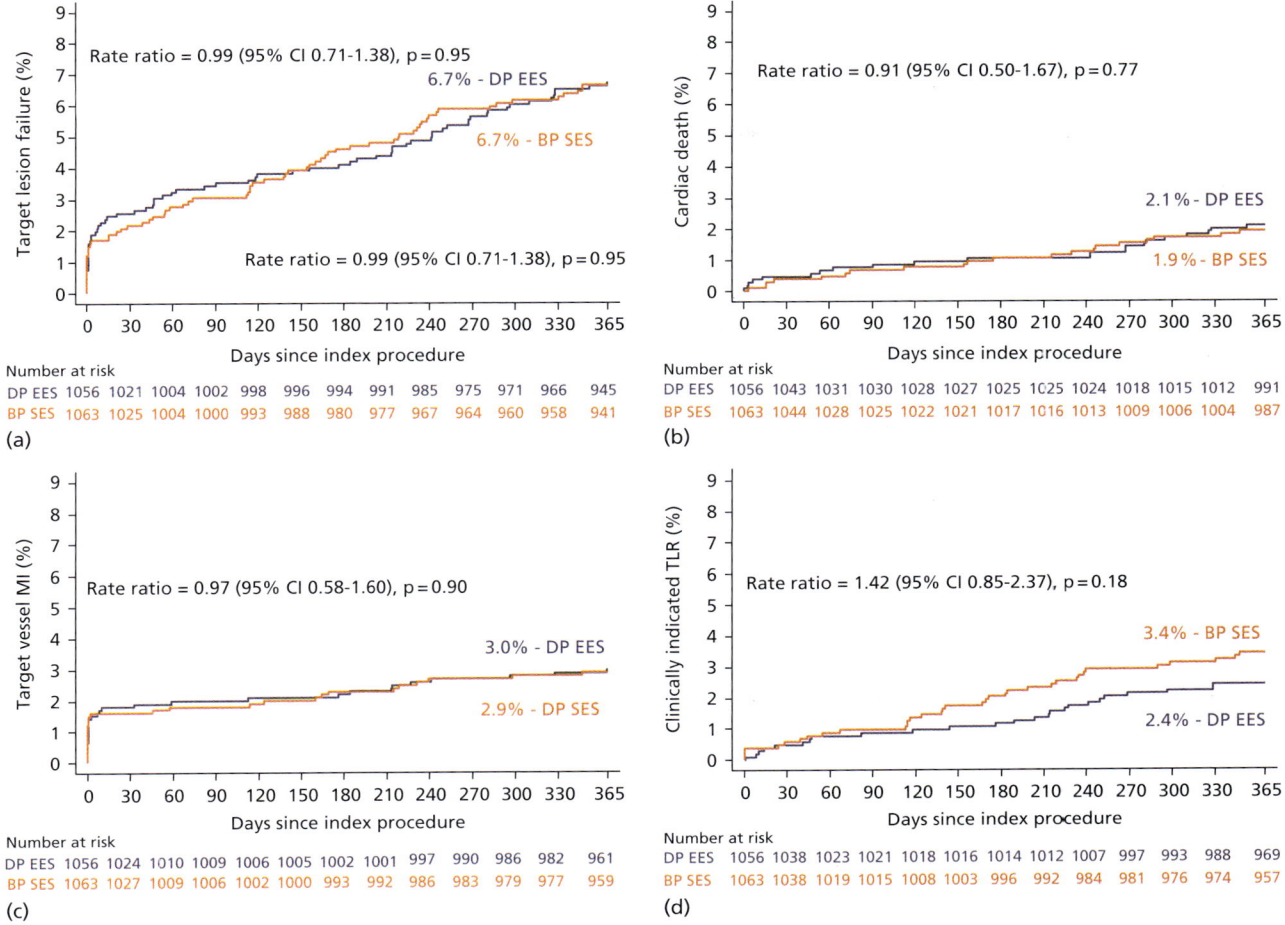

Figure 36.2 Results of the BIOSCIENCE trial. Time-to-event curves for the primary endpoint (target lesion failure) and the individual components of the primary endpoint up to 12 months follow-up. Target lesion failure (a), cardiac death (b), target vessel myocardial infarction (c), clinically indicated target lesion revascularization (d).

First-generation magnesium absorbable vascular scaffold

The balloon-expandable AMS-1 is composed of 93% magnesium and 7% rare earth metal. It is laser cut from a WE-43 magnesium alloy tube into sinusoidal in-phase hoops linked by straight bridges. Strut thickness is 165 μm; its crossing profile is 1.2 mm. It is radiolucent and does not contain radio-opaque markers. The device has a low elastic recoil (less than 5%) and a good initial radial strength with high collapse pressure (0.8 bar), similar to traditional stainless steel stents; however, it only provides radial support for 1–2 weeks. It is rapidly endothelialized and mostly degraded into inorganic ions within 60 days. However, this process does not induce a sustained inflammatory vessel reaction [25].

The PROGRESS AMS was a first-in-man, single arm study assessing the feasibility and the safety of the AMS-1 in 63 patients with single de novo coronary lesions. Although no event of death, MI, or ST was reported up to 1 year, the long-term patency was disappointing with a TLR rate of 23.8% at 4 months and 45% at 12 months. The LLL was 1.08 ± 0.49 mm and resulted from a faster than expected scaffold degradation resulting in an insufficient radial strength and vessel recoil. Intravascular imaging showed complete scaffold resorption at 4 months and the significant reduction of luminal dimensions were attributed for 45% to neointima formation, 42% to negative remodeling, and 13% to an increase in the plaque area outside the stent [27,28].

New magnesium absorbable vascular scaffolds

The findings of the PROGRESS AMS study prompted the development of ameliorated scaffolds to address the exaggerate vessel recoil by increasing the degradation time. The 6-Fr compatible, premounted AMS-2 featured a different alloy (with >90% magnesium, zirconium, yttrium, and rare earth metals) and a new design with a square cross-sectional shape of the strut (no more rectangular) and a reduced strut thickness (120 μm). The new alloy was slower resorbable and with a higher collapse pressure than AMS-1 (1.5 vs. 0.8 bar). The device showed prolonged mechanical integrity, improved radial strength and reduced neointimal proliferation in animal studies but was not tested in humans [29].

The AMS-3 (drug-eluting AMS, DREAMS) was coated with the poly(lactide-co-glycolide) (PLGA), a bioresorbable matrix (1 μm) for the controlled release of paclitaxel (0.07 μg/mm²). The best lactide to glycolide ratio for the PLGA polymer formulation, ensuring the optimal resorption time and drug elution, was established by experimental studies: 73 magnesium scaffolds with different combinations of lactide to glycolide and 36 control stents (18 TAXUS Liberté, 18 eucaTAX) were implanted in porcine coronary arteries.

Table 36.2 Absorbable magnesium scaffolds.

	AMS 1	AMS 2	AMS 3 (DREAMS 1G)	DREAMS 2G
Alloy	WE43	Refined WE43*	Refined WE43*	Refined WE43*
Drug (dose)	No	No	Paclitaxel (0.07 µg/mm²)	Sirolimus (1.4 µg/mm²)
Polymer	No	No	PLGA	PLLA
Scaffold design	4 crown/4 link	4 crown/4 link	6 crown/3 link	6 crown/2 link Two markers
Strut thickness (µm)	165	120	120	150
Magnesium absorption time (months)	1	2	3	12
Trials	PROGRESS AMS	No	BIOSOLVE-I	BIOSOLVE II (ongoing)
Late lumen loss (mm)	0.83±0.51 (at 4 months)	–	0.64±0.50 (at 6 months) 0.52±0.39 (at 12 months)	–

PLGA, Poly(lactide-co-glycolide); PLLA, Poly(L-lactic acid).
*>90% Magnesium, zirconium, yttrium, and rare earth metals.

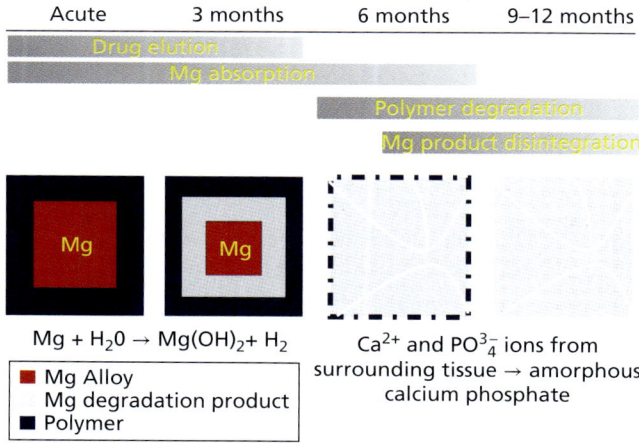

Acute   3 months   6 months   9–12 months

Drug elution
Mg absorption
Polymer degradation
Mg product disintegration

$Mg + H_2O \rightarrow Mg(OH)_2 + H_2$ Ca^{2+} and PO_4^{3-} ions from surrounding tissue → amorphous calcium phosphate

■ Mg Alloy
□ Mg degradation product
■ Polymer

Figure 36.3 Resorption rates of metal scaffolds. Drug release occurs within the first 3 months after device implantation. Magnesium (Mg) resorption starts early through hydrolysis whereas polymer biodegradation occurs at 6–12 months after implantation.

The formulation with 85 : 15 high-molecular-weight ratio was equivalent to TAXUS Liberté and superior to eucaTAX regarding LLL, intimal area, fibrin score, and endothelialization. The study allowed the identification of two phases in the resorption process of magnesium: (i) in the acute phase, the presence of water caused the formation of a mixture of magnesium hydroxide, oxygen, and magnesium carbonate; (ii) later, ions from surrounding tissue form a compound of amorphous calcium phosphate that fills the voids previously occupied by the dissolved struts (Figure 36.3).

The scaffold is balloon-expandable (semi-compliant) and is centered between two radio-opaque markers guiding proper positioning under fluoroscopy. It is available in the following dimensions: 3.25 or 3.5 mm in diameter and 16 mm in length.

The first-in-man BIOSOLVE-I trial assessed the safety and the performance of this device in 46 patients (47 lesions) enrolled at five European centers. Device and procedural success was 100%. The primary endpoint, target lesion failure (defined as a composite of cardiac death, target vessel MI, and clinically driven TLR) occurred in two patients (4%) at 6 months and three (7%) at 12 months (two clinically driven TLRs and one peri-procedural MI). No events of cardiac death or scaffold thrombosis were reported.

The in-scaffold LLL was 0.65±0.5 mm at 6 months and 0.52±0.39 mm at 12 months. Serial OCT performed in seven patients (5791 struts) showed 92.7% of apposed struts at 6 months and 99.8% at 12 months with only 0.1% persistent incomplete strut apposition and 0.1 late acquired incomplete strut apposition. A restoration of vessel geometry was also noted at 6 months, with the angulation of the treated segments reported to increase from 14.9±12.0 immediately post-procedure to 26.1±15.9 at late follow-up [30].

The second-generation DREAMS, DREAMS 2G, has a modified platform (WE43 alloy with 6-crown 2-link design and a strut thickness of 150 µm) with radio-opaque markers (tantalum) at both ends. The scaffold is coated with a bioresorbable polylactic acid polymer (7 µm) and elutes sirolimus at a dose of 1.4 µg/mm². It is currently being evaluated in the BIOSOLVE-II (NCT01960504), a prospective, multicenter trial aiming at the enrollment of 121 patients with de novo lesions in up to two coronary arteries. The primary endpoint is in-segment LLL at 6 months. Clinical outcomes will be assessed up to 3-year follow-up.

PK Papyrus stent

The PK Papyrus (Conformité Européenne (CE) marked in 2013) is a covered coronary stent system indicated for acute coronary artery perforations. It shares with the PRO-Kinetic and the Orsiro stent the common CoCr L-605 platform with the amorphous silicon carbide coating. Moreover, it has a unique single-layer coating made of 90 μm polyurethane membrane through an electrospinning process. The thin coating enables a 24% lower crossing profile in comparison with other covered devices. It is 5 Fr compatible and is available in a wide range of size (2.5–5.0 mm in diameter and 15–26 mm in length).

Interactive multiple choice questions are available for this chapter on www.wiley. com/go/dangas/cardiology

References

1 O'Brien BJ, Stinson JS, Larsen SR, Eppihimer MJ, Carroll WM. A platinum-chromium steel for cardiovascular stents. *Biomaterials* 2010; **31**(14): 3755–3761.

2 Kapnisis K, Constantinides G, Georgiou H, et al. Multi-scale mechanical investigation of stainless steel and cobalt-chromium stents. *J Mech Behav Biomed Mater* 2014; **40**: 240–251.

3 Mahmoodi M, Ghazanfari L. Fundamentals of biomedical applications of biomorphic SiC. In Gerhardt R. (ed.) Properties and Applications of Silicon Carbide. 2011. doi: 10.5772/14471. Available from: http://www.intechopen.com/books/properties-and-applications-of-silicon-carbide/fundamentals-of-biomedical-applications-of-biomorphic-sic (accessed May 2, 2016).

4 Kornowski R, Vaknin-Assa H, Ukabi S, Lev EI, Assali A. PRO-Kinetic: results from an "all-comers" single centre clinical experience. *EuroIntervention* 2009; **5**(1): 109–114.

5 Carrie D, Khalife K, Hamon M, et al. Initial and follow-up results of the Tenax coronary stent. *J Interv Cardiol* 2001; **14**(1): 1–5.

6 Hamm C. TENAX-XR a:SIC-H coated stent versus noncoated stents in 485 patients with acute coronary syndrome: 9- and 18-month follow-up: the TRUST trial. *J Am Coll Cardiol* 2002; **39**(s2): 310–310.

7 Dahm JB, Willems T, Wolpers HG, Nordbeck H, Becker J, Ruppert J. Clinical investigation into the observation that silicon carbide coating on cobalt chromium stents leads to early differentiating functional endothelial layer, increased safety and DES-like recurrent stenosis rates: results of the PRO-Heal Registry (PRO-Kinetic enhancing rapid in-stent endothelialisation). *EuroIntervention* 2009; **4**(4): 502–508.

8 Vermeersch P, Appelman Y, Horstkotte D, et al. Safety and efficacy of the cobalt chromium PRO-Kinetik coronary stent system: results of the MULTIBENE study. *Cardiovasc Revasc Med* 2012; **13**(6): 316–320.

9 Erbel R, Eggebrecht H, Roguin A, et al. Prospective, multi-center evaluation of a silicon carbide coated cobalt chromium bare metal stent for percutaneous coronary interventions: two-year results of the ENERGY Registry. *Cardiovasc Revasc Med* 2014; **15**(8): 381–387.

10 Lim SY, Park HW, Chung WY, et al. The efficacy and safety of PRO-kinetic metal alloy stent in hospitalized patients with acute ST-elevation myocardial infarction (The PROMETHEUS Study). *J Invasive Cardiol* 2012; **24**(6): 270–273.

11 Berlin T, Rozenbaum E, Arbel J, et al. Six- and twelve-month clinical outcomes after implantation of prokinetic BMS in patients with acute coronary syndrome. *J Interv Cardiol* 2010; **23**(4): 377–381.

12 Haine SE, Cornez BM, Jacobs JM, et al. Difference in clinical target lesion revascularization between a silicon carbide-coated and an uncoated thin strut bare-metal stent: the PRO-Vision study. *Can J Cardiol* 2013; **29**(9): 1090–1096.

13 Hamon M, Niculescu R, Deleanu D, Dorobantu M, Weissman NJ, Waksman R. Clinical and angiographic experience with a third-generation drug-eluting Orsiro stent in the treatment of single de novo coronary artery lesions (BIOFLOW-I): a prospective, first-in-man study. *EuroIntervention* 2013; **8**(9):1006–1011.

14 Windecker S, Haude M, Neumann FJ, et al. Comparison of a novel biodegradable polymer sirolimus-eluting stent with a durable polymer everolimus-eluting stent: results of the randomized BIOFLOW-II trial. *Circ Cardiovasc Interv* 2015; **8**(2): e001441.

15 Ruiz-Salmeron R. BIOFLOW-II: A randomized controlled trial Orsiro SES vs. Xience Prime EES – 24 months clinical results. Presented at TCT 2014.

16 Pilgrim T, Heg D, Roffi M, et al. Ultrathin strut biodegradable polymer sirolimus-eluting stent versus durable polymer everolimus-eluting stent for percutaneous coronary revascularisation (BIOSCIENCE): a randomised, single-blind, non-inferiority trial. *Lancet* 2014; **384**(9960): 2111–2122.

17 Franzone A, Pilgrim T, Heg D, et al. Clinical outcomes according to diabetic status in patients treated with biodegradable polymer sirolimus-eluting stents versus durable polymer everolimus-eluting stents. A pre-specified subgroup analysis of the BIOSCIENCE trial. *Circ Cardiovasc Interv* 2015; **8**(6): pii.

18 Waltenberger J. BIOFLOW-III an all comers registry with a Sirolimus eluting stent: presentation of 1-year TLF data in patients with complex lesions. Presented at EuroPCR, 2015.

19 Kiviniemi T. Early vascular healing of ORSIRO-SES vs RESOLUTE-ZES. HATTRICK-OCT trial. Presented at EuroPCR, 2013.

20 Lo J. Randomised comparison of a sirolimus-eluting stent with a biolimus-eluting stent in patients treated with PCI: the SORT OUT VII trial. EuroPCR, 2015.

21 Campos CM, Muramatsu T, Iqbal J, et al. Bioresorbable drug-eluting magnesium-alloy scaffold for treatment of coronary artery disease. *Int J Mol Sci* 2013; **14**(12): 24492–24500.

22 Sawyer PN, Srinivasan S. The role of electrochemical surface properties in thrombosis at vascular interfaces: cumulative experience of studies in animals and man. *Bull N Y Acad Med* 1972; **48**(2): 235–256.

23 Anstall HB, Hayward GH, Huntsman RG, Weitzman D, Lehmann H. The effect of magnesium on blood coagulation in human subjects. *Lancet* 1959; **1**(7077): 814–815.

24 Heublein B, Rohde R, Kaese V, Niemeyer M, Hartung W, Haverich A. Biocorrosion of magnesium alloys: a new principle in cardiovascular implant technology? *Heart* 2003; **89**(6): 651–656.

25 Waksman R, Pakala R, Kuchulakanti PK, et al. Safety and efficacy of bioabsorbable magnesium alloy stents in porcine coronary arteries. *Catheter Cardiovasc Interv* 2006; **68**(4): 607–17; discussion 18–19.

26 Zartner P, Cesnjevar R, Singer H, Weyand M. First successful implantation of a biodegradable metal stent into the left pulmonary artery of a preterm baby. *Catheter Cardiovasc Interv* 2005; **66**(4): 590–594.

27 Erbel R, Di Mario C, Bartunek J, et al. Temporary scaffolding of coronary arteries with bioabsorbable magnesium stents: a prospective, non-randomised multicentre trial. *Lancet* 2007; **369**(9576): 1869–1875.

28 Waksman R, Erbel R, Di Mario C, et al. Early- and long-term intravascular ultrasound and angiographic findings after bioabsorbable magnesium stent implantation in human coronary arteries. *JACC Cardiovasc Interv* 2009; **2**(4): 312–320.

29 Muramatsu T, Onuma Y, Zhang YJ, et al. Progress in treatment by percutaneous coronary intervention: the stent of the future. *Rev Esp Cardiol (Engl Ed)* 2013; **66**(6): 483–496.

30 Haude M, Erbel R, Erne P, et al. Safety and performance of the drug-eluting absorbable metal scaffold (DREAMS) in patients with de-novo coronary lesions: 12 month results of the prospective, multicentre, first-in-man BIOSOLVE-I trial. *Lancet* 2013; **381**(9869): 836–844.

CHAPTER 37

Novel Drug-Eluting Stent Systems

J. Ribamar Costa, Jr.[1,2], Adriano Caixeta[3,4], and Alexandre A.C. Abizaid[1,2,3]

[1] Instituto Dante Pazzanese de Cardiologia (IDPC), São Paulo, Brazil
[2] Hospital do Coração—Associação do Sanatório Sírio (HCor), São Paulo, Brazil
[3] Hospital Israelita Albert Einstein, São Paulo, Brazil
[4] Universidade Federal de São Paulo, São Paulo, Brazil

Drug-eluting stents (DES) were primarily conceived to reduce in-stent neointimal formation and therefore minimize the occurrence of restenosis, the major drawback of percutaneous coronary interventions (PCI) with plain old balloon angioplasty (POBA) and bare-metal stents (BMS) [1–4]. The development of DES has been pioneered through a combination of increased understanding of the biology of restenosis, the selection of drugs that target one or more pathways in the restenotic process, controlled-release drug delivery strategies, and the use of the stent as a delivery platform. Therefore, the clinical effects of DES are highly dependent on each of the components of the complex platform–drug–polymer, as well as the interactions among these elements.

Although first-generation DES Cypher (sirolimus-eluting stent; Cordis, Johnson & Johnson, Warren, NJ, USA) and Taxus (paclitaxel-eluting stent; Boston Scientific, Natick, MA, USA) have effectively achieved their main goal, reducing restenosis across virtually all lesions and patients subsets [5–11], their safety has been limited by suboptimal polymer biocompatibility, delayed stent endothelialization leading to late and very late thrombosis, and local drug toxicity [12–17], which ultimately prompted the development of biodegradable and polymer-free DES systems.

Additional improvements include the development of more modern platforms (e.g., better deliverability, radiopacity, flexibility, and radial strength) as well as the use of novel antiproliferative agents or reduced doses of current approved antiproliferative drugs.

It is important to highlight that the level of efficacy and long-term safety achieved with the current generation of durable and biodegradable polymer DES systems is very high and difficult to surpass. The current focus of metallic DES research is on the development of technologies to promote faster vessel healing allowing the shortening of dual antiplatelet therapy (DAPT) and therefore minimizing the bleeding risks associated with these medications [18,19].

This chapter briefly describes the main recent modifications in DES systems with emphasis on changes in metallic platforms, development of novel antiproliferative agents, and the ways to carry and control their distribution in the coronary artery, highlighting novel durable and biodegradable polymer coatings as well as non-polymeric DES systems.

Metallic platforms
Metallic alloys

Available DES platforms vary in metallic composition, strut design, and thickness. All these parameters have an important role. The main metallic alloys available for the stent platform include 316 L stainless steel, cobalt chromium (CoCr), platinum chromium (PtCr), nitinol, and tantalum.

For the first-generation of DES struts, including Cypher® and Taxus®, the predominant material used was 316 L stainless steel. This alloy has low elastic recoil (<5%), good radial strength, and excellent processing properties. Conversely, among its limitations, relatively low radio-opacity and flexibility as well as higher nickel content, which might trigger local inflammatory responses and restenosis, represent the major drawbacks of this alloy [20].

Most currently available DES systems use CoCr alloys (L605) in their platforms, which can provide superior radial force and better radio-opacity, with significantly thinner struts. CoCr appears to minimize the adverse proliferative response that accompanies the incorporation of other alloys (e.g., gold, nickel, molybdenum, and chromium), while enhancing visibility and flexibility. Although there is some evidence that the strut thickness of BMS can influence rates of restenosis and target lesion revascularization (TLR) [21–23], it is still unclear whether this association applies in a similar manner to DES. Recent experimental data suggested that strut thickness is positively correlated with less thrombus formation on the surface of the stent [24].

More recently, platinum alloys have been incorporated into clinical practice. As potential advantages, this metal is twice as dense as iron and cobalt, more malleable, corrosion and fracture-resistant, which allows the achievement of even thinner struts with equal or better radio-opacity. Also, the amount of nickel in platinum alloys is reduced, minimizing the potential disadvantages associated with this metal.

For novel self-expandable stents (e.g., Cardiomind™, Axxess™, STENTYS™), nitinol, an alloy of nickel and titanium, has been used as the predominant material because of its unique shape memory, biocompatibility, fatigue resistance, and superelastic properties.

Interventional Cardiology: Principles and Practice, Second Edition. Edited by George D. Dangas, Carlo Di Mario, and Nicholas N. Kipshidze.
© 2017 John Wiley & Sons, Ltd. Published 2017 by John Wiley & Sons, Ltd.

Stent and strut design

Basically, there are two stent designs: coil and slotted tube. However, platforms can also vary according to the percentage of metal coverage, number of struts, and strut thickness and morphology. Most of the currently used DES have a slotted tube and open cell design. While open cell stents tend to be easier to navigate in challenging coronary anatomies and also provide easier access to side branches, they also have less radial strength and less coverage of the lumen, which can impact drug distribution in tortuous anatomies. Additionally, to minimize edge barotrauma preventing dissections, current stents have round struts.

Medtronic has recently developed a novel non-slotted tube design consisting of a single, continuous strand of wire formed into sinusoid. The stent is then wrapped in a helical pattern to ensure maximum flexibility and conformability. This concept will be tested in their all-new polymer free drug-filled stent (DFS).

Delivery systems

Although the first metallic stent used in humans for PCI was a self-expanding Wallstent [25], the vast majority of current DES use balloon-expandable delivery technology.

None of the self-expanding stents has found broad application in the clinical scenario, mainly because of the drawbacks associated with this technology, such as the need to precisely match stent size to vessel size; different and sometimes technically challenging release mechanisms; and stent foreshortening during deployment. However, at present, a few dedicated self-expanding devices are being used in niche situations such as bifurcations (Axxess™, Stentys™, Capella™) [26–28], STEMI (Stentys™) [29], and small vessels (Cardiomind™) [30].

Antiproliferative agents

The ideal antiproliferative agent would be able to suppress excessive neointimal growth, with selectivity for suppression of smooth cell proliferation while maintaining endothelial cell proliferation and function. Additionally, it would have a wide therapeutic window and low inflammatory potential.

The antiproliferative efficacy of a drug is linked to its local pharmacokinetics and physicochemical properties (e.g., more lipophilic agents are non-soluble in water and tend to stay longer in the local tissue with better and more homogeneous distribution into the arterial wall) and to the stent strut configuration (e.g., open vs. closed-cell design, stent–artery coverage).

Most of the currently available DES use limus-related drugs, such as sirolimus, everolimus, Biolimus A9, zotarolimus, and novolimus. These agents bind to intracellular receptor FKBP-12 and inhibit the mammalian target of rapamycin (mTOR), blocking the cell cycle of the smooth muscle cell (SMC) from the G1 to S phase [31,32].

Sirolimus was the first member of the limus family to be successfully used to prevent restenosis after PCI. The other currently used limus agents are usually synthetic or semi-synthetic analogs of sirolimus with modification in the hydroxyl group at position C40 (everolimus and zotarolimus) or position 42-O (Biolimus A9), or by the removal of a methyl-group from carbon C16 (novolimus). Although these modifications impact their pharmacokinetics, these limus agents have been proven to be very effective antiproliferative agents in the clinical scenario.

An alternative to the limus agents is paclitaxel, which stabilizes the microtubules, thereby inhibiting cell division in the G0/G1 and G2/M phases. This agent has many favorable characteristics for local drug delivery, such as high degree of lipophilicity and long-lasting antiproliferative effects at relatively low concentrations. However, its beneficial anti-restenotic effects have been associated with local cytotoxicity and cell necrosis [33,34]. For this reason, limus family antiproliferative agents have been preferred.

Polymer coatings and alternative drug release technologies

Polymers serve as the interface between the stent and vascular tissue and function as the antiproliferative drug carrier, also controlling its release. Additional coating layers are found in many DES, and consist of either a top coating, to delay the drug release, or a base coating, to increase polymer adherence to the stent struts.

Both first-generation DES (Cypher and Taxus) used durable thick polymers to carry and control the release of their antiproliferative agents. The permanent presence of these polymers has been correlated to inflammatory responses and local toxicity in preclinical analysis [35–38]. Furthermore, durable polymers used in first-generation DES have been associated with mechanical complications (e.g., polymer delamination and "webbed" polymer surface leading to stent expansion issues) and non-uniform coating resulting in erratic drug distribution.

As a consequence, in recent years, the focus of clinical research has been on the development of novel drug carrier systems including more biocompatible durable polymers, biodegradable polymers, and non-polymeric stent surfaces.

Biodegradable polymers allow drug elution by drug diffusion or matrix degradation while durable polymers use particle dissolution. Conversely, non-polymeric DES systems incorporate alternative technologies such as reservoirs, surface modifications, and nanoparticles to carry and control the release of antiproliferative agents.

Current durable polymer DES

Although the current trend in DES development has moved toward biodegradable and polymer-free systems, three of the most used DES worldwide, Xience/Promus everolimus-eluting stent and Resolute zotarolimus-eluting stent, still follow the durable polymer concept. Both devices have built a strong body of scientific evidence, both in terms of efficacy and safety, and therefore have become the "gold standard" for novel technologies to be compared to.

Compared with the first generation of DES with durable polymers, these new devices not only incorporate more biocompatible materials such as acrylic and fluoro polymers but also change the metallic alloy on their platforms (from stainless steel to CoCr or PtCr) achieving thinner struts and lower crossing profiles to tackle more cumbersome anatomies. Their efficacy and safety has been tested in controlled trials in the most varied and complex patient profiles and coronary anatomies, with outstanding results. To summarize their clinical evidence, two recent meta-analyses showed their superiority over other clinically available devices.

Bangalore *et al.* [39], analyzing the outcomes of 258,544 patient-years of follow-up enrolled in 126 randomized trials showed that among all stent types, the newer generation durable polymer DES (zotarolimus-eluting stent Resolute, CoCr everolimus-eluting stents, and PtCr everolimus-eluting stents) were the most efficacious stents (lowest target vessel revascularization rates), and CoCr everolimus-eluting stents were the safest with significant reductions in definite stent thrombosis (rate ratio 0.35, 0.21–0.53), myocardial infarction (MI) (0.65, 0.55–0.75), and death (0.72, 0.58–0.90) compared with BMS [39].

Windecker *et al.* [40] investigated whether revascularization improves prognosis compared with medical treatment among patients with stable coronary artery disease. In order to achieve this, the authors built a Bayesian network meta-analysis to combine direct within-trial comparisons between treatments with indirect evidence from other trials while maintaining randomization. A total of 93,553 patients with 262,090 patient-years of follow-up were included from 100 randomized clinical trials. All PCI strategies, including POBA, BMS, and durable DES (first and newer generations) were included and compared with coronary artery bypass grafting (CABG) and medical treatment. They concluded that among patients with stable coronary artery disease, CABG reduces the risk of death, MI, and subsequent revascularization compared with medical treatment. All stent-based coronary revascularization technologies reduce the need for revascularization to a variable degree. However, only newer generation everolimus and zotarolimus-eluting stents improved survival compared with medical treatment [40].

Table 37.1 contains a brief description and angiographic performance of most currently used DES with durable polymers [41–45].

Biodegradable polymers DES

Since durable, thick polymers of first-generation DES seem to have a central role in perpetuating local vascular inflammatory reactions and potentially inducing the occurrence of late and very late stent thrombosis, the concept of a polymer that carries and controls the drug release during an proper period of time and then erodes and vanishes from the vascular surface seems to be very attractive.

Most of the systems presented in this section utilize poly-L-lactic acid (PLLA) and poly-D,L-lactide (PDLLA), which are progressively eroded by shortened ester bonds and ultimately degrade into lactic acid. Table 37.2 contains a brief description of the main components of the DES systems reviewed in this section [46–57]. It is beyond the scope of this chapter to detail all clinical trials with these devices; therefore, we focus mainly on the largest clinical studies with long-term clinical data available.

In the LEADERS trial, the BioMatrix™ stent was shown to be non-inferior to the first-generation durable polymer Cypher sirolimus-eluting stent, with respect to a composite endpoint of cardiac death, MI, and ischemia-driven target vessel revascularization at 12-month follow-up (BioMatrix 10.6% vs. Cypher 12.0%, p = 0.37) [46,58]. This non-inferiority has recently been confirmed at 5-year follow-up. Importantly, the BioMatrix stent showed a significantly lower incidence of definite very late stent thrombosis at 5-year follow-up (hazard ratio 0.26, 95% CI 0.10–0.68). The LEADERS trial not only provided the first evidence of improved clinical outcomes compared to first-generation DES, but is also the proof of concept in terms of biodegradable polymer DES.

A pooled data analysis of the randomized ISAR-TEST 3, ISAR-TEST 4, and LEADERS trials also showed that the DES with biodegradable polymers were associated with a lower risk of very late stent thrombosis as well as MI compared to the Cypher SES [59].

Based on the safety findings related to these devices, the Global LEADERS trial is currently recruiting patients to compare treatment with BioMatrix followed by the use of DAPT (aspirin + ticagrelor) for 1 month and than ticagrelor alone for additional 23 months with placebo. This study aimed to include 16,000 all-comer patients and was powered to compare the composite of all-cause mortality or non-fatal new Q-wave MI up to 2 years post-randomization.

However, the utility of biodegradable polymer stents in the context of excellent clinical outcomes with newer generation durable polymer stents still needs to be proven. A recent meta-analysis including 126 randomized trials and 258,544 patients treated with BMS, first- and second-generation durable polymer DES and biodegradable polymer DES failed to show the superiority of the biodegradable DES over new generation durable polymer DES. Indeed, newer generation durable polymer stents, and especially CoCr everolimus-eluting stents, presented the best combination of efficacy and safety in this meta-analysis [39].

It is important to highlight that not all biodegradable polymer DES are the same. While BioMatrix/Nobori are the most extensively evaluated devices in this category, they are still mounted on a thick (>120 μm) stainless steel platforms and their polymer erodes over 6–9 months, which is a long period of time compared to most recently developed biodegradable polymer systems such as Synergy or Orsiro.

Nevertheless, in the coming years we can expect much data on these devices because the majority of new DES programs are based on biodegradable polymer technology.

Non-polymeric DES

Non-polymeric DES have the potential to offer improved vascular healing avoiding the long-term negative effects of polymers. However, polymers in DES systems are intended not only to carry antiproliferative drugs, but also to control their release.

Most of the time, modifications in the surface of the platform are necessary to carry the antiproliferative agent (Figures 37.1 and 37.2). Alternatively, the drug can be directly attached to the stent surface by covalent bonds or crystallization/chemical precipitation or dissolved in a non-polymeric biodegradable carrier (e.g., nano particles) [60].

We will not go into detail on all clinical programs with these devices. Table 37.3 contains a brief description of the main components of the currently available (clinically or under investigation) polymer-free DES systems as well as the angiographic findings (late loss) in their first-in-man trials [61–63].

It is important to note that this is still an relatively new field in interventional cardiology and long-term data as well as larger controlled trials should be expected soon. Among the various promising polymer-free technologies, the BioFreedom™ stent deserves specific mention. Preclinical studies have reported lower injury scores; lower numbers of struts with fibrin, granulomas, and giant cells; significantly lower percentage of diameter stenosis; and greater endothelialization with the BioFreedom stent at 180-day follow-up compared to the Cypher SES. The first-in-man trial enrolled 182 patients who were randomized to receive either BioFreedom with standard dose (SD) Biolimus A9 (15.6 mg/mm), BioFreedom with low dose Biolimus A9 (7.8 mg/mm), or TAXUS Liberte PES. At 12 months, the in-stent LLL was 0.17 mm in the BioFreedom SD, which became the commercially available version.

Based on the enthusiastic initial findings, Biosensors initiated an audacious clinical trial, the LEADERS FREE, which had two primary objectives assessed by two separate primary endpoints: (i) to demonstrate in PCI candidates who are at high risk for bleeding and treated for 1 month with DAPT only, that the BioFreedom is non-inferior to the bare-metal comparator as measured by the a safety composite primary endpoint of cardiac death, MI, or stent thrombosis at 1 year; and (ii) to demonstrate superior efficacy of the BioFreedom by the incidence of clinically driven TLR at 1 year [64]. This trial recently completed enrollment and the primary endpoints will be presented soon.

Table 37.1 Main current durable polymer drug-eluting coronary stent systems.

Stent	Manufacturer	Anti-proliferative drug, dose and time of release	Platform alloy and thickness	Polymer type, thickness, location	Late-loss	Clinical trial
Endeavor™	Medtronic	Zotarolimus (10 µg/mm), 100% released in 2 weeks	CoCr, 91 µm	Phosphorilcoline (PC), 3 µm, abluminal	0.61 mm (12 months)	ENDEAVOR II[41]
DESyne™	Elixir Medical	Novolimus (5 µg/mm), 80% released in 3 months and 100% up to 6 months	CoCr, 80 µm	Poly n-butyl methacrylate (PBMA), < 3 µm, abluminal	0.11 mm (9 months)	Excella II[42]
Promus Element™	Boston Scientific	Everolimus (1 µg/mm²), 87% released in 3 months	PtCr, 81 µm	Copolymer of polyvinylidene fluoride co-hexafluoropropylene and Poly n-butyl methacrylate (PBMA), 6 µm, circumferential	0.17 mm (9 months)	PLATINUM QCA[43]
Resolute Integrity™	Medtronic	Zotarolimus (10 µg/mm), 85% released in 2 months	CoCr, 91 µm	BioLinx (C19 hydrophilic polymer/ polyvinyl pyrrolidinone/C10 hydrophobic polymer), 4.1 µm, abluminal	0.22 mm (9 months)	RESOLUTE FIM[44]
Xience V/Prime/ Expedition	Abbott Vascular	Everolimus (1 µg/mm²), 80% released in 1 month and 100% up to 3 months	CoCr, 81 µm	Copolymer of polyvinylidene fluoride co-hexafluoropropylene and Poly n-butyl methacrylate (PBMA), 7.6 µm, circumferential	0.10 mm	SPIRIT I[45]

CoCr, cobalt-chromium; PtCr, platinum-chromium

Table 37.2 Main current biodegradable polymer drug-eluting coronary stent systems.

Stent	Manufacturer	Anti-proliferative drug, dose and time of release	Platform alloy and thickness	Polymer type, thickness, location and duration of bioabsorption	Late-loss	Clinical trial
BioMatrix / NOBORI™	Biosensors / Terumo	Biolimus A9 (15.6 µg/mm) / 45% released in 1 month and 100% up to 3 months	SS, 112 µm	PLA, 10 µm, abluminal, absorption in 9 months	0.11 – 0.13 mm (9 months)	LEADERS[46]/ NOBORI I[47]
Biomime™	Meril Life Science	Sirolimus (1.25 µg/mm²), 100% released in 1 month	CoCr, 65 µm	PLLA/PLGA, 2 µm, abluminal, absorption N/A	0.15 mm (8 months)	MERIT I[48]
Combo™	OrbusNeich	EPC + Sirolimus(5 µg/mm) / 95% released in 3 months	SS, 100 µm	PLA/PLGA/CAP, 3-5 µm, abluminal, absorption in <3 months	0.39 mm (9 months)	REMEDEE[49]
DESyne BD™	Elixir Medical	Novolimus(5 µg/mm), 90% released in 3 months	CoCr, 81 µm	PLA, <3 µm, absorption in 6-9 months	0.16 mm (6 months)	EXCELLA BD*
Excel™	Biosensors	Sirolimus (195-376 µg) / release profile not informed	SS, 119 µm	PLA, 10-15 µm, absorption in 6-9 months	0.21 mm (6-12 months)	CREATE[50]
FIREHAWK™	MicroPort	Sirolimus (3.0 µm/mm), 75% released in 1 month and 90% up to 3 months	CoCr, 86 µm	PDLLA, abluminal (groove-filled), absorption in 9 months	0.13 mm (9 months)	TARGET I[51]
INSPIRON™	SCITECH	Sirolimus (1.4 µg/mm²), 80% released in 1 month	CoCr, 75 µm	PLA, PLGA, 5 µm, abluminal, absorption in 6-9 months	0.19 mm (6 months)	INSPIRON I[52]
MiStent™	Micell	Sirolimus (9 to 11 µg/mm), 100% released in 2 months	CoCr, 64 µm	PLGA, abluminal, thickness N/A, absorption in 3 months	0.08 mm (8 months)	DESSOLVE I[53]
ORSIRO™	Biotronik	Sirolimus (1.4 µg/mm²), 50% released in 1 month	CoCr, 60 µm	PLLA with silicon carbide layer, 7 µm, circumferential, absorption between 12 and 24 months	0.10 mm (9 months)	BIOFLOW II[54]
SYNERGY™	Boston Scientific	Everolimus (5.6 µg/mm), 50% released in 2 months	PtCr, 71 µm	PLGA, 4 µm, abluminal, absorption in 4 months	0.10 mm (6 months)	EVOLVE I[55]
Supralimus™	Sahajanand Medical	Sirolimus (6.6 µg/mm),	SS, 80 µm	Blend (PLLA-PLGA - PCL-PVP), 4-5 µm, abluminal, absorption in 7 months	0.09 mm (6 months)	SERIES I[56]
Ultimaster™	Terumo	Sirolimus (3.9 µm/mm), 100% in 3-4 months	CoCr, 80 µm	PDLLA/PCL, abluminal, absorption in 3-4 months. Polymer thickness not informed	0.04 mm (6 months)	CENTURY I[57]

CoCr, cobalt-chromium; N/A, not available; PCL, poly-L-lactide-co-e-caprolactone; PDLLA, poly-D, L-lactic acid; PLA, polylactic acid; PLGA, poly-lactide-co-glycolide; PLLA, poly-L-lactic acid; PtCr, platinum-chromium; PVP, poly-vinyl-pyrrolidone; SS, stainless steel.

* Data not published (only presented in international meetings).

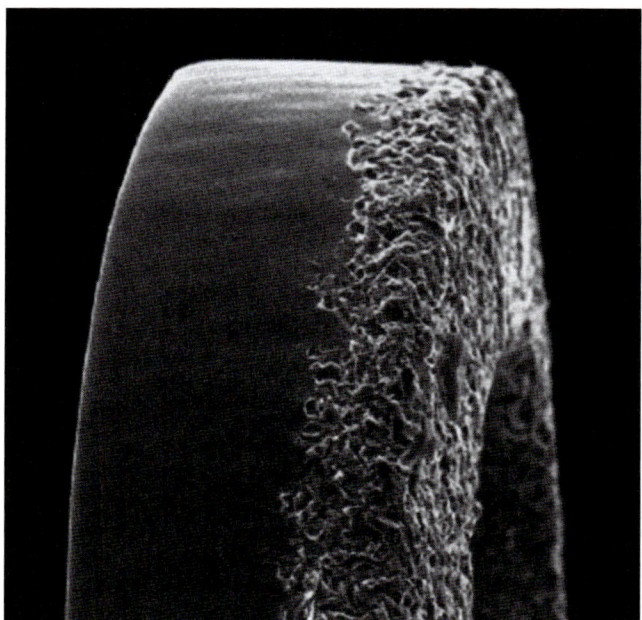

Figure 37.1 BioFreedom™ DCS system: A microscopic view of the stainless steel (316) BioFlex II stent, which has been modified with a proprietary surface treatment resulting in a selectively microstructured, abluminal surface to be loaded with Biolimus A9™. Source: Biosensors International. Reproduced with permission.

Future perspectives

PCI with bioabsorbable vascular scaffolds (BVS) has created interest because the need for mechanical support for the healing artery is temporary, and beyond the first few months there are potential disadvantages of a permanent metallic prosthesis. There are several potential advantages of this novel technology:

1 Reduction in the occurrence of special late and very late stent thrombosis. Once the antiproliferative drug and the temporary scaffold disappear, the possibility of thrombotic events in the site of PCI is considerably reduced.

2 Restoration of endothelial function. Once the "rigid" scaffold structure is removed, the shear stress is restored, favoring also late luminal increasing. Furthermore, the full patency of "jailed" side branches might be recovered.

3 Potential pediatric role because they allow vessel growth and do not need eventual surgical removal.

4 Possibility of vessel assessment with non-invasive imaging modalities such as coronary CT or MRI. The current technology of metallic stents results in excessive artifacts on angio CT, which precludes a definite non-invasive assessment of the stented segment. The absorbable scaffolds allow a clear visualization of the entire coronary tree from day one.

5 Possibility of further revascularization therapies in the treated segments. A current complaint is that the use of a "full metal jacket" to treat diffuse coronary disease might preclude CABG (or even repeat PCI) in case of future failure of PCI. As the BVS will be absorbed, in case of disease progression the surgeon would still have coronary segments to perform graft anastomosis.

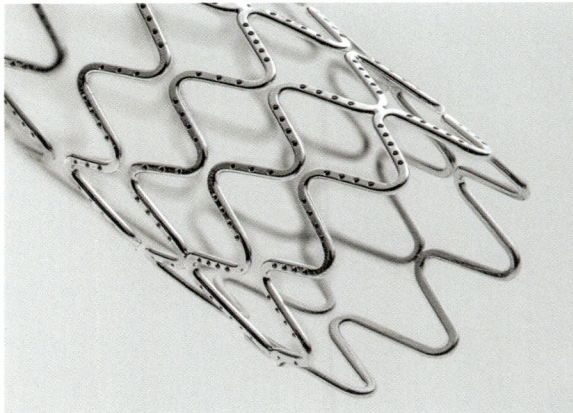

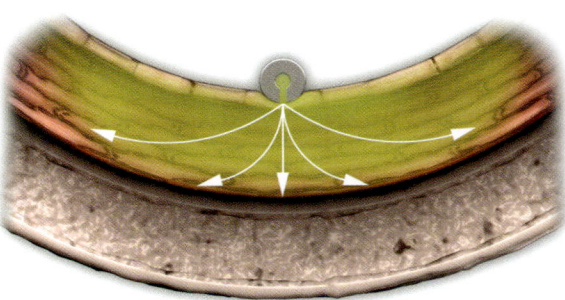

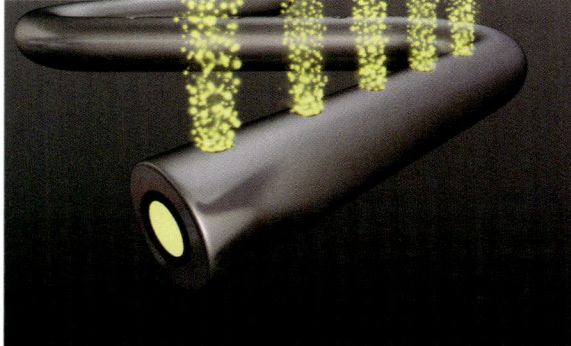

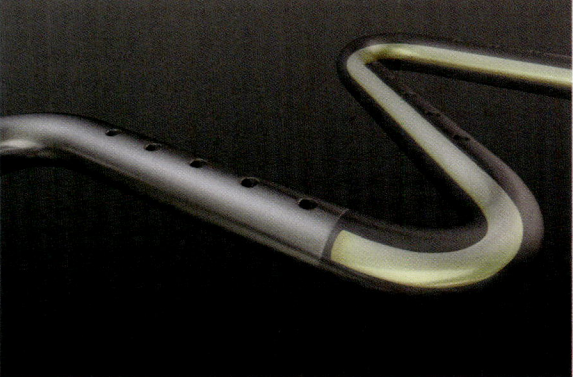

Figure 37.2 Drug-filled stent (DFS). Based on the continuous sinusoidal technology, this stent features a novel tri-layer wire design, with an outer cobalt chromium layer for strength, a middle tantalum layer for enhancing radiopacity, and an innermost core layer which is removed, creating a continuous strut lumen that is coated with drug. Sirolimus is eluted from the core upon implantation through holes on the abluminal surface of the stent, which allows for controlled and sustained polymer-free drug elution. Source: © Medtronic 2016. Reproduced with permission.

Table 37.3 Main current polymer-free drug-eluting coronary stent systems.

Stent	Manufacturer	Anti-proliferative drug, dose and time of release	Platform alloy and thickness	Surface modification	Late-loss	Clinical trial
Amazonia Pax™	Minvasys	Paclitaxel, 2.5 µg/mm², 98% released up to 1 month	CoCr, 73 µm	Abluminal micro-drop spray (crystallization process)	0.77 mm	PAX A*
BioFreedom™	Biosensors	Biolimus A9, 15.6 µg/mm; 90% released in 50 hours	SS, 119 µm	Abluminal microporous surface	0.17 mm (12 months)	BIOFREEDOM- FIM*
Cre8 ™	C.I.D	Sirolimus, 0.9 µg/mm², 100% released up to 3 months	CoCr, 80 µm	Abluminal reservoirs	0.14 mm (6 months)	NEXT[61]
Drug-filled stent (DFS)	Medtronic	Sirolimus, dose N/A, released up to 3 months	CoCr, 81 µm	Elution holes	N/A	N/A
FOCUS np™	Envision Scientific	Sirolimus, 6.75 µg/mm, 100% released up to 1 month	CoCr, 73 µm	Abluminal coating with encapsulated drug by nanoparticles	N/A	N/A
Nano™	Lepu Medical	Sirolimus, 2.2 mg/mm², 80% released up to 1 month	SS, 100 µm	Abluminal nanoporous surface	0.34 mm (9 months)	NANO – FIM[62]
Yukon Choice™	Translumina	Sirolimus, 11.7-21.9 µg (according to stent length), 100% released up to 25 days	SS, 87 µm	Abluminal microporous surface	0.48 mm (6 months)	ISAR test I[63]

Co-Cr, cobalt-chromium; SS, stainless steel.
* Data not yet published (presented in international meetings).

Conclusions

Current approaches to the development of DES are reviewed in this chapter. Although first-generation DES placed great emphasis on efficacy, long-term safety issues have arisen resulting in their replacement in clinical practice.

Newer metallic DES with durable and/or degradable polymer has been shown to decrease the risk of revascularization and ST events. However, the optimal stent design, the ideal polymers, antiproliferative drugs, and their degradation and release kinetics are still under investigation. Nevertheless, there is no doubt that DES will continue to play a pivotal part in the treatment of coronary artery disease, but future designs need to incorporate features that reduce thrombosis and promote endothelialization. Through the integration of mechanical, pharmacologic, and manufacturing endeavors, the development of an ideal DES is within reach.

Interactive multiple choice questions are available for this chapter on www.wiley.com/go/dangas/cardiology

References

1 Gruntzig AR, Senning A, Siegenthaler WE. Non-operative dilatation of coronary-artery stenosis: percutaneous transluminal coronary angioplasty. *N Engl J Med* 1979; **301**(2): 61–68.

2 Serruys PW, de Jaegere P, Kiemeneij F, *et al*. A comparison of balloon-expandable-stent implantation with balloon angioplasty in patients with coronary artery disease. Benestent Study Group. *N Engl J Med* 1994; **331**(8): 489–495.

3 Fischman DL, Leon MB, Baim DS, *et al*. A randomized comparison of coronary-stent placement and balloon angioplasty in the treatment of coronary artery disease. Stent Restenosis Study Investigators. *N Engl J Med* 1994; **331**(8): 496–501.

4 Brophy JM, Belisle P, Joseph L. Evidence for use of coronary stents: a hierarchical Bayesian meta-analysis. *Ann Intern Med* 2003; **138**(10): 777–786.

5 Morice MC, Serruys PW, Sousa JE, *et al*.; RAVEL Study Group. Randomized study with the sirolimus-coated Bx velocity balloon-expandable stent in the treatment of patients with de novo native coronary artery lesions: a randomized comparison of a sirolimus-eluting stent with a standard stent for coronary revascularization. *N Engl J Med* 2002; **346**(23): 1773–1780.

6 Moses JW, Leon MB, Popma JJ, *et al*.; SIRIUS Investigators. Sirolimus-eluting stents versus standard stents in patients with stenosis in a native coronary artery. *N Engl J Med* 2003; **349**(14): 1315–1323.

7 Stone GW, Ellis SG, Cox DA, *et al*.; TAXUS-IV Investigators. One-year clinical results with the slow-release, polymer-based, paclitaxel eluting TAXUS stent: the TAXUS-IV trial. *Circulation* 2004; **109**(16): 1942–1947.

8 Stone GW, Ellis SG, Cox DA, *et al*.; TAXUS-IV Investigators. A polymer-based, paclitaxel-eluting stent in patients with coronary artery disease. *N Engl J Med* 2004; **350**(3): 221–231.

9 Kastrati A, Dibra A, Spaulding C, *et al*. Meta-analysis of randomized trials on drug-eluting stents vs. bare-metal stents in patients with acute myocardial infarction. *Eur Heart J* 2007; **28**(22): 2706–2713.

10 Stettler C, Allemann S, Wandel S, *et al*. Drug eluting and bare metal stents in people with and without diabetes: collaborative network meta-analysis. *BMJ* 2008; **337**: a1331.

11 Kirtane AJ, Ellis SG, Dawkins KD, *et al*.. Paclitaxel eluting coronary stents in patients with diabetes mellitus: pooled analysis from 5 randomized trials. *J Am Coll Cardiol* 2008; **51**(7): 708–715.

12 Nakazawa G, Finn AV, Ladich E, *et al*. Drug-eluting stent safety: findings from preclinical studies. *Expert Rev Cardiovasc Ther* 2008; **6**: 1379–1391.

13 Nakazawa G, Finn AV, Joner M, *et al*. Delayed arterial healing and increased late stent thrombosis at culprit sites after drug-eluting stent placement for acute myocardial infarction patients: an autopsy study. *Circulation* 2008; **118**: 1138–1145.

14 Virmani R, Farb A, Guagliumi G, Kolodgie FD. Drug-eluting stents: caution and concerns for long-term outcome. *Coron Artery Dis* 2004; **15**: 313–318.

15 Feres F, de Ribamar Costa J Jr, Abizaid A. Very late thrombosis after drug-eluting stents. *Catheter Cardiovasc Interv* 2006; **68**: 83–88.

16 Cook S, Wenaweser P, Togni M, *et al*. Incomplete stent apposition and very late stent thrombosis after drug-eluting stent implantation. *Circulation* 2007; **115**: 2426–2434.

17 Siqueira DA, Abizaid AA, de Ribamar Costa J Jr, *et al*. Late incomplete apposition after drug-eluting stent implantation: incidence and potential for adverse clinical outcomes. *Eur Heart J* 2007; **28**: 1304–1309.

18 Palmerini T, Benedetto U, Bacchi-Reggiani L, *et al*. Mortality in patients treated with extended duration dual antiplatelet therapy after drug-eluting stent implantation: a pairwise and Bayesian network meta-analysis of randomised trials. *Lancet* 2015; **385**(9985): 2371–2382.

19 Palmerini T, Sangiorgi D, Valgimigli M, *et al*. Short- versus long-term dual antiplatelet therapy after drug-eluting stent implantation: an individual patient data pairwise and network meta-analysis. *J Am Coll Cardiol* 2015; **65**(11): 1092–1102.

20 Köster R, Vieluf D, Kiehn M, *et al*. Nickel and molybdenum contact allergies in patients with coronary in-stent restenosis. *Lancet* 2000; **356**(9245): 1895–1897.

21 Kastrati A, Mehilli J, Dirschinger J, *et al*. Intracoronary stenting and angiographic results: strut thickness effect on restenosis outcome (ISAR-STEREO) trial. *Circulation* 2001; **103**(23): 2816–2821.

22 Pache J, Kastrati A, Mehilli J, *et al*. Intracoronary stenting and angiographic results: strut thickness effect on restenosis outcome (ISAR-STEREO-2) trial. *J Am Coll Cardiol* 2003; **41**(8): 1283–1288.

23 Briguori C, Sarais C, Pagnotta P, *et al*. In-stent restenosis in small coronary arteries: impact of strut thickness. *J Am Coll Cardiol* 2002; **40**(3): 403–409.

24 Kolandaivelu K, Swaminathan R, Gibson WJ, *et al*. Stent thrombogenicity early in high-risk interventional settings is driven by stent design and deployment and protected by polymer-drug coatings. *Circulation* 2011; **123**(13): 1400–1409.

25 Sigwart U, Puel J, Mirkovitch V, Joffre F, Kappenberger L. Intravascular stents to prevent occlusion and restenosis after transluminal angioplasty. *N Engl J Med* 1987; **316**(12): 701–706.

26 Verheye S, Agostoni P, Dubois CL, *et al*. 9-month clinical, angiographic, and intravascular ultrasound results of a prospective evaluation of the Axxess self-expanding biolimus A9-eluting stent in coronary bifurcation lesions: the DIVERGE (Drug-Eluting Stent Intervention for Treating Side Branches Effectively) study. *J Am Coll Cardiol* 2009; **53**(12): 1031–1039.

27 Verheye S, Ramcharitar S, Grube E, *et al*. Six-month clinical and angiographic results of the STENTYS® self-apposing stent in bifurcation lesions. *EuroIntervention* 2011; **7**(5): 580–587.

28 Abizaid A, de Ribamar Costa J Jr, Alfaro VJ, *et al*. Bifurcated stents: giving to Caesar what is Caesar's. *EuroIntervention* 2007; **2**(4): 518–525.

29 Amoroso G, van Geuns RJ, Spaulding C, *et al*. Assessment of the safety and performance of the STENTYS self-expanding coronary stent in acute myocardial infarction: results from the APPOSITION I study. *EuroIntervention* 2011; **7**(4): 428–436.

30 Abizaid AC, de Ribamar Costa Jr J, Whitbourn RJ, Chang JC. The CardioMind coronary stent delivery system: stent delivery on a .014" guidewire platform. *EuroIntervention* 2007; **3**(1): 154–157.

31 Braun-Dullaeus RC, Mann MJ, Dzau VJ. Cell cycle progression: new therapeutic target for vascular proliferative disease. *Circulation* 1998; **98**(1): 82–89.

32 Marx SO, Marks AR. Bench to bedside: the development of rapamycin and its application to stent restenosis. *Circulation* 2001; **104**(8): 852–855.

33 Giannakakou P, Robey R, Fojo T, Blagosklonny MV. Low concentrations of paclitaxel induce cell type-dependent p53, p21 and G1/G2 arrest instead of mitotic arrest: molecular determinants of paclitaxel-induced cytotoxicity. *Oncogene* 2001; **20**(29): 3806–3813.

34 Blagosklonny MV, Darzynkiewicz Z, Halicka HD, *et al*. Paclitaxel induces primary and postmitotic G1 arrest in human arterial smooth muscle cells. *Cell Cycle* 2004; **3**(8): 1050–1056.

35 Kounis NG, Hahalis G, Theoharides TC. Coronary stents, hypersensitivity reactions, and the Kounis syndrome. *J Interv Cardiol* 2007; **20**: 314–323.

36 Pendyala LK, Li J, Shinke T, *et al*. Endothelium-dependent vasomotor dysfunction in pig coronary arteries with Paclitaxel-eluting stents is associated with inflammation and oxidative stress. *J Am Coll Cardiol Cardiovasc Interv* 2009; **2**: 253–262.

37 Luscher TF, Steffel J, Eberli FR, *et al*. Drug-eluting stent and coronary thrombosis: biological mechanisms and clinical implications. *Circulation* 2007; **115**: 1051–1058.

38 Finn AV, Nakazawa G, Joner M, *et al*. Vascular responses to drug eluting stents: importance of delayed healing. *Arterioscler Thromb Vasc Biol* 2007; **27**: 1500–1510.

39 Bangalore S, Toklu B, Amoroso N, *et al*. Bare metal stents, durable polymer drug eluting stents, and biodegradable polymer drug eluting stents for coronary artery disease: mixed treatment comparison meta-analysis. *BMJ* 2013; **347**: f6625.

40 Windecker S, Stortecky S, Stefanini GG, *et al*. Revascularisation versus medical treatment in patients with stable coronary artery disease: network meta-analysis. *BMJ* 2014; **348**: g3859.

41 Fajadet J, Wijns W, Laarman GJ, *et al*.; ENDEAVOR II Investigators. Randomized, double-blind, multicenter study of the Endeavor zotarolimus-eluting phosphoryl-

choline-encapsulated stent for treatment of native coronary artery lesions: clinical and angiographic results of the ENDEAVOR II trial. *Circulation* 2006; **114**(8): 798–806.

42 Serruys PW, Garg S, Abizaid A, *et al.* A randomised comparison of novolimus-eluting and zotarolimus-eluting coronary stents: 9-month follow-up results of the EXCELLA II study. *EuroIntervention* 2010; **6**(2): 195–205.

43 Meredith IT, Whitbourn R, Scott D, *et al.*. PLATINUM QCA: a prospective, multicentre study assessing clinical, angiographic, and intravascular ultrasound outcomes with the novel platinum chromium thin-strut PROMUS Element everolimus-eluting stent in de novo coronary stenoses. *EuroIntervention* 2011; **7**(1): 84–90.

44 Meredith IT, Worthley S, Whitbourn R, *et al.*; RESOLUTE Investigators. Clinical and angiographic results with the next-generation resolute stent system: a prospective, multicenter, first-in-human trial. *JACC Cardiovasc Interv* 2009; **2**(10): 977–985.

45 Serruys PW, Ong AT, Piek JJ, *et al.* A randomized comparison of a durable polymer Everolimus-eluting stent with a bare metal coronary stent: the SPIRIT first trial. *EuroIntervention* 2005; **1**(1): 58–65.

46 Windecker S, Serruys PW, Wandel S, *et al.* Biolimus-eluting stent with biodegradable polymer versus sirolimus-eluting stent with durable polymer for coronary revascularisation (LEADERS): a randomised non-inferiority trial. *Lancet* 2008; **372**(9644): 1163–1173.

47 Chevalier B, Serruys PW, Silber S, *et al* Randomised comparison of Nobori, biolimus A9-eluting coronary stent with a Taxus(R), paclitaxel-eluting coronary stent in patients with stenosis in native coronary arteries: the Nobori 1 trial. *EuroIntervention* 2007; **2**(4): 426–434.

48 Dani S, Costa RA, Joshi H, *et al.* First-in-human evaluation of the novel BioMime sirolimus-eluting coronary stent with bioabsorbable polymer for the treatment of single de novo lesions located in native coronary vessels: results from the meriT-1 trial. *EuroIntervention* 2013; **9**(4): 493–500.

49 Haude M, Lee SW, Worthley SG, *et al.* The REMEDEE trial: a randomized comparison of a combination sirolimus-eluting endothelial progenitor cell capture stent with a paclitaxel-eluting stent. *JACC Cardiovasc Interv* 2013; **6**(4): 334–343.

50 Han Y, Jing Q, Xu B, *et al.*; CREATE (Multi-Center Registry of Excel Biodegradable Polymer Drug-Eluting Stents) Investigators. Safety and efficacy of biodegradable polymer-coated sirolimus-eluting stents in "real-world" practice: 18-month clinical and 9-month angiographic outcomes. *JACC Cardiovasc Interv* 2009; **2**(4): 303–309.

51 Gao RL, Xu B, Lansky AJ, *et al.*; TARGET I Investigators. A randomised comparison of a novel abluminal groove-filled biodegradable polymer sirolimus-eluting stent with a durable polymer everolimus-eluting stent: clinical and angiographic follow-up of the TARGET I trial. *EuroIntervention* 2013; **9**(1): 75–83.

52 Ribeiro EE, Campos CM, Ribeiro HB, *et al.* First-in-man randomised comparison of a novel sirolimus-eluting stent with abluminal biodegradable polymer and thin-strut cobalt-chromium alloy: INSPIRON-I trial. *EuroIntervention* 2014; **9**(12): 1380–1384.

53 Ormiston J, Webster M, Stewart J, *et al.* First-in-human evaluation of a bioabsorbable polymer-coated sirolimus-eluting stent: imaging and clinical results of the DESSOLVE I Trial (DES with sirolimus and a bioabsorbable polymer for the treatment of patients with de novo lesion in the native coronary arteries). *JACC Cardiovasc Interv* 2013; **6**(10): 1026–1034.

54 Windecker S, Haude M, Neumann FJ, *et al.* Comparison of a novel biodegradable polymer sirolimus-eluting stent with a durable polymer everolimus-eluting stent: results of the randomized BIOFLOW-II trial. *Circ Cardiovasc Interv* 2015; **8**(2): e001441.

55 Meredith IT, Verheye S, Dubois CL, *et al.* Primary endpoint results of the EVOLVE trial: a randomized evaluation of a novel bioabsorbable polymer-coated, everolimus-eluting coronary stent. *J Am Coll Cardiol* 2012; **59**(15): 1362–1370.

56 Dani S, Kukreja N, Parikh P, *et al.* Biodegradable-polymer-based, sirolimus-eluting Supralimus stent: 6-month angiographic and 30-month clinical follow-up results from the series I prospective study. *EuroIntervention* 2008; **4**(1): 59–63.

57 Barbato E, Salinger-Martinovic S, Sagic D, *et al.* A first-in-man clinical evaluation of Ultimaster, a new drug-eluting coronary stent system: CENTURY study. *EuroIntervention* 2015; **11**(5): 541–548.

58 Serruys PW, Farooq V, Kalesan B, *et al.* Improved safety and reduction in stent thrombosis associated with biodegradable polymer-based biolimus-eluting stents versus durable polymer-based sirolimus-eluting stents in patients with coronary artery disease: final 5-year report of the LEADERS (Limus Eluted From A Durable Versus ERodable Stent Coating) randomized, noninferiority trial. *JACC Cardiovasc Interv* 2013; **6**(8): 777–789.

59 Stefanini GG, Byrne RA, Serruys PW, *et al.* Biodegradable polymer drug-eluting stents reduce the risk of stent thrombosis at 4 years in patients undergoing percutaneous coronary intervention: a pooled analysis of individual patient data from the ISAR-TEST 3, ISAR-TEST 4, and LEADERS randomized trials. *Eur Heart J* 2012; **33**(10): 1214–1222.

60 Chen W, Habraken TC, Hennink WE, Kok RJ. Polymer-free drug-eluting stents: an overview of coating strategies and comparison with polymer-coated drug-eluting stents. *Bioconjug Chem* 2015; **26**(7): 1277–1288.

61 Carrié D, Berland J, Verheye S, *et al.* A multicenter randomized trial comparing amphilimus- with paclitaxel-eluting stents in de novo native coronary artery lesions. *J Am Coll Cardiol* 2012; **59**(15): 1371–1376.

62 Zhang Y, Chen F, Muramatsu T, *et al.* Nine-month angiographic and two-year clinical follow-up of polymer-free sirolimus-eluting stent versus durable-polymer sirolimus-eluting stent for coronary artery disease: the Nano randomized trial. *Chin Med J (Engl)* 2014; **127**(11): 2153–2158.

63 Mehilli J, Kastrati A, Wessely R, *et al.*; Intracoronary stenting and angiographic restenosis: test equivalence between two drug-eluting stents (ISAR-TEST) Trial Investigators. Randomized trial of a nonpolymer-based rapamycin-eluting stent versus a polymer-based paclitaxel-eluting stent for the reduction of late lumen loss. *Circulation* 2006; **113**(2): 273–279.

64 Urban P, Abizaid A, Chevalier B, *et al.* Rationale and design of the LEADERS FREE trial: a randomized double-blind comparison of the BioFreedom drug-coated stent vs the Gazelle bare metal stent in patients at high bleeding risk using a short (1 month) course of dual antiplatelet therapy. *Am Heart J* 2013; **165**(5): 704–709.

PART II

Interventional Pharmacology

CHAPTER 38

Basics of Antiplatelet and Anticoagulant Therapy for Cardiovascular Disease

Piera Capranzano[1] and Dominick J. Angiolillo[2]

[1] Cardiovascular Department, Ferrarotto Hospital, University of Catania, Catania, Italy
[2] Department of Medicine, Division of Cardiology, University of Florida College of Medicine—Jacksonville, Jacksonville, FL, USA

Atherosclerotic cardiovascular disease comprises coronary artery disease (CAD), cerebrovascular disease, and peripheral artery disease (PAD). CAD manifestations include stable CAD and acute coronary syndromes (ACS), which embrace a spectrum of clinical presentations, ranging from unstable angina to non-ST-elevation myocardial infarction (NSTEMI), and ST-elevation MI (STEMI). The common pathophysiologic processes of these cardiovascular disease conditions and their clinical manifestations consist in atherosclerotic plaque progression, thrombosis, or embolization. Mural thrombus formation is the consequence either of the spontaneous disruption of an atherosclerotic plaque as in the setting of an ACS or of iatrogenic endothelial denudation as in the setting of a percutaneous coronary intervention (PCI) [1]. Indeed, spontaneous or iatrogenic erosion of the endothelial surface or rupture of atherosclerotic plaque triggers platelet and coagulation activation, leading to arterial thrombosis, which blocks blood flow and oxygen supply (ischemia) in the affected arteries [1,2]. The mechanisms of arterial thrombosis require a close interplay between platelets, endothelium, coagulation factors, and the extracellular matrix of the vessel wall. In particular, arterial thrombosis comprises three basic pathways: (i) platelet adhesion, activation, and aggregation; (ii) blood coagulation with fibrin formation; and (iii) fibrinolysis. This chapter reviews the pathophysiology of the arterial thrombosis cascade and provides a general overview of current and novel antiplatelet and anticoagulant agents.

Role of platelets and coagulation factors in thrombus formation

Platelet-activated thrombus formation proceeds in three stages:

1 An initiation phase involving platelet adhesion;
2 An extension phase including activation, additional recruitment, and aggregation of platelets; and
3 A perpetuation phase characterized by continued platelet stimulation and stabilization of clots [1,3].

Under physiologic conditions, endothelial cells exhibit antithrombotic properties. The endothelial discontinuity of endothelial barrier exposes the subendothelial layer, which contains thrombogenic components, such as collagen, von Willebrand factor (vWF), and other molecules (e.g., fibronectin), which bind to platelet receptors, inducing platelet adhesion [3,4]. This latter is mainly mediated by interaction between the glycoprotein (GP) Ib/V/IX receptor complex on the platelet surface to vWF, which is required for initiation of platelet adhesion under high shear rate conditions, and GP VI and Ia to collagen at sites of vascular injury [4]. These interactions allow the arrest and activation of adherent platelets (Figure 38.1) [5].

Platelet activation and aggregation in the extension phase can be induced by multiple pathways (Figure 38.2) [5–7]. When activated platelets adhere to sites of vascular injury, the local platelet-activating factors help to recruit additional circulating platelets to extend and stabilize the plug [4]. These platelet-activating factors include adenosine diphosphate (ADP), thromboxane A2 (TXA_2), serotonin, collagen, and thrombin [6]. ADP is one of the most important mediators of thrombosis. Platelets express two ADP-specific purinergic receptors: $P2Y_1$ and $P2Y_{12}$ [8]. Activation of the $P2Y_1$ receptor leads to signaling events that initiate a weak and transient phase of platelet aggregation [8]. In contrast, activation of the $P2Y_{12}$ receptor results in activation of the GPIIb/IIIa receptor, granule release, amplification of platelet aggregation, and stabilization of the platelet aggregate [8]. TXA_2 is a key platelet agonist, which derived from arachidonic acid through conversion by cyclo-oxygenase-1 (COX-1) and thromboxane synthase [9]. The binding of these agonists to their respective receptors ultimately activates the GP IIb/IIIa receptor, which promotes the interaction of adjacent platelets through fibrinogen (Figure 38.2) [7]. The perpetuation phase of thrombus formation is mediated by cell–cell, contact-dependent mechanisms, mostly intermediated by vWF under high shear stress conditions, which lead to changes in platelet morphology, expression of pro-coagulant and pro-inflammatory activities, and platelet aggregation [6].

Interventional Cardiology: Principles and Practice, Second Edition. Edited by George D. Dangas, Carlo Di Mario, and Nicholas N. Kipshidze.
© 2017 John Wiley & Sons, Ltd. Published 2017 by John Wiley & Sons, Ltd.

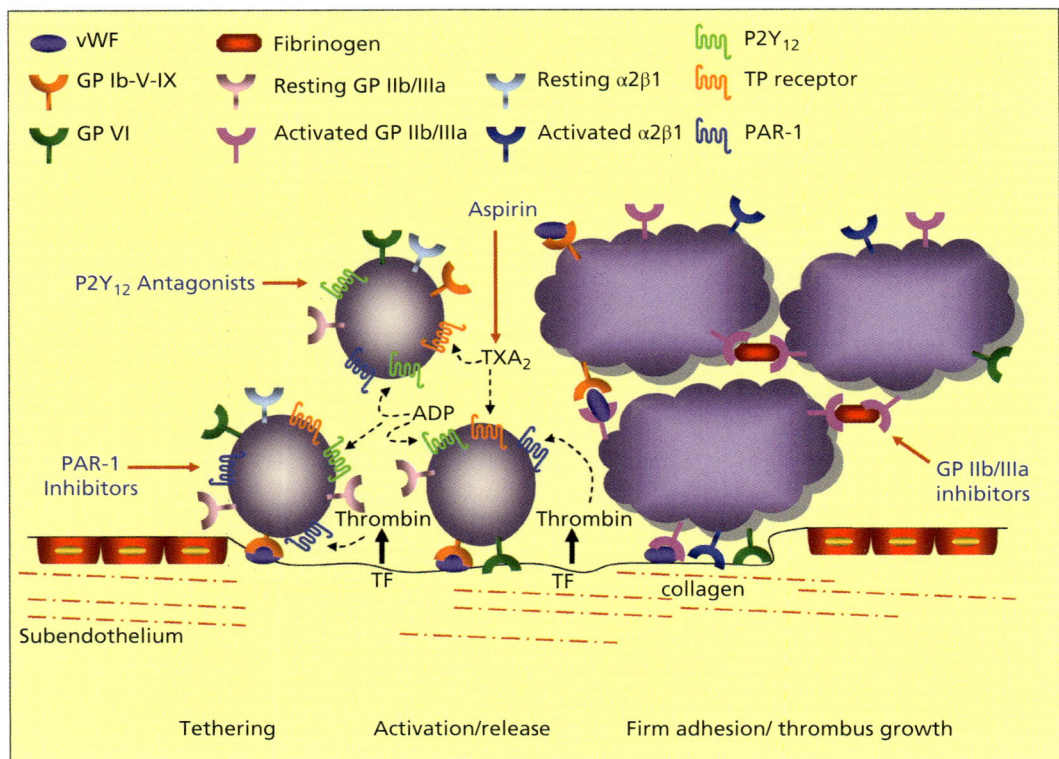

Figure 38.1 Platelet adhesion, activation, and aggregation. The interaction between glycoprotein (GP) Ib and von Willebrand factor (vWF) mediates platelets tethering, enabling subsequent interaction between GP VI and collagen. This triggers the shift of integrins to a high-affinity state and the release of adenosine diphosphate (ADP) and thromboxane A2 (TXA2) which bind to the P2Y12 and TP receptors, respectively. Tissue factor (TF) locally triggers thrombin formation, which contributes to platelet activation via binding to the platelet protease activated receptor (PAR-1). Source: Angiolillo DJ, *et al.* 2010 [5]. Reproduced with permission of the Japanese Circulation Society.

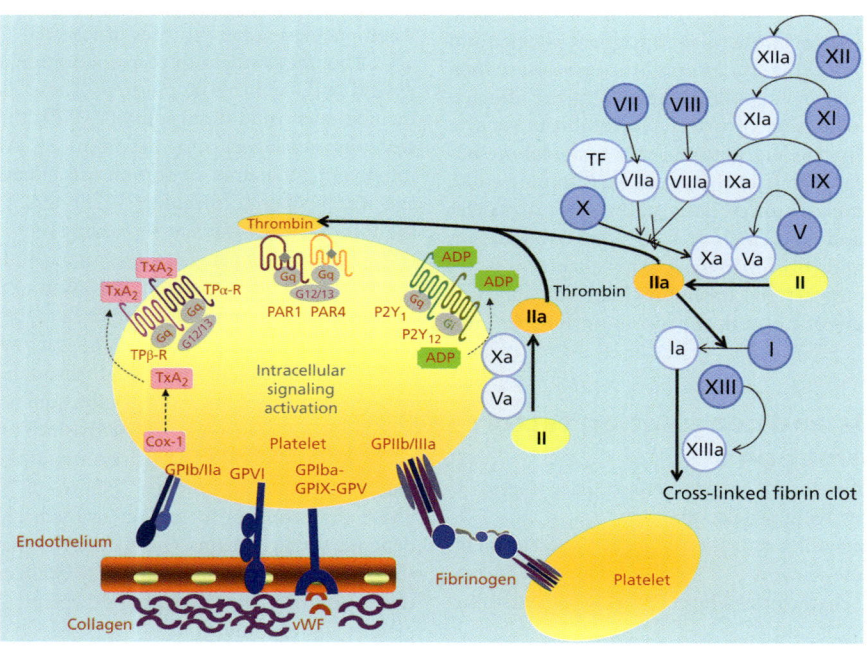

Figure 38.2 The platelet activation pathways and the coagulation cascade. Major platelet activation pathways are those stimulated by TXA2, ADP, and thrombin. These agonists bind and activate their respective receptors, which in turn stimulate the activation of associated G-proteins, ultimately activating GP IIb/IIIa and promoting the interaction of adjacent platelets within the clot. In addition to its role in platelet activation, thrombin generated through the activity of the coagulation cascade or by the prothrombinase complex (factor Xa–factor Va) on the surface of activated platelets converts fibrinogen to fibrin, which adds stability to the growing plug. TP, thromboxane receptor; vWF, von Willebrand factor. Source: Adapted from Angiolillo *et al.* 2013 [7]. Reproduced with permission of Springer.

The platelet clot is stabilized by fibrin derived from the coagulation cascade (Figure 38.2) [7]. Initiation of blood coagulation occurs mainly through tissue factor (TF), a membrane GP that following vessel wall injury becomes exposed to circulating blood and forms a complex with the zymogen factor VIIa [10]. The TF-factor VIIa complex activates factor X into factor Xa and factor IX into factor IXa (extrinsic pathway) [10]. Generated factor Xa initially converts limited amounts of prothrombin into thrombin (factor IIa) sufficient to activate factors VIII, V, and XI, thus amplifying the coagulation process. In addition, thrombin activates platelets triggering coagulation on the platelet surface, through complex formation between factor IXa and its cofactor factor VIIIa (intrinsic tenasease complex), where factor IX is activated to factor IXa by factor XIa via the intrinsic pathway [11]. Thus, Factors IXa and Xa represent points of convergence for the intrinsic and extrinsic pathways. Finally, factor Xa in complex with its cofactor factor Va (prothrombinase complex) activates prothrombin to thrombin ultimately resulting in the formation of a fibrin clot (Figure 38.2).

Thrombin is a very potent platelet agonist that activates platelets at extremely low concentrations (lower than those required for its anticoagulant effect; Figure 38.2) [12,13]. Thrombin-mediated platelet activation contributes to pathologic thrombosis, but preclinical studies suggest it may not be required for protective hemostasis [12–16]. Thrombin-mediated cleavage of fibrinogen into fibrin is more important for hemostasis than thrombin-mediated platelet activation [17]. Thrombin activates platelets by binding protease-activated receptor-1 (PAR-1) on the platelet surface, leading to several processes that enhance thrombus formation (Figure 38.2) [17,18].

Overview of antiplatelet agents for atherosclerotic diseases
Aspirin
Aspirin (ASA) permanently inactivate platelet COX-1, blocking the production of TXA_2 [19]. ASA is rapidly absorbed in the stomach and upper intestine. Peak plasma levels occur 30–40 minutes after ASA ingestion, and platelet inhibition is evident by 1 hour. In contrast, it can take up to 3–4 hours to reach peak plasma levels after the administration of enteric-coated ASA. ASA is the cornerstone of oral antiplatelet therapy for the prevention of atherothrombotic events [19]. Indeed, several large-scale clinical trials and meta-analyses have consistently demonstrated the benefit of ASA in significantly reducing fatal and non-fatal recurrent ischemic events in patients with a large spectrum of atherosclerotic disease manifestations [20]. Although ASA is recommended for secondary prevention in all patients who have experienced ischemic cerebrovascular events or ACS and/or undergoing PCI, it is associated with limitations [21,22]. These include a dose-dependent increased risk for bleeding and residual morbidity and mortality higher than those for more recently developed antiplatelet agents when used as monotherapy in different clinical settings [23]. In addition to clinical observations, measurements of platelet aggregation, activation, and bleeding time have suggested a wide interpatient variability in response to a given dose of ASA, and the decreased responsiveness is associated with a higher risk for atherothrombotic events [24].

P2Y$_{12}$ ADP receptor antagonists
These agents include currently available thienopyridines (ticlopidine, clopidogrel, and prasugrel), and a cyclopentyltriazolopyrimidine (ticagrelor), as well as several compounds in late development (cangrelor) (Table 38.1) [5,25]. These drugs exert their clinical benefit by selectively inhibiting ADP-induced platelet aggregation.

Clopidogrel, a second-generation thienopyridine, has largely replaced ticlopidine, a first-generation thienopyridine, because of its better safety profile and its ability to yield a more rapid antiplatelet effect through the administration of a loading dose [26,27]. The safety and efficacy of clopidogrel has been evaluated in several clinical trials, which have been performed in patients with different manifestations of atherothrombotic disease, including CAD, cerebrovascular disease, and PAD [28–35]. Reduction in the risk of ischemic events observed in trials of clopidogrel plus ASA in patients with ACS and/or undergoing PCI have led to the use of dual antiplatelet therapy as standard-of-care therapy in these patient populations [21,22]. However, dual antiplatelet therapy has been associated with increased bleeding risk. A large amount of evidence has demonstrated a wide variability of response to clopidogrel [36]. Importantly, inadequate inhibition of the ADP platelet-activation pathway increases risk for thrombotic events [36].

Prasugrel is a third-generation thienopyridine, which, as with clopidogrel, is orally administered as a prodrug, needing conversion to an active metabolite to irreversibly block the P2Y$_{12}$ receptor [37]. However, prasugrel is more efficiently metabolized than clopidogrel, reaching higher concentrations of its active metabolite more rapidly, resulting in faster onset of action, enhanced platelet inhibition, and lower interindividual response variability, even when compared with higher loading (600 mg) and maintenance doses (150 mg) of clopidogrel [37–39]. Prasugrel has been compared with clopidogrel in the TRITON-TIMI 38 trial in patients with ACS undergoing PCI, providing lower ischemic events, driven by a reduction in myocardial infarction (MI), and higher bleeding complications, but with a more favorable net clinical benefit [40]. Prasugrel was also compared with clopidogrel in the large spectrum of medically managed ACS patients in the TRILOGY-ACS trial, but failed to show superiority [41]. Prasugrel (60 mg loading dose and 10 mg/day maintenance dose) is currently approved for the prevention of atherothrombotic events in patients with ACS undergoing PCI. In patients with NSTEMI, prasugrel has to be given after coronary anatomy is known in patients undergoing PCI, as pretreatment with this drug did not reduce the 30-day rate of major ischemic events but increased the rate of major bleeding [42]. Contraindications to prasugrel include prior cerebrovascular events (CVA), high bleeding risk, and hypersensitivity. Dose modulation (prasugrel 5 mg) is suggested in older and low-weight patients.

Ticagrelor is a direct-acting oral agent, which provides higher and a more consistent degree of platelet inhibition than clopidogrel, and more rapid time to maximal platelet inhibition [43]. Several studies consistently showed that ticagrelor, in addition to antagonizing the P2Y$_{12}$ receptor, inhibits the cellular uptake of adenosine. The adenosine-mediated mode of action contributes to several specific effects of ticagrelor, including increase in coronary blood flow, improved endothelial function, reduced mortality in

Table 38.1 Properties of current and emerging P2Y$_{12}$ ADP receptor antagonists.

Agent	Class	Mechanism of action	Mode of administration	Frequency of maintenance dose administration	Approval/ development status
Ticlopidine	Thienopyridine (first generation)	Pro-drug, irreversible	Oral	Daily	Approved 1991
Clopidogrel	Thienopyridine (second generation)	Pro-drug, irreversible	Oral	Daily	Approved 1997
Prasugrel	Thienopyridine (third generation)	Pro-drug, irreversible	Oral	Daily	Approved 2009
Ticagrelor	Cyclopentyltria-zolopyrimidine	Direct-acting, reversible	Oral	Twice daily	Approved 2011
Cangrelor	ATP analog	Direct-acting, reversible	IV	n/a	Phase 3 CHAMPION-PLATFORM and CHAMPION-PCI trials terminated 2009; CHAMPION-PHOENIX terminated 2013
Elinogrel	Quinazolinedione	Direct-acting, reversible	IV and oral	Twice Daily	Phase 2 trials terminated

Source: Angiolillo DJ, et al. 2010 [5]. Reproduced with permission of the Japanese Circulation Society.

patients with ACS, increased incidence of ventricular pauses and of dyspnea, and increased creatinine levels [44]. Ticagrelor has been compared with clopidogrel in patients with ACS, both invasively and medically managed, in the PLATO trial, and was found to have superior efficacy, including lower cardiovascular mortality. Although overall major bleeding events were not increased, ticagrelor was associated with increased risk of spontaneous bleeding and higher rates of fatal intracranial hemorrhages [45]. Ticagrelor (180 mg loading dose and 90 mg twice daily maintenance dose) is currently approved for the prevention of atherothrombotic events in patients with ACS managed invasively or medically with no prior hemorrhagic stroke. Other contraindications include patients at high risk for bleeding, severe hepatic impairment, and hypersensitivity. There are several ongoing trials investigating ticagrelor in multiple therapeutic areas (e.g., secondary prevention, PAD, CVA, diabetes).

Cangrelor is a direct-acting, intravenously administered, highly selective P2Y$_{12}$ antagonist, with a short half-life (~2.6 minutes) [46]. It provides, in a dose-dependent manner, near-complete inhibition of ADP-induced platelet aggregation, with rapid onset and offset of action leading to recovery of platelet function within ~30–60 minutes after discontinuation [46]. Cangrelor has been compared with clopidogrel in three large-scale randomized trials in patients undergoing PCI, mostly for ACS. The first two trials (CHAMPION-PCI and PLATFORM), differing in the timing of study treatment start, failed to show any significant difference between the two treatments in ischemic events, probably in part because of a difficult adjudication of peri-procedural MI [47,48]. The recent CHAMPION-PHOENIX trial, using a more stringent definition of peri-procedural MI, has shown that cangrelor compared with clopidogrel significantly reduced ischemic events at 48 hours in about 11,000 patients undergoing PCI, including patients with stable CAD and ACS [49]. A pooled analysis of patient-level data from the three cangrelor trials, cangrelor compared with control (clopidogrel or placebo) reduced PCI peri-procedural thrombotic complications, at the expense of increased bleeding [50]. The pharmacologic profiles of cangrelor make it an attractive strategy for bridging therapy of patients on dual antiplatelet therapy who are scheduled for surgery. The BRIDGE trial compared cangrelor (0.75 μg/kg/min) with placebo for at least 48 hours, with the study drug discontinued ~1–6 hours before surgery, in patients with ACS (n = 210) on a thienopyridine scheduled for cardiac surgery [51]. Cangrelor compared with placebo was shown to consistently achieve and maintain adequate platelet inhibition at levels known to be associated with a low risk of thrombotic events, at the price of an increase in minor bleeding [51].

Glycoprotein IIb/IIIa inhibitors

GP IIb/IIIa inhibitors interfere with platelet cross-linking and clot formation, by competing with fibrinogen and vWF for GP IIb/IIIa binding [4]. GP inhibitors are only intravenously administered within the hospital setting in patients with ACS undergoing PCI and are not used in the long-term care of patients with atherothrombotic disease. Investigations of oral GP inhibitors have been halted as a result of negative results from several large trials. The three parenteral GP inhibitors in clinical use are abciximab, eptifibatide, and tirofiban.

Abciximab is a monoclonal antibody with a rapid onset and a short plasma half-life (<10 minutes) [52]. However, because of its high binding affinity for the receptor, it has a biologic half-life of 12–24 hours. An estimated 30% of GP IIb/IIIa receptors are still occupied by abciximab 8 days after completion of infusion [52]. The efficacy and safety of abciximab in patients undergoing PCI, including primary PCI for STEMI, have been evaluated in several trials, predating the use of clopidogrel [53–56]. Overall, these trials have shown that abciximab significantly improved PCI outcomes [53–56]. When abciximab was compared with placebo in patients undergoing PCI and receiving pretreatment (>2 hours) with clopidogrel 600 mg, additional benefits associated with abciximab were found only in high-risk patients with non-ST-elevation (NSTE) ACS with elevated levels of troponin, but not in those at low to intermediate risk undergoing elective PCI [57,58]. These observations suggest that when adequate inhibition of ADP-induced platelet aggregation is achieved, GP inhibitors should be restricted to high-risk ACS patients with positive cardiac markers. The issue of whether abciximab remains beneficial after adequate clopidogrel loading was tested also in patients (n = 800) with STEMI in the BRAVE 3 trial, showing no benefits in terms of infarct size prior to discharge [59]. However, the infarct size 30 days after primary PCI for anterior STEMI was reduced by the use of an intracoronary bolus of abciximab in the INFUSE-MI trial [60].

Eptifibatide is a small, reversible, and highly selective, synthetic heptapeptide with a rapid onset, a short plasma half-life (mean 1 hour), and a renal clearance accounting for 40% of total body clearance [52]. Recovery of platelet aggregation occurs within 2–4 hours after infusion discontinuation. Several randomized clinical trials have shown the efficacy and safety of eptifibatide in patients with NSTE-ACS or undergoing PCI [61–63]. The EARLY-ACS trial demonstrated that upstream administration of eptifibatide versus provisional eptifibatide after angiography resulted in similar 30-day rates of ischemic complications during PCI in patients with NSTE-ACS [64]. Major and minor bleeding events were significantly higher with early eptifibatide versus delayed eptifibatide [64]. Overall, these findings do not support the use of upstream rather than selective downstream GP inhibitors in patients with ACS undergoing PCI.

Tirofiban is a non-peptide, tyrosine-derived, highly selective inhibitor associated with a rapid onset, a short plasma half-life (about 2 hours), and a renal clearance in that range of 25–50% [52]. The efficacy and safety of tirofiban in patients with ACS/PCI have been investigated in several trials [65,66].

Phosphodiesterase inhibitors

Cilostazol is indicated for symptomatic relief of intermittent claudication from PAD and does not have an indication for treatment of patients with CAD although it has been studied extensively in adjunct to aspirin and clopidogrel. Cilostazol is an inhibitor of phosphodiesterase type III with both antiplatelet and vasodilatory effects [67] and is associated with more potent platelet inhibitory effects when added to aspirin and clopidogrel [68]. During PCI, cilostazol added to aspirin and clopidogrel ("triple therapy") was associated with a significantly reduced risk of stent thrombosis, angiographic restenosis, and clinical ischemic events without increased bleeding risk when compared with aspirin plus clopidogrel, especially among patients with diabetes [69]. An FDA warning indicates that cilostazol should be avoided in patients with congestive heart disease of any severity because of an increased mortality risk. Cilostazol is also frequently associated with headache, palpitations, and diarrhea.

Dipyridamole selectively inhibits the cyclic guanosine monophosphate (cGMP) phosphodiesterase type V enzyme, thus augmenting the antiplatelet effects of the NO–cGMP signaling pathway [70]. In a large ESPS II trial, dipyridamole with or without ASA effectively prevented stroke recurrence [71]. The ESPRIT trial demonstrated that dipyridamole plus ASA versus ASA alone may not only provide protection against stroke recurrence but also against MI or death from vascular causes [72]. Results of the PRoFESS trial showed that there was no significant difference in the risk of fatal or disabling stroke in patients receiving dipyridamole plus ASA when compared with clopidogrel [73].

PAR-1 antagonists

PAR-1 inhibitors block the binding of thrombin to PAR-1, thus inhibiting thrombin-induced platelet activation and aggregation. Preclinical observations showed PAR-1 receptor inhibition does not interfere with thrombin-mediated fibrin generation which is essential for hemostasis [14]. Two PAR-1 inhibitors are under clinical development for the prevention of arterial thrombosis: vorapaxar and atopaxar [74].

Vorapaxar is a highly selective, orally active, potent and competitive PAR-1 antagonist. Phase 1 and 2 studies have shown that adding vorapaxar to ASA plus clopidogrel does not significantly increase bleeding, but may have the potential for reducing ischemic events. These results set the rationale for two large-scale phase 3 trials: the TRACER and TRA 2°P-TIMI 50 [75,76]. The TRACER trial randomized 12,944 high-risk patients with NSTE ACS, mostly already on dual antiplatelet therapy, to vorapaxar or placebo, but was halted prematurely because of a lack of reduction in overall ischemic events and a significant increase in the risk of major bleeding, including intracranial hemorrhage, in the investigational arm [75]. In the TRA 2°P-TIMI 50 trial, vorapaxar (2.5 mg/day) compared with placebo significantly reduced ischemic events, at the cost of increased moderate or severe bleeding, including intracranial hemorrhage, in patients (n = 26,449) with a history of MI, ischemic stroke, or PAD [76]. Notably, after an interim analysis, the data and safety monitoring board recommended discontinuation of vorapaxar in patients with a history of stroke, because of an unacceptable risk of intracranial hemorrhage without an improvement in major vascular events, including ischemic stroke, as also shown by a subsequent subanalysis [77]. In contrast, another pre-specified subanalysis of the TRA 2°P-TIMI 50 showed that in patients with a history of MI, vorapaxar reduced ischemic events but increased the risk of moderate or severe bleeding [78]. Also, patients with PAD experienced less acute limb ischemia and peripheral arterial revascularization with vorapaxar, despite the higher risk of bleeding [79].

Clinical development of atopaxar is still in the early stage. Two phase 2 studies, LANCELOT-ACS and LANCELOT-CAD, have suggested a good safety profile of the drug in patients with ACS and CAD, respectively [80,81]. However, the highest doses of atopaxar compared with placebo were more commonly associated with QTc prolongation and transient liver enzymes elevation. Phase 3 investigations are not currently ongoing for atopaxar.

A meta-analysis of eight phase 2 and 3 trials of PAR-1 antagonists in patients (n = 41,647) with CAD highlighted a higher risk of major bleeding, including intracranial hemorrhage, with the novel agents over placebo, paralleled by a significantly lower risk of MI, which was consistently noted in studies of vorapaxar and atopaxar [82]. Interestingly, a significant interaction was found between bleeding with PAR-1 antagonists and the use of $P2Y_{12}$ inhibitors, suggesting that future studies on these novel agents in patients not receiving a $P2Y_{12}$ inhibitor or studies versus $P2Y_{12}$ inhibitors on a background of ASA therapy might be considered.

Other novel antiplatelet agents

Other agents are targeted to inhibit TXA_2-induced platelet activation mediated by TP receptors [83]. The rationale for the development of TP receptor antagonists (e.g., terutroban) is that platelets continue to be exposed to TXA_2 despite complete COX-1 blockade using ASA. Preclinical and clinical studies are currently ongoing for this family of platelet inhibitors as well as for other targets, including those targeted to inhibit serotonin and collagen receptors.

Overview of anticoagulant agents for atherosclerotic diseases

Anticoagulants are classified according to the target coagulation enzyme that is being inhibited (e.g., anti-factor IIa or antithrombins; anti-factor Xa; anti-factor IXa; Figure 38.3) [84]. They are further categorized based on whether inhibitory effects are direct or indirect (warranting a co-factor).

Thrombin inhibitors
Indirect thrombin inhibitors

Indirect thrombin inhibitors include unfractionated heparin (UFH) and low molecular weight heparins (LMWH). Thrombin has an active site and two exosites, one of which—exosite 1—binds to its fibrin substrate, orientating it toward the active site. UFH binds to exosite 2 on thrombin and also to antithrombin, forming a ternary complex, which is necessary for the inhibition of thrombin by antithrombin [85]. In contrast to thrombin inhibition, inactivation of factor Xa does not require the formation of the ternary complex. The ratio of anti-Xa to anti-IIa activity for UFH is equal to 1. LMWH derived from the fragmentation or the depolymerization of heparin by chemical or enzymatic process. Because most LMWH chains are not sufficiently long to form the ternary complex necessary for the inactivation of thrombin, their action is mainly directed against factor Xa, thereby the ratio of anti-IIa to anti-Xa activity varies from 1.9 to 3.8 (enoxaparin) [86].

The pharmacologic properties of UFH and LMWH are compared in Table 38.2. UFH has important limitations because of quite variable pharmacokinetic and pharmacodynamic profiles, significant non-specific protease binding, the inability to inhibit fibrin-bound thrombin, the prothrombotic effect on platelet activation and aggregation and, finally, the life-threatening risk of heparin-induced thrombocytopenia (HIT). Although to a less extent, part of these limitations are also associated with LMWH.

UFH and LMWH are routinely used in interventional practice as the standard anticoagulation for the treatment of patients with ACS and in the PCI setting [20,21]. In these populations, LMWH when compared with UFH has been found associated with a better overall efficacy profile and similar safety, while being more practical as, unlike UFH, it does not require anticoagulation monitoring and dose adjustment.

Direct thrombin inhibitors

Direct thrombin inhibitors (DTI) directly inhibit soluble and clot-bound thrombin without depending on antithrombin for anticoagulant activity. Indeed, they are physically small molecules that do not interact with exosite 2 but bind directly to the active site of thrombin and inhibit all its proteolytic activity without the need for antithrombin as an intermediary molecule. They have high specificity and potency for thrombin inhibition, and do not promote platelet aggregation. Given their potential benefits over heparins, parenteral DTIs have undergone extensive appraisal in patients with ACS or HIT, and those undergoing PCI. Three parenteral agents are currently available for clinical use in these populations: recombined hirudin (lepirudin), argatroban, and bivalirudin [87]. The oral agent dabigatran, while approved for clinical use as a replacement for warfarin in patients with atrial fibrillation (AF), clinical investigation has been halted in the setting of ACS after the very high bleeding rates observed in adjunct to dual antiplatelet therapy in the phase 2 RE-DEEM trial [88].

Lepirudin is a peptide that binds to the catalytic site and exosite 1 of thrombin with very high affinity. It has a half-life of 80 minutes

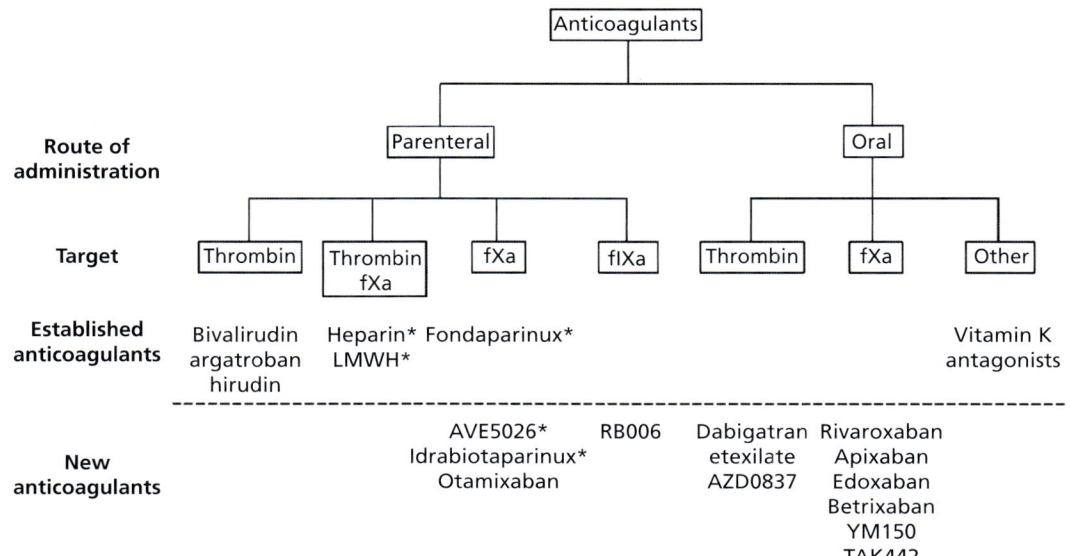

Figure 38.3 Established and new anticoagulants classified according to the target coagulation enzyme that is being inhibited. *Subcutaneously administered. Source: Eikelboom and Weitz 2010 [84]. Reproduced with permission of Wolters Kluwer Health.

Table 38.2 Comparison of pharmacologic properties of current anticoagulants.

Property	UFH	LMWH	Fondaparinux	Bivalirudin
Predictability in pharmacologic profile	–	++	+++	+++
Co-factor required	+++	+++	+++	–
Renal clearance	–	++	+++	++
Non-specific protein binding	+++	+	–	–
Platelect activation	+++	+	–	–
Rebound of thrombin generation after discontinuation	+++	+	–	–
Inhibition of bound thrombin	–	–	–	+++
Neutralization by platelet factor 4	+++	+	+	+
Inhibition of thrombin generation	+	++	++	+++

LMWH, low molecular weight heparin; UFH, unfractionated heparin.

and is cleared primarily by the kidneys. It is approved for treatment of patients with HIT. No studies have evaluated the role of lepirudin in contemporary PCI.

Argatroban is a synthetic peptide competitive inhibitor of thrombin, binding to a site near the catalytic site [87]. It has a short half-life (45 minutes) and is mainly metabolized by the liver, requiring dose adjustment in patients with hepatic dysfunction. It is approved for treatment of patients with HIT. A few small studies have evaluated the effects of argatroban during PCI, and it is approved in this setting as an alternative anticoagulant only in patients with HIT [21].

Bivalirudin (hirulog-1) is a 20-amino acid polypeptide and is a synthetic version of hirudin that binds to the catalytic site and exosite 1 of thrombin. This binding is reversible and is associated with the cleavage near the amino-terminal of bivalirudin by thrombin itself [89]. When bivalirudin is cleaved, the bond between exosite 1 and the amino-terminal of the bivalirudin segment is weakened, leading to the dissociation and to restoration of normal thrombin activity [89]. Bivalirudin has a half-life of 25 minutes, which is prolonged by renal insufficiency, and is primarily cleared via proteolysis, with renal excretion accounting for <20% of its degradation. The pharmacologic properties of bivalirudin compared with those of heparins are listed in Table 38.2.

Bivalirudin is currently the only DTI that has been extensively evaluated in several powered clinical trials with respect to its use in coronary intervention in patients with stable CAD and in those with ACS, including NSTEMI and STEMI [90–95]. Multicenter trials on bivalirudin are consistent in showing that bivalirudin compared with heparin plus GP inhibitors is associated with comparable ischemic outcomes and reduced major bleeding. Bivalirudin is currently approved for use during PCI as an alternative to UFH and in patients with HIT.

Factor Xa inhibitors
Indirect factor Xa inhibitors
Fondaparinux is the prototype of the indirect factor Xa inhibitor. Other agents are variants of fondaparinux and include idraparinux, idrabiotaparinux, and SR123781A. All these agents are

subcutaneously administrated. Only fondaparinux has been investigated in the setting of ACS/PCI.

Fondaparinux, a synthetic analog of the antithrombin-binding pentasaccharide sequence found in heparin, binds to antithrombin with very high specificity, enhancing the ability of antithrombin to neutralize factor Xa and hence the formation of thrombin. Fondaparinux has almost complete bioavailability after subcutaneous injection with rapid absorption, achieving a steady state after 3–4 daily doses. Its plasma half-life of approximately 17 hours allows once-daily administration at fixed dosages. It has a highly predictable anticoagulant effect and thus there is no need for laboratory monitoring. The pharmacologic properties of fondaparinux compared with those of heparins are listed in Table 38.2.

The efficacy and safety of fondaparinux (2.5 mg/day SC) compared to heparin were tested in patients with ACS [96–98]. In the NSTE-ACS population, fondaparinux was associated with superior net clinical benefit compared to enoxaparin [96–98]. In patients with STEMI, fondaparinux compared to UFH reduced the combined endpoint of death/MI in patients treated with thrombolysis, while those who underwent primary PCI had no significant benefit with fondaparinux [98]. Of concern, patients who underwent primary PCI with fondaparinux had more catheter-related thrombi, more coronary complications, and a trend toward higher death/MI compared to UFH. Fondaparinux is recommended for patients with NSTE-ACS in whom an early conservative or a delayed invasive strategy of management is considered and for STEMI patients receiving fibrinolytic therapy. Fondaparinux should not be used in patients with acute STEMI undergoing primary PCI. Despite guideline recommendations for the use of fondaparinux in ACS, fondaparinux is not approved for such use by the FDA in the USA.

Direct factor Xa inhibitors
Direct factor Xa inhibitors include parenteral agents, such as DX9065a and otamixaban, and several orally active drugs, including rivaroxaban, apixaban, edoxaban, darexaban, LY517717, and betrixaban. Only otamixaban, rivaroxaban, and apixaban have advanced to phase 3 clinical investigation in the setting of ACS/PCI.

Otamixaban is an intravenous, direct, reversible, selective inhibitor of factor Xa. It has an initial half-life of 30 minutes and rapid on–off anticoagulant activity. It is mainly cleared unchanged via the biliary system with no significant renal excretion (<25%), suggesting no need for dose modification in patients with renal insufficiency. Because of its predictable pharmacodynamics there is no need for anticoagulation monitoring. The SEPIA-ACS1 TIMI 42 trial showed a marked reduction in death/MI and similar bleeding rates with otamixaban at mid-range doses, compared with UFH plus eptifibatide [99]. These positive findings set the rationale for the investigation of otamixaban in phase 3 TAO randomized, double-blind, triple-dummy trial, in which otamixaban did not reduce the rate of ischemic events compared with UFH plus eptifibatide, but did increase bleeding in patients with NSTE ACS to be treated with dual oral antiplatelet therapy and an invasive strategy [100].

Rivaroxaban is an orally active oxazolidone derivative, which acts by directly and selectively inhibiting both free factor Xa and factor Xa bound in the prothrombinase complex. Rivaroxaban has a rapid and predictable anticoagulant effect with no need for dose adjustment or routine laboratory monitoring. The half-life is 9–13 hours and renal elimination accounts for 33%. It is approved for stroke prevention in patients with AF. A recent phase 3 trial (ATLAS ACS 2-TIMI 51) has evaluated rivaroxaban (2.5 or 5.0 mg twice daily) versus placebo on top of low-dose ASA (75–100 mg/day), with or without a thienopyridine, in 15,526 patients with ACS [101]. Rivaroxaban reduced the incidence of ischemic outcomes at the cost of increased bleeding. The 2.5 mg twice daily dose had the better risk–benefit balance, because of a lower bleeding risk than the 5 mg twice daily dose, with significant mortality reduction [101].

Apixaban is a potent direct inhibitor of both free and prothrombin-bound factor Xa, has a minimal affinity for factor IIa, a half-life of 8–15 hours, and is mainly eliminated via the fecal route (~75%). It is approved for stroke prevention in patients with AF. A recent phase 3 trial, APPRAISE-2, has evaluated apixaban 5 mg twice daily versus placebo on top of standard antiplatelet therapy in high-risk ACS patients [102]. The trial was stopped prematurely after recruiting 7392 of the preplanned 10,800 patients because an interim analysis showed that the increase of major bleeding with apixaban, including increases in fatal and intracranial bleeding, was not counterbalanced by the expected decrease in recurrent ischemic events compared with placebo. Importantly, the decrease in ischemic events was offset by an increase in bleeding both in patients taking only ASA and in those on dual antiplatelet therapy.

Other anticoagulants under clinical development

Investigations are ongoing on novel anticoagulants using recombinant proteins that are directed at the initiation of coagulation targeting tissue factor or factor VII. Another novel anticoagulant approach involves using RNA aptamer technology to target targeting coagulation factors (e.g., factor IXa). The advantage of this approach is the ability to initiate rapid anticoagulation that can be reversed immediately with a complementary RNA strand. The clinical safety and pharmacodynamic profiles of REG1, consisting of RB006 (drug), an injectable synthetic RNA aptamer that specifically binds and inhibits factor IXa, and RB007 (antidote), a complementary oligonucleotide that neutralizes the effect of RB006, have been evaluated in phase 1b and 2b studies in patients with stable CAD or ACS undergoing PCI and receiving standard antiplatelet therapy. In the phase 2b RADAR trial, the REG1 System with reversal from

50% to 100% compared to UFH or LMWH reduced major bleeding and ischemic events in 640 patients with ACS undergoing cardiac catheterization [103]. A large-scale phase 3 clinical investigation comparing REG1 with bivalirudin was interrupted because of serious adverse events related to allergic reactions.

Conclusions

Arterial thrombus formation is the common pathophysiologic process of different cardiovascular disease manifestations. Platelets and coagulation factors are key in this process. Identification of key targets within the platelet and coagulation cascade has been pivotal for the development of strategies aimed to reduce ischemic recurrences. Although recent advances in the field have yielded a greater reduction in ischemic events though their ability to achieve more potent blockade thrombotic processes, this has come at an increased risk of bleeding complications. Indeed, the future of antithrombotic therapies will rely on identifying treatment strategies that are able to find a fine balance between ischemic and bleeding risk. Emerging treatment regimens will represent a step forward toward reaching these goals.

> **Key points**
>
> - Arterial thrombus formation is the common pathophysiologic process of different cardiovascular disease manifestations. Platelets and coagulation factors are pivotal in this process.
> - Key targets within the platelet and coagulation cascade have been identified for the development of pharmacologic strategies aimed to reduce ischemic events.
> - Recently developed antiplatelet agents have yielded a greater reduction in ischemic events but associated with an increased risk of bleeding, especially in specific subgroups.
> - Recently developed anticoagulant agents have more favorable pharmacologic properties and better safety and efficacy profile.
> - New antithrombotic strategies are under development with the aim to find an optimal balance between ischemic and bleeding risk.

Disclosures

Dominick J. Angiolillo received payment as an individual for: (i) consulting fee or honorarium from Bristol Myers Squibb, Sanofi-Aventis, Eli Lilly, Daiichi-Sankyo, The Medicines Company, AstraZeneca, Merck, Abbott Vascular, and PLx Pharma; (ii) participation in review activities from CeloNova, Johnson & Johnson, St. Jude, and Sunovion; (iii) institutional payments for grants from Bristol Myers Squibb, Sanofi-Aventis, Glaxo Smith Kline, Eli Lilly, Daiichi-Sankyo, The Medicines Company, AstraZeneca. Piera Capranzano has no conflicts of interest.

Interactive multiple choice questions are available for this chapter on www.wiley.com/go/dangas/cardiology

References

1 Davi G, Patrono C. Platelet activation and atherothrombosis. *N Engl J Med* 2007; **357**: 2482–2494.
2 Libby P, Theroux P. Pathophysiology of coronary artery disease. *Circulation* 2005; **111**: 3481–3488.
3 Brass LF. Thrombin and platelet activation. *Chest* 2003; **124**: 18S–25S.
4 Varga-Szabo D, Pleines I, Nieswandt B. Cell adhesion mechanisms in platelets. *Arterioscler Thromb Vasc Biol* 2008; **28**: 403–12.

5 Angiolillo DJ, Ueno M, Goto S. Basic principles of platelet biology and clinical implications. *Circ J* 2010; **74**: 597–607.

6 Brass LF. Thrombin and platelet activation. *Chest* 2003; **124**: 18S–25S.

7 Angiolillo DJ, Ferrerio JL. Antiplatelet and anticoagulant therapy for atherothrombotic disease: the role of current and emerging agents. *Am J Cardiovasc Drugs* 2013; **13**: 233–250.

8 Dorsam RT, Kunapuli SP. Central role of the P2Y12 receptor in platelet activation. *J Clin Invest* 2004; **113**: 340–345.

9 Offermanns S. Activation of platelet function through G protein-coupled receptors. *Circ Res* 2006; **99**: 1293–1304.

10 Mackman N, Tilley RE, Key NS. Role of the extrinsic pathway of blood coagulation in hemostasis and thrombosis. *Arterioscler Thromb Vasc Biol* 2007; **27**: 1687–1693.

11 Monroe DM, Hoffman M, Roberts HF. Platelet and thrombin generation. *Arterioscler Thromb Vasc Biol* 2002; **22**: 1381–1389.

12 Brummel KE, Paradis SG, Butenas S, Mann KG. Thrombin functions during tissue factor-induced blood coagulation. *Blood* 2002; **100**: 148–152.

13 Mann KG. Thrombin formation. *Chest* 2003; **124**: 4S–10S.

14 Derian CK, Damiano BP, Addo MF, et al. Blockade of the thrombin receptor protease-activated receptor-1 with a small-molecule antagonist prevents thrombus formation and vascular occlusion in nonhuman primates. *J Pharmacol Exp Ther* 2003; **304**: 855–861.

15 Kato Y, Kita Y, Hirasawa-Taniyama Y, et al. Inhibition of arterial thrombosis by a protease-activated receptor 1 antagonist, FR171113, in the guinea pig. *Eur J Pharmacol* 2003; **473**: 163–169.

16 Vandendries ER, Hamilton JR, Coughlin SR, Furie B, Furie BC. Par4 is required for platelet thrombus propagation but not fibrin generation in a mouse model of thrombosis. *Proc Natl Acad Sci U S A* 2007; **104**: 288–292.

17 Coughlin SR. Protease-activated receptors in hemostasis, thrombosis and vascular biology. *J Thromb Haemost* 2005; **3**: 1800–1814.

18 Leger AJ, Covic L, Kuliopulos A. Protease-activated receptors in cardiovascular diseases. *Circulation* 2006; **114**: 1070–1077.

19 Patrono C. Aspirin as an antiplatelet drug. *N Engl J Med* 1994; **330**: 1287–1294.

20 Baigent C, Blackwell L, Collins R, et al. Aspirin in the primary and secondary prevention of vascular disease: collaborative meta-analysis of individual participant data from randomised trials. *Lancet* 2009; **373**: 1849–1860.

21 Wijns W, Kolh P, Danchin N, et al. Guidelines on myocardial revascularization. Task Force on Myocardial Revascularization of the European Society of Cardiology (ESC) and the European Association for Cardio-Thoracic Surgery (EACTS); European Association for Percutaneous Cardiovascular Interventions (EAPCI). *Eur Heart J* 2010; **31**: 2501–2555.

22 Levine GN, Bates ER, Blankenship JC, et al; American College of Cardiology Foundation; American Heart Association Task Force on Practice Guidelines; Society for Cardiovascular Angiography and Interventions 2011 ACCF/AHA/SCAI Guideline for Percutaneous Coronary Intervention. A report of the American College of Cardiology Foundation/American Heart Association Task Force on Practice Guidelines and the Society for Cardiovascular Angiography and Interventions. *J Am Coll Cardiol* 2011; **58**: e44–122.

23 Angiolillo DJ. The evolution of antiplatelet therapy in the treatment of acute coronary syndromes: from aspirin to the present day. *Drugs* 2012; **72**: 2087–2116.

24 Mason PJ, Jacobs AK, Freedman JE. Aspirin resistance and atherothrombotic disease. *J Am Coll Cardiol* 2005; **46**: 986–993.

25 Ferreiro JL, Angiolillo DJ. New directions in antiplatelet therapy. *Circ Cardiovasc Interv* 2012; **5**: 433–45.

26 Bertrand ME, Rupprecht HJ, Urban P, Gershlick AH; CLASSICS Investigators. Double-blind study of the safety of clopidogrel with and without a loading dose in combination with aspirin compared with ticlopidine in combination with aspirin after coronary stenting: the clopidogrel aspirin stent international cooperative study (CLASSICS). *Circulation* 2000; **102**: 624–629.

27 Cadroy Y, Bossavy JP, Thalamas C, Sagnard L, Sakariassen K, Boneu B. Early potent antithrombotic effect with combined aspirin and a loading dose of clopidogrel on experimental arterial thrombogenesis in humans. *Circulation* 2000; **101**: 2823–2828.

28 Yusuf S, Zhao F, Mehta SR, Chrolavicius S, Tognoni G, Fox KK. Effects of clopidogrel in addition to aspirin in patients with acute coronary syndromes without ST-segment elevation. *N Engl J Med* 2001; **345**: 494–502.

29 Chen ZM, Jiang LX, Chen YP, et al. Addition of clopidogrel to aspirin in 45,852 patients with acute myocardial infarction: randomised placebo-controlled trial. *Lancet* 2005; **366**: 1607–1621.

30 Sabatine MS, Cannon CP, Gibson CM, et al. Addition of clopidogrel to aspirin and fibrinolytic therapy for myocardial infarction with ST-segment elevation. *N Engl J Med* 2005; **352**: 1179–1189.

31 Mehta SR, Yusuf S, Peters RJ, et al. Effects of pretreatment with clopidogrel and aspirin followed by long-term therapy in patients undergoing percutaneous coronary intervention: the PCI-CURE study. *Lancet* 2001; **358**: 527–533.

32 Steinhubl SR, Berger PB, Mann JT 3rd, et al. Early and sustained dual oral antiplatelet therapy following percutaneous coronary intervention: a randomized controlled trial. *JAMA* 2002; **288**: 2411–2420.

33 A randomised, blinded, trial of clopidogrel versus aspirin in patients at risk of ischaemic events (CAPRIE). CAPRIE Steering Committee. *Lancet* 1996; **348**: 1329–1339.

34 Bhatt DL, Fox KA, Hacke W, et al. Clopidogrel and aspirin versus aspirin alone for the prevention of atherothrombotic events. *N Engl J Med* 2006; **354**: 1706–1717.

35 Bhatt DL, Flather MD, Hacke W, et al. Patients with prior myocardial infarction, stroke, or symptomatic peripheral arterial disease in the CHARISMA trial. *J Am Coll Cardiol* 2007; **49**: 1982–1988.

36 Ferreiro JL, Angiolillo DJ. Clopidogrel response variability: current status and future directions. *Thromb Haemost* 2009; **102**: 7–14.

37 Capranzano P, Ferreiro JL, Angiolillo DJ. Prasugrel in acute coronary syndrome patients undergoing percutaneous coronary intervention. *Expert Rev Cardiovasc Ther* 2009; **7**: 361–369.

38 Brandt JT, Payne CD, Wiviott SD, et al. A comparison of prasugrel and clopidogrel loading doses on platelet function: magnitude of platelet inhibition is related to active metabolite formation. *Am Heart J* 2007; **153**: 66.e9–16.

39 Wiviott SD, Trenk D, Frelinger AL, et al. Prasugrel compared with high loading-and maintenance-dose clopidogrel in patients with planned percutaneous coronary intervention: the Prasugrel in Comparison to Clopidogrel for Inhibition of Platelet Activation and Aggregation-Thrombolysis in Myocardial Infarction 44 trial. *Circulation* 2007; **116**: 2923–2932.

40 Wiviott SD, Braunwald E, McCabe CH, et al. Prasugrel versus clopidogrel in patients with acute coronary syndromes. *N Engl J Med* 2007; **357**: 2001–2015.

41 Roe MT, Armstrong PW, Fox KA, et al; TRILOGY ACS Investigators. Prasugrel versus clopidogrel for acute coronary syndromes without revascularization. *N Engl J Med* 2012; **367**: 1297–1309.

42 Montalescot G, Bolognese L, Dudek D, et al. Pretreatment with prasugrel in non-ST-segment elevation acute coronary syndromes. *N Engl J Med* 2013; **369**: 999–1010.

43 Capodanno D, Dharmashankar K, Angiolillo DJ. Mechanism of action and clinical development of ticagrelor, a novel platelet ADP P2Y12 receptor antagonist. *Expert Rev Cardiovasc Ther* 2010; **8**: 151–158.

44 Cattaneo M, Schulz R, Nylander S. Adenosine-mediated effects of ticagrelor: evidence and potential clinical relevance. *J Am Coll Cardiol* 2014; **63**: 2503–2509.

45 Wallentin L, Becker RC, Budaj A, et al. Ticagrelor versus clopidogrel in patients with acute coronary syndromes. *N Engl J Med* 2009; **361**: 1045–1057.

46 Ferreiro JL, Ueno M, Angiolillo DJ. Cangrelor: a review on its mechanism of action and clinical development. *Expert Rev Cardiovasc Ther* 2009; **7**: 1195–1201.

47 Harrington RA, Stone GW, McNulty S, et al. Platelet inhibition with cangrelor in patients undergoing PCI. *N Engl J Med* 2009; **361**: 2318–2329.

48 Bhatt DL, Lincoff AM, Gibson CM, et al; CHAMPION PLATFORM Investigators. Intravenous platelet blockade with cangrelor during PCI. *N Engl J Med* 2009; **361**: 2330–2341.

49 Bhatt DL, Stone GW, Mahaffey KW, et al. the CHAMPION PHOENIX Investigators. Effect of platelet inhibition with cangrelor during PCI on ischemic events. *N Engl J Med* 2013 **368**: 1303–1313.

50 Steg PG, Bhatt DL, Hamm CW, et al. Effect of cangrelor on periprocedural outcomes in percutaneous coronary interventions: a pooled analysis of patient-level data. *Lancet* 2013; **382**: 1981–1992.

51 Angiolillo DJ, Firstenberg MS, Price MJ, et al. Bridging antiplatelet therapy with cangrelor in patients undergoing cardiac surgery: a randomized controlled trial. *JAMA* 2012; **307**: 265–274.

52 Kleiman NS. Pharmacokinetics and pharmacodynamics of glycoprotein IIb-IIIa inhibitors. *Am Heart J* 1999; **138**: 263–275.

53 Randomised placebo-controlled and balloon-angioplasty-controlled trial to assess safety of coronary stenting with use of platelet glycoprotein-IIb/IIIa blockade. The EPISTENT Investigators. *Lancet* 1998; **352**: 87–92.

54 Use of a monoclonal antibody directed against the platelet glycoprotein IIb/IIIa receptor in high-risk coronary angioplasty. The EPIC Investigation. *N Engl J Med* 1994; **330**: 956–961.

55 Platelet glycoprotein IIb/IIIa receptor blockade and low-dose heparin during percutaneous coronary revascularization. The EPILOG Investigators. *N Engl J Med* 1997; **336**: 1689–1696.

56 Stone GW, Grines CL, Cox DA, et al. Comparison of angioplasty with stenting, with or without abciximab, in acute myocardial infarction. *N Engl J Med* 2002; **346**: 957–966.

57 Kastrati A, Mehilli J, Schuhlen H, et al. A clinical trial of abciximab in elective percutaneous coronary intervention after pretreatment with clopidogrel. *N Engl J Med* 2004; **350**: 232–238.

58 Kastrati A, Mehilli J, Neumann FJ, et al. Abciximab in patients with acute coronary syndromes undergoing percutaneous coronary intervention after clopidogrel pretreatment: the ISAR-REACT 2 randomized trial. *JAMA* 2006; **295**: 1531–1538.

59 Mehilli J, Kastrati A, Schulz S, *et al.*; Bavarian Reperfusion Alternatives Evaluation-3 (BRAVE-3) Study Investigators. Abciximab in patients with acute ST-segment-elevation myocardial infarction undergoing primary percutaneous coronary intervention after clopidogrel loading: a randomized double-blind trial. *Circulation* 2009; **119**: 1933–1940.

60 Stone GW, Maehara A, Witzenbichler B, *et al.*; INFUSE-AMI Investigators. Intracoronary abciximab and aspiration thrombectomy in patients with large anterior myocardial infarction: the INFUSE-AMI randomized trial. *JAMA* 2012; **307**: 1817–1826.

61 Randomised placebo-controlled trial of effect of eptifibatide on complications of percutaneous coronary intervention: IMPACT-II. Integrilin to Minimise Platelet Aggregation and Coronary Thrombosis-II. *Lancet* 1997; **349**: 1422–1428.

62 PURSUIT Trial Investigators. Inhibition of platelet glycoprotein IIb/IIIa with eptifibatide in patients with acute coronary syndromes: Platelet glycoprotein IIb/IIIa in unstable angina: receptor suppression using integrilin therapy. *N Engl J Med* 1998; **339**: 436–443.

63 ESPRIT Investigators. Novel dosing regimen of eptifibatide in planned coronary stent implantation (ESPRIT): a randomised, placebo-controlled trial. *Lancet* 2000; **356**: 2037–2044.

64 Giugliano RP, White JA, Bode C, *et al.* Early versus delayed, provisional eptifibatide in acute coronary syndromes. *N Engl J Med* 2009; **360**: 2176–2190.

65 Platelet Receptor Inhibition in Ischemic Syndrome Management in Patients Limited by Unstable Signs and Symptoms (PRISM-PLUS) Study Investigators. Inhibition of the platelet glycoprotein IIb/IIIa receptor with tirofiban in unstable angina and non-Q-wave myocardial infarction. *N Engl J Med* 1998; **338**: 1488–1497.

66 Topol EJ, Moliterno DJ, Herrmann HC, *et al.* Comparison of two platelet glycoprotein IIb/IIIa inhibitors, tirofiban and abciximab, for the prevention of ischemic events with percutaneous coronary revascularization. *N Engl J Med* 2001; **344**: 1888–1894.

67 Meadows TA, Bhatt DL. Clinical aspects of platelet inhibitors and thrombus formation. *Circ Res* 2007; **100**: 1261–1275.

68 Angiolillo DJ, Capranzano P, Goto S, *et al.* A randomized study assessing the impact of cilostazol on platelet function profiles in patients with diabetes mellitus and coronary artery disease on dual antiplatelet therapy: results of the OPTIMUS-2 study. *Eur Heart J* 2008; **29**: 2202–2211.

69 Lee S, Park S, Kim Y, *et al.* Drug-eluting stenting followed by cilostazol treatment reduces late restenosis in patients with diabetes mellitus the DECLARE-DIABETES Trial (A Randomized Comparison of Triple Antiplatelet Therapy with Dual Antiplatelet Therapy After Drug-Eluting Stent Implantation in Diabetic Patients). *J Am Coll Cardiol* 2008; **51**: 1181–1187.

70 Aktas B, Utz A, Hoenig-Liedl P, Walter U, Geiger J. Dipyridamole enhances NO/cGMP-mediated vasodilator-stimulated phosphoprotein phosphorylation and signaling in human platelets: in vitro and in vivo/ex vivo studies. *Stroke* 2003; **34**: 764–769.

71 Diener HC, Cunha L, Forbes C, Sivenius J, Smets P, Lowenthal A. European Stroke Prevention Study. 2. Dipyridamole and acetylsalicylic acid in the secondary prevention of stroke. *J Neurol Sci* 1996; **143**: 1–13.

72 Halkes PH, van Gijn J, Kappelle LJ, Koudstaal PJ, Algra A. Aspirin plus dipyridamole versus aspirin alone after cerebral ischaemia of arterial origin (ESPRIT): randomised controlled trial. *Lancet* 2006; **367**: 1665–1673.

73 Sacco RL, Diener HC, Yusuf S, *et al.* Aspirin and extended-release dipyridamole versus clopidogrel for recurrent stroke. *N Engl J Med* 2008; **359**: 1238–1251.

74 Angiolillo DJ, Capodanno D, Goto S. Platelet thrombin receptor antagonism and atherothrombosis. *Eur Heart J* 2010; **31**: 17–28.

75 Tricoci P, Huang Z, Held C, *et al*; the TRACER Investigators. Thrombin-receptor antagonist vorapaxar in acute coronary syndromes. *N Engl J Med* 2012; **366**: 20–33.

76 Morrow DA, Braunwald E, Bonaca MP, *et al*; TRA 2P–TIMI 50 Steering Committee and Investigators. Vorapaxar in the secondary prevention of atherothrombotic events. *N Engl J Med* 2012; **366**: 1404–1413.

77 Morrow DA, Alberts MJ, Mohr JP, *et al*; for the Thrombin Receptor Antagonist in Secondary Prevention of Atherothrombotic Ischemic Events–TIMI 50 Steering Committee and Investigators. Efficacy and safety of vorapaxar in patients with prior ischemic stroke. *Stroke* 2013; **44**(3): 691–698.

78 Scirica BM, Bonaca MP, Braunwald E, *et al*; TRA 2°P-TIMI 50 Steering Committee Investigators. Vorapaxar for secondary prevention of thrombotic events for patients with previous myocardial infarction: a prespecified subgroup analysis of the TRA 2°P-TIMI 50 trial. *Lancet* 2012; **380**: 1317–1324.

79 Bonaca MP, Morrow DA, Braunwald E. Vorapaxar for secondary prevention in patients with peripheral artery disease: results from the peripheral artery disease cohort of the TRA 2°P-TIMI 50 trial. American Heart Association Emerging Science Series Report. Available at http://my.americanheart.org/professional/Sessions/AdditionalMeetings/EmergingScienceSeries/2012-Emerging-Science-Series%C2%97-June-20-2012_UCM_441183_Article.jsp

80 O'Donoghue ML, Bhatt DL, Wiviott SD, *et al*; LANCELOT-ACS Investigators. Safety and tolerability of atopaxar in the treatment of patients with acute coronary syndromes: the lessons from antagonizing the cellular effects of Thrombin–Acute Coronary Syndromes Trial. *Circulation* 2011; **123**: 1843–1853.

81 Wiviott SD, Flather MD, O'Donoghue ML, *et al*; LANCELOT-CAD Investigators. Randomized trial of atopaxar in the treatment of patients with coronary artery disease: the lessons from antagonizing the cellular effect of Thrombin–Coronary Artery Disease Trial. *Circulation* 2011; **123**: 1854–1863.

82 Capodanno D, Bhatt DL, Goto S, *et al.* Safety and efficacy of protease-activated receptor-1 antagonists in patients with coronary artery disease: a meta-analysis of randomized clinical trials. *J Thromb Haemost* 2012; **10**: 2006–2015.

83 Chamorro A. TP receptor antagonism: a new concept in atherothrombosis and stroke prevention. *Cerebrovasc Dis* 2009; **27**(Suppl 3): 20–27.

84 Eikelboom JW, Weitz JI. New anticoagulants. *Circulation* 2010; **121**: 1523–1532.

85 Bjork I, Lindahl U. Mechanism of the anticoagulant action of heparin. *Mol Cell Biochem* 1982; **48**: 161–182.

86 Choay J, Petitou M, Lormeau JC, Sinay P, Casu B, Gatti G. Structure–activity relationship in heparin: a synthetic pentasaccharide with high affinity for antithrombin III and eliciting high anti-factor Xa activity. *Biochem Biophys Res Commun* 1983; **116**: 492–499.

87 Di Nisio M, Middeldorp S, Buller HR. Direct thrombin inhibitors. *N Engl J Med* 2005; **353**: 1028–1040.

88 Oldgren J, Budaj A, Granger CB, *et al*; RE-DEEM Investigators. Dabigatran vs. placebo in patients with acute coronary syndromes on dual antiplatelet therapy: a randomized, double-blind, phase II trial. *Eur Heart J* 2011; **32**: 2781–2789.

89 Witting JI, Bourdon P, Brezniak DV, Maraganore JM, Fenton JW 2nd. Thrombin-specific inhibition by and slow cleavage of hirulog-1. *Biochem J* 1992; **283**: 737–743.

90 Lincoff AM, Bittl JA, Harrington RA, *et al.* Bivalirudin and provisional glycoprotein IIb/IIIa blockade compared with heparin and planned glycoprotein IIb/IIIa blockade during percutaneous coronary intervention: REPLACE-2 randomized trial. *JAMA* 2003; **289**: 853–863.

91 Stone GW, McLaurin BT, Cox DA, *et al.* ACUITY Investigators. Bivalirudin for patients with acute coronary syndromes. *N Engl J Med* 2006; **355**: 2203–2216.

92 Stone GW, Witzenbichler B, Guagliumi G, *et al.* Bivalirudin during primary PCI in acute myocardial infarction. *N Engl J Med* 2008; **358**: 2218–2230.

93 Kastrati A, Neumann FJ, *et al*; ISAR-REACT 4 Trial Investigators. Abciximab and heparin versus bivalirudin for non-ST-elevation myocardial infarction. *N Engl J Med* 2011; **365**: 1980–1989.

94 Steg PG, van't Hof A, Hamm CW, *et al.* Bivalirudin started during emergency transport for primary PCI. *N Engl J Med* 2013; **369**: 2207–2217.

95 Shahzad A, Kemp I, Mars C, *et al.* Unfractionated heparin versus bivalirudin in primary percutaneous coronary intervention (HEAT-PPCI): an open-label, single centre, randomised controlled trial. *Lancet* 2014; **384**: 1849–1858.

96 Yusuf S, Mehta SR, Chrolavicius S, *et al.* Comparison of fondaparinux and enoxaparin in acute coronary syndromes. *N Engl J Med* 2006; **354**: 1464–1476.

97 Steg PG, Jolly SS, Mehta SR, et al. Low-dose vs standard-dose unfractionated heparin for percutaneous coronary intervention in acute coronary syndromes treated with fondaparinux: the FUTURA/OASIS-8 randomized trial. *JAMA* 2010; **304**: 1339–1349.

98 Yusuf S, Mehta SR, Chrolavicius S, *et al.* Effects of fondaparinux on mortality and reinfarction in patients with acute ST-segment elevation myocardial infarction: the OASIS-6 randomized trial. *JAMA* 2006; **295**: 1519–1530.

99 Sabatine MS, Antman EM, Widimsky P, *et al.* Otamixaban for the treatment of patients with non-ST-elevation acute coronary syndromes (SEPIA-ACS1 TIMI 42): a randomised, double-blind, active-controlled, phase 2 trial. *Lancet* 2009; **374**: 787–795.

100 Steg PG1, Mehta SR, Pollack CV Jr, *et al.* Anticoagulation with otamixaban and ischemic events in non-ST-segment elevation acute coronary syndromes: the TAO randomized clinical trial. *JAMA* 2013; **310**: 1145–1155.

101 Mega JL, Braunwald E, Wiviott SD, *et al.*; ATLAS ACS 2–TIMI 51 Investigators. Rivaroxaban in patients with a recent acute coronary syndrome. *N Engl J Med* 2012; **366**: 9–19.

102 Alexander JH, Lopes RD, James S, *et al.*; APPRAISE-2 Investigators. Apixaban with antiplatelet therapy after acute coronary syndrome. *N Engl J Med* 2011; **365**: 699–708.

103 Povsic TJ, Vavalle JP, Aberle LH, *et al.*; on behalf of the RADAR Investigators. A Phase 2, randomized, partially blinded, active-controlled study assessing the efficacy and safety of variable anticoagulation reversal using the REG1 system in patients with acute coronary syndromes: results of the RADAR trial. *Eur Heart J* 2013; **34**: 2481–2489.

CHAPTER 39

Balance of Ischemia and Bleeding in Selecting Antithrombotic Regimens

Bimmer E.P.M. Claessen and José P.S. Henriques
Department of Cardiology, Academic Medical Center – University of Amsterdam, Amsterdam, The Netherlands

In the USA, coronary revascularization by percutaneous coronary intervention (PCI) is performed over 1 million times annually [1]. However, PCI has only been associated with improved clinical outcomes when performed for acute coronary syndromes (ACS) [2,3]. In patients with stable coronary artery disease, there is an ongoing debate concerning the clinical usefulness of PCI. Although PCI is strongly associated with relief of anginal complaints and a reduction in the need for medication [4], no study to date has shown an improvement in terms of hard clinical endpoints (i.e., cardiac or all-cause mortality). Therefore, minimizing the number of ischemic and bleeding complications after PCI is an important priority for interventional cardiologists.

Rates of adverse outcomes after PCI vary widely. In general, adverse outcomes are more common after PCI for ACS compared with elective PCI. Moreover, rates of ischemic and bleeding complications tend to be lower in the selected patient populations of randomized clinical trials compared with unselected cohorts in observational studies. In this chapter, we aim to provide pharmacologic treatment strategies to optimize the safety and efficacy of PCI by minimizing the risk of ischemic and bleeding outcomes.

Definitions of the most common ischemic and bleeding outcomes

Uniform definitions of ischemic and bleeding complications of PCI are needed to adequately evaluate its safety and efficacy. However, there was a large variability in these definitions until as recently as 2007. In that year, an Academic Research Consortium (ARC) proposed definitions for a number of ischemic events which have subsequently been adopted across the world and are now being used in clinical research and practice [5]. Definitions of myocardial infarction (MI), restenosis, and stent thrombosis as proposed by the ARC are shown in Table 39.1. No definition for stroke was provided by the ARC; however, a useful definition was utilized in the HORIZONS-AMI (harmonizing outcomes with revascularization and stents in acute myocardial infarction) trial: "An acute neurologic deficit resulting in death or lasting for more than 24 hours, as classified by a physician, with supporting information, including brain images and neurologic/neurosurgical evaluation" [6].

Prior to 2011, when standardized bleeding definitions were proposed by the Bleeding Academic Research Consortium (BARC), a wide variety of different definitions for bleeding were used such as thrombolysis in myocardial infarction (TIMI) [7], global utilization of streptokinase and Tpa for occluded arteries (GUSTO) [8], global registry of acute coronary events (GRACE) [9], CRUSADE [10], and many others. The BARC proposed an objective, hierarchically graded classification for bleeding which is shown in Box 39.1. A growing number of randomized clinical trials and observational studies have adopted this bleeding definition, mostly reporting only BARC bleeding ≥3.

Outcomes after ischemic or bleeding complications

Both ischemic and bleeding complications are associated with an increased risk of mortality after PCI. A patient-pooled meta-analysis of three randomized trials comparing bivalirudin and heparin in PCI (n = 17,034) reported a hazard ratio for mortality of 4.2 and 2.9 after TIMI major bleeding and MI, respectively [11]. This study also showed that not all types of bleeding have similar effects on mortality as there was no increased risk of mortality after bleeding defined as a hematoma ≥5 cm at the arterial access site. This finding has also been reported by a number of other studies [12–14]. Interestingly, mortality is increased not only within the first 30 days after a bleeding event, but also thereafter. In contrast, some studies have suggested that MI is only associated with increased mortality within the first 30 days after the event [13]. The BARC bleeding definition has been validated in a patient-pooled analysis of six randomized trials of patients undergoing PCI [15]. BARC class ≥2 bleeding occurred in 9.9% of patients, and was associated with an increased 1-year mortality with an adjusted hazard ratio of 2.72. A retrospective analysis in over 2000 patients from an observational study in a large European tertiary care hospital indicated that the BARC bleeding classification can be used to identify STEMI patients at risk of 1-year mortality [16].

It remains unclear how a bleeding event contributes to an increased risk of mortality even beyond the first month after the event itself. A number of studies have reported suboptimal medical therapy in patients with bleeding events such as beta-blocker and statin therapy or a reduction in the use of antiplatelet agents, as has been reported in the PREMIER (prospective registry evaluating myocardial infarction: events and recovery) registry [17,18]. However, patient frailty and comorbidity have also been implicated as causal factors relating bleeding with an increased risk of mortality.

Interventional Cardiology: Principles and Practice, Second Edition. Edited by George D. Dangas, Carlo Di Mario, and Nicholas N. Kipshidze.
© 2017 John Wiley & Sons, Ltd. Published 2017 by John Wiley & Sons, Ltd.

Table 39.1 Definitions of myocardial infarction, restenosis, and stent thrombosis.

Classification	Biomarker criteria	Additional criteria
Myocardial infarction		
Peri-procedural MI PCI	Troponin >3 times URL or CKMB >3 times URL	Baseline value<URL
Peri-procedural MI CABG	Troponin >5 times URL or CKMB >5 times URL	Baseline value<URL and any of the following: new pathologic Q waves‡ or LBBB, new native or graft vessel occlusion, imaging evidence of loss of viable myocardium
Spontaneous	Troponin>URL or CKMB>URL	
Sudden death	Death before biomarkers obtained or before expected to be elevated	Symptoms suggestive of ischemia and any of the following: new ST elevation or LBBB, documented thrombus by angiography or autopsy
Reinfarction	Stable or decreasing values on two samples and 20% Increase 3–6 hours after second sample	If biomarkers increasing or peak not reached then insufficient data to diagnose recurrent MI

Angiographic restenosis
Diameter stenosis of ≥50%

Clinical restenosis
Diameter stenosis of ≥50% *and* one of the following

1. A positive history of recurrent angina pectoris, presumably related to the target vessel
2. Objective signs of ischemia at rest (ECG changes) or during exercise test (or equivalent), presumably related to the target vessel
3. Abnormal results of any invasive functional diagnostic test (e.g., coronary flow velocity reserve, fractional flow reserve <0.80; IVUS minimum cross-sectional area under 4 mm² (and <6.0 mm² for left main stem)
4. A TLR with a diameter stenosis ≥70% even in the absence of the above-mentioned ischemic signs or symptoms

Stent thrombosis

Definite stent thrombosis:
Angiographic confirmation of stent thrombosis

The presence of a thrombus that originates in the stent or in the segment 5 mm proximal or distal to the stent *and* at least one of the following within a 48-hour time window

- Acute onset of ischemic symptoms at rest
- New ischemic ECG changes that suggest acute ischemia
- Typical rise and fall in cardiac biomarkers

Pathologic confirmation of stent thrombosis

- Evidence of recent thrombus within the stent determined at autopsy or via examination of tissue retrieved following thrombectomy

Probable stent thrombosis
Any unexplained death within the first 30 days

Irrespective of the time after the index procedure, any MI that is related to documented acute ischemia in the territory of stent thrombosis and in the absence of any other obvious cause

Possible stent thrombosis
Any unexplained death from 30 days after intracoronary stenting

CABG, coronary artery bypass graft surgery; CKMB, creatine kinase MB; ECG, electrocardiogram; IVUS, intravascular ultrasound; LBBB, left bundle branch block; MI, myocardial infarction; PCI, percutaneous coronary intervention; TLR, target lesion revascularization; URL, upper range limit.

Box 39.1 Bleeding definition according to the Bleeding Academic Research Consortium.

Type 0: no bleeding

Type 1: bleeding that is not actionable and does not cause the patient to seek unscheduled performance of studies, hospitalization, or treatment by a healthcare professional; includes episodes leading to self-discontinuation of medical therapy by the patient without consulting a healthcare professional

Type 2: any overt, actionable sign of hemorrhage (e.g., more bleeding than would be expected for a clinical circumstance, including bleeding found by imaging alone) that does not fit the criteria for type 3, 4, or 5 but does meet at least one of the following criteria: (1) requiring non-surgical, medical intervention by a healthcare professional, (2) leading to hospitalization or increased level of care, or (3) prompting evaluation

Type 3a: Overt bleeding plus hemoglobin drop of 3 to <5 g/dL (provided hemoglobin drop is related to bleed)
Any transfusion with overt bleeding
Type 3b: Overt bleeding plus hemoglobin drop ≥5 g/dL (provided hemoglobin drop is related to bleed)
Cardiac tamponade
Bleeding requiring surgical intervention for control (excluding dental/nasal/skin/hemorrhoid)
Bleeding requiring intravenous vasoactive agents
Type 3c: Intracranial hemorrhage (does not include microbleeds or hemorrhagic transformation, does include intraspinal)
Subcategories confirmed by autopsy or imaging or lumbar puncture
Intraocular bleed compromising vision

Type 4: CABG-related bleeding
Perioperative intracranial bleeding within 48 h
Reoperation after closure of sternotomy for the purpose of controlling bleeding
Transfusion of ≥5 IU whole blood or packed red blood cells within a 48-hour period
Chest tube output ≥ 2 L within a 24-hour period

Type 5: Fatal bleeding
Type 5a: Probable fatal bleeding; no autopsy or imaging confirmation but clinically suspicious
Type 5b: Definite fatal bleeding; overt bleeding or autopsy or imaging confirmation

CABG, coronary artery bypass graft surgery.

Stent thrombosis (ST) is a dreaded complication of intracoronary stenting and is associated with high rates of morbidity and mortality [19–21]. Recent studies have suggested that the timing of the ST event (e.g., in-hospital vs. out-of-hospital, or early vs. late/very late) is correlated with the risk of mortality. Early stent thrombosis or stent thrombosis occurring in-hospital has been associated with worse clinical outcome than late/very late stent thrombosis [19,22,23].

Methods to assess the risk of ischemic and bleeding complications

Risk factors for ischemic and bleeding complications are known to overlap. A number of risk scores have been developed to individualize risk stratification for patients undergoing PCI. Pocock *et al.* [24] investigated predictors of bleeding and MI in 13,819 patients with ACS undergoing an early invasive strategy randomized to heparin plus a glycoprotein IIb/IIIa inhibitor (GPI), bivalirudin plus a GPI, or bivalirudin monotherapy. Predictors of both MI and bleeding included older age, ST-segment deviation ≥1 mm at baseline. Moreover, three predictors for MI were identified: elevated baseline cardiac biomarkers, family history of coronary artery disease, and a history of a prior MI. Finally, predictors of bleeding were female sex, baseline anemia, use of heparin plus a GPI compared with bivalirudin monotherapy, elevated baseline serum creatinine, elevated baseline white blood cell count, no history of a prior PCI, prior stroke, and treatment with heparin plus routine upstream GPI compared with deferred selective GPI use. Therefore, estimating an individual patient's risk to develop ischemic complications and bleeding complications permits personalized clinical decision making.

Currently, a large number of risk scores exist for MI, mortality, ST, and bleeding that can be used to assess the risk profile of an individual patient. The GRACE [25] and TIMI risk scores for non-ST segment elevation acute coronary syndromes [26] and for ST-segment myocardial infarction (STEMI) [27] can be easily accessed on the internet and are widely used in clinical practice to assess the risk of ischemic events. Additionally, Table 39.2 shows a risk score that can be used to predict the risk of stent thrombosis in patients with STEMI undergoing primary PCI with stent placement [28].

Two bleeding risk scores that are particularly useful in clinical practice are the REPLACE2/ACUITY/HORIZONS-AMI PCI bleeding risk score [11], and the HAS-BLED risk score, which can be useful in patients already treated with warfarin for atrial fibrillation [29]. Table 39.3 shows the variables of which these risk scores are composed.

Pharmacologic strategies to reduce ischemic and bleeding complications
Antithrombotic therapies

Antithrombotic therapy in PCI is focused on minimizing thrombotic complications while limiting the number of bleeding events. Figure 39.1 shows an overview of currently available antithrombotic drugs. At present, unfractionated heparin and bivalirudin (a direct thrombin inhibitor) are the most widely used antithrombotic drugs during PCI. A number of studies have shown a reduction in bleeding with bivalirudin compared with unfractionated heparin (with or without a GPI) [11,30–32]. Moreover, some studies have reported increased survival with bivalirudin

Table 39.2 Integer-based risk score for 1-year definite/probable stent thrombosis in patients with acute coronary syndromes.

Variable	Integer assignment for stent thrombosis	Risk score	Calculation
Type of acute coronary syndrome	NSTE-ACS w/o ST changes +1	NSTE-ACS with ST deviation +2	STEMI +4
Current smoker	Yes: +1		No: +0
Insulin-treated diabetes mellitus	Yes: +2		No: +0
History of PCI	Yes: +1		No: +0
Baseline platelet count	<250 K/μL: +0	250 K/μL–400 K/μL: +1	>400 K/μL: +2
Absence of early (pre-PCI) heparin *	Yes: +1		No: 0
Aneurysm or ulceration	Yes: +2		No: 0
Baseline TIMI flow grade 0/1	Yes: +1		No: 0
Final TIMI flow grade under 3	Yes: +1		No: 0
Number of vessels treated	1 vessel: +0	2 vessels: +1	3 vessels: +2

NSTE-ACS, non-ST-segment elevation acute coronary syndrome; PCI, percutaneous coronary intervention; TIMI, thrombolysis in myocardial infarction.
*Includes parenteral heparin or low molecular weight heparin.

monotherapy compared with heparin with or without a GPI [33–35]. Cavender and Sabatine [36] recently conducted a meta-analysis of 33,958 patients undergoing PCI from 16 randomized controlled trials comparing bivalirudin and heparin (with or without a GPI). This study showed that a bivalirudin-based anticoagulation regimen increased the risk of MI (risk ratio [RR] 1.09, 95% confidence interval [CI] 1.01–1.17; p = 0.02) and ST (RR 1.38, 95% CI 1.09–1.74; p = 0.007). Overall, bivalirudin significantly reduced the incidence of bleeding events (RR 0.62, 95% CI 0.49–0.78; p <0.0001). However, this reduction in bleeding was limited to trials comparing bivalirudin with provisional GPI use with heparin with protocol mandated GPI use (RR 0.53, 95% CI 0.47–0.61; p <0.0001), with no significant reductions in trials comparing bivalirudin with provisional GPI use and heparin with provisional GPI use (RR 0.78, 95% CI 0.51–1.19; p = 0.25) and trials comparing bivalirudin and heparin both with protocol mandated GPI use (RR 1.07, 95% CI 0.87–1.31; p = 0.53).

Fondaparinux, a pentasaccharide factor Xa inhibitor, was compared with unfractionated heparin in patients with STEMI in the 12,092-patient OASIS-6 (organization to assess strategies in acute ischemic syndromes) randomized trial [37]. In this trial, fondaparinux was associated with a reduction in death or reinfarction at 3–6 months' follow-up. However, this benefit was limited to patients not undergoing primary PCI. In patients undergoing PCI there was a higher rate of guiding catheter thrombosis and more coronary complications such as abrupt coronary artery closure, no reflow, dissection, or perforation. Therefore current guidelines state that fondaparinux should not be used as the sole anticoagulant to support PCI. The addition of an anticoagulant with anti-IIa activity is advised [38].

Antiplatet therapy
Aspirin and P2Y12 inhibitors
An aspirin loading dose of 325 mg orally or 500 mg intravenously is administered before PCI. There is no consensus on the optimal

dose of aspirin after PCI. However, a number of studies have shown a reduction in major bleeding when using a low maintenance dose of aspirin (i.e., <100 mg/day) [39–41]. This finding may be explained by the fact that doses of as little as 50 mg aspirin can sufficiently block the enzyme cyclo-oxygenase 1 (COX 1) in platelets to prevent platelet aggregation [42]. Higher doses of aspirin can increase the risk of developing gastrointestinal bleeding by inhibiting COX 1 in gastric mucosal cells which inhibits the production of protective prostaglandins [43].

Clopidogrel, prasugrel, and ticagrelor inhibit platelet activation by antagonizing the adenosine diphosphate receptor P2Y12. Clopidogrel and prasugrel irreversibly inhibit P2Y12 while its inhibition by ticagrelor is reversible. Current guidelines recommend a loading dose of either 600 mg clopidogrel, 60 mg prasugrel, or 180 mg ticagrelor before PCI [38]. After balloon angioplasty alone or bare metal stent (BMS) implantation P2Y12 inhibitors should be continued for 1 month. After drug-eluting stent (DES) implantation P2Y12 inhibitors should be continued for at least 12 months according to US guidelines and for 6 months according to European guidelines [38,44]. Therefore, BMS implantation may be preferred in patients at high risk of bleeding or likely not to be compliant.

Both prasugrel and ticagrelor have been associated with improved clinical outcomes as compared with clopidogrel [45,46]. Clopidogrel is a prodrug that requires transformation by cytochrome P-450 (CYP) enzymes to establish its antiplatelet effect. Variabilty in CYP activity by common polymorphisms resulting in a reduced function have been associated with reduced circulating levels of the active metabolite of clopidogrel, diminished platelet inhibition, and a higher rate of ST [47]. Prasugrel also requires conversion to an active metabolite to act as an antiplatelet agent. However, prasugrel inhibits platelet aggregation faster, more consistently, and to a greater extent than clopidogrel in patients undergoing PCI [48]. Prasugrel was compared with clopidogrel in the large randomized TRITON-TIMI 38 (trial to assess improvement in therapeutic outcomes by optimizing platelet inhibition

Table 39.3 The REPLACE-2/ACUITY/HORIZONS-AMI PCI bleeding risk score and the HAS-BLED bleeding risk score in patients with atrial fibrillation.

(a) REPLACE-2/ACUITY/HORIZONS-AMI PCI bleeding risk score

Serum creatinine (mg/dL)	<1.0 [0]		1.0-<1.2 [+2]	1.2-<1.4 [+4]	1.4-<1.6 [+6]	1.6-<1.8 [+8]	1.8-<2.0 [+10]	≥2.0 [+12]
Age (years)	<50 [0]		50-59 [+3]		60-69 [+6]		70-79[+9]	≥80 [+13]
Gender				Female [+5]				
White blood cell count (*10^9)	<10 [0]		10-<12 [+1]	12-<14 [+2]	14-<16 [+4]	16-<18 [+5]	18-<20 [+6]	≥20 [+8]
Presentation		Normal biomarkers (elective and NSTEMI) [0]		NSTEMI- raised biomarkers [+3]			STEMI [+6]	
Current cigarette smoker				Yes [+4]				
Antithrombotic medications	Heparin + GPI [0]					Bivalirudin monotherapy [-6]		

(b) HAS-BLED risk score

Hypertension	+1
Abnormal renal and liver function	+1 (for each)
Stroke	+1
Bleeding	+1
Labile INR	+1
Elderly	+1
Drugs or alcohol	+1 (for each)

ACUITY, Acute catheterization and urgent intervention triage strategy trial; HORIZONS-AMI, Harmonizing outcomes with revascularization and stents in acute myocardial infarction; INR, international normalized ratio; NSTEMI, non ST-segment elevation myocardial infarction; PCI, percutaneous coronary intervention; REPLACE-2, randomized evaluation of PCI linking angiomax to reduced clinical events 2; STEMI, ST-segment elevation myocardial infarction.

with prasugrel – thrombolysis in myocardial infarction) trial [48]. In this moderate–high risk ACS population, prasugrel was associated with a reduction in MI, urgent revascularization, and ST. However, prasugrel was associated with an excess in (fatal) bleeding. Subgroup analyses of TRITON TIMI 38 have suggested an increased benefit of prasugrel in diabetic patients and patients with STEMI undergoing PCI [49,50]. Prasugrel is contraindicated in patients with a history of prior stroke or transient ischemic attack, and is only recommended in patients >75 years if they have diabetes mellitus or a history of a prior MI.

Ticagrelor is not a prodrug but rather a direct-acting reversible P2Y12 inhibitor. It is dosed twice daily whereas clopidogrel and prasugrel are dosed once daily. The 18,624 patient PLATO (platelet inhibition and patient outcomes) trial comparing ticagrelor with clopidogrel in patients with ACS showed a reduction in death from vascular causes (ticagrelor group 4.0% vs. clopidogrel group 5.1%; p <0.001) and death from any cause (ticagrelor group 4.5% vs.

clopidogrel group 5.9%; p <0.001). Moreover, definite/probable stent thrombosis (2.2% vs. 2.9%) and MI (5.8% vs. 6.9%; p = 0.005) were lower in patients randomized to treatment with ticagrelor [45]. There were no differences in the rate of overall major bleeding. However, there was a higher rate of non-coronary artery bypass graft (CABG) related major bleeding with ticagrelor (4.5% vs. 3.8%). In patients undergoing PCI, the beneficial effects of ticagrelor were consistent with the overall results in the PLATO trial [51,52]. A post hoc analysis of the PLATO trial investigating patients with chronic kidney disease has suggested that ticagrelor compared with clopidogrel significantly reduces ischemic endpoints and mortality with similar rates of major bleeding [53].

Glycoprotein IIb/IIIa inhibitors

In the current era of dual antiplatelet therapy the role of GPIs is unclear, as most trials of GPIs in PCI were performed before the introduction of dual antiplatelet therapy. GPIs such as

Parenteral anticoagulants

Xa/IIa inhibitors:

Unfractionated heparin

Enoxaparin

Xa inhibitors:

Foundaparinux

Otamixaban

Direct thrombin inhibitors:

Argatroban

Bivalirudin

Hirudin

Parenteral antiplatelet agents

COX-I inhibitor:

IV aspirin (Aspegic)

Glycoprotein IIb/IIIA inhibitors:

Eptifibatide

Tirofiban

Abciximab

P2Y12 antagonists:

Cangrelor

Enteral anticoagulants

Direct thrombin inhibitors:

Dabigatran

Xa inhibitors:

Rivaroxaban

Apixaban

Edoxaban

Rivaroxaban

Enteral antiplatelet agents

COX-I inhibitor:

Aspirin

P2Y12 antagonists:

Clopidogrel

Prasugrel

Ticagrelor

PAR-1antagonists:

Vorapaxar

Figure 39.1 Overview of currently available antithrombotic drugs.

eptifibatide, tirofiban, and abciximab are intravenous antiplatelet agents that antagonize platelet aggregation by inhibiting the glycoprotein IIb/IIIa receptor. GPIs have been associated with an increased risk of bleeding and their use may therefore best be limited to patients not at high risk of developing bleeding complications [31,54]. Clinical trials in patients undergoing elective PCI pretreated with P2Y12 inhibitors have not shown any benefit of GPIs [55,56]. In patients with unstable angina or non-ST elevation ACS, GPIs may be associated with a reduction in ischemic outcomes [57]. Finally, in patients with STEMI the use of GPIs is generally limited to patients with large anterior MI or a large thrombus burden who have a high risk of ischemic events and a low risk of bleeding events. Moreover, bolus administration of GPIs can be considered as a bailout strategy in patients with a high risk of ischemic events but also a high risk of bleeding.

New oral anticoagulants after PCI

Novel oral anticoagulant drugs are also being investigated after PCI. The ATLAS ACS-TIMI 51 (Anti-Xa therapy to lower cardiovascular events in addition to standard therapy in subjects with acute coronary syndrome – thrombolysis in myocardial infarction) trial showed a reduction in death from cardiovascular causes, MI, or stroke in patients with a recent ACS with the addition of twice-daily 2.5 mg of the novel oral Xa inhibitor rivaroxaban [58]. The results of additional randomized clinical trials evaluating the use of oral anticoagulant drugs after PCI are eagerly awaited.

Low bleeding risk, low ischemic risk Preloading with: Aspirin and clopidogrel Anticoagulant therapy: Bivalirudin or unfractionated heparin Antithrombotic therapy at discharge: Aspirin, clopidogrel	**Low bleeding risk, high ischemic risk** Preloading with: Aspirin and prasugrel or ticagrelor* Anticoagulant therapy: Heparin plus a glycoprotein IIb/IIIa inhibitor Bivalirudin Antithrombotic therapy at discharge: Aspirin, prasugrel or ticagrelor, consider low-dose rivaroxaban
High bleeding risk, low ischemic risk Preloading with: Aspirin and clopidogrel Anticoagulant therapy: Bivalirudin Antithrombotic therapy at discharge: Aspirin, prasugrel or ticagrelor*	**High bleeding risk, high ischemic risk** Preloading with: Aspirin and clopidogrel, ticagrelor or prasugrel* Anticoagulant therapy: Bivalirudin Antithrombotic therapy at discharge: Aspirin, prasugrel or ticagrelor* Consider: low dose prasugrel (5 mg) and hybrid regimens with prasugrel or ticagrelor for 30 days before switching to clopidogrel
*General considerations to choose between prasugrel or ticagrelor ST-elevation myocardial infarction: prasugrel NON-ST-elevation acute coronary syndromes: ticagrelor Prior stroke, <60 kg, ≥75 years, creatinine clearance <60 mL/min: ticagrelor instead of prasugrel	

Figure 39.2 Algorithm suggesting antithrombotic strategies according to bleeding and ischemic risk.

Conclusions and recommendations for clinical practice

In general, a more aggressive anticoagulant regime will be associated with a reduction in ischemic events at the cost of an increased risk of bleeding. It is therefore paramount that all patients undergoing PCI should be evaluated for risk of bleeding. Patients at a low risk of bleeding will derive benefit from more aggressive antithrombotic therapy. However, patients at a high risk of bleeding will benefit from selective use of antithrombotic agents. On the other hand, the risk of developing ischemic complications should also be assessed, as patients undergoing PCI for ACS may benefit from more effective antithrombotic therapy (especially in STEMI) [38].

Figure 39.2 shows a treatment algorithm suggesting antithrombotic therapeutic options in patients undergoing PCI according to their bleeding and ischemic risks. Many new antithrombotic drugs are still being investigated and there is a large variety of antithrombotic drugs currently available, allowing extensive pharmacologic personalization (Figure 39.1).

Interactive multiple choice questions are available for this chapter on **www.wiley. com/go/dangas/cardiology**

References

1 DeFrances CJ, Lucas CA, Vuie VC, Golosinskiy A. *2006 National Hospital Discharge Survey*. Hyattsville, MD: National Center for Health Statistics: 2008.

2 Keeley EC, Boura JA, Grines CL. Primary angioplasty versus intravenous thrombolytic therapy for acute myocardial infarction: a quantitative review of 23 randomised trials. *Lancet* 2003; **361**(9351): 13–20.

3 Mehta SR, Cannon CP, Fox KA, *et al.* Routine vs selective invasive strategies in patients with acute coronary syndromes: a collaborative meta-analysis of randomized trials. *JAMA* 2005; **293**(23): 2908–2917.

4 Bucher HC, Hengstler P, Schindler C, Guyatt GH. Percutaneous transluminal coronary angioplasty versus medical treatment for non-acute coronary heart disease: meta-analysis of randomised controlled trials. *BMJ* 2000; **321**(7253): 73–77.

5 Cutlip DE, Windecker S, Mehran R, *et al.* Clinical end points in coronary stent trials: a case for standardized definitions. *Circulation* 2007; **115**(17): 2344–2351.

6 Mehran R, Brodie B, Cox DA, *et al.* The Harmonizing Outcomes with RevasculariZatiON and Stents in Acute Myocardial Infarction (HORIZONS-AMI) Trial: study design and rationale. *Am Heart J* 2008; **156**(1): 44–56.

7 Chesebro JH, Knatterud G, Roberts R, *et al.* Thrombolysis in Myocardial Infarction (TIMI) Trial, Phase I: A comparison between intravenous tissue plasminogen activator and intravenous streptokinase. Clinical findings through hospital discharge. *Circulation* 1987; **76**(1): 142–154.

8 GUSTO Investigators. An international randomized trial comparing four thrombolytic strategies for acute myocardial infarction. *N Engl J Med* 1993; **329**(10): 673–682.

9 Moscucci M, Fox KA, Cannon CP, *et al.* Predictors of major bleeding in acute coronary syndromes: the Global Registry of Acute Coronary Events (GRACE). *Eur Heart J* 2003; **24**(20): 1815–1823.

10 Subherwal S, Bach RG, Chen AY, *et al.* Baseline risk of major bleeding in non-ST-segment-elevation myocardial infarction: the CRUSADE (Can Rapid risk stratification of Unstable angina patients Suppress ADverse outcomes with Early implementation of the ACC/AHA Guidelines) Bleeding Score. *Circulation* 2009; **119**(14): 1873–1882.

11 Mehran R, Pocock S, Nikolsky E, *et al.* Impact of bleeding on mortality after percutaneous coronary intervention results from a patient-level pooled analysis of the REPLACE-2 (randomized evaluation of PCI linking angiomax to reduced clinical events), ACUITY (acute catheterization and urgent intervention triage strategy), and HORIZONS-AMI (harmonizing outcomes with revascularization and stents in acute myocardial infarction) trials. *JACC Cardiovasc Interv* 2011; **4**(6): 654–664.

12 White HD, Aylward PE, Gallo R, *et al.* Hematomas of at least 5 cm and outcomes in patients undergoing elective percutaneous coronary intervention: insights from the SafeTy and Efficacy of Enoxaparin in PCI patients, an internationaL randomized Evaluation (STEEPLE) trial. *Am Heart J* 2010; **159**(1): 110–116.

13 Mehran R, Pocock SJ, Nikolsky E, *et al.* A risk score to predict bleeding in patients with acute coronary syndromes. *J Am Coll Cardiol* 2010; **55**(23): 2556–2566.

14 Kikkert WJ, Delewi R, Ouweneel DM, *et al.* Prognostic value of access site and nonaccess site bleeding after percutaneous coronary intervention: a cohort study in ST-segment elevation myocardial infarction and comprehensive meta-analysis. *JACC Cardiovasc Interv* 2014; **7**(6): 622–630.

15 Ndrepepa G, Schuster T, Hadamitzky M, *et ai.* Validation of the Bleeding Academic Research Consortium definition of bleeding in patients with coronary artery disease undergoing percutaneous coronary intervention. *Circulation* 2012; **125**(11): 1424–1431.

16 Kikkert WJ, van Geloven N, van der Laan MH, *et al.* The prognostic value of bleeding academic research consortium (BARC)-defined bleeding complications in ST-segment elevation myocardial infarction: a comparison with the TIMI (Thrombolysis In Myocardial Infarction), GUSTO (Global Utilization of Streptokinase and Tissue Plasminogen Activator for Occluded Coronary Arteries), and ISTH (International Society on Thrombosis and Haemostasis) bleeding classifications. *J Am Coll Cardiol* 2014; **63**(18): 1866–1875.

17 Suh JW, Mehran R, Claessen BE, *et al.* Impact of in-hospital major bleeding on late clinical outcomes after primary percutaneous coronary intervention in acute myocardial infarction the HORIZONS-AMI (Harmonizing Outcomes With Revascularization and Stents in Acute Myocardial Infarction) trial. *J Am Coll Cardiol* 2011; **58**(17): 1750–1756.

18 Wang TY, Xiao L, Alexander KP, *et al.* Antiplatelet therapy use after discharge among acute myocardial infarction patients with in-hospital bleeding. *Circulation* 2008; **118**(21): 2139–2145.

19 Dangas GD, Claessen BE, Mehran R, *et al.* Clinical outcomes following stent thrombosis occurring in-hospital versus out-of-hospital: results from the HORIZONS-AMI (Harmonizing Outcomes with Revascularization and Stents in Acute Myocardial Infarction) trial. *J Am Coll Cardiol* 2012; **59**(20): 1752–1759.

20 de la Torre-Hernandez JM, Alfonso F, Hernandez F, *et al.* Drug-eluting stent thrombosis: results from the multicenter Spanish registry ESTROFA (Estudio ESpanol sobre TROmbosis de stents FArmacoactivos). *J Am Coll Cardiol* 2008; **51**(10): 986–990.

21 Iakovou I, Schmidt T, Bonizzoni E, *et al.* Incidence, predictors, and outcome of thrombosis after successful implantation of drug-eluting stents. *JAMA* 2005; **293**(17): 2126–2130.

22 Kimura T, Morimoto T, Kozuma K, *et al.* Comparisons of baseline demographics, clinical presentation, and long-term outcome among patients with early, late, and very late stent thrombosis of sirolimus-eluting stents: Observations from the Registry of Stent Thrombosis for Review and Reevaluation (RESTART). *Circulation* 2010; **122**(1): 52–61.

23 Lasala JM, Cox DA, Dobies D, *et al.* Drug-eluting stent thrombosis in routine clinical practice: two-year outcomes and predictors from the TAXUS ARRIVE registries. *Circ Cardiovasc Interv* 2009; **2**(4): 285–293.

24 Pocock SJ, Mehran R, Clayton TC, *et al.* Prognostic modeling of individual patient risk and mortality impact of ischemic and hemorrhagic complications: assessment from the Acute Catheterization and Urgent Intervention Triage Strategy trial. *Circulation* 2010; **121**(1): 43–51.

25 Granger CB, Goldberg RJ, Dabbous O, *et al.* Predictors of hospital mortality in the global registry of acute coronary events. *Arch Intern Med* 2003; **163**(19): 2345–2353.

26 Antman EM, Cohen M, Bernink PJ, *et al.* The TIMI risk score for unstable angina/non-ST elevation MI: A method for prognostication and therapeutic decision making. *JAMA* 2000; **284**(7): 835–842.

27 Morrow DA, Antman EM, Charlesworth A, *et al.* TIMI risk score for ST-elevation myocardial infarction: A convenient, bedside, clinical score for risk assessment at presentation: An intravenous nPA for treatment of infarcting myocardium early II trial substudy. *Circulation* 2000; **102**(17): 2031–2037.

28 Dangas GD, Claessen BE, Mehran R, *et al.* Development and validation of a stent thrombosis risk score in patients with acute coronary syndromes. *JACC Cardiovasc Interv* 2012; **5**(11): 1097–1105.

29 Lip GY, Frison L, Halperin JL, Lane DA. Comparative validation of a novel risk score for predicting bleeding risk in anticoagulated patients with atrial fibrillation: the HAS-BLED (Hypertension, Abnormal Renal/Liver Function, Stroke, Bleeding History or Predisposition, Labile INR, Elderly, Drugs/Alcohol Concomitantly) score. *J Am Coll Cardiol* 2011; **57**(2): 173–180.

30 Lee MS, Liao H, Yang T, *et al.* Comparison of bivalirudin versus heparin plus glycoprotein IIb/IIIa inhibitors in patients undergoing an invasive strategy: a meta-analysis of randomized clinical trials. *Int J Cardiol* 2011; **152**(3): 369–374.

31 De Luca G, Cassetti E, Verdoia M, Marino P. Bivalirudin as compared to unfractionated heparin among patients undergoing coronary angioplasty: a meta-analyis of randomised trials. *Thromb Haemost* 2009; **102**(3): 428–436.

32 Bertrand OF, Jolly SS, Rao SV, *et al.* Meta-analysis comparing bivalirudin versus heparin monotherapy on ischemic and bleeding outcomes after percutaneous coronary intervention. *Am J Cardiol* 2012; **110**(4): 599–606.

33 Lemesle G, De Labriolle A, Bonello L, *et al.* Impact of bivalirudin on in-hospital bleeding and six-month outcomes in octogenarians undergoing percutaneous coronary intervention. *Catheter Cardiovasc Interv* 2009; **74**(3): 428–435.

34 Bangalore S, Cohen DJ, Kleiman NS, *et al.* Bleeding risk comparing targeted low-dose heparin with bivalirudin in patients undergoing percutaneous coronary intervention: results from a propensity score-matched analysis of the Evaluation of Drug-Eluting Stents and Ischemic Events (EVENT) registry. *Circ Cardiovasc Interv* 2011; **4**(5): 463–473.

35 Stone GW, Witzenbichler B, Guagliumi G, *et al.* Bivalirudin during primary PCI in acute myocardial infarction. *N Engl J Med* 2008; **358**(21): 2218–2230.

36 Cavender MA, Sabatine MS. Bivalirudin versus heparin in patients planned for percutaneous coronary intervention: a meta-analysis of randomised controlled trials. *Lancet* 2014; **384**(9943): 599–606.

37 Yusuf S, Mehta SR, Chrolavicius S, *et al.* Effects of fondaparinux on mortality and reinfarction in patients with acute ST-segment elevation myocardial infarction: the OASIS-6 randomized trial. *JAMA* 2006; **295**(13): 1519–1530.

38 Levine GN, Bates ER, Blankenship JC, *et al.* 2011 ACCF/AHA/SCAI Guideline for Percutaneous Coronary Intervention. A report of the American College of Cardiology Foundation/American Heart Association Task Force on Practice Guidelines and the Society for Cardiovascular Angiography and Interventions. *J Am Coll Cardiol* 2011; **58**(24): e44–122.

39 Mahaffey KW, Wojdyla DM, Carroll K, *et al.* Ticagrelor compared with clopidogrel by geographic region in the Platelet Inhibition and Patient Outcomes (PLATO) trial. *Circulation* 2011; **124**(5): 544–554.

40 Jolly SS, Pogue J, Haladyn K, *et al.* Effects of aspirin dose on ischaemic events and bleeding after percutaneous coronary intervention: insights from the PCI-CURE study. *Eur Heart J* 2009; **30**(8): 900–907.

41 Yu J, Mehran R, Dangas GD, *et al.* Safety and efficacy of high- versus low-dose aspirin after primary percutaneous coronary intervention in ST-segment elevation myocardial infarction: the HORIZONS-AMI (Harmonizing Outcomes With Revascularization and Stents in Acute Myocardial Infarction) trial. *JACC Cardiovasc Interv* 2012; **5**(12): 1231–1238.

42 Montalescot G, Maclouf J, Drobinski G, Salloum J, Grosgogeat Y, Thomas D. Eicosanoid biosynthesis in patients with stable angina: beneficial effects of very low dose aspirin. *J Am Coll Cardiol* 1994; **24**(1): 33–38.

43 Campbell CL, Smyth S, Montalescot G, Steinhubl SR. Aspirin dose for the prevention of cardiovascular disease: a systematic review. *JAMA* 2007; **297**(18): 2018–2024.

44 Authors/Task Force members, Windecker S, Kolh P, Alfonso F, *et al.* 2014 ESC/EACTS Guidelines on myocardial revascularization: The Task Force on Myocardial Revascularization of the European Society of Cardiology (ESC) and the European Association for Cardio-Thoracic Surgery (EACTS) Developed with the special contribution of the European Association of Percutaneous Cardiovascular Interventions (EAPCI). *Eur Heart J* 2014; **35**(37): 2541–2619.

45 Wallentin L, Becker RC, Budaj A, *et al.* Ticagrelor versus clopidogrel in patients with acute coronary syndromes. *N Engl J Med* 2009; **361**(11): 1045–1057.

46 Wiviott SD, Braunwald E, McCabe CH, *et al.* Prasugrel versus clopidogrel in patients with acute coronary syndromes. *N Engl J Med* 2007; **357**(20): 2001–2015.

47 Mega JL, Close SL, Wiviott SD, *et al.* Cytochrome p-450 polymorphisms and response to clopidogrel. *N Engl J Med* 2009; **360**(4): 354–362.

48 Wiviott SD, Trenk D, Frelinger AL, *et al.* Prasugrel compared with high loading- and maintenance-dose clopidogrel in patients with planned percutaneous coronary intervention: the Prasugrel in Comparison to Clopidogrel for Inhibition of Platelet Activation and Aggregation-Thrombolysis in Myocardial Infarction 44 trial. *Circulation* 2007; **116**(25): 2923–2932.

49 Wiviott SD, Braunwald E, Angiolillo DJ, *et al.* Greater clinical benefit of more intensive oral antiplatelet therapy with prasugrel in patients with diabetes mellitus in the trial to assess improvement in therapeutic outcomes by optimizing platelet inhibition with prasugrel-Thrombolysis in Myocardial Infarction 38. *Circulation* 2008; **118**(16): 1626–1636.

50 Montalescot G, Wiviott SD, Braunwald E, *et al.* Prasugrel compared with clopidogrel in patients undergoing percutaneous coronary intervention for ST-elevation myocardial infarction (TRITON-TIMI 38): double-blind, randomised controlled trial. *Lancet* 2009; **373**(9665): 723–731.

51 Cannon CP, Harrington RA, James S, *et al.* Comparison of ticagrelor with clopidogrel in patients with a planned invasive strategy for acute coronary syndromes (PLATO): a randomised double-blind study. *Lancet* 2010; **375**(9711): 283–293.

52 Steg PG, James S, Harrington RA, *et al.* Ticagrelor versus clopidogrel in patients with ST-elevation acute coronary syndromes intended for reperfusion with primary percutaneous coronary intervention: A Platelet Inhibition and Patient Outcomes (PLATO) trial subgroup analysis. *Circulation* 2010; **122**(21): 2131–2141.

53 James S, Budaj A, Aylward P, *et al.* Ticagrelor versus clopidogrel in acute coronary syndromes in relation to renal function: results from the Platelet Inhibition and Patient Outcomes (PLATO) trial. *Circulation* 2010; **122**(11): 1056–1067.

54 Stone GW, Moliterno DJ, Bertrand M, *et al.* Impact of clinical syndrome acuity on the differential response to 2 glycoprotein IIb/IIIa inhibitors in patients undergoing coronary stenting: the TARGET Trial. *Circulation* 2002; **105**(20): 2347–2354.

55 Valgimigli M, Percoco G, Barbieri D, *et al.* The additive value of tirofiban administered with the high-dose bolus in the prevention of ischemic complications during high-risk coronary angioplasty: the ADVANCE Trial. *J Am Coll Cardiol* 2004; **44**(1): 14–19.

56 Kastrati A, Mehilli J, Schuhlen H, *et al.* A clinical trial of abciximab in elective percutaneous coronary intervention after pretreatment with clopidogrel. *N Engl J Med* 2004; **350**(3): 232–238.

57 Kastrati A, Mehilli J, Neumann FJ, *et al.* Abciximab in patients with acute coronary syndromes undergoing percutaneous coronary intervention after clopidogrel pretreatment: the ISAR-REACT 2 randomized trial. *JAMA* 2006; **295**(13): 1531–1538.

58 Mega JL, Braunwald E, Wiviott SD, *et al.* Rivaroxaban in patients with a recent acute coronary syndrome. *N Engl J Med* 2012; **366**(1): 9–19.

CHAPTER 40

Oral Antiplatelet Agents in PCI

Jonathan A. Batty[1,2], Joseph R. Dunford[1], George D. Dangas[3], and Vijay Kunadian[1,4]

[1] Institute of Cellular Medicine, Newcastle University, Newcastle upon Tyne, UK

[2] The Royal Victoria Infirmary, Newcastle upon Tyne NHS Foundation Trust, Newcastle upon Tyne, UK

[3] Department of Cardiology, Mount Sinai Medical Center, New York, NY, USA

[4] Freeman Hospital, Newcastle upon Tyne Hospital NHS Foundation Trust, Newcastle upon Tyne, UK

In addition to acting as the immediate effector of primary hemostasis, platelets are a critical mediator of atherothrombosis, following atherosclerotic plaque rupture in coronary artery disease (CAD). Oral antiplatelet therapy (APT) is a critical therapeutic strategy in the prevention and management of acute coronary syndrome (ACS; comprising non-ST-elevation ACS (NSTEACS) and ST-elevation myocardial infarction (STEMI)), and as an adjunct in percutaneous coronary intervention (PCI) [1,2]. The objectives of APT pharmacotherapy in PCI are twofold: (i) to mitigate the sequelae of iatrogenic plaque rupture in angioplasty or stenting; and (ii) to reduce the risk of intravascular and in-stent thrombus formation [3].

Oral antiplatelet agents recommended in the contexts of ACS and PCI operate by one of two major mechanisms: (i) inhibition of prostaglandin synthesis via cyclo-oxygenase isoform 1 antagonism (COX-1; e.g., aspirin); or (ii) inhibition of platelet aggregation, via adenosine diphosphate (ADP) $P2Y_{12}$-receptor antagonism (e.g., ticlopidine, clopidogrel, prasugrel, and ticagrelor). Although other classes of agent have been evaluated in clinical trials, dual antiplatelet therapy (DAPT) with aspirin and a $P2Y_{12}$-receptor antagonist remains the evidence-based mainstay of oral antiplatelet therapy in PCI. However, despite the benefits of this strategy, a considerable number of patients experience adverse, recurrent, peri- and postprocedural ischemic and atherothrombotic complications (e.g., reinfarction and stent thrombosis) [4–8]. As such, significant room for further optimization of antiplatelet therapy exists.

In general, greater potency platelet inhibition efficaciously translates into reduced risk of atherothrombotic and ischemic events, but at the expense of greater risks of bleeding. Indeed, even minor bleeding episodes can lead to non-compliance with therapy. As such, all decisions regarding the selection of APT must be in close collaboration with the patient; striving to achieve an optimal balance between safety and efficacy, maximizing prevention of ischemia and minimizing risk of hemorrhage.

The aim of this chapter is to summarize the clinical evidence regarding the optimization of oral antiplatelet therapy for patients undergoing PCI. It will consider the evolution of antiplatelet therapy as an adjunct to PCI, and explore emerging antiplatelet agents presently undergoing clinical development. The role of peri-procedural intravenous antiplatelet therapy, and combinations of antiplatelet and anticoagulant agents, is outside the scope of this review, and is considered elsewhere.

Methods

A series of structured searches of major biomedical databases (PubMed, Medline, Embase, and Web of Science) were performed on October 20, 2014, using the key terms "antiplatelet," "percutaneous coronary intervention," "acute coronary syndrome," "platelet function," "platelet reactivity," and "pharmacogenetics." Only articles published in English, between 1950 and 2014, were included. This is a synthesis of available clinical data regarding oral antiplatelet therapy during PCI.

Background
Platelet activation: pathophysiology and pharmacotherapeutic targets

During intra-arterial thrombosis, platelets become activated as a sequela of rupture, fissure, or erosion of a vulnerable, mural atherosclerotic plaque. The recruitment of platelets to the site of rupture results from complex interactions between specific platelet cell-surface receptors (e.g., platelet glycoprotein VI) and exogenous substrates (e.g., collagen, von Willebrand factor), which expose acidic phospholipids and induce conformational change in the platelet surface membrane. Following adhesion to the vessel wall, platelet–platelet aggregation occurs via synergistic adenosine diphosphate (ADP; $P2Y_1$, and $P2Y_{12}$) and glycoprotein (GP) IIb/IIIa receptor-mediated binding. Degranulation of a cocktail of pro-inflammatory mediators occurs, releasing thromboxane A_2 (TxA_2) and ADP, triggering further platelet activation and aggregation. The exposure of acidic phospholipids activates the coagulation cascade; thrombin-mediated cleavage of fibrinogen to insoluble fibrin culminates in the formation of an occlusive thrombus. Thrombin also interacts with platelets at protease-activated receptors (e.g., PAR-1), enhancing degranulation, and perpetuating further activation. Thus, the platelet is a complex structure, with numerous pharmacologic antithrombotic targets (Figure 40.1).

Interventional Cardiology: Principles and Practice, Second Edition. Edited by George D. Dangas, Carlo Di Mario, and Nicholas N. Kipshidze.
© 2017 John Wiley & Sons, Ltd. Published 2017 by John Wiley & Sons, Ltd.

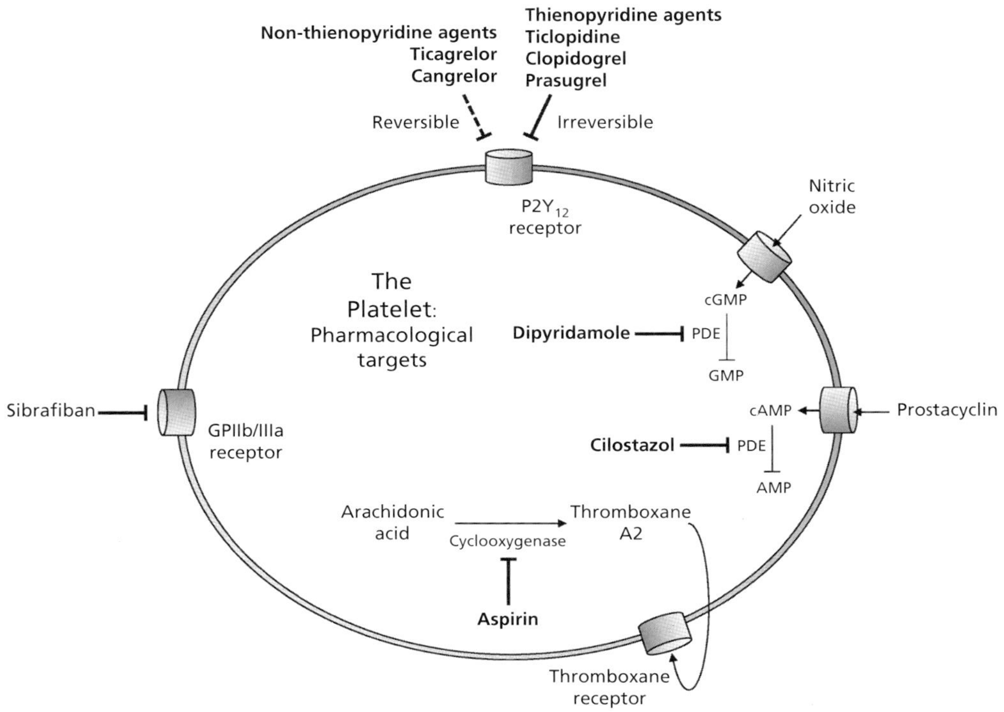

Figure 40.1 A simplified representation of the platelet and selected targets of oral antithrombotic agents.

Oral antiplatelet agents: pharmacology

Antiplatelet agents act via the inhibition of platelet recruitment, adhesion, aggregation, or activation. Aspirin is a ubiquitous, irreversible, non-specific inhibitor of COX, abrogating the downstream synthesis of TxA_2 from arachidonic acid, via selective acetylation of a serine residue at position 529. TxA_2 induces changes in platelet shape and enhances recruitment and aggregation, via binding to thromboxane and prostaglandin endoperoxide (TP) receptors. The thienopyridine-class agents (ticlopidine, clopidogrel, and prasugrel; first, second, and third generation, respectively) act via irreversible platelet ADP $P2Y_{12}$-receptor antagonism. Although both $P2Y_1$ and $P2Y_{12}$ cause aggregation, $P2Y_{12}$-mediated activation is the principal pathway. The thienopyridines are prodrugs; clopidogrel undergoes hepatic activation via a double-oxidation process mediated by the hepatic cytochrome (CYP) P450 system (predominantly CYP2C19) to an active metabolite, which inhibits the ADP $P2Y_{12}$ receptor for the lifespan of the platelet (7–10 days). Prasugrel has distinct pharmacokinetic advantages over clopidogrel: it undergoes more efficient hepatic biotransformation into the active form (with a single oxidation stage), has a more rapid onset of action, and demonstrates reduced variability in response, even compared to high-dose clopidogrel [9]. The non-thienopyridine, cyclopentyl-triazolopyrimidine agent ticagrelor is a reversible ADP $P2Y_{12}$-receptor antagonist, at an allosteric binding site. Unlike the thienopyridines, ticagrelor is administered in active form, and thus has a rapid onset of action, producing potent and consistent platelet inhibition. However, as ticagrelor has a plasma half-life of 8–12 hours, twice daily dosing is required (c.f. the previous agents, for which once daily dosing is sufficient). Additional oral antiplatelet drugs include sibrafiban, which acts to inhibit the GP IIb/IIIa receptor, and cilostazol, a selective phosphodiesterase-3 (PDE-3) inhibitor, which increases cyclic adenosine monophosphate (cAMP), leading to protein kinase A (PKA) activation and inhibition of platelet aggregation. Novel oral antiplatelet agents under development include antagonists of the TxA_2 and PAR-1 pathways.

Oral antiplatelet therapy and PCI

Since the first demonstration of human coronary angioplasty in 1978 [10], interventional cardiology techniques, equipment, peri- and post-procedural care has evolved significantly, leading to major improvements in therapeutic outcomes. Most significantly in the context of this chapter, the pharmacotherapy recommended during PCI has undergone many incremental and beneficial iterations. Antiplatelet therapy has emerged as a critical determinant of outcome following PCI, in both the management of stable CAD, and ACS. However, significant questions remain unanswered regarding the optimal agent(s), combination, and dosing regimen in oral antiplatelet therapy.

Aspirin (acetylsalicylic acid, ASA)

The role of aspirin in all patients with (or at high risk of) cardiovascular disease, is well defined. Evidence-based guidelines universally advocate that such patients should routinely and indefinitely receive low-dose (75–100 mg) aspirin, after an initial loading dose of 300–325 mg, in ACS [1,2]. A meta-analysis by the Antithrombotic Trialists' Collaboration of 287 studies of aspirin therapy in high-risk patients with cardiovascular disease (including over 135,000 patients) definitively established the benefits of such therapy; aspirin therapy reduced incidences of death, myocardial infarction (MI), and stroke by 25% [11]. However, a dose-dependent risk for (specifically, upper gastrointestinal) bleeding, with no bearing on efficacy, was observed. Thus, aspirin is routinely given to all patients with CAD, and was assumed to equally benefit those undergoing, and not undergoing, an invasive management strategy.

Early evidence regarding the benefits of aspirin in the specific context of coronary revascularization arose from ISIS-2, a double-blind, randomized, two-by-two factorial, placebo-controlled trial, which evaluated the effect of aspirin as an adjunct to thrombolysis (streptokinase) in the management of acute MI. This study, which randomized 17,187 patients, demonstrated that 1 month of aspirin, given alone or in combination with revascularization therapy, significantly improved outcome [12,13]. Contemporaneous insight into optimal aspirin dosing emerged from the CURRENT/OASIS-7 trial, in which 25,087 patients with ACS undergoing angiography were randomized to receive either open-label high (300–325 mg/day) versus low (75–100 mg/day, after initial 300 mg) dose aspirin for a month, in addition to high or standard dose of clopidogrel [14]. Although no differences between high and low dose aspirin were observed in overall efficacy (4.2% vs. 4.4%, hazard ratio (HR) 0.97, 95% confidence intervals (CI) 0.86–1.09; $p = 0.61$) or hemorrhage (2.3% vs. 2.3%, HR 0.99, 95% CI 0.84–1.17; $p = 0.90$), the high dose aspirin treatment was non-significantly associated with gastrointestinal bleeding (0.38% vs. 0.24%; $p = 0.051$) at 30 days. Further, a sub-study of the HORIZONS-AMI trial followed-up 2851 patients with STEMI who underwent primary PCI [15]. Of these, 2289 were discharged on low dose aspirin (≤200 mg/day) and 562 on high dose aspirin (>200 mg). Patients receiving high dose aspirin were more likely to have multiple cardiovascular risk factors and, accordingly, had greater 3-year rates of major adverse cardiovascular events (MACE) and significant bleeding. However, multivariate analysis demonstrated that high dose aspirin was significantly associated with a greater rate of major bleeding (HR 2.80, 95% CI 1.31–5.99; $p = 0.008$) but not MACE. These data demonstrate that after an appropriate loading dose prior to PCI (300 mg), which efficaciously improves peri-procedural outcomes, a low dose regimen (75 mg/day) is most appropriate for the long-term secondary prevention of cardiovascular events.

Subsequently, studies have established an association between poor responsiveness to aspirin (high on-aspirin platelet reactivity), and adverse outcomes peri- and post-PCI [16]. In studies that utilize robust COX-1-specific assays (e.g., serum TxA_2 quantification), the prevalence of the resistant phenotype is less than 5% of aspirin-treated patients [16]. A recent registry study of on-aspirin platelet reactivity, ISAR-ASPI, which quantified platelet function in 7090 PCI-treated patients, observed that high on-aspirin platelet reactivity was associated with a significantly increased risk of all-cause mortality or stent thrombosis at 30 days (2.5% vs. 1.1%, odds ratio (OR) 2.24, 95% CI 1.50–3.36) and 1-year (6.2% vs. 3.7%, OR 1.78, 95% CI 1.39–2.27; $p < 0.0001$) compared to those with normal platelet reactivity [17]. However, a major cause of apparent "aspirin resistance," and a major confounder, is poor patient compliance. Additional factors implicated include genetic polymorphism (e.g., in COX-1), and drug–drug interactions (e.g., with ibuprofen). These resistance phenotypes may require evaluation during post-PCI follow-up, in order to ensure treatment compliance and optimize lifelong aspirin dosing.

Thienopyridine P2Y$_{12}$ receptor antagonists
Ticlopidine
Dual antiplatelet therapy with ticlopidine and aspirin emerged as the standard of care after PCI in the mid-1990s, as a result of a number of trials demonstrating the superiority of this combination over aspirin monotherapy [18,19], and other available antithrombotic agents [19–22]. The addition of 250 mg ticlopidine twice daily was associated with fewer thrombotic and hemorrhagic complications. However, as a result of the delayed onset of action of ticlopidine, several days were required to achieve full antiplatelet effects, limiting immediate efficacy in ACS [23].

Clopidogrel
Following regulatory approval, clopidogrel rapidly superseded ticlopidine as the second antiplatelet of choice in PCI, as a result of a faster onset of action via administration of a loading dose [24]. The favorable safety profile of clopidogrel was first demonstrated in the CLASSICS trial, which randomized 1020 patients to receive 325 mg/day aspirin, and either: (i) 300 mg clopidogrel loading dose, followed by a 75 mg maintenance dose, (ii) 75 mg/day clopidogrel, or (iii) 250 mg twice daily dose of ticlopidine [25]. The primary endpoint was a composite of major bleeding complications, other significant side effects, or discontinuation of the study drug. At 28 days' follow-up, 4.6% clopidogrel-treated versus 9.1% ticlopidine-treated patients satisfied criteria for this endpoint (relative risk (RR) 0.50, 95% CI 95% CI 0.31–0.81; $p = 0.005$). The overall rate of MACE (cardiac death, MI, target lesion revascularization) remained comparable between groups (1.2 vs. 0.9 vs. 1.5 for groups (i), (ii), and (iii), respectively; p = not significant). However, CLASSICS randomized patients post-PCI; further studies were required to ascertain the effects of pretreatment clopidogrel.

Subsequent trials definitively demonstrated the incremental benefit of clopidogrel pretreatment, in reducing MACE during PCI, in ACS and stable angina [4–8]. First, the CURE trial randomized 12,562 patients in double-blind fashion to receive clopidogrel (300 mg pretreatment loading dose; 75 mg maintenance dose) or placebo [4]. A total of 2658 of these patients had NSTEACS and underwent PCI as part of the PCI-CURE sub-study [26]. The primary endpoint was a composite of cardiovascular death, MI, and target vessel revascularization, within 30 days of PCI. This endpoint was reached in 4.5% and 6.4% in the clopidogrel-treated and placebo-treated groups, respectively (RR 0.70, 95% CI 0.50–0.97; $p = 0.03$). This reduction in MACE was maintained to 9 months' follow-up ($p = 0.002$), with no differences in major bleeding ($p = 0.64$). This demonstrated that pretreatment with clopidogrel improved outcomes for invasively managed patients with NSTEACS, without significant risks of bleeding.

Further trials were performed to optimize the clopidogrel dosing regimen. The ARMYDA-2 trial randomized 255 patients scheduled to undergo PCI to receive either a 600 or 300 mg loading dose, given 4–8 hours pre-procedure [27]. At 30 days, the primary endpoint (death, MI, or target vessel revascularization) occurred in 4% and 12% of patients in the high and low-loading dose groups, respectively ($p = 0.041$). Multivariate analysis demonstrated a 50% risk reduction in MI associated with the high-loading dose (OR 0.48, 95% CI 0.15–0.97; $p = 0.044$). All safety endpoints (including bleeding) were similar between the two groups. Thus, this small trial indicated that a 600-mg loading dose was safe, and offered greater efficacy, compared to the conventional 300-mg loading dose, in patients undergoing PCI. The aforementioned CURRENT/OASIS-7 study also evaluated a high dose clopidogrel regimen (600 mg loading dose; 150 mg/day maintenance dose post-PCI days 2–7; 75 mg maintenance dose) versus the standard dose regimen, in ACS patients (n = 25,087), treated conservatively and invasively [14,28]. Overall, the efficacy of the high dose and conventional regimens was equivalent, with similar 30-day MACE rate (4.2% vs. 4.4%,

HR 0.94, 95% CI 0.83–1.06; p = 0.30), but increased major bleeding (1.7% vs. 1.3%, HR 1.26, 95% CI 1.03–1.54; p = 0.03). In prespecified subgroup analysis of invasively managed patients (n = 17,263), the high dose regimen led to fewer MACE (3.9 vs. 4.5, HR 0.86, 95% CI 0.74–0.99; p = 0.039), but greater major bleeding (1.6% vs. 1.1%; HR 1.41, 95% CI 1.09–1.83; p = 0.009).

Additional trials offered insight into the optimal timing of clopidogrel pre-treatment. CREDO randomized 2116 patients (scheduled for elective PCI) to receive 300 mg clopidogrel loading dose, or placebo, 3–24 hours pre-PCI, and 75 mg maintenance dose thereafter [5,29]. At 1 year, clopidogrel was associated with a significant reduction in the primary endpoint (composite of death, MI, stroke, and target vessel revascularization; RR 0.73, 95% CI 0.66–0.96; p = 0.02). Clopidogrel administration more than 6 hours pre-procedure (but not thereafter) was associated with significant benefit. Clopidogrel was not associated with a greater risk of major bleeding (8.8% vs. 6.7%; p = 0.07). Further to this, ARMYDA-5 PRELOAD evaluated the safety and efficacy of in-catheterization laboratory 600 mg pre-treatment, versus routine 6-hour pre-treatment, in 409 patients (39% with ACS) [30]. The primary endpoint was 30-day incidence of MACE. ARMYDA-5 PRELOAD demonstrated non-inferiority in primary endpoint between the pre-treatment and in-laboratory arms (8.8% vs. 10.3%; p = 0.72), with no increased risk of hemorrhage (5.4 vs. 7.8; p = 0.42). However, patients in the in-laboratory group demonstrated greater platelet reactivity at PCI, and 2 hours post-procedure (p = 0.043). Thus, an in-laboratory strategy was non-inferior to conventional pre-treatment—where unavoidable, high dose in-laboratory administration is a safe alternative. In the context of primary PCI for STEMI, the randomized CIPAMI trial evaluated the administration of clopidogrel in the pre-hospital phase of care [31]. Although terminated prematurely as a result of slow recruitment, CIPAMI reported a trend toward improved outcomes in the pre-hospital treatment group.

A meta-analysis of randomized and observational data has appraised the effect of pre-treatment with clopidogrel (vs. placebo, in addition to aspirin) on subsequent mortality and bleeding, in 37,814 patients undergoing PCI [32]. Clopidogrel pre-treatment was associated with improvements in the risk of MACE (OR 0.77, 95% CI 0.66–0.89; p <0.001) but without translation into improved mortality (OR 0.80, 95% CI 0.57–1.11). No differences were reported in major hemorrhage (OR 1.18, 95% CI 0.57–1.11). Although this analysis was limited by substantial interstudy heterogeneity (indications for PCI included stable and unstable angina, NSTEACS, and STEMI), the results suggest an inconsistent treatment effect exists across the spectrum of CAD presentations. The benefits of clopidogrel pre-treatment were greater with increasing severity of CAD (i.e., STEMI > NSTEMI > unstable angina > stable angina). Indeed, the authors report that clopidogrel pre-treatment did not improve outcomes in stable angina, and troublingly, was associated with a greater bleeding risk. A further meta-analysis by this group appraises the risks and benefits associated of thienopyridines pre-treatment in the context of 32,383 patients with NSTEACS (55% underwent PCI) [33]. Pre-treatment was associated with reduced MACE (OR 0.84, 95% CI 0.72–0.98; p = 0.02), driven by the inclusion of CURE and CREDO, but did not translate into improvements in mortality (OR 0.90, 95% CI 0.75–1.07; p = 0.24). No differences in MACE or mortality were observed in the subpopulation undergoing PCI. Significant excess bleeding (30–45%) was observed in all patients (OR 1.32, 95% CI 1.16–1.49; p <0.0001). Although these analyses included clopidogrel and prasugrel, analysis stratified by agent, or limited to randomized trial evidence, did not alter the findings.

Optimization of clopidogrel therapy

Despite the benefits of clopidogrel in the context of PCI, a significant number of patients experience recurrent, adverse, peri- and post-procedural atherothrombotic compilations, as a result of high on-treatment platelet reactivity [4–8]. This is hypothesized, in part, to be caused by the wide inter-individual variability in responsiveness to clopidogrel: a significant proportion of clopidogrel-treated patients have suboptimal inhibition of platelet function. The prevalence of this resistance phenotype ranges from 5% to 40%, dependent on the definition of resistance, platelet function assay, clopidogrel dosing regimen, and study population. One mechanism conferring inadequate clopidogrel responsiveness is the presence of loss-of-function alleles at the CYP2C19 locus; lack of expression of the CYP2C19 enzyme, and poor activation of clopidogrel [34]. Concomitant administration of agents that repress CYP2C19 activity (e.g., omeprazole) can also contribute to the resistance phenotype [35]. Indeed, these observations have prompted several regulatory agencies to issue warnings regarding the use of clopidogrel in such individuals. However, whether high PR represents a risk marker, or modifiable risk factor, remains a matter of contentious debate.

Several major studies have explored this issue, including GRAVITAS, which evaluated high-dose clopidogrel, in 2214 patients with stable CAD or NSTEACS undergoing PCI, with high on-clopidogrel PR [36]. Patients were randomized to high-dose (600 mg loading dose, 150 mg/day dose) or standard-dose clopidogrel (300 mg loading dose, 75 mg/day dose). At 6 months' follow-up, no differences in efficacy or safety endpoints were noted, differential clopidogrel dosing based on PR had no impact on clinical outcomes. In a further study, 429 ACS patients undergoing PCI with poor response to a 600-mg clopidogrel loading dose were randomized to receive either standard therapy, or up to three additional 600 mg clopidogrel loading doses, guided by PR, prior to PCI [37]. The authors observed that the rate of MACE was significantly lower in the PR-guided group than the control group (0.5 vs. 8.9%; p <0.001), with no difference in bleeding rates (2.8% vs. 3.7%; p=0.80), suggesting that PR-guided loading can be advantageous in the management of the clopidogrel resistance phenotype. The TRIGGER-PCI study specifically targeted higher potency thienopyridine pharmacotherapy to patients with the clopidogrel resistance phenotype [38]. Despite the pharmacodynamic superiority of the alternative agent, TRIGGER-PCI was stopped prematurely due to futility. The event rate was lower than predicted in both groups. The clinical utility of this strategy could not be determined.

In addition, trials have evaluated genotype-based dosing regimens. Most notably, the ELEVATE-TIMI-56 trial randomized 333 patients with stable CAD to receive CYP2C19 genotype-guided clopidogrel dosing regimens. Although this strategy successfully enabled patients with loss-of-function alleles to achieve levels of PR comparable to wild-type patients, this study was not powered to report clinical outcomes. Indeed, well-powered trials have thus far been performed in the context of PCI.

Thus, despite significant efforts, to date, differential dosing strategies, based on PR or pharmacogenetic testing, have had no beneficial impact on hard, clinical endpoints, in appropriately controlled, powered, randomized, and blinded trials. However, the development of greater potency P2Y$_{12}$-receptor antagonists, with less inter-individual variation, has proven highly fruitful.

Prasugrel

The third generation thienopyridine, prasugrel, has distinct pharmacokinetic advantages over clopidogrel: it has a more rapid onset of action, and demonstrates reduced variability in response. TRITON-TIMI-38 randomized 13,608 clopidogrel-naïve patients with moderate–high risk ACS undergoing PCI to receive either prasugrel (60 mg loading dose, 10 mg/day maintenance dose) or clopidogrel (300 mg loading dose, 70 mg maintenance dose) [39]. Randomization occurred following ascertainment of coronary anatomy, with the exception of patients undergoing primary PCI for STEMI. At 15 months' follow-up, the primary endpoint (composite of cardiovascular death, non-fatal MI, or stroke) occurred in 9.9% of prasugrel-treated and 12.1% of clopidogrel-treated patients (HR 0.81, 95% CI 0.73–0.90; p <0.001), driven by non-fatal MI (40% of which were peri-procedural) and stent thrombosis (HR 0.48, 95% CI 0.36–0.84; p <0.0001) [39,40]. This benefit was also observed at 30 days, and was independent of stent type. However, this was offset by a significant risk of major (2.4% vs. 1.8%, HR 1.32, 95% CI 1.03–1.68; p = 0.03) and fatal bleeding (0.4% vs. 0.1%, HR 4.19, 95% CI 1.58–11.11; p = 0.002) in the prasugrel-treated and clopidogrel-treated groups, respectively [39,41]. Pre-specified analysis demonstrated that prasugrel was associated with net benefit, despite bleeding risks (p = 0.004). Certain subgroups experienced greater benefits, including those with STEMI, and with diabetes mellitus, for whom the benefits far outweighed the risk of bleeding [42,43]. Conversely, no net benefit was observed in patients aged ≥75 years, weighing less than 60 kg, and with previous history of stroke or transient ischemic attack (TIA).

ACCOAST is the only placebo-controlled trial of prasugrel pre-treatment; randomizing 4033 NSTEACS patients (69% of whom underwent PCI) to receive 30 mg prasugrel, or placebo [44]. A supplementary 30-mg pre-PCI dose was administered following diagnostic angiography in the pre-treatment group, and 60 mg of prasugrel given to the placebo group. Pre-treatment was not associated with a reduced risk of MACE (HR 1.02, 95% CI 0.84–1.25; p = 0.81), although a higher rate of major bleeding was observed (HR 1.90, 95% CI 1.19–3.02; p = 0.006). Indeed, this rate of bleeding exceeding the a priori defined threshold, and the study was halted during enrolment.

Observational studies have also been undertaken to evaluate real-world prasugrel outcomes. Koshy et al. [45] recently reported a retrospective case series of 1688 primary PCI-treated patients with STEMI, who received pre-treatment with aspirin plus clopidogrel (n = 866) or prasugrel (n = 822) [45]. Patients were excluded if aged ≥75 years, weighed <60 kg or had active bleeding, cerebrovascular disease, or hepatic impairment. No differences were reported in the frequency of in-hospital bleeding complications, unadjusted in-hospital, 30-day or 1-year mortality, in prasugrel and clopidogrel-treated patients. Covariate-adjusted analysis demonstrated an association between prasugrel and reduced mortality at 1 year (HR 0.47, 95% CI 0.25–0.88; p = 0.018). However, several limitations of this study suggest caution in the interpretation of these findings, including the highly selected, retrospective population.

Recently, methodologically superior registry data has emerged, prospectively following 23,994 clopidogrel-treated and 2142 prasugrel-treated patients undergoing PCI [46]. Prasugrel was primarily used in patients with STEMI, without hemorrhagic risk factors. In patients presenting with ACS, lower mortality was observed in prasugrel-treated than the clopidogrel-treated patients; however, mortality remained equivocal in those undergoing elective angiography and PCI. In-hospital bleeding complications occurred less frequently in prasugrel-treated than clopidogrel-treated patients. These data suggest that when prasugrel is used in appropriately selected patients (i.e., those with ACS) and avoided in patients with characteristics indicating increased risk of hemorrhage, mortality and bleeding rates are acceptably low for both agents. These studies indicate that although prasugrel has a role in specific groups of high risk ACS patients, it should be used with caution in patients for whom the risks outweigh benefits.

Non-thienopyridine P2Y$_{12}$ receptor antagonists
Ticagrelor

The development of ticagrelor was impelled by the need for an agent that overcomes the limitations of the thienopyridines—the slow onset and wide inter-individual variability of clopidogrel, and the adverse safety profile of prasugrel. Preclinical and early phase clinical studies demonstrated that ticagrelor is characterized by rapid, extensive, and consistent antiplatelet activity, with favorable bleeding risks.

The landmark PLATO trial randomized 18,624 ACS patients to receive ticagrelor (180 mg loading dose, 90 mg twice daily maintenance dose) or clopidogrel (300–600 mg loading dose, 75 mg/day maintenance dose) [47]. Patients with moderate–high risk ACS received an additional, blinded loading dose of clopidogrel (total loading dose 600 mg) or placebo. In contrast to TRITON-TIMI-38, randomization occurred before angiography, and non-clopidogrel-naïve patients were eligible. At 12 months, ticagrelor significantly reduced the primary endpoint (cardiovascular death, non-fatal MI, or stroke; 9.8% vs. 11.7%, HR 0.84, 95% CI 0.77–0.92; p <0.0001), driven by reductions in cardiovascular mortality (4.0% vs. 5.1%, HR 0.79, 95% CI 0.69–0.91; p = 0.001), non-fatal MI (5.8% vs. 6.9%, HR 0.84, 95% CI 0.75–0.95; p = 0.005) and stent thrombosis (2.2% vs. 3.0%, HR 0.73, 95% CI 0.57–0.94; p = 0.014). Overall, no difference in bleeding was observed in ticagrelor-treated and clopidogrel-treated patients (11.6% vs. 11.2%, HR 1.04; p = 0.43). However, major bleeding was significantly higher in ticagrelor-treated patients (2.8% vs. 2.2%; p = 0.03; by TIMI criteria), including fatal intracranial hemorrhage (0.1% vs. 0.01%; p = 0.02), but not all-cause fatal bleeding (0.3% vs. 0.3%; p = 0.66). The absolute rate of major bleeding was similar to that in TRITON-TIMI-38. Several PLATO subgroup analyses demonstrate consistency of the benefits of ticagrelor in patients undergoing (i) coronary artery bypass graft surgery [48], (ii) planned PCI[49] and (iii) non-invasive, medical management [50]. Unlike prasugrel in TRITON-TIMI-38, there were no patient subgroups for which there was an excess frequency of bleeding, including those with cerebrovascular disease, or aged ≥75 years. However, several non-hematologic, off-target effects were observed; associated with discontinuation of the study drug including: (i) ventricular pauses, (ii) dyspnea, and (iii) elevated serum creatinine and uric acid. Although precise mechanisms remain to be definitively elucidated, these effects have not been proven to have any other demonstrable clinical impact. Additionally, subgroup analysis demonstrated worse outcomes in North American ticagrelor-treated patients, associated with the use of high dose daily aspirin (>100 mg) [51]. As such, the use of aspirin doses lower than 100 mg are recommended.

PLATO did not evaluate the use of a pre-treatment strategy compared with delayed administration; all patients received pre-treatment, irrespective of the intended (i.e., invasive or non-invasive) strategy. As such, the recently reported ATLANTIC study offers further insight on the optimal timing of administration; randomizing 1862 patients with STEMI in double-blind fashion to receive either pre-hospital or in-laboratory ticagrelor [52]. ATLANTIC recruited patients with ongoing STEMI of duration less than 6 hours; the median time difference between the two treatment arms (pre-hospital or in-hospital) was 31 minutes. No difference was observed in the proportion of patients achieving ≥70% resolution of ST-elevation prior to PCI, or TIMI flow grade 3 in the infarct-related artery at angiography. Thirty-day MACE rates did not significantly differ between the treatment arms, although the rate of stent thrombosis was lower in the pre-hospital group than the in-hospital group (0 vs. 0.8% at 24 hours, 0.2% vs. 1.2% at 30 days). The frequency of major bleeding was low and equivocal. Thus, administering ticagrelor in the pre-hospital setting does not improve outcomes (or increase risk) for patients with STEMI.

Until recently, there has existed a paucity of evidence regarding the long-term efficacy of treatment with ticagrelor post-MI and post-PCI. The multicenter PEGASUS-TIMI 54 trial randomized 21,162 patients (17,568 of whom had undergone previous PCI; 83.0%), 1–3 years post-MI, to receive ticagrelor 90 mg twice daily (high dose), ticagrelor 60 mg twice daily (low dose), or placebo, in addition to low dose aspirin, in double-blind fashion [53]. The primary efficacy endpoint (composite of cardiovascular death, MI, or stroke) was reduced in both the 90 and 60 mg groups, versus placebo (90 mg twice daily: HR 0.85, 0.75–0.96; p = 0.008; 60 mg twice daily: HR 0.84, 0.74–0.95; p = 0.004). However, there was no difference in the primary endpoint when comparing the low and high dose groups (p = NS). Patients receiving the low and high dose ticagrelor had a 2.3- and 2.7-fold greater risk of clinically significant bleeding, and a 3.0- and 3.7-fold greater need for transfusion, respectively, compared with placebo (all p <0.001). As such, the authors conclude that the long-term administration of 60 mg twice daily ticagrelor can offer the most attractive risk–benefit profile, in addition to low dose aspirin, following MI. Thus, the long-term administration of ticagrelor post-PCI, in carefully selected patients, offers significant improvements in patient outcomes.

Other oral antiplatelet agents

Despite significant progress in the development of oral antiplatelet agents as adjuncts to PCI, success has been far from universal. In particular, the development of the oral glycoprotein IIb/IIIa inhibitors has been fraught with difficulty: xemilofiban, orbofiban, and sibrafiban have all undergone extensive placebo-controlled phase 3 clinical trials in CAD [54–56]. Each of these trials failed to report benefits, and suggested increased off-target mortality associated with such therapy.

Other oral APT agents have received approval for clinical use in various clinical settings—including cilostazol, dypiridamole, and pentoxifylline—but are not indicated in PCI, because of an insufficient evidence of benefit. Several novel agents, targeting different pathways in the thrombotic pathway, are currently in development. These have emerged in response to the shortcomings of current APT, which include: (i) no available TxA_2 pathway inhibitor apart from aspirin, to which a significant proportion of patients are allergic, cannot tolerate, or demonstrate inadequate responses; and (ii) the slow offset of $P2Y_{12}$-receptor antagonists, an issue in patients with hemorrhagic complications.

Direct inhibition of the TxA_2 pathway poses several advantages over upstream COX-1 inhibition, including more potent platelet inhibition (via antagonism of endoperoxides at their receptors, or TxA_2 synthase) and less off-target effects (e.g., gastric mucosal erosion). TxA_2 inhibitors under development include picotamide, ridogrel, terutroban, ramatroban, EV077, and NCX4016. Although

TxA_2 inhibition remains a promising strategy, of the agents that have undergone clinical testing against aspirin (picotamide, ridogrel, terutroban), results have largely been underwhelming [57–59]. Elinogrel, a direct-acting, reversible ADP $P2Y_{12}$-receptor antagonist, available in both intravenous and oral forms, provides potent platelet inhibition, with rapid onset and offset of action [60]. Despite demonstrating early promise in preclinical and early clinical studies, a phase 2 trial of elinogrel as an adjunct to PCI demonstrated an unacceptable bleeding risk compared with clopidogrel (INNOVATE-PCI; HR 1.98, 95% CI 1.10–3.57) [61]. As a result, the development of elinogrel was terminated prior to phase 3 trials, in 2012.

Another potential avenue of antiplatelet therapy is inhibition of platelet PAR-1, which interacts with thrombin. Two candidate compounds are currently undergoing development; vorapaxar (which has undergone phase 3 trials) and atopaxar (which has undergone phase 2 trials). Two large-scale phase 3 trials of vorapaxar, TRACER and TRA 2°P-TIMI-50 both report that the agent is efficacious in preventing MACE, but at the expense of significant bleeding [62,63]. Indeed, both trials were terminated prematurely because of an unacceptable risk of hemorrhage. Phase 2 trials (LANCELOT-ACS, LANCELOT-CAD, and J-LANCELOT) demonstrated the favorable safety profile of atopaxar with regard to bleeding risk, in patients with both ACS and stable CAD [64–66]. However, other side effects (dose-related QTc prolongation, hepatic transaminase elevation) were observed. Although phase 3 trials are required to provide definitive answers, none are planned at present.

Additional potential oral agents in early, preclinical development, include nitric oxide donors (LA419, LA846), prostaglandin E receptor 3 (DG-041), and serotonin receptor antagonists (APD791). Further preclinical testing is required before the applications of these agents become apparent.

Clinical guidelines: oral antiplatelet therapy in PCI

Evidence-based clinical guidelines advise clinicians regarding the optimal antiplatelet pharmacotherapy in patients undergoing PCI. The latest European Society of Cardiology (ESC) and European Association for Cardiothoracic Surgery (EACTS) guidelines stratify optimal APT by indication for PCI: (i) stable CAD, (ii) NSTEACS, and (iii) STEMI (Table 40.1) [1]. In all indications for PCI, a 150–300 mg loading dose of aspirin, followed by 75–100 mg life-long daily maintenance dose, is recommended.

In PCI for stable CAD, 300–600 mg clopidogrel loading dose, followed by 75 mg/day, should be administered. Although no evidence of benefit exists for systematic clopidogrel preloading before diagnostic coronary angiography in stable CAD [32], a loading dose of 600 mg is recommended in patients scheduled for elective PCI if coronary anatomy has been pre-established. In PCI for NSTEACS, DAPT is recommended with a potent $P2Y_{12}$-receptor antagonist; either prasugrel (60 mg loading and 10 mg/day maintenance dose), ticagrelor (180 mg loading and 90 mg twice daily maintenance dose) or, when these are contraindicated or not available, clopidogrel (600 mg loading and 150 mg/day maintenance dose). In PCI for STEMI, DAPT with a potent $P2Y_{12}$-receptor antagonist is also recommended; either prasugrel (60 mg loading and 10 mg/day maintenance dose), or ticagrelor (180 mg loading and 90 mg twice daily maintenance dose). However, caution against the use of these agents is advised in patients with cerebrovascular disease, or moderate-to-severe hepatic impairment—clopidogrel (600 mg loading and

Table 40.1 Summary of current European (ESC/EACTS) guidelines regarding the use of oral antiplatelet agents in percutaneous coronary intervention (PCI).

Indication for PCI	Oral antiplatelet	Recommendations	Class	Level
Stable CAD	Aspirin	Indicated prior to elective stenting	I	B
		Pre-treatment with 150–300 mg loading dose if not on maintenance dose	I	C
		Life-long aspirin therapy recommended	I	A
	Clopidogrel	Treatment with 600 mg loading dose once anatomy known, and PCI is planned. Preferably ≥2 hours pre-procedure	I	A
		Consider pretreatment in patients at high probability for significant CAD	IIb	C
		In patients on 75 mg maintenance therapy, a new loading dose of 600 mg may be conisdered, once PCI is planned	IIb	C
		600 mg loading dose, 75 mg/day maintenance dose is recommended for elective stenting	I	A
		Continue for at least 1 month after BMS implantation	I	A
		Continue for at least 6 months after DES implantation	I	B
		Shorter duration (<6 months) can be considered after DES implantation for patients at high risk of bleeding	IIb	A
		Longer duration (>6 months) can be considered in patients at high ischemic risk and low bleeding risk	IIb	C
Non-ST-elevation ACS	Aspirin	Recommended in all patients without contraindications. 150–300 mg loading dose, 75–100 mg/day maintenance dose. To be continued indefinitely	I	A
	Prasugrel	60 mg loading dose, 10 mg/day maintenance dose, for patients in whom coronary anatomy is known and who are proceeding to PCI. Contraindicated in patients with prior TIA/stroke. Not recommended in patients >75 years of age. Consider lower maintenance dose in patients weighing <60 kg. Continue for 12 months, unless contraindications exist (excess bleeding risk)	I	B
	Ticagrelor	180 mg loading dose, 90 mg twice daily maintenance, for patients at moderate–high risk of ischemic events, regardless of initial treatment strategy including those pretreated with clopidogrel, if no contraindication. Continue for 12 months, unless contraindications exist (excess bleeding risk)	I	B
	Clopidogrel	600 mg loading dose, 75 mg/day dose, only when prasugrel or ticagrelor are not available or are contraindicated. Continue for 12 months, unless contraindications exist (excess bleeding risk)	I	B
ST-elevation MI	Aspirin	Recommended in all patients without contraindications. 150–300 mg loading dose, 75–100 mg/day maintenance dose. To be continued indefinitely	I	A
	Prasugrel	60 mg loading dose at first medical contact, 10 mg/day maintenance dose, unless contraindication. Contraindicated in patients with prior TIA/stroke. Not recommended in patients >75 years of age. Consider lower maintenance dose in patients weighing <60 kg. Continue for 12 months, unless contraindications exist (excess bleeding risk)	I	B
	Ticagrelor	180 mg loading dose at first medical contact, 90 mg twice daily maintenance, unless contraindication. Continue for 12 months, unless contraindications exist (excess bleeding risk)	I	B
	Clopidogrel	600 mg loading dose at first medical contact, 75 mg daily dose, only when prasugrel or ticagrelor are not available or are contraindicated. Continue for 12 months, unless contraindications exist (excess bleeding risk)	I	B

ACS, acute coronary syndrome; BMS, bare metal stent; CAD, coronary artery disease; DES, drug-eluting stent; MI, myocardial infarction; PCI, percutaneous coronary intervention.

Source: Adapted from: Kohl et al. (2014) [1].

Table 40.2 Summary of current North American (ACC/AHA/SCAI) guidelines regarding the use of oral antiplatelet agents in PCI.

Indication for PCI	Oral antiplatelet	Recommendations	Class	Level
ACS	Aspirin	Patients already taking daily aspirin therapy should take 81–325 mg before PCI	I	B
		Patients not on aspirin therapy should be given a loading dose of 325 mg before PCI	I	B
		After PCI, use of aspirin should be continued indefinitely	I	A
		After PCI, aspirin 81 mg/day should be used in preference to higher maintenance doses	IIa	B
	Clopidogrel	A loading dose of 600 mg of clopidogrel should be considered	I	B
		The clopidogrel loading dose for patients undergoing PCI post-fibrinolysis therapy should be: (i) 300 mg within 24 hours; or (ii) 600 mg >24 hours after receiving fibrinolysis	I	C
		In patients receiving a stent (either BMS or DES) during PCI, clopidogrel 75 mg/day should be given for at least 12 months	I	B
		If the risk of morbidity from bleeding outweighs the anticipated benefit afforded by a recommended duration of clopidogrel therapy after stent implantation, earlier discontinuation (e.g., <12 months) of clopidogrel inhibitor therapy is reasonable	IIa	C
	Prasugrel	A loading dose of 60 mg prasugrel should be considered	I	B
		In patients receiving a stent (either BMS or DES) during PCI, prasugrel 10 mg/day should be given for at least 12 months	I	B
		If the risk of morbidity from bleeding outweighs the anticipated benefit afforded by a recommended duration of prasugrel therapy after stent implantation, earlier discontinuation (e.g., <12 months) of prasugrel inhibitor therapy is reasonable	IIa	C
		Prasugrel should not be administered to patients with a prior history of stroke or transient ischemic attack	III	B
	Ticagrelor	A loading dose of 180 mg ticagrelor should be considered	I	B
		In patients receiving a stent (either BMS or DES) during PCI, ticagrelor 90 mg twice daily should be given for at least 12 months	I	B
		If the risk of morbidity from bleeding outweighs the anticipated benefit afforded by a recommended duration of clopidogrel therapy after stent implantation, earlier discontinuation (e.g., <12 months) of ticagrelor inhibitor therapy is reasonable	IIa	C
Non-ACS	Aspirin	Patients already taking daily aspirin therapy should take 81–325 mg before PCI	I	B
		Patients not on aspirin therapy should be given a loading dose of 325 mg before PCI	I	B
		After PCI, use of aspirin should be continued indefinitely	I	A
	Clopidogrel	A loading dose of 600 mg clopidogrel should be considered	I	B
		In patients receiving a stent (either BMS or DES) during PCI, clopidogrel should be given for a minimum of 1 month; ideally up to 12 months (unless bleeding risk increased—then it should be given for a minimum of 2 weeks)	I	B
	Prasugrel	If the risk of morbidity from bleeding outweighs the anticipated benefit afforded by a recommended duration of prasugrel therapy after stent implantation, earlier discontinuation (e.g., <12 months) of prasugrel inhibitor therapy is reasonable	IIa	C
		Prasugrel should not be administered to patients with a prior history of stroke or transient ischemic attack	III	B
	Ticagrelor	If the risk of morbidity from bleeding outweighs the anticipated benefit afforded by a recommended duration of clopidogrel therapy after stent implantation, earlier discontinuation (e.g., <12 months) of ticagrelor inhibitor therapy is reasonable	IIa	C

ACC, American College of Cardiology; ACS, acute coronary syndrome; AHA, American Heart Association; BMS, bare metal stent; CAD, coronary artery disease; DES, drug-eluting stent; PCI, percutaneous coronary intervention; SCAI, Society for Cardiac Angiography and Interventions.
Source: Adapted from Levine GN, et al. 2011 [2].

150 mg/day maintenance dose) should be substituted. In addition, all patients should be instructed not to prematurely discontinue oral APT without first consulting a physician, because of increased risks of recurrent MI and stent thrombosis [67].

The most recent American College of Cardiology (ACC) and American Heart Association (AHA) guidelines (Table 40.2) advocate broadly similar regimens [2]. An aspirin loading dose of 325 mg for aspirin-naïve patients, or 81–325 mg for patients previously receiving daily aspirin, is recommended, with low dose aspirin advocated indefinitely. Patients should also receive a loading dose of a $P2Y_{12}$-receptor antagonist; recommended options include: (i) clopidogrel (600 mg; ACS and non-ACS patients), (ii) prasugrel (60 mg; ACS patients), or ticagrelor (180 mg; ACS patients). Patients should be counseled on the need for, and risk of, DAPT in advance of stent placement, and alternatives pursued (i.e., balloon angioplasty) if patients are unwilling or unable to comply for the recommended duration. The guidelines advocate a holistic assessment of potential benefits and harms (thrombotic vs. bleeding risks), and pragmatic adjustment of the post-PCI antiplatelet regimen, accordingly.

Future perspectives

Despite significant progress, a number of questions remain unanswered regarding the optimization of oral antiplatelet therapy during PCI. Perhaps most importantly: how much scope remains for the further improvement of oral antiplatelet therapy in PCI, given the current status of such therapy, and recent improvements in intravenous antiplatelet agents (e.g., GP IIb/IIIa inhibitors, direct thrombin inhibitors). Insight from the PARIS registry, which prospectively studied 5018 patients undergoing PCI indicated that MACE following cessation of DAPT depend on the clinical circumstances of discontinuation, and attenuate over time [67]. Approximately half of all premature discontinuations within 2 years of PCI was physician-advised, and did not result in adverse outcomes. However, disruptions in antiplatelet therapy or non-compliance were associated with a significantly increased risk of MACE, which attenuated after 30 days. Surprisingly, the overall contribution of DAPT cessation was small—indeed, most MACE occurred while patients were receiving optimal DAPT (74%; 8.5% of overall study population). Although patients received mainly aspirin and clopidogrel DAPT, improvements in antiplatelet regimens may still yield improved outcomes in a large number of patients for whom existing therapy is ineffectual.

Despite a number of placebo- and clopidogrel-controlled studies, the relative efficacy and safety of prasugrel and ticagrelor remains uncertain: head-to-head comparisons, in prospective, randomized studies, are required. In the interim, subgroup and meta-analysis represents approaches by which these strategies can be indirectly compared, in different settings. A further concern is that of cost; the newer, more potent $P2Y_{12}$ inhibitors remain on-patent, and are thus greatly more expensive than clopidogrel, which has recently become available in a generic, inexpensive formulation in most countries. However, as the patents for prasugrel and ticagrelor expire in 2017 and 2018, respectively, generic forms could soon become available.

Conclusions

The evolution of antiplatelet strategies has yielded incremental improvements in peri- and post-PCI outcomes, as a direct result of demonstration of safety and efficacy in methodologically robust randomized clinical trials and prospective registries. However, despite notable advances and best-available antiplatelet regimens, a proportion of patients continue to experience adverse outcomes; both ischemic and from bleeding risks. As such, decisions regarding antiplatelet therapy must be patient-centered; holistically appraising the potential benefits and risks inherent with such treatment. Further optimization of present antiplatelet pharmacotherapeutic regimens, and the development of novel oral antiplatelet agents targeting novel pathways in the thrombotic pathway, will surely continue to improve outcomes following PCI.

Interactive multiple choice questions are available for this chapter on www.wiley. com/go/dangas/cardiology

References

1 Kolh P, Windecker S, Alfonso F, et al. 2014 ESC/EACTS Guidelines on myocardial revascularization: The Task Force on Myocardial Revascularization of the European Society of Cardiology (ESC) and the European Association for Cardio-Thoracic Surgery (EACTS)Developed with the special contribution of the European Association of Percutaneous Cardiovascular Interventions (EAPCI). *EurJ Cardiothorac Surg* 2014; **46**(4): 517–592.

2 Levine GN, Bates ER, Blankenship JC, et al. 2011 ACCF/AHA/SCAI Guideline for percutaneous coronary intervention: a report of the American College of Cardiology Foundation/American Heart Association Task Force on Practice Guidelines and the Society for Cardiovascular Angiography and Interventions. *J Am Coll Cardiol* 2011; **58**(24): e44–e122.

3 Rao SV, Ohman EM. Anticoagulant therapy for percutaneous coronary intervention. *Circ Cardiovasc Interv* 2010; **3**(1): 80–88.

4 Yusuf S, Zhao F, Mehta SR, et al. Effects of clopidogrel in addition to aspirin in patients with acute coronary syndromes without ST-segment elevation. *N Engl J Med* 2001; **345**(7): 494–502.

5 Steinhubl SR, Berger PB, Mann JT, 3rd, et al. Early and sustained dual oral antiplatelet therapy following percutaneous coronary intervention: a randomized controlled trial. *JAMA* 2002; **288**(19): 2411–2420.

6 Chen ZM, Jiang LX, Chen YP, et al. Addition of clopidogrel to aspirin in 45,852 patients with acute myocardial infarction: randomised placebo-controlled trial. *Lancet* 2005; **366**(9497): 1607–1621.

7 Sabatine MS, Cannon CP, Gibson CM, et al. Addition of clopidogrel to aspirin and fibrinolytic therapy for myocardial infarction with ST-segment elevation. *N Engl J Med* 2005; **352**(12): 1179–1189.

8 Bhatt DL, Fox KA, Hacke W, et al. Clopidogrel and aspirin versus aspirin alone for the prevention of atherothrombotic events. *N Engl J Med* 2006; **354**(16): 1706–1717.

9 Wiviott SD, Trenk D, Frelinger AL, et al. Prasugrel compared with high loading-and maintenance-dose clopidogrel in patients with planned percutaneous coronary intervention: the Prasugrel in Comparison to Clopidogrel for Inhibition of Platelet Activation and Aggregation–Thrombolysis in Myocardial Infarction 44 Trial. *Circulation* 2007; **116**(25): 2923–2932.

10 Gruntzig A. Transluminal dilatation of coronary-artery stenosis. *Lancet* 1978; **1**(8058): 263.

11 Antithrombotic Trialists' Collaboration. Collaborative meta-analysis of randomised trials of antiplatelet therapy for prevention of death, myocardial infarction, and stroke in high risk patients 2002; **324**: 71–86.

12 Randomised trial of intravenous streptokinase, oral aspirin, both, or neither among 17,187 cases of suspected acute myocardial infarction: ISIS-2. ISIS-2 (Second International Study of Infarct Survival) Collaborative Group. *Lancet* 1988; **2**(8607): 349–360.

13 Baigent C, Collins R, Appleby P, et al. ISIS-2: 10 year survival among patients with suspected acute myocardial infarction in randomised comparison of intravenous streptokinase, oral aspirin, both, or neither. The ISIS-2 (Second International Study of Infarct Survival) Collaborative Group. *BMJ* 1998; **316**(7141): 1337–1343.

14 Investigators C-O, Mehta SR, Bassand JP, et al. Dose comparisons of clopidogrel and aspirin in acute coronary syndromes. *N Engl J Med* 2010; **363**(10): 930–942.

15 Yu J, Mehran R, Dangas GD, et al. Safety and efficacy of high- versus low-dose aspirin after primary percutaneous coronary intervention in ST-segment elevation myocardial infarction: the HORIZONS-AMI (Harmonizing Outcomes With Revascularization and Stents in Acute Myocardial Infarction) trial. *JACC Cardiovasc Interv* 2012; **5**(12): 1231–1238.

16 Krasopoulos G, Brister SJ, Beattie WS, et al. Aspirin "resistance" and risk of cardiovascular morbidity: systematic review and meta-analysis. BMJ 2008; **336**(7637): 195–198.

17 Mayer K, Bernlochner I, Braun S, et al. Aspirin treatment and outcomes after percutaneous coronary intervention: results of the ISAR-ASPI Registry. J Am Coll Cardiol 2014; **64**(9): 863–871.

18 Hall P, Nakamura S, Maiello L, et al. A randomized comparison of combined ticlopidine and aspirin therapy versus aspirin therapy alone after successful intravascular ultrasound-guided stent implantation. Circulation 1996; **93**(2): 215–222.

19 Leon MB, Baim DS, Popma JJ, et al. A clinical trial comparing three antithrombotic-drug regimens after coronary-artery stenting. Stent Anticoagulation Restenosis Study Investigators. N Engl J Med 1998; **339**(23): 1665–1671.

20 Schomig A, Neumann FJ, Kastrati A, et al. A randomized comparison of antiplatelet and anticoagulant therapy after the placement of coronary-artery stents. N Engl J Med 1996; **334**(17): 1084–1089.

21 Bertrand ME, Legrand V, Boland J, et al. Randomized multicenter comparison of conventional anticoagulation versus antiplatelet therapy in unplanned and elective coronary stenting: the full anticoagulation versus aspirin and ticlopidine (fantastic) study. Circulation 1998; **98**(16): 1597–1603.

22 Urban P, Macaya C, Rupprecht HJ, et al. Randomized evaluation of anticoagulation versus antiplatelet therapy after coronary stent implantation in high-risk patients: the multicenter aspirin and ticlopidine trial after intracoronary stenting (MATTIS). Circulation 1998; **98**(20): 2126–2132.

23 Kuzniar J, Splawinska B, Malinga K, et al. Pharmacodynamics of ticlopidine: relation between dose and time of administration to platelet inhibition. Int J Clin Pharmacol Ther 1996; **34**(8): 357–361.

24 Cadroy Y, Bossavy JP, Thalamas C, et al. Early Potent antithrombotic effect with combined aspirin and a loading dose of clopidogrel on experimental arterial thrombogenesis in humans. Circulation 2000; **101**(24): 2823–2828.

25 Bertrand ME, Rupprecht H-J, Urban P, et al. Double-blind study of the safety of clopidogrel with and without a loading dose in combination with aspirin compared with ticlopidine in combination with aspirin after coronary stenting: the Clopidogrel Aspirin Stent International Cooperative Study (CLASSICS). Circulation 2000; **102**(6): 624–629.

26 Mehta SR, Yusuf S, Peters RJG, et al. Effects of pretreatment with clopidogrel and aspirin followed by long-term therapy in patients undergoing percutaneous coronary intervention: the PCI-CURE study. Lancet 2001; **358**(9281): 527–533.

27 Patti G, Colonna G, Pasceri V, et al. Randomized trial of high loading dose of clopidogrel for reduction of periprocedural myocardial infarction in patients undergoing coronary intervention: results from the ARMYDA-2 (Antiplatelet therapy for Reduction of MYocardial Damage during Angioplasty) study. Circulation 2005; **111**(16): 2099–2106.

28 Mehta SR, Tanguay JF, Eikelboom JW, et al. Double-dose versus standard-dose clopidogrel and high-dose versus low-dose aspirin in individuals undergoing percutaneous coronary intervention for acute coronary syndromes (CURRENT-OASIS 7): a randomised factorial trial. Lancet 2010; **376**(9748): 1233–1243.

29 Steinhubl SR, Berger PB, Brennan DM, et al. Optimal timing for the initiation of pre-treatment with 300 mg clopidogrel before percutaneous coronary intervention. J Am Coll Cardiol 2006; **47**(5): 939–943.

30 Di Sciascio G, Patti G, Pasceri V, et al. Effectiveness of in-laboratory high-dose clopidogrel loading versus routine pre-load in patients undergoing percutaneous coronary intervention: results of the ARMYDA-5 PRELOAD (Antiplatelet therapy for Reduction of MYocardial Damage during Angioplasty) randomized trial. J Am Coll Cardiol 2010; **56**(7): 550–557.

31 Zeymer U, Arntz HR, Mark B, et al. Efficacy and safety of a high loading dose of clopidogrel administered prehospitally to improve primary percutaneous coronary intervention in acute myocardial infarction: the randomized CIPAMI trial. Clin Res Cardiol 2012; **101**(4): 305–312.

32 Bellemain-Appaix A, O'Connor SA, Silvain J, et al. Association of clopidogrel pretreatment with mortality, cardiovascular events, and major bleeding among patients undergoing percutaneous coronary intervention: a systematic review and meta-analysis. JAMA 2012; **308**(23): 2507–2516.

33 Bellemain-Appaix A, Kerneis M, O'Connor SA, et al. Reappraisal of thienopyridine pretreatment in patients with non-ST elevation acute coronary syndrome: a systematic review and meta-analysis. 2014; **349**: g6269.

34 Simon T, Bhatt DL, Bergougnan L, et al. Genetic polymorphisms and the impact of a higher clopidogrel dose regimen on active metabolite exposure and antiplatelet response in healthy subjects. Clin Pharmacol Ther 2011; **90**(2): 287–295.

35 Angiolillo DJ, Gibson CM, Cheng S, et al. Differential effects of omeprazole and pantoprazole on the pharmacodynamics and pharmacokinetics of clopidogrel in healthy subjects: randomized, placebo-controlled, crossover comparison studies. Clin Pharmacol Ther 2011; **89**(1): 65–74.

36 Price MJ, Berger PB, Teirstein PS, et al. Standard- vs high-dose clopidogrel based on platelet function testing after percutaneous coronary intervention: the GRAVITAS randomized trial. JAMA 2011; **305**(11): 1097–1105.

37 Bonello L, Camoin-Jau L, Armero S, et al. Tailored clopidogrel loading dose according to platelet reactivity monitoring to prevent acute and subacute stent thrombosis. Am J Cardiol 2009; **103**(1): 5–10.

38 Trenk D, Stone GW, Gawaz M, et al. A randomized trial of prasugrel versus clopidogrel in patients with high platelet reactivity on clopidogrel after elective percutaneous coronary intervention with implantation of drug-eluting stents: results of the TRIGGER-PCI (Testing Platelet Reactivity In Patients Undergoing Elective Stent Placement on Clopidogrel to Guide Alternative Therapy With Prasugrel) study. J Am Coll Cardiol 2012; **59**(24): 2159–2164.

39 Wiviott SD, Braunwald E, McCabe CH, et al. Prasugrel versus clopidogrel in patients with acute coronary syndromes. N Engl J Med 2007; **357**(20): 2001–2015.

40 Wiviott SD, Braunwald E, McCabe CH, et al. Intensive oral antiplatelet therapy for reduction of ischaemic events including stent thrombosis in patients with acute coronary syndromes treated with percutaneous coronary intervention and stenting in the TRITON-TIMI 38 trial: a subanalysis of a randomised trial. Lancet 2008; **371**(9621): 1353–1363.

41 Antman EM, Wiviott SD, Murphy SA, et al. Early and late benefits of prasugrel in patients with acute coronary syndromes undergoing percutaneous coronary intervention: a TRITON-TIMI 38 (TRial to Assess Improvement in Therapeutic Outcomes by Optimizing Platelet InhibitioN with Prasugrel-Thrombolysis In Myocardial Infarction) analysis. J Am Coll Cardiol 2008; **51**(21): 2028–2033.

42 Wiviott SD, Braunwald E, Angiolillo DJ, et al. Greater clinical benefit of more intensive oral antiplatelet therapy with prasugrel in patients with diabetes mellitus in the trial to assess improvement in therapeutic outcomes by optimizing platelet inhibition with prasugrel: Thrombolysis in Myocardial Infarction 38. Circulation 2008; **118**(16): 1626–1636.

43 Montalescot G, Wiviott SD, Braunwald E, et al. Prasugrel compared with clopidogrel in patients undergoing percutaneous coronary intervention for ST-elevation myocardial infarction (TRITON-TIMI 38): double-blind, randomised controlled trial. Lancet 2009; **373**(9665): 723–731.

44 Montalescot G, Bolognese L, Dudek D, et al. Pretreatment with prasugrel in non-ST-segment elevation acute coronary syndromes. N Engl J Med 2013; **369**(11): 999–1010.

45 Koshy A, Balasubramaniam K, Noman A, et al. Antiplatelet therapy in patients undergoing primary percutaneous coronary intervention for ST-elevation myocardial infarction: a retrospective observational study of prasugrel and clopidogrel. Cardiovasc Ther 2014; **32**(1): 1–6.

46 Damman P, Varenhorst C, Koul S, et al. Treatment patterns and outcomes in patients undergoing percutaneous coronary intervention treated with prasugrel or clopidogrel (from the Swedish Coronary Angiography and Angioplasty Registry [SCAAR]). Am J Cardiol 2014; **113**(1): 64–69.

47 Wallentin L, Becker RC, Budaj A, et al. Ticagrelor versus clopidogrel in patients with acute coronary syndromes. N Engl J Med 2009; **361**(11): 1045–1057.

48 Held C, Asenblad N, Bassand JP, et al. Ticagrelor versus clopidogrel in patients with acute coronary syndromes undergoing coronary artery bypass surgery: results from the PLATO (Platelet Inhibition and Patient Outcomes) trial. J Am Coll Cardiol 2011; **57**(6): 672–684.

49 Cannon CP, Harrington RA, James S, et al. Comparison of ticagrelor with clopidogrel in patients with a planned invasive strategy for acute coronary syndromes (PLATO): a randomised double-blind study. Lancet 2010; **375**(9711): 283–293.

50 James SK, Roe MT, Cannon CP, et al. Ticagrelor versus clopidogrel in patients with acute coronary syndromes intended for non-invasive management: substudy from prospective randomised PLATelet inhibition and patient Outcomes (PLATO) trial. BMJ 2011; **342**: d3527.

51 Mahaffey KW, Wojdyla DM, Carroll K, et al. Ticagrelor compared with clopidogrel by geographic region in the platelet inhibition and patient outcomes (PLATO) trial. Circulation 2011; **124**(5): 544–554.

52 Montalescot G, van 't Hof AW, Lapostolle F, et al. Prehospital ticagrelor in ST-segment elevation myocardial infarction. N Engl J Med 2014; **371**(11): 1016–1027.

53 Bonaca MP, Bhatt DL, Cohen M, et al. Long-term use of ticagrelor in patients with prior myocardial infarction. N Engl J Med 2016; **pii**: S0735-1097(16)32403-2.

54 O'Neill WW, Serruys P, Knudtson M, et al. Long-term treatment with a platelet glycoprotein-receptor antagonist after percutaneous coronary revascularization. EXCITE Trial Investigators. Evaluation of oral xemilofiban in controlling thrombotic events. N Engl J Med 2000; **342**(18): 1316–1324.

55 Cannon CP, McCabe CH, Wilcox RG, et al. Oral glycoprotein IIb/IIIa inhibition with orbofiban in patients with unstable coronary syndromes (OPUS-TIMI 16) trial. Circulation 2000; **102**(2): 149–156.

56 Comparison of sibrafiban with aspirin for prevention of cardiovascular events after acute coronary syndromes: a randomised trial. The SYMPHONY Investigators. Sibrafiban versus aspirin to yield maximum protection from ischemic heart events post-acute coronary syndromes. Lancet 2000; **355**(9201): 337–345.

57 Neri Serneri GG, Coccheri S, Marubini E, *et al.* Picotamide, a combined inhibitor of thromboxane A2 synthase and receptor, reduces 2-year mortality in diabetics with peripheral arterial disease: the DAVID study. *Eur Heart J* 2004; **25**(20): 1845–1852.

58 van der Wieken LR, Simoons ML, Laarman GJ, *et al.* Ridogrel as an adjunct to thrombolysis in acute myocardial infarction. *Int J Cardiol* 1995; **52**(2): 125–134.

59 Bousser MG, Amarenco P, Chamorro A, *et al.* Terutroban versus aspirin in patients with cerebral ischaemic events (PERFORM): a randomised, double-blind, parallel-group trial. *Lancet* 2011; **377**(9782): 2013–2022.

60 Ueno M, Rao SV, Angiolillo DJ. Elinogrel: pharmacological principles, preclinical and early phase clinical testing. *Future Cardiol* 2010; **6**(4): 445–453.

61 Welsh RC, Rao SV, Zeymer U, *et al.* A randomized, double-blind, active-controlled phase 2 trial to evaluate a novel selective and reversible intravenous and oral P2Y12 inhibitor elinogrel versus clopidogrel in patients undergoing nonurgent percutaneous coronary intervention: the INNOVATE-PCI trial. *Circ Cardiovasc Interv* 2012; **5**(3): 336–346.

62 Tricoci P, Huang Z, Held C, *et al.* Thrombin-receptor antagonist vorapaxar in acute coronary syndromes. *N Engl J Med* 2012; **366**(1): 20–33.

63 Morrow DA, Braunwald E, Bonaca MP, *et al.* Vorapaxar in the secondary prevention of atherothrombotic events. *N Engl J Med* 2012; **366**(15): 1404–1413.

64 O'Donoghue ML, Bhatt DL, Wiviott SD, *et al.* Safety and tolerability of atopaxar in the treatment of patients with acute coronary syndromes: the lessons from antagonizing the cellular effects of Thrombin-Acute Coronary Syndromes Trial. *Circulation* 2011; **123**(17): 1843–1853.

65 Wiviott SD, Flather MD, O"Donoghue ML, *et al.* Randomized trial of atopaxar in the treatment of patients with coronary artery disease: the lessons from antagonizing the cellular effect of Thrombin-Coronary Artery Disease Trial. *Circulation* 2011; **123**(17): 1854–1863.

66 Goto S, Ogawa H, Takeuchi M, *et al.* Double-blind, placebo-controlled Phase II studies of the protease-activated receptor 1 antagonist E5555 (atopaxar) in Japanese patients with acute coronary syndrome or high-risk coronary artery disease. *Eur Heart J* 2010; **31**(21): 2601–2613.

67 Mehran R, Baber U, Steg PG, *et al.* Cessation of dual antiplatelet treatment and cardiac events after percutaneous coronary intervention (PARIS): 2 year results from a prospective observational study. *Lancet* 2013; **382**(9906): 1714–1722.

CHAPTER 41

Parenteral Anticoagulant Agents in PCI

Piera Capranzano[1], Corrado Tamburino[1], and George D. Dangas[2]

[1] Cardiovascular Department, Ferrarotto Hospital, University of Catania, Catania, Italy

[2] Department of Cardiology, Mount Sinai Medical Center, New York, NY, USA

Unfractionated heparin (UFH) has been the mainstay of anticoagulation in ischemic coronary disease for over a quarter of a century. However, pharmacologic treatment options have expanded rapidly over the past decade with the advent of low molecular weight heparins (LMWH), direct thrombin inhibitors, and factor Xa inhibitors. Discrete bodies of evidence have emerged to support the use of each of these agents across the spectrum of urgent or elective percutaneous coronary intervention (PCI). This chapter examines the data on the use of available anticoagulants in the setting of PCI for the different clinical presentations of coronary artery disease (CAD), and makes summary recommendations for best clinical practice.

Heparin
Structure and function

Heparin was fortuitously isolated from dog liver in 1916. Its structure was elucidated 20 years later at approximately the same time as it was introduced into clinical practice. UFH is a sulfated glycosaminoglycan composed of alternating uronate and glucosamine units that contain straight chain mucopolysaccharides of highly variable length. This complex heterogeneous substance has a molecular weight ranging 3–30 kDa with a mean of 15 kDa.

Heparin functions as an indirect thrombin inhibitor, exerting its effects through the endogenous serine protease antithrombin (AT) III (Table 41.1). As AT complexes with heparin it undergoes a conformational change, accelerating its enzymatic activity by 1000× to 4000×. This results in the rapid inhibition of factor IIA (thrombin), factor Xa, and, to a lesser extent, factors IXa and XIa (Figure 41.1). Heparin requires a specific pentasaccharide motif for AT binding and polysaccharide chains of at least 18 units of length for thrombin inactivation (ternary complex formation with AT and thrombin).

Guidelines recommendation

Despite the advent of new pharmacologic therapies and intracoronary interventions, UFH remains the standard of care for preventing thrombus formation and propagation in the setting of PCI. Indeed, it has a Class I indication for the use in PCI across the entire spectrum of clinical presentations of CAD, including stable CAD, non-ST-elevation acute coronary syndrome (NSTE-ACS), and ST-elevation myocardial infarction (STEMI) [1–3].

Dosing recommendation

Because of marked variability in UFH bioavailability, monitoring of its anticoagulant effect is required. Before PCI with no planned use of a glycoprotein IIb/IIIa inhibitor (GPI), UFH is administered as a 70–100 IU/kg bolus, to achieve a target activated clotting time (ACT) of 250–300 s for HemoTec and 300–350 s for Hemochron. If GPI use is planned, a 50–70 IU/kg bolus to achieve an ACT of 200–250 s is recommended. In patients with ACS, UFH can be initiated at presentation at an initial bolus of 60–70 IU/kg with a maximum of 5000 IU, followed by an initial infusion of 12–15 IU/kg/h, to a maximum of 1000 IU/h, maintaining an activated partial thromboplastin time (aPTT) level of 50–75 s, corresponding to 1.5–2.5 times the upper limit of normal. This narrow therapeutic window is due to the increased risk of bleeding complications, without further antithrombotic benefits at the higher aPTT values. In patients receiving prior UFH, at the time of PCI an additional UFH bolus is administered as needed (e.g., 2000–5000 IU) to achieve the ACT target level.

Heparin can be discontinued at the end of the PCI with few exceptions (left ventricular aneurysm and/or thrombus, atrial fibrillation, prolonged bed rest, deferred sheath removal).

Reversal

In the event of bleeding complications the anti-IIa effects of UFH can be reversed by the administration of protamine sulfate. Protamine should be given as a slow intravenous (IV) infusion administration of 1 mg protamine/100 units remaining circulating heparin. Patients should not receive a protamine bolus of >25–50 mg. Indeed, excessive protamine administration can lead to paradoxical anticoagulation. Those who have been previously exposed to protamine, including diabetic patients receiving insulin, have a 1% risk of a hypersensitivity or anaphylactic reaction.

Limitations

The use of UFH has a number of limitations (Table 41.1). Indeed, heparin is unable to bind clot-bound thrombin or factor Xa bound to platelets in the prothrombinase complex. It does bind non-specifically to platelets, macrophages, and endothelial cells, and can activate platelet function. These phenomena theoretically reduce the ischemic efficacy of heparin. Heparin also binds to cells and plasma proteins resulting in a variable dose–response relationship leading to

Interventional Cardiology: Principles and Practice, Second Edition. Edited by George D. Dangas, Carlo Di Mario, and Nicholas N. Kipshidze.
© 2017 John Wiley & Sons, Ltd. Published 2017 by John Wiley & Sons, Ltd.

Table 41.1 Comparison of antithrombotic agents.

Heparin	Enoxaparin	Direct thrombin inhibitors

• Indirect thrombin inhibitor
• Non-specific binding to:
  ○ Serine proteases
  ○ Endothelial cells
• Reduced effect in ACS
  ○ Inhibited by PF-4
  ○ Clot-bound thrombin
• Causes platelet aggregation
• Non-linear pharmacokinetics
• Risk of HIT
	• Indirect thrombin inhibitor
	• Less non-specific binding than UFH
	• Reduced effect in ACS
	  ○ Compared to UFH, markedly less inhibition by PF-4
	  ○ Clot-bound thrombin
	• Causes much less platelet aggregation than UFH
	• Predictable anticoagulation
	• Markedly reduced risk of HIT
		• Do not require a cofactor
		• Not inhibited by PF-4 or anti-heparin proteins
		• Effective against clot-bound thrombin
		• No platelet aggregation
		• Predictable anticoagulation
		• No thrombocytopenia

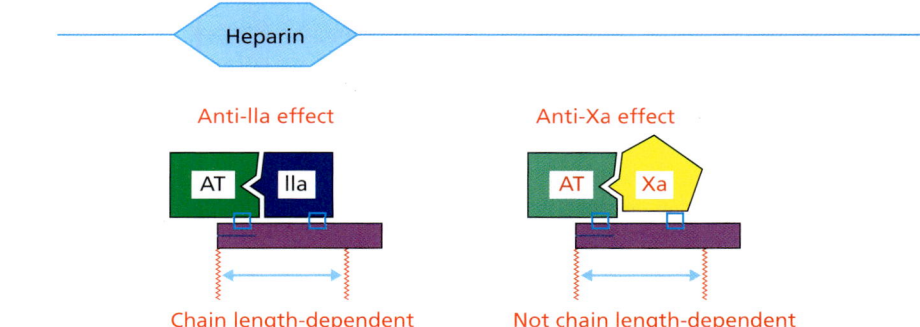

Figure 41.1 Schematic depiction of the anti-IIa and anti-Xa activities of unfractionated heparin (UFH).

a narrow therapeutic window, and to several side effects. Indeed, its interaction with platelet factor 4 can result in the production of antibodies that lead to heparin-induced thrombocytopenia (HIT). The XLM fraction (or "extra large" material >8 kDa heparin contains) also contributes to an increased risk of hemorrhagic complications.

Heparin-induced thrombocytopenia

As many as 20% of patients receiving UFH experience thrombocytopenia and/or >50% drop in their platelet count 48 hours after initiation of therapy. This thrombocytopenia is often benign, usually normalized even with continued heparin therapy, and is often referred to as HIT type 1.

In 0.2–0.3% of individuals receiving heparin, platelet counts will drop precipitously (thrombocytopenia with median count 60,000/μL, >50% drop in initial platelet count) after 4–10 days after initiation of heparin and will not reverse. Thrombocytopenia is often associated with thrombotic and rarely with hemorrhagic complications. This serious disorder is referred to as HIT type 2 (HIT-2). Rapid-onset HIT-2 occurs <24 hours after the initiation of heparin and is seen in the setting of previous heparin exposure within 3–4 months. Occasionally, thrombocytopenia can occur within days or weeks after cessation of heparin (delayed-onset HIT).

HIT-2 results from immunoglobulins G and M (IgG and IgM) antibody formation against a neoepitope created by the heparin–PF4 complex. Antibody formation leads to platelet consumption and often thrombosis; antibodies can also mediate heparin-induced skin necrosis. The heparin–PF4–antibody complex can bind platelet Fc-γ-RIIA, leading to platelet activation, PF4 release, and further propagation of platelet activation. The same complex can bind microvascular endothelial cells, leading to the release of platelet secretagogues and

adhesion molecules. Furthermore, the heparin–PF4–antibody complex can interact with monocytes to cause the release of tissue factor.

Thrombosis occurs in up to 75–90% of patients with HIT-2 and more commonly occurs in the venous (deep venous thrombosis/pulmonary embolism, gangrene, cerebral sinus thrombosis) as opposed to the arterial (myocardial infarction, stroke, acute limb ischemia, mesenteric ischemia) circulation.

HIT-2 is a clinical diagnosis but is aided by laboratory testing. Many hospitals use enzyme-linked immunosorbent assay (ELISA) to detect antibodies to the heparin–PF4 complex. This test is highly sensitive (>90–95% sensitivity) but much less specific (75–85% specificity) for HIT-2. Serotonin release and heparin-induced platelet aggregation have also been utilized to aid in making a diagnosis.

The first step in the treatment of HIT-2 is the immediate cessation of all heparin therapy including subcutaneous heparin and heparin flushes. Direct thrombin inhibitors (DTI), discussed later, are used to prevent primary or recurrent thrombosis. If a patient has thrombocytopenia but not thrombosis, a DTI is continued until the platelet count normalizes. Observation is reasonable if the patient is at high risk for bleeding but bear in mind that the patient is still at risk for thrombosis. If a patient requires ongoing anticoagulation for thrombosis or comorbidities (atrial fibrillation, mechanical valve) then a DTI is continued and overlapped for at least 5 days with warfarin therapy. Warfarin should be continued for 2–3 months or 3–6 months in the absence and in the presence of thrombosis, respectively. Heparin can be reintroduced for short periods of time (i.e., during cardiac surgery) in patients with history of HIT-2 (>4 months) who are clear of antibodies because the assumption is it would take approximately 3 days to mount an anamnestic response to repeated exposure.

Table 41.2 Comparison of low molecular weight heparins.

	Median molecular weight	Anti-Xa IU/mg	Anti-IIa IU/mg	Xa/IIa
Enoxaparin	4800	104	32	3.3
Dalteparin	5000	122	60	2.0
Nadroparin	4500	94	31	3.0
Tinzaparin	4500	90	50	1.8
Clivarine	3900	130	40	3.3

Low molecular weight heparin
Structure and function
Low molecular weight heparin is produced through the enzymatic or chemical (nitrous acid, alkaline) degradation of UFH. These processes result in smaller molecules containing shorter polysaccharide chains (Table 41.2). The molecular weight of LMWH ranges 2–9 kDa with an average of 4–5 kDa (Table 41.2). LMWH has a few theoretical advantages over UFH (Table 41.1). LMWH still acts through AT, but because many of its chains contain <18 monosaccharides they cannot form a ternary complex with AT and thrombin; therefore LMWH has preferential anti-Xa effect as opposed to antithrombin activity. LMWH has a complete bioavailability after subcutaneous administration, longer than twice the half-life of UFH (4.5–7 hours for enoxaparin) and a predictable dose–response relationship, not requiring anticoagulation monitoring (Table 41.1). LMWH incurs much less non-specific binding and therefore presents a lower risk of HIT-2 and results in less platelet activation than with UFH. LMWH is cleared predominantly by the kidneys but also by the reticulo-endothelial system. This becomes important for dosing in renal failure. Enoxaparin is the best studied LMWH for ischemic prophylaxis in CAD.

Enoxaparin in PCI for stable coronary artery disease
The role of enoxaparin in elective PCI for stable disease has been evaluated in the STEEPLE open-label trial which randomized 3528 patients to either IV enoxaparin 0.5 or 0.75 mg/kg or UFH [4]. The primary endpoint of non-CABG-related bleeding over 48 hours was significantly reduced for the lower dose (0.5 mg/kg) but not the higher dose (0.75 mg/kg) group. Major bleeding was significantly reduced in both enoxaparin groups, with similar efficacy compared with UFH. Enoxaparin provided more predictable anticoagulation. The enoxaparin low-dose arm was stopped prematurely because of a non-significant trend toward excess mortality not related to ischaemic events and not confirmed at 1 year of follow-up.

Based on this trial, enoxaparin should be considered as an alternative to UFH for elective PCI in patients with stable CAD according to European (Class IIa, B) and US (Class IIb, B) guidelines, respectively [1,5].

Enoxaparin in PCI for non-ST-elevation acute coronary syndrome
The SYNERGY study evaluated the safety and efficacy of enoxaparin within the context of an early invasive strategy in 10,027 patients with high risk ACS. Patients received either open-label enoxaparin (1 mg/kg) or UFH until anticoagulation was no longer required as judged by the patient's treating physician [6]. The majority of patients received contemporary pharmacologic therapy including aspirin (95%), thienopyridines (66%), and GPI (57%). Most patients (92%) underwent coronary angiography, 47% underwent PCI, and 19% bypass surgery. For those undergoing PCI who were assigned to enoxaparin, if the last enoxaparin dose was given <8 hours prior to the procedure no additional drug was given. If the last enoxaparin dose was given >8 hours prior to PCI an additional enoxaparin bolus of 0.3 mg/kg was administered prior PCI. Seventy-five percent of trial patients received antithrombin therapy prior to randomization. The enoxaparin group met non-inferiority criteria with respect to the primary efficacy composite endpoint of 30-day all-cause death or non-fatal myocardial infarction (MI). No significant differences were observed for ischemic events during PCI including abrupt closure, threatened abrupt closure, unsuccessful PCI, or emergency bypass surgery. There was a modest significant increase in bleeding complications with enoxaparin. However, a relative advantage of enoxaparin emerged when therapy crossovers were censored.

Based on this trial, enoxaparin should be considered for PCI in patients with NSTE-ACS pre-treated with subcutaneous enoxaparin according to European (Class IIa, B) and US (Class IIb, B) guidelines (Table 41.3) [1,2]. Crossover of UFH and LMWH is not recommended.

Enoxaparin in primary PCI for ST-elevation myocardial infarction
Enoxaparin (0.5 mg/kg intravenous bolus) was compared with UFH in the setting of primary PCI only in the ATOLL randomized, open-label trial, including 910 patients [7]. The 30-day primary

Table 41.3 European and US guidelines indications for the use of parenteral anticoagulant agents for percutaneous coronary intervention (PCI) in the setting of acute coronary syndrome.

	Enoxaparin		UFH		Bivalirudin	
NSTE-ACS (EU 2014) [1]	IIa*	B	I	C	I	A
NSTE-ACS (US 2011) [2]	IIb*	B	I	C	I	B
STEMI (EU 2014) [1]	IIa	B	I	C	IIa	A
STEMI (US 2013) [3]	–	–	I	C	I	B

*Enoxaparin should be considered for PCI in patients pre-treated with subcutaneous enoxaparin. Crossover of UFH and LMWH is not recommended. NSTE-ACS: non-ST-Elevation acute coronary syndrome; STEMI: ST-Elevation myocardial infarction; UFH: unfractionated heparin.

composite endpoint of death, complication of MI, procedural failure, or major bleeding was not significantly reduced in the enoxaparin arm. There was no signal of higher incidence of bleeding from use of enoxaparin over UFH. In the per-protocol analysis of the ATOLL trial—pertinent to more than 87% of the study population—enoxaparin was superior to UFH in reducing the primary endpoint, and also mortality and major bleedings, contributing to the improvement of the net clinical benefit [8].

Based on this trial, enoxaparin with or without GPI should be considered as an alternative to UFH for primary PCI in patients with STEMI according to the European guidelines (Class IIa, B; Table 41.3) [1]. There are no specific recommendations for the use of enoxaparin in the setting of primary PCI for STEMI in the US guidelines. According to these latter guidelines enoxaparin is recommended in Class I A as adjunctive antithrombotic therapy to support reperfusion in patients with STEMI treated with fibrinolytic therapy [3].

Dosing recommendations

In patients who have not received prior anticoagulant therapy a 0.5–0.75 mg/kg IV bolus is given before PCI. For prior treatment with enoxaparin, if the last subcutaneous dose was administered 8 hours earlier or if less than two therapeutic doses of enoxaparin have been administered, an additional intravenous dose of enoxaparin 0.3 mg/kg is given before PCI.

Enoxaparin dosage should be reduced to 1 mg/kg once daily in patients with a creatinine clearance <30 L/min and is contraindicated in dialysis. Also caution should be used when treating the elderly and patients at both extremes of the weight spectrum for fear of an unreliable dose–response and an increased risk of bleeding.

Protamine can reverse the anti-IIa effect of the higher molecular weight components of heparin but does not completely reverse the drug's anti-Xa activity. Protamine administered as 1 mg/100 units of circulating LMWH can reduce clinical bleeding. The dose should be reduced if LMWH was given >8 hours before the bleeding event.

Limitations of LMWH

LMWH can cause HIT-2, although the incidence is markedly decreased compared to UFH therapy. LMWH is also associated with bleeding complications without an ideal option for reversal, although protamine can inhibit anti-IIA effects.

Direct thrombin inhibitors

Direct thrombin inhibitors are small molecules that can bind and inactivate both circulating and clot-bound thrombin (Table 41.1). DTI do not interact with plasma proteins or cells; therefore DTI do not activate platelets and do not cause HIT. In fact, they are used for the treatment of HIT. DTI have a much more predictable dose response than UFH. The three available DTI are L-hirudin (lepirudin), argatroban, and bivalirudin.

Hirudin was initially isolated from *Hirudo medicinalis*, the medicinal leech, and was identified as an antithrombotic agent in 1884. Hirudin is a bivalent protein that binds irreversibly to thrombin. It is renally cleared and is relatively contraindicated in patients with renal insufficiency. Production of anti-hirudin antibodies is relatively common and can affect dosing, but there is only a 0.015% incidence of anaphylaxis with L-hirudin exposure and a 0.016% incidence with re-exposure.

Argatroban is a small, monovalent DTI that binds reversibly to thrombin. It has a half-life of 50 minutes and is hepatically cleared.

Argatroban is relatively contraindicated in patients with liver dysfunction. Argatroban is not immunogenic.

Bivalirudin is a bivalent 20 amino acid protein that reversibly inhibits thrombin. It has a half-life of 25 minutes and is cleared predominantly through proteolytic cleavage, with renal excretion accounting for <20% of its degradation. Bivalirudin is not immunogenic.

No studies have evaluated the role of lepirudin in contemporary PCI. A few small studies have evaluated the effects of argatroban during PCI, and it is approved in this setting as an alternative anticoagulant only in patients with HIT. Lepirudin and argatroban are approved only for the treatment of HIT. Bivalirudin can also be used in patients with HIT. Bivalirudin is currently the only DTI that has been extensively evaluated in several powered clinical trials with respect to its use in PCI across the broad spectrum of CAD [9].

Bivalirudin in PCI for stable coronary artery disease

ISAR-REACT-3 was the only randomized trial to compare bivalirudin (bolus 0.75 mg/kg; infusion 1.75 mg/kg/h) with UFH (140 IU/kg) in 4570 patients pre-treated with clopidogrel [10]. The trial showed similar net clinical outcomes (primary endpoint) between bivalirudin and UFH, with an excess of major bleeding in the UFH group, which could be attributable to the UFH dosage being higher than recommended. In the ISAR-REACT 3A trial the use of a reduced UFH bolus of 100 IU/kg in 2505 patients led to no differences between bivalirudin and UFH in terms of major bleeding, with a trend toward less ischemic events in the UFH arm [11]. In view of the ISAR-REACT 3 and 3A results with a trend toward a lower risk of MI, anticoagulation with UFH remains the standard anticoagulant treatment for elective PCI. According to the European guidelines, bivalirudin should be considered in place of UFH during elective PCI in patients at high-risk for bleeding (Class IIa, B) [3].

Bivalirudin in PCI for non-ST-elevation acute coronary syndrome

ACUITY was the first large-scale randomized trial to assess the use of bivalirudin as an alternative to UFH for anticoagulation in the contemporary treatment of NSTE-ACS [12]. It was found that 13,819 moderate to high risk patients with NSTE-ACS managed with contemporary pharmacotherapy and undergoing an early invasive strategy were randomized to UFH or enoxaparin plus planned GPI, bivalirudin plus planned GPI, or bivalirudin monotherapy. Therapy with GPI was randomized to downstream (in the catheterization laboratory) or upstream administration. Bivalirudin was started before angiography with an IV bolus of 0.1 mg/kg and an infusion of 0.25 mg/kg/h, followed before PCI by an additional IV bolus of 0.5 mg/kg and infusion of 1.75 mg/kg/h. The drug was stopped after PCI. Ninety-nine percent of patients underwent angiography within 19.6 hours following admission. Pre-treatment with clopidogrel was left to the discretion of the treating physician. Only 56% of patients received PCI through the femoral access, 11% received CABG, and 33% received medical therapy. Bivalirudin monotherapy met non-inferiority criteria with respect to the primary ischemic endpoint at 30 days (death, MI, or unplanned revascularization), with a significantly lower rate of major bleeding. Therefore, the 30-day net clinical outcome was significantly better with bivalirudin alone than with heparin plus GPI. Notably, this bivalirudin advantage was confirmed at 1-year follow-up and was not related to the timing of GPI administration (upstream or downstream).

In the ACUITY trial, major bleeding was an independent predictor of mortality at 30 days and 1 year [13,14]. Subgroup analysis suggested that while lack of clopidogrel pre-treatment did not affect the ischemic outcome for the two groups receiving GPI, it resulted in a significant increase in the ischemic endpoint for those receiving bivalirudin monotherapy.

The ACUITY PCI subanalysis analyzed outcomes for the 7789 patients in the PCI subgroup [15]. There was no difference in the primary ischemic endpoint or stent thrombosis, but bivalirudin monotherapy was associated with a significant reduction in major bleeding, minor bleeding, and transfusion requirements.

The safety and efficacy of bivalirudin monotherapy versus UFH plus GPI in NSTE-ACS patients undergoing PCI through the femoral access and pre-treated with clopidogrel were assessed in the more recent ISAR-REACT 4 trial [16]. At the time of PCI, patients in the bivalirudin group received a bolus dose of bivalirudin 0.75 mg/kg, followed by an infusion of 1.75 mg/kg/h for the duration of the procedure. Compared with ACUITY, the ISAR-REACT 4 trial:

1 Included only high risk patients with positive biomarkers undergoing PCI, whereas ACUITY also included patients with unstable angina;
2 UFH was the only heparin used in the control arm, whereas in ACUITY the use of enoxaparin was allowed in the heparin plus GPI arm;
3 GPIs were administered only after the guidewire had crossed the lesion, whereas in ACUITY patients assigned to heparin plus GPIs or bivalirudin plus GPIs were randomly assigned, in a two-by-two factorial design, to upstream or downstream treatment with GPIs);
4 Abciximab was the only GPI used in the control arm, whereas in ACUITY the use of tirofiban or eptifibatide was permitted;
5 Clopidogrel 600 mg was given before any study drug, whereas in ACUITY the initial dose and timing of clopidogrel were left to the discretion of the investigator;
6 The definition of major bleeding was less sensitive.

In the ISAR-REACT 4 trial the primary endpoint of death, recurrent MI, urgent target vessel revascularization, or major bleeding within 30 days was similar, but bivalirudin was associated with significantly less major bleeding, with the biggest difference between the two groups being in the access site bleeding.

Based on this latter trial, in the most recent 2014 European guidelines on myocardial revascularization, bivalirudin (0.75 mg/kg bolus, followed by 1.75 mg/kg/hour for up to 4 hours after the procedure) is recommended as alternative to UFH plus GPI during PCI in patients with NSTE-ACS (Class I A) [1], while UFH is recommended as anticoagulant for PCI in patients with NSTE-ACS, if patients cannot receive bivalirudin (Class I C; Table 41.4) [1]. Differently, in the most recent 2014 US guidelines on NSTE-ACS, there is no preference for one anticoagulation agent and both bivalirudin and UFH are indicated as anticoagulation options for PCI in NSTE-ACS in Class I B and I C, respectively, reflecting the higher number of evidences on bivalirudin (Table 41.3) [2]. According to the US guidelines, in patients with NSTE-ACS undergoing PCI who are at high risk of bleeding, it is reasonable to use bivalirudin monotherapy in preference to the combination of UFH and GPI (Class IIa B) [2].

Bivalirudin in primary PCI for ST-elevation myocardial infarction

The HORIZONS-AMI was the first large, multicenter, open-label trial, which randomized 3602 patients with STEMI undergoing primary PCI (93%) through the femoral access to bivalirudin or UFH plus planned GPI [17]. Bivalirudin was stopped at the end of PCI. This landmark trial showed that bivalirudin plus provisional GPI compared with UFH plus routine GPIs reduced major bleeding and the combined endpoint of all-cause death, reinfarction, repeat revascularization, definite stent thrombosis, stroke, or major bleeding both at 30 days and 1 year. In addition, bivalirudin was associated with improved overall and cardiac survival at 30 days and up to 3 years [18]. However, there was a higher incidence of acute stent thrombosis during the first 24 hours in the bivalirudin group (1.3% vs. 0.3%; p = 0.001), with no difference in stent thrombosis at 30 days. Pre-randomization use of UFH bolus and 600 mg clopidogrel loading dose were independent predictors of lower risk of acute and subacute stent thrombosis.

The EUROMAX multicenter, open-label trial compared outcomes of bivalirudin with UFH in STEMI patients (n = 2218) managed in a more contemporary practice setting, including prehospital initiation of study treatment in all patients, use of prasugrel and ticagrelor (59%) and radial artery access (47%) [19]. Planned GPI use was optional in both groups: in the bivalirudin arm upstream GPI (3.9%) was recommended only in the presence of a large thrombus, while in the UFH arm (58.5%) was left to the operator's preference. The GPI bailout use occurred in 7.9 % and 25.4 %, in the bivalirudin and UFG arms, respectively. Differently from in the HORIZONS-AMI trial, infusion of bivalirudin was to be continued for at least 4 hours after PCI, either at the higher dose used during PCI (1.75 mg/kg/h) or at the lower maintenance dose (0.25 mg/kg/h). The primary composite of death or major bleeding was significantly reduced by bivalirudin, driven by a significant reduction in major bleeding. However, the risk of acute stent thrombosis remained higher with bivalirudin (1.1% vs. 0.2%; p = 0.007). In a EUROMAX subanalysis, bivalirudin and UFH were compared according to the mode of GPI administration (routine [n = 649] vs. bailout [n = 460]) in the heparin arm [20]. The benefit of bivalirudin, driven by major bleeding reduction, was evident in both comparisons, versus heparin plus routine GPI, and versus heparin plus bailout GPI [20]. Similar to the main study, stent thrombosis was more frequent with bivalirudin, irrespective of GPI mode of use [20]. Although pre-specified, the conclusion of this subanalysis should be regarded only as hypothesis generating. Another subanalysis assessed the impact on outcomes of the bivalirudin infusion dose after PCI. The prolonged infusion of bivalirudin at the higher dose given during PCI (1.75 mg/kg/h) was associated with a rate of acute stent thrombosis (0.4%) similar to that in the UFH arm (0.2%) with or without GPI. Acute stent thrombosis was higher (1.6%) in the group continuing bivalirudin infusion at reduced dose (0.25 mg/kg/h) [21]. Major bleeding was lower with bivalirudin than with UFH, irrespective of the post-PCI infusion dose [21].

The HEAT-PPCI was a single-center study that challenged the benefit of bivalirudin in terms of reduced bleeding and improved net clinical outcomes [22]. Differently from previous bivalirudin trials, the HEAT-PPCI trial compared bivalirudin (n = 905) with UFH alone (n = 907), without routine use of GPI in the setting of primary PCI for STEMI. Indeed, GPIs were allowed only for bailout use in both treatment groups. Bivalirudin infusion was stopped at the end of PCI. Prasugrel and ticagrelor were used in about 90% of patients; radial access was used in 80%, and GPI were given to 13% and 15% of patients treated with bivalirudin and UFH, respectively. The 30-day primary composite endpoint of all-cause mortality, cerebrovascular accidents, recurrent infarction, urgent target vessel revascularization was significantly higher with bivalirudin, mostly driven by higher early MI. Definite or probable stent thrombosis, mostly acute, was significantly higher with bivalirudin (3.4% vs. 0.9%; p = 0.001). In disagreement with the other trials, there were no differences in major and minor bleeding between bivalirudin and UFH. The main concerns that have been raised in HEAT-PPCI include its open-label, single-center design and a possible under-dosing of bivalirudin.

Additional data on the comparative effectiveness of bivalirudin and UFH, with or without GPI in the setting of primary PCI, have been recently provided by the BRIGHT multicenter, open-label trial, which randomized Chinese patients with acute MI (90% STEMI) to bivalirudin alone (n = 735), UFH alone (n = 729), or UFH plus tirofiban (n = 730) [23]. Among patients treated with bivalirudin, a post-procedure infusion at the PCI dose of 1.75 mg/ kg/h was administered for a median of 180 minutes (IQR 148–240 minutes). The radial access was used in about 79% of patients. Net adverse clinical events at 30 days were lower in the bivalirudin group than both heparin groups, driven by reduction in major bleeding and no differences between treatments in the 30-day rates of major adverse cardiac or cerebral events. Moreover, there were no differences in 30-day stent thrombosis (0.6% in the bivalirudin, 0.9% in the heparin alone, and 0.7% in the heparin plus tirofiban group; p = 0.77) or in acute (<24 hour) stent thrombosis (0.3% in each group). Patients treated with UFH alone had similar ischemic outcomes compared with those treated with UFH plus tirofiban. At the 1-year follow-up, the results remained similar.

Based on the recent EUROMAX and HEAT-PCI trials casting doubts on the superior safety and efficacy balance of bivalirudin as compared with heparin plus GPI, the most recent 2014 European guidelines on myocardial revascularization have downgraded the recommendation for the use of bivalirudin in primary PCI for STEMI from Class I A to Class IIa A, while UFH is indicated in Class I C (Table 41.3) [1]. The recommended bivalirudin dosage is 0.75 mg/kg IV bolus followed by IV infusion of 1.75 mg/kg/h for up to 4 hours after the procedure [1]. This latter dose regimen seems effective and safe, with no excess in stent thrombosis and reduced bleeding compared to heparin with or without GPI, as demonstrated in the BRIGHT trial, which was published after the European guidelines release. In the most recent 2013 US guidelines on STEMI, both bivalirudin and UFH are indicated as anticoagulation options for primary PCI in Class I B and I C, respectively, reflecting the greater amount of evidence on bivalirudin (Table 41.3) [3]. These latter guidelines have been released before EUROMAX, HEAT-PCI, and BRIGHT trials and are based on the HORIZONS-AMI findings.

Factor Xa inhibitors

Factor Xa inhibitors are the most refined and lowest molecular weight heparin. They contain a pentasaccharide sequence that specifically binds factor Xa. Fondaparinux, the most well-studied and widely used of these agents, is a 1.7 KDa synthetic pentasaccharide that rapidly and reversibly binds AT, inducing a conformational change that accelerates AT–Xa interactions by >300-fold. Fondaparinux can be administered in a fixed dose (2.5 mg for creatinine clearance >30 L/minute) with no need for weight-based adjustment or routine monitoring. This drug does not significantly interact with any cells or other plasma proteins, and therefore does not affect platelet function or cause HIT.

In NSTE-ACS, fondaparinux with lower bleeding leads to lower 30-day mortality compared with enoxaparin and for this reason is the agent of choice for anticoagulation in this settings [24].

Because of higher catheter-related thrombosis, fondaparinux is not recommended for PCI, and the adjunctive use of UFH at the time of PCI in NSTE-ACS is recommended [25]. The addition of low or standard UFH dose at the time of PCI does not increase bleeding; low dose UFH was not superior to standard ACT-guided UFH dosing [25].

In patients with STEMI fondaparinux reduced death and MI in patients treated with thrombolysis, but increased ischemic events in primary PCI compared with UFH and thus is not recommended in this latter setting [26].

Interactive multiple choice questions are available for this chapter on www.wiley.com/go/dangas/cardiology

References

1 Kolh P, Windecker S, Alfonso F, et al. 2014 ESC/EACTS Guidelines on myocardial revascularization: The Task Force on Myocardial Revascularization of the European Society of Cardiology (ESC) and the European Association for Cardio-Thoracic Surgery (EACTS) Developed with the special contribution of the European Association of Percutaneous Cardiovascular Interventions (EAPCI). *Eur Heart J* 2014; **35**(37): 2541–2619.

2 Amsterdam EA, Wenger NK, Brindis RG, et al. 2014 AHA/ACC Guideline for the management of patients with non-ST-elevation acute coronary syndromes: a Report of the American College of Cardiology/American Heart Association Task Force on Practice Guidelines. *Circulation* 2014; **130**: e344–e426.

3 O'Gara PT, Kushner FG, Ascheim DD, et al. 2013 ACCF/AHA Guideline for the Management of ST-Elevation Myocardial Infarction A Report of the American College of Cardiology Foundation/American Heart Association Task Force on Practice Guidelines. *Circulation* 2013; **127**: e362–e425.

4 Montalescot G, White HD, Gallo R, et al. Enoxaparin versus unfractionated heparin in elective percutaneous coronary intervention. *N Engl J Med* 2006; **355**: 1006–1017.

5 Levine GN, Bates ER, Blankenship JC, et al. 2011 ACCF/AHA/SCAI Guideline for Percutaneous Coronary Intervention. A report of the American College of Cardiology Foundation/American Heart Association Task Force on Practice Guidelines and the Society for Cardiovascular Angiography and Interventions. *J Am Coll Cardiol* 2011; **58**: e44–e122.

6 Ferguson JJ, Califf RM, Antman EM, et al. Enoxaparin vs unfractionated heparin in high-risk patients with non-ST-segment elevation acute coronary syndromes managed with an intended early invasive strategy: primary results of the SYNERGY randomized trial. *JAMA* 2004; **292**: 45–54.

7 Montalescot G, Zeymer U, Silvain J, et al. Intravenous enoxaparin or unfractionated heparin in primary percutaneous coronary intervention for ST-elevation myocardial infarction: the international randomised open-label ATOLL trial. *Lancet* 2011; **378**: 693–703.

8 Collet JP, Huber K, Cohen M, et al. A direct comparison of intravenous enoxaparin with unfractionated heparin in primary percutaneous coronary intervention (from the ATOLL trial). *Am J Cardiol* 2013; **112**: 1367–1372.

9 Capodanno D, De Caterina R. Bivalirudin for acute coronary syndromes: premises, promises and doubts. *Thromb Haemost* 2015; **113**: 698–707.

10 Kastrati A, Neumann FJ, Mehilli J, et al. Investigators I-RT. Bivalirudin vs. unfractionated heparin during percutaneous coronary intervention. *N Engl J Med* 2008; **359**: 688–696.

11 Schulz S, Mehilli J, Neumann FJ, et al. ISAR-REACT 3A: a study of reduced dose of unfractionated heparin in biomarker negative patients undergoing percutaneous coronary intervention. *Eur Heart J* 2010; **31**: 2482–2491.

12 Stone GW, McLaurin BT, Cox DA, et al. Bivalirudin for patients with acute coronary syndromes. *N Engl J Med* 2006; **355**: 2203–2216.

13 Manoukian SV, Feit F, Mehran R, et al. Impact of major bleeding on 30-day mortality and clinical outcomes in patients with acute coronary syndromes: an analysis from the ACUITY trial. *J Am Coll Cardiol* 2007; **49**: 1362–1368.

14 Stone GW, Ware JH, Bertrand ME, et al. Antithrombotic strategies in patients with acute coronary syndromes undergoing early invasive management: one-year results from the ACUITY trial. *JAMA* 2007; **298**: 2497–2506.

15 Stone GW, White HD, Ohman EM, et al. Bivalirudin in patients with acute coronary syndromes undergoing percutaneous coronary intervention: a subgroup analysis from the Acute Catheterization and Urgent Intervention Triage strategy (ACUITY) trial. *Lancet* 2007; **369**: 907–919.

16 Kastrati A, Neumann FJ, Schulz S, *et al.* Abciximab and heparin vs. bivalirudin for non-ST-elevation myocardial infarction. *N Engl J Med* 2011; **365**: 1980–1989.

17 Stone GW, Witzenbichler B, Guagliumi G, *et al.* Bivalirudin during primary PCI in acute myocardial infarction. *N Engl J Med* 2008; **358**: 2218–2230.

18 Capranzano P, Dangas G. Bivalirudin for primary percutaneous coronary intervention in acute myocardial infarction: the HORIZONS-AMI trial. *Expert Rev Cardiovasc Ther* 2012; **10**: 411–422.

19 Steg PG, van 't HofAW, Hamm CW, *et al.* Bivalirudin started during emergency transport for primary PCI. *N Engl J Med* 2013; **369**: 2207–2217.

20 Zeymer U, van't Hof A, Adgey J, *et al.* Bivalirudin is superior to heparins alone with bailout GP IIb/IIIa inhibitors in patients with ST-segment elevation myocardial infarction transported emergently for primary percutaneous coronary intervention: a pre-specified analysis from the EUROMAX trial. *Eur Heart J* 2014; **35**: 2460–2467.

21 Clemmensen P, Wiberg S, Van't Hof A, *et al.* Acute stent thrombosis after primary percutaneous coronary intervention: insights from the EUROMAX trial (European Ambulance Acute Coronary Syndrome Angiography). *JACC Cardiovasc Interv* 2015; **8**: 214–220.

22 Shahzad A, Kemp I, Mars C, *et al.* Unfractionated heparin versus bivalirudin in primary percutaneous coronary intervention (HEAT-PPCI): an open-label, single centre, randomised controlled trial. *Lancet* 2014; **384**: 1849–5818.

23 Han Y, Guo J, Zheng Y, *et al.* Bivalirudin vs heparin with or without tirofiban during primary percutaneous coronary intervention in acute myocardial infarction: the BRIGHT randomized clinical trial. *JAMA* 2015; **313**: 1336–1346.

24 Yusuf S, Mehta SR, Chrolavicius S, *et al.* Comparison of fondaparinux and enoxaparin in acute coronary syndromes. *N Engl J Med* 2006; **354**: 1464–1476.

25 Steg PG, Jolly SS, Mehta SR, *et al.* Low-dose vs standard-dose unfractionated heparin for percutaneous coronary intervention in acute coronary syndromes treated with fondaparinux: the FUTURA/OASIS-8 randomized trial. *JAMA* 2010; **304**: 1339–1349.

26 Yusuf S, Mehta SR, Chrolavicius S, *et al.* Effects of fondaparinux on mortality and reinfarction in patients with acute ST-segment elevation myocardial infarction: the OASIS-6 randomized trial. *JAMA* 2006; **295**: 1519–1530.

CHAPTER 42
Parenteral Antiplatelet Agents in PCI

Piera Capranzano, Giuseppe Gargiulo, and Corrado Tamburino
Cardiovascular Department, Ferrarotto Hospital, University of Catania, Catania, Italy

Percutaneous coronary intervention (PCI) has a central role in the management of patients with stable or unstable coronary artery disease. To maintain the immediate results of PCI and prevent complications and recurrence of thrombotic events, inhibition of platelet activity is essential. Parenteral antiplatelet agents include glycoprotein IIb/IIIa inhibitors (GPI) and cangrelor, which is a reversible inhibitor of the platelet adenosine diphosphate receptor (P2Y$_{12}$). These agents have a useful pharmacologic profile because of their ability to reach rapid antiplatelet effect and overcome the limitations of oral antiplatelet agents.

This chapter examines the contemporary evidence on the use of parenteral antiplatelet agents in PCI, reporting current recommendations for best clinical practice [1–3].

Glycoprotein IIb/IIIa inhibitors

The IIb/IIIa integrin receptor on the surface of platelets binds preferentially to collagen and fibrinogen as well as fibronectin, vitronectin, and von Willebrand factor. IIb/IIIa activation triggers the final common pathway of platelet aggregation: fibrinogen cross-linking of platelets. Activation of the receptor also fosters platelet adhesion to the vascular endothelial surface. GPI abrogate the effects of the IIb/IIIa receptor on platelet aggregation and adhesion through reversible or irreversible inhibition (Figure 42.1). Three GPIs are commercially available: abciximab, eptifibatide, and tirofiban (Table 42.1).

Abciximab

This is a chimeric murine-human monoclonal antibody that consists of the Fab fragment of a murine glycoprotein IIb/IIIa antibody fused the constant region of human IgG. Abciximab binds to platelets with high affinity and irreversibly. It is a long-acting agent (>48 hours) but its effects are readily reversed with platelet transfusions. Abciximab has a rapid onset of action, a half-life of 30 minutes, and causes complete platelet inhibition within 2 hours of administration. Abciximab is eliminated by protease degradation. Patients sometimes produce anti-chimeric antibodies; however, hypersensitivity/anaphylactic reactions to abciximab are rare. Abciximab should be dosed as a bolus of 0.25 mg/kg followed by 0.125 µg/kg/min infusion (maximum 10 µg/min) which can be continued for 12 hours after PCI. There is no adjustment for renal insufficiency.

Eptifibatide

This is a non-immunogenic cyclic heptapeptide that reversibly inhibits the platelet IIb/IIIa receptor as a competitive inhibitor of the fibrinogen-binding site. Eptifibatide contains an active pharmacophore derived from barbourin, the primary component of southeastern pigmy rattlesnake poison. This agent is short acting (2–4 hours) and its effects are not reversible with platelet transfusions. Eptifibatide has a rapid onset, a half-life 2.5 hours, and causes high-level platelet inhibition within 2 hours of administration. Eptifibatide is cleared predominantly by the kidneys and should be dosed with caution in patients with renal insufficiency (infusion should be reduced by half if creatinine clearance is <50 mL/min and should be avoided in patients on hemodialysis). Eptifibatide should be dosed with a bolus of 180 µg/kg over 1–2 minutes, a second bolus of 180 µg/kg 10 minutes later, and an infusion of 2 µg/kg/min.

In the BRIEF-PCI trial, a single bolus dose plus a truncated infusion (<2 hours) of eptifibatide was used in low risk patients undergoing PCI and was found to have a similar incidence of death, myocardial infarction (MI), and target vessel revascularization (TVR), but with less incidence of major bleeding [4]. Accordingly, a recent retrospective study demonstrated that the catheterization laboratory-only regimen compared with prolonged infusion after PCI was associated with reduced bleeding complication in the absence of differences in death and MI [5].

Tirofiban

This is a reversible non-peptide GPI that acts as a competitive inhibitor of the fibrinogen-binding site. This agent is short acting (2–4 hours) and its effects are not reversible with platelet transfusions. When using tirofiban and eptifibatide approximately 4 hours are needed for the effects to wear off. Tirofiban is slower in onset than the other two GPIs, has a half-life of 2 hours, and causes high-level platelet inhibition within 2 hours of administration. Tirofiban is recommended for patients with STEMI at a high bolus dose of 25 µg/kg IV, then 0.15 µg/kg/min infusion. The bolus and infusion should be reduced by 50% in patients with a creatinine clearance of <30 mL/min.

Interventional Cardiology: Principles and Practice, Second Edition. Edited by George D. Dangas, Carlo Di Mario, and Nicholas N. Kipshidze.
© 2017 John Wiley & Sons, Ltd. Published 2017 by John Wiley & Sons, Ltd.

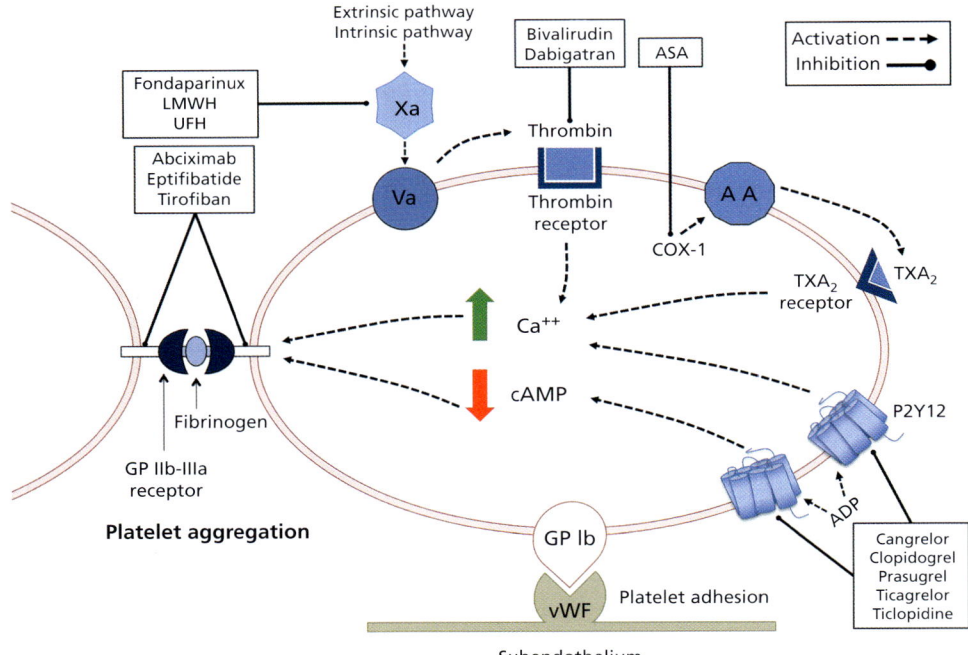

Figure 42.1 Platelet activation pathway and site of action of antiplatelet agents. AA, arachidonic acid; ADP, adenosine diphosphate; cAMP, cyclic adenosine monophosphate; ASA, acetylsalicylic acid (aspirin); COX-1, cyclo-oxygenase-1; GP, glycoprotein; LMWH, low molecular weight heparin; TXA_2, thromboxane A_2; UFH, unfractionated heparin; vWF, von Willebrand factor.

Table 42.1 Basic pharmacologic characteristics of glycoprotein IIb/IIIa inhibitors (GPI).

	Abciximab	**Eptifibatide**	**Tirofiban**
Type	Fab fragment of chimeric human-murine monoclonal antibody	Synthetic cyclic heptapeptide	Synthetic non-peptide
Molecular weight	Large molecule (47,515 Da)	Small molecule (832 Da)	Small molecule (496 Da)
Plasma half-life	10–30 minutes	2.5–2.8 hours	1.2–2 hours
Receptor binding	Minutes	Seconds	Seconds
Elimination route	Spleen	Renal 75%	Renal 65%; biliary 25%

Stable coronary artery disease

The evidence emerging from major clinical trials did not show additional benefit by administrating GPI after a loading dose of 600 mg clopidogrel [6–8]. Therefore, in the setting of elective PCI, GPI are not recommended except for "bailout" situations (intraprocedural thrombus formation, slow-flow, threatened vessel closure) in which they could be considered (Class IIa, level C of recommendation), as there is anecdotal experience suggesting potential benefits in these settings [1].

Non-ST-segment elevation acute coronary syndrome

Some older trials before the era of dual antiplatelet therapy showed that patients undergoing PCI experienced lower ischemic events, mainly driven by reduction in MI when receiving adequately dosed GPI combined with unfractionated heparin (UFH) instead of UFH alone [1,9]. Interestingly, the ISAR-REACT 2 trial, showed that the benefit in terms of composite primary endpoint (death, MI, or urgent TVR within 30 days) related to GPI use for PCI was still present even if clopidogrel pretreatment at loading dose of 600 mg was given in patients with NSTEMI, but not in those with unstable angina [10]. In the ACUITY trial, the combination of UFH plus GPI was compared with bivalirudin alone (with bailout GPI in 7.4%), demonstrating a significant benefit in terms of the composite of ischemic and bleeding complications (11.7% vs. 10.1% at 30 days; p = 0.02), mainly driven by decrease in major bleeding (5.7% vs. 3.0%; p <0.001) [11]. Notably, this bivalirudin advantage was confirmed at 1-year follow-up and was not related to the timing of GPI administration (upstream or downstream) [12]. In the latter trial, approximately 40% of the patients did not have elevated cardiac biomarkers, and more than 40% did not undergo PCI. The combination UFH plus abciximab was compared with bivalirudin alone in patients with NSTEMI undergoing PCI in the ISAR-REACT 4 trial [13]. In this latter study, no benefits have emerged in the primary composite endpoint (death, recurrent MI, urgent TVR, or major bleeding within 30 days), but significantly more major bleeding events were observed in the GPI group than in the bivalirudin group (4.6% vs. 2.6%; p = 0.02).

The use of upstream eptifibatide with or without clopidogrel pretreatment compared with downstream provisional eptifibatide in the EARLY-ACS trial was related to increased bleeding in the absence of ischemic benefits in patients with NSTE-ACS [14].

Finally, in the TRITON-TIMI 38 trial, ischemic and bleeding events of prasugrel versus clopidogrel were not influenced by GPI use: (i) the significant reduction of cardiovascular death, MI, or stroke by using prasugrel instead of clopidogrel remained significant in patients receiving GPI (n = 7414, 54.5% of overall study population) as was in patients not receiving GPI (p for interaction = 0.83); (ii) TIMI major or minor bleeding did not differ significantly between prasugrel and clopidogrel groups, irrespective of GPI use (p for interaction = 0.19) [15]. These data led to the following guidelines recommendations [1,2].

- European guidelines (on myocardial revascularization 2014):
  1 Current evidence does not support an additional benefit of routine upstream use of GPI in patients with NSTE-ACS undergoing coronary angiography (Class III, level A);
  2 GPI should be considered in bailout or thrombotic complications (Class IIa, level C);
- US guidelines (on NSTE-ACS management 2014):
  1 GPI use (abciximab, double-bolus eptifibatide or high-dose bolus tirofiban) is useful at the time of PCI in the case of NSTE-ACS with high-risk features (e.g., elevated troponin) but without adequate pre-treatment with clopidogrel or ticagrelor (Class I, level A);
  2 GPI use in upstream can be considered in patients treated with an early invasive strategy and dual antiplatelet therapy with intermediate/high risk features (e.g., positive troponin) (Class IIb, level B); and
  3 GPI use at the time of PCI could be reasonable in patients with NSTE-ACS and high-risk features (e.g., elevated troponin) treated with UFH and adequately pretreated with clopidogrel (Class IIa, level B). This latter recommendation should be reserved for those patients without high risk of bleeding complications and does not include prasugrel or ticagrelor because there are still insufficient data to make specific recommendations.

ST-segment elevation myocardial infarction

In the era before pre-loading with thienopyridines, several studies have shown that GPI, mainly abciximab, added to UFH in patients with STEMI treated with primary PCI is associated with improved outcomes [16–19]. In order to test if the early upstream administration of abciximab would improve outcomes compared with in catheterization laboratory administration, in the FINESSE trial [20], 2452 patients with STEMI undergoing primary PCI were randomly assigned to: (i) early upstream (at first medical contact) abciximab plus half-dose reteplase (combination-facilitated PCI); (ii) early upstream abciximab alone (abciximab-facilitated PCI), or (iii) abciximab administered immediately before the primary PCI. No significant differences emerged among the three groups in the primary endpoint (composite of all-cause death, ventricular fibrillation occurring more than 48 hours after randomization, cardiogenic shock, and congestive heart failure during the first 90 days after randomization; p = 0.55) and in 90-day mortality (p = 0.49). Importantly, subgroup analyses showed a survival benefit with the use of abciximab in patients presenting within 4 hours of symptom onset to non-PCI hospitals and requiring transfer for primary PCI [21].

In the On-TIME-2 trial including 936 patients with STEMI with a median time from onset of symptoms to diagnosis of 76 minutes, high-bolus dose tirofiban started during the pre-hospital phase and continued for up to 18 hours after the procedure provided significant improvements in surrogate markers of reperfusion

(ST-segment resolution) compared with placebo (only provisional use of tirofiban in catheterization laboratory) [22]. With upstream tirofiban, there was also a reduction in the composite secondary endpoint of death, recurrent MI, urgent TVR, and thrombotic bailout, although the difference was mainly caused by a decrease in the thrombotic bailout. These latter data were pooled together with those on 414 patients enrolled during the On-TIME-2 open-label run-in phase, comparing tirofiban with no tirofiban [23]. This protocol pre-specified pooled analysis of the two study phases showed that the rate of major adverse cardiac events at 30 days was significantly reduced by systematic high dose tirofiban versus no tirofiban or placebo, with also reduced mortality, in the absence of significant increase of major bleeding. Unfortunately, it was not clear if the benefits in On-TIME-2 were related to upstream versus downstream administration or related to systematic versus provisional administration. The differences of results between FINESSE and On-TIME-2 that should be considered are that the time from symptom onset to GPI administration was much shorter in On-TIME-2 [24], and, furthermore, in the FINESSE trial only a few patients were recruited by the ambulance system and only 40% of patients were transferred for PCI from centers without catheterization laboratories. The issue of whether abciximab remains beneficial after adequate clopidogrel loading was tested also in patients (n = 800) with STEMI in the BRAVE 3 trial, showing no benefits in terms of infarct size prior to discharge [25]. However, the infarct size 30 days after primary PCI for anterior STEMI was reduced by the systematic use of an intracoronary bolus of abciximab in the INFUSE-MI trial [26]. Therefore, there is no definitive answer regarding the current role of routine use of GPI in primary PCI, particularly when prasugrel or ticagrelor is used, and the value of starting upstream of PCI remains uncertain.

Finally, several studies have assessed the administration of abciximab as an intracoronary instead of intravenous bolus. Despite some small studies suggesting potential benefits of the intracoronary route, these observations were not confirmed in large randomized trials and in a recent meta-analysis pooling results of five randomized trials [27,28].

On this background the following guideline recommendations were set [1,3]:

- European guidelines (on myocardial revascularization 2014) [1]:
  1 Upstream use of GPI (versus in-lab use) can be considered only in high risk patients undergoing transfer for primary PCI (Class IIb, level B);
  2 In-lab use is reasonable for angiographic evidence of large thrombus, slow- or no-reflow, and other thrombotic complications as bailout therapy (Class IIa, level C), although this has not been tested in randomized trials.
- US guidelines (on STEMI management 2013) [3]:
  1 It is reasonable to begin treatment with an intravenous GPI such as abciximab (level of evidence A), high-bolus-dose tirofiban (level of evidence B), or double-bolus eptifibatide (level of evidence B) at the time of primary PCI (with or without stenting or clopidogrel pretreatment) in selected patients with STEMI who are receiving UFH (Class IIa).
  2 It may be reasonable to administer intravenous GPI in the pre-catheterization laboratory setting (e.g., ambulance, emergency department) to patients with STEMI for whom primary PCI is intended (Class IIb, level B of recommendation).
  3 It may be reasonable to administer intracoronary abciximab to patients with STEMI undergoing primary PCI (Class IIb, level B of recommendation).

Cangrelor

Cangrelor is an intravenous reversible P2Y$_{12}$ inhibitor. Chemically known as N-2-methylthio-ethyl-2-(3,3,3-trilflouroprpylthiol)-5′-adenyl acid, it is an analogue of adenosine triphosphate (ATP), the natural antagonist of the P2Y$_{12}$ receptor. It is dephosphorylated to the nucleoside and its primary metabolite is essentially inactive. It is characterized by a potent, predictable inhibition of ADP-induced inhibition of platelet aggregation that is virtually immediate (when administered as a bolus) and rapidly reversible. Cangrelor achieves almost complete and immediate inhibition of ADP-induced platelet aggregation when administered as a bolus of 30 µg/kg, and continuous infusion sustains the high degree of inhibition. The plasma half-life is approximately 3–5 minutes and platelet function is restored within 1 hour after cessation of infusion. Notably, cangrelor is not characterized by a significant renal or hepatic metabolism, a relevant difference when compared with oral P2Y$_{12}$ inhibitors that can be particularly attractive in the acute setting.

While the pivotal trials showed a satisfactory rate of major bleeding side effects, the highly potent cangrelor did not demonstrate a significant impact on adverse cardiac events. The initial promising results obtained in phase 2 studies have led the foundation for cangrelor phase 3 program, CHAMPION (Cangrelor versus standard tHerapy to Achieve optimal Management of Platelet InhibitiON). This program originally consisted of two randomized 1 : 1, double-blind, double-dummy trials: CHAMPION PCI and CHAMPION PLATFORM (Table 42.2) [29,30]. These trials tested

Table 42.2 Cangrelor phase 3 trials.

	CHAMPION PLATFORM	CHAMPION PCI	CHAMPION PHOENIX	BRIDGE
Number of patients	5295 (modified ITT)	8877 (ITT)	10,942 (modified ITT)	210
Patients included	Requiring PCI (with or without stent) in elective or ACS excluding STEMI and P2Y12 naive	Requiring PCI (with or without stent) in patients with ACS. Previous daily use of clopidogrel 75 mg allowed	Requiring either urgent or elective PCI and P2Y12 naive	ACS or treated with a coronary stent and receiving a thienopyridine awaiting CABG
Cangrelor protocol	30 µg/kg IV bolus and 4 µg/kg/minute IV infusion	30 µg/kg IV bolus and 4 µg/kg/minute IV infusion	30 µg/kg IV bolus and 4 µg/kg/minute IV infusion	Infusion of 0.75 µg/kg/minute IV on the basis of a stage I dose-finding study in 10 patients
Duration of treatment	Minimum infusion of 2 h and a maximum of 4 h, followed by clopidogrel 600 mg	Infusion at least 2 h or the duration of PCI, and a maximum of 4 h followed by clopidogrel 600 mg	Infusion at least 2 h or the duration of PCI, and a maximum of 4 h followed by clopidogrel 600 mg	Thienopyridines were stopped (clopidogrel 5 days before CABG, prasugrel 7 days) and cangrelor or placebo was administered for at least 48 h which was discontinued 1–6 h before CABG
Comparator	Clopidogrel 600 mg loading dose (end of PCI)	Clopidogrel 600 mg loading dose (before PCI)	Clopidogrel 300 or 600 mg loading dose (before PCI)	Placebo
Primary endpoint	Composite of death, MI, or IDR at 48 h	Composite of death from any cause, MI, or IDR at 48 h	Composite of death, MI, IDR, or ST at 48 h	Platelet reactivity assessed daily
Safety endpoint	Bleeding events at 48 h (single events and categorized events [ACUITY, GUSTO, TIMI criteria]	Bleeding events at 48 h (single events and categorized events [ACUITY, GUSTO, TIMI criteria]	Major/minor non-CABG related hemorrhage by clinically relevant criteria at 48 h (TIMI, GUSTO, others); Incidence of blood product transfusion until 48 h, categorized according to relationship with CABG	Excessive CABG surgery-related bleeding
Notes	Enrollment was stopped when a 70% interim analysis concluded that the trial would be unlikely to show superiority for the primary endpoint	Enrollment was stopped when a 70% interim analysis concluded that the trial would be unlikely to show superiority for the primary endpoint		

ACS, acute coronary syndromes; CABG, coronary artery bypass graft; IDR, ischemia-driven revascularization; ITT, intention-to-treat; MI, myocardial infarction; PCI, percutaneous coronary interventions; PRU, P2Y12 reaction unit; ST, stent thrombosis; STEMI, ST-segment elevation myocardial infarction.

the hypothesis that cangrelor, given during PCI, could reduce thrombotic events compared to clopidogrel administered at the beginning or at the end of PCI respectively, with an acceptable safety profile. The phase 3 CHAMPION-PCI and CHAMPION-PLATFORM trials compared cangrelor with clopidogrel 600 mg in patients with ACS scheduled for PCI, with the timing of the clopidogrel dose being the major difference between the trials. Both trials were prematurely discontinued because of insufficient evidence of the clinical effectiveness of cangrelor. However, there were reductions in stent thrombosis and death from any cause. Furthermore, the lack of overall demonstrable clinical benefit of cangrelor could be related to the definition of MI used, which made it difficult to adjudicate early ischemic events. The definition of MI used in CHAMPION PCI and PLATFORM did require biomarkers elevation but clinical judgment was applied to interpreting the relationship to the PCI or to the index event; that definition preceded the last update of universal definition of MI. According to the original definition, the presence of stable or falling biomarkers at the time of PCI was not required to define PCI-related MI endpoint. Two independent analyses of the CHAMPION dataset retrospectively applied the universal MI definition and consistently indicated a reduced number of PCI-related MI events and more favorable treatment effects for cangrelor.

On this background, the CHAMPION-PHOENIX study was designed with a careful evaluation of the MI definition [31]. Differing from the two previous studies, the CHAMPION-PHOENIX trial had the following characteristics: (i) the definition of MI as endpoint; (ii) the comparator arm was clopidogrel 300 or 600 mg, at the investigator's discretion; (iii) the primary endpoint was the composite of death, MI, ischemia-driven revascularization, or stent thrombosis (including intraprocedural) at 48 hours; and (iv) the population of interest was restricted to clopidogrel-naïve patients. The definition of MI used in PHOENIX was based on the Second Universal definition of MI for all types of MI but PCI-related (type 4a) MI, where this definition was expanded to include some elements (like angiographic complications) that were later included in the Third Universal MI definition. In PHOENIX PCI-related MI could be assessed using cardiac biomarkers only if troponin pre-PCI was normal or elevated but stable or falling according to at least two samples over 6 hours. As learned from CHAMPION PCI and PLATFORM, great emphasis was placed on an accurate assessment of baseline status: in PHOENIX, 98% of the enrolled patients had at least two troponin values before PCI. Patients with NSTE-ACS, with one or no biomarker assessment available or increasing biomarkers before PCI required additional evidence of MI. By definition, PCI-related MI was not adjudicated in patients with STEMI as entry diagnosis.

CHAMPION-PHOENIX (Table 42.2) was a randomized, double-blind, double-dummy trial that compared cangrelor with clopidogrel in 11,145 patients who had not previously received a P2Y$_{12}$ antagonist and required PCI, including patients with stable angina and ACS (with or without ST-segment elevation). The primary efficacy endpoint was a composite of death, MI, ischemia-driven revascularization, or stent thrombosis at 48 hours after randomization. The rate of the primary efficacy endpoint was lower in the cangrelor group than in the clopidogrel group (4.7% vs. 5.9%; p = 0.005), driven by the reduction in the rate of acute peri-procedural MI and by a reduced rate of stent thrombosis (0.8% vs. 1.4%; p = 0.01). The benefit from cangrelor was consistent across several pre-specified subgroups, except for diabetic patients, who represented 27.8% of the global population (p = 0.26). The rate of

the primary safety endpoint was 0.16% in the cangrelor group versus 0.11% in the clopidogrel group (p = 0.44). Overall, the data suggest a promising role for cangrelor, particularly for patients with ACS who could benefit from its pharmacologic rapidity in the onset–offset of action. However, future studies are needed to determine the optimal way to transition ACS PCI patients from cangrelor to prasugrel or ticagrelor; such patients represented only 43% of patients recruited in the CHAMPION-PHOENIX trial. The pre-specified pooled analysis of patient-level data from the three cangrelor trials confirmed the lower rates of PCI peri-procedural thrombotic complications (3.8% for cangrelor vs. 4.7% for control; p = 0.0007) and of stent thrombosis (0.5% vs. 0.8%; p = 0.0008) with no difference in major bleeding [32].

Because of its rapid on–off effect, cangrelor also has potential as a bridging agent in patients requiring surgery, by adequately preventing ischemic events while allowing rapid restoration of platelet function on therapy discontinuation in the event of bleeding. The BRIDGE study evaluated the efficacy of this strategy for patients taking clopidogrel who were scheduled for surgery (Table 42.2) [33]. A total of 210 patients taking thienopyridines for ACS or after stent placement, who were awaiting coronary artery bypass grafting (CABG), had their thienopyridine stopped and were then randomized to either cangrelor (0.75 µg/kg/min) or placebo for at least 48 hours. The study drug was discontinued 1–6 hours before CABG surgery. Patients randomized to cangrelor had lower levels of platelet reactivity throughout the treatment period compared with placebo. There was no significant difference in major bleeding prior to CABG surgery, although minor bleeding episodes were numerically higher with cangrelor. With the use of a surrogate endpoint (platelet reactivity as the primary endpoint) the findings of this trial must be interpreted with caution. However, it demonstrates the potential role of cangrelor in this not rare clinical setting.

Specific guidelines recommendations on the use of cangrelor are not available yet. Cangrelor has been approved in Europe for the reduction of thrombotic cardiovascular events in adult patients with coronary artery disease undergoing PCI who have not received an oral P2Y$_{12}$ inhibitor prior to the PCI procedure and in whom oral therapy with P2Y$_{12}$ inhibitors is not feasible or desirable. Recently, the FDA recommended approval for cangrelor for human use in the USA.

Interactive multiple choice questions are available for this chapter on www.wiley.com/go/dangas/cardiology

References

1 Kolh P, Windecker S, Alfonso F, *et al.* 2014 ESC/EACTS Guidelines on myocardial revascularization: The Task Force on Myocardial Revascularization of the European Society of Cardiology (ESC) and the European Association for Cardio-Thoracic Surgery (EACTS) Developed with the special contribution of the European Association of Percutaneous Cardiovascular Interventions (EAPCI). *Eur Heart J* 2014; **35**(37): 2541–2619.

2 Amsterdam EA, Wenger NK, Brindis RG, *et al.* 2014 AHA/ACC Guideline for the management of patients with non-ST-elevation acute coronary syndromes: a Report of the American College of Cardiology/American Heart Association Task Force on Practice Guidelines. *Circulation* 2014; **130**: e344–e426.

3 O'Gara PT, Kushner FG, Ascheim DD, *et al.* 2013 ACCF/AHA Guideline for the Management of ST-Elevation Myocardial Infarction A Report of the American College of Cardiology Foundation/American Heart Association Task Force on Practice Guidelines. *Circulation* 2013; **127**: e362–e425.

4 Fung AY, Saw J, Starovoytov A, *et al.* Abbreviated infusion of eptifibatide after successful coronary intervention the BRIEF-PCI (Brief Infusion of Eptifibatide Following Percutaneous Coronary Intervention) randomized trial. *J Am Coll Cardiol* 2009; **53**(10): 837–845.

5 Gurm HS, Hosman C, Bates ER, *et al.* Comparative effectiveness and safety of a catheterization laboratory-only eptifibatide dosing strategy in patients undergoing percutaneous coronary intervention. *Circ Cardiovasc Interv* 2015; **8**: e001880.

6 Valgimigli M, Percoco G, Barbieri D, *et al.* The additive value of tirofiban administered with the high-dose bolus in the prevention of ischemic complications during high-risk coronary angioplasty: the ADVANCE Trial. *J Am Coll Cardiol* 2004; **44**(1): 14–19.

7 Biondi-Zoccai G, Valgimigli M, Margheri M, *et al.* Assessing the role of eptifibatide in patients with diffuse coronary disease undergoing drug-eluting stenting: the INtegrilin plus STenting to Avoid myocardial Necrosis Trial. *Am Heart J* 2012; **163**(5): 835.e1–e7.

8 Kastrati A, Mehilli J, Schühlen H, *et al.* A clinical trial of abciximab in elective percutaneous coronary intervention after pretreatment with clopidogrel. *N Engl J Med* 2004; **350**(3): 232–238.

9 Boersma E, Harrington RA, Moliterno DJ, *et al.* Platelet glycoprotein IIb/IIIa inhibitors in acute coronary syndromes: a meta-analysis of all major randomised clinical trials. *Lancet* 2002; **359**(9302): 189–198.

10 Kastrati A, Mehilli J, Neumann FJ, *et al.* Abciximab in patients with acute coronary syndromes undergoing percutaneous coronary intervention after clopidogrel pretreatment: the ISAR-REACT 2 randomized trial. *JAMA* 2006; **295**(13): 1531–1538.

11 Stone GW, McLaurin BT, Cox DA, *et al.* Bivalirudin for patients with acute coronary syndromes. *N Engl J Med* 2006; **355**(21): 2203–2216.

12 Stone GW, Ware JH, Bertrand ME, *et al.* Antithrombotic strategies in patients with acute coronary syndromes undergoing early invasive management: one-year results from the ACUITY trial. *JAMA* 2007; **298**(21): 2497–2506.

13 Kastrati A, Neumann FJ, Schulz S, *et al.* Abciximab and heparin vs. bivalirudin for non-ST-elevation myocardial infarction. *N Engl J Med* 2011; **365**(21): 1980–1989.

14 Giugliano RP, White JA, Bode C, *et al.* Early vs. delayed, provisional eptifibatide in acute coronary syndromes. *N Engl J Med* 2009; **360**(21): 2176–2190.

15 O'Donoghue M, Antman EM, Braunwald E, *et al.* The efficacy safety of prasugrel with without a glycoprotein IIb/IIIa inhibitor in patients with acute coronary syndromes undergoing percutaneous intervention: a TRITON-TIMI 38 (Trial to Assess Improvement in Therapeutic outcomes by Optimizing Platelet Inhibition With Prasugrel-Thrombolysis In Myocardial Infarction 38) analysis. *J Am Coll Cardiol* 2009; **54**(8): 678–685.

16 Stone GW, Grines CL, Cox DA, *et al.* Comparison of angioplasty with stenting, with or without abciximab, in acute myocardial infarction. *N Engl J Med* 2002; **346**(13): 957–966.

17 De Luca G, Navarese E, Marino P. Risk profile and benefits from Gp IIb-IIIa inhibitors among patients with ST-segment elevation myocardial infarction treated with primary angioplasty: a meta-regression analysis of randomized trials. *Eur Heart J* 2009; **30**: 2705–2713.

18 Montalescot G, Barragan P, Wittenberg O, *et al.* Platelet glycoprotein IIb/IIIa inhibition with coronary stenting for acute myocardial infarction. *N Engl J Med* 2001; **344**(25): 1895–1903.

19 Neumann FJ, Kastrati A, Pogatsa-Murray G, *et al.* Evaluation of prolonged antithrombotic pretreatment ("cooling-off" strategy) before intervention in patients with unstable coronary syndromes: a randomized controlled trial. *JAMA* 2003; **290**(12): 1593–1599.

20 Ellis SG, Tendera M, de Belder MA, *et al.* Facilitated PCI in patients with ST-elevation myocardial infarction. *N Engl J Med* 2008; **358**(21): 2205–2217.

21 Herrmann HC, Lu J, Brodie BR, *et al.* Benefit of facilitated percutaneous coronary intervention in high-risk ST-segment elevation myocardial infarction patients presenting to nonpercutaneous coronary intervention hospitals. *JACC Cardiovasc Interv* 2009; **2**(10): 917–924.

22 Van't Hof AW, Ten Berg J, Heestermans T, *et al.* Ongoing Tirofiban In Myocardial infarction Evaluation 2 study group. Prehospital initiation of tirofiban in patients with ST-elevation myocardial infarction undergoing primary angioplasty (On-TIME 2): a multicentre, double-blind, randomised controlled trial. *Lancet* 2008; **372**(9638): 537–546.

23 en Berg JM, van't Hof AW, Dill T, *et al.* Effect of early, prehospital initiation of high bolus dose tirofiban in patients with ST-segment elevation myocardial infarction on short- and long-term clinical outcome. *J Am Coll Cardiol* 2010; **55**(22): 2446–2455.

24 Montalescot G. Mechanical reperfusion: treat well, treat on time too. *Lancet* 2008; **372**(9638): 509–510.

25 Mehilli J, Kastrati A, Schulz S, *et al.*; Bavarian Reperfusion Alternatives Evaluation-3 (BRAVE-3) Study Investigators. Abciximab in patients with acute ST-segment-elevation myocardial infarction undergoing primary percutaneous coronary intervention after clopidogrel loading: a randomized double-blind trial. *Circulation* 2009; **119**(14): 1933–1940.

26 Stone GW, Maehara A, Witzenbichler B, *et al.* Intracoronary abciximab and aspiration thrombectomy in patients with large anterior myocardial infarction: the INFUSE-AMI randomized trial. *JAMA* 2012; **307**(17): 1817–1826.

27 Thiele H, Wöhrle J, Hambrecht R, *et al.* Intracoronary vs. intravenous bolus abciximab during primary percutaneous coronary intervention in patients with acute ST-elevation myocardial infarction: a randomised trial. *Lancet* 2012; **379**(9819): 923–931.

28 Piccolo R, Eitel I, Iversen AZ, *et al.* Intracoronary versus intravenous bolus abciximab administration in patients undergoing primary percutaneous coronary intervention with acute ST-elevation myocardial infarction: a pooled analysis of individual patient data from five randomised controlled trials. *EuroIntervention* 2014; **9**(9): 1110–1120.

29 Bhatt DL, Lincoff AM, Gibson CM, *et al.* Intravenous platelet blockade with cangrelor during PCI. *N Engl J Med* 2009; **361**: 2330–2341.

30 Harrington RA, Stone GW, McNulty S, *et al.* Platelet inhibition with cangrelor in patients undergoing PCI. *N Engl J Med* 2009; **361**: 2318–2329.

31 Bhatt DL, Stone GW, Mahaffey KW, *et al.* Effect of platelet inhibition with cangrelor during PCI on ischemic events. *N Engl J Med* 2013; **368**: 1303–1313.

32 Steg PG, Bhatt DL, Hamm CW, *et al.* Effect of cangrelor on periprocedural outcomes in percutaneous coronary interventions: a pooled analysis of patient-level data. *Lancet* 2013; **382**(9909): 1981–1992.

33 Angiolillo DJ, Firstenberg MS, Price MJ, *et al.* Bridging antiplatelet therapy with cangrelor in patients undergoing cardiac surgery: a randomized controlled trial. *JAMA* 2012; **307**(3): 265–274.

CHAPTER 43

Role of Parenteral Agents in PCI for Stable Patients

Joanna Ghobrial, David A. Burke, and Duane S. Pinto
Beth Israel Deaconess Medical Center, Harvard Medical School, Boston, MA, USA

Optimal anticoagulation has proven to be a key component in the management of patients undergoing percutaneous coronary intervention (PCI). There has been a considerable evolution in the pharmacotherapy of PCI since the early days of balloon angioplasty. Medications with variable modes of action are used to reduce complications by inhibiting thrombin formation, platelet activation, and platelet aggregation. These medications have targeted different portions of the coagulation cascade, and newer synthetic agents have been developed to specifically target factor Xa or thrombin in an attempt to minimize ischemic and bleeding complications, goals that are often at odds with one another.

The principal aims of pharmacotherapy during PCI are to avoid the adverse consequences related to iatrogenic plaque rupture from balloon inflation or stent deployment after PCI and to reduce the risk of thrombus formation on intravascular PCI equipment during the procedure. Growing evidence supports use of a variety of agents in the setting of stable ischemic heart disease, unstable angina, non-ST-elevation myocardial infarction (NSTEMI), and ST-elevation myocardial infarction (STEMI).

Most data involving newer antithrombotic drugs focus on their use in acute coronary syndromes (ACS). However, the main aims of this review are to summarize the agents available for anticoagulation during elective PCI, to outline their mode of action, and to review the evidence supporting their use.

Antiplatelet therapy using glycoprotein IIb/IIIa inhibition

Platelet adherence to abnormal surfaces and aggregate is mediated by surface membrane glycoprotein receptors which are expressed in increasing numbers with platelet activation and are potential targets for antiplatelet therapies. The platelet glycoprotein IIb/IIIa receptor has a central role in platelet aggregation and so forms an attractive target for therapy.

Abciximab, tirofiban, and eptifibatide are currently available for clinical use. Abciximab is a monoclonal antibody directed against the glycoprotein receptor, while tirofiban and eptifibatide are high affinity non-antibody receptor inhibitors. The use of intravenous glycoprotein IIb/IIIa inhibitors (GPI) has been studied in patients with ACS and those undergoing intracoronary stent implantation and has been associated with improved outcomes (Figure 43.1).

The use of GPI among patients who are undergoing PCI depends upon on the clinical setting of PCI and patient risk for ischemic complications. The utility of GPI in "elective" PCI has been evaluated in the EPIC, EPILOG, and EPISTENT trials for abciximab [1–5], IMPACT-II and ESPRIT trials for eptifibatide [6,7], and the ADVANCE and TOPSTAR trials for tirofiban (Table 43.2) [8,9]. These trials were completed before the routine use of stents in patients undergoing PCI and before the use of clopidogrel prior to and/or at high dose before PCI and before development of more potent oral antiplatelet agents. The incremental benefit of GPI in patients pretreated with aspirin and clopidogrel was addressed in the ISAR-REACT series of randomized placebo-controlled trials. Among patients undergoing elective PCI, considered low to intermediate risk for ischemic complications, the ISAR-REACT trial found no benefit for GPI at 30 days or in subsequent follow-up at 1 year in patients who had received clopidogrel (600 mg) at least 2 hours prior to the procedure [10]. The same lack of benefit was apparent for GPI in a subgroup analysis of lower risk patients from the ESPRIT trial [11]. However, there is evidence that GPI did provide benefit among patients with ACS and high risk patients undergoing elective procedures who were pretreated with clopidogrel [10,12,13].

Based on available data, many operators limit use of GPI in elective PCI to those patients considered higher risk, or to those who have not already received appropriate pretreatment with antiplatelet therapy, those who have a suboptimal angiographic result or angiographic complications during the procedure, so-called bailout. There is marked variation in opinion regarding the optimal duration of GPI infusion following PCI.

Abciximab

Abciximab is the Fab fragment of the chimeric human-murine monoclonal antibody 7E3. With intravenous bolus, plasma concentrations decrease rapidly with an initial half-life of less than 10 minutes and second phase half-life of 30 minutes, likely related to rapid binding to the platelet glycoprotein receptor. At highest dose, 80% of platelet GP receptors are occupied in 2 hours, and platelet aggregation is completely inhibited. Upon cessation, free plasma concentrations rapidly fall over the first 6 hours, then at a slower rate.

When initially studied in ACS, patients invariably underwent angioplasty without stenting and thienopyridine therapy was not used.

Interventional Cardiology: Principles and Practice, Second Edition. Edited by George D. Dangas, Carlo Di Mario, and Nicholas N. Kipshidze.
© 2017 John Wiley & Sons, Ltd. Published 2017 by John Wiley & Sons, Ltd.

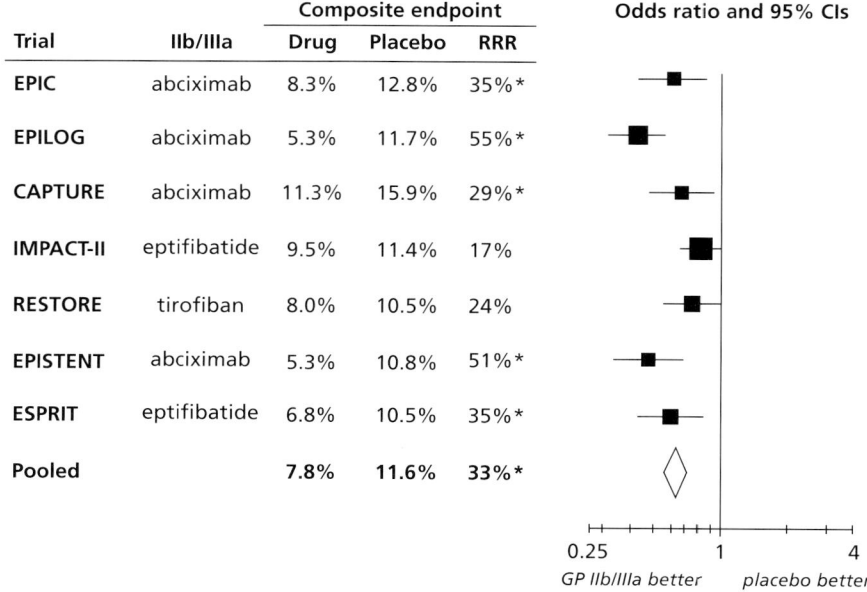

Trial	IIb/IIIa	Composite endpoint		
		Drug	Placebo	RRR
EPIC	abciximab	8.3%	12.8%	35%*
EPILOG	abciximab	5.3%	11.7%	55%*
CAPTURE	abciximab	11.3%	15.9%	29%*
IMPACT-II	eptifibatide	9.5%	11.4%	17%
RESTORE	tirofiban	8.0%	10.5%	24%
EPISTENT	abciximab	5.3%	10.8%	51%*
ESPRIT	eptifibatide	6.8%	10.5%	35%*
Pooled		7.8%	11.6%	33%*

Figure 43.1 Glycoprotein IIb/IIIa inhibitors in percutaneous coronary interventions. The composite endpoint is the risk of death, non-fatal myocardial infarction, or urgent revascularization at 30 days. * Indicates statistical significance at p <0.05. In EPIC, the abciximab bolus plus infusion group was compared with the placebo group. In EPILOG, the abciximab plus low dose heparin and the abciximab plus standard dose heparin groups were combined. In IMPACT-II, the low and high dose eptifibatide groups were combined. In EPISTENT, the stent plus abciximab group was compared with the stent plus placebo group. CIs, confidence intervals; GP, glycoprotein; RRR, relative risk reduction. Source: Sabatine MS, Jang I. The use of glycoprotein IIb/IIIa inhibitors in patients with coronary artery disease. Am J Med 2000; **109**(3): 224–237. Copyright 2000 Elsevier.

A number of randomized trials were performed and in a subsequent meta-analysis including over 5400 patients from the EPIC [1–3], EPILOG [4,14], RAPPORT [15], EPISTENT [5], and CAPTURE [16–20] studies who received percutaneous transluminal coronary angioplasty (PTCA), abciximab significantly reduced 30-day mortality and reinfarction (hazard ratio 0.52, 95% CI 0.41–0.65) [21]. A meta-analysis looking at patients with STEMI who underwent PCI with stenting with abciximab or placebo included the RAPPORT [15], ADMIRAL [22,23], ISAR REACT-2 [24], CADILLAC [25], and ACE studies [26]. Abciximab showed a significant reduction in mortality at 30 days (2.4% vs. 3.4% with placebo) and at 6–12 months (4.4% vs. 6.2%), with no increased bleeding seen in these patients [27].

In terms of patients with stable coronary heart disease undergoing PCI, the following trials evaluated outcomes comparing abciximab with placebo in predominantly stable patients and came to differing conclusions.

The EPILOG study examined a lower risk group of patients including approximately 30% with stable ischemia, and patients with unstable angina and ECG changes or acute myocardial infarction (MI) in the previous 24 hours were excluded. The trial randomized 2792 patients to undergo emergent or elective PCI with abciximab and either standard or low dose heparin versus placebo with standard dose heparin. The trial was terminated early at the first interim analysis for reaching its efficacy endpoint (death, MI, or urgent revascularization) at 30 days with greater than 50% relative reduction in both abciximab arms, standard and low dose heparin (composite event rates of 5.4% and 5.2%, respectively) compared with placebo (composite event rate of 11.7%). There was no difference in major bleeding between the groups [4]. Subsequently, the EPISTENT trial randomized 2399 patients undergoing elective (approximately 40%) or emergent PCI to stenting

alone, stenting with abciximab, or PTCA with abciximab [28,29]. All patients who received a stent were given aspirin and ticlopidine. Adverse events (death, MI, and urgent revascularization) at 30 days (10.8%, 5.3%, and 6.9%) and 6 months (11.4%, 5.6%, and 7.8%) were significantly lower in the abciximab groups, with the difference largely driven by reduced death and NSTEMI.

Conversely, the ISAR-REACT study consisted of 2159 patients with stable coronary artery disease undergoing PCI with stenting and treated with aspirin and thienopyridine, who were randomized to abciximab or placebo. The 30-day major adverse cardiac events (MACE) rates between abciximab and placebo were the same (both 4%), and major bleeding complications were comparable [10]. In the ISAR-REACT 2 trial, abciximab administration, among high risk patients with NSTEMI among receiving clopidogrel with a 600-mg loading dose, was associated with a lower incidence of death, MI, or urgent revascularization (8.9% vs. 11.9%, RR 0.75, 95% CI 0.58–0.97; p = 0.03), but the benefit was confined to those who with elevated troponin (13.1% vs. 18.3%, RR 0.71, 95% CI 0.54–0.95; p = 0.02) compared with those who had normal troponin level (4.6% vs. 4.6%, RR 0.99, 95% CI 0.56–1.76; p = 0.98) [13].

Tirofiban

Stable patients undergoing PCI were evaluated in the ADVANCE trial which aimed to assess the potential benefit of using a higher dose of tirofiban than had been used in trials assessing the drug in the setting of ACS (RESTORE, PRISM, and PRISM-PLUS trials) [30–32]. A total of 202 patients, pretreated with thienopyridines, were randomized to high dose bolus tirofiban (25 μg/kg/3 min, and infusion of 0.15 μg/kg/min for 24–48 hours) or to placebo [8]. At 6 months, adverse events (death, MI, target vessel revascularization (TVR), or bailout GPI) was significantly less frequent with tirofiban (20% vs. 35%, hazard ratio 0.51, 95% CI 0.29–0.88; p = 0.01), a difference driven by the incidence of MI and bailout GPI in the placebo group. In subgroup analysis, the benefit of tirofiban was significant among patients with ACS but not among those with stable angina.

A small study of 96 patients, the TOPSTAR (The Effect of Additional Temporary Glycoprotein IIb/IIIa Receptor Inhibition on Troponin Release in Elective Percutaneous Coronary Interventions after Pre-treatment with Aspirin and Clopidogrel) trial, was a randomized, double-blind, placebo-controlled study, and the first to observe that additional inhibition of platelet aggregation by tirofiban with aspirin and clopidogrel reduced peri-procedural troponin release and the composite endpoint (death, MI, and TVR) after 9 months (2.3% with tirofiban vs.13.0% with placebo; p <0.05) [9].

Eptifibatide

Eptifibatide is a hepapeptide of the glycoprotein IIb/IIIa receptor that inhibits platelet aggregation. The plasma half-life is 10–15 minutes, and it is predominantly renally excreted (75%) with the remainder via hepatic pathways (25%) (Table 43.1).

Over 4000 patients were enrolled in the IMPACT-II (Integrilin to Minimize Platelet Aggregation and Coronary Thrombosis-II) study (59% with stable coronary disease), which randomized patients to either placebo or one of two doses of eptifibatide [7]. At 30 days, there was no significant difference in the MACE rates between the groups, and eptifibatide did not increase rates of major bleeding or transfusion. By a treatment-received analysis, the lower dose regimen produced a significant reduction in the composite endpoint (11.6% vs. 9.1%; p = 0.035), with reduced rates of abrupt closure and ischemic events at 30 days, but the higher dose produced a less substantial reduction (11.6% vs. 10.0%; p = 0.18). The investigators believed that the doses studied appeared to be at the lower end of the efficacy–response curve, and that further investigation was needed.

The ESPRIT trial randomly assigned 2064 patients to placebo or eptifibatide immediately prior to elective PCI [6]. The trial was terminated prematurely because eptifibatide reduced the primary endpoint (48 hour death, MI, urgent revascularization, or bailout GPI) by 37% (6.6% vs. 10.5%; p = 0.0015).

The INSTANT trial attempted to examine the benefit of added eptifibatide to heparin versus heparin alone in stable patients undergoing complex PCI; however, the trial was stopped early because of slow enrollment and because it lacked statistical power, but there were favorable trends in the primary endpoint of abnormal post PCI creatine kinase-MB (CK-MB) (41% in eptifibatide and heparin group vs. 55% in the heparin alone group, RR 0.74; p = 0.169) [33] suggesting that further larger studies are warranted.

Comparisons between agents

The TARGET study was designed to test whether tirofiban was not inferior to abciximab in patients undergoing elective PCI, but demonstrated that tirofiban offered less protection from major ischemic events than did abciximab (30-day MACE 7.6% with tirofiban vs. 6.0% abciximab, HR 1.26, 95% CI 1.01–1.57; p = 0.038) [34]. The inferiority of tirofiban was thought to be to the result of an inadequate bolus regimen.

The TENACITY (Tirofiban Evaluation of Novel Dosing Versus Abciximab with Clopidogrel and Inhibition of Thrombin) trial sought to investigate a high dose tirofiban bolus regimen and randomized patients undergoing elective PCI to abciximab or tirofiban,

with all patients receiving aspirin and clopidogrel. Patients were additionally randomized to either unfractionated heparin (UFH) or bivalirudin. The planned enrollment of 8000 only reached 383 patients as a result of financial reasons. Results from this small group suggested that further study is warranted (30-day MACE, 8.8% with abciximab vs. 6.9% with tirofiban) [35].

A meta-analysis of eight prospective trials evaluating 14,644 patients undergoing PCI compared abciximab, tirofiban, and eptifibatide. Certain differences were noted between the agents, but these trials compared each drug with placebo so conclusions regarding comparative effectiveness is limited, especially because these trials largely included patients treated with PTCA only or those who did not receive thienopyridine treatment [36].

Unfractionated heparin

The most commonly used antithrombin agent for PCI has been UFH. UFH has been the gold standard for many years in the treatment of patients undergoing PCI because of its ease of administration, rapid onset, easily measurable efficacy (monitored by activated clotting time; ACT), and reversibility. It is a heterogeneous mixture of glycosaminoglycans of varying lengths with a high affinity for antithrombin. The antithrombin activity of UFH is dependent on antithrombin activation, which subsequently inactivates thrombin, and so UFH is considered an indirect antithrombin agent.

Elimination of UFH is initially through rapid metabolism within the endothelial cells and macrophages (zero-order kinetics), and then by a slower renal clearance (first-order kinetics). Plasma half-life is dependent on the dosage administered but is of the order of 1 hour at doses of 100 unit/kg. If necessary, the effects can be reversed with protamine sulfate.

UFH remains the mainstay anticoagulant worldwide in patients undergoing PCI. Despite its common use, there have been no prospective randomized comparisons demonstrating efficacy compared with placebo for obvious reasons, and the current dosing regimens are empiric because clinical experience and anecdotal evidence demonstrate clearly the need for some degree of anticoagulation with balloon and stent-mediated vascular wall injury. In a pooled analysis of data from randomized clinical trials utilizing UFH only, there was a gradient of benefit associated with increasing degrees of anticoagulation. At ACT levels >350 seconds there was an association with fewer ischemic events, although bleeding rates increased [37]. The STEEPLE (Safety and Efficacy of Intravenous Enoxaparin in Elective Percutaneous Coronary Intervention: An International Randomized Evaluation) Study [38] noted that bleeding increased significantly with ACT values >325 seconds, but ischemic events also increased when the ACT value was <325 seconds [38]. Available data do not support the use of prolonged heparin infusions after PCI where an excess in bleeding events and accompanying increase in the length of stay without a reduction in ischemic events has been observed with this approach.

Anticoagulation using UFH monotherapy appears insufficient to optimally protect against ischemic events such as peri-procedural MI in patients with ACS. Aggressive antiplatelet therapy is thought to prevent against embolization of platelet aggregates formed as a result of platelet activation induced by UFH. The use of high dose clopidogrel or GPI in elective PCI, or the use of both in patients with ACS undergoing PCI reduces peri-procedural ischemic complications with UFH [6,8,28].

The high ACT levels utilized in early studies are no longer thought to be required given the high prevalence of stent usage and

Table 43.1 Overview and dosing for antithrombin agents.

	Dose	Half-life	Clinical condition	Note	Trials
Heparins					
Unfractionated heparin	60 IU/kg IV bolus and 12 IU/kg infusion adjusted to maintain PTT 50–70 s Intermittent bolus dosing during PCI to maintain ACT >200–250 with GPI and >250–300 s for HemoTec or 300–350 s for Hemochron without GPI		Stable IHD UA NSTEMI conservative and invasive STEMI	Contraindicated with HIT Avoid switching to LMWH Continue if planned CABG Can use with fibrinolytic therapy though enoxaparin and fondaparinux superior	6 small randomized studies vs. placebo
Enoxaparin	1 mg/kg SQ twice daily up to 100 mg/dose For PCI, additional 0.3 mg/mg IV dose if last SQ dose >8 h or <2 doses administered but prior therapy administered With fibrinolysis and age >75 years, 30 mg IV followed 15 min later by 1 mg/kg subcutaneously every 12 h until hospital discharge for a maximum of 8 days. For age >75 years, eliminate IV bolus and reduce maintenance to 0.75 mg subcutaneously/twice daily and if CrCl <30 mL/min reduce subcutaneous dose frequency to daily irrespective of age	4.5 h	Stable IHD UA NSTEMI STEMI fibrinolysis	Reduce dose (1 mg/kg every 24 h) with renal failure (CrCl <30 mL/min) Avoid switch to UFH Avoid if CABG <24 h Discontinue 12–24 h before CABG and dose with UFH	ESSENCE/ TIMI-11B SYNERGY ACUTE-II INTERACT A to Z ExTRACT-TIMI 25
Dalteparin	120 IU/kg subcutaneously every 12 h (maximum 10,000 IU twice daily)	Approx 2–5 h	IV GPI planned: target ACT 200 s using UFH No IV GPI planned: target ACT 250–300 s for HemoTec; 300–350 s for Hemochron using UFH		FRISC FRIC
Glycoprotein IIb/IIIa inhibitors					
Abciximab	For PCI, 0.25 mg/kg IV bolus administered 10–60 min prior to PCI, followed by infusion of 0.125 µg/kg/min (max 10 µg/min) for 12 h	Approx 30 min	UA NSTEMI STEMI	No dose adjustment for renal or hepatic impairment	EPIC EPILOG RAPPORT EPISTENT CAPTURE RAPPORT ADMIRAL ISAR-REACT ISAR-2 CADILLAC
Tirofiban	(Off-label) for PCI: loading dose 25 µg/kg IV over 3 min at time of procedure. Infusion 0.15 µg/kg/min continued for 18–24 h UA/NSTEMI: initial rate 0.4 µg/kg/min IV for 30 min, then continued at 0.1 µg/kg/min. Dosing through procedure and for 12–24 h post-intervention	Approx 2 h	UA/NSTEMI in combination with heparin STEMI (off-label) Elective PCI (off-label)	Reduce dose to 50% normal rate with renal failure (CrCl <30 mL/min)	ADVANCE TOPSTAR

Drug	Dosing	Indications	Half-life	Cautions/Notes	Trials
Eptifibatide	PCI: bolus 180 µg/kg IV immediately before PCI, with infusion 2 µg/kg/min. Second bolus 180 µg/kg 10 min after first bolus. Infusion for 18–24h. Shorter infusion durations can be considered for non-emergent PCI in patients adequately pretreated with clopidogrel	Stable IHD, UA, NSTEMI, STEMI in combination with UFH	Approx 2.5h	Heparin infusion after PCI is discouraged. Discontinue >2–4h before CABG. Use with caution in renal impairment. Dialysis is a contraindication to use	ESPRIT, IMPACT-II

Direct thrombin inhibitors

Drug	Dosing	Indications	Half-life	Cautions/Notes	Trials
Bivalirudin	0.1 mg/kg IV bolus then 0.25 mg/kg/h IV. 0.75 mg/kg IV bolus then 1.75 mg/kg/h for PCI if no prior antithrombotic therapy administered	Stable IHD, UA, NSTEMI invasive, STEMI	Approx 25 min	Reduced with renal failure (0.25 mg/kg/h IV for hemodialysis). Caution with GFR <30 mL/h. Discontinue bivalirudin 3h before CABG and dose with UFH	HAS, ACUITY, REPLACE-2, ISAR-REACT-3, ISAR-REACT-4, HORIZONS-AMI, EUROMAX, NAPLES-III, BRIGHT, HEAT-PPCI
Argatroban	350 µg/kg IV over 3–5min then 25 µg/kg/min for PCI	Use in PCI in patients with HIT	Approx 50 min	Caution with hepatic impairment	

Factor XA inhibitors

Drug	Dosing	Indications	Half-life	Cautions/Notes	Trials
Fondaparinux	2.5 mg/day subcutaneously. With fibrinolysis, 2.5 IV followed 2.5 mg/day until hospital discharge for a maximum of 8 days	Medical, UA/NSTEMI conservative, STEMI fibrinolysis	17–21h	Contraindicated with renal failure (CrCl <30 mL/min). Significantly lower incidence of HIT compared with heparins. Discontinue enoxaparin 12–24h before CABG and dose with UFH	OASIS-5, OASIS-6, PENTUA
Rivaroxaban	Dose used in ATLAS ACS-TIMI 51 trial were 2.5 mg or 5 mg twice daily	**Not approved** for ACS or PCI in the USA	5–9h	Caution with hepatic impairment	ATLAS 2 ACS-TIMI 51

ACS, acute coronary syndrome; ACT, activated clotting time; CABG, coronary artery bypass grafting; CrCl, creatinine clearance; GFR, glomerular filtration rate; GPI, glycoprotein IIa/IIIb inhibitor; HIT, heparin-induced thrombocytopenia; IHD, ischemic heart disease; LMWH, low molecular weight heparin; NSTEMI, non-ST-elevation myocardial infarction; PCI, percutaneous coronary intervention; PTT, partial thromboplastin time; STEMI, ST-elevation myocardial infarction; UA, unstable angina; UFH, unfractionated heparin.

antiplatelet medications, nearly eliminating the complication of abrupt closure [39]. The optimal dosing regimen is not defined, but most practitioners utilize regimens of 40–60 IU/kg for goal ACT of >225 seconds when GPI is used and a goal ACT of >300 seconds when UFH is used alone (Table 43.1). A prospective single center trial of elective transfemoral PCI with low dose heparin at 40 IU/kg in 300 patients pretreated with aspirin and 600 mg clopidogrel showed low ischemic and bleeding complications [40], but a randomized trial has yet to be performed. The optimal dosing regimen with new oral antiplatelet agents, prasugrel and ticagrelor, also remains a matter of debate given variable times of pretreatment and the lack of supportive outcomes studies.

During PCI, major limitations of UFH include the narrow therapeutic window, unpredictable individual antithrombin response across patient populations and disease states, platelet activation, and an inability to bind to clot-bound thrombin. The latter is protected from inhibition by the heparin–antithrombin complex serving to propagate thrombus even while heparin is being administered, and it can act as a nidus for further thrombin activation upon discontinuation of heparin. There is also a risk of heparin-induced thrombocytopenia (HIT) and thrombosis syndrome (HITTS) [41]. The latter is rare in the setting of elective PCI, but can be seen with repeated exposures [42]. To address these limitations, other agents have been developed.

Low molecular weight heparins

Low molecular weight heparins (LMWH) are produced by chemical and enzymatic depolymerization of UFH resulting in fragments with a mean molecular weight of 3000–5000 Da. Specifically, these agents have a greater activity against factor Xa than against thrombin, a uniform and predictable anticoagulation action and lower incidence of HIT, addressing some of the limitations of UFH. LMWHs have a longer half-life than UFH, and clearance is by renal excretion. In patients with severe renal dysfunction (creatinine clearance <30 mL/min), the dosage is typically halved. Because it has greater anti-Xa activity, LMWH dosing cannot be reliably adjusted using the ACT (Table 43.1).

The most studied of the LMWHs is enoxaparin. An observational study of 803 patients with ACS treated with a twice daily dose of 1 mg/kg enoxaparin subcutaneously showed that 30-day mortality was closely linked with anti-Xa levels [43]. This study served as the basis of dosing for subsequent PCI studies where anti-Xa levels >0.5 IU/mL are considered therapeutic for enoxaparin [44]. However, anti-Xa levels are not commonly measured during PCI, though they are sometimes measured in medically treated patients.

One aspect of enoxaparin use is that the drug can be administered parenterally or subcutaneously. The subcutaneous route has been used for initial medical manananagement of ACS [45] and the parenteral route is used for PCI [44,46].

Experience with enoxaparin in PCI included a series of studies performed by the National Investigators Collaborating on Enoxaparin (NICE) group. The NICE-1 registry consisted of 828 patients receiving intravenous enoxaparin before coronary intervention at time of elective or urgent PCI. All patients received aspirin, and clopidogrel pretreatment at that time was left to operator discretion. The composite endpoint of death, MI, and urgent revascularization at 30 days was seen in 7.7%, with MI in 5.4% [47].

NICE-4 evaluated PCI with enoxaparin and compared these patients with historic data from the EPILOG and EPISTENT studies where UFH and a GPI (abciximab) were used. NICE-4 adopted

a protocol where 818 patients received enoxaparin 0.75 mg/kg and abciximab 0.25 mg/kg bolus followed by 0.125 µg/kg/min infusion. The 30-day composite endpoint of death, MI, or urgent revascularization occurred in 6.8%, suggesting that enoxaparin can confer a similar efficacy and safety to UFH when used with abciximab [47].

The SYNERGY (Superior Yield of the New Strategy of Enoxaparin, Revascularization and Glycoprotein IIb/IIIa Inhibitors) trial randomized 10,027 patients with ACS to either subcutaneous enoxaparin or intravenous UFH. Enoxaparin proved non-inferior to UFH with the primary endpoint of death or MI at 30 days. For PCI, there was no difference in rates of unsuccessful PCI, abrupt closure, or emergency coronary artery bypass grafting (CABG) between groups. There was a significantly higher rate of thrombolysis in myocardial infarction (TIMI) major bleeding among patients receiving enoxaparin, but no significant difference in the rate of GUSTO severe bleeding, TIMI minor bleeding, or blood transfusions between enoxaparin or UFH groups [46]. The SYNERGY data were not blinded and there was significant crossover between UFH and enoxaparin; an occurrence associated with worse bleeding outcomes compared with no crossover.

Though not the primary intent of the study, the EXTRACT-TIMI-25 (Enoxaparin and Thrombolysis Reperfusion for Acute Myocardial Infarction Treatment, Thrombolyis in MI-Study 25) reported on the role of enoxaparin for elective PCI after STEMI. PCI occurred at a median of 109–122 hours following fibrinolysis [48]. The 2272 patients on enoxaparin undergoing PCI had a significant reduction in 30-day death or MI (10.7% vs. 13.8%; p = 0.001) without an increase in TIMI major bleeding, providing indirect evidence that enoxaparin is superior to UFH in reducing ischemic complications during STEMI and for elective PCI after fibrinolysis.

The CRUISE trial randomized 261 patients undergoing elective or urgent PCI to intravenous enoxaparin 1 mg/kg or UFH, with all patients also receiving eptifibatide. There was no difference in bleeding complications or angiographic complications (6.3% vs. 6.2%; p = NS) during the procedure, and no differences in ischemic endpoints at 48 hours or 30 days.

The STEEPLE trial evaluated 3528 patients with PCI who were randomized to enoxaparin (0.5 or 0.75 mg/kg) or UFH adjusted according to ACT, and stratified according to the use or non-use of GPI [44]. GPI and thienopyridines were used in 40% and 95% of patients, respectively, and 16% of cases required multivessel intervention. The lowest rate of non-CABG-related bleeding at 48 hours was seen in the 0.5 mg/kg enoxaparin arm (5.9% vs. 8.5%; p = 0.01), but the 0.75 mg/kg enoxaparin dose was not significantly different (6.5% vs. 8.5%; p = 0.051). Patients in the 0.5 mg/kg group achieved a therapeutic level of anticoagulation 78.8% of the time compared with 91.8% in the 0.75 mg/kg group. Only 19.7% of patients in the UFH arm achieved therapeutic anticoagulation (p <0.001 for either enoxaparin dose vs. UFH) [22]. The trial was not large enough to provide a definitive comparison of efficacy in prevention of ischemic events.

A meta-analysis of 13 trials comparing intravenous LMWH with UFH showed that a strategy of intravenous LMWH was associated with significant reduction in major bleeding (odds ratio 0.57, 95% CI 0.40–0.82), with no difference in death, MI, or TVR [49]. Overall, the use of intravenous enoxaparin during elective PCI is associated with a better safety profile than weight-adjusted UFH with no additional risk of ischemic events. The possibility of improved outcomes compared with UFH among patients undergoing elective PCI with aggressive intravenous or oral antiplatelet therapy remains unproven. Coupled with an inability to easily monitor therapeutic levels during PCI, complex dosing regimens, and the need for dose adjustment among patients with impaired renal function, enoaxaparin is not frequently utilized during elective PCI.

Dalteparin

Supportive data for the LMWH dalteparin are limited. While dalteparin was utilized in 2457 patients undergoing PCI in ACS, the subjection of this study was comparing an early invasive to conservative approach to PCI in ACS rather than a comparison of anticoagulation strategies [50]. Use of dalteparin in elective PCI has not been adequately studied. A dose-ranging study of 107 patients with all patients receiving aspirin and abciximab led to early unblinding of the study and the decision to terminate the lower dose 40 unit/kg arm. The composite endpoint of death, MI, and urgent revascularization was observed in 15.5% of patients, and major bleeding and transfusion each occurred in 2.8% of patients. Despite the fact that the study was inadequately powered to evaluate the agent fully in this setting, the high clinical event rates resulted in limited uptake.

Fondaparinux

In the attempt to overcome the limitations of the heparins, newer agents have been developed to specifically inhibit factor Xa. Fondaparinux, a pentasaccharide, is a synthetic indirect inhibitor of factor Xa that mimics the action of heparin through its interaction with antithrombin. Its half-life is approximately 20 hours, allowing once daily dosing. Action upstream from thrombin in the coagulation cascade is an attractive feature during PCI, and HIT is extremely rare [51]. It is contraindicated with renal insufficiency because of primarily renal excretion (Table 43.1).

Phase 2 experience proved promising with fondaparinux during PCI in the ASPIRE study (Arixtra Study in Percutaneous Coronary Intervention: A Randomized Evaluation) which randomized 350 patients undergoing elective or urgent PCI to two doses intravenously (2.5 and 5.0 mg) or weight-adjusted UFH. There was no difference compared with UFH in terms of total bleeding (7.7% UFH vs. 6.4% fondaparinux; p = 0.61) and the composite of MACE (death, MI, urgent TVR, or use of bailout GPI) (6.0% UFH vs. 6.0% fondaparinux; p = 0.97) [51].

The OASIS-5 (Organization to Assess Strategies in Acute Ischemic Syndromes) trial was the only study to evaluate patients undergoing PCI. Over 20,000 patients with ACS were randomized to enoxaparin or fondaparinux. There were no differences in ischemic complications, but there was benefit in respect of bleeding events with fondaparinux as compared with the LMWH (enoxaparin 8.8% vs. fondaparinux 3.3%; p <0.001). A substantial number of patients received UFH in both arms of the trial, and the protocol was actually modified during the course of the study to ensure use of UFH with fondaparinux because of a significantly higher rate of catheter-related thrombosis (enoxaparin 0.5% vs. fondaparinux 1.3%; p = 0.001). The concerns of the study were corroborated in the subsequent OASIS-6 trial in patients with STEMI. Primary PCI with fondaparinux resulted in significantly higher 30-day mortality and reinfarction than in patients with UFH [52]. As a result, guidelines recommend the addition of agents with activity against factor IIa during PCI in patients treated with fondaparinux. As such, this medication is suggested for use among patients being treated medically for ACS and has a limited role in elective PCI (Table 43.2).

Direct antithrombin agents

The most studied direct thrombin inhibitor in PCI is bivalirudin. It is a small molecule, consisting of 20 amino acids, and is a bivalent synthetic direct thrombin inhibitor. It binds directly to thrombin in both its fluid phase and also its clot-bound form, unlike heparin-based drugs, which bind only to free (unbound) thrombin. Bivalirudin inactivates thrombin directly and does not require laboratory monitoring to assess effect. Half-life is approximately 25 minutes and it does not cause HIT. Thrombin-induced platelet aggregation is essentially obliterated by bivalirudin (Table 43.1).

There is a large body of evidence in support of bivalirudin use in patients with ACS, including those with unstable angina, NSTEMI, and STEMI [53–59]. In the ACUITY trail [56], bivalirudin monotherapy in an early invasive PCI strategy in patients with unstable angina and NSTEMI provided superior 30-day clinical outcomes compared with a heparin and GPI regimen, and ACUITY scale major bleeding was reduced by 47% with bivalirudin at 30 days (3.0% vs. 5.7%, RR 0.53, 95% CI 0.43–0.65; p <0.001) [56]. HORIZONS-AMI, one of the largest trial assessing bivalirudin in STEMI, reported a mortality benefit at 30 days in the bivalirudin monotherapy group compared with a heparin plus GPI strategy (cardiac death 1.8% vs. 2.9%; p = 0.03; all cause mortality 2.1% vs. 3.1%; p = 0.047). The 30-day rate of net adverse clinical events including a lower rate of major bleeding was lower with bivalirudin alone (4.9% vs. 8.3%, RR 0.60; p <0.001) [56].

Bivalirudin use in ACS has recently become a controversial topic in light of the HEAT-PPCI trial, a randomized controlled trial, where 1812 patients undergoing emergency PCI received either bivalirudin or heparin, with similar rate of use of GPI in both arms (13% and 15%, respectively). The primary efficacy endpoint (all-cause mortality, cerebrovascular accident, reinfarction, target lesion revascularization) occurred in 8.7% of the bivalirudin group and 5.7% of the heparin group (absolute risk difference 3.0%; p = 0.01), and the primary safety outcome (major bleeding) occurred in 3.5% of the bivalirudin group and 3.1% in the heparin group, showing that heparin monotherapy relative to bivalirudin monotherapy reduced ischemic events with no difference in major bleeding [60].

Stent thrombosis associated with bivalirudin treatment has been noted now in several trials including HORIZONS-AMI, HEAT-PPCI, and EUROMAX [55]; this effect was mitigated in the BRIGHT trial where they used a prolonged infusion of bivalirudin post PCI of approximately 4 hours. In BRIGHT, 2194 patients with acute MI were randomized to bivalirudin, heparin alone, or heparin with tirofiban. Primary endpoint (death, MI, TVR, stroke, any bleeding at 30 days) occurred in 8.8% of the bivalirudin group, 13.2% of the heparin only group, and 17% of the heparin and tirofiban group (p <0.001); this difference was driven completely by the reduction in bleeding complications, with no difference in MACE [61].

In patients with stable coronary disease undergoing elective PCI, there have been two randomized trials supporting the use of bivalirudin. The REPLACE-2 (Randomized Evaluation of PCI Linking Angiomax to Reduced Clinical Events-2) study was a multicenter, double-blind, triple dummy randomized trial in patients with a low to moderate risk for ischemic complications undergoing PCI (56% elective cases). Patients were randomized to heparin with planned GPI (abciximab, or eptifibatide) or bivalirudin with provisional GPI. At 30 days, there was no significant difference in MACE (death, MI, urgent revascularization, or major bleeding) between the groups (9.2% in bivalirudin group vs. 10.0% in heparin plus GPI). In-hospital major bleeding rates were significantly reduced by bivalirudin (2.4% vs. 4.1%; p <0.001).

Table 43.2 Recommendations for antithrombin use.

	Recommendation	Class of recommendation	Level of evidence	Guideline
Unfractionated heparin	UFH should not be given to patients already receiving therapeutic subcutaneous enoxaparin	III (Harm)	B	PCI
	For patients with UA/NSTEMI in whom an initial conservative strategy is selected, enoxaparin or fondaparinux is preferable to UFH as anticoagulant therapy, unless CABG is planned within 24 h	IIa	B	UA/NSTEMI
	For patients with UA/NSTEMI who are managed conservatively and do not develop an indication for catheterization continue UFH for 48 h if managed without PCI or CABG; otherwise discontinue	I	A	UA/NSTEMI
Enoxaparin	For PCI, additional 0.3 mg/mg IV dose if last SQ dose >8–12 h or <2 doses administered	I	B	PCI
	PCI with enoxaparin can be reasonable in patients either treated with "upstream" subcutaneous enoxaparin for UA/NSTEMI or who have not received prior antithrombin therapy and are administered IV enoxaparin at the time of PCI	IIa	B	PCI
	For patients with UA/NSTEMI in whom an initial conservative strategy is selected, enoxaparin or fondaparinux is preferable to UFH as anticoagulant therapy, unless CABG is planned within 24 h	I	A	UA/NSTEMI
	Continue enoxaparin for duration of hospitalization, up to 8 days, if given before diagnostic angiography and no PCI or CABG	I	A	UA/NSTEMI
Bivalirudin	For patients undergoing PCI, bivalirudin is useful as an anticoagulant with or without prior treatment with UFH	I	B	PCI
	Either discontinue bivalirudin or continue at 0.25 mg/kg/h for up to 72 h at the physician's discretion if given before diagnostic angiography and no PCI or CABG	I	B	UA/NSTEMI
	With HIT, it is recommended that bivalirudin or argatroban be used to replace UFH	I	B	PCI
Fondaparinux	Fondaparinux should not be used as the sole anticoagulant to support PCI	III (Harm)	C	PCI
	For UA/NSTEMI patients in whom an initial conservative strategy is selected, enoxaparin or fondaparinux is preferable to UFH as anticoagulant therapy, unless CABG is planned within 24 h	I	A	UA/NSTEMI
	Continue fondaparinux for duration of hospitalization, up to 8 days, if given before diagnostic angiography and no PCI or CABG	I	A	UA/NSTEMI
	With a conservative strategy, in those patients who have an increased risk of bleeding, fondaparinux is preferable	I	B	UA/NSTEMI
Argatroban	With HIT, it is recommended that bivalirudin or argatroban be used to replace UFH	I	B	PCI
Glycoprotein IIb/IIIa inhibitors	Elective PCI patients treated with UFH and not pretreated with clopidogrel, GPI can be used (abciximab, double-bolus eptifibatide, or high-bolus dose of tirofiban)	IIa	B	PCI
	If pretreated with clopidogrel, in elective patients using UFH, the level of evidence is less compelling	IIb	B	PCI

The ISAR-REACT-3 (Intracoronary Stenting and Anti-thrombotic Regimen – Rapid Early Action for Coronary Treatment) trial evaluated 4570 troponin-negative patients treated with aspirin and clopidogrel (600 mg loading dose) at least 2 hours prior to planned PCI. Patients were randomized to 140 IU/kg UFH or bivalirudin in what was a placebo-controlled trial. The primary endpoint of MACE at 30 days (death, MI, urgent TVR, or major bleeding) was not different (UFH 8.7% vs. bivalirudin 8.3%, RR 0.94, 95% CI 0.77–1.15; p = 0.57). There was a significant reduction in major bleeding (4.6% vs. 3.1%; p = 0.008) and minor bleeding (9.9% vs. 6.8%; p = 0.001) with bivalirudin, but one criticism is that UFH dosing was higher than used in contemporary practice [58,62]. Thus, the patients in the UFH arm may have had higher bleeding rates, resulting in the apparent advantage for bivalirudin.

The NAPLES-III trial showed no difference between bivalirudin and UFH use in elective PCI in patients with high bleeding risk. The study randomized 837 patients with stable and unstable angina and high predicted risk of bleeding to receiving either bivalirudin or heparin therapy (WITHOUT concomitant GPI) during elective transfemoral PCI. The primary endpoint of in-hospital bleeding was similar between the bivalirudin and heparin arms (3.3% vs. 2.6%; p = 0.54). Clinical endpoints at 30 days were also similar between the two arms with regard to MACE (6.5% vs. 4.3%; p = 0.17), death (2.4% vs. 1.4%), MI (0.2% vs. 0%), stent thrombosis (0.5% vs. 0.5%), and 1 year outcomes were likewise similar. The use of dual antiplatelet therapy (DAPT) was not clarified in this trial [63]. Notably, heparin dosing in NAPLES-III was similar current practice at 70 IU/kg, rather than the higher dose of 140 IU/kg used in ISAR-REACT 3.

A 2014 meta-analysis, including data from 16 trials with 33,958 patients, including elective PCI reported an increase in the risk of MACE with bivalirudin-based regimens compared with heparin-based regimens (risk ratio 1.09; p = 0.02), which was largely driven by increases in MI and revascularization. Bivalirudin increased the risk of stent thrombosis (risk ratio 1.38; p = 0.0074). Furthermore, while bivalirudin lowered the risk of major bleeding, this varied largely depending on whether GPI were used with heparin (risk ratio 0.53; p <0.0001) or provisionally planned in both arms (risk ratio 0.78, p = 0.25; risk ratio 1.07, p = 0.53) [64]. Needless to say, there are a wide array of varying of protocols and patients included in this meta-analysis, which limits its applicability.

Taken together, these trials indicate that bivalirudin is a reasonable alternative to UFH alone or in combination with GPI in patients undergoing elective PCI, especially in patients with high bleeding risk. However, there is a consistent signal in ACS trials of acute stent thrombosis associated with bivalirudin use which may be mitigated by prolonging the infusion or more potent platelet inhibition, issues that warrant further study.

Other agents

Argatroban is a direct thrombin inhibitor approved by the Food and Drug Administration (FDA) in 2000 for use in prophylaxis or treatment of thrombosis in patients with HIT. In 2002, it was approved for use during PCI in patients who have HIT or are at risk of developing it. It is given intravenously, has a half-life of 50 minutes, and is metabolized in the liver. It can be used in the setting of renal failure, but not in those with significant hepatic dysfunction (Table 43.1). Another direct thrombin inhibitor, lepirudin, had been available for HIT patients. A business decision was made by the manufacturer to discontinue production of this agent in May 2012. More evidence is still needed to clarify the role of novel oral anticoagulants such as rivaroxaban, dabigatran, and apixaban in elective PCI.

Intravenous antiplatelet therapy

Until recently, glycoprotein IIb/IIIa receptor antagonists were the only intravenous antiplatelet medications approved for use in the USA until cangrelor was approved in June 2015. Cangrelor is an intravenous $P2Y_{12}$ receptor antagonist with near immediate effect. It has a half-life of 2.6–3.3 minutes, and normal platelet function is restored within 1 hour of discontinuation. The medication was evaluated in a series of trials. The Cangrelor versus Standard Therapy to Achieve Optimal Management of Platelet Inhibition (CHAMPION)-PCI and CHAMPION-PLATFORM studies yielded disappointing results. The two trials were stopped prematurely, after interim analyses indicated that demonstration of a benefit for the primary endpoint would be unlikely [65,66]. Secondary endpoints, from the CHAMPION-PLATFORM trial, indicated that PCI patients receiving cangrelor had fewer stent thromboses compared with delayed administration of clopidogrel. As such, the CHAMPION-PHOENIX trial was designed comparing cangrelor at the time of PCI to clopidogrel administration after PCI [67]. In approximately 11,000 patients undergoing PCI, the primary endpoint of all-cause mortality, MI, ischemia-driven revascularization, or stent thrombosis at 48 hours was lower with cangrelor than clopidogrel (4.7% vs. 5.9%, OR 0.78, 95% CI 0.66–0.93; p = 0.005). This difference was largely attributable to a difference in the rate of stent thrombosis at 48 hours (0.8% vs. 1.4%, OR 0.62, 95% CI 0.43–0.90; p = 0.01), of which most were intraprocedural stent thromboses (0.6% vs. 1.0%, OR 0.65, 95% CI 0.42–0.99; p = 0.04). These differences persisted to 30 days. ACUITY major bleeding was more frequent with cangrelor (4.3% vs. 2.5%, OR 1.72, 95% CI 1.39–2.13; p <0.001). Cangrelor is approved for PCI amongst patients who have not received GPI or adequate pretreatment with oral antiplatelet medications.

Conclusions

Anticoagulation strategies have rapidly evolved over recent decades and numerous agents are now available. An improved understanding of the coagulation cascade and the interplay between thrombin and platelet activation has led to the development of agents specifically targeting key components of the coagulation cascade. Along with improvements in PCI technique, expanded use of these agents has led to impressive reductions in ischemic outcomes and more recently in bleeding events. While the magnitude of benefit of these agents in clinical trials over UFH is smaller or non-existent in elective PCI compared with PCI in ACS, there are certainly a number of patients at high bleeding risk or who have contraindications to UFH and can benefit from these agents.

The mainstay for anticoagulation in PCI for patients with stable disease remains UFH, with selective use of additional intravenous or oral antiplatelet agents, but LMWH and direct thrombin inhibitors, either alone or in combination with heparins, have a variety of benefits. Whether more aggressive DAPT, especially prasugrel, ticagrelor, or cangrelor, improves ischemic outcomes with UFH, LMWH, or bivalirudin without an increase in bleeding complications remains unknown and whether the benefits demonstrated in patients with ACS can be generalized to stable patients remains a

Key points

- Despite significant improvements, it remains important to select anticoagulant agents carefully in the percutaneous treatment of coronary disease with the dual goal of decreasing ischemic events and minimizing bleeding complications.
- In the "elective" population, glycoprotein IIb/IIIa receptor inhibitors tend to be reserved for higher risk patients, for those not adequately pretreated with thienopyridines, or for those with a suboptimal procedural outcome.
- Unfractionated heparin (UFH) continues to be a mainstay in the elective PCI population because of its ease of use, simple monitoring, and reversibility.
- Enoxaparin has been shown to have reduced bleeding outcomes, with comparable ischemic events to UFH in patients undergoing PCI, but the inability to easily monitor the level of anticoagulation has limited its use.
- Bivalirudin is a reasonable alternative to UFH, especially in patients with high bleeding risk.

matter of debate. Finally, personalizing the optimal antithrombin in combination with the optimal antiplatelet agent for a patient based on individual hematologic, genetic, angiographic, and comorbid factors has the potential to improve outcomes dramatically but remains an enormously challenging task for future investigation.

Interactive multiple choice questions are available for this chapter on www.wiley.com/go/dangas/cardiology

References

1 Use of a monoclonal antibody directed against the platelet glycoprotein IIb/IIIa receptor in high-risk coronary angioplasty: the EPIC Investigation. *N Engl J Med* 1994; **330**: 956–961.

2 Topol EJ, Califf RM, Weisman HF, *et al*. Randomised trial of coronary intervention with antibody against platelet IIb/IIIa integrin for reduction of clinical restenosis: results at six months. The EPIC Investigators. *Lancet* 1994; **343**: 881–886.

3 Topol EJ, Ferguson JJ, Weisman HF, *et al*. EPIC Investigator Group. Long-term protection from myocardial ischemic events in a randomized trial of brief integrin beta3 blockade with percutaneous coronary intervention: evaluation of platelet IIb/IIIa inhibition for prevention of ischemic complication. *JAMA* 1997; **278**: 479–484.

4 EPILOG Investigators. Platelet glycoprotein IIb/IIIa receptor blockade and low-dose heparin during percutaneous coronary revascularization. *N Engl J Med* 1997; **336**: 1689–1696.

5 Topol EJ, Mark DB, Lincoff AM, *et al*. Outcomes at 1 year and economic implications of platelet glycoprotein IIb/IIIa blockade in patients undergoing coronary stenting: results from a multicentre randomised trial. EPISTENT Investigators. Evaluation of Platelet IIb/IIIa Inhibitor for Stenting. *Lancet* 1999; **354**: 2019–2024.

6 ESPRIT Investigators. Enhanced Suppression of the Platelet IIb/IIIa Receptor with Integrilin Therapy. Novel dosing regimen of eptifibatide in planned coronary stent implantation (ESPRIT): a randomised, placebo-controlled trial. *Lancet* 2000; **356**: 2037–2044.

7 Randomised placebo-controlled trial of effect of eptifibatide on complications of percutaneous coronary intervention: IMPACT-II. Integrilin to Minimise Platelet Aggregation and Coronary Thrombosis-II. *Lancet* 1997; **349**: 1422–1428.

8 Valgimigli M, Percoco G, Barbieri D, *et al*. The additive value of tirofiban administered with the high-dose bolus in the prevention of ischemic complications during high-risk coronary angioplasty: the ADVANCE Trial. *J Am Coll Cardiol* 2004; **44**: 14–19.

9 Bonz AW, Lengenfelder B, Strotmann J, *et al*. Effect of additional temporary glycoprotein IIb/IIIa receptor inhibition on troponin release in elective percutaneous coronary interventions after pretreatment with aspirin and clopidogrel (TOPSTAR trial). *J Am Coll Cardiol* 2002; **40**: 662–668.

10 Kastrati A, Mehilli J, Schuhlen H, *et al*. A clinical trial of abciximab in elective percutaneous coronary intervention after pretreatment with clopidogrel. *N Engl J Med* 2004; **350**: 232–238.

11 Puma JA, Banko LT, Pieper KS *et al*. Clinical characteristics predict benefits from eptifibatide therapy during coronary stenting: insights from the Enhanced Suppression of the Platelet IIb/IIIa Receptor With Integrilin Therapy (ESPRIT) trial. *J Am Coll Cardiol* 2006; **47**: 715–718.

12 Kandzari DE, Berger PB, Kastrati A, *et al*. Influence of treatment duration with a 600-mg dose of clopidogrel before percutaneous coronary revascularization. *J Am Coll Cardiol* 2004; **44**: 2133–2136.

13 Kastrati A, Mehilli J, Neumann FJ, *et al*. Abciximab in patients with acute coronary syndromes undergoing percutaneous coronary intervention after clopidogrel pretreatment: the ISAR-REACT 2 randomized trial. *JAMA* 2006; **295**: 1531–1538.

14 Lincoff AM, Tcheng JE, Califf RM, *et al*. Sustained suppression of ischemic complications of coronary intervention by platelet GP IIb/IIIa blockade with abciximab: one-year outcome in the EPILOG trial. Evaluation in PTCA to Improve Long-term Outcome with abciximab GP IIb/IIIa blockade. *Circulation* 1999; **99**: 1951–1958.

15 Brener SJ, Barr LA, Burchenal JE, *et al*. Randomized, placebo-controlled trial of platelet glycoprotein IIb/IIIa blockade with primary angioplasty for acute myocardial infarction. ReoPro and Primary PTCA Organization and Randomized Trial (RAPPORT) Investigators. *Circulation* 1998; **98**: 734–741.

16 Simoons ML, de Boer MJ, van den Brand MJ, *et al*. Randomized trial of a GPIIb/IIIa platelet receptor blocker in refractory unstable angina. European Cooperative Study Group. *Circulation* 1994; **89**: 596–603.

17 Randomised placebo-controlled trial of abciximab before and during coronary intervention in refractory unstable angina: the CAPTURE Study. *Lancet* 1997; **349**: 1429–1435.

18 van den Brand M, Laarman GJ, Steg PG, *et al*. Assessment of coronary angiograms prior to and after treatment with abciximab, and the outcome of angioplasty in refractory unstable angina patients: angiographic results from the CAPTURE trial. *Eur Heart J* 1999; **20**: 1572–1578.

19 Klootwijk P, Meij S, Melkert R, Lenderink T, Simoons ML. Reduction of recurrent ischemia with abciximab during continuous ECG-ischemia monitoring in patients with unstable angina refractory to standard treatment (CAPTURE). *Circulation* 1998; **98**: 1358–1364.

20 Hamm CW, Heeschen C, Goldmann B, *et al*. Benefit of abciximab in patients with refractory unstable angina in relation to serum troponin T levels. c7E3 Fab Antiplatelet Therapy in Unstable Refractory Angina (CAPTURE) Study Investigators. *N Engl J Med* 1999; **340**: 1623–1629.

21 Bhatt DL, Lincoff AM, Califf RM, *et al*. The benefit of abciximab in percutaneous coronary revascularization is not device-specific. *Am J Cardiol* 2000; **85**: 1060–1064.

22 Montalescot G, Barragan P, Wittenberg O, *et al*. Platelet glycoprotein IIb/IIIa inhibition with coronary stenting for acute myocardial infarction. *N Engl J Med* 2001; **344**: 1895–1903.

23 Three-year duration of benefit from abciximab in patients receiving stents for acute myocardial infarction in the randomized double-blind ADMIRAL study. *Eur Heart J* 2005; **26**: 2520–2523.

24 Neumann FJ, Kastrati A, Schmitt C, *et al*. Effect of glycoprotein IIb/IIIa receptor blockade with abciximab on clinical and angiographic restenosis rate after the placement of coronary stents following acute myocardial infarction. *J Am Coll Cardiol* 2000; **35**: 915–921.

25 Stone GW, Grines CL, Cox DA, *et al*. Comparison of angioplasty with stenting, with or without abciximab, in acute myocardial infarction. *N Engl J Med* 2002; **346**: 957–966.

26 Antoniucci D, Rodriguez A, Hempel A, *et al*. A randomized trial comparing primary infarct artery stenting with or without abciximab in acute myocardial infarction. *J Am Coll Cardiol* 2003; **42**: 1879–1885.

27 De Luca G, Suryapranata H, Stone GW, *et al*. Abciximab as adjunctive therapy to reperfusion in acute ST-segment elevation myocardial infarction: a meta-analysis of randomized trials. *JAMA* 2005; **293**: 1759–1765.

28 Randomised placebo-controlled and balloon-angioplasty-controlled trial to assess safety of coronary stenting with use of platelet glycoprotein-IIb/IIIa blockade. *Lancet* 1998; **352**: 87–92.

29 Lincoff AM, Califf RM, Moliterno DJ, *et al*. Complementary clinical benefits of coronary-artery stenting and blockade of platelet glycoprotein IIb/IIIa receptors. Evaluation of Platelet IIb/IIIa Inhibition in Stenting Investigators. *N Engl J Med* 1999; **341**: 319–327.

30 Effects of platelet glycoprotein IIb/IIIa blockade with tirofiban on adverse cardiac events in patients with unstable angina or acute myocardial infarction undergoing coronary angioplasty. The RESTORE Investigators. Randomized Efficacy Study of Tirofiban for Outcomes and REstenosis. *Circulation* 1997; **96**: 1445–1453.

31 Platelet Receptor Inhibition in Ischemic Syndrome Management (PRISM) Study Investigators. A comparison of aspirin plus tirofiban with aspirin plus heparin for unstable angina. *N Engl J Med* 1998; **338**: 1498–1505.

32 Platelet Receptor Inhibition in Ischemic Syndrome Management in Patients Limited by Unstable Signs and Symptoms (PRISM-PLUS) Study Investigators. Inhibition of the platelet glycoprotein IIb/IIIa receptor with tirofiban in unstable angina and non-Q-wave myocardial infarction. *N Engl J Med* 1998; **338**: 1488–1497.

33 Biondi-Zoccai G, Valgimigli M, Margheri M, *et al.* Assessing the role of eptifibatide in patients with diffuse coronary disease undergoing drug-eluting stenting: the INtegrilin plus STenting to Avoid myocardial Necrosis Trial. *Am Heart J* 2012; **163**: 835 e1–7.

34 Topol EJ, Moliterno DJ, Herrmann HC, *et al.* Comparison of two platelet glycoprotein IIb/IIIa inhibitors, tirofiban and abciximab, for the prevention of ischemic events with percutaneous coronary revascularization. *N Engl J Med* 2001; **344**: 1888–1894.

35 Moliterno DJ. A randomized two-by-two comparison of high-dose bolus tirofiban versus abciximab and unfractionated heparin versus bivalirudin during percutaneous coronary revascularization and stent placement: the tirofiban evaluation of novel dosing versus abciximab with clopidogrel and inhibition of thrombin (TENACITY) study trial. *Catheter Cardiovasc Interv* 2011; **77**: 1001–1009.

36 Brown DL, Fann CS, Chang CJ. Meta-analysis of effectiveness and safety of abciximab versus eptifibatide or tirofiban in percutaneous coronary intervention. *Am J Cardiol* 2001; **87**: 537–541.

37 Chew DP, Bhatt DL, Lincoff AM, *et al.* Defining the optimal activated clotting time during percutaneous coronary intervention: aggregate results from 6 randomized, controlled trials. *Circulation* 2001; **103**: 961–966.

38 Montalescot G, Cohen M, Salette G, *et al.* Impact of anticoagulation levels on outcomes in patients undergoing elective percutaneous coronary intervention: insights from the STEEPLE trial. *Eur Heart J* 2008; **29**: 462–471.

39 Brener SJ, Moliterno DJ, Lincoff AM, Steinhubl SR, Wolski KE, Topol EJ. Relationship between activated clotting time and ischemic or hemorrhagic complications: analysis of 4 recent randomized clinical trials of percutaneous coronary intervention. *Circulation* 2004; **110**: 994–998.

40 Lee MS, Oyama J, Iqbal Z, Tarantini G. Low-dose heparin for elective percutaneous coronary intervention. *J Interv Cardiol* 2014; **27**: 58–62.

41 Hirsh J, Fuster V. Guide to anticoagulant therapy. Part 1: Heparin. *Circulation* 1994; **89**: 1449–1468.

42 Warkentin TE. Drug-induced immune-mediated thrombocytopenia: from purpura to thrombosis. *N Engl J Med* 2007; **356**: 891–893.

43 Montalescot G, Collet JP, Tanguy ML, *et al.* Anti-Xa activity relates to survival and efficacy in unselected acute coronary syndrome patients treated with enoxaparin. *Circulation* 2004; **110**: 392–8.

44 Montalescot G, White HD, Gallo R, *et al.* Enoxaparin versus unfractionated heparin in elective percutaneous coronary intervention. *N Engl J Med* 2006; **355**: 1006–1017.

45 Cohen M, Demers C, Gurfinkel EP, *et al.* A comparison of low-molecular-weight heparin with unfractionated heparin for unstable coronary artery disease. Efficacy and Safety of Subcutaneous Enoxaparin in Non-Q-Wave Coronary Events Study Group. *N Engl J Med* 1997; **337**: 447–452.

46 Ferguson JJ, Califf RM, Antman EM, *et al.* Enoxaparin vs unfractionated heparin in high-risk patients with non-ST-segment elevation acute coronary syndromes managed with an intended early invasive strategy: primary results of the SYNERGY randomized trial. *JAMA* 2004; **292**: 45–54.

47 Kereiakes DJ, Grines C, Fry E, *et al.* Enoxaparin and abciximab adjunctive pharmacotherapy during percutaneous coronary intervention. *J Invasive Cardiol* 2001; **13**: 272–278.

48 Gibson CM, Murphy SA, Montalescot G, *et al.* Percutaneous coronary intervention in patients receiving enoxaparin or unfractionated heparin after fibrinolytic therapy for ST-segment elevation myocardial infarction in the ExTRACT-TIMI 25 trial. *J Am Coll Cardiol* 2007; **49**: 2238–2246.

49 Dumaine R, Borentain M, Bertel O, *et al.* Intravenous low-molecular-weight heparins compared with unfractionated heparin in percutaneous coronary intervention: quantitative review of randomized trials. *Arch Intern Med* 2007; **167**: 2423–2430.

50 Rich MW. Multidisciplinary interventions for the management of heart failure: where do we stand? *Am Heart J* 1999; **138**: 599–601.

51 Mehta SR, Steg PG, Granger CB, *et al.* Randomized, blinded trial comparing fondaparinux with unfractionated heparin in patients undergoing contemporary percutaneous coronary intervention: Arixtra Study in Percutaneous Coronary Intervention: a Randomized Evaluation (ASPIRE) Pilot Trial. *Circulation* 2005; **111**: 1390–1397.

52 Yusuf S, Mehta SR, Chrolavicius S, *et al.* Effects of fondaparinux on mortality and reinfarction in patients with acute ST-segment elevation myocardial infarction: the OASIS-6 randomized trial. *JAMA* 2006; **295**: 1519–1530.

53 Patti G, Pasceri V, D'Antonio L, *et al.* Comparison of safety and efficacy of bivalirudin versus unfractionated heparin in high-risk patients undergoing percutaneous coronary intervention (from the Anti-Thrombotic Strategy for Reduction of Myocardial Damage During Angioplasty-Bivalirudin vs Heparin study). *Am J Cardiol* 2012; **110**: 478–484.

54 Hamon M, Nienaber CA, Galli S, *et al.* Bivalirudin in percutaneous coronary intervention: the EUROpean BiVaIIrudin UtiliSatION in Practice (EUROVISION) Registry. *Int J Cardiol* 2014; **173**: 290–294.

55 Steg PG, van't Hof A, Hamm CW, *et al.* Bivalirudin started during emergency transport for primary PCI. *N Engl J Med* 2013; **369**: 2207–2217.

56 Stone GW, McLaurin BT, Cox DA, *et al.* Bivalirudin for patients with acute coronary syndromes. *N Engl J Med* 2006; **355**: 2203–2216.

57 Lincoff AM, Bittl JA, Harrington RA, *et al.* Bivalirudin and provisional glycoprotein IIb/IIIa blockade compared with heparin and planned glycoprotein IIb/IIIa blockade during percutaneous coronary intervention: REPLACE-2 randomized trial. *JAMA* 2003; **289**: 853–863.

58 Stone GW, Witzenbichler B, Guagliumi G, *et al.* Bivalirudin during primary PCI in acute myocardial infarction. *N Engl J Med* 2008; **358**: 2218–2230.

59 Bittl JA, Strony J, Brinker JA, *et al.* Treatment with bivalirudin (Hirulog) as compared with heparin during coronary angioplasty for unstable or postinfarction angina. Hirulog Angioplasty Study Investigators. *N Engl J Med* 1995; **333**: 764–769.

60 Shahzad A, Kemp I, Mars C *et al.* Unfractionated heparin versus bivalirudin in primary percutaneous coronary intervention (HEAT-PPCI): an open-label, single centre, randomised controlled trial. *Lancet* 2014; **384**: 1849–1858.

61 Han Y. Bivalirudin versus heparin monotherapy and glycoprotein IIb/IIIa plus heparin for patients with AMI undergoing coronary stenting (BRIGHT). China Interventional Therapeutics (CIT 2014); Shanghai, China; March 21, 2014.

62 Schulz S, Mehilli J, Ndrepepa G, *et al.* Bivalirudin vs. unfractionated heparin during percutaneous coronary interventions in patients with stable and unstable angina pectoris: 1-year results of the ISAR-REACT 3 trial. *Eur Heart J* 2010; **31**: 582–587.

63 Briguori C, Visconti G, Focaccio A, *et al.* Novel Approaches for Preventing or Limiting Events (NAPLES III) Trial: randomised comparison of bivalirudin versus unfractionated heparin in patients at high risk of bleeding undergoing elective coronary stenting throught the femoral approach. rationale and design. *Cardiovasc Drug Ther* 2014; **28**: 273–279.

64 Cavender MA, Sabatine MS. Bivalirudin versus heparin in patients planned for percutaneous coronary intervention: a meta-analysis of randomised controlled trials. *Lancet* 2014; **384**: 599–606.

65 Bhatt DL, Lincoff AM, Gibson CM, *et al.* Intravenous platelet blockade with cangrelor during PCI. *N Engl J Med* 2009; **361**: 2330–2341.

66 Harrington RA, Stone GW, McNulty S. *et al.* Platelet inhibition with cangrelor in patients undergoing PCI. *N Engl J Med* 2009; **361**: 2318–2329.

67 Bhatt DL, Stone GW, Mahaffey KW, *et al.* Effect of platelet inhibition with cangrelor during PCI on ischemic events. *N Engl J Med* 2013; **368**: 1303–1313.

CHAPTER 44

Vasoactive and Antiarrhythmic Drugs During PCI

Bimmer E.P.M. Claessen and José P.S. Henriques

Department of Cardiology, Academic Medical Center – University of Amsterdam, Amsterdam, The Netherlands

Patients undergoing percutaneous coronary intervention (PCI) are administered a large variety of pharmacologic agents during this procedure. In addition to antithrombotic drugs to minimize the risk of thrombotic complications of the mechanical intervention performed during PCI, patients are sometimes administered sedatives, analgesics, vasodilators, antiarrhythmic agents, vasopressors, and inotropes. Sedative and analgesic drugs are used to increase patient well-being during the procedure. Vasodilators can be administered for a variety of indications, for example to facilitate standardized and accurate vessel size measurements, treatment of the no-reflow phenomenon after PCI, treatment of arterial spasm during PCI, or inducing maximal hyperemia to facilitate measurement of fractional flow reserve (FFR). Antiarrhythmic drugs are indicated for recurrent ventricular fibrillation, ventrical tachycardia, or to prevent ventricular extrasystoles during ventriculography. Moreover, several drugs should be interrupted before coronary angiography or PCI such as metformin, diuretics, and angiotensin converting enzyme (ACE) inhibitors.

Vasodilators during PCI

Vasodilators are used during PCI to treat arterial or coronary spasm or no-reflow, to accurately assess the diameter of coronary arteries before stent implantation, or to induce hyperemia during invasive coronary physiology measurements. Nitroglycerine, verapamil, and adenosine are frequently used during PCI to achieve vasodilatation. Nitroglycerin was discovered by Asciano Sobrero in 1847, who first noted a violent headache after administering a small quantity of nitroglycerine on his tongue [1]. He also discovered its explosive properties and was badly scarred on the face after a nitroglycerine explosion. Nitroglycerine (glycerine trinitrate) is an organic nitrate that releases nitric oxide (NO) through an enzymatic reaction [2]. Nitroglycerine causes vasodilatation without a reduction in blood pressure in doses up to 200 μg. However, when doses exceeding 250 μg are administered, hypotension can result without a further increase in coronary vasodilatation [3]. Direct NO donors such as nitroprusside and molsidomine release NO directly without the need for activation by molecular metabolism [4,5].

Verapamil, a calcium channel blocker, is a class IV antiarrhythmic agent according to the Vaughan Williams classification. Verapamil has negative chronotropic effects by decreasing the electrical impulse conduction in the atrioventricular (AV) node, where there is a high concentration of calcium channels [6]. By blocking calcium channels in the smooth muscle of coronary arteries, verapamil also induces vasodilatation [7]. Because of the different mechanisms by which verapamil and nitroglycerin cause coronary artery vasodilatation, they are often combined and administered together as an intracoronary "cocktail." Because of its negative chronotropic properties, verapamil is contraindicated in patients with severe bradycardia. Furthermore, verapamil is contraindicated in patients with left ventricular dysfunction because of its negative inotropic properties. Diltiazem, another calcium channel blocker, has stronger vasodilating and weaker negative chronotropic effects than verapamil [8].

Adenosine is a purine nucleoside that can bind to purinergic receptors in different cell types. Vasodilatation results by binding to adenosine type 2A (A_{2a}) receptors in vascular smooth muscle cells. Moreover, adenosine inhibits calcium entry into the cell through L-type calcium channels which are present in vascular smooth muscle cells and also in the sinoatrial and the AV nodes resulting in negative chronotropic and dromotropic effects [9]. Adenosine is used to induce hyperemia to accurately assess the severity of intermediate coronary artery stenoses by FFR [10]. Adenosine can be administered by both intracoronary or intravenous infusion.

Vasodilators in the treatment of no-reflow

The no-reflow phenomenon is caused by vasospasm and downstream embolization of debris during PCI or suboptimal reperfusion of an infarct artery attributed to endothelial injury in addition to embolization and vasospasm [11]. Most studies investigating the utility of vasoactive drugs to treat or prevent no-reflow have been conducted in the setting of PCI for acute coronary syndromes (ACS). A recent meta-analysis of 3821 patients from 10 randomized controlled trials undergoing PCI for ACS investigated whether adjunct therapy with adenosine was associated with a reduction in no-reflow and subsequently clinical outcomes [12]. Compared with placebo, adenosine was significantly associated with a reduction of post-procedural no-reflow with an odds ratio of 0.25 (95% confidence interval 0.08–0.73; p = 0.01). However, adenosine failed to reduce mortality, reinfarction, symptoms of heart failure, and

Interventional Cardiology: Principles and Practice, Second Edition. Edited by George D. Dangas, Carlo Di Mario, and Nicholas N. Kipshidze.

© 2017 John Wiley & Sons, Ltd. Published 2017 by John Wiley & Sons, Ltd.

ST-segment resolution. Nicorandil and nitroprusside have also been associated with improved coronary flow [13,14], again without a benefit in terms of hard clinical endpoints. Therefore, these agents are not commonly used in everyday clinical practice. The administration of an intracoronary vasodilator to treat PCI-related no-reflow carries a Class IIa recommendation with a level of evidence B in the current interventional guidelines [11].

Vasodilators in the treatment of arterial spasm
Vascular access is associated with fewer bleeding complications when compared with the femoral approach and is rapidly becoming the standard of care for coronary angiography and percutaneous PCI [15]. However, radial artery spasm (RAS) causes reduced success rates and patient discomfort during cardiac catheterization via the radial approach in approximately 10% of patients [16]. Risk factors for the development of RAS include smaller diameter radial arteries, female gender, larger sheath size, and operator inexperience [17]. RAS can be prevented and treated by using intra-arterial nitroglycerin or a cocktail of vasodilating agents (i.e., $100\,\mu g$ nitroglycerine with 1.25 mg verapamil) [18].

Antiarrhythmic drugs in PCI
Ischemia or pain during PCI results in an increased sympathoadrenal tone that can induce a rise in heart rate, blood pressure, and myocardial contractility, resulting in increased oxygen demand. Beta-blockers decrease myocardial oxygen demand by lowering heart rate and blood pressure [19]. A number of animal studies have shown that the administration of beta-blockers can reduce myocardial injury in animal models of myocardial infarction [20,21]. Moreover, clinical studies established that the administration of intracoronary beta-blockers during PCI may reduce adverse clinical events and myocardial injury after PCI [22–24]. For example, the METOCARD-CNIC (the effect of metoprolol in cardioprotection during an acute myocardial infarction) trial randomized 270 consecutive patients with an anterior ST-elevation myocardial infarction (STEMI) to treatment with intravenous metoprolol or nothing before reperfusion [25]. The investigators showed a significant reduction in infarct size, assessed by magnetic resonance imaging (MRI) at 5–7 days after the infarction. Currently, larger clinical trials powered for clinical endpoints are being conducted that investigate whether the promising results of early metoprolol administration before reperfusion in patients with STEMI can be confirmed.

Other antiarrhythmic drugs are sporadically used during PCI. Lidocaine is not only used as a local anesthetic, but also acts as a Class Ib antiarrhythmic drug, blocking the rapid influx of sodium ions during the depolarization of cardiac myocytes. Class Ib antiarrhythmics primarily affect the His–Purkinje system and are used to treat ventricular tachycardias. Ventricular extrasystoles occur frequently during left ventriculography. Sporadically, sustained ventricular tachycardia ensues. A bolus of intravenous lidocaine can be injected to stop ventricular tachycardia.

Peri-procedural sedation
During PCI, peri-procedural sedation is sometimes applied to achieve a minimally depressed state of consciousness without compromising the airway and by allowing the patient to respond to verbal comments [26]. Usually, benzodiazepines are used to achieve conscious sedation. Benzodiazepines such as oxazepam, midazolam, and diazepam have sedative, hypnotic, muscle relaxant, and anxiolytic effects by selectively enhancing the inhibitory activity of gamma-aminobutyric acid (GABA) by binding to the benzodiazepine site of the $GABA_a$ receptor in the central nervous system [27]. Anterograde amnesia can sometimes be a welcome side effect of benzodiazepines, causing patients to forget any unpleasantness during the procedure.

A potential complication when using procedural sedation is the possibility that a level of sedation deeper than desired is induced. For this reason, current guidelines recommend that level of consciousness, respiratory rate, blood pressure, and oxygen saturation should be monitored [11]. Additionally, catheterization laboratories should be outfitted with oxygen and suction ports and a resuscitation cart. Other, less frequently used drugs used for peri-procedural sedation include the opioid fentanyl, and the hypnotic propofol [11]. Table 44.1 shows an overview of commonly used short-acting drugs used in peri-procedural sedation.

Which drugs should be discontinued before PCI?
Contrast-induced acute kidney injury (CI-AKI) can result as a side effect of using contrast agents in PCI and is associated with prolonged hospital stay. CI-AKI is an infrequent complication in non-diabetic patients with normal renal function (~2%) [28]. However, CI-AKI has been reported to occur in up to 50% of patients with diabetic nephropathy and a mean serum creatinine of 5.9 mg/dL [29]. An association between CI-AKI and an increased incidence of myocardial infarction, target vessel revascularization, and death after PCI has been reported [30,31]. Although the mechanism causing CI-AKI is currently incompletely understood, direct cytotoxicity of iodineated contrast agents and disturbances in renal hemodynamics have been identified to be contributing factors (Table 44.2) [32].

Patients undergoing PCI will often use medication that is associated with an increased risk of CI-AKI such as diuretics, non-steroidal anti-inflammatory drugs (NSAIDs), and angiotensin-converting enzyme inhibitors (ACEI), angiotensin II receptor blockers, and direct renin inhibitors. These drugs may cause prerenal kidney insufficiency and are routinely discontinued 24–48 hours prior to

Table 44.1 Overview of short-acting drugs used in peri-procedural sedation.

Class	Drugs	Effects	Onset (min)	Duration (min)	Reversal agents
Benzodiazepines	Midazolam	Sedative, anxiolytic	2–3	45–60	Flumazenil
Opioids	Fentanyl	Analgesic	3–5	30–60	Arexate
Other	Propofol	Sedative, anxiolytic	<1	5–15	None

Table 44.2 Drugs that should be stopped prior to PCI.

Class	Drugs	Reason to discontinue
Diuretics	Furosemide, bumetanide, hydrochlorothiazide, chlorthalidone	Can cause prerenal kidney injury
Angiotensin-converting enzyme inhibitors	Captopril, enalapril, ramipril, lisinopril	Can cause prerenal kidney injury
Angiotensin II receptor blockers	Valsartan, candesartan, irbesartan	Can cause prerenal kidney injury
Direct renin inhibitors	Aliskiren	Can cause prerenal kidney injury
Non-steroidal anti-inflammatory drugs	Ibuprofen, diclofenac, naproxen	Can cause prerenal kidney injury
Aminoglycoside antibiotics	Gentamicin, amikacin, tobramycin	Nephrotoxicity by inhibiting protein synthesis in renal cells. Nephrotoxicity is increased in patients with liver failure
Biguanides	Metformin	Increased risk of lactate acidosis

PCI and restarted after 24–48 hours after PCI. However, no clinical trials have investigated whether discontinuation of ACEI or diuretics is associated with reduction in CI-AKI and subsequently a reduction in clinical outcome. Interestingly, it was once thought that prophylactic treatment with diuretics during PCI could prevent CI-AKI by inducing and maintaining diuresis and blocking of the oxygen-demanding active ionic transport processes in the loop of Henle. Solomon et al. [33] randomized 78 patients with chronic renal insufficiency who underwent cardiac angiography to receive saline alone, saline plus mannitol, or saline plus furosemide during a period of 12 hours before and 12 hours after angiography. The incidence of CI-AKI, defined as a rise in serum creatinine of 0.5 mg/dL within 48 hours after angiography, was 11%, 28%, and 40% in the saline, mannitol, and furosemide groups, respectively (p = 0.05). Prehydration with saline became the standard of care after the publication of this landmark trial.

Metformin, an antidiabetic agent from the class of biguanides, is associated with the incidence of potentially lethal lactate acidosis [34]. The risk of lactate acidosis is increased in patients with acute renal insufficiency, therefore metformin is usally discontinued 24–38 hours after PCI and restarted 48 hours after the procedure after renal function has been assessed.

High-dose statin treatment to reduce the risk of peri-procedural MI

Peri-procedural myocardial injury, assessed by a rise in cardiac biomarkers after PCI, remains a common complication. Pretreatment with high doses of hydroxymethyl-glutaryl-CoA reductase inhibitors, commonly known as statins, is known to reduce the incidence of peri-procedural myocardial injury. A study by Pasceri et al. [35] randomized 153 patients with chronic stable angina undergoing elective PCI to pretreatment with atorvastatin 40 mg once daily versus placebo. In this study, the detection of cardiac biomarkers above the upper limit of normal was significantly reduced with statin pretreatment compared with placebo (20% vs. 48% for troponin I; p = 0.0004). A single loading dose of 80 mg atorvastatin or 40 mg rosuvastatin has also been found to reduce peri-procedural myocardial injury [36,37].

A small number of other studies and meta-analyses have confirmed the protective effects of statin pretreatment before PCI [38,39]. The exact mechanism by which statins reduce peri-procedural myocardial injury is not well understood. These effects of statins occur before significant lipid lowering has occurred, therefore it is hypothesized that pleitropic effects of statins such as anti-inflammatory effects, a reduction in oxidative stress, or improvement of endothelial function are involved.

Vasopressors and inotropes during PCI

Vasopressors and inotropes are sometimes used to treat patients who are hemodynamically unstable during PCI in whom short- or medium-term recovery is expected. Many of the vasopressors and inotropes are a member of the family of catecholamines. These catecholamines, such as adrenaline, noradrenaline, dopamine, dobutamine, isoproterenol, and phenylephrine, act by stimulating alfa- or beta-adrenergic receptors. Simply put, beta-receptor stimulation results in positive chronotropy, positive inotropy, and vasodilatation. Alfa-adrenergic stimulation results in vasoconstriction. As vasodilatation by agents with primarily beta-adrenergic receptor stimulating properties can cause blood pressure to fall, inotropes such as noradrenaline (with predominantly alfa-adrenergic activity) and phenylephrine (selective alfa-adrenergic activity) are often used in combination with vasopressors. Important complications of catecholamines include tachycardias, both supraventricular and ventricular [40]. Finally, stress dose glycocorticoids (cortisol 100 mg every 8 hours intravenously) should be considered in refractory hypotension and in patients thought to be at risk for adrenal insufficiency under stress (e.g., those on high maintenance dose of oral steroids).

Conclusions

A large number of adjunct drugs are used during PCI for a variety of indications. The use of a variety of sedative, vasoactive, antiarrhythmic, vasopressive, inotropic, and risk-factor modifying drugs during PCI are sometimes used. Moreover, some types of drugs must be temporarily stopped when performing PCI. Decision on which adjunct drugs to use during PCI and which drugs to stop during PCI should be made carefully, and should be tailored to the specific needs of individual patients.

Interactive multiple choice questions are available for this chapter on www.wiley.com/go/dangas/cardiology

References

1 Marsh N, Marsh A. A short history of nitroglycerine and nitric oxide in pharmacology and physiology. *Clin Exp Pharmacol Physiol* 2000; **27**(4): 313–319.

2 Mayer B, Beretta M. The enigma of nitroglycerin bioactivation and nitrate tolerance: news, views and troubles. *Br J Pharmacol* 2008; **155**(2): 170–184.

3 Jost S, Nolte CW, Sturm M, Hausleiter J, Hausmann D. How to standardize vasomotor tone in serial studies based on quantitation of coronary dimensions? *Int J Card Imaging* 1998; **14**(6): 357–372.

4 Ignarro LJ, Lippton H, Edwards JC, *et al.* Mechanism of vascular smooth muscle relaxation by organic nitrates, nitrites, nitroprusside and nitric oxide: evidence for the involvement of S-nitrosothiols as active intermediates. *J Pharmacol Exp Ther* 1981; **218**(3): 739–749.

5 Rosenkranz B, Winkelmann BR, Parnham MJ. Clinical pharmacokinetics of molsidomine. *Clin Pharmacokinet* 1996; **30**(5): 372–384.

6 Katz AM. Calcium channel diversity in the cardiovascular system. *J Am Coll Cardiol* 1996; **28**(2): 522–529.

7 Braun LT. Calcium channel blockers for the treatment of coronary artery spasm: rationale, effects, and nursing responsibilities. *Heart Lung* 1983; **12**(3): 226–232.

8 Fugit MD, Rubal BJ, Donovan DJ. Effects of intracoronary nicardipine, diltiazem and verapamil on coronary blood flow. *J Invasive Cardiol* 2000; **12**(2): 80–85.

9 Martynyuk AE, Kane KA, Cobbe SM, Rankin AC. Role of nitric oxide, cyclic GMP and superoxide in inhibition by adenosine of calcium current in rabbit atrioventricular nodal cells. *Cardiovasc Res* 1997; **34**(2): 360–367.

10 Park SJ, Ahn JM, Kang SJ. Paradigm shift to functional angioplasty: new insights for fractional flow reserve- and intravascular ultrasound-guided percutaneous coronary intervention. *Circulation* 2011; **124**(8): 951–957.

11 Levine GN, Bates ER, Blankenship JC, *et al.* 2011 ACCF/AHA/SCAI Guideline for Percutaneous Coronary Intervention. A report of the American College of Cardiology Foundation/American Heart Association Task Force on Practice Guidelines and the Society for Cardiovascular Angiography and Interventions. *J Am Coll Cardiol* 2011; **58**(24): e44–122.

12 Navarese EP, Buffon A, Andreotti F, *et al.* Adenosine improves post-procedural coronary flow but not clinical outcomes in patients with acute coronary syndrome: a meta-analysis of randomized trials. *Atherosclerosis* 2012; **222**(1): 1–7.

13 Ito H, Taniyama Y, Iwakura K, *et al.* Intravenous nicorandil can preserve microvascular integrity and myocardial viability in patients with reperfused anterior wall myocardial infarction. *J Am Coll Cardiol* 1999; **33**(3): 654–660.

14 Amit G, Cafri C, Yaroslavtsev S, *et al.* Intracoronary nitroprusside for the prevention of the no-reflow phenomenon after primary percutaneous coronary intervention in acute myocardial infarction: a randomized, double-blind, placebo-controlled clinical trial. *Am Heart J* 2006; **152**(5): 887 e9–14.

15 Romagnoli E, Biondi-Zoccai G, Sciahbasi A, *et al.* Radial versus femoral randomized investigation in ST-segment elevation acute coronary syndrome: the RIFLE-STEACS (Radial Versus Femoral Randomized Investigation in ST-Elevation Acute Coronary Syndrome) study. *J Am Coll Cardiol* 2012; **60**(24): 2481–2489.

16 Gorgulu S, Norgaz T, Karaahmet T, Dagdelen S. Incidence and predictors of radial artery spasm at the beginning of a transradial coronary procedure. *J Interv Cardiol* 2013; **26**(2): 208–213.

17 Kiemeneij F. Prevention and management of radial artery spasm. *J Invasive Cardiol* 2006; **18**(4): 159–160.

18 Ho HH, Jafary FH, Ong PJ. Radial artery spasm during transradial cardiac catheterization and percutaneous coronary intervention: incidence, predisposing factors, prevention, and management. *Cardiovasc Revasc Med* 2012; **13**(3): 193–195.

19 Viskin S, Kitzis I, Lev E, *et al.* Treatment with beta-adrenergic blocking agents after myocardial infarction: from randomized trials to clinical practice. *J Am Coll Cardiol* 1995; **25**(6): 1327–1332.

20 Miura M, Thomas R, Ganz W, *et al.* The effect of delay in propranolol administration on reduction of myocardial infarct size after experimental coronary artery occlusion in dogs. *Circulation* 1979; **59**(6): 1148–1157.

21 Reimer KA, Rasmussen MM, Jennings RB. Reduction by propranolol of myocardial necrosis following temporary coronary artery occlusion in dogs. *Circ Res* 1973; **33**(3): 353–363.

22 Zalewski A, Goldberg S, Dervan JP, Slysh S, Maroko PR. Myocardial protection during transient coronary artery occlusion in man: beneficial effects of regional beta-adrenergic blockade. *Circulation* 1986; **73**(4): 734–739.

23 Sharma SK, Kini A, Marmur JD, Fuster V. Cardioprotective effect of prior beta-blocker therapy in reducing creatine kinase-MB elevation after coronary intervention: benefit is extended to improvement in intermediate-term survival. *Circulation* 2000; **102**(2): 166–172.

24 Park H, Otani H, Noda T, *et al.* Intracoronary followed by intravenous administration of the short-acting beta-blocker landiolol prevents myocardial injury in the face of elective percutaneous coronary intervention. *Int J Cardiol* 2013; **167**(4): 1547–1551.

25 Ibanez B, Macaya C, Sanchez-Brunete V, *et al.* Effect of early metoprolol on infarct size in ST-segment-elevation myocardial infarction patients undergoing primary percutaneous coronary intervention: the Effect of Metoprolol in Cardioprotection During an Acute Myocardial Infarction (METOCARD-CNIC) trial. *Circulation* 2013; **128**(14): 1495–1503.

26 Venneman I, Lamy M. Sedation, analgesia and anesthesia for interventional radiological procedures in adults. Part II. Recommendations for interventional radiologists. *JBR-BTR* 2000; **83**(3): 116–120.

27 Barnard EA, Skolnick P, Olsen RW, *et al.* International Union of Pharmacology. XV. Subtypes of gamma-aminobutyric acidA receptors: classification on the basis of subunit structure and receptor function. *Pharmacol Rev* 1998; **50**(2): 291–313.

28 Rihal CS, Textor SC, Grill DE, *et al.* Incidence and prognostic importance of acute renal failure after percutaneous coronary intervention. *Circulation* 2002; **105**(19): 2259–2264.

29 Manske CL, Sprafka JM, Strony JT, Wang Y. Contrast nephropathy in azotemic diabetic patients undergoing coronary angiography. *Am J Med* 1990; **89**(5): 615–620.

30 Lindsay J, Apple S, Pinnow EE, *et al.* Percutaneous coronary intervention-associated nephropathy foreshadows increased risk of late adverse events in patients with normal baseline serum creatinine. *Catheter Cardiovasc Interv* 2003; **59**(3): 338–343.

31 Lindsay J, Canos DA, Apple S, Pinnow E, Aggrey GK, Pichard AD. Causes of acute renal dysfunction after percutaneous coronary intervention and comparison of late mortality rates with postprocedure rise of creatine kinase-MB versus rise of serum creatinine. *Am J Cardiol* 2004; **94**(6): 786–789.

32 Heyman SN, Rosen S, Brezis M. Radiocontrast nephropathy: a paradigm for the synergism between toxic and hypoxic insults in the kidney. *Exp Nephrol* 1994; **2**(3): 153–157.

33 Solomon R, Werner C, Mann D, D'Elia J, Silva P. Effects of saline, mannitol, and furosemide to prevent acute decreases in renal function induced by radiocontrast agents. *N Engl J Med* 1994; **331**(21): 1416–1420.

34 Kajbaf F, Lalau JD. The criteria for metformin-associated lactic acidosis: the quality of reporting in a large pharmacovigilance database. *Diabet Med* 2013; **30**(3): 345–348.

35 Pasceri V, Patti G, Nusca A, Pristipino C, Richichi G, Di Sciascio G. Randomized trial of atorvastatin for reduction of myocardial damage during coronary intervention: results from the ARMYDA (Atorvastatin for Reduction of MYocardial Damage during Angioplasty) study. *Circulation* 2004; **110**(6): 674–678.

36 Briguori C, Visconti G, Focaccio A, *et al.* Novel approaches for preventing or limiting events (Naples) II trial: impact of a single high loading dose of atorvastatin on periprocedural myocardial infarction. *J Am Coll Cardiol* 2009; **54**(23): 2157–2163.

37 Yun KH, Jeong MH, Oh SK, *et al.* The beneficial effect of high loading dose of rosuvastatin before percutaneous coronary intervention in patients with acute coronary syndrome. *Int J Cardiol* 2009; **137**(3): 246–251.

38 Zhang F, Dong L, Ge J. Effect of statins pretreatment on periprocedural myocardial infarction in patients undergoing percutaneous coronary intervention: a meta-analysis. *Ann Med* 2010; **42**(3): 171–177.

39 Winchester DE, Wen X, Xie L, Bavry AA. Evidence of pre-procedural statin therapy a meta-analysis of randomized trials. *J Am Coll Cardiol* 2010; **56**(14): 1099–1109.

40 Overgaard CB, Dzavik V. Inotropes and vasopressors: review of physiology and clinical use in cardiovascular disease. *Circulation* 2008; **118**(10): 1047–1056.

CHAPTER 45

The Optimal Duration of Dual Antiplatelet Therapy After PCI

Mikkel Malby Schoos[1], Roxana Mehran[2], and George D. Dangas[2]

[1] Zealand University Hospital, Denmark

[2] Department of Cardiology, Mount Sinai Medical Center, New York, NY, USA

Rationale and evolution behind dual antiplatelet therapy after stent implantation

The first coronary angioplasty was performed in 1977. It was soon realized that occlusion and restenosis were the most common reasons for transluminal balloon angioplasty to fail to provide long-term benefit and an intravascular mechanical support was therefore developed with the aim of preventing restenosis and sudden closure. Almost a decade later, in 1986, following the first implantation of a coronary stent, its usefulness was promptly established in a case series published in the *New England Journal of Medicine* in 1987 [1]. However, in this very first report, the risk of thrombotic stent occlusion was described. In early clinical trials, around 1990, the rate of stent thrombosis was approaching 20% [2], which led to the adoption of anticoagulant (heparin followed by oral warfarin) and antiplatelet regimens including oral aspirin and dipyridamole. The incorporation of this antithrombotic strategy was subsequently tested in randomized clinical trials in the mid-1990s, comparing stent implantation with balloon angioplasty, and demonstrated a reduced risk of acute and subacute stent thrombosis of approximately 3.5% [3,4]. In 1998, Leon *et al.* [5] published a landmark trial establishing that in comparison with aspirin alone and the combination of aspirin and warfarin, a treatment strategy with aspirin and ticlopidine resulted in a lower rate of stent thrombosis, although there were more hemorrhagic complications than with aspirin alone at 30 days' follow-up. This regimen of a thienopyridine derivative added to aspirin has been the mainstay of antiplatelet therapy after coronary stenting ever since and introduced the concept of dual antiplatelet therapy (DAPT) in patients undergoing percutaneous coronary intervention (PCI). In 2001, the CURE trial tested another thienopyridine derivative, clopidogrel, on top of aspirin, and lately new P2Y12 inhibitors have been introduced—prasugrel [6] in 2007 and ticagrelor [7] in 2009—which have further improved the outcome of DAPT regimens in patients with stents.

In parallel with the evolution of the DAPT regimen, stent technology has matured from bare metal stents (BMS) over first generation to now second generation drug-eluting stents (DES) and improvements in stent technology have direct implications for the clinical strategy of DAPT.

Longstanding controversy about the safety of first generation DES, because of their delayed stent strut neoendothelialization preventing restenosis but promoting thrombosis on the exposed stent struts compared to BMS, was fueled by concerns of late (beyond 30 days) and very late (beyond 1 year) stent thrombosis (ST) in patients discontinuing DAPT [8–11], and annual accrual rates of ST events up to 4 years [12].

In comparison with older platforms, second generation DES differ by a stent platform of a cobalt-chromium or platinum-chromium alloy which enables thinner strut configurations, rendering the stent more deliverable. Newer generation DES also have improved polymer technology with enhanced drug deliverability which generates less vascular inflammatory response and more rapid vessel healing by faster endothelial coverage of stent struts, as well as less vessel remodeling, persistent fibrin and platelet deposition, and premature neoatherosclerosis [13]. Consequently, trials investigating second generation DES have consistently shown lower rates of target lesion revascularization (TLR), myocardial infarction (MI), and ST than first generation DES [14,15].

Early cessation of DAPT has been known to increase the risk of thrombotic events after PCI with first generation DES [16]; however, randomized studies suggest that shorter durations are safe with newer stent platforms. Faster vessel healing after stent implantation results in a decreased need for antithrombotic protection. Recently, strategies with DAPT of only 3 months' duration have proven successful [17].

The use of newer generation DES has rapidly increased and is currently implanted in approximately 85% of patients undergoing PCI. In a nationwide cohort study from Sweden, the use of new-generation DES increased from 10% in 2009 to 85% in 2012. In the meantime, the use of BMS decreased from 50% in 2007 to 15% in 2012, while the use of older generation DES decreased from 50% in 2007 to 0.1% in 2012 [18].

This constantly evolving stent technology affects international guidelines on myocardial revascularization, which have recently been altered with regard to the relevant antiplatelet therapy after implantation of second generation DES.

Interventional Cardiology: Principles and Practice, Second Edition. Edited by George D. Dangas, Carlo Di Mario, and Nicholas N. Kipshidze.
© 2017 John Wiley & Sons, Ltd. Published 2017 by John Wiley & Sons, Ltd.

International guidelines on the duration of dual antiplatelet therapy

In patients with stable coronary artery disease, the latest European guidelines on myocardial revascularization released by the European Society of Cardiology and the European Association for Cardio-Thoracic Surgery (ESC/EACTS) recommend DAPT for at least 1 month after BMS implantation and 6 months after DES implantation. Shorter DAPT duration (<6 months) can be considered in patients at high risk of bleeding. Furthermore, lifelong single antiplatelet therapy (usually aspirin) is indicated. Finally, DAPT can be used for longer than 6 months in patients with high ischemic risk and low bleeding risk.

In patients with acute coronary syndrome (ACS) undergoing PCI, the ESC/EACTS guidelines recommend that a P2Y12 inhibitor is maintained over 12 months in addition to aspirin, unless there are contraindications such as excessive risk of bleeding. Treatment options are prasugrel (60 mg loading dose, 10 mg/day) and ticagrelor (180 mg loading dose, 90 mg twice daily) clopidogrel (600 mg loading dose, 75 mg/day) should only be used when prasugrel or ticagrelor are not available or are contraindicated [19].

The American guidelines differ in that they do not differentiate the duration of DAPT according to ACS presentation in patients with stents and generally suggest longer DAPT duration than the ECS/EACTS. The latest ACCF/AHA/SCAI guidelines recommend DAPT to be continued for up to 12 months in non-invasively treated patients with non-ST segment elevation (NSTE) ACS and for at least 12 months in all ACS and non-ASC patients undergoing PCI with DES [20,21].

The interest of the shortest possible DAPT regimen lies primarily in the optimal balance between preventing ischemic events after PCI and avoiding the bleeding complications inherent to antiplatelet treatment. Two landmark trials have provided solid evidence that the occurrence of major bleeding after PCI increases mortality. In both the HORIZONS-AMI (The Harmonizing Outcomes with RevasculariZatiON and Stents in Acute Myocardial Infarction) [22] and OASIS-5 (Organization for the Assessment of Strategies for Ischemic Syndromes) [23] trials, the ischemic endpoints between the treatment groups were similar but major bleeding differed significantly, resulting in a mortality benefit associated with reduced bleeding. Since then, several other substudies in cohorts originating from randomized clinical trials have confirmed that major bleeding is a powerful independent predictor of short and long-term mortality [24,25]. Short DAPT regimes that do not compromise the ischemic protective benefit will also provide substantial savings in healthcare expenses.

Trials behind the guidelines for best evidence-based clinical practice

Seminal trials have delineated the current recommendations on DAPT in patients with and without ACS [26–30]. The Clopidogrel for the Reduction of Events During Observation (CREDO) trial evaluated the benefit of long-term (12-month) treatment with the addition of clopidogrel to aspirin after elective PCI (65% had a recent MI or unstable angina) and found a significant 27% relative reduction in the combined risk of death, MI, or stroke in the clopidogrel group [30].

The Clopidogrel in Unstable Angina to Prevent Recurrent Events (CURE) trial enrolled ACS patients without ST-segment elevation to receive clopidogrel on top of aspirin for 3–12 months; the mean duration of treatment was 9 months. The primary outcome, a composite of death from cardiovascular causes, non-fatal MI, or stroke, was relatively reduced at 20%. This benefit was driven by fewer MI in the clopidogrel group, while there was no isolated effect on cardiovascular death, and this came at the price of a 1.3-fold increased risk of major bleeding [26].

In the CURE-PCI trial, which investigated patients with ACS undergoing PCI and receiving aspirin, the addition of clopidogrel pretreatment followed by an 8-month regimen led to a 31% reduction in cardiovascular death or MI compared with placebo. There was no isolated effect on mortality [28].

The CLARITY–TIMI 28 trial (Addition of Clopidogrel to Aspirin and Fibrinolytic Therapy for Myocardial Infarction with ST-Segment Elevation) demonstrated that the addition of clopidogrel improved the patency rate of the infarct-related artery and reduced ischemic complications at 30 days' follow-up in patients with STEMI and who were treated with aspirin and a standard fibrinolytic regimen [29].

The COMMIT trial demonstrated that in patients with acute MI, clopidogrel added to aspirin during hospital admission and up to 4 weeks after the index event reduced both mortality and major vascular events in hospital. In both trials, bleeding was not increased [27].

In the context of these guideline referenced trials, the American recommendation of DAPT for at least 12 months in patients with ACS undergoing PCI might seem arbitrary, as none of these trials specifically investigated the recommended 12 month DAPT duration in an exclusive ACS population. Meanwhile, this recommendation has been sustained for over a decade because of repeated reports of early DAPT discontinuation and ACS predicting late coronary stent thrombosis [8,9,31].

Conversely, the latest European guidelines on DAPT duration after implanting second generation stents in patients with stable coronary artery disease recommend a 6-month DAPT duration [19], demonstrating the current controversy of differing needs for antiplatelet therapy for patients with ACS and those without the condition.

Parallels of stent technology evolution and shorter DAPT regimen

Randomized controlled trials (RCT) suggest that shorter durations of DAPT are safe with newer stent platforms. In a recent meta-analysis, the clinical impact of extended DAPT duration >12 months versus short DAPT duration (6 months) in all-comer PCI with predominantly second generation DES did not reduce ischemic events, but increased major bleeding [32], lending support to previous findings in patients with first generation DES [33,34].

This ongoing area of controversy was recently tested by Vahrenhorst et al. [35] in a prospective cohort of 56,440 unselected new-onset and clopidogrel-naïve patients with ACS (40% STEMI) from the SWEDEHART registry, predominantly treated with BMS. In extensively adjusted analyses, DAPT >6 months was associated with a 25% lower risk of all-cause death, stroke, or reinfarction but more bleeding at 1 year compared with treatment for 6 months. Only event-free patients within the first 6 months were considered. The demographics illustrated how contemporary treatment decisions are steered by patient comorbidities such as previous PCI, insulin-treated diabetes, stent type, count and length, as well as atrial fibrillation, anticoagulant treatment, and bleeding risk. This study indicated that DAPT for >6 months in patients with ACS reduces ischemic endpoints irrespective of patient characteristics, supporting the current guidelines for ACS treatment [35].

These results have to be interpreted in the light of two pivotal studies that were conducted in primarily non-ACS patients treated with first generation stents, showing that the vast majority (up to 80%) of definite or probable ST occur in the first 6 months after DES implantation and, additionally, the median time interval from thienopyridine therapy discontinuation to ST increases from several days to several months after the first 6 months, weakening the idea of a direct relationship between DAPT cessation and the occurrence of ST beyond 6 months after PCI [33,36].

DAPT cessation is traditionally classified using a binary, on–off approach that ignores the clinical reasons and underlying context in which antiplatelet treatment is discontinued. An alternative approach was recently offered by the PARIS (Patterns of Non-adherence to Anti-platelet Regiments In Stented Patients) trial, classifying DAPT cessation according to the clinical circumstance of DAPT withdrawal, which directly influenced adverse cardiac outcome after stenting and was related to whether the patient discontinued therapy by physician recommendation, interrupted for surgery, or disrupted because of non-adherence or bleeding [37].

It is likely that the optimal duration of DAPT is the dependent on patient's risk profile. To date, specific recommendations on DAPT duration according to risk subset have not been given in international guidelines; however, contemporary clinical practice undoubtedly modifies duration of DAPT after PCI by risk profile assessment based on patient demographics and procedural characteristics.

High risk patients

The clinical practice of extended DAPT duration in high risk patients is based on landmark studies such as the CHARISMA (Clopidogrel for High Atherothrombotic Risk and Ischemic Stabilization, Management, and Avoidance) and CAPRIE (Clopidogrel versus Aspirin in Patients at Risk of Ischaemic Events) trials, in which only the subset of patients enrolled based on previously documented coronary or peripheral atherosclerotic artery disease derived benefit of extended clopidogrel in terms of a reduction in the composite of MI, stroke, or death from cardiovascular causes [38,39]. In addition, Eisenstein et al. [40] showed in a large observational study that event-free patients at 6 and 12 months post PCI landmark analyses benefited from extended DAPT at up to 2 years' follow-up.

In a more contemporary setting, the PEGASUS-TIMI 54 study investigated the efficacy and safety of ticagrelor beyond 1 year after MI. In a double-blind 1 : 1 : 1 fashion, 21,162 patients who had had an MI 1–3 years earlier, were randomly assigned to ticagrelor at a dose of 90 mg twice daily, ticagrelor at a dose of 60 mg twice daily, or placebo. All the patients were to receive low-dose aspirin and were followed for a median of 33 months. The treatment with ticagrelor in both doses significantly reduced the risk of cardiovascular death, MI, or stroke but increased the risk of major bleeding [41].

This message was recently expanded to non-high risk patients: the DAPT (Dual Antiplatelet Therapy) study enrolled all-comer patients after they had undergone a coronary stent procedure in which a first generation DES was placed in over 30% of subjects. After 12 months of treatment with a thienopyridine drug (clopidogrel or prasugrel) and aspirin, patients were randomly assigned to continue receiving thienopyridine treatment or to receive placebo for another 18 months. In almost 10,000 patients, DAPT beyond 1 year significantly reduced the risks of ST and major cardiovascular and cerebrovascular events but was associated with an increased risk of bleeding [42].

This is disputed in a randomized controlled trial by Lee et al. [43], who reported that in event-free patients at 12 months after PCI, predominantly with first generation DES (65%), an additional 24 months of DAPT versus aspirin alone did not reduce the risk of the composite endpoint of death from cardiac causes, MI, or stroke.

The RESET Trial (REal Safety and Efficacy of 3-month dual antiplatelet Therapy following Endeavor zotarolimus-eluting stent implantation) [44] randomly assigned study participants to receive either the Endeavour zotarolimus stent followed by 3 months of DAPT or another currently available DES followed by 12 months of DAPT. The Endeavour zotarolimus + 3-month DAPT regimen was non-inferior to the standard therapy with respect to cardiovascular death, MI, stent thrombosis, TVR, or bleeding at 1 year. Importantly, there was no positive interaction for treatment effect by predefined subgroups, being diabetes mellitus (DM) but also >65 years of age, gender, ACS, congestive heart failure, stent length, multivessel disease, and vessel diameter, all factors considered characteristics defining a high risk patient profile. These results indicate that in patients treated with second generation DES, DAPT duration is not influenced by risk profile, although the combined endpoint of ischemic and bleeding outcome and the limited power of the subgroup analyses have to be kept in mind.

Nevertheless, the Prolonging Dual Antiplatelet Treatment After Grading Stent-Induced Intimal Hyperplasia Study (PRODIGY) confirmed the RESET results. A regimen of 24 months of clopidogrel therapy in patients who had received a balanced mixture of DES and BMS was not more effective than a 6-month clopidogrel regimen in reducing the composite of death from any cause, MI, or stroke [45]. Again, these results were found to be consistent across risk subgroups of age (>65 years), ACS, and DM.

Baber et al. [46] recently showed that associations between either chronic kidney disease (CKD) or DM alone and high residual platelet reactivity were attenuated after covariate adjustment while the odds for platelet reactivity associated with both CKD and DM remained significant with an approximate 2.5-fold increased risk. Consequently, the presence of both CKD and DM seem to confer a synergistic impact on residual platelet reactivity when compared with either condition alone.

Whether more potent platelet inhibitors improve outcomes among patients with risk factors is controversial and warrants investigation.

In a prespecified subgroup analysis of the PCI-CURE trial [21], the addition of clopidogrel to aspirin in patients with NSTE-ACS undergoing PCI significantly reduced cardiovascular death or MI in non-diabetic patients but had no beneficial effect in patients with diabetes. This finding could lead to the speculation that clopidogrel does not provide sufficient ischemic protection in patients with DM. In a prespecified substudy of the TRITON-TIMI 38 trial [6], subjects with DM had a greater reduction in recurrent MI than patients without DM when treated with prasugrel compared to clopidogrel, without an observed increase in major bleeding. This implies that patients with DM could benefit from the more intensive antiplatelet effect provided by prasugrel [47]. Angiolillo et al.[48] confirmed these findings in patients with type 2 DM and CAD. Standard-dose prasugrel was associated with greater platelet inhibition during both the loading and maintenance periods when compared with double-dose clopidogrel [22]. Conversely, in the PLATO trial, ticagrelor reduced ischemic events in patients with ACS in comparison with clopidogrel, irrespective of diabetic status, glycemic control, and insulin treatment [15]. Recently, a small, single center, open-label study randomized 100 patients with DM and undergoing PCI for an ACS to receive either prasugrel or ticagrelor. Platelet reactivity assessed between 6 and 18 hours postloading dose with ticagrelor showed significantly lower platelet reactivity than prasugrel. Whether this signal of higher potency of ticagrelor could translate into a clinical benefit is unknown [23].

Hence, the clinical necessity of intensified platelet inhibition in patients with DM remains unclear and beneficial effects might be specific to the various P2Y12 compounds. Alternatively, the different findings of prasugrel and ticagrelor in diabetic populations could relate to variations in patient profiles. In fact, a recent clinical report suggests that higher on-treatment platelet reactivity is prevalent among obese patients, although the signal was confined to those who also had the metabolic syndrome [24]. Whether an increased body mass index (BMI) by itself is associated with platelet reactivity is controversial [25].

The matter of prolonged DAPT duration might be summarized as it was stated in the conclusion of a recent meta-analysis. Findings were that short DAPT duration had overall lower rates of bleeding yet higher rates of ST compared with longer DAPT duration, with the latter effect being significantly attenuated with the use of second generation DES. There was a trend of higher all-cause mortality, which was numerically higher with longer DAPT durations but without reaching statistical significance. Prolonging DAPT therefore requires careful assessment of the trade-off between ischemic and bleeding complications [49]. The recent DAPT study offers some insight into the mechanisms of increased all-cause mortality with longer duration of DAPT [42]. While there was no significant difference between the randomized treatments (thienopyridine vs. placebo for 18 months after 1 year of treatment with clopidogrel or prasugrel and aspirin after DES) with respect to severe bleeding (GUSTO criteria) or with respect to fatal bleeding, non-cardiovascular death was increased with prolonged DAPT treatment, in part explained by bleeding related non-cardiovascular deaths caused by trauma [42].

DAPT duration in patients in need of surgery

The length of a planned DAPT regimen after PCI can influence or in some cases even postpone or inhibit other treatments needed by the patient.

Surgery is a frequent cause of DAPT cessation in patients following PCI, with approximately 5% of patients with stents undergoing cardiac or non-cardiac surgery within the first year of PCI [50–52]. Surgery is associated with platelet activation [53] and coronary artery thrombus is a likely mechanism of peri-operative MI [54], which in turn is the most common major vascular complication after surgery and independently associated with 30-day mortality [55–57].

Nevertheless, there is ongoing controversy over the optimal timing and peri-operative strategy of oral antiplatelet treatment in patients undergoing both cardiac and non-cardiac surgery. Currently, the ACCF/AHA/SCAI (American College of Cardiology Foundation/American Heart Association/Society for Cardiac Angiography and Interventions) guidelines regarding revascularization before non-cardiac surgery hold a IIa benefit > risk recommendation (level of evidence B) for balloon angioplasty or BMS implantation followed by 4–6 weeks of DAPT [20]. This grace period after BMS implantation relates to the increased thrombogenicity in the immediate postoperative phase, inherent to the prothrombotic effect of surgery. In the earlier days of coronary

angioplasty with BMS, catastrophic outcomes of very elevated rates of death and MI, with ST accounting for most of the fatal events, were reported when patients underwent surgery within the first 2–5 weeks [58,59], a timeframe that corresponds accurately with the 4-week period of vascular healing with complete stent strut coverage after BMS implantation [60]. Since then, studies conducted in patients with first generation DES showed that non-cardiac surgery within the first year after PCI was an independent predictor of adverse ischemic events. Rates were higher when surgery was performed within 6 months of PCI but stabilized thereafter [61,62], which, in comparison to BMS, was most likely a function of the delayed vessel healing because of the antiproliferative drugs eluted and the polymer coating in first generation DES implants [8,9,13].

Parallel results from recent stent trials indicate that a 3-month grace period after PCI with second generation DES implantation is probably advisable before recommending interruption of DAPT for surgery [17,63].

In the event of surgery, guidelines hold a Class IIa recommendation for discontinuation of DAPT, with continuous aspirin treatment if possible and restart of P2Y12 inhibitors in the immediate postoperative period. However, the level of evidence in support of this recommendation is scarce (level C), with the limited data available relying on expert consensus [20]. The recent results from the large RCT POISE-2 (PeriOperative ISchemic Evaluation-2) have questioned this clinical practice, as the administration of aspirin (100 mg/day after a 200-mg loading dose) before non-cardiac surgery and throughout the early post-surgical period had no significant effect on the rate of a composite of death or non-fatal MI but increased the risk of major bleeding [64]. The American Society of Regional Anesthesia Guidelines for peri-operative management of patients on antiplatelet therapy even recommends that all elective surgery after DES implantation should be postponed for 12 months [65]. Therefore, a tendency exists toward BMS implantation if surgery is planned. In the event that elective surgery can be postponed for 3 months, these guideline precautions might be unnecessary and possibly even disadvantageous as the patient will not benefit from the lower revascularization rates of second generation DES over BMS [15].

Atrial fibrillation

It is estimated that 5–7% of patients undergoing PCI have atrial fibrillation (AF) [6]. Warfarin has been the standard of care for several decades and has been considered superior to DAPT in preventing stroke and thromboembolism in patients with AF who do not undergo PCI [7]. Conversely, in patients in need of PCI, DAPT with aspirin and thienopyridine has been shown to be more beneficial in preventing ST than oral anticoagulation alone [66].

The current AHA guidelines on AF for patients undergoing PCI are non-specific as they recommend "BMS may be considered to minimize the required duration of DAPT" and "It may be reasonable to use clopidogrel concurrently with OAC but without ASA" [67]. One European and one North American recent consensus paper state that triple therapy (TT) with warfarin, aspirin, and thienopyridine should be preferred for patients with AF undergoing PCI with stenting and CHADS2 > 1 [68,69]. The length of triple therapy in these patients is dependent on stent type and the assessment of ischemic and bleeding risk. After BMS implantation, TT should be limited to 1 month, 3 months after limus stents, and 6 months after paclitaxel stents. For DES, warfarin plus either clopidogrel or aspirin (100 mg) with concomitant proton pump inhibitor treatment should be continued for up to 12 months after PCI. Hereafter warfarin alone should be continued lifelong. It is well recognized that the benefits of TT come with a significant bleeding risk (threefold increase compared to warfarin monotherapy; five-fold increase compared to DAPT), which further increases with longer durations of TT [70,71]. In patients with high bleeding risk, the recommendation is to avoid DES altogether. However, with the recent results from pooled analyses from the RESULTE programs considering zotarolimus stents [63], the recommendation of avoid-ing DES implantation in patients with AF could be obsolete with the latest generation scaffolds and polymer coatings.

These consensus statements have recently been challenged by the WOEST trial which found that in patients undergoing PCI and on an anticoagulant (69% indication AF, 88% CHADS2 > 1), the use of clopidogrel without aspirin was associated with a significant reduc-tion in bleeding complications and no increase in the rate of throm-botic events compared to TT [72]. These results were confirmed by a recent Danish nationwide retrospective study based on dispensed drug prescriptions in patients with AF hospitalized with an MI and/or undergoing PCI, in whom oral anticoagulants and clopidogrel was equal or better than TT on both benefit and safety outcomes [73].

Future directives

Several large RCTs studying the duration of DAPT after PCI are currently enrolling. The Ticagrelor With Aspirin or Alone in High-Risk Patients After Coronary Intervention (TWILIGHT) trial has the primary objective to determine in 9000 patients undergoing PCI the impact of antiplatelet monotherapy with ticagrelor alone versus DAPT with ticagrelor plus aspirin for 12 months in reducing clinically relevant bleeding (efficacy) among high risk patients undergoing PCI who have completed a 3-month course of aspirin plus ticagrelor (NCT02270242). An upcoming trial is the Short Duration of Dual antiplatElet Therapy With SyNergy II Stent in Patients Older Than 75 Years Undergoing Percutaneous Coronary Revascularization (SENIOR) study in patients with stable angina, silent ischemia (1 month DAPT), or ACS (6 months DAPT) (NCT02099617).

Finding the right balance in patients with AF undergoing PCI, which minimizes bleeding risk and maintains anti-ischemic effi-cacy, remains a complex and controversial clinical dilemma in these unique patients. The arrival of novel antiplatelet agents and anticoagulants on the scene has led to an exponential increase in the combinations that can be employed by clinicians in real-life situations. At present, four approved oral anticoagulant options for AF (vitamin K antagonist, dabigatran, rivaroxaban, and apixaban) and edoxaban (imminent approval awaited), as well as four com-monly used oral antiplatelet options (aspirin, clopidogrel, ticagre-lor, prasugrel). There is little evidence on this topic and currently the PIONEER-AF trial is enrolling patients with AF undergoing PCI, randomizing participants to rivaroxaban 2.5 mg twice daily + one P2Y12 inhibitor, rivaroxaban 15 mg once daily + one P2Y12 inhibitor, or vitamin K antagonist (VKA) + one P2Y12 inhibitor and aspirin (PIONEER-AF; NCT01830543), with an inclusion period projected to run until July 2015. A trial with dabi-gatran (RE-DUAL PCI) is on the horizon, planning to randomize participants to either Pradaxa 110 mg twice daily + APT, Pradaxa 150 mg twice daily + APT or VKA + DAPT. The sheer number of combinations means that the best APT and anticoagulant combina-tion and duration based on solid randomized data will not be known for many years.

Interactive multiple choice questions are available for this chapter on www.wiley.com/go/dangas/cardiology

References

1 Sigwart U, Puel J, Mirkovitch V, Joffre F, Kappenberger L. Intravascular stents to prevent occlusion and re-stenosis after transluminal angioplasty. *N Engl J Med* 1987; **316**: 701–706.

2 Serruys PW, Strauss BH, Beatt KJ, *et al.* Angiographic follow-up after placement of a self-expanding coronary-artery stent. *N Engl J Med* 1991; **324**: 13–7.

3 Fischman DL, Leon MB, Baim DS, *et al.* A randomized comparison of coronary-stent placement and balloon angioplasty in the treatment of coronary artery disease. *N Engl J Med* 1994; **331**: 496–501.

4 Serruys PW, de Jaegere P, Kiemeneij F, *et al.* A comparison of balloon-expandable-stent implantation with balloon angioplasty in patients with coronary artery disease. *N Engl J Med* 1994; **331**: 489–495.

5 Leon MB, Baim DS, Popma JJ, *et al.* A clinical trial comparing three antithrom-botic-drug regimens after coronary-artery stenting. *N Engl J Med* 1998; **339**: 1665–1671.

6 Wiviott SD, Braunwald E, McCabe CH, *et al.* Prasugrel versus clopidogrel in patients with acute coronary syndromes. *N Engl J Med* 2007; **357**: 2001–2015.

7 Wallentin L, Becker RC, Budaj A, *et al.* Ticagrelor versus clopidogrel in patients with acute coronary syndromes. *N Engl J Med* 2009; **361**: 1045–1057.

8 Camenzind E, Steg PG, Wijns W. A cause for concern. *Circulation* 2007; **115**: 1440–1455.

9 Ong ATL, McFadden EnP, Regar E, *et al.* Late angiographic stent thrombosis (last) events with drug-eluting stents. *J Am Coll Cardiol* 2005; **45**: 2088–2092.

10 McFadden EnP, Stabile E, Regar E, *et al.* Late thrombosis in drug-eluting coro-nary stents after discontinuation of antiplatelet therapy. *Lancet* 1923; **364**: 1519–1521.

11 van Werkum JW, Heestermans AA, Zomer AC, *et al.* Predictors of coronary stent thrombosis: The Dutch Stent Thrombosis Registry. *J Am Coll Cardiol* 2009; **53**: 1399–1409.

12 Wenaweser P, Daemen J, Zwahlen M, *et al.* Incidence and correlates of drug-eluting stent thrombosis in routine clinical practice: 4-year results from a large 2-institutional cohort study. *J Am Coll Cardiol* 2008; **52**: 1134–1140.

13 Stefanini GG, Holmes DR. Drug-Eluting coronary-artery stents. *N Engl J Med* 2013; **368**: 254–265.

14 Baber U, Mehran R, Sharma SK, *et al.* Impact of the everolimus-eluting stent on stent thrombosis: a meta-analysis of 13 randomized trials. *J Am Coll Cardiol* 2011; **58**: 1569–1577.

15 Palmerini T, Biondi-Zoccai G, la Riva D, *et al.* Clinical outcomes with drug-eluting and bare-metal stents in patients with ST-segment elevation myocardial infarction: evidence from a comprehensive network meta-analysis. *J Am Coll Cardiol* 2013; **62**: 496–504.

16 Faxon DP, Lawler E, Young M, Gaziano M, Kinlay S. Prolonged clopidogrel use after bare metal and drug-eluting stent placement: The Veterans Administration Drug-Eluting Stent Study. *Circ Cardiovasc Interv* 2012; **5**: 372–380.

17 Feres F, Costa RA, Abizaid A. Three vs twelve months of dual antiplatelet therapy after zotarolimus-eluting stents: the OPTIMIZE randomized trial. *JAMA* 2013; **310**: 2510–2522.

18 Sarno G, Lagerqvist B, Nilsson J, *et al.* Stent thrombosis in new-generation drug-eluting stents in patients with STEMI undergoing primary PCI: a report from SCAAR. *J Am Coll Cardiol* 2014; **64**: 16–24.

19 Windecker S, Kohl P, Alfonso F, *et al.* 2014 ESC/EACTS Guidelines on myocardial revascularization: The Task Force on Myocardial Revascularization of the European Society of Cardiology (ESC) and the European Association for Cardio-Thoracic Surgery (EACTS)Developed with the special contribution of the European Association of Percutaneous Cardiovascular Interventions (EAPCI). *Eur Heart J* 2014; **35**: 2541–2619.

20 Levine GN, Bates ER, Blankenship JC, *et al.* 2011 ACCF/AHA/SCAI guideline for percutaneous coronary intervention. *Cathet Cardiovasc Intervent* 2013; **82**: E266–E355.

21 Writing Committee, Jneid H, Anderson JL, Wright RS, *et al.* 2012 ACCF/AHA focused update of the guideline for the management of patients with unstable angina/non-ST-elevation myocardial infarction (Updating the 2007 Guideline and Replacing the 2011 Focused Update): A Report of the American College of Cardiology Foundation/American Heart Association Task Force on Practice Guidelines. *Circulation* 2012; **126**: 875–910.

22 Stone GW, Witzenbichler B, Guagliumi G, *et al.* Bivalirudin during primary PCI in acute myocardial infarction. *N Engl J Med* 2008; **358**: 2218–2230.

23 Fifth Organization to Assess Strategies in Acute Ischemic Syndromes Investigators, Yusuf S, Mehta SR, Chrolavicius S, *et al.* Comparison of fondaparinux and enoxaparin in acute coronary syndromes. *N Engl J Med* 2006; **354**: 1464–1476.

24 Manoukian SV, Feit F, Mehran R, *et al.* Impact of major bleeding on 30-day mortality and clinical outcomes in patients with acute coronary syndromes: an analysis from the ACUITY trial. *J Am Coll Cardiol* 2007; **49**: 1362–1368.

25 Mehran R, Pocock S, Nikolsky E, *et al.* Impact of bleeding on mortality after percutaneous coronary intervention: results from a patient-level pooled analysis of the REPLACE-2 (Randomized Evaluation of PCI Linking Angiomax to Reduced Clinical Events), ACUITY (Acute Catheterization and Urgent Intervention Triage Strategy), and HORIZONS-AMI (Harmonizing Outcomes With Revascularization and Stents in Acute Myocardial Infarction) Trials. *JACC Cardiovasc Interv* 2011; **4**: 654–664.

26 Yusuf S, Zhao F, Mehta SR, Chrolavicius S, Tognoni G, Fox KK; Clopidogrel in Unstable Angina to Prevent Recurrent Events Trial Investigators. Effects of clopidogrel in addition to aspirin in patients with acute coronary syndromes without ST-Segment elevation. *N Engl J Med* 2001; **345**: 494–502.

27 Chen ZM, Jiang LX, Chen YP, *et al.* Addition of clopidogrel to aspirin in 45,852 patients with acute myocardial infarction: randomised placebo-controlled trial. *Lancet* 2005; **366**: 1607–1621.

28 Mehta SR, Yusuf S, Peters RJ, *et al.* Effects of pretreatment with clopidogrel and aspirin followed by long-term therapy in patients undergoing percutaneous coronary intervention: the PCI-CURE study. *Lancet* 2001; **358**: 527–533.

29 Sabatine MS, Cannon CP, Gibson CM, *et al.* Addition of clopidogrel to aspirin and fibrinolytic therapy for myocardial infarction with ST-segment elevation. *N Engl J Med* 2005; **352**: 1179–1189.

30 Steinhubl SR, Berger PB, Mann IJ. Early and sustained dual oral antiplatelet therapy following percutaneous coronary intervention: a randomized controlled trial. *JAMA* 2002; **288**: 2411–2420.

31 D'Ascenzo F, Bollati M, Clementi F, *et al.* Incidence and predictors of coronary stent thrombosis: Evidence from an international collaborative meta-analysis including 30 studies, 221,066 patients, and 4276 thromboses. *Int J Cardiol* 2013; **167**: 575–584.

32 Cassese S, Byrne RA, Tada T, King LA, Kastrati A. Clinical impact of extended dual antiplatelet therapy after percutaneous coronary interventions in the drug-eluting stent era: a meta-analysis of randomized trials. *Eur Heart J* 2012; **33**: 3078–3087.

33 Schulz S, Schuster T, Mehilli J, *et al.* Stent thrombosis after drug-eluting stent implantation: incidence, timing, and relation to discontinuation of clopidogrel therapy over a 4-year period. *Eur Heart J* 2009; **30**: 2714–2721.

34 Dangas GD, Claessen BE, Mehran R, Xu K, Stone GW. Stent thrombosis after primary angioplasty for STEMI in relation to non-adherence to dual antiplatelet therapy over time: results of the HORIZONS-AMI trial. *EuroIntervention* 2013; **8**: 1033–1039.

35 Varenhorst C, Jensevik K, Jernberg T, *et al.* Duration of dual antiplatelet treatment with clopidogrel and aspirin in patients with acute coronary syndrome. *Eur Heart J* 2014; **35**: 969–978.

36 Airoldi F, Colombo A, Morici N, *et al.* Incidence and predictors of drug-eluting stent thrombosis during and after discontinuation of thienopyridine treatment. *Circulation* 2007; **116**: 745–754.

37 Mehran R, Baber U, Steg PG, *et al.* Cessation of dual antiplatelet treatment and cardiac events after percutaneous coronary intervention (PARIS): 2 year results from a prospective observational study. *Lancet* 1923; **382**: 1714–1722.

38 CAPRIE Steering Committee. A randomised, blinded, trial of clopidogrel versus aspirin in patients at risk of ischaemic events (CAPRIE). *Lancet* 1996; **348**: 1329–1339.

39 Bhatt DL, Fox KAA, Hacke W, *et al.* Clopidogrel and aspirin versus aspirin alone for the prevention of atherothrombotic events. *N Engl J Med* 2006; **354**: 1706–1717.

40 Eisenstein EL, Anstrom KJ, Kong DF. Clopidogrel use and long-term clinical outcomes after drug-eluting stent implantation. *JAMA* 2007; **297**: 159–168.

41 Bonaca MP, Bhatt DL, Cohen M, *et al.* Long-term use of ticagrelor in patients with prior myocardial infarction. *N Engl J Med* 2015; **372**: 1791–1800.

42 Mauri L, Kereiakes DJ, Yeh RW, *et al.* Twelve or 30 months of dual antiplatelet therapy after drug-eluting stents. *N Engl J Med* 2014; **371**: 2155–2166.

43 Lee CW, Ahn JM, Park DW, *et al.* Optimal duration of dual antiplatelet therapy after drug-eluting stent implantation: a randomized, controlled trial. *Circulation* 2014; **129**: 304–312.

44 Kim BK, Hong MK, Shin DH, *et al.* A new strategy for discontinuation of dual antiplatelet therapy: the RESET Trial (REal Safety and Efficacy of 3-month dual antiplatelet Therapy following Endeavor zotarolimus-eluting stent implantation). *J Am Coll Cardiol* 2012; **60**: 1340–1348.

45 Valgimigli M, Campo G, Monti M, *et al.* Short- versus long-term duration of dual-antiplatelet therapy after coronary stenting: a randomized multicenter trial. *Circulation* 2012; **125**: 2015–2026.

46 Baber U, Bander J, Karajgikar R, *et al.* Combined and independent impact of diabetes mellitus and chronic kidney disease on residual platelet reactivity. *Thromb Haemost* 2013; **110**: 118–123.

47 Wiviott SD, Braunwald E, Angiolillo DJ, *et al.* for the TRITON-TIMI. Greater clinical benefit of more intensive oral antiplatelet therapy with prasugrel in patients with diabetes mellitus in the trial to assess improvement in therapeutic outcomes by optimizing platelet inhibition with prasugrel–Thrombolysis in Myocardial Infarction 38. *Circulation* 2008; **118**: 1626–1636.

48 Angiolillo DJ, Badimon JJ, Saucedo JF *et al.* A pharmacodynamic comparison of prasugrel vs. high-dose clopidogrel in patients with type 2 diabetes mellitus and coronary artery disease: results of the Optimizing anti-Platelet Therapy In diabetes MellitUS (OPTIMUS)-3 Trial. *Eur Heart J* 2011; **32**: 838–846.

49 Giustino G, Baber U, Sartori S, *et al.* Duration of dual antiplatelet therapy after drug-eluting stent implantation: a systematic review and meta-analysis of randomized controlled trials. *J Am Coll Cardiol* 2015; **65**: 1298–1310.

50 Berger PB, Kleiman NS, Pencina MJ, *et al.* Frequency of major noncardiac surgery and subsequent adverse events in the year after drug-eluting stent placement: results from the EVENT (Evaluation of Drug-Eluting Stents and Ischemic Events) Registry. *JACC Cardiovasc Interv* 2010; **3**: 920–927.

51 Ferreira-González I, Marsal JR, Ribera A, *et al.* Background, incidence, and predictors of antiplatelet therapy discontinuation during the first year after drug-eluting stent implantation. *Circulation* 2010; **122**: 1017–1025.

52 Rossini R, Capodanno D, Lettieri C, *et al.* Prevalence, predictors, and long-term prognosis of premature discontinuation of oral antiplatelet therapy after drug eluting stent implantation. *Am J Cardiol* 2011; **107**: 186–194.

53 Dahl OE. Mechanisms of hypercoagulability. *Thromb Haemost* 1999; **82**: 902–906.

54 Gualandro DM, Campos CA, Calderaro D, *et al.* Coronary plaque rupture in patients with myocardial infarction after noncardiac surgery: frequent and dangerous. *Atherosclerosis* 2012; **222**: 191–195.

55 Botto F, Alonso-Coello P, Chan MTV, *et al.* Myocardial injury after noncardiac surgery: a large, international, prospective cohort study establishing diagnostic criteria, characteristics, predictors, and 30-day outcomes. *Anesthesiology* 2014; **120**: 564–578.

56 Devereaux PJ, Xavier D, Pogue J, *et al.* Characteristics and short-term prognosis of perioperative myocardial infarction in patients undergoing noncardiac surgery: a cohort study. *Ann Intern Med* 2011; **154**: 523–528.

57 Devereaux PJ, Chan MT, Alonso-Coello P, *et al.* Association between postoperative troponin levels and 30-day mortality among patients undergoing noncardiac surgery. *JAMA* 2012; **307**: 2295–2304.

58 Kaluza GL, Joseph J, Lee JR, Raizner ME, Raizner AE. Catastrophic outcomes of noncardiac surgery soon after coronary stenting. *J Am Coll Cardiol* 2000; **35**: 1288–1294.

59 Wilson SH, Fasseas P, Orford JL, *et al.* Clinical outcome of patients undergoing non-cardiac surgery in the two months following coronary stenting. *J Am Coll Cardiol* 2003; **42**: 234–240.

60 Joner M, Nakazawa G, Finn AV, *et al.* Endothelial cell recovery between comparator polymer-based drug-eluting stents. *J Am Coll Cardiol* 2008; **52**: 333–342.

61 Schouten O, van Domburg RT, Bax JJ, *et al.* Noncardiac surgery after coronary stenting: early surgery and interruption of antiplatelet therapy are associated with an increase in major adverse cardiac events. *J Am Coll Cardiol* 2002; **49**: 122–124.

62 van Kuijk JP, Flu WJ, Schouten O, *et al.* Timing of noncardiac surgery after coronary artery stenting with bare metal or drug-eluting stents. *Am J Cardiol* 2009; **104**: 1229–1234.

63 Silber S, Kirtane AJ, Belardi JA, *et al.* Lack of association between dual antiplatelet therapy use and stent thrombosis between 1 and 12 months following resolute zotarolimus-eluting stent implantation. *Eur Heart J* 2014; **35**: 1949–1956.

64 Devereaux PJ, Mrkobrada M, Sessler DI, *et al.* Aspirin in patients undergoing noncardiac surgery. *N Engl J Med* 2014; **370**: 1494–1503.

65 Horlocker TT, Wedel DJ, Rowlingson JC, *et al.* Regional anesthesia in the patient receiving antithrombotic or thrombolytic therapy: American Society of Regional Anesthesia and Pain Medicine Evidence-Based Guidelines (Third Edition). *Reg Anesth Pain Med* 2010; **35**: 64–101

66 Andersen LV, Vestergaard P, Deichgraeber P, Lindholt JS, Mortensen L, Frost L. Warfarin for the prevention of systemic embolism in patients with non-valvular atrial fibrillation: a meta-analysis. *Heart* 2008; **94**: 1607–1613.

67 January CT, Wann LS, Alpert JS, *et al.* 2014 AHA/ACC/HRS Guideline for the Management of Patients With Atrial Fibrillation: A Report of the American College of Cardiology/American Heart Association Task Force on Practice Guidelines and the Heart Rhythm Society. *J Am Coll Cardiol* 2014; **64**: e1–e76.

68 Faxon DP, Eikelboom JW, Berger PB, *et al.* Consensus Document: Antithrombotic therapy in patients with atrial fibrillation undergoing coronary stenting. *A North-American perspective. Thromb Haemost* 2011; **106** 572–584.

69 Lip GYH, Huber K, Andreotti F, *et al.* Management of antithrombotic therapy in atrial fibrillation patients presenting with acute coronary syndrome and/or undergoing percutaneous coronary intervention/ stenting. A Consensus Document of the European Society of Cardiology Working Group on Thrombosis, endorsed by the European Heart Rhythm Association [EHRA] and the European Association of Percutaneous Cardiovascular Interventions [EAPCI]. *Thromb Haemost* 2010; **103**: 13–28.

70 Lamberts M, Olesen JB, Ruwald MH, *et al.* Bleeding after initiation of multiple antithrombotic drugs, including triple therapy, in atrial fibrillation patients following myocardial infarction and coronary intervention: A Nationwide Cohort Study. *Circulation* 2012; **126**: 1185–1193.

71 Gage BF, Waterman AD, Shannon W, Boechler M, Rich MW, Radford MJ. Validation of clinical classification schemes for predicting stroke: results from the national registry of atrial fibrillation. *JAMA* 2001; **285**: 2864–2870.

72 Dewilde WJ, Oirbans T, Verheugt FW, *et al.* Use of clopidogrel with or without aspirin in patients taking oral anticoagulant therapy and undergoing percutaneous coronary intervention: an open-label, randomised, controlled trial. *Lancet* 1930; **381**: 1107–1115.

73 Lamberts M, Gislason GH, Olesen JB, *et al.* Oral anticoagulation and antiplatelets in atrial fibrillation patients after myocardial infarction and coronary intervention. *J Am Coll Cardiol* 2013; **62**: 981–989.

CHAPTER 46

Triple Antiplatelet Therapy and Combinations with Oral Anticoagulants After PCI

Jonathan A. Batty[1,2], Joseph R. Dunford[1], Roxana Mehran[3], and Vijay Kunadian[1,4]

[1] Institute of Cellular Medicine, Newcastle University, Newcastle upon Tyne, UK

[2] The Royal Victoria Infirmary, Newcastle upon Tyne NHS Foundation Trust, Newcastle upon Tyne, UK

[3] Department of Cardiology, Mount Sinai Medical Center, New York, NY, USA

[4] Freeman Hospital, Newcastle upon Tyne Hospital NHS Foundation Trust, Newcastle upon Tyne, UK

Dual antiplatelet therapy (DAPT), comprising aspirin and a $P2Y_{12}$-receptor antagonist, is recommended following stent implantation during percutaneous coronary intervention (PCI), by European [1,2] and North American [3,4] guidelines. Although DAPT efficaciously improves peri- and post-procedural outcomes, a significant proportion of patients experience stent thrombosis, reinfarction, and cardiac-related death [5]. In order to further improve patient outcomes, several studies have been conducted to determine the efficacy and safety of administering a further antithrombotic agent, such as an anticoagulant or an additional antiplatelet agent. However, such antithrombotic regimens can lead to an increased risk of bleeding. There remains a great deal of heterogeneity between studies, and so the clinical utility of such therapies is still debated.

Up to 10% of patients undergoing PCI also have a prior indication for long-term oral anticoagulation (OAC), such as atrial fibrillation (AF) or a mechanical heart valve *in situ*. This proportion is set to rise markedly, because of the increasing prevalence of comorbidity, AF, and valvular heart disease; a sequela of population aging [6–11]. Although vitamin K antagonists (VKAs; e.g., warfarin) remain the mainstay of OAC, novel non-vitamin K antagonist oral anticoagulants (NOACs; e.g., apixaban, rivaroxaban and dabigatran) have been developed with potentially advantageous pharmacologic properties and improved safety profiles [12]. Conventional wisdom has held that co-administration of DAPT and OAC (triple antithrombotic therapy; TATT) significantly reduces thromboembolic events, at the expense of increased major bleeding. Because of the narrow margin between the risks and benefits of triple therapy regimens, it is imperative that such strategies are evidence-based and patient-centered, and balance the thromboembolic and hemorrhagic risk factors of the patient [13]. Recent randomized and observational evidence has emerged to offer insight into the net benefits and risks of this strategy, in the settings of PCI and acute coronary syndrome (ACS), and has led to changes to best practice guidelines [14,15].

This chapter reviews the safety and efficacy of triple antiplatelet and antithrombotic regimens, following PCI. It examines the preliminary data regarding novel oral anticoagulants, summarizes the latest evidence-based clinical guidelines, and addresses questions that remain unanswered regarding the optimal clinical use of such antithrombotic regimens.

Methods

A series of structured searches of major biomedical databases (PubMed, Medline, Embase, and Web of Science) were performed, using the key terms; "triple therapy," "percutaneous coronary intervention," "stent implantation," "antiplatelet," "anticoagulation," and "novel anticoagulant agents." Only articles published in English, between 1950 and 2014, were included. This is a synthesis of all available clinical data regarding TATT following PCI.

Platelet activation and the pathophysiology of arterial thrombosis

The primary trigger of intra-arterial thrombosis is rupture of a vulnerable atherosclerotic plaque, which develops from the progressive accumulation of lipid-laden macrophages in the arterial wall. Following rupture, platelet recruitment occurs via the interaction of cell-surface receptors (e.g., glycoprotein VI) with collagen and von Willebrand factor. Following platelet adhesion to the vessel wall, adenosine diphosphate (ADP; $P2Y_1$ and $P2Y_{12}$) and glycoprotein IIb/IIIa (GP IIb/IIIa) receptor-mediated binding of additional platelets occurs, causing aggregation. Degranulation of a cocktail of pro-inflammatory mediators from the platelet releases thromboxane A_2 (TxA_2) and adenosine diphosphate (ADP) which, in turn, propagate further activation. Simultaneously, tissue factor exposed from the denuded plaque activates the clotting cascade via the extrinsic pathway, activating factor VII. This sequentially activates factor X, V, and the final common pathway, activating thrombin. Thrombin cleaves soluble fibrinogen to fibrin monomers, which polymerize to form an insoluble meshwork in which platelets and red blood cells become trapped and so a thrombus is formed. Thrombin interacts with platelets at protease-activated receptors (e.g., PAR-1) to further enhance degranulation, perpetuating further platelet activation. Thus, arterial thrombosis is dependent on activation of both platelets and the clotting cascade; pharmacotherapeutic strategies targeting these pathways are critical in preventing adverse outcomes following PCI.

Interventional Cardiology: Principles and Practice, Second Edition. Edited by George D. Dangas, Carlo Di Mario, and Nicholas N. Kipshidze.

© 2017 John Wiley & Sons, Ltd. Published 2017 by John Wiley & Sons, Ltd.

Mechanisms of antithrombotic pharmacotherapy

Antithrombotic drugs are classified in two main categories: (i) antiplatelet agents, which act via inhibition of platelet recruitment, adhesion, aggregation, or activation, and (ii) anticoagulant agents, which act via inhibition of critical components of the coagulation cascade. Aspirin is a ubiquitous, irreversible, non-specific inhibitor of cyclo-oxygenase (COX), abrogating downstream TxA_2 production; clopidogrel, prasugrel, and ticagrelor act via antagonism of the ADP $P2Y_{12}$ receptor. The traditional anticoagulants, such as warfarin, reduce vitamin K-dependent clotting factor (II, VII, IX, and X) synthesis, via inhibition of vitamin K epoxide reductase subunit C1 (VKORC1). This impairs both the intrinsic and extrinsic clotting pathways. The NOACs directly act on critical components of the final common pathway of the coagulation cascade: apixaban, rivaroxaban, and edoxaban inhibit free/platelet-bound factor Xa (as opposed to low molecular weight heparins and fondaparinux, which bind to Xa via antithrombin III). Dabigatran directly inhibits free/platelet-bound thrombin, abrogating the conversion of fibrinogen to fibrin.

Triple antiplatelet therapy following PCI
Phosphodiesterase-3 inhibitors

Many randomized trials have evaluated the benefits and risks of cilostazol in addition to DAPT following PCI. The largest study randomized 1212 patients to receive either DAPT alone (aspirin and clopidogrel), or with the addition of cilostazol [16]. The addition of cilostazol reduced the composite endpoint of major adverse cardiovascular events (MACE; cardiac death, non-fatal myocardial infarction, stroke, or target vessel revascularization; 0.3 vs. 15.1%; p = 0.01), without increasing the risk of major bleeding (0.0 vs. 0.2%; p = 0.50). To date, 10 further randomized controlled trials have assessed the incremental benefits of cilostazol, randomizing 5096 patients to receive either DAPT (aspirin and clopidogrel) or triple antiplatelet therapy (TAPT; aspirin, clopidogrel, and cilostazol) following PCI [16–25]. Although the sample size of individual trials is relatively low (n = 84–1212 patients), with many reporting equivocal results, meta-analysis demonstrates that cilostazol reduces MACE (odds ratio [OR] 0.56, 95% confidence intervals [CI] 0.47–0.68; p <0.00001), without increasing bleeding (OR 1.42, 95% CI 0.52–3.85; p = 0.49) [26–29].

Registry studies of cilostazol-treated patients have provided additional insights. The DECREASE registry (n = 3099) evaluated DAPT (aspirin and clopidogrel) versus TAPT (aspirin, clopidogrel, and cilostazol), reporting that TAPT was associated with reduced risk of subsequent MI (hazard ratio [HR] 0.23, 95% CI 0.08–0.70; p = 0.01) and stent thrombosis (HR 0.14, 95% CI 0.04–0.52; p = 0.004), with no differences in major hemorrhage (HR 0.97, 95% CI 0.44–2.12; p = 0.94) at 12 months [30]. However, no difference in mortality was observed (HR 0.76, 95% CI 0.40–1.45; p = 0.41). The COBIS-II registry (n = 2756) evaluated TAPT versus DAPT in patients with coronary bifurcation lesions [31]. Although patients who received TAPT had more cardiovascular comorbidities, there were no significant differences in DAPT versus TAPT in terms of MI, stent thrombosis, mortality, or bleeding complications.

Despite these promising results, a study by Yang et al. [32] demonstrated that DAPT regimens containing the third-generation thienopyridine prasugrel induced superior platelet inhibition compared to a TAPT regimen of aspirin, clopidogrel, and cilostazol (VerifyNow-$P2Y_{12}$ assay; 72.1 ± 12.2 vs. 57.5 ± 23.5, respectively; p = 0.020) [32]. Although clinical data are not presented, this highlights the complexity associated with comparing permutations of antiplatelet agents in higher order regimens. A subsequent meta-analysis, which indirectly compares the efficacy of different DAPT regimens with cilostazol-containing TAPT, reports that TAPT significantly reduced MACE rate, compared with prasugrel- and ticagrelor-based DAPT (prasugrel: OR 0.70, 95% CI 0.56–0.87; p = 0.0012; ticagrelor: OR 0.67, 95% CI 0.55–0.83; p = 0.0003) [29]. Furthermore, TAPT with cilostazol did not increase the frequency of major bleeding (OR 1.42, 95% CI 0.52–3.85; p = 0.49) or overall bleeding (OR 1.16, 95% CI: 0.79–1.69; p = 0.45).

Glycoprotein IIb/IIIa inhibitors

The oral platelet GP IIb/IIIa inhibitors xemilofiban, orbofiban, and sibrafiban have undergone extensive phase 3 clinical trials [33–35]. The placebo-controlled EXCITE trial evaluated xemilofiban 10 and 20 mg, administered three times daily for 2 weeks, followed by twice-daily dosing, for up to 6 months following PCI, in 7232 patients [33]. All patients received aspirin therapy; patients receiving stents in the placebo group also received the first generation $P2Y_{12}$-receptor antagonist, ticlopidine. This trial failed to achieve reductions in its primary endpoint (a composite of death, recurrent MI, and revascularization), demonstrating no benefit of xemilofiban at 6 months at a 10 mg (HR 1.03, 95% CI 0.86–1.23; p = 0.82) or 20 mg (HR 0.94, 95% CI 0.78–1.13; p = 0.36) dose. The OPUS-TIMI 16 trial randomized 10,302 patients presenting with ACS to either 50 mg orbofiban twice daily for 6 months, 50 mg orbofiban twice daily for 30 days followed by 30 mg twice daily for 5 months, or placebo [34]. All patients received aspirin therapy; placebo-treated patients receiving stents received ticlopidine. OPUS-TIMI was halted prematurely because of significantly increased mortality in the orbofiban arm (5.1 vs. 3.7% in the 50/30 mg orofiban-treated vs. placebo-treated group; p = 0.008). Bleeding was dose-dependently higher in orofiban-treated patients, occurring in 2.0%, 3.7%, and 4.5% in the placebo, 50/30, and 50/50 groups, respectively (p <0.0001). The SYMPHONY trial studied weight- creatinine-individualized sibrafiban therapy versus aspirin in 9233 ACS patients [35]. The primary endpoint (death, reinfarction, or severe ischemia) did not differ between aspirin, low, or high dose sibrafiban-treated patients, but major bleeding was more common in sibrafiban-treated patients (OR 1.34, 95% CI 1.05–1.71) compared to aspirin alone. Enrolment of second SYMPHONY, comparing low dose sibrafiban with aspirin, high dose sibrafiban without aspirin, or aspirin alone, was terminated prematurely, following analysis of SYMPHONY [36]. In those randomized (6671 of a planned 9000 patients) a major bleeding risk was also observed in sibrafiban-treated patients.

Each phase 3 oral GP IIb/IIIa inhibitor trial reported significant harms associated with such therapy. Subsequent meta-analysis confirmed this phenomenon, demonstrating significant excess mortality, regardless of aspirin co-administration or dosage [37]. However, trials of intravenous GP IIb/IIIa inhibitors (abciximab, eptifibatide, and tirofiban) demonstrate significant benefits as adjuncts to PCI during the management of ACS, and stable CAD [38,39]. The unfavorable safety profile of oral agents precluded their usage in clinical practice.

Antiplatelet combinations with oral anticoagulants following PCI
Vitamin K antagonists

Although the beneficial effects of warfarin in reducing morality and preventing reinfarction post-MI have been ascertained in several placebo-controlled, randomized studies, these predate the widespread implementation of mechanical reperfusion strategies and DAPT, and as such have uncertain relevance to contemporary practice [40,41]. In the context of multiagent regimens, a large meta-analysis demonstrated that there was no mortality benefit associated with the routine co-administration of warfarin and DAPT versus DAPT alone (OR 1.20, 95% CI 0.63–2.27; p = 0.56); reductions in the incidence of ischemic events (OR 0.29, 95% CI 0.15–0.58; p = 0.0004) were counterbalanced by a twofold increased risk of bleeding (OR 2.00, 95% CI 1.41–2.83; p <0.0001) [42]. The use of OACs in combination with DAPT for specific, high risk patient groups, such as those with comorbid AF and *in situ* mechanical heart valves, is further evaluated in this chapter.

Non-vitamin K antagonist oral anticoagulants

Direct thrombin inhibitors

Impelled by the advent of NOACs, renewed interest has emerged in routine combination antithrombotic therapy following PCI [43]. However, phase 3 clinical trials exploring the use of NOACs in AF systematically excluded patients with recent stent implantation, and conversely, recent trials of ACS management have excluded patients on novel anticoagulants. The placebo-controlled, dose-escalation RE-DEEM study randomized 1861 patients with ACS to receive standard DAPT (aspirin and clopidogrel, or another thienopyridine) alone, or with dabigatran, following PCI [44]. Patients were randomized to receive placebo or dabigatran 50, 75, 110, or 150 mg (each twice daily). Although the study was not adequately powered to assess efficacy, because of multiple-group comparisons and the small event rates within each group (1.7–3.8%), it was able to detect differences in major bleeding (the primary study outcome). A dose-dependent relationship with bleeding risk was robustly observed in dabigatran-treated patients, compared with placebo-treated controls (50 mg: HR 1.77, 95% CI 0.70–4.50; 75 mg: HR 2.17, 95% CI 0.88–5.31; 110 mg: HR 3.92, 95% CI 1.72–8.95; and 150 mg: HR 4.27, 95% CI 1.86–9.81), with equivocal antithrombotic benefit.

Direct factor Xa inhibitors

The APPRAISE study randomized 1715 patients with ST-elevation or non-ST-elevation MI to evaluate the incremental effects of apixaban in addition to DAPT [45]. Patients received placebo or apixaban 2.5 mg (twice daily), 10 mg (once daily), 10 mg (twice daily), or 20 mg (once daily). The high dose groups (20 mg/day) were later discontinued, following early reports of excessive clinically significant bleeding among patients receiving these regimens (7.8% and 7.3% of patients administered 10 mg twice daily and 20 mg once daily, respectively). Among patients receiving the lower dose regimens, the risk of clinically significant bleeding remained greater than that of placebo-treated controls (2.5 mg twice daily: HR 1.78, 95% CI 0.91–3.48; p = 0.09; 10 mg once daily: HR 2.45, 95% CI 1.31–4.61; p = 0.005). The apixaban-treated groups experienced a reduced rate of further cardiovascular events compared to the placebo-treated group (2.5 mg twice daily: HR 0.73, 95% CI 0.19–0.56; 10 mg once daily: HR 0.61, 95% CI 0.04–0.65). However, the observed increase in bleeding risk was more pronounced, and reductions in ischemic events less evident, in patients taking aspirin plus clopidogrel, compared to those taking aspirin alone. Subsequently, the APPRAISE-2 trial was prematurely terminated following recruitment of 7392 (of target enrolment of 10,848) patients, randomized to receive 5 mg twice daily apixaban (based on the optimal dosing profile identified in APPRAISE) or placebo, in

addition to aspirin and a P2Y$_{12}$-receptor antagonist [46]. Significant increases in major bleeding were observed with apixaban treatment compared to the control group (HR 2.59, 95% CI 1.50–4.46; p = 0.001). During apixaban therapy, a greater number of these episodes were intracranial or fatal, compared to placebo. No differences in the rates of MACE were observed (7.9 vs. 7.5%, respectively; p = 0.51), at 8 months' follow-up. These data indicate that the use of apixaban, even at the 5 mg dose determined in APPRAISE to offer the greatest risk–benefit profile, increased major hemorrhage, without reducing incident cardiovascular events. Although the authors suggest the inclusion of patients with extensive comorbidities, such as advanced age, diabetes mellitus, heart failure, and renal impairment, could have increased the rate of bleeding, these factors were distributed equally throughout both groups, and should not have deleteriously impacted upon outcomes.

The ATLAS-ACS-TIMI 46 study aimed to identify the optimal dosage regimen of rivaroxaban, in ACS patients receiving aspirin with or without a thienopyridine [47]. This trial randomized 3491 patients (2730 on DAPT) to either a receive placebo, or rivaroxaban at daily doses of 5, 10, 15, and 20 mg, administered in a single or divided doses. This study reported a daily dose-dependent, increased risk of clinically significant bleeding with rivaroxaban versus placebo (5 mg: HR 2.21, 95% CI 1.25–3.91; 10 mg: HR 3.35, 95% CI 2.31–4.87; 15 mg: HR 3.60, 95% CI 2.32–5.58; and 20 mg: HR 5.06, 95% CI 3.45–7.42; p <0.0001). However, rivaroxaban treatment efficaciously reduced mortality and MACE, compared with placebo (doses combined: HR 0.69, 95% CI 0.50–0.96; p = 0.027). Twice daily rivaroxaban 2.5 and 5 mg achieved the optimum balance between minimization of bleeding risk, and maximization of benefit. The phase III ATLAS-ACS-2-TIMI-51 study then randomized 15,526 patients to either placebo, twice daily rivaroxaban 2.5 or 5 mg (in addition to aspirin and a thienopyridine) [48]. At 13 months' follow-up, rivaroxaban therapy reduced the risk of a composite endpoint of MI, stroke, and death (doses combined: HR 0.84, 95% CI 0.74–0.96; p = 0.008), with greater risk reductions amongst those receiving twice daily 5 mg compared with twice daily 2.5 mg dosage (8.8% vs. 9.1%). Although rivaroxaban was associated with an increased risk of major bleeding (doses combined: HR 3.96, 95% CI 2.46–6.38; p <0.001), fatal hemorrhage remained equal (HR 1.19, 95% CI 0.54–2.59; p = 0.66). Thus, rivaroxaban may represent a useful adjunct to DAPT following PCI.

Although development was later discontinued, the efficacy of darexaban was evaluated in a multicenter, double-blind, randomized trial, RUBY-1 [49]. This trial randomized 1279 patients with ACS to receive one of six darexaban regimens (10–60 mg/day, in once-only or divided dose regimens) or placebo, in addition to DAPT. At 6 weeks' follow-up, darexaban was associated a significant dose-dependent risk of bleeding (overall HR 2.28, 95% CI 1.13–4.60; p = 0.022). Although underpowered to definitively provide insight into clinical efficacy, no differences in mortality or adverse cardiac events were noted between the darexaban and placebo-treated groups.

A meta-analysis of seven phase 2 and 3 studies of NOACs in ACS (n = 30,866; 26,731 on DAPT) demonstrates that the addition of a NOAC to standard therapy, as indicated, reduced the incidence of MACE (HR 0.87, 95% CI 0.80–0.95), but doubled the risk of significant bleeding (HR 2.34, 95% CI 2.06–2.66) [50]. The analyses were robust; with low interstudy heterogeneity, and equivalent outcomes when limited to phase 3 studies. Thus, the results of this meta-analysis, in line with the individual trials, demonstrate that while NOACs can offer incremental efficacy over DAPT regimens, this may be outweighed by associated excess bleeding.

Achieving improved outcomes following PCI: a role for a third agent?

At present, insufficient evidence of an acceptable risk–benefit balance exists to recommend the routine use of a third antithrombotic agent in the post-PCI setting [1,3,4,51]. The addition of cilostazol to present TAPT regimens may be associated with improved outcomes, particularly for patients known to be at high risk of recurrent adverse events following PCI [52,53]. However, limited evidence of benefits on absolute endpoints and uncertain efficacy in comparison to contemporary DAPT regimens have precluded the inclusion of cilostazol in guidelines. Although the use of intravenous GP IIb/IIIa inhibitors has become the standard of care for certain patients during revascularization, the adverse safety profile of oral agents precludes their further development as adjunct to DAPT. The routine administration of OACs with DAPT remains controversial; any antithrombotic benefits of VKAs are counterbalanced by increased risk of hemorrhage and pragmatic limitations associated with maintaining therapeutic anticoagulation. Although early evidence suggests NOACs can reduce the risk of post-procedure adverse cardiovascular events, a significant risk of bleeding, high cost, and difficulties in reversal limits routine administration. As such, DAPT remains the mainstay of treatment following ACS. The routine use of additional antithrombotic agents poses significant risks, without proven benefit. Antithrombotic regimens should be reserved for specific cases, in which there is proven clinical benefit.

Triple antithrombotic therapy following PCI with prior indications for OAC
Vitamin K antagonists

As a consequence of population aging, an increasing number of patients presenting for PCI have comorbid indications for long-term OAC, such as AF, *in situ* mechanical heart valves, or intramural thrombus [54]. However, in AF, it remains challenging to identify patients who would benefit from long-term OAC. The CHADS$_2$ (congestive heart failure, hypertension, age over 75 years, diabetes mellitus, and transient ischemic attack or stroke) and CHA$_2$DS$_2$-VASc (CHADS$_2$ factors, vascular disease, age over 65 years, and female sex) tools aid clinicians in making recommendations regarding the appropriateness of OAC [55,56]. Each factor scores one, apart from those indicated with subscript characters. A CHADS$_2$ or CHA$_2$DS$_2$-VASc score ≥ 1 should prompt consideration of OAC (antithromboembolic benefits outweigh risk of hemorrhage). The HAS-BLED (hypertension, abnormal renal/liver function, stroke, bleeding predisposition, labile international normalized ratio [INR], elderly, and drug history) score is used to ascertain bleeding risk; scores ≥ 3 indicate high risk of bleeding, and suggest caution when considering OAC [57]. HAS-BLED also has clinical utility in combination with antithrombotic regimens, predicting bleeding risk with moderate accuracy during combination antithrombotic pharmacotherapy. The development and validation of further scores may better guide decisions regarding the use of novel antithrombotic regimens following PCI.

For patients who have prior indications for both OAC and undergo PCI, the most common therapeutic regimen consists of warfarin, aspirin, and a thienopyridine (OAC + DAPT). However, is such a strategy rigorously evidence-based? A retrospective, nationwide study (n = 11,480), demonstrates that patients treated with warfarin, aspirin, and clopidogrel are at increased risk of spontaneous (and fatal) hemorrhage, compared to patients treated with DAPT alone (10.2 vs. 3.2; p = 0.01) [58]. Outcomes are compared in patients treated with: (i) all agents (n = 1,495), (ii) warfarin plus either aspirin (n = 1,310) or clopidogrel (n = 527), (iii) aspirin and clopidogrel (n = 3144), and (iv) antiplatelet or anticoagulant monotherapy (n = 5004). Patients receiving OAC + DAPT had high rates of clinically significant bleeding during the first 30 days (22.6 per 100 patient-years), reducing over 2 months (20.2), to approximately half at 3 months (10.7), indicating no safe therapeutic window exists. The bleeding risk in patients receiving DAPT + OAC remained greater than a single antiplatelet agent and OAC, at 3 months (HR 1.47, 95% CI 1.04–2.08) and 1 year (HR 1.36, 95% CI 0.95–1.95). Notably, no significant difference in thromboembolic risk was observed for DAPT + OAC versus a single antiplatelet agent and OAC (HR 1.15, 95% CI 0.95–1.40), calling into question the use of multiple antiplatelet agents. The findings of multiple, small, observational studies with regard to bleeding risk are in agreement. Rogacka *et al.* [59] also noted that amongst patients receiving DAPT + OAC following PCI (n = 127), most bleeding (67%) occurs within the first month. The AVIATOR registry prospectively followed 425 patients with AF receiving PCI because of ACS. On discharge, patients received OAC + DAPT (n = 185), or DAPT (n = 240; aspirin and clopidogrel) [60]. At 1 year, the risk of MACE was similar in both groups (14% vs. 16%, HR 0.90; p = 0.78), although the risk of bleeding was greater in those receiving OAC + DAPT (13% vs. 6%; HR 2.05; p = 0.03). Yu *et al.* [61] report a contemporary cohort of n = 367 patients with AF undergoing drug-eluting stent implantation; 154 received OAC + DAPT, 213 received DAPT alone. At 2 years, the OAC + DAPT group experienced a greater rate of major bleeding (16.7% vs. 4.6%; p <0.001), without significant increases in MACE (22.1% vs. 17.7%; p = 0.31).

Although informative observational studies are limited by selection bias, and the lack of a control group, precluding definitive conclusions regarding the safety and efficacy of triple antithrombotic therapy in patients at risk of thromboembolism, further interventional studies were required. The seminal WOEST trial randomized 573 patients receiving OAC and undergoing PCI, to receive either clopidogrel alone, or with aspirin, in addition to their pre-existing VKA, using an open-label design [62]. PCI was primarily elective; drug-eluting stents were used in 65% of cases. AF (with CHADS$_2$ ≥ 1) was the most frequent indication for anticoagulation. At 1 year, bleeding was significantly less in patients receiving OAC plus clopidogrel, compared with those receiving OAC + DAPT (HR 0.36, 95% CI 0.26–0.50; p <0.0001). Although inadequately powered to demonstrate non-inferiority, the absolute MACE rate was lower with OAC plus clopidogrel versus OAC + DAPT (11.1% vs. 17.6%, HR 0.60, 95% CI 0.38–0.94; p = 0.025). Thus, the removal of aspirin significantly reduces the risk of bleeding by more than 50%, without increases in MACE. The authors hypothesize that inhibition of thrombin (factor IIa; a powerful platelet activator) with VKA OACs, and the P2Y$_{12}$ receptor (which has a major role in amplifying the effects of TxA$_2$) with clopidogrel, reduces the importance of COX inhibition in the protection against thromboembolic events.

The findings of WOEST were supported by the observational data in the Danish National Registry, which included 12,165 patients with AF, receiving multiple antithrombotic regimens following PCI [63]. At 1 year, no increased risk of MACE was observed for OAC plus clopidogrel in comparison to OAC + DAPT (HR 0.69,

95% CI 0.48–1.00), OAC plus aspirin (HR 0.96, 95% CI 0.77–1.19) or aspirin plus clopidogrel (HR 1.17, 95% CI 0.96–1.42), supporting the notion that OAC plus clopidogrel reduces MACE to an equivalent extent as OAC+DAPT. The bleeding risk for OAC plus clopidogrel was lower than for OAC+DAPT, albeit non-significantly (HR 0.78, 95% CI 0.55–1.12). There was a similar rate of all-cause mortality in OAC plus clopidogrel and OAC+DAPT, but greater rates for OAC plus aspirin, and DAPT alone. Thus, the Danish registry is the second major study to suggest the lack of efficacy of aspirin in antithrombotic regimens with OAC and clopidogrel.

Further observational studies have confirmed the safety and efficacy of OAC plus clopidogrel following PCI in patients with AF. Seivani *et al.* [64] report a registry of 221 patients receiving prior OAC and different antithrombotic regimens, following drug-eluting stent implantation. Patients received 6–12 months of clopidogrel therapy, followed by OAC monotherapy alone. The combination of OAC and clopidogrel was safe and efficacious; however, a sharp rise in MACE following clopidogrel cessation was noted, particularly in patients with sub-therapeutic anticoagulation. More recently, the non-randomized prospective AFCAS registry followed 975 patients

receiving DAPT, OAC+DAPT and OAC plus clopidogrel, in order to evaluate clinical safety and efficacy [65]. However, at 1 year, no significant intergroup differences in terms of occurrence of MACE, or frequency of bleeding, in both crude and propensity score-adjusted analysis, were observed.

Further insights into the risks associated with the inclusion of aspirin arose from the CORONOR registry, which prospectively enrolled 4184 patients with stable CAD, with no MI or revascularization for 1 year before enrolment [66]. Although the majority received antiplatelet monotherapy (n=2798), a significant proportion received DAPT (aspirin and clopidogrel; n=861) or an OAC (n=461). Among these, 342 patients received VKA and an antiplatelet agent (aspirin, n=308; clopidogrel, n=34). At 2 years, the use of a VKA was not associated with significantly increased risk of bleeding (HR 1.69, 95% CI 0.39–7.30); however, this was highly significant in those receiving aspirin concomitantly (HR 7.30, 95% CI 3.91–13). This study extends the insights of WOEST into the excess risk associated with the inclusion of aspirin in multiple antithrombotic regimens. Figure 46.1 summarizes the evidence regarding combinations of antithrombotic agents, in patients with AF undergoing PCI.

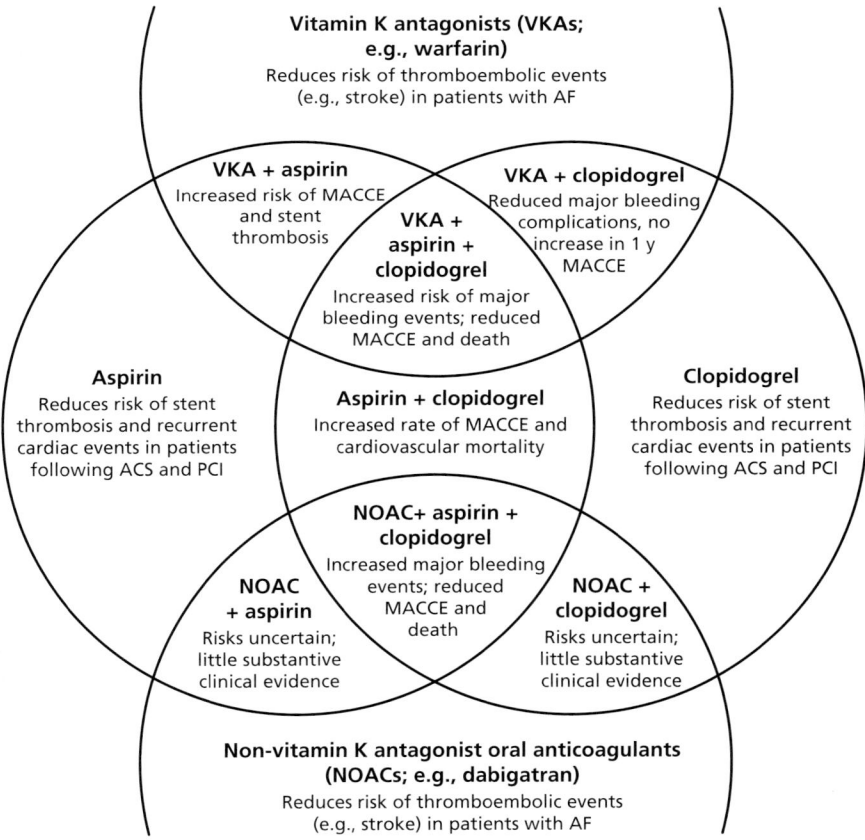

Figure 46.1 A summary of the risks and benefits of different combinations of antithrombotic agents for patients with indications for both oral anticoagulation and dual antiplatelet therapy. For patients with AF whom undergo PCI, the number of possible combinations of antiplatelet agents is significant. This modified Venn diagram briefly summarizes the clinical evidence regarding each regimen. Antithrombotic combinations for patients with indications for an anticoagulant following PCI for ACS recommended by the ESC/ACC are dependent on bleeding and stroke risk, but include initial triple antithrombotic therapy with OAC (VKA or NOAC) + aspirin + clopidogrel, followed by OAC (VKA or NOAC) + clopidogrel (for up to 12 months post-procedure), and life-long OAC (VKA or NOAC). AF, atrial fibrillation; MACCE, major adverse cardiac and cerebrovascular events; MI, myocardial infarction; NOAC, non-vitamin K antagonist oral anticoagulants; OAC, oral anticoagulants; PCI, percutaneous coronary intervention; VKA, vitamin K antagonists; y, year.

Until recently, significant uncertainty prevailed regarding the optimal length for OAC + DAPT therapy following stent implantation. The recent ISAR-TRIPLE trial randomized 614 patients to either a 6-week or 6-month OAC + DAPT therapy regimen, following drug-eluting stent implantation [67]. Aspirin and OAC were continued indefinitely; only the duration of clopidogrel therapy changed. At 9 months' follow-up, no difference was noted in composite clinical outcomes between groups (9.8% vs. 8.8%, HR 1.14, 95% CI 0.68–1.91; p = 0.63). Thus, shortening the duration of OAC + DAPT neither reduced major bleeding (p = 0.44), nor increased the incidence of ischemic events (p = 0.87), and appears safe.

Non-vitamin K antagonist oral anticoagulants

Given the non-inferior clinical efficacy, favorable safety profile, and numerous pragmatic benefits of NOACs, co-administration with DAPT could represent an advantage over VKAs among patients requiring triple antithrombotic therapy. Several studies explored the role of the NOACs in this context. The RE-LY trial evaluated 18,113 patients with AF who were administered either warfarin (according to INR), or dabigatran (110 or 150 mg, twice daily) [68]. *Post hoc* subgroup analysis of patients co-administered antiplatelet therapy at baseline (n = 6952) has been performed. Of these, 5789 received aspirin monotherapy, 351 received clopidogrel monotherapy, and 812 received DAPT [69]. Patients receiving concurrent low dose dabigatran and antiplatelet agents had a reduced risk of bleeding, compared with patients administered warfarin and antiplatelet agents (HR 0.82, 95% CI 0.67–1.00), despite a similar risk of cerebrovascular and systemic embolism (HR 0.93, 95% CI 0.70–1.25). Patients receiving high dose dabigatran were at similar risk of bleeding and embolism compared with warfarin (HR 0.93, 95% CI 0.76–1.12 and HR 0.80, 95% CI 0.59–1.08, respectively). This suggests that low dose dabigatran represents an alternative therapeutic option to warfarin, with equivocal thromboembolic benefits, and reduced bleeding risk.

In the ATLAS studies, and the first APPRAISE trial, an indication for ongoing anticoagulation was amongst the exclusion criteria, and so the safety of apixaban and rivaroxaban was not evaluated amongst patients with AF; however, the doses used in these studies were previously demonstrated to provide effective thromboprophylaxis for patients with AF [70,71], suggesting that in this setting TATT with these drugs could have a role. However, further study is clearly needed.

Clinical guidelines: DAPT in combination with OAC in AF

European Joint Society guidelines address issues associated with managing patients with AF who require treatment for ACS [72,73]. These provide detailed recommendations on the evidence-based optimal management strategy, based on the nature of the stent used during PCI, and achieving an equilibrium between risk factors associated with bleeding, reinfarction, stent thrombosis, and adverse cardiac, cerebrovascular, and thromboembolic events. Updated in 2014 (Table 46.1) [73] to reflect the clinical evidence that has emerged since the 2010 version [72], these guidelines emphasize formal assessment of hemorrhagic risk (i.e., using the HAS-BLED score) and stroke risk (CHA_2DS_2-VAS_C), and vary depending on the setting of PCI (stable CAD or ACS). For example, in patients with a low baseline bleeding risk (HAS-BLED 0-2), and significant risk of stroke (CHA_2DS_2-$VAS_C \geq 2$), undergoing elective PCI, at least 4 weeks (and no longer than 6 months) of OAC + DAPT,

followed by OAC and clopidogrel alone until 12 months post-procedure, and lifelong OAC thereafter. These guidelines no longer differ between drug-eluting and bare metal stents. Furthermore, European ACS guidelines [1,2] do not advocate routine post-procedural oral anticoagulant therapy, except when a specific indication exists (AF, mechanical valve, or left ventricular thrombus). In such patients, the guidelines advocate that triple antithrombotic therapy should be continued for the minimal possible time (to reduce bleeding risk), until stent endothelialization is complete. Importantly, while long-term OAC is to be used in conjunction with DAPT, the target INR should be reduced, to 2.0–2.5. For patients at high risk of gastrointestinal bleeds, gastric protection (i.e., a proton pump inhibitor) should be initiated.

North American guidelines are largely in line with their European counterparts [74,75]. Updated in 2014, guidance from the American Joint Societies regarding PCI in patients with AF advocate consideration of BMS implantation to minimize the duration of OAC + DAPT. For patients at high risk of stroke (CHA_2DS_2-VAS_c $\geq$2), the use of OAC + DAPT is advocated for either 1 or 3–6 months, depending on the type of the stent, followed by an OAC and clopidogrel (but without aspirin) until 12 months post-procedure. Following 12 months of antiplatelet therapy, antiplatelet therapy should be stopped, and OAC continued, as required. If the stroke risk is low (CHA_2DS_2-VAS_c 0–1) DAPT is recommended for 12 months, before returning to regular AF treatment. The target INR should remain at 2.0–3.0 (Table 46.2).

Though the European and American guidelines differ in how they stratify patients for antithrombotic therapy (European by bleeding and stroke risk, and clinical setting of PCI; American by stroke risk and the nature of the implanted stent), both recommend a role for triple therapy in certain patient subgroups, in the early period following PCI. Although no robust guidelines exist regarding the role of triple anticoagulant therapy for other indications (i.e., mechanical valve prostheses, intramural thrombus, or DVT) the AF guidelines should translate to such cases, as bleeding risk remains clinically determinable.

Unanswered questions and future perspectives

A significant number of questions remain unanswered considering the efficacy of TAPT and the use of OAC following PCI. Many of the trials occurred before contemporary proton pump inhibitor (PPI) therapy was routinely recommended as the standard of care with DAPT, efficaciously reducing major gastrointestinal bleeding [76]. Although studies have reported that combining the PPI omeprazole and clopidogrel can lead to diminished antiplatelet efficacy, via impairment of the formation of the active metabolite of clopidogrel, this has not had reported clinical consequences [77,78]. The COGENT trial randomized 3873 75 mg clopidogrel-treated ACS patients to receive either omeprazole 20 mg or placebo [79]. The addition of omeprazole proved superior to placebo in reducing the rate of overt gastrointestinal bleeding (HR 0.13, 95% CI 0.03–0.56; p = 0.001), with no significant differences in the risk of adverse cardiovascular events (HR 0.99, 95% CI 0.68–1.44; p = 0.96). Subsequent reports have advocated that PPI should be encouraged during multiple antiplatelet pharmacotherapy [78]. Indeed, such therapy can abrogate the risk of bleeding that has thus far precluded the addition of additional antithrombotic agents to DAPT regimens; further study, both in the form of new trials and post hoc analysis of completed trials, is warranted.

Table 46.1 2014 ESC guidelines for the recommended antithrombotic strategies following PCI in patients with AF a moderate to high stroke risk.

Bleeding risk (HAS-BLED)	Stroke risk (CHA$_2$DS$_2$-VAS$_c$)	Clinical setting	Treatment recommendation	Evidence class/level
Low or moderate (0–2)	Moderate (1 in males)	Stable CAD	≥4 weeks (≤6 months): OAC + aspirin + clopidogrel Up to 12 months: OAC + clopidogrel (or aspirin) Lifelong: OAC	IIa / C IIb / C I / B
	High (≥2)	Stable CAD	≥ 4 weeks (≤6 months): OAC + aspirin + clopidogrel Up to 12 months: OAC + clopidogrel (or aspirin) Lifelong: OAC	IIa / C IIb / C I / B
	Moderate (1 in males)	ACS	6 months: OAC + aspirin + clopidogrel Up to 12 months: OAC + clopidogrel (or aspirin) Lifelong: OAC	IIa / C IIb / C I / B
	High (≥2)	ACS	6 months: OAC + aspirin + clopidogrel Up to 12 months: OAC + clopidogrel (or aspirin) Lifelong: OAC	IIa / C IIb / C I / B
High (≥3)	Moderate (1 in males)	Stable CAD	12 months: OAC + clopidogrel Lifelong: OAC	IIa / C I / B
	High (≥2)	Stable CAD	4 weeks: OAC + aspirin + clopidogrel Up to 12 months: OAC + clopidogrel (or aspirin) Lifelong: OAC	IIa / C IIb / C I / B
	Moderate (1 in males)	ACS	4 weeks: OAC + aspirin + clopidogrel Up to 12 months: OAC + clopidogrel (or aspirin) Lifelong: OAC	IIa / C IIb / C I / B
	High (≥2)	ACS	4 weeks: OAC + aspirin + clopidogrel Up to 12 months: OAC + clopidogrel (or aspirin) Lifelong: OAC	IIa / C IIb / C I / B

No differentiation in guidelines regarding whether OAC is preferentially a VKA or NOAC. If warfarin is the OAC of choice, INR should be maintained at 2.0–2.5 while on DAPT, and 2.0–3.0 otherwise. NOACs should be administered at the lower tested dose in AF (dabigatran 110 mg twice daily, rivaroxaban 15 mg once daily. or apixaban 2.5 mg twice daily. PPI should be considered in all patients. Newer generation drug-eluting stents are preferred over bare metal stents in patients at low baseline bleeding risk.

ACS, acute coronary syndrome; AF, atrial fibrillation; CAD, coronary artery disease; DAPT, dual antiplatelet therapy; ESC, European Society of Cardiology; INR, international normalized ratio; NOAC, non-vitamin K antagonist oral anticoagulant; OAC, oral anticoagulant agent; PCI, percutaneous coronary intervention; VKA, vitamin K antagonist.

Source: Adapted from Task Force members, Lip GY, et al. [73].

Patients with AF requiring PCI tend to be of advanced age, and have high rates of comorbidity. Many are octogenarians, a group that is frequently under-represented (or actively excluded from) randomized trials of antiplatelet and triple therapy. As such, it is uncertain whether present guidelines can be safely applied to this group. By definition, such patients will have a high CHA$_2$DS$_2$-VAS$_c$ score, in addition to a greater risk of bleeding when administered OACs. In this group, the importance of even minor bleeding should not be underestimated—even minor and non-clinically significant bleeds can lead to poor compliance with, and discontinuation of, therapy, with the potential for catastrophic thrombotic and thromboembolic complications. Thus, in addition to the routine inclusion of older patients in future studies, specific evaluation of approaches to the management of this challenging group are required.

Many further studies exploring the risks and benefits of triple antithrombotic therapy following PCI are presently ongoing with objectives relevant to this chapter, include the PIONEER AF-PCI, RE-DUAL PCI, MUSICA-2, and LASER studies. The PIONEER AF-PCI (NCT01830543) study is designed to evaluate rivaroxaban at two separate doses versus vitamin K antagonist anticoagulants, in addition to antiplatelet monotherapy, or various DAPT combinations. The projected enrolment is n = 2,169, and the study is scheduled for completion in 2016. Similarly, the multicenter RE-DUAL PCI study (NCT02164864) is designed to compare dabigatran at two dosage levels, plus a single, non-aspirin oral antiplatelet versus warfarin plus DAPT, in patients with AF undergoing PCI. The trial has an a priori defined primary endpoint of death, MI, and stroke, hopes to recruit 8520 patients, and is expected to complete in 2017. The MUSICA-2 trial (NCT01141153) is a smaller study, investigating the safety and efficacy of the triple antithrombotic regimen of the vitamin K antagonist acenocoumarol, in addition to aspirin and clopidogrel in 304 patients, expected to report in 2016. A further

Table 46.2 2012 ACCP guidelines for the recommended antithrombotic strategies following PCI in patients with AF.

Stroke risk (CHADS$_2$)	Stent type	Treatment recommendation	Evidence class/level
High (≥2)	BMS	4 weeks: OAC + aspirin + clopidogrel	IIa / C
		Up to 12 months: OAT + clopidogrel	IIb / C
		Lifelong: OAT	I / B
	DES	3–6 months: OAT + aspirin + clopidogrel (depending on stent type)	IIa / C
		Up to 12 months: OAT + clopidogrel	IIb / C
		Lifelong: OAT	I / B
	None	Up to 12 months: OAT + clopidogrel	IIb / C
		Lifelong: OAT	I / B
Low (0–1)	BMS or DES	Up to 12 months: aspirin + clopidogrel	IIb / C
		Lifelong: OAT or aspirin + clopidogrel, as indicated	I / B
	None	Up to 12 months: aspirin + clopidogrel	IIb / C
		Lifelong: OAT or aspirin + clopidogrel, as indicated	I / B

BMS, bare metal stent; DES, drug-eluting stent; OAT, oral anticoagulant agent.
OAT may be a VKA or NOAC, depending on clinical factors.
Source: Adapted from You *et al.* [74].

ongoing, non-randomized, observational study, the prospective, multicenter LASER (NCT00865163) registry, with nested case–control design, is following 2000 patients following PCI; half have prior indications for VKAs, half do not. It is hoped that the results of the LASER registry will offer insight into the rates of clinically relevant bleeding events associated with anticoagulation in contemporary PCI.

Conclusions

Despite numerous robust randomized controlled trials and meta-analyses, the safety of triple antiplatelet and antithrombotic therapy remains controversial. Although the evidence of clinical benefit is insufficient to advocate the routine use of such regimens following PCI or ACS, patients at high risk of further thrombotic or thromboembolic events could stand to benefit from these high intensity treatment regimens. Novel anticoagulant agents demonstrate significant promise in providing additional protection against recurrent infarction and stent thrombosis, with safety profiles non-inferior to traditional oral anticoagulants. It remains conceivable that these agents offer the greatest balance of risk and benefit in high risk patients, although further prospective evaluation is required. Whenever higher order antithrombotic agents are to be combined, careful elucidation and consideration of bleeding risk must be weighed up against the potential benefits of such therapy.

Interactive multiple choice questions are available for this chapter on www.wiley.com/go/dangas/cardiology

References

1 Hamm CW, Bassand JP, Agewall S, *et al.* ESC Guidelines for the management of acute coronary syndromes in patients presenting without persistent ST-segment elevation: The Task Force for the management of acute coronary syndromes (ACS) in patients presenting without persistent ST-segment elevation of the European Society of Cardiology (ESC). *Eur Heart J* 2011; **32**(23): 2999–3054.

2 Steg PG, James SK, Atar D, *et al.* ESC Guidelines for the management of acute myocardial infarction in patients presenting with ST-segment elevation. *Eur Heart J* 2012; **33**(20): 2569–2619.

3 American College of Emergency Physicians, Society for Cardiovascular Angiography Interventions, O'Gara PT, *et al.* 2013 ACCF/AHA guideline for the management of ST-elevation myocardial infarction: executive summary: a report of the American College of Cardiology Foundation/American Heart Association Task Force on Practice Guidelines. *J Am Coll Cardiol* 2013; **61**(4): 485–510.

4 Amsterdam EA, Wenger NK, Brindis RG, *et al.* 2014 AHA/ACC Guideline for the Management of Patients With Non-ST-Elevation Acute Coronary Syndromes: Executive Summary: A Report of the American College of Cardiology/American Heart Association Task Force on Practice Guidelines. *Circulation* 2014; **130**(25): 2354–2394.

5 Mulukutla SR, Marroquin OC, Vlachos HA, *et al.* Benefit of long-term dual antiplatelet therapy in patients treated with drug-eluting stents: from the NHLBI Dynamic Registry. *Am J Cardiol* 2013; **111**(4): 486–492.

6 Faxon DP, Eikelboom JW, Berger PB, *et al.* Consensus document: antithrombotic therapy in patients with atrial fibrillation undergoing coronary stenting. A North-American perspective. *Thromb Haemost* 2011; **106**(4): 572–584.

7 Wang TY, Robinson LA, Ou FS, *et al.* Discharge antithrombotic strategies among patients with acute coronary syndrome previously on warfarin anticoagulation: physician practice in the CRUSADE registry. *Am Heart J* 2008; **155**(2): 361–368.

8 Oudot A, Steg PG, Danchin N, *et al.* Impact of chronic oral anticoagulation on management and outcomes of patients with acute myocardial infarction: data from the RICO survey. *Heart* 2006; **92**(8): 1077–1083.

9 Lane DA, Raichand S, Moore D, *et al.* Combined anticoagulation and antiplatelet therapy for high-risk patients with atrial fibrillation: a systematic review. *Health Technol Assess* 2013; **17**(30): 1–188.

10 Kralev S, Schneider K, Lang S, *et al.* Incidence and severity of coronary artery disease in patients with atrial fibrillation undergoing first-time coronary angiography. *PLoS One* 2011; **6**(9): e24964.

11 Barnett K, Mercer SW, Norbury M, *et al.* Epidemiology of multimorbidity and implications for health care, research, and medical education: a cross-sectional study. *Lancet* 2012; **380**(9836): 37–43.

12 Ruff CT, Giugliano RP, Braunwald E, *et al.* Comparison of the efficacy and safety of new oral anticoagulants with warfarin in patients with atrial fibrillation: a meta-analysis of randomised trials. *Lancet* 2014; **383**(9921): 955–962.

13 Mega J, Carreras ET. Antithrombotic therapy: triple therapy or triple threat? *Hematology* 2012; **2012**: 547–552.

14 Lip GYH, Windecker S, Huber K, *et al.* Management of antithrombotic therapy in atrial fibrillation patients presenting with acute coronary syndrome and/or undergoing percutaneous coronary or valve interventions: a joint consensus document of the European Society of Cardiology Working Group on Thrombosis, European Heart Rhythm Association (EHRA), European Association of Percutaneous

Cardiovascular Interventions (EAPCI) and European Association of Acute Cardiac Care (ACCA) endorsed by the Heart Rhythm Society (HRS) and Asia-Pacific Heart Rhythm Society (APHRS). *Eur Heart J* 2014; **35**(45): 3155–3179.

15 January CT, Wann LS, Alpert JS, *et al.* 2014 AHA/ACC/HRS Guideline for the Management of Patients With Atrial Fibrillation: Executive Summary. A Report of the American College of Cardiology/American Heart Association Task Force on Practice Guidelines and the Heart Rhythm Society. *J Am Coll Cardiol* 2014; **64**(21): 2305–2307.

16 Han Y, Li Y, Wang S, *et al.* Cilostazol in addition to aspirin and clopidogrel improves long-term outcomes after percutaneous coronary intervention in patients with acute coronary syndromes: a randomized, controlled study. *Am Heart J* 2009; **157**(4): 733–739.

17 Wang SL, Sun F, Zhao X, *et al.* [Effect of percutaneous coronary intervention timing and cilostazol use on left ventricular remodeling in patients with non-ST elevation myocardial infarction]. *Zhonghua Xin Xue Guan Bing Za Zhi* 2010; **38**(10): 870–874.

18 Suh JW, Lee SP, Park KW, *et al.* Multicenter randomized trial evaluating the efficacy of cilostazol on ischemic vascular complications after drug-eluting stent implantation for coronary heart disease: results of the CILON-T (influence of CILostazol-based triple antiplatelet therapy ON ischemic complication after drug-eluting stenT implantation) trial. *J Am Coll Cardiol* 2011; **57**(3): 280–289.

19 Kim YH, Park SW, Lee SW, *et al.* Sirolimus-eluting stent versus paclitaxel-eluting stent for patients with long coronary artery disease. *Circulation* 2006; **114**(20): 2148–2153.

20 Lu YL, Chen YD, Lu SZ. [Effects of intensive antiplatelet therapy in patients with high platelet aggregability after percutaneous coronary intervention]. *Zhonghua Xin Xue Guan Bing Za Zhi.* 2007; **35**(9): 793–796.

21 Lee SW, Park SW, Kim YH, *et al.* A randomized, double-blind, multicenter comparison study of triple antiplatelet therapy with dual antiplatelet therapy to reduce restenosis after drug-eluting stent implantation in long coronary lesions: results from the DECLARE-LONG II (Drug-Eluting Stenting Followed by Cilostazol Treatment Reduces Late Restenosis in Patients with Long Coronary Lesions) trial. *J Am Coll Cardiol* 2011; **57**(11): 1264–1270.

22 Lee SW, Chun KJ, Park SW, *et al.* Comparison of triple antiplatelet therapy and dual antiplatelet therapy in patients at high risk of restenosis after drug-eluting stent implantation (from the DECLARE-DIABETES and -LONG Trials). *Am J Cardiol* 2010; **105**(2): 168–173.

23 Gao W, Zhang Q, Ge H, *et al.* Efficacy and safety of triple antiplatelet therapy in obese patients undergoing stent implantation. *Angiology* 2013; **64**(7): 554–558.

24 Chen YD, Lu YL, Jin ZN, *et al.* A prospective randomized antiplatelet trial of cilostazol versus clopidogrel in patients with bare metal stent. *Chin Med J (Engl)* 2006; **119**(5): 360–366.

25 Ahn CM, Hong SJ, Park JH, *et al.* Cilostazol reduces the progression of carotid intima-media thickness without increasing the risk of bleeding in patients with acute coronary syndrome during a 2-year follow-up. *Heart Vessels* 2011; **26**(5): 502–510.

26 Ding XL, Xie C, Jiang B, *et al.* Efficacy and safety of adjunctive cilostazol to dual antiplatelet therapy after stent implantation: an updated meta-analysis of randomized controlled trials. *J Cardiovasc Pharm Ther* 2012; **18**(3): 222–228.

27 Geng DF, Liu M, Jin DM, *et al.* Cilostazol-based triple antiplatelet therapy compared to dual antiplatelet therapy in patients with coronary stent implantation: a meta-analysis of 5,821 patients. *Cardiology* 2012; **122**(3): 148–157.

28 Jang JS, Jin HY, Seo JS, *et al.* A meta-analysis of randomized controlled trials appraising the efficacy and safety of cilostazol after coronary artery stent implantation. *Cardiology* 2012; **122**(3): 133–143.

29 Chen Y, Zhang Y, Tang Y, *et al.* Long-term clinical efficacy and safety of adding cilostazol to dual antiplatelet therapy for patients undergoing PCI: a meta-analysis of randomized trials with adjusted indirect comparisons. *Curr Med Res Opin* 2014; **30**(1): 37–49.

30 Lee SW, Park SW, Yun SC, *et al.* Triple antiplatelet therapy reduces ischemic events after drug-eluting stent implantation: Drug-Eluting stenting followed by Cilostazol treatment REduces Adverse Serious cardiac Events (DECREASE registry). *Am Heart J* 2010; **159**(2): 284–291 e1.

31 Song PS, Song YB, Yang JH, *et al.* Triple versus dual antiplatelet therapy after percutaneous coronary intervention for coronary bifurcation lesions: results from the COBIS (COronary BIfurcation Stent) II Registry. *Heart Vessels* 2015; **30**(4): 458–468.

32 Yang TH, Jin HY, Choi KN, *et al.* Randomized comparison of new dual-antiplatelet therapy (aspirin, prasugrel) and triple-antiplatelet therapy (aspirin, clopidogrel, cilostazol) using P2Y12 point-of-care assay in patients with STEMI undergoing primary PCI. *Int J Cardiol* 2012; **168**(1): 207–211.

33 O'Neill WW, Serruys P, Knudtson M, *et al.* Long-term treatment with a platelet glycoprotein-receptor antagonist after percutaneous coronary revascularization. EXCITE Trial Investigators. Evaluation of Oral Xemilofiban in Controlling Thrombotic Events. *N Engl J Med* 2000; **342**(18): 1316–1324.

34 Cannon CP, McCabe CH, Wilcox RG, *et al.* Oral glycoprotein IIb/IIIa inhibition with orbofiban in patients with unstable coronary syndromes (OPUS-TIMI 16) trial. *Circulation* 2000; **102**(2): 149–156.

35 SYMPHONY Investigators. Comparison of sibrafiban with aspirin for prevention of cardiovascular events after acute coronary syndromes: a randomised trial. Sibrafiban versus Aspirin to Yield Maximum Protection from Ischemic Heart Events Post-acute Coronary Syndromes. *Lancet* 2000; **355**(9201): 337–345.

36 Second SI. Randomized trial of aspirin, sibrafiban, or both for secondary prevention after acute coronary syndromes. *Circulation* 2001; **103**(13): 1727–1733.

37 Chew DP, Bhatt DL, Sapp S, *et al.* Increased mortality with oral platelet glycoprotein IIb/IIIa antagonists: a meta-analysis of phase III multicenter randomized trials. *Circulation* 2001; **103**(2): 201–206.

38 Winchester DE, Wen X, Brearley WD, *et al.* Efficacy and safety of glycoprotein IIb/IIIa inhibitors during elective coronary revascularization: a meta-analysis of randomized trials performed in the era of stents and thienopyridines. *J Am Coll Cardiol* 2011; **57**(10): 1190–1199.

39 Geeganage C, Wilcox R, Bath PM. Triple antiplatelet therapy for preventing vascular events: a systematic review and meta-analysis. *BMC Med* 2010; **8**: 36.

40 Hurlen M, Abdelnoor M, Smith P, *et al.* Warfarin, aspirin, or both after myocardial infarction. *N Engl J Med* 2002; **347**(13): 969–974.

41 Smith P. Long-term anticoagulant treatment after acute myocardial infarction. *The Warfarin Re-Infarction Study. Ann Epidemiol* 1992; **2**(4): 549–552.

42 Gao F, Zhou YJ, Wang ZJ, *et al.* Meta-analysis of the combination of warfarin and dual antiplatelet therapy after coronary stenting in patients with indications for chronic oral anticoagulation. *Int J Cardiol* 2011; **148**(1): 96–101.

43 Costopoulos C, Niespialowska-Steuden M, Kukreja N, *et al.* Novel oral anticoagulants in acute coronary syndrome. *Int J Cardiol* 2013; **167**(6): 2449–2455.

44 Oldgren J, Budaj A, Granger CB, *et al.* Dabigatran vs. placebo in patients with acute coronary syndromes on dual antiplatelet therapy: a randomized, double-blind, phase II trial. *Eur Heart J* 2011; **32**(22): 2781–2789.

45 Alexander JH, Becker RC, Bhatt DL, *et al.* Apixaban, an oral, direct, selective factor Xa inhibitor, in combination with antiplatelet therapy after acute coronary syndrome: results of the Apixaban for Prevention of Acute Ischemic and Safety Events (APPRAISE) trial. *Circulation* 2009; **119**(22): 2877–2885.

46 Alexander JH, Lopes RD, James S, *et al.* Apixaban with antiplatelet therapy after acute coronary syndrome. *N Engl J Med* 2011; **365**(8): 699–708.

47 Mega JL, Braunwald E, Mohanavelu S, *et al.* Rivaroxaban versus placebo in patients with acute coronary syndromes (ATLAS ACS-TIMI 46): a randomised, double-blind, phase II trial. *Lancet* 2009; **374**(9683): 29–38.

48 Mega JL, Braunwald E, Wiviott SD, *et al.* Rivaroxaban in patients with a recent acute coronary syndrome. *N Engl J Med* 2012; **366**(1): 9–19.

49 Steg PG, Mehta SR, Jukema JW, *et al.* RUBY-1: a randomized, double-blind, placebo-controlled trial of the safety and tolerability of the novel oral factor Xa inhibitor darexaban (YM150) following acute coronary syndrome. *Eur Heart J* 2011; **32**(20): 2541–2554.

50 Oldgren J, Wallentin L, Alexander JH, *et al.* New oral anticoagulants in addition to single or dual antiplatelet therapy after an acute coronary syndrome: a systematic review and meta-analysis. *Eur Heart J* 2013; **34**(22): 1670–1680.

51 Task Force on the management of ST-segment elevation acute myocardial infarction of the European Society of Cardiology (ESC), Steg PG, James SK, Atar D, *et al.* ESC Guidelines for the management of acute myocardial infarction in patients presenting with ST-segment elevation. *Eur Heart J* 2012; **33**(20): 2569–2619.

52 Lee SW, Park SW, Kim YH, *et al.* Drug-eluting stenting followed by cilostazol treatment reduces late restenosis in patients with diabetes mellitus the DECLARE-DIABETES Trial (A Randomized Comparison of Triple Antiplatelet Therapy with Dual Antiplatelet Therapy After Drug-Eluting Stent Implantation in Diabetic Patients). *J Am Coll Cardiol* 2008; **51**(12): 1181–1187.

53 Gao W, Zhang Q, Ge H, Guo Y, Zhou Z. Efficacy and safety of triple antiplatelet therapy in obese patients undergoing stent implantation. *Angiology* 2013; **64**(7): 554–558.

54 Schwalm JD, Ahmad M, Salehian O, *et al.* Warfarin after anterior myocardial infarction in current era of dual antiplatelet therapy: a randomized feasibility trial. *J Thromb Thrombolysis* 2010; **30**(2): 127–132.

55 Gage BF, Waterman AD, Shannon W, *et al.* Validation of clinical classification schemes for predicting stroke: results from the National Registry of Atrial Fibrillation. *JAMA* 2001; **285**(22): 2864–2870.

56 Lip GY, Nieuwlaat R, Pisters R, *et al.* Refining clinical risk stratification for predicting stroke and thromboembolism in atrial fibrillation using a novel risk factor-based approach: the Euro heart survey on atrial fibrillation. *Chest* 2010; **137**(2): 263–272.

57 Pisters R, Lane DA, Nieuwlaat R, *et al.* A novel user-friendly score (HAS-BLED) to assess 1-year risk of major bleeding in patients with atrial fibrillation: the Euro Heart Survey. *Chest* 2010; **138**(5): 1093–1100.

58 Lamberts M, Olesen JB, Ruwald MH, *et al.* Bleeding after initiation of multiple antithrombotic drugs, including triple therapy, in atrial fibrillation patients following

myocardial infarction and coronary intervention: a nationwide cohort study. *Circulation* 2012; **126**(10): 1185–1193.

59 Rogacka R, Chieffo A, Michev I, *et al.* Dual antiplatelet therapy after percutaneous coronary intervention with stent implantation in patients taking chronic oral anticoagulation. *JACC Cardiovasc Interv* 2008; **1**(1): 56–61.

60 Christodoulidis G, Mennuni MG, Sartori S, *et al.* TCT-474 triple vs. dual antithrombotic therapy in patients with atrial fibrillation and acute coronary syndromes: The AVIATOR Registry. *J Am Coll Cardiol* 2014; **64**(11S).

61 Yu CW, Kang DO, Cho JY, *et al.* TCT-475 triple antithrombotic therapy versus dual antiplatelet therapy in patients with atrial fibrillation undergoing drug-eluting stent implantation. *J Am Coll Cardiol* 2014; **64**(11S).

62 Dewilde WJ, Oirbans T, Verheugt FW, *et al.* Use of clopidogrel with or without aspirin in patients taking oral anticoagulant therapy and undergoing percutaneous coronary intervention: an open-label, randomised, controlled trial. *Lancet* 2013; **381**: 1107–1115.

63 Lamberts M, Gislason GH, Olesen JB, *et al.* Oral anticoagulation and antiplatelets in atrial fibrillation patients after myocardial infarction and coronary intervention. *J Am Coll Cardiol* 2013; **62**(11): 981–989.

64 Seivani Y, Abdel-Wahab M, Geist V, *et al.* Long-term safety and efficacy of dual therapy with oral anticoagulation and clopidogrel in patients with atrial fibrillation treated with drug-eluting stents. *Clin Res Cardiol* 2013; **102**(11): 799–806.

65 Rubboli A, Schlitt A, Kiviniemi T, *et al.* One-year outcome of patients with atrial fibrillation undergoing coronary artery stenting: an analysis of the AFCAS registry. *Clin Cardiol* 2014; **37**(6): 357–364.

66 Lemesle G, Lamblin N, Meurice T, *et al.* Dual antiplatelet therapy in patients with stable coronary artery disease in modern practice: prevalence, correlates, and impact on prognosis (from the Suivi d'une cohorte de patients CORONariens stables en region NORd-Pas-de-Calais study). *Am Heart J* 2014; **168**(4): 479–486.

67 Fiedler KA, Maeng M, Mehilli J, *et al.*, eds. *TCT-014 Duration of triple therapy in patients requiring oral anticoagulation after drug-eluting stent implantation (ISAR-TRIPLE Trial).* Transcatheter Cardiovascular Therapeutics; 2014; Washington DC, United States.

68 Connolly SJ, Ezekowitz MD, Yusuf S, *et al.* Dabigatran versus warfarin in patients with atrial fibrillation. *N Engl J Med* 2009; **361**(12): 1139–1151.

69 Dans AL, Connolly SJ, Wallentin L, *et al.* Concomitant use of antiplatelet therapy with dabigatran or warfarin in the randomized evaluation of long-term anticoagulation therapy (RE-LY) trial. *Circulation* 2013; **127**(5): 634–640.

70 Granger CB, Alexander JH, McMurray JJ, *et al.* Apixaban versus warfarin in patients with atrial fibrillation. *N Engl J Med* 2011; **365**(11): 981–992.

71 Patel MR, Mahaffey KW, Garg J, *et al.* Rivaroxaban versus warfarin in nonvalvular atrial fibrillation. *N Engl J Med* 2011; **365**(10): 883–891.

72 Lip GY, Huber K, Andreotti F, *et al.* Antithrombotic management of atrial fibrillation patients presenting with acute coronary syndrome and/or undergoing coronary stenting: executive summary--a Consensus Document of the European Society of Cardiology Working Group on Thrombosis, endorsed by the European Heart Rhythm Association (EHRA) and the European Association of Percutaneous Cardiovascular Interventions (EAPCI). *Eur Heart J* 2010; **31**(11): 1311–1318.

73 Task Force members, Lip GY, Windecker S, *et al.* Management of antithrombotic therapy in atrial fibrillation patients presenting with acute coronary syndrome and/or undergoing percutaneous coronary or valve interventions: a joint consensus document of the European Society of Cardiology Working Group on Thrombosis, European Heart Rhythm Association (EHRA), European Association of Percutaneous Cardiovascular Interventions (EAPCI) and European Association of Acute Cardiac Care (ACCA) endorsed by the Heart Rhythm Society (HRS) and Asia-Pacific Heart Rhythm Society (APHRS). *Eur Heart J* 2014; **35**(45): 3155–3179.

74 You JJ, Singer DE, Howard PA, *et al.* Antithrombotic therapy for atrial fibrillation: Antithrombotic Therapy and Prevention of Thrombosis, 9th ed: American College of Chest Physicians Evidence-Based Clinical Practice Guidelines. *Chest* 2012; **141**(2 Suppl): e531S–75S.

75 January CT, Wann LS, Alpert JS, *et al.* 2014 AHA/ACC/HRS Guideline for the Management of Patients With Atrial Fibrillation. A Report of the American College of Cardiology/American Heart Association Task Force on Practice Guidelines and the Heart Rhythm Society. *J Am Coll Cardiol* 2014; **64**(21): e1–76.

76 Moukarbel GV, Signorovitch JE, Pfeffer MA, *et al.* Gastrointestinal bleeding in high risk survivors of myocardial infarction: the VALIANT Trial. *Eur Heart J* 2009; **30**(18): 2226–2232.

77 Gilard M, Arnaud B, Cornily JC, *et al.* Influence of omeprazole on the antiplatelet action of clopidogrel associated with aspirin: the randomized, double-blind OCLA (Omeprazole CLopidogrel Aspirin) study. *J Am Coll Cardiol* 2008; **51**(3): 256–260.

78 Focks JJ, Brouwer MA, van Oijen MG, *et al.* Concomitant use of clopidogrel and proton pump inhibitors: impact on platelet function and clinical outcome: a systematic review. *Heart* 2013; **99**(8): 520–527.

79 Bhatt DL, Cryer BL, Contant CF, *et al.* Clopidogrel with or without omeprazole in coronary artery disease. *N Engl J Med* 2010; **363**(20): 1909–1917.

CHAPTER 47

Peri-procedural Platelet Function Testing in Risk Stratification and Clinical Decision Making

Paul A. Gurbel[1], Fang Liu[2], Gailing Chen[2], and Udaya S. Tantry[1]

[1] Inova Center for Thrombosis Research and Drug Development, Inova Heart and Vascular Institute, Falls Church, VA, USA
[2] Sinai Center for Thrombosis Research, Cardiac Catheterization Laboratory, Baltimore, MD, USA

Myocardial infarction (MI) and stent thrombosis are catastrophic events that occur in patients with coronary artery disease (CAD) undergoing percutaneous coronary intervention (PCI). Overwhelming evidence exists that thrombus generation resulting from platelet activation and aggregation at the sites of plaque rupture is the primary process involved in the occurrence of the latter clinical events. Although thromboxane A2 and adenosine diphosphate (ADP) act synergistically during platelet aggregation, the ADP-P2Y$_{12}$ receptor interaction has a central role in sustaining the activation of glycoprotein IIb/IIIa receptors by amplifying the response to agonists. P2Y$_{12}$ activation also modulates platelet procoagulant activity, P-selectin expression, and inflammation (Figure 47.1) [1].

The clinical efficacy of dual antiplatelet therapy (DAPT) of aspirin and a P2Y$_{12}$ receptor blocker in preventing MI and stent thrombosis has been demonstrated in a wide range of high risk CAD patients [1]. However, clopidogrel therapy, the most widely used P2Y$_{12}$ receptor blocker, is associated with widely variable pharmacodynamic response where approximately one in three clopidogrel-treated patients will have high platelet reactivity (HPR). The HPR measured peri-procedurally has been strongly linked to PCI ischemic event occurrence in observational studies of thousands of patients. Despite the fundamental importance of unblocked P2Y$_{12}$ receptors in the genesis of thrombosis, the clear demonstration of clopidogrel non-responsiveness, and their strong link to increased post-PCI ischemic risk, cardiologists largely do not determine platelet function in their high risk patients treated with clopidogrel. In comparison to the objective assessments and adjustments frequently made during treatment with most other cardiovascular drugs, this "non-selective" or "one-size-fits-all" approach to clopidogrel, the most widely used P2Y$_{12}$ inhibitor to prevent a catastrophic thrombotic event occurrence, is paradoxical [1–3].

There has been a long-term reluctance to assess platelet function because of the potential introduction of artifacts by laboratory methods, incomplete reflection of the actual *in vivo* thrombotic process, and failure to establish unequivocally a causal relation between the results of the test and thrombotic event occurrence [4]. In the last decade, the understanding of platelet receptor physiology has markedly improved, more potent P2Y$_{12}$ receptor blockers which

can overcome some of the limitations of clopidogrel have been developed, and cheaper generic clopidogrel is available. In addition, more user-friendly platelet function assays which can reliably determine the antiplatelet effect of P2Y$_{12}$ receptor blockers have stimulated great interest in therapy monitoring and personalized therapy [5,6].

Initial evidence for HPR to ADP as a risk factor

In 2003, the response variability and resistance of clopidogrel was first demonstrated using conventional platelet aggregometry and flow cytometry studies in patients undergoing PCI who had received a 300-mg loading dose followed by 75 mg/day maintenance dose of clopidogrel [7]. Since then, numerous similar observations using various assays to measure ADP-induced platelet reactivity have been made in subsequent studies involving thousands of PCI patients, which indicate clopidogrel non-responsiveness where a substantial percentage of patients (up to 35%) exhibit either negligible or no antiplatelet response to clopidogrel [5,6].

Most translational research studies linking ADP-induced platelet aggregation during clopidogrel administration to clinical outcomes were performed in patients undergoing PCI. Barragan *et al.* [8] reported an association between post-treatment P2Y$_{12}$ reactivity measured by vasodilator-stimulated phosphoprotein phosphorylation (VASP-P) assay and the occurrence of stent thrombosis in a case–control study of PCI patients. Matetzky *et al.* [9] observed that patients undergoing primary PCI for ST-segment elevation myocardial infarction (STEMI) who were in the lowest quartile of clopidogrel responsiveness (measured by aggregometry) had the highest rates of ischemic events during follow-up.

Given the interindividual variability in baseline ADP-induced platelet aggregation, the measurement of clopidogrel responsiveness (absolute or relative changes in platelet aggregation from baseline) may overestimate ischemic risk in non-responders with low pre-treatment reactivity as well as underestimating risk in responders who remain with high platelet reactivity after treatment [10,11]. Therefore, the absolute level of platelet reactivity during treatment

Interventional Cardiology: Principles and Practice, Second Edition. Edited by George D. Dangas, Carlo Di Mario, and Nicholas N. Kipshidze.
© 2017 John Wiley & Sons, Ltd. Published 2017 by John Wiley & Sons, Ltd.

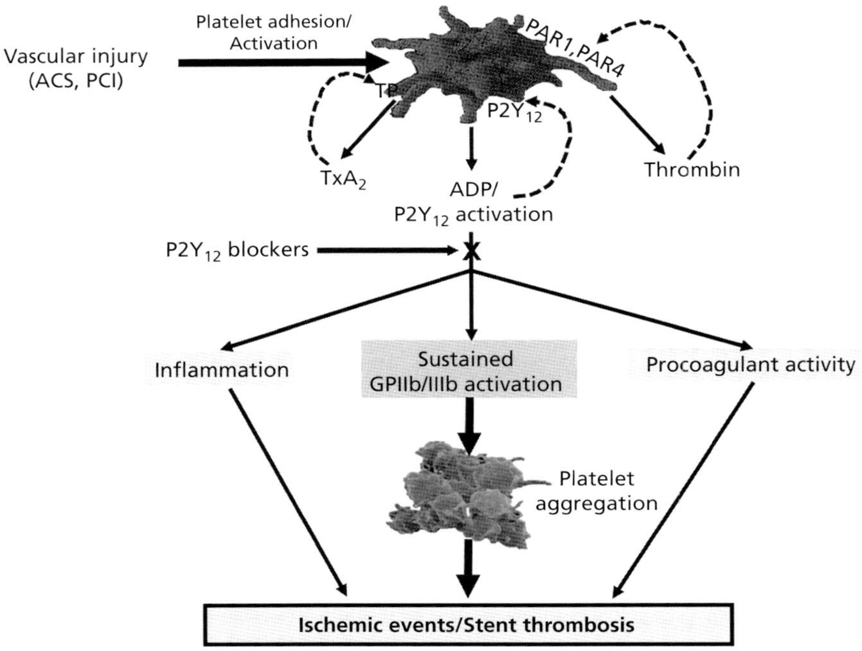

Figure 47.1 Central role of ADP-P2Y$_{12}$ interaction in platelet aggregation and ischemic event occurrence during percutaneous coronary intervention.

(i.e., on-treatment platelet reactivity) has been proposed as a better measure of thrombotic risk than responsiveness to clopidogrel. Subsequent studies based on aggregometry demonstrated that a threshold of ~50% maximal peri-procedural aggregation (20 µmol ADP) was strongly associated with 6-month ischemic event occurrence; ~40% aggregation (20 µmol ADP) was associated with stent thrombosis occurrence and ~46% pre-procedural platelet aggregation (5 µmol ADP) among patients before stenting was associated with 24 month post-PCI ischemic event occurrence [12–14]. Using the VerifyNow P2Y$_{12}$ assay, it was demonstrated that patients with post-treatment reactivity ≥235 PRU (upper quartile) had significantly higher rates of cardiovascular death (2.8% vs. 0%; p = 0.04) and stent thrombosis (4.6% vs. 0%; p = 0.004) [15]. Low responders as indicated by upper quintile (~416 AU*min) using the Multiplate analyzer, had a significantly higher risk of definite stent thrombosis and a higher mortality rate within 30 days compared with normal responders [16]. These initial studies stimulated a great interest in platelet function testing (PFT) in patients undergoing PCI during DAPT in identifying patients at high risk for recurrent ischemic event occurrences.

HPR cut-off values defined by receiver operating characteristic curve analysis

Receiver operating characteristic (ROC) curve analysis was used to define a threshold or cut-point of on-treatment platelet reactivity associated with the optimal combination of sensitivity and specificity to identify thrombotic and/or ischemic risk. A consensus statement was proposed with HPR cut-off values based on ROC curve analysis for various platelet function assays [5,6].

In a time-dependent covariate Cox regression analysis of on-treatment platelet reactivity in the GRAVITAS (Gauging Responsiveness with A VerifyNow assay—Impact on Thrombosis And Safety) study (n = 2214), HPR defined as a P2Y$_{12}$ reaction units (PRU) <208 was an independent predictor of event-free survival at 60 days (hazard ratio

[HR] 0.23; p = 0.047) and strongly trended to be an independent predictor at 6 months (HR 0.54; p = 0.06) [17]. In the multinational prospective registry study ADAPT-DES (Assessment of Dual AntiPlatelet Therapy with Drug-Eluting Stents) involving >8500 patients (~50% of patients with ACS), 43% of patients met the criteria of HPR (>208 PRU) and PRU >208 was independently associated with an ~4.0, 1.5, and 1.8-fold increase in the risk of definite or probable stent thrombosis at 0–30 days (HR 3.90, 95% confidence interval [CI] 1.90–8.00; p <0.0001), 30 days to 1 year (HR 1.55, 95% CI 0.76–3.18; p = 0.23), and 2 years (HR 1.84; p = 0.009), respectively. PRU >208 identified the risk for definite or probable stent thrombosis in 35% of patients [18,19]. The relationship between HPR and ischemic event occurrences was more pronounced in patients with ACS than patients with stable CAD (adjusted HR 2.60, p <0.005 and HR 1.44, p = 0.47, respectively). Finally, in a recent meta-analysis of 20 observational studies comprising a total of 9187 PCI patients, HPR (>208 PRU) was demonstrated to be a strong predictor of myocardial infarction, stent thrombosis, and the composite endpoint of reported ischemic events (odds ratio [OR] 3.0, 4.1, and 4.9, respectively; p < 0.00001 for all cases) [20].

Randomized trials of platelet function testing

In the GRAVITAS trial, primarily stable and low risk PCI patients with HPR (≥230 PRU) were randomized to 75 mg/day standard or 150 mg/day high clopidogrel dosing. High dose clopidogrel treatment was ineffective in reducing 6-month composite ischemic event occurrence and there was an unexpectedly low event rate (2.3%) in both groups [21]. The pharmacodynamic effect of high dose clopidogrel was relatively modest (~40% of the patients still had HPR) and unlikely to influence clinical outcomes in an overall low risk population [22]. In support of this hypothesis, in the ELEVATE-TIMI 51 trial, up to 225 mg/day clopidogrel dose was required to overcome HPR [23].

In the TRIGGER-PCI trial, the effects of a more potent active arm (prasugrel) compared with standard dose clopidogrel in low risk patients with HPR (>208 PRU) undergoing non-urgent PCI was investigated [24]. This trial was prematurely terminated because of a very low incidence of cardiovascular events. Finally, in the ARCTIC study, 2440 low risk patients (27% NST-ACS vs. 73% patients with stable CAD) scheduled for planned coronary stenting were randomly assigned to a strategy of platelet-function monitoring and drug adjustment or to a conventional strategy without monitoring. In the monitoring arm, one-third of patients had HPR (>235 PRU or <15% inhibition) before stent implantation and 80% of these patients received additional clopidogrel loading dose for PCI while only 2.3% received prasugrel loading doses. The primary endpoint was not different in the monitoring arm compared to the conventional arm (34.6% vs. 31.1%, HR 1.13; p = 0.10) [25]. In totality, these recent studies that included low risk patients undergoing PCI with low event rates demonstrate that high dose clopidogrel is not an optimal strategy to overcome HPR and suggest that future personalized antiplatelet therapy trials should focus on enrolling high risk patients undergoing PCI and treating patients with HPR with prasugrel or ticagrelor. In addition, potent $P2Y_{12}$ receptor blocker should be administered as soon as possible—even before PCI—to prevent early events.

While the results of the latter three randomized trials were negative, smaller studies have suggested that the PFT-directed approach may be effective with proper implementation. In two small multicenter studies, a strategy of tailoring incremental loading doses of clopidogrel to reduce on-treatment platelet reactivity below the HPR cut-off based on the VASP-P before PCI was associated with significantly reduced adverse event occurrence, including early stent thrombosis without increasing thrombolysis in myocardial infarction (TIMI) major or minor bleeding [26,27]. Similarly, two other studies have suggested that the selective administration of a glycoprotein IIb/IIIa receptor inhibitor to patients undergoing elective PCI who were identified as poor responders to acetylsalicylic acid or clopidogrel was effective in reducing both 30-day and 1-year post-PCI ischemic events without increasing bleeding rates [28,29]. In a recent study, Aradi *et al.* [30] demonstrated that patients with ACS undergoing successful PCI and identified as having HPR during clopidogrel therapy using the multiplate device and switching to prasugrel exhibited reduced thrombotic and bleeding events to a level similar to that of those without HPR treated with clopidogrel.

A meta-analysis of nine randomized trials demonstrated a significant reduction in cardiovascular mortality and stent thrombosis in HPR patients when intensified antiplatelet therapy was used [31]. Of interest, the benefit was mostly observed in high risk patients, suggesting that other factors, including demographic, clinical, and angiographic factors, must also be taken into consideration to identify the patients at greatest risk. For this purpose, recent studies have suggested that adding clinical variables and genotype to platelet reactivity measurements (a combined risk factor) could improve risk prediction [32,33].

Relation between low on-treatment platelet reactivity and bleeding: the therapeutic window concept

In addition to the upper threshold for ischemic risk (i.e., HPR), small translational research studies have suggested a relation between low on-treatment platelet reactivity (LPR) with bleeding

(Table 47.1) [34–40]. Unlike arterial ischemic events that are mainly platelet-centric, the underlying mechanisms of bleeding during PCI are more complex and heterogeneous in origin. The role that platelet function has in these different types of bleeding might vary, and it might be related to the extent of impaired hemostatic potential and possibly a higher degree of platelet inhibition. The concept of a "therapeutic window" of $P2Y_{12}$ receptor reactivity associated with both ischemic event occurrence (upper threshold, HPR) and bleeding risk (lower threshold, LPR) has been proposed [41]. Based on observational studies, various cut-offs for HPR and LPR are presented in Table 47.2 [35,37,38,40]. These cut-offs could be used in future studies of personalized antiplatelet therapy. This approach is more meaningful while titrating the dose of more potent $P2Y_{12}$ receptor blockers that are known to be associated with increased incidences of bleeding.

Relation of platelet reactivity to bleeding during surgery

In patients undergoing coronary artery bypass grafting (CABG), withdrawal of a $P2Y_{12}$ receptor blocker treatment for 5–7 days is recommended by the guidelines to avoid excessive peri-operative bleeding by allowing platelet function recovery [42,43]. As clopidogrel therapy is associated with response variability and nonresponsiveness, it was suggested that an objective measurement of the antiplatelet effect of clopidogrel before surgery can obviate the need for the recommended waiting period in a substantial percentage of patients. In support of this hypothesis, in the prospective Time Based Strategy to Reduce Clopidogrel Associated Bleeding During CABG (TARGET CABG) study, clopidogrel response was measured by thrombelastography with platelet mapping and surgery was scheduled with no delay in those with ADP-induced maximum amplitude (MA_{ADP}) >50 mm, within 3–5 days in those with MA_{ADP} = 35–50 mm, and after 5 days in those with MA_{ADP} <35 mm. This study demonstrated that stratifying clopidogrel-treated patients to specific waiting periods based on a preoperative assessment of clopidogrel response resulted in similar peri-operative bleeding compared to clopidogrel-naïve patients undergoing elective first time on-pump CABG [44]. Despite the absence of evidence from a large-scale prospective trial, in the 2012 Society of Thoracic Surgeons Guideline for cardiovascular surgeons, it was stated that "For patients on dual antiplatelet therapy, it is reasonable to make decisions about surgical delay based on tests of platelet inhibition rather than arbitrary use of a specified period of surgical delay. Class IIa (Level B)" [45].

HPR in patients with STEMI during prasugrel and ticagrelor therapy

An accumulating body of data suggests that drug absorption in patients with ACS is impaired, particularly in patients with STEMI. Impaired bioavailability of clopidogrel in patients with STEMI, resulting in suboptimal platelet inhibition compared with healthy controls, has been demonstrated [46]. In a recent prospective, single-blind study, 55 STEMI patients undergoing PCI were randomized to either ticagrelor or prasugrel; platelet reactivity measured by VerifyNow did not differ significantly between ticagrelor and prasugrel therapy at 1 hour. However, HPR at 2 hours persisted in a significant percentage of patients in both groups and again differ from the findings in stable, non-PCI patients where the frequency of high on-treatment platelet reactivity

Table 47.1 Relation between platelet function measurement and bleeding in patients treated with PCI.

Study	Patients (n) and P2Y$_{12}$ treatment	Platelet function test(s)	Bleeding criteria	Outcome
Cuisset et al. [34]	NSTE-ACS (n = 597), clopidogrel	LTA preheparin ADP-induced aggregation and VASP-PRI	Non-CABG, TIMI major and minor	<40% aggregation associated with higher risk of 30 days post-discharge bleeding
Sibbing et al. [35]	PCI (n = 2533) clopidogrel	Multiplate analyzer, ADP-induced aggregation	Procedure-related non-CABG TIMI major bleeding	<19 AU/min associated with 3.5× bleeding
Mokhtar et al. [36]	PCI (n = 346) Clopidogrel, retrospective analysis	VASP Assay	Non-CABG TIMI minor and major	Low on treatment PRI independent predictor of bleedings
Gurbel et al. [37]	PCI (n = 225) clopidogrel	MA-ADP TEG platelet mapping assay		≤31 MA-ADP associated with post-PCI bleeding
Campo et al. [38]	PCI (n = 300), Clopidogrel	VerifyNow P2Y$_{12}$ assay	TIMI bleeding	<85 PRU was associated with bleeding events >238 PRU was associated with ischemic events
Parodi et al. [39]	PCI (n = 298) prasugrel	LTA	Entry site bleeding	LPR associated with bleeding
Bonello et al. [40]	ACS patients undergoing PCI (n = 301) prasugrel	VASP Assay	Major and minor TIMI bleeding	VASP-PRI <16% associated with major bleedings

ADP, adenosine diphosphate; AU, arbitrary aggregation units; CAD, coronary artery disease; DAPT, dual antiplatelet therapy; DES, drug-eluting stent; LTA, light transmittance aggregometry; MA, maximum amplitude; NSTE-ACS, non-ST-segment elevation acute coronary syndrome; PA, platelet aggregation; PCI, percutaneous coronary intervention; TIMI, thrombolysis in myocardial infarction.

Table 47.2 Platelet reactivity cut-off associated with ischemic and bleeding events (therapeutic window).

	Cut-off associated with ischemic event occurrences	Cut-off associated with bleeding event occurrences [ref]
VerifyNow P2Y$_{12}$ Assay (PRU)	>208	<85 [18,38]
Multiplate Analyzer ADP-induced aggregation (AU)	>46	<19 [35]
Vasodilator Stimulated Phosphoprotein Phosphorylation-Platelet Reactivity Index (%)	≥50%	<16% [40]
Thrombelastography Platelet Mapping Assay ADP-induced Platelet-fibrin clot strength (mm)	>47	<31 [37]

was negligible [47]. In another study of 50 patients with STEMI undergoing primary PCI on bivalirudin monotherapy, patients were randomly treated with 60 mg prasugrel loading dose or 180 mg ticagrelor loading dose. Both prasugrel and ticagrelor therapy was only effective in inhibiting platelet reactivity in ~50% of patients at 2 hours. At least 4 hours were required to achieve effective platelet inhibition in ~80% of patients. Interestingly, morphine use was associated with a delayed activity of both agents [48]. In a subsequent study of healthy volunteers, morphine use was associated with delayed clopidogrel absorption and reduced clopidogrel active metabolite levels which were accom-

panied by delayed maximum platelet inhibition (up to 4 hours) [49]. At this time, the clinical significance of HPR in patients with STEMI during prasugrel or ticagrelor therapy is unknown.

Conclusions

Currently, there is conclusive pharmacodynamic evidence that clopidogrel has a suboptimal effect in a substantial proportion of patients and HPR is strongly associated with poorer clinical outcomes in high risk clopidogrel-treated patients who have undergone PCI. Most of the studies linking HPR to thrombotic event occurrence have employed a peri-procedural platelet reactivity measurement. HPR may be most predictive of event occurrence in high risk patients. Recent data indicate that prasugrel and ticagrelor therapy is also associated with non-responsiveness, particularly soon after stenting in high risk patients (although <10%). The primary goal of PFT is to identify the patient who is suboptimally responsive and to adjust therapy accordingly to reduce the risk for the catastrophic events of MI and stent thrombosis. Genotyping predicts who is at risk of being suboptimally responsive but does not replace PFT.

Recent prospective, randomized trials have failed to demonstrate that personalized antiplatelet therapy based on platelet function is effective in reducing ischemic event occurrences. It should be acknowledged that randomized trials of personalized antiplatelet therapy are associated with major limitations, such as the enrollment of low risk patients, which resulted in low event rates and lack of power—and the use of high dose clopidogrel, which is not an optimal strategy to overcome HPR and to improve clinical outcomes. Therefore, the results of these randomized trials should not be used to refute the utility of PFT or personalized antiplatelet therapy strategies.

Treatment with more potent $P2Y_{12}$ receptor blockers, such as prasugrel and ticagrelor, is associated with faster and greater platelet inhibition than clopidogrel therapy and is a credible alternative strategy to overcome HPR during clopidogrel therapy. Therefore, a reasonable strategy is to assess platelet function in high risk clopidogrel-treated patients (e.g., patients with current or prior ACS, a history of stent thrombosis and target vessel revascularization, poor left ventricular function, multivessel stenting, complex anatomy (bifurcation, long, small stents), high body mass index, diabetes mellitus, and patients co-treated with proton pump inhibitors) and use of more potent $P2Y_{12}$ receptor therapy selectively in the patient with HPR. Unselected therapy with the new $P2Y_{12}$ receptor blockers is associated with increased bleeding. It is also important to note that clopidogrel results in an adequate $P2Y_{12}$ receptor inhibition in about two-thirds of the patients undergoing PCI. Selectively treating these patients with generic clopidogrel rather than treating all patients with new and potent $P2Y_{12}$ inhibitors might provide significant cost savings.

Moreover, rather than ischemic events alone, both ischemic and bleeding events (net clinical outcome) should be considered as a primary composite endpoint. This will not only increase the event rate, but also improve overall clinical outcome in the presence of more potent $P2Y_{12}$ receptor blocker therapies that are known to be associated with increased bleeding events. It is crucial to capture early events that are platelet-centric and that are significantly influenced by improved treatment strategies. It was also suggested that serial PFT can facilitate the modification of treatment strategies over time and improve net clinical outcomes. Currently, two large-scale studies of personalized antiplatelet therapy (ANTARCTIC [NCT01538446] and TROPICAL-ACS [NCT01959451]) are under way.

In the absence of evidence from a superiority trial, at this time we must rely on the guidelines and the existing observational data while fully keeping in mind the role that platelet physiology has in catastrophic event occurrence in the stented patient. Finally, it is not practical and wise to ignore the strong evidence that:

1 HPR is associated with post-PCI ischemic event occurrences;
2 User-friendly and reliable assays are available to assess platelet function;
3 More potent $P2Y_{12}$ receptor blockers are available to overcome HPR in 35% of patients;
4 Nearly 65% of patients without HPR can be optimally treated with less expensive generic clopidogrel; and
5 Excessive bleeding can be avoided and net clinical outcome can be improved by utilizing serial PFT in patients treated with the more potent $P2Y_{12}$ receptor blockers.

The therapeutic window concept for the $P2Y_{12}$ receptor blocker therapy can facilitate the balance between reducing ischemic events and avoiding bleeding events, thereby improving net clinical outcome. PFT can have a role to monitor: (i) efficacy when clopidogrel is the chosen therapy; and (ii) safety of the long-term use of new, more potent drugs, especially in low risk patients and in patients with high bleeding risk. Finally, platelet reactivity should not be regarded as an absolute and sole prognostic marker, instead platelet reactivity should be evaluated in combination with demographic variables associated with risk, the time of platelet reactivity testing with respect to the time of PCI and the presence of ACS.

Disclosures

Dr. Gurbel reports serving as a consultant, receiving fees/honoraria from Daiichi Sankyo, Lilly, Bayer, AstraZeneca, Merck, Boehringer, Janssen, and CSL; receiving grants from the National Institutes of Health, Daiichi Sankyo/Lilly, CSL, AstraZeneca, Harvard Clinical Research Institute, Bayer, Haemonetics, Duke Clinical Research Institute, Sinnowa, Coramed, and Accumetrics. Other authors report no conflict of interest.

Interactive multiple choice questions are available for this chapter on www.wiley.com/go/dangas/cardiology

References

1 Gurbel PA, Tantry US. Do platelet function testing and genotyping improve outcome in patients treated with antithrombotic agents?: platelet function testing and genotyping improve outcome in patients treated with antithrombotic agents. *Circulation* 2012; **125**: 1276–1287.

2 Gurbel PA, Tantry US. Combination antithrombotic therapies. *Circulation* 2010; **121**: 569–583.

3 Gurbel PA, Rafeedheen R, Tantry US. Update: acute coronary syndromes (V). Personalized antiplatelet therapy. *Rev Esp Cardiol* 2014; **67**: 480–487.

4 Hirsh J. Hyperactive platelets and complications of coronary artery disease. *N Engl J Med* 1987; **316**: 1543–1544.

5 Bonello L, Tantry US, Marcucci R, et al. Working Group on high on treatment platelet reactivity: consensus and future directions on the definition of high on treatment platelet reactivity to adenosine diphosphate. *J Am Coll Cardiol* 2010; **56**: 919–933.

6 Tantry US, Bonello L, Aradi D, et al. Working Group on On-Treatment Platelet Reactivity. Consensus and update on the definition of on-treatment platelet reactivity to adenosine diphosphate associated with ischemia and bleeding. *J Am Coll Cardiol* 2013; **62**: 2261–2273.

7 Gurbel PA, Bliden KP, Hiatt BL, et al. Clopidogrel for coronary stenting: response variability, drug resistance, and the effect of pretreatment platelet reactivity. *Circulation* 2003; **107**: 2908–2913.

8 Barragan P, Bouvier JL, Roquebert PO, et al. Resistance to thienopyridines: clinical detection of coronary stent thrombosis by monitoring of vasodilator-stimulated phosphoprotein phosphorylation. *Catheter Cardiovasc Interv* 2003; **59**: 295–302.

9 Matetzky S, Shenkman B, Guetta V, et al. Clopidogrel resistance is associated with increased risk of recurrent atherothrombotic events in patients with acute myocardial infarction. *Circulation* 2004; **109**: 3171–3175.

10 Samara WM, Bliden KP, Tantry US, et al. The difference between clopidogrel responsiveness and posttreatment platelet reactivity. *Thromb Res* 2005; **115**: 89–94.

11 Michelson AD, Linden MD, Furman MI, et al. Evidence that pre-existent variability in platelet response to ADP accounts for "clopidogrel resistance." *J Thromb Haemost* 2007; **5**: 75–81.

12 Gurbel PA, Bliden KP, Guyer K, *et al.* Platelet reactivity in patients and recurrent events post-stenting: results of the Prepare Poststenting Study. *J Am Coll Cardiol* 2005; **46**: 1820–1826.

13 Gurbel PA, Bliden KP, Samara W, *et al.* The clopidogrel Resistance and Stent Thrombosis (CREST) study. *J Am Coll Cardiol* 2005; **46**: 1827–1832.

14 Gurbel PA, Antonino MJ, Bliden KP, *et al.* Platelet reactivity to adenosine diphosphate and long-term ischemic event occurrence following percutaneous coronary intervention: a potential antiplatelet therapeutic target. *Platelets* 2008; **19**: 595–604.

15 Price MJ, Endemann S, Gollapudi RR, *et al.* Prognostic significance of post-clopidogrel platelet reactivity assessed by a point-of-care assay on thrombotic events after drug-eluting stent implantation. *Eur Heart J* 2008; **29**: 992–1000.

16 Sibbing D, Braun S, Morath T, *et al.* Platelet reactivity after clopidogrel treatment assessed with point-of-care analysis and early drug-eluting stent thrombosis. *J Am Coll Cardiol* 2009; **53**: 849–56.

17 Price MJ, Angiolillo DJ, Teirstein PS, *et al.* Platelet reactivity and cardiovascular outcomes after percutaneous coronary intervention: a time-dependent analysis of the Gauging Responsiveness with a VerifyNow P2Y12 assay: Impact on Thrombosis and Safety (GRAVITAS) trial. *Circulation* 2011; **124**: 1132–1137.

18 Stone GW, Witzenbichler B, Weisz G, *et al.,* for the ADAPT-DES Investigators. Platelet reactivity and clinical outcomes after coronary artery implantation of drug-eluting stents (ADAPT-DES): a prospective multicentre registry study. *Lancet* 2013; **382**: 614–623.

19 Stuckey TD, Kirtane AJ, Brodie BR, *et al.* for the ADAPT-DES investigators. *ADAPT-DES two-year results: relation between high platelet reactivity on clopidogrel and outcomes after DES implantation: two year results from the ADAPT-DES study.* Presented at 25th TCT meetings; Washington DC; 2013.

20 Aradi D, Komócsi A, Vorobcsuk A, *et al.* Prognostic significance of high on-clopidogrel platelet reactivity after percutaneous coronary intervention: systematic review and meta-analysis. *Am Heart J* 2010; **160**: 543–551.

21 Price MJ, Berger PB, Teirstein PS, *et al.* GRAVITAS Investigators. Standard- vs high-dose clopidogrel based on platelet function testing after percutaneous coronary intervention: the GRAVITAS randomized trial. *JAMA* 2011; **305**: 1097–1105.

22 Gurbel PA, Tantry US. An initial experiment with personalized antiplatelet therapy: the GRAVITAS trial. *JAMA* 2011; **305**: 1136–1137.

23 Mega JL, Hochholzer W, Frelinger AL 3rd, *et al.* Dosing clopidogrel based on CYP2C19 genotype and the effect on platelet reactivity in patients with stable cardiovascular disease. *JAMA* 2011; **306**: 2221–2228.

24 Trenk D, Stone GW, Gawaz M, *et al.* A randomized trial of prasugrel versus clopidogrel in patients with high platelet reactivity on clopidogrel after elective percutaneous coronary intervention with implantation of drug-eluting stents: results of the TRIGGER-PCI (Testing Platelet Reactivity In Patients Undergoing Elective Stent Placement on Clopidogrel to Guide Alternative Therapy With Prasugrel) study. *J Am Coll Cardiol* 2012; **59**: 2159–2164.

25 Collet JP, Cuisset T, Rangé G, *et al.* ARCTIC Investigators. Bedside monitoring to adjust antiplatelet therapy for coronary stenting. *N Engl J Med* 2012; **367**: 2100–2109.

26 Bonello L, Camoin-Jau L, Arques S, *et al.* Adjusted clopidogrel loading doses according to vasodilator-stimulated phosphoprotein phosphorylation index decrease rate of major adverse cardiovascular events in patients with clopidogrel resistance: a multicenter randomized prospective study. *J Am Coll Cardiol* 2008; **51**: 1404–1411.

27 Bonello L, Camoin-Jau L, Armero S, *et al.* Tailored clopidogrel loading dose according to platelet reactivity monitoring to prevent acute and subacute stent thrombosis. *Am J Cardiol* 2009; **103**: 5–10.

28 Valgimigli M, Campo G, de Cesare N, *et al.;* Tailoring Treatment With Tirofiban in Patients Showing Resistance to Aspirin and/or Resistance to Clopidogrel (3T/2R) Investigators. Intensifying platelet inhibition with tirofiban in poor responders to aspirin, clopidogrel, or both agents undergoing elective coronary intervention: results from the double-blind, prospective, randomized Tailoring Treatment with Tirofiban in Patients Showing Resistance to Aspirin and/or Resistance to Clopidogrel study. *Circulation* 2009; **119**: 3215–3222.

29 Cuisset T, Frere C, Quilici J, *et al.* Glycoprotein IIb/IIIa inhibitors improve outcome after coronary stenting in clopidogrel nonresponders: a prospective, randomized study. *JACC Cardiovasc Interv* 2008; **1**: 649–653.

30 Aradi D, Tornyos A, Pintér T, *et al.* Optimizing P2Y12 receptor inhibition in patients with acute coronary syndrome on the basis of platelet function testing: impact of prasugrel and high-dose clopidogrel. *J Am Coll Cardiol* 2014; **63**: 1061–1070.

31 Aradi D, Komócsi A, Price MJ, *et al.,* for the Tailored Antiplatelet Treatment Study Collaboration. Efficacy and safety of intensified antiplatelet therapy on the basis of platelet reactivity testing in patients after percutaneous coronary intervention: systematic review and metaanalysis. *Int J Cardiol* 2013; **167**: 2140–2148.

32 Geisler T, Grass D, Bigalke B, *et al.* The Residual Platelet Aggregation After Deployment of Intracoronary Stent (PREDICT) score. *J Thromb Haemost* 2008; **6**: 54–61.

33 Fontana P, Berdagué P, Castelli C, *et al.* Clinical predictors of dual aspirin and clopidogrel poor responsiveness in stable cardiovascular patients from the ADRIE study. *J Thromb Haemost* 2010; **8**: 2614–2623.

34 Cuisset T, Cayla G, Frere C, *et al.* Predictive value of post-treatment platelet reactivity for occurrence of post-discharge bleeding after non-ST elevation acute coronary syndrome. Shifting from antiplatelet resistance to bleeding risk assessment? *EuroIntervention* 2009; **5**: 325–329.

35 Sibbing D, Schulz S, Braun S, *et al.* Antiplatelet effects of clopidogrel and bleeding in patients undergoing coronary stent placement. *J Thromb Haemost* 2010; **8**: 250–256.

36 Mokhtar OA, Lemesle G, Armero S, *et al.* Relationship between platelet reactivity inhibition and non-CABG related major bleeding in patients undergoing percutaneous coronary intervention. *Thromb Res* 2010; **126**: 147–149.

37 Gurbel PA, Bliden KP, Navickas IA, *et al.* Adenosine diphosphate-induced platelet-fibrin clot strength: a new thrombelastographic indicator of long-term poststenting ischemic events. *Am Heart J* 2010; **160**: 346–354.

38 Campo G, Parrinello G, Ferraresi P, *et al.* Prospective evaluation of on-clopidogrel platelet reactivity over time in patients treated with percutaneous coronary intervention relationship with gene polymorphisms and clinical outcome. *J Am Coll Cardiol* 2011; **57**: 2474–2483.

39 Parodi G, Bellandi B, Venditti F, *et al.* Residual platelet reactivity, bleedings, and adherence to treatment in patients having coronary stent implantation treated with prasugrel. *Am J Cardiol* 2012; **109**: 214–218.

40 Bonello L, Mancini J, Pansieri M, *et al.* Relationship between posttreatment platelet reactivity and ischemic and bleeding events at 1-year follow-up in patients receiving prasugrel. *J Thromb Haemost* 2012; **10**: 1999–2005.

41 Gurbel PA, Becker RC, Mann KG, *et al.* Platelet function monitoring in patients with coronary artery disease. *J Am Coll Cardiol* 2007; **50**: 1822–1834.

42 Hamm CW, Bassand JP, Agewall S, *et al.* ESC Guidelines for the management of acute coronary syndromes in patients presenting without persistent ST-segment elevation: the task force for the management of acute coronary syndromes (ACS) in patients presenting without persistent ST-segment elevation of the European Society of Cardiology (ESC). *Eur Heart J* 2011; **32**: 2999–3054.

43 Levine GN, Bates ER, Blankenship JC, *et al.* American College of Cardiology Foundation; American Heart Association Task Force on Practice Guidelines; Society for Cardiovascular Angiography and Interventions. 2011 ACCF/AHA/ SCAI Guideline for Percutaneous Coronary Intervention. A report of the American College of Cardiology Foundation/American Heart Association Task Force on Practice Guidelines and the Society for Cardiovascular Angiography and Interventions. *J Am Coll Cardiol* 2011; **58**: e44–122.

44 Mahla E, Suarez TA, Bliden KP, *et al.* Platelet function measurement-based strategy to reduce bleeding and waiting time in clopidogrel-treated patients undergoing coronary artery bypass graft surgery: the timing based on platelet function strategy to reduce clopidogrel-associated bleeding related to CABG (TARGET-CABG) Study. *Circ Cardiovasc Interv* 2012; **5**: 261–269.

45 Ferraris VA, Saha SP, Oestreich JH, *et al.* Society of Thoracic Surgeons. 2012 update to the Society of Thoracic Surgeons guideline on use of antiplatelet drugs in patients having cardiac and noncardiac operations. *Ann Thorac Surg* 2012; **94**: 1761–1781.

46 Heestermans AA, van Werkum JW, Taubert D, *et al.* Impaired bioavailability of clopidogrel in patients with a ST-segment elevation myocardial infarction. *Thromb Res* 2008; **122**: 776–781.

47 Alexopoulos D, Xanthopoulou I, Gkizas V, *et al.* Randomized assessment of ticagrelor versus prasugrel antiplatelet effects in patients with ST-segment-elevation myocardial infarction. *Circ Cardiovasc Interv* 2012; **6**: 797–804.

48 Parodi G, Valenti R, Bellandi B, *et al.* Comparison of prasugrel and ticagrelor loading doses in ST-segment elevation myocardial infarction patients: RAPID (Rapid Activity of Platelet Inhibitor Drugs) primary PCI study. *J Am Coll Cardiol* 2013; **61**: 1601–1606.

49 Hobl EL, Stimpfl T, Ebner J, *et al.* Morphine decreases clopidogrel concentrations and effects: a randomized, double blind, placebo-controlled trial. *J Am Coll Cardiol* 2014; **63**: 630–635.

CHAPTER 48

Genetics and Pharmacogenetics in Interventional Cardiology

Hillary Johnston-Cox, Johan L.M. Björkegren, and Jason C. Kovacic
Icahn School of Medicine at Mount Sinai, New York, NY, USA

Heritability accounts for the number of observed differences in a disease trait because of inherited genetic differences between people. While other mechanisms like epigenetic modification of deoxyribonucleic acid (DNA) likely also contribute to inheritance, most inherited differences are thought to be carried by changes to the nucleotide DNA sequence (i.e., A, T, C, and G; Figure 48.1). Although environmental and genetic influences were initially thought to be independent factors contributing to disease, it is now appreciated that the interaction of genetic and environmental factors is a major element contributing to an ultimate clinical disease phenotype such as coronary artery disease (CAD). As we elaborate later, it now appears that the absence or presence of environmental factors, such as presence of smoking or lack of exercise, can determine if a genetic factor will contribute to the pathogenesis of disease. As becomes evident in this chapter, the redirecting of our scientific efforts toward understanding aspects of CAD, such as the biologic intersection point of genetics–genomics and environmental influences using systems genetics, is potentially of very high yield in terms of advancing our understanding of the causality of this disease. This chapter focuses on reviewing the genetics of CAD as relevant to interventional cardiology, discussing limitations to genomewide association studies (GWAS) and the knowledge gained so far, and finally proposing future directions for identifying the presently unknown genetic aspects of CAD and how this knowledge might be useful in the clinic and catheterization laboratory.

Initial focus on human genetics: rare single-gene disorders

The heritability of traits that are passed between generations is thought to be predominantly carried in DNA, manifested as alterations in DNA that include single nucleotide polymorphisms (SNPs), deletions, insertions, and copy number variants. A component of heritability that is independent of DNA [1,2] can be mediated via epigenetic mechanisms that generally involve changes in either the methylation status of DNA or in histone changes that impact DNA transcription [3]. However, epigenetic mechanisms are beyond the scope of this chapter.

Rare single-gene disorders generally arise by a single change in a DNA coding region that typically follows a known pattern of inheritance (Mendelian inheritance) between generations. Common inheritance patterns for single-gene disorders include autosomal dominant, autosomal recessive, and X-chromosome-linked inheritance. However, not all carriers of a single-gene variant that is associated with a Mendelian disorder will develop that disease, thus penetrance (the proportion of persons carrying a mutation or genetic change that develop the clinical disease) is generally <100%. Penetrance is also is a time-dependent component of disease development. For example, in cystic fibrosis (CF) and Huntington's disease (HD), these two diseases are generally 100% penetrant; CF presents in infancy and HD presents generally in late adulthood. Other single-gene disorders, like the *BRCA1* gene, have "incomplete penetrance" (<100% of persons carrying the disease-causing *BRCA1* gene develop the relevant diseases) and a lifetime penetrance risk, suggesting that there are other elements of risk including environmental and other genetic predispositions that contribute to the development of the disease. This also suggests that there are resistance variants that protect individuals from developing single-gene disorders [4], which is relevant when risk stratifying patients for management and addressing preventative measures for a disease. As further defining features of single-gene disorders and in contrast to CAD, although the penetrance of many single-gene disorders is high, the occurrence of these disorders is less than 1% in the general population. Furthermore, the frequency and phenotypic expression of these genes varies in different populations as a result of differences in genetic ancestry in those communities.

Through the study of "classic" disease phenotypes that arise with single-gene disorders and their patterns of inheritance, initial DNA-based pedigree and linkage studies were first used to understand causative variants for rare disorders showing Mendelian inheritance [5]. In summary, these techniques involve very careful clinical phenotyping of family members, and then searching for DNA changes that are apparent in the affected versus non-affected family members. The first single-gene cardiovascular disorder to be extensively studied using these techniques was familial hypertrophic cardiomyopathy, with the subsequent discovery of the missense mutation within the cardiac beta-myosin heavy chain gene. Following this, other genetic mutations for many other generally single-gene cardiovascular disorders were identified, including long QT syndrome, dilated cardiomyopathy, Wolf–Parkinson–White

Interventional Cardiology: Principles and Practice, Second Edition. Edited by George D. Dangas, Carlo Di Mario, and Nicholas N. Kipshidze.
© 2017 John Wiley & Sons, Ltd. Published 2017 by John Wiley & Sons, Ltd.

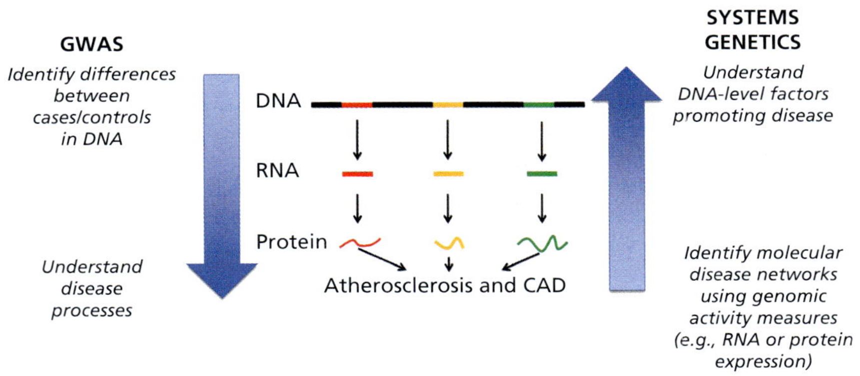

Figure 48.1 Overview of differing approaches of genomewide association studies (GWAS) versus systems genetics. Fundamentally, GWAS begins with an analysis of DNA and then attempts to define molecular processes. Systems genetics begins by studying genomic activity measures reflecting disease-relevant molecular processes (e.g., RNA or protein levels) to understand biologic disease networks that ultimately permit DNA-level changes driving these processes to be revealed.

syndrome, Brugada syndrome, and arrhythmogenic right ventricular dysplasia. Subsequent studies of other rare single-gene disorders led to the identification of mutated genes including those involved in familial hypercholesterolemia, such as mutations in the low density lipoprotein receptor (LDL-R).

While these approaches used to study single-gene disorders were highly successful and opened the door to our understanding of the genetic basis of disease, this type of approach for common complex disorders such as CAD and atherosclerosis is not broad enough to encompass the relevant biologic processes and multiple causative genes involved in the pathogenesis of these diseases [6].

Realm of GWAS: understanding the genetics of common complex disorders

Unlike single-gene disorders like those discussed above, the genetics of CAD is fundamentally more complex. CAD is one of many "polygeneic" or "common complex disorders." Unlike single-gene disorders which are rare, run in families, and are also highly heritable (i.e., they are genetically driven by typically one or only a few genes), the etiology of common complex disorders typically involves significant contributions from both genetic and environmental risk factors and their interactions. As a consequence, complex disorders are far more prevalent in the community ("common"), and are not limited to specific families. Furthermore, unlike single-gene disorders where the effect of each disease-causing genetic alteration is typically quite large, in common complex disorders the effect of each disease-relevant genetic alteration is only minimal to modest, and there are typically also many genetic alterations implicated in disease pathogenesis. Other examples of common complex disorders are diabetes, obesity, hypertension, and stroke.

The widespread prevalence and diversity of risk factors of the common complex diseases made linkage analysis of family pedigrees (as applied to single-gene disorders) inappropriate to study CAD. In addition, from the outset of investigations there was a notion that common complex disorders are driven by many genetic factors, each with weaker effects. As a consequence, a research tool allowing for the analysis of a multitude of genetic markers in thousands of individuals in the general population across families in case–control association studies was proposed to better study common complex

disorders; this was the beginning of the era of genomewide association studies (GWAS) [7]. In summary, GWAS design involves collecting large numbers of subjects with the disease ("cases") and controls without the disease and then looking for changes in DNA that are present in the cases and not the controls. Ideally, cases and controls are matched for as many non-disease-related features as possible (age, gender, race/ethnicity, and other comorbidities).

The study of CAD using GWAS first began in the Wellcome Trust Case Control Consortium, which identified the famous 9p21 locus that is associated with CAD [7–9]. Since this initial study, 153 suggestive DNA variants have been identified with GWAS, with 50 being replicated in meta-analyses of GWAS datasets [10]. These variants are prevalent in the general population but the observed effect of the variants is weak, with each conferring a minimal to modest average increase in relative risk of ~18% [7]. The ability of this approach to identify numerous genetic markers and isolate many previously unknown disease-causing genes is impressive and notable. Nevertheless, the 153 CAD-associated variants that have been identified by GWAS are responsible for only approximately 10.6% of the genetic variation of CAD in the general population [10]. Indeed, not only for CAD but for most other complex diseases, about 90% of their heritability is not explained by loci identified so far by GWAS, despite including very large GWAS sample sizes [10].

To place this information in context, it is important to also appreciate the overall contribution of the traditional risk factors versus genetics to the development of CAD. Seminal studies performed several decades ago defined that the genetic variance in CAD is 40–60% [11]. In other words, heritable factors are thought to account for about 50% of the likelihood of developing CAD, with the remaining ~50% of risk thought to be attributable to environmental and lifestyle-related risk factors such as smoking, sedentary lifestyle, obesity, salt intake, diet, and other factors. Therefore, with 50% heritability, the 153 loci identified by the GWAS explain ~5% of the overall likelihood of developing CAD (Figure 48.2). Accordingly, further study regarding independent genetic risk factors and how they are influenced by environmental factors to contribute to CAD heritability is warranted [12].

The development of more complete DNA sequencing techniques, such as whole exome/whole genome sequencing (WES/WGS) generally applied to case–control cohorts as in GWAS, could be used as a tool to identify additional rare risk variants that might have more

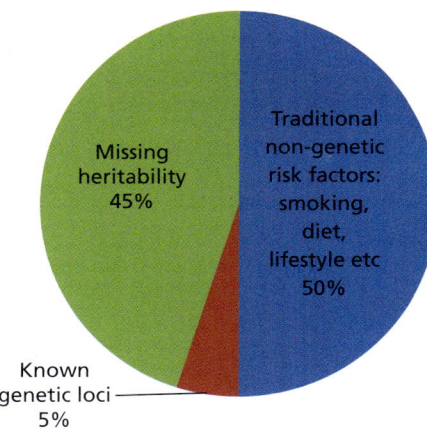

Figure 48.2 Current understanding of coronary artery disease (CAD). While traditional risk factors likely account for ~50% of the likelihood of developing CAD and ~5% is attributable to known CAD risk loci, approximately 45% of the likelihood of developing CAD is thought to be caused by currently unknown genetic factors: the "missing heritability" of CAD.

effect on heritability [13]. Preliminary findings from WES indicate, however, that the number of SNPs in coding regions (i.e., exomes) that potentially contribute to some fraction of the missing heritability of CAD is sparse. The lack of coding region SNPs associated with CAD, as discussed in more detail later, underscores the notion indicated from studies like ENCODE that risk SNPs identified by GWAS are largely situated in regulatory regions of the genome rather than in protein-coding regions [14]. Nevertheless, the next section specifically evaluates CAD and the role for genes identified in GWAS so far, and we argue that it is likely that these genes belong to a group of genes that are mostly important at specific intervals in the protracted course of the pathogenesis of CAD. We argue that those identified by GWAS might not necessarily be involved in the final culmination of CAD leading to clinical events. Thus, we believe complementary approaches beyond GWAS will be required to explain the full heritability of CAD and particularly to explain the occurrence of clinical events.

Identification and characterization of genetic risk variants for CAD and MI

Since the discovery in 2007 of the 9p21 CAD risk variant using GWAS [9,15], initial efforts focused on increasing sample sizes, defining new variants, and then replicating and confirming these findings [16]. Eventually, in order to detect risk variants with low frequency and minimal effect, large collaborative groups were founded to provide for larger sample sizes, one of which being the Coronary Artery Disease Genome-Wide Replication and Meta-Analysis (CARDIoGRAM). This meta-analysis confirmed 10 previously described risk variants as well as the identification of 13 new risk variants for CAD [17–19]. These genetic risk variants for CAD are common but with a relative risk that is usually minimal to moderate. The currently known CAD genetic risk variants are presented in Table 48.1.

Of the genetic risk variants identified for CAD, 35 of the 50 act through currently unknown mechanisms and many of these are in non-coding DNA regions, suggesting that there are several pathways that contribute to the pathogenesis of CAD that have yet to be

described. Other genetic variants have been linked to established risk factors for CAD, including those involved in lipid metabolism, such as variants related to LDL cholesterol, lipoprotein-a, apolipoprotein-B, LDL-R, apolipoprotein-E, and ABCG5. A new variant not previously associated with LDL-C includes a SNP associated with Sortilin1 (SORT1), which is thought to modulate LDL-C secretion [20]. In addition, the discovery of the PCSK9 variant has led to the development of novel agents to reduce LDL cholesterol levels (PCSK9 inhibitors) that are now in advanced stages of clinical testing [21,22].

As a relevant aspect of CAD and myocardial infarction (MI), an MI is typically caused by an occlusive thrombus that is superimposed on an atherosclerotic plaque. The acute rupture of this plaque is what precipitates the formation of a thrombus. However, the presence of CAD is the result of typically decades of slow progression of this disease process. Importantly therefore, the biology of plaque development and acute plaque rupture with thrombus formation are distinct, and consequently the genetic variants contributing to thrombus formation are distinct from those that contribute to the protracted development of atherosclerosis. The variant 9p21 is associated with both processes but likely mostly accounted for in CAD [23,24]. However, it is particularly notable that the only genetic risk variant currently associated with MI is the ABO blood group locus [24]. Multiple studies have suggested and confirmed an association between the ABO blood groups at locus 9q34.2 and MI, including CARDIoGRAM, which demonstrated an increased risk of 20% for MI with A and B risk variants [19]. Blood groups A and B encode for a protein that transfers a carbohydrate on von Willebrand factor (alpha-1-3-N-acetylgalactoseaminyltransferase); this results in a prolonged half-life of von Willebrand factor with predisposition to coronary thrombosis and subsequent MI [25]. In the Nurse's Health Study, the blood group A or B was associated with a 10% increased frequency of MI, the combination of A and B blood groups increased the risk to 20% [26]. Clearly, much remains to be understood regarding the molecular mechanisms whereby these risk loci promote CAD.

Relevance of CAD pathogenesis and clinical manifestations from a genetics perspective

It is becoming increasingly clear that the development of atherosclerotic lesions and CAD is profoundly influenced by genetic factors. While atherosclerotic biology is comprehensively covered in other chapters of this book, here we very briefly summarize what we perceive to be the key aspects related to atherosclerosis and CAD as relevant to genetic factors.

Atherosclerotic lesion development within the coronary vessels generally follows a sigmoidal-shaped (S-shaped) model, with the caveat that the late stage of atherosclerosis with plaque development and progression can be variable and include further rapid progression [27,28]. In detail, studies in both humans and mice have supported the notion that atherosclerosis develops over a long period of time, but with a period of rapid progression before a later final period of generally slowed growth [29–32]. Plaque development is initiated by retention of circulating plasma lipoproteins, predominantly LDL, at sites in the vasculature that are regions of turbulent blood flow. Some LDL particles remain within the subendothelial space and are modified by redox processes. The endothelium is activated by oxidized LDL via the expression of adhesion molecules,

Table 48.1 Fifty genetic variants currently verified as associated with coronary artery disease (CAD) or myocardial infarction (MI) by genomewide association studies (GWAS).

Nearby gene (allele)	Chromosome location	SNP	Odds ratio
Associated with LDL cholesterol			
LPA	6q25.3	rs3798220	1.92 (1.48–2.49)
APOB	2p24.1	rs515135	1.03
SORT1	1p13.3	rs599839	1.29 (1.18–1.40)
LDLR	19p13.2	rs1122608	1.14 (1.09–1.19)
APOE	19q13.32	rs2075650	1.14 (1.09–1.19)
ABCG5-ABCG8	2p21	rs6544713	1.07 (1.04–1.11)
PCSK9	1p32.3	rs11206510	1.15 (1.10–1.21)
Associated with HDL cholesterol			
ANKS1A	6p21.31	rs12205331	1.04
Associated with triglycerides			
TRIB1	8q24.13	rs10808546	1.08 (1.04–1.12)
ZNF259, APOA5-A4-C3-A1	11q23.3	rs964184	1.13 (1.10–1.16)
Associated with hypertension			
SH2B3	12q24.12	rs3184504	1.13 (1.08–1.18)
CYP127A1, CNNM2, NT5C2	10q24.32	rs12413409	1.12 (1.08–1.16)
GUCYA3	4q31.1	rs7692387	1.13
FURIN-FES	15q26.1	rs17514846	1.04
Associated with myocardial infarction			
ABO*	9q34.2	rs579459	1.10 (1.07–1.13)
Mechanism of risk unknown			
CDKN2A, CDKN2B	9p21.3	rs4977574	1.25 (1.18–1.31) to 1.37 (1.26–1.48)
MIA3	1q41	rs17465637	1.20 (1.12–1.30)
CXCL12	10q11.21	rs1746048	1.33 (1.20–1.48)
WDR12	2q33.1	rs6725887	1.16 (1.10–1.22)
PHACTR1	6p24.1	rs12526453	1.13 (1.09–1.17)
MRPS6	21q22.11	rs9982601	1.19 (1.13–1.27)
MRAS	3q22.3	rs2306374	1.15 (1.11–1.19)

Table 48.1 (Continued)

Nearby gene (allele)	Chromosome location	SNP	Odds ratio
KIAA1462	10p11.23	rs2505083	1.07 (1.04–1.09)
PPAP2B	1p32.2	rs17114036	1.17 (1.13–1.22)
IL5	5q31.1	rs2706399	1.02 (1.01–1.03)
TCF21	6q23.2	rs12190287	1.08 (1.06–1.10)
BCAP29	7q22.3	rs10953541	1.08 (1.05–1.11)
ZC3HC1	7q32.2	rs11556924	1.09 (1.07–1.12)
LIPA	10q23.31	rs1412444	1.09 (1.07–1.12)
PDGF	11q22.3	rs974819	1.07 (1.04–1.09)
COL4A1, COL4A2	13q34	rs4773144	1.07 (1.05–1.09)
HHIPL1	14q32.2	rs2895811	1.07 (1.05–1.10)
ADAMTS7	15q25.1	rs3825807	1.08 (1.06–1.10)
SMG6, SRR	17p13.3	rs216172	1.07 (1.05–1.09)
RASD1, SMCR3, PEMT	17p11.2	rs12936587	1.07 (1.05–1.09)
UBE2Z, GIP, ATP5G1, SNF8	17q21.32	rs46522	1.06 (1.04–1.08)
IRX1, ADAMTS16	5p13.3	rs11748327	1.25 (1.18–1.33)
BTN2A1	6p22.1	rs6929846	1.51 (1.28–1.77)
C6orf105	6p24.1	rs6903956	1.65 (1.44–1.90)
HCG27 and HLA-C	6p21.3	rs3869109	1.15
IL6R	1q21	rs4845625	1.09
EDNRA	Chr4	rs1878406	1.09
HDAC9	7p21.1	rs2023938	1.13
VAMP5-VAMP8	2p11.2	rs1561198	1.07
ZEB2-AC074093.1	Chr2	rs2252641	1
SLC22A4-SLC22A5	Chr5	rs273909	1.11
KCNK5	6p21	rs10947789	1.01
PLG	6q26	rs4252120	1.07
LPL	8p22	rs264	1.06
FLT1	13q12	rs9319428	1.1

CAD, coronary artery disease; CI, confidence interval; HDL, high density lipoprotein; LDL, low density lipoprotein; MI, myocardial infarction; SNP, single nucleotide polymorphism.

* Risk variant located on 9q34.2 only associated with MI, not CAD.

Source: Adapted from Roberts R. Genetics of coronary artery disease. *Circ Res* 2014; **114**: 1890–1903.

leading to transendothelial migration of leukocytes (predominantly monocytes). Within the subendothelial space and the intima, monocytes differentiate into macrophages. These macrophages uptake oxidized LDL particles, initiating foam cell formation, a key process of atherosclerosis. The accumulation of foam cells in the intima manifests as the appearance of fatty streaks on histologic examination. Aggregation of multiple foam cells leads to formation of small atherosclerotic plaques with well-defined borders [32].

The second phase of atherosclerosis involves the rapid expansion of the small plaques across the arterial wall and into the lumen of the blood vessel, leading to compromise of blood flow. Through the use of ^{14}C dating of human plaques, this rapid phase is thought to occur less than 10 years prior to clinical symptoms [30].

The third and final stage can be variable. In about 30% of the cases, rapid progression of lesions occurs over 12 months to a fibroatheroma, with encapsulation of the lipid-rich core by a thin or thick cap. The most unstable lesions are the thin-cap atheromas that lead to an acute MI. In the span of 12 months, 75% of thin-cap fibroatheromas stabilize, while 5% of the thick-cap atheromas will develop high risk features [28,33]. The rupture of a complex plaque is influenced by an interplay of multiple factors including: extent and degree of necrosis of the deposited lipid core mediated by proliferating macrophages within the plaque area; the de novo migration/emigration of monocytes; extent of luminal stenosis; plaque burden; vessel remodeling into the lumen of the vessel; and the thickness of the fibrous cap [34]. An occlusive thrombus leads to reduced perfusion of the myocardium which results in an acute coronary syndrome or sudden cardiac death.

Specific limitations of GWAS and presently identified CAD risk loci

While the achievements regarding the genetics of CAD thus far using GWAS cannot be gainsaid, there are several inherent limitations to the GWAS study design that we believe are responsible for skewing the nature of the genetic loci identified. This idea is supported by three conventions underlying development and phenotypic expression of complex diseases: shifting environments, time, and case–control overlap.

Shifting environments

The DNA code in each individual is established at conception. Therefore, DNA variants that function independent of environmental factors are most likely to reach significance in a GWAS because these are not reliant on any specific environmental factor to be present for their effect to become manifest. On the other hand, DNA variants that are dependent on environmental stimuli or factors are unlikely to reach the same significance in a GWAS because the additional element of the requisite environmental influence is needed, which may or may not occur in a given individual. The context-dependent or environmentally influenced risk modifiers of genetic risk in CAD include lifestyle factors such as smoking, diet, salt intake, and sedentary lifestyle, or coexisting comorbidities including obesity, diabetes, hypertension, and inflammatory driven diseases. Other risk factors include environmental pollution and highly stressful events [35,36], but these are even harder to account for in an individual patient. However, environmental factors that decide whether a genetic factor will influence CAD development or not can also be local in a given tissue. As an example, fatty liver can induce a number of genes in the liver that influence the genetic risk of CAD which are absent or insignificant in the normal liver. Such

context-dependent or environmentally influenced genetic factors may be identifiable in GWAS datasets, but current analytic approaches have failed to do so [37]. In summary, genetic variants modifying gene expression in CAD that are dependent on environmental contexts is a phenomenon that has been confirmed to be common and strong experimentally [38–41]. The reanalysis of GWAS datasets seeking to identify such context-dependent variants is potentially a very fruitful line of investigation which several groups are now actively pursuing.

Time

DNA variants involved in the regulation of disease processes over a long period of time (and which remain operative despite changing environmental and other influences) are more likely to reach genomewide significance in GWAS in comparison to those that regulate processes over a short period of time. Therefore, the DNA variants that are found to have genomewide significance in GWAS are most likely to be implicated in the early phase of disease pathogenesis where the initial growth phase is slow and spread over more time in comparison to the rapid growth phase or late phases. The pathogenesis of early CAD is likely driven more by genetic predisposition in comparison to the later stages of the disease and is less likely to be influenced by the factors that likely drive later stages of the disease, including diabetes, obesity, and different inflammatory states. The later stages of the disease are also more complex given that there are generally additional disease processes acting in parallel across organ systems (i.e., CAD includes the liver and pancreas in diabetes, adipose stores in obesity or systemic immune modulation). Late modulators of disease are complex and involve multiple systemic cofactors that are related to environmental or stimulus-dependent DNA variants that are unlikely to be of genomewide significance in a GWAS.

Case–control overlap

In the control populations sampled in GWAS studies for common complex disorders such as CAD, who did not have clinically manifest CAD or MI, it is inevitable that many had subclinical atherosclerotic disease and CAD. Therefore, using a GWAS study design, the power to detect subtle variants associated with CAD was almost certainly eroded because of the inclusion of persons with significant but subclinical CAD in the control population. In the absence of rigorous screening methods such as angiography, which is clearly impractical when recruiting many thousands of healthy controls as required for GWAS, it is impossible to exclude this confounding effect.

These limitations to the GWAS design, namely case–control overlap, lack of accounting for environmental factors, and bias toward genetic variants with a protracted period of effect, have implications for how we interpret the CAD risk alleles identified using GWAS. For example, because the GWAS design favors the identification of genes that have a role during early CAD development, these early phase genes are likely to be best suited to develop preventative measures for patients with these loci in addition to the development of disease therapies targeted toward inhibiting early disease development. A key limitation of identifying genes that are involved early in disease pathogenesis includes not being able to identify risk factors for secondary prevention and lack of development of therapies targeted toward the later, more rapidly progressive phases of CAD implicated in clinical manifestations such as MI and stroke.

Analysis of the validated genes linked to the CAD GWAS loci (Table 48.1) further confirms this outlook [10]. Of the 50 genes identified, 10 are involved in regulating lipid levels, including high density lipoprotein and triglycerides (Table 48.1) [7]. Circulating lipids have a major role in early atherosclerosis development; this supports the notion that targeting of the loci identified in GWAS would be most useful in primary prevention, also supported by data demonstrating that LDL lowering leads to regression of atherosclerosis more significantly in early than in advanced lesions [29]. Other CAD risk loci identified so far include genes related to hypertension (Table 48.1), which contributes to early endothelial cell activation and with hypertension having little impact on disease progression in the later phases of atherosclerosis. Indeed, most of CAD-associated loci identified by GWAS have been implicated in early CAD development with the exception of the ABO locus (Table 48.1), highlighting that context- and environmental-dependent variants and those operative late in the disease process are likely to be under-represented.

Integration of GWAS findings into future models of disease: systems genetics to identify networks mediating pathogenesis of disease and key regulatory pathways

Given the complexity of CAD and that GWAS tends to identify genes and loci associated with the early phases of disease development, the next question that arises is how to best identify later phase genetic loci that are dependent on environmental contexts and that are activated over a shorter course of time. Systems genetics is rapidly coming to the forefront as a potential solution to this issue [42–45]. Systems genetics works to identify key drivers of disease through the use of network models of interacting molecular pathways by integrating the analyses of both DNA and genomic (e.g., RNA, protein) datasets. Systems genetics data can be enriched by integration with GWAS datasets, and then ultimately used to identify and characterize DNA variants that contribute to the pathogenesis of late phases of complex diseases. The expectation is that systems genetics will also facilitate the development of diagnostic tools and the identification of new treatment targets for these complex diseases, with the goal of prevention of further remodeling and perhaps regression of current disease.

For common complex diseases such as CAD, the mere isolated effect of the individual genetic variants and/or genes as identified by GWAS does not explain the intrinsic complexity of the molecular disease processes. These diseases have polygenic regulation that involves the interaction of multiple genes within a complex and dynamic biologic network. These types of networks are sparse, with most genes (denoted as nodes) having a limited number of interactions with other genes (edges), with a small number of highly interconnected nodes acting as hubs given their multiple interactions (Figure 48.3) [46]. By studying measures of gene activity and creating network models of disease, systems genetics can identify these highly interconnected nodes [47]. Particularly important nodes can be considered as key drivers of any given disease process. By applying these approaches and the development of new technologies for screening genomes and studying genomic activity, and the

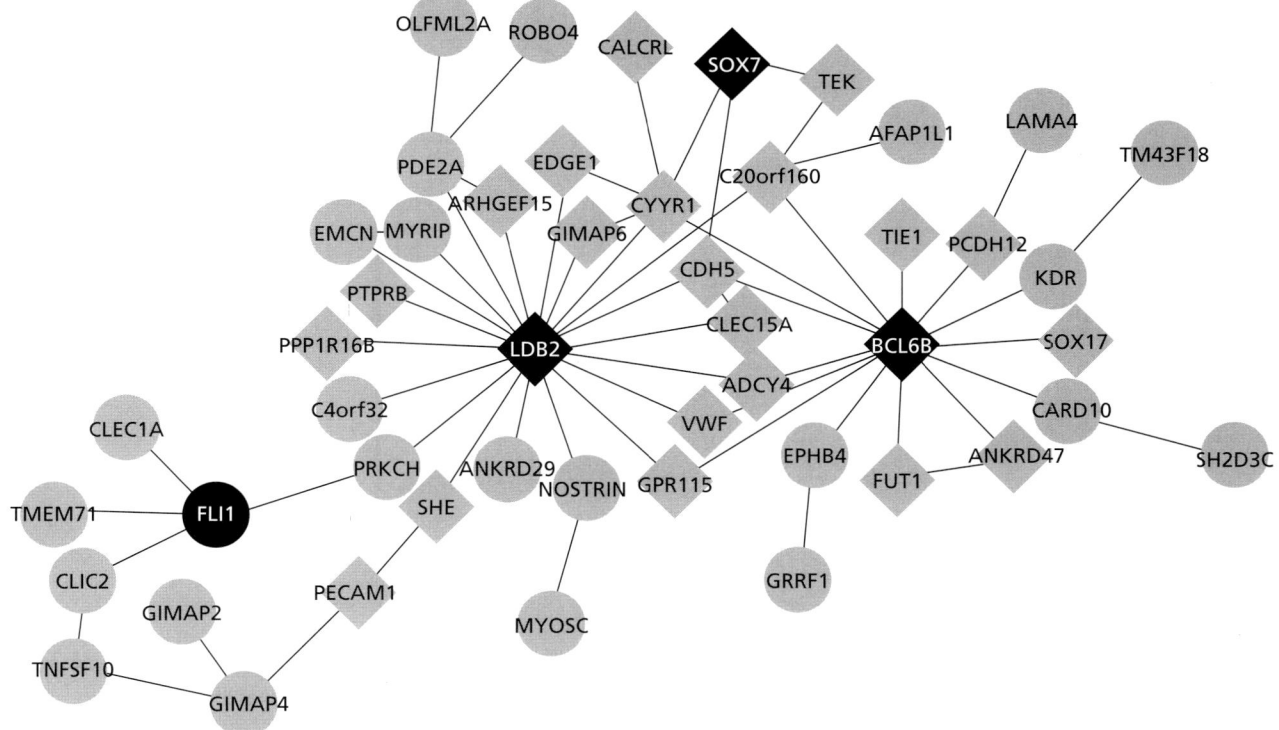

Figure 48.3 CAD regulatory network. This CAD regulatory network was identified by the team in the STAGE study. Regulatory genes are shown in black. Of these, Lim-domain binding 2 (LDB2) was found to be a high-hierarchy regulator of the transendothelial migration of leukocytes (TEML) pathway in atherosclerosis development, with a functional LDB2 variant (eQTL rs 10939673) linked to an increased risk for CAD [6,92]. Source: Hagg *et al.* 2009 [6]. Reproduced under the Creative Commons Attribution (CC BY) license.

advancement of computational analysis of growing datasets, we now appear poised for the large-scale application of system genetics to biology, medicine, and healthcare.

An example of this includes the STAGE (Stockholm Atherosclerosis Gene Expression) [6] and STARNET (Stockholm-Tartu Atherosclerosis Reverse Network Engineering Task) studies (Figure 48.3). With STAGE as the pilot forerunner study, STARNET is a landmark genetics-of-RNA-expression study comprising 925 CAD cases who had coronary artery bypass graft surgery and 207 controls without CAD who had open-thorax surgery. Each subject underwent DNA sampling, clinical characterization, angiographic assessment of CAD burden, and RNA isolation from up to nine CAD-relevant tissues: atherosclerotic (aorta) and non-atherosclerotic (internal mammary artery) arterial wall, liver, abdominal and subcutaneous fat, skeletal muscle, whole blood, and macrophages and foam cells differentiated from primary monocytes *in vitro*. RNA from these samples was then sequenced and extensive expression datasets were generated. The utility of these datasets includes: (i) to identify causal regulatory factors that potentially drive molecular mechanisms behind disease processes made possible through the study of multiple tissues involved in the pathogenesis of CAD; and (ii) to identify DNA variants that are involved in controlling gene expression in these networks. Furthermore, as these studies are primarily based on RNA expression data reflecting both genetic and environmental influences, this type of approach should permit the study of complex diseases in the later stages of disease pathogenesis, where the regulatory factors are more likely to be dependent on environmental contexts, including multiorgan cross-regulation. The STAGE/STARNET dataset can be used to identify expression quantitative trait loci (eQTLs) in CAD [48–52]; eQTLs are generally DNA variants, usually SNPs, that regulate gene expression levels. eQTLs are determined by linking the alleles of SNPs discovered by genotyping patient's DNA with gene expression levels from the different tissues. Thus, SNP alleles can be associated with different gene expression levels of tissues and can be identified as eQTLs. It is expected that this approach will help elucidate the large fraction of unknown heritability behind complex diseases and contribute to the development of novel molecular diagnostics and individually tailored therapies in healthcare.

Pharmacogenomics and interventional cardiology
Clopidogrel pharmacogenetics

Moving away from the genetics of CAD and to other relevant situations in the catheterization laboratory where pharmacogenetics has a key role, in recent times a large amount of data has emerged to highlight the importance that genetic influences have in the individual response to clopidogrel therapy. Indeed, despite the fact that clopidogrel remains the current cornerstone of antiplatelet therapy for patients undergoing percutaneous coronary intervention (PCI) for stable CAD, approximately 4–30% of patients do not respond adequately to this agent [53,54]. This is supported by pharmacologic studies that demonstrated *ex vivo* ADP-stimulated platelet reactivity (a surrogate marker of clopidogrel response) varies substantially in patient populations treated with clopidogrel [53,55]. Patients who have undergone recent stent implantation who receive clopidogrel and who exhibit high on-treatment platelet reactivity (HTPR) are more likely to develop a recurrent adverse clinical event [56]. While several clinical and demographic factors affect clopidogrel efficacy, the contribution of these factors is relatively modest

[57]. However, genetic studies have revealed several SNPs that significantly influence clopidogrel response. Specifically, genetic variants in genes responsible for clopidogrel transport and bioavailability (ATP-binding cassette subfamily B member 1 (*ABCB1*) [58–63], hepatic metabolism (CYP enzymes) [64–66], paraoxonase 1 (*PON1*) [67–70], carboxylesterase 1 (*CES1*) [71,72], and receptor interaction/activation (*P2Y12*) [73–75]) have been shown to have a role in clopidogrel pharmacodynamics, pharmacokinetics, and subsequent cardiovascular event rates. While it is possible to perform testing for these genetic variants, at present such testing has not been shown to be clinically efficacious and is currently given a IIb recommendation (level of evidence C) by the AHA/ACC, with the comment: "Genotyping for a CYP2C19 loss of function variant in patients with UA/NSTEMI (or, after ACS and with PCI) on P2Y12 receptor inhibitor therapy might be considered if results of testing may alter management" [76]. The TAILOR-PCI study is a multisite, prospective, randomized study that is currently recruiting patients and which seeks to use genetic testing for the *2 and *3 CYP2C19 alleles to determine whether choosing clopidogrel versus ticagrelor based on these genotype data will influence major adverse cardiovascular events. It is hoped that this study will give definitive proof as to whether genetic testing for likely responsiveness to clopidogrel has a role in the care of patients post-PCI requiring antiplatelet therapy.

Warfarin pharmacogenetics

Warfarin is widely used for the treatment and prevention of thromboembolic diseases, but is characterized by its narrow therapeutic index, individual variability in response, high rates of adverse events, and requirement for cautious patient selection and frequent adjustment for therapeutic dosing [77–79]. Standard dosing for warfarin is 2–6 mg/day; however, the effective daily dose varies from 0.5 to more than 30 mg in the general population. Subtherapeutic dosing results in a risk of failing to control blood clotting, whereas supratherapeutic dosing can lead to excessive and uncontrolled bleeding. Genetic polymorphisms of a number of enzymes involved in the mechanism of action and pharmacokinetics of warfarin have been demonstrated to be pivotal in determining the individual variability in response to warfarin therapy. Those studied include polymorphisms of *VKORC1* and *CYP2C9* [80–84], as well as genes that indirectly influence warfarin anticoagulation: *GGCX* [85], *CALU* [86], and *PROC* [87]. Of these, *VKORC1* polymorphisms account for approximately 25% of the variability in warfarin dosage and many studies have consistently shown that *VKORC1* genotype is the single biggest predictor of warfarin dose [88]. Those that carry the 1173 T/T allele of *VKORC1* require approximately 30–50% less warfarin daily dose than patients with wild-type 1173C/C allele, while polymorphisms in the coding regions of *VKORC1* lead to varying degrees of drug resistance. Patients who carry the CYP2C9*2 and -*3 alleles have a reduced capacity for metabolizing (S)-warfarin, resulting in supratherapeutic levels. However, variability in warfarin efficacy is a complex issue that involves more than just the genotypes of *CYP2C9* and *VKORC1*. Other factors, including age, gender, diet, drugs, and BMI, contribute another 20% (reviewed in [89,90]). Beyond these factors, there still exist further unidentified factors that account for almost 50% of variability of response to warfarin. Potentially, this complexity in the genetics and other factors that influence warfarin efficacy led to the failure of the much anticipated COAG study to find a benefit of genetic testing to aid in the initial choice of warfarin dose [91]. In the COAG study, over 1000 patients who were being initiated on warfarin were assigned to receive an initial dose using an algorithm based on genotype plus clinical data versus clinical data only. Unfortunately, genotype-guided warfarin dosing did not improve anticoagulation control during the first 4 weeks of therapy and at the current time there is no clinical indication for such testing. Nevertheless, although the newer novel oral anticoagulant medications have rapidly displaced warfarin as the agent of choice in eligible patients, the continued need for warfarin in specific patient subsets and its far lower cost appear to support further studies to identify important networks responsible for variability in drug response. These data would potentially help in improving therapeutic response, reduce adverse effects, and assist in reducing overall healthcare costs.

Conclusions

GWAS have played a critical part in identifying risk variants that partially explain the heritability of common complex diseases such as atherosclerosis and CAD. These risk variants have facilitated the identification of new molecular pathways that are involved in the pathogenesis of disease. However, the GWAS design appears to have limitations, and in particular it likely overlooks context-dependent risk variants (i.e., those that only exert risk when a specific environmental stimulus or factor is also present). These environment or context-dependent factors are likely to be most influential during the later and complex stages of common complex disease development and are therefore thought to exert a significant effect on molecular processes that are active in short timeframes during the later stages of CAD, such as the events in the weeks leading up to plaque rupture and MI. As we move into a new era of genetic studies where systems genetics assumes a major role in our investigative approach, further study of disease-causing networks is expected to uncover key biologic pathways involved in the pathobiology of common complex diseases, including CAD. In turn, it is anticipated that our improved understanding of these causal disease networks will permit the development of improved diagnostic tools, enhanced risk stratification, and novel therapeutic applications. Specific to the catheterization laboratory, as we unravel the causal molecular pathways that promote CAD and adverse vascular remodeling, it is certainly possible that novel stent platforms and adjunctive pharmacotherapies will also be developed which leverage this improved genetic and biologic knowledge.

Interactive multiple choice questions are available for this chapter on www.wiley. com/go/dangas/cardiology

References

1 Hughes V. Epigenetics: the sins of the father. *Nature* 2014; **507**: 22–24.
2 Cortijo S, Wardenaar R, Colome-Tatche M, et al. Mapping the epigenetic basis of complex traits. *Science* 2014; **343**: 1145–1148.
3 Holliday R. DNA methylation and epigenetic mechanisms. *Cell Biophys* 1989; **15**: 15–20.
4 Friend SH, Schadt EE. Translational genomics: clues from the resilient. *Science* 2014; **344**: 970–972
5 Ku CS, Naidoo N, Pawitan Y. Revisiting Mendelian disorders through exome sequencing. *Hum Genet* 2011; **129**: 351–370.
6 Hagg S, Skogsberg J, Lundstrom J, et al. Multi-organ expression profiling uncovers a gene module in coronary artery disease involving transendothelial migration of leukocytes and lim domain binding 2: The Stockholm atherosclerosis gene expression (stage) study. *PLoS Genet* 2009; **5**: e1000754.
7 Roberts R. Genetics of coronary artery disease. *Circ Res* 2014; **114**: 1890–1903.
8 Samani NJ, Erdmann J, Hall AS, et al. Genomewide association analysis of coronary artery disease. *N Engl J Med* 2007; **357**: 443–453.
9 McPherson R, Pertsemlidis A, Kavaslar N, et al. A common allele on chromosome 9 associated with coronary heart disease. *Science* 2007; **316**: 1488–1491.
10 Deloukas P, Kanoni S, Willenborg C, et al. Large-scale association analysis identifies new risk loci for coronary artery disease. *Nat Genet* 2013; **45**: 25–33.
11 Marenberg ME, Risch N, Berkman LF, Floderus B, de Faire U. Genetic susceptibility to death from coronary heart disease in a study of twins. *N Engl J Med* 1994; **330**: 1041–1046.
12 Schadt EE, Bjorkegren JL. NEW: network-enabled wisdom in biology, medicine, and health care. *Sci Transl Med* 2012; **4**: 115rv111.
13 Manolio TA, Collins FS, Cox NJ, et al. Finding the missing heritability of complex diseases. *Nature* 2009; **461**: 747–753.
14 Gerstein MB, Kundaje A, Hariharan M, et al. Architecture of the human regulatory network derived from encode data. *Nature* 2012; **489**: 91–100.
15 Helgadottir A, Thorleifsson G, Manolescu A, et al. A common variant on chromosome 9p21 affects the risk of myocardial infarction. *Science* 2007; **316**: 1491–1493.
16 Dandona S, Stewart AF, Roberts R. Genomics in coronary artery disease: past, present and future. *Can J Cardiol* 2010; **26**(Suppl A): 56A–59A.
17 Coronary Artery Disease (C4D) Genetics Consortium. A genome-wide association study in Europeans and South Asians identifies five new loci for coronary artery disease. *Nat Genet* 2011; **43**: 339–344.
18 Preuss M, Konig IR, Thompson JR, et al. Design of the coronary artery disease genome-wide replication and meta-analysis (cardiogram) study: a genome-wide association meta-analysis involving more than 22 000 cases and 60 000 controls. *Circ Cardiovasc Genet* 2010; **3**: 475–483.
19 Samani NJ, Deloukas P, Erdmann J, et al. Large scale association analysis of novel genetic loci for coronary artery disease. *Arterioscler Thromb Vasc Biol* 2009; **29**: 774–780.
20 Musunuru K, Strong A, Frank-Kamenetsky M, et al. From noncoding variant to phenotype via sort1 at the 1p13 cholesterol locus. *Nature* 2010; **466**: 714–719.
21 Roberts R. Genetics of premature myocardial infarction. *Curr Atheroscler Rep* 2008; **10**: 186–193.
22 Ni YG, Di Marco S, Condra JH, et al. A pcsk9-binding antibody that structurally mimics the EGF(a) domain of LDL-receptor reduces LDL cholesterol in vivo. *J Lipid Res* 2011; **52**: 78–86.
23 Dandona S, Stewart AF, Chen L, et al. Gene dosage of the common variant 9p21 predicts severity of coronary artery disease. *J Am Coll Cardiol* 2010; **56**: 479–486.
24 Reilly MP, Li M, He J, et al. Identification of adamts7 as a novel locus for coronary atherosclerosis and association of abo with myocardial infarction in the presence of coronary atherosclerosis: two genome-wide association studies. *Lancet* 2011; **377**: 383–392.
25 Gill JC, Endres-Brooks J, Bauer PJ, Marks WJ Jr, Montgomery RR. The effect of ABO blood group on the diagnosis of von Willebrand disease. *Blood* 1987; **69**: 1691–1695.
26 He M, Wolpin B, Rexrode K, et al. ABO blood group and risk of coronary heart disease in two prospective cohort studies. *Arterioscler Thromb Vasc Biol* 2012; **32**: 2314–2320.
27 Allaby M. *A Dictionary of Zoology*. New York: Oxford University Press: 1999.
28 Narula J, Kovacic JC. Putting TCFA in clinical perspective. *J Am Coll Cardiol* 2014; **64**: 681–683.
29 Bjorkegren JL, Hagg S, Talukdar HA, et al. Plasma cholesterol-induced lesion networks activated before regression of early, mature, and advanced atherosclerosis. *PLoS Genet* 2014; **10**: e1004201.
30 Hagg S, Salehpour M, Noori P, et al. Carotid plaque age is a feature of plaque stability inversely related to levels of plasma insulin. *PloS One* 2011; **6**: e18248.
31 Lusis AJ. Atherosclerosis. *Nature* 2000; **407**: 233–241.
32 Skogsberg J, Lundstrom J, Kovacs A, et al. Transcriptional profiling uncovers a network of cholesterol-responsive atherosclerosis target genes. *PLoS Genet* 2008; **4**: e1000036.
33 Kubo T, Maehara A, Mintz GS, et al. The dynamic nature of coronary artery lesion morphology assessed by serial virtual histology intravascular ultrasound tissue characterization. *J Am Coll Cardiol* 2010; **55**: 1590–1597.
34 Bentzon JF, Otsuka F, Virmani R, Falk E. Mechanisms of plaque formation and rupture. *Circ Res* 2014; **114**: 1852–1866.
35 Peters MN, Moscona JC, Katz MJ, et al. Natural disasters and myocardial infarction: the six years after hurricane Katrina. *Mayo Clinic Proc* 2014; **89**: 472–477.
36 Chan C, Elliott J, Troughton R, et al. Acute myocardial infarction and stress cardiomyopathy following the Christchurch earthquakes. *PloS One* 2013; **8**: e68504.
37 Lusk CM, Dyson G, Clark AG, et al. Validated context-dependent associations of coronary heart disease risk with genotype variation in the chromosome 9p21 region: the atherosclerosis risk in communities study. *Hum Genet* 2014; **133**: 1105–1116.
38 Smith EN, Kruglyak L. Gene–environment interaction in yeast gene expression. *PLoS Biol* 2008; **6**: e83.
39 Smirnov DA, Morley M, Shin E, Spielman RS, Cheung VG. Genetic analysis of radiation-induced changes in human gene expression. *Nature* 2009; **459**: 587–591.

40 Romanoski CE, Lee S, Kim MJ, *et al*. Systems genetics analysis of gene-by-environment interactions in human cells. *Am J Hum Genet* 2010; **86**: 399–410.

41 Orozco LD, Bennett BJ, Farber CR, *et al*. Unraveling inflammatory responses using systems genetics and gene–environment interactions in macrophages. *Cell* 2012; **151**: 658–670.

42 Kidd BA, Peters LA, Schadt EE, Dudley JT. Unifying immunology with informatics and multiscale biology. *Nat Immunol* 2014; **15**: 118–127.

43 Lusis AJ, Weiss JN. Cardiovascular networks: systems-based approaches to cardiovascular disease. *Circulation* 2010; **121**: 157–170.

44 Civelek M, Lusis AJ. Systems genetics approaches to understand complex traits. *Nat Rev Genet* 2014; **15**: 34–48.

45 Dirac MA, Horan KL, Doody DR, *et al*. Environment or host?: a case–control study of risk factors for *Mycobacterium avium* complex lung disease. *Am J Respir Crit Care Med* 2012; **186**: 684–691.

46 Barabasi AL, Oltvai ZN. Network biology: understanding the cell's functional organization. *Nat Rev Genet* 2004; **5**: 101–113.

47 Schadt EE. Molecular networks as sensors and drivers of common human diseases. *Nature* 2009; **461**: 218–223.

48 Hubner N, Wallace CA, Zimdahl H, *et al*. Integrated transcriptional profiling and linkage analysis for identification of genes underlying disease. *Nat Genet* 2005; **37**: 243–253.

49 Cookson W, Liang L, Abecasis G, Moffatt M, Lathrop M. Mapping complex disease traits with global gene expression. *Nat Rev Genet* 2009; **10**: 184–194.

50 Nicolae DL, Gamazon E, Zhang W, Duan S, Dolan ME, Cox NJ. Trait-associated SNPS are more likely to be EQTLS: annotation to enhance discovery from GWAS. *PLoS Genet* 2010; **6**: e1000888.

51 Kang HP, Morgan AA, Chen R, Schadt EE, Butte AJ. Coanalysis of GWAS with EQTLS reveals disease-tissue associations. *AMIA Jt Summits Transl Sci Proc* 2012; **2012**: 35–41.

52 Westra HJ, Peters MJ, Esko T, *et al*. Systematic identification of trans eqtls as putative drivers of known disease associations. *Nat Genet* 2013; **45**: 1238–1243.

53 Gurbel PA, Bliden KP, Hiatt BL, O'Connor CM. Clopidogrel for coronary stenting: response variability, drug resistance, and the effect of pretreatment platelet reactivity. *Circulation* 2003; **107**: 2908–2913.

54 Gurbel PA, Cummings CC, Bell CR, Alford AB, Meister AF, Serebruany VL. Onset and extent of platelet inhibition by clopidogrel loading in patients undergoing elective coronary stenting: the plavix reduction of new thrombus occurrence (pronto) trial. *Am Heart J* 2003; **145**: 239–247.

55 Serebruany VL, Steinhubl SR, Berger PB, Malinin AI, Bhatt DL, Topol EJ. Variability in platelet responsiveness to clopidogrel among 544 individuals. *J Ame Coll Cardiol* 2005; **45**: 246–251.

56 Bonello L, Tantry US, Marcucci R, *et al*. Consensus and future directions on the definition of high on-treatment platelet reactivity to adenosine diphosphate. *J Am Coll Cardiol* 2010; **56**: 919–933.

57 Frelinger AL 3rd, Bhatt DL, Lee RD, *et al*. Clopidogrel pharmacokinetics and pharmacodynamics vary widely despite exclusion or control of polymorphisms (cyp2c19, abcb1, pon1), noncompliance, diet, smoking, co-medications (including proton pump inhibitors), and pre-existent variability in platelet function. *J Am Coll Cardiol* 2013; **61**: 872–879.

58 Ameyaw MM, Regateiro F, Li T, *et al*. Mdr1 pharmacogenetics: frequency of the c3435t mutation in exon 26 is significantly influenced by ethnicity. *Pharmacogenetics* 2001; **11**: 217–221.

59 Taubert D, von Beckerath N, Grimberg G, *et al*. Impact of p-glycoprotein on clopidogrel absorption. *Clin Pharmacol Ther* 2006; **80**: 486–501.

60 Ferrieres J, Bataille V, Leclercq F, *et al*. Patterns of statin prescription in acute myocardial infarction: the French registry of acute ST-elevation or non-ST-elevation myocardial infarction (FAST-MI). *Atherosclerosis* 2009; **204**: 491–496.

61 Mega JL, Close SL, Wiviott SD, *et al*. Genetic variants in abcb1 and cyp2c19 and cardiovascular outcomes after treatment with clopidogrel and prasugrel in the triton-timi 38 trial: a pharmacogenetic analysis. *Lancet* 2010; **376**: 1312–1319.

62 Luo M, Li J, Xu X, Sun X, Sheng W. Abcb1 c3435t polymorphism and risk of adverse clinical events in clopidogrel treated patients: a meta-analysis. *Thromb Res* 2012; **129**: 754–759.

63 Su J, Xu J, Li X, *et al*. Abcb1 c3435t polymorphism and response to clopidogrel treatment in coronary artery disease (CAD) patients: a meta-analysis. *PloS One* 2012; **7**: e46366.

64 Varenhorst C, James S, Erlinge D, *et al*. Genetic variation of cyp2c19 affects both pharmacokinetic and pharmacodynamic responses to clopidogrel but not prasugrel in aspirin-treated patients with coronary artery disease. *Eur Heart J* 2009; **30**: 1744–1752.

65 Collet JP, Hulot JS, Anzaha G, *et al*. High doses of clopidogrel to overcome genetic resistance: the randomized crossover clovis-2 (clopidogrel and response variability investigation study 2). *JACC Cardiovasc Interv* 2011; **4**: 392–402.

66 Hulot JS, Collet JP, Cayla G, *et al*. Cyp2c19 but not pon1 genetic variants influence clopidogrel pharmacokinetics, pharmacodynamics, and clinical efficacy in post-myocardial infarction patients. *Circ Cardiovasc Interv* 2011; **4**: 422–428.

67 Bouman HJ, Schomig E, van Werkum JW, *et al*. Paraoxonase-1 is a major determinant of clopidogrel efficacy. *Nat Med* 2011; **17**: 110–116.

68 Lewis JP, Fisch AS, Ryan K, *et al*. Paraoxonase 1 (pon1) gene variants are not associated with clopidogrel response. *Clin Pharmacol Ther* 2011; **90**: 568–574.

69 Reny JL, Combescure C, Daali Y, Fontana P. Influence of the paraoxonase-1 q192r genetic variant on clopidogrel responsiveness and recurrent cardiovascular events: a systematic review and meta-analysis. *J Thromb Haemost* 2012; **10**: 1242–1251.

70 Li X, Zhang L, Chen X, *et al*. Pon1 q192r genotype influences clopidogrel responsiveness by relative platelet inhibition instead of on-treatment platelet reactivity. *Thromb Res* 2013; **132**: 444–449.

71 Lewis JP, Horenstein RB, Ryan K, *et al*. The functional g143e variant of carboxylesterase 1 is associated with increased clopidogrel active metabolite levels and greater clopidogrel response. *Pharmacogenet Genom* 2013; **23**: 1–8.

72 Zhu HJ, Wang X, Gawronski BE, Brinda BJ, Angiolillo DJ, Markowitz JS. Carboxylesterase 1 as a determinant of clopidogrel metabolism and activation. *J Pharmacol Exp Ther* 2013; **344**: 665–672.

73 Simon T, Verstuyft C, Mary-Krause M, *et al*. Genetic determinants of response to clopidogrel and cardiovascular events. *N Engl J Med* 2009; **360**: 363–375.

74 Bura A, Bachelot-Loza C, Ali FD, Aiach M, Gaussem P. Role of the p2y12 gene polymorphism in platelet responsiveness to clopidogrel in healthy subjects. *J Thromb Haemost* 2006; **4**: 2096–2097.

75 Lev EI, Patel RT, Guthikonda S, Lopez D, Bray PF, Kleiman NS. Genetic polymorphisms of the platelet receptors p2y(12), p2y(1) and GP IIIa and response to aspirin and clopidogrel. *Thromb Res* 2007; **119**: 355–360.

76 Jneid H, Anderson JL, Wright RS, *et al*. 2012 accf/aha focused update of the guideline for the management of patients with unstable angina/non-st-elevation myocardial infarction (updating the 2007 guideline and replacing the 2011 focused update): a report of the American College of Cardiology Foundation/American Heart Association Task Force on Practice Guidelines. *J Am Coll Cardiol* 2012; **60**: 645–681.

77 Klein TE, Altman RB, Eriksson N, *et al*. Estimation of the warfarin dose with clinical and pharmacogenetic data. *N Engl J Med* 2009; **360**: 753–764.

78 Budnitz DS, Lovegrove MC, Shehab N, Richards CL. Emergency hospitalizations for adverse drug events in older Americans. *N Engl J Med* 2011; **365**: 2002–2012.

79 Pirmohamed M, James S, Meakin S, *et al*. Adverse drug reactions as cause of admission to hospital: prospective analysis of 18 820 patients. *BMJ* 2004; **329**: 15–19.

80 Johnson JA, Cavallari LH. Pharmacogenetics and cardiovascular disease: implications for personalized medicine. *Pharmacol Rev* 2013; **65**: 987–1009.

81 Fung E, Patsopoulos NA, Belknap SM, *et al*. Effect of genetic variants, especially cyp2c9 and vkorc1, on the pharmacology of warfarin. *Semin Thromb Hemost* 2012; **38**: 893–904.

82 Johnson JA, Cavallari LH, Beitelshees AL, Lewis JP, Shuldiner AR, Roden DM. Pharmacogenomics: application to the management of cardiovascular disease. *Clin Pharmacol Ther* 2011; **90**: 519–531.

83 Lee MT, Klein TE. Pharmacogenetics of warfarin: challenges and opportunities. *J Hum Genet* 2013; **58**: 334–338.

84 Jorgensen AL, FitzGerald RJ, Oyee J, Pirmohamed M, Williamson PR. Influence of cyp2c9 and vkorc1 on patient response to warfarin: a systematic review and meta-analysis. *PloS One* 2012; **7**: e44064.

85 Wadelius M, Chen LY, Downes K, *et al*. Common VKORC1 and GGCX polymorphisms associated with warfarin dose. *Pharmacogenet J* 2005; **5**: 262–270.

86 Voora D, Koboldt DC, King CR, *et al*. A polymorphism in the VKORC1 regulator calumenin predicts higher warfarin dose requirements in African Americans. *Clin Pharmacol Ther* 2010; **87**: 445–451.

87 Wadelius M, Chen LY, Eriksson N, *et al*. Association of warfarin dose with genes involved in its action and metabolism. *Hum Genet* 2007; **121**: 23–34.

88 Owen RP, Gong L, Sagreiya H, Klein TE, Altman RB. VKORC1 pharmacogenomics summary. *Pharmacogenet Genom* 2010; **20**: 642–644.

89 Ma Q, Lu AY. Pharmacogenetics, pharmacogenomics, and individualized medicine. *Pharmacol Rev* 2011; **63**: 437–459.

90 Shahabi P, Dube MP. Cardiovascular pharmacogenomics; state of current knowledge and implementation in practice. *Int J Cardiol* 2015; **184**: 772–795.

91 Kimmel SE, French B, Kasner SE, *et al*. A pharmacogenetic versus a clinical algorithm for warfarin dosing. *N Engl J Med* 2013; **369**: 2283–2293.

92 Shang MM, Talukdar HA, Hofmann JJ, *et al*. Lim domain binding 2: a key driver of transendothelial migration of leukocytes and atherosclerosis. *Arterioscler Thromb Vasc Biol* 2014; **34**: 2068–2077.

CHAPTER 49

Monitoring and Reversal of Anticoagulation and Antiplatelet Agents

Gregory W. Yost[1] and Steven R. Steinhubl[2]

[1] Geisinger Medical Center, Danville, PA, USA

[2] Scripps Translational Science Institute, San Diego, CA, USA

Closure of a coronary vessel has been the biggest concern with performing interventions since the beginnings of percutaneous transluminal coronary angioplasty (PTCA). Thrombosis remains a prominent concern despite the advances in percutaneous coronary intervention (PCI), especially with stenting. Thrombogenic potential exists in a newly placed stent until there is complete endothelialization [1], after ~28 days for bare metal stent and longer for drug-eluting stents because of delayed neointimal proliferation [2,3]. There is extensive clinical evidence that the use of antithrombotic therapy lowers the risk of vessel closure during and after PCI. Anticoagulation and dual antiplatelet therapy with stent placement is a standard of treatment with Class I indication according to current practice guidelines [4]. Anticoagulation has been used since before the stent era and, although not as rigorously studied as antiplatelets in PCI, it remains a routine part of therapy for two major reasons: preventing arterial thrombus formation and reducing thrombogenicity of catheters and guidewires used during the invasive procedures [5].

Since PTCA was first described [6,7], and the breakthrough studies on the role of stents [8,9], the evolution in anticoagulation and antiplatelet therapy used during PCI has led to reductions in periprocedural ischemic events and stent thrombosis [10]. There is a significant trade-off with higher risk of major and minor bleeding when using greater combinations and doses of anticoagulation and antiplatelet for protection against thrombogenic and embolic events [11]. This chapter describes each of the commonly used antiplatelet and anticoagulants used at time of PCI with specific focus on drug monitoring and reversal, if applicable.

Anticoagulants

Exposure of clotting factors to disrupted endothelium, catheters, and guidewires predisposes to thrombosis during catheterization. Anticoagulation therapy is used to minimize thrombus propagation on the endovascular surface and formation of new thrombi from PCI equipment use [5,12]. Ideal anticoagulation would effectively prevent thrombus formation, have low risk of bleeding, a safe monitoring profile, short duration of effect (half-life), and could be reversed if necessary. Anticoagulants used during PCI include unfractionated heparin (UFH), low molecular weight heparin (LMWH), direct thrombin inhibitors, and indirect factor Xa inhibitors (Table 49.1) [12,13].

Unfractionated heparin

Thrombus propagation occurs when thrombin is produced on the surface of activated platelets, converting fibrinogen to fibrin. Fibrin is cross-linked with factor XIIIa reinforcing platelet aggregation and culminating in clot formation. Heparin combines with antithrombin to indirectly inactivate thrombin, factors Xa, and intrinsic pathway factors XIIa, XIa, and IXa [14,15]. UFH has been proven to be beneficial in the treatment of unstable angina or myocardial infarction (MI; not treated with thrombolytic therapy) [16–18]. While anticoagulants have been shown to inactivate von Willebrand factor there may be differences between anticoagulants in curbing its release. Enoxaparin lessens the release more than UFH. This can be important in patients with unstable angina when there may be an early rise of von Willebrand factor. This early release of von Willebrand factor is associated with worse outcomes [19,20].

Use of intravenous (IV) UFH given before PCI to prevent intracoronary thrombosis was started at the time of the very first percutaneous intervention by Andreas Gruntzig and has remained the gold standard through the current age of routine stenting and use of dual antiplatelets [5]. In the early phases of PTCA the vessel closure rate during or after dilatation was 2–11% [21]. Use of UFH lowered these rates but there remained a risk for closure because there was no clear consensus for proper dosing. Changes in heparin dosing recommendations and the increasing use of radial artery access have reduced the incidence of ischemia and bleeding events when UFH is used in preference to alternative anticoagulants [12,22]. Unfractionated heparin remains the most commonly used anticoagulant despite the availability of newer medications.

Despite UFH being the most widely used anticoagulant there are several limitations to its use beyond the risk of bleeding seen in all anticoagulants. UFH has a less predictable pharmacologic profile.

This article updates Yost GW, Steinhubl SR, Monitoring and reversal of anticoagulation and antiplatelets. *Interventional Cardiology Clinics* 2015; **4**: 643–663, with permission of the publisher.

Interventional Cardiology: Principles and Practice, Second Edition. Edited by George D. Dangas, Carlo Di Mario, and Nicholas N. Kipshidze.
© 2017 John Wiley & Sons, Ltd. Published 2017 by John Wiley & Sons, Ltd.

IIIa inhibitors. This corresponded with peak anti-Xa levels of 0.86 ± 0.11 $(0.69–1.14)$ U/mL for enoxaparin alone group and 0.78 ± 0.12 $(0.61–1.10)$ U/mL for the enoxaparin plus GP IIb/IIIa group. Despite the corresponding lower levels in presence of GP IIb/IIIa, the anti-Xa levels remained within the recommended therapeutic ranges of 0.6–1.8 U/mL at time of PCI. There were similar decreases in HEMONOX CT and anti-Xa levels at 30 and 60 minutes following administration of enoxaparin in both treatment groups. Although this was a small observational study, the significant correlation between HEMONOX CT and anti-Xa levels during PCI support its potential use as a POCT for enoxaparin [63].

Monitoring is not indicated in all situations but may be warranted in certain populations that may be at higher risk of bleeding (e.g., increased age, history of gastrointestinal bleeding, renal insufficiency) [58]. The clearance of LMWH's anti-Xa effect is largely correlated with creatinine clearance and its decreased clearance poses greater risk for major bleeding events [66]. Monitoring and dosing of different LMWH agents in obese patients have been studied. Anti-factor Xa activity levels increased to appropriate levels when administered based on body weight up to 144 kg for enoxaparin, 190 kg for dalteparin, and 165 kg for tinazaparin [37]. Until there is a universally accepted recommendation for monitoring, the guidelines advocate additional dosing of LMWH before PCI to be dependent on timing of the most recent dose. No additional anticoagulation therapy is needed if the last dose of enoxaparin was less than 8 hours prior to PCI. If the last dose of enoxaparin was 8–12 hours prior to PCI, a 0.3 mg/kg bolus of IV enoxaparin at time of PCI is recommended. If the last dose of enoxaparin was more than 12 hours prior to PCI then conventional anticoagulation therapy is advised [67].

Reversal

The half-life of LMWH is 3–6 hours after subcutaneous administration but is longer in patients with kidney disease. A major concern for most clinicians in using LMWH is that there is no proven reversal agent. Protamine sulfate only partially reverses the effects of LMWH because while it neutralizes the anti-factor IIa activity, it has little to no effect on the anti-Xa activity [68]. When immediate reversal is needed, it is generally recommended to give 1 mg protamine sulfate per 100 anti-Xa units of LMWH given in the last 8 hours (where 1 mg enoxaparin equals 100 anti-Xa units). A second dose of 0.5 mg protamine sulfate per 100 anti-Xa units (or per 1 mg enoxaparin administered) can be given if bleeding continues. The maximum single dose of protamine sulfate is 50 mg [69].

Pentasaccharides (fondaparinux)

Fondaparinux is a synthetic derivative of the natural pentasaccharide sequence found in heparin. This works through antithrombin to inhibit factor Xa with greater specificity than UFH and LMWH. Fondaparinux does not directly inhibit thrombin because it is a short molecule and unable to form a bridging complex between antithrombin and thrombin. Fondaparinux is subcutaneously injected, reaches peak levels in 2 hours, and is excreted in urine with a half-life of 17 hours in a younger population and ~21 hours in the elderly. Like LMWH, fondaparinux has less binding to other plasma proteins as seen with UFH. It is typically administered once daily without monitoring because of its long half-life, bioavailability, and predictable anticoagulant response. It is contraindicated in renal insufficiency (creatinine clearance less than 30 mL/min) [13,35,37].

Several studies have supported fondaparinux as a safe and effective alternative for anticoagulation in setting of ACS and PCI.

The PENTALYSE study revealed that administration of pentasaccharide inhibiting factor Xa with alteplase can be as safe and effective at revascularizing as UFH with alteplase in patients with STEMI. There were similar coronary patency rates seen by angiography after 90 minutes but a trend toward lower re-occlusions in the culprit coronary artery and less revascularizations after 5–7 days [70]. The PENTUA study suggested that fondaparinux has similar safety and efficacy to enoxaparin when used for treatment of ACS without ST-elevation and not undergoing revascularization within 48 hours. This study showed no significant dose responses between different doses of fondaparinux (2.5, 4, 8, and 12 mg once daily). There were no significant differences in fondaparinux plasma concentrations between groups with primary endpoints (i.e., death, MI, and recurrent ischemia) and those without primary endpoints. Similarly, non-significant differences in plasma concentrations were seen in groups with bleeding versus those without bleeding. The lowest primary event rate was seen in the fondaparinux 2.5 mg dose group. Also, no major bleeding events occurred in the fondaparinux 2.5 mg and enoxaparin groups [71]. OASIS 5 held up the notion that fondaparinux was non-inferior to enoxaparin in the subsequent 9 day endpoint outcomes of death, MI, and refractory ischemia when used for treatment of high risk unstable angina or NSTEMI. Fondaparinux was superior to enoxaparin in respect to significant reductions in major bleeding at 9 days, deaths at 30 days, and deaths at 180 days [72]. The results from the ASPIRE study showed fondaparinux was just as efficacious and safe as using UFH for patients undergoing elective or urgent PCI, regardless whether or not a GP IIb/IIIa inhibitor was being used. In this trial, fondaparinux was given in 2.5 or 5 mg doses. There were no significant differences in bleeding complications between the two doses but there was a trend for lower incidences with the 2.5 mg dose. The procedural success rate was high in all groups with a slightly better percentage in the higher dose fondaparinux group: 96.3% for UFH; 96.5% for fondaparinux 2.5 mg; and 98.4% for fondaparinux 5 mg [73]. In patients with STEMI treated conservatively and not undergoing PCI, OASIS 6 showed reductions in death and recurrent infarction without increased risk of bleeding events when using fondaparinux compared to UFH [74].

Further pooled analysis into OASIS 5 and 6 trials supported the net clinical outcomes favoring fondaparinux over heparin therapies, which was mainly driven by reduction in bleeding events. Despite this positive finding there was higher rate of catheter-related thrombosis in OASIS 5 and likewise in OASIS 6 when fondaparinux was not used with UFH. OASIS 6 study showed a significantly higher 30-day rate of death or reinfarction when fondaparinux is used alone during primary PCI as part of therapy for STEMI, compared with the UFH group. This risk of catheter-related thrombus with fondaparinux was minimized without an increase in major bleeding when UFH (50–60 IU/kg) was given in the catheterization laboratory immediately before PCI [75]. Based on these findings, current guidelines recommend use of additional agents with activity against factor IIa when using fondaparinux for primary PCI [4].

Monitoring

Monitoring for fondaparinux is not routinely recommended. A fondaparinux specific anti-Xa assay can be used when needed but there is no clearly established therapeutic range, unlike LMWH. Peak steady state when using therapeutic doses of fondaparinux (e.g., 7.5 mg) should be 1.20–1.26 mg/L 3 hours after dosing [37]. Currently, there is no point of care test available for use during PCI [13].

Reversal

Despite the reductions in major bleeding rates identified in previous trials, there remains a concern for bleeding complications because of its long half-life. Fondaparinux does not bind to protamine sulfate, unlike UFH and LMWH [37]. Recombinant factor VIIa is recommended for uncontrolled bleeding attributed to fondaparinux. Recombinant factor VIIa is able to overcome thrombin inhibition by fondaparinux and has been shown to normalize the prolongation of aPTT and prothrombin time (PT) [76].

Direct thrombin inhibitors (bivalirudin, argatroban)

Use of direct thrombin inhibitors has shown benefit in preventing ischemic complications from PCI [77,78]. Direct thrombin inhibitors do not require antithrombin as a cofactor, unlike UFH, LMWH, and fondaparinux. Direct thrombin inhibitors are able to directly inhibit both circulating thrombin and clot-bound thrombin. They are also more predictable than heparins because they do not activate platelets (thus not neutralized by platelet factor 4 when platelets are activated) and do not bind to plasma proteins [79]. Without platelet activation there is no interaction with platelet factor 4, thus eliminating the possibility of immune-mediated heparin-induced thrombocytopenia (HIT). This makes direct thrombin inhibitors a safe alternative to heparin for PCI in patients with HIT [80]. The direct thrombin inhibitors currently available for use during PCI are bivalirudin and argatroban.

Bivalirudin

Bivalirudin is a synthetic analogue of hirudin that is slowly cleaved by thrombin and only transiently inhibits thrombin. Its quick onset of action achieving therapeutic ACT within 5 minutes and a short half-life of approximately 25 minutes contribute to its safe profile with lower risk of bleeding, making it attractive for use during PCI [79,81]. Bivalirudin has been extensively studied since its development. Studies have shown reduced incidences of bleeding compared with heparin when used as treatment with a thrombolytic agent for acute MI and unstable angina. After proving that it was a safe alternative to heparin in the setting of balloon angioplasty it was later suggested to lower ischemic complications in addition to a lower risk of bleeding [77,78,82–84]. These initial studies of bivalirudin were carried out in the era before use of GP IIb/IIIa inhibitors. The REPLACE-2 trial tested the safety and efficacy of using bivalirudin compared to heparin with planned use of GP IIb/IIIa inhibitors during PCI. The results showed that bivalirudin was noninferior to heparin plus a GP IIb/IIIa antagonist with significantly less bleeding in the bivalirudin group. The secondary triple composite endpoint of death, MI, or urgent revascularization was nonsignificantly lower in the heparin plus GP IIb/IIIa group [85]. ISAR-REACT 4 trial showed similar rates of death, MI, or revascularization between bivalirudin and heparin plus GP IIb/IIIa inhibitor groups when used during PCI in patients with NSTEMI. However, the outcomes showed an increased risk of bleeding in the heparin plus GP IIb/IIIa inhibitor group [86]. The ACUITY investigators studied the outcomes of treating moderate to high risk ACS patients. Groups were divided as follows: UFH or enoxaparin with GP IIb/IIIa inhibitor; bivalirudin with GP IIb/IIIa inhibitor; or bivalirudin alone. Results showed bivalirudin had similar rates of ischemia whether or not it was used with GP IIb/IIIa inhibitors but had significantly lower rates of bleeding when used alone when compared with the heparin (or enoxaparin) plus GP IIb/IIIa

inhibitor group [87]. This was further expanded on by the HORIZONS-AMI trial investigators who compared outcomes of patients with STEMI treated with either bivalirudin alone or heparin plus GP IIb/IIIa inhibitors. Interestingly, there was a higher rate of stent thrombosis within 24 hours (1.3% vs. 0.3%; p <0.001) but significantly reduced 30-day mortality (2.1% vs. 3.1%, P = 0.047) in the bivalirudin arm. The reduced 30-day event rate was largely because of the significantly lower rate of major bleeding with bivalirudin than heparin plus GP IIb/IIIa inhibitors (4.9% vs. 8.3%; p <0.001) [88]. These studies were carried out in the era mostly using a femoral artery approach and were limited in almost exclusively comparing bivalirudin alone with heparin plus a GP IIb/IIIa antagonist but never with UFH alone. Several more recent studies have attempted to overcome this limitation. The radial artery approach has been increasingly used and is associated with less risk of bleeding, while dual oral antiplatelet therapy has become routine, diminishing the antithrombotic benefit of GP IIb/IIIa antagonists. A recent large randomized trial in a primary PCI STEMI population compared UFH alone with bivalirudin and found heparin alone was better at reducing ischemic events, including stent thrombosis, with no difference in bleeding complications [22].

Monitoring

Bivalirudin can typically be given immediately prior to PCI with 0.75 mg/kg IV bolus then 1.75 mg/kg/hour continuous infusion. It is renally excreted; however, no adjustments need to be made until creatinine clearance (CrCl) is less than 30. If the CrCl is 10–29 mL/minute then the infusion rate should be decreased to 1 mg/kg/hour; and decreased to 0.25 mg/kg/hour if the patient is on hemodialysis. This can be continued for up to 4 hours after the PCI procedure at the discretion of the physician [89]. Bivalirudin can cause elevations in multiple coagulation assays: aPTT, PT, INR, and ACT. Routine monitoring is not required with use of bivalirudin but can be performed with ACT. In REPLACE-2, the median ACT 5 minutes after a bolus infusion (0.75 mg/kg) followed by continuous infusion (1.75 mg/kg/hr) was 358 s. If ACT is <225 s after first bolus, then an additional bivalirudin bolus of 0.3 mg/kg should be given. If ACT is >225 s, then no further monitoring is required as infusion dose should maintain appropriate ACT levels. Because of the short half-life of bivalirudin (~25 minutes), an ACT is also not required before sheath removal [85,89,90].

Argatroban

Argatroban is a small, synthetically derived, direct thrombin inhibitor that reversibly binds to the active site of thrombin. It is metabolized through the liver and has a half-life of approximately 45 minutes [81]. Use of argatroban in combination with thrombolytic therapy compared with heparin with thrombolytic therapy has shown better rates of TIMI III flow on angiography at 90 minutes. Despite potentially better TIMI III flow rates there have been no differences in total mortality, recurrent MI, revascularization, or ischemic stroke. There was a non-significant lower incidence of bleeding in the argatroban group [91].

The prospective ARG-E04 trial tested three different doses of argatroban in comparison with UFH during PCI. In this study, argatroban rapidly and consistently achieved sufficient ACT prolongation to allow for shortened time to initiate PCI compared with patients receiving UFH (ACT target parameter of 250 s used for anticoagulation). There were no significant differences in angiographic success rates, composite endpoints (death, MI, or revascularization), or incidence of bleeding. This study proved that argatroban dose-dependently achieved ACT prolongation more effectively than UFH in patients undergoing elective PCI with dual antiplatelet therapy (aspirin and clopidogrel). Importantly, this study provides evidence that argatroban has a predictable anticoagulant effect and can be used in patients undergoing PCI with dual antiplatelet therapy (only studied with aspirin and clopidogrel). Particular settings where argatroban may be most attractive is in patients with HIT or renal dysfunction when undergoing PCI [80,92].

Monitoring

Like bivalirudin, argatroban can cause elevations in multiple monitoring assays: aPTT, PT, ACT, and ecarin clotting time (ECA-T) which is sensitive only to direct thrombin inhibitors. There seems to be a consistent dose–effect relationship with using argatroban, regardless of the assay used. In contrast to UFH, argatroban causes a faster response in all coagulation parameters—quicker rise after initiation and normalization after stopping medication. ACT is the most appropriate method for monitoring the effect of argatroban in patients undergoing PCI [93].

Argatroban is given intravenously with bolus dose of 350 μg/kg followed by initial infusion rate of 25 μg/kg/minute. ACT should be checked within 10 minutes and can proceed with PCI if ACT >300 s. If ACT <300 s, give an additional 150 μg/kg bolus and increase the infusion rate to 30 μg/kg/minute. If ACT >450 s, decrease the infusion rate to 15 μg/kg/minute. An ACT level should be obtained within 10 minutes after any change to the infusion rate of argatroban [94].

Reversal of direct thrombin inhibitors (bivalirudin, argatroban)

There are no specific reversal agents available for direct thrombin inhibitors. In normal healthy subjects with normal kidney function, coagulation times will return to normal within 1 hour of discontinuing the infusion. Recombinant factor VIIa can reduce some of the bleeding effect from these agents. Hemodialysis can remove approximately 25% of bivalirudin or argatroban [37].

Antiplatelets

Platelets have a key role in arterial thrombotic events. Once normal endothelium is compromised, platelet adhesion, activation, and aggregation lead to thrombus formation. Adhesion of platelets to the site of vessel wall injury occurs via von Willebrand factor and other glycoprotein cell receptors (GP Ib/IX/V, GP IV, GP VI, GP Ia/IIa). Platelet activation occurs following adhesion which initiates further activation of surrounding platelets through secretion of platelet granules from agonists (adenosine diphosphate, collagen, thrombin), synthesis of thromboxane A2, and increased expression of activated GP IIb/IIIa receptors on the platelet surface. The activation also facilitates binding of factors Va and VIIIa. Platelet aggregation occurs via fibrinogen acting as a bridge between GP IIb/IIIa receptors on neighboring platelets. Platelet aggregation leads to formation of a platelet plug which is further anchored by fibrin mesh developed from the coagulation cascade [14,95]. This important cascade of events leads to the serious complications of MI and stroke. Steps of the cascade can be interrupted by different classes of antiplatelet agents in order to minimize the risk of arterial thrombosis. Aspirin irreversibly inhibits the production of thromboxane A2 by acetylating cyclo-oxygenase-1 (COX-1). This reduces platelet activation and recruitment to the site of injury. Thienopyridines (ticlopidine, clopidogrel, prasugrel) and other adenosine diphosphate

(ADP) antagonists (ticagrelor, cangrelor) inhibit the P2Y12 receptor, a key ADP receptor on the platelet surface. Ticlopidine, clopidogrel, and prasugrel irreversibly inhibit P2Y12, whereas ticagrelor and cangrelor are reversible inhibitors of P2Y12. GP IIb/IIIa inhibitors (abciximab, eptifibatide, tirofiban) inhibit platelet aggregation by preventing fibrinogen and von Willebrand factor from binding to activated GP IIb/IIIa [35]. Antiplatelet therapy is the standard of care, not only in patients undergoing PCI, but also in the acute and long-term management of ACS (Table 49.2) [95–97].

Aspirin

Aspirin (ASA) has long been recognized for its protective effect of thrombotic occlusive events and its importance in reducing incidence of death, MI, and stroke as seen in the large meta-analysis carried out by the Antithrombotic Trialists' Collaboration [98]. ASA has also been shown to significantly decrease mortalities in the setting of acute STEMI and severe cardiovascular complications in patients undergoing PCI. Since the benefit of ASA has been widely established, it is now the standard of therapy in clinical practice and routine background therapy when studying possible additive benefits of other agents used in treatment of ACS or during PCI [14].

Several studies have attempted to define the "optimal" dose of ASA. A dose of 75 mg achieves complete inactivation of COX-1 [35]. When comparing ASA 75 mg/day with high doses up to 1500 mg/day there has been no proven benefit but rather there is increased risk of bleeding (particularly gastrointestinal). There is less conclusive evidence on the benefit of doses less than 75 mg [99–101]. In situations where an immediate antithrombotic event is needed (i.e., ACS, ischemic stroke), a higher dose of aspirin (160–325 mg) should be given as either a chewed pill, solution, or even intravenously where available. Current PCI guidelines recommend giving ASA 325 mg at least 2 hours and preferably 24 hours prior to PCI [4,98]. Low doses of ASA (75–150 mg/day) are recommended for long-term prevention of vascular events in high risk patients with less risk of bleeding events [102].

Monitoring

Although not routinely utilized in the clinical setting, multiple methods of monitoring platelet function have been developed over time. These monitoring methods have been developed and studied in the setting of ASA therapy and in the evaluation of bleeding diatheses without antiplatelet therapy. Ideally, platelet monitoring assays would identify whether a patient who had an occlusive event (MI or ischemic stroke) while on ASA therapy was caused by treatment failure or treatment resistance, or prospectively identify the risk of a patient developing severe bleeding, especially in the setting of surgery.

The bleeding time was the initial and is still the only *in vivo* test of platelet function. Initially developed as a measure of bleeding diatheses and the influence of platelet count, but after decades of broad clinical use it was subsequently found not to be predictive of clinical bleeding in the setting of surgery or antiplatelet therapy [103]. Several point-of-care antiplatelet assays have been developed and studied in research settings; however, similar to bleeding time, there has been no clinical evidence that shows the clinical benefit of these monitoring methods. Light transmittance aggregometry (LTA) is the historic gold standard of platelet function testing which has shown a significantly higher risk of thrombotic events in patients with increased aggregation in the setting of ASA therapy. However, this test is labor intensive and technically demanding,

Table 49.2 Types and properties of common antiplatelet agents.

	Mechanism of action	Time of onset (half-life)	Recommended point-of-care test	Platelet function test available	Reversal for bleeding
Aspirin	Irreversibly inhibits COX-1,2 and thromboxane-A2	1–2 hours (~3 hours for doses up to 325 mg)	None	LTA	Platelets, Desmopressin
Clopidogrel	Thienopyridine; Irreversibly blocks P2Y12 receptor	20–30% platelet inhibition at 6 hours, 300–600 mg (6 hours); 50–60% platelet inhibition at 5–7 days, 50–100 mg	None	LTA, VerifyNow®, ImpactR®, TEG®, VASP, Multiplate	Platelets, Desmopressin
Prasugrel		<30 minutes, 60 mg (7 hours)	None	LTA, VerifyNow®, ImpactR®, TEG®, VASP, Multiplate	Platelets, Desmopressin
Ticagrelor	Non-thienopyridine; reversibly inhibiting P2Y12 receptors	41% platelet inhibition <30 minutes, 180 mg (6–12 hours)	None	LTA, VerifyNow®, ImpactR®, TEG®, VASP, Multiplate	Platelets, Desmopressin
Cangrelor		Rapid onset (3–6 minutes)	None	LTA, VerifyNow®, ImpactR®, TEG®, VASP, Multiplate	Platelets, Desmopressin
Abciximab	Near irreversible, GP IIb/IIIa inhibition	<10 minutes (15–30 minutes)	None	LTA, VerifyNow®, PFA-100®	Platelets, Desmopressin
Eptifibatide	Reversible GP IIb/IIIa inhibition	<60 minutes (2–3 hours)	None	LTA, VerifyNow®, PFA-100®	Hemodialysis, Platelets, Desmopressin
Tirofiban	Reversible GP IIb/IIIa inhibition	<30 minutes (1.5–2 hours)	None	LTA, VerifyNow®, PFA-100®	Hemodialysis, Platelets, Desmopressin

COX, cyclo-oxygenase; GP, glycoprotein; LTA, light transmission aggregometry; PFA-100®, platelet function analyzer; VASP, vasodilator-stimulated phosphoprotein phosphorylation.

preventing its routine application in clinical practice. Simpler, point-of-care devices such as the VerifyNow aspirin assay have been developed and shown to correlate well with LTA. Studies using the VerifyNow aspirin assay found that patients with elevated platelet agglutination while receiving ASA had higher elevations of cardiac biomarkers (CK-MB, troponin I) when undergoing elective PCI. Unlike the LTA, the VerifyNow aspirin assay has less processing time and is easier to use. Despite these findings, there have been no studies to suggest change of therapy, based on point-of-care ASA assays, would have a benefit on clinical outcomes or cost efficiency [95,104,105].

Reversal

The antiplatelet effect of ASA lasts 5–10 days. Rarely does the antiplatelet effect of aspirin need to be reversed, with the exception of intracranial bleeding. However, if bleeding from aspirin needs to be reversed immediately, platelet concentrate can be administered, although banked platelets are also functionally diminished. Desmopressin, or DDAVP, can also be used to correct the antiplatelet effect of aspirin. Dosing is similar when used for hemophilia or von Willebrand disease: 0.3 μg/kg in 100 mL infused over 30 minutes [69].

P2Y12 inhibitors (clopidogrel, prasugrel, ticagrelor, cangrelor)

Inhibiting P2Y12 receptors for ADP provide additional antiplatelet therapy to ASA. Some studies suggest even synergistic platelet inhibition provides enhanced protection from thrombotic complications during PCI. The role of dual antiplatelet therapy beyond the setting of PCI is less clear and may be agent specific [100].

Clopidogrel received FDA approval in 1998 following the results of the CAPRIE trial which compared ASA only with clopidogrel alone. The clopidogrel group of patients had a statistically significant (p = 0.043) lower risk of MI, ischemic stroke, or vascular death (9.8%) compared with the ASA group (10.7%). This study showed that clopidogrel is a safe and effective alternative to aspirin [106]. The CURE Trial was the first large-scale prospective trial of dual antiplatelet therapy versus ASA alone which found that when used for patients with unstable angina or NSTEMI, clopidogrel plus ASA reduces ischemic events relative to ASA, regardless of whether invasive or non-invasive therapy. There was a higher incidence of major bleeding events, with an increased risk of CABG-related bleeding limited to those who underwent surgery sooner than 5 days after discontinuing clopidogrel. The subanalysis of the PCI cohort, PCI-CURE, showed that ASA with clopidogrel pretreatment (median 6 days) followed by long-term therapy after PCI had a 31% reduction in cardiovascular death or MI at 30 days and 9 months (p = 0.002) when compared to no pretreatment and short-term dual therapy (4 weeks after PCI). There was no significant difference in major bleeding between the groups [107]. The CREDO trial studied the benefits of pretreatment and long-term treatment (1 year) with clopidogrel and ASA in the setting of non-urgent PCI. The results showed a 26.9% relative risk reduction for combined incidence of death, MI, or stroke (p = 0.02) at 1 year, although only a trend toward benefit at 30 days as a result of pretreatment [96]. A post hoc analysis of the results suggested that a longer interval between the loading dose of clopidogrel and PCI can further reduce peri-procedural thrombotic events. Patients receiving 300 mg clopidogrel at least 10–12 hours prior to PCI experienced a significant reduction in the combined 30-day endpoint [108]. Giving a loading dose of 600 mg clopidogrel to patients undergoing PCI raises the plasma concentration of the clopidogrel-active metabolite and causes greater suppression of ADP-induced platelet aggregation. Further aggregation suppression was not significant with doses higher than 600 mg (i.e., 900 mg) [109]. Using a loading dose of 600 mg prior to PCI in comparison with 300 mg showed a significant reduction in the primary endpoints of death, MI, and target vessel revascularization at 30 days (4% vs. 12%, respectively; p = 0.041). The 600 mg loading dose was associated with a lower incidence of peri-procedural MI (OR 0.48, 95% CI 0.15–0.97; p = 0.044) [110,111].

Use of clopidogrel in setting of acute STEMI treated with a primary non-invasive strategy gained acceptance following the results of CLARITY-TIMI 28 and COMMIT trials [112,113]. Patients with STEMI initially treated with a thrombolytic who then received clopidogrel prior to PCI showed reductions in death, recurrent MI, and stroke without increased bleeding [114]. The CURRENT-OASIS 7 trial was a large multicenter international study that showed benefit of using a double dose of clopidogrel for 7 days starting with a loading dose of 600 mg followed by 150 mg in comparison to the standard dose of 300 mg loading dose then 75 mg/day. There was a lower incidence in the primary outcomes of cardiovascular death, MI, or stroke when using a double dose of clopidogrel versus the standard dose (3.9% vs. 4.5%, respectively; adjusted HR 0.74–0.99; p = 0.039). Lower incidence of MI was the main reason for this difference as there were similar rates of cardiovascular deaths and stroke between the two groups. Stent thrombosis was also much lower in the double dose group [115]. The GRAVITAS trial showed that a prolonged course of double dose clopidogrel at 150 mg/day versus 75 mg/day had no reduction in cardiovascular death, MI, or stent thrombosis even in patients with high platelet reactivity [116].

Prasugrel is a new thienopyridine proven to be beneficial in the treatment of patients with ACS undergoing PCI. Similar to clopidogrel, prasugrel irreversibly binds to the P2Y12 receptor. Prasugrel is rapidly absorbed and nearly completely activated. In contrast, clopidogrel is more slowly absorbed and only ~15% undergoes metabolic activation [35]. The quick onset of action for prasugrel makes it attractive to use at the time of PCI, especially in the setting of ACS. Prasugrel 60 mg achieves high levels of platelet inhibition by 30 minutes as opposed to clopidogrel 300 and 600 mg doses which require 4–6 hours. The duration of platelet inhibition for both clopidogrel and prasugrel lasts for at least 5–7 days because of its irreversible binding of P2Y12 receptors [117–119]. In patients with ACS scheduled to undergo PCI, TRITON-TIMI 38 proved prasugrel to be superior in both loading and maintenance doses (60 and 10 mg) to clopidogrel (300 and 75 mg) in preventing death, MI, ischemic stroke, urgent revascularization, and stent thrombosis (9.9% vs. 12.1%, hazard ratio 0.81; p < 0.001). There was a significantly higher risk of major bleeding, specifically in patients aged >75 years, weight <60 kg, or with a history of stroke or TIA. The overall benefit with prasugrel is strengthened after excluding these patients (HR 0.74, 95% CI 0.66–0.84; p < 0.001) [120–122].

Ticagrelor is a novel, non-thienopyridine, reversible P2Y12 inhibitor that has a rapid onset of action within 30 minutes to peak platelet inhibition within 2 hours. Because of its reversible receptor binding properties, ticagrelor has a short half-life of 6–12 hours and requires twice daily dosing [117]. The PLATO investigators showed superiority of ticagrelor compared with clopidogrel in patients with ACS with or without STEMI, all on a background of ASA. Patients in the ticagrelor group had significantly lower rates of death from vascular causes, MI, or stroke without an increase in the rate of major bleeding. The benefits were evident at 30 days and persisted at 1-year follow-up [123]. Early administration of ticagrelor (pre-hospital vs. in-hospital) prior to PCI has been shown to be safe and to reduce the incidence of stent thrombosis at 24 hours and 30 days [124].

Cangrelor is an intravenously administered non-thienopyridine that reversibly inhibits the P2Y12 receptor, achieving high levels of platelet inhibition *in vitro* and *ex vivo*. It is notable for its very rapid onset of action and short half-life (3–6 minutes) [125]. Normalization of platelet function occurs within 60 minutes after discontinuing cangrelor. Prior large-scale randomized trials did not find cangrelor to be superior to placebo or clopidogrel 600 mg when used in patients with ACS or stable angina when given prior to PCI in terms of reducing composite endpoints (death, MI, or revascularization) [126,127]. More recently, a study has shown promise in the use of cangrelor when compared with clopidogrel loading doses at time of PCI for stable angina, ACS without ST-segment elevation, or STEMI. Patients receiving cangrelor had lower composite endpoint rates of death from any cause, MI, revascularization, or stent thrombosis at 48 hours (4.7% vs. 5.9%, OR 0.78, 95% CI 0.66–0.93; p = 0.005) with peri-procedural MI driving most of the benefit. There was a non-significant increase in bleeding with cangrelor by some definitions [128]. Cangrelor is potentially an alternative agent in patients unable to take or adequately absorb enteral medications; however, at this time it is not commercially available.

Current guideline recommendations are to give a loading dose of a P2Y12 inhibitor (i.e., clopidogrel 600 mg, prasugrel 60 mg, ticagrelor 180 mg) prior to PCI in ACS and non-ACS settings followed by maintenance dual antiplatelet therapy with ASA and a P2Y12 inhibitor (clopidogrel 75 mg/day, prasugrel 10 mg/day, ticagrelor 90 mg twice daily) for at least 1 month after bare metal stent placement and at least 1 year after drug-eluting stent placement [4,129].

Monitoring

Tailored antiplatelet therapy based on platelet reactivity and responsiveness has been theorized to potentially improve outcomes. One theory regarding the concern of antiplatelet resistance is that there is actual platelet hyper-reactivity in the setting of the acute thrombotic event, although whether it is a cause or effect is not clear [130]. Several studies using the VerifyNow P2Y12 assay have shown a correlation between higher platelet reactivity based on the assay and adverse cardiovascular outcomes including death [131]. The GRAVITAS trial aimed to evaluate whether tailoring clopidogrel after PCI would improve outcomes based on point-of-care platelet function assays but found no improvement in outcomes with higher dose antiplatelet therapy based on higher platelet reactivity [116]. Similarly, the ARCTIC trial found no differences in major adverse cardiac events (MACE) when antiplatelet therapy was tailored both before and after stent placement based on platelet function monitoring using the VerifyNow P2Y12 assay (Accumetrics Corporation, San Diego, CA, USA) compared with standard treatment without monitoring [132]. The vasodilator-stimulated phosphoprotein (VASP) phosphorylation analysis is highly specific for P2Y12 inhibitors showing strong correlation between platelet reactivity and clinical outcomes but it is not useful as a point-of-care method during PCI [133,134]. Another method of monitoring is using multiple electrode platelet aggregometry with the Multiplate analyzer (Roche, Basel, Switzerland). A study using the Multiplate point-of-care method was able to show a strong correlation amongst patients considered poor responders to clopidogrel (evident by higher platelet reactivity) with higher incidence of stent thrombosis [135]. Further, a study used the Multiplate analyzer to adjust antiplatelet

therapy in patients 12–36 hours after PCI and who were pretreated with clopidogrel. Patients found to have high platelet reactivity based on Multiplate analyzer results were randomized to either prasugrel or higher dose clopidogrel. This tailoring of therapy showed not only significantly more platelet inhibition, but lower incidence of death, MI, stent thrombosis, or stroke in the prasugrel group compared with the high dose clopidogrel group. The prasugrel group had a similarly lower risk than patients without high platelet reactivity. There was also less bleeding when switched to prasugrel [136]. Despite efforts made to identify an accurate and reliable point-of-care assay for P2Y12 inhibitors at time of PCI and for tailored antiplatelet therapy, there is insufficient evidence that point-of-care platelet function testing for P2Y12 inhibitors would be beneficial [137,138]. The ongoing TROPICAL-ACS trial, with an anticipated enrollment of 2600 using the Multiplate analyzer, will be one of the largest and definitive studies of the potential benefit of tailored antiplatelet therapy based on monitoring [139].

Reversing P2Y12 antagonists

Bleeding while on dual antiplatelet therapy remains a difficult situation to manage. Patients who have undergone recent stent implantation are still at high risk of stent thrombosis until complete endothelialization occurs. Besides cangrelor, all P2Y12 antagonists require days off therapy before platelet function is normalized. If the decision is made to reverse bleeding induced by P2Y12 inhibitors, it is recommended to administer platelet concentrate. Desmopressin (DDAVP) can also be used to correct the effect on platelet aggregation [69].

Glycoprotein IIb/IIIa inhibitors (abciximab, eptifibatide, tirofiban)

Vessel trauma by PCI can lead to adhesion, followed by activation and aggregation of platelets. GP IIb/IIIa inhibitors offer additional protection from thrombus formation by preventing platelet aggregation and reducing risk of intracoronary thrombosis [140]. Currently, three GP IIb/IIIa inhibitors are available for use during PCI: abciximab, eptifibatide, and tirofiban. These agents block fibrinogen from binding to GP IIb/IIIa receptors. Meta-analysis of GP IIb/IIIa inhibitors during PCI has shown a 30-day mortality benefit in addition to fewer incidences of non-fatal MI and urgent repeat revascularizations. The strongest data supporting the use of GP IIb/IIIa inhibitors comes from trials studying abciximab [141]. The EPILOG and EPISTENT trials demonstrated sustained benefits in these endpoints up to 1 year whereas EPIC reported benefit at 3 years [10,142–144]. Select populations especially experience a protective effect during PCI with GP IIb/IIIa inhibitors: high risk ACS, diabetic patients, and those with chronic kidney disease [145].

The first developed GP IIb/IIIa inhibitor, abciximab, is a human-murine chimeric monoclonal antibody with high affinity for GP IIb/IIIa receptors leading to near-irreversible inhibition, although its plasma half-life is short. Approximately 50% platelet inhibition remains 24 hours after discontinuing abciximab. The EPIC trial first showed its clinical benefit during PCI with a 35% reduction in rate of primary endpoints (death from any cause, non-fatal MI, CABG, or repeat PCI for acute ischemia; placement of intra-aortic balloon pump to relieve refractory ischemia); a 10% reduction was observed after abciximab bolus alone [142,146]. The breakthrough trials EPIC, EPILOG, and EPISTENT demonstrated that treatment with abciximab and UFH (abciximab continued after procedure) was superior to UFH alone in reducing major adverse cardiac events following PCI without significant differences in bleeding complications between the treatment groups [142–144].

Abciximab administration can improve outcomes in PCI for patients with STEMI. The ADMIRAL trial randomized patients to receive abciximab plus stenting or placebo plus stenting for treatment of STEMI. Abciximab improved coronary patency and left ventricular function with fewer incidences of reinfarction and recurrent ischemia. Although not statistically significant, there remained a mortality benefit from 30 days to 3 years after PCI treatment of STEMI in patients who received abciximab. In this 3-year follow-up period there was a 30% relative risk reduction of the composite endpoint of death and MI [147]. The CADILLAC trial randomized 2082 patients presenting with STEMI to treatment groups of balloon angioplasty alone, balloon angioplasty plus abciximab, stenting alone, or stenting plus abciximab. Use of abciximab showed significant improvements (p <0.001) in the primary composite endpoint of death, reinfarction, stroke, and ischemia-driven target vessel revascularization. The endpoint occurrences were balloon angioplasty alone 20%, balloon angioplasty plus abciximab 16.5%, bare metal stent alone 11.5%, and bare metal stent plus abciximab 10.2%. These endpoints were mainly driven by revascularization as there were no significant differences between the groups treated with stents in terms of rates of death, stroke, or reinfarction [148]. Antoniucci et al. [149] similarly demonstrated a reduction in composite endpoint of death, reinfarction, target vessel revascularization, and stroke at 1 month when comparing bare metal stent plus abciximab to bare metal stent alone (4.5% vs. 10.5%, respectively; p = 0.023). There was also smaller infarct size on technetium-99 m sestamibi scintigraphy at 1 month. Abciximab is recommended for STEMI and high risk patients undergoing PCI. Abciximab is not recommended for low risk patients or non-invasive treatment for ACS [150,151].

There has been less convincing evidence for eptifibatide and tirofiban. Both are smaller molecules than abciximab. Eptifibatide is a synthetic heptapeptide (<1000 Da) that reversibly binds to a beta subunit of GP IIb/IIIa receptor, causing platelet inhibition correlating to the plasma level of the drug. It is metabolized by the kidneys with half-life of ~2–3 hours. Tirofiban is a tyrosine derivative non-peptide that is metabolized by the biliary system (30–40%) and primarily excreted by the kidneys (60–70%). Tirofiban half-life is ~1.5–2 hours [152].

The IMPACT-II trial randomized patients undergoing elective, urgent, or emergency PCI to one of three treatment arms: placebo, eptifibatide 135 µg/kg bolus followed by 0.5 µg/kg/min infusion, or eptifibatide 135 µg/kg bolus followed by 0.75 µg/kg/min infusion. There was no significant difference between the eptifibatide groups compared with placebo in the composite endpoint of death, MI, unplanned surgical or repeat percutaneous revascularization, or coronary stent implantation for abrupt closure. Additionally, there was no difference in outcomes between the eptifibatide groups [153]. It has been hypothesized that the doses used in this trial may have been insufficient to provide adequate platelet inhibition [14]. The PURSUIT trial investigators used higher doses of eptifibatide in patients with ACS, but without STEMI. Those patients undergoing early PCI (<72 hours) treated with eptifibatide 180 µg/kg bolus followed by 2.0 µg/kg/min infusion had a significantly lower 30-day composite endpoint of death or non-fatal MI than the placebo group (11.6% vs. 16.7; p = 0.01) [154]. The ESPRIT trial randomized 2064 patients undergoing PCI to receive a high dose regimen of eptifibatide or placebo. The eptifibatide group received two boluses of 180 µg/kg administered 10 minutes apart followed by 2.0 µg/kg/

min infusion for 18–24 hours. Both groups also received ASA, heparin, and a thienopyridine as part of standard therapy. The primary endpoint was composite of death, MI, urgent target vessel revascularization, and thrombotic bailout GP IIb/IIIa inhibitor therapy within 48 hours after randomization. The trial was terminated early because of significant efficacy findings: primary endpoint reduced from 10.5% in placebo group to 6.6% in eptifibatide group (p = 0.0015). Although not frequent, major bleeding occurred more often in the eptifibatide group (1.3% vs. 0.4%; p = 0.027). This trial proved that pretreatment with eptifibatide as a GP IIb/IIIa inhibitor significantly reduces ischemic complications during PCI [155], and provided the recommended eptifibatide dosing in current guidelines for patients undergoing PCI treated with UFH [4].

Tirofiban showed a non-significant trend toward reduced endpoints of death, MI, revascularization in the balloon angioplasty-based RESTORE trial; however, there was also higher rates of major bleeding than with placebo [156]. Later, the PRISM-PLUS investigators demonstrated greater efficacy in patients with ACS treated with UFH plus tirofiban over UFH alone. The endpoint of death, MI, or refractory ischemia was reduced from 17.9% in the UFH alone group to 12.9% in the UFH plus tirofiban at 30 days (p = 0.004). Subgroup analysis of patients who underwent PCI provided further evidence that the combination of tirofiban with UFH compared with UFH alone reduced the endpoint incidence from 15.3% to 8.8% (risk ratio 0.55, CI 95% 0.32–0.94) [157]. In the TARGET trial, tirofiban was compared head-to-head against abciximab in a non-inferiority trial in ~5000 patients undergoing PCI. Surprisingly, tirofiban was found to be inferior to abciximab [158]. Subsequent studies suggested that the dose of tirofiban studied in TARGET was too low. Smaller trials have studied higher doses with encouraging results [159]. Current PCI guidelines recommend administration of GP IIb/IIIa inhibitors with UFH in patients with high risk ACS when not treated with bivalirudin and not adequately pretreated with a thienopyridine [4].

Monitoring

Although the GP IIb/IIIa inhibitors are beneficial during PCI, there is a narrow therapeutic window. Earlier studies on GP IIb/IIIa inhibitors showed higher risk of bleeding and thrombocytopenia (especially with abciximab). There is variability amongst GP IIb/IIIa inhibitors as a result of pharmacologic differences. For example, the plasma level of eptifibatide correlates closely with platelet inhibition, whereas abciximab does not provide good correlation because it has high affinity to the receptors and is cleared rapidly from plasma [160]. This brings up the important question as to how to best tailor GP IIb/IIIa therapy, not only during PCI, but also for the return of normal platelet function. The theoretical benefit of tailored therapy based on monitoring is met with the real-life limitations such as technical experience, expensive equipment, and transferring what is found in vitro to the clinical situation. It remains to be proven whether an assay can provide the most reliable results and be translated into clinical practice [161].

Light transmission aggregometry has historically been the gold standard of platelet function testing. Although it is based on the fibrinogen–GP IIb/IIIa aggregation, its poor reproducibility between laboratories, long sampling time, and labor-intensive requirements make it less appealing during PCI.

The best study to date correlating the efficiency of platelet inhibition through GP IIb/IIIa inhibitors with clinical outcomes was the GOLD multicenter study. This study used the point-of-care Ultegra-rapid platelet function assay (RPFA), known as the

VerifyNow assay. The VerifyNow assay provides a quick and simple means of monitoring GP IIb/IIIa inhibitors with results that correlate well with aggregometry and receptor-binding assays [162]. In this study, 485 patients were evaluated for the primary endpoint of MACE: death, MI, or urgent target vessel revascularization in hospital or within 7 days of PCI. The predominant GP IIb/IIIa inhibitor used was abciximab (84%), others received tirofiban (9%) or eptifibatide (7%). The dosing regimens for each medication were based on previously described trials showing potential benefit of their use in PCI. Platelet inhibition was achieved at high percentages in the initial 10 minutes (96±9%), 1 hour (95±8%), and 8 hours (91±11%) after initiating therapy. However, at 24 hours the mean inhibition decreased to 73±20% with wide variability. The patients in the lowest quartile of platelet inhibition (<95%) at 10 minutes after GP IIb/IIIa bolus had a substantially higher incidence (14.4%) of MACE compared with those with >95% platelet inhibition (6.4%; p = 0.006). This study confirmed higher incidences of MACE are associated with lower levels of platelet inhibition but was not designed to demonstrate that altering therapy to achieve higher levels of inhibition improved outcomes. The study did not find a correlation between the level of platelet inhibition and major bleeding complications when using the point-of-care assay. However, an increased procedural ACT correlated with major bleeding [163,164].

Reversing GP IIb/IIIa inhibitors

Platelet monitoring for return to normal function is helpful in nonemergent situations; however, immediate reversal is warranted when major bleeding occurs or emergency CABG is needed. The pharmacodynamics of each GP IIb/IIIa inhibitor affect how they can be reversed in emergent situations. No direct antidote is available for any of the three available GP IIb/IIIa receptor antagonists.

Despite the long dissociation half-life from GP IIb/IIIa receptors of abciximab (up to 6–12 hours), it has a short plasma half-life (15–30 minutes) meaning that little of the medication remains in the plasma once discontinued. Platelet transfusion after discontinuing abciximab decreases the platelet receptor occupancy which is related to platelet function inhibition. Platelet transfusion leads to redistribution of abciximab from platelets saturated with the medication to transfused cells. This causes a "dilution" of bound GP IIb/IIIa receptors by abciximab with little hemostatic defect [165,166]. In addition to platelet transfusion, administration of desmopressin (DDAVP) can also have an additive effect in normalizing platelet function following GP IIb/IIIa inhibition [99].

Platelet transfusion is ineffective for the smaller molecule GP IIb/IIIa inhibitors (i.e., eptifibatide and tirofiban) because of their high plasma levels. The pharmacokinetic effect is dose dependent. The biologic half-life is ~2.5 hours for these agents based on the adjusted dosing for CrCl [146]. Reversal of the antiplatelet effect from eptifibatide and tirofiban occurs within 2–4 hours after discontinuation. It is typically considered safe to proceed with surgical procedure after the allotted time [166]. In patients with advanced renal insufficiency, where the time to reversal may be longer, hemodialysis can hasten the reversal of platelet inhibition induced by these agents [167,168].

Conclusions

Anticoagulation and antiplatelet therapy have been extensively studied since their inception. While certain agents have advantages and disadvantages relative to others, there will likely never be a "one size fits all" medication. Therapies require tailoring based on the unique needs of the patient. This holds true during PCI where certain presentations or pre-existing comorbidities make one anticoagulant or antiplatelet agent better than another. It is important not only to understand which therapies are available but when one is preferable over another, what are their unique limitations, and what other tools are needed to achieve optimal use of the medication. Understanding how to monitor (if possible) the therapy and how to manage emergency situations (major bleeding) is as crucial as the technical skills required during PCI.

Interactive multiple choice questions are available for this chapter on www.wiley.com/go/dangas/cardiology

References

1 Kolandaivelu K, Swaminathan R, Gibson WJ, et al. Stent thrombogenicity early in high-risk interventional settings is driven by stent design and deployment and protected by polymer-drug coatings/clinical perspective. *Circulation* 2011; **123**(13): 1400–1409.

2 Van Belle E, Tio FO, Couffinhal T, Maillard L, Passeri J, Isner JM. Stent endothelialization. *Circulation* 1997; **95**(2): 438–448.

3 Xie Y, Takano M, Murakami D, et al. Comparison of neointimal coverage by optical coherence tomography of a sirolimus-eluting stent versus a bare-metal stent three months after implantation. *Am J Cardiol* 2008; **102**(1): 27–31.

4 Writing Committee Members, Levine GN, Bates ER, et al. 2011 ACCF/AHA/SCAI guideline for percutaneous coronary intervention. *Circulation* 2011; **124**(23): e574–e651.

5 Popma JJC, Weitz J, Bittl JA, et al. Antithrombotic therapy in patients undergoing coronary angioplasty. *Chest* 1998; **114**(5, Suppl): 728S–741S.

6 Gruntzig A. Transluminal dilatation of coronary-artery stenosis. *Lancet* 1978; **1**(8058): 263.

7 Gruntzig A, Hirzel H, Goebel N, et al. [Percutaneous transluminal dilatation of chronic coronary stenoses. first experiences]. *Schweiz Med Wochenschr* 1978; **108**(44): 1721–1723.

8 Fischman DL, Leon MB, Baim DS, et al. A randomized comparison of coronary-stent placement and balloon angioplasty in the treatment of coronary artery disease. *N Engl J Med* 1994; **331**(8): 496–501.

9 Serruys PW, Jaegere P, Kiemeneij F, et al. A comparison of balloon-expandable-stent implantation with balloon angioplasty in patients with coronary artery disease. *N Engl J Med* 1994; **331**(8): 489–495.

10 Harding SA, Walters D, Palacios I, Oesterle SN. Adjunctive pharmacotherapy for coronary stenting. *Curr Opin Cardiol* 2001; **16**(5): 293–299.

11 Hochholzer W, Wiviott SD, Antman EM, et al. Predictors of bleeding and time dependence of association of bleeding with mortality/clinical perspective. *Circulation* 2011; **123**(23): 2681–2689.

12 Rao SV, Ohman E, Magnus. Anticoagulant therapy for percutaneous coronary intervention. *Circ Cardiovasc Interv* 2010; **3**(1): 80–88.

13 O'Neill BP, Shaw ES, Cohen MG. Anticoagulation in percutaneous coronary intervention. *Interv Cardiol* 2010; **2**(4): 559–577.

14 Garg R, Uretsky BF, Lev EI. Anti-platelet and anti-thrombotic approaches in patients undergoing percutaneous coronary intervention. *Catheter Cardiovasc Interv* 2007; **70**(3): 388–406.

15 Hirsh JA, Sonia S, Halperin JL, Fuster V. Guide to anticoagulant therapy: heparin. A statement for healthcare professionals from the American Heart Association. *Circulation* 2001; **103**(24): 2994–3018.

16 Cohen MA, , Parry PC, Xiong G, et al.; Valentin Antithrombotic Therapy in Acute Coronary Syndromes Research Group. Combination antithrombotic therapy in unstable rest angina and non-Q-wave infarction in nonprior aspirin users: primary end points analysis from the ATACS trial. *Circulation* 1994; **89**(1): 81–88.

17 Oler A, Whooley MA, Oler J, Grady D. Adding heparin to aspirin reduces the incidence of myocardial infarction and death in patients with unstable angina: a meta-analysis. *JAMA* 1996; **276**(10): 811–815.

18 Neri Serneri GG, Rovelli F, Gensini GF, Pirelli S, Carnovali M, Fortini A. Effectiveness of low-dose heparin in prevention of myocardial reinfarction. *Lancet* 1987; **1**(8539): 937–942.

19 Li Y,b, Rha S, Chen K, et al. Low-molecular-weight heparin versus unfractionated heparin in acute ST-segment elevation myocardial infarction patients undergoing primary percutaneous coronary intervention with drug-eluting stents. *Am Heart J* 2010; **159**(4): 684–690e1.

20 Montalescot G, Collet JP, Lison L, et al. Effects of various anticoagulant treatments on von Willebrand factor release in unstable angina. J Am Coll Cardiol 2000; **36**(1): 110–114.

21 de Feyter PJ, van den Brand M, Laarman GJ, et al. Acute coronary artery occlusion during and after percutaneous transluminal coronary angioplasty: frequency, prediction, clinical course, management, and follow-up. Circulation 1991; **83**(3): 927–936.

22 Shahzad A, Kemp I, Mars C, et al. Unfractionated heparin versus bivalirudin in primary percutaneous coronary intervention (HEAT-PPCI): an open-label, single centre, randomised controlled trial. Lancet 2014; **384**(9957): 1849–1858.

23 Young E, Prins M, Levine MN, Hirsh J. Heparin binding to plasma proteins, an important mechanism for heparin resistance. Thromb Haemost 1992; **67**(6): 639–643.

24 Marciniak E. Factor-xa inactivation by antithrombin. 3. Evidence for biological stabilization of factor xa by factor V-phospholipid complex. Br J Haematol 1973; **24**(3): 391–400.

25 Hirsh J, Warkentin TE, Raschke R, Granger C, Ohman EMBC, Dalen JE. Heparin and low-molecular-weight heparin: mechanisms of action, pharmacokinetics, dosing considerations, monitoring, efficacy, and safety. Chest 1998; **114**(5, Suppl): 489S–510S.

26 Xiao Z, Theroux P. Platelet activation with unfractionated heparin at therapeutic concentrations and comparisons with a low-molecular-weight heparin and with a direct thrombin inhibitor. Circulation 1998; **97**(3): 251–256.

27 D'Angelo A, Seveso MP, D'Angelo SV, Gilardoni F, Dettori AG, Bonini P. Effect of clot-detection methods and reagents on activated partial thromboplastin time (APTT): implications in heparin monitoring by APTT. Am J Clin Pathol 1990; **94**(3): 297–306.

28 McGarry TF Jr, Gottlieb RS, Morganroth J, et al. The relationship of anticoagulation level and complications after successful percutaneous transluminal coronary angioplasty. Am Heart J 1992; **123**(6): 1445–1451.

29 Ferguson JJ, Dougherty KG, Gaos CM, Bush HS, Marsh KC, Leachman DR. Relation between procedural activated coagulation time and outcome after percutaneous transluminal coronary angioplasty. J Am Coll Cardiol 1994; **23**(5): 1061–1065.

30 Narins CR, Hillegass WB Jr, Nelson CL, et al. Relation between activated clotting time during angioplasty and abrupt closure. Circulation 1996; **93**(4): 667–671.

31 Chew DPBS, Bhatt DL, Lincoff AM, et al. Defining the optimal activated clotting time during percutaneous coronary intervention: aggregate results from 6 randomized, controlled trials. Circulation 2001; **103**(7): 961–966.

32 Brener SJ, Moliterno DJ, Lincoff AM, et al. Relationship between activated clotting time and ischemic or hemorrhagic complications: analysis of 4 recent randomized clinical trials of percutaneous coronary intervention. Circulation 2004; **110**(8): 994–998.

33 Montalescot G, Cohen M, Salette G, et al. Impact of anticoagulation levels on outcomes in patients undergoing elective percutaneous coronary intervention: Insights from the STEEPLE trial. Eur Heart J 2008; **29**(4): 462–471.

34 Doherty TM, Shavelle RM, French WJ. Reproducibility and variability of activated clotting time measurements in the cardiac catheterization laboratory. Catheter Cardiovasc Interv 2005; **65**(3): 330–337.

35 Weitz JI. Blood coagulation and anticoagulant, fibrinolytic, and antiplatelet drugs. In: Brunton LL, Chabner BA, Knollmann BC(), eds. Goodman & Gilman's The Pharmacological Basis of Therapeutics, 12th edn. New York: McGraw-Hill, 2011.

36 Wakefield TW, Hantler CB, Wrobleski SK, Crider BA, Stanley JC. Effects of differing rates of protamine reversal of heparin anticoagulation. Surgery 1996; **119**(2): 123–128.

37 Garcia DA, Baglin TP, Weitz JIFCCP, Samama MM. Parenteral anticoagulants: antithrombotic therapy and prevention of thrombosis, 9th edn: American College of Chest Physicians evidence-based clinical practice guidelines. Chest 2012; **141**(2) (Suppl): e24S–e43S.

38 Harenberg J. Pharmacology of low molecular weight heparins. Semin Thromb Hemost 1990; **16**(Suppl): 12–18.

39 Kadakia RA, Baimeedi SR, Ferguson JJ. Low-molecular-weight heparins in the cardiac catheterization laboratory. Texas Heart Inst J 2004; **31**(1): 72–83.

40 Kleinschmidt K, Charles R. Pharmacology of low molecular weight heparins. Emerg Med Clin North Am 2001; **19**(4): 1025–1049.

41 Antman EM. The search for replacements for unfractionated heparin. Circulation 2001; **103**(18): 2310–2314.

42 Weitz JI. Low-molecular-weight heparins. N Engl J Med 1997; **337**(10): 688–699.

43 Ferguson JJ, Antman EM, Bates ER, et al. Combining enoxaparin and glycoprotein IIb/IIIa antagonists for the treatment of acute coronary syndromes: final results of the national investigators collaborating on enoxaparin-3 (NICE-3) study. Am Heart J 2003; **146**(4): 628–634.

44 Gurfinkel EP, Manos EJ, Mejail RI, et al. Low molecular weight heparin versus regular heparin or aspirin in the treatment of unstable angina and silent ischemia. J Am Coll Cardiol 1995; **26**(2): 313–318.

45 Klein W, Buchwald A, Hillis SE, et al. Comparison of low-molecular-weight heparin with unfractionated heparin acutely and with placebo for 6 weeks in the management of unstable coronary artery disease: fragmin in unstable coronary artery disease study (FRIC). Circulation 1997; **96**(1): 61–68.

46 Cohen M, Demers C, Gurfinkel EP, et al. A comparison of low-molecular-weight heparin with unfractionated heparin for unstable coronary artery disease. N Engl J Med 1997; **337**(7): 447–452.

47 Antman EMFACC, The Thrombolysis in Myocardial InfarctionB Trial Investigators. TIMI 11B. enoxaparin versus unfractionated heparin for unstable angina or non-Q-wave myocardial infarction: a double-blind, placebo-controlled, parallel-group, multicenter trial. rationale, study design, and methods. Am Heart J 1998; **135**(6, Part 3): S353–S360.

48 Antman EM, Cohen M, Radley D, et al. Assessment of the treatment effect of enoxaparin for unstable angina/non-Q-wave myocardial infarction: TIMI 11B-ESSENCE meta-analysis. Circulation 1999; **100**(15): 1602–1608.

49 SYNERGY Trial Investigators. Enoxaparin vs unfractionated heparin in high-risk patients with non-ST-segment elevation acute coronary syndromes managed with an intended early invasive strategy: primary results of the SYNERGY randomized trial. JAMA 2004; **292**(1): 45–54.

50 Drouet L, Bal dit Sollier C, Martin J. Adding intravenous unfractionated heparin to standard enoxaparin causes excessive anticoagulation not detected by activated clotting time: results of the STACK-on to ENOXaparin (STACKENOX) study. Am Heart J 2009; **158**(2): 177–184.

51 Montalescot G, White HD, Gallo R, et al. Enoxaparin versus unfractionated heparin in elective percutaneous coronary intervention. N Engl J Med 2006; **355**(10): 1006–1017.

52 Kereiakes DJ, Grines C, Fry E, et al. Enoxaparin and abciximab adjunctive pharmacotherapy during percutaneous coronary intervention. J Invasive Cardiol 2001; **13**(4): 272–278.

53 Bhatt DL, Lee BI, Casterella PJ, et al. Safety of concomitant therapy with eptifibatide and enoxaparin in patients undergoing percutaneous coronary intervention: results of the coronary revascularization using integrilin and single bolus enoxaparin study. J Am Coll Cardiol 2003; **41**(1): 20–25.

54 Dumaine R, Borentain M, Bertel O, et al. Intravenous low-molecular-weight heparins compared with unfractionated heparin in percutaneous coronary intervention: quantitative review of randomized trials. Arch Intern Med 2007; **167**(22): 2423–2430.

55 Gallo R, Steinhubl SR, White, Harvey D, for the STEEPLE Investigators. Impact of anticoagulation regimens on sheath management and bleeding in patients undergoing elective percutaneous coronary intervention in the STEEPLE trial. Catheter Cardiovasc Interv 2009; **73**(3): 319–325.

56 Henry TD, Satran D, Knox LL, Iacarella CL, Laxson DD, Antman EM. Are activated clotting times helpful in the management of anticoagulation with subcutaneous low-molecular-weight heparin? Am Heart J 2001; **142**(4): 590–593.

57 Linkins L, Julian JA, Rischke J, Hirsh J, Weitz JI. In vitro comparison of the effect of heparin, enoxaparin and fondaparinux on tests of coagulation. Thromb Res 2002; **107**(5): 241–244.

58 Abbate R, Gori AM, Farsi A, Attanasio M, Pepe G. Monitoring of low-molecular-weight heparins in cardiovascular disease. Am J Cardiol 1998; **82**(5, Suppl 2): 33L–36L.

59 Choussat Ré, Montalescot G, Collet JP, et al. A unique, low dose of intravenous enoxaparin in elective percutaneous coronary intervention. J Am Coll Cardiol 2002; **40**(11): 1943–1950.

60 Collet JP, Montalescot G, Golmard JL, et al. Percutaneous coronary intervention after subcutaneous enoxaparin pretreatment in patients with unstable angina pectoris. Circulation 2001; **103**(5): 658–663.

61 Montalescot G, Collet JP, Tanguy ML, et al. Anti-xa activity relates to survival and efficacy in unselected acute coronary syndrome patients treated with enoxaparin. Circulation 2004; **110**(4): 392–398.

62 Martin JL, Fry ETA, Sanderink GCM, et al. Reliable anticoagulation with enoxaparin in patients undergoing percutaneous coronary intervention: the pharmacokinetics of enoxaparin in PCI (PEPCI) study. Catheter Cardiovasc Interv 2004; **61**(2): 163–170.

63 Rouby SE, Cohen M, Gonzales A, et al. Point-of-care monitoring of enoxaparin in the presence of GPIIb/IIIa combined therapy during percutaneous coronary interventions. Point of Care 2005; **4**(1): 30–35.

64 Moliterno DM, Mukherjee D. Applications of monitoring platelet glycoprotein IIb/IIIa antagonism and low molecular weight heparins in cardiovascular medicine. Am Heart J 2000; **140**(6, Suppl): S136–S142.

65 Moliterno DJ, Hermiller JB, Kereiakes DJ, et al. A novel point-of-care enoxaparin monitor for use during percutaneous coronary intervention: results of the evaluating enoxaparin clotting times (ELECT) study. J Am Coll Cardiol 2003; **42**(6): 1132–1139.

66 Lim W, Dentali F, Eikelboom JW, Crowther MA. Meta-analysis: low-molecular-weight heparin and bleeding in patients with severe renal insufficiency. Ann Intern Med 2006; **144**(9): 673–684.

67 Popma JJ, Berger P, Ohman E, Harrington RA, Grines C, Weitz JI. Antithrombotic therapy during percutaneous coronary intervention: the seventh ACCP conference on antithrombotic and thrombolytic therapy. *Chest* 2004; **126**(3, Suppl): 576S–599S.

68 Lindblad B, Borgstrom A, Wakefield TW, Whitehouse WM Jr, Stanley JC. Protamine reversal of anticoagulation achieved with a low molecular weight heparin. the effects on eicosanoids, clotting and complement factors. *Thromb Res* 1987; **48**(1): 31–40.

69 Levi M, Eerenberg E, Kamphuisen PW. Bleeding risk and reversal strategies for old and new anticoagulants and antiplatelet agents. *J Thromb Haemost* 2011; **9**(9): 1705–1712.

70 Coussement PK, Bassand JP, Convens C, *et al.* A synthetic factor-xa inhibitor (ORG31540/SR9017A) as an adjunct to fibrinolysis in acute myocardial infarction: the PENTALYSE study. *Eur Heart J* 2001; **22**(18): 1716–1724.

71 Simoons ML, Bobbink IW, Boland J, *et al.* A dose-finding study of fondaparinux in patients with non-ST-segment elevation acute coronary syndromes: the pentasaccharide in unstable angina (PENTUA) study. *J Am Coll Cardiol* 2004; **43**(12): 2183–2190.

72 Fifth Organization to Assess Strategies in Acute Ischemic Syndromes,Investigators, Yusuf S, Mehta SR, *et al.* Comparison of fondaparinux and enoxaparin in acute coronary syndromes. *N Engl J Med* 2006; **354**(14): 1464–1476.

73 Mehta SR, Steg PG, Granger CB, *et al.* Randomized, blinded trial comparing fondaparinux with unfractionated heparin in patients undergoing contemporary percutaneous coronary intervention. Arixtra study in percutaneous coronary intervention. A randomized evaluation (ASPIRE) pilot trial. *Circulation* 2005; **111**(11): 1390–1397.

74 Yusuf S, Mehta SR, Chrolavicius S, *et al.* Effects of fondaparinux on mortality and reinfarction in patients with acute ST-segment elevation myocardial infarction: the OASIS-6 randomized trial. *JAMA* 2006; **295**(13): 1519–1530.

75 Mehta SR, Boden WE, Eikelboom JW, *et al.* Antithrombotic therapy with fondaparinux in relation to interventional management strategy in patients with ST- and non-ST-segment elevation acute coronary syndromes: An individual patient-level combined analysis of the fifth and sixth organization to assess strategies in ischemic syndromes (OASIS 5 and 6) randomized trials. *Circulation* 2008; **118**(20): 2038–2046.

76 Bijsterveld NR, Moons AH, Boekholdt SM, *et al.* Ability of recombinant factor VIIa to reverse the anticoagulant effect of the pentasaccharide fondaparinux in healthy volunteers. *Circulation* 2002; **106**(20): 2550–2554.

77 Topol EJ, Bonan R, Jewitt D, *et al.* Use of a direct antithrombin, hirulog, in place of heparin during coronary angioplast. *Circulation* 1993; **87**(5): 1622–1629.

78 Bittl JA, Strony J, Brinker JA, *et al.* Treatment with bivalirudin (hirulog) as compared with heparin during coronary angioplasty for unstable or postinfarction angina. *N Engl J Med* 1995; **333**(12): 764–769.

79 Bates SM, Weitz JI. The mechanism of action of thrombin inhibitors. *J Invasive Cardiol* 2000; **12**(Suppl F): 27 F–32.

80 Lewis BE, Hursting MJ. Direct thrombin inhibition during percutaneous coronary intervention in patients with heparin-induced thrombocytopenia. *Exp Rev Cardiovasc Ther* 2007; **5**(1): 57–68.

81 Lee CJ, Ansell JE. Direct thrombin inhibitors. *Br J Clin Pharmacol* 2011; **72**(4): 581–592.

82 White HD, Aylward PE, Frey MJ, *et al.* Randomized, double-blind comparison of hirulog versus heparin in patients receiving streptokinase and aspirin for acute myocardial infarction (HERO). *Circulation* 1997; **96**(7): 2155–2161.

83 Kong DF, Topol EJ, Bittl JA, *et al.* Clinical outcomes of bivalirudin for ischemic heart disease. *Circulation* 1999; **100**(20): 2049–2053.

84 Bittl JA, Chaitman BR, Feit F, Kimball W, Topol EJ. Bivalirudin versus heparin during coronary angioplasty for unstable or postinfarction angina: final report reanalysis of the bivalirudin angioplasty study. *Am Heart J* 2001; **142**(6): 952–959.

85 Lincoff A, Michael Bittl JA, Harrington RA, *et al.* Bivalirudin and provisional glycoprotein IIb/IIIa blockade compared with heparin and planned glycoprotein IIb/IIIa blockade during percutaneous coronary intervention: REPLACE-2 randomized trial. *JAMA* 2003; **289**(7): 853–863.

86 Kastrati A, Neumann F, Schulz S, *et al.* Abciximab and heparin versus bivalirudin for non-ST-elevation myocardial infarction. *N Engl J Med* 2011; **365**(21): 1980–1989.

87 Stone GW, McLaurin BT, Cox DA, *et al.* Bivalirudin for patients with acute coronary syndromes. *N Engl J Med* 2006; **355**(21): 2203–2216.

88 Stone GW, Witzenbichler B, Guagliumi G, *et al.* Bivalirudin during primary PCI in acute myocardial infarction. *N Engl J Med* 2008; **358**(21): 2218–2230.

89 The Medicines Company. Angiomax. 2000. Available at: http://www.themedicinescompany.com/products/us-marketed-products (accessed May 12, 2016).

90 Moen MD, Keating GM, Wellington K. Bivalirudin: a review of its use in patients undergoing percutaneous coronary intervention. *Drugs* 2005; **65**(13): 1869–1891.

91 Wong C, White HD. Direct antithrombins: mechanisms, trials, and role in contemporary interventional medicine. *Am J Cardiovasc Drug* 2007; **7**(4): 249–257.

92 Rossig L, Genth-Zotz S, Rau M, *et al.* Argatroban for elective percutaneous coronary intervention: the ARG-E04 multi-center study. *Int J Cardiol* 2011; **148**(2): 214–219.

93 Akimoto K, Klinkhardt U, Zeiher A, Niethammer M, Harder S. Anticoagulation with argatroban for elective percutaneous coronary intervention: population pharmacokinetics and pharmacokinetic-pharmacodynamic relationship of coagulation parameters. *J Clin Pharmacol* 2011; **51**(6): 805–818.

94 GlaxoSmithKline. Argatroban Injection. 2000. Available at: https://www.gsksource.com/argatroban (accessed May 12, 2016).

95 van Werkum JW, Hackeng CM, Smit JJ, van't Hof AWJ, Verheugt FWA, ten Berg JM. Monitoring antiplatelet therapy with point-of-care platelet function assays: a review of the evidence. *Future Cardiol* 2008; **4**(1): 33–55.

96 Steinhubl SR, Berger PB, Mann JT 3rd, *et al.*; CREDO Investigators. Clopidogrel for the Reduction of Events During Observation. Early and sustained dual oral antiplatelet therapy following percutaneous coronary intervention: a randomized controlled trial. *JAMA* 2002; **288**: 2411–2420.

97 Becker R, Meade T, Berger P, *et al.* The primary and secondary prevention of coronary artery disease: American College of Chest Physicians Evidence-based Clinical Practice Guidelines (8th edn). *Chest* 2008; **133**: 776S–814S.

98 Antithrombotic Trialists' Collaboration. Collaborative meta-analysis of randomised trials of antiplatelet therapy for prevention of death, myocardial infarction, and stroke in high risk patients. *BMJ* 2002; **324**: 71–86.

99 Reiter RA, Jilma B. Platelets and new antiplatelet drugs. *Therapy* 2005; **2**(3): 465–502.

100 Holmes DR Jr, Kereiakes DJ, Kleiman NS, Moliterno DJ, Patti G, Grines CL. Combining antiplatelet and anticoagulant therapies. *J Am Coll Cardiol* 2009; **54**(2): 95–109.

101 Campbell CL, Smyth S, Montalescot G, Steinhubl SR. Aspirin dose for the prevention of cardiovascular disease: a systematic review. *JAMA* 2007; **297**(18): 2018–2024.

102 Peters RJ, Mehta SR, Fox KA, *et al.* Effects of aspirin dose when used alone or in combination with clopidogrel in patients with acute coronary syndromes: observations from the clopidogrel in unstable angina to prevent recurrent events (CURE) study. *Circulation* 2003; **108**: 1682–1687.

103 Steinhubl SR. Historical observations on the discovery of platelets, platelet function testing and the first antiplatelet agent. *Curr Drug Targets* 2011; **12**(12): 1792–1804.

104 Polena S, Zazzali KMDO, Shaikh HDO, *et al.* Comparison of a point-of-care platelet function testing to light transmission aggregometry in patients undergoing percutaneous coronary intervention pretreated with aspirin and clopidogrel. *Point of Care* 2011; **10**(1): 35–39.

105 Hezard N, TessierMarteau A, Macchi L. New insight in antiplatelet therapy monitoring in cardiovascular patients: from aspirin to thienopyridine. *Cardiovasc Hematol Disord Drug Targets* 2010; **10**(3): 224–233.

106 CAPRIE Steering Committee. A randomised, blinded, trial of clopidogrel versus aspirin in patients at risk of ischaemic events (CAPRIE). *Lancet* 1996; **348**: 1329–1339.

107 Mehta SR, Yusuf S, Peters RJ, *et al.* Effects of pretreatment with clopidogrel and aspirin followed by long-term therapy in patients undergoing percutaneous coronary intervention: the PCI-CURE study. *Lancet* 2002; **359**: 527–533.

108 Steinhubl SR, Berger PB, Brennan DM, Topol EJ, CREDO I. Optimal timing for the initiation of pre-treatment with 300 mg clopidogrel before percutaneous coronary intervention. *J Am Coll Cardiol* 2006; **47**(5): 939–943.

109 von Beckerath N, Taubert D, Pogatsa-Murray G, Schömig E, Kastrati A, Schömig A. Absorption, metabolization, and antiplatelet effects of 300-, 600-, and 900-mg loading doses of clopidogrel: results of the ISAR-CHOICE (intracoronary stenting and antithrombotic regimen: Choose between 3 high oral doses for immediate clopidogrel effect) trial. *Circulation* 2005; **112**(19): 2946–2950.

110 Patti G, Colonna G, Pasceri V, Pepe LL, Montinaro A, Di Sciascio G. Randomized trial of high loading dose of clopidogrel for reduction of periprocedural myocardial infarction in patients undergoing coronary intervention: Results from the ARMYDA-2 (antiplatelet therapy for reduction of MYocardial damage during angioplasty) study. *Circulation* 2005; **111**(16): 2099–2106.

111 Levine GN, Bates ER, Blankenship JC, *et al.* 2011 ACCF/AHA/SCAI guideline for percutaneous coronary intervention: a report of the American College of Cardiology Foundation/American Heart Association task force on practice guidelines and the society for cardiovascular angiography and interventions. *J Am Coll Cardiol* 2011; **58**(24): e44–122.

112 Sabatine MS, Cannon CP, Gibson CM, *et al.* Addition of clopidogrel to aspirin and fibrinolytic therapy for myocardial infarction with ST-segment elevation. *N Engl J Med* 2005; **352**: 1179–1189.

113 Chen ZM, Jiang LX, Chen YP, *et al.* Addition of clopidogrel in 45,852 patients with acute myocardial infarction: randomised placebo-controlled trial. *Lancet* 2005; **366**: 1607–1621.

114 Sabatine MS, Cannon CP, Gibson CM, *et al.* Effect of clopidogrel pretreatment before percutaneous coronary intervention in patients with ST-elevation myocardial infarction treated with fibrinolytics: the PCI-CLARITY study. *JAMA* 2005; **294**(10): 1224–1232.

115 Mehta SR, Tanguay J, Eikelboom JW, *et al.* Double-dose versus standard-dose clopidogrel and high-dose versus low-dose aspirin in individuals undergoing percutaneous coronary intervention for acute coronary syndromes (CURRENT-OASIS 7): a randomised factorial trial. *Lancet* 2010; **376**(9748): 1233–1243.

116 Price MJ, Berger PB, Teirstein PS, *et al.* Standard- vs high-dose clopidogrel based on platelet function testing after percutaneous coronary intervention: the GRAVITAS randomized trial. *JAMA* 2011; **305**(11): 1097–1105.

117 Wong YW, Prakash R, Chew DP. Antiplatelet therapy in percutaneous coronary intervention: recent advances in oral antiplatelet agents. *Curr Opin Cardiol* 2010; **25**: 305–311.

118 Angiolillo DJ. The evolution of antiplatelet therapy in the treatment of acute coronary syndromes: from aspirin to the present day. *Drugs* 2012; **72**(16): 2087–2116.

119 Wiviott SD, Trenk D, Frelinger AL, *et al.* Prasugrel compared with high loading- and maintenance-dose clopidogrel in patients with planned percutaneous coronary intervention: the prasugrel in comparison to clopidogrel for inhibition of platelet activation and aggregation-thrombolysis in myocardial infarction 44 trial. *Circulation* 2007; **116**(25): 2923–2932.

120 Antman EM, Wiviott SD, Murphy SA, *et al.* Early and late benefits of prasugrel in patients with acute coronary syndromes undergoing percutaneous coronary intervention: a TRITON-TIMI 38 (TRial to assess improvement in therapeutic outcomes by optimizing platelet InhibitioN with prasugrel-thrombolysis in myocardial infarction) analysis. *J Am Coll Cardiol* 2008; **51**: 2028–2033.

121 Montalescot G, Wiviott SD, Braunwald E, *et al.* Prasugrel compared with clopidogrel in patients undergoing percutaneous coronary intervention for ST-elevation myocardial infarction (TRITON-TIMI 38): double-blind, randomised controlled trial. *Lancet* 2009; **373**(9665): 723–731.

122 Tcheng JE, Mackay SM. Prasugrel versus clopidogrel antiplatelet therapy after acute coronary syndrome: matching treatments with patients. *Am J Cardiovasc Drugs* 2012; **12**(2): 83–91.

123 Wallentin L, Becker RC, Budaj A, *et al.* Ticagrelor versus clopidogrel in patients with acute coronary syndromes. *N Engl J Med* 2009; **361**: 1045–1057.

124 Montone RA, Hoole SP, West NE. Prehospital ticagrelor in ST-segment elevation myocardial infarction. *N Engl J Med* 2014; **371**: 2338–2339.

125 Akers WS, Oh JJ, Oestreich JH, Ferraris S, Wethington M, Steinhubl SR. Pharmacokinetics and pharmacodynamics of a bolus and infusion of cangrelor: a direct, parenteral P2Y12 receptor antagonist. *J Clin Pharmacol* 2010; **50**(1): 27–35.

126 Bhatt DL, Lincoff AM, Gibson CM, *et al.* Intravenous platelet blockade with cangrelor during PCI. *N Engl J Med* 2009; **361**: 2330–2341.

127 Harrington RA, Stone GW, McNulty S, *et al.* Platelet inhibition with cangrelor in patients undergoing PCI. *N Engl J Med* 2009; **361**: 2318–2329.

128 Bhatt DL, Stone GW, Mahaffey KW, *et al.* Effect of platelet inhibition with cangrelor during PCI on ischemic events. *N Engl J Med* 2013; **368**(14): 1303–1313.

129 Amsterdam EA, Wenger NK, Brindis RG, *et al.* 2014 AHA/ACC guideline for the management of patients with non-ST-elevation acute coronary syndromes: a report of the American College of Cardiology/American Heart Association Task Force on Practice Guidelines. *Circulation* 2014; **64**: e139–228.

130 Linden MD, Tran H, Woods R, Tonkin A. High platelet reactivity and antiplatelet therapy resistance. *Semin Thromb Hemost* 2012; **38**(2): 200–212.

131 Price MJ, Kalyanasundaram A, Berger PB. The evidence base for platelet function testing in patients undergoing percutaneous coronary intervention. *Circ Cardiovasc Interv* 2010; **3**(3): 277–283.

132 Collet J, Cuisset T, Rangé G, *et al.* Bedside monitoring to adjust antiplatelet therapy for coronary stenting. *N Engl J Med* 2012; **367**(22): 2100–2109.

133 Bonello L, Paganelli F, Arpin-Bornet M, *et al.* Vasodilator-stimulated phosphoprotein phosphorylation analysis prior to percutaneous coronary intervention for exclusion of postprocedural major adverse cardiovascular events. *J Thromb Haemost* 2007; **5**(8): 1630–1636.

134 Gorog DA, Fuster V. Platelet function tests in clinical cardiology: unfulfilled expectations. *J Am Coll Cardiol* 2013; **61**(21): 2115–2129.

135 Sibbing D, Braun S, Morath T, *et al.* Platelet reactivity after clopidogrel treatment assessed with point-of-care analysis and early drug-eluting stent thrombosis. *J Am Coll Cardiol* 2009; **53**(10): 849–856.

136 Aradi D, Tornyos A, Pinter T, *et al.* Optimizing P2Y12 receptor inhibition in patients with acute coronary syndrome on the basis of platelet function testing: impact of prasugrel and high-dose clopidogrel. *J Am Coll Cardiol* 2014; **63**(11): 1061–1070.

137 Steinhubl SR. The illusion of "optimal" platelet inhibition. *JACC Cardiovasc Interv* 2012; **5**(3): 278–280.

138 Aradi D, Storey RF, Komocsi A, *et al.* Expert position paper on the role of platelet function testing in patients undergoing percutaneous coronary intervention. *Eur Heart J* 2014; **35**(4): 209–215.

139 Klinikum der Universitaet Muenchen. Testing responsiveness to platelet inhibition on chronic antiplatelet treatment for acute coronary syndromes trial (TROPICAL-ACS). 2000. Available at: https://clinicaltrials.gov/ct2/show/NCT01959451 (accessed May 12, 2016).

140 Dangas G, Colombo A. Platelet glycoprotein IIb/IIIa antagonists in percutaneous coronary revascularization. *Am Heart J* 1999; **138**(1, Suppl): 16–23.

141 Kong DF, Hasselblad V, Harrington RA, *et al.* Meta-analysis of survival with platelet glycoprotein IIb/IIIa antagonists for percutaneous coronary interventions. *Am J Cardiol* 2003; **92**(6): 651–655.

142 EPIC Investigators. Use of a monoclonal antibody directed against the platelet glycoprotein IIb/IIIa receptor in high-risk coronary angioplasty. *N Engl J Med* 1994; **330**(14): 956–961.

143 EPILOG Investigators. Platelet glycoprotein IIb/IIIa receptor blockade and low-dose heparin during percutaneous coronary revascularization. *N Engl J Med* 1997; **336**(24): 1689–1696.

144 EPISTENT Investigators. Randomised placebo-controlled and balloon-angioplasty-controlled trial to assess safety of coronary stenting with use of platelet glycoprotein-IIb/IIIa blockade: evaluation of platelet IIb/IIIa inhibitor for stenting. *Lancet* 1998; **352**(9122): 87–92.

145 Zimarino M, De Caterina R. Glycoprotein IIb-IIIa antagonists in non-ST elevation acute coronary syndromes and percutaneous interventions: From pharmacology to individual patient's therapy: Part 1: The evidence of benefit. *J Cardiovasc Pharmacol* 2004; **43**(3): 325–332.

146 Nguyen CM, Harrington RA. Glycoprotein IIb/IIIa receptor antagonists: a comparative review of their use in percutaneous coronary intervention. *Am J Cardiovasc Drug* 2003; **3**(6): 423–436.

147 ADMIRAL Investigators. Three-year duration of benefit from abciximab in patients receiving stents for acute myocardial infarction in the randomized double-blind ADMIRAL study. *Eur Heart J* 2005; **26**(23): 2520–2523.

148 Stone GW, Grines CL, Cox DA, *et al.* Comparison of angioplasty with stenting, with or without abciximab, in acute myocardial infarction. *N Engl J Med* 2002; **346**(13): 957–966.

149 Antoniucci D, Rodriguez A, Hempel A, *et al.* A randomized trial comparing primary infarct artery stenting with or without abciximab in acute myocardial infarction. *J Am Coll Cardiol* 2003; **42**(11): 1879–1885.

150 GUSTO IV-ACS Investigators. Effect of glycoprotein IIb/IIIa receptor blocker abciximab on outcome in patients with acute coronary syndromes without early coronary revascularisation. *Lancet* 2001; **357**(9272): 1915–1924.

151 Kastrati A, Mehilli J, Neumann F, *et al.* Abciximab in patients with acute coronary syndromes undergoing percutaneous coronary intervention after clopidogrel pretreatment: the ISAR-REACT 2 randomized trial. *JAMA* 2006; **295**(13): 1531–1538.

152 Koutouzis M, Grip L. Glycoprotein IIb/IIIa inhibitors during percutaneous coronary interventions. *Interv Cardiol* 2010; **2**(3): 301–318.

153 IMPACT-II Investigators. Randomised placebo-controlled trial of effect of eptifibatide on complications of percutaneous coronary intervention: IMPACT-II. integrilin to minimise platelet aggregation and coronary thrombosis-II. *Lancet* 1997; **349**: 1422–1428.

154 PURSUIT Trial Investigators. Inhibition of platelet glycoprotein IIb/IIIa with eptifibatide in patients with acute coronary syndromes. *N Engl J Med* 1998; **339**: 436–443.

155 ESPRIT Investigators. Novel dosing regimen of eptifibatide in planned coronary stent implantation (ESPRIT): a randomised, placebo-controlled trial. *Lancet* 2000; **356**: 2037–2044.

156 RESTORE Investigators. Effects of platelet glycoprotein IIb/IIIa blockade with tirofiban on adverse cardiac events in patients with unstable angina or acute myocardial infarction undergoing coronary angioplasty. *Circulation* 1997; **96**: 1445–1453.

157 Platelet Receptor Inhibition in Ischemic Syndrome Management in Patients Limited by Unstable Signs and SYmptoms (PRISM-PLUS) Study Investigators. Inhibition of the platelet glycoprotein IIb/IIIa receptor with tirofiban in unstable angina and non-Q-qave myocardial infarction. *N Engl J Med* 1998; **338**: 1488–1497.

158 Topol EJ, Moliterno DJ, Herrmann HC, *et al.* Comparison of two platelet glycoprotein IIb/IIIa inhibitors, tirofiban and abciximab, for the prevention of ischemic events with percutaneous coronary revascularization. *N Engl J Med* 2001; **344**(25): 1888–1894.

159 Moliterno DJ; TENACITY Steering Committee and Investigators. A randomized two-by-two comparison of high-dose bolus tirofiban versus abciximab and unfractionated heparin versus bivalirudin during percutaneous coronary revascularization and stent placement: the tirofiban evaluation of novel dosing versus abciximab with clopidogrel and inhibition of thrombin (TENACITY) study trial. *Catheter Cardiovasc Interv* 2011; **77**(7): 1001–1009.

160 Warltier DC, Kam P, Egan M. Platelet glycoprotein IIb/IIIa antagonists: pharmacology and clinical developments. *Anesthesiology* 2002; **96**(5): 1237–1249.

161 Coller BS. Monitoring platelet GP IIb/IIIa antagonist therapy. *Circulation* 1998; **97**(1): 5–9.

162 Wheeler GL, Braden GA, Steinhubl SR, *et al.* The ultegra rapid platelet-function assay: comparison to standard platelet function assays in patients undergoing percutaneous coronary intervention with abciximab therapy. *Am Heart J* 2002; **143**(4): 602–611.

163 Steinhubl SR, Talley J, David Braden GA, *et al.* Point-of-care measured platelet inhibition correlates with a reduced risk of an adverse cardiac event after percutaneous coronary intervention: results of the GOLD (AU-assessing ultegra) multicenter study. *Circulation* 2001; **103**(21):2572–2578.

164 Tamberella M, Bhatt D, Chew D, *et al.* Relation of platelet inactivation with intravenous glycoprotein IIb/IIIa antagonists to major bleeding (from the GOLD study). *Am J Cardiol* 2002; **89**: 1429–1431.

165 Mascelli M, Lance E, Damaraju L, Wagner C, Weisman H, Jordan R. Pharmacodynamic profile of short-term abciximab treatment demonstrates prolonged platelet inhibition with gradual recovery from GP IIb/IIIa receptor blockade. *Circulation* 1998; **97**: 1680–1688.

166 Tcheng J. Clinical challenges of platelet glycoprotein IIb/IIIa receptor inhibitor therapy: bleeding, reversal, thrombocytopenia, and retreatment. *Am Heart J* 2000; **139**: s38–s45.

167 Schroeder WS., Gandhi PJ. Emergency management of hemorrhagic complications in the era of glycoprotein IIb/IIIa receptor antagonists, clopidogrel, low molecular weight heparin, and third-generation fibrinolytic agents. *Curr Cardiol Rep* 2003; **5**: 310–317.

168 Sperling RT, Pinto DS, Ho KK, Carrozza JP Jr. Platelet glycoprotein IIb/IIIa inhibition with eptifibatide: prolongation of inhibition of aggregation in acute renal failure and reversal with hemodialysis. *Catheter Cardiovasc Interv* 2003; **59**: 459–462.

PART III

Hypertension and Structural Heart Disease

CHAPTER 50

Right Heart Catheterization and Pulmonary Hemodynamics

P. Christian Schulze

Friedrich-Schiller-University Jena, Jena, Germany

Right heart catheterization using floating catheters allows the analysis of right atrial, right ventricular, pulmonary artery, and pulmonary capillary wedge pressures, determination of cardiac output using the Fick principle, and thermodilution and analysis of blood oxygenation levels. Further, detailed screening for cardiac shunts and structural defects can be performed.

Risks during flotation catheter placement, invasive hemodynamics, and subsequent monitoring are very low. Most common are insertion-site hematomas. Central cardiac complications are extremely rare. Temporary cardiac arrhythmias during the procedure are common and usually self-terminating. When placed for long-term monitoring, line infection and sepsis can develop.

Balloon flotation catheters

Balloon flotation catheters are the established intravascular monitoring devices for the assessment of right heart (RH) function and hemodynamics. There are various types of balloon flotation catheter, which are all characterized by a soft, flexible, fluoroscopically visible structure with an inflatable balloon at the distal tip (Figure 50.1). The balloon allows floating of the device with the bloodstream from the right atrium into the right ventricle and further into the pulmonary artery. Thermistors allow thermodilution cardiac output measurements to be obtained. Further, through pressure sensors, cardiac pressures can be monitored. Internal lumens allow blood collections for Fick cardiac output measurements and shunt analysis.

Technique

Placement of flotation catheters can be performed through the internal jugular vein, most commonly on the right side, but other central sites including the left neck and through the subclavian veins are possible access sites. Further, peripheral right or left femoral vein access, in particular during standard left heart catheterization procedures, and through the brachial veins are common access sites. However, femoral access is limited by the inability of the patient to move and has been associated with higher rate of infections and site complications such as bleeding.

Standard placement technique follows a modified Seldinger technique. A 21-gauge guide needle is used to find and access the vein. Using the guide needle, a larger needle is used to enter the vein followed by advancement of a short guidewire. The needles are removed and a 7-Fr sheath is introduced into the vessel with an internal dilator. The dilator is then removed with the placement wire and stable blood flow through the lateral port confirmed followed by flushing of the sheath and the ports. With the sheath in place, the balloon flotation catheter is advanced into the vein and advanced by around 20 cm. At this point, the balloon is inflated allowing easy advancement of the balloon tip into the right atrium for measurement of right atrial pressure. Attention should be paid to the curvature of the catheter which is designed to be advanced from the neck with a tip pointing toward the left to facilitate crossing of the tricuspid valve from the right atrium. With further advancement, the tricuspid valve is crossed and the balloon placed in the right ventricle for pressure analysis. At this point, the catheter has to be redirected to point upwards with clockwise rotation and advancement into the right ventricular outflow track for crossing through the pulmonic valve into the main pulmonary artery. Once placed in the pulmonary artery, the catheter can be further advanced into a distal pulmonary artery and into the wedge position. Most commonly, the catheter floats into the right pulmonary artery and distally into a segmental artery in the right middle or lower lobe.

During the advancement of the catheter, deep inspiration maneuvers can be used to facilitate the movement of the balloon via the the increased cardiac return and pulmonary flow during inspiration. If unable to move the balloon tip from a distal position in the right ventricle, which is more common during procedures from the femoral access sites because of the preformed structure and curving, a conventional 0.035-inch guidewire can be used to stabilize the catheter. An alternative technique for advancing the flotation catheter is by forming a loop in the right atrium with a lateral pointing of the balloon tip. With further advancement, the tip will point downwards and can be moved through the tricuspid valve into the right ventricle.

Placement of the flotation catheter in the cardiac chambers has to be confirmed by changes in specific waveforms and pressures

---

Interventional Cardiology: Principles and Practice, Second Edition. Edited by George D. Dangas, Carlo Di Mario, and Nicholas N. Kipshidze.
© 2017 John Wiley & Sons, Ltd. Published 2017 by John Wiley & Sons, Ltd.

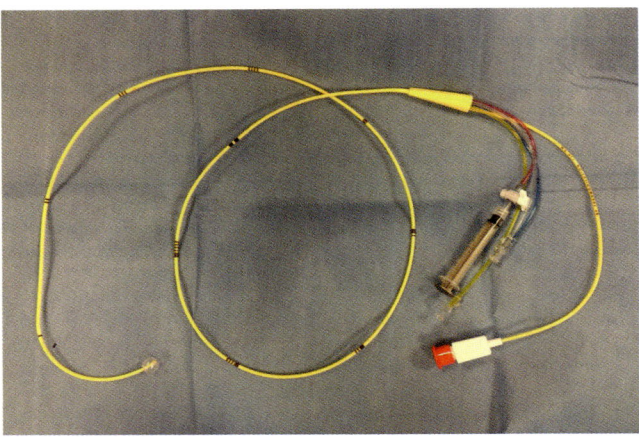

Figure 50.1 Swan–Ganz catheter with inflated balloon at the distal tip.

(Figure 50.2). Once a stable wedge position has been reached and the measurement has been achieved, the balloon should be deflated and the catheter be retracted by several inches for stable placement in the larger branches of the pulmonary artery to avoid accidental perforation. Prolonged positioning in the wedge position is to be avoided. Removal of the catheter requires deflation of the balloon, which has to be confirmed before retraction.

Pulmonary hemodynamics
Normal cardiac and pulmonary hemodynamics
Normal pulmonary hemodynamics are shown in Table 50.1 and illustrated in Figure 50.2. Cardiac and pulmonary hemodynamics are directly related to cardiac venous return and preload. Respiratory variation in inspiration with decreased intrathoracic pressure and increase venous return and in expiration with increased intrathoracic pressures and reduced venous return play an important part in the definition of cardiac pressures, filling, and hemodynamics. Of note, in intubated patients, these hemodynamics are reversed because of the positive end-expiratory pressures and respiratory dynamics associated with positive pressure ventilation. Normal cardiac filling pressures and hemodynamics with normal cardiac output are associated with central venous mixed saturations of >65%. Cardiac output can be calculated by the formula according to Fick:

$$CO = \text{oxygen consumption} / Hg\left(g/dL\right) \times 1.34 \times$$
$$\left(\text{arterial } O_2 \text{ saturation} - \text{mixed venous } O_2 \text{saturation}\right)$$

(Hg – hemoglobin; O2 – oxygen). Cardiac index is cardiac output corrected for body surface area (BSA):

$$CI = CO / BSA.$$

An important parameter of cardiopulmonary hemodynamics is systemic and pulmonary vascular resistance. Systemic vascular resistance (SVR) is calculated as follows:

$$SVR = \left(\text{mean arterial blood pressure} - RA \text{ pressure}\right)/\text{cardiac output}.$$

SVR is found elevated in circumstances of increased vascular tone such as in hypertension and decompensated heart failure.

Pulmonary vascular resistance (PVR) is defined as:

$$PVR = \left(\text{mean PAP} - PCWP\right)/\text{cardiac output}.$$

Elevated PCR is a marker of lung disease and is found to be fixed and non-reversible in interstitial lung diseases, chronic obstructive pulmonary disease (COPD), and several forms of pulmonary hypertension. Reversible increases in PVR are typical for pulmonary hypertension caused by left heart failure or elevated filling pressures from volume overload. Pharmacologic testing for these changes are described later.

Heart failure and low cardiac output
The main indication for the analysis of cardiac filling pressures and hemodynamics is the suspicion of a low cardiac output state in the setting of heart failure with dilated or ischemic cardiomyopathy, valvular heart disease, and to diagnose cardiac or pulmonary causes of shortness of breath and fatigue. A low cardiac output state is characterized as cardiac output below normal (CO <4 L/min or CI <2 L/min/m² BSA). Associated filling pressures can be elevated, normal, or low depending on the fluid status of the patient. The MVO$_2$ is typically decreased leading to the diagnosis of a low cardiac output state. The Fick formula for calculation of cardiac output allows a more reliable method than the thermodilation method which can be affected by severe tricuspid regurgitation, not uncommon in severe heart failure.

Left heart failure
Central hemodynamics in patients with isolated left heart failure are characterized primarily by elevated left-sided filling pressures with notable increases in pulmonary capillary wedge pressure (PCPW) with or without elevated pulmonary arterial pressures (PAPs). Reduced cardiac output is shown by reduced MVO$_2$. Severe left heart failure induces all changes of right heart failure caused by increased right-sided filling pressures from impaired flow and the associated volume overload of the right ventricle.

Right heart failure
Right heart failure is most commonly a secondary phenomenon of left heart failure. Isolated right heart failure can occur acutely after right ventricular infarction and, rarely, caused by genetic right ventricular cardiomyopathies. Further, it occurs in 30–35% of patients following implantation of a left ventricular assist device because of the inability of the right ventricle to respond to the increased preload following surgery. Hemodynamics are characterized by increased right atrial pressures (>8 mmHg) with inappropriately "normal" or elevated pulmonary artery pressures.

Pulmonary hypertension
Pulmonary hypertension is defined as a mean pulmonary artery pressure of >25 mmHg. Many clinicians consider a mPAP of 21–24 mmHg as borderline pulmonary hypertension. The underlying type of pulmonary hypertension (WHO 1–5) defines the associated cardiac filling pressures. Group 1 PH (pulmonary arterial hypertension) is characterized by normal capillary wedge pressures (<15 mmHg) while group 2 PH (pulmonary hypertension with left heart disease) is defined by the presence of elevated capillary wedge pressures (>25 mmHg).

Shunt diagnostics
Cardiac shunt diagnostics is based on changes in the oxygen saturation caused by the mixture of oxygen-rich blood after lung passage with oxygen-depleted blood from the periphery. At any point,

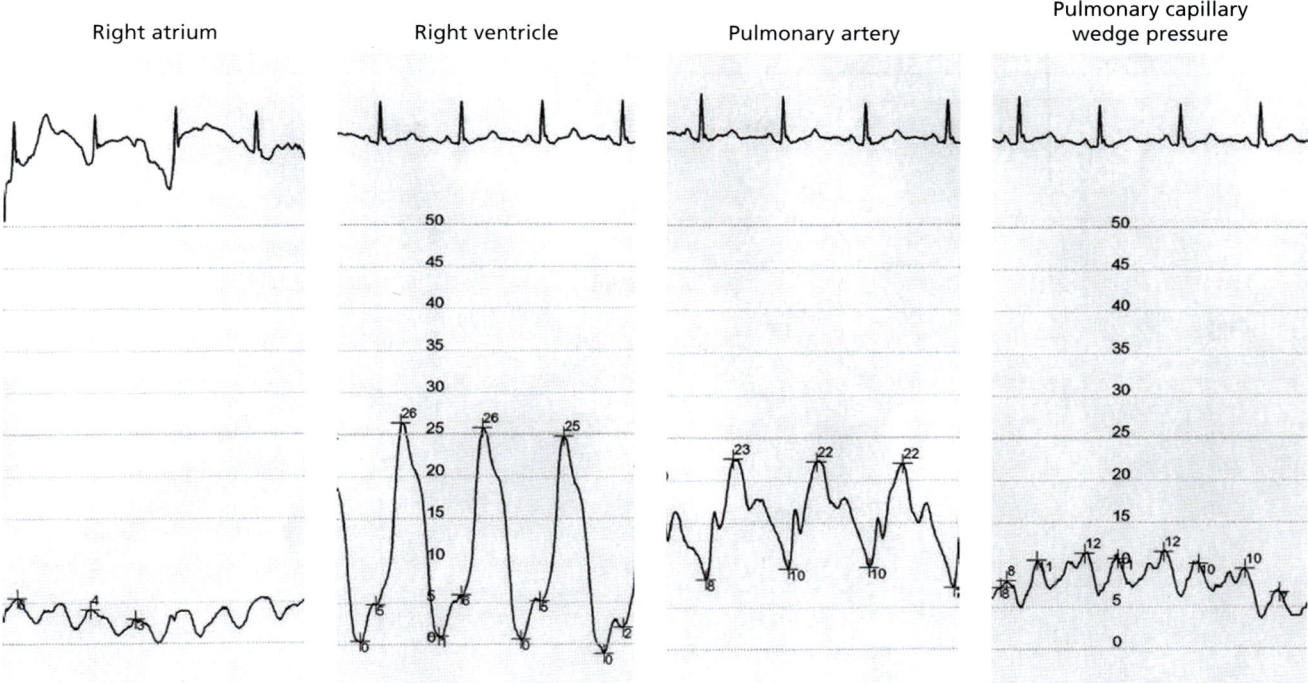

Figure 50.2 Normal hemodynamics.

Table 50.1 Normal and pathologic cardiac hemodynamics and filling pressures.

	Right atrium	Right ventricle	Pulmonary artery	Pulmonary capillary wedge pressure	MVO$_2$
Normal	<5	<30/5	<30/10 (<25)	<12	>65
Pulmonary hypertension	Normal or elevated	Normal or elevated	>25	Normal or elevated	Normal or reduced
Left heart failure	Normal or elevated	Normal or elevated	Normal or elevated	>15	Reduced
Right heart failure	>5–8	"Normal" or elevated	"Normal" or elevated	Normal	Normal or reduced

All pressures are in mmHg.
MVO$_2$, mixed venous oxygen saturation.

blood samples can be collected through the internal lumen of the catheter. Typically, sampling occurs in the superior vena cava, the inferior vena cava, the right atrium and ventricle at various positions as needed to specify positions of suspected defects, in the main as well as the left and right pulmonary artery.

Pharmacologic drug testing

Pharmacologic drug testing is a standard procedure in the catheterization laboratory and allows the characterization of elevated filling pressures, definition of right heart or left heart failure, and the definition of pulmonary hypertension as a primary or secondary phenomenon.

Inotropic drug testing using PDE5 inhibitors such as milrinone or beta-adrenergic stimulation using dobutamine is performed to test the contractile response in patients with reduced ejection fraction and reduced cardiac output. A continuous infusion of the drug with continuous measurement of cardiac filling pressures and central oxygen saturations (MVO$_2$) are performed. Many centers define a positive response as an increase in cardiac output by >20% or a decrease in PCWP by >20%. Typical protocols allow increased doses of inotropes every 3–5 minutes with a full set of hemodynamics and MVO$_2$. Of note, cardiac hemodynamics might not change immediately, in particular in the setting of biventricular failure and volume overload, and a positive response might require testing not only acutely in the catheterization laboratory but also retesting after 24 hours.

Another role for pharmacologic drug testing is in the characterization of abnormal pulmonary artery pressure, elevated transpulmonary gradients (TPG), and increased PVR. This is of utmost importance for the evaluation of patients before heart transplantation as an increased TPG and PVR has been associated with the occurrence of right ventricular failure and increased morbidity and

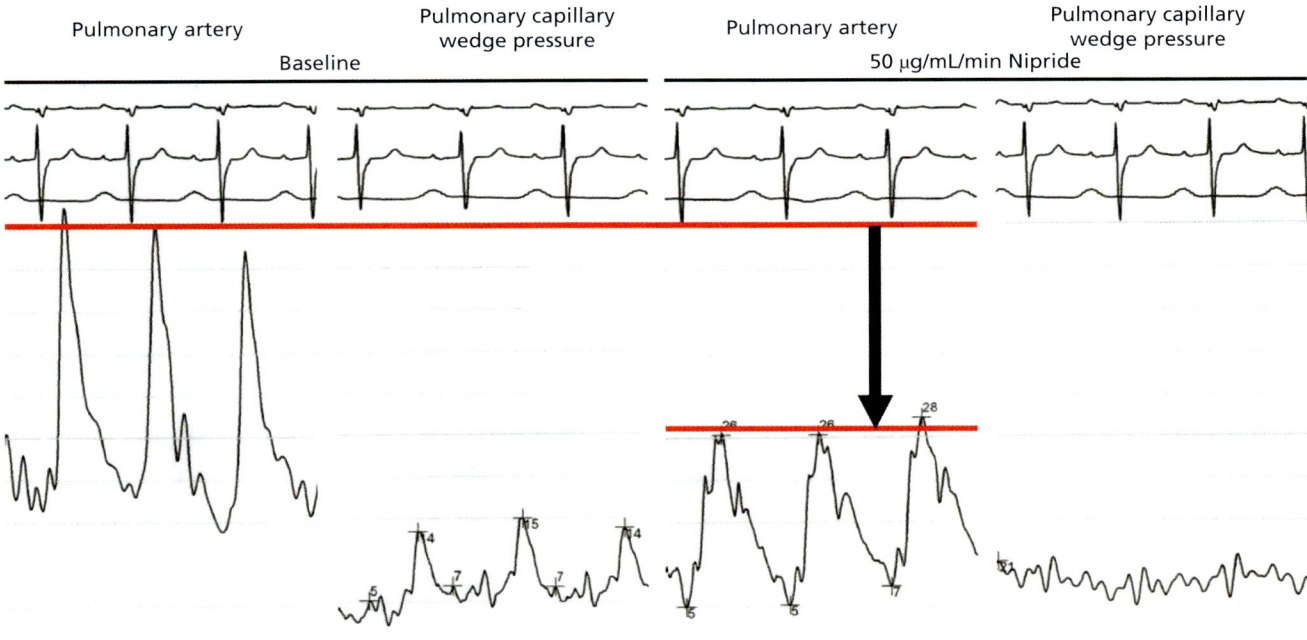

Figure 50.3 Right heart catheterization and pharmacologic drug testing for the assessment of pulmonary hypertension. With continuous infusion of sodium nitroprusside (50 μg/mL/min), pulmonary artery pressure decreased from 50/18 to 26/7 mmHg. Pulmonary capillary wedge pressure (PCWP) remained stable at 7–9 mmHg. Note the v-waves at baseline which resolved in response to vasodilator infusion.

mortality after heart transplantation. Standard right heart catheterization is used as a first step. In the normotensive patient in the setting of elevated PCWP and increased PAP, pulmonary and systemic vasodilators can safely be tested. Most established is short-term infusion of sodium nitroprusside (nipride) with subsequent decrease in SVR and PVR as a result of the direct vasodilatory effect of nitric oxide on vascular smooth muscle cells. After baseline measurements, the dosage of sodium nitropusside is increased stepwise from 25 μg/L/min by 25 μg/mL/min steps as illustrated in Figure 50.3. A positive response is defined as a decrease in PVR by >20%.

Invasive hemodynamics and cardiac filling pressure measurements are helpful in the characterization of patients with pulmonary hypertension for their response to pulmonary vasodilators and supplemental oxygen. A standard test involves a baseline right heart catheterization with definition of cardiac filling pressures and hemodynamics. High dose nasal oxygen is first applied to the patient and the direct pulmonary vasodilatory response is assessed after 3–5 minutes using a full set of cardiac hemodynamics and systemic oxygen saturation measurements. In patients with normal PCWP, pure pulmonary vasodilators such as inhaled nitric oxide, epoprostenol (flolane), or iloprost (ventaxis) can be tested. Of note, such testing is contraindicated in patients with elevated PCWP because of the risk of inducing pulmonary edema caused by poor left heart function leading to worsening of pulmonary congestion. The response is monitored by continuous assessment of pulmonary artery pressure and repeated measurements of cardiac output. A positive response is defined as a decrease of mean PAP by >10 mmHg to reach an absolute value of 40 mmHg or lower.

Interactive multiple choice questions are available for this chapter on www.wiley. com/go/dangas/cardiology

CHAPTER 51

Treatment of Pulmonary Embolism: Medical, Surgical, and Percutaneous

Ian del Conde and Barry T. Katzen
Miami Cardiac and Vascular Institute, Miami, FL, USA

Pulmonary embolism (PE) presents in a continuum of severity that spans from incidentally discovered subsegmental PE to massive PE resulting in cardiogenic shock and death. The main cause of death in patients with large PE is right ventricular failure, cardiogenic shock, and refractory hypoxemia. Therefore, rapid recanalization of the pulmonary arteries is the ultimate goal of all therapies for acute PE, regardless if pharmacologic (anticoagulation or systemic fibrinolysis), surgical, or catheter-based.

Risk stratification and patient selection

All patients presenting with PE should be risk-stratified with the goal of: (i) identifying patients who are at high risk of dying if they do not receive treatment with thrombolysis or surgical embolectomy; and (ii) identifying patients who are likely to develop chronic thromboembolic pulmonary hypertension (CTEPH). Whereas a number of well-validated risk stratification tools help identify patients at increased risk of death or clinical deterioration from PE, identifying patients who are more likely to develop CTEPH is more challenging. CTEPH occurs in 2–4% of patients after acute PE, and is mostly diagnosed in patients who are in their forties [1,2]. Recurrent PE, larger perfusion defects, and younger age at presentation appear to be some of the strongest predictors for the development of CTEPH [3]. Whether thrombolysis (systemic or catheter-based) or thrombectomy decrease the risk of developing CTEPH is not known, but there are small studies that suggest that aggressive revascularization of the pulmonary arteries in large PEs is associated with lower pulmonary pressures than in patients who receive anticoagulation therapy alone [4].

There are three main risk categories in patients with PE [5,6]. Each category carries a specific definition and has important implications regarding prognosis and treatment considerations:

1 *Massive PE*: PE that results in persistent hypotension (systolic blood pressure <90 mmHg for over 15 minutes), vasopressor requirement, or in profound bradycardia (heart rate <40 b.p.m.). The short-term mortality in these patients can be as high as 50–65%.

2 *Submassive PE*: diagnosed in patients with acute PE who have a normal blood pressure, but who have evidence of right ventricular (RV) dysfunction, which can be detected on physical examination, cardiac biomarkers, electrocardiography (ECG),

echocardiography, and chest computed tomography (CT) [6,7]. Patients are usually tachycardic, with an elevated jugular venous pressure. If the RV is significantly dilated, a right parasternal heave can be palpated. ECG findings of acute PE with RV strain include sinus tachycardia, incomplete or complete right bundle-branch block, T-wave inversions in leads V1 through V4, and the combination of an S wave in lead I, Q wave in lead III, and T-wave inversion in lead III (S1Q3T3).

Normotensive patients with acute PE who have any of the following factors at presentation are at increased risk of death and clinical deterioration: (i) RV systolic dysfunction, usually determined by echocardiography; (ii) RV dilatation, which can be demonstrated either by echocardiography or chest CT angiography, (iii) elevated plasma levels of brain natriuretic peptide (BNP) or N-terminal pro-BNP (NT-ProBNP); or (iv) evidence of myocardial injury, as assessed by elevated levels of troponin T and I [8–11]. Although patients with submassive PE have in-hospital mortality rates of around 2–3%, which is much lower than that of patients with massive PE [7,12], they are at increased risk of death or escalation of therapy (e.g., need for endotracheal intubation, cardiopulmonary resuscitation, thrombolysis). Consequently, these patients are often considered for thrombolysis.

RV dilatation is defined as the right ventricular diameter to left ventricular diameter ratio greater than 0.9 [13–15]. This ratio can be measured by echocardiography in the apical four-chamber view, measuring the maximal ventricular diameters at end-diastole. More commonly, however, the measurement is made on PE-protocol chest CT angiography. The RV/LV short-axis diameters are measured at the valvular plane. Maximal ventricular diameters are obtained by measuring the distance between the free ventricular wall and the interventricular septum, perpendicular to the septum. When making the RV measurements, contrast within the LV should be seen. Non-gated, axial images are sufficient for the accurate measurement of the maximal ventricular diameters, and reformatted four-chamber views are not required [16].

3 *Low-risk PE*: patients with no high-risk features (i.e., normotensive with no evidence of RV dilatation or dysfunction, and with normal levels of pro-BNP and troponin I or T) have low mortality rates and generally do well with anticoagulation alone [17,18].

Interventional Cardiology: Principles and Practice, Second Edition. Edited by George D. Dangas, Carlo Di Mario, and Nicholas N. Kipshidze.
© 2017 John Wiley & Sons, Ltd. Published 2017 by John Wiley & Sons, Ltd.

Therapies for acute PE

Patients with low-risk PE who have no contraindications to anti-coagulation should be treated with anticoagulation alone [17,18]. Patients with massive PE are at high risk of death and should be considered for emergent systemic intravenous thrombolysis, which can be quickly administered in the emergency room or a hospital ward. Surgical embolectomy can also be considered if it can be performed quickly. Most contemporary catheter-based therapies take at least a few hours to achieve meaningful revascularization of the pulmonary arteries, and are therefore generally not the preferred strategy for most patients with massive PE who are hemodynamically unstable. Whether patients with submassive PE should be managed with anti-coagulation alone, systemic thrombolysis, or catheter-based throm-bolysis is still being hotly debated. Patients with submassive PE with a low or acceptable bleeding risk, and with evidence of severe RV dysfunction or myonecrosis can benefit from catheter-based thera-pies or even systemic thrombolysis. Surgical embolectomy is almost never performed in hemodynamically stable patients.

Medical therapy

Anticoagulation

Anticoagulation therapy remains a cornerstone in the management of patients with acute PE. Patients who have no low-risk PE can be considered for initial treatment with one of the new oral anticoagu-lants, potentially avoiding the need for initial parenteral heparin or low molecular weight heparins (LMWH). The preferred parenteral options for therapeutic anticoagulation include LMWH or fonda-parinux [17]. For patients with end-stage renal disease, unfraction-ated heparin is an option. If heparin-induced thrombocytopenia is suspected, argatroban or bivalirudin can be used. If the patient is being considered for systemic or catheter-based thrombolysis, a short-acting intravenous anticoagulant, such as unfractionated heparin, is preferred because it can be discontinued and reversed rapidly. Short-acting intravenous anticoagulants should also be considered in patients with acute PE who are at high risk of bleed-ing (e.g., in the early postoperative period).

The new oral anticoagulants, including the factor Xa antagonists, rivaroxaban, apixaban and edoxaban, and the direct thrombin inhibitor, dabigatran, have now been studied in approximately 27,000 patients with venous thromboembolism (VTE) enrolled in phase 3 clinical trials [19–24]. These agents have similar efficacy to

standard anticoagulation (initial heparin/LMWH bridge to a vitamin K antagonist), but are associated with fewer bleeding complications, including a ~45–55% reduction in the risk of fatal bleeding or intracranial hemorrhage [25,26]. Another significant advantage of the new oral anticoagulants is that in contrast to coumadin, they are not cumbersome to take: all of these agents use fixed dosing and monitoring is not required; there are no significant food–drug interactions, and they have fewer drug–drug interactions than vitamin K antagonists. Table 51.1 summarizes the basic pharmaco-logic properties and FDA-approved doses for these drugs.

Systemic thrombolysis

The only FDA-approved fibrinolytic drug for the treatment of acute PE is recombinant tissue plasminogen activator (rt-PA, or alteplase). The standard, FDA-approved dose of rt-PA consists of a 100-mg intravenous infusion over 2 hours. Systemic thrombolysis is the first-line therapy in patients with massive PE and cardiovascular collapse, who have no contraindications to fibrinolysis, because it can be administered without significant delay, which may not be the case for interventional or surgical therapies. Table 51.2 lists absolute and relative contraindications to thrombolysis.

The main evidence derived from a randomized controlled trial to support thrombolysis in patients with massive PE comes from a very small trial in which patients with acute PE, hypotension, and heart failure were randomized to pharmacologic thrombolysis with 1,500,000 IU streptokinase infused in 1 hour followed by heparin, or to heparin alone [27]. The trial was stopped after the first eight patients were enrolled. All patients in the anticoagulation-alone arm died from heart failure whereas all patients in the thrombolysis group survived. Consistent with these findings, a meta-analysis of five trials suggested that systemic thrombolytic therapy in patients with massive PE resulted in a 55% reduction in the risk of death or recurrent PE (9.4% vs. 19.0%; odds ratio 0.45) compared with heparin alone [28]. Based on these data, it is generally accepted that patients with massive PE should be considered for emergent thrombolysis or revascularization of the pulmonary arteries, either surgically or through a catheter-based procedure [6,29,30]. The ninth American College of Chest Physicians (ACCP) and the American Heart Association (AHA) / American College of Cardiology (ACC) guidelines give a Class 2 C (very weak recommendation) and IIa (weight of evidence/opinion is in favor of usefulness) recommendations, respectively, to thromboly-sis in massive PE [6,17]. The weak strength of these recommendations

Table 51.1 Novel oral anticoagulants for the treatment of acute venous thromboembolism.

Drug	Mechanism of action	Approved dose*	Half-life	Renal excretion	Pivotal VTE trials [ref]
Dabigatran etexilate	Direct thrombin inhibitor	CrCl >30 mL/min: 150 mg PO BID after 5–10 days of initial parenteral anticoagulation	12–17 hours	85%	RECOVER I and II [23,24]
Rivaroxaban	Direct factor Xa inhibitor	15 mg PO BID x 21 days with food, then 20 mg/day PO	5–13 hours	33%	EINSTEIN [21,22]
Apixaban	Direct factor Xa inhibitor	10 mg PO BID for 7 days, then 5 mg PO BID	9–14 hours	27%	AMPLIFY [19]
Edoxaban	Direct factor Xa inhibitor	60 mg PO once daily after 5–10 days of initial parenteral anticoagulation†	9–10 hours	50%	HOKUSAI-VTE [20]

BID, twice daily; CrCl, creatinine clearance; PO, per os (orally); VTE, venous thromboembolism.
* Dose approved by the US Food and Drug Administration for the treatment of acute venous thromboembolism.
† Edoxaban dose reduction: 30 mg once daily in patients with CrCl 15–50 mL/min, weight ≤60 kg, or if taking certain concomitant P-GP inhibitor medications.

is a reflection of the absence of high quality data (e.g., large randomized controlled clinical trials) to guide management in these patients rather than evidence of marginal clinical benefit.

Systemic thrombolysis in patients with submassive PE has also been studied. In the MAPPET study, 256 patients with submassive PE were randomized to alteplase plus heparin, or heparin plus placebo [12]. The primary endpoint, consisting of in-hospital death or clinical deterioration that required escalation of therapy (defined as need for catecholamine infusion, secondary thrombolysis, endotracheal intubation, cardiopulmonary rescucitation, or surgical or

Table 51.2 Contraindications to systemic thrombolysis.

Absolute	Relative
Any intracranial hemorrhage	TIA in the preceding 6 months
	Oral anticoagulation
Known intracranial lesions that predispose to bleeding (e.g., malignancy, aneurysms, or arteriovenous malformations)	Pregnancy of first postpartum week
	Non-compressible puncture sites
	Traumatic resuscitation
Ischemic stroke in the previous 3 months	Uncontrolled hypertension (SBP >180 mmHg)
Major trauma or surgery in the preceding 3 weeks	Advanced liver disease
Active bleeding	Age >75 years
	Infective endocarditis
	Active peptic ulcer

SBP, systolic blood pressure; TIA, transient ischemic attack.

catheter thrombectomy) was significantly reduced and the patient to receive thrombolysis, from 24.6% (heparin plus placebo) to 11% (alteplase plus heparin) (p = 0.006). However, most of this benefit was driven not by decreased mortality, but by decreased rates of escalation of therapy. Although rates of major bleeding were higher in the thrombolysis group (3.6% vs. 0.8%), there was only one case of fatal bleeding and no cases of hemorrhagic stroke in patients treated with thrombolysis. More recently, in the PEITHO trial, 1006 patients with submassive PE were randomized to the fibronolytic drug, tenecteplase, or placebo [31]. All patients received therapeutic anticoagulation with heparin. Death or hemodynamic decompensation (the primary outcome) occurred in 13 of 506 patients (2.6%) in the tenecteplase group compared with 28 of 499 (5.6%) in the placebo group, representing a 66% risk reduction (p = 0.02). Similar to MAPPET [12], thrombolysis had no effect on mortality, and the difference in the primary outcome was primarily driven by lower rates of hemodynamic decompensation. These findings support the premise that rapid recanalization of the pulmonary arteries in submassive PE results in decreased hemodynamic decompensation. However, the cost of these benefits was a substantial increase in the risk of major bleeding, including hemorrhagic stroke (11.5% of patients who received tenecteplase experienced major bleeding, compared to 2.4% in the placebo group). Intracranial hemorrhage occurred in 2% of patients who received tenecteplase and 0.2% of patients who received placebo. The current ACCP and AHA/ACC guidelines give a Class 2C and IIB (usefulness/efficacy is less well established) recommendations, respectively, to the use of thrombolysis in patients with submassive PE [6,17].

Surgical embolectomy

Surgical embolectomy is a safe and effective technique in the treatment of acute PE when performed by an experienced cardiothoracic surgeon (Figure 51.1). Surgical embolectomy requires a median sternotomy and cardiopulmonary bypass. Although different surgical techniques have been described, an incision into the main pulmonary artery is usually made, allowing thrombus to be

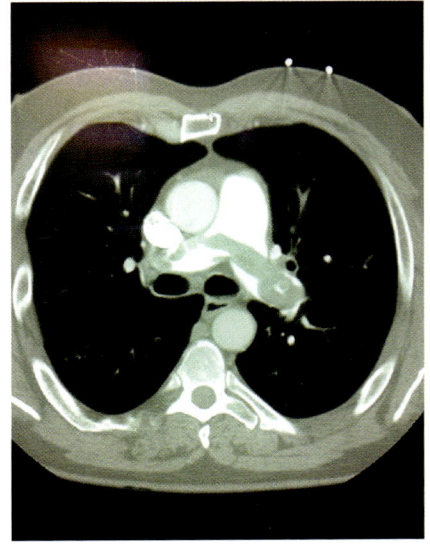
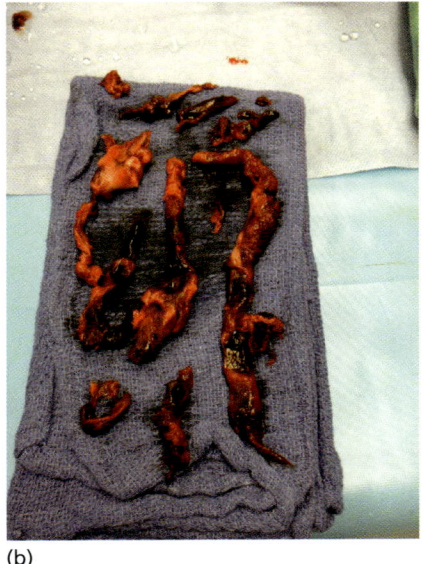
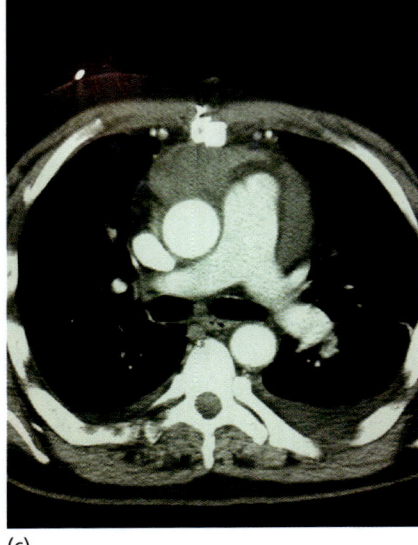

(a)   (b)   (c)

Figure 51.1 Surgical embolectomy. The patient presented with massive pulmonary embolus (PE), with persistent hypotension. (a) Chest CT angiogram demonstrated a large, almost occlusive saddle embolus, with a severely dilated right ventricle. The patient underwent surgical embolectomy. (b) Large emboli (up to 10 cm in length) were retrieved. (c) Postoperative CT angiogram showed minimal residual emboli. Source: Photographs courtesy of Dr. Marco Bologna, Miami Cardiac and Vascular Institute, Miami, FL, USA.

removed. The incision can be extended into the distal pulmonary arteries when necessary. The degree of revascularization of the pulmonary arteries that can be achieved surgically is generally much more significant than with catheter therapies. Surgical embolectomy is most effective in patients with large central or saddle pulmonary emboli. Peri-operative mortality for patients undergoing surgical embolectomy has declined over the last two decades. Survival rates among patients with massive PE treated with surgical embolectomy have been reported to be as high as 75–86% [32,33].

Catheter-based therapies

Contemporary catheter-based treatment of acute PE offers significant versatility which can be advantageous for tailoring therapy to the individual patient. Techniques are based primarily on mechanical removal or fragmentation of the thrombus or a hybrid approach (pharmacomechanical therapy) which combines a mechanical approach with local thrombolysis. The mechanical component allows rapid recanalization of the pulmonary artery and increases exposure of the thrombus to the fibrinolytic agent. The pharmacologic component allows a steady reduction in thrombus burden via a longer catheter-delivered infusion of a fibrinolytic agent at a dosage that is typically a fraction of that used in systemic thrombolysis. An important principle is that in contrast to catheter-directed thrombectomy in other vascular territories (e.g., coronary arteries, lower extremities, or vascular grafts), interventional treatment of PE should be aimed at improving hemodynamic status rather than obtaining optimal angiographic results. Revascularization of the pulmonary arteries with contemporary devices and techniques is somewhat limited, and generally requires several hours. Therefore, catheter-based techniques are generally used in patients with submassive PE rather than in hemodynamically unstable patients.

Catheter-directed thrombolysis

In catheter-directed thrombolysis access is usually obtained through a femoral vein or the right internal jugular vein. A multi-holed infusion catheter is advanced into the pulmonary artery.

The catheter tip is positioned within or just proximal to the embolus. Although there are no standardized thrombolytic infusion protocols, common regimens include alteplase 0.5–1.0 mg/hour over a period of 12–24 hours. If two (i.e., bilateral) catheters are used, the dose in each of the catheters is halved. Typical total doses of alteplase are 20–30 mg over 24 hours. Whether anticoagulation should be continued during the infusion of the fibrinolytic agent is a matter of some debate. Most interventionalists hold full-dose anticoagulation during fibrinolysis, and instead infuse a reduced dose of heparin (e.g., 300–500 U/hour) through the sidearm of the access sheath. In otherwise young and healthy patients deemed at very low risk of bleeding, and who have significant thrombus burden, full-dose anticoagulation with a short-acting drug (e.g., unfractionated heparin) can be continued during the infusion of the fibrinolytic. Some interventionalists follow fibrinogen levels during the infusion of the fibrinolytic because it has been suggested (though not conclusively demonstrated) that significant drops in fibrinogen levels predict bleeding complications. Fibrinogen levels are determined at baseline, and then at 4–6 hour intervals. If the fibrinogen levels fall to 30–40% of their level at baseline (or an absolute level <100–150 mg/dL), then the dose of the fibrinolytic infusion rate can be reduced.

Ultrasound-assisted thrombolysis

The EkoSonic Endovascular System (EKOS Corporation, Bothwell, WA, USA) (Figures 51.2 and 51.3) is the only catheter at this time to have been cleared by the Food and Drug Administration (FDA) for use in treating patients with acute PE. The device consists of two endovascular devices: an Intelligent Drug Delivery Catheter (IDDC), which is a 5.2 Fr multi-lumen infusion catheter, and a MicroSonic Device (MSD) containing several evenly spaced ultrasound transducers positioned along the treatment zone. The EkoSonic device is capable of simultaneously infusing a fibrinolytic drug within the pulmonary artery, and of emitting low-power, high-frequency (2.2 MHz) ultrasound that "loosens" the thrombus, increasing penetration of the fibrinolytic drug into the

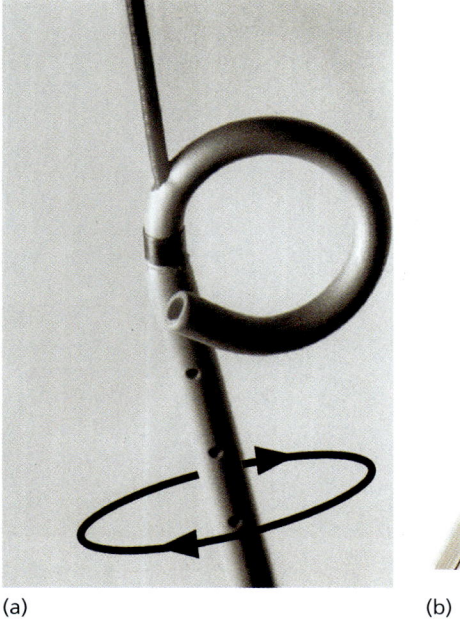
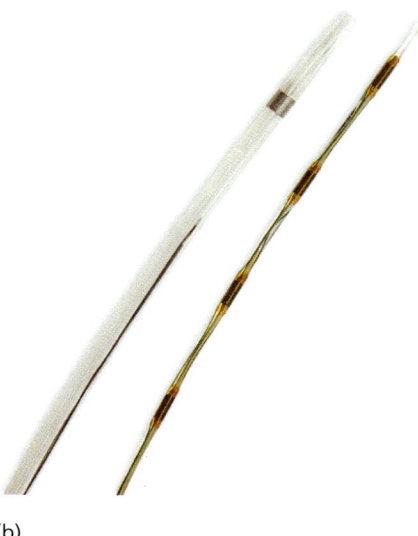

(a)   (b)

Figure 51.2 (a) Rotatable pigtail catheter. (b) EkoSonic Endovascular System. See text for details.

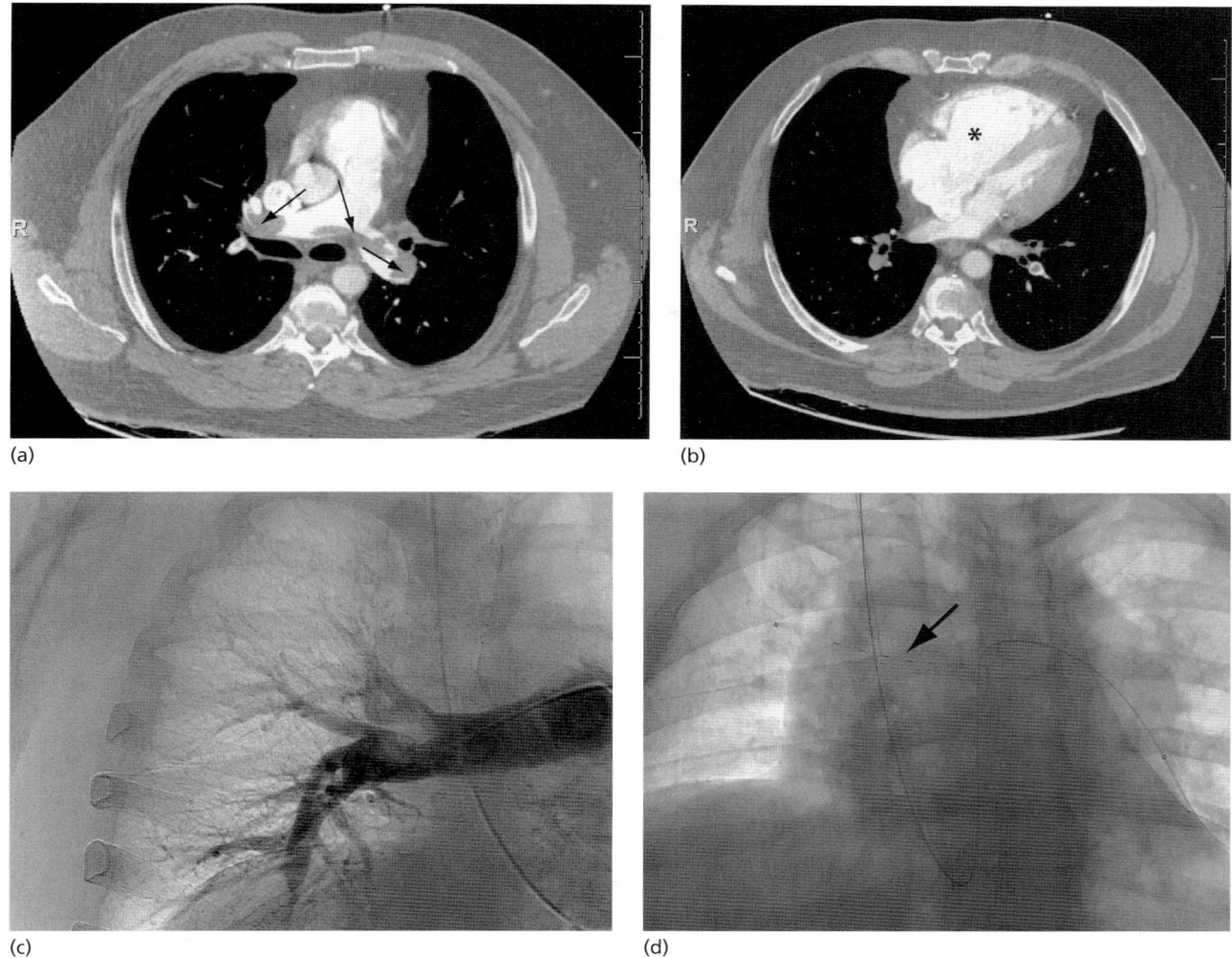

Figure 51.3 Catheter-based therapy for a patient with submassive PE. (a) Saddle embolus extending into the bilateral main pulmonary arteries (arrows). (b) Marked right ventricular (RV) dilatation (asterisk) with a RV : LV ratio of 1.7. (c) Pulmonary angiogram shows a large filling defect within the right pulmonary artery. (d) An EkoSonic catheter was placed in the bilateral pulmonary arteries. Tissue plasminogen activator (tPA) was infused at a rate of 0.5 mg/hour through each catheter for approximately 12 hours.

thrombus, and (theoretically) accelerating thrombolysis. This is one of the best studied modern devices for the catheter-based treatment of acute PE. The SEATTLE-II trial was a prospective, single arm trial that evaluated the efficacy and safety of the EkoSonic catheter to reverse right ventricular dilatation on chest CT angiography in 150 patients presenting acute PE with an RV : LV ratio ≥0.9 [34]. Of enrolled patients, 79% had submassive PE, while 20.7% met criteria for massive PE. The alteplase dose protocol was 1 mg/hour for 24 hours with the use of a unilateral catheter, and 1 mg/hour/catheter for 12 hours in patients receiving bilateral catheters. Successful device placement was achieved in 97.5% of patients. The mean total dose of alteplase administered was approximately 24 mg. At 48 hours, there was a 30% decrease in the RV : LV ratio, from 1.55 pre-procedure, to 1.13 (p <0.0001). Similarly, pulmonary artery systolic pressures dropped from 51 mmHg pre-procedure to 37 mmHg at 48 hours. Major bleeding was experienced by 11.4% of patients within 30 days, but there were no cases of intracranial hemorrhage.

Suction embolectomy

The AngioVac System (AngioVac, Vortex Medical, MA, USA) is a suction device that allows the suction of intravascular material (e.g., thrombus, myxoma, and vegetation) while maintaining extracorporeal circulation. This option can be attractive in patients with large central PE [35], or those who are ineligible for thrombolysis. The system consists of two components: the AngioVac Cannula catheter, and the AngioVac Circuit (Figure 51.4). The 25-Fr catheter has a balloon-expandable funnel at the tip that functions as a cannula. The catheter can be advanced percutaneously or through a surgical cutdown, usually through groin access, although some interventionalists have used this system through the right internal jugular vein. An adjustable amount of suction (up to 80 mmHg) is applied at the cannula to suction the unwanted material; blood is filtered and then returned via another sheath to a contralateral large peripheral vein. The Circuit system has features of a cardiopulmonary bypass circuit and requires a trained perfusionist for its operation. The limited flexibility and maneuverability of the 25-Fr

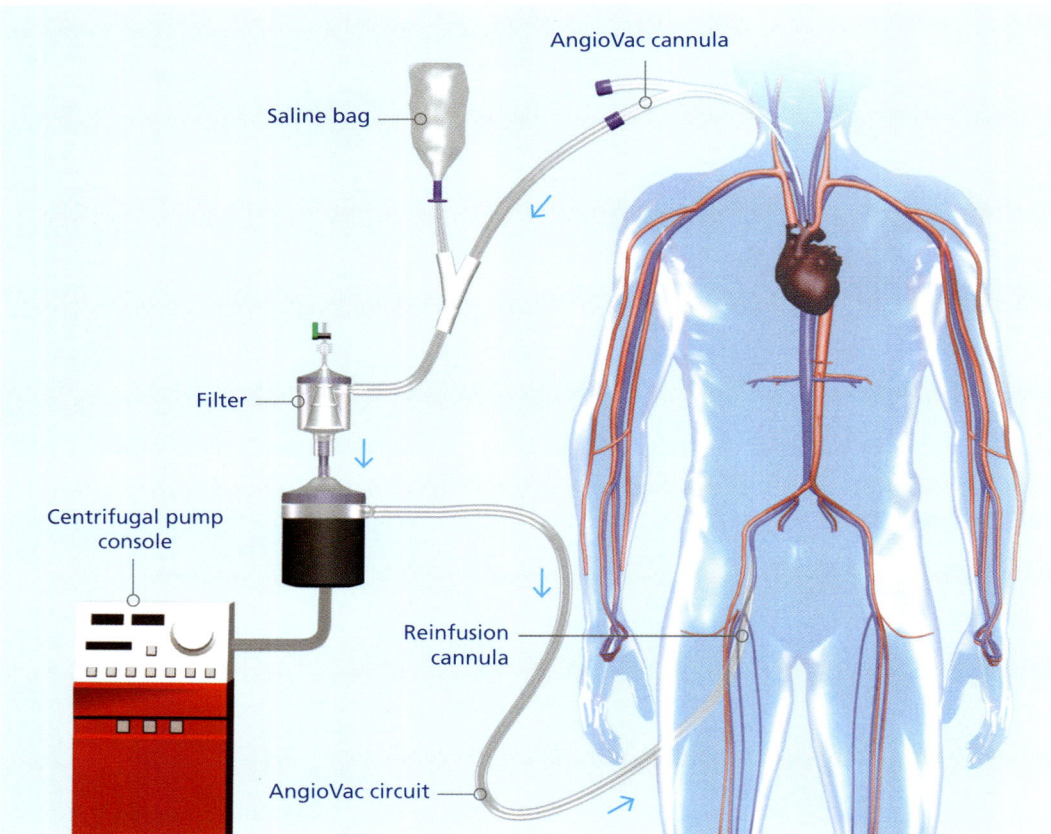

Figure 51.4 The AngioVac System. Unwanted intravascular material is aspirated with the AngioVac cannula. Blood is filtered, and then reinfused into a large peripheral vein.

catheter is an important limitation of this system in the treatment of patients with PE.

Right ventricular assist device

Although experience with right ventricular assist devices (RVAD) for the treatment of massive PE is extremely limited, there are case reports that suggest they can be a life-saving intervention in carefully selected cases. As opposed to extracorporeal membrane oxygenation (ECMO), which bypasses the entire pulmonary circulation, RVAD only bypasses the RV. RVADs can be placed surgically, or percutaneously. In at least one recent case report of a 48-year-old patient with acute massive PE and persistent cardiogenic shock, bypassing the acutely failing RV, but not the pulmonary circulation, with a percutaneous RVAD stabilized the patient and led to a full recovery [36,37].

Rotatable pigtail catheter

This is an early technique in catheter-directed therapies for PE [4,38,39]. A high-torque 5-Fr pigtail catheter is advanced over the wire and wedged within the thrombus. The catheter has a radiopaque tip, 10 side holes, and an oval side hole in the outer tangential plane of the loop that allows straight passage of the guidewire (Figure 51.2). Once positioned within the thrombus, the loop is rapidly spun around the axis formed by the catheter and guidewire, fragmenting the thrombus. This is a purely mechanical form of thrombolysis which can be considered in patients with massive or submassive PE, with contraindications to pharmacologic thrombolysis, and who are not candidates for other surgical or catheter-based therapies.

Aspirex

The Aspirex device (Straub Medical, Wangs, Switzerland) has three components: the catheter (usually 6, 8, or 10 Fr), a control unit, and an electric motor (drive). At the tip of the catheter there is a helix-like driveshaft inside the catheter tubing, creating negative pressure that allows thrombus aspiration through a distal aspiration port. Although the device has been extensively tested in animals, and there are a numerous published small case series that suggest its efficacy and safety, it has not been approved by the FDA, and is not available in the USA.

Rheolytic thrombectomy (AngioJet)

The AngioJet device (Medrad Interventional, PA, USA) consists of a double-lumen catheter that generates high-pressure saline jets at the catheter tip, creating a vacuum that allows thrombus aspiration. There are numerous reports of the development of severe bradyarrhythmias (including high-degree AV block and asystole) and death developing within seconds of activating the system [40–42]. These concerns have prompted the FDA to issue a black-box warning regarding intrapulmonary interventions with the AngioJet system.

Inferior vena cava filters

The only indication for an inferior vena cava (IVC) filter use in patients with acute PE that all major societies agree with is in patients who have contraindications to anticoagulation (AHA/ACC class I recommendation, level of evidence B). Other more controversial indications include patients with acute PE who have poor cardiopulmonary reserve and who are deemed to be at high risk of death if they develop another PE (Class IIb recommendation, level of evidence C). Most patients with massive or submassive PE fall into this category. In a recent analysis from a Nationwide Inpatient Sample that included over 2 million patients who were discharged with a diagnosis of PE, IVC filter use was associated with lower in-hospital mortality in patients with massive PE, and in stable PE patients who underwent thrombolysis [43]. IVC filter placement has been shown to reduce the incidence of recurrent PE, but not to lower long-term mortality. IVC filters do not prevent continued thrombus formation, and can increase the risk of deep venous thrombosis. Patients who receive removable IVC filters should be re-evaluated periodically for retrieval of the filter as soon as deemed safe.

Conclusions

All patients with acute PE should be risk-stratified as soon as the diagnosis of PE is made. Patients who meet criteria for massive PE should receive systemic thrombolysis, unless there are any contraindications. Surgical embolectomy is also an option if it can be performed quickly. Because revascularization of the pulmonary arteries with catheter-based therapies generally takes at least a few hours, these strategies are rarely used in hemodynamically unstable patients. However, catheter-based therapies should be considered in patients with submassive PE who do not have increased bleeding risk, especially if there is evidence of significant RV dilatation or dysfunction, or myonecrosis. Currently, there are no standard protocols for catheter-based therapies for PE, and the strength of recommendations for this strategy are overall weak. The catheter or device used is usually determined by institutional experience and resources. The strongest indication for IVC filter use is in patients with acute PE who are ineligible for anticoagulation. However, selected patients with submassive or massive PE can also benefit from placement of a retrievable IVC filter, even if they are candidates for anticoagulation.

Interactive multiple choice questions are available for this chapter on www.wiley.com/go/dangas/cardiology

References

1 Becattini C, Agnelli G, Pesavento R, *et al.* Incidence of chronic thromboembolic pulmonary hypertension after a first episode of pulmonary embolism. *Chest* 2006; **130**: 172–175.

2 Pengo V, Lensing AW, Prins MH, *et al.* Incidence of chronic thromboembolic pulmonary hypertension after pulmonary embolism. *N Engl J Med* 2004; **350**: 2257–2264.

3 Piazza G, Goldhaber SZ. Chronic thromboembolic pulmonary hypertension. *N Engl J Med* 2011; **364**: 351–360.

4 Nakazawa K, Tajima H, Murata S, Kumita SI, Yamamoto T, Tanaka K. Catheter fragmentation of acute massive pulmonary thromboembolism: distal embolisation and pulmonary arterial pressure elevation. *Br J Radiol* 2008; **81**: 848–854.

5 Casazza F, Becattini C, Bongarzoni A, *et al.* Clinical features and short term outcomes of patients with acute pulmonary embolism. The Italian Pulmonary Embolism Registry (IPER). *Thromb Res* 2012; **130**: 847–852.

6 Jaff MR, McMurtry MS, Archer SL, *et al.* Management of massive and submassive pulmonary embolism, iliofemoral deep vein thrombosis, and chronic thromboembolic pulmonary hypertension: a scientific statement from the American Heart Association. *Circulation* 2011; **123**: 1788–1830.

7 Piazza G. Submassive pulmonary embolism. *JAMA* 2013; **309**: 171–180.

8 Piazza G, Goldhaber SZ. Management of submassive pulmonary embolism. *Circulation* 2010; **122**: 1124–1129.

9 Konstantinides S, Geibel A, Olschewski M, *et al.* Importance of cardiac troponins I and T in risk stratification of patients with acute pulmonary embolism. *Circulation* 2002; **106**: 1263–1268.

10 Becattini C, Casazza F, Forgione C, *et al.* Acute pulmonary embolism: external validation of an integrated risk stratification model. *Chest* 2013; **144**: 1539–1545.

11 Trujillo-Santos J, den Exter PL, Gomez V, *et al.* Computed tomography-assessed right ventricular dysfunction and risk stratification of patients with acute non-massive pulmonary embolism: systematic review and meta-analysis. *J Thromb Haemost* 2013; **11**: 1823–1832.

12 Konstantinides S, Geibel A, Heusel G, *et al.* Heparin plus alteplase compared with heparin alone in patients with submassive pulmonary embolism. *N Engl J Med* 2002; **347**: 1143–1150.

13 Reid JH, Murchison JT. Acute right ventricular dilatation: a new helical CT sign of massive pulmonary embolism. *Clin Radiol* 1998; **53**: 694–698.

14 Schoepf UJ, Kucher N, Kipfmueller F, Quiroz R, Costello P, Goldhaber SZ. Right ventricular enlargement on chest computed tomography: a predictor of early death in acute pulmonary embolism. *Circulation* 2004; **110**: 3276–3280.

15 van der Meer RW, Pattynama PM, van Strijen MJ, *et al.* Right ventricular dysfunction and pulmonary obstruction index at helical CT: prediction of clinical outcome during 3-month follow-up in patients with acute pulmonary embolism. *Radiology* 2005; **235**: 798–803.

16 Lu MT, Demehri S, Cai T, *et al.* Axial and reformatted four-chamber right ventricle-to-left ventricle diameter ratios on pulmonary CT angiography as predictors of death after acute pulmonary embolism. *AJR Am J Roentgenol* 2012; **198**: 1353–1360.

17 Kearon C, Akl EA, Comerota AJ, *et al.* Antithrombotic therapy for VTE disease: Antithrombotic Therapy and Prevention of Thrombosis, 9th edn. *American College of Chest Physicians Evidence-Based Clinical Practice Guidelines. Chest* 2012; **141**: e419S–94S.

18 Guyatt GH, Akl EA, Crowther M, *et al.* Executive summary: Antithrombotic Therapy and Prevention of Thrombosis, 9th ed: American College of Chest Physicians Evidence-Based Clinical Practice Guidelines. *Chest* 2012; **141**: 7S–47S.

19 Agnelli G, Buller HR, Cohen A, *et al.* Oral apixaban for the treatment of acute venous thromboembolism. *N Engl J Med* 2013; **369**: 799–808.

20 Hokusai VTEI, Buller HR, Decousus H, *et al.* Edoxaban versus warfarin for the treatment of symptomatic venous thromboembolism. *N Engl J Med* 2013; **369**: 1406–1415.

21 EINSTEIN–PE Investigators, Bauersachs R, Berkowitz SD, *et al.* Oral rivaroxaban for symptomatic venous thromboembolism. *N Engl J Med* 2010; **363**: 2499–2510.

22 EINSTEIN–PE Investigators, Buller HR, Prins MH, *et al.* Oral rivaroxaban for the treatment of symptomatic pulmonary embolism. *N Engl J Med* 2012; **366**: 1287–1297.

23 Schulman S, Kakkar AK, Goldhaber SZ, *et al.* Treatment of acute venous thromboembolism with dabigatran or warfarin and pooled analysis. *Circulation* 2014; **129**: 764–772.

24 Schulman S, Kearon C, Kakkar AK, *et al.* Dabigatran versus warfarin in the treatment of acute venous thromboembolism. *N Engl J Med* 2009; **361**: 2342–2352.

25 Chai-Adisaksopha C, Crowther M, Isayama T, Lim W. The impact of bleeding complications in patients receiving target-specific oral anticoagulants: a systematic review and meta-analysis. *Blood* 2014; **124**: 2450–2458.

26 Yeh CH, Gross PL, Weitz JI. Evolving use of new oral anticoagulants for treatment of venous thromboembolism. *Blood* 2014; **124**: 1020–1028.

27 Jerjes-Sanchez C, Ramirez-Rivera A, de Lourdes Garcia M, *et al.* Streptokinase and heparin versus heparin alone in massive pulmonary embolism: a randomized controlled trial. *J Thromb Thrombolysis* 1995; **2**: 227–229.

28 Wan S, Quinlan DJ, Agnelli G, Eikelboom JW. Thrombolysis compared with heparin for the initial treatment of pulmonary embolism: a meta-analysis of the randomized controlled trials. *Circulation* 2004; **110**: 744–749.

29 Kucher N, Goldhaber SZ. Management of massive pulmonary embolism. *Circulation* 2005; **112**: e28–32.

30 Kucher N, Rossi E, De Rosa M, Goldhaber SZ. Massive pulmonary embolism. *Circulation* 2006; **113**: 577–582.

31 Meyer G, Vicaut E, Danays T, *et al.* Fibrinolysis for patients with intermediate-risk pulmonary embolism. *N Engl J Med* 2014; **370**: 1402–1411.

32 Dauphine C, Omari B. Pulmonary embolectomy for acute massive pulmonary embolism. *Ann Thoracic Surg* 2005; **79**: 1240–1244.

33 Leacche M, Unic D, Goldhaber SZ, *et al.* Modern surgical treatment of massive pulmonary embolism: results in 47 consecutive patients after rapid diagnosis and aggressive surgical approach. *J Thoracic Cardiovasc Surg* 2005; **129**: 1018–1023.

34 Piazza G. Multicenter trial of ultrasound-facilitated, low-dose fibrinolysis for acute massive and submassive pulmonary embolism (SEATTLE II). 2014 American College of Cardiology meeting, 2014.

35 Dudiy Y, Kronzon I, Cohen HA, Ruiz CE. Vacuum thrombectomy of large right atrial thrombus. *Catheter Cardiovasc Interv* 2012; **79**: 344–347.

36 Geller BJ, Morrow DA, Sobieszczyk P. Percutaneous right ventricular assist device for massive pulmonary embolism. *Circ Cardiovasc Interv* 2012; **5**: e74–75.

37 Kaltenbock F, Gombotz H, Tscheliessnigg KH, Matzer C, Winkler G, Auer T. [Right ventricular assist device (RVAD) in septic, fulminating pulmonary artery embolism]. *Der Anaesthesist* 1993; **42**: 807–810.

38 Eid-Lidt G, Gaspar J, Sandoval J, *et al.* Combined clot fragmentation and aspiration in patients with acute pulmonary embolism. *Chest* 2008; **134**: 54–60.

39 Schmitz-Rode T, Janssens U, Duda SH, Erley CM, Gunther RW. Massive pulmonary embolism: percutaneous emergency treatment by pigtail rotation catheter. *J Am Coll Cardiol* 2000; **36**: 375–380.

40 Bonvini RF, Righini M, Roffi M. Angiojet rheolytic thrombectomy in massive pulmonary embolism: locally efficacious but systemically deleterious? *J Vasc Interv Radiol* 2010; **21**: 1774–1776; author reply 1776–1777.

41 Karnabatidis D, Katsanos K, Kagadis GC, Siablis D. Re: Bradyarrhythmias during use of the angiojet system. *J Vasc Interv Radiol* 2007; **18**: 937; author reply 938.

42 Divekar AA, Scholz T, Fernandez JD. Novel percutaneous transcatheter intervention for refractory active endocarditis as a bridge to surgery: angiovac aspiration system. *Catheteri Cardiovasc Interv* 2013; **81**: 1008–1012.

43 Stein PD, Matta F, Keyes DC, Willyerd GL. Impact of vena cava filters on in-hospital case fatality rate from pulmonary embolism. *Am J Med* 2012; **125**: 478–484.

Renal Denervation for Resistant Hypertension

Hitesh C. Patel[1], Carl Hayward[1], Sebastian Ewen[2], and Felix Mahfoud[2,3]

[1] National Institute of Health Research (NIHR), Royal Brompton & Harefield NHS Foundation Trust, London, UK

[2] Universitätsklinikum des Saarlandes, Homburg-Saar, Germany

[3] Harvard-MIT Biomedical Engineering, Institute of Medical Engineering and Science, Cambridge, MA, USA

Hypertension is a common condition with an estimated 1 billion individuals affected worldwide [1]. In 2010, it was the leading single risk factor for mortality and accounted for 9.4 million deaths worldwide [2]. Worryingly, its prevalence is increasing and it is estimated that over the next two decades hypertension will affect approximately half of the world's population [1].

A meta-analysis of almost 1 million patients confirmed a linear relationship between blood pressure and vascular mortality [3]. This linear dose–response relationship serves to remind us that not only are those patients with higher blood pressure at greater risk of cardiovascular events, but also that any reduction in blood pressure will help reduce this risk. Indeed, a 2-mmHg reduction in systolic blood pressure is expected to reduce stroke mortality by 10% [3].

Despite an awareness of hypertension and its harmful consequences being described in texts dating back to ancient China (2600 BC), effective therapies were not first reported until the 1900s [4]. Two therapeutic options were available: the low sodium Kempner diet and surgical sympathectomy. Though sometimes efficacious, neither was well tolerated by patients and both fell out of favor in the 1950s when the first effective antihypertensive medications were developed [4].

Therapeutic options have progressed since then. The most recent international guidelines on the management of hypertension (from the European Society of Cardiology) [5], suggest that following diagnosis patients should implement lifestyle changes which include sodium restriction, moderation of alcohol consumption, dietary changes, weight reduction, regular physical exercise, and smoking cessation. In conjunction with this, medications are also required and currently the available classes of antihypertensives include: angiotensin-converting enzyme inhibitors, angiotensin II receptor antagonists, calcium-channel blockers, and diuretics. Further treatment strategies include aldosterone-receptor antagonists, adrenoreceptor (α or β) blockers, and centrally acting agents.

Resistant hypertension

Amongst treated hypertensive patients, only 50% will achieve adequate control [4]. Those who do not are either not compliant with medications, are under-medicated, or are misdiagnosed and have white coat hypertension [6]. Up to 20% of patients with uncontrolled hypertension develop secondary (and thereby potentially curable) forms of hypertension [7]. Those that remain are classified as having resistant hypertension, defined as blood pressure consistently >140/90 mmHg despite compliance with at least three classes of antihypertensives (one of which is a diuretic) at maximally tolerated doses [6].

The resistant hypertension cohort tends to have a longer duration of hypertension, greater end-organ damage, and a greater mortality rate than non-resistant hypertensive patients [6]. As such, this high-risk patient group would benefit from intensive treatment. However, the evidence-base guiding management of resistant hypertension is sparse; there are fewer than 10 randomized, controlled, and blinded studies involving patients with resistant hypertension. There has been resurgence of interest in the management of this condition driven by the development of novel non-pharmacologic therapies. In this chapter, we review one of these therapies, renal denervation, and summarize its journey from bench to bedside.

Rationale of targeting the renal sympathetic nervous system

An important factor underlying several forms of hypertension is an elevated level of sympathetic nerve activity. Neurogenic control of blood pressure is evidenced by the increase in blood pressure in patients with hypertension when waking up, coincident with the morning surge in sympathetic activity [8]. The role of the sympathetic nervous system in hypertension has further been conclusively demonstrated in animal and human studies using complementary techniques [9,10]. A dose–response relationship has been demonstrated, in that those individuals with higher blood pressure also display evidence of greater sympathetic activation [11]. It is the sympathetic efferents and sensory afferents of the kidney that are particularly important for the development and progression of hypertension [12].

Sympathetic nerve fibres originating from the brainstem supply the renal vasculature, tubules, and juxtaglomerular apparatus via the thoracic sympathetic ganglia (T10–12) [13]. Activation of the nerves at each of these sites is associated with reduced renal blood flow, salt and water retention, and activation of the renin–angiotensin–aldosterone

Interventional Cardiology: Principles and Practice, Second Edition. Edited by George D. Dangas, Carlo Di Mario, and Nicholas N. Kipshidze.

© 2017 John Wiley & Sons, Ltd. Published 2017 by John Wiley & Sons, Ltd.

system, which all promote hypertension [13]. Furthermore, afferent nerves originating predominantly from the renal pelvic wall travel to the brain and contralateral kidney via the dorsal root ganglia. The role of these nerves in hypertension is less well defined. Animal studies have demonstrated that electrical stimulation of these afferent nerves can produce sympathetic activation and augment blood pressure, though contradictory findings have also been published [14]. There is some evidence that sensory signals from the kidney can augment whole body sympathetic tone thereby not only activating renal efferents, but also efferent fibres to the heart and peripheral vasculature [15]. In animal models of hypertension, surgical denervation of the renal sympathetics (afferent and efferent) significantly reduces blood pressure [16].

However, the relationship between blood pressure and the sympathetic nervous system is complex and is not the panacea for blood pressure control. First, using the noradrenaline spillover technique it has been shown that the sympathetic nervous system in hypertensive patients is most activated in those aged 20–39 years and that with increasing age this effect attenuates [17]. This suggests that in the majority of patients with hypertension (i.e., those older than 40 years), the renal sympathetic nervous system is not as important a target. Second, hypertension is not always neurogenic in origin (e.g., patients have secondary causes of hypertension). Finally, even less is known about the role of the sympathetic nervous system in those with resistant hypertension and interestingly there is some evidence to suggest that sympathetic activity in resistant hypertension could be related to prescribed drugs, notably diuretics and vasodilators [8]. Others have shown that the level of sympathetic activity in patients with resistant hypertension is similar to healthy non-hypertensive elderly individuals [8].

Surgical sympathetic denervation

Prior to the advent of effective antihypertensive medications, patients with malignant hypertension (hypertension with papilledema) had a mortality rate of 100% at 5 years [4]. There was already data in that era to suggest that the sympathetic nerves were important for the genesis of hypertension and it was in this climate that surgeons were spurred to perform sympathectomies for hypertension.

The surgical technique involved either a selective renal sympathectomy (renal decapsulation or cautery/transection of the renal sympathetic nerve) or a non-selective ganglionectomy. Large series of patients with severe hypertension, including individuals with end-organ damage, experienced a reduction of BP accompanied by an improvement of mortality after sympathetic splanchnicectomy [18–20]. Interestingly, an improvement of mortality was also observed in patients who did not exhibit a meaningful BP reduction [19,20]. Responses to this therapy were variable and frequently there was a constellation of associated non-desirable autonomic side effects [18]. With the development of the first antihypertensive medications, surgical denervation was removed from the physician's armoury as a treatment for hypertension.

More recently, the value of surgical denervation has been realized in a sub-selected group of patients within renal transplant medicine. In patients who remain hypertensive after renal transplantation, native nephrectomy (which involves interruption of the renal sympathetic nerves) has been shown to improve blood pressure control and improve allograft perfusion by attenuating the heightened neurohumoral activation from the diseased kidneys [21].

Percutaneous denervation

With the maturation of percutaneous intervention and radiofrequency ablation for the treatment of cardiac arrhythmias, it was not a large theoretical leap to conceive a device and technique to ablate the renal sympathetic nerves. To take this step, an understanding of the anatomic relationship between the lumen of the renal artery and the sympathetic nerves is required, as is an understanding of the effect of radiofrequency energy on the tissue around the ablation catheter tip.

Anatomy of the renal sympathetic nerves

Initial work in human cadavers lent support to the feasibility of renal denervation using ablation through the renal artery lumen. These data suggested that over 90% of the renal nerves (afferents and efferents) were located circumferentially within 2 mm of the lumen wall of the renal artery in the adventitia, making them amenable to disruption with ablation [22].

This work has since been surpassed by Sakakura and colleagues who performed a human autopsy study with key differences: they examined a larger number of individuals and nerves (20 patients with 10,320 nerves vs. 5 patients with 956 nerves); they used a perfusion-fixed technique under physiologic pressure; and histologic analysis was performed of the whole peri-renal tissue as opposed to the first 2.5 mm of peri-vascular tissue [23]. They demonstrated that while there was a greater density of nerves in the proximal and mid segment of the renal artery, the nerves in the distal segment were closer to the renal artery lumen and hence more accessible to ablation. In a small subset they also found that there was no difference in nerve anatomy between hypertensive and non-hypertensive subjects.

Accessory renal arteries were also shown to be associated with sympathetic nerves. They confirmed that renal arteries are surrounded by both afferent and efferent nerves, though the latter are more numerous. In contrast to the earlier work they discovered that 28% of the sympathetic nerves are more than 4 mm away from the artery lumen, suggesting that a significant proportion of nerves are not accessible to current ablation technology (Figure 52.1). What remains unknown is the proportion of nerves that need to be interrupted to produce physiologic changes and clinical benefit.

Ablation catheter technology and the biophysics of ablation

There are six CE marked renal denervation catheters commercially available (Table 52.1). Five deliver radiofrequency energy (RF) while the other uses ultrasound. RF and ultrasound are forms of energy that exist on the electromagnetic spectrum. Both techniques lead to tissue damage through a process of resistive heating as consequence of energy being deposited in the area of interest (ablation is not synonymous with cautery). As the target tissue heats up, this then conducts heat to the surrounding tissues leading to expansion of the ablation lesion [24].

Ablation lesion size is determined by the power and duration of energy delivery, tissue contact of the catheter (this is important for RF only) and electrode cooling/tissue temperature [24]. As such, it cannot be assumed that each of the available catheters creates comparable lesions. The duration of energy delivery for each catheter varies between 10 to 120 seconds, but is usually less than 2 minutes per application. The latest generation multi-electrode catheters enable all electrodes to be activated simultaneously thereby reducing overall procedure time and radiation exposure. Cooling of the lumen wall is an important feature of ablation as this enables greater

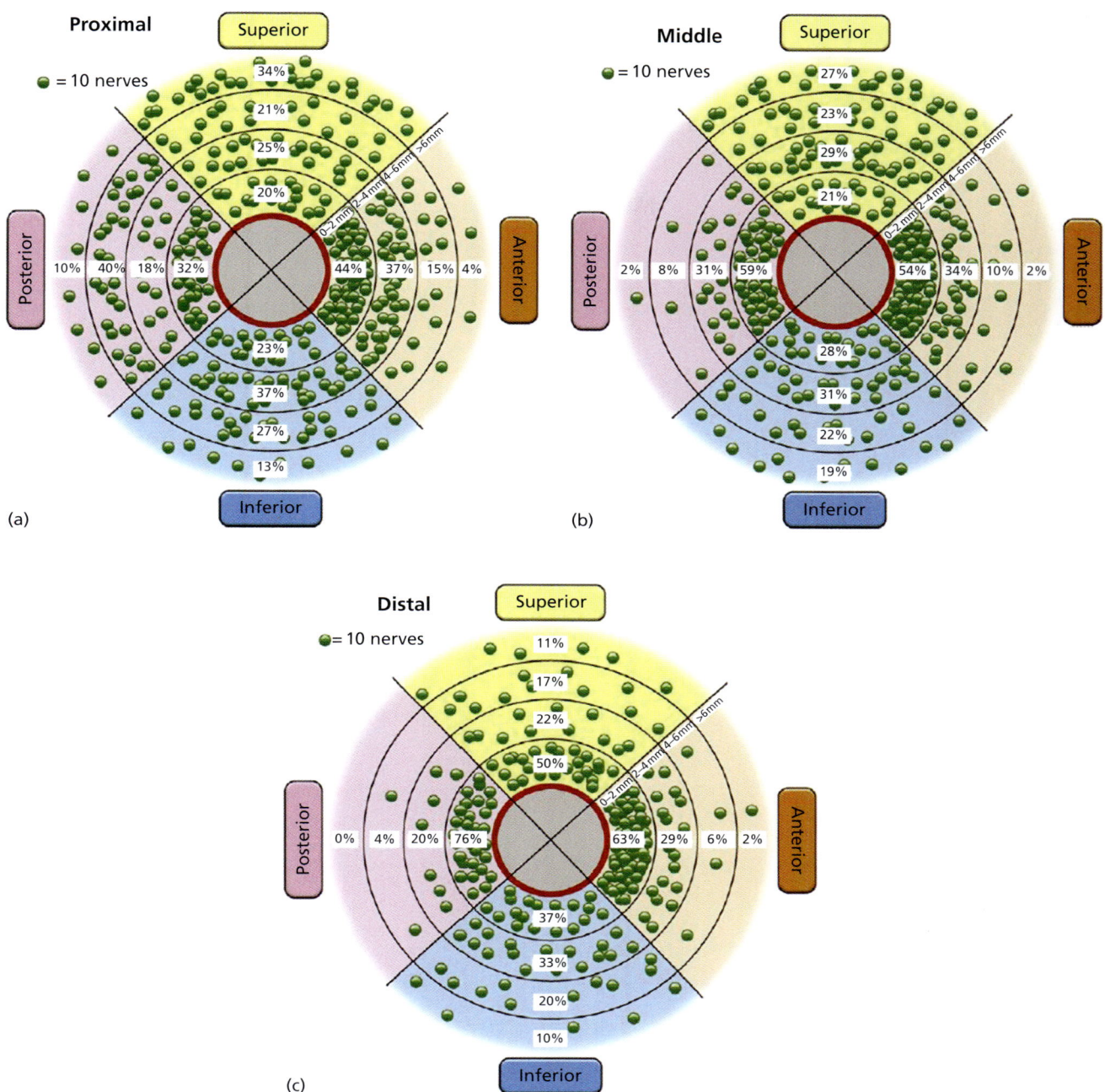

Figure 52.1 The distribution and density of renal nerves in the proximal (a), middle (b), and distal (c) portion of the renal artery. Each green dot represents 10 nerves. Source: Mahfoud F, *et al.* 2014 [44]. Copyright 2014 Elsevier.

energy deposition along with reduced surface damage. The current catheter systems rely either on renal artery blood flow or irrigation to cool the endothelial surface of the artery. Although each system is tested on large mammals as part of the approval process, the results of these investigations are not widely available making it difficult to compare the depth of lesion created by each technology. A recent case report of a postmortem of a 36-year-old woman who had undergone renal denervation showed that the ablation did not extend further than 2 mm from the lumen [25].

Trial evidence

The first-in-man experience of renal denervation therapy was reported in the pilot study, SYMPLICITY HTN I, which used the Medtronic single electrode Flex catheter [26]. A series of safety measures were built into this pilot study. First, all participants were at the severe end of the spectrum of resistant hypertension with entry criteria mandating a systolic blood pressure of 160 mmHg or greater. Second, the first 10 patients underwent a staged procedure with the first procedure treating one renal artery followed by a

Table 52.1 The currently available renal denervation catheters with CE mark.

Catheter		Energy	Electrode	Balloon (sizes)	Cooling	Lesion	Ablation T	Max power (W)	Size (Fr)	OTW
Symplicity Flex (Medtronic)		RF	Unipolar, single	No	Blood	Operator dependent	>480 s per artery (120 s per site)	8	6	N
Symplicity Spyral (Medtronic)		RF	Unipolar, multiple (4)	No	Blood	Helical	60 s per artery	8	6	Y
Vessix (Boston Scientific)		RF	Bipolar, multiple (4–8)	Yes (4, 5, 6, 7 mm)	None	Helical	30 s per artery	1	7	Y
EnligHTN (St. Jude)		RF	Unipolar, multiple (4)	No (basket size 16/18 mm)	Blood	Helical	60 s per artery	6	8	N
Iberis (Terumo)		RF	Unipolar, single	No	Blood	Operator dependent	>480 s per artery	8	4	N
Paradise (Recor)		US	NA	Yes (5, 6, 7, 8 mm)	Closed irrigation	Circumferential	10 s per artery	30	6	N

OTW, over the wire; R, radiofrequency; U, ultrasound.

second procedure a month later to treat the other kidney. A third angiogram was performed 2 weeks after the second procedure. The renal arteries were assessed once more at 6 months with a magnetic resonance angiogram. Following the original publication (n = 88), the study was extended and data are now available for 111 patients with 3-year follow-up [27].

There were no major safety concerns from this pilot study and at 1-month follow-up there was a 21/10 mmHg reduction in office blood pressure. The patients who completed 3 years' follow-up displayed a further reduction in blood pressure at 32/14 mmHg below baseline. The results of this trial must be interpreted within the constraints of first-in-man study design: a single-arm, open labeled trial that ultimately should be viewed as showing no evidence of undue harm and a strong signal for efficacy. Similar first-in-man studies have reported efficacy and safety with the other catheter designs [28,29].

This was followed-up by two more SYMPLICITY studies in which the same catheter system was used. SYMPLICITY HTN-2 was a multicenter, randomized, open label trial [30]. Fifty-two patients were allocated to renal denervation and 54 were allocated to control (usual medical therapy; there was no sham procedure). At 6 months there was a significant reduction in blood pressure in the active arm by 32/12 mmHg on office readings, whereas there was a small increase in blood pressure in the control arm of 1/0 mmHg. In a subset of 20 patients who underwent ambulatory blood pressure monitoring the blood pressure reduction in the active arm was more modest at 11/7 mmHg and there was a small, statistically insignificant, reduction in the control arm of 3/1 mmHg.

These results captured the imagination of both interventionalists and hypertension specialists alike. Renal denervation for resistant hypertension was offered on an individual patient basis in Europe, Asia, and Australasia. The findings of the majority of the subsequently published reports echoed the impressive blood pressure effects seen in the first two SYMPLICITY trials.

However, the absence of a blinded sham procedure in the control arm raised theoretical concerns about bias and the reliability of these studies [31]. An additional concern about the conduct of these studies was the absence of ambulatory blood pressure monitoring to exclude white coat hypertension. A European study in 346 patients with uncontrolled hypertension undergoing renal denervation addressed the concern about white coat hypertension by using ambulatory monitoring to dichotomize patients into true resistant hypertension (both office and ambulatory measures elevated, n = 303) and pseudoresistant hypertension (office measurement elevated but ambulatory measures normal, n = 43) [32]. Renal denervation was performed on both groups and although there was a similar reduction in office blood pressure measurements in both, only the true resistant cohort demonstrated a reduction in ambulatory measures.

The US Food and Drug Administration required that a further trial be conducted before endorsing renal denervation as a licensed therapy for resistant hypertension. To this end, the SYMPLICITY HTN-3 trial was launched which is, to date, the only trial of renal denervation with a sham-control and a blinded design [33]. It was performed across 88 centers in the USA. Ambulatory blood pressure monitoring was mandated not only to exclude white coat hypertension at screening, but also to assess response to therapy as a secondary endpoint.

SYMPLICITY HTN-3 randomized 535 patients, making it to date the largest single trial conducted in this field. In the renal denervation group, the office systolic blood pressure dropped significantly at 6 months by 14 mmHg and the ambulatory systolic blood pressure by 7 mmHg. However, these falls were not significantly different from the large blood pressure reductions observed in the sham arm. In sub-group analysis there was a signal that the denervation was more effective in Caucasians than African-Americans. As a consequence of the findings of SYMPLICITY HTN-3 the clinical role of renal denervation in the treatment of resistant hypertension has been challenged. Protagonists of renal denervation and the authors themselves have raised concerns that the procedural performance in the three trials may not have been equivalent as the operators in SYMPLICITY HTN-3 were less experienced with the technique. Indeed, only 26 of 111 interventionalists in SYMPLICITY HTN-3 had performed five or more renal denervations. In a *post hoc* multivariate analysis of the blood pressure response in the trial, number of ablation attempts was associated with a greater blood pressure drop.

The majority of the trial data of renal denervation in resistant hypertension is based upon the Symplicity Flex catheter system, which was first on the market. Newer catheter systems have evolved to provide complete circumferential ablations and work is still ongoing to determine if renal denervation using different technologies is effective.

The procedure
Patient selection
According to the current European Hypertension Guidelines, renal denervation represents a last resort treatment option for patients with resistant hypertension, in whom medical therapy fails to control blood pressure values <160/<110 mmHg. Those centers that wish to perform renal denervation (currently in a research context) ought to embrace a multidisciplinary team approach for each patient. A dedicated hypertension specialist should be involved in their management [5].

The renal denervation trials specified certain anatomic features as exclusion criteria, though there have been reports of the procedure being safely performed even in the presence of some of these:
1 The renal arteries ought to be greater than 4 mm in diameter to accommodate the ablation catheter and minimize complications.
2 The presence of any accessory or polar arteries must be sought.
3 A length of at least 20 mm of renal artery must be available for ablation prior to any branches.
4 Significant renal artery stenosis or fibromuscular dysplasia is a contraindication to the procedure.

Computerized tomography, magnetic resonance angiography, or renal duplex ultrasound of the renal arteries and kidneys are the preferred imaging modalities to determine this anatomy as they allow complete visualization of the vessels, which is not always feasible with ultrasound. In particular they can identify accessory arteries (these are arteries that enter the kidney via the hilum alongside the main renal artery) and polar arteries (which enter the kidney away from the hilum; Figure 52.2). Accessory arteries are found in 20% of the general population. Furthermore, cross-sectional imaging can identify branches of the main renal artery that supply important other organs (adrenal gland, testes, ovaries), whose ostia should not be put at risk.

Patients with renal artery stents have been excluded from renal denervation trials. However, there are reports of ablations being performed to the renal artery wall distal to a stent [34]. It is likely that ablation will be ineffective in segments, which have stents *in situ*, but appears to be safe and effective when performed distal to stented segments [35].

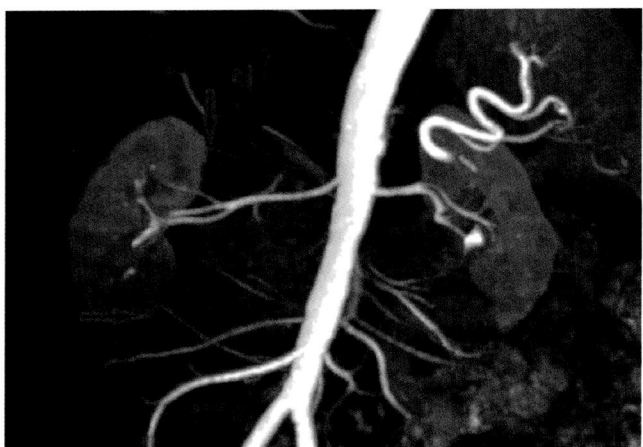

Figure 52.2 Magnetic resonance angiography of the renal arteries. Polar arteries to the right kidney are highlighted with blue arrows. An accessory artery entering at the hilum is highlighted with a red arrow.

Estimated glomerular filtration rate ought to be greater than 45 mL/min/1.73 m². While it may be feasible to perform the procedure when the renal function is worse, this is not recommended outside of a clinical trial and in cooperation with a nephrologist as part of a multidisciplinary team.

Patient preparation

When ablation is applied to the renal artery lumen, nocioceptors are stimulated resulting in visceral pain. General anesthesia is rarely required but analgesia (morphine and/or fentanyl) and sedation (midazolam) are mandatory. To reduce the risk of gastric aspiration the patient should be in a fasting state.

As shown on optical coherence tomography, renal denervation can induce thrombus formation at ablation sites [36]. Heparin should therefore be administered during the procedure and titrated to maintain the activated clotting time (ACT) >250 s. It is also suggested that antiplatelet agents (e.g., acetylsalicylic acid 75–100 mg/day) should be administered for 4 weeks following the procedure to further reduce the risk of thrombus (though there is no definitive trial evidence for this recommendation).

As for all procedures using contrast medium, it is advisable to withhold certain medications that can increase the risk of contrast nephropathy. These include metformin, non-steroidal anti-inflammatory drugs, and inhibitors of the renin–angiotensin–aldosterone system. Pre-hydration with intravenous fluid is also recommended. Centers that have performed renal denervation in patients with an estimated glomerular filtration rate <30 mL/min/1.73 m² have used carbon dioxide angiography to reduce the risk of contrast nephropathy, though this is not widely available.

Vascular access and renal angiogram

Continuous monitoring of heart rate, blood pressure, and oxygen saturation is mandatory after administration of analgesics and sedatives. Currently, Terumo's Iberis system and Recor's Paradise system can be deployed via the radial artery but all other systems require femoral arterial access (Table 52.1). The size of femoral sheath depends on the type of catheter used and can vary from 5 to 8 Fr. The first step of the intervention (in patients with preserved renal function) is to obtain angiographic images of the renal artery with an automated aortogram (to identify accessory arteries and origin of each artery). Typically, 30 mL of contrast at 20 mL/s is delivered by an autoinjector. The tip of the pigtail is positioned at the level of the L1 vertebra (using the 12th rib as a landmark) and an image is acquired in the anterioposterior (AP) plane. A selective angiogram of each target artery is then acquired to confirm suitability for ablation and exclusion of significant renal artery stenosis. Intra-arterial nitrates are helpful to dilate the renal artery fully. The usual choice of guiding catheter is either the internal mammary guide (IMA) or the renal double curve (RDC1). For femoral approach cases it is important to remember to use the shorter length catheters. For radial approach, long multipurpose or steerable guiding catheters are ideal. At the end of the procedure the sheath can be removed and the puncture site either manually compressed or an appropriate closure device used.

Ablation

Ablation is preferentially applied in a helical pattern (as opposed to circumferentially in one cross-sectional plane) to ensure as many branches of the sympathetic nerves are targeted as possible but minimizing the risk of inducing renal artery stenosis. This is particularly important with the single electrode catheters (Medtronic Flex and Terumo Iberis) as this pattern is created by the operator whereas the multi-electrode systems create this pattern automatically with a single ablation. The Paradise system, which utilizes ultrasound energy, is the only system that applies energy in a circular pattern.

The power output (Watts) of each catheter system is adjusted automatically by propietary algorithms built into the generators and is predominately determined by sensed impedance (Ohms), electrode temperature (°C) and rate of temperature increase. Cell death occurs instantly at 50 °C [24]. For effective and safe ablation, target tissue temperature should be 60–80 °C. A gradual decline in impedance (5–20%) suggests good tissue contact and position. A rapid decline suggests loss of tissue contact, whereas a rapid increase might indicate coagulum formation. Some generators terminate the ablation prematurely if these parameters are detected.

Certain practical pointers are important with all of the ablation systems. First, proper electrode contact with the vessel wall is important with RF energy [24]. This can be assessed using fluoroscopy and the detection of appropriate impedance readings. Second, the catheter position should be stable and this can be confirmed with both fluoroscopy and the presence of stable impedance measurements (variations <20 Ohms). To improve stability and vessel apposition some of the systems provide rotation and flexion control (Flex, Iberis), some require balloon inflation (Vessix, Paradise), while others have a preformed spiral or basket design (Spyral, EnligHTN). Third, ablations should be performed in the distal main artery first followed by further ablations as the catheter is withdrawn and rotated to a new more proximal segment. This is mandatory with the single electrode systems (Flex, Iberis, at least four ablations per artery) and suggested for the other multi-electrode systems.

When this procedure was first pioneered in humans it was suggested that the last ablation should be applied close to the renal artery origin in a superior position. The histology data do not entirely support this assertion and suggest that the nerve density is greater proximally and ventrally but the nerves are closer to the lumen distally [23]. Theoretically, one would assume that the more unique sites at which energy can be safely delivered, the greater the probability of interruption of the sympathetic nerves.

A major limitation of renal denervation remains the lack of intraprocedural markers of efficacy, thus remaining an entirely anatomically driven procedure. Blood pressure and heart rate response to renal sympathetic nerve stimulation before and after denervation are a potential method to assess efficacy of the procedure. There are some preliminary human [37] and animal data [38] to suggest that there is a dampened blood pressure and heart rate response to renal nerve stimulation after successful denervation.

Complications

Early complications of the procedure include those of any angiographic or ablation procedure: vascular access site damage; infection; skin burns; and contrast nephropathy. It is important to perform a selective renal artery angiogram at the end of the procedure. Spasm or edema of treated renal arteries is considered normal and should resolve within hours of ablation. There is a risk of renal artery dissection or rupture either caused by trauma from the renal denervation catheter, guidewires, or the ablation itself. This would be identified during the procedure and hence could be promptly treated with angioplasty and stenting (bare or covered).

There are case reports to suggest that renal denervation can induce renal artery stenosis, especially if the procedure is performed adjacent to existing plaque [39]. However, this is an uncommon complication with an incidence estimated to be <1%. Evidence from trial and registry data does not suggest that renal denervation accelerates renal dysfunction. However, patients who undergo renal denervation should be followed up long term and in those who display worsening renal function, rebound hypertension or episodes of acute heart failure, iatrogenic renal artery stenosis should be excluded. In addition to renal artery stenosis another cause of rebound hypertension is regeneration and reconnection of the renal sympathetic nerves, which has been shown to occur in animal models [40].

Unlike surgical sympathectomy for hypertension, which commonly resulted in profound orthostatic dysfunction or chronotropic incompetence, there is no evidence to suggest that percutaneous denervation is associated with these adverse effects [41,42].

The future

Renal denervation remains a relatively safe procedure, but there remain questions to be answered as to its efficacy, which can only be achieved by well-designed and well-conducted trials. Useful lines of enquiry include:

1 What percentage of renal nerves need to be ablated to show clinical benefit?

2 Are the newer multi-electrode catheters more effective in causing denervation but as safe?

3 How can success of renal sympathetic denervation be confirmed during the procedure?

4 Should patients be selected for the procedure on the basis of an elevated blood pressure *and* evidence of an elevated sympathetic nerve activity?

So far, renal denervation has been investigated predominantly in patients with resistant hypertension, a condition characterized by high cardiovascular morbidity and mortality. However, renal denervation could be particularly beneficial in other conditions associated with high sympathetic activity. There have already been some early studies investigating its role in heart failure [43] and atrial fibrillation [37]. More studies are needed to understand the role of this interesting treatment approach in different disease states.

Interactive multiple choice questions are available for this chapter on www.wiley.com/go/dangas/cardiology

References

1 Kearney P, Whelton M, Reynolds K, *et al.* Global burden of hypertension: analysis of worldwide data. *Lancet* 2005; **365**: 217–23.

2 Kintscher U. The burden of hypertension. *Eurointervention* 2013; **9**: R12–15.

3 Prospective Studies Colloboration. Age-specific relevance of usual blood pressure to vascular mortality: a meta-analysis of individual data for one million adults in 61 prospective studies. *Lancet* 2002; **360**: 1903–1913.

4 Patel HC, di Mario C. Renal denervation for hypertension: where are we now? *Br J Cardiol* 2013; **20**: 142–147.

5 Mancia G, Fagard R, Narkiewicz K, *et al.* 2013 ESH/ESC Guidelines for the management of arterial hypertension of the European Society of Hypertension (ESH) and of the European Society of Cardiology (ESC). *Eur Heart J* 2013; **34**: 2159–2219.

6 Calhoun D, Jones D, Textor S, *et al.* Resistant hypertension: diagnosis, evaluation, and treatment: a scientific statement from the American Heart Association Professional Education Committee of the Council for High Blood Pressure Research. *Hypertension* 2008; **51**: 1403–1419.

7 Tsioufis C, Kordalis A, Flessas D, *et al.* Pathophysiology of resistant hypertension: the role of sympathetic nervous system. *Int J Hypertens* 2011; doi:10.4061/2011/642416.

8 Floras J. Renal denervation for drug-resistant hypertension: suffering its original sin, seeking redemption. *Canadian J Cardiol* 2014; **30**: 476–478.

9 Mancia G, Grassi G, Giannattasio C, Seravalle G. Sympathetic activation in the pathogenesis of hypertension and progression of organ damage. *Hypertension* 1999; **34**: 724–728.

10 Grassi G. Role of the sympathetic nervous system in human hypertension. *J Hypertens* 1998; **16**: 1979–1987.

11 Grassi G, Cattaneo BM, Seravalle G, *et al.* Baroreflex control of sympathetic nerve activity in essential and secondary hypertension. *Hypertension* 1998; **31**: 68–72.

12 Di Bona G. Sympathetic nervous system and the kidney in hypertension. *Curr Opin Nephrol Hypertens* 2002; **11**: 197–200.

13 Myat A, Redwood S, Qureshi A, *et al.* Renal sympathetic denervation therapy for resistant hypertension. A contemporary synopsis and future implications. *Circ Cardiovasc Interv* 2013; **6**: 184–197.

14 Katholi R, Rocha-Singh K, Goswami N, Sobotka P. Renal nerves in the maintenance of hypertension: a potential therapeutic target. *Curr Hypertens Rep* 2010; **12**: 196–204.

15 De Jager R, Blankestij P. Pathophysiology I: the kidney and the sympathetic nervous system. *Eurointervention* 2013; **9**: R42–47.

16 Schlaich M, Sobotka P, Krum H, *et al.* Renal denervation as a therapeutic approach for hypertension: novel implications for an old concept. *Hypertension* 2009; **54**: 1195–1201.

17 Esler M, Jennings G, Biviano B, Lambert G, Hasking G. Mechanism of elevated plasma noradrenaline in the course of essential hypertension. *J Cardiovasc Pharm* 1986; **8**: S39–43.

18 Allen E. Sympathectomy for essential hypertension. *Circulation* 1952; **6**: 131–140.

19 Smithwick RH, Thompson JE. Splanchnicectomy for essential hypertension; results in 1,266 cases. *JAMA* 1953; **152**: 1501–1504.

20 Peet MM, Woods WW, Braden S. The surgical treatment of hypertension. *JAMA* 1940; **115**: 1875–1885.

21 Curtis J, Luke R, Diethelm A, Whelchel J, Jones P. Benefits of removal of native kidneys in hypertension after renal transplantation. *Lancet* 1985; **8458**: 739–742.

22 Atherton D, Deep N, Mendelsohn F. Micro-anatomy of the renal sympathetic nervous system: a human post-mortem histologic study. *Clin Anat* 2012; **25**: 628–633.

23 Sakakura K, Ladich E, Cheng Q, *et al.* Anatomic assessment of sympathetic periarterial renal nerves in man. *J Am Coll Cardiol* 2014; **64**: 635–643.

24 Patel HC, Dhillon P, Mahfoud F, *et al.* The biophysics of renal sympathetic denervation using radiofrequency energy. *Clin Res Cardiol* 2014; **103**: 337–344.

25 Vink E, Goldschmeding R, Vink A, *et al.* Limited destruction of renal nerves after catheter-based renal denervation: results of a human case study. *Nephrol Dial Transplant* 2014; **29**: 1608–1610.

26 Krum H, Schlaich M, Whitbourn R, *et al.* Catheter-based renal sympathetic denervation for resistant hypertension: a multicentre safety and proof-of-principle cohort study. *Lancet* 2009; **373**: 1275–1281.

27 Krum H, Schlaich M, Sobotka P, *et al.* Percutaneous renal denervation in patients with treatment-resistant hypertension: final 3-year report of the Symplicity HTN-1 study. *Lancet* 2014; **383**: 622–629.

28 Worthley S, Tsioufis C, Worthley M, *et al.* Safety and efficacy of a multi-electrode renal sympathetic denervation system in resistant hypertension: the EnligHTN I trial. *Eur Heart J* 2013; **34**: 2132–2140.

29 Mabin T, Sapoval M, Cababe V, Stemmett J, Iyer M. First experience with endovascular ultrasound renal denervation for the treatment of resistant hypertension. *EuroIntervention* 2012; **8**: 57–61.

30 Simplicity HTN-2 Investigators. Renal sympathetic denervation in patients with treatment-resistant hypertension (The Simplicity HTN-2 Trial): a randomised controlled trial. *Lancet* 2010; **376**: 1903–1909.

31 Howard JP, Nowbar AN, Francis DP. Size of blood pressure reduction from renal denervation: insights from metaanalysis of antihypertensive drug trials of 4121 patients with a focus on trial design: the CONVERGE report. *Heart* 2013; **99**: 1579–1587.

32 Mahfoud F, Ukena C, Schmieder R, et al. Ambulatory blood pressure changes after renal sympathetic denervation in patients with resistant hypertension. *Circulation* 2013; **128**: 132–140.

33 Bhatt DL, Kandzari DE, O'Neill WW, et al.; SYMPLICITY HTN-3 Investigators. A controlled trial of renal denervation for resistant hypertension. *N Engl J Med* 2014; **370**: 1393–1401.

34 Ziegler A, Franke J, Bertog S. Renal denervation after renal artery stenting. *Catheter Cardiovasc Interv* 2013; **81**: 342–375.

35 Mahfoud F, Tunev S, Ruwart J, et al. Efficacy and safety of catheter-based radiofrequency renal denervation in stented renal arteries. *Circ Cardiovasc Interv* 2014; **7**: 813–820.

36 Templin C, Jaguszewski M, Ghadri J, et al. Vascular lesions induced by renal nerve ablation as assessed by optical coherence tomography: pre- and post- procedural comparison with the Simplicity and the EnligHTN multi-electrode renal denervation catheter. *Eur Heart J* 2013; **34**: 2141–2148.

37 Pokushalov E, Romanov A, Corbucci G, et al. A randomized comparison of pulmonary vein isolation with versus without concomitant renal artery denervation in patients with refractory symptomatic atrial fibrillation and resistant hypertension. *J Am Coll Cardiol* 2012; **60**: 1163–1170.

38 Chinushi M, Izumi D, Iijima K, et al. Blood pressure and autonomic responses to electrical stimulation of renal arterial nerves before and after ablation of the renal artery. *Hypertension* 2013; **61**: 450–456.

39 Kaltenback B, Id D, Franke J, et al. Renal artery stenosis after renal sympathetic denervation. *J Am Coll Cardiol* 2012; **60**: 2694–2695.

40 Mulder J, Hokfelt T, Knuepfer M, Kopp U. Renal sensory and sympathetic nerves reinnervate the kidney in a similar time-dependent fashion after renal denervation in rats. *Am J Physiol Regul Integr Comp Physiol* 2013; **304**: R675–682.

41 Lenski M, Mahfoud F, Razouk A, et al. Orthostatic function after renal sympathetic denervation in patients with resistant hypertension. *Int J Cardiol* 2013; **169**: 418–424.

42 Ukena C, Mahfoud F, Kindermann I, et al. Cardiorespiratory response to exercise after renal sympathetic denervation in patients with resistant hypertension. *J Am Coll Cardiol* 2011; **58**: 1176–1182.

43 Patel H, Rosen D, Lindsay A, et al. Targeting the autonomic nervous system: measuring autonomic function and novel devices for heart failure management. *Int J Cardiol* 2013; **170**: 107–117.

44 Mahfoud F, Edelman E, Bohm M. Catheter-based renal denervation is no simple matter: lessons to be learned from our anatomy. *J Am Coll Cardiol* 2014; **64**: 644–646.

CHAPTER 53

Antithrombotic Strategies in Valvular and Structural Heart Disease Interventions

Mikkel Malby Schoos[1], Davide Capodanno[2], and George D. Dangas[3]

[1] Zealand University Hospital, Denmark

[2] Ferrarotto Hospital, University of Catania, Italy

[3] Department of Cardiology, Mount Sinai Medical Center, New York, NY, USA

Intervention for valvular and structural heart disease is an exponentially growing field within interventional cardiology. Transcatheter therapies for both valvular and congenital heart disease imply the introduction of large and potentially thrombogenic instruments through the venous or arterial system to the site of the intervention, as well as the implantation of devices that require time for full endothelization. In addition, a proportion of these patients have a greater propensity for hemodynamic compromise, which increases the risk of ischemic stroke. For these reasons, the use of antithrombotic drugs for reducing the risk of stroke, systemic embolism, or valve/device thrombosis in the early and mid-term period is key to achieving successful procedural results and improving the overall outcomes of transcatheter procedures. However, drugs and regimens for antiplatelet and anticoagulant therapy for valvular and structural interventions are mostly empirical in daily practice and typically administered at the operator's discretion. The objectives of this chapter are: (i) to review the current evidence supporting the rationale for antithrombotic management of patients undergoing transcatheter aortic valve implantation (TAVI), percutaneous mitral valve repair with the Mitraclip system, patent foramen ovale (PFO), atrial septal defect (ASD) closure, and left atrial appendage closure (LAAC); (ii) to describe common strategies for managing antiplatelet and anticoagulant therapy in patients with valvular and structural heart disease undergoing transcatheter procedures; and (iii) to provide insights on future directions and research lines in this field.

Embolism and thrombosis in valvular and structural transcatheter interventions

Embolic stroke is one of the most feared complications of interventional catheter procedures, being associated not only with increased acute mortality, but also with increased morbidity and physical disability.

Transcatheter aortic valve implantation

Cerebral silent embolic events have been reported post-TAVI by magnetic resonance imaging (MRI) in 68–84% of cases (Figure 53.1) [1–5]. Intriguingly, however, the vast majority of lesions had no remaining signal in follow-up MRI and cognitive function stayed unaffected [4]. On a more clinical level, randomized controlled trials (Table 53.1) and most registries report stroke rates after transcatheter aortic valve replacement (TAVR) in the range of 2–6% at 30 days' follow-up. A weighted meta-analysis of 53 studies including a total of 10,037 patients estimated the incidence of peri-procedural stroke and subsequent outcomes in patients undergoing transfemoral, transapical, or trans-subclavian TAVI. Pooled rates of stroke within 24 hours and 30 days were $1.5 \pm 1.4\%$ and $3.3 \pm 1.8\%$, and six of every seven stroke events were classified as major strokes. Not surprisingly, patients who experienced a stroke also experienced a 3.5-fold increased risk of mortality at 30 days ($25.5 \pm 21.9\%$ vs. $6.9 \pm 4.2\%$) [6]. Similarly, another weighted meta-analysis using Valve Academic Research Consortium (VARC) definitions reported a 3.2% (95% confidence interval (CI) 2.1–4.8%) risk of major stroke at 30 days [7]. Of note, the incidence of stroke peaks within 2 days, but continues slightly afterwards, reflecting the high baseline risk of patients who are currently referred for TAVI (Figure 53.2) [8]. Valve thrombosis is estimated at a non-negligible weighted rate of 1.2% (95% CI 0.3–2.2%) [7].

MitraClip

In the EVEREST II (Endovascular Valve Edge-to-Edge Repair Study), the only randomized trial to date reporting data of MitraClip versus surgical mitral repair or replacement, two strokes occurred within 30 days in the interventional arm (1.1% vs. 2.1% in the surgical arm; p = 0.89) [9]. Observational series with different baseline case-mix reported major strokes in 0–2.6% of cases [10–15]. A weighted meta-analysis could meaningfully increase the precision of this risk estimate, given the small number of patients enrolled in the studies, mostly reflecting the early experience of single institutions with percutaneous mitral valve repair. In the EVEREST II trial, clip thrombosis was uncommon, being detected in 1 of 184 cases (0.5%). However, a recent large national registry from Germany described an in-hospital stroke incidence of 0.4%, but an additional 1% transient ischemic attack (TIA) and a 0.3% systemic embolism rate, yielding an almost 2% occurrence of potential thromboembolic events [16].

Interventional Cardiology: Principles and Practice, Second Edition. Edited by George D. Dangas, Carlo Di Mario, and Nicholas N. Kipshidze.
© 2017 John Wiley & Sons, Ltd. Published 2017 by John Wiley & Sons, Ltd.

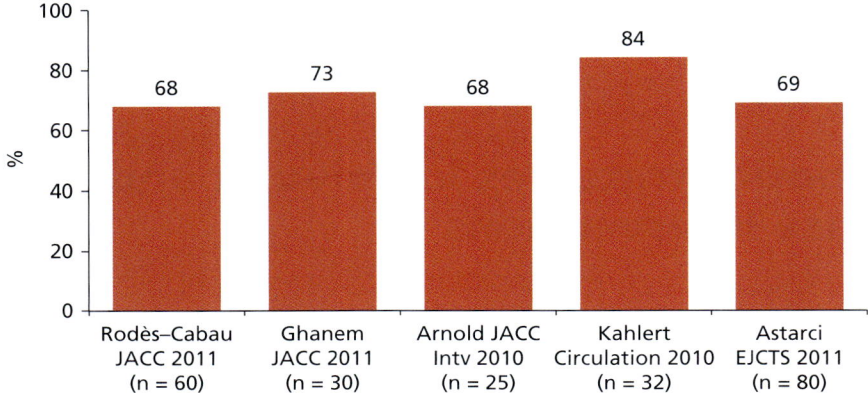

Figure 53.1 New cerebral ischemic lesions post-transcatheter aortic valve implantation (TAVI) as detected by magnetic resonance imaging.

Patent foramen ovale and atrial septal defect closure

The options for secondary prevention of cryptogenic embolism in patients with PFO are administration of antithrombotic medications or percutaneous closure of the PFO. Whether closure is superior to medical therapy is still unsettled, as recent results of a multinational trial investigating closure of a PFO for secondary prevention of cryptogenic embolism did not result in a significant reduction in the risk of recurrent embolic events or death as compared with medical therapy, although there was a non-significant numerical benefit of device closure and the study was possibly underpowered [17].

Data on peri-procedural stroke as the consequence of percutaneous closure of a PFO or an ASD cannot be easily disconnected from the underlying risk of recurrent stroke owing to suboptimal sealing of the shunt area or cerebrovascular embolism from alternative sources. In addition, closure devices differ in terms of thrombogenicity and the incidence of new-onset conditions at high embolic potential, including atrial fibrillation [18–22]. In 499 patients from the Amplatzer PFO closure device arm of the RESPECT (Randomized Evaluation of Recurrent Stroke Comparing PFO Closure to Established Current Standard of Care Treatment) trial, one ischemic stroke (0.2%) occurred 1 week post-implant and another one 5 months post-implant with finding of severe shunting related to previously undiagnosed sinus venosus defect, requiring surgical closure [22]. No thrombus was detected on any implanted device. In observational series, thromboembolic events while on antiplatelet treatment have been reported in 1.6–8.2% of patients within 1 year after PFO closure [23–29]. Also, many cases of device thrombosis have been reported within the first months after ASD device implantation, with an incidence of up to 7%, depending on the device [30,31].

Conversely, in the trial by Meier *et al.* [17], where endpoint adjudication was performed blinded to the study group assignments (medical therapy vs. device closure), stroke (0.5%), TIA (2.5%), and systemic embolism incidence (0%) remained numerically lower than in medically treated patients and the incidence curves only diverged late (after 6 months post-procedure). The likelihood of a substantial procedure-related thromboembolism occurrence is therefore controversial.

Left atrial appendage closure

In patients with non-valvular atrial fibrillation and absolute contraindications to anticoagulation therapy, LACC with the WATCHMAN or AMPLATZER device is an emergent interventional treatment option to reduce the risk of cardiac thromboembolisms [32–34]. Procedure-related stroke rates were 1.1% and 0.7% in the PROTECT AF [33] and PREVAIL [34] trials, respectively. Preliminary results in small series suggest that the risk of device thrombosis is very low. Urena *et al.* [32] reported on patients having the AMPLATZER Cardiac Plug device implanted followed by dual or single antiplatelet therapy and showed a low rate of embolic and bleeding events after a mean follow-up of 20 months.

Pathophysiology of stroke and systemic embolism in valvular and structural transcatheter interventions

Not surprisingly, embolism of thrombotic material is more commonly detected in left heart catheterization procedures, which require advancing the catheter through the aorta, thus increasing the risk of embolization by scraping of aortic plaques with subsequent direct embolization of debris to the brain. Indeed, scraping of aortic plaques occurs more commonly with large catheters, such as those employed for TAVI. Embolic stroke also theoretically occurs in the setting of right heart catheterization in patients with PFO or ASD, or following transeptal puncture in patients undergoing Mitraclip implantation.

Transcatheter aortic valve implantation

The time distribution of strokes is inherently correlated to the underlying pathophysiology. Strokes occurring in the acute (<24 hours) and sub-acute early (<30 days) post-TAVR period are strongly related to procedural factors, whereas late events (1–12 months) are mostly connected to patient and disease factors [35].

Pathophysiologic mechanisms of early stroke after TAVR

Van Mieghem *et al.* [36] recently examined the histopathology of embolic debris captured in an embolic protection device following TAVR. Macroscopic debris was found in 30 (75%) patients and, out of those, 27% had amorphous calcium or valve tissue likely to originate from degenerated aortic leaflets, and 43% had evidence of collagenous tissue coming from either the valve or the aortic wall. Importantly, about half (55%) of patients had thrombotic tissue debris.

Several pathophysiologic mechanisms account for this macroscopic debris. First, the aortic arch is recognized as a source of embolic material. In fact, retrograde progression of atheroma from

Table 53.1 The risk of stroke in patients undergoing transcatheter aortic valve implantation (TAVI).

	30 days			1 year			2 years		
Balloon expandable valve (Sapien)									
Partner A [83]	Surgery (n=351)	TAVR (n=348)	p	Surgery (n=351)	TAVR (n=348)	p	Surgery (n=351)	TAVR (n=348)	p
TIA	1 (0.3)	3 (0.9)	0.33	4 (1.5)	8 (2.6)	0.32	5 (2.0)	10 (3.6)	0.26
Minor stroke	1 (0.3)	3 (0.9)	0.34	2 (0.7)	3 (0.9)	0.84	14 (4.9)	24 (7.7)	0.17
Major Stroke	7 (2.1)	13 (3.8)	0.2	8 (2.4)	17 (5.1)	0.07			
Balloon expandable valve (Sapien)									
Partner B [84]	Standard Tx (n=179)	TAVR (n=179)	p	Standard Tx (n=179)	TAVR (n=179)	p	Standard Tx (n=179)	TAVR (n=179)	p
TIA	0	0	–	0	1 (0.6)	0.37	N/A	N/A	N/A
Minor stroke	1 (0.6)	3 (1.7)	0.62	1 (0.6)	4 (2.2)	0.37	8 (5.5)	22 (13.8)	0.01
Major Stroke	2 (1.1)	9 (5.0)	0.06	7 (3.9)	14 (7.8)	0.18			
Self-expandable valve (CoreValve)									
Adams et al. [85]	Surgery (n=357)	TAVR (n=390)	p	Surgery (n=357)	TAVR (n=390)	p	Surgery (n=357)	TAVR (n=390)	p
TIA	1 (0.3)	3 (0.8)	0.36	5 (1.6)	6 (1.6)	0.93	N/A	N/A	N/A
Minor stroke	12 (3.4)	4 (1.0)	0.03	20 (6.0)	11 (3.0)	0.05	N/A	N/A	N/A
Major Stroke	11 (3.1)	15 (3.9)	0.55	23 (7.0)	22 (5.8)	0.59	N/A	N/A	N/A
Self-expandable valve (CoreValve)									
Popma et al. [86]	Surgery	TAVR (n=489)	p	Surgery	TAVR (n=489)	p	Surgery	TAVR	p
TIA	N/A	3 (0.6)	N/A	N/A	5 (1.1)	N/A	N/A	N/A	N/A
Minor stroke	N/A	9 (1.9)	N/A	N/A	14 (3.2)	N/A	N/A	N/A	N/A
Major Stroke	N/A	11 (2.3)	N/A	N/A	19 (4.3)	N/A	N/A	N/A	N/A

N/A, not applicable; TAVR, transcatheter aortic valve replacement; TIA, transient ischemic attack; Tx, therapy.

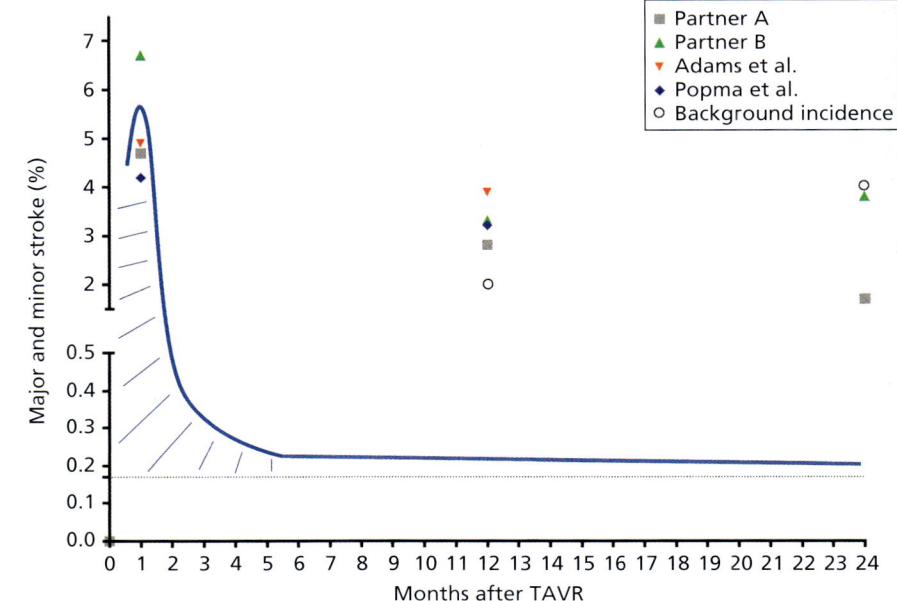

Figure 53.2 Stroke incidence is estimated to be ≈5.5% at 30 days and ≈8–9% at 1 year, based on the PARTNER and the CoreValve programs. Approximately half of the strokes at 30 days occur within the first 24 hours, amounting to 2.5–3% from days 2–30. Additionally, the large majority (>75%) of strokes within 1 year occur in the first 6 months, amounting to additional ~3.5% in the period 1–6 months [80]. The symbols mark the cumulative incidence at the given time point based on landmark trials. The clear circle indicates the cumulative incidence of the background population (2% per year in patients over 80 years of age) and the dotted line the monthly stroke incidence rate (0.17%) of the background population based on the European epidemiologic study by Truelsen et al. [81] and the stroke incidence meta-analysis by Russo et al. [82].

the descending aorta to the arch has been shown to correlate significantly with presence of cardiovascular risk factors and advanced age, conditions that are frequently encountered in patients referred for TAVI [37]. Retrograde crossing of a stenotic aortic valve during diagnostic catheterization results in new focal cerebral lesions in 22% of patients [38].

Second, initial balloon aortic valvuloplasty (BAV) not only results in the fracture of valvular tissue leading to embolism of overlying calcium deposits, but also increases the risk of thrombogenic complications. Stenotic valves host large amounts of localized tissue factor and thrombin covered by vascular endothelium. BAV, by means of endothelial denudation and fracture of the valve, exposes these factors to blood circulation, which in turn triggers coagulation cascades and platelet activation resulting in increased inflammation and recurrent thrombogenicity [39]. Therefore, thromboemboli can arise from the bioprosthesis before endothelialization is complete. Aggregation of platelet and fibrin has been known to occur on valve leaflet within a few hours after implantation [8]. It has been suggested that the balloon expandable valve produces emboli during positioning of the valve on the annulus, whereas the self-expanding valve does so during valve deployment, as manifested by simultaneous transcranial Doppler studies [40,41].

Furthermore, the interaction of the newly deployed stent valve with the aortic annulus over the displaced natural valve can cause additional embolic debris. Additional possible mechanisms are prosthetic valve surface exposure, flow turbulence, and exposure of stents struts to the circulation [42]. Blood stasis in the perivalvular space "outside" the metallic stent of a undersized or underexpanded prosthetic valve, where the irregularly crushed native aortic valve cusps persist, could also generate thrombi with subsequent events.

Given these pathoanatomic considerations mainly related to the aortic arch, the choice of the arterial access has a pivotal role in the determination of embolic risk with the potential advantage of non-transfemoral approaches. The transapical approach offers an option in patients hosting a high degree of aortic atheroma with potential reduction of the risk caused by aorta manipulation and anterograde valve access. The transapical access has previously been associated with the lowest risk [6]. However, the transapical approach is limited by the risk of air embolisms, given the large catheter used and the direct communication of the left ventricle to the external air space [43] and the transapical approach is considered the more invasive procedure. Furthermore, no differences in the rates of in-hospital stroke were noted in a propensity-matched comparison between the subclavian and transfemoral access from the Italian registry of the self-expanding Medtronic CoreValve (Medtronic Inc., Minneapolis, MN, USA; 2.1% vs. 2.1%; p = 0.99) [44]. Spurring the controversy are results showing that despite propensity matching, peripheral artery disease, a marker of more advanced and extended atherosclerosis, was still more prevalent in patients from the Italian CoreValve registry treated via the subclavian approach than those treated transfemorally (85% vs. 21%; p <0.0001) and therefore the advantages of non-transfemoral accesses in this kind of comparison are likely underestimated. Variables that are more specifically linked with the TAVI procedure include device manipulation in the arch, the possibility to dislocate plaque or calcium particles while crossing the native valve, and the act of deploying/post-dilating the prosthesis. A transcranial Doppler study during TAVI showed that the majority of procedural embolic events occurred during balloon valvuloplasty, manipulation of catheters across the aortic valve, and valve implantation [45]. Differences in the risk of stroke could be theoretically attributable to different mechanisms of valve deployment (self-expanding vs. balloon-expandable) and characteristics of the available systems. There are currently no conclusive data suggesting differences in the stroke rate of the two types of valves. Ideally, this hypothesis should be investigated in the setting of a large head-to-head randomized comparison. In a propensity-matched comparison of the self-expanding Medtronic CoreValve and the balloon-expandable Edwards SAPIEN/SAPIEN XT (Edwards Lifesciences, Irvine, CA, USA) transcatheter heart valves from the PRAGMATIC Plus (Pooled-RotterdAm-MilAno-Toulouse In Collaboration) initiative, the rates of stroke were numerically higher with the CoreValve system but did not significantly differ at 30 days, likely as the reflection of the small sample size (2.9% vs. 1.0%, odds ratio [OR] 3.06, 95% CI 0.61–15.35; p = 0.17) [46]. In contrast, the recent randomized CHOICE trial showed a numerical difference in stroke incidence at 30 days between the balloon and self-expandable valves (5.8% vs. 2.6%; p = 0.33) [47]. Although these results are based on small event numbers and the result of chance, they could point to another potential, yet unconfirmed, mechanism of ischemic injury during TAVR. Hypoperfusion could occur during BAV and balloon expandable valve deployment because of repeated rapid ventricular pacing which is necessary for positioning and deployment resulting in transiently reduced cardiac output. This technique could therefore induce ischemia to watershed areas localized in the border zones between the territories of two major arteries in the brain, where cerebral blood flow can be additionally impaired as a result of decreased washout of dislodged microemboli [48]. These mechanisms are particularly likely in the elderly population of patients undergoing TAVI.

Finally, operator's experience plays a major part. This includes a meticulous technique and proper management of antiplatelet and anticoagulant therapy. A list of potential explanations for the risk of stroke in patients undergoing TAVI is shown in Table 53.2.

Pathophysiologic mechanisms of late stroke after TAVR

There is a range of other explanations for peri-procedural stroke in TAVI patients. First, elderly patients present with a higher prevalence of comorbidities of embolic potential, such as hypertension, atrial fibrillation, and carotid stenosis, which is why the stroke risk 6 months after TAVR is believed to approach the basis risk of the age-matched background population. New onset atrial fibrillation (NOAF) is a common complication after cardiac surgery with inflammatory factors acting as mediators. Patients undergoing TAVR are mainly octogenarians, representing a population with an even higher baseline risk for NOAF because of diastolic dysfunction and left atrium enlargement as a consequence of aortic stenosis [49]. Instrumentation during the TAVR procedure is another likely mechanism of NOAF. The increased prevalence of atrial fibrillation after TAVR is a likely cause of the elevated stroke risk during the first 6 months after TAVR.

Mitraclip

Embolic stroke is uncommon in the setting of right heart catheterization. However, blood clots can form in and around catheters inside the venous system in patients who are not adequately anticoagulated. The execution of a trans-septal puncture during the procedure determines a transient direct communication between the venous and the arterial circulation, thereby creating the premises of paradoxical embolism. Reasons for clot formation vary according to host factors, catheter characteristics, cannulation site, and

Table 53.2 Stroke determinants in patients undergoing transcatheter aortic valve implantation (TAVI).

Patient related	Age
	Aortic atherosclerosis
	Smaller aortic valve area
	Atrial fibrillation
	Carotid artery disease
	Cerebral artery atherosclerosis
	Watershed phenomenon
	Peripheral vascular disease
	Non-transfemoral candidate
Procedure related	Device manipulation
	Crossing of the native valve
	Fracture of the native valve
	Pacing during valve deployment
	Prosthesis deployment
	Post-dilatation
	Bio-prosthesis dislodgment/embolization
	Access related
	Operator's experience
	Valve thrombosis
Device related	Valve
	Frame
Post-procedure related	Antiplatelet therapy
	Anticoagulation therapy

antithrombotic prophylaxis. Right and left heart thromboemboli in the setting of Mitraclip procedures rarely include thrombi that may develop within the cardiac chambers on injured endothelium and implanted devices.

Patent foramen ovale and atrial septal defect closure

Adding to thrombotic mechanisms described earlier for the Mitraclip procedure, transcatheter closure of PFO has been shown to induce significant activation of the coagulation system, which reaches maximal levels 7 days after device deployment, gradually returning to baseline by day 90 [50]. However, implantation of the device does not seem to be associated with any increase in platelet activation in aspirin-treated patients. These findings are similar to those obtained after transcatheter closure of ASD [51].

Antithrombotic strategies in patients undergoing valvular and structural percutaneous interventions

The approach to antithrombotic prophylaxis against valve or device-related thromboembolic complications in valvular and structural transcatheter intervention is currently empiric. Disadvantages of antithrombotic therapy include the risk of bleeding, especially in elderly patients like those undergoing valvular procedures [52].

Transcatheter aortic valve implantation
Pre- and intraprocedural antithrombotic treatment

Antithrombotic treatment is believed to be a cornerstone for the prevention of ischemic strokes during and post-TAVR. Albeit

Table 53.3 Recommendations for antithrombotic agents and strategies after transcatheter aortic valve replacement (TAVR).

	ACC/AHA/STS [77]	ESC [78]	CCS statement [62]	ACCP [55]
Procedural	Unfractionated heparin Goal ACT: 300s Reversal with protamine recommended			
Post-procedural	Aspirin 81 mg indefinitely Clopidogrel 75 mg for 3–6 months If VKA indicated, no clopidogrel	ASA or clopidogrel indefinitely ASA and clopidogrel early after TAVI If VKA indicated, no antiplatelet therapy	Indefinite low-dose aspirin + P2Y$_{12}$ for 1–3 months If OAC is indicated, avoid triple Tx unless definite indication exists	Aspirin (50–100 mg/day) + clopidogrel (75 mg/day) over VKA for 3 months

ACC, American College of Cardiology; ACCP, American College of Chest Physicians; ACT, activated clotting time; AHA, American Heart Association; ASA, acetylsalicylic acid; CCS, Canadian Cardiovascular Society; ESC, European Society of Cardiology; OAC, oral anticoagulant; P2Y$_{12}$, thienopyridine; TAVI, transcatheter aortic valve implantation; VKA, vitamin K antagonists.

TAVR procedures have been performed for more than a decade, little is known about optimal antiplatelet and anticoagulation therapy. There is no consensus on the optimal duration of dual antiplatelet therapy after TAVI and current recommendations for antithrombotic agents and strategies for TAVR (Table 53.3) and are not based on large controlled randomized studies. Thus, there is an unmet need for better antithrombotic therapies given the fact that the incidence of major stroke has not declined significantly over time.

Intraprocedural anticoagulation with weight-adjusted unfractionated heparin (UFH) has been a well-established standard of care in all major published registries of TAVI, although clinical practice regarding dosing is variable. In the PARTNER trial, heparin was used for procedural anticoagulation (5000 IE bolus loading dose) with a target of activated clotting time (ACT) >250 s, whereas guidelines recommend a target time of 300 s. Using UFH and protamine sulfate to reverse the anticoagulant effect at the end of the procedure has the advantage of being intuitive, relatively economical, and broadly familiar in the interventional and surgical setting. On the downside, this approach suffers from ample variability in pharmacokinetics and pharmacodynamics of heparin, resulting in wide interindividual response. In addition, late anticoagulant effects of heparin, which dissociates from cells and proteins, and protamine, with rebound bleeding, have been described. Finally, rapid reversal of anticoagulation can lead to prothrombotic rebound with detrimental clinical consequences. (Clinical research in this area of TAVR is described in the section on Future directions.)

Similarly, dual antiplatelet therapy (loading dose, maintaining dose, duration) after TAVR has not been explicitly defined. For example, the PARTNER (Placement of Aortic Transcatheter Valves) trial recommendations were 75–100 mg/day aspirin, a 300 mg clopidogrel loading dose and 75 mg/day for 6 months following TAVR [53]. In the large FRANCE-2 (French Aortic National CoreValve and Edwards) registry [54], patients were on aspirin (≤160 mg/day) and clopidogrel (300 mg loading dose, then 75 mg/ day) before the procedure and aspirin alone after 1 month of dual therapy. In general, it seems that most centers adopt a strategy of low-dose aspirin and a short to intermediate period with a thienopyridine. The American College of Chest Physicians (ACCP) practice guidelines for antithrombotic and thrombolytic therapy in valvular heart disease support this strategy, but with a low grade of recommendation and level of evidence [55]. The recommendations for antithrombotic agents and strategies in patients undergoing TAVR are summarized in Table 53.3.

Post-procedural antithrombotic treatment

The underlying rationale for adding clopidogrel to aspirin derives from the initial TAVI experience, when extracorporeal bypass for hemodynamic support was used during the procedure. Grube *et al.* [56] observed two cases of prolonged and severe post-procedural thrombocytopenia in patients who were not treated with clopidogrel, likely as the reflection of platelet activation processes and consumption. TAVI is now performed mostly under local anesthesia and/or light sedation with no need for extracorporeal circulatory support, and very infrequent cases of mild and transient thrombocytopenia have been reported [57]. The need for a course of dual antiplatelet therapy is theoretically supported by the delay of time needed for incorporation of the prosthesis within the aortic wall for neointimal tissue growth and endothelialization. This process begins with early fibrin deposition, linked to inflammatory response and foreign body reactions. Three months later, smooth muscle cells and endothelial cells replace fibrin [58]. While these findings derive from histopathologic studies of CoreValve explants, clinical evidence for the benefit of dual antiplatelet therapy after TAVI remains elusive. Clopidogrel loading dose or treatment duration or are not specifically defined in guidelines, and lately the general usefulness of clopidogrel on top of aspirin in TAVR patients has been questioned [59,60]. In two studies comparing DAPT with mono-antiplatelet therapy (aspirin or clopidogrel), dual antiplatelet therapy did not reduce the incidence of new strokes but was associated with a significantly higher rate of major and life-threatening bleeding complications.

Ussia *et al.* [59] reported in a small single center study on 79 patients randomized to either dual antiplatelet therapy with a 300-mg loading dose of clopidogrel on the day before TAVI followed by a 3-month maintenance dose of 75 mg/day on a background of aspirin 100 mg or aspirin alone. The primary efficacy endpoint, a composite of major cardiac and cerebrovascular events, including overall mortality, myocardial infarction, major stroke, urgent or emergency conversion to surgery, or life-threatening bleeding, occurred with a similar frequency between the two groups both at 30 days (13% vs. 15%; p = 0.71) and 6 months (18% vs. 15%; p = 0.85). There were no differences in VARC-defined major and minor bleeding between the two strategies. Although limited by the small sample size, this study does not seem to support a strategy of short-term adjunctive use of clopidogrel added to aspirin after TAVI. These findings were essentially confirmed by Durand et al. [60] in a recent prospective observational study. As it is unclear whether thrombi produced during and after TAVR are of platelet or thrombin-based origin, the latter does not favor clopidogrel as an effective agent in these patients and more investigations are needed.

Controversy also exists for patients with a history of pre-existing atrial fibrillation. There is no consensus or evidence from trials regarding treatment with triple therapy, warfarin with one antiplatelet or warfarin alone, although American and Canadian guidelines discourage the use of triple therapy (Table 53.3) [61,62].

In a recent report, serial imaging of bioprosthetic aortic valves implanted either surgically or with a TAVR procedure were found to exhibit leaflet thrombosis in 15–20% which was associated with leaflet motion abnormality and less frequently with adverse neurologic events and disappeared with oral anticoagulation [63]. This finding concurs with an earlier report of successful treatment of bioprosthetic valve thrombosis with anticoagulation [64]. These observations have increased the medical awareness around this phenomenon and has initiated the clinical investigation on leaflet thrombosis, leaflet motion imaging, and their possible relationship with neurological overt or silent abnormalities. This field is expected to evolve over the following years.

MitraClip

The manufacturer leaves antithrombotic management of Mitraclip to the discretion of the operator, because of a lack of specific investigations comparing different treatment strategies after percutaneous mitral valve repair. Indicatively, in the EVEREST II trial, patients were treated with heparin during the procedure, and a combination of aspirin (at a dose of 325 mg/day) for 6 months and clopidogrel (at a dose of 75 mg/day) for 30 days after the procedure. While no definite device thrombosis was identified in the EVEREST trial, several cases of large thrombus formation after Mitraclip procedure in clinical practice have been reported. Bekeredjian et al. [65] published a case report on thrombus in the posterolateral wall of the left atrium and on the right atrial side of the septum on day 5 after Mitraclip implantation, and the authors reported a note of caution on the need for a course of anticoagulation in patients undergoing percutaneous mitral valve repair. Hamm et al. [66] reported a 3-week post-procedural cardioembolic stroke caused by thrombus formation on the MitraClip, despite the patient receiving dual platelet therapy. Overall, evidence on peri-procedural antithrombotic regimens is very sparse, but Alsidawi and Effat [67] recently published a set of recommendations; however, these can neither be interpreted as a consensus paper nor as guidelines. They state that patients not being treated with antiplatelets should be started on aspirin 325 mg and clopidogrel 75 mg immediately after the procedure for 6 months to 1 year. Anticoagulation should be interrupted at least 5 days before the procedure. Only patients with high risk for thrombosis (previous mitral valve prosthesis, caged-ball or tilting disc aortic valve, stroke, TIA or venous thromboembolism within 6 months, CHADS2 ≥ 5, rheumatic valvular heart disease, or severe thrombophilia) should be bridged regardless of their risk of bleeding. The management of patients with moderate risk for thrombosis should be individualized depending on their bleeding risk and informed decision. Heparin should be bolused

right after successful trans-septal puncture (ACT around 250) and bivalirudin is not recommended. Patients in whom anticoagulation was interrupted before the procedure should be started back on their anticoagulation regimen. If needed, heparin infusion can be started 6 hours after the access sheath is removed. Post-procedural anticoagulation is currently not recommended if no other indication for anticoagulation exists; however, the above case reports call for more studies addressing this issue and caution is warranted.

Patent foramen ovale and atrial septal defect closure

There are no studies on the most appropriate antithrombotic therapy after transcatheter closure of PFO/ASD, and the choice of antithrombotic drugs after these procedures has been empirically determined, with aspirin as the agent most frequently used. In the CLOSURE-1 (A Prospective, Multicenter, Randomized Controlled Trial to Evaluate the Safety and Efficacy of the STARFlex® Septal Closure System Versus Best Medical Therapy in Patients With a Stroke and/or Transient Ischemic Attack Due to Presumed Paradoxical Embolism Through a Patent Foramen Ovale) trial, after PFO closure with the StarFlex device, all patients were given a standard antiplatelet regimen including clopidogrel (75 mg/day) for 6 months, and aspirin (81–325 mg/day) for 2 years. Experimental studies have demonstrated that the Amplatzer PFO occluder is partially endothelialized 1 month after implantation and completely covered by neoendothelial cells at 3 months [68]. Thus, the first weeks after PFO closure constitute a vulnerable window with newer devices, in which the closure system is potentially more thrombogenic [69,70]. Remarkably, most of the patients who experience device thrombosis are receiving antiplatelet treatment, and most of them are successfully treated with heparin or warfarin. Therefore, some operators advocate short-term anticoagulation (1–3 months) after PFO/ASD closure. Once device endothelialization is completed and no residual shunt is observed, anticoagulant treatment is then switched to antiplatelet therapy or no antithrombotic treatment.

Left atrial appendage closure

In order to prvent to prevent large thrombus formation on the device during its endothelialization, patients were treated with warfarin and aspirin (81 mg) for 45 days after implantation, in both the PROTECT AF and PREVAIL trials [32,34]. Furthermore, these study designs dictated that if the 45-day transesophageal echocardiography documented either complete closure of the left atrial appendage, or if residual peri-device flow was <5 mm in width and there was no definite visible large thrombus on the device, warfarin was discontinued. After discontinuation of warfarin, only clopidogrel 75 mg/day and aspirin 81–325 mg/day were prescribed until the 6-month follow-up visit, at which time clopidogrel was discontinued and aspirin alone was continued indefinitely.

Future directions and conclusions

Bivalirudin is a direct selective inhibitor of the activated coagulation factor II (thrombin). Direct thrombin inhibitors have some advantages over the heparins, such as lack of dependence on plasma protein, which results in a more predictable response and makes them very attractive for use in populations at high risk of bleeding (Table 53.4). Bivalirudin was shown to be efficacious in BAV patients in the BRAVO (Effect of Bivalirudin on Aortic Valve Intervention Outcomes) trial [71]. Bivalirudin is evaluated for its assumed beneficial bleeding profile but concerns over reversibility

Table 53.4 Pharmacologic properties of heparin and bivalirudin.

	UFH	Bivalirudin
Bioavailability (%)	35	100
Action independent of antithrombin III	No	Yes
Non-specific protease binding	Yes	No
Predictable PK-PD	No	Yes
Inhibits fibrin-bound thrombin	No	Yes
Activates/aggregates platelet	Yes	No
Half-life (minutes)	60–90	25

PK-PD, pharmacokinetic–pharmacodynamic; UFH, unfractionated heparin.

of its activity exist in the case of life-threatening bleeding/vascular complications. Additionally, it is a strictly procedural agent (parenteral administration) which can only impact acute events.

Bivalirudin was recently evaluated against procedural heparin during TAVR in the BRAVO 2/3 (Effect of Bivalirudin on Aortic Valve Intervention Outcomes 2/3) trial, which is an ongoing international, multicenter, open-label, randomized controlled trial of bivalirudin in patients undergoing transfemoral TAVI. A total of 802 patients were randomly assigned to either standard dosing of bivalirudin (bolus 0.75 mg/kg plus infusion) or UFH (targeting an activated coagulation time ≥250 s) as control (UFH with possible protamine reversal). Use of antiplatelet agents pre-, during, and post-procedure, and possibly oral anticoagulants post-procedure, will be according to the sites' standard practice. The primary endpoint was major bleeding defined as Bleeding Academic Research Consortium (BARC) type ≥3 at 48 hours or hospital discharge, whichever occurred first [72]. Based on the final results of the BRAVO3 trial [73], direct thrombin inhibition with bivalirudin during TAVI did not significantly reduce major bleeding at 48 hours and was found non-inferior to heparin with respect to the net adverse clinical event rate at 30-days post-TAVI. Despite the absence of an immediate antidote (which was a safety concern for this approach early on), rates of adverse events were in fact arithmetically lower with bivalirudin. This indicated that the percent of anticoagulant reversal in case of life-threatening complications does not have an overwhelming clinical impact. If one takes into account the cost of bivalirudin, heparin (with possible reversal with heparin) remains the main anticoagulant for TAVI. Anticoagulation with bivalirudin is safe and feasible in patients who undergo TAVI and cannot receive heparin. Further research with antithrombin agents is expected to evolve in this field.

The clustering of thromboembolic risk factors in TAVI populations such as renal failure (10%), atrial fibrillation (40%), severe chronic obstructive pulmonary disease (15%), coronary artery disease (70%), peripheral vascular disease (30%), and moderate to severe mitral regurgitation(30%), implies that long-term anticoagulation therapy (beyond 12 months) after TAVR is of value. Whether such a strategy would provide benefit is currently unknown [74].

Importantly however, >50% of post-procedural strokes are of a likely thromboembolic nature. To that end, the prescription of a mid-term (up to 6–12 months) anticoagulation therapy might have

a significant role in the reduction of subacute and late strokes [75]. Currently, anticoagulation treatment after TAVI is only recommended if other indications for anticoagulation exist.

Triple therapy after TAVI should be avoided in those patient cohorts with a high inherent bleeding risk. Furthermore, data show no difference in stroke rates in mono-antiplatelet versus dual antiplatelet therapy, and the combination of one oral anticoagulant with one antiplatelet has recently shown better safety results without excess ischemic events in comparison to triple therapy in patients with atrial fibrillation [76]. The exact regimen and duration remain to be determined in a prospective manner. Modifiable risk factors of late strokes such as hypertension, diabetes, dyslipidemia, and smoking, should undergo aggressive treatment attempts. The pharmacology-oriented guidelines of the TAVI field are expected to evolve over time based on evidence generated from trials [77,78].

A number of relatively novel antiplatelet (i.e., prasugrel, ticagrelor) and anticoagulant (dabigatran, rivaroxaban, apixaban) agents have recently entered the cardiologist's armamentarium in Europe and the USA. None of these drugs is currently approved from European or US regulatory agencies for antithrombotic management of patients undergoing valvular or structural percutaneous intervention. Randomized clinical trials remain the most appropriate setting to establish the safety and efficacy of a drug for any novel indication. Several studies for patients undergoing TAVI are underway. The currently enrolling POPular-TAVI trial investigates 1000 patients divided in two cohorts, one with (cohort A) and one without (cohort B) a pre-existing oral anticoagulation indication (atrial fibrillation, previous systemic embolism, mitral valve prosthesis) (NCT02247128). Patients in cohort A are randomized to aspirin monotherapy versus sspirin + clopidogrel and patients in cohort B are randomized to oral anticoagulation vs. oral anticoagulation + clopidogrel. Another ongoing trial is the ARTE study (n = 300), which randomizes TAVI patients to aspirin monotherapy versus DAPT for at least 6 months (NCT01559298).

The safety and efficacy of the current approach for TAVI, Mitraclip implantation, and PFO/ASD closure, mostly using a short to intermediate term combination of aspirin and clopidogrel after the procedure, and UFH during the procedure, has never been prospectively investigated in a randomized clinical trial. Therefore, at present, the apparent superiority of any antithrombotic approach over another remains speculative. Research questions include which antiplatelet anticoagulant agents to use after valvular and structural interventions, when they should be administered, at which doses, and for how long. Careful and tailored risk–benefit assessment is needed for any antithrombotic combination in patients undergoing valvular or structural transcatheter interventions [79].

Interactive multiple choice questions are available for this chapter on www.wiley.com/go/dangas/cardiology

References

1 Rodés-Cabau J, Dumont E, Boone RH, *et al*. Cerebral embolism following transcatheter aortic valve implantation: comparison of transfemoral and transapical approaches. *J Am Coll Cardiol* 2011; **57**: 18–28.

2 Ghanem A, Müller A, Nähle CP, *et al*. Risk and fate of cerebral embolism after transfemoral aortic valve implantation: a prospective pilot study with diffusion-weighted magnetic resonance imaging. *J Am Coll Cardiol* 2010; **55**: 1427–1432.

3 Arnold M, Schulz-Heise S, Achenbach S, *et al*. Embolic cerebral insults after transapical aortic valve implantation detected by magnetic resonance imaging. *JACC Cardiovasc Interv* 2010; **3**: 1126–1132.

4 Kahlert P, Al-Rashid F, Döttger P, *et al*. Cerebral embolization during transcatheter aortic valve implantation: a transcranial Doppler study. *Circulation* 2012; **126**: 1245–1255.

5 Astarci P, Glineur D, Kefer J, *et al*. Magnetic resonance imaging evaluation of cerebral embolization during percutaneous aortic valve implantation: comparison of transfemoral and trans-apical approaches using Edwards Sapiens valve. *Eur J Cardiothorac Surg* 2011; **40**: 475–479.

6 Eggebrecht H, Schmermund A, Voigtländer T, *et al*. Risk of stroke after transcatheter aortic valve implantation (TAVI): a meta-analysis of 10,037 published patients. *EuroIntervention* 2012; **8**: 129–138.

7 Généreux P, Head SJ, Van Mieghem NM, *et al*. Clinical outcomes after transcatheter aortic valve replacement using valve academic research consortium definitions: a weighted meta-analysis of 3,519 patients from 16 studies. *J Am Coll Cardiol* 2012; **59**: 2317–2326.

8 Tay EL, Gurvitch R, Wijesinghe N, *et al*. A high-risk period for cerebrovascular events exists after transcatheter aortic valve implantation. *JACC Cardiovasc Interv* 2011; **4**: 1290–1297.

9 Feldman T, Foster E, Glower DD, *et al*. EVEREST II Investigators. Percutaneous repair or surgery for mitral regurgitation. *N Engl J Med* 2011; **364**: 1395–1406.

10 Franzen O, Baldus S, Rudolph V, *et al*. Acute outcomes of MitraClip therapy for mitral regurgitation in high-surgical-risk patients: emphasis on adverse valve morphology and severe left ventricular dysfunction. *Eur Heart J* 2010; **31**: 1373–1381.

11 Tamburino C, Ussia GP, Maisano F, *et al*. Percutaneous mitral valve repair with the MitraClip system: acute results from a real world setting. *Eur Heart J* 2010; **31**: 1382–1389.

12 Rudolph V, Knap M, Franzen O, *et al*. Echocardiographic and clinical outcomes of MitraClip therapy in patients not amenable to surgery. *J Am Coll Cardiol* 2011; **58**: 2190–2195.

13 Baldus S, Schillinger W, Franzen O, *et al*. MitraClip therapy in daily clinical practice: initial results from the German transcatheter mitral valve interventions (TRAMI) registry. *Eur J Heart Fail* 2012; **14**: 1050–1055.

14 Grasso C, Capodanno D, Scandura S, *et al*. One- and twelve-month safety and efficacy outcomes of patients undergoing edge-to-edge percutaneous mitral valve repair (from the GRASP Registry). *Am J Cardiol* 2013; **111**: 1482–1487.

15 Whitlow PL, Feldman T, Pedersen WR, *et al*. Acute and 12-month results with catheter-based mitral valve leaflet repair: the EVEREST II (Endovascular Valve Edge-to-Edge Repair) High Risk Study. *J Am Coll Cardiol* 2012; **59**: 130–139.

16 Schillinger W, Hünlich M, Baldus S, *et al*. MitraClip-therapy in highly aged patients: results from the German TRAnscatheter Mitral valve Interventions (TRAMI) Registry. *EuroIntervention* 2013; **9**: 84–90.

17 Meier B, Kalesan B, Mattle HP, *et al*. Percutaneous closure of patent foramen ovale in cryptogenic embolism. *N Engl J Med* 2013; **368**: 1083–1091.

18 Taaffe M, Fischer E, Baranowski A, *et al*. Comparison of three patent foramen ovale closure devices in a randomized trial (Amplatzer versus CardioSEAL-STARflex versus Helex occluder). *Am J Cardiol* 2008; **101**: 1353–1358.

19 Krumsdorf U, Ostermayer S, Billinger K, *et al*. Incidence and clinical course of thrombus formation on atrial septal defect and patent foramen ovale closure devices in 1,000 consecutive patients. *J Am Coll Cardiol* 2004; **43**: 302–309.

20 Furlan AJ, Reisman M, Massaro J, *et al*. Closure or medical therapy for cryptogenic stroke with patent foramen ovale. *N Engl J Med* 2012; **366**: 991–999.

21 Windecker S. The PC trial: Percutaneous closure of patent foramen ovale versus medical treatment in patients with cryptogenic embolism. Paper presented at Transcatheter Therapeutics; October 25, 2012; Miami, FL.

22 Carroll JD. The RESPECT trial: A randomized evaluation of recurrent stroke comparing PFO closure to established current standard of care treatment. Paper presented at Transcatheter Therapeutics; October 25, 2012; Miami, FL.

23 Martín F, Sánchez PL, Doherty E, *et al*. Percutaneous transcatheter closure of patent foramen ovale in patients with paradoxical embolism. *Circulation* 2002; **106**: 1121–1126.

24 Windecker S, Wahl A, Chatterjee T, *et al*. Percutaneous closure of patent foramen ovale in patients with paradoxical embolism: long-term risk of recurrent thromboembolic events. *Circulation* 2000; **101**: 893–898.

25 Braun M, Fassbender D, Schoen SP, *et al*. Transcatheter closure of patent foramen ovale in patients with cerebral ischemia. *J Am Coll Cardiol* 2002; **39**: 2019–2025.

26 Braun M, Gliech V, Boscheri A, *et al*. Transcatheter closure of patent foramen ovale (PFO) in patients with paradoxical embolism: periprocedural safety and mid-term follow-up results of three different device occluder systems. *Eur Heart J* 2004; **25**: 424–430.

27 Windecker S, Wahl A, Nedeltchev K, *et al*. Comparison of medical treatment with percutaneous closure of patent foramen ovale in patients with cryptogenic stroke. *J Am Coll Cardiol* 2004; **44**: 750–758.

28 Beitzke A, Schuchlenz H, Gamillscheg A, Stein J, Wendelin G. Catheter closure of the persistent foramen ovale: mid-term results in 162 patients. *J Interv Cardiol* 2001; **14**: 223–230.

29 Wahl A, Meier B, Haxel B, *et al*. Prognosis after percutaneous closure of patent foramen ovale for paradoxical embolism. *Neurology* 2001; **57**: 1330–1332.

30 Sherman JM, Hagler DJ, Cetta F, et al. Thrombosis after septal closure device placement: a review of the current literature. *Catheter Cardiovasc Interv* 2004; **63**: 486–489.

31 Krumsdorf U, Ostermayer S, Billinger K, *et al*. Incidence and clinical course of thrombus formation on atrial septal defect and patent foramen ovale closure devices in 1,000 consecutive patients. *J Am Coll Cardiol* 2004; **43**: 302–309.

32 Urena M, Rodés-Cabau J, Freixa X, *et al*. Percutaneous left atrial appendage closure with the AMPLATZER cardiac plug device in patients with nonvalvular atrial fibrillation and contraindications to anticoagulation therapy. *J Am Coll Cardiol* 2013; **62**: 96–102.

33 Holmes DR, Reddy VY, Turi ZG, *et al*. Percutaneous closure of the left atrial appendage versus warfarin therapy for prevention of stroke in patients with atrial fibrillation: a randomised non-inferiority trial. *Lancet* 2015; **374**: 534–542.

34 Holmes J, Kar S, Price MJ, *et al*. Prospective randomized evaluation of the watchman left atrial appendage closure device in patients with atrial fibrillation versus long-term warfarin therapy: The PREVAIL Trial. *J Am Coll Cardiol* 2014; **64**: 1–12.

35 Stortecky S, Windecker S. Stroke: an infrequent but devastating complication in cardiovascular interventions. *Circulation* 2012; **126**(25): 2921–2924.

36 Van Mieghem NM, Schipper ME, Ladich E, *et al*. Histopathology of embolic debris captured during transcatheter aortic valve replacement. *Circulation* 2013; **127**(22): 2194–2201.

37 Di Tullio MR, Sacco RL, Savoia MT, Sciacca RR, Homma S. Aortic atheroma morphology and the risk of ischemic stroke in a multiethnic population. *Am Heart J* 2000; **139**: 329–336.

38 Omran H, Schmidt H, Hackenbroch M, *et al*. Silent and apparent cerebral embolism after retrograde catheterisation of the aortic valve in valvular stenosis: a prospective, randomised study. *Lancet* 2003; **361**(9365): 1241–1246.

39 Marechaux S, Corseaux D, Vincentelli A, *et al*. Identification of tissue factor in experimental aortic valve sclerosis. *Cardiovascular pathology : the official journal of the Society for Cardiovascular Pathology*. 2009 Mar–Apr; **18**(2): 67–76.

40 Erdoes G, Basciani R, Huber C, *et al*. Transcranial Doppler-detected cerebral embolic load during transcatheter aortic valve implantation. *Eur J Cardiothorac Surg* 2012; **41**(4): 778–783; discussion 783–784.

41 Kahlert P, Al-Rashid F, Dottger P, *et al*. Cerebral embolization during transcatheter aortic valve implantation: a transcranial Doppler study. *Circulation* 2012; **126**(10): 1245–1255.

42 Sun JC, Davidson MJ, Lamy A, Eikelboom JW. Antithrombotic management of patients with prosthetic heart valves: current evidence and future trends. *Lancet* 2009; **374**(9689): 565–576.

43 Rodes-Cabau J, Dumont E, Boone RH, *et al*. Cerebral embolism following transcatheter aortic valve implantation: comparison of transfemoral and transapical approaches. *J Am Coll Cardiol* 2011; **57**(1): 18–28.

44 Petronio AS, De Carlo M, Bedogni F, *et al*. 2-year results of CoreValve implantation through the subclavian access: a propensity-matched comparison with the femoral access. *J Am Coll Cardiol* 2012; **60**: 502–507.

45 Drews T, Pasic M, Buz S, *et al*. Transcranial Doppler sound detection of cerebral microembolism during transapical aortic valve implantation. *Thorac Cardiovasc Surg* 2011; **59**: 237–242.

46 Chieffo A, Buchanan GL, Van Mieghem NM, *et al*. Transcatheter aortic valve implantation with the Edwards SAPIEN versus the Medtronic CoreValve Revalving System Devices. A Multicenter Collaborative Study: The PRAGMATIC Plus Initiative (Pooled-RotterdAm-Milano-Toulouse In Collaboration) *J Am Coll Cardiol* 2013; **61**: 830–836.

47 Abdel-Wahab M, Mehilli J, Frerker C, *et al*. Comparison of balloon-expandable vs self-expandable valves in patients undergoing transcatheter aortic valve replacement: the CHOICE randomized clinical trial. *JAMA* 2014; **311**: 1503–1514.

48 Hynes BG, Rodes-Cabau J. Transcatheter aortic valve implantation and cerebrovascular events: the current state of the art. *Ann N Y Acad Sci* 2012; **1254**: 151–163.

49 Stortecky S, Windecker S. Stroke: an infrequent but devastating complication in cardiovascular interventions. *Circulation* 2012; **126**(25): 2921–2924.

50 Bédard E, Rodés-Cabau J, Houde C, *et al*. Enhanced thrombogenesis but not platelet activation is associated with transcatheter closure of patent foramen ovale in patients with cryptogenic stroke. *Stroke* 2007; **38**: 100–104.

51 Rodés-Cabau J, Palacios A, Palacio C, *et al*. Assessment of the markers of platelet and coagulation activation following transcatheter closure of atrial septal defects. *Int J Cardiol* 2005; **98**: 107–112.

52 Capodanno D, Angiolillo DJ. Antithrombotic therapy in the elderly. *J Am Coll Cardiol* 2010; **56**: 1683–1692.

53 Smith CR, Leon MB, Mack MJ, *et al.* Transcatheter versus surgical aortic-valve replacement in high-risk patients. *N Engl J Med* 2011; **364**: 2187–2198.

54 Gilard M, Eltchaninoff H, Iung B, *et al.* Registry of transcatheter aortic-valve implantation in high-risk patients. *N Engl J Med* 2012; **366**: 1705–1715.

55 Whitlock RP, Sun JC, Fremes SE, Rubens FD, Teoh KH; American College of Chest Physicians. Antithrombotic and thrombolytic therapy for valvular disease: Antithrombotic Therapy and Prevention of Thrombosis, 9th ed: American College of Chest Physicians Evidence-Based Clinical Practice Guidelines. *Chest* 2012; **141**: e576S–600S.

56 Grube E, Laborde JC, Gerckens U, *et al.* Percutaneous implantation of the CoreValve self-expanding valve prosthesis in high-risk patients with aortic valve disease: the Siegburg first-in-man study. *Circulation* 2006; **114**: 1616–1624.

57 Ussia GP, Scarabelli M, Mulè M, *et al.* Postprocedural management of patients after transcatheter aortic valve implantation procedure with self-expanding bioprosthesis. *Catheter Cardiovasc Interv* 2010; **76**: 757–766.

58 Noble S, Asgar A, Cartier R, Virmani R, Bonan R. Anatomo-pathological analysis after CoreValve Revalving system implantation. *EuroIntervention* 2009; **5**: 78–85.

59 Ussia GP, Scarabelli M, Mulè M, *et al.* Dual antiplatelet therapy versus aspirin alone in patients undergoing transcatheter aortic valve implantation. *Am J Cardiol* 2011; **108**: 1772–1776.

60 Durand E, Blanchard D, Chassaing S, *et al.* Comparison of two antiplatelet therapy strategies in patients undergoing transcatheter aortic valve implantation. *Am J Cardiol* 2014; **113**(2): 355–360.

61 Holmes DR Jr, Mack MJ, Kaul S, *et al.* 2012 ACCF/AATS/SCAI/STS expert consensus document on transcatheter aortic valve replacement. *J Am Coll Cardiol* 2012; **59**: 1200–1254.

62 Webb J, Rodes-Cabau J, Fremes S, *et al.* Transcatheter aortic valve implantation: a Canadian Cardiovascular Society position statement. *Can J Cardiol* 2012; **28**: 520–528.

63 Makkar RR, Fontana G, Jilaihawi H, *et al.* Possible subclinical leaflet thrombosis in bioprosthetic aortic valves. *N Engl J Med* 2015; **373**: 2015–2024.

64 Cota L, Stabile E, Agrusta M, *et al.* Bioprostheses "thrombosis" after transcatheter aortic valve replacement. *J Am Coll Cardiol* 2013; **61**: 789–791.

65 Bekeredjian R, Mereles D, Pleger S, *et al.* Large atrial thrombus formation after MitraClip implantation: is anticoagulation mandatory? *J Heart Valve Dis* 2011; **20**: 146–148.

66 Hamm K, Barth S, Diegeler A, *et al.* Stroke and thrombus formation appending to the MitraClip™: what is the appropriate anticoagulation regimen? *J Heart Valve Dis* 2013; **22**: 713–715.

67 Alsidawi S, Effat M. Peri-procedural management of anti-platelets and anticoagulation in patients undergoing MitraClip procedure. *J Thromb Thrombolysis* 2014; **38**: 416–419.

68 Han YM, Gu X, Titus JL, *et al.* New self-expanding patent foramen ovale occlusion device. *Cathet Cardiovasc Interv* 1999; **47**: 370–376.

69 Cenni E, Ciapetti G, Cervellati M, *et al.* Activation of the plasma coagulation system induced by some biomaterials. *J Biomed Mater Res* 1996; **31**: 145–148.

70 Hong J, Azens A, Ekdahl KN, *et al.* Material-specific thrombin generation following contact between metal surfaces and whole blood. *Biomaterials* 2005; **26**: 1397–1403.

71 Kini A, Yu J, Cohen MG, *et al.* Effect of bivalirudin on aortic valve intervention outcomes study: a two-centre registry study comparing bivalirudin and unfractionated heparin in balloon aortic valvuloplasty. *EuroIntervention* 2014; **10**: 312–319.

72 Sergie Z, Lefevre T, Van Belle E, *et al.* Current periprocedural anticoagulation in transcatheter aortic valve replacement: could bivalirudin be an option? Rationale and design of the BRAVO 2/3 studies. *J Thromb Thrombolysis* 2013; **35**(4): 483–493.

73 Dangas GD, Lefèvre T, Kupatt C, *et al.* Bivalirudin versus heparin anticoagulation in transcatheter aortic valve replacement: a randomized phase 3 trial. *J Am Coll Cardiol* 2015; **66**: 2860–2868.

74 Mack MJ, Brennan J, Brindis R, *et al.* OUtcomes following transcatheter aortic valve replacement in the united states. *JAMA* 2013; **310**(19): 2069–2077.

75 Merie C, Kober L, Skov Olsen P, *et al.* Association of warfarin therapy duration after bioprosthetic aortic valve replacement with risk of mortality, thromboembolic complications, and bleeding. *JAMA* 2012; **308**(20): 2118–2125.

76 Dewilde WJ, Oirbans T, Verheugt FW, *et al.* Use of clopidogrel with or without aspirin in patients taking oral anticoagulant therapy and undergoing percutaneous coronary intervention: an open-label, randomised, controlled trial. *Lancet* 2013; **381**(9872): 1107–1115.

77 Holmes DR Jr, Mack MJ, Kaul S, *et al.* 2012 ACCF/AATS/SCAI/STS expert consensus document on transcatheter aortic valve replacement. *J Am Coll Cardiol* 2012; **59**(13): 1200–1254.

78 Vahanian A, Alfieri O, Andreotti F, *et al.* Guidelines on the management of valvular heart disease (version 2012): the Joint Task Force on the Management of Valvular Heart Disease of the European Society of Cardiology (ESC) and the European Association for Cardio-Thoracic Surgery (EACTS). *Eur J Cardiothorac Surg* 2012; **42**(4): S1–44.

79 Giustino G, Dangas GD. Stroke prevention in valvular heart disease: from the procedure to long-term management. *EuroIntervention* 2015; **11**(Suppl W): 26–31.

80 Nombela-Franco L, Webb JG, de Jaegere PP, *et al.* Timing, predictive factors, and prognostic value of cerebrovascular events in a large cohort of patients undergoing transcatheter aortic valve implantation. *Circulation* 2012; **126**: 3041–3053.

81 Truelsen T, Piechowski-Jóźwiak B, Bonita R, Mathers C, Bogousslavsky J, Boysen G. Stroke incidence and prevalence in Europe: a review of available data. *Eur J Neurol* 2006; **13**: 581–598.

82 Russo T, Felzani G, Marini C. Stroke in the very old: a systematic review of studies on incidence, outcome, and resource use. *J Aging Res* 2011; **2011**: 108785.

83 Kodali SK, Williams MR, Smith CR, *et al.* Two-year outcomes after transcatheter or surgical aortic-valve replacement. *N Engl J Med* 2012; **366**: 1686–1695.

84 Makkar RR, Fontana GP, Jilaihawi H, *et al.* Transcatheter aortic-valve replacement for inoperable severe aortic stenosis. *N Engl J Med* 2012; **366**: 1696–1704.

85 Adams DH, Popma JJ, Reardon MJ, *et al.* Transcatheter aortic-valve replacement with a self-expanding prosthesis. *N Engl J Med* 2014; **370**: 1790–1798.

86 Popma JJ, Adams DH, Reardon MJ, *et al.* Transcatheter aortic valve replacement using a self-expanding bioprosthesis in patients with severe aortic stenosis at extreme risk for surgery. *J Am Coll Cardiol* 2014; **63**: 1972–1981.

Alcohol Septal Ablation for Hypertrophic Obstructive Cardiomyopathy

Amir-Ali Fassa[1], George D. Dangas[2], and Ulrich Sigwart[3]

[1] La Tour Hospital, Geneva, Switzerland

[2] Department of Cardiology, Mount Sinai Medical Center, New York, NY, USA

[3] Geneva University Hospitals, Geneva, Switzerland

Left-ventricular outflow tract obstruction is seen in approximately 25% of patients with hypertrophic cardiomyopathy under resting conditions, and is an independent predictor of poor prognosis [1,2]. Although negative inotropic drugs can efficiently alleviate symptoms in many cases, 5–10% of patients with hypertrophic obstructive cardiomyopathy (HOCM) remain refractory to drug therapy [3]. Surgical myectomy (also known as the Morrow operation) has been performed since the 1960s, and has been shown to reduce outflow gradients. Nevertheless, some patients are not regarded as favorable candidates for this major intervention because of factors such as advanced age, concomitant medical conditions, or previous cardiac surgery [4,5]. In 1994, a catheter treatment (known under a variety of abbreviations listed in Box 54.1) using absolute alcohol to induce a localized myocardial infarction to the interventricular septum was introduced as an alternative to surgery [6]. Alcohol-induced septal branch ablation had been previously described for therapy of ventricular tachycardia [7]. This technique was applied to HOCM after clinical observations of improvement in a patient with septal hypertrophy who developed an anterior myocardial infarction and also the transient reduction in left-ventricular outflow pressure gradients observed with temporary septal artery balloon occlusion. Since its introduction, there has been growing enthusiasm for this technique. Indeed, over 800 procedures were performed during the first 5 years [8], and the number to date is probably more than 5000 [9,10]. Although initially confined to Europe and North America, this technique is now being performed worldwide [11].

Selection of patients

Patient selection for alcohol septal ablation (ASA) should be based on a careful individual evaluation of the clinical symptoms, associated comorbidities, and echocardiographic and angiographic parameters [5,9,12]. The primary indications for the procedure are New York Heart Association (NYHA) or Canadian Cardiovascular Score (CCS) Class III or IV symptoms despite adequately tolerated drug therapy with a documented left ventricular outflow tract (LVOT) gradient variably defined as ≥50 mmHg at rest or after exercise, or >30 mmHg at rest or ≥60 mmHg under stress. Likewise, selected patients with advanced NYHA or CCS Class II symptoms (e.g., those with syncope and severe pre-syncope) and a resting gradient >50 mmHg or >30 mmHg at rest and ≥100 mmHg with stress can also be considered for the procedure (Box 54.2). However, a septal wall thickness <18 mm should be taken as a contraindication for ASA because of the risk of septal perforation.

Mechanisms of treatment efficacy

In HOCM, obstruction is caused by protrusion of the hypertrophied interventricular septum into the outflow tract and by systolic anterior movement of the mitral valve due to a Venturi phenomenon and a drag effect [5,13].

ASA induces a well-demarcated subaortic necrosis, corresponding to approximately 10% of the post-ablation total left ventricle mass (or 31% of the septal myocardial mass), as assessed by various imaging techniques (such as single-photon emission computed tomography, positron emission tomography, and contrast-enhanced magnetic resonance imaging) [14–18]. However, with the use of smaller ethanol doses nowadays, septal necrosis is probably less.

The hemodynamic response to the induced reduction of septal myocardium is usually triphasic [5,19]. Immediately after ASA, there is a marked reduction of the LVOT gradient. Proposed mechanisms involved in the acute benefit are improvement in left ventricular relaxation and compliance via a reduction in regional asynchrony, resulting in an increase in left ventricular passive filling and a reduction in left atrial size and left ventricular ejection force [20–23]. This initial relief is usually followed during the following days by a rise of the LVOT gradient to about 50% of the pre-procedure level, possibly in relation to some degree of recovery from stunning or to edema caused by the infarct, which subsequently disappears [19,24]. Finally, within the following weeks to months, there is a new decrease in LVOT gradient back to the post-ablation level. It is believed that long-term benefit results from the creation of localized septal infarction and scarring, which increase LVOT diameter as a result of septal thinning and "therapeutic remodeling" [14,20,25,26]. The overall effect is an increase in left ventricular

Interventional Cardiology: Principles and Practice, Second Edition. Edited by George D. Dangas, Carlo Di Mario, and Nicholas N. Kipshidze.

© 2017 John Wiley & Sons, Ltd. Published 2017 by John Wiley & Sons, Ltd.

Box 54.1 Common abbreviations for alcohol septal ablation.

ASA	Alcohol septal ablation
ASR	Alcohol septal reduction
NSMR	Non-surgical myocardial reduction
NSRT	Non-surgical septal reduction therapy
PTSMA	Percutaneous transluminal septal myocardial ablation
TAA	Transcoronary alcohol ablation
TASH	Transcoronary ablation of septal hypertrophy

Box 54.2 Criteria for selection of patients for alcohol septal ablation.

- Symptoms refractory to adequate tolerated drug therapy
- NYHA or CCS Class III or IV with a resting gradient of >30 mmHg or ≥60 mmHg under stress or ≥50 mmHg at rest and/or with provocation
- NYHA or CCS Class II in selected patients (e.g., those with syncope or severe pre-syncope) with a resting gradient >50 mmHg or >30 mmHg at rest and ≥100 mmHg with stress
- Basal septal wall thickness ≥18 mm
- Adequately sized septal perforator supplying the area of the systolic anterior motion-septum contact
- High risk of surgical morbidity and mortality
- Absence of concomitant cardiac disease requiring surgery (such as extensive coronary artery disease that would be treated surgically, organic valvular disease, morphologic abnormalities of the mitral valve and papillary muscles)

CCS, Canadian Cardiovascular Society; NYHA, New York Heart Association.

size, a decrease in left ventricular mass and hypertrophy [15,25,26], and alteration of septal activation, resulting in incoordination of contraction [27]. The regression of hypertrophy in areas remote from the basal septum after ASA indicates that myocardial hypertrophy in HOCM is in part afterload dependent and is not entirely caused by the genetic defect [25,26]. Furthermore, changes in diastolic function resulting from ASA also seem to contribute to long-term improvement in hemodynamics [28]. This effect might be brought about by more favorable relaxation as well as a reduction in left ventricular stiffness secondary to regression of hypertrophy [22,23,25,29,30], decrease in interstitial collagen, and expression of tumor-necrosis factor [31].

The technique
Assessment of outflow gradient
Although some centers only measure the gradient non-invasively using echocardiography, most operators use hemodynamic measurement of outflow gradient during the procedure to confirm the gradient. A 5 Fr pigtail or multipurpose catheter with side holes situated close to the tip can be used to measure pre-stenotic pressure. Many operators prefer to introduce the catheter retrogradely via a controlateral femoral arterial puncture, rather than perform trans-septal puncture with a Brockenbrough catheter as described initially [6]. It is essential to place the catheter close to the apex particularly in cases with mid-ventricular hypertrophy. A J-wire is sometimes used to advance the catheter further toward the apex. Attention should be paid to avoid entrapment in the myocardium, as this can exaggerate the gradient. This is achieved by injecting a small volume of contrast via the catheter, and checking for proper clearance of the dye.

A 7 or 8 Fr guiding catheter (e.g., short tip Judkins type which allows deep intubation of the vessel if necessary) is placed in the ascending aorta to measure the post-stenotic pressure. A 6 Fr catheter can cause excessive pressure damping with concomitant use of a balloon catheter required for alcohol injection later during the procedure, and should therefore not be used. After exclusion of a valvular gradient, the peak-to-peak intraventricular gradient should be measured at rest, during isoproterenol infusion, and after extrasystoles (Figure 54.1). Isoproterenol infusion is particularly useful to reveal a gradient in sedated patients and can be administered by diluting 200 µg in 50 mL saline, with injection of a bolus of 1–3 mL followed by additional boluses until a heart rate of 100–120 b.p.m. is reached.

In order to ensure backup pacing in the advent of complete atrioventricular (AV) block, a temporary pacing wire should be placed in the right ventricle. If extrasystoles are not observed spontaneously, the pacing wire may also serve to measure the post-extrasystolic gradient by programmed stimulation (with coupling intervals of approximately 370 ms). Any beta-blocker therapy should be discontinued because of the increased risk of heart block and also in order to assess the underlying outflow gradient optimally.

Placement and testing of the balloon catheter
An angiogram of the left coronary artery is performed (Figure 54.2a). Milking of the septal perforators that supply the hypertrophied segments, which is often observed, is a good indicator for identifying the target vessel. Placing the guidewire in the septal branch can occasionally be challenging because of a steep take-off angle. It can be helpful to pre-shape the guidewire with two angles through a needle as shown in Figure 54.3 (rather than a curve). A floppy guidewire should be tried first, and advanced distally into the septal perforator in order to ensure stability. Stiffer guidewires (intermediate, or in rare cases a standard wire) are sometimes needed to make the balloon go through steep angles. Exceptionally, a 4 Fr catheter with a sharp angle (e.g., an internal mammary catheter) can be used as an inner catheter to pre-select septal branches with extremely steep takeoffs for placing the 0.014-inch guidewire. Nonetheless, catheters should be manipulated with extreme caution to avoid dissection. Ultimately, another balloon catheter can also be briefly inflated just distally to the septal branch, and the 0.014-inch guidewire bounced off into the targeted vessel.

The targeted septal branch should have a diameter of at least 1.5 mm. After administration of intravenous heparin, the shortest available balloon catheter (a 10 × 2 mm balloon is suitable for most cases) is placed as proximally as possible in a stable position. The balloon should be adapted to the dimension of the vessel and slightly oversized (usually 2–3 mm). Although balloons dedicated to this procedure have been developed, standard angioplasty balloons can be used. If there is early proximal branching of the septal perforator, a very short balloon (5 mm) can be used. Consequently, the guiding catheter should be positioned more deeply to give more support for the balloon catheter and avoid recoil during injection. The balloon should be inflated with a pressure of 4–6 bar, and proper positioning should be verified by injection of contrast agent into the left coronary artery (Figure 54.2b), and then distally via the lumen of the balloon catheter using about 1 mL dye (Figure 54.2c). Absence of retrograde leakage and stability of balloon position (especially with shorter balloons) should be verified cautiously. A key point is to inject the contrast *forcefully* via the inflated balloon catheter when testing for stability. In addition, the extent of

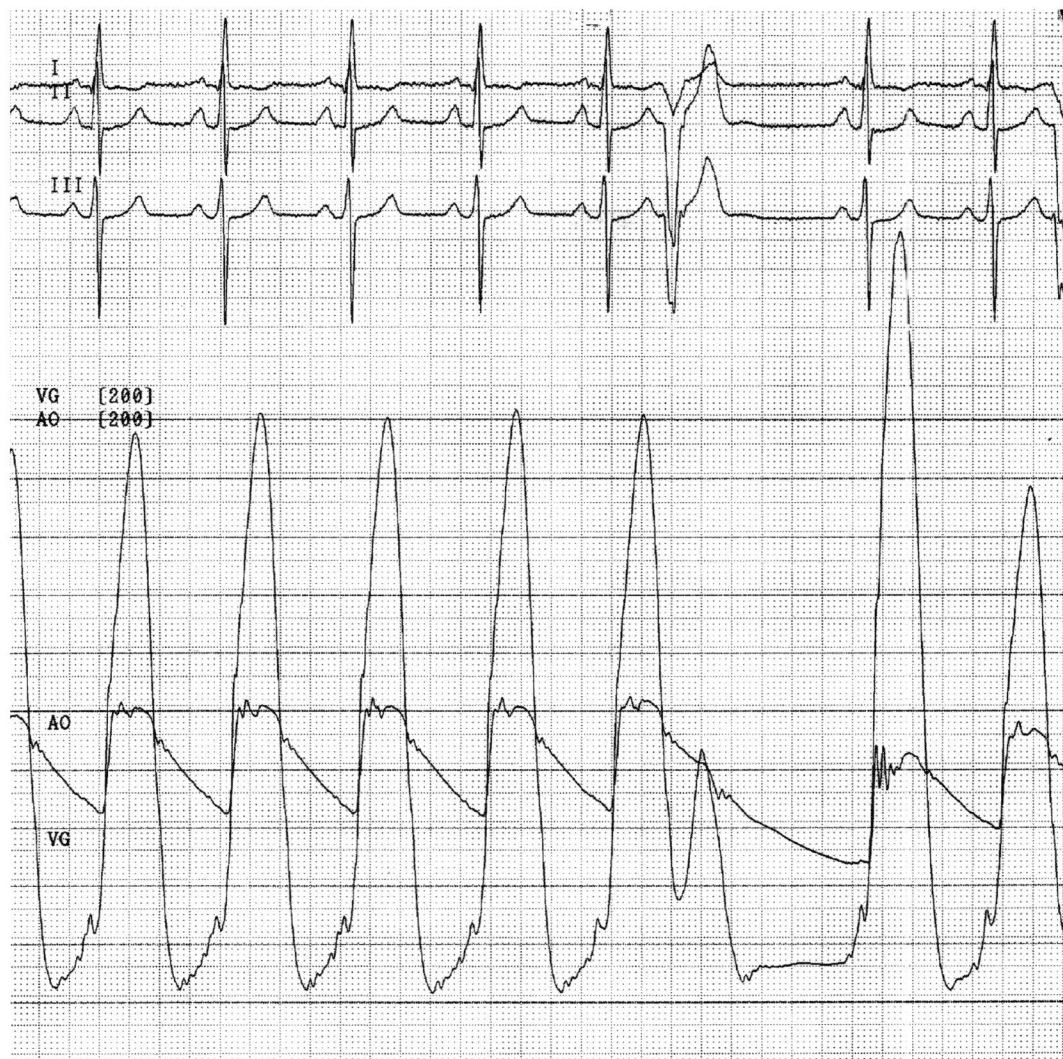

Figure 54.1 Hemodynamic monitoring with a resting peak-to-peak gradient of 100 mmHg and a post extrasystolic gradient of approximately 170 mmHg.

myocardium supplied by the septal branch and shunting of flow to non-targeted regions can also be analyzed, preferably using two different projections. The injection of contrast agent also increases ischemia to the territory of the septal branch. The outflow gradient should be monitored constantly, and within 5 minutes of balloon occlusion, a drop in the resting gradient by >30 mmHg or the post-extrasystolic gradient by >50 mmHg should be observed. In a significant proportion of patients, these criteria are not met [30]. Nowadays most operators prefer echocardiographic criteria using echo contrast to delineate the target area. If necessary, the balloon catheter can be positioned in another septal branch. The target vessel occasionally originates from an intermediate or diagonal branch [32], or from the posterior descending artery in case of a dominant right coronary artery [12].

Guidance by myocardial contrast echocardiography (MCE) has proved to be particularly useful, and can influence the interventional strategy in 15–20% of cases either by changing the target vessel or aborting the procedure. In addition, MCE allows increased success

rates despite reduced infarct size, which in turn reduces complications [20,32]. Before injecting alcohol, 1–2 mL echo contrast (e.g., Sonovue®, Levovist®, Optison®, Albunex®) is injected via the inflated balloon catheter under transthoracic echocardiography in the apical four- and five-chamber views (Figure 54.4a). This will ascertain whether the opacified myocardium is adjacent to the region where the anterior mitral leaflet comes into contact with the septum, and allows withholding of alcohol administration where there is a suboptimal perfusion pattern, such as if the right side of the interventricular septum is predominantly opacified [33]. This technique also allows the delineation of the infarct zone and rules out any retrograde leakage or involvement of myocardium distant from the expected target region such as the ventricular free wall or papillary muscles [16,32,34]. With echo contrast volumes of more than 1 mL, transcapillary leakage of the contrast medium into the ventricles occurs, more often the right than the left (Figure 54.4b). When echo contrast is not available, echocardiography can also be performed by using agitated regular contrast dye injection in the septal

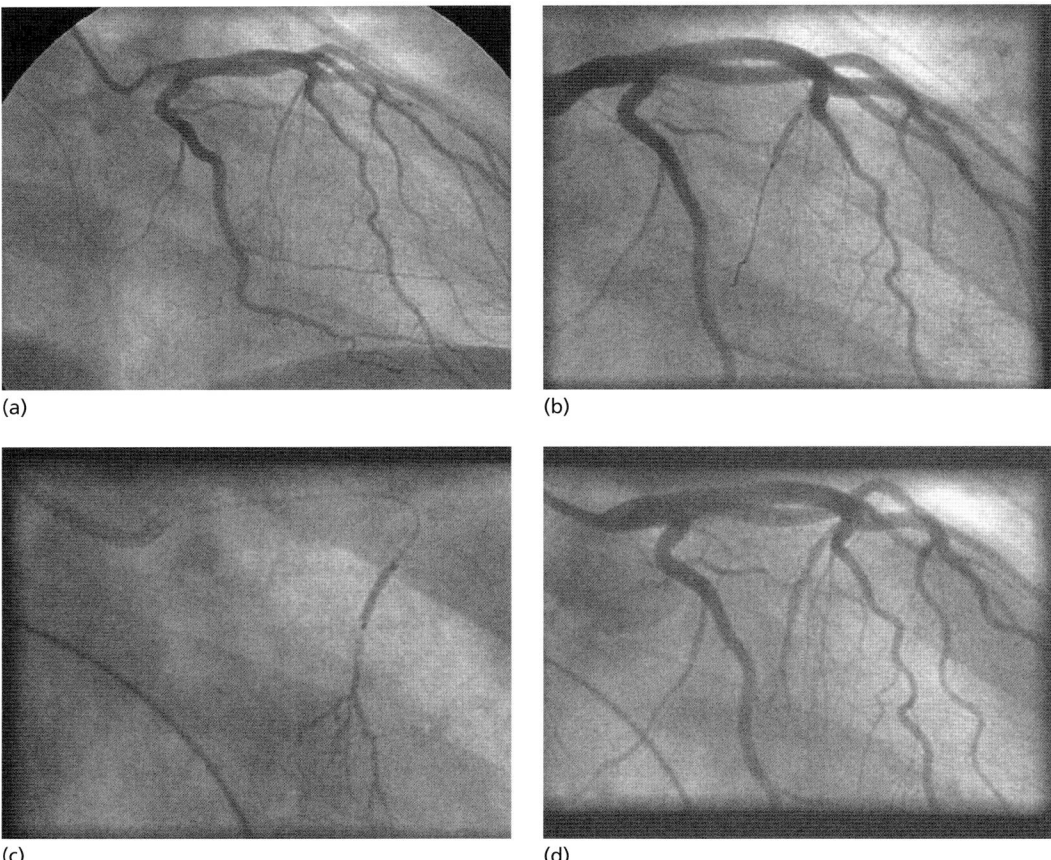

Figure 54.2 Angiography of the left coronary artery (a). Right anterior oblique view (b). Balloon catheter inflated and placed in the first septal branch over a 0.014-inch guidewire (c). Contrast medium is injected via the balloon catheter to confirm the absence of retrograde leakage (d). Angiogram after alcohol injection. Note that the first septal branch is patent.

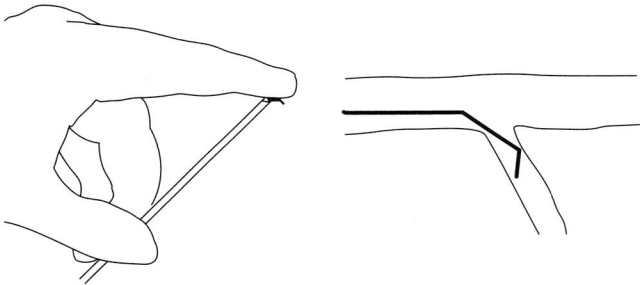

Figure 54.3 Pre-shaping the 0.014-inch guidewire with two angles through a blunt needle (left) and positioning of the guidewire in a septal branch (right).

perforator via the occluded balloon catheter. Furthermore, contrast dye injections through the inflated balloon should not be carried out before echographic imaging (e.g., when testing for balloon stability), as this can opacify the myocardium and make interpretation of the images more difficult during subsequent injections.

Alcohol injection

Once the septal perforator is deemed suitable and the balloon position is stable without any retrograde spilling, 0.7–3 mL 96% alcohol is injected through the inflated balloon catheter. Before

this, analgesia can be administered for pain control. The volume injected depends on the dimension of the vessel and the volume of the targeted myocardium. The speed of delivery is subject to debate, as the alcohol may be either injected slowly over 1–5 minutes or as a bolus. We prefer the latter technique, as this allows more efficient dissipation of the alcohol over a larger volume of myocardium and avoids preferential streaming to a single region. However, it can be argued that slow injection allows for longer contact of the alcohol with the myocardium (for instance, by initially inducing capillary leakage which subsequently allows more alcohol extravasations into the interstitial tissue). Nonetheless, recent animal studies have shown that it is not the speed of alcohol injection, but the amount of alcohol injected that determines the resultant infarct size [35,36]. Therefore, during recent years, there has been a tendency to reduce the volume of alcohol injected to a maximum of 2 mL [14,30,37], which reduces complications. During injection, the electrocardiogram should be closely monitored, and the injection aborted if AV block develops. The balloon should remain inflated during at least 5 minutes in order to enhance contact of alcohol with the tissue and avoid reflux into the left anterior descending artery. Angiography of the left coronary artery should be repeated following balloon deflation in order to confirm patency of the left anterior descending artery (Figure 54.2d). The target septal vessel is not necessarily occluded, although flow usually appears sluggish. It is not

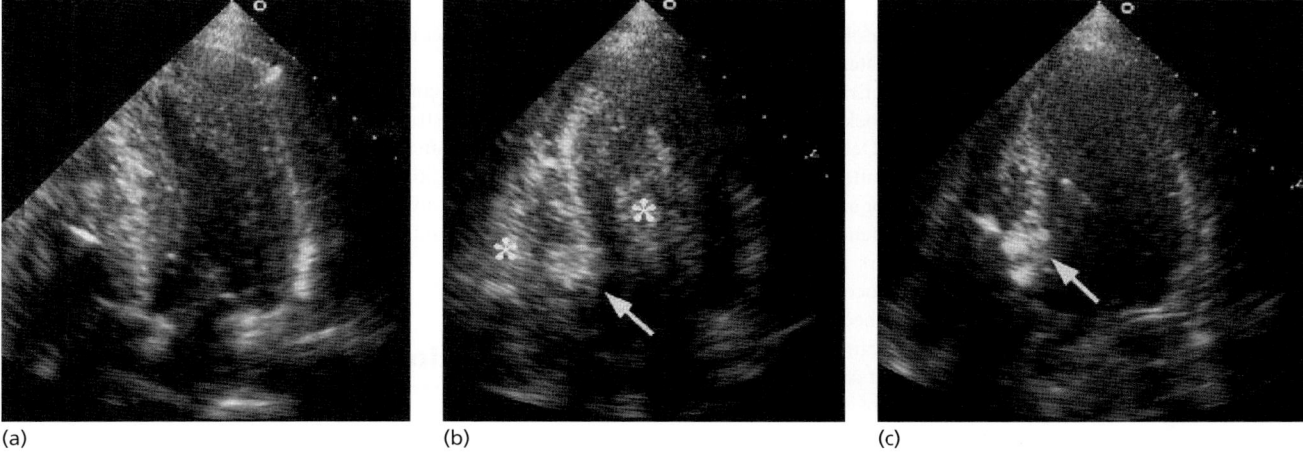

(a)   (b)   (c)

Figure 54.4 (a) Apical four-chamber echocardiogram showing the hypertrophied septum (b). Injection of echo contrast via the occluded balloon catheter positioned in the first septal perforator, with opacification of the basal septum (arrow). Note the presence of echo contrast (asterisks) within both ventricles due to transcapillary passage (c). After alcohol injection, the area of necrosis becomes echodense (arrow).

known whether this has any impact on treatment efficacy. Echocardiographically, the injection of alcohol results in a marked contrast effect, which is much stronger than currently available echo contrast agents (Figure 54.4c).

The hemodynamic objective is a decrease of the gradient to <10 mmHg at rest in patients with resting gradients >30 mmHg, or a decrease by >50% of a significant provokable gradient [12]. If there is a significant residual gradient after a period of 5–10 minutes following the last injection, a new alcohol injection can be attempted by placing the balloon more proximally inside the same septal branch, or using a shorter balloon if branches of the septal perforator were occluded by the balloon inflation during the first injection. Alternatively, a second septal perforator can be targeted using the same procedure as for the first branch. Most patients require one target perforator branch only, especially since the advent of MCE. Furthermore, a residual gradient of <30 mmHg is often acceptable, as it has been shown that outflow gradient can further decrease over time [19]. Some operators therefore prefer a "one vessel per session" approach, and it is still unclear whether more than a single septal perforator should be targeted initially.

Post-procedural management

Vascular sheaths can be removed after normalization of coagulation parameters. Heparin at therapeutic levels does not need to be pursued after the procedure. Furthermore, all patients should receive aspirin (e.g., 100 mg/day) before the procedure, which should be continued for 1 month to prevent mural thrombosis resulting from the infarct. Creatinine kinase (CK) levels should be assessed every 4 hours in order to measure peak values. Peak rises are commonly in the range of 750–1500 U/L. Patients should be observed in the coronary care unit for 48 hours, with removal of the transvenous pacemaker at the end of this period in the absence of AV block. The patient can then be transferred to a monitored step-down unit for the remainder of the hospital stay (which is usually 1 day). Inotropic and chronotropic therapy, especially beta-blockers, can be resumed—possibly at lower doses—if there are no significant bradyarrhythmias [12].

Treatment efficacy

Although no randomized controlled trial comparing ASA with surgical myectomy has been performed, the general consensus is that in centers with appropriate expertise, operative risks, hemodynamic benefits, and initial symptomatic benefits are broadly comparable with either technique [38]. Evidence from non-randomized trials also indicate that ASA is similar to myectomy with respect to hemodynamic and functional improvement [39–41]. Pooled results of published studies on ASA show acute reductions in mean resting LVOT gradients from 65 to 17 mmHg and mean post-extrasystolic gradients from 125 to 53 mmHg, with persistence of the reduction after 12 months (16 and 32 mmHg, respectively) [42]. In addition, there is a significant improvement at 12 months of functional class (NYHA Class 2.9–1.2, CCS 1.9–0.4), peak oxygen consumption (17.8–23.6 mL/kg/min), and exercise capacity (86.2–122.8 W). Procedure success is achieved in 89% of cases. Repeat procedures despite initial success are required because of recurring gradient and symptoms in 7% of patients. Reported predictors of procedural failure are total peak CK<1300 U/L and immediate residual LVOT gradient ≥25 mmHg [43].

Adverse events

Early mortality (occurring during or up to 30 days after the procedure) is low, with a mean value of 1.5% reported [42], which is similar to that for surgical myectomy. Causes of early mortality include left anterior descending dissection, ventricular fibrillation, cardiac tamponade, cardiogenic shock, and pulmonary embolism. Late all-cause mortality is reported at 0.5%, the most frequent causes being sudden cardiac death, pulmonary embolism, congestive heart failure, and other non-cardiac causes. Other reported adverse events include coronary dissection and spasm (1.8% and 1.4%, respectively), stroke (1.1%), and pericardial effusion (0.6%).

Spontaneous ventricular fibrillation in the immediate peri-procedural period is not frequent (2.2%), and sustained ventricular tachycardia is extremely rare (only three cases reported in current literature) [42,44].

The most frequent complication of ASA is complete AV block requiring permanent pacemaker implantation. Occurrence of acute complete AV block during the procedure varies between 21% and 70% of patients [45–49]. Yet there is recovery of AV conduction in most cases (41–100%) before leaving the catheterization laboratory, and in two-thirds of patients within the first 3 days [46,47]. Disappearance of procedural complete AV block has been reported as late as 13 days after the procedure [46]. Delayed complete AV block can also develop later during hospitalization in patients without previous procedural complete AV block or as a recurrence after recovery from acute complete AV block. Depending on the definition used, delayed complete AV block occurs in 1–25% of cases, after a mean period of 36 hours post-procedure, and usually requires permanent pacemaker implantation because of persistence of the conduction defect [47,49]. The block can appear sometimes as late as 96 hours after the procedure [50]. It is thought that transient procedural conduction abnormalities are likely caused by the acute effects of alcohol on the myocardium and conduction system (ischemia, edema, and inflammation), while permanent conduction abnormalities are probably caused by necrosis, scarring and, possibly, remodeling [47]. Ultimately, around 10% of patients require permanent pacemaker implantation after ASA [42].

Several studies have sought to determine predictors of development of delayed complete AV block, with conflicting results [43,47,49,51]. Overall, the most consistent predictors of subsequent permanent pacing implantation appear to be baseline left bundle branch block (LBBB), baseline first-degree AV block, and procedural complete AV block [43,47–49,51]. Some authors suggest elective permanent pacemaker implantation prior to ASA in patients with baseline LBBB [48]. Furthermore, an earlier study showed that use of MCE limits infarct size and reduces the need for permanent pacemaker implantation from 17% to 7%, subsequently leading to widespread use of MCE during ASA [45]. Other parameters reported as significant predictors of complete AV block development are new intraventricular conduction defects, pre- or post-procedure prolongation of QRS duration, retrograde AV nodal block (assessed by simultaneous electrophysiologic investigation), advanced age, female gender, bolus injection of alcohol, and injection of more than one septal artery. However, none of these parameters were systematically confirmed across different studies [43,47–49,51]. Based on several of these predictors, some groups have elaborated specific management strategies based on risk of complete AV block occurrence [48,49]. We and others implant a pacemaker if the block persists for >48–72 hours, although AV conduction recovers in many patients with longer observation [43].

New right bundle branch block (RBBB) is seen approximately in half of patients [42]. This finding is not surprising, because the right bundle is a discrete structure that is vascularized by septal branches from the left anterior coronary artery in 90% of patients, whereas the left bundle is fan-like and receives a dual blood supply from perforator branches of both the left anterior descending and posterior descending arteries. The left conduction system can nevertheless be involved, and new left anterior fascicular block is reported in 6% of procedures [42]. Furthermore, a cardiac magnetic resonance study reported a greater left ventricular mass reduction following ASA in patients who developed new RBBB compared with those without RBB [52].

Despite the creation of a septal infarct, new Q-waves in the septal leads are rarely seen after ASA. Baseline Q waves even tend to disappear following the procedure [53].

In patients with permanent pacemakers undergoing ASA, loss of capture occurs if the ventricular lead is placed near the septum [54]. Increasing pacing to maximum output during the first days following the procedure might therefore be prudent in these patients.

Finally, although concern has been raised about creation of an arrhythmogenic substrate by ASA [10,55], there is currently no evidence that indicates an increase in incidence of ventricular arrhythmias or sudden death during follow-up, as assessed by serial electrophysiologic studies before and after the procedure [30,56] or by analysis of implantable cardioverter-defibrillator intervention rate [57].

Future directions

Since the original description in 1995, the procedure has undergone several modifications and improvements that have led to optimization of the results and minimization of complications, most importantly through the reduction of the effective dose of alcohol and the use of MCE. Recently, use of intracardiac echocardiography has been described as a way to provide continuous imaging of the treated segment of the septum during the whole procedure [58,59]. Facilitation of septal artery cannulation by magnetic navigation has also been reported [60]. Other novelties include use of polyvinyl alcohol foam particles, absorbable gelatin sponge, or septal coil embolization as alternatives to alcohol, which can further reduce the incidence of complete heart block [61–63]. Finally, reduction of septum by radiofrequency catheter ablation and cryoablation are currently under investigation [64,65].

Clinical investigation and expert consensus documents have produced more clinical outcomes data regarding this interventional procedure and have attempted to put in perspective the other two ways to approach hypertrophic cardiomyopathy: conservative medical therapy and surgical myomectomy. The importance of a comprehensive evaluation with clinical, imaging, genetics, interventional and surgeon specialists has become widely accepted and the arrhythmic risk of all these patients warrants additional evaluation with electrophysiology point of view. Reviewing these data, we deduce that different types of patients are treated with different therapeutic approaches and none of the studies employed prospective randomization. Therefore, the nature of the observations does not allow a fair comparison among the three treatment strategies [66–70].

Conclusions

Although surgical myectomy has set the standard of therapy for drug-resistant HOCM, ASA is an alternative that may be considered in many patients. Data indicate that functional and hemodynamic success is high and similar to that of surgery, with the advantage that it may be performed in patients in whom major surgery is considered unsuitable. Benefits in comparison to myectomy also include shorter hospital stay, minimum pain, and avoidance of complications associated with surgery and cardiopulmonary bypass. Nevertheless, ASA has an important learning curve, with potentially serious complications, the most frequent of which is complete AV block requiring permanent pacemaker implantation in approximately 10% of patients. Although these rates are declining with continuing experience, the advent of imaging techniques such as MCE and use of lower alcohol doses, the procedure should be performed only by experienced operators and on carefully selected patients.

Interactive multiple choice questions are available for this chapter on www.wiley. com/go/dangas/cardiology

References

1 Maron BJ, Olivotto I, Spirito P, *et al*. Epidemiology of hypertrophic cardiomyopathy-related death: revisited in a large non-referral-based patient population. *Circulation* 2000; **102**: 858–864.

2 Maron MS, Olivotto I, Betocchi S, *et al*. Effect of left ventricular outflow tract obstruction on clinical outcome in hypertrophic cardiomyopathy. *N Engl J Med* 2003; **348**: 295–303.

3 Maron BJ, Bonow RO, Cannon RO III, *et al*. Hypertrophic cardiomyopathy. Interrelations of clinical manifestations, pathophysiology, and therapy. *N Engl J Med* 1987; **316**: 780–789.

4 Maron BJ. Hypertrophic cardiomyopathy: a systematic review. *JAMA* 2002;. **287**: 1308–1320.

5 Maron BJ, McKenna WJ, Danielson GK, *et al*. American College of Cardiology/ European Society of Cardiology clinical expert consensus document on hypertrophic cardiomyopathy. A report of the American College of Cardiology Foundation Task Force on Clinical Expert Consensus Documents and the European Society of Cardiology Committee for Practice Guidelines. *Eur Heart J* 2003; **24**: 1965–1991.

6 Sigwart U. Non-surgical myocardial reduction for hypertrophic obstructive cardiomyopathy. *Lancet* 1995; **346**: 211–214.

7 Brugada P, de Swart H, Smeets JL, *et al*. Transcoronary chemical ablation of ventricular tachycardia. *Circulation* 1989; **79**: 475–482.

8 Spencer WH III, Roberts R. Alcohol septal ablation in hypertrophicobstructive cardiomyopathy: the need for a registry. *Circulation* 2000; **102**: 600–601.

9 Roberts R, Sigwart U. Current concepts of the pathogenesis and treatment of hypertrophic cardiomyopathy. *Circulation* 2005; **112**: 293–296.

10 Marron B. Controversies in cardiovascular medicine: surgical myectomy remains the primary treatment option for severely symptomatic patients with obstructive hypertrophic cardiomyopathy. *Circulation* 2007; **116**: 196–206.

11 Li ZQ, Cheng TO, Zhang WW, *et al*. Percutaneous transluminal septal myocardial ablation for hypertrophic obstructive cardiomyopathy: the Chinese experience in 119 patients from a single center. *Int J Cardiol* 2004; **93**: 197–202.

12 Holmes DR Jr, Valeti US, Nishimura RA. Alcohol septal ablation for hypertrophic cardiomyopathy: indications and technique. *Catheter Cardiovasc Interv* 2005; **66**: 375–389.

13 Jiang L, Levine RA, King ME, *et al*. An integrated mechanism for systolic anterior motion of the mitral valve in hypertrophic cardiomyopathy based on echocardiographic observations. *Am Heart J* 1987; **113**: 633–644.

14 Kuhn H, Gietzen FH, Schafers M, *et al*. Changes in the left ventricular outflow tract after transcoronary ablation of septal hypertrophy (TASH) for hypertrophic obstructive cardiomyopathy as assessed by transoesophageal echocardiography and by measuring myocardial glucose utilization and perfusion. *Eur Heart J* 1999; **20**: 1808–1817.

15 Lakkis NM, Nagueh SF, Kleiman NS, *et al*. Echocardiography-guided ethanol septal reduction for hypertrophic obstructive cardiomyopathy. *Circulation* 1998; **98**: 1750–1755.

16 Nagueh SF, Lakkis NM, He ZX, *et al*. Role of myocardial contrast echocardiography during nonsurgical septal reduction therapy for hypertrophic obstructive cardiomyopathy. *J Am Coll Cardiol* 1998; **32**: 225–229.

17 van Dockum WG, ten Cate FJ, ten Berg JM, *et al*. Myocardial infarction after percutaneous transluminal septal myocardial ablation in hypertrophic obstructive cardiomyopathy: evaluation by contrast-enhanced magnetic resonance imaging. *J Am Coll Cardiol* 2004; **43**: 27–34.

18 Valeti US, Nishimura RA, Holmes DR Jr, *et al*. Comparison of surgical septal myectomy and alcohol septal ablation with cardiac magnetic resonance imaging in patients with hypertrophic obstructive cardiomyopathy. *J Am Coll Cardiol* 2007; **49**: 350–357.

19 Yoerger DM, Picard MH, Palacios IF, *et al*. Time course of pressure gradient response after first alcohol septal ablation for obstructive hypertrophic cardiomyopathy. *Am J Cardiol* 2006; **97**: 1511–1514.

20 Flores-Ramirez R, Lakkis NM, Middleton KJ, *et al*. Echocardiographic insights into the mechanisms of relief of left ventricular outflow tract obstruction after nonsurgical septal reduction therapy in patients with hypertrophic obstructive cardiomyopathy. *J Am Coll Cardiol* 2001; **37**: 208–214.

21 Park TH, Lakkis NM, Middleton KJ, *et al*. Acute effect of nonsurgical septal reduction therapy on regional left ventricular asynchrony in patients with hypertrophic obstructive cardiomyopathy. *Circulation* 2002; **106**: 412–415.

22 Nagueh SF, Lakkis NM, Middleton KJ, *et al*. Changes in left ventricular diastolic function 6 months after nonsurgical septal reduction therapy for hypertrophic obstructive cardiomyopathy. *Circulation* 1999; **99**: 344–347.

23 Nagueh SF, Lakkis NM, Middleton KJ, *et al*. Changes in left ventricular filling and left atrial function six months after nonsurgical septal reduction therapy for hypertrophic obstructive cardiomyopathy. *J Am Coll Cardiol* 1999; **34**: 1123–1128.

24 Baggish AL, Smith RN, Palacios I, *et al*. Pathological effects of alcohol septal ablation for hypertrophic obstructive cardiomyopathy. *Heart* 2006; **92**: 1773–1778.

25 Mazur W, Nagueh SF, Lakkis NM, *et al*. Regression of left ventricular hypertrophy after nonsurgical septal reduction therapy for hypertrophic obstructive cardiomyopathy. *Circulation* 2001; **103**: 1492–1496.

26 van Dockum WG, Beek AM, ten Cate FJ, *et al*. Early onset and progression of left ventricular remodeling after alcohol septal ablation in hypertrophic obstructive cardiomyopathy. *Circulation* 2005; **111**: 2503–2508.

27 Henein MY, O'Sullivan CA, Ramzy IS, *et al*. Electromechanical left ventricular behavior after nonsurgical septal reduction in patients with hypertrophic obstructive cardiomyopathy. *J Am Coll Cardiol* 1999; **34**: 1117–1122.

28 Jassal DS, Neilan TG, Fifer MA, *et al*. Sustained improvement in left ventricular diastolic function after alcohol septal ablation for hypertrophic obstructive cardiomyopathy. *Eur Heart J* 2006; **27**: 1805–1810.

29 Sitges M, Shiota T, Lever HM, *et al*. Comparison of left ventricular diastolic function in obstructive hypertrophic cardiomyopathy in patients undergoing percutaneous septal alcohol ablation versus surgical myotomy/myectomy. *Am J Cardiol* 2003; **91**: 817–821.

30 Boekstegers P, Steinbigler P, Molnar A, *et al*. Pressure-guided nonsurgical myocardial reduction induced by small septal infarctions in hypertrophic obstructive cardiomyopathy. *J Am Coll Cardiol* 2001; **38**: 846–853.

31 Nagueh SF, Stetson SJ, Lakkis NM, *et al*. Decreased expression of tumor necrosis factor-alpha and regression of hypertrophy after nonsurgical septal reduction therapy for patients with hypertrophic obstructive cardiomyopathy. *Circulation* 2001; **103**: 1844–1850.

32 Faber L, Seggewiss H, Welge D, *et al*. Echo-guided percutaneous septal ablation for symptomatic hypertrophic obstructive cardiomyopathy: 7 years of experience. *Eur J Echocardiography* 2004; **5**: 347–355.

33 Okayama H, Sumimoto T, Morioka N, *et al*. Usefulness of selective myocardial contrast echocardiography in percutaneous transluminal septal myocardial ablation: a case report. *Jpn Circ J* 2001; **65**: 842–844.

34 Harada T, Ohtaki E, Sumiyoshi T, *et al*. Papillary muscles identified by myocardial contrast echocardiography in preparation for percutaneous transluminal septal myocardial ablation. *Acta Cardiol* 2002; **57**: 25–27.

35 Li ZQ, Cheng TO, Liu L, *et al*. Experimental study of relationship between intracoronary alcohol injection and the size of resultant myocardial infarct. *Int J Cardiol* 2003; **91**: 93–96.

36 Cheng TO. In percutaneous transluminal septal myocardial ablation for hypertrophic obstructive cardiomyopathy, it is not the speed of intracoronary alcohol injection but the amount of alcohol injected that determines the resultant infarct size. *Circulation* 2004; **110**: e23.

37 Veselka J, Prochazkova S, Duchonova R, *et al*. Alcohol septal ablation for hypertrophic obstructive cardiomyopathy: lower alcohol dose reduces size of infarction and has comparable hemodynamic and clinical outcome. *Catheter Cardiovasc Interv* 2004; **63**: 231–235.

38 Watkins H, McKenna WJ. The prognostic impact of septal myectomy in obstructive hypertrophic cardiomyopathy. *J Am Coll Cardiol* 2005; **46**: 477–479.

39 Nagueh SF, Ommen, SR, Lakkis, NM, *et al*. Comparison of ethanol septal reduction therapy with surgical myectomy for the treatment of hypertrophic obstructive cardiomyopathy. *J Am Coll Cardiol* 2001; **38**: 1701–1706.

40 Qin JX, Shiota T, Lever HM, *et al*. Outcome of patients with hypertrophic obstructive cardiomyopathy after percutaneous transluminal septal myocardial ablation and septal myectomy surgery. *J Am Coll Cardiol* 2001; **38**: 1994–2000.

41 Firoozi S, Elliott PM, Sharma S, *et al*. Septal myotomy–myectomy and transcoronary septal alcohol ablation in hypertrophic obstructive cardiomyopathy. *Eur Heart J* 2002; **23**: 1617–1624.

42 Alam M, Dokainish H, Lakkis N. Alcohol septal ablation for hypertrophic obstructive cardiomyopathy: a systematic review of published studies. *J Interven Cardiol* 2006; **19**: 319–327.

43 Chang SM, Lakkis NM, Franklin J, *et al*. Predictors of outcome after alcohol septal ablation therapy in patients with hypertrophic obstructive cardiomyopathy. *Circulation* 2004; **109**: 824–827.

44 Simon RDB, Crawford FA III, Spencer WH III, *et al*. Sustained ventricular tachycardia following alcohol septal ablation for hypertrophic obstructive cardiomyopathy. *Pacing Clin Electrophysiol* 2005; **28**: 1354–1356.

45 Faber L, Seggewiss H, Gleichmann U. Percutaneous transluminal septal myocardial ablation in hypertrophic obstructive cardiomyopathy: results with respect to intraprocedural myocardial contrast echocardiography. *Circulation* 1998; **98**: 2415–2421.

46 Reinhard W, Ten Cate FJ, Scholten M, *et al.* Permanent pacing for complete atrioventricular block after nonsurgical (alcohol) septal reduction in patients with obstructive hypertrophic cardiomyopathy. *Am J Cardiol* 2004; **93**: 1064–1066.

47 Chen AA, Palacios IF, Mela T, *et al.* Acute predictors of subacute complete heart block after alcohol septal ablation for obstructive hypertrophic cardiomyopathy. *Am J Cardiol* 2006; **97**: 264–269.

48 Faber L, Welge D, Fassbender D, *et al.* Percutaneous septal ablation for symptomatic hypertrophic obstructive cardiomyopathy: managing the risk of procedure-related AV conduction disturbances. *Int J Cardiol* 2007; **119**: 163–167.

49 Lawrenz T, Lieder F, Bartelsmeier M, *et al.* Predictors of complete heart block after transcoronary ablation of septal hypertrophy. Results of a prospective electrophysiological investigation in 172 patients with hypertrophic obstructive cardiomyopathy. *J Am Coll Cardiol* 2007; **49**: 2356–2363.

50 Wykrzykowska JJ, Kwaku K, Wylie J, *et al.* Delayed occurrence of unheralded phase IV complete heart block after ethanol septal ablation for symmetric hypertrophic obstructive cardiomyopathy. *Pacing Clin Electrophysiol* 2006; **29**: 674–678.

51 Talreja DR, Nishimura RA, Edwards WD, *et al.* Alcohol septal ablation versus surgical septal myectomy: comparison of effects on atrioventricular conduction tissue. *J Am Coll Cardiol* 2004; **44**: 2329–2332.

52 McCann GP, Van Dockum WG, Beek AM, *et al.* Extent of myocardial infarction and reverse remodeling assessed by cardiac magnetic resonance in patients with and without right bundle branch block following alcohol septal ablation for obstructive hypertrophic cardiomyopathy. *Am J Cardiol* 2007; **99**: 563–567.

53 Runquist LH, Nielsen CD, Killip D, *et al.* Electrocardiographic findings after alcohol septal ablation therapy for obstructive hypertrophic cardiomyopathy. *Am J Cardiol* 2002; **90**: 1020–1022.

54 Valettas N, Rho R, Beshai J, *et al.* Alcohol septal ablation complicated by complete heart block and permanent pacemaker failure. *Catheter Cardiovasc Interv* 2003; **58**: 189–193.

55 Maron BJ, Dearani JA, Ommen SR, *et al.* The case for surgery in obstructive hypertrophic cardiomyopathy. *J Am Coll Cardiol* 2004; **44**: 2044–2053.

56 Gietzen FH, Leuner CJ, Raute-Kreinsen U, *et al.* Acute and long-term results after transcoronary ablation of septal hypertrophy (TASH): catheter interventional treatment for hypertrophic obstructive cardiomyopathy. *Eur Heart J* 1999 **20**: 1342–1354.

57 Lawrenz T, Obergassel L, Lieder F, *et al.* Transcoronary ablation of septal hypertrophy does not alter ICD intervention rates in high risk patients with hypertrophic obstructive cardiomyopathy. *Pacing Clin Electrophysiol* 2005; **28**: 295–300.

58 Pedone C, Vijayakumar M, Ligthart JM, *et al.* Intracardiac echocardiography guidance during percutaneous transluminal septal myocardial ablation in patients with obstructive hypertrophic cardiomyopathy. *Int J Cardiovasc Intervent* 2005; **7**: 134–137.

59 Alfonso F, Martín D, Fernández-Vázquez F, *et al.* Intracardiac echocardiography guidance for alcohol septal ablation in hypertrophic obstructive cardiomyopathy. *J Invasive Cardiol* 2007; **19**: E134–E136.

60 Bach RG, Leach C, Milov SA, *et al.* Use of magnetic navigation to facilitate transcatheter alcohol septal ablation for hypertrophic obstructive cardiomyopathy. *J Invasive Cardiol* 2006; **18**: E176–E178.

61 Gross CM, Schulz-Menger J, Kramer J, *et al.* Percutaneous transluminal septal artery ablation using polyvinyl alcohol foam particles for septal hypertrophy in patients with hypertrophic obstructive cardiomyopathy: acute and three-year outcomes. *J Endovasc Ther* 2004; **11**: 705–711.

62 Llamas-Espero GA, Sandoval-Navarrete S. Percutaneous septal ablation with absorbable gelatin sponge in hypertrophic obstructive cardiomyopathy. *Catheter Cardiovasc Interv* 2006; **69**: 231–235.

63 Durand E, Mousseaux E, Coste P, *et al.* Non-surgical septal myocardial reduction by coil embolization for hypertrophic obstructive cardiomyopathy: early and 6 months follw-up. *Eur Heart J* 2008; **29**: 348–355.

64 Lawrenz T, Kuhn H. Endocardial radiofrequency ablation of septal hypertrophy: a new catheter-based modality of gradient reduction in hypertrophic obstructive cardiomyopathy. *Z Kardiol* 2004; **93**: 493–499.

65 Keane D, Hynes B, King G, *et al.* Feasibility study of percutaneous transvalvular endomyocardial cryoablation for the treatment of hypertrophic obstructive cardiomyopathy. *J Invasive Cardiol* 2007; **19**: 247–251.

66 Veselka J, Krejčí J, Tomašov P, Zemánek D. Long-term survival after alcohol septal ablation for hypertrophic obstructive cardiomyopathy: a comparison with general population. *Eur Heart J* 2014; **35**(30): 2040–2045.

67 Maron BJ, Maron MS. Hypertrophic cardiomyopathy. *Lancet* 2013; **381**(9862): 242–245.

68 Almasood A, Garceau P, Woo A, Rakowski H, Schwartz L, Overgaard CB. Time to significant gradient reduction following septal balloon occlusion predicts the magnitude of final gradient response during alcohol septal ablation in patients with hypertrophic obstructive cardiomyopathy. *JACC Cardiovasc Interv* 2011; **4**(9): 1030–1034.

69 Quintana E, Sabate-Rotes A, Maleszewski JJ, *et al.* Septal myectomy after failed alcohol ablation: does previous percutaneous intervention compromise outcomes of myectomy? *J Thorac Cardiovasc Surg* 2015; **150**(1): 159–216.

70 Maron BJ, Nishimura RA. Surgical septal myectomy versus alcohol septal ablation: assessing the status of the controversy in 2014. *Circulation* 2014; **130**(18): 1617–1624.

CHAPTER 55

Left Atrial Appendage Exclusion

Jorge G. Panizo and Jacob S. Koruth

Helmsley Electrophysiology Center, Mount Sinai Hospital, New York, NY, USA

The relationship between thromboembolic events and atrial fibrillation (AF) has been convincingly established in numerous studies [1,2]. Prevention of these embolic events has traditionally been based on chronic oral anticoagulation with either warfarin or one of the newer oral anticoagulant agents (NOAC) [3]. The left atrial appendage (LAA) has been identified to be the site of thrombus formation in most patients in this setting [4]. Based on this, percutaneous and/or surgical exclusion of the LAA has been demonstrated to be an effective approach to reduce the thromboembolic risk associated with AF.

Surgical LAA exclusion has been performed for many decades as part of cardiac surgical procedures like mitral valve surgery. However, this approach is limited by complications such as peri-operative stroke and/or bleeding, incomplete LAA closure, laceration, and so on. Because of its invasive nature and the morbidity associated with surgical exclusion, non-surgical approaches have gained considerable momentum. This chapter provides an overview primarily addressing catheter-based devices that are currently available or being investigated for LAA exclusion. Most of these are designed to obstruct the LAA orifice mechanically from the endocardial aspect (e.g., Watchman and Amplatzer cardiac plug: endocardial devices). The Lariat procedure, however, uses a combined endo-epicardial access to suture ligate the base of the LAA from its epicardial aspect (epicardial device). The chapter includes a general description of implant technique, procedural tips, and recommendations post-implantation.

Indication for LAA exclusion

Endocardial devices

The only endocardial device approved in the USA is the Watchman device which is indicated for patients at risk for embolic events (CHA2DS-VASC2 > 1) who have been deemed to be suitable for anticoagulation *and* have an appropriate rationale to seek a non-pharmacologic alternative:

- History of major or recurrent bleeding on anticoagulation therapy;
- High risk of major bleeding secondary to trauma related to lifestyle, occupation, frequent falls or fall risk, where the benefits of anticoagulation outweigh the risk of major bleeding; and
- Inability to maintain a stable INR or comply with INR monitoring (and unable to take a NOAC).

The reader should note that these are the only approved indications that are supported by randomized data [5].

However, endocardial devices may be also considered as *options* for certain other patients. One must keep in mind that these indications are not approved in the USA, are not supported by randomized data but are derived from observational studies, and involve the use of antiplatelet agents that themselves carry a significant bleeding risk:

- Patients with absolute contraindications to anticoagulation such as history of a significant bleeding event such as intracranial or life-threatening bleed, the source of which cannot be eliminated;
- Increased bleeding risk: HAS-BLED score ≥3;
- Requiring prolonged triple therapy (aspirin, clopidogrel, and warfarin/NOAC) such as patients with AF with recent coronary stenting [6];
- Conditions such as chronic inflammatory bowel disease, thrombocytopenia, or cancer that increase bleeding risk (not reflected by HAS-BLED score).

Epicardial devices

This approach is currently only available using the Lariat device. The typical patient offered this approach has an absolute contraindication to anticoagulation. Outside the USA, if dual antiplatelet therapy is allowable, endocardial devices are still often used; however, if antiplatelet therapy is also contraindicated then this remains the only available option.

Endocardial devices: design and technical details

Watchman LAA Occlusion device

The Watchman device (Boston Scientific, Natick, MA, USA) (Figure 55.1a) is a nitinol-nickel and titanium alloy based device with 10 active fixation anchors around its perimeter frame designed to engage the LAA wall. The nitinol frame expands radially to maintain its position within the LAA. In addition, it has a membranous cap made of polyethylene terephthalate that functions as a filter to block emboli from exiting the LAA. It is available in five different sizes: 21, 24, 27, 30, and 33 mm. The Watchman device is supported by evidence that includes nearly 6000 patient-years of

Interventional Cardiology: Principles and Practice, Second Edition. Edited by George D. Dangas, Carlo Di Mario, and Nicholas N. Kipshidze.
© 2017 John Wiley & Sons, Ltd. Published 2017 by John Wiley & Sons, Ltd.

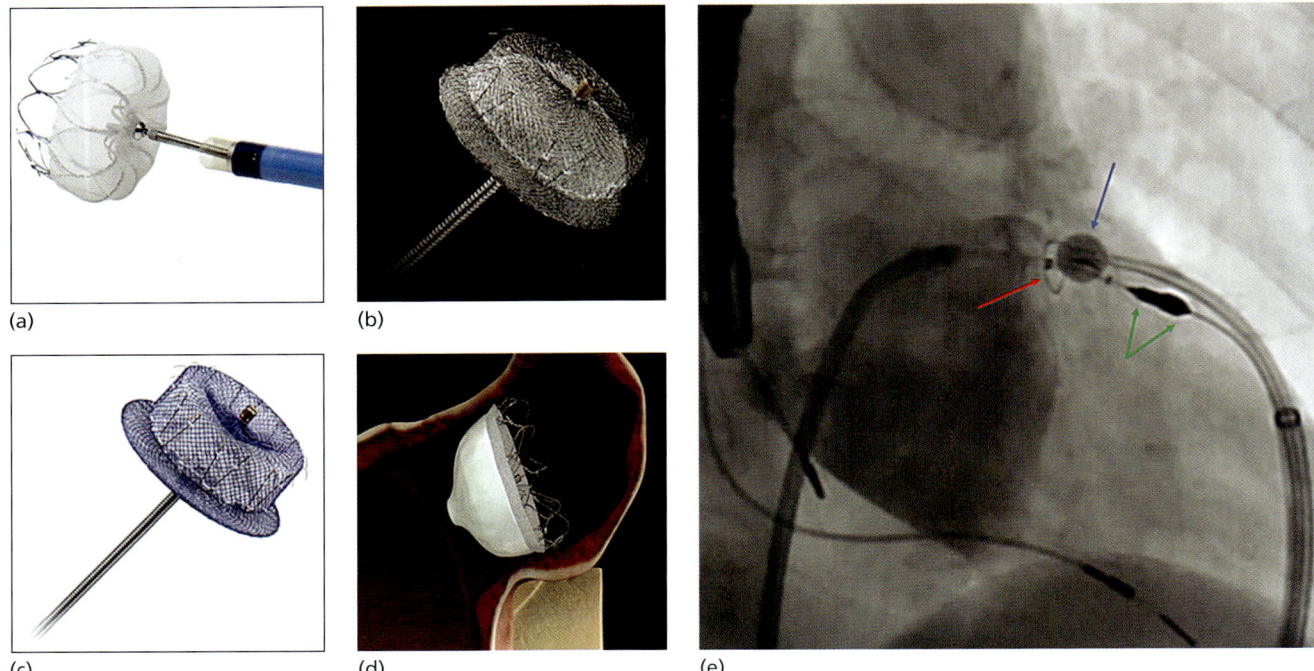

Figure 55.1 (a) Watchman device. (b) Amplatzer Cardiac Plug. (c) Amulet device. (d) WaveCrest device. (e) Fluoroscopic image of left atrial appendage (LAA) closure using the Lariat device: endo- and epicardial magnet-tipped are connected from both sides of LAA apex (green arrows); the endocardial balloon is seen inflated at the level of the LAA ostium (blue arrow) and the epicardial suture is seen as it is tightened around the LAA ostium (red arrow). The left atrium can be seen outlined by iodinated contrast. Sources: (a) Boston Scientific. Reproduced with permission. (b) St. Jude Medical, Cardiology Division. Reproduced with permission. (d) Coherex Medical. Reproduced with permission.

follow-up and is currently the only device approved by the US Food and Drug Administration for LAA exclusion [5,7–9].

Amplatzer Cardiac Plug

The first generation of the Amplatzer Cardiac Plug (ACP 1) device (St. Jude Medical, Minneapolis, MN, USA) consists of a self-expandable cylindrical nitinol "lobe" connected to a nitinol "disk" by a short flexible waist that facilitates positioning and conformation to different LAA shapes (Figure 55.1b). This design was made for sealing the body and ostium of the LAA, respectively. Unlike the Watchman, its length is shorter than its diameter which has advantages for certain LAA shapes [10].

The new generation Amplatzer Cardiac Plug (ACP 2, Amulet device; Figure 55.1c) is designed to accommodate the highly variable anatomy of the LAA and reduce complications [11]. It is available in eight sizes ranging from 16 to 34 mm and has a bigger proximal lobe, a longer waist, recessed proximal end screw, and more stabilizing wires than older models.

WaveCrest LAA Occlusion system

The WaveCrest system (Coherex Medical, Salt Lake City, UT, USA) is a nitinol structure without any exposed metal (Figure 55.1d). Its independent fixation anchors are separately actionable and radially positioned to stabilize the device once the right position is attained. The current generation offers three sizes: 22, 27, and 32 mm. It has been designed for more proximal placement and provides an alternative for very short LAAs.

Procedural aspects for implantation

In the following section we describe the implantation technique primarily of the Watchman and ACP devices. Implantation is typically performed under general anesthesia, based on the need for continuous use of transesophageal echocardiography (TEE) and the potential risk of tamponade or device embolization from inadvertent patient movement during the procedure. Operators should be prepared to identify and treat complications such as cardiac tamponade, air, and device embolism, and so on. Developing protocols for the management of these, including the availability of emergent cardiac surgical backup, are necessary. Fluoroscopy and continuous TEE assessment by an experienced echocardiographer are required. Invasive arterial pressure monitoring is optional.

Imaging

Initially, the echocardiographer rules out thrombus within the left atrium (LA) and LAA. Once the decision to proceed with the implant is made, unilateral femoral venous access is obtained. Although pre-procedural imaging (CT/MRI) can be useful, intra-procedural TEE assessment is usually sufficient. In general, the Watchman and ACP are sized such that they are 15–20% larger than the diameter of the landing zone within the LAA to allow for stable positioning. The most useful TEE views to assess LAA anatomy are the mid-esophageal views at 0°, 45°, 90°, and 135° (Figure 55.2) [12].

The following measurements are usually obtained:
- *LAA ostium*: this measurement is taken from the level of the left circumflex artery to a point 1 cm from the tip of the left superior

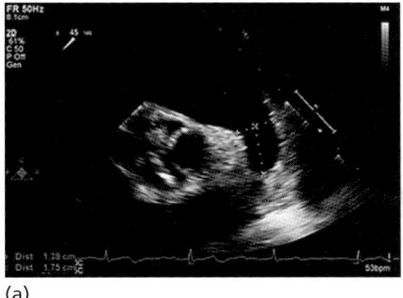

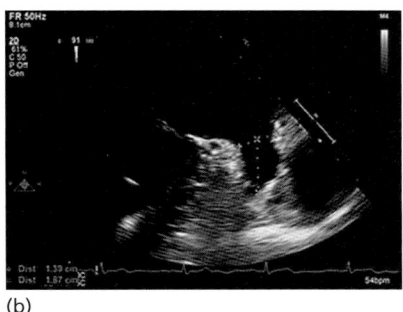

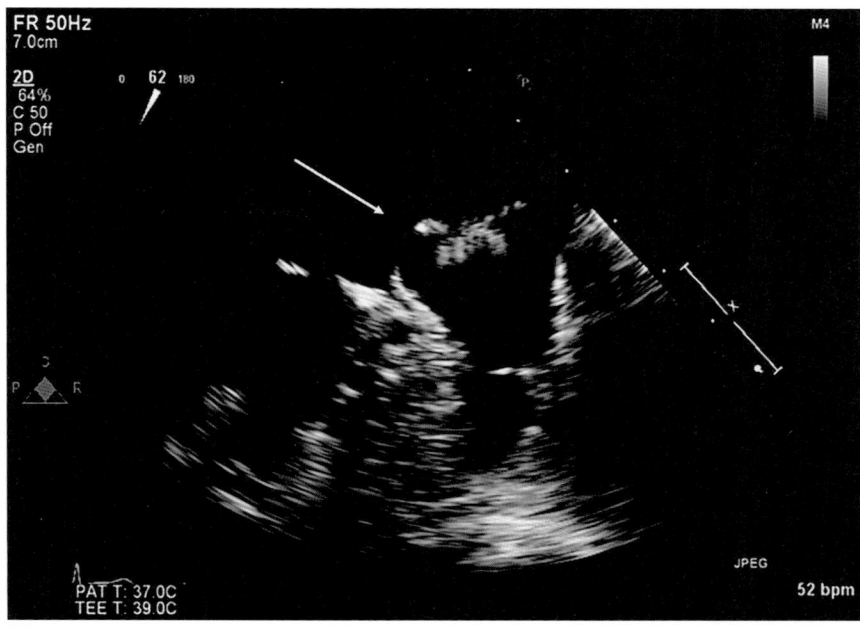

Figure 55.2 (a) LAA measurements in the standard transesophageal echocardiography (TEE) view at 45° and 90° (b). (c) TEE image showing a Watchman device already implanted in the LAA (white arrow).

pulmonary vein limbus (0° view) or from the mitral annulus to a point 1 cm from the limbus (45°, 90°, and 135° views). The Watchman can be implanted if the maximum LAA ostium measures between 17 and 31 mm. The ACP1 device is restricted to ostia less than 29 mm. For larger diameters, the Amulet device is a reasonable alternative.

- *Depth*: measured from the ostial line to LAA apex. A depth that is smaller than the width of the ostium can result in unstable positioning of some devices. In this situation the WaveCrest device is an alternative.

Transeptal access

Anticoagulation with heparin to achieve activated clotting times of 250–300 seconds is required. Access is then obtained under fluoroscopic and/or TEE guidance. It is very important to perform the septal puncture in the inferior portion of the posterior septum, as this allows for direct alignment of the delivery sheath with the LAA. A suboptimal puncture often forces the operator to perform unnecessary manipulation of the delivery sheath during device deployment increasing the risk of potential complications. LA pressures are obtained and if <10 mmHg infusing saline avoids underestimation of LAA size. Device specific sheaths are then placed within the LA for device delivery.

LAA angiography

An adequate outline of LAA is essential to visualize the landing zone. This is usually performed by placing a 4–6 Fr pigtail catheter within the LAA. The best fluoroscopic views to visualize the landing zone for the Watchman is right anterior oblique (RAO) 30° with 30° caudal angulation; for the ACP and WaveCrest devices, RAO with 30° cranial angulation is most useful.

Sizing and positioning

The size of the Watchman device chosen should be 15–20% larger than the diameter of the landing zone within the LAA to prevent dislodgement. For the Watchman device, there are three radio-opaque marker bands on the access sheath that serve as additional guides to assess the depth of the LAA. The Watchman device should be avoided if the LAA depth is less than the device diameter and/or LAA ostium is <17 or >31 mm. For ACP devices, ACP1 must be avoided if the landing zone diameter is >29 mm and/or LAA depth <10 mm. The Amulet must be avoided if the landing zone diameter is >31 mm and/or LAA depth <7.5 mm. The device is typical upsized by 3–5 mm for ACP1 and 2–4 mm for the Amulet (based on landing zone/neck of LAA). Finally, the WaveCrest was designed to cover LAA ostia between 18 and 30 mm.

Deployment

Once angiography is performed, the pigtail catheter is used as a non-traumatic rail over which the delivery sheath is advanced into the LAA. From this point onwards, the patient can be made apneic (if under general anesthesia) as this minimizes the risk of trauma to the LAA wall by the sheath device. Generous "back-bleeding" from the sheath and maintaining "fluid–fluid" connection while loading the device into the delivery sheath are critical for reducing the risk of air embolism.

For the Watchman, once the constrained device is inserted all the way to the tip of the access sheath, the sheath is retracted so that the device is exposed within the LAA resulting in deployment. This is confirmed by TEE imaging. For the ACP, the delivery sheath is placed 1.5 cm within the LAA and the "lobe" of the device is delivered by retracting the sheath followed by deployment of the "disk" upon retracting the sheath further. Following deployment, respiration can be resumed if apnea was used.

Confirmation and release

Watchman release criteria:

1 *Position*: the plane of the maximum diameter should be at or just distal to the LAA ostium. If it too distal within the LAA, partial/full recapture may be required for repositioning.
2 *Anchor*: a fluoroscopic "tug test" is performed to demonstrate proper anchoring.
3 *Size*: the widest plane of the device should be compressed to 80–92% of its original size. This confirms the correct choice of size.
4 *Seal*: ensure that all LAA lobes are distal to the device and confirm that there is complete occlusion of the LAA ostium. Color Doppler is used to detect leaks. Partial or full recapture can be performed until residual jets are minimized.

ACP release criteria:

1 Proper alignment and adequate compression of the lobe. Absence of compression suggests proximal position or undersizing.
2 Lobe position (at least two-thirds) distal to left circumflex artery on TEE.
3 Slight concave shape of disk.
4 Separation of the disk from the lobe.

Once all criteria are met and there is no leak noted on TEE, the device can be released. A gentle tug test is occasionally used to establish stability.

The Lariat system: a combined endocardial–epicardial approach

The Lariat system (SentreHeart, Redwood City, CA, USA) involves obtaining epicardial access followed by placing an epicardial suture that is then tightened around the base of the LAA, excluding it from the LA. This system combines trans-septal access (endocardial) followed by the placement of a magnet-tipped 0.025-inch wire within the LAA apex. This magnetically connects itself with a second magnet-tipped epicardial wire introduced on to the epicardial aspect of the LAA apex (Figure 55.1e). The endocardial wire has a compliant 15-mm balloon that when inflated allows identification of the LAA os. A lasso suture is then delivered over the connected wire and then ligated at the LAA os. LAA closure is confirmed by TEE and the pre-tied suture is released. TEE is performed in follow-up to demonstrate absence of any LA–LAA communication.

The Lariat can be considered as an alternative when LAA diameters are too large for either Watchman or ACP devices (although the upper limit for Lariat is 40 mm). However, this approach is contraindicated in patients with prior heart surgery because of the presence of pericardial adhesions. This device should also be avoided in patients with superiorly oriented LAA or if the LAA apex is behind the pulmonary artery. The existing literature provides little insight into its effectiveness as an approach to reducing stroke or its safety relative to other approaches [13].

Post-implantation consideration and follow-up

Endocardial devices

After femoral venous sheath removal, adequate hemostasis can be obtained by manual compression or by placing a subcutaneous non-absorbable figure-of-eight stitch around the tract of the sheath

[14]. The "stitch" approach allows for adequate hemostasis by bringing the subcutaneous tissue together over the vein puncture site. Patients should be observed overnight and it is especially important that nursing staff are familiar with identifying complications that are known to occur with these procedures. Transthoracic echocardiogram (TTE) is often performed to rule out pericardial effusion prior to discharge, although this may not be necessary in experienced centers.

Anticoagulation considerations

For the Watchman device, warfarin is continued post-procedurally (INR 2.0–3.0) along with aspirin 81–100 mg/day.

After 6 weeks, a TEE is performed to confirm exclusion of the LAA:

- (i) Complete occlusion or (ii) residual leak less than 5 mm wide: warfarin can be stopped and replaced with clopidogrel 75 mg/day with increase in dose of aspirin to 300–325 mg/day. This dual antiplatelet therapy (DAT) should be continued for a total of 6 months. Thereafter, long-term aspirin at 300–325 mg is recommended.
- (iii) Leak greater than 5 mm in width or (iv) presence of thrombus over the device: the patient should be maintained on warfarin and return in 4–6 weeks for repeat imaging.

The Watchman was approved for clinical use in the USA on the basis of continued use of warfarin after device implantation and the above protocols are followed in clinical practice. However, the ASAP trial [15] investigated the use of 1–6 months of DAT—aspirin and clopidogrel daily—followed by long-term aspirin only, as an alternative to the warfarin strategy. This study demonstrated that the Watchman could be safely implanted without peri-procedural warfarin therapy with an acceptable ischemic stroke rate of 1.7% (compared to 2.2% stroke rate seen in the PROTECT-AF trial). This strategy, although not supported by randomized data, has a role in some specific clinical situations.

The ACP devices have a low thrombogenicity profile and 6 months of DAT without concomitant oral anticoagulant therapy is thought to be sufficient [16,17]. Of note, although many successful implants have been performed outside the USA using this strategy, there are no randomized data available.

Other considerations

Given that endocardial devices are prosthetic materials placed within the circulatory system, endocarditis prophylaxis for the 6 months following implantation should be prescribed when indicated. Continuing prophylaxis beyond this point is left to the physician's discretion.

Epicardial devices (Lariat)

With regards to epicardial access, a pigtail catheter is placed within the pericardial space for drainage overnight prior to removal. It is mandatory to perform a TTE before discharge to rule out pericardial effusion.

Anticoagulation considerations

Although this is typically performed in patients who cannot receive antiplatelet or anticoagulation therapy, in practice there is a marked heterogeneity in the use of these agents. Continuation of agents when possible is a reasonable strategy to prevent acute post-procedural thrombus formation [18].

Areas for future research

Except for the Watchman device, none of the other devices have been evaluated by randomized controlled trials and device-specific trials are needed to allow the use of these devices clinically with confidence. Although comparisons with warfarin have been made, further studies evaluating LAA closure techniques against NOACs are needed. In addition, enhancements in delivery techniques, device design, and device thrombogenicity will ultimately lead to improved efficacy and safety of this approach to stroke prevention.

Interactive multiple choice questions are available for this chapter on www.wiley.com/go/dangas/cardiology

References

1 Watson T, Shantsila E, Lip GY. Mechanisms of thrombogenesis in atrial fibrillation: Virchow's triad revisited. *Lancet* 2009; **373**: 155–166.

2 January CT, L. Wann S, Alpert JS, *et al.* 2014 AHA/ACC/HRS Guideline for the management of patients with atrial fibrillation: a report of the American College of Cardiology/American Heart Association Task Force on Practice Guidelines and the Heart Rhythm Society. *J Am Coll Cardiol* 2014; **64**: e1–76.

3 Granger CB, Armaganijan LV. Newer oral anticoagulants should be used as first-line agents to prevent thromboembolism in patients with atrial fibrillation and risk factors for stroke or thromboembolism. *Circulation* 2012; **125**: 159–164.

4 Holmes DR, Reddy VY, Turi ZG, *et al.* Percutaneous closure of the left atrial appendage versus warfarin therapy for prevention of stroke in patients with atrial fibrillation: a randomised non-inferiority trial. *Lancet* 2009; **374**: 534–542.

5 Holmes DR Jr, Kar S, Price MJ, *et al.* Prospective randomized evaluation of the Watchman Left Atrial Appendage Closure device in patients with atrial fibrillation versus long-term warfarin therapy: the PREVAIL trial. *J Am Coll Cardiol* 2014; **64**(1): 1–12.

6 Faxon D, Eikelboom J, Berger P, *et al.* Consensus document: antithrombotic therapy in patients with atrial fibrillation undergoing coronary stenting: a North American perspective. *Thromb Haemost* 2011; **106**: 572–584.

7 Fountain RB, Holmes DR, Chandrasekaran K, *et al.* The PROTECT AF (WATCHMAN Left Atrial Appendage System for Embolic PROTECTion in Patients with Atrial Fibrillation) Trial. *Am Heart J* 2006; **151**: 956–961.

8 Reddy VY, Holmes D, Doshi SK. The safety of percutaneous left atrial appendage closure: results from PROTECT AF and the Continued Access Registry. *Circulation* 2011; **123**: 417–424.

9 Reddy VY, Doshi SK, Sievert H, *et al.* Percutaneous left atrial appendage closure for stroke prophylaxis in patients with atrial fibrillation: 2.3-year follow-up of the PROTECT AF (Watchman Left Atrial Appendage System for Embolic Protection in Patients With Atrial Fibrillation) trial. *Circulation* 2013; **127**: 720–729.

10 Urena M, Rodés-Cabau J, Freixa X, *et al.* Percutaneous left atrial appendage closure with the AMPLATZER cardiac plug device in patients with nonvalvular atrial fibrillation and contraindications to anticoagulation therapy. *J Am Coll Cardiol* 2013; **62**(2): 96–102.

11 Freixa X1, Chan JL, Tzikas A, Garceau P, Basmadjian A, Ibrahim R. The Amplatzer™ Cardiac Plug 2 for left atrial appendage occlusion: novel features and first-in-man experience. *EuroIntervention* 2013; **8**(9): 1094–1098.

12 Meier B, Blaauw Y, Khattab AA, *et al.* EHRA/EAPCI expert consensus statement on catheter-based left atrial appendage occlusion. *Europace* 2014; **16**: 1397–1416.

13 Shetty R, Leitner J, Zhang M. Percutaneous catheter-based left atrial appendage ligation and management of periprocedural left atrial appendage perforation with the LARIAT suture delivery system. *J Invasive Cardiol* 2012; **24**: E289–293.

14 Cilingiroglu M, Salinger M, Zhao D, Feldman T. Technique of temporary subcutaneous "figure-of-eight" sutures to achieve hemostasis after removal of large-caliber femoral venous sheaths. *Catheter Cardiovasc Interv* 2011; **78**(1): 155–160.

15 Reddy VY, Möbius-Winkler S, Miller MA, *et al.* Left atrial appendage closure with the Watchman device in patients with a contraindication for oral anticoagulation: ASA Plavix Feasibility Study with Watchman Left Atrial Appendage Closure Technology (ASAP Study). *J Am Coll Cardiol* 2013; **61**: 2551–2556.

16 Park J, Bethencourt A, Sievert H, *et al.* Left atrial appendage closure with Amplatzer Cardiac Plug in atrial fibrillation: initial European experience. *Catheter Cardiovasc Interv* 2011; **77**: 700–706.

17 Krumsdorf U, Ostermayer S, Billinger K, *et al.* Incidence and clinical course of thrombus formation on atrial septal defect and patient foramen ovale closure devices in 1,000 consecutive patients. *J Am Coll Cardiol* 2004; **43**: 302–309.

18 Pillarisetti J, Reddy YM, Gunda S, *et al.* Endocardial (Watchman) versus epicardial (Lariat) left atrial appendage exclusion devices: understanding the differences in the location and type of leaks and their clinical implications. *Heart Rhythm* 2015; **12**: 1501–1507.

CHAPTER 56

Cryptogenic Stroke, Patent Foramen Ovale, and ASD Closure

Barry Love

Mount Sinai Medical Center, New York, NY, USA

Excluding bicuspid aortic valve, atrial septal defect (ASD) is the most common congenital defect first recognized in adulthood while a patent foramen ovale (PFO) is found in 20–30% of normal adults. Hemodynamically significant ASDs should be closed to treat symptoms and to prevent the sequelae of long-term left-to-right shunt. Most ASDs are of the secundum type and 80–90% can be closed percutaneously [1] with equivalent safety and efficacy to surgery in the properly selected patient [2,3]. PFO closure is more controversial. PFOs can be closed as secondary prevention after a stroke or transient ischemic attack (TIA) although the effectiveness of this strategy remains an area of controversy.

Types of ASD and PFO

The most common type of ASD is the ostium secundum type. Ostium secundum (or simply secundum) ASDs are defects that result from excessive resorbtion of septum primum during development. The "secundum" refers not to the septum, but to this being the second hole that is seen in the septum during development.

Ostium primum ASD is less common. It results as a failure of the growing septum primum to reach the AV valves and is a persistence of the first hole to be seen in the septum. Ostium primum ASD is always associated with a defect in the AV valves and is found more commonly in patients with Down syndrome. These defects cannot be closed percutaneously as the defect is contiguous with the AV valves. Other types of atrial septal defects including sinus venosus ASD and sinoseptal defects are much less common, and are not amenable to percutaneous closure.

The foramen ovale is the flap valve that persists between septum secundum to the right and septum primum to the left. Normally, the two septae fuse in the months and years after birth; however, in 20–30% of adults, the potential "trapdoor" remains. The distance that septum primum extends beyond the inferior limit of septum secundum is referred to as the tunnel, which can be quite long. Redundancy of septum primum is called an atrial septal aneurysm defined as excursion of >1 cm. Septum secundum is sometimes quite thickened (lipomatous) in older adults.

Cryptogenic stroke and its relation to PFO

Ischemic stoke is common. In older adults, the etiology is usually attributed to carotid stenosis, intracranial stenosis associated with hypertension, and cardioembolic from atrial fibrillation. Typical risk factors include age, hypertension, smoking, hypercholesterolemia, and family history.

In younger patients without these factors, stroke is much less common and the usual mechanism is referred to as cryptogenic. In patients with cryptogenic stroke, especially those younger than 55 years, a patent foramen ovale is found more often than is found in the general population (~40% compared with 20–30% in the general population) [4,5]. There is presumptive evidence that small venous thromboemboli that would be harmlessly filtered out in the lungs can pass from the right atrium to the left atrium and then pass unfiltered to the brain causing transient ischemic attack or stroke.

In a patient without a prior history of stroke or TIA and the presence of a PFO, there is generally no indication for PFO closure. The risk of a first neurologic event with a PFO is extremely low and cannot be shown to be higher than the baseline risk [6]. However, in a patient who has had a prior stroke or TIA and also has a PFO, the data suggest a risk of 1–5% per year of recurrent stroke [7]. The risk appears to be on the higher end of the range (3–5% per year) for those who have an atrial septal aneurysm in addition to the PFO [7]. In those patients, secondary prevention becomes an important goal.

To date, there have been three large randomized clinical trials, none of which showed a statistically benefit to PFO closure over medical therapy alone. Having said that, there were significant issues with these trials that may have masked a true benefit to the therapy of PFO closure in young patients with cryptogenic stroke and PFO.

The first randomized controlled trial was the Closure I trial which randomized over 900 patients with stroke or TIA to PFO closure using the Cardioseal occluder against medical therapy with warfarin or antiplatelet therapy [8]. There was not a statistically significant difference in outcome of device closure patients versus

Interventional Cardiology: Principles and Practice, Second Edition. Edited by George D. Dangas, Carlo Di Mario, and Nicholas N. Kipshidze.
© 2017 John Wiley & Sons, Ltd. Published 2017 by John Wiley & Sons, Ltd.

either medical arm and no difference between coumadin and antiplatelet therapy; however, the medical therapy arm was not randomized. The major criticism of this trial was poor patient selection in that it was felt in retrospect that many patients with other causes of stroke and TIA were not properly screened out of enrollment, leading to a higher incidence of stroke than expected in both treatment arms and lack of treatment efficacy for PFO closure.

The PC trial, published in March 2013, was a multinational, multicenter trial that randomized 414 patients with PFO and stroke, TIA, or peripheral embolization to medical therapy or device closure with an Amplatzer PFO occluder. Over 4 years, a recurrent event occurred in 3.4% of the closure group and 5.2% of the medically treated group (hazard ratio (HR) 0.62; p = 0.34). [9]. The study had difficulty enrolling especially because PFO closure was being practiced extensively outside the USA and was underpowered to detect a difference.

Published simultaneously with the PC trial was the most rigorous trial to date, the RESPECT trial comparing the Amplatzer PFO Occluder to medical therapy (warfarin or antiplatelet therapy) in patients with stroke (not TIA) [10]. The RESPECT trial enrolled 980 patients randomized 1 : 1 and completion of the trial occurred after 25 stroke events. Entry criteria were more rigorous than Closure I and the mean age of the patients was 45.9 years. In the intention-to-treat analysis over the course of the trial, there were 16 strokes in the medical therapy group and 9 in the closure group equaling a 51% risk reduction of device therapy but the p value of this difference was only 0.08 – not quite reaching statistical significance. However, on further analysis, three of the patients in the closure group did not have a device in place at the time of their stroke. When those three patients were excluded and the data analyzed on an "as-treated" basis, the risk reduction increased to 73% (p = 0.007). Subgroup analysis shows an even stronger benefit to closure in patients with atrial septal aneurysm, substantial shunt on bubble study, and to those treated with antiplatelet therapy versus anticoagulation. The risk of PFO closure was low with a 2.4% incidence of procedure-related events and a 2% incidence of device-related events—none fatal.

Based on these data, the trial sponsor (St. Jude Medical) has submitted an application to the FDA for the Amplatzer PFO occluder for secondary prevention of stroke in patients with PFO. However, despite the data being published for more than 2 years, the FDA has yet to make a determination. The significance of the study results are debated in the medical literature [11,12]. PFO closure is being performed outside the USA using various occluders, and in the USA off-label using the Amplatzer™ Cribriform Septal Occluder, and also with the Gore® Helex® Occluder/Cardioform. A third randomized trial is underway comparing the Gore Helex/Cardioform Occluder to medical therapy but enrollment has been difficult.

Our practice has been to offer PFO closure to patients with PFO and cryptogenic stroke after a full disclosure of the state of the science and discussion of the small risk of the procedure. The usual patient is between 18 and 60 years of age with a PFO demonstrated by transesophageal echocardiography (TEE), with positive bubble study, and a prior stroke or TIA with no other cause demonstrated. The stroke work-up is ideally undertaken in partnership with a stroke neurologist to exclude other etiologies for stroke that will not be helped by PFO closure.

The presence of an atrial septal aneurysm and strongly positive bubble study makes the case for closure more compelling and, in our opinion, a reasonable option for patients. There is certainly

no benefit to having a PFO, and so the arguments against closure are the risk of the procedure (low), and the cost. Insurance coverage for off-label PFO closure has been variable in the USA, with some insurers outright refusing to cover the procedure and others willing to pay for the procedure based on the available data.

A rare indication for PFO closure absent stroke or TIA is the patient with orthodeoxia-platypnea syndrome as a result of right to left flow at the atrial septal defect. This unusual circumstance can be seen following a pulmonary lobectomy in a patient with a PFO. In this instance, upright positioning directs the inferior vena cava (IVC) flow across the PFO resulting in significant right to left shunt and desaturation (orthodeoxia) and shortness of breath (platypnea) in the upright position. These patients have a very large bubble shunt seen on echocardiography – worse in the upright position. PFO closure in these patients is curative [13].

Patients with PFO closed for secondary stroke/TIA prevention have reported an improvement or even cure of recurrent migraine symptoms that were present prior to closure. Patients with migraine and aura are more likely to have a PFO (40–60%) than found in the general population (20–30%) [14]. Despite initial enthusiasm, only a single trial of prospective studies to assess PFO closure as a therapy for recurrent migraine in patients without stroke or TIA has been completed, with disappointing results [15].

Atrial septal defect
Physiology
Although ASD is usually diagnosed in childhood, it is also the most commonly diagnosed congenital condition in adulthood (excluding bicuspid aortic valve). It is not uncommon to see an adult patient with a significant ASD with only subtle physical examination findings. In addition, flow across an ASD is dependent on the *relative* diastolic compliances between the right and left ventricles. With increasing age, the left ventricle becomes less compliant, increasing the flow across an ASD that had otherwise gone undetected. Symptoms of shortness of breath on exertion can start to appear in middle age onwards as a result of the increased flow. Atrial fibrillation as a result of chronic left and right atrial stretch from volume starts to be seen in the fourth and fifth decade onwards.

Indications for closure
ASDs that have a shunt fraction of ≥ 1.5 : 1 should be closed as these have been shown to be enough of a hemodynamic burden to increase the risk of right heart failure, arrhythmias (mainly atrial fibrillation), and pulmonary hypertension (PAH) with time [16]. In addition, exercise capacity is increased in patients undergoing closure for hemodynamically significant ASD [17]. Severe PAH, especially in a younger patient, is a relative contraindication to closure and can hasten their demise. Advanced PAH therapy should be considered and these patients should be managed in conjunction with an experienced PAH center. Some benefit from ASD closure if they respond to treatment [18]. Milder pulmonary hypertension in older patients (<½ systemic pressure) is common and usually improves with closure as pressure = flow/resistance. When the flow across the pulmonary bed is reduced, the corresponding pressure will decrease as well.

The size of an ASD in the adult that can lead to a significant shunt is usually one that is larger than 6 mm. Smaller ASDs in the adult are not associated with enough left to right shunt to warrant closure on a hemodynamic basis.

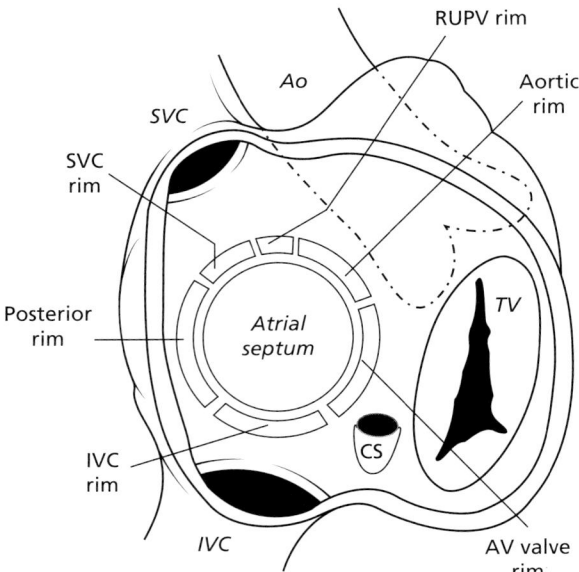

Figure 56.1 Atrial septum defect (ASD) rims. Atrial septum as viewed from the right atrial surface. The rim that is usually deficient to some degree is the antero-superior or aortic rim. Large defects often have limited inferior vena cava (IVC) rim for a distance and are called IVC confluent.

ASD transcatheter closure: patient selection

For patients with ASD, a TEE showing a secundum ASD and right ventricular dilatation is required. Further anatomic information can be obtained with a pre-procedural TEE but this step can also be obtained at the time of closure if the transthoracic images are good. A good device candidate is one where the defect is large enough to warrant closure, but not so large as to make closure unlikely to be successful. The usual "window" where this falls is a defect of 6–26 mm in diameter. The occluder size needed for closure will be several millimeters larger than the static dimension measured on echocardiography. Smaller than 6 mm is unlikely to require closure and larger than 26 mm becomes less likely that a device will be able to close the defect without embolization. The largest ASD occluder is a 40-mm Amplatzer Septal Occluder (38 mm in the USA); however, devices this large are rarely used and are best limited to centers with extensive ASD closure experience. There is always discussion about adequacy of atrial septal "rims" for closure (Figure 56.1). The minimum rim is frequently quoted as 5 mm; however, in practice, many patients have deficiency especially of the anterior rim and can have a successful implantation provided the remainder of the rims are adequate and the device is not oversized [19].

Closure of ASD and PFO

In 1995, the Amplatzer Septal Occluder was first introduced for human study for closure of atrial septal defect and gained CE mark in 1998 and FDA approval in 2001. The Gore Helex Occluder was FDA approved in 2006 and has been recently supplanted by the newer Gore Cardioform Occluder that was FDA approved in 2015. Gore has ceased manufacturing the Helex occluder since mid 2015. There are no devices yet approved for PFO closure in the USA.

The Amplatzer Septal Occluder (ASO) is made from a winding of nitinol wire creating two disks and a central waist with polyester

fabric disks sewn into the mesh to create an occluding surface. This device was the first approved device to close ASDs and gained widespread popularity owing to its simple design, ease of use, and excellent closure characteristics. The device is sized according to the central waist ranging from 4 to 40 mm (38 mm in the USA) (Table 56.1).

The Amplatzer Cribiform Septal Occluder is a modified version of the ASO designed to close multifenestrated atrial septal defects. This occluder is different from the ASO in that the central waist is narrow and closure relies on the disks of the occluder. The Cribiform occluder is available in four sizes: 18, 25, 30, and 35 mm which corresponds to the size of the disks. The cribiform occluder is very similar to the PFO occluder used in the RESPECT study; however, the PFO occluder has a uniform 18 mm left atrial disk and the right atrial disk is 18, 25, or 35 mm in diameter. Owing to the design, the cribiform occluder is most used for off-label PFO closure in the USA.

The Gore Helex occluder is a winding of a nitinol wire frame with a Goretex (ePTFE) bag that, when extruded from the delivery catheter, creates two disks of equal size. Unlike the Amplatzer, the device size refers to the size of the disks. The device sizes are available from 15 to 35 mm in 5-mm increments. The Helex occluder has been supplanted by the newly approved Gore Septal Occluder (renamed the Gore Cardioform). The Cardioform is a multilobed nitinol frame with a Goretex bag. The device is superior to the Helex in that the multilobed design is more rigid and less prone to embolization. The simple delivery handle system is also an improvement over the clumsy push–pull technique needed for the Helex. The Cardioform is available in sizes from 15 to 30 mm in 5-mm increments with a recommended 1.7 : 1 sizing ratio also making the device best suited to small and medium-sized defects up to 17 mm.

Contraindications to ASD and PFO closure

The usual considerations of active infection or left atrial thrombus would preclude patients from a closure procedure. Defects other than PFO or secundum ASD cannot be closed with current device technology. The presence of a temporary IVC filter is sometimes encountered in patients undergoing PFO closure. Venography should be undertaken in those patients to ensure that there is not a large thrombus on the filter that could be dislodged with paradoxical embolization. Congenitally interrupted IVC with azygous continuation is rarely encountered but makes closure from the femoral approach impossible. Transhepatic access for closure or an superior vena cava (SVC) approach could be attempted by experienced operators in settings where the IVC approach is contraindicated.

Technique

ASD and PFO closure are similar. We will begin the discussion with the elements that are common to both and diverge for the differences.

Premedication

Aspirin 81 mg is usually started 3–5 days beforehand. For patients with aspirin sensitivity, clopidogrel 75 mg/dly can be used instead.

Femoral venous access provides the preferred angle for ASD and PFO closure. ASD and PFO closure is difficult from the SVC approach owing to the sharp angle needed to cross back from right atrium to left atrium with a relatively large, stiff sheath. Arterial access is not usually performed unless concomitant coronary angiography is required. For patients > 50 years of age in whom

Table 56.1 Comparison of devices available for atrial septal defect (ASD) and patent foramen ovale (PFO) closure.

Device	Device image	Indications	Labeled sizes (mm)	Central waist (mm)	Right atrial disk	Left atrial disk	Delivery sheath
Amplatzer Septal Occluder		ASD closure	4–40 (38 in USA)	= labeled size	Central waist + 8 mm for sizes up to 10 mm Central waist + 12 mm for sizes ≥11 mm	Central waist + 10 mm for sizes up to 10 mm Central waist + 14 mm for sizes ≥11 mm. (+16 mm for sizes ≥34 mm)	7–12 Fr
Amplatzer Cribiform Septal Occluder		Multiply fenestrated ASD PFO*	18 25 30 35	2	= labeled size	= labeled size	8 Fr
Amplatzer PFO Occluder		PFO closure (outside USA)	18 25 35	2	= labeled size	18 mm for all	8 Fr

(Continued)

Table 56.1 (Continued)

Device	Device image	Indications	Labeled sizes (mm)	Central waist (mm)	Right atrial disk	Left atrial disk	Delivery sheath
Gore Helex		ASD and PFO* No longer manufactured	15 20 25 30 35	None	= labeled size	= labeled size	9 Fr without guidewire 12 Fr with guidewire
Gore Cardioform		ASD and PFO*	15 20 25 30	None	= labeled size	=labeled size	9 Fr without guidewire 12 Fr with guidewire

* Denotes off-label use in USA.

there is a large ASD and risk of device embolization, we perform coronary angiography routinely prior to attempting ASD closure in case surgery is required.

For atrial septal defect, a right heart catheterization is performed to assess cardiac pressures and shunt fraction. For PFO, unless there are other issues, we usually do not assess hemodynamics.

Heparinization is achieved with 100 U/kg heparin to a maximum of 5000 units with an activated clotting time (ACT) goal of ≥250 s.

Imaging for ASD and PFO closure

Single plane fluoroscopy is sufficient for ASD and PFO closure and echocardiographic imaging is required for both.

TEE is most commonly used for ASD closure, while intracardiac echocardiography (ICE) is a good alternative for PFO closure and also for smaller ASDs. For TEE, the echocardiographer or anesthesiologist will be an indispensable ally in assessment of the atrial septum, device selection, and assessment of device positioning across the atrial septum. Two-dimensional imaging is usually better than three-dimensional imaging for assessing defect size and rims (Figure 56.2).

For ICE, the interventionalist usually also interprets the images. The advantage of ICE is that the procedure can be performed with minimal sedation without the use of anesthesia and with a faster post-procedure recovery. TEE generally provides a better view of the atrial septum and we prefer this imaging for larger ASDs. ICE probes are disposable and cost in the range of $2500 each. There are companies that will resterilize used probes and sell them back (usually at about half the cost of a new probe) for up to three times of use.

Intracardiac echocardiography

Two ICE imaging systems are available: Seimens AcuNav and St Jude Viewflex. The Siemens probes are available in 8 and 10 Fr and the St. Jude catheter needs a 10 Fr introducer. Unlike intravascular ultrasound (IVUS), ICE has a "forward looking" array rather than a circumferential array to give a two-dimensional view of the anatomy. Both ICE probes have handles that allow for two degrees of freedom of movement of the tip—forward and backward in the plane of the array and side-to-side—and also have color Doppler for assessment of flow. Access for the additional catheter is usually performed in the same femoral vein as access for the catheterization a few millimeters inferior to the first needle entry.

The ICE catheter is advanced to the right atrium. Often this needs to be done under fluoroscopy as the catheter tends to "snag" in venous tributaries and patients complain of back pain when it occurs. The atrial septum is best viewed by retroflexing the catheter and turning the catheter clockwise past the aorta to view the septum in a "long axis" view (Figure 56.2, Aa). The foramen ovale is seen in this view. Color Doppler interrogation can be performed to assess for ASD and the catheter should be rotated clockwise and counterclockwise to "sweep" the atrial septum for ASD. The catheter can then be further retroflexed and rotated rightward to view the septum in a "short axis" view (Figure 56.2, Bb). The aortic rim of tissue is best viewed in this plane to assess for deficiency. The ASD should be measured in both planes. For patients with PFO, a bubble study can be performed at this point to assess for right to left bubble shunt. The patient can be instructed to perform a Valsalva to bring out right to left shunt not observable at rest.

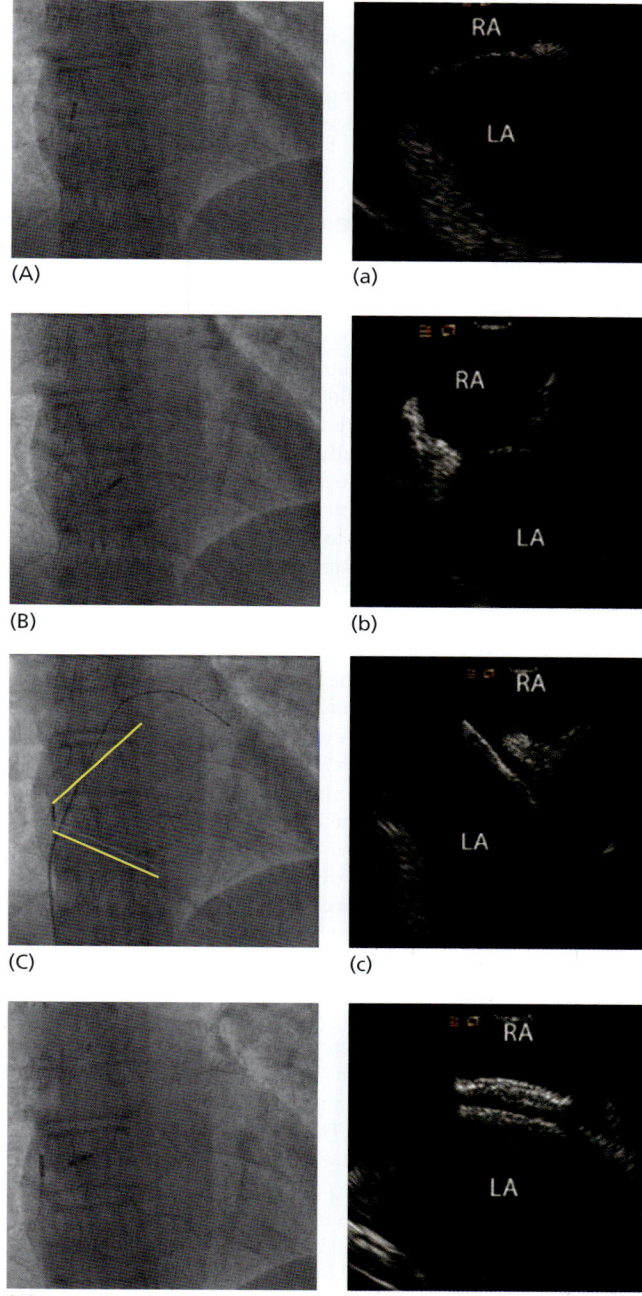

Figure 56.2 Intracardiac echocardiogram and corresponding fluoroscopic images during patent foramen ovale (PFO) closure. Note that unlike transesophageal echocardiography, the right atrium (RA) is the closest chamber to the probe. A: ICE catheter in RA retroflexed to view atrial septum in long axis (a). B: ICE catheter further retroflexed and turned clockwise to view atrial septum in short axis (b). C: Crossing PFO with multipurpose catheter and Magic Torque wire. Note that wire crosses the septum at the level of the catheter imaging the PFO. The wire tip is in the left atrial appendage (c) wire crossing PFO. D: Following placement of a 25 mm Amplatzer™ Cribiform Occluder, the device is visualized in the long-axis with ICE (d).

Once the defect is crossed and closure is underway, the septum can be viewed as the left atrial disk contacts the septum and after the right atrial disk is formed. Final device position and a postprocedure color Doppler interrogation for ASD or bubble study for PFO can then be performed (Figure 56.2, Dd).

ASD and PFO closure precedure

After access and interrogation of the atrial septum with ICE or TEE, the ASD/PFO is crossed in preparation for closure. The easiest catheter and wire combination in our experience is a 6 Fr Multipurpose catheter and a 0.035–260 cm Magic Torque wire (Boston Scientific). The advantage of this wire is that it is very directable, the floppy tip avoids damage to cardiac structures, and the relatively stiff shaft can be used as the guidewire over which the delivery sheath is advanced for PFO closure without the need to exchange guidewires. The multipurpose catheter is positioned in the lower one-third of the right atrium and the tip is directed to the patient's left and then turned clockwise. Clockwise rotation points the tip posteriorly where the atrial septum lies. The atrial septum is probed with the wire and entry to the left atrium is confirmed when the wire crosses to the left of the spine without ventricular ectopy. If ventricular ectopy is encountered, the wire is in the right ventricle and needs to be withdrawn and probing continued more posteriorly (more clockwise rotation of the catheter). One "trick" that can be used to help cross the PFO/ASD is that with ICE or TEE, the ultrasound array that is imaging the PFO/ASD must be at the same superior/inferior location as the PFO for the imaging. Under fluoroscopy, the array can be visualized and probing aimed at that level (Figure 56.2, Cc). In our experience, the ultrasound image itself is not particularly helpful in probing for the defect as the part of the wire that is seen tantalizingly near to the defect may be the shaft and not the tip.

Once the PFO/ASD is crossed, the tip of the wire will often lie in the left atrial appendage (LAA) (Figure 56.2, C) The wire is seen to be at the left upper heart border, and usually curls back to the LA. This is not a good wire position as the thin LAA can be perforated with a wire or the device delivery system. It is best to have wire position in a left pulmonary vein. This is accomplished by advancing the MP catheter over the wire to the middle of the spine, withdrawing the wire, turning clockwise (posterior), and probing for the pulmonary vein. The wire will pass beyond the heart border when it is in a left pulmonary vein.

Some advocate a trans-septal puncture to close PFOs with a long tunnel. In order perform a trans-septal puncture, septum primum needs to be entered quite a bit more inferior than normal or the trans-septal needle will just ride up the septum and cross the PFO. A device placed lower in the septum may not then adequately close the PFO. In our experience, we have only rarely needed to consider a trans-septal puncture to adequately close a PFO. For long tunnels, the Amplatzer Cribiform Occluder is better at closing the defect than the Gore occluders.

ASD sizing

The ASD is first sized by TEE or ICE in the static dimension in orthogonal planes and the rims are assessed. The retroaortic rim is usually this most important and is most often deficient (i.e., less

than 5 mm). If the rim is deficient for only a small distance, then device implantation is probably safe. A large distance of "bare" aorta, however, with no rim should alert the implanter to use caution in device selection and consider avoiding the Amplatzer Septal Occluder because of the risk of device erosion. Balloon-sizing the defect is important in device selection in all but the smallest of ASDs. A 24 or 34 mm compliant sizing balloon (St. Jude Medical) is used for this purpose. The initial guidewire used to cross the ASD is exchanged for an Amplatz Super Stiff Guidewire (Boston Scientific) with a short (2 cm) floppy tip with the tip placed in a left pulmonary vein. The balloon is inflated under fluoroscopy using dilute contrast (20% contrast, 80% saline) across the ASD until there is no longer flow seen crossing the defect under echocardiography (the so called "stop-flow" diameter). At this point, a small indentation or "waist" is seen fluoroscopically on the balloon (Figure 56.3d) A short cine run is taken and a note made of the exact amount of volume remaining in the syringe used to inflate the balloon. The balloon is then deflated and removed. The balloon is then reinflated outside the body to the same volume stopping at the same point where stop-flow point was encountered. A sizing plate (St. Jude Medical) can then be used to compare the indentation on the balloon seen fluoroscopically with a similar indentation formed when the balloon is placed through varying sizes on a sizing plate. When the same amount of indentation is found, this is the "stop-flow" diameter. This size can also be calculated from the cine image using the marker bands for sizing and it can also be performed by echocardiography; however, we find these two methods to be less reliable than the sizing plate method.

ASD device selection

If the stop-flow diameter is up to 17 mm, both the Gore Cardioform or Amplatzer Septal Defect Occluder can be considered. Larger defects are only suitable for the Amplatzer Septal Occluder. Practically speaking, even the largest Cardioform is much less likely to deploy satisfactorily if the stop-flow is larger than 15 mm.

If there is minimal retroaortic rim, the Cardioform may be advantageous in reducing the risk of device erosion (Figure 56.3a). However, from a practical standpoint, device erosion has been reported mainly for Amplatzer occluder sizes >18 mm and so the risk reduction for the Gore occluder may be overstated.

For Amplatzer sizing, a device at, or 1–2 mm larger than the stop-flow diameter is chosen, keeping in mind that the central waist is the labeled diameter for the Amplatzer occluders. For the Gore Cardioform Occluder, a device at least 1.7× and preferably 2× the the stop-flow diameter is chosen. In our experience, almost all adults with an ASD suitable for the Cardioform occluder receive the 30 mm occluder.

PFO device selection

Although some advocate balloon-sizing for PFO closure, in our experience this has not proved helpful or necessary. The vast majority of PFOs are closed with a 25 mm Amplatzer Cribiform Occluder, or a 20 or 25 mm Helex or Cardioform Occluder. For a very aneurysmal septum, we find a 30 mm Amplatzer Cribiform Occluder is better at stabilizing more of the septum.

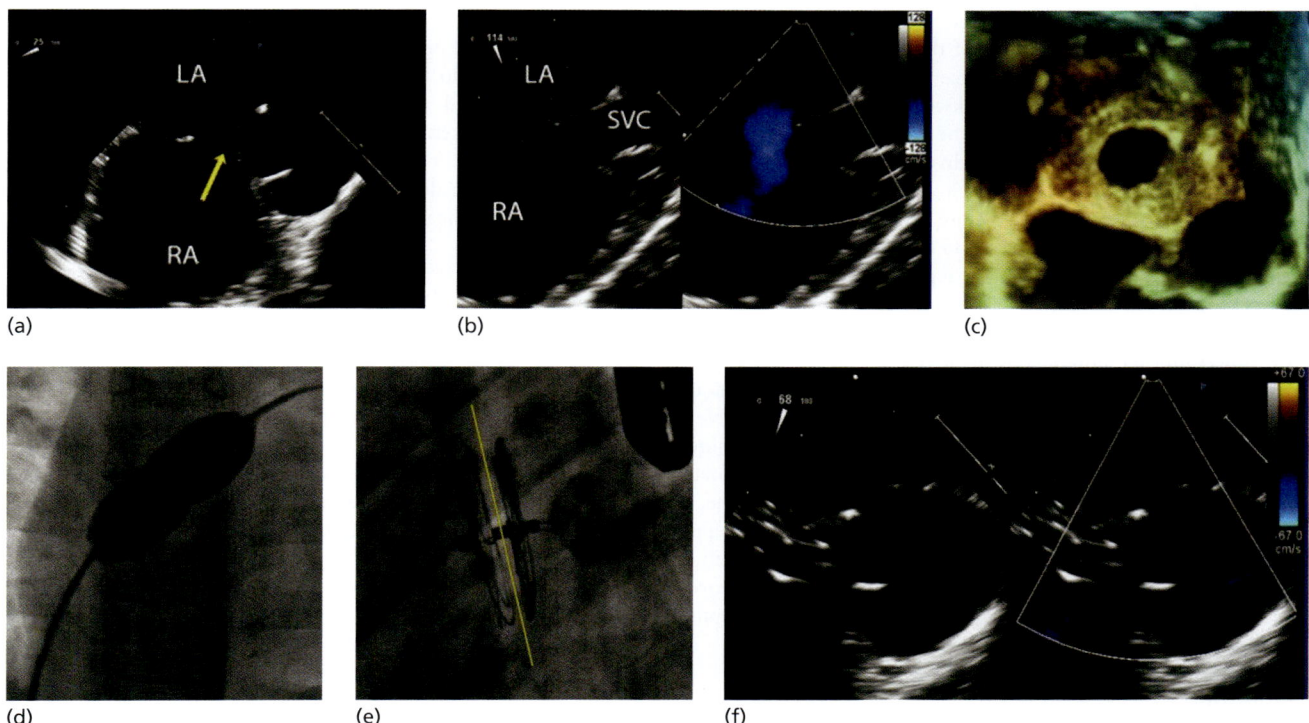

Figure 56.3 ASD closure with a Gore® Cardioform. (a) TEE short axis view of the ASD showing 12 mm defect in that plane with minimal retroaortic rim (arrow). (b) TEE long axis view of the septum showing also 12 mm defect in the orthogonal plane. Note the relatively short distance as well to the superior vena cava (SVC). (c) 3D TEE from the left atrial view showing the ASD. Although the 3D image confirms that the ASD is circular, the relationship to the other cardiac structures is not well seen in 3D. (d) Balloon-sizing of th ASD showing a 15 mm "stop-flow" diameter. (e) Following device release the 30 mm Gore Cardioform Occluder is viewed in a steep LAO view. Note the separation of the disks when the LA and RA disks are on their respective sides (yellow line). (f) TEE post-device release shows good device position and no residual color flow across the ASD.

Device delivery

Amplatzer Cribiform and Amplatzer Septal Occluder

The Amplatzer devices use a long sheath as part of the delivery system. For all sizes of the Cribiform, an 8 Fr delivery system is acceptable. For the Septal occluder, delivery systems ranging 7–12 Fr are used depending on the size of the device. The device is screwed on to the delivery cable that has been put through the loader. Care is taken not to screw the device on too tight on the cable otherwise release can prove challenging. The device is then withdrawn into the loader submerged in a bowl of saline. The device is advanced just to the tip of the loader. Any residual air is flushed from the loader by squeezing about 20 mL saline through the side port of the loader while tapping the loader to disengage any bubbles.

The short sheath is then removed and the delivery sheath passed over the wire. The long sheath positioned in the left atrium over the wire with the dilator approaching but not entering the left pulmonary vein. The sheath is then advanced off the dilator to the tip. The wire and dilator are then removed. The next step is critical. Especially in a spontaneously breathing patient (i.e., when using ICE instead of TEE), the left atrial pressure in young patients without left-sided disease often phasically dips below 0 mmHg—especially if the patient is snoring. If care is not taken, a large air embolism can be entrained through the long sheath into the left atrium with potentially catastrophic results. A minor air embolism is usually noted by ST elevation in the inferior leads because of embolization to the right coronary artery. If that occurs, administration of 100% oxygen and elevation of the systemic arterial pressure with vasoconstrictors usually resolves the issue within a few minutes. To avoid this problem, the tip of the sheath should be covered with a finger immediately once the dilator is removed and a syringe attached quickly to the hub. To remove any air in the sheath, 10–20 mL of freely aspirated blood should be withdrawn. The loader is then connected to the hub while continually flushing saline through the loader to ensure a "bubble-free" connection.

The device is advanced to the tip of the delivery sheath by advancing the delivery cable. The delivery sheath is pulled back to the middle of the left atrium and the left atrial disk is then delivered by pushing the device out of the sheath. The entire apparatus is then withdrawn until the left atrial disk is opposed to the septum. This is felt by gentle resistance on the delivery cable and also by visualizing the left atrial disk against the septum on the echocardiogram. The delivery cable is then held fixed against the table and the sheath is withdrawn uncovering the central waist and right atrial disk in the case of a Septal occluder or just the right atrial disk in the case of a Cribiform occluder. The delivery cable is then advanced to form the right atrial disk against the septum. A gentle push–pull of the delivery cable ensures that the device is correctly opposed to the septum. If the device is not in a good position, the device can be recaptured into the delivery sheath and delivery reattempted. If the device is recaptured in the right atrium, the delivery sheath is sufficiently curved to allow crossing of the atrial septum with the device at the tip of the delivery sheath; however, this should be performed very cautiously as inadvertent cardiac perforation could occur if not at the atrial septum.

The device position is re-evaluated by echocardiography and if both disks are on the correct side of the septum and there is not deformation of the aorta by the device, the device can be released. This is accomplished by counterclockwise unscrewing of the delivery cable using the torque tool on the back of the delivery cable. Once the device releases from the delivery cable, it will reorient on the septum as the torque from the delivery cable is removed.

Larger ASDs can be difficult to close because the leading edge of the left atrial disk tends to cross over to the right of the aortic rim as the device is withdrawn against the septum. In that instance, one can try to deploy the central waist and right atrial disk more leftward but that often results in the entire device deploying on the left atrial side. Multiple attempts at deployment and recapturing the device are sometimes required. There have been many techniques described to overcome this difficulty; however, the most reliable in our experience has been the right upper pulmonary vein technique. After the left atrial disk is deployed, the delivery system is rotated clockwise until the left atrial disk orients in a horizontal plane. At that moment, the left atrial disk is in the mouth of the right upper pulmonary vein. The device is withdrawn until resistance is felt on the septum and the central waist and right atrial disk are deployed. The device will usually "snap" into position across the atrial septum with this maneuver.

Cardioform

The Cardioform device is first prepared outside the body by submerging the occluder in saline, flushing the delivery system, and then withdrawing the device inside the catheter. The delivery catheter for all sizes is 9 Fr but a 12 Fr sheath is necessary to pass the delivery system with the use of a guidewire. We find this most advantageous and the small increase in sheath size is not problematic. The delivery system is then advanced to the middle of the left atrium over the guidewire and the wire is then withdrawn. The left atrial disk is then formed with a simple forward motion of the slider until the left atrial disk is completely formed. The delivery catheter is then withdrawn against the septum and the right atrial disk is formed by completing the forward motion of the slider. A gentle push–pull of the delivery catheter can be performed to ensure stable position against the atrial septum. The device is evaluated by ultrasound and good position with each disk on the correct side of the atrial septum is ensured. If the device is not in satisfactory position, the device can be recaptured by simply retracting the slider and the process can be repeated.

When the device is in good position, the lock loop is set by pinching and sliding the release mechanism. The device usually reorients a fair bit on the atrial septum when the tension of the delivery system is removed. The frontal camera should be moved to a steep LAO to see both left and right atrial disks perpendicular to each other. When the device is in a good position, a straight line can be drawn between the disks that does not cross any of the "petals" of the frame (Figure 56.3, E). If this cannot be done, one needs to suspect that the device is not in a good position across the septum and consideration should be given to removing the device and reattempting placement with a new occluder.

When the lock loop is set and device position is satisfactory, the retrieval cord is removed by lifting up the red retrieval cord handle and applying gentle smooth traction on the cord. This needs to be done gently as too much force risks dislodging the device. Once the retrieval cord is removed, the delivery system can be removed from the body. A final examination of the device is performed with echocardiography (Figure 56.3f).

Once the lock loop is set, device placement is committed. However, the device can still be removed if needed at this point using the retrieval cord. To do this, the outer sheath as part of the delivery system is unscrewed, and the device is withdrawn into the sheath. Care needs to be taken with the maneuver as the device is being held by only the retrieval cord. Overly aggressive pulling can break this safety cable making device removal more complex, necessitating a snare and a larger sheath and risking embolization.

Completing the procedure

The device is reassessed using echocardiographic imaging and a final bubble study performed if the indication was PFO closure. The delivery sheath and ICE probe are removed and the sheaths are removed. Hemostasis is obtained with manual pressure. We do not reverse heparin as it can lead to thrombosis on the device. As the access is venous only, hemostasis usually takes just a few minutes. The tracking forms for device implantation need to be completed and returned to the manufacturer as required by the FDA.

Adverse events

Serious adverse events are reported in 0.3–0.5% of all implants [20,21]. Of these, perforation/tamponade and embolization predominate. Device embolization generally occurs during the procedure or within the first 12 hours post-procedure. If the device embolizes to the aorta or pulmonary artery, transcatheter retrieval is feasible. To retrieve an embolized device, the screw (Amplatzer) or end (Helex or Cardioform) needs to be firmly grasped using a snare, and the device withdrawn into a sheath at least 2 Fr sizes larger than the size used to place the device. The device should be fully withdrawn into a long sheath prior to pulling the device through the heart. If the device is lodged in the right or left ventricle, it is inadvisable to attempt catheter removal as this risks tearing the chordae of the tricuspid or mitral valve. This is then best left to the surgeon to remove and close the defect at the same time.

Other rare risks of device closure include endocarditis, stroke, thrombus on the device, air embolism, and device erosion. The risk of erosion has been reported only with the Amplatzer occluder and occurs in 1–3/1000 implants [22]. Device oversizing has been implicated as risk factor as has implantation with retroaortic rim <2 mm. The risk of "insufficient rim," however, has not been clearly established and at least 40% of secundum ASDs have some measure of deficient rim. This has therefore been labeled a "warning" and not a contraindication for device placement. We feel that careful assessment of the aorta is indicated after device placement and if the device appears to impinge on the aorta, we consider device removal and either reattempting with a smaller device or abandoning the procedure. Device erosion usually occurs within the first few months after closure but late reports of erosion beyond a year have been known to occur. If a patient complains of chest pain following ASD closure, they should be evaluated by echocardiography. If a new pericardial effusion is present, consideration should be given to an erosion event and cardiac surgical consultation obtained promptly.

Arrhythmias—mainly atrial fibrillation—occurs in about 0.5% of patients [2]. Older age is a risk factor. Patients with longstanding shunt from ASD are at risk for atrial fibrillation. Once established, atrial fibrillation will not be improved by ASD closure. In some patients, we have referred for ablation or left atrial appendage occlusion prior to ASD closure.

Headaches are seen in some patients following closure with the Amplatzer Septal Occluder. This seems to occur more frequently in patients with a history of migraine. It is felt to be caused by platelet activation and changing the antiplatelet regimen to clopidogrel from aspirin seems to resolve the symptoms promptly in most patients [23].

There are rare reports of patients experiencing persistent symptoms of chest pain, palpitations, and shortness of breath following Amplatzer Septal Occluder implantation that are thought to be a result of nickel allergy [24]. In some patients, symptoms improve following surgical explant. This phenomenon is very rare, however, compared with the prevalence of nickel sensitivity in the general population (~8%) and we do not routinely test for nickel sensitivity prior to implantation.

Aftercare

Patients undergoing PFO or small ASD closure are usually discharged the same day, whereas we keep patients with larger ASDs overnight to assess for embolization with a transthoracic echocardiogram the following morning. Outpatient follow-up visits with a transthoracic echocardiogram are recommended at 1 week, 1 month, 6 months, and then yearly thereafter. Because the risk of erosion is low and no known methods are able to predict this in follow-up, we feel that unless there are ongoing concerns, follow-up can be generally discontinued after a year and patients instructed that if they experience cardiac symptoms they should be re-evaluated.

Antiplatelet therapy for ASD and PFO closure (aspirin 81 mg or clopridogrel 75 mg) is continued for 6 months until the device is fully endothelialized. At this point, antiplatelet therapy is stopped for ASD patients. However, for PFO patients, we feel that continuing ASA 81 mg/day is a reasonable recommendation based on a "belt and suspenders" approach—that is, some of the strokes that occur in patients undergoing PFO closure are related to other factors and aspirin is helpful to decrease the risk of recurrent events in those patients.

Endocarditis prophylaxis is recommended for dental visits for 6 months following device placement and can then be discontinued. For practical purposes, we recommend that patients avoid routine dental work for 6 months.

The devices are all MRI compatible.

Future directions

The FDA are to decide in the near future if the RESPECT data warrants a device-specific approval for PFO closure in cryptogenic stroke. The Gore REDUCE trial will complete enrollment as another randomized trial comparing device with medical closure in the management of cryptogenic stroke and TIA. New devices continue to be developed to improve on closing larger ASDs while minimizing the risk of complications. Gore currently has a next generation Cardioform in development with self-centering properties to allow larger defects to be closed. Without a PFO market, companies are wary of investing significant resources in new ASD closure designs as the risks are high and the rewards are limited given the smaller population of patients with ASD than with other diseases.

Interactive multiple choice questions are available for this chapter on www.wiley.com/go/dangas/cardiology

References

1 Butera G, Romagnoli E, Carminati M, *et al.* Treatment of isolated atrial septal defects: impact of age and defect morphology in 1013 consecutive patients. *Am Heart J* 2008; **156**: 706–712.

2 Du ZD, Hijazi ZM, Kleinman CS, *et al.*; Amplatzer Investigators. Comparison between transcatheter and surgical closure of secundum atrial septal defect in children and adults: results of a multicenter nonrandomized trial. *J Am Coll Cardiol* 2002; **39**: 1836–1844.

3 Jones TK, Latson A, Zahn E, *et al.* Results of the US Multicenter pivotal study of the HELEX septal occluder for percutaneous closure of secundum atrial septal defects. *J Am Coll Cardiol* 2007; **49**: 2215–2221.

4 Hagen PT, Scholz DG, Edwards WD. Incidence and size of patent foramen ovale during the first 10 decades of life: an autopsy study of 965 normal hearts. *Mayo Clin Proc* 1984; **59**: 17–20.

5 Lechat P, Mas JL, Lascault G, *et al.* Prevalence of patent foramen ovale in patients with stroke. *N Engl J Med* 1988; **318**(10): 1148–1152.

6 Di Tullio MR, Sacco RL, Sciacca RR, *et al.* Patent foramen ovale and the risk of ischemic stroke in a multiethnic population. *J Am Coll Cardiol* 2007; **49**: 797–802.

7 Mas JL, Arquizan C, Lamy C, *et al.* Recurrent cerebrovascular events associated with patent foramen ovale, atrial septal aneurysm, or both. *N Engl J Med* 2001; **345**: 1740–1746.

8 Furlan AJ, Reisman M, Massaro J, *et al.* Closure or medical therapy for cryptogenic stroke with patent foramen ovale. *N Engl J Med* 2012; **366**: 991–9.

9 Meier B, Kalesan B, Mattle HP, *et al.* percutaneous closure of patent foramen ovale in cryptogenic embolism. *N Engl J Med* 2013; **368**: 1083–1091.

10 Carroll JD, Saver JL, Thaler DE, *et al.* Closure of patent foramen ovale versus medical therapy after cryptogenic stroke. *N Engl J Med* 2013; **368**: 1092–1100.

11 Calvet D, Mas JL. Closure of patent foramen ovale in cryptogenic stroke: a never ending story. *Curr Opin Neurol* 2014; **27**(1): 13–19.

12 Nietlispach F, Meier B. Percutaneous closure of patent foramen ovale: safe and effective but underutilized. *Expert Rev Cardiovasc Ther* 2015; **13**(2): 121–123.

13 Cheng TO. Transcatheter closure of patent foramen ovale: a definitive treatment for playpnea-orthodeoxia. *Catheter Cardiovasc Interv* 2000; **51**: 120.

14 Del Sette M, Angeli S, Leandri M, *et al.* Migraine with aura and right-to-left shunt on transcranial Doppler: a case–control study. *Cerebrovasc Dis* 1998; **8**: 327–330.

15 Dowson A, Mullen MJ, Peatfield R, *et al.* Migraine Intervention with StarFlex Technology (MIST) Trial. *Circulation* 2008; **117**: 1397–1404.

16 Murphy JG, Gersh BJ, McGoon MD, *et al.* Long-term outcome after surgical repair of isolated atrial septal defect: follow-up at 27 to 32 years. *N Engl J Med* 1990; **323**: 1645–1650.

17 Brochu MC, Baril JF, Dore A, *et al.* Improvement in exercise capacity in asymptomatic and mildly symptomatic adults after percutaneous atrial septal defect closure. *J Am Coll Cardiol* 2001; **37**: 2108–2113.

18 Frost AE, Quinones MA, Zoghbi WA, *et al.* Reversal of pulmonary hypertension and subsequent repair of atrial septal defect after treatment with continuous intravenous epoprostenol. *J Heart Lung Transplant* 2005; **25**: 501–503.

19 Zhong-Dong D, Koenig P, Qi-Ling C, *et al.* Comparison of transcatheter closure of secundum atrial septal defect using the Amplatzer Septal Occluder associated with deficient versus sufficient rims. *Am J Cardiol* 2002; **90**(8): 865–869.

20 Omeish A, Hijazi ZM. Transcatheter closure of atrial septal defects in children and adults using the Amplatzer Septal Occluder. *J Interv Cardiol* 2001; **14**: 37–44.

21 Majunke N, Bialkowski J, Wilson N. Closure of atrial septal defect with the Amplatzer Septal Occluder in adults. *Am J Cardiol* 2009; **103**: 550–554.

22 Letter from St. Jude Medical to Implanters of the AMPLZTER Septal Occluder January 17, 2013.

23 Kato Y, Kobayashi T, Ishido H, *et al.* Migraine attacks after transcatheter closure of atrial septal defect. *Cephalagia* 2013; **33**(15):1229–1237.

24 Rabkin DG, Whitehead KJ, Michaels AD, *et al.* Unusual presentation of nickel allergy requiring explantation of an Amplatzer Atrial Septal Occluder device. *Clin Cardiol* 2009; **32**(8): E55–57.

CHAPTER 57

Paravalvular Leak Closure and Ventricular Septal Defect Closure

Saurabh Sanon[1], Mackram F. Eleid[1], Allison K. Cabalka[2], and Charanjit S. Rihal[1]

[1] Division of Cardiovascular Diseases, Mayo Clinic College of Medicine, Rochester, MN, USA
[2] Division of Pediatric Cardiology, Mayo Clinic College of Medicine, Rochester, MN, USA

Transcatheter paravalvular leak closure

Upon long-term follow-up after prosthetic valve replacement, up to 17% of prosthetic mitral valves and 10% of prosthetic aortic valves develop peri-prosthetic regurgitation [1–3]. Furthermore, the incidence of moderate or severe peri-prosthetic regurgitation after transcatheter aortic valve replacement has been reported to range from 15% to 20% [4]. While most such patients remain asymptomatic, at least in the short term, 1–3% eventually develop symptoms necessitating intervention [5,6]. Because the underlying anatomic substrate that predisposes to development of peri-prosthetic regurgitation remains, and because re-operation carries significant morbidity and mortality, transcatheter closure of peri-prosthetic regurgitation becomes an attractive treatment option. This chapter discusses the fundamental principles of paravalvular regurgitation evaluation and percutaneous closure.

Pathophysiology

The most common etiologies implicated in the development of paravalvular regurgitation include:

1 Underlying tissue friability resulting from senescence, prior endocarditis, or a systemic inflammatory condition with or without corticosteroid use;
2 Extensive annular calcification, especially asymmetric calcification; and
3 Previous valvular surgery (multiple valvular re-do procedures) [7,8]. Technical aspects of the surgical procedure, such as suture technique and shape of the implant used, are also known to be associated with development of paravalvular regurgitation. While early development of paravalvular regurgitation is usually related to the relative shape of the implant compared with the annulus and underlying annular calcification, later development of paravalvular regurgitation is usually related to tissue friability and suture dehiscence.

Clinical features

Mild paravalvular regurgitation can often be asymptomatic; however, more severe degrees of paravalvular regurgitation can present with signs and symptoms of congestive heart failure. In some cases, even modest volume paravalvular regurgitation can lead to profound symptoms of heart failure becuase of regurgitation into a non-compliant chamber, either left atrium (LA) or left ventricle (LV). Patients also develop hemolysis from shear stress on red blood cells (RBCs), and present with fatigue, conjunctival and palmar crease pallor, jaundice, hematuria, and petechiae. Patients with aortic paravalvular regurgitation can present with a diastolic decrescendo murmur over the left sternal border, and patients with mitral paravalvular regurgitation often present with a pansystolic murmur over the mitral area with radiation incumbent on the direction of the major jet. Other classic signs of congestive heart failure can also occur, including elevated jugular venous pressure (JVP), dependent edema, orthopnea, paroxysmal nocturnal dyspnea, and cardiac cachexia.

Diagnostic evaluation
Laboratory findings

Basic laboratory testing should be performed to assess presence, severity, and mechanism of anemia including markers of hemolysis. These should include hemoglobin, hematocrit, reticulocyte count, mean corpuscular volume, reticulocyte count, haptoglobin, lactate dehydrogenase, iron, folic acid, total and direct bilirubin, and peripheral smear examination for the presence of schistocytes. The following findings typically suggest hemolysis: undetectable haptoglobin level, lactate dehydrogenase >500 units, >1% schistocytes on peripheral smear, and >5% reticulocytes.

Imaging

Transthoracic echocardiography (TTE) is usually the first line imaging modality to detect paravalvular regurgitation. While anterior aortic paravalvular regurgitation is easily detected using this modality, detection of posterior leaks is often hampered because of acoustic shadowing from prosthetic valves. Furthermore, the phenomenon of "garden-hosing," which is caused when a strong color flow Doppler signal emanates from a small defect and fans out to occupy a relatively small left ventricular outflow tract, makes accurate assessment of the severity of the paravalvular regurgitation by color flow difficult. Real-time three-dimensional transesophageal echocardiography (TEE) overcomes some of these challenges and allows accurate detection of the location and severity of paravalvular regurgitation. This modality is particularly useful for mitral paravalvular regurgitation. Intracardiac imaging, although not commonly used, can assist with procedural imaging, especially posteriorly located aortic paravalvular regurgitation which can be imaged using an intracardiac imaging catheter positioned in the

Interventional Cardiology: Principles and Practice, Second Edition. Edited by George D. Dangas, Carlo Di Mario, and Nicholas N. Kipshidze.
© 2017 John Wiley & Sons, Ltd. Published 2017 by John Wiley & Sons, Ltd.

right ventricular outflow tract. Aortography can allow accurate assessment of the severity of aortic paravalvular regurgitation in the absence of intravalvular regurgitation. EKG-gated cardiac computed tomography with volume-rendering reconstruction provides invaluable information for peri-procedural planning including accurate detection of paravalvular defect location, shape, and size. It also allows identification of orthogonal angles of AP and lateral imaging intensifiers that would facilitate crossing the paravalvular defect.

Localization

Aortic paravalvular regurgitation is typically localized using the transthoracic aortic short axis view and identifying the regurgitation in relation to one of six sectors each equaling 60°, based on position on the valve leaflets. This is then correlated with a corresponding position on the left anterior oblique (LAO) caudal view. The echocardiographic view of the valve is known to be rotated clockwise by 120° compared with the fluoroscopic LAO caudal view.

In our practice, mitral paravalvular regurgitation localization is performed using a triangulation system utilizing the following landmarks: the anteriorly located aortic valve, the anterolaterally located left atrial appendage, and the medially located atrial septum. Others recommend using a clock face system to localize the paravalvular regurgitation.

These nomenclature systems allow accurate and effective communication between the echocardiographer and structuralist, which is essential to the success of transcatheter paravalvular leak occlusion.

Transcatheter paravalvular regurgitation occlusion
Indications

The recent American College of Cardiology/American Heart Association guidelines for the management of valvular heart disease give percutaneous repair of paravalvular prosthetic valve regurgitation a Class IIa indication for patients with intractable hemolysis or New York Heart Association (NYHA) class III or IV heart failure who are at high risk for surgery and have anatomic features suitable for catheter-based therapy, when performed in centers with expertise in this procedure [9]. The common indications for transcatheter paravalvular regurgitation occlusion include:

1 Clinically and/or hemodynamically significant paravalvular regurgitation as evidenced by symptoms and signs of congestive heart failure or hemolytic anemia;
2 Stable prosthetic valve function; and
3 Defect size involving less than one-quarter valve circumference.

Contraindications include active infection or endocarditis, and unstable prosthesis and regurgitation involving more than one-third of the circumference of the prosthetic annulus.

Devices

Currently, there are no FDA-approved devices for paravalvular leak occlusion. Amplatzer™ Vascular Plug (AVP; AVP II, or IV), Amplatzer™ Duct Occluder, Amplatzer™ Septal Occluder, and Amplatzer™ Muscular VSD Occluder (all manufactured by St. Jude Medical, St. Paul, MN, USA) have been used to occlude paravalvular leaks. We recommend using the AVP II or AVP IV because these devices have a finer and softer nitinol mesh that lowers incidence of hemolysis compared with the other devices. The AVP III has an oblong cross-sectional shape that is particularly suited for paravalvular leak occlusion; this device is available in Europe but not in the USA.

With any device, extreme care must be taken to avoid interference with prosthetic valve leaflet motion or interaction with surrounding structures prior to device deployment.

Techniques
Aortic transcatheter paravalvular regurgitation occlusion

We recommend approaching aortic paravalvular defects using a retrograde aortic approach. For most anteriorly located defects, TTE is sufficient to guide the procedure. This also allows the use of moderate sedation, as opposed to general anesthesia, which is required for prolonged TEE procedural guidance. Posteriorly located defects often require TEE guidance, or intracardiac imaging (ICE) from the right ventricular outflow tract. The fluoroscopy gantries are oriented to visualize the sewing ring on its side on the right anterior oblique (RAO) view and en face on the LAO caudal view. We utilize a "5-in-6" telescoping, coaxial catheter system (125 cm 5 Fr multipurpose diagnostic coronary catheter inside a 6 Fr 100 cm multipurpose guiding catheter) and a 0.035-inch stiff angled glide wire to cannulate the defect. Alternatively, in larger aortic roots, an AL1 catheter can be used to provide directionality to the glidewire. Once the defect is cannulated the 5 Fr multipurpose catheter is used to cross the defect followed by the 6 Fr multipurpose guide. An exchange length 0.032-inch Amplatz Extra-stiff guidewire (Cook Medical, Bloomington, IN, USA) with a preformed LV curve is then positioned in the LV (the anchor wire technique; Figure 57.1a). Alternatively, the stiff angled glide wire can be extruded out through the native/bioprosthetic aortic valve and snared in the ascending aorta to be exteriorized via the contralateral femoral artery forming a stable arterio-arterial rail (modified anchor wire technique). Care must be taken to closely monitor hemodynamics while using this technique, because hemodynamically significant aortic regurgitation can develop secondary to the rail. For smaller defects necessitating deployment of a single closure device this may not be required; however, for planned deployment of multiple devices either an anchor wire or formation of a rail becomes necessary. Once the anchor wire or arterio-arterial rail is in place the guiding catheter can be replaced with a 90 cm Cook Flexor Shuttle sheath to facilitate device delivery. Knowledge of the compatibility of combinations of catheters, wires, and closure devices is crucial to ensure success.

Mitral transcatheter paravalvular regurgitation occlusion

An antegrade tranvenous trans-septal approach is commonly used for mitral paravalvular defects; however, retrograde aortic and LV apical approaches are necessary when cannulation of the defect is unsuccessful using the former approach. This might occur in the case of medial defects, which can be challenging to cannulate because of proximity to the interatrial septum. TEE guidance and general anesthesia are essential. Gantry setup is similar to that described for aortic paravalvular leaks. TEE and fluoroscopic guidance is used for trans-septal puncture. For medial defects a posterior location of interatrial puncture with the superior–inferior plane at the level of the defect is recommended as this provides the ability to maneuver catheters toward the defect along the mitral annular plane. After obtaining access to the LA, the interatrial septum is dilated using an Inoue dilator and an 8.5 or 11 Fr Agilis NxT Steerable guiding catheter (St. Jude Medical, St. Paul, MN, USA) is introduced over an Inoue wire into the LA. Meticulous care is required to maintain an activated clotting time ≥300 s to avoid development of thrombosis. A 5-in-6 telescoping catheter system and exchange length 0.032-inch stiff angled glide wire are used

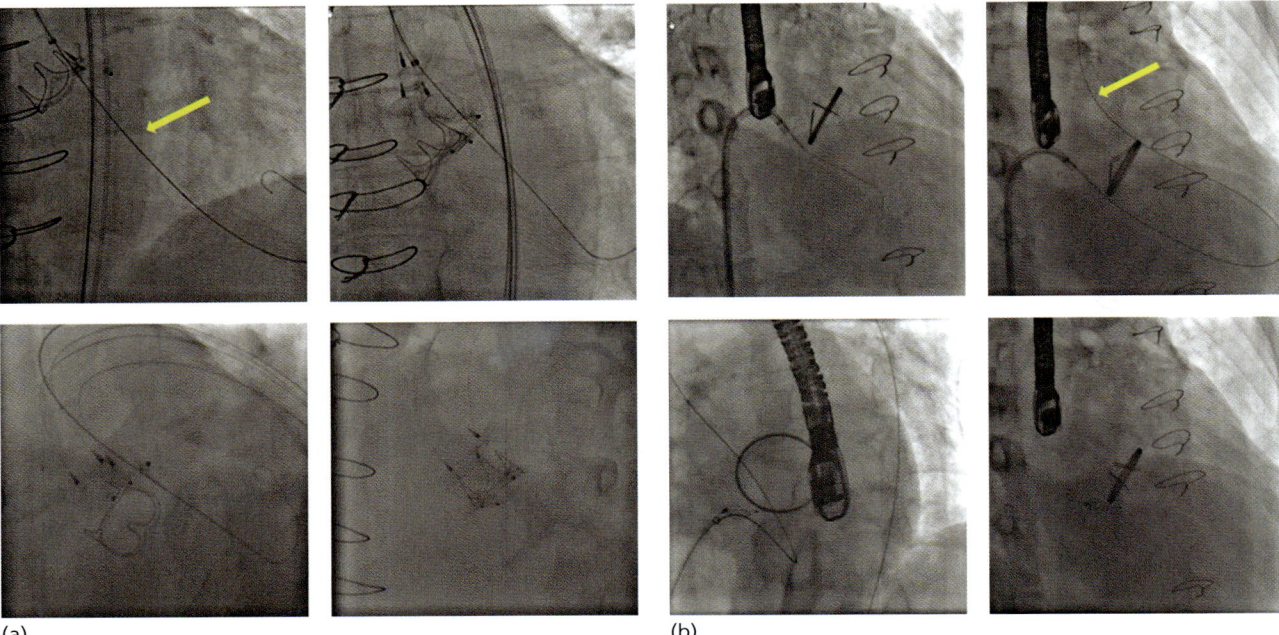

Figure 57.1 (a) Transcatheter aortic paravalvular leak closure. Top left: LV anchor wire (arrow) through an aortic paravalvular defect. Top right, bottom left: right anterior oblique and left anterior oblique views of nested Amplatzer vascular plugs with anchor wire in place. Bottom right: Amplatzer vascular plugs ready for deployment, yet still attached to their delivery cables. (b) Transcatheter mitral paravalvular leak closure. Top left: Agilis catheter with telescoping catheters, and a still angled Glide wire cannulated through a mitral paravalvular defect. Top right: arrow demonstrates the modified anchor wire technique (arteriovenous loop). Bottom left: an Amplatzer vascular plug being deployed with arteriovenous loop in place. Bottom right: deployed Amplatzer vascular plug.

through the Agilis catheter to cannulate the defect. The 5 and 6 Fr multipurpose catheters are then sequentially advanced into the LV. Depending on the size of the defect one or more devices are required, and can be deployed as described in the subsequent sections.

Sequential deployment technique using the Anchor wire

An 0.032-inch exchange length extrastiff Amplatz guidewire with an LV curve is carefully positioned in the LV and the multipurpose guide is replaced by a appropriately sized Cook Flexor Shuttle Sheath in the LV. Once the first closure device has been successfully deployed, the Shuttle sheath is removed over the guidewire and then reloaded on to the guidewire, leaving the device cable outside of the sheath to facilitate delivery of additional devices using the same sequence. This allows sequential deployment of multiple devices without losing access to the LV.

Sequential deployment technique using an arteriovenous rail or transapical rail (modified Anchor wire)

When additional support is required, the hydrophilic guidewire can be snared in the ascending aorta and exteriorized (Figure 57.1b). An appropriately sized Flexor Shuttle sheath is used as described earlier. With the arteriovenous guidewire rail in position, the first closure device can be placed through the shuttle sheath alongside the existing exteriorized guidewire rail. The Shuttle sheath is then removed and reloaded over the arteriovenous rail, leaving the device delivery cable outside the sheath. Multiple devices can be placed using this sequence while maintaining complete control on wire tension, and allowing device delivery at the end of the

procedure. An attractive aspect of this technique is the ability to reverse course and remove all devices at the very end of the procedure.

Simultaneous deployment technique (double wire technique)

In this technique two or more 0.032-inch Amplatz ExtraStiff Guide Wires are used to make LV loops through the 6 Fr guiding catheter. A large 20 Fr venous sheath is often used. The guiding catheter is removed over the guidewires and two separate 5-in-6 catheter systems are loaded on the guidewires and advanced into the ventricle. The 5 Fr diagnostic catheters are then removed and the 6 Fr guides are used to deploy devices simultaneously.

Complications

Procedural complications include bleeding (5.2%), prosthetic leaflet impingement (4%), device embolization (<1%), and need for emergency surgery (0.9%). Thirty-day complication rates have been described by our group at 8.7% (sudden and unexplained death 1.7%; stroke 2.6%; emergency surgery 0.9%; bleeding 5.2%) [10].

Follow-up

We recommend close follow-up of the patient to monitor resolution of hemolysis and/or heart failure symptoms. No additional antiplatelet or anticoagulation therapy is necessary from the standpoint of the occluder device(s) placed. Serial screening imaging with TTE is recommended during follow-up visits to assess residual paravalvular regurgitation.

Conclusions

In high surgical risk patients with hemolysis or heart failure symptoms secondary to paravalvular regurgitation, transcatheter paravalvular leak occlusion has emerged as a promising and effective therapy when performed in centers with experienced operators.

Transcatheter VSD closure

Ventricular septal defects (VSD) can be divided into congenital (comprising up to 20% of congenital heart defects) and acquired etiologies resulting from either myocardial infarct or post-surgical changes. VSDs are classified as muscular, peri-membranous, or supracristal according to their location within the interventricular septum. Among congenital causes, peri-membranous VSD are the most common (70%) whereas pure muscular VSDs account for 15% and supracristal 5% of congenital VSDs. Catheter VSD closure in indicated for heart failure symptoms, left heart chamber enlargement/volume overload, and previous endocarditis [11]. In the setting of left heart chamber enlargement, VSD closure can prevent the development of pulmonary hypertension, ventricular dysfunction, aortic regurgitation, and arrhythmias. While surgical closure is considered the gold standard treatment, it may be associated with morbidity and mortality, prompting development of less invasive percutaneous transcatheter techniques. Since the first percutaneous VSD closure was performed in 1988 [12], improvements in technique including smaller sheath size and availability of newer dedicated Amplatzer (St. Jude Medical, St. Paul, MN, USA) devices, transcatheter VSD closure has become an increasingly safe and effective procedure.

Patient selection

Transcatheter VSD closure is an especially attractive option in patients with increased surgical risk, multiple previous surgical interventions, "Swiss cheese" type VSDs where multiple defects are present, and poorly accessible muscular VSDs. Anatomic characteristics that favor transcatheter VSD closure over surgical closure include defect location that is remote from the tricuspid valve and aorta, in order to minimize device interference with these structures [11].

Important exclusion criteria to transcatheter VSD closure include:
1 Presence of other cardiac lesion requiring surgical repair;
2 Irreversible pulmonary vascular disease (pulmonary vascular resistance index >6–8 WU/m²);
3 Contraindication to antiplatelet therapy;
4 Uncontrolled infection; and
5 Anatomic features that make transcatheter closure unfavorable (concomitant subaortic rim <2 mm from peri-membranous VSD, close proximity to tricuspid valve).

Procedural techniques

Several devices are available for transcatheter VSD closure including the muscular Amplatzer VSD occluder, membranous Amplatzer VSD occluder (not available in the USA), ASD Amplatzer occluder. Amplatzer ASD and VSD occluder devices are made of self-expanding nitinol, consisting of two umbrellas and middle "waist." Polyester fabric inserts aid in closing the defect by providing a foundation for tissue growth over the device after deployment. Maximum umbrella size for the 18 mm muscular VSD occluder is 26 mm, 54 mm for the 28 mm ASD occluder, and 32 mm for the

24 mm Amplatzer muscular post-infarct VSD occluder. Devices are secured to a delivery cable and inserted into a delivery sheath ranging 6–10 Fr in size. Device sizes are selected based on two-dimensional echocardiographic measurements; generally the waist of the device should be 1–2 mm larger than the defect size (Table 57.1). Longer waist lengths are required as interventricular septum thickness increases, for instance in adults. Additionally, post-myocardial infarction VSD closure requires longer device waists because of the unique nature of these defects.

Pre-procedural antibiotic prophylaxis (typically, intravenous cefazolin) is administered as well as aspirin (325 mg) and intravenous heparin (100 U/kg). In many patients, the procedure can be performed using conscious sedation. Patients who are better suited for general anesthesia are those in which TEE use is planned, internal jugular vein access is used for device delivery, or in the setting of post-myocardial infarction VSD.

VSD closure

Femoral arterial access is performed with insertion of a 6 Fr sheath and either femoral venous or internal jugular (IJ) venous access obtained with a 7 Fr sheath depending on the planned approach for closure. Femoral access is usually preferred for defects in the more superior portion of the septum (i.e., membranous) whereas IJ more commonly used for other locations. If ICE is planned, an additional 10 Fr sheath is placed in the femoral vein. The VSD is then crossed retrogradely from the LV using fluoroscopic and echocardiographic guidance (TTE, TEE, or ICE) with either a diagnostic right Judkins or a multipurpose catheter and an exchange-length stiff angled glidewire. After the defect is crossed, the wire is typically advanced into the pulmonary artery (PA). A balloon-tipped end-hole catheter is then used to cross the tricuspid valve from the right side with the balloon inflated, in order to avoid entrapment of the chordal apparatus during later placement of the device. This catheter is advanced into the PA and an exchange length guidewire is positioned through the end-hole catheter over which the guide for the snare is positioned. The glide wire is then snared and exteriorized through the venous access site, establishing an arteriovenous rail. If desired, a sizing balloon can be used to help in the assessment of the VSD size by stop-flow method and to delineate the VSD boundaries more accurately; however, echocardiographic guidance is sufficient in most cases (Figure 57.2).

The appropriate sized delivery sheath is then advanced through the venous access site, over the wire rail, into the LV (if one elects to leave the wire rail in place during device delivery a larger sheath will be needed). The wire and dilator are then removed and the loaded device is advanced through the sheath, across the defect, and into the LV. The device is then extruded from the sheath into the LV until the left-sided umbrella is expanded, being careful not to deploy the device into the mitral apparatus. The delivery catheter is then drawn back into the right ventricle until the left-sided umbrella is against the septum, as guided by fluoroscopic and echocardiographic imaging. Finally, the right-sided umbrella is released by withdrawing the sheath, thus covering the defect. The device is then tested for stability by gentle pulling and pushing under fluoroscopic and echocardiographic guidance. Doppler color-flow is used to determine the presence and degree of residual shunting as well as potential interference with surrounding structures such as the tricuspid and aortic valves. Once device position is determined to be stable and there is a significant reduction in shunt (≤ mild residual shunt), the device is released.

Table 57.1 Transcatheter ventricular septal defect (VSD) closure devices.

Device	Device size/waist diameter (mm)	Disc diameter (mm)	Waist length (mm)	Min. sheath size (Fr)
Amplatzer Muscular VSD Occluder	4	9	7	6
	6	14	7	6
	8	16	7	6
	10	18	7	6
	12	20	7	7
	14	22	7	8
	16	24	7	8
	18	26	7	9
Amplatzer ASD Occluder	4–10	RA 12–18; LA 16–22	3	6
	11–17	RA 21–27; LA 25–31	4	7
	18–24	RA 28–34; LA 32–38	4	9
	26–30	RA 36–40; LA 40–44	4	10
	32–38	RA 42–48; LA 46–54	4	12
Amplatzer Membranous VSD Occluder*	4–12	RV 8–16; LV 10–18	N/A	7
	13–14	RV 17–18; LV 19–20	N/A	8
	15–18	RV 19–22; LV 21–24	N/A	9
Amplatzer Post-Infarct VSD Occluder *	16	26	10	9
	18	28	10	9
	20	30	10	10
	22	32	10	10
	24	34	10	10

ASD, atrial septal defect; LA, left atrium; LV, left ventricle; RA, right atrium; RV, right ventricle; VSD, ventricular septal defect.
* Devices not available in the USA.
Source: Data obtained from St. Jude Medical Corporation, St. Paul, MN, USA.

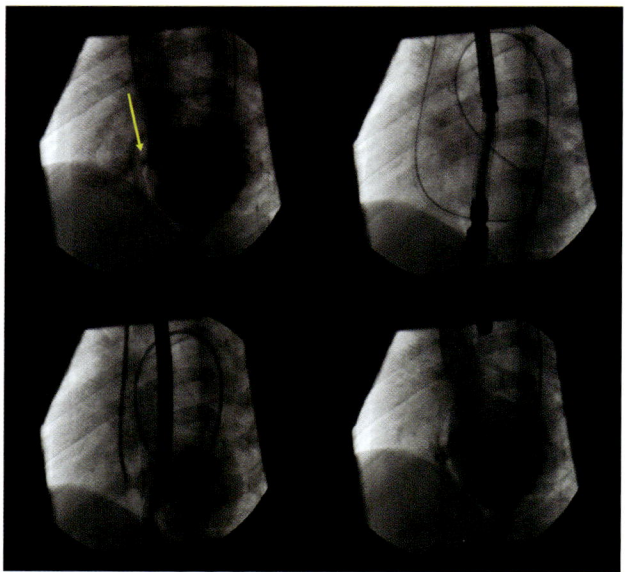

Figure 57.2 Transcatheter ventricular septal defect (VSD) closure. Top left: left anterior oblique left ventricle (LV) angiogram demonstrating muscular VSD with communication from left to right ventrile (arrow). Top right: an arteriovenous rail from femoral artery to internal jugular vein is established. Bottom left: muscular VSD device prior to release with LV angiogram showing no residual shunting. Bottom right: device is released with stable position and minimal residual shunt.

Efficacy and complications

Procedural success rates for transcatheter closure are approximately 90–95% for congenital and post-surgical peri-membranous and muscular defects. Complete VSD closure is achieved in 40–50% of patients immediately post-procedure and 80–90% at 1 year [13]. Residual shunting is usually trivial or mild in degree, with <1% of patients having severe residual shunt requiring surgery [13]. Complications have been reported in up to 10% of patients, including 3–4% risk of rhythm and conduction disturbances, <1% risk of device embolism, <1% risk of major vascular complications, <1% of infection, development of new aortic or tricuspid regurgitation (3–6% of patients, usual of trivial or mild degree), hypotension, and blood loss [13,14].

In contrast, closure of post-infarct VSD has a much lower success rate, in part because of the tendency of the defect to grow over time because of ongoing necrosis and the critically ill state of such patients. Closure performed in the acute setting is associated with a significantly less successful longer term result. While initial procedural success can be as high as 86% [15], the procedural complication rate is 41% including major residual shunting, left ventricular rupture, and device embolization. When cardiogenic shock is present at baseline, despite an 80% procedural success rate, long-term mortality is 93%, reflecting the extreme critical illness present in this population.

Conclusions

Transcatheter VSD closure has emerged as an effective and safe treatment in selected patients with appropriate indications. Advances in catheter-based techniques, imaging, and device technology continue to expand the use of percutaneous transcatheter VSD closure.

Interactive multiple choice questions are available for this chapter on www.wiley.com/go/dangas/cardiology

References

1 Ionescu A, Fraser AG, Butchart EG. Prevalence and clinical significance of incidental paraprosthetic valvar regurgitation: a prospective study using transoesophageal echocardiography. *Heart* 2003; **89**: 1316–1321.

2 Hammermeister K, Sethi GK, Henderson WG, Grover FL, Oprian C, Rahimtoola SH. Outcomes 15 years after valve replacement with a mechanical versus a bioprosthetic valve: final report of the Veterans Affairs randomized trial. *J Am Coll Cardiol* 2000; **36**: 1152–1158.

3 Genoni M, Franzen D, Vogt P, et al. Paravalvular leakage after mitral valve replacement: improved long-term survival with aggressive surgery? *Eur J Cardiothorac Surg* 2000; **17**: 14–19.

4 Sinning JM, Hammerstingl C, Vasa-Nicotera M, et al. Aortic regurgitation index defines severity of peri-prosthetic regurgitation and predicts outcome in patients after transcatheter aortic valve implantation. *J Am Coll Cardiol* 2012; **59**: 1134–1141.

5 Miller DL, Morris JJ, Schaff HV, Mullany CJ, Nishimura RA, Orszulak TA. Reoperation for aortic valve periprosthetic leakage: identification of patients at risk and results of operation. *J Heart Valve Dis* 1995; **4**: 160–165.

6 Jindani A, Neville EM, Venn G, Williams BT. Paraprosthetic leak: a complication of cardiac valve replacement. *J Cardiovasc Surg (Torino)* 1991; **32**: 503–508.

7 Wasowicz M, Meineri M, Djaiani G, et al. Early complications and immediate postoperative outcomes of paravalvular leaks after valve replacement surgery. *J Cardiothorac Vasc Anesth* 2011; **25**: 610–614.

8 Rallidis LS, Moyssakis IE, Ikonomidis I, Nihoyannopoulos P. Natural history of early aortic paraprosthetic regurgitation: a five-year follow-up. *Am Heart J* 1999; **138**: 351–357.

9 Nishimura RA, Otto CM, Bonow RO, et al. 2014 AHA/ACC Guideline for the Management of Patients With Valvular Heart Disease: a report of the American College of Cardiology/American Heart Association Task Force on Practice Guidelines. *Circulation* 2014; **129**: e521–643.

10 Sorajja P, Cabalka AK, Hagler DJ, Rihal CS. Percutaneous repair of paravalvular prosthetic regurgitation: acute and 30-day outcomes in 115 patients. *Circ Cardiovasc Interv* 2011; **4**: 314–321.

11 Warnes CA, Williams RG, Bashore TM, et al. ACC/AHA 2008 Guidelines for the Management of Adults with Congenital Heart Disease: a report of the American College of Cardiology/American Heart Association Task Force on Practice Guidelines (writing committee to develop guidelines on the management of adults with congenital heart disease). *Circulation* 2008; **118**: e714–833.

12 Lock JE, Block PC, McKay RG, Baim DS, Keane JF. Transcatheter closure of ventricular septal defects. *Circulation* 1988; **78**: 361–368.

13 Carminati M, Butera G, Chessa M, et al. Transcatheter closure of congenital ventricular septal defects: results of the European Registry. *Eur Heart J* 2007; **28**: 2361–2368.

14 Holzer R, Balzer D, Cao QL, Lock K, Hijazi ZM. Device closure of muscular ventricular septal defects using the Amplatzer muscular ventricular septal defect occluder: immediate and mid-term results of a US registry. *J Am Coll Cardiol* 2004; **43**: 1257–1263.

15 Thiele H, Kaulfersch C, Daehnert I, et al. Immediate primary transcatheter closure of postinfarction ventricular septal defects. *Eur Heart J* 2009; **30**: 81–88.

CHAPTER 58

Aortic Valvuloplasty and Large-Bore Percutaneous Arterial Access

Matthew I. Tomey, Annapoorna S. Kini, Samin K. Sharma, and Jason C. Kovacic

The Zena and Michael A. Wiener Cardiovascular Institute, and The Marie-Josée and Henry R. Kravis Cardiovascular Health Center, Icahn School of Medicine at Mount Sinai, New York, NY, USA

Near-abolition of rheumatic heart disease in developed countries has transformed the demography of aortic stenosis (AS), which today results primarily from age-associated calcific degeneration [1]. Once common in the sixth decade of life, onset of AS today occurs most commonly in the eighth decade of life. Among older adults, AS is common, with moderate or severe valvular AS documented in 2.8% of US adults over age 75 [2]. Accordingly, with aging of the population [3], incidence is rising.

In the absence of aortic valve replacement (AVR), symptomatic severe AS portends a high risk of mortality that has remained largely unchanged despite advances in medical therapy [4–6]. And yet, with shift in the onset of AS to later years of life, its natural history has been transposed to an age with greater burdens of frailty and medical comorbidities, complicating management. Before the recent advent of transcatheter AVR (TAVR), only half of older adults with severe AS would ever visit a cardiothoracic surgeon, and fewer still would ultimately undergo AVR. Common reasons for this gap included advanced age, comorbidities, high operative risk, perceived lack of symptoms, and refusal by patients or family members [7]. TAVR today offers a lifesaving option for many patients at high or extreme risk for surgical AVR [8–10], and an emerging alternative for those at intermediate risk [10a].

Percutaneous balloon aortic valvuloplasty (BAV) is a minimally invasive structural intervention for management of symptomatic severe valvular AS which emerged in the 1980s, first used in children with congenital AS [11] and subsequently in adults with bicuspid aortic valve disease, rheumatic heart disease, and calcific AS [12,13]. The technique found particular application among patients who were too ill to undergo surgery [14]. With a minimally invasive approach, it was possible to achieve immediate reduction in the transvalvular aortic gradient, increase in calculated aortic valve area, and often improvement in left ventricular function [15–17]. Enthusiasm for these acute benefits and accompanying symptom relief [18] was tempered, however, by recognition of their lack of durability. Three-quarters of patients exhibit hemodynamic evidence of restenosis at 6-month follow-up after BAV [19–21], and indeed, reductions in transvalvular gradient can begin to regress within days after the procedure [22]. Correspondingly, BAV has

been found to yield no benefit for event-free or actuarial survival above and beyond that expected with medical management of AS alone [23,24]. With appreciation that BAV, though less invasive than surgery, was not without risk [25], the procedure was largely dismissed as a standard treatment for symptomatic severe AS, and rather relegated to the roles of palliation in selected cases or occasional temporization prior to surgical AVR [26].

TAVR has disrupted the field of AS management, however, and accordingly, BAV is receiving a second look [27]. The TAVR movement has renewed attention to the many patients with AS previously deprived of intervention because of advanced age or comorbidities. Implementation of percutaneous transfemoral TAVR has required teaching and learning skills shared with BAV and, in particular, techniques for safe large-bore femoral arterial access and closure. Indications for BAV have emerged before and during the TAVR procedure. In several centers, the introduction of a TAVR program brought with it an increase in utilization of BAV [28,29]. This chapter provides a comprehensive reassessment of BAV and large-bore arterial access for adult patients with calcific AS in the era of TAVR.

Basic principles and mechanisms of action

Broadly, BAV entails large-bore vascular access, typically via the femoral artery; placement of a stiff guidewire across the aortic valve; delivery of a non-compliant balloon over the guidewire to the level of the aortic valve; balloon inflation; device removal; and arteriotomy closure. For each element, there exist specialized equipment, essential technique, and opportunities for failure and complications.

Inflation and deflation of a non-compliant balloon placed properly across the stenosed aortic valve produces an immediate increase in valvular effective orifice area via three major mechanisms: fracture of calcium deposits, rupture of commissural fusion, and, to a lesser degree, stretch of valve and annular tissue [13,30–32]. This increase in effective orifice area, typically 50% above baseline upon immediate reassessment [33], confers an acute reduction in transvalvular pressure gradient and left ventricular afterload. Accordingly, immediately post-BAV, patients characteristically

Interventional Cardiology: Principles and Practice, Second Edition. Edited by George D. Dangas, Carlo Di Mario, and Nicholas N. Kipshidze.
© 2017 John Wiley & Sons, Ltd. Published 2017 by John Wiley & Sons, Ltd.

experience a fall in left ventricular peak systolic pressure, left ventricular end-diastolic pressure, and pulmonary capillary wedge pressure. Correction of afterload mismatch [34] can be associated with an increase in calculated cardiac output and improvement in left ventricular ejection fraction, particularly among those with left ventricular systolic dysfunction at baseline [17,33]. In the absence of a change in stroke volume, improvement in left ventricular performance can be evident in a decrease in ejection time, particularly in the later decelerative phase of systole [35]. Additional salutary effects of BAV include attenuation of sympathetic nervous system and renin–angiotensin–aldosterone system activation and mitigation of hemostatic dyscrasias associated with AS, typified by shearing of von Willebrand factor multimers [36,37].

Effects of BAV on aortic valve area, hemodynamics, and left ventricular performance are short-lived. Regression begins quickly: within 2–4 days after BAV patients can expect a 20% increase in mean and peak instantaneous pressure gradient, with 80% of patients experiencing a rise in peak instantaneous pressure gradient of at least 10% [22]. This rebound in pressure gradient can be explained in part by a small but measurable increase in stroke volume via reduction in afterload mismatch. Inflammation and fibrosis of the valve following traumatic injury mediate a structural remodeling response that also contributes to restenosis. In the early weeks following BAV, there is evidence of hemorrhage and inflammation at sites of calcium fracture, with a neutrophilic predominance [38]. By 2 months, microfractures persist but with a transition in associated inflammation to a heavier infiltrate of lymphocytes, plasma cells, granulation, and mesenchymal tissue [38]. In the months that follow, the acute inflammatory response gives way to mesenchymal cell proliferation, hyalinization, myxoid change, and dystrophic calcification and scarring [39]. By 6 months, approximately half of patients experience restenosis back to their baseline level of valvular stenosis [18,40,41].

Indications and evidence for use

Although TAVR has inspired re-examination of BAV, the essential transience of the benefits of BAV remains unchanged, and this informs contemporary indications for its use. In older patients with calcific AS, the primary indication for BAV is to provide temporary relief of transvalvular pressure gradient and symptoms in well-selected patients in anticipation of definitive therapy with surgical AVR or TAVR. Current American College of Cardiology (ACC)/American Heart Association (AHA) guidelines issue a single recommendation for BAV: "Percutaneous aortic balloon dilation may be considered as a bridge to surgical AVR or TAVR in patients with severe symptomatic AS" (Class IIb, level of evidence C) [42].

In clinical practice, this "bridging" role has been applied in several scenarios. For patients acutely ill with symptomatic, severe AS who are too unstable to undergo either surgical AVR or TAVR, BAV facilitates partial recovery en route to subsequent definitive therapy [28,29,43]. In other patients with symptomatic, severe AS, particularly those with evidence of a low cardiac output, low left ventricular ejection fraction, and/or low transvalvular gradient, BAV serves a diagnostic purpose to assess the likelihood of improved left ventricular performance in response to afterload reduction. In certain patients requiring urgent surgery, BAV is sometimes used as a short-term measure with intent to reduce the cardiovascular risk of non-cardiac surgery [44–47]. High quality evidence for this approach is lacking and current guidelines do not endorse it [42]. Finally, in patients who cannot undergo either

surgical AVR or TAVR, BAV remains useful as a palliative measure for temporary symptom relief in select patients. Among inoperable patients randomized to standard therapy in the Placement of Aortic Transcatheter Valves (PARTNER) trial, the 73% of patients who underwent BAV post-randomization enjoyed a significant improvement in quality of life at 30 days that was sustained to 6 months but gone by 1 year [43].

As a new role for BAV, it has become an integral step during TAVR in many centers. The purpose of performing BAV as the step immediately prior to the deployment of a percutaneous valve during TAVR is to ensure the aortic valve leaflets open adequately to permit the passage of the valve across the calcified and disease aortic valve apparatus. However, this indication for BAV continues to evolve as the crossing and deployment profiles of the various TAVR valves improves. Typically, operator preference has a significant role in the decision to perform BAV immediately prior to valve deployment during TAVR.

In children and young adults with congenital AS, BAV maintains an important role. As discussion of BAV in the young exceeds the scope of this chapter, we direct our readers elsewhere for further review [48].

Patient selection and contraindications to BAV

In appreciation of both the temporary benefits and the significant risks of BAV, contemplation of the procedure must obey the principle of *primum non nocere*. The assessment of benefits and risks is inherently individualized. It is nonetheless important to highlight a few relative if not absolute contraindications to BAV: moderate to severe valvular aortic insufficiency; lack of a safe means for percutaneous vascular access and closure; eligibility for primary surgical AVR or TAVR; and, conversely, lack of likelihood to benefit from mechanical relief of AS.

Analysis of the TAVR experience has made apparent a subset of patients with symptomatic, severe AS who do not benefit from correction of AS, even by AVR. At 1 year follow-up of the PARTNER trial, 30% of inoperable patients assigned to TAVR were dead, and half were either dead or devoid of even moderate improvement in functional status or quality of life [8,49]. Clinical predictors of increased risk in the setting of severe AS are presented in Box 58.1 [50].

A final word of caution is warranted concerning risks and benefits of repeated BAV. Given the predictable eventual recurrence of

> **Box 58.1** Adverse prognostic indicators for balloon aortic valvuloplasty
>
> - Severe left ventricular dysfunction, as evidenced by low flow (stroke volume index <35 mL/m²), low gradient (resting mean gradient <20 mmHg), and/or low ejection fraction with lack of contractile reserve (increase in stroke volume ≥20%) on dobutamine stress echocardiography [51]
> - Severe myocardial fibrosis, as assessed by cardiac magnetic resonance imaging [52]
> - Severe concurrent mitral [53,54] or tricuspid [55] valve regurgitation
> - Severe pulmonary hypertension [56]
> - Severe liver, kidney, or lung disease, particularly when associated with oxygen dependence
> - Severe elevation in global risk scores such as the Society for Thoracic Surgeons risk score (>15%) [57] and the logistic EuroSCORE [58]
> - Geriatric factors, including frailty, malnutrition, impaired cognition, mood disturbance, social isolation, disability, impaired mobility, fall tendency, and polypharmacy [59–61]

stenosis and symptoms after initial BAV, in selected surviving patients with symptomatic, severe AS, repeated BAV can be considered. It is important to recognize that hemodynamic benefits of repeat BAV may be more modest than those achieved with initial balloon dilatation [43], and durability of benefits may be reduced [62]. For a given patient, the probability of experiencing a serious complication of BAV increases with repeated exposure to the procedure. Risks are particularly elevated on the third and fourth occasions [62].

Approach to the procedure

BAV, like its descendant TAVR, can be accomplished either via an anterograde or retrograde approach, described as the direction in which the balloon crosses the aortic valve relative to the direction of blood flow.

An *anterograde approach*, in which the balloon approaches the valve via the left ventricle, can be accomplished either via left ventricular apical access or via venous access with accompanying trans-septal or caval–aortic [63] puncture. The major advantage of an anterograde approach is avoidance of the arterial system, which is affected by a substantial and sometimes prohibitive burden of atherosclerosis in many candidates (Table 58.1). Transvenous access, in particular, offers the putative advantage of reduced access site bleeding and vascular complications in association with large-bore vascular access. A transvenous approach was indeed used for the first case of TAVR in humans [64]. Transapical access, which was studied in the context of TAVR in the PARTNER trial [8,9], offers the added advantages of a shorter distance from the access point to the aortic valve, avoidance of the aortic arch with the device, coaxial wire positioning across the aortic valve, and secure access site closure under direct visualization, at the expense of a mini-thoracotomy [65]. Somewhat surprisingly, expected benefits of the transapical approach for stroke avoidance were not observed in the PARTNER trial. Potential explanations include residual confounding from vasculopathy influencing selection for the transapical approach in the PARTNER trial [66] and the likelihood that many if not all intraprocedural strokes during TAVR occur during device positioning and deployment at the level of the aortic valve, irrespective of approach [67]. Importantly, while anterograde BAV is still performed in association with anterograde TAVR, given the more invasive nature of this approach it is difficult to conceive of any situation in which anterograde BAV would be performed as a stand-alone procedure in the current era. The remainder of this chapter exclusively considers the retrograde approach.

A *retrograde approach* has been traditionally favored for BAV. In this approach, access is obtained via a large artery (typically, the common femoral artery), and equipment is advanced over guidewires to the left heart via retrograde passage through the aorta. In most cases, transfemoral access permits a totally percutaneous approach. Challenges particular to the transfemoral retrograde approach include risks of vascular complications, bleeding, often tortuous aortoiliac anatomy, and a long distance from the access point to the aortic valve (70–100 cm), creating opportunities for wire bias, slack, and non-coaxial device positioning across the aortic valve [65]. In the following sections, we discuss the optimal approach to large-bore arterial access and retrograde percutaneous transfemoral BAV, acknowledging that there exist inter-institutional and inter-operator differences in technique, preference, and style.

Large-bore arterial access

Safe femoral arterial access is a fundamental step in BAV and TAVR, with important implications for procedural success, safety, and patient satisfaction. Indeed, there are numerous other indications for large-bore percutaneous arterial access in the modern catheterization laboratory, such as left ventricular hemodynamic support devices [72,73]. The techniques described are equally applicable across all of these applications.

Table 58.1 Atherosclerotic disease burden in high-risk patients with severe aortic stenosis.

Citation	Year	Description	n	CAD (%)	CVD (%)	PAD (%)
Leon et al. [8]	2010	PARTNER trial (extreme risk cohort)	179	67.6	27.4	30.3
Rodes-Cabau et al. [56]	2010	Canadian registry	339	69.0	22.7	35.4
Smith et al. [9]	2011	PARTNER trial (high risk cohort)	348	74.9	29.3	43.0
Moat et al. [68]	2011	British registry	870	47.6	–	29.0
Gilard et al. [58]	2012	French registry	3195	47.9	10.0	20.8
Mack et al. [69]	2013	STS/ACC TVT registry	7710	68.9	13.0	31.3
Adams et al. [10]	2014	US CoreValve trial	394	75.4	12.9	41.7
Abdel-Wahab et al. [70]	2014	CHOICE trial	241	63.1	19.9	17.4
Hamm et al. [71]	2014	German registry	3875	54.4	13.2	20.1

Percentages reflect investigator-reported rates of disease at baseline per study definitions.
ACC, American College of Cardiology; CAD, coronary artery disease; CVD, cerebrovascular disease or stroke; PAD, peripheral artery disease; PARTNER, Placement of Aortic Transcatheter Valves; STS, Society of Thoracic Surgeons; TVT, transcatheter valve therapy.

Successful arterial access provides a sufficiently large channel to permit both insertion and removal of necessary devices such as a BAV balloon; an unobstructed pathway from the access point to the aortic annulus and heart; an "exit strategy" for safe closure and hemostasis at procedure conclusion; and minimization of pain, bleeding, and vascular complications. With effective percutaneous access and closure, a patient can be mobilized within hours of BAV, or even TAVR, with little to show other than a small incision and a bandage.

Candidates for large-bore arterial access, however, often represent a particularly vulnerable subset of patients with severe AS with a disproportionate burden of frailty, comorbidity, and instability, limiting tolerance for complications. The femoral and iliac arteries are commonly affected by atherosclerosis, as shown in Table 58.1, with associated tortuosity, calcification, and luminal narrowing. Sheaths required for BAV are large, ranging from 9 to 12 Fr (3–4 mm) in diameter, while access for TAVR requires access from 14 up to 22–24 Fr. Vascular complications of BAV remain common, affecting 5–10% of patients in the TAVR era [74]. The stakes of vascular complications are high. In patients undergoing transcatheter aortic valve interventions including BAV, major vascular complications are associated with higher rates of bleeding, transfusion, renal failure, and mortality [74,75]. Accordingly, meticulous planning and technique for femoral arterial access and closure for BAV and TAVR are required.

Access planning

Increasingly, computed tomography angiography (CTA) is performed prior to contemplating large bore arterial access for the purpose of access planning. This exercise is mandatory prior to arterial access for TAVR. Selected recent recommendations for this imaging from the Society for Cardiovascular Computed Tomography [76] are presented in Box 58.2. When CTA is available, it is essential that the primary operator responsible for access reviews the primary imaging data in advance of the procedure. Nevertheless, in many cases, a comprehensive, appropriately protocolled CTA may not be available at the time of BAV. Attention should be paid in these cases to iliofemoral angiography performed in the context of cardiac catheterization.

Key observations on pre-procedure CTA, if available, and prior iliofemoral angiography include the size, tortuosity, plaque burden, and calcification of the left and right iliac and femoral arteries.

Special note should be made of the location of the common femoral bifurcation, particular areas of heavy plaque or calcification, anomalies and anatomic variants, and any evidence of vascular injury or soft tissue pathology secondary to prior procedures. Based on these observations, the operator should form a strategy for the laterality, precise cranio-caudal position, and caliber of the femoral arteriotomy.

Sheath selection

Sheath sizes appropriate for transfemoral BAV range in caliber 9–22 Fr, with requirements that vary based on balloon selection (Table 58.2). Sheath selection for TAVR is dependent on the valve being implanted, and ranges 14–22 Fr. As mentioned, there are three principal factors to consider in terms of suitability of vascular access for large-bore sheath insertion: minimum diameter, tortuosity, and degree of calcification. While not the only factor to be considered, experience with TAVR has demonstrated the danger of sheath oversizing. A sheath-to-femoral artery ratio exceeding 1.05 predicts increased risks of not only vascular complications but also short-term mortality [77].

In addition to sheath caliber, it is important to tailor sheath length to vascular anatomy. For most patients, standard short sheaths measuring 10–12 cm in length are sufficient to provide secure arterial access and support for BAV. In selected patients with significant iliofemoral plaque, calcification, or tortuosity, a longer sheath is desired to facilitate torque control and smooth device advancement and retrieval. A 25 cm sheath is usually adequate to bypass the iliac arteries, whereas a 45–55 cm sheath will typically terminate comfortably in the descending thoracic aorta. In rare cases with extreme aortoiliac tortuosity, longer sheaths are considered. For TAVR, in most cases using a percutaneous transfemoral approach, a 25–40 cm sheath is used which terminates in the mid-descending aorta.

Pre-closure

Successful use of a percutaneous suture-mediated closure device dramatically simplifies large-bore arterial access site management. In published observational data, the use of a percutaneous suture-mediated closure "pre-close" technique has been associated with improved vascular and bleeding outcomes. In the Effect of Bivalirudin on Aortic Valve Intervention Outcomes (BRAVO)

Box 58.2 Recommendations for use of CTA in TAVR access planning

- CTA should be performed in the evaluation process of patients who are under consideration for TAVR unless there is a contraindication
- CTA datasets should be interpreted jointly with a member of the TAVR procedural team or reviewed with the operator before the procedure
- Slice thickness should be ≤1.0 mm
- Imaging of the aorta and peripheral vessels should extend from the aortic arch (and preferably subclavian artery) to below the groin
- Imaging of the abdominal aorta and peripheral vessels does not need to be ECG gated
- CTA examinations should be performed with iodinated contrast medium. Contrast agent exposure can be an issue in patients who are often of advanced age and may have renal impairment. Contrast reduction and adherence to protocols for prevention of contrast-induced nephropathy is recommended
- Qualitative assessment of vascular tortuosity should be performed
- Qualitative assessment of vascular calcification should be performed
- Consideration to varied thresholds of vessel size (sheath : femoral artery ratio) should be contemplated, depending on the presence and extent of vascular calcification
- The left ventricle should be evaluated for the presence of thrombus and, if a transapical access route is planned, for geometry and position of the apex
- The entire aorta should be imaged and evaluated, unless a transapical access is planned
- Severe elongation and kinking of the aorta, dissection, and obstructions caused by thrombus or other material should be reported

CTA, computed tomography angiography; ECG, electrocardiogram; TAVR, transcatheter aortic valve replacement.

Source: Selected recommendations from the Society for Cardiovascular Computed Tomography, adapted from Achenbach *et al.* 2012 [76]. Copyright 2012, with permission from Elsevier.

Table 58.2 Selected aortic valvuloplasty balloons and recommended sheath sizes.

Balloon	Manufacturer	Diameter (mm)	Length (cm)	Sheath size (Fr)	Illustration
Z-MED™	B. Braun	18	4	10	
		20	4	12	
		22	4	12	
		25	4	12	
Z-MED™ II	B. Braun	18	3, 4, or 6	10	
		20	4	12	
		22	4	12	
		23	4	14	
		25	4 or 5	14	
Tyshak®	B. Braun	18	3 or 5	8	
		20	3, 4, or 6	8	
		22	4	9	
		25	4	9	
Tyshak II®	B. Braun	18	3, 4, 5, or 6	8	
		20	3, 4, 5, or 6	8	
		22	4, 5, or 6	8	
		23	4 or 5	9	
		25	4, 5, or 6	9	
NuCleus-X™	B. Braun	18	4, 5, or 6	10	
		20	4, 5, or 6	12	
		22	4, 5, or 6	12	
		25	4, 5, or 6	12	
Vida® PTV Dilatation Catheters	C.R. Bard, Inc.	18	2, 4, or 6	8 or 9	
		20	2 or 4	9	
		22	2 or 4	10	
		24	2 or 4	10	
Bard® True Dilatation® Balloon Valvuloplasty Catheters	C.R. Bard, Inc.	20	4.5	11	
		22	4.5	12	
		24	4.5	12	

Z-MED, Tyshak and NuCleus-X are trademarks and/or registered trademarks of B. Braun Interventional Systems, Inc. (Bethlehem, PA, USA). Bard, True Dilatation, and Vida are trademarks and/or registered trademarks of C.R. Bard, Inc. (New Providence, NJ, USA). Braun balloon images: Reproduced with permission from B. Braun Interventional Systems. Bard balloon images: Copyright 2015 C.R. Bard, Inc. Used with permission.

registry of 428 patients undergoing BAV between 2005 and 2011, patients treated with pre-closure technique (n = 269) experienced a significantly lower rate of not only major bleeding (5.6% vs. 14.5%; p = 0.01), but also a composite of major bleeding, myocardial infarction, stroke, and all-cause mortality (10% vs. 24.5%; p <0.001) [78]. It is important when interpreting such observational data to acknowledge the influence of atherosclerotic disease burden on patient eligibility for vascular closure device use and likelihood of device success.

Anterior wall calcification and vascular fibrosis are key predictors of closure device failure [79]. In addition to providing a plausible explanation for an increase in closure device failure, local access site bleeding, and vascular complications [56], iliofemoral atherosclerosis

has been shown to predict incident cardiovascular events attributable to other vascular beds [80].

Pre-closure technique can be accomplished using either of two commercially available suture-mediated closure systems marketed by Abbott Vascular (Redwood, CA, USA): Prostar® XL and Perclose ProGlide®. Both systems can be used for primary closure at the conclusion of a transfemoral procedure ("post-closure"), with the Prostar XL device indicated for closure of arteriotomies of 8.5–10 Fr and the Perclose ProGlide device indicated for closure of arteriotomies of 5–8 Fr. With a pre-closure technique, sutures are partially deployed prior to maximal dilatation of the arteriotomy, permitting more certain grasping of peri-arteriotomy arterial tissue and the ability to close larger holes. For closure of very large arteriotomies, multiple devices can be used in conjunction. In published literature, a single Prostar XL device has been used successfully to pre-close arteriotomies as large as 18 or 19 Fr, and a pair of devices has been used successfully to close arteriotomies measuring 22 or 24 Fr in the context of TAVR [81]. With the Perclose ProGlide device, a combination of two devices can be used to close arteriotomies measuring 8.5–24 Fr. In our practice, we have observed that pre-closure with a single Perclose ProGlide device can sometimes be adequate to achieve closure of 9 or 10 Fr arteriotomies.

One study has compared the Prostar XL with Perclose ProGlide devices for the purpose of pre-closure prior to TAVR. In the multicenter retrospective ClOsure device iN TRansfemoral aOrtic vaLve implantation (CONTROL) study, which included 3138 patients undergoing percutaneous transfemoral TAVR, propensity-matched comparison of 944 patients assigned to pre-closure with either device revealed a significant excess of major vascular complications in Prostar XL-treated patients (7.4% vs. 1.9%; p <0.001) [82]. Additionally, Prostar XL-treated patients experienced higher rates of major bleeding and acute kidney injury and had longer hospital stays. Differences in outcomes between the two devices perhaps reflect differences in device design. Whereas the Prostar XL delivers four needles on each end of two sutures, all delivered simultaneously outward from the arterial lumen, the Perclose ProGlide delivers two needles on each end of one suture, with two devices typically deployed in sequence via a cross-hair approach [82]. Failure of the Prostar XL is total, whereas one of two Perclose ProGlide sutures can accomplish partial or even complete success.

It is clear that experience matters. There is a demonstrable learning curve with percutaneous suture-mediated closure systems, with success rates improving from 85% to over 95% in seasoned operators [81]. When performed by experienced operators, percutaneous suture-mediated closure is furthermore associated with substantial reduction in total and major vascular complications, including iliac complications, and shorter stays in the intensive care unit after TAVR [81]. We strongly advocate that operators in training gain experience with use of a percutaneous suture-mediate closure system of choice in cases with smaller arteriotomies prior to application in BAV or TAVR.

The above data have been progressively incorporated in contemporary practice, and our perception is that most operators now prefer pre-closure with Perclose ProGlide devices. For illustration of the steps in device use, readers are encouraged to view a manufacturer video demonstrating recommended technique which is freely available online (http://www.abbottvascular.com/us/video/proglide-lhc-video.html).

Pre-closure with Perclose ProGlide®

As a critical first step, pre-procedure review of available iliofemoral imaging data is mandatory. While for TAVR ileofemoral assessment is primarily performed by CTA, for BAV CTA data may not be available, in which case the operator must rely on careful examination of the groin and iliofemoral anatomy by inspection, palpation, and fluoroscopic assessment. A prior history of multiple catheterizations via the right femoral artery should also be considered, which typically leads to scarring of the arterial access site which makes pre-closure more challenging. In this case a left femoral approach can be preferable. If a CTA is available, it is essential to pay close attention to the common femoral arteries, to identify vascular diameter and areas of calcification, the site of the bifurcation

of the common femoral artery, and to relate these data to bony landmarks such as the femoral head that can then be used as a reference for accurate arteriotomy.

On inspection, identify the inguinal crease and make note of any superficial scars, wounds, and fungal infections that could interfere with access. On palpation, identify the inguinal ligament and the point of maximal impulse of the femoral arterial pulse, scanning cranially and caudally, paying attention to areas of a diffuse or split impulse, which may reflect the bifurcation of the femoral artery into its superficial and deep branches. If the pulse is diminished or absent, be suspicious of significant aortoiliac atherosclerosis. It is important also to recognize qualities of the soft tissue overlying the femoral artery, such as scarring and depth of adipose tissue, which can impede delivery of larger sheaths or percutaneous sutures. On fluoroscopic assessment, evaluate the appearance of the unopacified femoral artery in the anteroposterior projection with particular attention to zones of dense calcification. Real-time fluoroscopy during left–right rotation of the camera provides additional three-dimensional perspective of vascular calcification, in particular permitting recognition of anterior wall calcium. A radio-opaque object such as a hemostat can be placed at this time to mark a desired location for arterial puncture.

Given the frailty and hemodynamic tenuousness of many patients undergoing large-bore arterial access, aim to use minimal necessary doses of parenteral anxiolytics and narcotics, instead favoring thorough local anesthesia, typically with 1% lidocaine. Next proceed with arterial puncture. Many techniques are possible here, and typically the "optimal" technique for any individual operator will be closely related to what they usually perform for small-bore access. A popular approach is to initial "micro-access" using a 21-gauge needle and compatible wire, then confirming position by contrast injection through a 1–2 Fr microsheath. An anterior wall puncture of the common femoral artery in an area of minimal calcification and plaque is required to permit pre-closure technique. Accordingly, in the event of a suboptimal puncture, it is easy to remove the microsheath and abort the arteriotomy, obtain manual hemostasis, and reattempt access. Once satisfactory arteriotomy is achieved, exchange the micro-access system for an 0.035-inch wire and proceed with pre-closure.

Other popular techniques for accurate arteriotomy include first accessing the contralateral common femoral artery and then placing a small catheter in the ipsilateral external iliac artery and then performing an angiogram to precisely delineate the ideal access point on the desired side for the large-bore sheath. As a variation on this, 4–5 Fr pigtail catheter can be placed from the contralateral common femoral artery into the precise position in the ipsilateral common femoral artery that is desirable to access (guided by contrast injections and angiography through the pigtail as needed), with the operator then accessing the ipsilateral common femoral artery under fluoroscopy by aiming the tip the arteriotomy needle directly at the center of the pigtail.

Once suitable ipsilateral access has been initially secured by any of these techniques, to facilitate successful pre-closure and subsequent large sheath delivery, it is advantageous to prepare the tissue track by blunt dissection. This can be performed before or after arterial puncture. The optimal tissue track should be large enough to accommodate the main sheath without being unnecessarily broad; free of clots, fat, skin tags, and fibrinous strands; and straight. Serpentine tracks significantly increase the difficulty of sheath insertion and closure.

Next advance a first Perclose ProGlide device over the 0.035-inch guidewire into the femoral artery until pulsatile flow is observed from the device's marker lumen. Next, rotate the device 30–45° clockwise prior to deploying its suture in usual fashion. Then lower the footplate and withdraw the device, harvesting the sutures and re-establishing wire access to the vessel. It is important at this point to secure the lock and rail ends of the suture using a hemostat, taking care to avoid any tension in the suture (which would prematurely tighten the knot). Repeat the process using a second Perclose ProGlide device, instead rotating the device 30–45° counterclockwise prior to deploying the suture. If a single device is used, this can be deployed at 0°. Following pre-closure, access is re-established using an 0.035-inch guidewire. In a stepwise fashion, sequentially dilate the tissue track and arteriotomy from 8 Fr up to the desired sheath size (usually using only one or perhaps two dilation size increments) and finally insert the main sheath.

Contralateral safety wire

While less commonly used now because of decreasing TAVR sheath sizes, an optional technique is to deliver a "safety wire" from the contralateral common femoral artery down the ipsilateral ileofemoral arterial system. Typically, a stiff 0.018-inch guidewide is used for this purpose, which is performed using standard iliac crossover techniques. The wire is delivered down to the ipsilateral distal superficial femoral or proximal popliteal artery, and remains in place throughout the entire procedure. The safety wire can be delivered prior to pre-closure, with a small risk of entanglement in the Perclose sutures, or after pre-close, with the possibility of some difficulty navigating around the sheath and Perclose sutures that will then be in place in the ipsilateral common femoral artery. This safety wire provides secure access to the true lumen of the access vessel, and can be used to deliver an adjunctive balloon for inflation in the external iliac artery or at the arteriotomy site to assist with access site closure. In the advent of ileofemoral dissection, rupture, or perforation, a safety wire can be a lifesaving method to deliver a covered stent or other device. In contemporary practice, a safety wire is rarely if ever used for stand-alone BAV, but is typically still used for larger TAVR sheaths.

Performing balloon aortic valvuloplasty

Prior to proceeding with BAV, if not previously performed, it is advisable to perform a comprehensive right and left heart catheterization in the standard fashion, including hemodynamic assessment and coronary angiography. Aortography is also performed in the left anterior oblique 30° projection to assess baseline severity of aortic insufficiency.

Anticoagulation during BAV

Anticoagulation is indicated during BAV to reduce risk of procedure-related thrombosis and arterial thromboembolism. This is usually with a low dose of unfractionated heparin or bivalirudin – typically, half the dose that would normally be administered for coronary intervention.

Historically, the preference during BAV was to use unfractionated heparin, with variable application of protamine at procedure conclusion for reversal of anticoagulation. Recently, there has been interest in using bivalirudin as an alternative to heparin for BAV and TAVR. Putative advantages of bivalirudin include predictable anticoagulant effect, avoidance of heparin-induced thrombocytopenia, and a proven track record of bleeding avoidance in the setting of percutaneous coronary intervention [83]. Potential disadvantages include irreversibility, reliance on renal clearance, and cost. To date, no randomized trials have compared the two agents for use in BAV. In the Effect of Bivalirudin on Aortic Valve Intervention Outcomes (BRAVO) registry, which retrospectively studied 427 patients undergoing BAV at two high-volume centers, patients receiving bivalirudin (n = 223; 52.2%) experienced a lower rate of major bleeding (4.9% vs. 13.2%; p = 0.003) that remained significant after multivariate analysis [84]. Observed reduction in bleeding was driven by both access site related bleeding (3.6% vs. 7.8%; p = 0.06) and non-access site related bleeding (1.3% vs. 5.4%; p = 0.02), which included pericardial bleeding. Stroke was rare, with two major strokes documented in the heparin group and none in the bivalirudin group.

Crossing the aortic valve

Multiple techniques are available for crossing the aortic valve. Often preferred is an Amplatz right 2 (AR2) catheter with careful advance of a stiff, straight-tipped hydrophilic guide wire in the left anterior oblique projection. For different aortic configurations, other catheters may be preferable to optimize alignment of wire advance with the axis of the aortic annulus. For dilated aortic roots, an Amplatz left 1 catheter may be more appropriate. A to-and-fro motion of the catheter tip with the cardiac cycle can indicate alignment of the catheter with the turbulent jet of left ventricular outflow and improved likelihood of success. If wire crossing is unsuccessful after 2–3 minutes, it is usual to withdraw and clean the wire and flush the catheter prior to reattempt.

Once the wire crosses the aortic valve into the left ventricle, extreme care must be taken. Excessive advance of the slippery, sharp, stiff hydrophilic wire can easily perforate the left ventricle, precipitating pericardial hemorrhage and cardiac tamponade [85]. Mechanical irritation of the often hypertrophied left ventricular myocardium can precipitate ventricular tachyarrhythmias, poorly tolerated in the setting of severe AS. Once intracavitary position is confirmed, the hydrophilic wire is carefully exchanged for the soft-tipped catheter and removed.

Wires

After measuring and recording the transaortic valve pressure gradient, the next step is to exchange the catheter for a stiff wire to support BAV. This can either be done directly, or by first placing an exchange-length soft wire and changing the AR2 catheter for a pigtail catheter, and then introducing the stiff wire via the pigtail. The latter two-step approach is preferable for operators less experienced in handling the very stiff wires required for BAV and TAVR that can also perforate the ventricle.

Several wires are suitable to support BAV, such as the J-tipped Amplatz Extra Stiff, the straight 1 cm floppy tip Amplatz Super Stiff™, and Lunderquist® wires (all from Cook Medical, Bloomington, IN, USA), in progressive order of increasing stiffness and support. If there are no mitigating factors such as vascular tortuosity, it is usually advisable to use the least stiff wire from among these options. Some of these wires require shaping prior to use, in which case either a pigtail bend (for the Amplatz Super Stiff), or a larger V-shaped bend (for the Amplatz Extra Stiff) are usually created. Appropriate positioning of this wire at the left ventricular apex is essential to minimize the risk of lacerating the ventricle during the procedure. Exchange and replacement of the stiff wire using a pigtail catheter can help to ensure central wire positioning, free from the mitral apparatus.

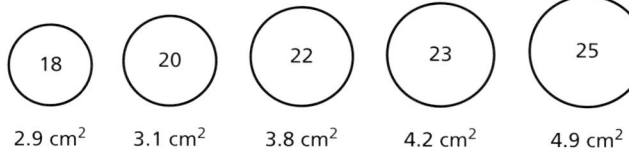

Figure 58.1 Valvuloplasty balloon sizes and corresponding cross-sectional area.

BAV balloons

A selection of BAV balloons is presented in Table 58.2. Balloons vary with respect to length and size; shape, with some balloons featuring a central "waist"; profile and associated sheath size requirement; speed of inflation and deflation; radiographic markers for placement; materials; and compliance. Choice of a specific balloon for an individual patient is influenced by annular size, availability, operator comfort, and limitations on safe sheath sizing.

With respect to balloon sizing, it is advisable to favor a balloon to aortic annulus diameter ratio of <1 : 1. Typically, most operators use an initial size range of 18–23 Fr for most patients. It is important to also note that whereas balloons expand to become circular in cross-section (Figure 58.1), the aortic annulus is rarely circular but is usually elliptical [86,87]. Annular size tends to be smaller in women [87] and larger in patients with bicuspid aortic valves [88]. In patients with very severe AS or heavy calcification of the valve apparatus, initial inflation with a balloon sized 1 : 1 with the aortic annulus may not be feasible or safe.

Balloons used in aortic valvuloplasty, sized with respect to diameter in millimeters, expand to become circular in cross-section, with a corresponding area equal to π times the radius squared. As discussed later, the feared complication of BAV, especially if performed as a stand-alone procedure not in association with TAVR, is severe aortic regurgitation. This concern means it is always advisable to be conservative in balloon selection for BAV. Sequential dilatation with a larger balloon is always an option, in which case it is possible to assess the degree of aortic regurgitation and ensure there has been no increase, prior to upsizing to a large balloon.

Pacing

Rapid ventricular pacing (at 180–200 b.p.m.) at the time of balloon inflation acutely decreases stroke volume and cardiac motion. This facilitates precise balloon placement and reduces likelihood of balloon slippage or to-and-fro movement. To the extent that such to-and-fro motion can transform the balloon and wire into a spear and a saw, avoidance of this motion might reduce likelihood of ventricular perforation, pericardial hemorrhage, and cardiac tamponade during BAV. Whether rapid ventricular pacing should be performed routinely is controversial, with uncertainty about its deleterious hemodynamic effects and limited data concerning safety and efficacy [89]. In published observational literature [90], rapid ventricular pacing was helpful in balloon placement and safe even in high risk BAV patients. In order to minimize any added ischemic insult, it is important to minimize the duration of pacing. To accomplish this, close teamwork between operators and trained laboratory technical staff is essential.

Procedural conclusion

Following balloon inflation and deflation, the balloon is withdrawn from the body. Hemodynamic measurements are repeated to assess interval change in aortic valve gradient and area, and aortography is repeated to assess interval change in aortic regurgitation. Close monitoring is essential during this time, as new onset hypotension can be indicative of one of several life-threatening complications. If the patient remains stable and the result is acceptable, it is appropriate to proceed to arteriotomy closure. If a significant gradient remains, it is possible to consider repeat BAV using a larger balloon. In the decision to use a second, larger balloon, it is critical to weigh the potential risks, which of course increase with larger balloon size, against the benefits. For many frail elderly patients undergoing BAV as a stand-alone palliative or temporizing procedure, the risk often outweighs the possible benefit. While an "acceptable" result from stand-alone BAV varies according to the patient and their indication to undergo the procedure, typically a reduction in peak gradient by 50–70% is considered successful. Attempting to achieve a more substantial reduction in aortic gradient is unrealistic and potentially dangerous.

Arteriotomy closure and troubleshooting

If pre-closure technique was successful, the pre-deployed sutures can then be used to close the arteriotomy. Usually during TAVR, but rarely for BAV due to smaller sheath sizes and lack of contralateral access, the large-bore sheath is first retracted to the external iliac artery, and digital subtraction angiography (DSA) of the ipsilateral common and external iliac arteries is performed to ensure no arterial perforation or dissection. If there is no vascular injury, at this time the stiff wire is usually swapped for a softer wire, because withdrawing the stiff wire used for BAV/TAVR (especially if it has a large loop at the end) through the arteriotomy can damage the femoral artery. If a safety wire was placed, a conservatively sized peripheral balloon can be inflated in the distal external iliac artery to decrease flow. As the large-bore access sheath is removed from the body, the Perclose sutures are tightened in sequence, in the same order in which they were initially deployed. A guidewire can be left in place during this step, maintaining access to the vessel and allowing reinsertion of a hemostatic sheath in the event that suture-mediated closure is unsuccessful. Again, if a safety wire was placed, a low pressure inflation at the arteriotomy site is usually performed to aid with hemostasis. If contralateral access was obtained, a final DSA is then performed, and the procedure completed. Often, despite successful pre-closure, 5–15 minutes of additional manual groin compression is needed to achieve complete hemostasis.

For BAV using up to 12 Fr sheaths, if pre-closure fails and there was no contralateral access, sustained manual compression is usually attempted to obtain hemostasis. If pre-closure fails with larger sheath sizes where there is typically contralateral access, sustained balloon inflation at the arteriotomy site is performed. Ideally, this is via the safety wire that was placed at the beginning of the procedure. If a safety wire was not placed, then it may be necessary to consider wiring across the arteriotomy site from the contralateral femoral access site. Technically, this can range from being relatively simple if the issue is an unacceptable residual stenosis of the large-bore access arteriotomy, to exceptionally challenging if there is a complex dissection, perforation, avulsion or significant hemorrhage from the large-bore arteriotomy site. Obviously, if any of these more serious complications arise, more advanced salvage techniques such as covered stent placement are required. If covered stent placement is needed, this is best performed on the ipsilateral wire for common and external iliac complications, but for major complications at the large-bore arteriotomy site, a wire from the contralateral side is required. Complex iliac anatomy (calcification, stenosis, tortuosity) in BAV/TAVR patients can add significant procedural challenge to the management of any vascular complication.

Complications of BAV and their management

Complications are common and can be life-threatening. A list of key complications of BAV is presented in Table 58.3, with frequencies as reported in the recent BRAVO registry [84].

Vascular complications are a particular concern, and patients having BAV or TAVR are at heightened risk because of comorbid atherosclerosis and large-bore sheaths. Valve Academic Research Consortium criteria for major and minor vascular complications are presented in Box 58.3.

Structural complications particular to BAV merit special consideration. Acute reduction in left ventricular afterload can induce development of a dynamic intracavitary gradient, particularly in patients with left ventricular hypertrophy, small chamber size, and any pre-existing left ventricular outflow tract obstruction. Arterial pressure recordings can reveal hypotension and new onset of a spike-and-dome waveform. In rare cases, reported chiefly in the setting of TAVR [92], this can manifest fulminantly as cardiovascular collapse, earning the appellation of "suicide left ventricle." Management consists of volume resuscitation and pure vasopressors (e.g., phenylephrine) without beta-adrenergic agonist properties.

Acute aortic insufficiency (~1%) [93] is a devastating complication of BAV which is best avoided by careful patient selection and balloon sizing. Clinical manifestations of acute aortic insufficiency include hypotension, a widened pulse pressure, flash pulmonary edema, cardiovascular collapse and arrest usually with pulseless electrical activity. Left ventricular pressure recordings show a steep rise in left ventricular diastolic pressure, equaling aortic diastolic pressure prior to end-diastole in the setting of severe aortic regurgitation. By contrast aortography, severe aortic insufficiency is evidenced by instantaneous opacification of the left ventricle. Acute management, complicated by coexisting AS, consists of diuretics, arterial vasodilators, fast ventricular pacing, and surgical consultation if appropriate.

Patients with very severe AS and associated extensive aortic annular calcification are at risk for annular rupture (0.3%) [93]. Extreme caution is warranted in these cases. This catastrophic, rare complication of BAV is rapidly fatal, and the prognosis of emergent cardiac surgery is poor.

Cardiac perforation results in pericardial hemorrhage and cardiac tamponade (0.3–1.2%) [84,93]. Causes of perforation include the temporary venous pacing wire, the hydrophilic wire used to cross the aortic valve, the stiff wire used to support BAV, and the balloon itself. Clinical presentation can be insidious as blood gradually accumulates in the pericardium, not becoming clinically manifest as hypotension until several minutes later. Fluoroscopy reveals a pericardial shadow. Echocardiography confirms the diagnosis of pericardial effusion and can show evidence of tamponade physiology. Treatment is emergent pericardiocentesis and discontinuation of anticoagulation with protamine administration if heparin was

Table 58.3 Complications of balloon aortic valvuloplasty.

Complication	Frequency (%)
Mortality (in-hospital)	6
Bleeding:	
Major (BARC 3, 4, or 5)	9
Minor (BARC 1 or 2)	4
Vascular complications:	
Major	2
Minor	5
Acute kidney injury	10
Myocardial infarction	3
Major stroke	0.5

Frequencies reflect reported event rates as adjudicated according to VARC and BARC criteria in the Effect of Bivalirudin on Aortic Valve Intervention Outcomes (BRAVO) registry [84].
BARC, Bleeding Academic Research Consortium; VARC, Valve Academic Research Consortium.

Box 58.3 Vascular access site and access-related complications

Major vascular complications:
- Any thoracic aortic dissection
- Access site or access-related vascular injury (dissection, stenosis, perforation, rupture, arteriovenous fistula, pseudoaneurysm, hematoma, irreversible nerve injury, or compartment syndrome) leading to either death, need for significant blood transfusions (≥4 U), unplanned percutaneous or surgical intervention, or irreversible end-organ damage (e.g., hypogastric artery occlusion causing visceral ischemia or spinal artery injury causing neurologic impairment)
- Distal embolization (non-cerebral) from a vascular source requiring surgery or resulting in amputation or irreversible end-organ damage

Minor vascular complications:
- Access site or access-related vascular injury (dissection, stenosis, perforation, rupture, arteriovenous fistula or pseudoaneuysms requiring compression or thrombin injection therapy, or hematomas requiring transfusion of ≥2 but, 4 U) *not* requiring unplanned percutaneous or surgical intervention, and *not* resulting in irreversible end-organ damage
- Distal embolization treated with embolectomy and/or thrombectomy and *not* resulting in amputation or irreversible end-organ damage
- Failure of percutaneous access site closure resulting in interventional (e.g., stent graft) or surgical correction and not associated with death, need for significant blood transfusions (≥4 U), or irreversible end-organ damage

Current definitions according to the Valve Academic Research Consortium.

Source: Leon MB, *et al.* 2011 [91]. Copyright 2011, with permission from Elsevier.

used. Depending on the site and size of perforation, bleeding sometimes ceases spontaneously; in other cases, limited cardiac surgery with patch placement is required to obtain hemostasis.

Conclusions, recommendations, and future directions

The advent of TAVR has renewed interest in BAV and reminded us of its limitations. For patients once untreated for a deadly disease, BAV offers a minimally invasive option for temporary mechanical relief of severe AS and its symptoms. Yet, while minimally invasive, BAV still exposes patients to mortal risks. Though alleviating symptoms, BAV confers no durable benefit for longevity. Patients considering palliative BAV must still ask: "Am I willing to risk death for a chance at an improved quality of life?" For some, the answer is yes. Honest, open, patient-centered conversations are mandatory to establish a plan of care tailored to an individual. For many patients under consideration for BAV, adjunctive consultation with palliative care services are useful to facilitate broader conversations about goals of care.

Recognition of the persistently high rates of major complications of BAV reminds us of the need for further improvement in safety. Opportunities for improvement include research and development of lower profile balloon systems with smaller sheath requirements; atraumatic wires to cross the valve and support BAV; and bleeding avoidance strategies, including closure devices and different anticoagulant regimens.

Finally, as TAVR matures, miniaturizes, and streamlines, the question becomes: are there any remaining candidates for standalone BAV, or is the only appropriate mechanical treatment for severe AS an AVR? We foresee a continuing role for BAV for some time to come but predict that accessibility and availability of TAVR will only continue to increase.

Interactive multiple choice questions are available for this chapter on www.wiley.com/go/dangas/cardiology

References

1 Rose AG. Etiology of valvular heart disease. *Curr Opin Cardiol* 1996; **11**: 98–113.
2 Mozaffarian D, Benjamin EJ, Go AS, *et al.* Heart disease and stroke statistics—2015 update: a report from the American Heart Association. *Circulation* 2015; **131**: e29–322.
3 Kovacic JC, Moreno P, Hachinski V, Nabel EG, Fuster V. Cellular senescence, vascular disease, and aging: Part 1 of a 2-part review. *Circulation* 2011; **123**: 1650–1660.
4 Braunwald E. On the natural history of severe aortic stenosis. *J Am Coll Cardiol* 1990; **15**: 1018–1020.
5 Ross J Jr, Braunwald E. Aortic stenosis. *Circulation* 1968; **38**: 61–67.
6 Carabello BA. Introduction to aortic stenosis. *Circ Res* 2013; **113**: 179–185.
7 Bach DS. Prevalence and characteristics of unoperated patients with severe aortic stenosis. *J Heart Valve Dis* 2011; **20**: 284–291.
8 Leon MB, Smith CR, Mack M, *et al.* Transcatheter aortic-valve implantation for aortic stenosis in patients who cannot undergo surgery. *N Engl J Med* 2010; **363**: 1597–1607.
9 Smith CR, Leon MB, Mack MJ, *et al.* Transcatheter versus surgical aortic-valve replacement in high-risk patients. *N Engl J Med* 2011; **364**: 2187–2198.
10 Adams DH, Popma JJ, Reardon MJ, *et al.* Transcatheter aortic-valve replacement with a self-expanding prosthesis. *N Engl J Med* 2014; **370**: 1790–1798.
10a Leon MB, Smith CR, Mack MJ, *et al.* Transcatheter or surgical aortic valve replacement in intermediate risk patients. *N Engl J Med* 2016; **374**: 1609–1620.
11 Lababidi Z. Aortic balloon valvuloplasty. *Am Heart J* 1983; **106**: 751–752.
12 Cribier A, Savin T, Saoudi N, Rocha P, Berland J, Letac B. Percutaneous transluminal valvuloplasty of acquired aortic stenosis in elderly patients: an alternative to valve replacement? *Lancet* 1986; **1**: 63–67.
13 McKay RG, Safian RD, Lock JE, *et al.* Balloon dilatation of calcific aortic stenosis in elderly patients: postmortem, intraoperative, and percutaneous valvuloplasty studies. *Circulation* 1986; **74**: 119–125.
14 Cribier A, Savin T, Berland J, *et al.* Percutaneous transluminal balloon valvuloplasty of adult aortic stenosis: report of 92 cases. *J Am Coll Cardiol* 1987; **9**: 381–386.
15 Harpole DH, Davidson CJ, Skelton TN, Kisslo KB, Jones RH, Bashore TM. Changes in left ventricular systolic performance immediately after percutaneous aortic balloon valvuloplasty. *Am J Cardiol* 1990; **65**: 1213–1218.
16 McKay RG. The Mansfield Scientific Aortic Valvuloplasty Registry: overview of acute hemodynamic results and procedural complications. *J Am Coll Cardiol* 1991; **17**: 485–491.
17 Percutaneous balloon aortic valvuloplasty: acute and 30-day follow-up results in 674 patients from the NHLBI Balloon Valvuloplasty Registry. *Circulation* 1991; **84**: 2383–2397.
18 Scherer HE, Lindner K, Wosnoik W, Engel HJ. [Hemodynamic and clinical results following percutaneous aortic valve valvuloplasty in adults]. *Z Kardiol* 1990; **79**: 489–498.
19 Harrison JK, Davidson CJ, Leithe ME, Kisslo KB, Skelton TN, Bashore TM. Serial left ventricular performance evaluated by cardiac catheterization before, immediately after and at 6 months after balloon aortic valvuloplasty. *J Am Coll Cardiol* 1990; **16**: 1351–1358.
20 Bashore TM, Davidson CJ. Follow-up recatheterization after balloon aortic valvuloplasty. Mansfield Scientific Aortic Valvuloplasty Registry Investigators. *J Am Coll Cardiol* 1991; **17**: 1188–1195.
21 Harpole DH, Davidson CJ, Skelton TN, Kisslo KB, Jones RH, Bashore TM. Early and late changes in left ventricular systolic performance after percutaneous aortic balloon valvuloplasty. *Am J Cardiol* 1990; **66**: 327–332.
22 Davidson CJ, Harpole DA, Kisslo K, *et al.* Analysis of the early rise in aortic transvalvular gradient after aortic valvuloplasty. *Am Heart J* 1989; **117**: 411–417.
23 Lieberman EB, Bashore TM, Hermiller JB, *et al.* Balloon aortic valvuloplasty in adults: failure of procedure to improve long-term survival. *J Am Coll Cardiol* 1995; **26**: 1522–1528.
24 Otto CM, Mickel MC, Kennedy JW, *et al.* Three-year outcome after balloon aortic valvuloplasty: insights into prognosis of valvular aortic stenosis. *Circulation* 1994; **89**: 642–650.
25 Di Mario C, Serruys PW, Luijten HE, *et al.* Percutaneous balloon valvuloplasty in adult aortic stenosis: a palliative treatment but not without risk. *Cardiologia* 1987; **32**: 535–543.
26 Dauterman KW, Michaels AD, Ports TA. Is there any indication for aortic valvuloplasty in the elderly? *Am J Geriatr Cardiol* 2003; **12**: 190–196.
27 Hara H, Pedersen WR, Ladich E, *et al.* Percutaneous balloon aortic valvuloplasty revisited: time for a renaissance? *Circulation* 2007; **115**: e334–338.
28 Hui DS, Shavelle DM, Cunningham MJ, Matthews RV, Starnes VA. Contemporary use of balloon aortic valvuloplasty in the era of transcatheter aortic valve implantation. *Tex Heart Inst J* 2014; **41**: 469–476.
29 Saia F, Marrozzini C, Ciuca C, *et al.* Emerging indications, in-hospital and long-term outcome of balloon aortic valvuloplasty in the transcatheter aortic valve implantation era. *EuroIntervention* 2013; **8**: 1388–1397.
30 Safian RD, Mandell VS, Thurer RE, *et al.* Postmortem and intraoperative balloon valvuloplasty of calcific aortic stenosis in elderly patients: mechanisms of successful dilation. *J Am Coll Cardiol* 1987; **9**: 655–660.
31 Kennedy KD, Hauck AJ, Edwards WD, Holmes DR Jr, Reeder GS, Nishimura RA. Mechanism of reduction of aortic valvular stenosis by percutaneous transluminal balloon valvuloplasty: report of five cases and review of literature. *Mayo Clin Proc* 1988; **63**: 769–776.
32 Letac B, Gerber LI, Koning R. Insights on the mechanism of balloon valvuloplasty in aortic stenosis. *Am J Cardiol* 1988; **62**: 1241–1247.
33. McKay RG, Safian RD, Lock JE, *et al.* Assessment of left ventricular and aortic valve function after aortic balloon valvuloplasty in adult patients with critical aortic stenosis. *Circulation* 1987; **75**: 192–203.
34 Ross J Jr. Afterload mismatch in aortic and mitral valve disease: implications for surgical therapy. *J Am Coll Cardiol* 1985; **5**: 811–826.
35 Ferguson JJ 3rd, Bush HS, Riuli EP. Effect of balloon aortic valvuloplasty on the dynamics of left ventricular ejection. *Cathet Cardiovasc Diagn* 1989; **18**: 73–78.
36 Loscalzo J. From clinical observation to mechanism: Heyde's syndrome. *N Engl J Med* 2012; **367**: 1954–1956.
37 Bander J, Elmariah S, Aledort LM, *et al.* Changes in von Willebrand factor-cleaving protease (ADAMTS-13) in patients with aortic stenosis undergoing valve replacement or balloon valvuloplasty. *Thromb Haemost* 2012; **108**: 86–93.
38 Farb A, Moses JW, Wallerson DC, Gold JP, Subramanian VA. Valve injury and repair in balloon aortic valvuloplasty. *Cathet Cardiovasc Diagn* 1989; **18**: 90–95.

39 Serruys PW, Di Mario C, Essed CE. Restenosis 3 months after successful percutaneous aortic valvoplasty: a clinicopathological report. *Int J Cardiol* 1987; **17**: 210–213.

40 Block PC, Palacios IF. Clinical and hemodynamic follow-up after percutaneous aortic valvuloplasty in the elderly. *Am J Cardiol* 1988; **62**: 760–763.

41 Safian RD, Berman AD, Diver DJ, *et al.* Balloon aortic valvuloplasty in 170 consecutive patients. *N Engl J Med* 1988; **319**: 125–130.

42 Nishimura RA, Otto CM, Bonow RO, *et al.* 2014 AHA/ACC guideline for the management of patients with valvular heart disease: a report of the American College of Cardiology/American Heart Association Task Force on Practice Guidelines. *J Am Coll Cardiol* 2014; **63**: e57–185.

43 Kapadia S, Stewart WJ, Anderson WN, *et al.* Outcomes of inoperable symptomatic aortic stenosis patients not undergoing aortic valve replacement: insight into the impact of balloon aortic valvuloplasty from the PARTNER trial (Placement of AoRTic TraNscathetER Valve trial). *JACC Cardiovasc Interv* 2015; **8**: 324–333.

44 Coverstone E, Korenblat K, Crippin JS, Chapman WC, Kates AM, Zajarias A. Aortic balloon valvuloplasty prior to orthotopic liver transplantation: a novel approach to aortic stenosis and end-stage liver disease. *Case Rep Cardiol* 2014; **2014**: 325136.

45 Kalarickal P, Liu Q, Rathor R, Ishag S, Kerr T, Kangrga I. Balloon aortic valvuloplasty as a bridge to liver transplantation in patients with severe aortic stenosis: a case series. *Transplant Proc* 2014; **46**: 3492–3495.

46 Kogoj P, Devjak R, Bunc M. Balloon aortic valvuloplasty (BAV) as a bridge to aortic valve replacement in cancer patients who require urgent non-cardiac surgery. *Radiol Oncol* 2014; **48**: 62–66.

47 Fukunaga H, Higashitani M, Tobaru T, Mahara K, Takanashi S, Takayama M. Emergent balloon aortic valvuloplasty as a bridge to transcatheter aortic valve implantation with marked risk reduction of perioperative and postoperative mortality. *Cardiovasc Interv Ther* 2016; **31**: 151–155.

48 Feltes TF, Bacha E, Beekman RH 3rd, *et al.* Indications for cardiac catheterization and intervention in pediatric cardiac disease: a scientific statement from the American Heart Association. *Circulation* 2011; **123**: 2607–2652.

49 Reynolds MR, Magnuson EA, Lei Y, *et al.* Health-related quality of life after transcatheter aortic valve replacement in inoperable patients with severe aortic stenosis. *Circulation* 2011; **124**: 1964–1972.

50 Lindman BR, Alexander KP, O'Gara PT, Afilalo J. Futility, benefit, and transcatheter aortic valve replacement. *JACC Cardiovasc Interv* 2014; **7**: 707–716.

51 Tribouilloy C, Levy F, Rusinaru D, *et al.* Outcome after aortic valve replacement for low-flow/low-gradient aortic stenosis without contractile reserve on dobutamine stress echocardiography. *J Am Coll Cardiol* 2009; **53**: 1865–1873.

52 Weidemann F, Herrmann S, Stork S, *et al.* Impact of myocardial fibrosis in patients with symptomatic severe aortic stenosis. *Circulation* 2009; **120**: 577–584.

53 Toggweiler S, Boone RH, Rodes-Cabau J, *et al.* Transcatheter aortic valve replacement: outcomes of patients with moderate or severe mitral regurgitation. *J Am Coll Cardiol* 2012; **59**: 2068–2074.

54 Bedogni F, Latib A, De Marco F, *et al.* Interplay between mitral regurgitation and transcatheter aortic valve replacement with the CoreValve Revalving System: a multicenter registry. *Circulation* 2013; **128**: 2145–2153.

55 Barbanti M, Binder RK, Dvir D, *et al.* Prevalence and impact of preoperative moderate/severe tricuspid regurgitation on patients undergoing transcatheter aortic valve replacement. *Catheter Cardiovasc Interv* 2015; **85**: 677–684.

56 Rodes-Cabau J, Webb JG, Cheung A, *et al.* Transcatheter aortic valve implantation for the treatment of severe symptomatic aortic stenosis in patients at very high or prohibitive surgical risk: acute and late outcomes of the multicenter Canadian experience. *J Am Coll Cardiol* 2010; **55**: 1080–1090.

57 Makkar RR, Fontana GP, Jilaihawi H, *et al.* Transcatheter aortic-valve replacement for inoperable severe aortic stenosis. *N Engl J Med* 2012; **366**: 1696–1704.

58 Gilard M, Eltchaninoff H, Iung B, *et al.* Registry of transcatheter aortic-valve implantation in high-risk patients. *N Engl J Med* 2012; **366**: 1705–1715.

59 Stortecky S, Schoenenberger AW, Moser A, *et al.* Evaluation of multidimensional geriatric assessment as a predictor of mortality and cardiovascular events after transcatheter aortic valve implantation. *JACC Cardiovasc Interv* 2012; **5**: 489–496.

60. Schoenenberger AW, Stortecky S, Neumann S, *et al.* Predictors of functional decline in elderly patients undergoing transcatheter aortic valve implantation (TAVI). *Eur Heart J* 2013; **34**: 684–692.

61 Green P, Woglom AE, Genereux P, *et al.* The impact of frailty status on survival after transcatheter aortic valve replacement in older adults with severe aortic stenosis: a single-center experience. *JACC Cardiovasc Interv* 2012; **5**: 974–981.

62 Agarwal A, Kini AS, Attanti S, *et al.* Results of repeat balloon valvuloplasty for treatment of aortic stenosis in patients aged 59 to 104 years. *Am J Cardiol* 2005; **95**: 43–47.

63 Greenbaum AB, O'Neill WW, Paone G, *et al.* Caval-aortic access to allow transcatheter aortic valve replacement in otherwise ineligible patients: initial human experience. *J Am Coll Cardiol* 2014; **63**: 2795–2804.

64 Cribier A, Eltchaninoff H, Bash A, *et al.* Percutaneous transcatheter implantation of an aortic valve prosthesis for calcific aortic stenosis: first human case description. *Circulation* 2002; **106**: 3006–3008.

65 Walther T, Kempfert J. Transapical vs. transfemoral aortic valve implantation: which approach for which patient, from a surgeon's standpoint. *Ann Cardiothorac Surg* 2012; **1**: 216–219.

66 Blackstone EH, Suri RM, Rajeswaran J, *et al.* Propensity-matched comparisons of clinical outcomes after transapical or transfemoral transcatheter aortic valve replacement: a placement of aortic transcatheter valves (PARTNER)-I trial substudy. *Circulation* 2015; **131**: 1989–2000.

67 Kahlert P, Al-Rashid F, Dottger P, *et al.* Cerebral embolization during transcatheter aortic valve implantation: a transcranial Doppler study. *Circulation* 2012; **126**: 1245–1255.

68 Moat NE, Ludman P, de Belder MA, *et al.* Long-term outcomes after transcatheter aortic valve implantation in high-risk patients with severe aortic stenosis: the UK TAVI (United Kingdom Transcatheter Aortic Valve Implantation) Registry. *J Am Coll Cardiol* 2011; **58**: 2130–2138.

69 Mack MJ, Brennan JM, Brindis R, *et al.* Outcomes following transcatheter aortic valve replacement in the United States. *JAMA* 2013; **310**: 2069–2077.

70 Abdel-Wahab M, Mehilli J, Frerker C, *et al.* Comparison of balloon-expandable vs self-expandable valves in patients undergoing transcatheter aortic valve replacement: the CHOICE randomized clinical trial. *JAMA* 2014; **311**: 1503–1514.

71 Hamm CW, Mollmann H, Holzhey D, *et al.* The German Aortic Valve Registry (GARY): in-hospital outcome. *Eur Heart J* 2014; **35**: 1588–1598.

72 Kovacic JC, Nguyen HT, Karajgikar R, Sharma SK, Kini AS. The Impella Recover 2.5 and TandemHeart ventricular assist devices are safe and associated with equivalent clinical outcomes in patients undergoing high-risk percutaneous coronary intervention. *Catheter Cardiovasc Interv* 2013; **82**: E28–37.

73 Kovacic JC, Kini A, Banerjee S, *et al.* Patients with 3-vessel coronary artery disease and impaired ventricular function undergoing PCI with Impella 2.5 hemodynamic support have improved 90-day outcomes compared to intra-aortic balloon pump: a sub-study of the PROTECT II trial. *J Interv Cardiol* 2015; **28**: 32–40.

74 Ben-Dor I, Pichard AD, Satler LF, *et al.* Complications and Outcome of balloon aortic valvuloplasty in high-risk or inoperable patients. *JACC Cardiovasc Interv* 2010; **3**: 1150–1156.

75 Genereux P, Webb JG, Svensson LG, *et al.* Vascular complications after transcatheter aortic valve replacement: insights from the PARTNER (Placement of AoRTic TraNscathetER Valve) trial. *J Am Coll Cardiol* 2012; **60**: 1043–1052.

76 Achenbach S, Delgado V, Hausleiter J, Schoenhagen P, Min JK, Leipsic JA. SCCT expert consensus document on computed tomography imaging before transcatheter aortic valve implantation (TAVI)/transcatheter aortic valve replacement (TAVR). *J Cardiovasc Comput Tomogr* 2012; **6**: 366–380.

77 Toggweiler S, Gurvitch R, Leipsic J, *et al.* Percutaneous aortic valve replacement: vascular outcomes with a fully percutaneous procedure. *J Am Coll Cardiol* 2012; **59**: 113–118.

78 O'Neill B, Singh V, Kini A, *et al.* The use of vascular closure devices and impact on major bleeding and net adverse clinical events (NACE) in balloon aortic valvuloplasty: a sub-analysis of the BRAVO study. *Catheter Cardiovasc Interv* 2014; **83**: 10.1002/ccd.24892.

79 Eisenack M, Umscheid T, Tessarek J, Torsello GF, Torsello GB. Percutaneous endovascular aortic aneurysm repair: a prospective evaluation of safety, efficiency, and risk factors. *J Endovasc Ther* 2009; **16**: 708–713.

80 Davidsson L, Fagerberg B, Bergstrom G, Schmidt C. Ultrasound-assessed plaque occurrence in the carotid and femoral arteries are independent predictors of cardiovascular events in middle-aged men during 10 years of follow-up. *Atherosclerosis* 2010; **209**: 469–473.

81 Hayashida K, Lefèvre T, Chevalier B, *et al.* True percutaneous approach for transfemoral aortic valve implantation using the Prostar XL Device: impact of learning curve on vascular complications. *JACC Cardiovasc Interv* 2012; **5**: 207–214.

82 Barbash IM, Barbanti M, Webb J, *et al.* Comparison of vascular closure devices for access site closure after transfemoral aortic valve implantation. *Eur Heart J* 2015; **36**: 3370–3379.

83 Dauerman HL, Rao SV, Resnic FS, Applegate RJ. Bleeding avoidance strategies. Consensus and controversy. *J Am Coll Cardiol* 2011; **58**: 1–10.

84 Kini A, Yu J, Cohen MG, *et al.* Effect of bivalirudin on aortic valve intervention outcomes study: a two-centre registry study comparing bivalirudin and unfractionated heparin in balloon aortic valvuloplasty. *EuroIntervention* 2014; **10**: 312–319.

85 Holmes JDR, Nishimura R, Fountain R, Turi ZG. Iatrogenic pericardial effusion and tamponade in the percutaneous intracardiac intervention era. *JACC Cardiovasc Interv* 2009; **2**: 705–717.

86 Piazza N, de Jaegere P, Schultz C, Becker AE, Serruys PW, Anderson RH. Anatomy of the aortic valvar complex and its implications for transcatheter implantation of the aortic valve. *Circ Cardiovasc Interv* 2008; **1**: 74–81.

87 Buellesfeld L, Stortecky S, Kalesan B, *et al.* Aortic root dimensions among patients with severe aortic stenosis undergoing transcatheter aortic valve replacement. *JACC Cardiovasc Interv* 2013; **6**: 72–83.

88 Philip F, Faza NN, Schoenhagen P, *et al.* Aortic annulus and root characteristics in severe aortic stenosis due to bicuspid aortic valve and tricuspid aortic valves: implications for transcatheter aortic valve therapies. *Catheter Cardiovasc Interv* 2015; **86**: E88–98.

89. Carroll JD. Optimizing technique and outcomes in structural heart disease interventions: Rapid pacing during aortic valvuloplasty? *Catheter Cardiovasc Interv* 2010; **75**: 453–454.

90 Witzke C, Don CW, Cubeddu RJ, *et al.* Impact of rapid ventricular pacing during percutaneous balloon aortic valvuloplasty in patients with critical aortic stenosis: should we be using it? *Catheter Cardiovasc Interv* 2010; **75**: 444–452.

91 Leon MB, Piazza N, Nikolsky E, *et al.* Standardized endpoint definitions for Transcatheter Aortic Valve Implantation clinical trials: a consensus report from the Valve Academic Research Consortium. *J Am Coll Cardiol* 2011; **57**: 253–269.

92 Suh WM, Witzke CF, Palacios IF. Suicide left ventricle following transcatheter aortic valve implantation. *Catheter Cardiovasc Interv* 2010; **76**: 616–620.

93 Eltchaninoff H, Durand E, Borz B, *et al.* Balloon aortic valvuloplasty in the era of transcatheter aortic valve replacement: acute and long-term outcomes. *Am Heart J* 2014; **167**: 235–240.

CHAPTER 59

Transfemoral Aortic Valve Implantation: Preparation, Implantation, and Complications

Brandon M. Jones[1], Samir R. Kapadia[1], Amar Krishnaswamy[1], Stephanie Mick[1], and E. Murat Tuzcu[2]

[1]Cleveland Clinic, Cleveland, OH, USA
[2]Cleveland Clinic, Abu Dhabi, United Arab Emirates

Calcific aortic stenosis is an increasingly common problem in developed countries, with an estimated prevalence of 2–4% among adults over 65 years old [1]. After the onset of symptoms, severe aortic stenosis is associated with a median survival of approximately 2 years without intervention [2]. Surgical aortic valve replacement (SAVR) has long been the standard of care for managing symptomatic aortic stenosis in the absence of significant comorbidities [3]. Unfortunately, in practice, at least 30% of such patients do not undergo SAVR because of risk factors that are felt to put them at prohibitive surgical risk [4]. Initially, attempts to manage inoperable patients with balloon aortic valvuloplasty (BAV) showed short-term improvement in symptoms, but a high rate of stenosis recurrence and no improvement in survival [5]. Similarly, medical therapy has not been shown to significantly impact the disease process. Therefore, there continued to be a great need for novel therapies to treat patients without surgical options for aortic valve replacement. The result was the development of transcatheter aortic valve replacement (TAVR), which was first performed in a human patient by Cribier et al. in 2002 [6].

Several pivotal trials were subsequently conducted to study the safety and efficacy of TAVR [7–10]. Because of the success of these clinical trials, TAVR has become an established therapy for inoperable and high-risk patients with severe aortic stenosis, shown excellent safety in certain intermediate risk populations, and grown from a technologic standpoint to include multiple valve designs, vascular access approaches, and unique procedural considerations (Figure 59.1) [11]. Generally speaking, TAVR has been divided into procedures that can be performed through adequate peripheral vascular access (most commonly from the femoral artery), and those requiring direct access to the thoracic cavity, either through the left ventricle (LV) apex via a mini-thoracotomy (transapical) or through the ascending aorta via a mini-sternotomy (transaortic). For specific patients in whom neither the transfemoral nor traditional chest access approaches are considered feasible, operators have successfully implanted the valve using access at the subclavian artery, axillary artery, carotid artery, or femoral vein (via a transseptal or transcaval approach). This chapter discusses the steps required to evaluate a patient for transfemoral (TF) TAVR, outlines the interventional technique for performing both balloon-expandable and self-expandable TAVR, and discusses the identification and management of procedural complications.

Indications and candidacy for TAVR

Currently, TAVR is indicated for inoperable and high-risk patients with symptomatic, severe aortic stenosis, as determined by the existing guidelines on management of valvular heart disease [3]. In the USA, the Edwards SAPIEN-XT and S3 (Edwards Life Sciences, Inc., Irvine, CA, USA) balloon expandable valves and the Medtronic self-expanding CoreValve® and Evolute-R® (Medtronic, Inc., Minneapolis, MN, USA) are currently approved by the Food and Drug Administration (FDA) for commercial use. In Europe, there are additional devices that have obtained the Conformité Européenne (CE) mark of approval. As the technology grows, the populations in whom it is appropriate to offer TAVR continues to evolve, and recently published studies involve patients that are at intermediate surgical risk [12]. Currently, TAVR with the Medtronic, self-expanding CoreValve is also an approved strategy for patients with severe, bioprosthetic valve degeneration, commonly referred to as "valve-in-valve TAVR." TAVR is not currently approved for patients with severe aortic regurgitation without stenosis. The lack of appropriate devices for a frequently non-calcified aortic valve and large annulus will need to be resolved before this technique can be widely applied to pure aortic regurgitation cases.

The most essential aspect of evaluating a patient for TAVR is the heart team approach, which focuses on a multidisciplinary assessment of each patient with the collaboration of cardiac surgeons, interventional cardiologists, imaging specialists, other experts from different disciplines, nurses, and other support staff. A careful assessment of comorbid conditions, both cardiovascular and non-cardiovascular, is important in determining each patient's risk for a traditional surgical valve replacement (SAVR), and evaluation by a cardiac surgeon experienced in SAVR is a requirement to determine surgical risk category. Traditionally, these categories have been defined as low, intermediate, high, and extreme (not suitable for SAVR or "inoperable"). While the Society of Thoracic Surgeons (STS) risk calculator has often been used to set more quantifiable ranges for each of these categories, especially in the setting of randomized clinical trials, there are certain factors that are not accounted for in the established surgical risk calculators that have an especially large impact on surgical candidacy. These factors include the presence of a porcelain aorta (evaluated by chest CT), chest wall deformities, severe lung disease (evaluated by pulmonary function

Interventional Cardiology: Principles and Practice, Second Edition. Edited by George D. Dangas, Carlo Di Mario, and Nicholas N. Kipshidze.
© 2017 John Wiley & Sons, Ltd. Published 2017 by John Wiley & Sons, Ltd.

SAPIEN (Edwards)
*no longer available

SAPIEN XT (Edwards)
*commercially available

S3 (Edwards)
*commercially available

Balloon
Expandable

CoreValve (Medtronic)
*commercially available

CoreValve Evolut R
*commercially available

Portico™ transcatheter
aortic heart valve
(St. Jude Medical)

Self
Expandable

Lotus (Boston Scientific)

Direct Flow Valve (Direct Flow Medical)

Other
Designs

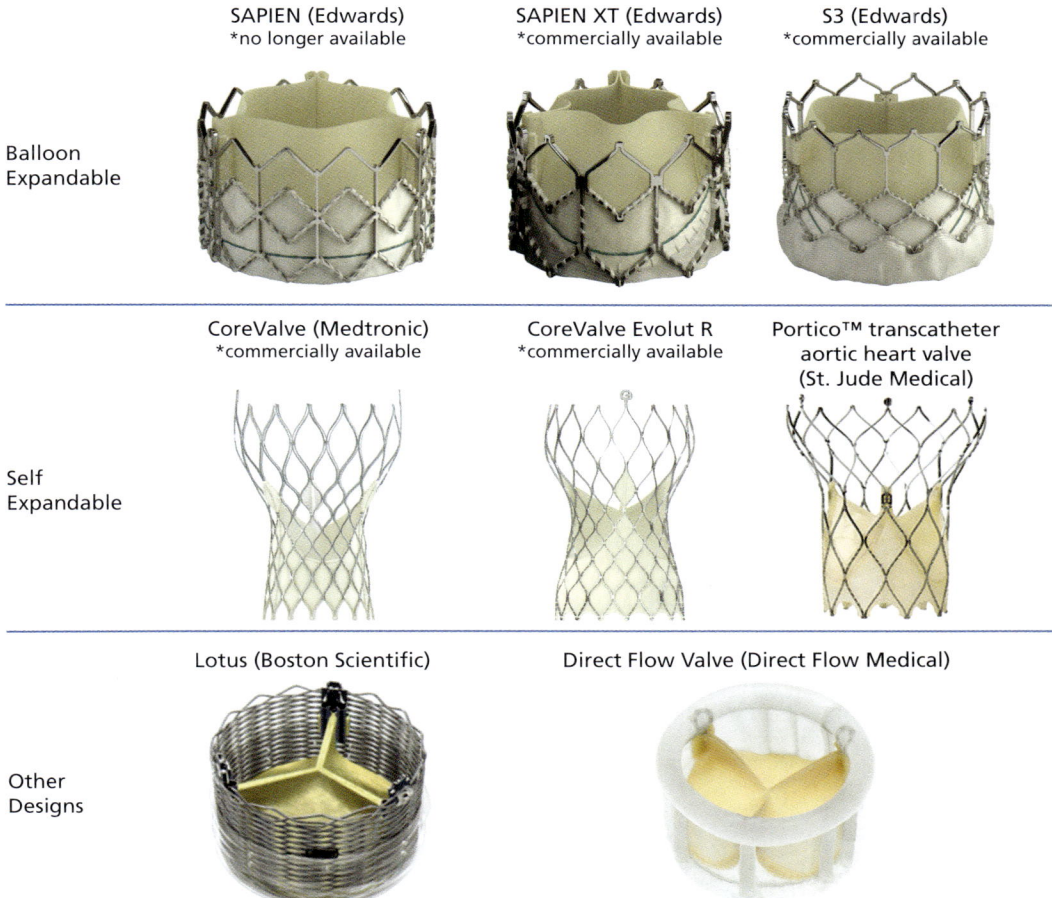

Figure 59.1 Commercially available and investigational TAVR devices in the USA. Sources: Top row: Images used with permission of Edwards Lifesciences LLC, Irvine, CA. Edwards, Edwards Lifesciences, Edwards SAPIEN, SAPIEN, SAPIEN XT, and SAPIEN 3 are trademarks of Edwards Lifesciences Corporation. Middle row (left and middle): CoreValve® images used with permission by Medtronic © 2016. (right): Portico™ Transcatheter Aortic Heart Valve. Portico and St. Jude Medical are trademarks of St. Jude Medical, Inc. or its related companies. Reproduced with permission of St. Jude Medical, © 2016. All rights reserved. Bottom row (left): Image provided courtesy of Boston Scientific. © 2016 Boston Scientific Corporation or its affiliates. All rights reserved. (right): DirectFlow valve image used with permission of DirectFlow.

tests), cirrhosis, prior radiation to the chest, prior bypass graft anatomy complicating re-do sternotomy, or significant frailty [13]. Thus, the heart team approach is absolutely essential to ensure that the best possible options are made available to each individual patient.

Contraindications to TAVR

In some situations, despite elevated surgical risk, TAVR is not the most appropriate option. TAVR is often a less appropriate option for patients with multivalve disease requiring additional surgical replacement and/or repair, concomitant aortopathy, concomitant significant coronary artery disease not amenable to PCI, no or minimally calcified aortic valve disease in which the device may be less secure, and in some congenitally malformed valves. When the annulus is too small or too large to accommodate a transcatheter device, surgery is sometimes the only option. Finally, in some instances it is clear that the patient's symptoms and life expectancy are limited by factors outside of their severe AS, and it is important not to offer a procedure that is unlikely to improve functional status or survival. It is inappropriate to offer TAVR to individuals

with a severely limited life expectancy because of non-cardiac, comorbid conditions [13].

Evaluating the patient for transfemoral TAVR

The most common route for TAVR is via the common femoral artery, termed the transfemoral (TF) approach. Other options include the transapical (TA) approach which is performed via a small left anterior thoracotomy, passing the catheter through the apex of the LV, and the transaortic (TAo) approach which is commonly performed via a partial sternotomy, allowing direct access to the ascending aorta (discussed separately). Some operators perform the TAo approach via right thoracotomy or manubriotomy.

TF-TAVR has the obvious benefit of being minimally invasive by obviating the need for sternotomy or thoracotomy, and in many cases can be completed using local anesthesia and conscious sedation. The primary requirement for TF candidacy is adequate iliofemoral artery access. Many patients with calcific AS also possess significant peripheral arterial disease, and a careful evaluation of

Table 59.1 Commercially available and investigational transcatheter aortic valve replacement (TAVR) devices in the USA.

Valve	Available sizes (diameter in mm)	Fits native annulus size (mm)	Sheath size (inner diameter Fr)	Minimum femoral artery diameter* (mm)	State of technology
Commercially available					
Edwards SAPIEN XT	23	18-22	16	6.0	CE Mark
	26	21-25	18	6.5	FDA Approved
	29	24-27	20	7.0	
Edwards S3	20	16-19	14	5.5	CE Mark
	23	18-22	14	5.5	FDA Approved
	26	21-25	14	5.5	S3i Trial (intermediate risk)
	29	24-28	16	6.0	
Medtronic CoreValve	23	18-20	18	6.0	CE Mark
	26	20-23	18	6.0	FDA approved
	29	23-27	18	6.0	
	31	26-29	18	6.0	
Medtronic Evolut R	23	18-20	14 Equivalent	5.0	CE Mark
	26	20-23		5.0	FDA Approved
	29	23-26		5.0	SURTAVI Trial (intermediate risk)
Investigational devices					
St. Jude Portico	23	19-21	18	6.0	CE Mark
	25	21-23	18	6.0	US trials ongoing
Boston Scientific Lotus	23	20-23	18	6.0	CE Mark
	25	23-25	18	6.0	REPRISE III Trial (USA)
	27	25-27	20	6.5	enrollment complete
Direct Flow Valve (DF Medical)	23	19-21	18	6.0	CE Mark
	25	21-24	18	6.0	SALUS Trial (USA) ongoing
	27	24-26	18	6.0	
	29	26-28	18	6.0	

* Based on manufacturer labeling where available. In practice, most valves that require an 18 Fr sheath can be placed through a minimal luminal diameter of 6 mm, and with the 14 Fr S3 sheath, as low as 5 mm, but individual practices differ.

the arterial anatomy is essential. Fortunately, there have been significant improvements in the size of the delivery sheaths needed for TAVR from the first generation devices to the present day, and in the recently completed PARTNER II continued access registry involving the Edwards S3 valve, 84% of high-risk patients and 89% of intermediate risk patients were able to undergo TAVR via the TF approach.

All patients being considered for TAVR should undergo a contrast enhanced computed tomography(CT) scan of the chest, abdomen, and pelvis. The chest CT should be gated (images acquired at the same point in the cardiac cycle to limit artifact) to accurately determine the size of the aortic annulus, which dictates the size of the valve that the patient requires. The annulus is rarely a circular structure but frequently elliptical, so valve sizing based on single-diameter echocardiographic measurements can lead to significant error. Gaining a precise measurement of the aortic annulus is very important in reducing valve undersizing which is a significant risk factor for paravalvular regurgitation, and CT has been shown to reduce the degree of undersizing when compared with transthoracic or transesophageal echocardiography [14,15]. Tomographic

assessment of the aortic root is also important to evaluate the distance between the annulus and the coronary artery ostia.

After obtaining the CT of the chest, imaging is continued through the abdomen and pelvis to evaluate the iliofemoral anatomy. The required iliofemoral diameter is dependent on the type and size of valve that is used. Table 59.1 shows the various available valve designs, sizes, corresponding sheath sizes, and minimal luminal diameter needed to accommodate the vascular sheath. The decision regarding adequate iliofemoral access is comprehensive and must take into account not only the size of the artery, but the presence of calcification, whether the calcification is circumferential, and the presence of significant tortuosity. Calcific arteries are less compliant and pose a higher risk for vascular complications, especially when the luminal diameter is borderline and calcification is circumferential [16].

When renal function is deemed insufficient to tolerate a normal contrast CT, alternative ways to obtain the required information must be considered. One such strategy is to obtain annular measurements by cardiac magnetic resonance imaging (MRI) or three-dimensional transesophageal echocardiography (3D-TEE), and subsequently obtain a CT of the abdomen and pelvis by direct intra-aortic injection of 10–15 mL contrast via a pigtail catheter. The pigtail catheter is placed and positioned under fluoroscopy via the common femoral artery in the cardiac catheterization laboratory, and the patient is then transported to the CT scanner for a direct, arterial contrast CT, which can be performed with minimal contrast.

Alternative vascular access has been an area of significant investigation as some patients have significant iliofemoral disease and are at prohibitive risk for TAo or TA TAVR. The subclavian and axillary arteries have been utilized in small groups of patients receiving the Edwards SAPIEN and Medtronic CoreValve devices, and appear both safe and feasible [17–19]. The carotid artery has also been used in small series of patients [20]. A venous, transseptal approach has been reported in small series as well, involving passage of the device from the femoral vein to the right atrium, across the intra-atrial septum, into the LV, and across the valve in an antegrade fashion [21,22]. Finally, a transcaval approach has been described that involves gaining access to the femoral vein, and crossing from the inferior vena cava (IVC) to the descending aorta in the abdomen [23]. A closure device is then used to repair the arteriovenous fistula that is created at the conclusion of the procedure.

Management of cardiovascular comorbidities pre-TAVR

Patients with senile, calcific aortic stenosis often have coexisting coronary artery disease, and commonly require concomitant coronary artery bypass grafting at the time of surgical AVR. In patients who are selected to undergo TAVR, similar efforts to achieve revascularization prior to the valve procedure are also important to consider. The impact of unrevascularized coronary artery disease on outcomes after TAVR has been difficult to quantify, however, as this is typically an exclusion criteria for clinical trials and retrospective analysis has its inherent biases. One prospective registry study considered the pre-TAVR SYNTAX score (and for patients who were revascularized the residual SYNTAX score), and showed that the severity of CAD prior to TAVR was associated with an increase in cardiovascular mortality [24]. In general, severe stenosis in the presence of symptoms or large areas of ischemia that are amenable to percutaneous coronary intervention (PCI) should be considered for PCI prior to TAVR. However, chronic occlusions, especially those with adequate collateral flow, are permissible to be approached less aggressively, but each case must be considered individually. Finally, in our experience, conservative management of certain asymptomatic but angiographically evident stenoses did not compromise the success of TAVR.

Carotid artery disease is also commonly found in patients with severe aortic stenosis, and must be carefully considered prior to TAVR. When severe carotid artery stenosis is discovered, particularly if the patient is symptomatic, carotid artery stenting (CAS) or carotid endarterectomy (CEA) should be considered [25]. Intermediate lesions must be considered on a case-by-case basis, but situations in which carotid intervention would be especially important to consider prior to TAVR include patients with complete occlusion of the contralateral internal carotid artery (unprotected carotid stenosis), or patients who are likely to have a prolonged period of hypotension or hemodynamic instability during TAVR.

Electrical conduction system abnormalities must also be considered, especially as they relate to LV function and the selection of balloon-expandable versus self-expandable TAVR devices. Patients with symptomatic LV dysfunction and significant left bundle-branch block (LBBB) need to be evaluated for cardiac resynchronization therapy either before or after TAVR. It is important not to overlook the possibility of a LBBB cardiomyopathy superimposed upon a decline in LV function from valvular heart disease. Also, a proportion of patients undergoing TAVR develop additional AV conduction disease during or after the procedure. This is more common with self-expanding valves, but irrelevant in patients who are already pacemaker dependent.

Certainly, it is important to optimize a patient's hemodynamic status prior to any invasive procedure, and in more tenuous patients, Swan–Ganz catheter guided management to ensure adequate optimization of pre-load and after-load in the days leading up to TAVR can be important. Optimal management of non-cardiovascular comorbid conditions is often equally important including chronic obstructive pulmonary disease (COPD), chronic kidney disease, and diabetes mellitus.

Interventional technique for TF-TAVR

There can be considerable variation from institution to institution with regard to the facilities, personnel, and equipment that are involved in the procedure. While most hospitals perform TAVR in a "hybrid" suite that has the capability to be used as a catheterization laboratory as well as an operating room, some perform the procedure in a dedicated cardiac catheterization suite. While TF-TAVR does not routinely require surgical access to the thorax, it is prudent to be prepared for any potential complications that would require emergency thoracotomy or sternotomy and cardiopulmonary bypass, and many institutions complete a full surgical preparation of the chest in the unlikely event that conversion to an open heart procedure is required [26]. Additionally, at most institutions the procedure is performed with the active participation of both interventional cardiologists and cardiac surgeons for similar reasons.

A decision must next be made with regard to the type of anesthesia used. During the early experience, it was almost universally accepted that patients be placed under general anesthesia during TF-TAVR to allow for careful cardiopulmonary monitoring and to more easily facilitate continuous TEE during the procedure. As the procedure has become more refined, however, and with the significant reductions in paravalvular leak (PVL) seen with newer generation devices, there has been less need for intra-procedural TEE, although the impact of this strategy on PVL-related outcomes is still unknown. Also, some patients undergoing TF-TAVR have significant lung disease that makes endotracheal intubation undesirable. As a result, many institutions have transitioned to performing selected procedures under conscious sedation with excellent results [27,28]. That said, there are clear benefits to the involvement of anesthesiologists during TAVR, and rapid access to both general anesthesia and TEE is essential in case they are needed.

The following workflow describes the routine procedural steps in our institution. Once the patient is prepared and appropriate sedation administered, the next step is to obtain vascular access for the procedure. One arterial sheath is placed in the common femoral artery at the location where the TAVR sheath will eventually be placed. This should be on the side with the most favorable anatomy as determined by pre-op evaluation. Given that this site will need to accommodate the largest arterial access sheath, exact placement of

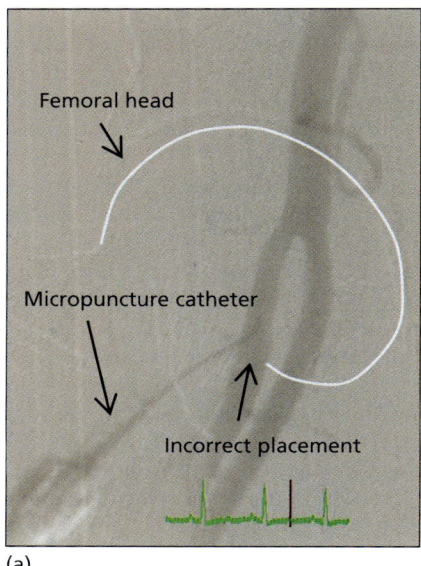

(a)

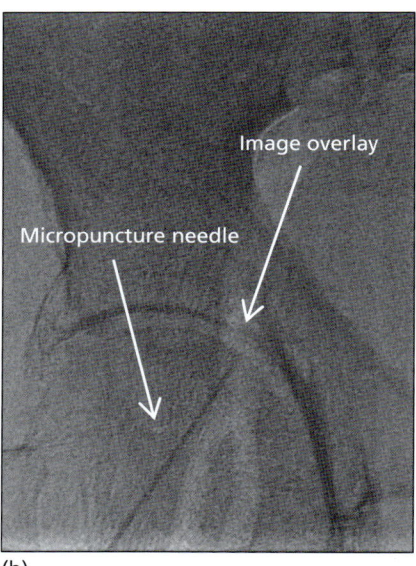

(b)

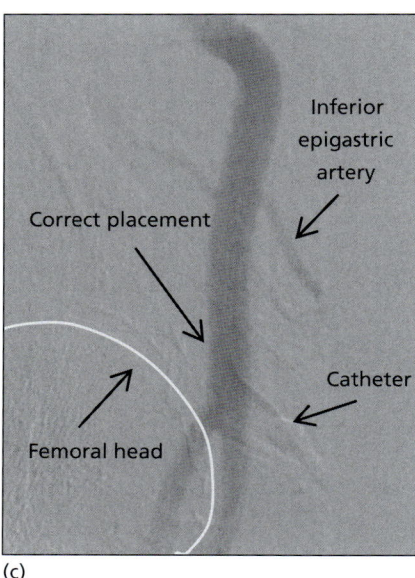

(c)

Figure 59.2 Technique for confirming correct femoral arteriotomy site by fluoroscopy. In this example, the femoral artery bifurcation is much higher than usual, above the mid-femoral head. The initial arteriotomy was found to be incorrectly placed in the superficial femoral artery (a). The micropuncture sheath was therefore removed and access re-attempted under fluoroscopy with image overlay (b). Correct placement is achieved and confirmed to be located above the bifurcation and below the inferior epigastric artery (c).

the needle stick is essential. One way to ensure the correct placement of the arteriotomy is to confirm the relationship between the femoral artery bifurcation and the femoral head by either pre-op CT or angiography, and then gain access to the artery with fluoroscopic guidance utilizing a micropuncture needle. Alternatively, using ultrasound guidance to identify the bifurcation can also be very useful. These strategies ensure that the artery is accessed at the desired location, which can be confirmed by a small injection of diluted contrast through the micropuncture sheath, best visualized with digital subtraction angiography (DSA) in an ipsilateral projection of approximately 40° which shows the femoral artery bifurcation (Figure 59.2). Once the correct arteriotomy location is confirmed, the micropuncture sheath is exchanged for a short 5 Fr sheath. Contralateral arterial access is obtained in a similar manner, and this sheath is used to place a 5 Fr pigtail catheter in the aortic root for angiography during valve position/deployment. While this can instead be placed from a radial approach, we prefer the femoral arterial access so that endovascular repair of any delivery sheath complications can be accomplished. Venous access is obtained with a sheath large enough to accommodate a temporary pacemaker wire. If desired, a second venous access can be used for a pulmonary artery (Swan–Ganz) catheter, although this is usually performed from the neck if necessary.

Once the appropriate arterial and venous access has been obtained, the next step is preclosure of the TAVR sheath site. This is accomplished by sequentially deploying two Perclose ProGlide® (Abbott Vascular, Minneapolis, MN, USA) suture-mediated closure systems at the 10 and 2-o'clock positions. This stepwise process requires the replacement of the wire to hold arterial position during each sheath and Perclose exchange. The Perclose strings are then pulled gently away and secured with a clamp on the adjacent drape, taking care not to lock the knot. The ProStar XL (Abbott Vascular) system can also be used for preclosure of the arteriotomy, although this has become less common. The use of preclosure devices has

reduced the need for surgical cutdown and primary repair in the vast majority of cases [29,30]. Surgical cutdown can still be considered in cases of extreme calcification around the puncture site or the presence of aorto-femoral grafting, and when necessary, an axillary or femoral graft can be utilized.

Next, a temporary pacemaker wire is placed into the right ventricle (RV) apex and appropriate capture is tested at a rate of 180–220 beats per minute. When the risk for permanent pacemaker is high, a screw-in lead from the internal jugular vein may be preferred. The high incidence of conduction system abnormalities after CoreValve placement must be considered, and at our institution it is routine to place an active fixation temporary pacemaker wire that is left in place for 72 hours after the procedure. In cases where the patient has a pre-existing permanent pacemaker, a passive fixation wire can be used peri-procedurally for more modest RV pacing (rate in the 100–120 range) if necessary to assist with CoreValve deployment or for rapid RV pacing if valve post-dilation is necessary.

Intravenous heparin is then administered to achieve a therapeutic activated clotting time (ACT) >300 seconds, and the TAVR sheath is carefully upsized over a stiff wire (e.g., Lunderquist). A 5–6 Fr angled pigtail catheter is advanced to the non-coronary cusp, and the fluoroscopic projection demonstrating the perpendicular annular plane is established, and all three inferior margins precisely superimposed [31]. The valve is then crossed utilizing a 5-Fr Amplatz left-1 (AL-1) diagnostic catheter and a 0.035-inch straight-tip guidewire. Care should be taken not to cross through the mitral subvalvular apparatus. After advancing the AL-1 into the LV, it is exchanged for a pigtail catheter to record simultaneous pressure measurements across the aortic valve. Next, an Amplatz Extra-stiff 0.035-inch guidewire is shaped with a large curve at the distal end, and the belly of the curve is placed carefully into the apex of the LV. When placing a CoreValve, an Amplatz Super Stiff™ guidewire is utilized (rather than the Extra-Stiff) to obtain additional support for stabilizing the position of the delivery system. However, it is felt that the Super Stiff guidewire can bias the delivery system of the SAPIEN devices too far to the posterior aortic wall or hold back the prosthetic valve leaflet after deployment (causing valvular aortic regurgitation).

BAV is often performed at this point with the intent of preparing the native valve to accommodate the prosthesis. As device technology has progressed, however, BAV has been utilized with decreasing frequency in balloon expandable TAVR, and is not commonly used with self-expandable valves. Finally, the prosthetic valve is loaded onto the delivery device, and advanced into the aortic position, coaxial to the annulus. The device should be positioned at the appropriate height, taking the annular anatomy and position of the coronary ostia into account. Both root angiography and TEE (when utilized) can be used to position the valve. The balloon-expandable valves are typically positioned with the lower third of the device in the annulus and the remainder of the device above the valve level. The technique for positioning of the CoreValve involves placing the device slightly lower in the left ventricular outflow tract (LVOT) and then withdrawing the device to the desired height.

When ready to implant the balloon expandable valve, respirations are held, rapid pacing from the temporary pacemaker wire is initiated, and the valve is deployed under fluoroscopy (Figure 59.3a, b). It is important to deflate the balloon completely prior to the cessation of RV pacing so the valve does not become dislodged as the balloon is ejected. Comparatively, the self-expandable valve does not require rapid pacing, but often a rate of 100–110 bpm is used to decrease the cardiac output modestly. The valve is then unsheathed starting with the LVOT portion, withdrawn to the desired height in the annulus, and fully deployed (Figure 59.3c–f). The position and function of all valves should then be evaluated angiographically, echocardiographically, and hemodynamically. If the valve is positioned too high or too low, a second valve can be considered if needed. Post-dilatation of an underexpanded valve can be done when there is significant perivalvular regurgitation, or a second valve can be deployed within the first. While the balloon-expandable SAPIEN valves cannot be moved once deployed, the CoreValve can be partially deployed and pulled back slightly if needed. This is because of the unsheathing mechanism involved in deploying the CoreValve, but once partially unsheathed, the device cannot be resheathed to be recovered. Some newer generation devices including the Boston Scientific Lotus and the Direct Flow Medical valve have the advantage of being fully retrievable. The Medtronic Evolut R system, an iteration of the CoreValve, is retrievable when it is partially, but not fully, deployed.

When the procedure is considered complete, the access sheath is removed, and the pre-closure devices secured. It is important to maintain wire position during closure in the event that one of the sutures fails. Also, proximal balloon occlusion of the iliac artery via the contralateral arterial access can assist in preventing blood loss during sheath removal and suture securement. A final angiographic picture through the contralateral arterial access can confirm the absence of occult bleeding or other vascular complications prior to removal of the smaller arterial sheath.

Valve designs that have the CE mark for use in Europe, and are under investigation but not currently approved for use by the US FDA, include the self-expandable Portico valve (St. Jude Medical, St. Paul, Minnesota, MN, USA), and the uniquely designed Lotus Valve (Boston Scientific) and Direct Flow Valve (Direct Flow Medical, Santa Rosa, CA, USA).

Complications of TF-TAVR

There are a number of peri-procedural and post-procedural complications that must be considered in patients undergoing TAVR. The Valve Academic Research Consortium (VARC-2) has outlined criteria to standardize the definitions for these complications in clinical practice and in the setting of outcomes adjudication for clinical trials [13]. Procedural complications have become less common in more contemporary series, likely because of a combination of device improvements and operator experience. Complications lead to significant morbidity, mortality, and account for approximately 25% on non-implant-related hospital costs associated with TAVR [32]. Complications that are particularly important to consider in patients undergoing TAVR include vascular and access site complications, bleeding, stroke, conduction system disease, cardiac tamponade, annular rupture, peri-valvular aortic regurgitation, and device malpositioning or embolization (Table 59.2).

The most common complications of TF-TAVR relate to issues with the vascular access site. Vascular complications can be as simple as VARC-2 minor bleeding, but given the relatively large sheaths that are required, more serious complications such as rupture, dissection, or occlusion sometimes occur. Major vascular complications have been reported in up to 16% of patients undergoing TF-TAVR, but appear to be significantly declining, occurring in only 8% of the non-randomized continued access registry patients in the PARTNER trial, and <6% of TF patients in the PARTNER II trial using the S3 valve [33,34]. Vascular complications are more common in patients with calcific, small caliber, or tortuous arteries. When severe bleeding is identified, an endovascular balloon can be inflated to achieve temporary hemostasis, or a covered stent placed. Minor bleeding at the arteriotomy or venipuncture site can usually be controlled by applying external pressure. In cases where there is ongoing bleeding after the pre-closure sutures are tightened, another Perclose or an Angio-Seal device (St. Jude Medical) can be advanced over the wire and subsequently deployed to help close the residual hole.

Late bleeding complications can also occur after TAVR, which was seen with an incidence of 5.9% and at a median of 132 days in the PARTNER cohort/registries [35]. The cause of late bleeding was most commonly found to be gastrointestinal complications (40.8%), neurologic complications (15.5%), or traumatic falls (7.8%), and were more common in patients with low baseline hemoglobin, atrial fibrillation or flutter, moderate or severe paravalvular leak, or larger LV mass. Bleeding has been defined in the VARC-2 document as either minor, major (associated with a drop in hemoglobin ≥3 g/dL or requiring ≥2 units of whole blood/RBC transfusion), or life-threatening (drop in hemoglobin >5 g/dL or >4 units transfusion, involving a critical organ, leading to shock requiring surgery or vasopressors, or fatal) [13].

Stroke is an uncommon but dreaded complication of any cardiovascular procedure. While the initial results of the PARTNER 1A and 1B randomized cohorts raised concern for an elevated risk of stroke with TAVR compared with SAVR or medical therapy, more recent studies have shown significant improvements, and no elevated risk with TAVR compared with surgery [7,10]. Most neurologic events associated with TAVR are felt to be embolic in nature, and the 30-day incidence of clinical stroke or TIA in a large meta-analysis of 10,037 TAVR patients was 3.3 ± 1.8% [36]. Studies utilizing diffusion weighted MRI, however, have shown a high incidence of subclinical events in both TAVR and SAVR patients, so there has been considerable focus on finding strategies to protect the cerebral vasculature [37]. Much of this focus has been

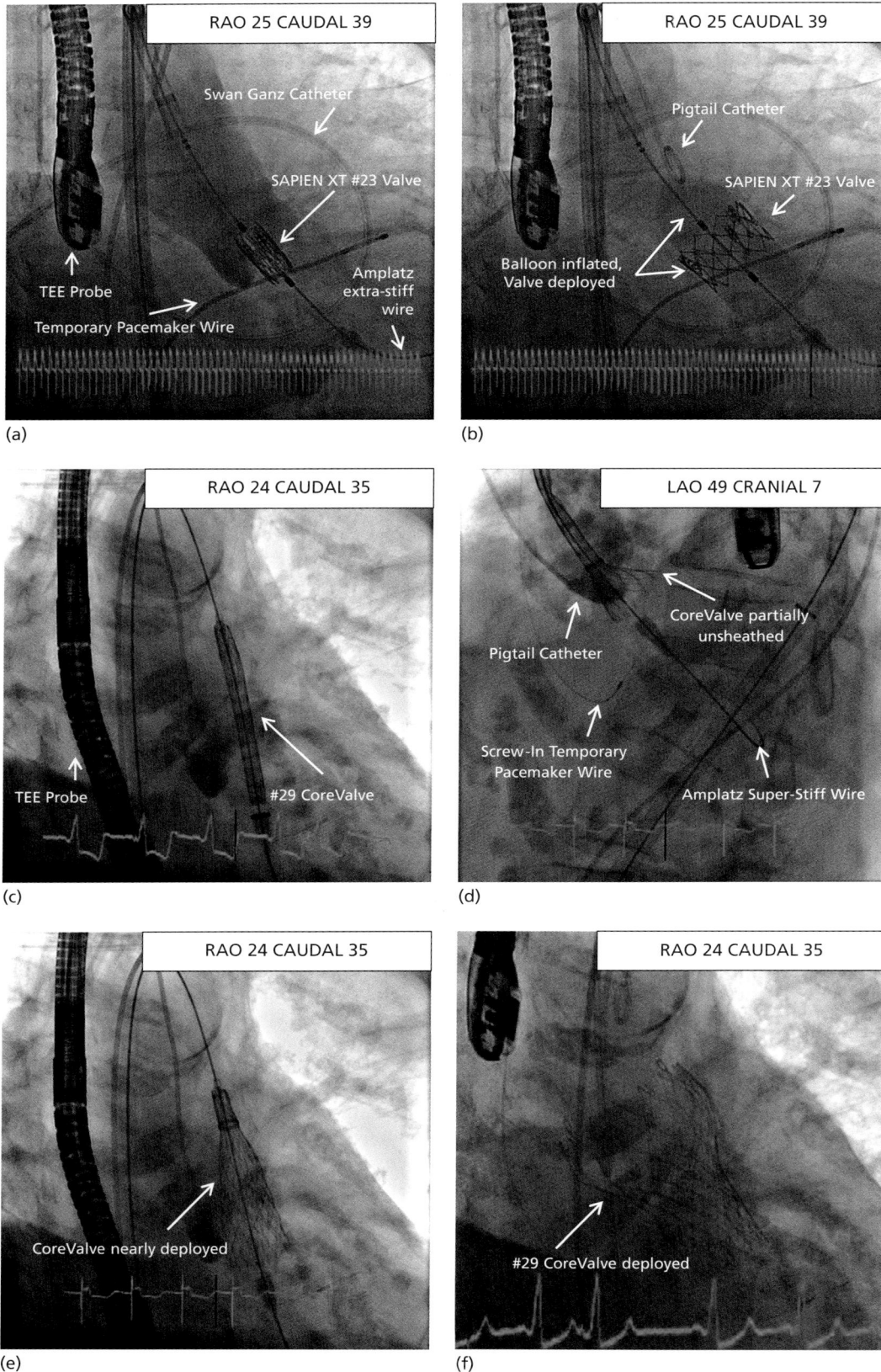

Figure 59.3 Positioning and deployment of the SAPIEN XT (a, b) and CoreValve (c–f) TAVR devices.

Table 59.2 Complications of transcatheter aortic valve replacement (TAVR).

Complication	Risk factors	Ways to mitigate/resolve
Vascular complications	Small femoral artery luminal diameter Calcified arteries, especially circumferential	Careful pre-procedural planning and evaluation of arterial access Confirm correct femoral artery placement (above bifurcation, below inferior epigastric) prior to large sheath dilatation Pre-closure of the arteriotomy site Iliac angiography at conclusion of the case Prompt endovascular or surgical repair of vascular injuries
Stroke	Older age, female, prior cerebrovascular or peripheral vascular disease, diabetes, hypertension, prior cardiac surgery Need for balloon post-dilatation No clear differences in TAVR route or device design Post-TAVR atrial fibrillation	Appropriate heparinization during procedure Appropriate pharmacologic treatment post-procedure Anticoagulation when needed for atrial fibrillation Minimize unnecessary manipulations of the device in the aortic root Cerebral embolic protection devices (under investigation) Alternative antiplatelet and anticoagulant regimens (under investigation)
Conduction system disease	Pre-existing conduction system disease Pre-existing right bundle branch block Valve oversizing Low valve implantation Self-expandable devices Calcified annulus	Consider active fixation, temporary pacemaker for high-risk cases and for self-expandable devices Carefully monitor patients post-procedure for conduction system disease Permanent pacemaker implantation when indicated Limit device oversizing (must be weighed against risk of paravalvular regurgitation)
Cardiac tamponade	Temporary pacemaker perforation Guidewire perforation Annular rupture during BAV or valve deployment (more common in oversized valves, calcified annulus, with post-dilatation, and with balloon-expandable valves)	Careful wire management Limit device oversizing (must be weighed against risk of paravalvular regurgitation) Prompt diagnosis and management in the setting of hemodynamic instability Consider self-expanding device (less risk of annular rupture) for severely calcified annulus
Aortic regurgitation	Asymmetric, calcified annulus Device undersizing	Annular sizing and valve measurement by multidetector CT, cardiac MRI, or 3D transesophageal echocardiogram rather than single dimension sizing by 2D transthoracic echocardiogram Post-dilatation or placement of a second valve (must be weighed against risk of stroke or annular rupture) Central regurgitation requires placement of a second valve if not resolving
Valve malpositioning or embolization	Deployment of the valve too high or too low Valve undersizing	Careful pre-procedural evaluation including annular size, and distance from annulus to coronary ostia Prompt intervention for coronary artery ostial occlusion with PCI or CABG

BAV, balloon aortic valvuloplasty; CABG, coronary artery bypass grafting; CT, computed tomography; MRI, magnetic resonance imaging; PCI, percutaneous coronary intervention.

turned to the study of embolic protection devices, of which there have been several systems under investigation including the Claret Sentinel Cerebral Protection System, and the Triguard Cerebral Protection Device (Figure 59.4). Further studies are also underway to evaluate the optimal anticoagulant strategies for TAVR. Current guidelines support the use of procedural heparin, then aspirin (50–100 mg/day) plus clopidogrel (75 mg/day) for 3 months after

TAVR followed by aspirin monotherapy (Grade 2C) [13,38]. Ongoing trials are studying the use of bivalirudin compared with unfractionated heparin, the use of the vitamin K antagonist acenocoumarol after TAVR, and the use of dual antiplatelet therapy versus aspirin alone.

Conduction system disturbances can also occur after TAVR, sometimes resulting in the need for permanent pacemaker

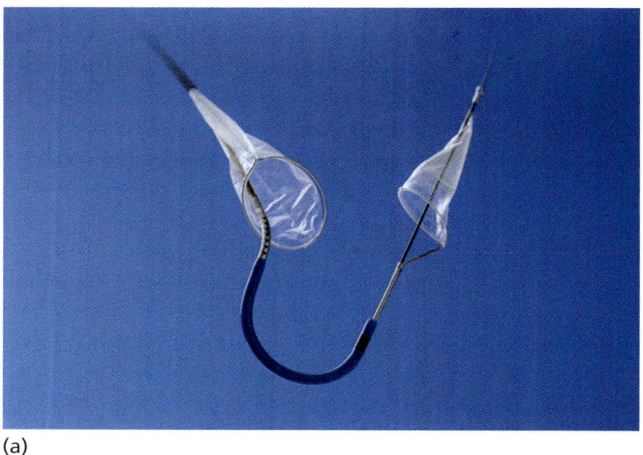

(a)

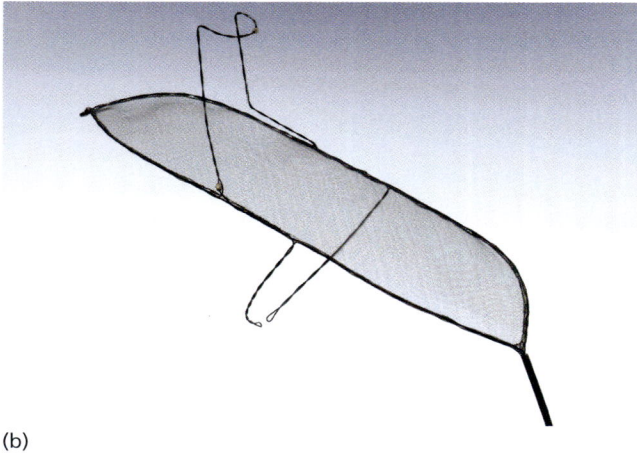

(b)

Figure 59.4 Embolic protection devices used in transfemoral TAVR. Embolic protection devices that are under investigation for use during transfemoral TAVR. (a) The Claret Sentinel® Cerebral Protection System. (b) The Triguard Cerebral Protection Device. Sources: (a) Courtesy of Claret Medical®, Santa Rosa, CA, USA; (b) Courtesy of Keystone heart, Herzliya Pituach, Israel.

implantation (PPI). The mechanism for conduction abnormalities is thought to be mechanical compression of the conductive tissues, and the left bundle is particularly vulnerable. Thus, pre-existing RBBB is significantly associated with the need for PPI after TAVR, as is lower implantation of the prosthesis in the LVOT, calcified annulus, or a significantly oversized prosthesis [39,40]. Perhaps the strongest association with the need for post-TAVR PPI is the use of a self-expanding prosthesis. In the GARY registry, there was a significantly higher incidence of PPI with the Medtronic CoreValve (25.2%) than the Edwards SAPIEN device (5.0%). At our institution, we maintain an active fixation temporary pacemaker for 72 hours after CoreValve placement for this reason. When needed, pacemaker implantation has no adverse associations with short or long-term outcomes in TAVR patients, and is protective against unexpected death [41].

Cardiac tamponade is a rare complication of TF-TAVR. This can occur because of RV perforation from a temporary pacemaker wire, LV perforation from guidewires used to cross the aortic valve or support the TAVR device, or from annular rupture. Annular rupture is rare, but has been reported in 1% of TAVR procedures, and contained asymptomatic rupture may occur more frequently without detection [42]. Rupture can occur at the supra-annular, intra-annular, or sub-annular level, and sometimes involves multiple levels of the annulus and aortic root. Injury can occur during balloon pre-dilatation of the aortic valve, prosthetic valve deployment, or post-dilatation to reduce paravalvular leak. Annular rupture is not typically observed in self-expanding valves, unless post-dilatation is required. Rupture occurs more frequently when the valve is oversized ≥20% and when the LVOT is calcified and subsequently less compliant [43]. Rupture often leads to immediate hemodynamic instability from tamponade, but presentation can sometimes be delayed or even occult in a contained rupture or hematoma. Generally, the presence of a hemopericardium should lead to suspicion for annular rupture, which can be confirmed by echocardiography or aortic root angiography. Treatment of less severe situations involve pericardial drainage and careful observation, but many cases will require emergency cardiopulmonary bypass and surgical correction. The mortality in patients who undergo open heart surgery because of annular rupture is very high at approximately 50%, and the outcome in patients who are observed more conservatively is not known [42].

Paravalvular aortic regurgitation after TAVR has also been extensively studied. There is a higher incidence of aortic regurgitation after TAVR than surgical AVR, which is not surprising considering that the prosthesis must be expanded to fit in an asymmetric annulus which is often heavily calcified. Several studies have shown an increase in mortality among patients with moderate or severe aortic regurgitation after TAVR, and even mild aortic regurgitation can be associated with worse outcomes [44,45]. When significant aortic regurgitation is identified at the time of TAVR, additional balloon inflation of the valve can be attempted to reduce paravalvular leak, although this can predispose to an increase in central regurgitation if the valve is over-distended. In some cases, a second valve is placed inside the first valve in attempts to reduce the severity of regurgitation. Unfortunately, both of these techniques are associated with a small, but not insignificant, increase in the risk of further embolic stroke, or injury to the annulus or conduction system. Fortunately, however, newer TAVR device designs have been specifically designed to reduce the incidence of paravalvular regurgitation. For example, the direct-flow valve is designed with two inflatable cuffs on the superior and inferior aspect of the valve apparatus that attempt to create a tighter seal between valve and annulus. Similarly, the Edwards S3 valve is designed with a skirt on the outer aspect of the inferior portion of the prosthesis. It is to be hoped that, with these and other technologic advances, there will be a significant reduction in aortic regurgitation after TAVR in the future. It remains to be seen whether these reductions in aortic regurgitation will correlate with similar improvements in clinical outcomes.

Conclusions

TAVR is an exciting therapy for patients with severe, symptomatic aortic stenosis who are at elevated risk for surgery, and the technology continues to evolve to include new valve designs, vascular access strategies, lower profile devices, and adjunctive methods to reduce the risk of procedural complications. It is to be hoped that, with these efforts, cardiologists and cardiac surgeons will be increasingly empowered to offer the best possible strategy for aortic valve therapy to each individual patient, as the burden of calcific aortic stenosis continues to grow among our aging population.

Case study

The patient is an 85-year-old male who is referred for evaluation of severe aortic stenosis. He has a past medical history of hypertension, coronary artery disease with three-vessel bypass surgery 10 years ago, chronic kidney disease with a baseline creatinine of 2.2 g/dL (GFR 26 mL/min/1.73 m²), mild COPD due to a remote history of smoking, and insulin-dependent diabetes mellitus. He has progressive dyspnea on exertion with New York Heart Association Class III symptoms. One year ago he was able to walk 2 miles at a slow pace approximately three times per week, but currently he is unable to walk for more than 10 minutes without having to stop to catch his breath. He also notes difficulty with breathing while sleeping at night and requires three pillows to prop up his head. He denies chest pain either at rest or on exertion.

The physical examination is notable for an elderly-appearing man who is well developed and with no labored breathing at rest. There is no distention of the jugular veins and no carotid bruits. The lungs are clear to auscultation bilaterally except for faint bibasilar crackles on inspiration. The heart sounds are regular with a III/VI systolic murmur that is late peaking. The abdomen is soft and non-tender without organomegaly. The extremities are notable for 2/2 bilateral radial and pedal pulses without pitting edema.

A transthoracic echocardiogram is obtained and reveals normal left ventricular size with a mildly reduced left ventricular ejection fraction of 45%, mild mitral and tricuspid regurgitation, and severe aortic stenosis with a peak/mean gradient of 76/46 mmHg, and calculated aortic valve area of 0.76 cm².

The patient undergoes a left heart catheterization showing severe, native coronary artery disease, but patent bypass grafts to the left anterior descending, first obtuse marginal, and posterior descending arteries. Due to his baseline renal dysfunction, a cardiac MRI is carried out to evaluate annular size, and found to be 24 mm in average diameter. A CT scan with direct arterial contrast injection via a pigtail catheter is completed and the minimal luminal diameter of the left iliofemoral system is 6 mm and the right iliofemoral system is 9 mm with mild bilateral calcification.

The patient is evaluated by the heart team including a cardiac surgeon and an interventional cardiologist and it is determined that he is at high risk for re-do open heart surgery for aortic valve replacement with a calculated STS score of 9.4% for risk of mortality. It is determined that the patient is an appropriate candidate for transfemoral TAVR, and the patient undergoes implantation of a commercially available, 26 mm Edwards SAPIEN XT valve via the right femoral artery. After the procedure, the patient has no apparent complications, begins ambulating slowly on post-procedure day 1, and is discharged from the hospital on post-TAVR day 3.

Interactive multiple choice questions are available for this chapter on www.wiley.com/go/dangas/cardiology

References

1 Freeman RV, Otto CM. Spectrum of calcific aortic valve disease: pathogenesis, disease progression, and treatment strategies. *Circulation* 2005; **111**(24): 3316–3326.

2 Sarin RK, Ross AM, Rose LI, Rios JC, Massumi RA. Combined supravalvular aortic and pulmonary artery stenosis. *Angiology* 1968; **19**(5): 293–298.

3 Nishimura RA, Otto CM, Bonow RO, et al. 2014 AHA/ACC guideline for the management of patients with valvular heart disease: a report of the American College of Cardiology/American Heart Association Task Force on Practice Guidelines. *J Thorac Cardiovasc Surg* 2014; **148**(1): e1–e132.

4 Iung B, Cachier A, Baron G, et al. Decision-making in elderly patients with severe aortic stenosis: why are so many denied surgery? *Eur Heart J* 2005; **26**(24): 2714–2720.

5 O'Neill WW. Predictors of long-term survival after percutaneous aortic valvuloplasty: report of the Mansfield Scientific Balloon Aortic Valvuloplasty Registry. *J Am Coll Cardiol* 1991 ; **17**(1): 193–198.

6 Cribier A, Eltchaninoff H, Bash A, et al. Percutaneous transcatheter implantation of an aortic valve prosthesis for calcific aortic stenosis: first human case description. *Circulation* 2002; **106**(24): 3006–3008.

7 Leon MB, Smith CR, Mack M, et al. Transcatheter aortic-valve implantation for aortic stenosis in patients who cannot undergo surgery. *N Engl J Med* 2010; **363**(17): 1597–1607.

8 Adams DH, Popma JJ, Reardon MJ, et al. Transcatheter aortic-valve replacement with a self-expanding prosthesis. *N Engl J Med* 2014; **370**(19): 1790–1798.

9 Popma JJ, Adams DH, Reardon MJ, et al. Transcatheter aortic valve replacement using a self-expanding bioprosthesis in patients with severe aortic stenosis at extreme risk for surgery. *J Am Coll Cardiol* 2014; **63**(19): 1972–1981.

10 Smith CR, Leon MB, Mack MJ, et al. Transcatheter versus surgical aortic-valve replacement in high-risk patients. *N Engl J Med* 2011; **364**(23): 2187–2198.

11 Piazza N, Kalesan B, van Mieghem N, et al. A 3-center comparison of 1-year mortality outcomes between transcatheter aortic valve implantation and surgical aortic valve replacement on the basis of propensity score matching among intermediate-risk surgical patients. *JACC Cardiovasc Interv* 2013; **6**(5): 443–451.

12 Leon MB, Smith CR, Mack MJ, et al. Transcatheter or surgical aortic-valve replacement in intermediate-risk patients. *N Engl J Med* 2016; **374**(17): 1609–1620.

13 Holmes DR Jr, Mack MJ, Kaul S, et al. 2012 ACCF/AATS/SCAI/STS expert consensus document on transcatheter aortic valve replacement. *J Am Coll Cardiol* 2012; **59**(13): 1200–1254.

14 O'Brien B, Schoenhagen P, Kapadia SR, et al. Integration of 3D imaging data in the assessment of aortic stenosis: impact on classification of disease severity. *Circ Cardiovasc Imaging* 2011; **4**(5): 566–573.

15 Jilaihawi H, Doctor N, Kashif M, et al. Aortic annular sizing for transcatheter aortic valve replacement using cross-sectional 3-dimensional transesophageal echocardiography. *J Am Coll Cardiol* 2013; **61**(9): 908–916.

16 Krishnaswamy A, Parashar A, Agarwal S, et al. Predicting vascular complications during transfemoral transcatheter aortic valve replacement using computed tomography: a novel area-based index. *Catheter Cardiovasc Interv* 2014; **84**(5): 844–851.

17 Bruschi G, De Marco F, Fratto P, et al. Alternative approaches for trans-catheter self-expanding aortic bioprosthetic valves implantation: single-center experience. *Eur J Cardiothorac Surg* 2011; **39**(6): e151–158.

18 Al Kindi AH, Salhab KF, Roselli EE, Kapadia S, Tuzcu EM, Svensson LG. Alternative access options for transcatheter aortic valve replacement in patients with no conventional access and chest pathology. *J Thorac Cardiovasc Surg* 2014; **147**(2): 644–651.

19 Ciuca C, Tarantini G, Latib A, Gasparetto V, et al. Trans-subclavian versus transapical access for transcatheter aortic valve implantation: a multicenter study. *Catheter Cardiovasc Interv* 2016; **87**(2): 332–338.

20 Thourani VH, Li C, Devireddy C, et al. High-risk patients with inoperable aortic stenosis: use of transapical, transaortic, and transcarotid techniques. *Ann Thorac Surg* 2015; **99**(3): 817–823; discussion 823–825.

21 Cohen MG, Singh V, Martinez CA, et al. Transseptal antegrade transcatheter aortic valve replacement for patients with no other access approach: a contemporary experience. *Catheter Cardiovasc Interv* 2013; **82**(6): 987–993.

22 Chi Lam SC, Bertog S, Sievert H. Transseptal strategy in retrograde transcatheter valve-in-valve implantation for failed surgical aortic bioprosthesis. *Catheter Cardiovasc Interv* 2014; **83**(5): 817–821.

23 Greenbaum AB, O'Neill WW, Paone G, et al. Caval-aortic access to allow transcatheter aortic valve replacement in otherwise ineligible patients: initial human experience. *J Am Coll Cardiol* 2014; **63**(25 Pt A): 2795–2804.

24 Stefanini GG, Stortecky S, Cao D, et al. Coronary artery disease severity and aortic stenosis: clinical outcomes according to SYNTAX score in patients undergoing transcatheter aortic valve implantation. *Eur Heart J* 2014; **35**(37): 2530–2540.

25 Brott TG, Halperin JL, Abbara S, et al. 2011 ASA/ACCF/AHA/AANN/AANS/ACR/ASNR/CNS/SAIP/SCAI/SIR/SNIS/SVM/SVS guideline on the management of patients with extracranial carotid and vertebral artery disease: a report of the American College of Cardiology Foundation/American Heart Association Task Force on Practice Guidelines, and the American Stroke Association, American Association of Neuroscience Nurses, American Association of Neurological Surgeons, American College of Radiology, American Society of Neuroradiology, Congress of Neurological Surgeons, Society of Atherosclerosis Imaging and Prevention, Society for Cardiovascular Angiography and Interventions, Society of Interventional Radiology, Society of NeuroInterventional Surgery, Society for Vascular Medicine, and Society for Vascular Surgery. *Circulation*. 2011; **124**(4): e54–130.

26 Roselli EE, Idrees J, Mick S, et al. Emergency use of cardiopulmonary bypass in complicated transcatheter aortic valve replacement: importance of a heart team approach. *J Thorac Cardiovasc Surg* 2014; **148**(4): 1413–1416.

27 Petronio AS, Giannini C, De Carlo M, et al. Anaesthetic management of transcatheter aortic valve implantation: results from the Italian CoreValve registry. *EuroIntervention* 2015; **10**(11): pii.

28 Babaliaros V, Devireddy C, Lerakis S, et al. Comparison of transfemoral transcatheter aortic valve replacement performed in the catheterization laboratory (minimalist approach) versus hybrid operating room (standard approach): outcomes and cost analysis. *JACC Cardiovasc Interv* 2014; **7**(8): 898–904.

29 Haulon S, Hassen Khodja R, Proudfoot CW, Samuels E. A systematic literature review of the efficacy and safety of the Prostar XL device for the closure of large femoral arterial access sites in patients undergoing percutaneous endovascular aortic procedures. *Eur J Vasc Endovasc Surg* 2011; **41**(2): 201–213.

30 Nakamura M, Chakravarty T, Jilaihawi H, et al. Complete percutaneous approach for arterial access in transfemoral transcatheter aortic valve replacement: a comparison with surgical cut-down and closure. *Catheter Cardiovasc Interv* 2014; **84**(2): 293–300.

31 Kasel AM, Cassese S, Leber AW, von Scheidt W, Kastrati A. Fluoroscopy-guided aortic root imaging for TAVR: "follow the right cusp" rule. *JACC Cardiovasc Imaging* 2013; **6**(2): 274–275.

32 Arnold SV, Lei Y, Reynolds MR, et al. Costs of periprocedural complications in patients treated with transcatheter aortic valve replacement: results from the placement of aortic transcatheter valve trial. *Circ Cardiovasc Interv* 2014; **7**(6): 829–836.

33 Genereux P, Head SJ, Van Mieghem NM, et al. Clinical outcomes after transcatheter aortic valve replacement using valve academic research consortium definitions: a weighted meta-analysis of 3,519 patients from 16 studies. *J Am Coll Cardiol* 2012; **59**(25): 2317–2326.

34 Fearon WF, Kodali S, Doshi D, et al. Outcomes after transfemoral transcatheter aortic valve replacement: a comparison of the randomized PARTNER (Placement of AoRTic TraNscathetER Valves) trial with the NRCA (Nonrandomized Continued Access) registry. *JACC Cardiovasc Interv* 2014; **7**(11): 1245–1251.

35 Genereux P, Cohen DJ, Mack M, et al. Incidence, predictors, and prognostic impact of late bleeding complications after transcatheter aortic valve replacement. *J Am Coll Cardiol* 2014; **64**(24): 2605–2615.

36 Eggebrecht H, Schmermund A, Voigtlander T, Kahlert P, Erbel R, Mehta RH. Risk of stroke after transcatheter aortic valve implantation (TAVI): a meta-analysis of 10,037 published patients. *EuroIntervention* 2012; **8**(1): 129–138.

37 Spaziano M, Francese DP, Leon MB, Genereux P. Imaging and functional testing to assess clinical and subclinical neurological events after transcatheter or surgical aortic valve replacement: a comprehensive review. *J Am Coll Cardiol* 2014; **64**(18): 1950–1963.

38 Whitlock RP, Sun JC, Fremes SE, Rubens FD, Teoh KH. Antithrombotic and thrombolytic therapy for valvular disease: Antithrombotic Therapy and Prevention of Thrombosis, 9th edn: American College of Chest Physicians Evidence-Based Clinical Practice Guidelines. *Chest* 2012; **141**(2 Suppl): e576S–600S.

39 Erkapic D, Kim WK, Weber M, et al. Electrocardiographic and further predictors for permanent pacemaker requirement after transcatheter aortic valve implantation. *Europace* 2010; **12**(8): 1188–1190.

40 Houthuizen P, van der Boon RM, Urena M, et al. Occurrence, fate and consequences of ventricular conduction abnormalities after transcatheter aortic valve implantation. *EuroIntervention* 2014; **9**(10): 1142–1150.

41 Urena M, Webb JG, Tamburino C, et al. Permanent pacemaker implantation after transcatheter aortic valve implantation: impact on late clinical outcomes and left ventricular function. *Circulation* 2014; **129**(11): 1233–1243.

42 Pasic M, Unbehaun A, Buz S, Drews T, Hetzer R. Annular rupture during transcatheter aortic valve replacement: classification, pathophysiology, diagnostics, treatment approaches, and prevention. *JACC Cardiovasc Interv* 2015; **8**(1 Pt A): 1–9.

43 Barbanti M, Yang TH, Rodes Cabau J, et al. Anatomical and procedural features associated with aortic root rupture during balloon-expandable transcatheter aortic valve replacement. *Circulation* 2013; **128**(3): 244–253.

44 Tamburino C, Capodanno D, Ramondo A, et al. Incidence and predictors of early and late mortality after transcatheter aortic valve implantation in 663 patients with severe aortic stenosis. *Circulation* 2011; **123**(3): 299–308.

45 Athappan G, Patvardhan E, Tuzcu EM, et al. Incidence, predictors, and outcomes of aortic regurgitation after transcatheter aortic valve replacement: meta-analysis and systematic review of literature. *J Am Coll Cardiol* 2013; **61**(15): 1585–1595.

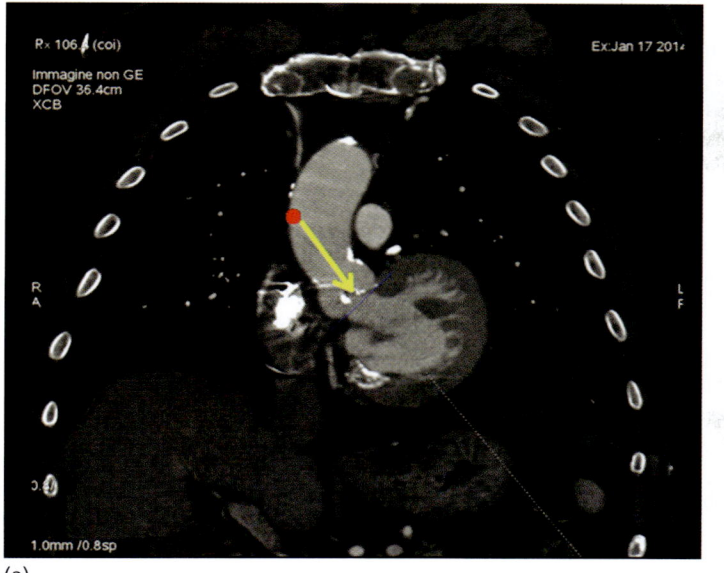
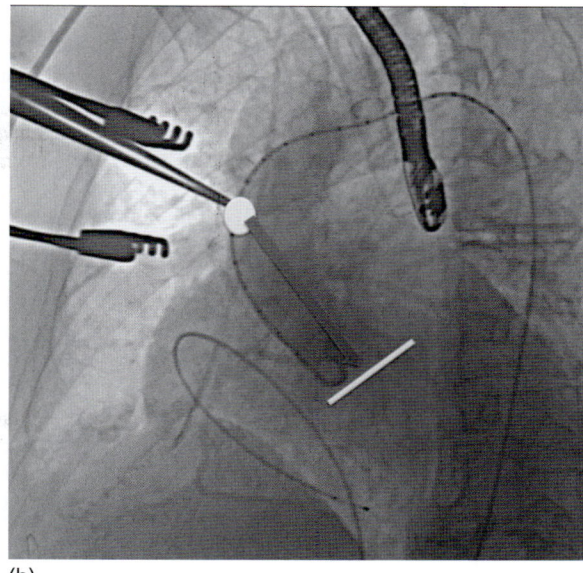

(a)   (b)

Figure 60.2 Site of aortic access and purse-string position. (a) The TAo zone or the ideal site for purse-string is evaluated on multislice computed tomography; this varies slightly depending on the valve and delivery system. (b) Aortogram identifying the valve deployment view as well as confirm the distance between the aortic annulus and site of purse-string (at least 6 cm) and evaluate implant trajectory.

mini-sternotomy, as this gives the operator more control. Re-confirmation of the site of the purse-string should be made by fluoroscopy before they are placed to evaluate distance from aortic annulus and implant trajectory (Figure 60.2). A suture ring or bumper should be used to stabilize the sheath. A Seldinger technique should be used to cannulate the aorta. If the aorta is thin, a small knife can be preferred to insert the sheath. The wire position should be similar to that for the TF approach, with a large loop in the left ventricle free of kinks with the tip free to avoid trauma.

The TAo approach is now a well-established approach and can essentially be used for any TAVI device that can be implanted through a TF approach. A large body of experience exists in the TAo approach for SAPIEN and CoreValve, and there is emerging experience for other devices including the Engager (Medtronic, Minneapolis, MN, USA), Lotus (Boston Scientific, Natick, MA, USA), and Direct Flow (Direct Flow Medical Inc., Santa Rosa, CA, USA).

Edwards SAPIEN XT and SAPIEN 3

Several groups have reported on their experience with implanting the SAPIEN XT and more recently SAPIEN 3 (Edwards LifeSciences) via a TAo approach. The largest XT series comprised 83 patients with unfavorable peripheral access by Hayashida *et al.* [19]. All procedures were performed with the Ascendra 2 or older generations of the Ascendra system (Edwards LifeSciences), which did not have a nose cone. Device success rate was 92.6%, paravalvular leak ≥2/4 was seen in 7.4%, conversion to open chest surgery was required in 5.3% (three aortic dissections, one valve migration, and one left main stem occlusion), and 30-day mortality was 7.4%. Lardizabal *et al.* [20] published a single-center series of 44 patients who underwent SAPIEN TAVI via TAo, and compared them with a non-randomized cohort who underwent TA from the same institution. Results showed equivalent 30-day combined safety endpoints, but significantly lower rate of major bleeding and vascular

complications, as well as intensive care stay in the TAo group. Published literature on the SAPIEN 3 is limited but a small number of procedures were performed in the initial CE mark study [21].

CoreValve

Following the first clinical procedure this approach was developed at the Niguarda Ca' Granda hospital in Milan [11,12,18]. Since then multiple single center and multicenter experiences have been reported [22]. The largest series of CoreValve direct aortic implantation was presented by Bruschi *et al.* at the 46th annual ANMCO meeting [23]. The EURyDICE Registry: EURopean DIrect Aortic Corevalve Experience, is a multicenter experience that comprises patients treated in 20 centers in nine countries in Europe and in Israel, between June 2008 and January 2014. A total of 519 cases have been collected. Mean age of the population was 81.3 ± 6.3 years, 48% were female, mean logistic EuroSCORE was 25.8 ± 15.8; 429 patients were in New York Heart Association (NYHA) Class ≥ III (83%). Peripheral vasculopathy was the principal exclusion criterion from transfemoral TAVI and was present in 330 patients (64%); 306 patients had coronary artery disease (59%) and 109 patients had undergone previous coronary artery bypass surgery. TAVI procedure was performed in 224 of cases (43%) through a right anterior mini-thoracotomy in the second intercostal space or via an upper hemi-sternotomy in the other 295 patients. A size 29 mm CoreValve was implanted in 228 patients (44%). Procedural success was achieved in 509 patients (98%). Four patients required a second valve implanted and two patients had more than moderate para-valvular regurgitation; 30-day mortality was 8%. Seven patients experienced stroke (1.4%) and 72 patients (14%) required a new permanent pacemaker; 93% of patients had aortic regurgitation <2+/4+. Median postoperative hospitalization was 9 days. Low access site complications and low stroke rate were two obvious highlights of these data.

Engager

The Engager™ aortic valve bioprosthesis (Medtronic, Inc., Minneapolis, MN, USA) consists of bovine pericardium mounted in a self-expanding nitinol frame. The stents consist of a main frame and a support frame. The control arms of the support frame are designed to be placed into the sinus of the aortic root and capture the native leaflets to aim to achieve an anatomically correct position in a defined height of implantation to minimize the risk of coronary obstruction, with a valve design that is also intended to minimize paravalvular regurgitation. The prosthesis is available in two sizes (23 and 26 mm) covering annulus diameters of 21–27 mm. The delivery system is 29 Fr with a 32 Fr crossing profile.

The Engager bioprosthesis has been evaluated in first-in-man, feasibility studies, as well as a European pivotal trial [24–26]. All of the published literature has been for the TA access, but Bapat et al. (personal communication) have successfully implanted this device TAo, with excellent procedural and short- to medium-term outcomes. This demonstrates that the TAo procedure remains robust despite larger sheath sizes.

Direct Flow

The Direct Flow Medical TAVI (Direct Flow Medical Inc., Santa Rosa, CA, USA) is the first aortic transcatheter valve device that is not based on a metallic frame technology. The Direct Flow is a bovine pericardial valve with an expandable Dacron polyester double ring design containing non-compliant angioplasty balloon technology. The upper (aortic) and lower (ventricular) ring balloons, interconnected by a tubular bridging system, can be pressurized independently through position-fill lumens. This inflatable and deflatable support structure allows precise positioning, retrieval, and assessment of valve performance before final fixation with a durable polymer. An 18-Fr sheath is used for all valve sizes. Early clinical results have shown excellent short-term results with 99% freedom from all-cause mortality at 30 days in the Prospective Multicenter Evaluation Direct Flow Study [27].

The first instance of Direct Flow TAVI made through a right anterior mini-thoracotomy was reported by Bruschi et al. [28], in a 78-year-old patient affected by severe aortic stenosis and severe peripheral vasculopathy, who had previously undergone CABG with bilateral mammary artery grafts. The standard technique to implant the device by "inner curve technique" was modified to treat this patient, where pulling on the portion directed to the outer side of the aorta was done before realigning the device at the annulus "outer curve technique." The conclusions to be drawn from this are that with Direct Flow it is possible to perform a direct aortic approach even if the distance between the entry site and aortic annulus is <5 cm, (i.e., due to right mammary course), and that the angle between the sheath and ascending aorta is not a problem with Direct Flow. So, differently from other TAVI devices, it should be possible to choose any entry site on the ascending aorta, because coaxial alignment of the device is independent from entry site and perfect Direct Flow implantation is obtained by pulling on the three positioning wires.

Lotus

Lotus Valve (Boston Scientific) is a second-generation transcatheter heart valve device with two unique features: it is repositionable and retrievable, and it has an adaptive seal to reduce paravalvular leak.

It is implanted using a dedicated TF delivery system, which has a "pre-curve" to accommodate the curve of the aortic arch. Early clinical results have shown excellent short-term results [29]. First-in-man implantation of this device by TAo has been reported by Bapat et al. [30]. The valve is delivered using a delivery system, which is introduced through a dedicated sheath (20 or 22 Fr outer diameter). As the pre-curve in the delivery system, which was designed to facilitate a TF approach, cannot be overcome with any available sheath, it is important to choose an ideal site of the aortic puncture so as to achieve a coaxial placement of the Lotus valve. The site chosen should be at least 7 cm from the aortic annulus and on the anterior wall of the ascending aorta. For SAPIEN and CoreValve, the preferred site of the purse-string would be a lateral portion of the aorta to get a coaxial alignment of the device to the annulus but for the Lotus, because of the pre-curve, the purse-string should be placed anterior or slightly to the left of the ascending aorta. Amongst the currently available sheaths, we found that the Ascendra sheath (Edwards Life Sciences) was optimal as it has internal (tip) and external distance markers and it is not hydrophilic. A fluoroscopic marker at the tip for the delivery system is important as it allows the operator to visualize how far the tip is in the aorta and its relationship with the delivery system so as to allow complete expansion of the device and avoid pop-out. This is particularly important for Lotus deployment as the sheath tends to move inwards in the first half of the deployment and outwards during the latter.

TAo: comparison with other approaches

Across the world, the TA approach remains the default non-TF approach, and the majority of data available are therefore for TA compared with TF. There are no randomized data comparing TA with TF, but virtually all studies report better outcomes in those undergoing TF, but this is largely because of the higher underlying risk and comorbidities of patients who undergo TA. However, there are identifiable features of the TA approach that increase risk:

1 Access site problems, including apical rupture and delayed pseudoaneurysm formation [31,32];
2 Interference with postoperative respiratory dynamics because of thoracotomy;
3 Effects of left ventricular function because of the disruption and suturing of the left ventricular apex [33].

A TAo approach can potentially overcome each of these issues. There is no surgical interference of cardiac structures— the ventricular cavity–and mitral valve; it avoids the arch, which potentially reduces the risk of stroke. A mini-sternotomy without accessing the pelural cavities provides the best non-TF option in those with poor respiratory function. Indeed, its advantages over a full sternotomy are well described, including reduced postoperative FiO_2 requirement, pain, and lengths of intensive care and hospital stay [34]. There are also technical aspects including improved tactile feedback because of the proximity to the aortic annulus as well as an ability to perform hybrid procedures.

Contraindications

The only contraindications for this approach are a complete porcelain aorta where there is presence of calcium in the TAo zone, although the advent of cardiac CT technology has shown that this is quite a rare occurrence, and when the ascending aorta is not accessible as a result of anatomic deformity of the chest wall.

Rare types of access for high risk inoperable TAVI

As described earlier, TA access was part of the first large TAVI trial because of an anatomically intuitive direct cardiac exposure with a minimally extensive lateral thoracotomy [35–37]. However, it was realized that this approach and the patients selected for it had many inherent limitations: the severe calcification of the arterial system ("porcelain ascending aorta") or otherwise extensive subocclusive disease of the aorta, the subclavian and the iliac arteries, frail status, severe kyphoscoliosis, possible injury to the coronaries during apex suturing, suboptimal apex hemostasis because of frail myocardium, stroke, and infection [9,31–33,37]. Notably, the valve delivery, positioning, and implantation was the least complicated part of this entire procedure. Although dedicated valve delivery equipment has been made available, most of these risks are related to unfavorable patient comorbidities; hence, this type of access was reserved only for patients completely unsuitable for any alternative. Research initiatives to develop minimally invasive or even percutaneous closure devices/techniques for the left ventricular apex have been incomplete thus far. Accordingly, TA access TAVI remains currently feasible but with an ever-shrinking clinical application.

Another type of "heroic" TAVI access has been developed in response to the high complication rate of TA TAVI. Again, patients without any feasible aortic, subclavian, or iliofemoral access for TAVI are the target patient population. Transcaval abdominal aortic access has been described [38] and can be performed after a careful anatomic plan has been developed based on the CT aortography review [39]. Adequate access through either one of the iliofemoral veins and the inferior vena cava is available for the TAVI delivery system. The "tricky" part in planning this procedure is to identify an area of the abdominal aorta appropriate to receive the large-bore device at an area adjacent to the cava (because a transseptal needle would be used to obtain wire access from the cava to the aorta) and away from important arterial branches in such a way that the aorto-caval communication can be sealed with an intracardiac closure device before sheath retrieval following successful TAVI. However, there are still patients for whom this approach cannot be performed as a result of "porcelain" abdominal aorta or other extreme anatomic unsuitability.

Such high risk patients can be approached with antegrade transmitral access [40] provided that the angle of mitral and aortic annulus is not extremely sharp and the left ventricular cavity is of sufficient size to allow passage of the bulky TAVI delivery system without myocardial rupture or ripping of the anterior mitral valve leaflet (both imminently fatal complications). Notably, this was the very first way TAVI was implanted but was quickly abandoned because of the frequency of these two major complications.

Interestingly, transcarotid TAVI delivery [41] has also been described in high risk TAVI candidates who are obviously inoperable otherwise and have no other mode of access.

Conclusions

The TAo approach using the majority of the currently available TAVI devices is feasible and safe. It is less invasive than the TA approach, provides an access route that is considerably more familiar to cardiac surgeons which improves the learning curve, and provides the option of performing hybrid procedures. Although randomized head-to-head comparisons with TA have not yet been published, the available data suggest more favorable outcomes for TAo. Dedicated delivery options for the newer devices should make what is already a very straightforward procedure even easier, resulting in shorter procedure times as well as improved outcomes.

Disclosure

V. Bapat is a Consultant for Edwards Lifesciences, Medtronic Inc., St. Jude Medical, Boston Scientific and Symetis. G. Bruschi is a Consultant for Medtronic Inc. and Direct Flow. K. Asrress has no conflicts of interest to declare.

Interactive multiple choice questions are available for this chapter on www.wiley. com/go/dangas/cardiology

References

1 Cribier A, Eltchaninoff H, Tron C, et al. Early experience with percutaneous transcatheter implantation of heart valve prosthesis for the treatment of end-stage inoperable patients with calcific aortic stenosis. *J Am Coll Cardiol* 2004; **43**(4): 698–703.

2 Cribier A, Eltchaninoff H, Bash A, et al. Percutaneous transcatheter implantation of an aortic valve prosthesis for calcific aortic stenosis: first human case description. *Circulation* 2002; **106**(24): 3006–3008.

3 Vahanian A, Alfieri O, Al-Attar N, et al. Transcatheter valve implantation for patients with aortic stenosis: a position statement from the European Association of Cardio-Thoracic Surgery (EACTS) and the European Society of Cardiology (ESC), in collaboration with the European Association of Percutaneous Cardiovascular Interventions (EAPCI). *Eur Heart J* 2008; **29**(11): 1463–1470.

4 Thomas M, Schymik G, Walther T, et al. Thirty-day results of the SAPIEN aortic bioprosthesis european outcome (SOURCE) registry: a European registry of transcatheter aortic valve implantation using the Edwards SAPIEN valve. *Circulation* 2010; **122**(1): 62–69.

5 Wendler O, Walther T, Nataf P, et al. Trans-apical aortic valve implantation: univariate and multivariate analyses of the early results from the SOURCE registry. *Eur J Cardiothorac Surg* 2010; **38**(2): 119–127.

6 Piazza N, Grube E, Gerckens U, et al. Procedural and 30-day outcomes following transcatheter aortic valve implantation using the third generation (18 Fr) corevalve revalving system: results from the multicentre, expanded evaluation registry 1-year following CE mark approval. *EuroIntervention* 2008; **4**(2): 242–249.

7 Leon MB, Smith CR, Mack M, et al. Transcatheter aortic-valve implantation for aortic stenosis in patients who cannot undergo surgery. *N Engl J Med* 2010; **363**(17): 1597–1607.

8 Webb JG. Transcatheter valve in valve implants for failed prosthetic valves. *Catheter Cardiovasc Interv* 2007; **70**(5): 765–766.

9 Ye J, Cheung A, Lichtenstein SV, et al. Six-month outcome of transapical transcatheter aortic valve implantation in the initial seven patients. *Eur J Cardiothorac Surg* 2007; **31**(1): 16–21.

10 Latsios G, Gerckens U, Grube E. Transaortic transcatheter aortic valve implantation: a novel approach for the truly "no-access option" patients. *Catheter Cardiovasc Interv* 2010; **75**(7): 1129–1136.

11 Bauernschmitt R, Schreiber C, Bleiziffer S, et al. Transcatheter aortic valve implantation through the ascending aorta: an alternative option for no-access patients. *Heart Surg Forum* 2009; **12**(1): E63–64.

12 Bruschi G, Fratto P, De Marco F, et al. The trans-subclavian retrograde approach for transcatheter aortic valve replacement: single-center experience. *J Thorac Cardiovasc Surg* 2010; **140**(4): 911–915, 915.e1–2.

13 Asgar AW, Mullen MJ, Delahunty N, et al. Transcatheter aortic valve intervention through the axillary artery for the treatment of severe aortic stenosis. *J Thorac Cardiovasc Surg* 2009; **137**(3): 773–775.

14 Moynagh AM, Scott DJA, Baumbach A, et al. CoreValve transcatheter aortic valve implantation via the subclavian artery: comparison with the transfemoral approach. *J Am Coll Cardiol* 2011; **57**(5): 634–635.

15 Bapat V, Thomas M, Hancock J, et al. First successful trans-catheter aortic valve implantation through ascending aorta using Edwards SAPIEN THV system. *Eur J Cardiothorac Surg* 2010; **38**(6): 811–813.

16 Bapat V, Attia R, Redwood S, et al. Use of transcatheter heart valves for a valve-in-valve implantation in patients with degenerated aortic bioprosthesis: technical considerations and results. *J Thorac Cardiovasc Surg* 2012; **144**(6): 1372–1379; discussion 1379–1380.

17 Etienne PY, Papadatos S, El Khoury E, *et al.* Transaortic transcatheter aortic valve implantation with the Edwards SAPIEN valve: feasibility, technical considerations, and clinical advantages. *Ann Thorac Surg* 2011; **92**(2): 746–748.

18 Bruschi G, de Marco F, Botta L, *et al.* Direct aortic access for transcatheter self-expanding aortic bioprosthetic valves implantation. *Ann Thorac Surg* 2012; **94**(2): 497–503.

19 Hayashida K, Romano M, Lefèvre T, *et al.* The transaortic approach for transcatheter aortic valve implantation: a valid alternative to the transapical access in patients with no peripheral vascular option. A single center experience. *Eur J Cardiothorac Surg* 2013; **44**(4): 692–700.

20 Lardizabal JA, O'Neill BP, Desai HV, *et al.* The transaortic approach for transcatheter aortic valve replacement: initial clinical experience in the United States. *J Am Coll Cardiol* 2013; **61**(23): 2341–2345.

21 Webb J, Gerosa G, Lefèvre T, *et al.* Multicenter evaluation of a next-generation balloon-expandable transcatheter aortic valve. *J Am Coll Cardiol* 2014; **64**(21): 2235–2243.

22 Alegría-Barrero E, Chan PH, Di Mario C, *et al.* Direct aortic transcatheter aortic valve implantation: a feasible approach for patients with severe peripheral vascular disease. *Cardiovasc Revasc Med* 2012; **13**(3): 201.e5–7.

23 Bruschi G, Chevalier B, De Marco F, *et al.* EURyDICE registry: European direct aortic corevalve experience. *G Ital Cardiol* 2015; **16**(Suppl 1): e12–24.

24 Falk V, Walther T, Schwammenthal E, *et al.* Transapical aortic valve implantation with a self-expanding anatomically oriented valve. *Eur Heart J* 2011; **32**(7): 878–887.

25 Sündermann SH, Grünenfelder J, Corti R, *et al.* Outcome of patients treated with Engager transapical aortic valve implantation: one-year results of the feasibility study. *Innovations (Phila)* 2013; **8**(5): 332–336.

26 Sündermann SH, Holzhey D, Bleiziffer S, Treede H, Falk V. Medtronic Engager™ bioprosthesis for transapical transcatheter aortic valve implantation. *EuroIntervention* 2013; **9**(Suppl): 97–100.

27 Schofer J, Colombo A, Klugmann S, *et al.* Prospective multicenter evaluation of the direct flow medical transcatheter aortic valve. *J Am Coll Cardiol* 2014; **63**(8): 763–768.

28 Bruschi G, Merlanti B, Barosi A, *et al.* Direct aortic direct flow implantation via right anterior thoracotomy in a patient with patent bilateral mammary artery coronary grafts. *Int J Cardiol* 2015; **185**: 22–24.

29 Meredith IT, Worthley SG, Whitbourn RJ, *et al.* Transfemoral aortic valve replacement with the repositionable lotus valve system in high surgical risk patients: the REPRISE I study. *EuroIntervention* 2014; **9**(11): 1264–1270.

30 Bapat VN, Asrress KN, Boix R, *et al.* Transaortic transcatheter aortic valve implantation using LOTUS valve: first-in-man experience. *EuroIntervention* 2015; **11**(7): pii.

31 Al-Attar N, Ghodbane W, Himbert D, *et al.* Unexpected complications of transapical aortic valve implantation. *Ann Thorac Surg* 2009; **88**(1): 90–94.

32 Wong DR, Ye J, Cheung A, *et al.* Technical considerations to avoid pitfalls during transapical aortic valve implantation. *J Thorac Cardiovasc Surg* 2010; **140**(1): 196–202.

33 Astarci P, Glineur D, Kefer J, *et al.* "Ring pledget": a new concept for secure apex closure during transapical aortic valve implantation. *Innovations (Phila)* 2010; **5**(2): 136–137.

34 Bonacchi M, Prifti E, Giunti G, *et al.* Does ministernotomy improve postoperative outcome in aortic valve operation? A prospective randomized study. *Ann Thorac Surg* 2002; **73**(2): 460–465; discussion 465–466.

35 Blackstone EH, Suri RM, Rajeswaran J, *et al.* Propensity-matched comparisons of clinical outcomes after transapical or transfemoral transcatheter aortic valve replacement: a placement of aortic transcatheter valves (PARTNER)-I trial substudy. *Circulation* 2015; **131**(22): 1989–2000.

36 Mack MJ, Leon MB, Smith CR; PARTNER 1 Trial Investigators. 5-year outcomes of transcatheter aortic valve replacement or surgical aortic valve replacement for high surgical risk patients with aortic stenosis (PARTNER 1): a randomised controlled trial. *Lancet* 2015; **385**(9986): 2477–2484.

37 Dewey TM, Bowers B, Thourani VH, *et al.* Transapical aortic valve replacement for severe aortic stenosis: results from the nonrandomized continued access cohort of the PARTNER trial. *Ann Thorac Surg* 2013; **96**(6): 2083–2089.

38 Greenbaum AB, O'Neill WW, Paone G, *et al.* Caval-aortic access to allow transcatheter aortic valve replacement in otherwise ineligible patients: initial human experience. *J Am Coll Cardiol* 2014; **63**(25 Part A): 2795–2804.

39 Lederman RJ, Chen MY, Rogers T, *et al.* Planning transcaval access using CT for large transcatheter implants. *JACC Cardiovasc Imaging* 2014; **7**(11): 1167–1171.

40 Cohen MG, Singh V, Martinez CA, *et al.* Transseptal antegrade transcatheter aortic valve replacement for patients with no other access approach: a contemporary experience. *Catheter Cardiovasc Interv* 2013; **82**(6): 987–993.

41 Thourani VH, Li C, Devireddy C, *et al.* High-risk patients with inoperative aortic stenosis: use of transapical, transaortic, and transcarotid techniques. *Ann Thorac Surg* 2015; **99**(3): 817–823.

CHAPTER 61

New Aortic Valve Technologies

Dimytri Alexandre Siqueira[1] and Alexandre A.C. Abizaid[1,2,3]

[1] Dante Pazzanese Institute of Cardiology, São Paulo, Brazil
[2] Hospital do Coração—Associação do Sanatório Sírio (HCor), São Paulo, Brazil
[3] Hospital Israelita Albert Einstein, São Paulo, Brazil

First performed in 2002 [1], transcatheter aortic valve replacement (TAVR) allows implantation of a prosthetic heart valve within the diseased native aortic valve without the need for open heart surgery and cardiopulmonary bypass, offering an established therapeutic option to elderly patients considered at high surgical risk or with contraindications to surgery. Despite the excellent outcomes observed with the balloon-expandable devices SAPIEN™/SAPIEN XT™ (Edwards Lifesciences, Irvine, CA, USA) [2,3] and with the self-expandable system Medtronic CoreValve® (Medtronic, Minneapolis, MN, USA) [4], the first devices approved globally, the occurrence of adverse events such as paravalvular regurgitation, valve malpositioning, vascular complications, and conduction disorders need to be addressed in order to further improve the prognosis of high risk patients with aortic stenosis and potentially expand the indications of TAVR to lower risk individuals.

Development of newly transcatheter aortic bioprosthesis is aimed to facilitate the procedure and underscores the need to: (i) reduce delivery catheter diameter, preventing vascular complications: (ii) to ensure accurate annular positioning, allowing the retrieval, recapture, and re-implantation of the device in cases of prosthesis misplacement; and (iii) to incorporate innovative design features that reduce the occurrence of paravalvular leaks, conduction disturbances, and coronary occlusion. Currently, some different percutaneous aortic valves—"second-generation TAVR devices"—are commercially available in Europe and others are gaining early clinical evaluation [5,6]. In this chapter, the unique features and the initial clinical results of new aortic valve technologies are reviewed.

SAPIEN 3

The balloon-expandable SAPIEN 3 transcatheter heart valve system™ (Edwards Lifesciences Inc.) has several new features intended to ensure a more precise implantation and to reduce the occurrence of paravalvular leak and vascular complications [5,6]. The SAPIEN 3™ (S3) valve is composed of modified bovine pericardial tissue leaflets sutured in a cobalt-chromium stent design, which permitted a further downsizing in profile (Figure 61.1a). Like the SAPIEN XT™ (Edwards Lifesciences Inc.) device, the inflow of the S3 is covered by an internal polyethylene terephthalate (PET) skirt; an additional outer PET sealing cuff was incorporated to prevent paravalvular regurgitation. Four sizes are available (20, 23, 26, and 29 mm), covering annulus sizes between 16 and 28 mm.

The new transfemoral delivery system is called Commander™ (Figure 61.1b) and has a smaller profile (14 Fr) and a higher flexibility than the previous NovaFlex™ delivery catheter (Edwards Lifesciences Inc.). Therefore, navigation through tortuosities is facilitated and the S3 can be positioned more coaxial to the native valve in challenging anatomies, such as horizontal aorta. A complementary wheel has been added in the delivery handle, and the height of the implant can be adjusted precisely, providing accurate and more reproducible valve positioning and further preventing paravalvular leak, conduction disturbances, and permanent pacemaker need. During balloon inflation, the stent frame of the crimped valve foreshortens predominantly from below, so this movement should be anticipated when positioning the device.

The S3 system is compatible with a 14 Fr expandable eSheath™ (Edwards Lifesciences Inc.), which transiently expands as the prosthesis passes through the sheath. With the improved profile, the incidence of vascular and hemorrhagic complications is reduced, and a broader proportion of patients can be treated by transfemoral access (a minimum vessel diameter of 5.5 mm ileofemoral arteries is required). The profile of the transapical Edwards Certitude delivery system™ (Edwards Lifesciences Inc.) has also been downsized to 18 Fr (for S3 23–26 mm) and 21 Fr (S3 29 mm).

In the first-in-human experience with the SAPIEN 3™, 15 patients with symptomatic, severe aortic stenosis were treated by transfemoral approach [7]. All the devices were successfully implanted, and the aortic valve area and the mean transaortic gradient improved from 0.7 ± 0.2 to 1.5 ± 0.2 cm^2 (p <0.001) and from 42.2 ± 10.3 to 11.9 ± 5.3 mmHg (p <0.001), respectively. None of the patients had moderate or severe paravalvular aortic regurgitation. In the PARTNER II S3 trial, 1076 patients considered intermediate risk for surgical aortic valve replacement and 583 patients deemed high risk or inoperable were treated with the SAPIEN 3™ valve [8]. In the high risk cohort, the mortality rate at 30 days was 2.2% and the stroke occurred in 1.5% of patients; the rate of moderate–severe aortic regurgitation was 2.9%. For the intermediate risk patients, all-cause mortality was 1.1%, and 2.6% had a stroke at 30 days; the rate of moderate and severe paravalvular regurgitation was 4.2% in this cohort.

Interventional Cardiology: Principles and Practice, Second Edition. Edited by George D. Dangas, Carlo Di Mario, and Nicholas N. Kipshidze.
© 2017 John Wiley & Sons, Ltd. Published 2017 by John Wiley & Sons, Ltd.

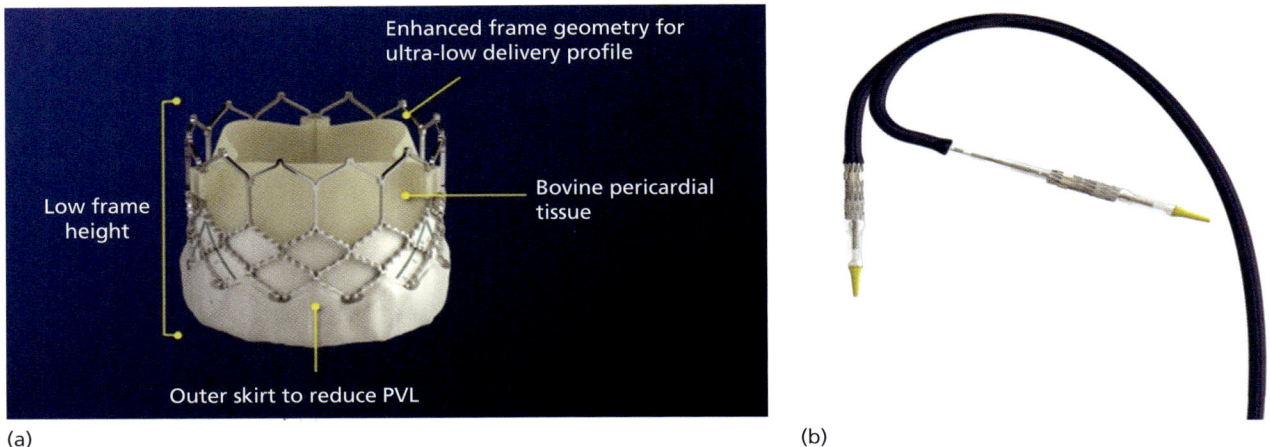

(a)   (b)

Figure 61.1 (a) SAPIEN 3: composed of bovine pericardial tissue leaflets in a cobalt-chromium stent design; the inflow has an outer sealing cuff to prevent paravalvular regurgitation. (b) Commander™ delivery system: with small profile (14 Fr) and high flexibility, facilitates navigation through tortuosities and assures coaxiality to aortic annulus. Balloon-expandable devices SAPIEN™/SAPIEN XT™. Reproduced with permission from Edwards Lifesciences, Irvine, CA, USA.

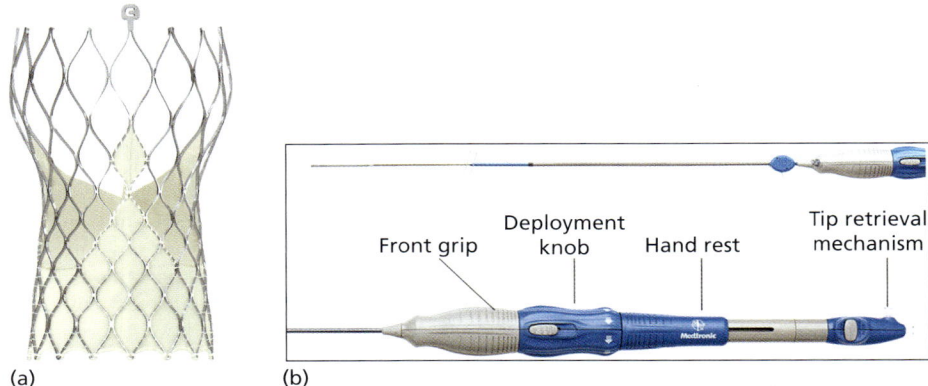

(a)   (b)

Figure 61.2 (a) CoreValve™ Evolut R: composed of self-expanding nitinol stent frame, porcine leaflets and an extended pericardial skirt – reducing the risk of paravalvular leaks. (b) InLine™ sheath: with a 14 Fr profile (true outer 18 Fr) allows for a sheathless procedure, reducing vascular complications. CoreValve® images used with permission by Medtronic © 2016.

CoreValve Evolut R

The major improvements of the new Medtronic CoreValve system–CoreValve Evolut R™ (Medtronic, Minneapolis, MN, USA) were developed to provide stable and controlled deployment of the prosthesis at the desired level of the aortic annulus and to prevent paravalvular regurgitation, making the procedure more predictable [9]. The fully repositioning and recapture properties enables accurate positioning and minimizes the risks of paravalvular leakage, mitral anterior leaflet compromise, valve embolization, and conduction disturbances requiring permanent pacemaker. Although several other features of the previous CoreValve™ system (like the self-expanding nitinol stent frame, the porcine leaflets, and the supra-annular functioning of the valve leaflets) have been preserved, the distal inflow portion has been redesigned for an extended pericardial skirt, further reducing the risk of paravalvular aortic regurgitation (Figure 61.2a). The outflow portion is 10 mm shorter than the previous version, aimed to optimize fit in angulated anatomy. The Evolut R ™ is available in four sizes (23, 26, 29, and 31 mm), covering aortic annuli from 18 to 30 mm. The new delivery system (Enveo R™) guarantees a rapid, precise interaction between deployment knob rotation and prosthesis unsheathing and resheathing (Figure 61.2b). It has a reinforced nitinol capsule for resheathing and an integrated sheath, mounted in the catheter and named InLine™. The InLine™ sheath has a 14 Fr profile (true outer 18 Fr), which allows for a sheathless procedure, further reducing the rate of vascular complications.

Initial clinical outcomes for CoreValve Evolut R system™ were reported in a first-in-man experience, multicenter study with 60 patients [10]. Transfemoral access was possible in all but one patient (98.3%) and a correct valve position with one device in place was achieved in 98.3%. All resheathing and recapture attempts (22 in 15 patients) were performed safely and successfully. Post-dilatation was required in 21.7% of cases, and mean aortic gradient decreased from 49.1 mmHg at baseline to 8.1 mmHg post-procedure; moderate or severe aortic regurgitation were observed in 3.4% of patients at 30 days. No incidents of death or stroke were observed at 30 days, and the pacemaker rate was 11.7%.

Lotus™ valve system

The Lotus™ valve system (Boston Scientific, Natick, MA, USA) [11] is designed to ensure a precise positioning, minimizing paravalvular regurgitation. The valve is comprised of bovine pericardial leaflets within a braided, single nitinol wire in a self-expanding frame. A radio-opaque marker is located centrally in the frame to aid in positioning. The valve frame is surrounded in its inflow (ventricular) portion by an outer sleeve membrane (Adaptative Seal™), which can potentially occupy remaining gaps between the valve and aortic annulus, thus preventing paravalvular aortic regurgitation (Figure 61.3a). Inside its delivery catheter, the Lotus™ valve is stretched to 70 mm length, and shortens to approximately 19 mm after deployment. It is available in three sizes (23, 25, and 27 mm), which permits the treatment of patients with aortic annulus from 19 to 27 mm. The valve is pre-attached to the delivery system and is deployed in a controlled mechanical fashion, which enables proper leaflets function early in the expansion phase—mitigating hemodynamic instability during this part of the procedure—and allows for helpful evaluation of positioning and performance before final release (Figure 61.3b). In cases of significant paravalvular leakage, coronary compromised or severe conduction disturbances, the special property of resheathing the Lotus™ valve permits repositioning and retrievable maneuvers. The delivery system of the Lotus™ has a 18–20 French size, is pre-curved, and covered with a hydrophilic coating, which ensures a better trackability in diseased and tortuous vessels and for adjustment to the angulation of the aortic arch.

Successful implantation of the Lotus valve was first reported in Germany in 2007 [12]. After refinement of the initial design, the valve underwent clinical testing. In the REPRISE I trial and feasibility study to assess the acute safety and performance of the Lotus™ valve, 11 high-surgical risk patients with symptomatic, severe aortic stenosis were treated [13]. In all patients, the valve was successfully deployed in the first attempt. Partial resheathing was required and successfully performed in four patients; none required full retrieval. A successful implantation without residual gradient and major adverse cardiovascular or cerebrovascular events was achieved in nine patients (82%), with no in-hospital major adverse cardiac and coronary events (MACCE) in 10 patients. One patient suffered a major stroke and other patient had a mean gradient above 20 mmHg at discharge. The hemodynamic performance of the Lotus™ valve was sustained: mean aortic gradient decreased from 53.9 ± 20.9 mmHg at baseline to 15.4 ± 4.6 mmHg (p <0.001) at 1 year and valve area increased from 0.7 ± 0.2 to 1.5 ± 0.2 cm^2 (p <0.001). After adjudication by an independent core laboratory, paravalvular aortic regurgitation was mild (n = 2), trivial (n = 1), or absent (n = 8) as assessed by echocardiography. Four patients (36.3%) required a permanent pacemaker post-procedure.

In the prospective, single-arm, multicenter REPRISE II trial, 120 patients considered to be at high surgical risk by a heart team were selected [14]. The valve was successfully implanted using transfemoral access in all patients; complications such as valve embolization, ectopic valve deployment, or additional valve implantation were not observed. All required attempts of repositioning (n = 26) and retrieval (n = 6) the valve were successful; 34 patients (28.6%) received a permanent pacemaker. The primary device performance endpoint (30-day mean pressure gradient by echocardiography) was met, and the mean gradient improved from 46.4 ± 15.0 to 11.5 ± 5.2 mmHg; mean effective orifice area increased from 0.7 ± 0.2 to 1.7 ± 0.4 cm^2 post-procedure. At 30 days, the mortality rate was 4.2% and major stroke occurred in

1.7%. Only one (1.0%) patient had moderate paravalvular regurgitation, and none had a severe paravalvular leak. The ongoing REPRISE III is a randomized, multicenter, controlled trial that aims to assess the safety and effectiveness of the Lotus system, as compared to the self-expandable CoreValve™; more than 1000 patients were expected to be enrolled in 60 centers.

ACURATE valve system

The Symetis Acurate™ transcatheter valve (Symetis SA, Ecublens, Switzerland) is a self-expanding nitinol device, with supra-annular porcine leaflets and a unique stent arquitecture [15]. The stent frame is divided into three parts, released in sequential steps from the aorta to left ventricle (Figure 61.4):

1 The "upper crown" is first deployed in a subcoronary position and provides fixation to the annulus, capturing the native leaflets and reducing the occurrence of coronary obstruction.

2 Three aortic stabilization arches, designed for self-alignment and coaxiality, are then released and prevent tilting of the device during deployment; up to this point the valve can still be repositioned and retrieved.

3 The "lower crown" has good radial force and after unsheathing, protrudes minimally in the left ventricular outflow tract, which favorably impacts post-procedure pacemaker rate.

The upper crown is fenestrated, and the stent body and lower crown have internal and external pericardial skirts, also preventing paravalvular leak. The Acurate valve™ is available in three sizes, covering aortic annulus sizes from 21 to 27 mm (ACURATE™ S 21–23 mm, M 23–25 mm, and L 25–27 mm).

In a multicenter post-market study, 250 high risk, elderly patients with severe aortic stenosis were treated with the ACURATE TA™ (transapical) bioprosthesis (Symetis SA, Ecublens, Switzerland) [16]. Mean STS and logistic Euroscore were $8.0 \pm 5.9\%$ and $22.3 \pm 12.7\%$, respectively. The procedural success rate was 98% (n = 245) with two valve-in-valve procedures and three conversions to open-heart surgery. Moderate paravalvular regurgitation was detected in 2.3% of patients, and none had a severe aortic regurgitation. A new pacemaker implantation was required in 10% of patients and 30-day mortality rate was 6.8%. Well-grounded in the ACURATE TA™ experience, a transfemoral version of the device was developed: ACURATE Neo™ (Symetis SA, Ecublens, Switzerland). The ACURATE Neo™ has a very flexible delivery catheter compatible with a 18 Fr sheath. The first-in-man trial enrolled 20 patients in Brazil and Germany between February and August 2012 [15]. Patients were 84.8 ± 4.5 years old with a mean logistic EuroSCORE of $26.5 \pm 8.0\%$. The procedural success was 95% (n = 19) and one patient had to be treated with a valve-in-valve procedure because of low (too ventricular) placement. The effective orifice area improved from 0.7 to 1.8 cm^2 and all except one patient have more-than-mild paravalvular regurgitation. The pacemaker rate was 10% (n = 2).

Direct Flow

The Direct Flow™ transcatheter heart valve (Direct Flow Medical Inc., Santa Rosa, California, USA) differs from the other new aortic valve technologies already in clinical use, as it consists in a non-metallic, trileaflet bovine pericardial valve attached to an inflatable, polyester fabric cuff [5,6]. Two circular balloons—one proximal (aortic) and the other distal (ventricular)—were connected by vertical tubular supports and inflated independently and sequentially with a solidified polymer that hardens the non-metallic frame,

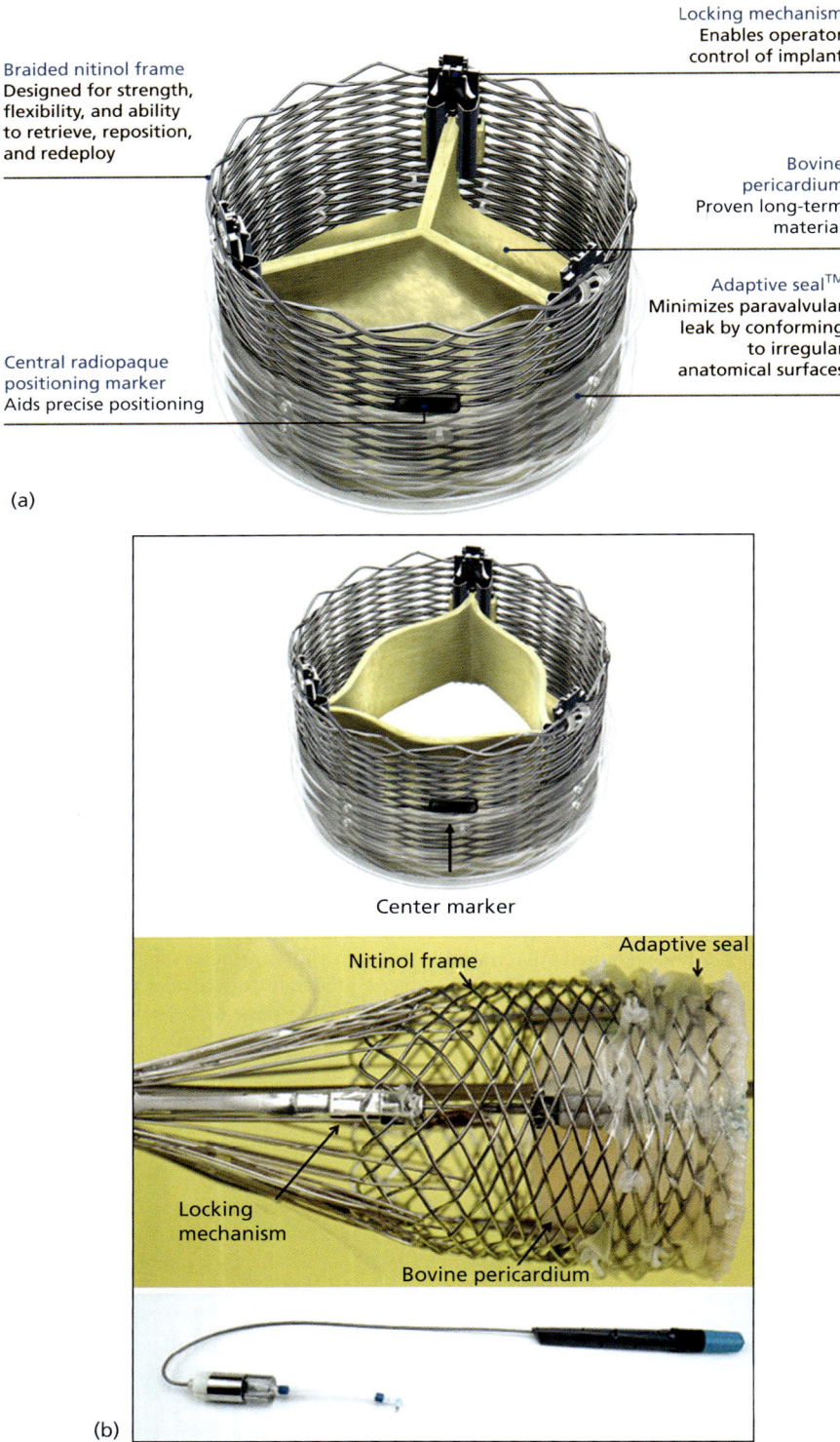

Figure 61.3 (a) Lotus valve: composed of bovine pericardial leaflets within a braided, single nitinol wire in a self-expanding frame; an outer sleeve membrane in its inflow portion prevents paravalvular leak. (b) Lotus valve: pre-attached to the delivery system and deployed mechanically. Property of resheathing permits repositioning and retrievable attempts. The delivery system is pre-curved and covered with a hydrophilic coating. Images used with permission of Boston Scientific Corporation.

encircling the annulus and anchoring the bioprosthesis at the annular level (Figure 61.5). The device is fully repositionable and retrievable through the introducer prior to final deployment, allowing for accurate and controlled deployment to ensure perfect sealing and reduced risk of paravalvular aortic regurgitation. Other technical advantages of the Direct Flow™ system includes its flexibility due to the non-metallic design, an important feature in tortuous anatomies; maintenance of hemodynamic stability throughout the

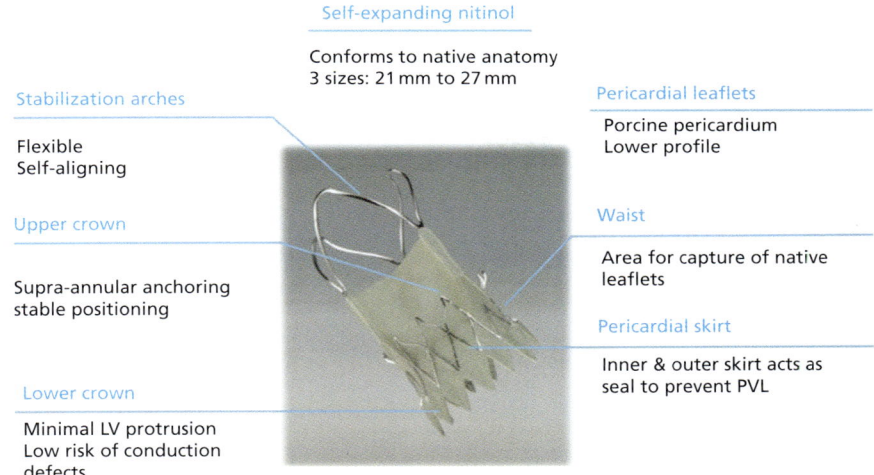

Self-expanding nitinol

Conforms to native anatomy
3 sizes: 21 mm to 27 mm

Stabilization arches

Flexible
Self-aligning

Upper crown

Supra-annular anchoring
stable positioning

Lower crown

Minimal LV protrusion
Low risk of conduction
defects

Pericardial leaflets

Porcine pericardium
Lower profile

Waist

Area for capture of native
leaflets

Pericardial skirt

Inner & outer skirt acts as
seal to prevent PVL

Figure 61.4 Symetis Acurate Neo™ valve: self-expanding nitinol device, with supra-annular porcine leaflets. The stent frame is divided into three parts, released in sequential steps: the upper crown, the stabilization arches, and the lower crown. Image used with permission of Symetis SA.

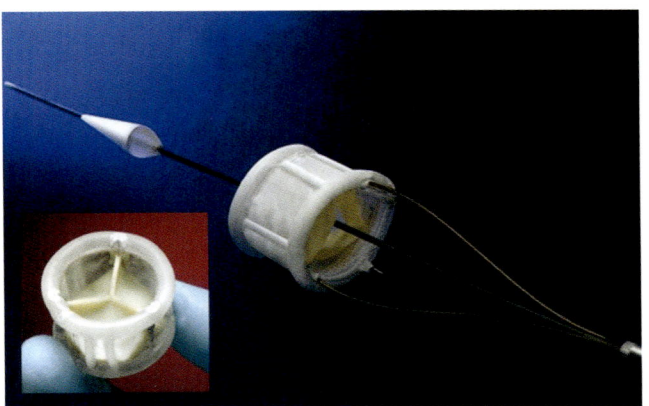

Figure 61.5 The Direct Flow Medical® Transcatheter Aortic Valve consists of a trileaflet bovine pericardial valve attached to a non-metallic, inflatable, polyester fabric cuff. Image used with permission of Direct Flow Medical.

deployment, because transaortic blood flow is preserved and rapid pacing is not required during positioning and implantation; and, finally, the inflatable polyester cuff conforms to the native aortic annulus, minimizing further the risk of paravalvular regurgitation. The Direct Flow™ bioprosthesis is available in four sizes (23, 25, 27, and 29 mm), for aortic annulus sizes between 19 and 28 mm. The delivery system is 18 Fr-compatible for all valve sizes.

The safety and efficacy of Direct Flow Medical system™ were evaluated in a prospective, multicenter, non-randomized trial with 100 high surgical risk patients with severe aortic stenosis [17]. All procedures were performed transfemorally, and all patients underwent balloon valvuloplasty before valve implantation to ensure expansion of the stenotic leaflets and annulus; the mean time for valve positioning, assessment, and deployment was 14 minutes. Freedom from all-cause mortality at 30 days (the pre-specified primary endpoint) was 99%, and overall device success was 93%. The mean aortic valve gradient decreased from 45.9 ± 9.6 to 12.6 ± 7.1 mmHg post-procedure, and the effective orifice area increased from 0.65 ± 0.18 cm^2 at baseline to 1.50 ± 0.56 cm^2 at 30 days. Total aortic regurgitation was mild or less in 98.6%, and no patient had severe aortic regurgitation. Paravalvular regurgitation was none in 70.3%, mild in 28.4%, and moderate in 1 (1.4%). Stroke rate was 2.7%, and 16% required a new, permanent pacemaker.

Because of the non-metallic design, concerns about durability and recoil of the Direct Flow Medical valve™ have been raised. So far, 2-year data from the very first patients (n = 16)—treated with an older version of the device—revealed that there were no changes in the position, diameter, or orifice area of the prosthesis over time with no evidence of recoil, as assessed by multislice computed tomography. Hemodynamic performance were also stable by echocardiography, with absent and mild aortic regurgitation in 73% and 27% of patients, respectively [18].

Engager

The Medtronic Engager™ aortic bioprosthesis (Medtronic Inc.) is designed for a transapical, antegrade approach and combines a self-expanding nitinol frame and bovine pericardium trileaflets [5,6,19]. The nitinol stent consists of a central frame, which houses the leaflets, and a support frame, with control arms designed to stabilize the device in the sinuses of Valsalva, obtain anatomic orientation and positioning. The prosthesis has a polyester sleeve sutured to the main frame to reduce the risk of paravalvular regurgitation (Figure 61.6). The Engager™ is available in two sizes, 23 and 26 mm, for an annulus range between 21 and 27 mm. The first step of the implantation procedure consists in locating the support arms into the sinuses of Valsalva. Correct subcoronary positioning is mandatory, and should be verified by angiography. Repositioning (if necessary with recapture of the support arms) could be performed at this stage. The commissural posts are then released, and final deployment is ideally performed under rapid ventricular pacing for stability and accuracy of positioning.

The Engager™ underwent first-in-man implantation in 2008 [19]. The feasibility study with the new Engager® system was conducted in 10 patients at high risk for surgery (mean age 82.5 ± 3.6 years, mean logistic EuroSCORE 24.6 ± 13.6%). Implantation was successful in all patients, and no complications related to the device were reported. Aortic regurgitation caused by paravalvular leakage was absent or trivial ($\leq$grade 1) in the majority (90%) of patients, and two required required permanent pacemaker implantation for complete atrioventricular block.

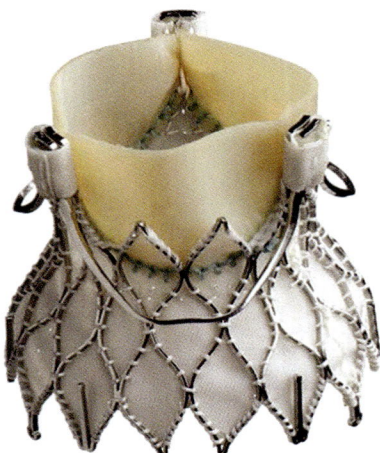

Figure 61.6 Medtronic Engager™ bioprosthesis. Designed for a transapical approach, is composed by a self-expanding nitinol frame, bovine pericardium trileaflets, and a polyester sleeve to reduce the risk of paravalvular regurgitation. Image used with permission by Medtronic ©2016. Note added in proof: The Engager bioprosthesis has been discontinued.

In a published, interim analysis of the multicenter Engager® pivotal trial, 61 patients with mean age of 81.9 years and mean logistic EuroSCORE of 18.9% were selected. Overall device success, defined by modified VARC criteria, was achieved in 94.3%, without conversions to surgery, second valve implantation, device malposition, aortic annular rupture, or coronary obstruction. All-cause mortality was 9.9% at 30 days and 16.9% at 6 months. Mean aortic valve gradient improved from 43.7 ± 16.7 to 11.5 ± 5.0 mmHg at 30 days, and there was no paravalvular regurgitation greater than mild through 6 months [20].

Portico

The Portico™ valve (St. Jude Medical, USA) consists of bovine pericardial tissue mounted on a nitinol, self-expandable stent (Figure 61.7). Although similar in appearance to the CoreValve™, the Portico™ prosthesis has several and distinct features aimed at reducing potential complications:

1 The inflow portion is covered by a porcine pericardium cuff designed to minimize paravalvular leaks.
2 The leaflets are located lower on the support frame, minimizing device protrusion into the left ventricular outflow tract and therefore conduction disturbances.
3 The valve is resheathable and can be repositioned before deployment, provided the stent has not been fully released.
4 A large stent cell design guarantees easier access to coronaries and results in a low crimped profile; the large cell area also potentially minimizes the risk of paravalvular leak by allowing valve tissue to conform around calcific nodules at the annulus.

The valve uses Linx® anti-calcification technology [21].

In the first-in-man experience, the Portico™ valve was implanted in 10 patients with severe aortic stenosis using transfemoral access [22]. Device implantation was successful in all patients. Prosthesis recapture and repositioning was required in four patients, and one patient underwent a second transcatheter valve implantation because of intermittent prosthetic leaflet dysfunction. Mean transaortic gradient decreased from 44.9 ± 16.7 to 10.9 ± 3.8 mmHg (p <0.001), and valve area increased from 0.6 ± 0.1 to 1.3 ± 0.2 cm² (p <0.001). Moderate paravalvular regurgitation was detected in one patient (10%). No major strokes, major vascular complications, major bleeds, need of permanent

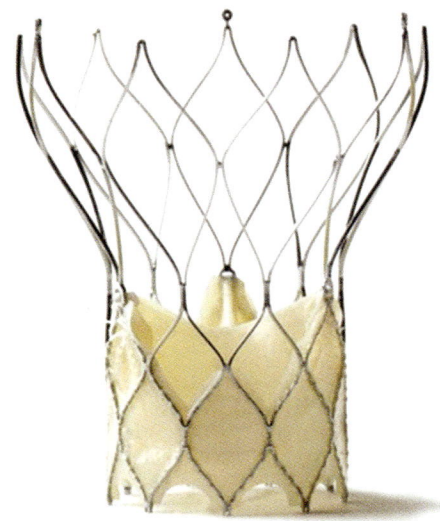

Figure 61.7 Portico™ valve. Bovine pericardial tissue mounted on a nitinol, self-expandable stent, with inflow portion covered by a porcine pericardium cuff to minimize paravalvular leaks. Valve is resheathable and can be repositioned before deployment. Source: Portico and St. Jude Medical are trademarks of St. Jude Medical, Inc. or its related companies. Reproduced with permission of St. Jude Medical, ©2016. All rights reserved.

pacemaker, or deaths were reported. The feasibility of transapical implantation of the Portico® valve has been investigated in Canada and Europe [23]. A total of seven cases were successfully performed, with procedure successes in 100% according to VARC II definition. Paravalvular regurgitation was mild or trace in all patients. The 24 Fr delivery system used is one of the smallest used for transapical access, and could, in particular, be safer in patients with left ventricular dysfunction.

JenaValve

The JenaValve® prosthesis (JenaValve Technology GmbH, Munich, Germany) consists of a porcine root valve mounted on a low profile, self-expanding nitinol frame [5,6,24]. Initially a transapical-only system, which included a sheathless 32 Fr delivery catheter (Cathlete; JenaValve Technology GmbH), the prosthesis is available in three sizes (23, 25, and 27 mm), covering aortic valve annuli from 21 to 27 mm. The self-expanding stent has three feelers, which should be placed in the left, right, and non-coronary cusps before deployment (Figure 61.8). The purpose is to position the commissures of the prosthesis precisely on the commissures of the native aortic valve. After the feelers have been placed in the correct orientation, the catheter is pulled back up until a tactile feedback indicates the contact of the feelers with the proper cusps; the lower part of the JenaValve® is then released. Rapid pacing is not required during prosthesis positioning, and hemodynamic flow is maintained during prosthesis placement. Patients' native valve leaflets are hence clipped between the feelers and the base of the prosthesis. This clipping mechanism firmly anchors the prosthesis independently of the amount calcium at the aortic annulus or leaflets, providing active fixation and resistance to migration. At this point the bioprosthesis is competent and functioning but still repositionable and retrievable. After releasing the base, the last step in deployment is the opening of the upper part of the nitinol frame. Because of the clipping mechanism, the JenaValve® is the only transcatheter heart valve with a CE

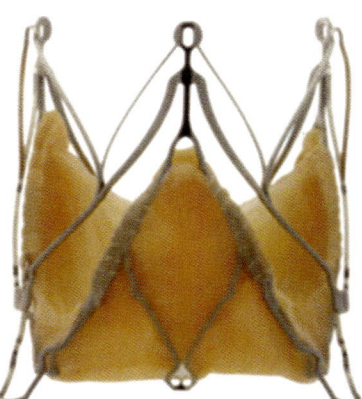

Figure 61.8 JenaValve prosthesis. Composed of porcine root valve mounted on a low-profile, self-expanding nitinol frame, it has three feelers to be placed in the native aortic cusps before deployment. Image used with permission of JenaValve Technology, Inc.

Mark indication for symptomatic, severe pure aortic regurgitation. A transfemoral concept has been presented.

The safety and efficacy of transapical implantation of the JenaValve® were evaluated in two multicenter, prospective trials [25]. In the first trial, 67 patients with severe aortic stenosis considered high-risk surgical candidates (mean age 83.1 ± 3.9 years, mean logistic EuroSCORE 28.4 ± 6.5%) underwent transapical implantation of the device. The procedural success rate was 89.6% (60/67 patients). Mortality at 30 days was 7.6%, and conversion to open heart surgery was required in four patients (6%). Stroke occurred in two patients (3%), and permanent pacemaker implantation was necessary in eight patients (12%). After the procedure, patients had a reduction in mean transvalvular gradient (40.6 ± 15.9 to 10.0 ± 7.2 mmHg) and an increase in valve area (0.7 ± 0.2 to 1.7 ± 0.6 cm², respectively). None of the treated patients had moderate to severe (>grade 2+) paravalvular aortic regurgitation. In the second trial, 31 patients with severe aortic regurgitation considered high-risk surgical candidates (mean age 73.8 ± 9.7 years, mean logistic EuroSCORE 23.6 ± 14.5%) underwent transapical implantation of the device [26]. The procedural success rate was 96.8% (30/31 patients). Mortality at 30 days was 12.9%, and no conversion to open heart surgery was required. No stroke occurred, and permanent pacemaker implantation was necessary in two patients (6.4%). After the procedure, mean transvalvular gradient was low (7.9 ± 4.0 mmHg), and none of the treated patients had moderate or worse paravalvular aortic regurgitation. More recently, clinical and valve performance results from a multicenter, prospective postmarket registry including both aortic stenosis and aortic regurgitation patients have been reported.

Conclusions

TAVI has become a feasible and effective therapeutic option for inoperable or high surgical risk patients with severe aortic stenosis. Despite the impressive and positive clinical results with the first-generation devices, there are many challenges to be addressed for further improvement in outcomes and, potentially, to expand the indications to lower risk patients. New valve technologies are characterized by repositionable and/or retrievable properties, lower profile, and innovative features designed to prevent complications such as paravalvular leaks, vascular complications, and conduction disturbances. Further studies are necessary to evaluate if the theoretical benefits of the second-generation valves will result in better clinical outcomes.

Interactive multiple choice questions are available for this chapter on www.wiley.com/go/dangas/cardiology

References

1 Cribier A, Eltchaninoff H, Bash A, *et al.* Percutaneous transcatheter implantation of an aortic valve prosthesis for calcific aortic stenosis: first human case description. *Circulation* 2002; **106**: 3006–3008.

2 Leon MB, Smith CR, Mack M, *et al.* Transcatheter aortic-valve implantation for aortic stenosis in patients who cannot undergo surgery. *N Engl J Med* 2010; **363**: 1597–1607.

3 Smith CR, Leon MB, Mack MJ, *et al.* Transcatheter versus surgical aortic-valve replacement in high-risk patients. *N Engl J Med* 2011; **364**: 2187–2198.

4 Adams DH, Popma JJ, Reardon MJ, *et al.* Transcatheter aortic-valve replacement with a self-expanding prosthesis. *N Engl J Med* 2014; **370**: 1790-1798.

5 Tchetche D, Van Mieghem NM. New-generation TAVI devices: description and specifications. *EuroIntervention* 2014; **10**: U90–U100.

6 Taramasso M, Pozzol A, Latib A, *et al.* New devices for TAVI: technologies and initial clinical experiences. *Nat Rev Cardiol* 2014; **11**: 157–167.

7 Binder RK, Rodés-Cabau J, Wood DA, *et al.* Transcatheter aortic valve replacement with the SAPIEN3: a new balloon-expandable transcatheter heart valve. *JACC Cardiovasc Interv* 2013; **6**(3): 293–300. doi:10.1016/j.jcin.2012.09.019.

8 Kodali SH. Clinical and echocardiographic outcomes at 30 days with the SAPIEN 3 TAVR system in inoperable, high-risk and intermediate-risk aortic stenosis patients. Presented at ACC Scientifc Sessions, March 2015. Available at: http://www.acc.org/about-acc/press-releases/2015/03/15/14/04/sapien-3-improves-30-day-outcomes-for-major-endpoints (accessed May 17, 2016).

9 Sinning JM, Werner N, Nickenig G, Grube E. Medtronic CoreValve Evolut R with EnVeo R. *EuroIntervention* 2013; **9**: S97–S100.

10 Meredith IT, Walton T, Brecker S, Pasupati S, Blackman D, Manoharan G. Early results from the CoreValve Evolut R Study. *J Am Coll Cardiol* 2015; **65**(10 S). doi:10.1016/S0735-1097(15)61782-X.

11 Meredith I, Hood K, Haratani N, Allocco D, Dawkins K. Boston Scientific Lotus valve. *EuroIntervention* 2012; **8**: Q70–Q74.

12 Buellesfeld L, Gerckens U, Grube E. Percutaneous implantation of the first repositionable aortic valve prosthesis in a patient with severe aortic stenosis. *Catheter Cardiovasc Interv* 2008; **71**: 579–584.

13 Meredith IT, Worthley SG, Whitbourn RJ, *et al.* Transfemoral aortic valve replacement with the repositionable Lotus Valve System in high surgical risk patients: the REPRISE I study. *EuroIntervention* 2013; **9**: 1264–1270.

14 Meredith IT, Walters DL, Dumonteil N, *et al.* Transcatheter aortic valve replacement for severe symptomatic aortic stenosis using a repositionable valve system: 30-day primary endpoint results from the REPRISE II Study. *J Am Coll Cardiol* 2014; **64**(13): 1339–1348. doi:10.1016/j.jacc.2014.05.067.

15 Mollmann H, Diemert P, Grube E, Baldus S, Kempfert J, Abizaid A. Symetis ACURATE TF aortic bioprosthesis. *EuroIntervention* 2013; **9**: S107–110.

16 Kempfert J, Holzhey D, Hofmann S, *et al.* First registry results from the newly approved ACURATE TA™ TAVI system. *Eur J Cardiothorac Surg* 2015; **48**: 137–141. doi:10.1093/ejcts/ezu367.

17 Schofer J, Colombo A, Klugmann S, *et al.* Prospective multicenter evaluation of the Direct Flow medical transcatheter aortic valve. *J Am Coll Cardiol* 2014; **63**(8): 763–768. doi:10.1016/j.jacc.2013.10.013.

18 Bijuklic K, Tuebler T, Reichenspurner H, *et al.* Midterm stability and hemodynamic performance of a transfemorally implantable nonmetallic, retrievable, and repositionable aortic valve in patients with severe aortic stenosis: up to 2-year follow-up of the direct-flow medical valve: a pilot study. *Circ Cardiovasc Interv* 2011; **4**: 595–601.

19 Sündermann SH, Holzhey D, Bleiziffer S, Treede H, Falk V. Medtronic Engager™ bioprosthesis for transapical transcatheter aortic valve implantation. *Eurointervention* 2013; **9**: S97–S100.

20 Holzhey D, Linke A, Treede H, *et al.* Intermediate follow-up results from the multicenter Engager European pivotal trial. *Ann Thorac Surg* 2013; **96**(6): 2095–100. doi: 10.1016/j.athoracsur.2013.06.089. Epub 2013 Sep 7.

21 Manoharan G, Spence M, Rodés-Cabau J, Webb J. St Jude Medical Portico valve. *EuroIntervention* 2012; **8**: Q97–Q101.

22 Willson AB, Rodès-Cabau J, Wood DA, *et al.* Transcatheter aortic valve replacement with the St. Jude Medical Portico valve: first-in-human experience. *J Am Coll Cardiol* 2012; **60**(7): 581–586. doi:10.1016/j.jacc.2012.02.045.

23 Cheung A, Makkar R, Fontana GP. St. Jude Medical Portico™ transapical technology. *EuroIntervention* 2013; **9**: S101–S102.

24 Rudolph T, Baldus S, Cheung A, Fontana G. JenaValve: transfemoral technology. *EuroIntervention* 2013; **9**: S103–S106.

25 Treede H, Mohr FW, Baldus S, *et al.* Transapical transcatheter aortic valve implantation using the JenaValveTM system: acute and 30-day results of the multicentre CE-mark study. *Eur J Cardiothorac Surg* 2012; **41**: e131–e138.

26 Seiffert M, Bader R, Kappert U, *et al.* Initial German experience with transapical implantation of a second-generation transcatheter heart valve for the treatment of aortic regurgitation. *J Am Coll Cardiol Cardiovasc Interv* 2014; **7**: 1168–1177.

CHAPTER 62

Transseptal Puncture

Alec Vahanian, Dominique Himbert, Fabrice Extramiana, Gregory Ducrocq, and Eric Brochet

Hôpital Bichat-Claude Bernard, Paris, France

Transseptal catheterization (TS) remains an integral yet specialized technique for interventional cardiologists and electrophysiologists. It was introduced in the late 1950s [1]. Initially seldom used, mostly because of lack of experience and trepidation, this relatively complex technique has had a revival with the introduction of new percutaneous electrophysiologic and structural, especially valvular, interventions (Box 62.1) [2–8].

This chapter describes the technical aspects of the procedure, including guidance by imaging, then addresses the specific aspects related to specific interventions performed for which TS is the first step.

Training

The presence of a learning curve has been well described [2,3]. Thus, training in transseptal catheterizations involves the acquisition of specialist skills [9]. However, currently there are no specific data regarding the minimum numbers needed for initial training and maintenance of competency.

Physicians performing transseptal catheterization must have a good knowledge of the pathoanatomy of the heart, hemodynamics, and echocardiography. Interventionists must be able to recognize and manage complications such as tamponade and stroke. Training in transseptal catheterization is expected to derive benefit from simulator training before clinical training during specific courses on the technique [10].

Echocardiographic guidance

Echocardiographic examination performed before TS catheterization must carefully look for abnormalities of the interatrial septum such as very thick septum, calcifications, aneurysmal deformation, and presence of a patent foramen ovale, which should be taken into account when performing the procedure. In addition, the presence of even mild to moderate pericardial effusion should be described in the echocardiography report in order to serve as a comparator if hemopericardium is suspected during the procedure.

The goal of the guidance of TS puncture is to puncture the fossa ovalis which is composed mainly of thin and fibrous tissue and is the easiest and safest part of the septum for a standard puncture. In valve disease, the position of the fossa ovalis can be altered because, when the LA is enlarged, the fossa ovalis tends to be displaced inferiorly.

Both transesophageal echocardiography (TEE) and intracardiac echocardiography (ICE) provide excellent imaging of the interatrial septum, which is useful to guide the orientation of the catheter and needle in the fossa ovale, to show proper positioning and tenting of the septum, and monitor the crossing of the septum. Drawbacks of echocardiographic guidance are the need for anesthesia, or at least analgesia, in most patients when TEE is performed; the cost of the devices and the need for a second femoral access are the drawbacks for ICE. The recent introduction of real time 3D TEE further improves imaging of the septum [11,12].

During electrophysiologic interventions or percutaneous mitral balloon commissurotomy, in experienced teams, echocardiographic guidance, using either TEE or ICE, is restricted to patients in whom there are anticipated difficulties, such as severe thoracic deformity, or when unexpected difficulties occur. ICE is widely used in the USA as demonstrated by the fact that approximately 50% of the experts involved in the 2007 consensus statement on atrial fibrillation ablation routinely used ICE to facilitate the transseptal procedure or to guide catheter ablation [18]. TEE guidance is mandatory for the technical steps needed after transseptal catheterization in most structural interventions and is therefore systematically used in such procedures. It is also a useful adjunct in the early part of the operator's experience. Effective echocardiographic guidance requires specialized training for the echocardiographer, without which may result in a false impression of security. Finally, successful echocardiographic guidance requires good understanding and collaboration between the interventionist and the echocardiographist, as well as the use of similar definitions, to optimize the performance of the procedure.

Transthoracic echocardiographic (TTE) guidance is seldom used because it is difficult to perform at the same time as fluoroscopic imaging. However, it could be helpful in experienced hands.

Interventional Cardiology: Principles and Practice, Second Edition. Edited by George D. Dangas, Carlo Di Mario, and Nicholas N. Kipshidze.
© 2017 John Wiley & Sons, Ltd. Published 2017 by John Wiley & Sons, Ltd.

Finally, isolated case reports have described the feasibility of transseptal puncture on echocardiographic guidance alone, without fluoroscopy, in emergency cases [13]. However, this approach cannot be recommended at the present time.

Equipment

The Brockenbrough needle is the most commonly used transseptal needle, which is 70 cm long, has a curved tip, and tapers distally. A hub arrow on the proximal part indicates the direction of the needle. The stylet inside the needle should be removed before use [14].

The most commonly used catheters comprise a dilator and a sheath, and are 8 Fr [15]. This allows the introduction of another catheter, such as a floating balloon, in the left atrium (LA) after penetration and withdrawal of the dilator (Figure 62.1). A variety of dilator shapes are available in order to adapt to the requirements of the procedure. The most commonly used are the Mullins sheath or the St. Jude SL 0 or SL 1 sheaths. The conventional Mullins sheath is advised when aiming to cross the mitral valve using another catheter. The St. Jude type devices are advisable when catheterization of the superior pulmonary vein is planned for mitral clip or left atrial appendage closure, for example (Figure 62.2).

Before performing transseptal catheterization, it is necessary to carefully check: (i) that the proximal arrow is aligned with the needle tip, and (ii) to measure the distance (in fingers) between the proximal part of the catheter and the proximal arrow when the tip of the needle is advanced to lie just inside the dilator to avoid inadvertent puncture during manipulation (Figure 62.3).

Procedure

Before starting the procedure, the patient must be lying flat for better anatomic landmarks. This could be difficult in emergency cases such as pulmonary edema, which requires a semi-supine position. In such cases, the procedure should only be performed by an experienced operator.

A 5 Fr pigtail should be positioned retrogradely from the femoral artery to the right aortic coronary sinus for identification of the aorta and systemic pressure monitoring. However, left heart catheterization can be omitted by experienced operators, but is useful otherwise when only fluoroscopic guidance is used.

Percutaneous venous access is via a puncture of the right femoral vein as this offers a direct approach from the inferior vena cava

Box 62.1 Indications for transseptal puncture during interventional procedures

Structural interventions:
- Percutaneous mitral balloon commissurotomy
- Percutaneous edge-to-edge mitral repair
- Antegrade aortic balloon valvuloplasty
- Transcatheter aortic valve implantation
- Patent foramen ovale closure
- Percutaneous occlusion of the left atrial appendage
Electrophysiologic studies and catheter ablation:
- Left-sided accessory pathways
- Pulmonary vein ablation for paroxysmal atrial fibrillation
- Left atrial tachycardia
- Atypical left atrial flutters
- Left ventricular tachycardia
Circulatory support:
- Percutaneous left ventricular assist device

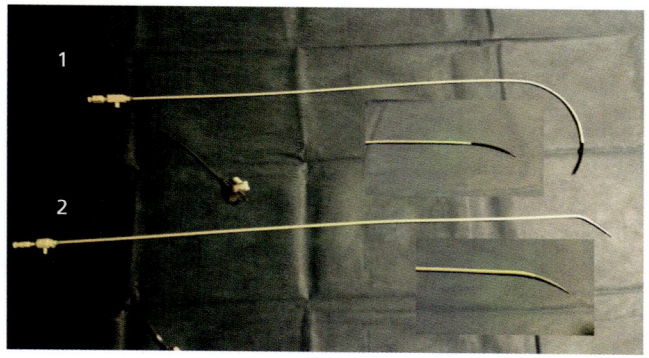

Figure 62.2 Different shapes of dilator and sheaths used for transseptal catheterization. 1. This curved shape enables catheterization of the left ventricle afterward through the mitral valve. 2. The straighter shape facilitates the catheterization of the upper pulmonary vein, which is useful during MitraClip or left atrial occlusion procedures.

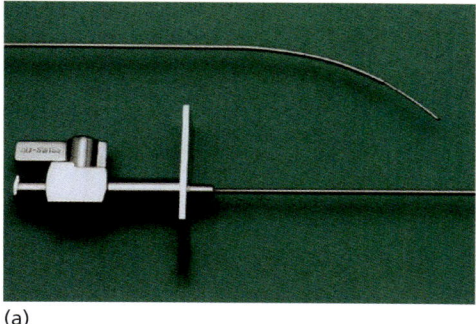

(a)

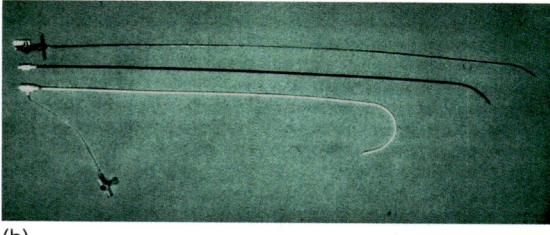

(b)

Figure 62.1 Equipment. (a) The needle: proximal tip with an arrow and a tap; distal tip which is tapered. (b) Transseptal needle, alongside the Mullins dilator and sheath.

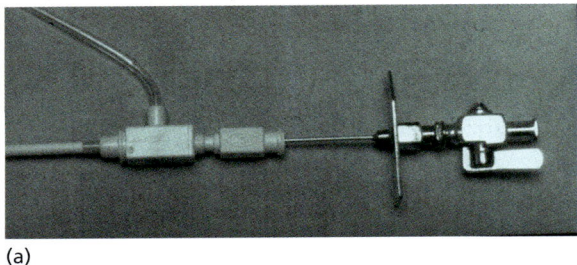

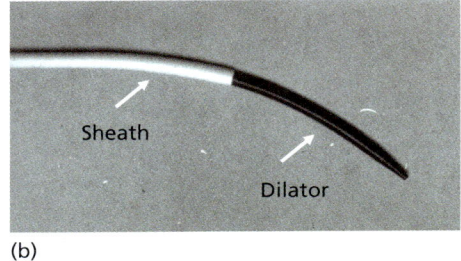

(a)   (b)

Figure 62.3 Measurements of the landmarks between needle and catheter. Measurement of the distance between the proximal of the needle arrow and the proximal part of the catheter (a) necessary to position the needle just inside the catheter (b).

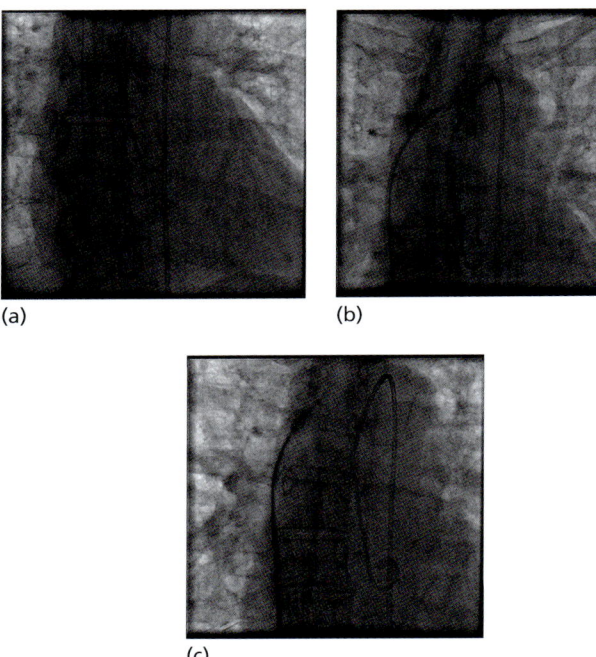

(a)   (b)

(c)

Figure 62.4 Procedure I: Positioning in antero-posterior view. (a) Pigtail catheter placed on the aortic cusps. The dilator is advanced into the superior vena cava. (b) The guidewire is removed. (c) The needle is advanced through the dilator. Courtesy of Professor A. Cribier.

to the interatrial septum at the fossa ovalis. If right access is not possible, left femoral access can be attempted but this renders the procedure more difficult, and can be painful for the patient and lead to a vagal reaction. In very rare cases, transseptal catheterization has been performed using a transjugular or transhepatic approach [16].

A 0.032–0.035-inch J-tipped guidewire is advanced into the superior vena cava, up to the origin of the left innominate vein, in anteroposterior view. It is important to avoid forcing the guidewire into the right atrial appendage, as this is a fragile structure. The catheter is advanced over the guidewire into the superior vena cava and the guidewire is removed (Figure 62.4).

The Brockenbrough needle is connected to a pressure line, which is continuously flushed, and inserted into the dilator just inside the distal end under fluoroscopic guidance and using the predetermined measurement. The needle is allowed to rotate freely while being advanced. If resistance is felt, the proximal hub arrow should be gently rotated until the needle can be advanced without resistance. In the very rare cases where difficulties persist, it could be helpful to push the needle over a 0.0014 angioplasty guidewire. This latter modification seems more useful than the stylet provided with the needle.

When the needle reaches the desired position inside the catheter the flush is stopped and pressure is continuously monitored. From then on, it is necessary to hold the needle and the catheter firmly and to move them as a unit. Initially, the tip of the catheter is orientated toward the right shoulder of the patient in anteroposterior view. Then, under continuous fluoroscopic and pressure monitoring, both the catheter and needle are withdrawn downward and rotated counterclockwise until contact with the septum is felt.

Other techniques initially orientate the catheter toward the left shoulder (innominate vein) and perform a clockwise rotation. In such cases, when the system is withdrawn three sequential bumps can be felt representing (i) the right atrium–superior vena cava junction; (ii) movement over the ascending aorta of which pulsations can be felt; and (iii) the passage over the limbus to enter the fossa ovalis. Whatever method is used, the proximal arrow and the tip of the needle have a posteromedial position of 4–6 o'clock, looking from bottom to top in anteroposterior view (Figure 62.5). The angle is chosen according to the size of the LA (4 o'clock in normal size; up to 6 o'clock in a large atrium).

The selection of an adequate puncture site varies according to the imaging modality used for its guidance. If the procedure is fluoroscopy guided, in anteroposterior view, the correct position of the tip of the needle is usually mid-way between the pigtail and the right atrial border in the horizontal axis and slightly below the horizontal line at the level of the pigtail. It is recommended that a complementary view is used to provide further information on the orientation of the needle in the anteroposterior axis before puncturing the septum (Figures 62.6 and 62.7). This could be a lateral view with a target zone at the mid-part of the line between the pigtail and the spina, or right anterior oblique 30° with a target zone vertically in the middle of the line between the pigtail and the spina and below a horizontal line at the level of the pigtail. With both methods, the puncture site is posterior and inferior to the aortic plane.

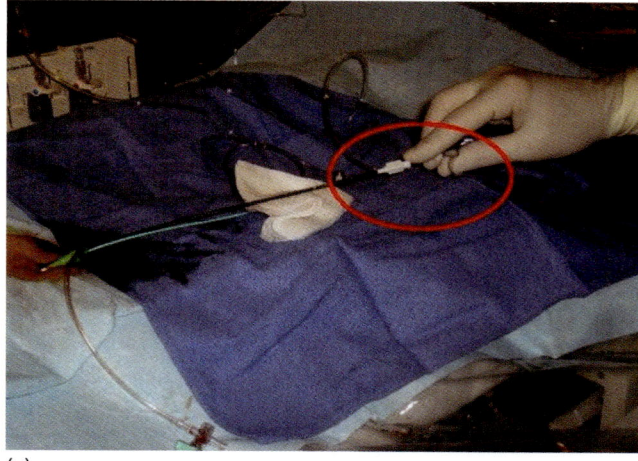

(a)

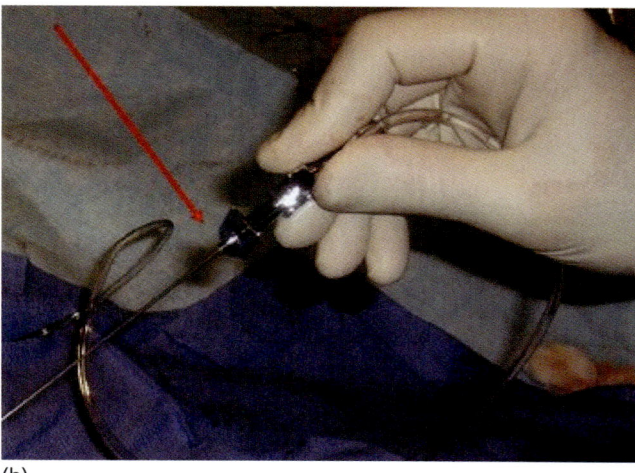

(b)

Figure 62.5 Procedure II: Positioning of the needle. (a) The catheter and the needle are moved as a unit, keeping in mind the predetermined distance necessary to avoid protrusion of the needle out of the catheter. (b) The needle is rotated so that the arrow is oriented to 5 o'clock (red arrow).

If the TS is guided by echocardiography (Figure 62.8), three two-dimensional TEE planes are sequentially used to define the preferred puncture site precisely [11]:

1 Short axis view at the base (30–50°) which allows for anterior–posterior orientation;

2 Long axis view (bicaval) at 90–120° which allows for superior–inferior orientation;

3 Four-chamber view (0°) is used to determine the correct height above the mitral valve which is mandatory when performing the MitraClip and other mitral procedures.

The position of the TS needle can be identified by a tent-like doming of the interatrial septum toward the LA (tenting; Figure 62.9). Successful crossing of the septum is confirmed by the abrupt loss of tenting. Thee-dimensional X-plane imaging facilitates the TS puncture by presenting a short and a long axis view simultaneously, thus providing anteroposterior and superior–inferior orientation in a single view.

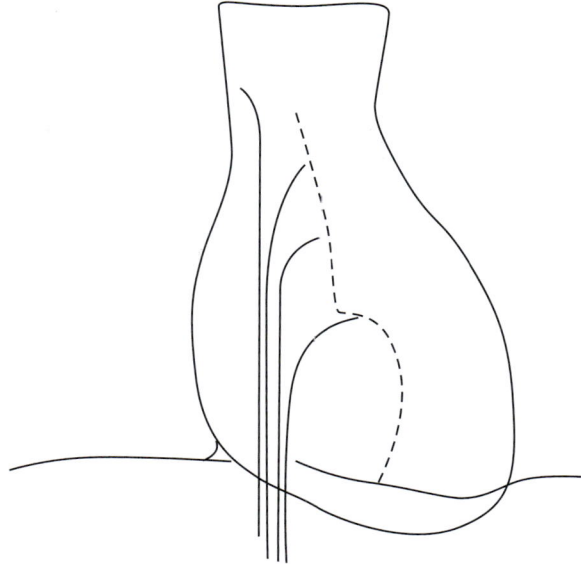

Figure 62.6 Procedure III: Reaching the fossa ovale. The catheter and needle are moved downward to the fossa ovale. Courtesy of Dr. S. Shaw.

When using ICE imaging, tenting of the interatrial septum should be identified in the long axis view and clear visualization of the point of maximal tenting should be obtained before puncturing. Relationship with the aortic root can be obtained by counterclockwise rotation of the ICE catheter. Confirmation of the location of the ICE catheter in the LA can be obtained by injection of non-agitated saline or contrast during ICE imaging or the presence of a left-to-right shunt with color Doppler. In addition to visual guidance, it is important to feel a sensation of more or less elastic resistance through the catheter, which happens in most cases.

If the previous stage is successfully performed, the catheter may pass into the LA without puncture by the needle which is shown by the LA pressure recording. This can occur in cases with patent foramen ovale but also in its absence [17]. If this is the case, the catheter and the needle are gently pushed without resistance and the needle is withdrawn.

However, in most cases it is necessary to puncture the septum. The needle is gently advanced. Entry into the LA is indicated by changes in pressure tracing. If no changes are perceived this can be a result of:

1 Problems with pressure recording, or problems with the permeability of the needle. In the latter case, as opposed to forceful flushing, it is recommended to gently aspirate blood, which will be red if the needle is in the LA.

2 If the position seems adequate, but there is still resistance to penetration, it may be because of a thick or fibrous septum, especially in children or in patients with previous cardiac surgery, or a "receding septum" feeling, which can be because of an aneurysm of the septum requiring the application of additional pressure.

3 Incorrect positioning which requires re-puncture at another site. In such cases, the catheter and needle should not be re-advanced upward, and the maneuver should be restarted.

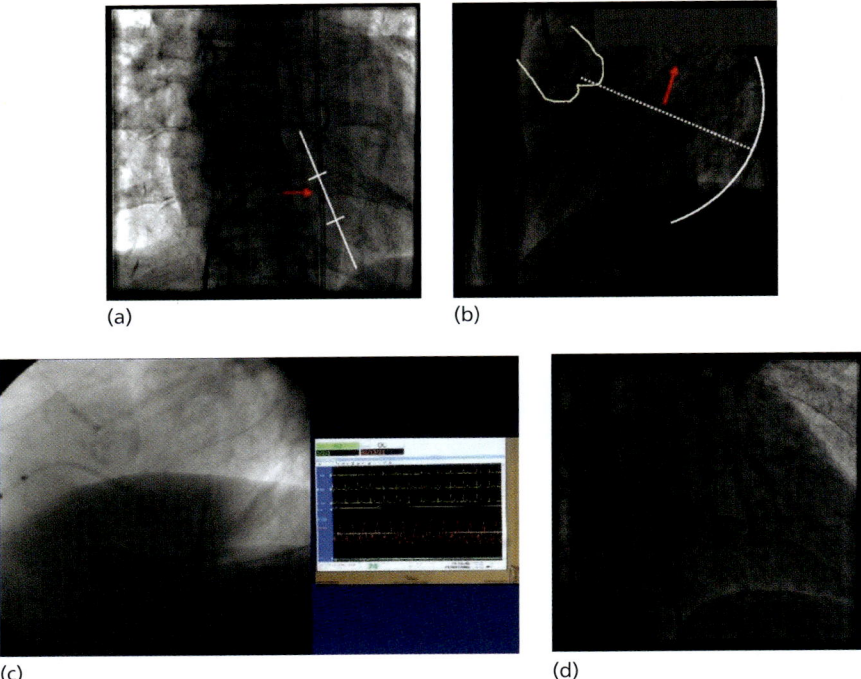

(a) (b)

(c) (d)

Figure 62.7 Procedure IV: Transseptal puncture. (a) Antero-posterior view. The catheter and needle are at the level of the fossa ovale, below and lateral to the pigtail. (b) Lateral view. The catheter and needle are below and posterior to the pigtail catheter. (c) The needle is advanced and left atrial pressure is obtained. Courtesy of Professor A. Cribier. (d) The position of the puncture in right anterior oblique 30° is also inferior and posterior to the aortic cusps.

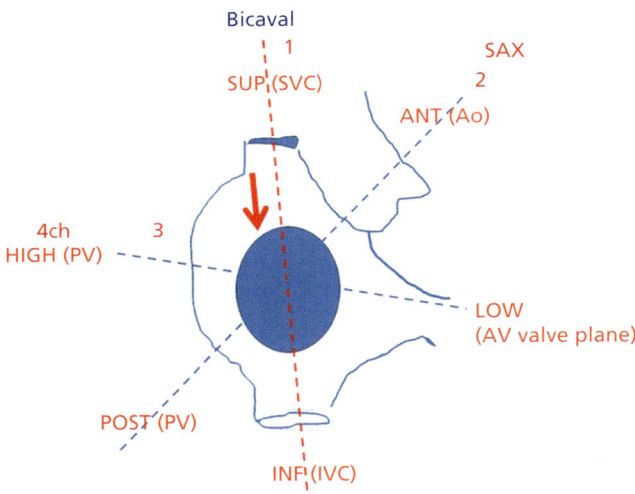

Figure 62.8 Guidance of transseptal puncture by echocardiography. Transesophageal echocardiographic views. 1: Bicaval view shows the position: superior directed toward the superior vena cava versus inferior toward the inferior vena cava. 2: Short axis view: anterior directed toward the aorta versus posterior. 3: Four-chamber view: low, close to the atrioventricular plane versus high at a distance.

The entire system is withdrawn into the inferior vena cava, the needle is withdrawn, and the J-tipped guidewire is advanced through the catheter and repositioned in the superior vena cava. The catheter should be advanced into the LA only when assurance is obtained that the needle has crossed the septum.

Before advancing the catheter it is recommended to return to the anteroposterior view, which provides a better view of the borders of the LA, to avoid damage to the neighboring structures (i.e., LA wall, left atrial appendage, or pulmonary veins when using fluoroscopic guidance only).

Before moving forward it is necessary to be sure that the X-ray table is fixed and will not move during the following maneuvers. It is now even more important to move the needle and the catheter as a unit because the needle is protruding into the LA. Continuous pressure is applied with the right hand at the proximal part of the needle while the left hand holds the catheter at the groin and provides counter-resistance if necessary.

When both the needle and the catheter have crossed the septum, the needle is withdrawn. The LA pressure is then recorded. It is necessary to ensure that both the needle and the catheter have crossed the septum before removing the needle because too early removal of the needle can lead to backward movement of the catheter into the RA. When using a dilator and a sheath after crossing of the septum, the needle is withdrawn into the dilator. The dilator and the sheath are then advanced into the LA. The needle and the dilator are removed and the sheath is carefully flushed before connection to the pressure line.

Heparin, usually with a target activated clotting time (ACT) of 250–300 s, is given when the catheter is securely positioned in the LA.

Specificities in transseptal puncture
Anatomic variations
Large right or left atrium
In patients with enlarged atrial cavities the ideal puncture site is slightly below this line but not too posteriorly. It should be stressed

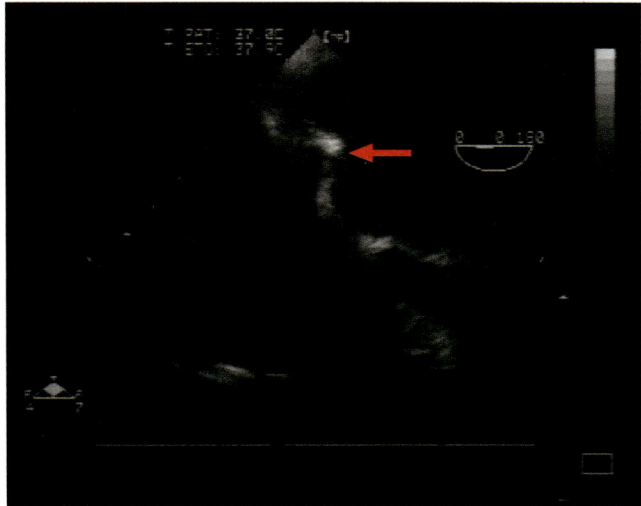

(a)

(b)

Figure 62.9 Transesophageal echocardiography showing the tenting of the interatrial septum during the septal puncture. (a) 2D echo; (b) 3D echo.

that a too posterior puncture, outside the boarders of the fossa ovale, should be avoided in order to avoid a perforation into the pericardial space between the two atria. In such cases, the convexity of the septum as a result of LA enlargement can cause catheter slippage and, thus, can impede adequate contact with the septum. In addition, in patients with severely enlarged RA it is useful to slightly bend the needle at 10 cm from the tip to facilitate contact with the septum.

Resistant septum

This can occur in re-do interventions [18], either after cardiac surgery or multiple electrophysiologic interventions or in older patients, after thoracic radiation. If resistance to crossing the septum with the needle occurs, pressure must be continuously applied until crossing has been achieved. If crossing is still not possible, it may be useful to introduce an inverted exchange angioplasty 0.014 guidewire into the needle [19]. A more sophisticated variant is the SafeSept® wire (Pressure Products, San Pedro, CA, USA) where a 0.014 coronary guidewire is advanced through the TS needle lumen

and as soon as the wire enters the LA it takes a J shape to avoid damaging the LA wall [20]. Recent alternatives have been developed using radiofrequency, which does not require mechanical force [21,22]; this can be carried out using dedicated catheters such as the Baylis (Baylis Medical, Montreal, Canada). However, radiofrequency can also be used by a standard electrosurgical cautery generator via the TS needle, brief pulses being applied to the hub of the TS needle by direct contact [23].

If the needle can cross but not the catheter, it may be useful to introduce an exchange angioplasty 0.018 guidewire into the needle (Steelcore, Abbott Vascular) up to the superior pulmonary vein and use it as support for both the needle and the catheter. If this maneuver fails, an exchange angioplasty 0.014 guidewire can be introduced into the needle, to withdraw both the needle and the catheter and insert an angioplasty balloon (2 mm) to dilate the septum before re-advancing the transseptal catheter over this guidewire [24]. This latter technique is difficult and not always successful. Finally, it can be necessary to re-do the puncture at another site, as the first attempt was likely not at the fossa but at a thicker part of the septum.

Subsequent interventional procedure
Percutaneous mitral commissurotomy

When performing the Inoue technique the preferred site for the transseptal puncture is usually in the lower part of the fossa ovale if the LA is severely enlarged. However, if crossing the mitral valve is not possible using this puncture location, it can be necessary to re-do the transseptal puncture in a slightly higher position and more posteriorly [5].

Percutaneous mitral valve repair or replacement

The most common mitral valve repair technique used today is the edge-to-edge technique using the MitraClip. The transseptal puncture is performed under echocardiographic guidance, which is subsequently necessary for the performance of the procedure [25]. The determination of the optimal puncture site is of major importance for a MitraClip procedure.

The puncture must be performed in the superior–posterior part of the fossa ovalis and at an adequate distance from the mitral valve (Figure 62.10). The optimal height above the mitral valve differs for primary and secondary mitral regurgitation (MR). In cases with primary MR the puncture site should be 4–5 cm above the mitral annulus, thus providing enough space to maneuver the delivery system adequately within the LA. In patients with secondary MR, important valve tethering results most often in a shift in position of the line of coaptation to below the mitral annulus. Subsequently, TS puncture needs to be lower, approximately 3.5 cm above the annular plane or 4–4.5 cm above the coaptation of both leaflets in order to be able to advance the catheter more deeply into the LA.

An inadequate puncture site will lead to the following complications: aortic hugging if the puncture is too anterior, for example through a patent foramen ovale; inability to cross the mitral valve in a too high puncture; inability to pull back the clip and tether the leaflets after a too low puncture; and, finally, risk of perforation if the puncture is too posterior.

The stability of the position of the needle should be carefully checked before pushing the sheath over the needle. For this purpose the use of radiofrequency energy could be a useful adjunct by avoiding the potential slippage of the needle while applying force to cross the septum.

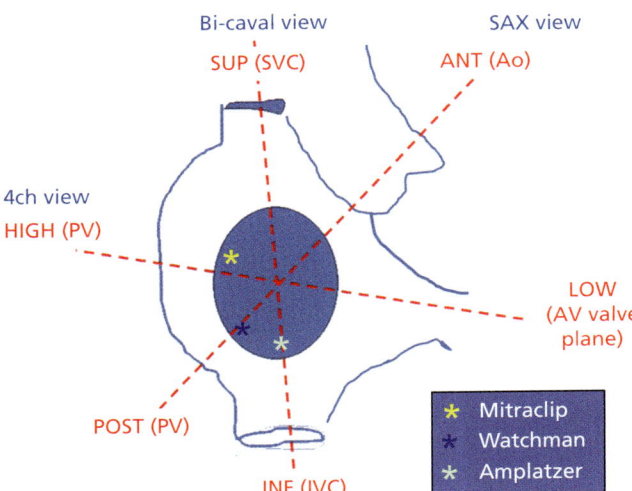

Figure 62.10 Optimal location of the transseptal puncture site in selected structural interventions: Mitraclip, left atrial occlusion using the Watchman or Amplatzer devices. Ant, anterior; Ao, aorta; AV, aortic valve; IVC, inferior vena cava; PV, pulmonary veins; 4 ch, four-chamber view; SAX, short axis view.

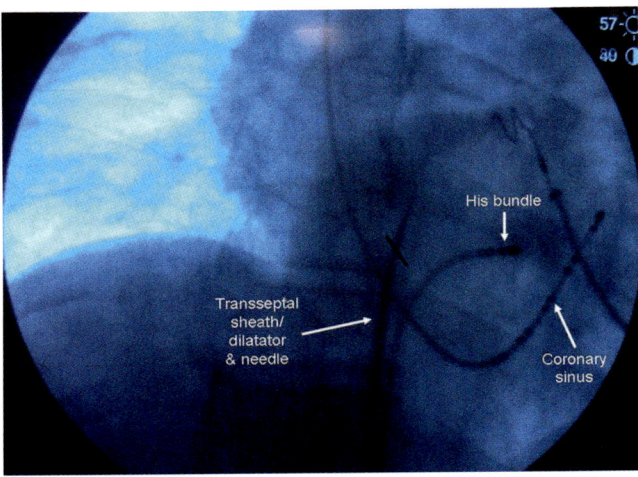

Figure 62.11 Transseptal catheterization in electrophysiologic interventions: electrophysiology and ablation catheters as landmarks. Catheter position during the transseptal puncture. RAO 30° view. The black line indicates the position of the fossa ovalis.

There are no precise recommendations concerning the transseptal technique for other mitral interventions such as "valve-in-a-valve" or "valve-in-a-ring" or direct annuloplasty because the number of cases performed is still limited [8,26]. As a general rule, the TS puncture for these procedures shares most of the characteristics of that used for the MitraClip technique (i.e., a superior and posterior puncture in order to allow for sufficient maneuverability in the LA and crossing of the mitral valve).

Left atrial appendage closure

Transseptal puncture is also the first step of the percutaneous left atrial closure techniques. Here again the location of the transseptal puncture is important and somewhat dependent on the particular characteristics of the device to be implanted in order to facilitate coaxial alignment and reduce the risk of complications such as tamponade or embolization. When using the Watchman device, the ideal location is in the middle portion of the posterior fossa which allows a coaxial engagement of the appendage. The TS puncture is ideally slightly more anterior and inferior with the Amplatzer device (Figure 62.10).

Patent foramen ovale closure

The presence of a long funnel-shaped patent foramen ovale is challenging for the placement of most closure devices. A TS puncture of the most cephalad aspect of the septum primum at the level of the fossa ovalis allows placement of the device which can then "sandwich" both the septum primum and secundum and effectively close the tunnel [27].

Electrophysiology

Interventional electrophysiologists have used TS since the 1980s as an alternative or complementary approach to the retro-aortic route to ablate left-sided accessory pathways. However, the spread of the technique in the electrophysiology laboratory has followed the development of left atrial ablation to treat atrial fibrillation.

The techniques of TS have similarities whether used in the electrophysiology laboratory or in the hemodynamic or structural intervention laboratory but some specific features deserve to be emphasized [3,4,18,22,28–31]. Specific features of TS in the electrophysiology laboratory include the following.

1 *Electrophysiology and ablation catheters as landmarks* The position of the His bundle indicates the level of the most inferior aspect of the non-coronary cusp. The catheter placed in the coronary sinus provides information on coronary sinus ostium location as well as on the position of the lower portion of the mitral annulus. On a 30° right anterior oblique view, the fossa ovalis is located midway between the His bundle and the right atrial posterior wall on the anterior–posterior axis and below or at the level of the His bundle on the superior–inferior axis (Figure 62.11).

2 *The double transseptal technique* In most cases, more than one catheter is used for left atrial ablation. This is done using either a double TS puncture or a single puncture. In the former, a guidewire is placed in the left superior pulmonary vein through the first sheath and dilator which are then pulled back into the right atria. Next, the ablation catheter (through a second sheath) is positioned (under fluoroscopy and/or TEE or ICE) in the fossa ovalis and pushed into the left atria following the guidewire direction. Finally, the first sheath and dilator are pushed over the wire into the LA (Figure 62.12). An alternative method for the double transseptal technique with a single puncture has also been described [32].

3 Resistant septum in cases of re-do procedure and thrombotic issues have been addressed earlier.

Circulatory support

Transseptal catheterization can also be used during percutaneous left ventricular assist device implantation.

The Tandem Heart (Cardiac Assist Technologies Inc., Pittsburg, PA, USA) is a transseptal left atrial to femoral arterial assist device that provides left heart bypass designed for short-term circulatory support. The inflow transseptal cannula is a 21 Fr polyurethane catheter with a large end hole and 14 side holes to facilitate left atrial decompression [33].

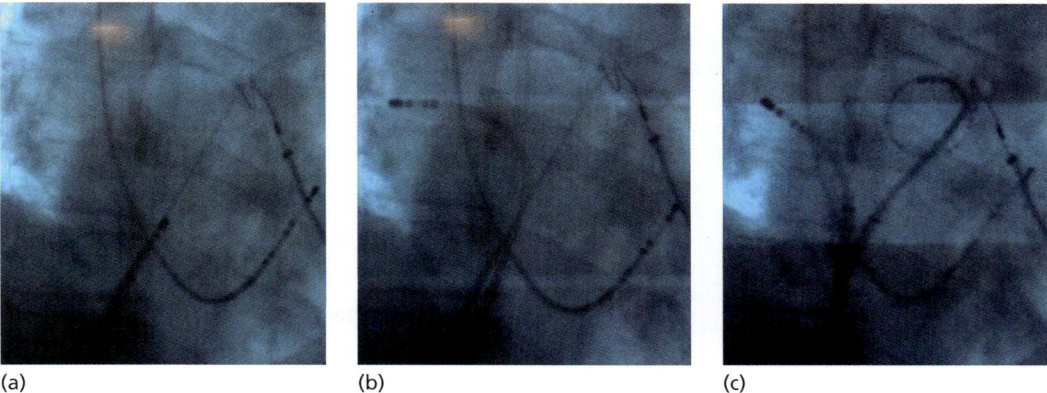

(a)   (b)   (c)

Figure 62.12 Transseptal catheterization in electrophysiologic interventions: the double transseptal technique. (a) Guidewire in the left superior pulmonary vein and ablation catheter on the right side of the transseptal puncture. (b) Guidewire in the left superior pulmonary and ablation catheter in the right superior pulmonary vein. (c) Ablation catheter in the right superior pulmonary vein and lasso catheter at the ostium of the left superior pulmonary vein.

Table 62.1 Complications of transseptal catheterization.

	n	Death (%)	Tamponade (%)	Embolism (%)
Roelke *et al.* [2]	1279	0.08	1.2	0.08
Fagundes *et al.* [30]	1150	0	1	0.4
De Ponti *et al.* [3]	5520	0.008	0.1	0.008
Michowitz *et al.* [31]*	34,943	0.8	0.08†	NA

* Catheter ablation of atrial fibrillation.
† Related to transseptal puncture.

Transseptal catheterization can also be used to unload the LA in patients with persisting pulmonary edema after implantation of a femoro-femoral Extra-Corporeal Membrane Oxygenator.

Complications

Although generally safe, transseptal catheterization is associated with an incidence of complications, albeit low, if performed carefully following the rules described earlier (Table 62.1) [2,3,30,31,34–37]. The failure rate is usually 1–2% and fatality is the exception.

Heart perforation related to transseptal puncture concerns the free wall of the RA, LA, left atrial appendage, or a puncture going from the RA to the LA via the pericardium, or the aorta. It mostly occurs when the operator is less experienced. Unfavorable patient characteristics such as severe atrial enlargement or thoracic deformity also increase risk. Perforation of the heart can result in mild pericardial effusion without clinical consequences, but hemopericardium usually has immediate clinical consequences resulting in tamponade. Its incidence is around 1% but can be as high as 4% in centers with limited experience. It should always be suspected as a potential cause when hypotension occurs during transseptal catheterization. The potential consequences of this complication necessitate the immediate availability of echocardiography whenever transseptal catheterization is performed.

Puncture of the aorta by the needle only is usually without consequences when it is recognized immediately by pressure monitoring. It requires close monitoring and avoidance of heparin administration. On the other hand, advancement of the catheter in such cases can lead to massive hemopericardium. If hemopericardium is suspected, echocardiography should be performed urgently before deterioration occurs. Hemopericardium requires immediate pericardiocentesis, ideally performed under echocardiographic guidance after reversal of anticoagulation if already given. In most cases, hemopericardium from transseptal catheterization can be managed by pericardiocentesis, especially when it results from a puncture by the transseptal needle only. If this is successful, the planned procedure can then be continued but the patient should be closely monitored.

Embolism can be caused by a pre-existing thrombus, usually in the left atrial appendage, or one developed during the procedure. The TS puncture in itself is seldom responsible for this complication which is mostly related to the lengthy procedures performed afterwards [38]. Cerebral embolism usually results in stroke. Less frequently, coronary embolism leads to transient ST segment elevation. The treatment of cerebral embolism should be in collaboration with a stroke center. Cerebral imaging should be performed on an emergency basis to rule out hemorrhage, then intra-arterial fibrinolytic therapy should be administered early in the absence of contraindications.

In the case of persistent ST segment elevation, coronary angiography should be performed. ST segment elevation in the inferior leads accompanied by diaphoresis, hypotension, and chest discomfort with normal coronary angiogram has been occasionally observed after transseptal catheterization as is also the case after other intracardiac manipulations. They can be neutrally mediated as a Bezold–Jarish-like reflex and are responsive to atropine [37]. In the very rare cases where a coronary occlusion is present, coronary angioplasty can be performed, while thrombo-aspiration could be an appealing alternative. Inferior vena cava perforation and retroperitoneal hematoma could be the consequences of pushing the needle extruded from the catheter during its positioning in the vena cava.

Atrial tachyarrhythmias are possible but are rare and usually transient. Persistent interatrial shunts are not observed after the performance of transseptal catheterization in isolation.

Contraindications

To avoid these complications, any of the following contraindications must be eliminated. The performance of TEE is recommended in the days just preceding transseptal catheterization to disclose left atrial thrombosis as the technique is contraindicated in patients with a thrombus floating in the LA cavity or on the atrial septum. No consensus has been reached regarding patients with thrombosis in the LA appendage. In such cases, TS can only be indicated in patients who are candidates for urgent intervention but not surgery, or if intervention is not required urgently and when oral anticoagulation can be given for at least 2 months, and new TEE shows the thrombus has disappeared. LA myxoma also constitutes a contraindication.

TS should not be performed in patients with bleeding disorders, especially caused by too high anticoagulation (INR >1.5), in particular in patients who have not undergone previous cardiac operation. When intravenous heparin is used, it should be discontinued 4 hours before and can be restarted 2 hours after the procedure. This rule has been recently challenged in two circumstances where the risk of thrombosis resulting from the withdrawal of anticoagulation in lengthy procedures was felt to be superior to that of bleeding: (i) in MitraClip implantation when it is performed by experienced operators under TEE it is possible to perform TS with an INR >2 [39]; (ii) the same opinion is shared by electrophysiologists planning TS before atrial fibrillation (AF) ablation because of the long duration of the procedure, the presence of AF, and the thrombotic effect of radiofrequency lesion, clotting in the left atria and/or on the TS sheath and ensuing stroke are always feared. Hence, most echocardiography centers now perform TS and catheter ablation of AF without warfarin discontinuation and with heparin on top of vitamin K antagonists, which reduces the occurrence of peri-procedural stroke and minor bleeding complications. During AF ablation procedures, heparin is administered prior to or immediately following TS and adjusted to achieve an ACT of 300–400 s throughout the procedure [28,38].

Thoracic deformity, such as cyphoscoliosis, is a contraindication if severe. In practice, the level of acceptable deformity depends on operator experience and the availability of echocardiographic guidance.

Complex congenital diseases are also considered contraindicative because of the altered anatomic landmarks.

Transseptal catheterization can be performed in dextrocardia by experienced operators using left femoral access, inversion of the X-ray image, and echocardiographic guidance [40].

Obstruction of the vena cava is a classic contraindication for femoral access but membranous obstruction of the vena cava can be dilated. The presence of a filter in the vena cava is not an absolute contraindication if it is permeable.

Another contraindication is agenesis of the vena cava associated with azygos return. This latter condition should be diagnosed by X-ray before the procedure or, if during the procedure the catheter has an unusually posterior position behind the heart, confirmed by venous angiography in the RA [41]. In such circumstances TS can be performed using a transjugular approach if absolutely necessary.

Presence of an interatrial patch [24], or even atrial septal occluder [42], is not an absolute contraindication but may render the crossing of the interatrial septum difficult.

Conclusions

Transseptal catheterization has had a revival since it is the first step for several structural interventions as well as in interventional electrophysiology. Imaging guidance by echocardiography has considerably eased the performance of the procedure. However, it remains a demanding procedure and requires specific expertise. A stepwise and cautious technique is the key to limiting complications. It is hoped that further refinements in the technique will result from the evaluation of new technologies and better guidance by multi-imaging modalities.

Interactive multiple choice questions are available for this chapter on www.wiley. com/go/dangas/cardiology

References

1 Ross J Jr, Braunwald E, Morrow AG. Transseptal left atrial puncture; new technique for the measurement of left atrial pressure in man. *Am J Cardiol* 1959; **3**: 653–655.

2 Roelke M, Smith AJ, Palacios IF. The technique and safety of transseptal left heart catheterization: the Massachusetts General Hospital experience with 1,279 procedures. *Cathet Cardiovasc Diagn* 1994; **32**: 332–339.

3 De Ponti R, Cappato R, Curnis A, et al. Trans-septal catheterization in the electrophysiology laboratory: data from a multicenter survey spanning 12 years. *J Am Coll Cardiol* 2006; **47**(5): 1037–1042.

4 Haïssaguerre M, Jaïs P, Shah DC, et al. Spontaneous initiation of atrial fibrillation by ectopic beats originating in the pulmonary veins. *N Engl J Med* 1998; **339**: 659–666.

5 Vahanian A, Palacios IF. Percutaneous approaches to valvular disease. *Circulation* 2004; **109**: 1572–1579.

6 Feldman T, Foster E, Glower DD, et al; EVEREST II Investigators. Percutaneous repair or surgery for mitral regurgitation. *N Engl J Med* 2011; **364**: 1395–1406.

7 Holmes DR, Reddy VY, Turi ZG, et al.; PROTECT AF Investigators. Percutaneous closure of the left atrial appendage versus warfarin therapy for prevention of stroke in patients with atrial fibrillation: a randomised non-inferiority trial. *Lancet* 2009; **374**: 534–542.

8 Bouleti C, Fassa AA, Himbert D, et al. Transfemoral implantation of transcatheter heart valves after deterioration of mitral bioprosthesis or surgical repair. *JACC Cadiovasc Interv* 2015; **8**: 83–91.

9 Ruiz CE, Feldman TE, Hijazi ZM, et al. Interventional fellowship in structural and congenital heart disease for adults. *JACC Cadiovasc Interv* 2010; **3**: e1–15.

10 De Ponti R, Marazzi R, Ghiringhelli S, et al. Superiority of simulator-based training compared with conventional training methodologies in the performance of transseptal catheterization. *J Am Coll Cardiol* 2011; **58**: 359–363.

11 Wunderlich N, Franke J, Wilson N, Sievert H. 3D echo-guidance for structural heart interventions. *Interv Cardiol* 2009; **4**: 16–20.

12 Lang RM, Badano LP, Tsang W, et al. EAE/ASE Recommendations for image aquisition and display using three-dimensional echocardiography. *J Am Soc Echocardiogr* 2012; **25**: 3–46.

13 Trehan VK, Nigam A, Mukhopadhyay S, et al. Bedside percutaneous transseptal mitral commissurotomy under sole transthoracic echocardiographic guidance in a critically ill patient. *Echocardiography* 2006; **23**: 312–314.

14 Brockenbrough EC, Braunwald E, Ross J Jr. Transseptal left heart catheterization: a review of 450 studies and description of an improved technic. *Circulation* 1962; **25**: 15–21.

15 Mullins CE. Transseptal left heart catheterization: experience with a new technique in 520 pediatric and adult patients. *Pediatr Cardiol* 1983; **4**: 239–245.

16 Cheng TO. All roads lead to Rome: transjugular or transfemoral approach to percutaneous transseptal balloon mitral valvuloplasty? *Catheter Cardiovasc Interv* 2003; **59**: 266–267.

17 Wang Y, Xue YM, Mohanty P, et al. Dilator method and needle method for atrial transseptal puncture: a retrospective study from a cohort of 4443 patients. *Europace* 2012; **14**: 1450–1456.

18 Marcus GM, Ren X, Tseng ZH, et al. Repeat transseptal catheterization after ablation for atrial fibrillation. *J Cardiovasc Electrophysiol* 2007; **18**: 55–59.

19 Hildick-Smith D, McCready J, de Giovanni J. Transseptal puncture: use of an angioplasty guidewire for enhanced safety. *Catheter Cardiovasc Interv* 2007; **69**: 519–521.

20 Wadehra V, Buxton AE, Antoniadis AP, et al. The use of a novel nitinol guidewire to facilitate transseptal puncture and left atrial catheterization for catheter ablation procedures. *Europace* 2011; **13**: 1401–1405.

21 Sherman W, Lee P, Hartley A, Love B. Transatrial septal catheterization using a new radiofrequency probe. *Catheter Cardiovasc Interv* 2005; **66**: 14–17.

22 Hsu JC, Badhwar N, Gerstenfeld EP, et al. Randomised trial of conventional transseptal needle versus radiofrequency energy needle puncture for left atrial access (the TRAVERSE-LA Study). *J Am Heart Assoc* 2013; **2**: e000428.

23 Maisano F, La Canna G, Latib A, et al. Transseptal access for MitraClip® procedures using surgical diathermy under echocardiographic guidance. *EuroIntervention* 2012; **8**: 579–586.

24 Triantafyllou K, Brochet E, Himbert D, et al. Coronary angioplasty tools to facilitate percutaneous mitral commissurotomy following surgical closure of ostium secundum atrial septal defect. *Eurointervention* 2007; **10**: Case 2. http://www.europcronline.com/eurointervention/10th_issue/case2/.

25 Wunderlich NC, Siegel RJ. Peri-interventional echo assessment for the MitraClip procedure. *Eur Heart J* 2013; **14**: 935–949.

26 Maisano F, La Canna G, Latib A, et al. First-in-man transseptal implantation of a "surgical-like" mitral valve annuloplasty device for functional mitral regurgitation. *JACC: Cardiovasc Interv* 2014; **7**: 1326–1328.

27 Ruiz CE. The puncture technique: a new method for transcatheter closure of patent foramen ovale. *Catheter Cardio Interv* 2001; **53**: 369–372.

28 2012 HRS/EHRA/ECAS Expert Consensus Statement on Catheter and Surgical Ablation of Atrial Fibrillation. *Europace* 2012; **14**: 528–606.

29 HRS/EHRA/ECAS Expert Consensus Statement on Catheter and Surgical Ablation of Atrial Fibrillation: recommendations for personnel, policy, procedures and follow-up. *Europace* 2007; **9**: 335–379.

30 Fagundes RL, Mantica M, De Luca L, et al. Safety of single transseptal puncture for ablation of atrial fibrillation: retrospective study from a large cohort of patients. *J Cardiovasc Electrophysiol* 2007; **18**: 1277–1281.

31 Michowitz Y, Rahkovich M, Oral H, et al. Effects of sex on the incidence of cardiac tamponade after catheter ablation of atrial fibrillation: results from a worldwide survey in 34943 atrial fibrillation ablation procedures. *Circ Arrhythm Electrophysiol* 2014; **7**: 274–280.

32 Fisher WG, Ro AS. Trans-septal catheterization. In Huang SKS, Wood MA (eds) *Catheter Ablation of Cardiac Arrhythmias*. Saunders, 2006: 635–648.

33 Glassman E, Chinitz LA, Levite HA, Slater J, Winer H. Percutaneous left atrial to femoral arterial bypass pumping for circulatory support in high-risk coronary angioplasty. *Cathet Cardiovasc Diagn* 1993; **29**: 210–216.

34 Liu TJ, Lai HC, Lee WL, et al. Immediate and late outcomes of patients undergoing transseptal left-sided heart catheterization for symptomatic valvular and arrhythmic diseases. *Am Heart J* 2006; **151**: 235–241.

35 Lew AS, Harper RW, Federman J, Anderson ST, Pitt A. Recent experience with transeptal catheterization. *Cathet Cardiovasc Diagn* 1983; **9**: 601–609.

36 O'Keefe JH Jr, Vlietstra RE, Hanley PC, et al. Revival of the transseptal approach for catheterization of the left atrium and ventricle. *Mayo Clin Proc* 1985; **60**(11): 790–795.

37 Hildick-Smith DJ, Ludman PF, Shapiro LM. Inferior ST-segment elevation following transseptal puncture for balloon mitral valvuloplasty is atropine-responsive. *J Invasive Cardiol* 2004; **16**: 1–2.

38 Di Biase L, Burkhardt JD, Santangeli P, et al. Periprocedural stroke and bleeding complications in patients undergoing catheter ablation of atrial fibrillation with different anticoagulation management: results from the Role of Coumadin in Preventing Thromboembolism in Atrial Fibrillation (AF) Patients Undergoing Catheter Ablation (COMPARE) randomized trial. *Circulation* 2014; **129**: 2638–2644.

39 Boekstegers P, Hausleiter J, Baldus S, et al. Percutaneous interventional mitral regurgitation treatment using the Mitra-Clip system. *Clin Res Cardiol* 2014; **103**: 85–96.

40 Nallet O, Lung B, Cormier B, et al. Specifics of technique in percutaneous mitral commissurotomy in a case of dextrocardia and situs inversus with mitral stenosis. *Cathet Cardiovasc Diagn* 1996; **39**: 85–88.

41 Attias D, Himbert D, Redheuil A, et al. Piège du cathétérisme trans-septal pour commissurotomie mitral percutanée: l'interruption de la veine cave inférieure avec continuation azygos: a propos d'un cas et revue littérature. *Arch Mal Coeur Vaiss* 2007; **100**: 64–67.

42 Cook S, Meier B, Windecker S. Transseptal tandem heart implantation through an Amplatzer atrial septal occluder. *J Invasive Cardiol* 2007; **19**: 198–199.

CHAPTER 63

Principles of Carpentier's Reconstructive Surgery in Degenerative Mitral Valve Disease

Farzan Filsoufi[1] and Alain Carpentier[2]

[1] Icahn School of Medicine at Mount Sinai, New York, NY, USA

[2] Hôpital Européen, Georges-Pompidou, Paris, France

Degenerative mitral valve disease has become the predominant cause of mitral regurgitation (MR) in developed countries during the last four decades mainly because of the eradication of rheumatic fever and the aging population. Several confusing terminologies (myxomatous valve disease, mitral valve prolapse, floppy valve, flail leaflet, and so on) have been used in the literature to describe degenerative mitral valve disease. The understanding of valve pathology is facilitated by the use of the "pathophysiologic triad" [1].

Pathophysiology and functional classification

The pathophysiologic triad is composed of etiology (cause of the disease), valve lesions (resulting from the disease), and valve dysfunction (resulting from the lesion) [1]. These distinctions are relevant because long-term prognosis depends on etiology, whereas treatment strategy and surgical techniques depend on valve dysfunctions and lesions, respectively (Table 63.1).

Carpentier's functional classification is used to describe the mechanism of MR (Figure 63.1) [1]. This classification is based on the opening and closing motions of the mitral leaflets. Patients with type I dysfunction have normal leaflet motion. MR in these patients is caused by annular dilatation or leaflet perforation.

There is increased leaflet motion in patients with type II dysfunction with the free edge of the leaflet overriding the plane of the annulus during systole (leaflet prolapse). The most common lesions responsible for type II dysfunction are chordae elongation or rupture, and papillary muscle elongation or rupture. Patients with degenerative mitral valve regurgitation often present with type II dysfunction.

Patients with type IIIa dysfunction have a restricted leaflet motion during both diastole and systole. The most common lesions are leaflet thickening and/or retraction, chordae thickening and/or shortening or fusion, and commissural fusion. MR is most often associated with some degrees of mitral stenosis. The most common corresponding etiologies are rheumatic valve disease, mitral calcification, and carcinoid valve disease.

The mechanism of MR in type IIIb dysfunction is restricted leaflet motion during systole. Left ventricular enlargement with apical papillary muscle displacement causes this type of valve dysfunction. The two most frequent etiologies are ischemic and dilated cardiomyopathy.

The functional classification is further refined by the introduction of segmental analysis which allows the precise localization of leaflet dysfunction, which is of critical importance while performing reconstructive surgery [2].

The mitral valve is separated into eight segments (Figure 63.2). Anterolateral and posteromedial commissures are two segments. Two indentations on the posterior leaflet divide this structure into three anatomically individualized scallops. The three scallops of the posterior leaflet are identified as P1 (anterior scallop), P2 (middle scallop), and P3 (posterior scallop). The three corresponding segments of the anterior leaflet are A1 (anterior segment), A2 (middle segment), and A3 (posterior segment).

Application of pathophysiologic triad in patients with degenerative mitral valve disease

Etiologies of degenerative mitral disease include Barlow's disease and fibroelastic deficiency. Marfan's disease, the third etiology, is encountered in a minority of patients. In about 10–20% of patients, although the valve displays some pathologic features compatible with either Barlow's disease or fibroelastic deficiency, it is difficult to determine the exact etiology, leading our group to suggest the concept of "spectrum of degenerative mitral valve disease." The mechanism of MR is often leaflet prolapse (type II dysfunction) resulting from chordae rupture or elongation. Barlow's disease is the most common condition affecting up to 5% of the population whereas fibroelastic deficiency is observed with increasing frequency as the age of the population increases.

Barlow's disease

Barlow's disease appears early in life, and patients typically have a long history of a systolic murmur [3,4]. Most patients who require surgery for MR are referred for surgery in their fourth or fifth decades of life. The valve is billowing with typically thick leaflets and with marked excess tissue (Figure 63.3a). The chordae are thickened, elongated, and may be ruptured. Papillary muscles are also

Interventional Cardiology: Principles and Practice, Second Edition. Edited by George D. Dangas, Carlo Di Mario, and Nicholas N. Kipshidze.
© 2017 John Wiley & Sons, Ltd. Published 2017 by John Wiley & Sons, Ltd.

Table 63.1 Pathophysiologic triad.

Dysfunction	Lesions	Etiology
Type I Normal leaflet motion	Annular dilatation Leaflet perforation/tear	Dilated cardiomyopathy Endocarditis

Type II
Excess leaflet motion
(leaflet prolapse)
	Elongation/rupture chordae
	
	Elongation/rupture of papillary muscle
		Degenerative valve disease
		    Fibroelastic deficiency
		    Barlow's disease
		    Marfan disease
		Endocarditis
		Trauma
		Ischemic cardiomyopathy

Type IIIa Restricted leaflet motion (Diastole and Systole)	Leaflet thickening/retraction Leaflet calcification Chordal thickening/retraction/fusion Commissural fusion	Rheumatic heart disease Carcinoid heart disease
Type IIIb Restricted leaflet motion (Systole)	Left ventricular dilatation/aneurysm Papillary muscle displacement Chordae tethering	Ischemic/Dilated cardiomyopathy

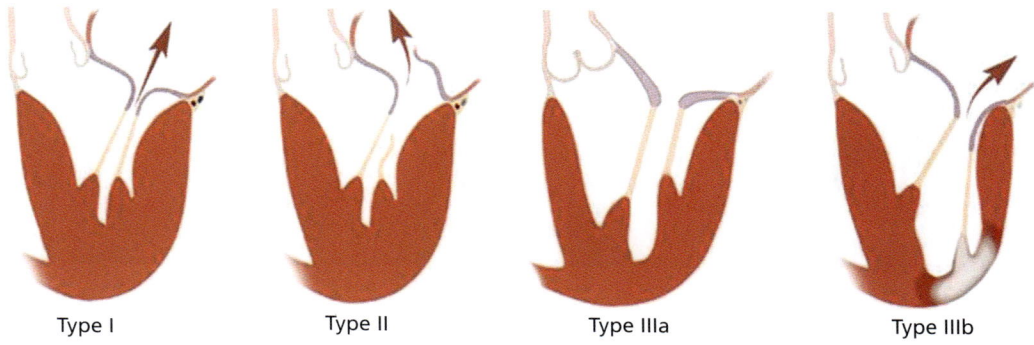

Type I   Type II   Type IIIa   Type IIIb

Figure 63.1 Carpentier's functional classification. Source: Carpentier A, *et al.* 2010 [14]. Copyright 2010 Saunders/Elsevier.

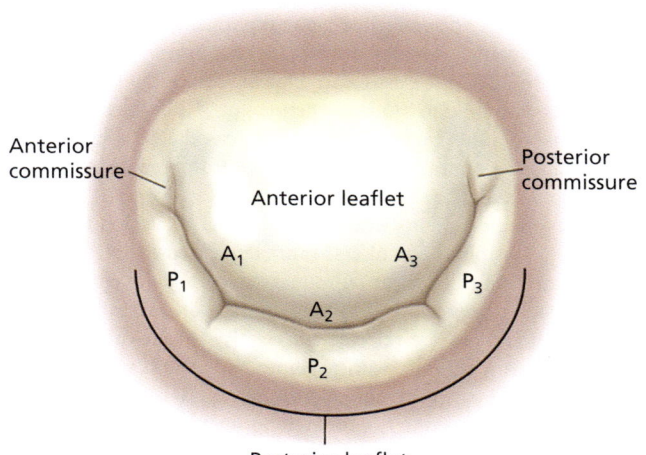

Figure 63.2 Segmental valve analysis. Source: Carpentier A, *et al.* 2010 [14]. Copyright 2010 Saunders/Elsevier.

occasionally elongated. The annulus is dilated and sometimes calcified. Most patients with Barlow's valve present with the prolapse of multiple segments of the valve. Bileaflet prolapse is present in about 30% of patients. Histologically, there is extensive myxoid degeneration with destruction of the normal three-layer leaflet tissue architecture.

Fibroelastic deficiency

Fibroelastic deficiency is most common in elderly patients (>65 years) with a relatively short history of MR [4]. Valve analysis typically shows transparent leaflets with no excess tissue except in the prolapsing segment, and elongated, thin, frail, and often ruptured chordae (Figure 63.3b). The annulus is often dilated, and may be calcified. Most these patients present with isolated P2 prolapse. An important feature of fibroelastic deficiency is the development of secondary lesions at the level of prolapsing segment with myxoid degeneration, excess tissue, and leaflet thickening which may entertain the confusion with the diagnosis of Barlow's disease on echocardiography or histologic analysis.

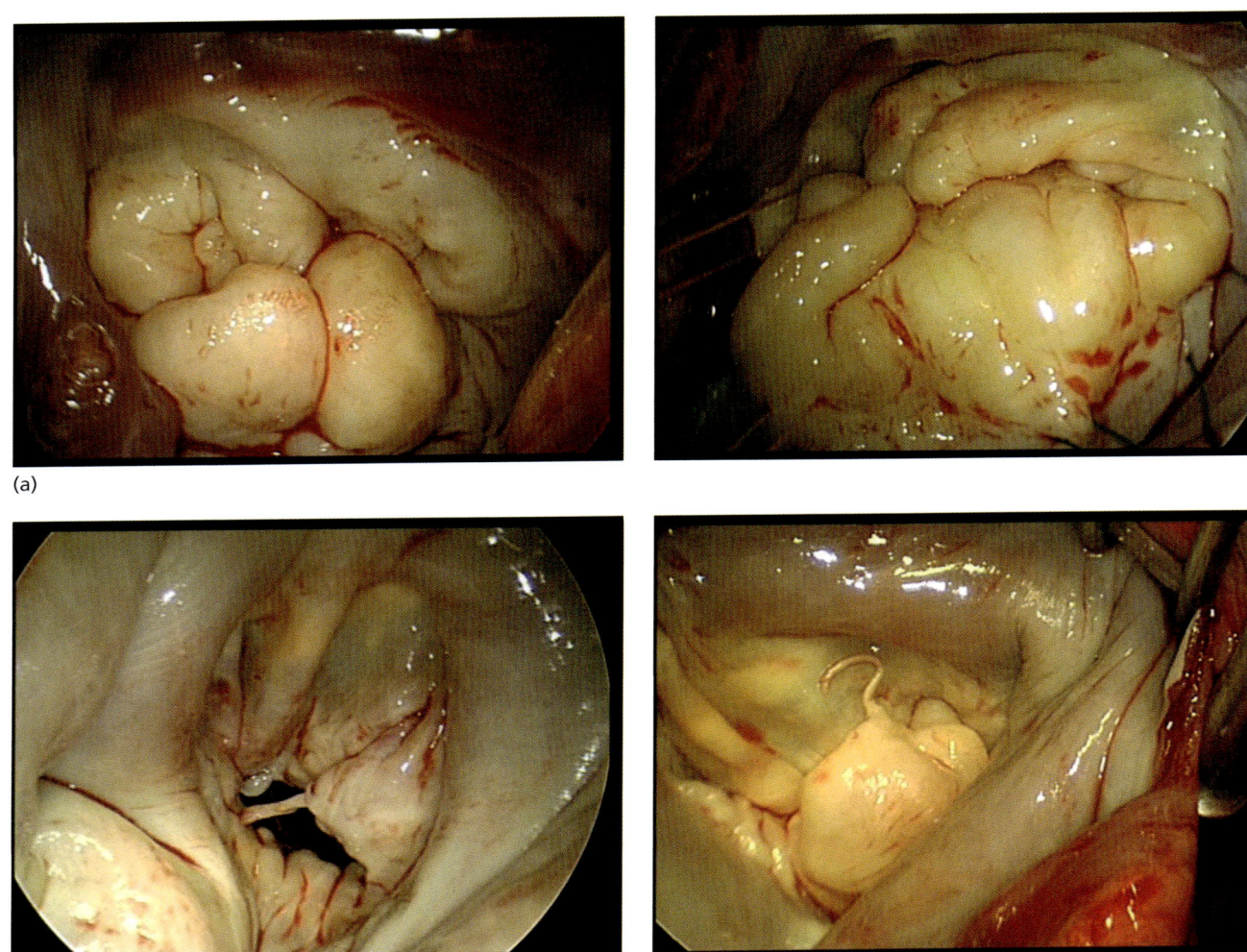

Figure 63.3 (a) Barlow's disease. (b) Fibroelastic deficiency.

Marfan's disease

Marfan's disease with MR is characterized by excess leaflet tissue, which can be thickened (without myxoid degeneration), and a dilated annulus that is rarely calcified [5].

Surgical indications

In patients with degenerative mitral disease, the very low operative mortality (less than 0.5%) and morbidity combined with the excellent long-term results of mitral valve reconstruction have considerably modified the indications of surgery during the last decade.

Several variables such as clinical symptoms, atrial fibrillation, severity of MR, left ventricular ejection fraction, left ventricular end-systolic diameter, pulmonary hypertension, and the overall surgical risk profile (age, comorbid factors) should be taken into consideration for decision-making with regard to the indications of surgery.

All symptomatic patients with moderate to severe MR should be referred for surgical intervention. It is preferable to operate on patients early in their symptomatic course, as long-term survival following mitral valve reconstruction is less favorable in patients with New York Heart Association Class III or IV symptoms or left ventricular ejection fraction <60%. It is important to stress that

in patients with degenerative mitral disease with New York Heart Association Class I or II and ejection fraction >60%, the life expectancy following mitral valve reconstruction is similar to that of an age- and gender-matched general population. As Carpentier stated, "following valvular reconstruction most patients with degenerative valve disease are cured for the rest of their lives."

Patients with mild to moderate degrees of MR in the presence of symptoms will often be found to have increased MR or inadequate increase in ejection fraction on stress echocardiography and should also be considered for surgical treatment.

Asymptomatic patients with left ventricular dilatation (left ventricular end-systolic diameter >45 mm), decreased ejection fraction (<60%), atrial fibrillation or pulmonary hypertension (pulmonary artery systolic pressure >50 mmHg at rest or >60 mmHg with exercise) should also be referred for elective mitral valve surgery. When following patients with asymptomatic moderate to severe MR, one should pay particular attention to serial ejection fraction, as a drop to <60% confers poorer long-term survival even with successful mitral valve reconstruction.

The decision to refer or accept an asymptomatic patient for mitral valve surgery should also take into consideration one important factor, which is the likelihood of valve reconstruction which depends mainly on: (i) the etiology of MR (Barlow's disease vs. fibroelastic deficiency); and (ii) surgeon's skill and experience in valve reconstruction. For example, patients with Barlow's disease and bileaflet prolapse, which often require a complex operative procedure, should be referred to centers where reconstructive surgery can be performed with a great certainty.

Principles of mitral valve surgery
Perioperative management

Standard techniques of monitoring (e.g., arterial line, central venous access, Foley catheter) are used in patients undergoing mitral valve reconstructive surgery. A Swan–Ganz catheter should be placed in cases of complex mitral valve reconstructive surgery, multivalve surgery, combined mitral and coronary artery bypass grafting (CABG) surgery, and in patients with increased operative risk (e.g., left ventricular dysfunction, pulmonary hypertension, reoperation). Initially, a transesophageal echocardiography (TEE) should be performed in all patients. TEE is important to determine the mechanism and severity of MR, to assess left ventricular function, quality of reconstruction, and de-airing of the cardiac cavities at the completion of the procedure. An external defibrillator is placed in reoperation and minimally invasive approaches. A double lumen endotracheal tube is necessary in right thoracotomy incisions [6]. An epiaortic scanning of the ascending aorta is recommended in elderly patients with associated atherosclerotic risk factors, and those undergoing a combined mitral valve and CABG surgery prior to arterial cannulation.

Surgical incisions and cardiopulmonary bypass

A small skin incision and a midline sternotomy remain the most commonly performed surgical approach in mitral valve reconstructive surgery. It provides an excellent access to all cardiac structures allowing for central cannulation using the ascending aorta and the superior and inferior vena cava.

Mini-invasive, direct vision mitral surgery is performed through the partial upper or lower hemisternotomy. A 6 cm skin incision is performed in both cases. The sternum is partially divided from the sternal notch to the left fourth intercostal space (upper hemisternotomy) and from the xyphoide to the second right intercostal space (lower hemisternotomy) [7]. Central arterial and venous cannulations are often possible with these approaches. Video-directed [8] and robotic mitral valve surgeries are performed through a right mini-thoracotomy at the fourth intercostal space.

Multiport access is obtained by additional keyhole incisions. Peripheral vessels are used to initiate cardiopulmonary bypass. Additional adjunctive techniques such as port access instrumentation, CO_2 insufflation, and vacuum-assisted venous drainage are frequently used to facilitate these surgical procedures.

Myocardial protection is achieved with intermittent antegrade or a combined antegrade and retrograde administration of high potassium cold blood cardioplegia. Further myocardial protection can be obtained by moderate systemic hypothermia at 28–30 °C. The myocardial temperature should be assessed continuously during the procedure and maintained below 15 °C. If it exceeds 15°, additional administration of cardioplegic solution is necessary.

Mitral valve exposure and intraoperative valve analysis

Perfect exposition of the mitral valve is essential before undertaking mitral valve reconstructive surgery. We favor the interatrial approach through the Sondergaard's groove. The interatrial groove is incised and the two atria are dissected and divided up to the fossa ovalis. This dissection exposes the roof of the left atrium, which is opened close to the mitral valve [2]. In patients with a small left atrium, the inferior extension of the left atrial incision between the right inferior pulmonary vein and inferior vena cava optimizes the mitral valve exposure.

The entire mitral valve apparatus must be carefully examined to confirm the mechanism of MR, to assess the feasibility of reconstruction, and to plan the exact operative strategy. The endocardium of the left atrium is examined for jet lesions, which indicate opposite leaflet prolapse. The mitral annulus is examined to assess the severity of annular dilatation, and the presence and extent of calcification. The valvular apparatus is examined with a nerve hook in order to assess the severity and the extent of leaflet prolapse according to the segmental valve analysis [2]. The anterior paracommissural scallop of the posterior leaflet (P1) is often intact and rarely prolapsing in patients with degenerative disease. The P1 segment constitutes the reference point [2]. Applying traction to the free edge of other valvular segments and comparing them to P1 determines the severity and the extent of leaflet prolapse.

Fundamentals of mitral valve reconstructive surgery

The goals of reconstructive surgery are preservation or restoration of normal leaflet motion, creation of a large surface of coaptation, and stabilization of the entire annulus with a remodeling annuloplasty (Figure 63.4) [1]. Current surgical techniques allow surgeons to perform reconstructive surgery in almost all patients

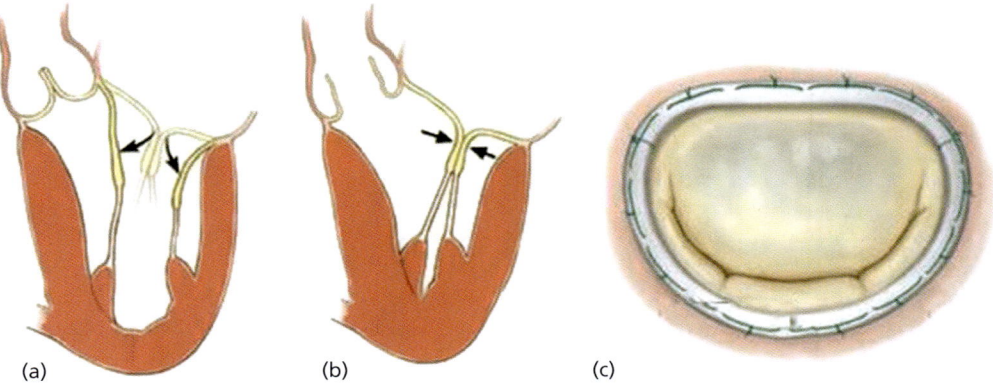

(a)   (b)   (c)

Figure 63.4 Principles of reconstructive surgery. Source: Carpentier A, *et al.* 2010 [14]. Copyright 2010 Saunders/Elsevier.

with degenerative mitral disease, provided that these guidelines are followed carefully.

Posterior leaflet prolapse

Limited posterior leaflet prolapse is best treated by a triangular resection. Extensive posterior leaflet prolapse is treated by a quadrangular resection of the prolapsed area. Stay sutures are placed around the normal chordae in order to determine the prolapsed area. The prolapsed segment is then removed by performing a perpendicular incision from the free edge toward the annulus, resecting a quadrangular portion of the leaflet. Plication sutures are placed along the posterior annulus in the resected area. Finally, direct sutures of the leaflet remnants restore valve continuity without tension (Figure 63.5).

When excessive posterior leaflet tissue is present, such as in Barlow's disease, it is important to reduce the height of the posterior leaflet to less than 15 mm to prevent postoperative systolic anterior motion (SAM) [9]. A sliding leaflet technique is performed following quadrangular resection. The P1 and P3 segments are detached from the annulus; compression sutures are then placed in the posterior segment of the annulus. A sliding plasty of the P1 and P3 segments is performed and the gap between the two scallops is closed with interrupted sutures. In Barlow's valve with significant excess tissue of posterior leaflet, an additional triangular resection at the base of P1 and P3 may be necessary prior to proceeding with the sliding leaflet plasty.

Sliding plasty is also indicated if a large segment of the posterior leaflet is resected. Plication of a large segment of the posterior

annulus must be avoided because of the increased risk of circumflex artery kinking.

Anterior leaflet prolapse

Several techniques are described to correct anterior leaflet prolapse depending upon the extent of the prolapse and the lesions responsible (chordae elongation versus rupture).

Triangular resection

Limited prolapse of the anterior leaflet with excess tissue can be treated by a small triangular resection of the prolapsed area followed by direct closure with interrupted monofilament sutures. The triangular resection must not be extended to the body of the anterior leaflet and should not involve more than 10% of the anterior leaflet surface area. Large resection of the anterior leaflet distorts the geometry and reduces the coaptation area. In addition, it compromises leaflet mobility considerably and is incriminated as a risk factor for repair failure.

Chordae transposition

Chordae transposition from the secondary position to the free margin of the anterior leaflet is the most preferable technique. A strong and normal secondary chordae adjacent to the prolapsing area is identified. This chordae is detached at 2 mm from its origin on the body of the anterior leaflet. If the chordae is cut at its base, this will likely cause leaflet perforation. It is then attached to the free margin of the anterior leaflet in the prolapsed area with a figure-of-eight suture. In case of a large prolapsed area, several secondary chordae

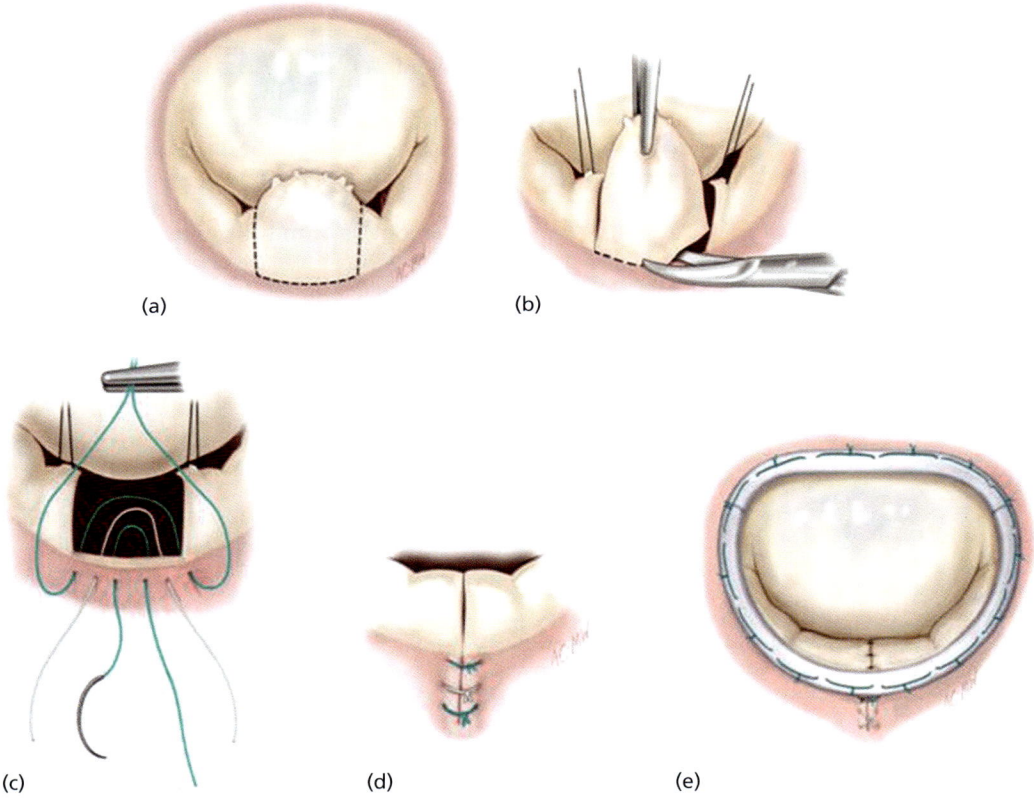

(a)   (b)

(c)   (d)   (e)

Figure 63.5 Posterior leaflet quadrangular resection with annular plication. Source: Carpentier A, *et al.* 2010 [14]. Copyright 2010 Saunders/Elsevier.

should be transferred to the free margin with a maximum 5 mm interval between two adjacent chordae.

In the absence of normal secondary chordae, chordae transposition from the posterior leaflet to the anterior leaflet should be considered. If marginal chordae of the posterior segment opposite to the prolapsed area of the anterior leaflet is normal, it can be used for chordae transposition. A small segment of the posterior leaflet with its marginal chordae is detached and then reattached to the free margin of the anterior leaflet at the site of prolapse. Interrupted sutures are used to close the defect in the posterior leaflet.

If these two techniques can not be applied, the use of artificial chordae is a valuable alternative.

Papillary muscle sliding plasty

This technique is convenient for anterior leaflet prolapse caused by elongation (<5 mm) of multiple chordae arising from a papillary muscle. The portion of the papillary muscle supporting the elongated chordae is split longitudinally and re-sutured to the other portion at a lower level. This downward displacement of papillary muscle corrects leaflet prolapse.

Papillary muscle shortening

Papillary muscle elongation or chordae elongation involving a group of chordae can also be treated by papillary muscle shortening. A triangular wedge at the base of the papillary muscle is resected. This defect is then closed by direct suture resulting in a reduced height of the papillary muscle and correction of chordae length. Papillary muscle shortening not only corrects the leaflet prolapse, but also reduces considerably the billowing of the leaflet body. This procedure is typically indicated in Barlow's disease with bileaflet prolapse.

Commissural prolapse

Commissural prolapse is best treated by resection of the prolapsed area followed by annular plication (limited prolapse) or sliding plasty of the paracommissural area (extensive prolapse) (e.g., A1 and P1 sliding plasty for anterolateral commissural prolapse). Additional inverting sutures should be placed in the newly created commissure in order to avoid residual minimal regurgitation. Occasionally, a patient presents with a papillary muscle with two heads. The rupture of one head can lead to commissural prolapse, which can be corrected by reattachment of the latter to the remnant papillary muscle. If extensive commissural and paracommissural prolapse resulting from chordae elongation are present, papillary muscle sliding plasty or papillary muscle shortening are valuable alternative options.

Remodeling ring annuloplasty

In patients with a normal mitral valve, the ratio between anteroposterior (septolateral) and transverse diameter of the mitral annulus is 3 : 4 during systole. This ratio is inverted in patients with degenerative mitral valve disease and annular dilatation [1]. The remodeling ring annuloplasty restores the physiologic ratio with maximal orifice area during systole. Therefore the prosthetic ring restores not only the size, but also the shape of the annulus. Remodeling annuloplasty provides increased leaflet coaptation area without causing any valvular stenosis. Furthermore, it prevents late annular dilatation and preserves leaflet mobility. Appropriate ring sizing is based on the intercommissural distance and the surface area of the anterior leaflet, measured with an obturator (Figure 63.6). If the surgeon hesitates between two sizes, in patients with degenera-

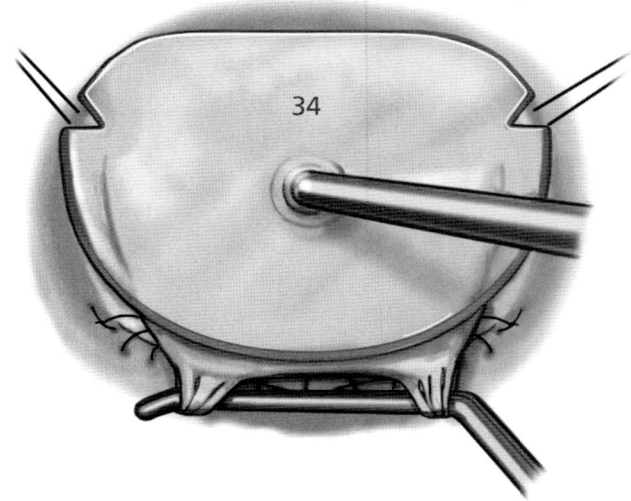

Figure 63.6 Ring selection based on sizing of the mitral valve: (i) measure of inter-commissural distance, (ii) measure of the anterior leaflet surface area.

tive mitral valve disease the selection of the greater size is recommended in most instances [2]. In Barlow's valve, the typical size of the prosthetic ring is 36–40 mm [10]. The choice of a too small ring increases significantly the risk of post-repair SAM [11].

Sutures are placed circumferentially through the mitral annulus. These sutures are equally spaced in the area between the two commissures and the corresponding segment of the selected prosthetic ring. In the remaining portion of the annulus, the spacing is set to conform the annulus to the shape and size of the prosthetic ring. When the ring sutures are tied, the ring reshapes the annulus in its normal systolic position.

Saline test and post bypass TEE

The quality of the repair must be evaluated at the completion of the reconstruction and before tying the ring to the annulus with a saline test. Saline is injected into the ventricular cavity through the mitral valve with a syringe while the aortic root is vented to prevent air emboli into the coronary arteries. A symmetric line of coaptation, parallel to the posterior aspect of the annulus, and at distance from the left ventricular outflow tract (3/4 to 1/4 ratio of anterior to posterior leaflet) indicates a satisfactory result. An asymmetrical line of coaptation indicates the presence of residual leaflet prolapse or restricted leaflet motion, which must be corrected. If the posterior leaflet occupies half or more of the orifice area its height should be reduced (less than 15 mm) to minimize the risk of SAM. Two hooks should also be used to determine the length of the coaptation which is ideally greater than 10 mm. At the completion of cardiopulmonary bypass, the quality of reconstruction is assessed by TEE. This examination should carefully evaluate leaflet motion, the competency of the valve and rule out the presence of post-valvuloplasty SAM in patients with excess leaflet tissue. In the presence of residual regurgitation, TEE is crucial to determine the severity and the mechanism of regurgitation which can justify a second look. No patient should leave the operating room with more than 1+ residual MR. In patients with ≥2+ MR, a second bypass run is necessary to reanalyze the valve and correct a residual valvular dysfunction.

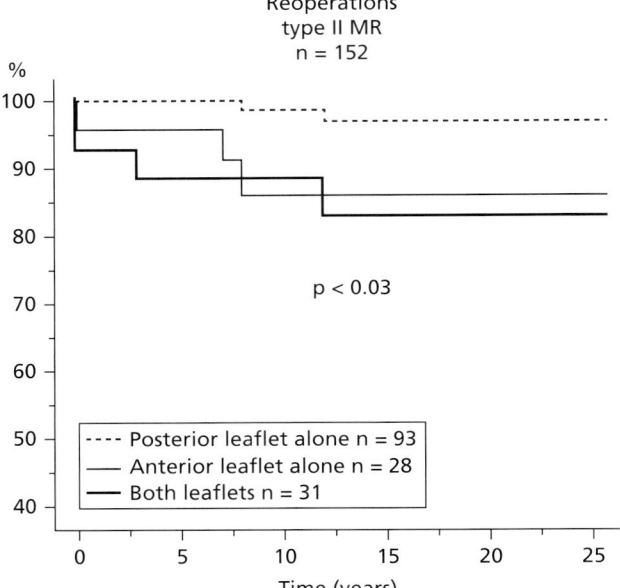

Figure 63.7 Reoperation according to leaflet prolapse.
Source: Braunberger E, *et al.* 2001 [12]. Reproduced with permission of Wolters Kluwer Health.

Results

Patients with degenerative mitral valve disease are the most suitable for reconstructive surgery [12–14]. Operative mortality in this group of patients is less than 0.5% in experienced centers [10] with a repair rate of near 100% [13]. In patients with severe MR, reconstructive surgery should be carried out before the occurrence of clinical symptoms, atrial fibrillation, pulmonary hypertension, and left ventricular dysfunction or enlargement.

The long-term survival of patients with preserved left ventricular function following reconstructive surgery is similar to that of an age and gender-matched population.

Our group was among the first to publish the very long-term results (>20 years) of mitral reconstructive surgery [12]. This observational study, which consisted of 162 consecutive patients operated on between 1970 and 1984, was mostly composed of patients with degenerative disease (90%). The main mechanism of MR was type II dysfunction in 152 (94%) patients. Posterior, anterior, and bileaflet prolapse were present in 93 (61%), 28 (19%), and 31 (20%) patients, respectively. All patients underwent annuloplasty; valve resection was done in 126 patients, and shortening or transposition of the chordae in 46 patients. The linearized rate of reoperation was 0.4% per patient year. Freedom from reoperation was 97%, 86%, and 83%

for posterior, anterior, and bileaflet prolapse, respectively, at 20 years (Figure 63.7). The increased rate of early reoperation in the anterior leaflet prolapse group was attributed to technical failure. The widespread use of intraoperative TEE and improved surgical techniques (chordae transposition) have most likely contributed in reducing the incidence of early failure in the last two decades. However, the freedom from reoperation was unchanged at 10, 20, and 25 years of follow-up. These excellent and stable results confirm the predictability and durability of mitral valve reconstruction in degenerative disease. Today, reconstructive valve surgery allows patients to enjoy a normal life and to be cured for the rest of their life [14].

Interactive multiple choice questions are available for this chapter on www.wiley.com/go/dangas/cardiology

References

1 Carpentier A. Cardiac valve surgery: the "French correction." *J Thorac Cardiovasc Surg* 1983; **86**(3): 323–337.
2 Carpentier AF, Lessana A, Relland JY, *et al.* The "physio-ring": an advanced concept in mitral valve annuloplasty. *Ann Thorac Surg* 1995; **60**(5): 1177–1185; discussion 1185–1186.
3 Barlow JB, Bosman CK, Pocock WA, Marchand P. Late systolic murmurs and non-ejection ("mid-late") systolic clicks: an analysis of 90 patients. *Br Heart J* 1968; **30**(2): 203–218.
4 Carpentier A, Chauvaud S, Fabiani JN, *et al.* Reconstructive surgery of mitral valve incompetence: ten-year appraisal. *J Thorac Cardiovasc Surg* 1980; **79**(3): 338–348.
5 Fuzellier JF, Chauvaud SM, Fornes P, *et al.* Surgical management of mitral regurgitation associated with Marfan's syndrome. *Ann Thorac Surg* 1998; **66**(1): 68–72.
6 Adams DH, Filsoufi F, Byrne JG, Karavas AN, Aklog L. Mitral valve repair in redo cardiac surgery. *J Card Surg* 2002; **17**(1): 40–45.
7 Loulmet DF, Carpentier A, Cho PW, *et al.* Less invasive techniques for mitral valve surgery. *J Thorac Cardiovasc Surg* 1998; **115**(4): 772–729.
8 Casselman FP, Van Slycke S, Dom H, Lambrechts DL, Vermeulen Y, Vanermen H. Endoscopic mitral valve repair: feasible, reproducible, and durable. *J Thorac Cardiovasc Surg* 2003; **125**(2): 273–282.
9 Jebara VA, Mihaileanu S, Acar C, *et al.* Left ventricular outflow tract obstruction after mitral valve repair: results of the sliding leaflet technique. *Circulation* 1993; **88**(5 Pt 2): 1130–1134.
10 Adams DH, Anyanwu AC, Rahmanian PB, Abascal V, Salzberg SP, Filsoufi F. Large annuloplasty rings facilitate mitral valve repair in Barlow's disease. *Ann Thorac Surg* 2006; **82**(6): 2096–2100; discussion 2101.
11 Mihaileanu S. Outflow tract obstruction and failed mitral repair. *Circulation* 1994; **90**(2): 1107–1108.
12 Braunberger E, Deloche A, Berrebi A, *et al.* Very long-term results (more than 20 years) of valve repair with Carpentier's techniques in nonrheumatic mitral valve insufficiency. *Circulation* 2001; **104**(12 Suppl 1): 8–11.
13 Castillo JG, Anyanwu AC, Fuster V, Adams DH. A near 100% repair rate for mitral valve prolapse is achievable in a reference center: implications for future guidelines. *J Thorac Cardiovasc Surg* 2012; **144**(2): 308–312.
14 Carpentier A, Adams DH, Filsoufi F. *Carpentier's Reconstructive Valve Surgery*. Philadelphia; Saunders/Elsevier: 2010.

CHAPTER 64

Mitral Valve Repair: MitraClip and Emerging Techniques

Ted Feldman[1], Mohammad Sarraf[1], Mayra Guerrero[1], and Francesco Maisano[2]

[1] NorthShore University HealthSystem, Evanston, IL, USA
[2] University Hospital Zurich, Zurich, Switzerland

Percutaneous mitral valve repair has emerged as an alternative to surgery for patients with significant symptomatic mitral regurgitation (MR) and prohibitive risk for surgical mitral repair or replacement. The first MR surgical treatment concept to be adapted for percutaneous use was the double-orifice or edge-to-edge repair [1]. The surgical technique was developed in the early 1990s [2]. The free edges of the mitral leaflets are sewn together along the coaptation surface of the mid segments of the anterior and posterior mitral leaflets to create a double orifice valve. This technique was used initially for patients with focal anterior leaflet mitral prolapse [3]. The initial description of the surgical technique specifically suggested that "the concept introduced by this type of repair can open the perspective of percutaneous correction of MR."

Percutaneous mitral leaflet repair with MitraClip

The edge-to-edge repair concept led to the development of the MitraClip [4]. This device replicates the surgical repair by mechanically grasping the mitral leaflet free edges. The device is introduced into the left atrium via transseptal puncture, positioned and opened above the mitral leaflets, passed beyond the leaflets tips into the left ventricle (LV), and then slowly pulled back toward the atrium to grasp the leaflets (Figure 64.1). The clip is then closed to create a double orifice valve, and the effect on reduction of MR is assessed. The MitraClip can be reopened and repositioned, or removed completely, up to the point that it is released.

The MitraClip system consists of three major components: a 24-Fr steerable guiding catheter, the clip delivery system (CDS), and the MitraClip device. The CDS has a steering mechanism for the clip and controls to manage the opening and closing of the clip, the lock, and the "gripper," which is a barbed element to help affix the mitral leaflets to the clip arms. The clip is covered in polyester fabric. The deployment is completely reversible and it is possible to grasp the mitral leaflets and ultimately choose to release them and remove the clip safely when needed (Figures 64.2 and 64.3).

The first procedures were carried out in July 2003. After demonstrating feasibility in the EVEREST I trial [5], the MitraClip was evaluated in a randomized trial comparing the MitraClip with conventional surgery for patients deemed good surgical candidates, EVEREST II

(Figure 64.4) [6]. The majority of the patients randomized in the EVEREST II trial were patients with degenerative mitral regurgitation (DMR). About one-fourth had functional MR (FMR).

At 1 year of follow-up, the major findings of EVEREST II trial were that the MitraClip was less successful at reducing MR than surgery, but led to similar improvements in favorable LV remodeling and clinical outcomes including functional class and quality of life scores. Subgroup analysis showed that the patients who derived the greatest improvement with MitraClip were older, had FMR, and had poor LV function. This latter finding has contributed to the broader use of the MitraClip in this clinical setting in global practice, and the subsequent development of the EVEREST REALISM Registry. In the first 6 months after MitraClip therapy in the EVEREST II trial, almost 20% of patients required surgery. Almost half of these were because of initially unsuccessful procedures with an inability to either implant a clip successfully, or inadequate reduction in MR. Almost 9% of these patients who had single leaflet detachment from the MitraClip device. In this instance, a single leaflet is noted to have escaped from the clips typically at the 30-day follow-up visit. No occurrences of complete embolization occurred in this experience. Single leaflet detachment was not associated with clinical events, but obviously led to a failure to reduce MR adequately. After the initial 6-month period, when the early procedure failures are noted, comparisons of MitraClip and surgery in the EVEREST II randomized trial show equivalent outcomes in terms of reoperation, mortality, and LV remodeling.

At 5 years, the outcomes from the MitraClip therapy in EVEREST II trial are remarkably stable [7]. The durability of LV remodeling and stability of the mitral annular dimensions suggest that after initially successful therapy, the procedure results are durable for at least 5 years.

It has been recognized that during this randomized trial, many patients who might have benefited from MitraClip had too high surgical risk to be enrolled. This led to a high risk registry [8]. Ultimately, 351 high risk patients were prospectively enrolled [9].

The global experience with MitraClip in the ensuing decade of experience has witnessed a dramatic improvement in acute procedure success with rates approaching 100%. In addition, single leaflet detachment now occurs in about only 1% of patients. Thus, most of the failures seen in the first 6 months in EVEREST II would not occur in current practice.

Interventional Cardiology: Principles and Practice, Second Edition. Edited by George D. Dangas, Carlo Di Mario, and Nicholas N. Kipshidze.
© 2017 John Wiley & Sons, Ltd. Published 2017 by John Wiley & Sons, Ltd.

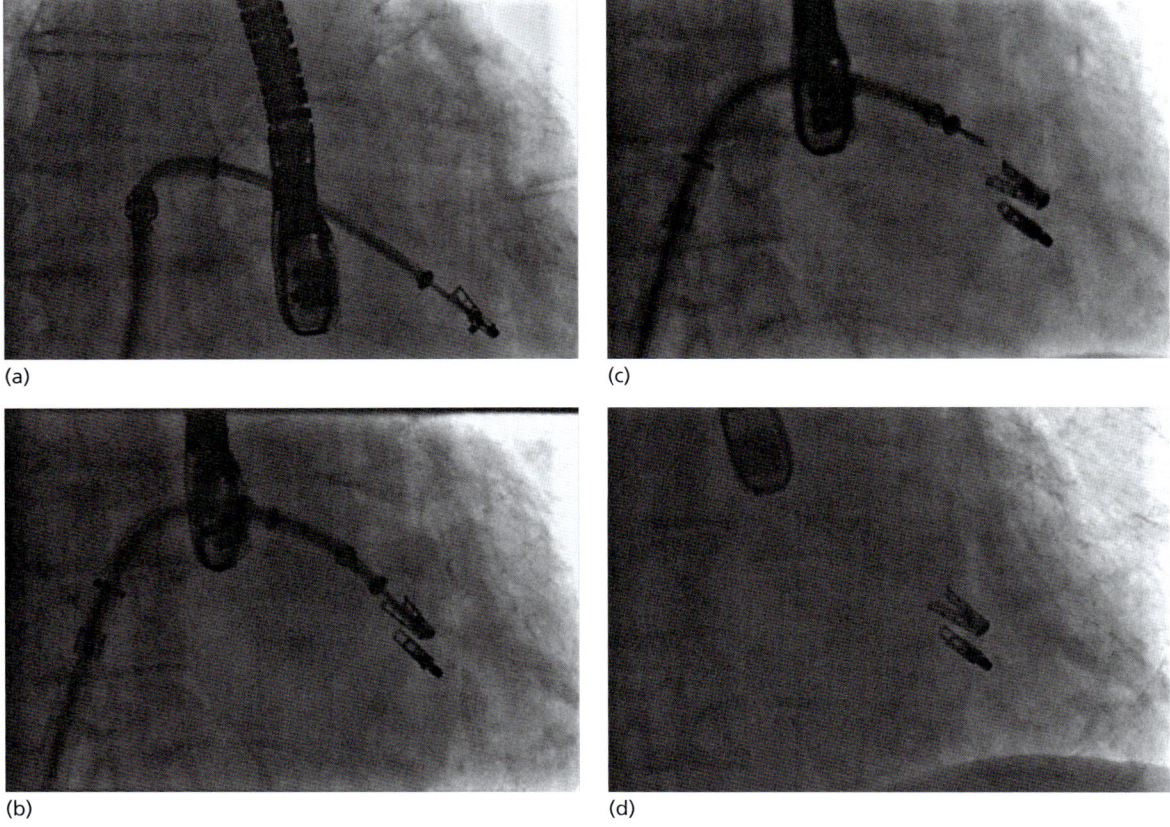

Figure 64.1 Fluoroscopic images of a MitraClip procedure. (a) A single MitraClip has been advanced into the left ventricle beyond the mitral leaflets. The open clip will be pulled back to grasp the leaflets, and then released. (b) After placement of the first clip a second clip is placed. (c) Release of the second clip. (d) Final appearance of two clips. Note the transesophageal echocardiography (TEE) probe in all of the images. Two clips are placed on the mitral leaflets in about half of cases, and one clip in half.

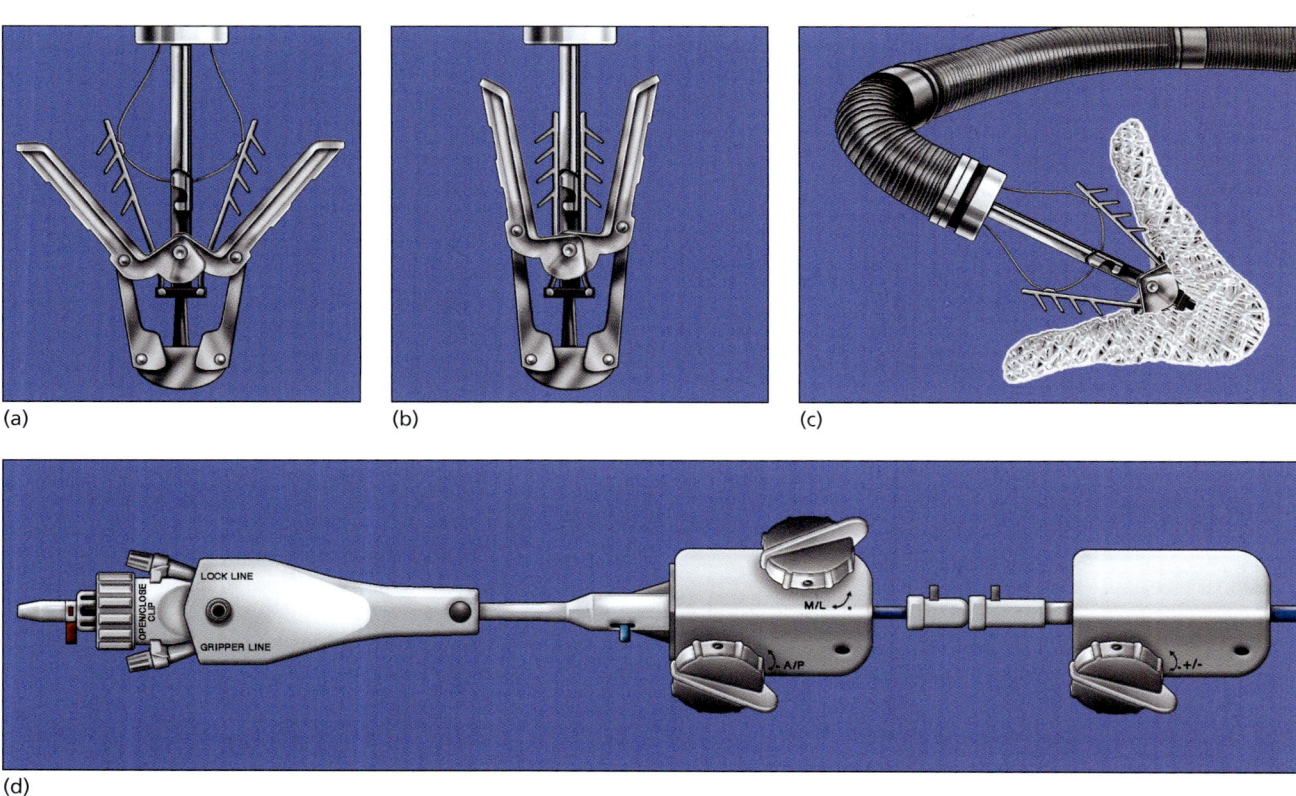

Figure 64.2 The MitraClip System. (a) The partially open MitraClip device is shown without its fabric covering. A fine wire runs through the barbed "grippers," which is used to raise the grippers. (b) The device in closed configuration. (c) The MitraClip is attached to the clip delivery system (CDS), which protrudes from the steerable guide catheter. (d) Control knobs allow deflection of the guide and CDS to steer the system through the left atruim and position the MitraClip above the mitral orifice. Source: Feldman T, Young A. *J Am Coll Cardiol* 2014; **63**: 2057–2068.

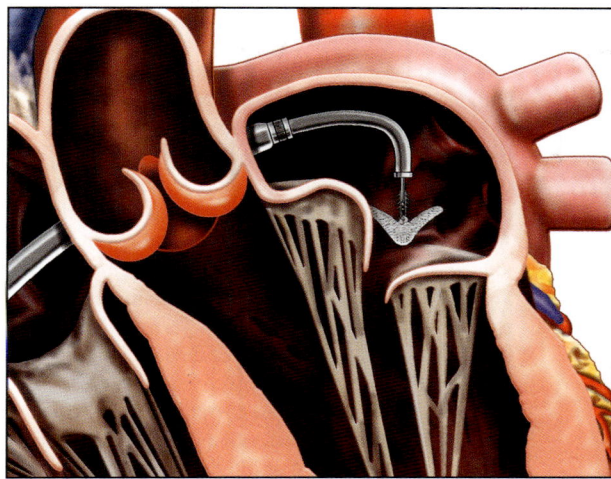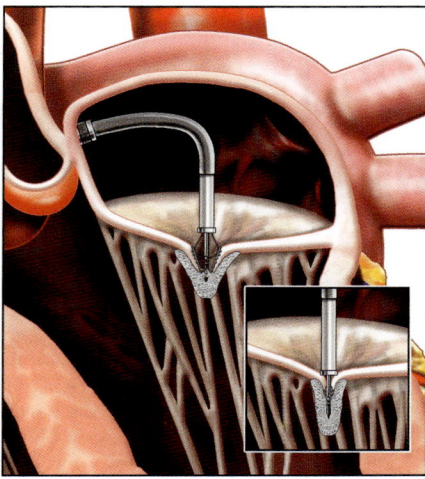

Figure 64.3 To introduce the clip, the Clip Delivery System (CDS) is advanced through the guide into the left atrium (left). Under echocardiographic and fluoroscopic guidance, the clip is aligned perpendicular to the valve plane, with the clip arms perpendicular to the line of coaptation. It is then advanced into the left and then slowly retracted to grasp the leaflets (right). The clip is closed (right, inset), and if reduction of mitral regurgitation is satisfactory, it is released. Source: Feldman T, Young A. *J Am Coll Cardiol* 2014; **63**: 2057–2068. Artwork by Craig Skaggs.

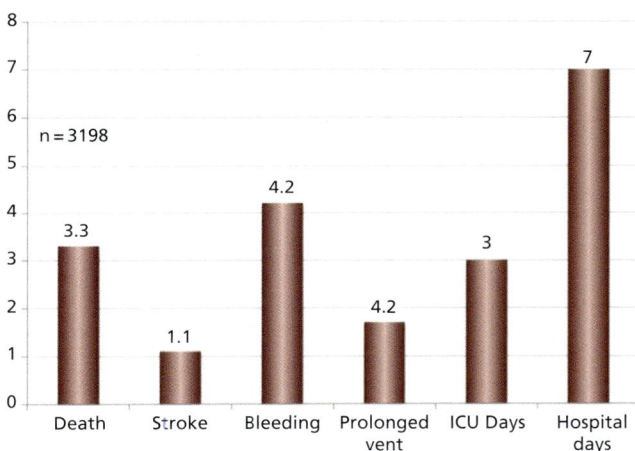

Figure 64.4 A recent review highlights the procedural safety of MitraClip leaflet repair. In a meta-analysis including over 3000 patients from 21 studies, 30-day outcomes for high risk patients showed low morbidity and mortality. Source: Philip F, *et al.* 2014 [10]. Reproduced with permission of John Wiley & Sons.

One of the striking findings from the EVEREST II trial is the safety of the MitraClip procedure. The procedure can be performed with remarkable hemodynamic stability, despite the fact that a large caliber device is manipulated in the mitral apparatus of the beating heart. In the randomized EVEREST II comparison with surgery, the MitraClip procedure was, as anticipated, significantly safer. There was virtually no procedure mortality, and the most frequent event was bleeding from the access site. Recent global experience with the device in high-risk patients has reinforced the safety profile of the therapy. Recent meta-analysis in over 3000 patients with an estimated STS risk of 10% or greater showed a 30-day mortality of only 3.3%, and a stroke rate of 1.1% within 30 days [10]. In the EVEREST REALISM high risk DMR subset, the actual 30-day mortality was 6.3% compared to a predicted mortality for this patient group with multiple comorbidities of >13% [11]. In the meta-analysis, the number of ICU days and

hospital stay were significantly shorter than in matched surgical patients. In fact, in the contemporary experience with the therapy, over 85% of patients are typically discharged directly to home without need for rehabilitation or an extended hospital stay, despite significant age and comorbidities [12].

MitraClip has been widely used internationally since CE Mark approval in 2008, based on the EVEREST I feasibility trial. The path to FDA approval has been significantly more protracted. Approval ultimately came from a subanalysis of the REALISM High Risk Registry. Of the 351 patients in the registry, a total of 127 patients were thought to have both prohibitive risk for surgery and DMR as the underlying etiology for their MR. These patients were selected by a panel of cardiovascular surgeons who felt that they had prohibitive risk for mitral valve surgery. The resultant population had a mean age of 82 years and a STS mortality risk of 13%. They had multiple comorbidities including coronary artery disease in 73%, prior cardiovascular surgery in 48%, atrial fibrillation in 71%, diabetes in 30%, and moderate to severe renal disease in 28%. Despite this very aged and complex population, the average hospital length of stay was only 2.9 days. Eighty-seven percent of these patients were discharged directly home. The safety of the procedure was reflected in a 30-day observed mortality of 6.3%, which is significantly lower when compared with the predicted mortality of 13.2%. The most important finding from this analysis was a reduction in hospitalizations for heart failure in the year after MitraClip therapy compared to the year prior, with a 73% decrease in the re-hospitalization rate (Figure 64.5). This led to the FDA approval of the MitraClip system in October 2013. The indication for use of the MitraClip delivery system is for the "percutaneous reduction of significant symptomatic MR due to primary abnormality of the mitral apparatus (degenerative MR) in patients who have been determined to have a prohibitive risk for mitral valve surgery by a heart team, which includes a cardiac surgeon experienced in mitral valve surgery and a cardiologist experienced in mitral valve disease, and in whom existent comorbidities would not preclude the expected benefit from reduction of the MR." The approved indication is thus for prohibitive surgical risk patients with DMR. In the first year after approval of the device in the USA, about 800 procedures were performed at almost 70 sites.

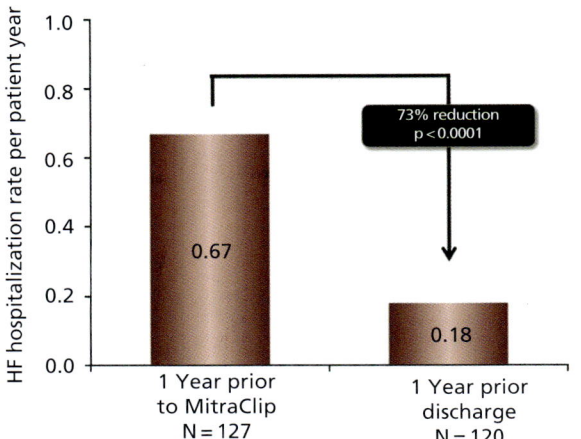

Figure 64.5 Heart failure hospitalizations were reduced by 73% after MitraClip, comparing the year prior with the year after treatment. Source: Lim DS, Reynolds MR, Feldman T, et al. 2014 [11].

While the labeled indication for use in the USA is for DMR, the preponderance of global use of the MitraClip is among patients who have FMR. As FMR is a disease of the LV, most commonly in high surgical risk patients and often associated with ischemic LV dysfunction, treating the FMR without addressing the underlying LV dysfunction might not have a favorable impact on mortality. The benefit in this setting has yet to be shown in randomized trials. Observational and retrospective surgical series have shown mixed results from mitral repair. There has been favorable LV remodeling in some studies, but also high rates of recurrent MR and no impact on mortality. In addition, the commercial international experience with MitraClip for FMR has been accrued without a systematic approach for patient selection. Therefore, the reports on this experience are from heterogenous groups, including mixed etiologies and widely varied levels of LV systolic function. The EVEREST II randomized trial subgroup analysis showed the best outcomes in patients with older age, poor LV function, and functional MR. This might have driven the preponderance of use in this setting in clinical practice. Nonetheless, the benefit of MitraClip compared with optimal medical therapy including cardiac resynchronization therapy has not been studied in a randomized clinical trial. For this reason, the FDA has not approved its use in this setting.

The benefit of the MitraClip in patients with FMR is being evaluated in the Clinical Outcomes Assessment of the MitraClip Percutaneous Therapy for High Surgical Risk Patients (COAPT) trial in the USA. The COAPT trial will randomize 430 patients in a 1 : 1 comparison of MitraClip with guideline-directed medical therapy. The safety endpoint is the composite of death, stroke, worsening renal function, left ventricular assist device (LVAD) implant, or heart transplant at 12 months. The primary effectiveness endpoint is recurrent heart failure hospitalizations. Enrollment started in 2013 and is currently ongoing.

Percutaneous indirect and direct annuloplasty

While the MitraClip therapy has been used in more than 18,000 patients worldwide, several other percutaneous repair technologies are at an earlier stage of development. Currently, approaches that include direct and indirect annuloplasty make up the other entrants into the percutaneous mitral repair field. Indirect annuloplasty can be accomplished with the Carillon Mitral Contour System (Cardiac Dimensions, Inc., Kirkland, Washington, USA). This is the next most frequently used mitral repair technology after MitraClip. Indirect annuloplasty is performed via device placement in the coronary sinus. The device is a wire structure made of nitinol. One of the most attractive features of this approach is the ease of use. A 9-Fr guide catheter is placed in the coronary sinus via internal jugular venous access. A left coronary catheter is used for monitoring of the left coronary system for potential circumflex branch compression during device insertion. Transesophageal echocardiogram is utilized to assess the effect of device cinching on MR during the procedure. The distal anchor is released in the distal coronary sinus, and then the guide catheter is pulled back to cinch the coronary sinus and shorten the posterior annular circumference. Assessments of coronary circulation and reductions in MR can be made at that point. If the results appear satisfactory, the device can be released (Figure 64.6).

Two prospective registries, TITAN I and II, have been evaluated [13]. The findings suggest significant reductions in indices of MR severity, and improvements in LV chamber dimensions and clinical parameters such as New York Heart Association (NYHA) Functional Class and 6 minute walk test. One of the concerns with this device is compression of the circumflex coronary branches, because the coronary sinus frequently crosses over these vessels [14]. While this limited the therapy during early experience, it appears that in most cases the position of the device can be adjusted to relieve coronary compression. Among patients with functional MR, approximately 90% are good candidates for this therapy based on their anatomy. A unique observation with Carillon in the TITAN trials is progressive improvements in MR reduction and LV chamber dimensions over the first year after device implantation, with associated improvement in clinical status. This observation needs to be verified in a larger trial. There have been no direct comparisons of Carillon with MitraClip, but overall the reductions in MR and improvements in clinical status with Carillon seem similar to the outcomes seen with MitraClip.

Several technologies implant a device directly into the mitral annulus to reduce the annulus circumference. Access to the annulus can be either antegrade through transseptal puncture or retrograde through the aortic valve and LV.

The Mitralign Percutaneous Annuloplasty System (Mitralign, Tewksbury, MA, USA) is predicated on surgical annular suture plication [15]. A deflectable transaortic catheter is advanced to the LV and used to deliver pledgeted anchors through the posterior annulus (Figure 64.7). These anchors can be tethered together resulting in a segmental posterior annuloplasty to shorten the annulus up to 17 mm. In 15 patients treated in a phase 1 trial, the 1-year results demonstrated at least 1+ MR reduction that was associated with improved NYHA function class and reduction in tenting area and depth. A CE approval trail has completed enrollment and is awaiting follow-up.

The Accucinch system (Guided Delivery Systems, Santa Clara, CA, USA) is based on suture annuloplasty. A retrograde femoral arterial approach to gain access to the LV aspect of the mitral annulus is used. A catheter is placed under the posterior mitral leaflet next to the anterior trigone, adjacent to the annular tissue beneath the valve (Figure 64.8). Using this catheter, up to 20 anchors can be placed from the anterior to posterior commissures along the posterior mitral annulus. These anchors are connected

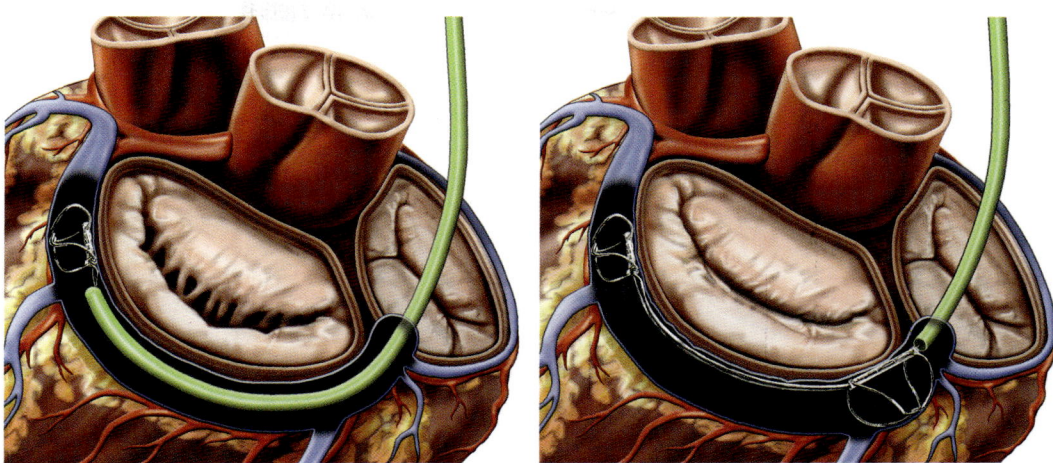

Figure 64.6 Coronary sinus annuloplasty: the Cardiac Dimensions Carillon Device: The guide catheter is introduced through jugular venous access. The device is delivered in the distal coronary sinus andf the distal anchor is released (left), and then the guide catheter is pulled back to release the proximal anchor in the coronary sinus ostium. The wireform, made of nitinol wire, after release in the coronary sinus (right). Cinching of the mitral annulus results in compression of the septal–lateral dimension and thus the regurgitant orifice. Source: Feldman T, Young A. *J Am Coll Cardiol* 2014; **63**: 2057–2068. Artwork by Craig Skaggs.

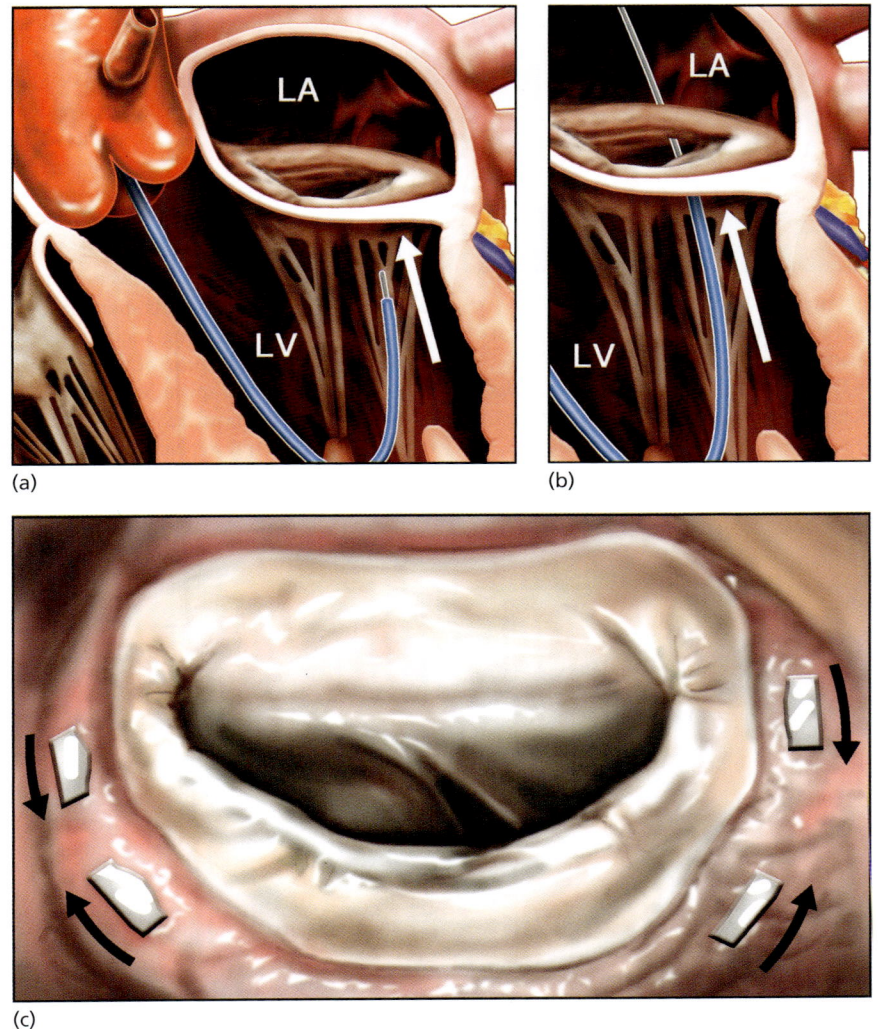

Figure 64.7 Mitralign annular plication: (a) shows the retrograde guide catheter in the LV, with the distal catheter tip under the mitral annulus, behind the posterior leaflet (arrow). A wire has been passed from the left ventricle (LV) through the annulus and into the left atrium (LA) in (b). Two pairs of wires are used to place pledgets near both commissures, shown from the left atrial side in (c). The pledgets are drawn together (arrows) to decrease the mitral annular circumference. Source: Feldman T, Young A. *J Am Coll Cardiol* 2014; **63**: 2057–2068. Artwork by Craig Skaggs.

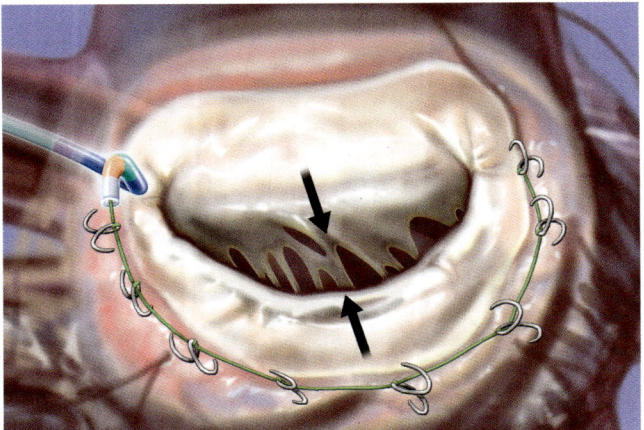

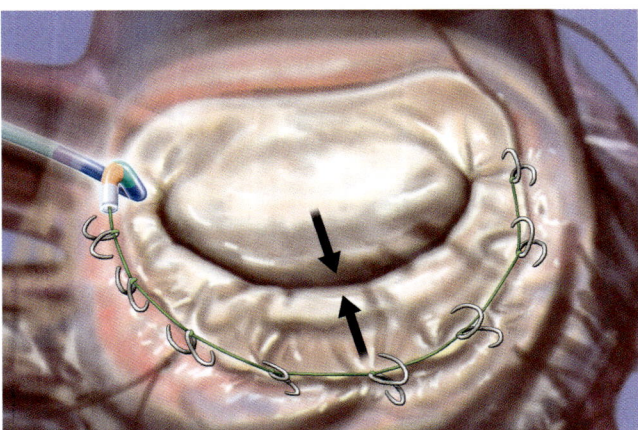

Figure 64.8 Direct annuloplasty: the Guided Delivery Systems Accucinch device is delivered through retrograde catheterization of the left ventricle (top). The arrows highlight the separation of the leaflet edges, which define the regurgitant orifice. Anchors are placed in the posterior mitral annulus and connected with a "drawstring" to cinch the annular circumference. When the cord is tightened the basilar myocardium and annulus draw the mitral leaflets together to decrease the regurgitant orifice (bottom). Source: Feldman T, Young A. *J Am Coll Cardiol* 2014; **63**: 2057–2068. Artwork by Craig Skaggs.

by a suture that can plicate the annulus to reduce the mitral annular circumference and MR.

The Cardioband (Valtech, Or Yehuda, Israel) most closely resembles a surgical annuloplasty ring [16]. It utilizes transseptal percutaneous placement of a series of small corkscrew anchors on the atrial side of the left atrium by transesophageal echocardiogram. The anchors are connected by a Dacron sleeve that can be subsequently tensioned and reduce the mitral annular circumference (Figure 64.9). Preclinical studies in a swine model have shown excellent outcomes in short term and up to 90 days. Early results in patients are promising and a CE approval trial is underway.

Another developing technique is chordal replacement. This is challenging to accomplish by completely percutaneous methods, and early work has been via LV apical access during a beating heart surgery [17,18].

Transcatheter mitral valve replacement

Transcatheter mitral valve replacement (TMVR) as a therapy for FMR is also developing, with several different devices having first in human experience in the last 2 years. The effort to develop TMVR is just beginning, with the total number of treated patients in low double-digits at the time of this writing. Early experience with valve-in-valve implants of transcatheter aortic valve replacement (TAVR) devices for degenerated mitral bioprosthetic valves and native calcific mitral stenosis have demonstrated proof of concept for TMVR [19,20]. The obvious appeal of replacement is the elimination of residual MR and the potential for recurrence of MR that is common with percutaneous repair devices. The challenges facing development of these devices include larger area and asymmetrical "D" shape of the mitral valve, lack of calcium for anchoring, and more complicated delivery route compared to TAVR. The large mitral area and annuls diameter necessitates bulkier, larger profile devices. Anchoring requires special valve frame features dedicated to the purpose. Delivery in the early development has been mostly transapical, with the hope that transseptal delivery will eventually be most frequent. The question is often asked: will transcatheter mitral replacement eliminate the need for repair approaches? Transcatheter mitral repair and replacement interventions will become complementary solutions to accommodate the variability of the disease. Algorithms for patient-specific approach

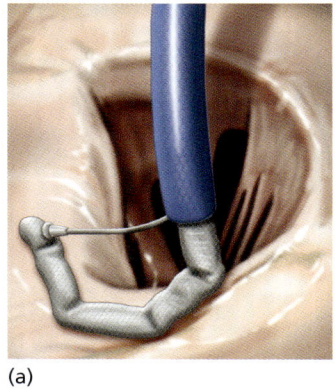

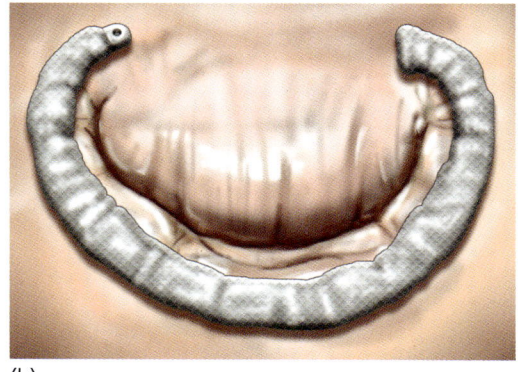

(a)   (b)

Figure 64.9 Valtech CardioBand. (a) A transseptal guide catheter delivering the annuloplasty ring in segments. Each segment is sequentially anchored into the annulus. (b) The final annuloplasty ring encircling the posterior leaflet. Source: Feldman T, Young A. *J Am Coll Cardiol* 2014; **63**: 2057–2068. Artwork by Craig Skaggs.

will evolve as outcomes in the several patient subpopulations become available. Imaging screening and guidance will have a fundamental role in determining the relative role of these procedures in the future.

Interactive multiple choice questions are available for this chapter on www.wiley. com/go/dangas/cardiology

References

1 Alfieri O, Maisano F, De Bonis M, *et al.* The double-orifice technique in mitral valve repair: a simple solution for complex problems. *J Thorac Cardiovasc Surg* 2001; **122**: 674–681.

2 Alfieri O, De Bonis M. Genesis of the surgical edge-to-edge repai. In Feldman T, St. Goar F. (eds) *Percutaneous Mitral Leaflet Repair.* Informa, London: 2012; 173–178.

3 Maisano F, Schreuder JJ, Oppizzi M, Fiorani B, Fino C, Alfieri O. The double-orifice technique as a standardized approach to treat mitral regurgitation due to severe myxomatous disease: surgical technique. *Eur J Cardiothroac Surg* 2000; **17**: 201–205.

4 St. Goar F. Development of percutaneous edge-to-edge repair: The MitraClip® story. In Feldman T, St. Goar F. (eds) *Percutaneous Mitral Leaflet Repair.* Informa, London: 2012; 31–35.

5 Feldman T, Wasserman HS, Herrmann HC, *et al.* Percutaneous mitral valve repair using the edge-to-edge technique: six-month results of the EVEREST Phase I Clinical Trial. *J Am Coll Cardiol* 2005; **46**: 2134–2140.

6 Feldman T, Foster E, Glower D, *et al.;* EVEREST II Investigators. Percutaneous repair or surgery for mitral regurgitation. *N Engl J Med* 2011; **364**: 1395–1406.

7 Mauri L, Glower DG, Apruzzese P, *et al.;* EVEREST II Investigators. Four-year results of a randomized controlled trial of percutaneous repair versus surgery for mitral regurgitation. *J Am Coll Cardiol* 2013; **62**: 317–328.

8 Whitlow P, Feldman T, Pedersen W, *et al.* The EVEREST II High Risk Study: acute and 12 month results with catheter based mitral valve leaflet repair. *J Am Coll Cardiol* 2012; **59**: 130–139.

9 Glower D, Kar S, Lim DS, *et al.* Percutaneous MitraClip device therapy for mitral regurgitation in 351 patients: high risk subset of the EVEREST II Study. *J Am Coll Cardiol* 2014; **64**: 172–181.

10 Philip F, Athappan G, Tuzcu EM, Svensson LG, Kapadia SR. MitraClip for severe symptomatic mitral regurgitation in patients at high surgical risk: a comprehensive systematic review. *Catheter Cardiovasc Interv* 2014; **84**: 581–590.

11 Lim DS, Reynolds MR, Feldman T, *et al.* Improved functional status and quality of life in prohibitive surgical risk patients with degenerative mitral regurgitation following transcatheter mitral valve repair with the MitraClip system. *J Am Coll Cardiol* 2014; **64**: 182–192.

12 Schillinger W, Hünlich M, Baldus S, *et al.* Acute outcomes after MitraClip(R) therapy in highly aged patients: results from the German TRAnscatheter Mitral valve Interventions (TRAMI) Registry. *EuroIntervention* 2013; **9**: 84–90.

13 Siminiak T, Wu JC, Haude M, *et al.* Treatment of functional mitral regurgitation by percutaneous annuloplasty: results of the TITAN Trial. *Eur J Heart Fail* 2012; **14**(8): 931–938.

14 Choure AJ, Garcia MJ, Hesse B, *et al.* In vivo analysis of the anatomical relationship of coronary sinus to mitral annulus and left circumflex coronary artery using cardiac multidetector computed tomography: implications for percutaneous coronary sinus mitral annuloplasty. *J Am Coll Cardiol* 2006; **48**: 1938–1945.

15 Mandinov L, Bullesfeld L, Kuck KH, Grube E. Early insight into Mitralign direct annuloplasty for treatment of functional mitral regurgitation. *Interv Cardiol Rev* 2011; **6**: 170–172.

16 Maisano F, Vanermen H, Seeburger J, *et al.* Direct access transcatheter mitral annuloplasty with a sutureless and adjustable device: preclinical experience. *Eur J Card Thorac* 2012; **42**: 524–529.

17 Seeburger J, Leontjev S, Neumuth M, *et al.* Trans-apical beating-heart implantation of neo-chordae to mitral valve leaflets: results of an acute animal study. *Eur J Card Thorac Surg* 2012; **41**: 173–176.

18 Bajona P, Katz WE, Daly RC, Zehr KJ, Speziali G. Beating-heart, off-pump mitral valve repair by implantation of artificial chordae tendineae: an acute in vivo animal study. *J Thorac Cardiovasc Surg* 2009; **137**: 188–193.

19 Guerrero M, Greenbaum A, O'Neill W. First in human percutaneous implantation of a balloon expandable transcatheter heart valve in a severely stenosed native mitral valve. *Catheter Cardiovasc Interv* 2014; **83**: E287–291.

20 Himbert D, Bouleti C, Iung B, *et al.* Transcatheter valve replacement in patients with severe mitral valve disease and annular calcification. *J Am Coll Cardiol* 2014; **64**: 2557–2558.

CHAPTER 65

Balloon Mitral Valvuloplasty

C.N. Manjunath[1], Nagaraja Moorthy[1], and Upendra Kaul[2]
[1]Sri Jayadeva Institute of Cardiovascular Sciences and Research, Bangalore, India
[2]Fortis Escorts Heart Institute, New Delhi, India

Although the prevalence of rheumatic fever has greatly decreased in the Western world, mitral stenosis (MS) still results in significant morbidity and mortality especially in developing countries. Rheumatic heart disease is responsible for valvular MS in nearly almost all cases. MS occurs when stenosis of the valve occurs from leaflet thickening, commissural fusion (Figure 65.1), and chordal shortening or fusion restricting blood flow from the left atrium to the left ventricle during diastole. This ultimately results in increased pulmonary capillary wedge pressure, an elevated pulmonary vascular resistance, and right ventricular dysfunction. Echocardiography has a major role in decision-making for MS, allowing confirmation of diagnosis, quantification of stenosis severity and its hemodynamic consequences, and guides management options.

Anatomic considerations

The mitral valve (MV) apparatus is a complex structure consisting of annulus fibrosus, mitral leaflets, chordae tendinae, papillary muscles, and the posterior wall of the left ventricle. All these components should be considered functionally as a single unit, because derangements of any one can affect overall MV performance.

The normal mitral valve area (MVA) is 4.0–6.0 cm². An MVA of >1.5 cm² usually does not produce symptoms. As the severity of MS increases, cardiac output becomes subnormal at rest and fails to increase during exercise. This is the main reason for considering MS significant when MVA is ≤1.5 cm². When the MVA is reduced to 1.5 cm² or less, symptoms become severe and complications develop.

Balloon mitral valvuloplasty
Historical aspect

The treatment of MS has been revolutionized since the development of balloon mitral valvuloplasty (BMV). In 1982, Kanji Inoue, a Japanese cardiac surgeon, first developed the idea that a degenerated mitral valve could be inflated using a balloon with differential compliance [1]. In India, Lock *et al.* [2] first reported the use of a cylindrical balloon for mitral valvuloplasty. Subsequently, the idea of a double-balloon technique was introduced from Saudi Arabia [3] as a potential alternative method for balloon commissurotomy. The double balloon

technique requires that two guidewires be positioned in the left ventricular apex, through which two floating balloon catheters are then advanced across the mitral valve orifice. However, the double-balloon technique is technically more demanding and thus often requires a longer procedure time, which can lead to inadvertent complications. The guidewire positioned in the left ventricular apex sometimes induces perforation of the apex, leading to cardiac tamponade. Therefore, Inoue's single-balloon technique has become the most popular method for performing BMV in most parts of the world. The mechanism of BMV is the same as the already abandoned closed mitral commissurotomy [4]. Pathologic studies have disclosed that the main mechanism of successful BMV is a split of the commissures. Before 1984, when Inoue *et al.* [1] first described the clinical application of percutaneous BMV, surgical mitral commissurotomy was the preferred option for patients who had severe MS. Since its introduction, percutaneous mitral commissurotomy has demonstrated good immediate and mid-term results [5,6] and has replaced surgical mitral commissurotomy as the preferred treatment of rheumatic MS in appropriate candidates.

Indications and recommendations for percutaneous balloon mitral valvuloplasty

Indications for BMV have been formulated by the American College of Cardiology (ACC) and the American Heart Association (AHA) [7,8].

Class I recommendations

1 BMV is recommended for symptomatic patients with severe MS (mitral valve area ≤1.5 cm², stage D) and favorable valve morphology in the absence of left atrial thrombus or moderate–severe mitral regurgitation (MR) (level of evidence A).

2 BMV is effective for asymptomatic patients with moderate or severe MS and valve morphology that is favorable for BMV who have pulmonary hypertension (pulmonary artery systolic pressure greater than 50 mmHg at rest or greater than 60 mmHg with exercise) in the absence of left atrial thrombus or moderate to severe MR (level of evidence C).

Interventional Cardiology: Principles and Practice, Second Edition. Edited by George D. Dangas, Carlo Di Mario, and Nicholas N. Kipshidze.
© 2017 John Wiley & Sons, Ltd. Published 2017 by John Wiley & Sons, Ltd.

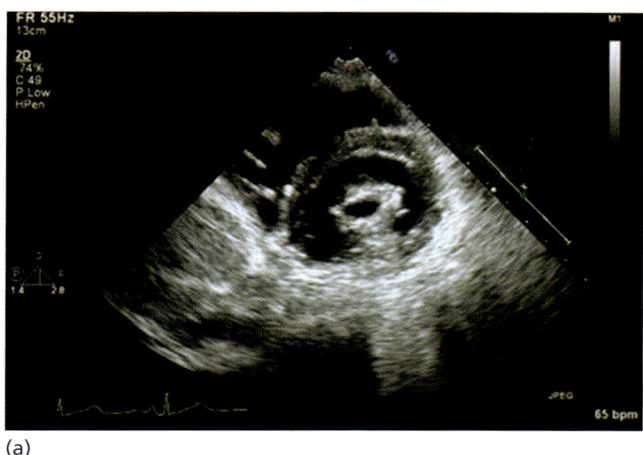
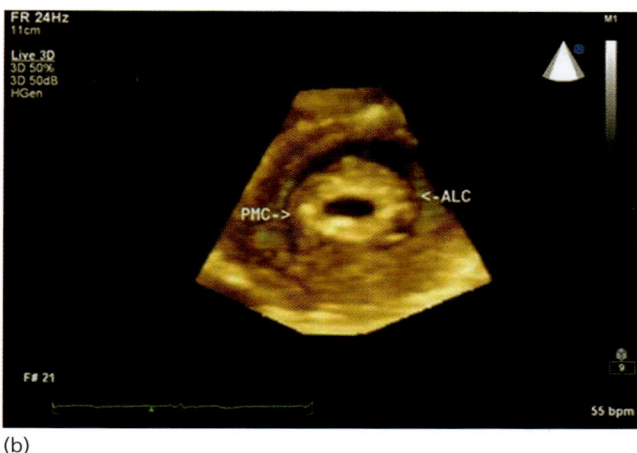

Figure 65.1 (a) Transthoracic 2D; and (b) 3D echocardiogram showing thickened mitral valve with bicommissural fusion giving "fish-mouth" appearance.

Class IIa recommendations

1 BMV is reasonable for asymptomatic patients with very severe MS (mitral valve area ≤1.0 cm², stage C) and favorable valve morphology in the absence of left atrial thrombus or moderate–severe MR (level of evidence C).

Class IIb recommendations

1 BMV can be considered for asymptomatic patients with severe MS (mitral valve area ≤1.5 cm², stage C) and valve morphology favorable for BMV in the absence of left atrial thrombus or moderate–severe MR who have new onset of atrial fibrillation (AF) (level of evidence C).

2 BMV can be considered for symptomatic patients with MVA greater than 1.5 cm² if there is evidence of hemodynamically significant MS based on pulmonary artery wedge pressure greater than 25 mmHg or mean mitral valve gradient greater than 15 mmHg during exercise (level of evidence C).

3 BMV can be considered for severely symptomatic patients (NYHA Class III–IV) with severe MS (mitral valve area ≤1.5 cm², stage D) who have a suboptimal valve anatomy and who are not candidates for surgery or at high risk for surgery (level of evidence C).

Contraindications

The following are contraindications for BMV (i.e., Class III recommendations).

1 BMV is not indicated for patients with mild MS (level of evidence C).

2 BMV should not be performed in patients with moderate–severe MR or left atrial body thrombus, bicommissural calcium (level of evidence C). However, using a modified over-the-wire technique, BMV can be safely carried out in patients with types Ia, Ib, and II or LA/LAA thrombus after 8–10 weeks of anticoagulation.

Peri-procedural care

Preprocedural planning

Physical examination is an important initial step in assessing the pliability of the valve. Accentuation of the first heart sound (S1) occurs when the mitral valve leaflets are pliable. Marked calcification or thickening of the mitral valve leaflets reduces the amplitude

of S1, probably because of diminished motion of the leaflets. The opening snap of the mitral valve is caused by a sudden tensing of the valve leaflets after the valve cusps have completed their opening excursion. It is most readily audible at the apex; if present, it indicates that the mitral valve has at least some mobility.

The likelihood of hemodynamic benefit and the risk of complications with BMV are predicted by the morphologic features of the valve leaflets and subvalvular structures. With rigid, thickened valves that exhibit extensive subvalvular fibrosis and calcification, results will be suboptimal [7].

Role of echocardiography in BMV: valve assessment and case selection

Echocardiography is the primary modality of evaluation for patients who are planned for BMV. It is essential for the preprocedural evaluation of patients, case selection, intraprocedural monitoring, and the post-procedural assessment and follow-up (Box 65.1). The primary aim of echocardiographic assessment is to find the suitable valve for BMV and identify high risk echocardiographic features that may result in complications. The echocardiographic scoring system developed by Wilkins *et al.* [9] is useful for estimating likely outcomes of BMV (Table 65.1).

In this system, points are given for leaflet mobility, valve thickening, subvalvular thickening, and valvular calcification. The final score is determined by adding the points for each of the components (maximum, 16 points). A score of 8 or lower is usually associated with excellent immediate and long-term results for BMV, whereas scores higher than 8 are associated with less impressive results, including the risk of development of MR. However, in our institution, 30–35% patients undergoing BMV have Wilkins scores of 8–12, and this group of patients have optimal immediate and long-term results with comparable complications.

An important factor in determining the suitability of the valve for BMV is the presence of commissural calcification, assessed by means of a two-dimensional echocardiography in short-axis view. The presence or absence of severe calcification of one or both commissures is an independent determinant of near-term success during the procedure, as well as long-term outcome [10]. In asymmetric involvement of the commissures, in which one commissure is heavily fibrosed or calcified, splitting can occur in the opposite commissure. However, calcification of both commissures is considered as absolute contraindication for BMV as it poses increased risk of leaflet tear. The presence of predominant subvalvular fibrosis and calcification results in suboptimal results from BMV because it is unclear that balloon dilatation is able to split chordal fusion.

Several echocardiographic scoring systems have been proposed as a guide to the selection of patients for BMV. Although studies using these methods have been shown to correlate with the immediate results, no single parameter is able to predict success or complications independently. Therefore, these criteria should be used only as a guide to the severity of the individual morphologic variables of the mitral valve.

BMV is now the procedure of choice for selected MS patients. Optimally, a team comprising an interventionalist and a cardiac imaging expert collaborates during the preprocedural and peri-

procedural assessment. Targeted echocardiography not only is critical to the selection of candidates for BMV but also can be of great value in guiding the procedure and assessing the results [11]. Simultaneous echocardiography (transthoracic, transesophageal, or intracardiac echocardiography) directly illustrates the relation of the catheter to myocardial structures.

In patients whose anatomy is distorted by an enlarged LA or kyphoscoliosis, echocardiography can be used to ensure that the catheter crosses the atrial septum at the level of the fossa ovalis. Catheter crossing elsewhere can give rise to complications, and through the muscular portion of the septum can result in difficult manipulation of the balloon catheter into left ventricle. Echocardiography is useful for directing the catheter across the mitral valve; the balloon initially tends to position itself toward the lateral annulus in the left atrium. Finally, hemodynamic evaluation of the transmitral gradient and the severity of MR is easily performed by means of Doppler echocardiography [11].

Patient preparation

Usually, BMV is carried out with the patient under local anaesthesia and moderate sedation. The patient remains in the supine position during the procedure.

Techniques
Approach

Retrograde (transarterial) and antegrade (transvenous) approaches to BMV have been described. The retrograde approach eliminates the risk of atrial septal defect but carries a risk of potential arterial damage; because of its complexity, it has now been largely abandoned [12]. Currently, the antegrade approach with transseptal catheterization is more widely used. It is usually performed through the femoral vein or, exceptionally, through the jugular vein [13].

Choice of technique
Double-balloon technique

In this approach, after transseptal catheterization, a balloon-tipped catheter is advanced into the left ventricle. One or two exchange guidewires are advanced through the lumen of the balloon-tipped

---

Box 65.1 Role of two-dimensional Doppler echocardiography in the evaluation of patients undergoing balloon mitral valvotomy.

Preprocedural evaluation:
- Severity of valve disease
- Mitral valve gradient
- Mitral valve area
- Severity of mitral regurgitation
- Left atrial/LA appendage thrombus
- Subvalvular apparatus
- Valvular/commissural calcification
- Interatrial septal bulge/aneurysm
- Associated other valvular disease
- Preprocedural pulmonary artery pressure and right ventricular function

During balloon mitral valvotomy:
- Assistance in transseptal puncture
- Changes in valve area or gradient
- Changes in mitral regurgitation
- Complications (pericardial effusion, tamponade, atrial septal defect, etc.)

Post-procedural follow-up and long-term results:
- Restenosis
- Changes in mitral regurgitation grade
- Residual atrial septal defects
- Pulmonary artery pressure
- Ventricular size and function
- Progress of other valve disease

Table 65.1 Echocardiography scoring system (Wilkins score) to predict outcome of mitral balloon valvuloplasty.

Grade	Mobility	Thickening	Calcification	Subvalvular thickening
1	Highly mobile valve with only leaflet tips restricted	Leaflets near normal in thickness (4–5 mm)	A single area of increased echo brightness	Minimal thickening just below the mitral leaflets
2	Leaflet mid and base portions have normal mobility	Midleaflets normal, considerable thickening of margins (5–8 mm)	Scattered areas of brightness confined to leaflet margins	Thickening of chordal structures extending to one-third of the chordal length
3	Valve continues to move forward in diastole, mainly from the base	Thickening extending through the entire leaflet (5–8 mm)	Brightness extending into the mid-portions of the leaflets	Thickening extended to distal third of the chords
4	No or minimal forward movement of the leaflets in diastole	Considerable thickening of all leaflet tissue (>8–10 mm)	Extensive brightness throughout much of the leaflet tissue	Extensive thickening and shortening of all chordal structures extending down to the papillary muscles

The total score is the sum of the four items and ranges between 4 and 16.

catheter and positioned in the apex of the left ventricle or, less frequently, in the ascending aorta.

The balloon-tipped catheter is withdrawn over the guidewires, and the interatrial septum is dilated with the use of a peripheral angioplasty balloon (6–8 mm in diameter). Finally, the valvotomy balloons (15–20 mm in diameter) are advanced over the guidewires and positioned across the mitral valve and dilated [12].

Multitrack technique

Bonhoeffer *et al.* [14] have described the use of the multitrack system, which is a refinement of the double-balloon technique that employs a monorail system requiring only one guidewire. This technique allows easier dilatation than the standard technique; however, clinical experience with the multitrack system is still limited.

Metallic commissurotomy

Cribier *et al.* [15] introduced the metallic commissurotomy in the 1990s. This procedure is as efficacious as balloon commissurotomy, but it is more demanding on the operator than the Inoue technique and appears to carry a higher risk of pericardial effusion and tamponade as a consequence of the presence of a stiff guidewire in the left ventricle. The potential advantage of the procedure is its cost-effectiveness.

Inoue balloon technique

The Inoue balloon technique, first described in 1984 [1], is still the most commonly employed technique today. Wide experience has now been acquired by a number of groups worldwide. In developing countries, Inoue prototype Accura Balloon (Vascular Concepts) is routinely used with comparable success rates.

Vascular access

A 7 Fr sheath is inserted in the right femoral vein for transseptal access; a 5 Fr sheath is placed in the right or left femoral artery for left heart catheterization. Two pressure transducers are required for simultaneous left atrial, left ventricular pressures. A pigtail catheter is placed in the aortic root (left/non-coronary sinus), and aortic pressures are obtained.

Transseptal puncture

Transseptal catheterization is a vital component of BMV. The goal of transseptal catheterization is to cross from the right atrium to the left atrium through the fossa ovalis. Puncture of the fossa ovalis itself is safe; the danger of the transseptal approach lies in the possibility that the needle and catheter will puncture an adjacent structure (e.g., the coronary sinus, the posterior wall of the right atrium, or the aortic root). To minimize the risk of complications, the operator must have a detailed knowledge of the regional anatomy of the atrial septum.

Equipment for septal puncture Essential instruments include a pre-shaped transseptal sheath with introducer (Mullins sheath) and a pre-shaped transseptal puncture needle (Brockenbrough needle).

Landmarks for septal puncture Transseptal puncture if usually carried out under fluoroscopic guidance. There are certain fluoroscopic landmarks that are used to identify the location of fossa ovalis. The pigtail marks the location of aortic valve. In anteroposterior view, the fossa ovalis lies inferior and medial to the aortic valve. To select the optimal transseptal puncture site, two imaginary lines are drawn: (i) the vertical midline; and (ii) the horizontal M line. The point of intersection of vertical "midline" and horizontal "M line" locates the site of septal puncture.

As seen in Figure 65.2a, a horizontal line is drawn from the tip of the pigtail catheter placed in the non-coronary sinus of the aortic root and the lateral border of the left atrium. The vertical line drawn from the midpoint of this line is the *vertical midline*. The *horizontal M line* is the line crossing the center of the mitral annulus. It is derived from a diastolic stop frame of diagnostic left ventriculography obtained in right anterior oblique (RAO) 30° projection (Figure 65.2b). The plane of the mitral annulus is obtained by joining fulcrum points of the mitral valve. From the midpoint of this line, a horizontal line is drawn toward the vertebral body. This is referenced to a vertebral body. The ideal puncture site is the intersection of the vertical midline and the M line. Usually, the intersection point will be half to one vertebral body below the horizontal line drawn from the aortic root in the vertical midline.

In most institutions the septal puncture is carried out in left anterior oblique (LAO) 40°, or in left lateral projection as shown in Figure 65.2c. In these projections the ideal septal puncture site corresponds to the midpoint between the pigtail catheter placed in aortic sinus and the spine. The position should also be confirmed in RAO 30° projection (Figure 65.2d).

The procedural technique (see Video 65.1)

The procedure is always performed via a femoral approach with a 8–9 Fr sheath in the femoral vein and a 5 Fr sheath in the femoral artery, with the patient under light sedation. After bolus administration of 1000 U heparin, right heart catheterization is performed. The Mullins sheath is advanced over a 0.032-inch guidewire into the superior vena cava, preferably into left innominate vein. The pigtail catheter is placed in the aortic root in the non-coronary cusp. A standard Brockenbrough needle is then advanced into the Mullins sheath about 2–3 cm short of the tip. It is useful to keep a finger between the base of the Brockenbrough needle and hub of the Mullins sheath to prevent inadvertent advancement of the needle. While most operators attach a 2 mL contrast-filled syringe, preferable with a Luer lock, it is also possible to attach the needle to a pressure transducer. The entire assembly of the Mullins sheath with the needle is then gradually withdrawn in the AP projection under fluoroscopy into the right atrium, taking care that the Brockenbrough needle points at the 4 o'clock position. The assembly first descends from the superior vena cava into the right atrium and then along the thick part of the interatrial septum. The entire assembly is then withdrawn slowly until it reaches the level of the aortic valve. During this manoeuvre, care is taken that needle continues to point at 4 o'clock position. It is then gradually withdrawn further below the level of the aortic valve about half to one vertebral space, to lie along the interatrial septum at the expected location of the fossa ovalis. The position of the needle is then confirmed in RAO 30°, LAO 45° or dead lateral.

In RAO 30°, the interatrial septum is generally enface and the needle tip should point away from the operator, and also the needle should lie posterior and inferior to the plane of the aorta. In the lateral view, the needle should be facing posteriorly toward the spine and should be halfway from pigtail to spine. The needle should not be too low. The position of the needle needs to be confirmed in all three views for a safe and optimal septal puncture. Transesophageal (TEE) or intracardiac echocardiography (ICE) can be useful in identifying the anatomic location of the interatrial septum relative to the right atrium. The septal indentation by Brockenbrough needle guides the intended site of septal puncture. Echocardiography also helps in early detection of complications such as pericardial effusion, perforation, and tamponade. However, in the authors' institution, TEE/ICE is not routinely used during

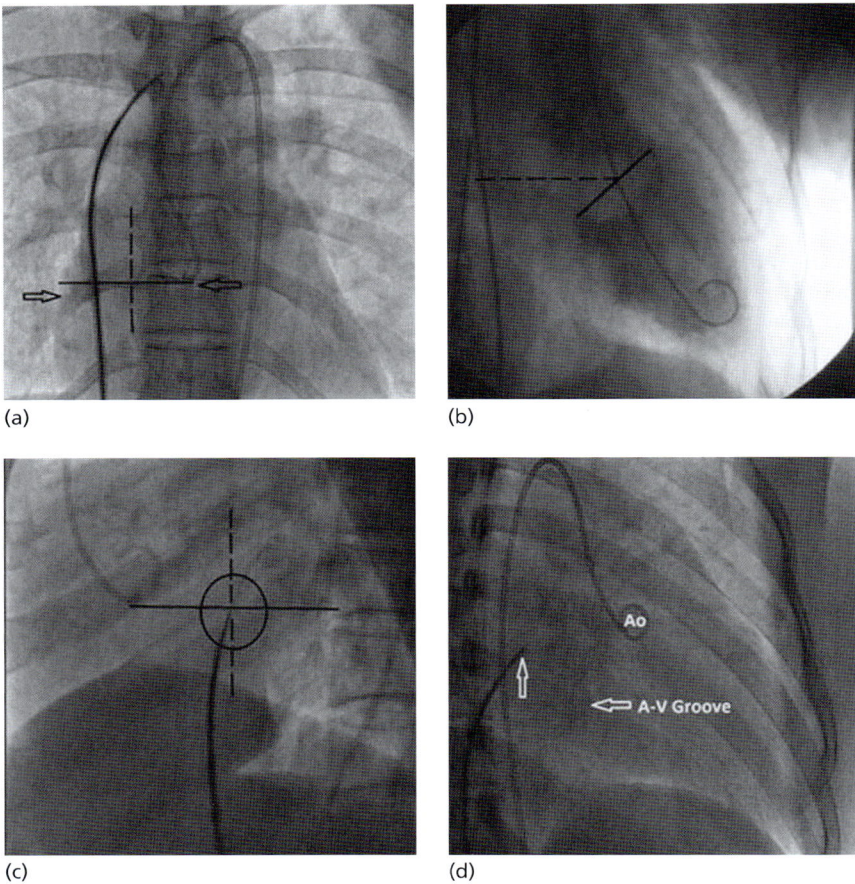

Figure 65.2 Fluroscopic landmarks for septal puncture. (a) An imaginary horizontal line is drawn from point T to point L where the line intersects the lateral border of the left atrium. The dotted vertical line crossing the midpoint between T and L is the midline. (b) The M line is obtained using the left ventriculogram with a stop frame RAO view. The target site for septal puncture is located at the intersecting point of the vertical midline and the horizontal M line. (c) Fluoroscopic landmark for septal puncture in LAO projection and (d) in RAO projection.

septal puncture. Transthoracic echocardiography is sufficient in majority of patients with good echo window to guide and confirm site of septal puncture and to recognize early tamponade. A gentle probing in this area may often permit left atrium entry through the stretched fossa ovalis without an actual need for needle puncture.

Successful entry into the left atrium should be confirmed both by recording a left atrial pressure waveform and by withdrawing oxygenated blood or by demonstrating the typical fluoroscopic appearance of the left atrium during a small contrast injection through the needle. Once the catheter is safely placed in the left atrium, heparin (usually 100 U/kg) is administered for anticoagulation. Anticoagulation time is monitored during the procedures to maintain appropriate levels of anticoagulation. Box 65.2 summarizes the steps of the septal puncture procedure.

Dilatation of interatrial septal puncture site

After advancing the Brockenbrough needle, a coiled-tip guidewire is placed into the left atrium through the Brockenbrough sheath. The septal dilator (14 Fr polyethylene tube with a thinner tip 70 cm in length) is advanced over the coiled-tip wire to facilitate the entry of an Inoue balloon catheter.

> **Box 65.2** Steps of septal puncture
>
> Step 1 Mullins sheath with Brockenbrough needle positioned in superior vena cava. Pigtail catheter positioned in aorta at the level of aortic valve
> Step 2 Mullins sheath with Brockenbrough needle withdrawn into the right atrium to lie half to one vertebra below the level of the pigtail catheter in AP projection
> Step 3 Brockenbrough needle rotated to 4–5 o'clock position. Optimal position confirmed in AP, RAO, and lateral/LAO projection. (Refer above described fluoroscopic landmarks)
> Step 4 Left atrial (LA) entry by probing around fossa ovalis site with tip of Mullins sheath or septal puncture performed by protruding the Brockenbrough needle slightly beyond the Mullins sheath
> Step 5 Confirm left atrial entry by withdrawal of oxygenated blood , pressure recording showing LA pressure tracing and by contrast injection into LA chamber

Selection of balloon catheter

The most commonly used balloon catheters during BMV are the triple lumen Inoue balloon catheter (Toray International America Inc.) and the double lumen Accura balloon catheter (Vascular Concepts, Halstead, UK). Both Accura and Inoue mitral valvotomy balloons are effective in providing relief from hemodynamically significant MS in terms of gain in valve area and reduction in transmitral gradient. Both have similar procedural success and complication rates, restenosis, and follow-up events at 1 year [16,17]. A balloon catheter system for accomplishing BMV consists of the following devices: Inoue/Accura balloon catheter, metallic stiffening cannula (18 gauge, 80 cm in length) for stretching and stiffening the Inoue balloon catheter, guidewire for BMV (0.028 inches in diameter, 180 cm in length), dilator (14 Fr polyethylene tube with a thinner tip 70 cm in length) for dilating the puncture site of the femoral vein and atrial septum, and a stylet (wire with J-shaped tip, 0.038 inches in diameter, 80 cm in length) for directing the Inoue balloon toward the mitral orifice.

The balloon diameter size is chosen on the basis of the patient's weight, height, and body surface area. Most commonly, the reference size of the balloon is calculated according to Hung's formula [18]: the patient's height (in cm) is rounded to the nearest zero and divided by 10 and 10 added to the ratio to yield the reference size (in mm), for example, if the patient's height is 158 cm, then reference diameter will be 160/10 + 10 = 26 mm.

In case of pliable, non-calcified valves with mitral regurgitation of ≤1+, a balloon catheter with a nominal reference size calculated according to Hung's formula can be used. In contrast in patients with high risk features of developing severe MR (valvular calcification, severe subvalvular stenosis, and non-pliable valves), a balloon catheter two size smaller than reference size is selected. However, after each dilatation, echocardiography should be reviewed for new appearance of significant MR or worsening of pre-existing MR before the next inflation.

At the authors' institution, initial inflation is carried out at 2 mm less than the reference diameter and size is upgraded after carefully assessing hemodynamics and MR. The balloon catheter upsizing should be *guided, graded, and gated* to achieve optimal results.

Crossing the mitral valve

In the next step, the Inoue/Accura balloon catheter is advanced over the coiled-tip wire. Once the balloon catheter has crossed the interatrial septum, the catheter should be placed in the left atrium so that the catheter forms a loop with the tip facing toward the mitral valve orifice. Several techniques are described for entering mitral valve: (i) vertical method, (ii) direct method, (iii) sliding method, (iv) posterior loop method, and (v) modified over-the-wire technique. The stylet is inserted in the balloon catheter, and the stylet is given 2–3 anticlockwise rotations so that the balloon catheter with stylet is moved together toward the mitral valve orifice. In RAO view, the deflated Inoue balloon catheter is advanced until the tip of the catheter has crossed the mitral valve into the left ventricle. Once the balloon is close to the valve, a bobbing movement or "woodpecking sign" of the balloon can be observed. Once the balloon catheter is across the valve orifice, a fall in the aortic pressure may be noticed. ECG showing ventricular ectopic indicates that the balloon is in the left ventricle.

Once the balloon catheter has been inserted into the left ventricle, the distal portion of the balloon is inflated with contrast media (diluted 1 : 1) using a specially graduated syringe. The catheter is then pulled until resistance is felt when the balloon catheter aligns across the mitral valve. Once this happens, inflate the balloon fully to expand the proximal part of the balloon. The valve will be stretched and the commissures will give way. Figure 65.3 shows a step-by-step demonstration of the BMV procedure.

During inflation of the balloon, the appearance of a deformed distal balloon (balloon impasse sign/balloon compression sign) suggests entrapment in the subvalvular apparatus as shown in Figure 65.4. In this situation, further inflation should not be performed and the balloon should be repositioned to a location that is more proximal to the mitral orifice to avoid trauma to the subvalvular apparatus.

After each dilatation, the operator should obtain the left atrial pressure through the middle port of the Inoue catheter and the left ventricular pressure through the pigtail catheter simultaneously. If the pressure gradient between the left atrial pressure and the simultaneously obtained left ventricular pressure does not decrease, the balloon size is increased in 1-mm increments until the pressure gradient decreases or substantial worsening of mitral regurgitation occurs. In addition, two-dimensional echocardiographic observations are performed after each dilatation. To assess mitral valve orifice area after each dilatation, planimetry of the valve orifice with two-dimensional echocardiography should be adopted rather than the pressure half-time method on continuous Doppler waveform, because pressure half-time-derived orifice area might be inaccurate in this acute setting [19].

If one of the three following events is encountered—decrease in the pressure gradient between the left atrium and the left ventricle, occurrence of significant mitral regurgitation, or substantial splitting of the commissure—further dilatation is not performed (Box 65.3; Figure 65.5) [20].

BMV in difficult scenarios

BMV in LA/LAA clot

Left atrial thrombus occurs in 3–13% of patients with MS and its presence is generally considered as a contraindication for BMV. Systemic embolization occurs in 0.3–0.8% of patients during or shortly after the procedure and represents a potentially devastating complication. TEE is recommended before the procedure to determine the presence of left atrial thrombus, with specific attention paid to the left atrial appendage. If a thrombus is found, 3 months of anticoagulation with warfarin can result in resolution of the thrombus.

Left atrial thrombus in patients with MS has long been regarded as a contraindication for BMV. In selected patients with MS with left atrial thrombus (types Ia, Ib, and IIa) (Figure 65.6) [21], BMV can be performed safely with the modified over-the-wire technique (Figure 65.7) [22]. Systemic thromboembolism, technical failures, and other complications are very rare when performed by experienced operators.

Our modification of the over-the-wire technique is safe, effective, and does not require any additional accessories. Using this technique, BMV can be performed, even in difficult cases wherein the conventional method of crossing the mitral valve has failed. This technique involves direct positioning of a coiled Inoue wire into the left ventricle through the Mullin sheath followed by introduction of an Inoue catheter over the wire as illustrated in Figure 65.7.

BMV in giant left atrium/interatrial septal aneurysm

The size of the left atrium with or without interatrial septal (IAS) aneurysm has been noted to have a significant influence on outcome as in patients with large left atria, technical difficulties can be encountered in performing the transseptal puncture and crossing the MV orifice. In such situations increasing the curvature of the Brockenbrough needle or probing around the fossa ovalis assists in safe septal puncture. When difficulty is encountered in crossing

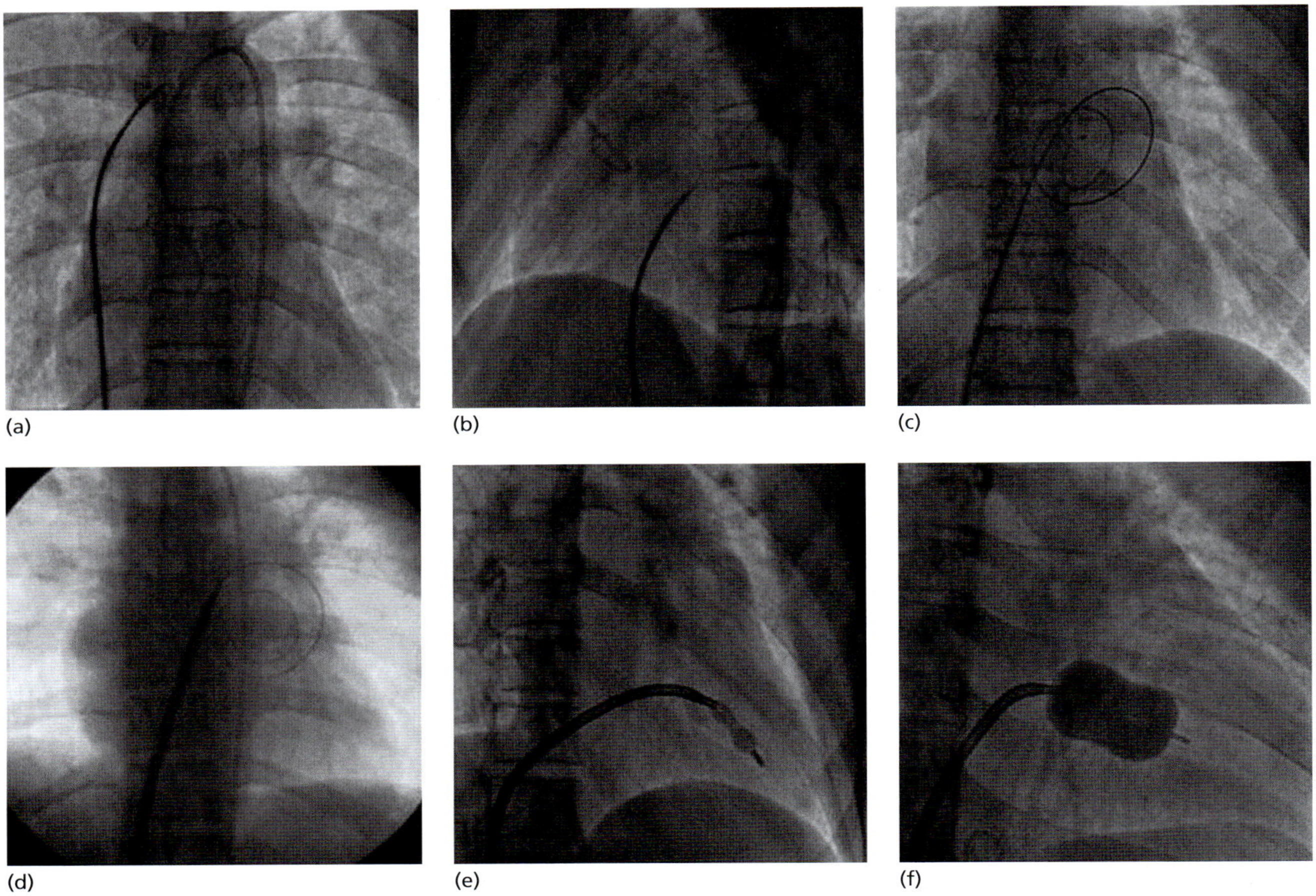

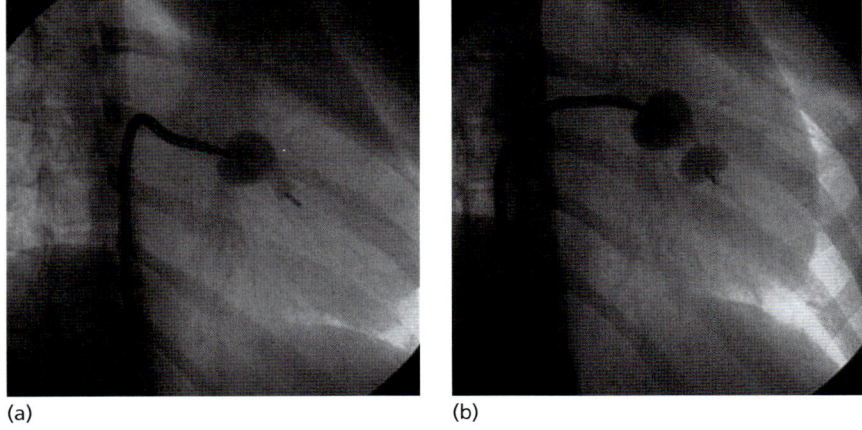

Figure 65.3 Salient steps of balloon mitral valvuloplasty (BMV). (a) Pigtail catheter in aorta; (b) septal puncture using Brockenbrough needle; (c) coiled wire in LA after septal puncture; (d) septal dilatation with 14 Fr dilator; (e) Inoue balloon LA entry assisted with stylet; (f) fully inflated Inoue balloon across mitral valve.

Figure 65.4 Distorted shape of Inoue balloon inside left ventricle showing impasse sign (a) and compression sign (b) suggestive of severe submitral stenosis.

Box 65.3 Definition of successful balloon mitral valvuloplasty

1 ≥50% increase in the mitral valve area
2 Increase in mitral valve area to ≥1.5 cm²
3 Significant fall in left atrial pressure and transmitral gradient (Figure 65.5)
4 Mitral regurgitation not more than Grade II
5 At least one of the commissures is split
6 No major complications

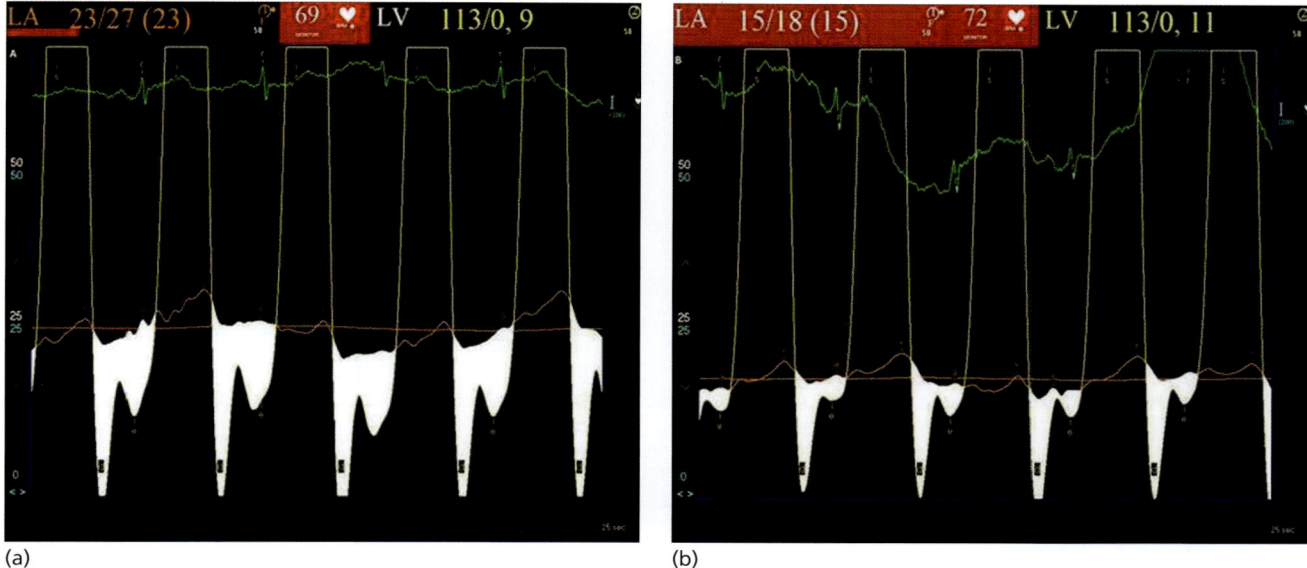

Figure 65.5 The images depict simultaneous tracings of pulmonary capillary wedge pressure and left ventricular pressure in a patient with mitral stenosis before and after valvuloplasty. The preprocedural peak transmitral gradient was 24 mmHg and end diastolic gradient was 14 mmHg; post-procedural peak gradient was 4 mmHg and end diastolic gradient was1 mmHg.

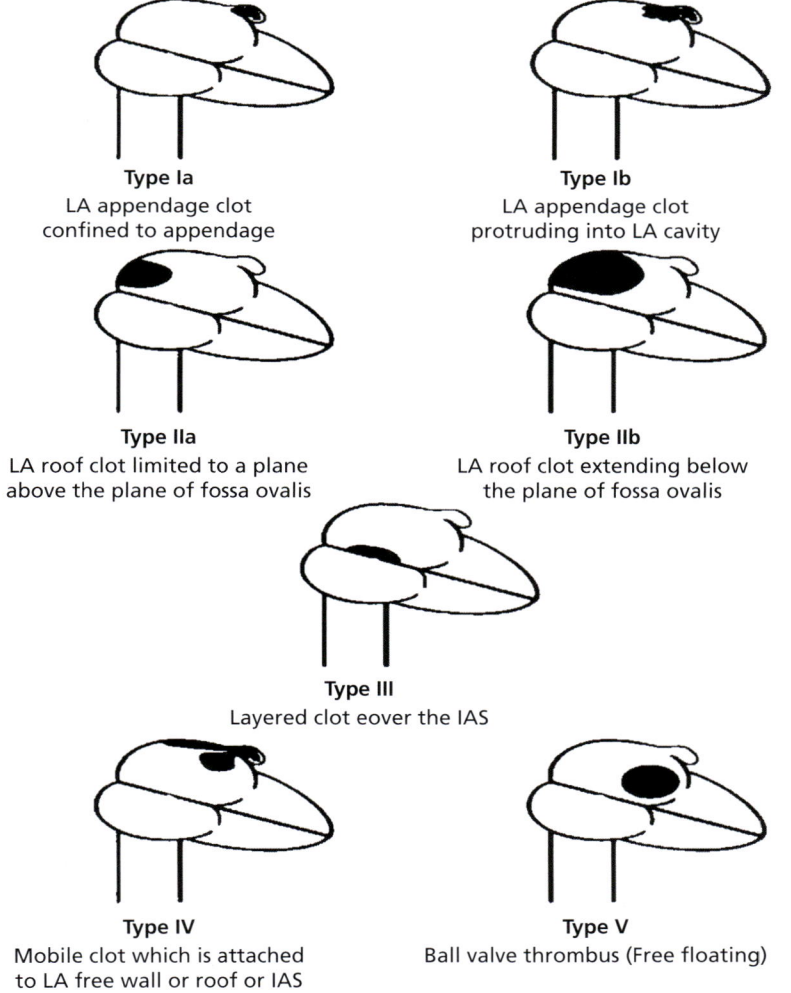

Type Ia
LA appendage clot
confined to appendage

Type Ib
LA appendage clot
protruding into LA cavity

Type IIa
LA roof clot limited to a plane
above the plane of fossa ovalis

Type IIb
LA roof clot extending below
the plane of fossa ovalis

Type III
Layered clot eover the IAS

Type IV
Mobile clot which is attached
to LA free wall or roof or IAS

Type V
Ball valve thrombus (Free floating)

Figure 65.6 Classification of left atrial clot. Source: Manjunath CN, *et al.* 2009 [21]. Copyright © 2009 Wiley-Liss, Inc.

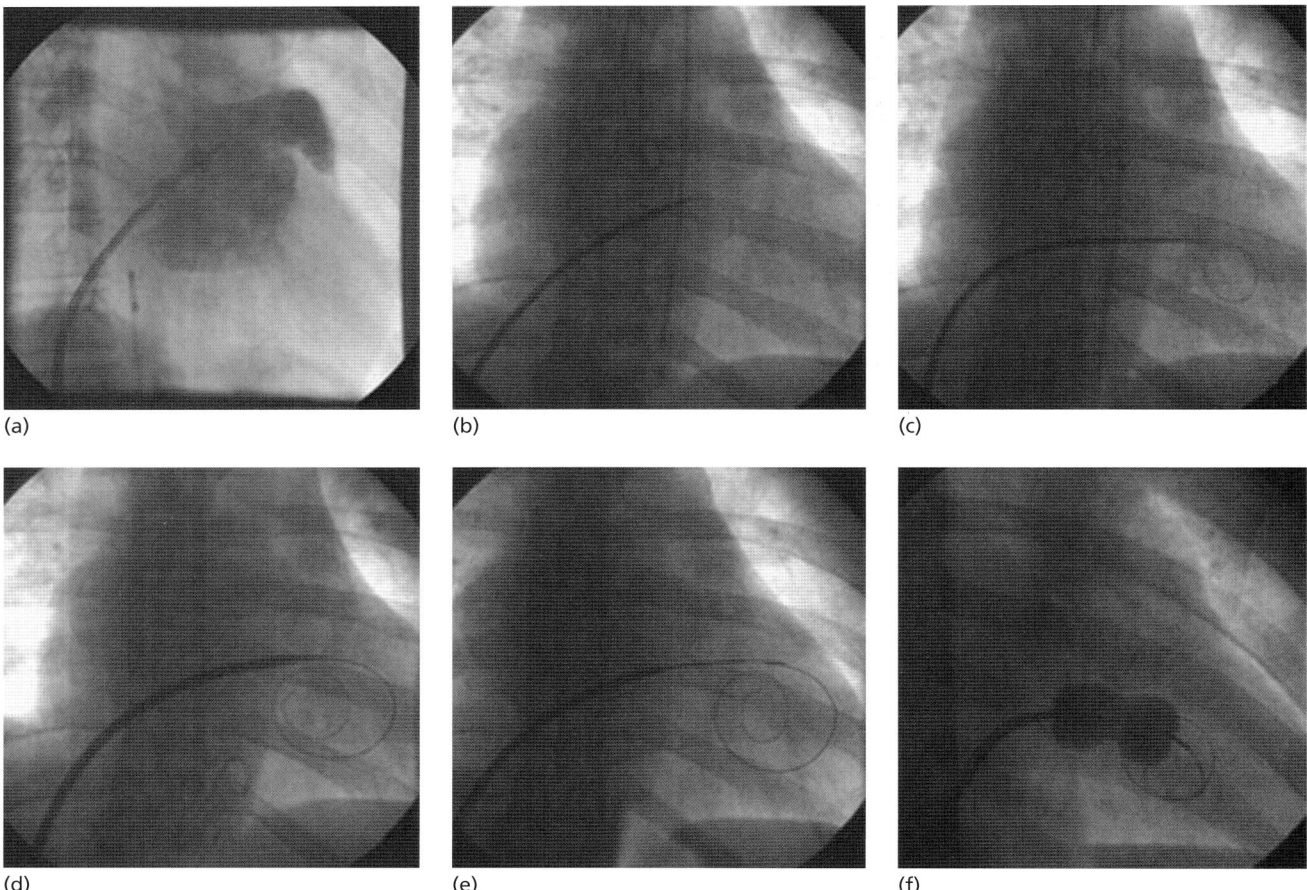

Figure 65.7 Over-the-wire technique described by Manjunath *et al.* [22]. Cine recordings showing the position of LA appendage and the steps involved in modified over-the-wire technique. (a) Position of the left atrial appendage. (b) Mullins sheath near the mitral valve. (c) Coiled guidewire directly introduced into left ventricle. (d) Septal dilatation over the coiled guidewire. (e) Accura balloon over the coiled guidewire crossing the mitral valve. (f) Accura balloon inflation.

the mitral valve, either changing the shape of the stylet, reverse loop entry, modified over-the-wire technique (Figure 65.7), balloon flotation catheter-assisted entry, or deliberate low septal puncture methods can be used to enter the left ventricle.

BMV in severe subvalvular disease

In severe submitral stenosis, balloon entry into left ventricle can be difficult. Severe subvalvular stenosis can affect immediate procedural results as well as increase the incidence of acute severe MR. Severe subvalvular stenosis also causes difficulty in entering the Inoue balloon into the left ventricle. In such situations, predilating and releasing submitral apparatus stenosis using peripheral angioplasty balloon (short length balloons with 6–8 mm in diameter) facilitates subsequent entry of a 12 Fr Inoue balloon catheter. This can be achieved either through an antegrade or retrograde approach. However, utmost care should be taken not to cause chordal or papillary muscle rupture.

BMV in IVC interruption/IVC anomalies through IJV approach

In the vast majority of patients, BMV can be successfully performed using femoral venous access; however, certain congenital or acquired anomalies of the inferior vena cava (IVC) or iliofemoral veins preclude this option and necessitate the use of alternative access

routes. The transjugular approach to transseptal BMV is a useful alternative in patients with venous anomalies that preclude the conventional femoral venous approach. Landmarks for septal puncture are derived from Inoue's angiographic method in frontal projection. Alternatively, levophase injection of pulmonary arteriogram can be utilized to delineate the interatrial septum. The appropriate site of septal puncture is 2 cm below the left atrial roof. Deliberate high atrial puncture facilitates balloon crossing into the left ventricle in jugular approach. However, very high puncture should be avoided because it is associated with high incidence of cardiac tamponade. If the septal puncture is low or at fossa ovalis, the over-the-wire technique can be helpful in delivering the balloon through the mitral valve orifice. Other than a Inoue balloon, a single balloon technique can be applied for mitral valve dilatation. The procedure-related complications, including cardiac tamponade, emergency surgery, acute severe MR, and embolization, are similar to the transfemoral approach. However, the transjugular approach is technically challenging but can be considered as an alternative to the femoral approach when the anatomic variations warrant it.

BMV in juvenile mitral stenosis

In comparison with adults, children and adolescents with rheumatic mitral stenosis more often have severe pulmonary hypertension and very high transmitral gradient but less often have atrial fibrillation and left atrial dilatation. Although the mitral valves in these younger patients are typically more pliable, with less calcification and lower echocardiographic scores than in older populations [23,24] we frequently encounter young patients with mitral stenosis who have severe subvalvular disease and grossly thickened leaflets, indicative of the fulminant course of the disease in this population.

Careful attention to procedural details—use of a balloon diameter smaller than the typically recommended size, stepwise increases in balloon diameter, meticulous pressure gradient measurement, and watch for MR after each dilatation—is important in these young patients. BMV in young patients is effective, safe, and provides better immediate results than in adults particularly with regard to acute complications. Although indexed MVA was larger than in adults, freedom from restenosis and from clinical events at 10 years was no different from adult populations [25].

BMV in pregnancy

The majority of patients with moderate to severe MS worsen during pregnancy because of increased intravascular volume and increases in heart rate. Symptoms occur in 25% of patients, become apparent by 20 weeks' gestation, and aggravate at the time of labor and delivery. Without intervention, maternal mortality is significantly higher (6.8%) for those in NYHA Classes III and IV, particularly during labor and delivery [26]. Optimal timing of BMV is the end of the second trimester or the beginning of the third trimester during which radiation risk to the fetus is negligible.

BMV should be performed by experienced operators with abdominal and pelvic shielding and with minimum radiation exposure and should be avoided during the first trimester. With these precautions, BMV can be safely performed in pregnancy. Esteves *et al.* [27] reported optimal immediate and long-term results in pregnant patients who underwent BMV during the second trimester of their pregnancy.

Complications of BMV

Most of the adverse complications relevant to this procedure occur during the procedure (i.e., during the process of interatrial septum puncture, manipulation of the Inoue balloon catheter in the left atrium, and commissurotomy of the mitral valve by Inoue balloon catheter). Major complications with regard to the Brockenbrough puncture are related to penetration of the Brockenbrough needle into the adjacent structure (i.e., ascending aorta and the post-atrium pericardial space). Procedural mortality is in the range of 0–3% in most series. Table 65.2 lists complications during BMV.

Pericardial effusion and tamponade

The most common serious complication is hemopericardium, with an incidence of 0–2.0% [28]. When hemopericardium or rupture into the space surrounding the aortic root occurs, protamine sulfate should be administered to promote spontaneous hemostasis unless urgent surgical intervention is necessary.

Although relatively rare, unintended perforation by the tip of the Inoue catheter or guidewires while being manipulated in the cardiac chambers might occur in the left atrial appendage, the pulmonary veins, or the left ventricular apex because of the vulnerability of these structures.

When hemopericardium or rupture into the space surrounding the aortic root occurs, protamine sulfate should be administered to promote spontaneous hemostasis unless urgent surgical intervention is necessary.

Acute mitral regurgitation

An increase in mitral regurgitation is another possible complication after commissurotomy; however, in most cases, the degree of mitral regurgitation slightly increases after BMV without requiring surgical intervention. The mechanism of the increase or new appearance of mitral regurgitation is reported to be excessive tearing of the commissure(s) or the posterior/anterior leaflet at non-commissural part, incomplete closure of a calcified leaflet, and localized rupture of the subvalvular apparatus. The mechanism of post-BMV mitral regurgitation is reported to be closely related to long-term prognosis. Severe mitral regurgitation is relatively rare, with a frequency ranging from 1.3% to 19% in different series [29–32]. Surgical findings [29,33] suggest that this complication is related to non-commissural tearing of the posterior or anterior leaflet and chordal rupture. Additionally, with significant asymmetric commissural calcification, the non-calcified commissure can tear, causing severe MR.

The incidence of acute severe MR following BMV in our study is 1.3% [29]. Clinically, hypotension and hypoxia are the predominant manifestations of acute severe MR. Anterior mitral leaflet tear is the most common cause for severe MR (Figure 65.8). The severity of submitral disease which is underestimated by 2D-TTE appears to

Table 65.2 Complications during balloon mitral valvuloplasty

Complications	Incidence (%)	Management
Pericardial effusion/tamponade	0.5–12.0	1. Pericardiocentesis 2. Reversal of heparin with protamine 3. Autotransfusion 4. BMV through second puncture to reduce LA pressure 5. Surgical closure of perforation when conservative strategy fails
Acute severe MR requiring surgery	0.9–2.0	Early MVR, preferably within 24 hours, is recommended for optimal outcome
Acute embolism or stroke	0.5–5.0	Conservative management ? Intra-arterial lysis
Residual atrial septal defect	At 48 hours: 60–70 At 6 months: 8–10	Conservative in almost all cases

BMV, balloon mitral valvuloplasty; LA, left atrium; MR, mitral regurgitation; MVR, mitral valve replacement.

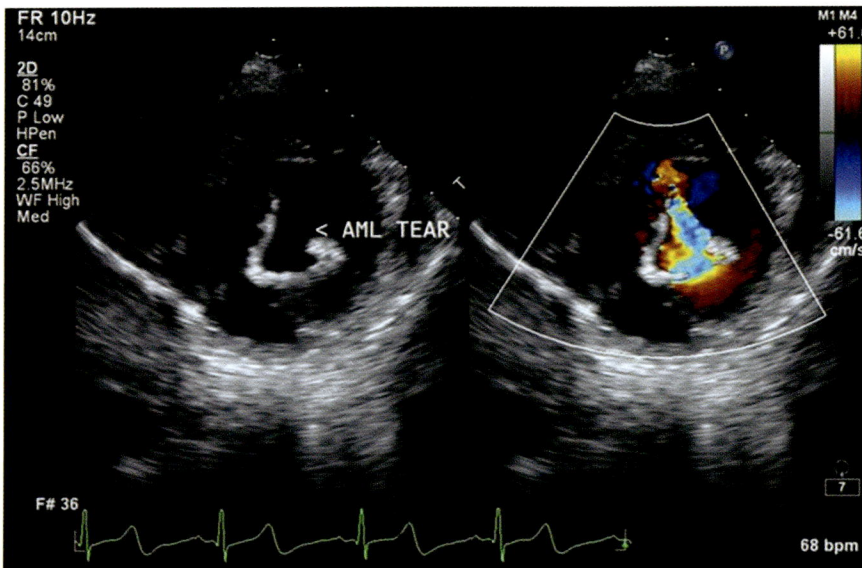

Figure 65.8 Transthoracic echocardiography showing post BMV anterior mitral leaflet tear and severe mitral regurgitation.

be one of the important risk factors predisposing to severe MR. A strategy of early MVR, preferably within 24 hours of onset of severe MR, is recommended for optimal outcome.

Stroke and embolism

Detachment of undetected microthrombi in the left atrium or left atrial appendage by the catheter or guidewire tip can occasionally occur. To avoid these mechanical complications, gentle manipulation of the guidewires and catheters are required, and the Inoue catheter should be formed using the stylet, with the tip of the catheter properly directed toward the mitral valve orifice.

The frequency of embolic events related to mitral valvuloplasty is in the range of 0.5–5.0%. On rare occasions, such events cause of permanent severe disability and even death. In view of the severe potential consequences of this complication, it is critical for the operators to take all possible precautions to prevent it.

Residual atrial septal defect

The frequency of atrial septal defects after mitral valvuloplasty is in the range of 10–90% in different series. These are typically small and restrictive shunts. Significant right-to-left shunts occur on rare occasions in patients who had pulmonary hypertension and elevated right heart pressures. In our study [34], incidence of residual atrial septal defect within 48 hour of percutaneous transmitral commissurotomy (PTMC) by TEE color flow Doppler imaging is 66.5%. These defects are hemodynamically significant only in 4.3% of patients. Surrogate markers of elevated left atrial pressures do not determine the development of atrial septal defect after PTMC. Most of the defects close spontaneously and a residual defect is observed in 8.7% patients at 6 months.

Results of BMV

Immediate results

The binary endpoint of immediate procedural success is most often a final valve area >1.50 cm² without moderate or severe mitral regurgitation. After BMV, mitral valve area approximately

doubles in most successful cases. Mitral valve anatomy as assessed by two-dimensional echocardiography is a strong predictor of the immediate results of BMV. The previously described Wilkins score has a discriminant cut-off point of 8 according to analyses of the immediate results of BMV. Whatever echocardiographicc scoring system is used, older age, smaller valve area, previous commissurotomy, or baseline mitral regurgitation should be considered as potential predictors for poor immediate outcome with a similar predictive strength as valve calcification [30]. In clinical practice, young patients (<50 years) with favorable valve anatomy have usually shown particularly good immediate results [35,36].

Long-term results

Most patients with initial procedural success report significant functional improvement. When immediate results are suboptimal, the patient's functional status does not improve or improves only transiently.

The best results of BMV are observed in young patients who have MS with favorable anatomic characteristics (i.e., pliable non-calcified valves and moderate impairment of the subvalvular apparatus). Published series from India and Tunisia have clearly demonstrated the safety and efficacy of BMV in such patients [37,38]. After BMV, at least 90% of patients are alive without intervention on the mitral valve and with few or no symptoms 5–7 years after the procedure. Randomized trials conducted in these young populations show that 3- and 7-year results after BMV are as good as those obtained with open-heart commissurotomy and better than those with closed-heart commissurotomy.

Suboptimal immediate results lead to relatively early intervention, which explains the presence of an early drop in event-free survival rates after the procedure. Post-BMV mitral restenosis is defined as a valve area <1.5 cm² or a >50% loss of the initial gain in valve area [39]. The incidence of restenosis after a successful procedure ranges from 2% to 40% in different studies, at time intervals ranging from 3 to 10 years. Reportedly, the freedom from restenosis rates were 85% at 5 years, 70% at 10 years, and 44% at 15 years and were significantly higher (i.e., 92% at 5 years,

85% at 10 years, and 65% at 15 years) for patients with optimal morphology [40,41]. Depending on the anatomy, restenosis can be treated either with repeat MBV or with surgical mitral valve replacement. Repeat BMV should be proposed as first-line therapy if the patient had symptoms related to MS and showed only mild mitral regurgitation based on the observational evidence that the mechanism of mitral restenosis is primarily commissural refusion.

Conclusions

Although the incidence of rheumatic fever and the prevalence of rheumatic heart disease as sequelae are decreasing in most Asian countries, a small but substantial occurrence of rheumatic MS exists in Asia. Since its introduction, percutaneous mitral commissurotomy has demonstrated good immediate and mid-term results and has replaced surgical mitral commissurotomy as the preferred treatment of rheumatic MS in appropriate candidates. Aadequate understanding of indications, BMV procedures, complications, and assessment of results are key factors.

Interactive multiple choice questions are available for this chapter on www.wiley. com/go/dangas/cardiology

References

1 Inoue K, Owaki T, Nakamura T, Kitamura F, Miyamoto N. Clinical application of transvenous mitral commissurotomy by a new balloon catheter. *J Thorac Cardiovasc Surg* 1984; **87**: 394–402.

2 Lock JE, Khalilullah M, Shrivastava S, Bahl V, Keane JF. Percutaneous catheter commissurotomy in rheumatic mitral stenosis. *N Engl J Med* 1985; **313**: 1515–1518.

3 Al Zaibag M, Ribeiro PA, Al Kasab S, Al Fagih MR. Percutaneous double-balloon mitral valvctomy for rheumatic mitral-valve stenosis. *Lancet* 1986; **1**: 757–761.

4 Hogan K, Ramaswamy K, Losordo DW, Isner JM. Pathology of mitral commissurotomy performed with the Inoue catheter: implications for mechanisms and complications. Cathet Cardiovasc Diagn 1994; Suppl 2: 42–51.

5 Rahman F, Akhter N, Anam K, et al. Balloon mitral valvuloplasty: immediate and short term haemodynamic and clinical outcome. *Mymensingh Med J* 2010; **19**(2): 199–207.

6 Zhao Q, Hu X. Systematic comparison of the effectiveness of percutaneous mitral balloon valvotomy with surgical mitral commissurotomy. *Swiss Med Wkly* 2011; **141**: w13180.

7 Nishimura RA, Otto CM, Bonow RO, et al. 2014 AHA/ACC guideline for the management of patients with valvular heart disease: executive summary: a report of the American College of Cardiology/American Heart Association Task Force on Practice Guidelines. *Circulation* 2014; **129**(23): e521–643.

8 Bonow RO, Carabello BA, Chatterjee K, et al. ACC/AHA 2006 guidelines for the management of patients with valvular heart disease: a report of the American College of Cardiology/American Heart Association Task Force on Practice Guidelines (Writing Committee to Develop Guidelines for the Management of Patients With Valvular Heart Disease. *J Am Coll Cardiol* 2006; **48**(3): e1–148.

9 Wilkins GT, Weyman AE, Abascal VM, et al. Percutaneous balloon dilatation of the mitral valve: an analysis of echocardiographic variables related to outcome and the mechanism of dilatation. *Br Heart J* 1988; **60**: 299–308.

10 Cannan CR, Nishimura RA, Reeder GS, et al. Echocardiographic assessment of commissural calcium: a simple predictor of outcome after percutaneous mitral balloon valvotomy. *J Am Coll Cardiol* 1997; **29**(1): 175–180.

11 Hilliard AA, Nishimura RA. The interventional cardiologist and structural heart disease: the need for a team approach. *JACC Cardiovasc Imaging* 2009; **2**(1): 1–7.

12 Topol EJ. Mitral valvuloplasty. In: *Textbook of Interventional Cardiology*, 5th edn. Saunders Elsevier: 2008; 50.

13 Joseph G, Chandy S, George P, et al. Evaluation of a simplified transseptal mitral valvuloplasty technique using over-the-wire single balloons and complementary femoral and jugular venous approaches in 1,407 consecutive patients. *J Invasive Cardiol* 2005; **17**(3): 132–138.

14 Bonhoeffer P, Esteves C, Casal U, et al. Percutaneous mitral valve dilatation with the Multi-Track System. *Catheter Cardiovasc Interv* 1999; **48**(2): 178–183.

15 Cribier A, Eltchaninoff H, Koning R, et al. Percutaneous mechanical mitral commissurotomy with a newly designed metallic valvulotome: immediate results of the initial experience in 153 patients. *Circulation* 1999; **99**(6): 793–799.

16 Nair KK, Pillai HS, Thajudeen A, et al. Comparative study on safety, efficacy, and midterm results of balloon mitral valvotomy performed with triple lumen and double lumen mitral valvotomy catheters. *Catheter Cardiovasc Interv* 2012; **80**(6): 978–986.

17 Manjunath CN, Dorros G, Srinivasa KH, et al. The Indian experience of percutaneous transvenous mitral commissurotomy: comparison of the triple lumen (Inoue) and double lumen (Accura) variable sized single balloon with regard to procedural outcome and cost savings. *J Interv Cardiol* 1998; **11**: 107–112.

18 Hung JS, Lau KW. Pitfalls and tips in Inoue balloon mitral commissurotomy. *Catheter Cardiovasc Diagn* 1996; **37**: 188–199.

19 Thomas JD, Wilkins GT, Choong CY, et al. Inaccuracy of mitral pressure half-time immediately after percutaneous mitral valvotomy: dependence on transmitral gradient and left atrial and ventricular compliance. *Circulation* 1988; **78**: 980–993.

20 Vahanian A. How to do a mitral valvuloplasty. *Int J Cardiol* 1996; **55**: 1–7.

21 Manjunath CN, Srinivasa KH, Ravindranath KS, et al. Balloon mitral valvotomy in patients with mitral stenosis and left atrial thrombus. *Catheter Cardiovasc Interv* 2009; **74**(4): 653–661.

22 Manjunath CN, Srinivasa KH, Patil CB, Venkatesh HV, Bhoopal TS, Dhanalakshmi C. Balloon mitral valvuloplasty: our experience with a modified technique of crossing the mitral valve in difficult cases. *Cathet Cardiovasc Diagn* 1998; **44**: 23–26.

23 Bahl VK, Chandra S, Kothari SS, et al. Percutaneous transvenous mitral commissurotomy using Inoue catheter in juvenile rheumatic mitral stenosis. *Catheter Cardiovasc Diagn* 1994; **Suppl 2**: 82–86.

24 Harikrishnan S, Nair K, Tharakan JM, Titus T, Kumar VK, Sivasankaran S. Percutaneous transmitral commissurotomy in juvenile mitral stenosis: comparison of long term results of Inoue balloon technique and metallic commissurotomy. *Catheter Cardiovasc Interv* 2006; **67**(3): 453–459.

25 Gamra H, Betbout F, Ben Hamda K, et al. Balloon mitral commissurotomy in juvenile rheumatic mitral stenosis: a ten year clinical and echocardiographic actuarial results. *Eur Heart J* 2003; **24**(14): 1349–1356.

26 de Souza JA, Martinez EE Jr, Ambrose JA, et al. Percutaneous balloon mitral valvuloplasty in comparison with open mitral valve commissurotomy for mitral stenosis during pregnancy. *J Am Coll Cardiol* 2001; **37**: 900–903.

27 Esteves CA, Munoz JS, Braga S, et al. Immediate and long-term follow-up of percutaneous balloon mitral valvuloplasty in pregnant patients with rheumatic mitral stenosis. *Am J Cardiol* 2006; **98**: 812–816.

28 Martinez-Rios MA, Tovar S, Luna J, Eid-Lidt G. Percutaneous mitral commissurotomy. *Cardiol Rev* 1999; **7**: 108–116.

29 Nanjappa MC, Ananthakrishna R, Hemanna Setty SK, et al. Acute severe mitral regurgitation following balloon mitral valvotomy: echocardiographic features, operative findings, and outcome in 50 surgical cases. *Catheter Cardiovascular Interv* 2013; **81**(4): 603–608.

30 Iung B, Cormier B, Ducimetière P, et al. Immediate results of percutaneous mitral commissurotomy: a predictive model on a series of 1514 patients. *Circulation* 1996; **94**(9): 2124–2130.

31 Iung B, Nicoud-Houel A, Fondard O, et al. Temporal trends in percutaneous mitral commissurotomy over a 15-year period. *Eur Heart J* 2004; **25**(8): 701–707.

32 Varma PK, Theodore S, Neema PK, et al. Emergency surgery after percutaneous transmitral commissurotomy: operative versus echocardiographic findings, mechanisms of complications, and outcomes. *J Thorac Cardiovasc Surg* 2005; **130**(3): 772–776.

33 Choudhary SK, Talwar S, Venugopal P. Severe mitral regurgitation after percutaneous transmitral commissurotomy: underestimated subvalvular disease. *J Thorac Cardiovasc Surg* 2006; **131**(4): 927.

34 Manjunath CN, Panneerselvam A, Srinivasa KH, et al. Incidence and predictors of atrial septal defect after percutaneous transvenous mitral commissurotomy: a transesophageal echocardiographic study of 209 cases. *Echocardiography* 2013; **30**(2): 127–130.

35 Nobuyoshi M, Hamasaki N, Kimura T, et al. Indications, complications, and short-term clinical outcome of percutaneous transvenous mitral commissurotomy. *Circulation* 1989; **80**: 782–792.

36 Neumayer U, Schmidt HK, Fassbender D, Mannebach H, Bogunovic N, Horstkotte D. Early (three-month) results of percutaneous mitral valvotomy with the Inoue balloon in 1,123 consecutive patients comparing various age groups. *Am J Cardiol* 2002; **90**: 190–193.

37 Ben Farhat M, Ayari M, Maatouk F, *et al.* Percutaneous balloon versus surgical closed and open mitral commissurotomy: seven-year follow-up results of a randomized trial. *Circulation* 1998; **97**: 245–250.

38 Arora R, Kalra GS, Singh S, *et al.* Percutaneous transvenous mitral commissurotomy: immediate and long-term follow-up results. *Catheter Cardiovasc Interv* 2002; **55**: 450–456.

39 Hernandez R, Banuelos C, Alfonso F, *et al.* Long-term clinical and echocardiographic follow-up after percutaneous mitral valvuloplasty with the Inoue balloon. *Circulation* 1999; **99**: 1580–1586.

40 Fawzy ME, Shoukri M, Al Buraiki J, *et al.* Seventeen years' clinical and echocardiographic follow up of mitral balloon valvuloplasty in 520 patients, and predictors of long-term outcome. *J Heart Valve Dis* 2007; **16**: 454–460.

41 Fawzy ME, Shoukri M, Hassan W, Nambiar V, Stefadouros M, Canver CC. The impact of mitral valve morphology on the long-term outcome of mitral balloon valvuloplasty. *Catheter Cardiovasc Interv* 2007; **69**: 40–46.

CHAPTER 66

Pulmonary Artery and Valve Catheter-Based Interventions

Kasey Chaszczewski[1], Damien Kenny[2], and Ziyad M. Hijazi[3]

[1] Rush University Medical Center, Chicago, IL, USA
[2] Our Lady's Children's Hospital, Dublin, Ireland
[3] Sidra Medical and Research Center, Doha, Qatar

Advancement within interventional cardiology hinges upon the continued development of less invasive procedures that aim to achieve the same efficacy as primary surgical repair. This continuous pursuit, obstacle identification, and further innovation is perhaps best exemplified by the progressive advancement of pulmonary artery and valve-based interventions.

Pulmonary artery and pulmonary valve stenosis are common features of many forms of congenital heart disease. Each results in the elevation of right ventricular pressure, right ventricular hypertrophy, and eventually right ventricular dilatation and failure. Previously, surgical valvotomy had been the sole option to relieve these forms of obstruction. However, the development of pulmonary balloon valvuloplasty, over three decades ago, provided an alternative that avoided cardiopulmonary bypass and has now replaced surgical repair as the preferred intervention.

Yet it is essential to recognize that valvuloplasty is not without its own disadvantages. It is understood that in relieving stenosis the dilatation inherently causes damage to the valve leaflets and can result in a degree of pulmonary regurgitation. Previously, a significant degree of pulmonary regurgitation was deemed an expected and acceptable outcome of the procedure. Such was also the case for patients with tetralogy of Fallot who had undergone transannular patching. However, as significantly more patients are surviving and thriving to adulthood, the resultant consequences have become more apparent and in turn less acceptable. Now these patients require further intervention to address the right ventricular overload, ventricular dysfunction, and ventricular arrhythmias caused by their pulmonary regurgitation. Until just over a decade ago, surgical reintervention had remained the sole treatment option available. However, the advent of transcatheter pulmonary valve replacement (tPVR) has become a realistic alternative.

This chapter details the indications, complications, and outcomes of the primary catheter-based interventions of the right ventricular outflow tract, the pulmonary valve, and the pulmonary arteries.

Balloon pulmonary artery angioplasty

Pulmonary artery stenosis occurs both as a feature of congenital heart disease as well as a sequela of its repair. Typically, congenital pulmonary artery stenosis occurs in conjunction with pulmonary valve stenosis, ventricular septal defects, and tetralogy of Fallot. There is also a well-established association with multiple genetic syndromes including Williams syndrome, Noonan syndrome, Alagille syndrome, and Ehlers–Danlos syndrome.

Alternatively, acquired stenosis occurs as a result of scarring at sites of surgical intervention. Some of the most common sites are at the point of conduit insertion, along the surgical connection of an aortopulmonary shunt, following arterial switch operation for transposition of the great arteries, and after placement of pulmonary bands to control excessive pulmonary blood flow [1].

Indications

Branch pulmonary artery stenosis is the most common indication for balloon angioplasty in pediatric patients. Angioplasty can acutely relieve significant areas of stenosis; however, there are high rates of recurrence in these stenotic regions [2]. Therefore, balloon angioplasty without stent implantation is typically reserved for severe stenosis in very small patients who require prompt intervention or patients with complex arterial anatomy. More satisfactory results can be obtained with the use of cutting balloons.

The primary indications for angioplasty in patients with stenosis based on recent pediatric interventional guidelines are:

- Measurable gradient greater than 20–30 mmHg across the stenosis;
- Right ventricular pressure greater than 50% systemic;
- Evidence of right ventricular failure; and
- Relative flow discrepancy of less than 35%/65% between lungs [3].

While these criteria appear clear and succinct there are frequently difficulties in assessing the gradient across stenotic segments. In some patient cohorts, particularly those with Glenn and Fontan physiology, significant pressure gradients do not exist and therefore angiographic assessment of the relative narrowing is also important. Three-dimensional rotational angiography can prove beneficial in achieving a complete evaluation of the vessel diameter and thus guiding intervention [4].

Procedural technique

Access is typically achieved through the femoral vein and a guidewire is then advanced through the right heart into the pulmonary arteries, and beyond the area of stenosis. Angiography and accurate vessel measurements can be performed prior to this or following

Interventional Cardiology: Principles and Practice, Second Edition. Edited by George D. Dangas, Carlo Di Mario, and Nicholas N. Kipshidze.
© 2017 John Wiley & Sons, Ltd. Published 2017 by John Wiley & Sons, Ltd.

good wire placement with a multitrack catheter. The chosen balloon catheter should be approximately 3–4 times the diameter of the stenotic vessel but not more than 2 mm greater than the diameter of the adjacent normal vessel. In order to achieve a successful dilatation there must be a degree of tearing of the intima of the vessel. For this reason, it is imperative to inflate to a high enough pressure to remove the waist, as lesser pressures are associated with a significantly higher rate of recurrence [2,5].

Generally, a longer sheath is advisable when using cutting balloons. The microtomes of the device score the vessel wall and in doing so disrupt the fibrous connections contributing to stenosis and can cause damage to surrounding structures when removed. The cutting balloon diameter should not exceed the normal vessel diameter in order to minimize risk for vessel rupture [6,7]. In larger children with severe localized stenosis the cutting balloon diameter can be smaller than the normal vessel diameter and can be followed with a high pressure balloon for maximum effect. Each balloon dilatation attempt should be followed by angiography to ensure there is no vessel wall damage.

Complications

Typically, the pulmonary arteries are extremely compliant vessels and are able to tolerate dilatation to greater than three times their stenotic diameter. As previously noted, though, successful dilatation hinges on causing controlled damage to the intima of the vessels. Segments of stenosis, both congenital and iatrogenic, represent areas of abnormal tissue that are inherently less compliant and therefore at increased risk of rupture. Pulmonary vessel rupture can cause a hemothorax and, depending on the severity of the injury and bleeding, can lead to death [8].

Outcomes

Balloon angioplasty typically results in excellent acute improvement with up to a 50% increase in vessel diameter and a 50% decrease in gradient. However, because of the high frequency of restenosis, balloon angioplasty alone often does not provide long-term benefit without the use of an endovascular stent [4,8].

A multicenter prospective randomized trial comparing the use of high-pressure balloon dilatation with cutting balloon devices found the latter to demonstrate superior efficacy. In each case, an attempt was made to dilate the vessel using a low-pressure balloon (<8 atm). In the event this did not eliminate the waist (71% of attempts), either cutting balloon deployment followed by repeat low-pressure balloon dilatation or high-pressure balloon dilatation (15–22 atm) was performed. Cutting balloon dilatation resulted in an improvement in vessel diameter by 85% compared with only 52% in the high-pressure arm [7]. There were no serious adverse events and the authors concluded that cutting balloon therapy is more effective than high-pressure balloon angioplasty for pulmonary artery stenosis not responsive to low pressure balloons.

Pulmonary artery endovascular stenting
Indications

The primary indications for endovascular stent placement are the same as those for pulmonary artery balloon angioplasty with the addition that balloon angioplasty alone has not or likely will not provide an adequate response. Ideal stent placement occurs when the child's vessels are large enough to accommodate a stent with adult-sized potential, which is usually not feasible in neonates and small infants. Thus, endovascular stenting in these patients

should be reserved for patients requiring urgent intervention when angioplasty, including the use of cutting balloons, has not provided adequate relief.

Procedural technique

Venous access is achieved in a similar fashion to balloon angioplasty and a catheter is advanced to the pulmonary arteries. Good wire position is vital and, once achieved, a long sheath is advanced across the stenosis to ensure the stent will pass freely across the stenosis. Stent advancement without the use of a long sheath has been described in smaller children [9]; however, there is a risk of the stent migrating from the balloon during advancement with this approach. Adequate stent crimping over an appropriate-sized balloon can mitigate against stent movement off the balloon when advancing through the longer sheath. When the stent is in correct position, as confirmed by angiograms through the side-arm of the long sheath, the delivery sheath is fully retracted from the balloon, the balloon is inflated, and the stent is fixed within the vessel. This technique is utilized to deliver single, tandem, or bifurcating stents.

Unlike balloon angioplasty, dilatation beyond the desired vessel diameter is typically unnecessary, as the stent will provide the required support upon deflation of the delivery balloon. Similarly, pre-dilatation of the stenotic region is typically unnecessary except for a few specific circumstances. The primary indication for pre-dilatation is that the degree of stenosis is so significant that the sheath and delivery catheter cannot be advanced beyond the affected area [3].

Small patients, refractory to balloon angioplasty, are challenging because the smaller caliber of their vessels may not tolerate the necessary larger, stiffer catheters. In this circumstance the use of a pre-mounted stent can be preferable as it precludes the need for a longer sheath and provides a significant degree of flexibility [10]. An evolving number of lower profile pre-mounted stents that are dilatable to 5–18 mm are now available and are very attractive for use in this circumstance [11,12].

Complications

The implantation of endovascular stents requires larger, stiffer guidewires and delivery systems, thus increasing the risk for vascular damage. Damage to the intima may be reduced as there is more support for the vessel wall with less need for over-dilatation and hence less risk for artery rupture [13]. Either way, it is advisable to have a covered stent available for use should arterial damage be encountered.

Many of the primary complications associated with endovascular stent placement focus on stent migration and poor positioning following placement. In the event that the stent is improperly sized, the stent can undergo embolization in a retrograde fashion to the main pulmonary artery or the right ventricle [13].

Outcomes

The outcomes of stent implantation for pulmonary artery stenosis have been quite good. Significant restenosis of single vessel pulmonary artery stents occurs in less than 7% of patients [13]. There are typically two primary mechanisms by which restenosis of the vessel occurs. The first is the continued growth of the patient and their vasculature as the stent itself remains fixed. In these cases, redilatation of the stent has proven to be safe and effectively reduces the gradient [14]. The second is intimal hyperplasia, particularly at the edges of stents or areas of overlap. The rates of restenosis secondary to intimal hyperplasia have declined with continued experience and associated attempts to avoid stent overlap and severe angulation between the vessel wall and stent [15].

Pulmonary artery stenting has also proven effective in adults with congenital heart disease. Typically, these patients require bilateral or multiple stents. One retrospective study demonstrated a reduction in mean systolic gradient from 24 to 3 mmHg [16].

Balloon pulmonary valvuloplasty

Pulmonary valvular stenosis is a common feature of a wide array of congenital heart diseases which can present in a plethora of fashions. Patients with mild to moderate obstruction often remain asymptomatic until adolescence at which point they begin to develop exercise intolerance, as their right ventricular output can no longer compensate for their increased demands. Occasionally, mild–moderate stenosis improves through childhood and does not require intervention. Alternatively, critical pulmonary stenosis causes significant cyanosis in the neonatal period, and patients are dependent upon a patent ductus arteriosus to provide adequate pulmonary blood flow. Regardless of the severity of the obstruction, balloon valvuloplasty has become the treatment of choice for valvular pulmonary stenosis [17].

Indications

Balloon pulmonary valvuloplasty is indicated for any symptomatic patient following diagnosis of valvar stenosis. Timing is particularly important for neonates with critical stenosis as these patients are typically maintained on prostaglandin infusions to ensure patency of the ductus arteriosus.

Indications for intervention in asymptomatic patients are customarily guided by their degree of obstruction on echocardiogram or resting gradients across the valve during diagnostic catheterization. Typically, a peak instantaneous gradient of 40 mmHg or right ventricular systolic pressures greater than 50% systemic on echocardiogram serve as sufficient criteria to pursue intervention [18].

It is important to note that transcatheter valvotomy and valvuloplasty are contraindicated in patients with right ventricle dependent coronary circulation, in the setting of pulmonary atresia with intact ventricular septum, as these patients have been noted to have significantly higher mortality [19].

Procedural technique

Following assessment of the pressure gradient and right ventricular angiography to evaluate the annular diameter, a guidewire is placed into one of the branch pulmonary arteries. An appropriately sized balloon catheter is placed over the wire and advanced to the midpoint of the valvular obstruction. The balloon is fully inflated, assessing for disappearance of the waist. Following dilatation, the gradient across the valve should be reassessed, with success considered improvement to less than 30 mmHg.

Generally accepted recommendations advocate the use of devices with a balloon to annulus ratio of 1.2–1.4 : 1 in children [3,20]. Inflation of the balloon effectively separates the inappropriately fused valve cusps, thus reducing the degree of stenosis. However, by rupturing the fused cusps, the procedure also inherently places the patient at risk of developing or worsening valvular regurgitation. To minimize the risk and degree of regurgitation, certain groups have recommended balloon selection with a ratio closer to 1.2–1.25 [21]. In neonates with critical pulmonary stenosis, a balloon to annulus ratio closer to 1 : 1 may be preferable.

Balloon pulmonary valvuloplasty has also been effectively utilized in adult patients. Balloon diameter selection is more challenging in adults, as there are significantly fewer data available. Best available data suggest that balloon diameter approximately 1 mm larger than the annulus is effective [22,23]. In larger patients, achieving a balloon diameter of this size with conventional balloons has often necessitated the use of double and triple balloon techniques. However, the introduction of Inoue balloons has provided an effective alternative, permitting single balloon dilatation [23].

Complications

Pulmonary artery tears, rupture of tricuspid valve papillary muscles, and right ventricular outflow tract rupture have all been documented; however, all have decreased significantly in frequency with continued experience and improvement in device technology.

Hypertrophy of the infundibulum is a common response to pulmonary stenosis. Therefore, not unexpectedly, the incidence of infundibular obstruction following the procedure remains high, occurring in approximately 30% of cases [24]. With time, the hypertrophy decreases and the degree of obstruction abates. However, if the gradient across the right ventricular outflow tract (RVOT) is greater than 50 mmHg acutely following intervention, patients transiently require beta-blockade to augment right ventricular output [24].

Outcomes

Large studies of pulmonary valvuloplasty have routinely demonstrated effective relief of pulmonary stenosis. A study of 533 patients found that of those with normal valve morphology, 85% maintained a gradient <36 mmHg and were free from reintervention during a median follow-up of 33 months. Results were less impressive for patients found to have dysplastic valve morphology, with only 65% demonstrating a similar outcome [25]. These findings have been consistent across studies and have been notably less successful in patients with Noonan syndrome who classically exhibit thickened, dysplastic valve leaflets. However, given the relative low rate of severe complications compared with surgical repair, valvuloplasty is still typically attempted [26].

Expansion of the balloon across the patient's annulus intrinsically increases the risk of developing pulmonary regurgitation with an incidence of 10–40% [27]. A study of 41 patients who had undergone balloon valvuloplasty for isolated valvar pulmonary stenosis utilized cardiac magnetic resonance imaging (MRI) and exercise testing to assess the degree and effect of valvar insufficiency at a median follow-up of 13 years. Based on cardiac MRI findings, 34% of patient had a regurgitant fraction >15%, 10% of patients had a fraction >30%, and 5% with a fraction >40%. This study excluded individuals with other forms of congenital heart disease, those with residual valvar stenosis, and those requiring interim valve replacements. However, it suggests that while valvar insufficiency following balloon dilatation is prevalent and more likely when larger balloon to annulus ratios are used, the frequency of severe regurgitation may not be as high as previously assumed [28].

Right ventricular outflow tract stenting

Neonates with tetralogy of Fallot present a unique challenge as they classically demonstrate an anterior and cephalad deviation of their infundibular septum, producing a muscular subvalvar narrowing. Combined with infundibular hypertrophy, this can result in severe RVOT obstruction. These patients will inevitably require definitive surgical repair; however, delaying surgical intervention until the patient is 3–4 months of age has been associated with improved clinical outcomes [29]. Therefore, the goal of immediate therapy is to reduce the patient's obstruction, improve pulmonary blood flow, and in turn stimulate catch-up growth of their hypoplastic pulmonary arteries.

In those patients with severe RVOT obstruction, options to restore adequate pulmonary artery blood flow include a systemic to pulmonary artery (modified Blalock–Taussig) shunt or a complete neonatal repair. A review of the Society of Thoracic Surgeons Database revealed that both are associated with relatively high mortality rates, 6.2% and 7.8%, respectively, during the first month of life [29]. Stenting of the RVOT can provide a significant reduction in cyanosis and allow time for pulmonary artery growth prior to surgical repair.

Indications

RVOT stenting is indicated in patients with severely narrowed RVOT causing profound desaturations and in those requiring continuous prostaglandin infusion to maintain adequate pulmonary blood flow. At this time there are no consensus guidelines that establish criteria for intervention.

Procedural technique

Biplane angiography of the right ventricle is utilized to better define the patient's underlying anatomy and extent of RVOT obstruction. Pre-dilatation of the pulmonary valve with balloon valvuloplasty can be performed to improve ease of access across the valve. The use of a guidewire with markers is helpful given the likelihood of foreshortening in standard angiographic projections leading to potential underestimation of the length of obstruction. Either a pre-mounted coronary or peripheral vascular stent can be deployed depending on the patient's size. Peripheral vascular stents provide the benefit of potential for progressive dilatation as the child grows, whereas the maximal diameter of coronary stents is inherently limited.

Ideally, the stent is not placed across the pulmonary valve so as to avoid or minimize pulmonary regurgitation. However, in the event this is not possible relief of RVOT obstruction is preferable. Placement of a stent across the pulmonic valve produces the same physiology as a non-valved right ventricle to pulmonary artery conduit, which is generally well tolerated prior to definitive surgical repair. In the event that the stent does not cross the pulmonary valve, simultaneous balloon valvuloplasty addresses the fact that obstruction is typically seen at multiple levels of the right ventricle.

Complications

RVOT stenting carries with it a risk profile similar to other stent-related interventions. Specifically, patients can experience perforation of the pulmonary artery or RVOT with associated hemopericardium, cardiac tamponade, and death. Another significant risk is the dislodgement of the stent with possible embolization. For this reason close attention should be paid to appropriately sizing the device prior to deployment. Finally, RVOT stenting carries the theoretical risk of coronary compression and thus this must be considered when evaluating these patients.

Of note, multiple small to medium-sized case studies have demonstrated complication rates less than those associated with a Blalock–Taussig shunt [30–32], therefore suggesting that RVOT stenting should be considered the preferred first step in palliation.

Outcomes

Effective stenting of the RVOT in neonates with significant desaturations has demonstrated significant improvement in oxygen saturation, pulmonary blood flow, pulmonary artery growth, and delay to definitive surgical repair. A study of 55 patients demonstrated a median improvement in oxygen saturation of 20% following intervention and the ability to remove all but one patient (11 of 12) from continuous prostaglandin infusion [30]. Perhaps even more importantly, given the implications for surgical repair, is that stenting improved median pulmonary artery Z scores by 2 [30,31]. Subsequent surgical repair has not been shown to be associated with significant morbidity as a consequence of the pre-existing stent.

Transcatheter pulmonary valve implantation

As detailed throughout this chapter there are a multitude of congenital and acquired abnormalities of the pulmonary valve, which eventually necessitate surgical replacement of the valve. The three types of valves typically utilized for surgical replacement are homografts from cadavers, valved conduits, or bioprosthetic valves implanted directly in the RVOT [3], the choice of which is dictated by the patient's size and the nature of the RVOT disease. In each case, the typical mechanism of non-native valve failure is caused by progressive stenosis of the valve with or without concomitant insufficiency. The primary mechanisms contributing to failure are a combination of external compression, internal calcification, development of fibrotic intimal peel, and patient outgrowth [33]. The combination of these factors necessitates reintervention of conduits in about 25% of smaller patients by approximately 4–5 years after homograft placement [34]. In an effort to address this, balloon dilatation of the conduit has been performed, but has demonstrated minimal improvement in the long-term utility of the conduit [35]. Following this failure, RVOT stent implantation across the valve was employed, thus reducing the degree of stenosis but permitting free regurgitation. This strategy has been shown to postpone surgical repair [36]; however, it places the patient at significant risk of right ventricular dilatation and progressive failure. Most recently, the development of a pulmonary valve that can be deployed via catheterization has effectively produced a reduction in both stenosis and regurgitation across the valve. In doing so, tPVR has reduced right ventricular pressures, improved biventricular function, and reduced arrhythmogenic electrical remodeling, thus becoming the therapy of choice for repair of stenotic RVOT conduits. With evolving technology, tPVR may also soon compete with surgical valve replacement for chronic severe native outflow regurgitation.

Indications

Given the relatively recent development and utilization of tPVR, precise indications for and timing of intervention have yet to be firmly established. Theoretically, ideal timing is prior to the point at which replacement of a competent valve can no longer re-establish normalization of ventricular volumes and function. Consensus guidelines for intervention in pediatric cardiac disease advocate use in patients with a right ventricle to pulmonary conduit and associated moderate to severe pulmonary regurgitation or stenosis, provided the patient meets inclusion and exclusion criteria for the available valve (Melody™; Medtronic, Minneapolis, MN, USA and SAPIEN™; Edwards Lifesciences LLC, Irvine, CA, USA) [3]. The Melody trial also included a mean RVOT gradient of ≥35 mmHg as an indication to intervene [37]. As a source of comparison, surgical guidelines suggest that surgical replacement is typically indicated for patients with a right ventricular end diastolic volume (RVEDV) greater than 150 mL/m^2 on cardiac MRI [38]. These guidelines reflect the different cohort of patients with predominant pulmonary regurgitation that are usually assessed for surgical valve replacement. In each case, cardiac MRI provides accurate assessments of ventricular volumes, function, and regurgitant fraction. However, MRI is time-consuming, uncomfortable for patients, and may require sedation in young patients with tenuous ventricular function.

As a result of these disadvantages of cardiac MRI, the US Melody clinical trial investigated the reliability and accuracy of right heart evaluation via echocardiography and the results were striking. Assessment of RVOT obstruction with Doppler echocardiography correlates closely with gradient evaluation by catheterization and three-point severity scale assessment of valve regurgitation was consistent with cardiac MRI derived regurgitant fraction. Perhaps most notably, patients with an indexed apical diastolic area >30 cm^2/m^2 by echocardiography correlated extremely well with patients with RVEDV >160 mL/m^2 by cardiac MRI. These results suggest that echocardiography, a significantly less cumbersome imaging modality, can be utilized as a screening modality for tPVR candidates [37]. The primary limitations of echocardiography in this setting are that it does not provide detailed imaging of the RVOT and branch pulmonary arteries, assessment of the degree of conduit calcification, or adequate evaluation of the relationship of coronary arteries to the conduit. However, in this setting cardiac computed tomography (CT) has the capacity to provide superior temporal and spatial resolution than cardiac MRI for these indices.

In addition to the degree of conduit dysfunction and right ventricular dysfunction, increased propensity for arrhythmia also guides intervention with tPVR. Significant pulmonary valve regurgitation that results in right ventricular dilatation also produces a significant degree of electrical remodeling and in turn an increased propensity for ventricular arrhythmias. A 10-year follow-up demonstrated that a prolonged QRS duration >180 ms is associated with a 42-fold increased risk of developing sustained ventricular tachycardia and a 2.2-fold increased risk of sudden cardiac death [39]. With resolution of significant pulmonary regurgitation, tPVR has been demonstrated to reduce QRS duration [40], and in doing so reduce the risk of ventricular arrhythmia and sudden cardiac death.

Procedural technique

Prior to intervention it is imperative to assess the proximity of the coronary vessels to the RVOT, as coronary compression is a well-documented complication reported in approximately 4% of cases [41]. Once this relationship is established, pre-stenting of the conduit should be performed. Pre-stenting of the conduit serves to minimize the degree of residual stenosis as well as decrease the rate of stent fracture, seen predominantly with the Melody valve [42].

Once coronary assessment and pre-stenting is completed, tPVR proceeds with one of two currently available valves. Delivery of each valve requires a delivery sheath that is at least 22 Fr, although refinements in SAPIEN valve technology and delivery sheaths for transcatheter aortic valve replacement can benefit those requiring tPVR. The significant sheath size requirement has precluded the use of transfemoral access in smaller patients (typically <30 kg). In such cases, access through the internal jugular vein or via a right ventricular free wall approach can be utilized [43].

The Melody valve is a bovine jugular vein sewn inside a Cheatham-Platinum stent that is hand-crimped onto a balloon-in-balloon angioplasty balloon catheter. The valve's companion delivery system, the Ensemble delivery system, and Melody valve are introduced into the access vein and advanced to the RVOT. When proper placement has been achieved, the inner and then outer balloon system are inflated, thus securing the valve in place (Figure 66.1). Alternatively, the SAPIEN valve is formed from an arrangement of three bovine pericardial leaflets sewn inside a stainless steel stent. The valve is crimped onto the delivery balloon by a crimper and then advanced in a similar fashion. In both cases, wire position and stiffness are vital to creating enough, but not too much, support to advance the large and stiff valve system around the right heart.

The newer Edwards valve, SAPIEN XT, made of cobalt chromium, and new delivery catheter, NovaFlex, can be inserted via a larger 18–20 Fr expandable sheath (eSheath).

Complications

The complications associated with tPVR can be divided into those seen peri-procedurally and those seen commonly at follow-up. First, conduit rupture has been documented as a consequence of balloon dilatation of the homograft during pre-stenting [44]. Such cases typically occur as a consequence of dilatation of severely calcified homografts with significantly reduced compliance, although the exact mechanisms are unclear and hence deciphering a risk profile for each patient has not been possible to date. Balloon dilatation of the RVOT is essential to assess for potential coronary artery compression. This assessment is often one of the subtlest yet most important aspects of the procedure, as one must decide how aggressive to be in relation to ruling out coronary compression. In either case, it is imperative to have covered stents available to address potential conduit rupture [45].

Following deployment of the new valve, patients may demonstrate valve dislodgement and resultant device embolization. The valve typically embolizes in a retrograde fashion to the right ventricle where percutaneous retrieval is possible though technically challenging. In the event percutaneous retrieval is not feasible, the stent must then be retrieved surgically [46]. Finally, coronary artery compression is a complication that can be avoided with adequate pre-intervention surveillance. The importance of monitoring is reiterated by the fact that US Melody cohort study demonstrated that 4.4% of included patients demonstrated unfavorable coronary anatomy [47].

Following intervention, the most common complication and indication for reintervention is stent fracture. The incidence of stent fracture with the Melody valve has been quite significant, with documented incidence as high as 22% [44,47]. Stent fracture can result in the recurrence of significant RVOT obstruction and resultant elevation in right ventricular pressures. However, a more recent study with a pre-stenting of 95% demonstrated a stent fracture rate of less than 5% [48], suggesting that this measure is able to significantly reduce this troubling complication. Endocarditis, particularly with the Melody valve, is also a concern. Close observation of the true rates of endocarditis is warranted.

Outcomes

Post-procedural evaluation of both the Melody and SAPIEN valves has demonstrated significant reduction in indicators of pulmonary valve dysfunction with low rates of morbidity and valve failure. Lurz et al. [44] demonstrated improvement in right ventricle to pulmonary artery gradient from a mean of 37 to 17 mmHg and right ventricle systolic pressure from 63 to 45 mmHg with the use of the

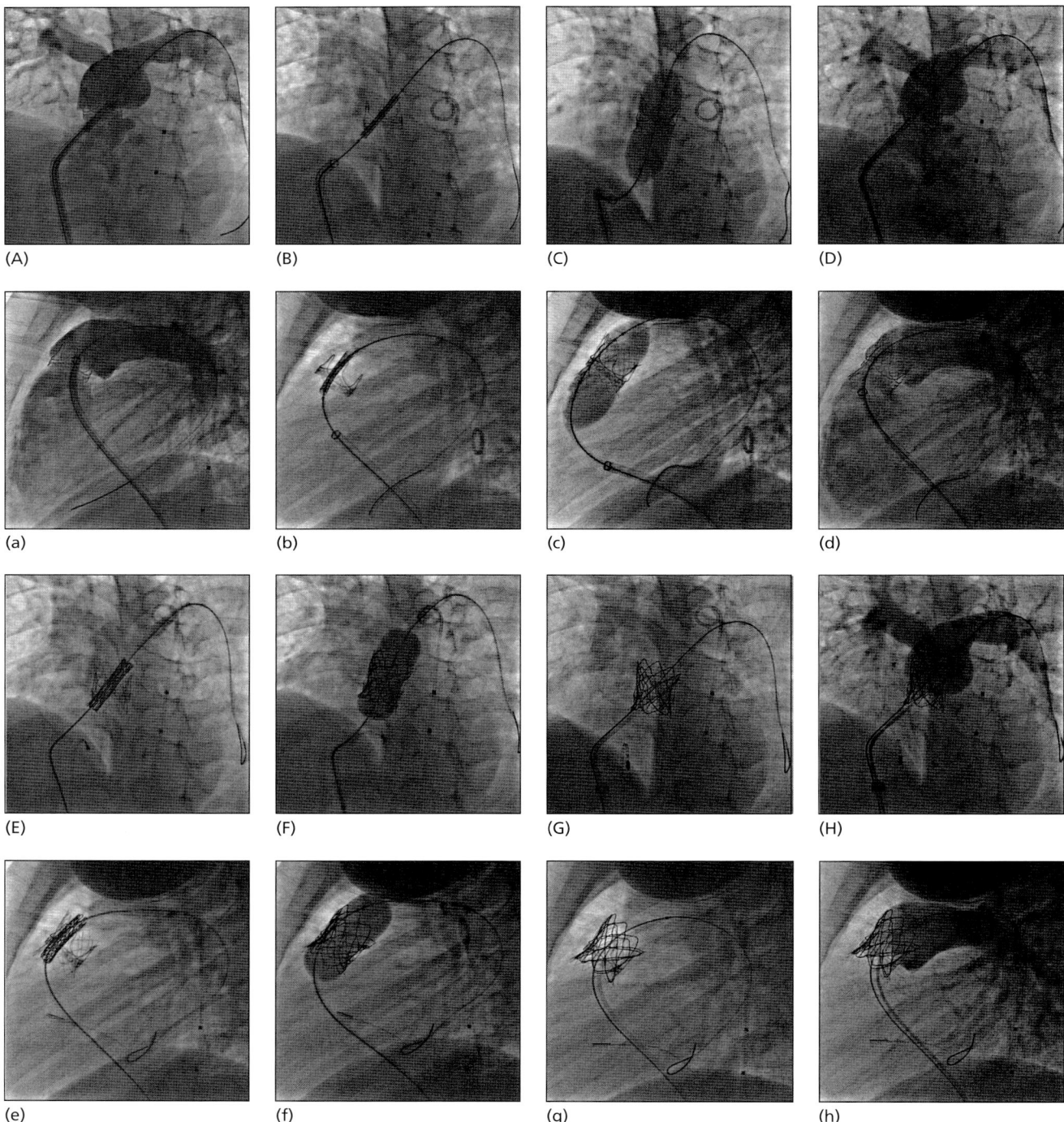

Figure 66.1 Fluoroscopic images demonstrating implantation of Melody® valve (Antero-posterior view, capital letters; lateral views, lowercase). A: Angiography distal to the bioprosthetic valve demonstrates some RVOT narrowing with concomitant pulmonary regurgitation. B: Delivery and (C) balloon inflation of pre-stent, followed by (D) angiography without evidence of damage to RVOT. E: Delivery and (F) balloon inflation of the Melody valve within the pre-stented RVOT. G: Appropriate positioning of the Melody valve, and (H) final angiography without evidence of pulmonary regurgitation. Coronary angiography was performed prior to pre-stenting and demonstrated remote take-off and course of the left coronary artery. Compression is deemed to be less likely in the setting of a pre-existing bioprostheis.

Melody valve [44]. McElhinney *et al.* [47] demonstrated similar results of tPVR with Melody valve with mean gradient reduction from 28.1 to 12.7 mmHg, and right ventricle systolic pressure reduction from 61.6 to 47.2 mmHg. Investigation of the SAPIEN valve has yielded comparable results with an effective reduction of gradient from 27 to 12 mmHg [49].

At this time direct comparisons between surgical valve revision and tPVR are not available; however, tPVR outcomes have demonstrated low valve failure rates. As further experience is gained the incidence of adverse events continues to decline and has been cited at approximately 5% [44,47]. Similarly, mean freedom from reintervention at 1 year had been documented as high as 94% [47] and as high as 70% at 70 months [44].

The future

Although tPVR is evolving into an acceptable alternative to surgery, much uncertainty exists as longer term data are lacking. It appears that initial benefits on right ventricular remodeling occur within the first 6 months with limited further changes in RVEDV or ejection fraction as measured by MRI at 1 year [50]. However, this is likely to mirror surgical data, and concerns should be targeted less toward continued right ventricle remodeling than valve and stent durability. There is every reason to believe that valve durability will be at least as good as surgical valve replacement, as reports have demonstrated pulmonary regurgitant fractions ≥30% at 1 year in 7% of surgical valve replacement patients [38]. However, it may be difficult to recruit patients into a randomized clinical trial to prove this considering patient preference for tPVR. A recent meta-analysis of PVR after tetralogy of Fallot repair in 3118 patients from 48 studies revealed pooled 5-year re-replacement of the pulmonary valve of 4.9% [51] and mirroring this in the shorter

term must be a targeted goal. Although risk factors for re-intervention are being identified [52], the exact pathologic mechanisms of valve degeneration in a host of different conduits have only been postulated on through case reports [53]. One attractive option with tPVR is the potential for further valve replacement with the valve-in-valve technique, extending the number of repeat percutaneous valve replacements to an as yet undefined number [54].

Strategies for the future should be threefold: The first should be consolidating and improving upon current techniques to minimize procedural risk and simplify follow-up protocols thus reducing cost, which is not inconsiderable [55,56], and inconvenience to the patient. Intracardiac echocardiography has provided excellent imaging of valve function in the acute phase confirming valve competency, which can be otherwise distorted by catheters required for post-deployment angiography and can provide more accurate post-deployment assessment of valve function.

The second endeavor should be aimed at further valve development to extend technology to those with native RVOTs. Although deployment of balloon expandable stents in native outflow tracts is evolving with larger valve systems, SAPIEN XT is available in 29 mm, and has been deployed in the pulmonary position [57], it is likely a self-expanding system will gain wider clinical acceptance. Clinical reports of a new valve sewn into a self-expanding nitinol frame have been described (Figure 66.2) [58];

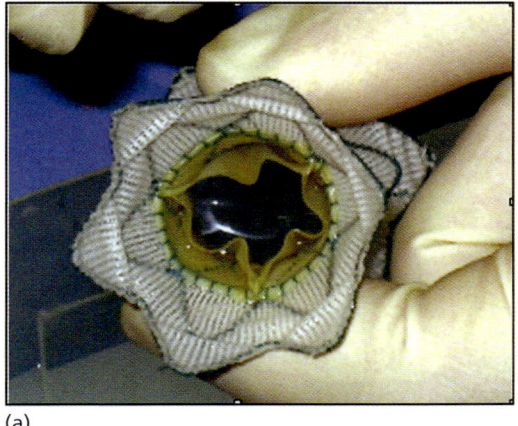

(a)

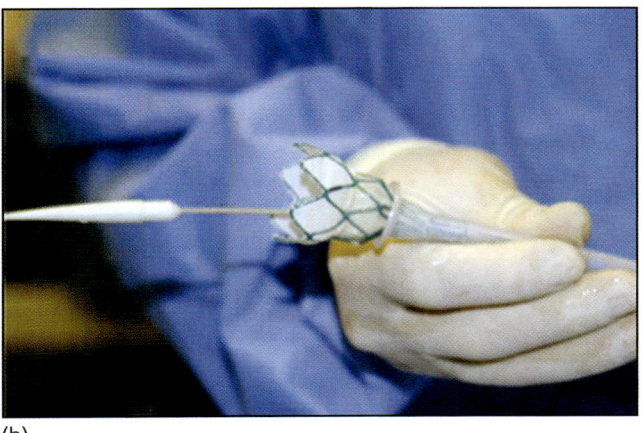

(b)

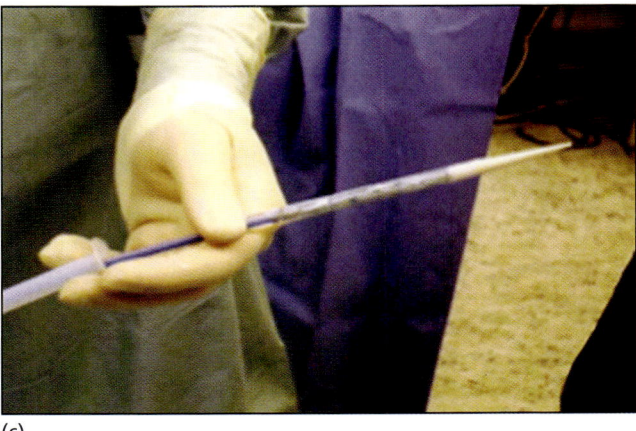

(c)

Figure 66.2 Self-expanding Medtronic Atlas valve and delivery system, currently being developed for native RVOT implantation. (a) Valve as viewed from short axis; (b) being loaded into delivery system; and (c) completely loaded and ready for delivery.

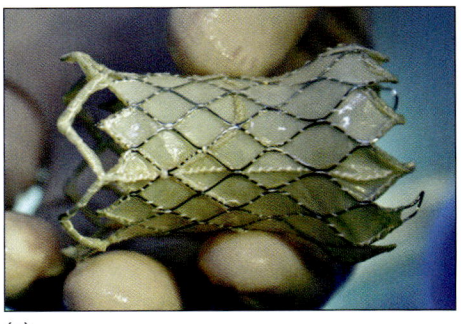
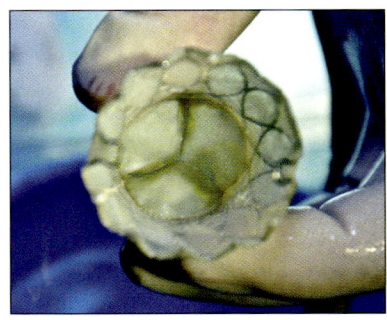

(a)

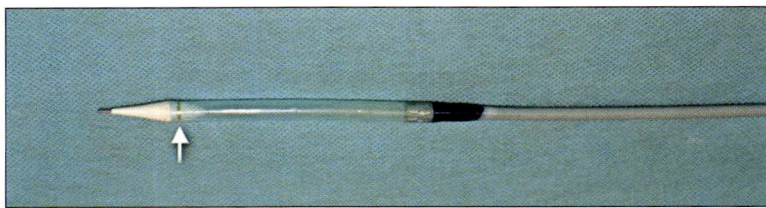

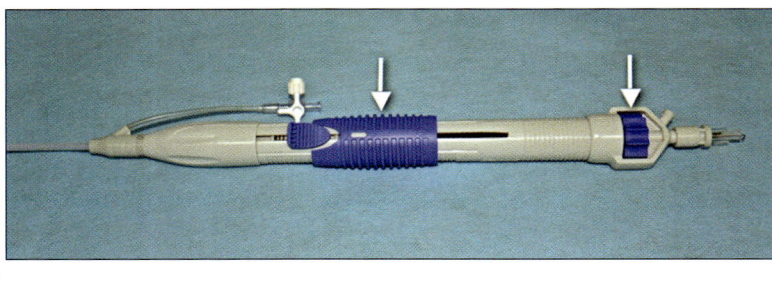

(b)

Figure 66.3 (a) Venus P valve viewed from long (left) and short axis (right). Note the flared, uncovered distal aspect of the valve which serves to anchor the device and decrease the likelihood of migration. (b) Venus P valve delivery system. Note the tapered distal end of the delivery system (top). The proximal end of the delivery system (bottom) has a controlled release handle which allows both slow and fast valve deployment.

however, applicability of this technology over the anatomic and dynamic variability that exists within the RVOT [59] remains questionable and further modifications may be necessary. The outcomes of a small feasibility trial in 20 patients using this valve are awaited. Other self-expanding valve systems are in development.

The Venus Pulmonary Valve (Venus Medtech, Shanghai, China) is a self-expandable nitinol multilevel support frame with a tri-leaflet porcine pericardial tissue valve (Figure 66.3a) with a 19–24Fr delivery catheter (Figure 66.3b). The entire stent is covered, except the distal cells, by porcine pericardial tissue. A flared uncovered outflow end secures anchoring at the distal (pulmonary artery bifurcation) end with radio-opaque markers indicating the distal anchoring position and the valve location. The proximal end is also flared but covered allowing conformability within the dilated RVOT. Stent valve diameters range from 24–36 mm (in 2-mm increments) with each diameter available in 25 and 30 mm straight sections lengths. Early clinical experience is promising with excellent early valve function and right ventricle remodeling reported [60].

The last endeavor should be to merge these approaches with tissue engineering technologies to provide living autologous valve replacements with regenerative and growth potential. This approach has been described in an animal model [61], and although representing the longer term goal of valve replacement, this may be some way off as yet.

Interactive multiple choice questions are available for this chapter on www.wiley.com/go/dangas/cardiology

References

1 Davies R, Radtke W, Klenk D, *et al*. Bilateral pulmonary arterial banding results in an increased need for subsequent pulmonary artery interventions. *J Thorac Cardiovasc Surg* 2014; **147**: 706–712.

2 Bush D, Hoffman T, Del Rosario J, *et al*. Frequency of restenosis after balloon pulmonary arterioplasty and its causes. *Am J Cardiol* 2000; **86**: 1205–1209.

3 Feltes TF, Bacha E, Beekman RH 3rd, *et al*; on behalf of the American Heart Association Congenital Cardiac Defects Committee of the Council on Cardiovascular Disease in the Young, Council on Clinical Cardiology, and Council on Cardiovascular Radiology and Intervention. Indications for cardiac catheterization and intervention in pediatric cardiac disease: a scientific statement from the American Heart Association. *Circulation* 2011; **123**: 2607–2652.

4   Berman DP, Khan DM, Gutierrez Y, Zahn EM. The use of three-dimensional rotational angiography to assess the pulmonary circulation following cavo-pulmonary connection in patients with single ventricle. *Catheter Cardiovasc Interv* 2012; **80**(6): 922–930.

5   Gentles TL, Lock JE, Perry SB. High pressure balloon angioplasty for branch pulmonary artery stenosis: Early experience. *J Am Coll Cardiol* 1993; **22**: 867–872.

6   Butera G, Antonio LT, Massimo C, Mario C. Expanding indications for the treatment of pulmonary artery stenosis in children by using cutting balloon angioplasty. *Catheter Cardiovasc Interv* 2006; **67**: 460–465.

7   Bergersen L, Gauvreau K, Justino H, *et al.* Randomized trial of cutting balloon compated with high-pressure angioplasty for the treatment of resistant pulmonary artery stenosis. *Circulation* 2011; **124**: 2388–2396.

8   Kan JS, Marvin WJ, Bass JL, *et al.* Balloon angioplasty branch pulmonary artery stenosis: results from the Valvuloplasty and Angioplasty of Congenital Anomalies Registry. *Am J Cardiol* 1990; **65**: 798–801.

9   Moszura T, Michalak KW, Dryzek P, *et al.* One center experience in pulmonary artery stenting without long vascular sheath. *Cardiol J* 2010; **17**(2): 149–156.

10 Sreeram N, Emmel M, Ben Mime L, Brockmeier K, Bennink G. Perioperative placement of stents for relief of proximal pulmonary arterial stenoses in infants. *Cardiol Young* 2008; **18**: 158–164.

11 Stern HJ, Baird CW. A premounted stent that can be implanted in children and re-dilated to 20 mm: Introducing the Edwards Valeo Lifestent. *Catheter Cardiovasc Intervent* 2009; **74**: 905–912.

12 Sharma N, Goreczny. The role of the new Valeo stent in treating pulmonary artery stenoses in children with complex cardiac malformations: a report of two cases. *Am J Case Rep* 2014; **15**: 275–279.

13 Shaffer KM, Mullins CE, Grifka RG, *et al.* Intravascular stents in congenital heart disease: short- and long-term results from a large single-center experience. *J Am Coll Cardiol* 1998; **31**: 661–667.

14 Schneider MB, Zartner P, Duveneck K, Lange PE. Various reasons for repeat dilatation of stented pulmonary arteries in paediatric patients. *Heart* 2002; **88**: 505–509.

15 McMahon CJ, El-Said HG, Grifka RG, Fraley JK, Nihill MR, Mullins CE. Redilation of endovascular stents in congenital heart disease: factors implicated in the development of restenosis and neointimal proliferation. *J Am Coll Cardiol* 2001; **38**: 521–526.

16 Kenny D, Amin Z, Slyder S, Hijazi ZM. Medium-term outcomes for peripheral pulmonary artery stenting in adults with congenital heart disease. *J Interv Cardiol* 2011; **24**(4): 373–377.

17 Stanger P, Cassidy SC, Girod DA, Kan JS, Lababidi Z, Shapiro SR. Balloon pulmonary valvuloplasty: results of the Valvuloplasty and Angioplasty of Congenital Anomalies Registry. *Am J Cardiol* 1990; **65**: 775–783.

18 Silvilairat S, Cabalka AK, Cetta F, Hagler DJ, O'Leary PW. Echocardiographic assessment of isolated pulmonary valve stenosis: which outpatient Doppler gradient has the most clinical validity? *J Am Soc Echocardiogr* 2005; **18**: 1137–1142.

19 Giglia TM, Mandell VS, Connor AR, Mayer JE Jr, Lock JE. Diagnosis and management of right ventricle-dependent coronary circulation in pulmonary atresia with intact ventricular septum. *Circulation* 1992; **86**: 1516–1528.

20 Radtke W, Keane JF, Fellows KE, *et al.* Percutaneous balloon valvotomy of congenital pulmonary stenosis using oversized balloons. *J Am Coll Cardiol* 1986; **8**: 909–915.

21 Rao P. Percutaneous balloon pulmonary valvuloplasty: state of the art. *Cathet Cardiovasc Intervent* 2007; **69**: 747–763.

22 Teupe CHJ, Burger W, Schrader R, Zeiher A. Late (five to nine years) follow-up after balloon dilatation of valvar pulmonary stenosis in adults. *Am J Cardiol* 1997; **80**: 240–242.

23 Bahl VK, Chandra S, Goel A, Goswami KC, Wasir HS. Versatility of Inoue balloon catheter. *Int J Cardiol* 1997; **59**: 75–83.

24 Thapar MK, Rao PS. Significance of infundibular obstruction following balloon valvuloplasty for valvar pulmonic stenosis. *Am Heart J* 1989; **118**: 99–103.

25 McCrindle BW. Independent predictors of long-term results after balloon pulmonary valvuloplasty. *Circulation* 1994; **89**: 1751–1759.

26 Ballerini L, Mullins CE, Cifarelli A, *et al.* Percutaneous balloon valvuloplasty of pulmonary valve stenosis, dysplasia, and residual stenosis after surgical valvotomy for pulmonary atresia with intact ventricular septum: long-term results. *Cathet Cardiovasc Diagn* 1990; **19**: 165–169.

27 Masura J, Burch M, Deanfield JE, Sullivan ID. Five-year follow-up after balloon pulmonary valvuloplasty. *J Am Coll Cardiol* 1993; **21**: 132–136.

28 Harrild D, Powell A, Trang T, *et al.* Long-term pulmonary regurgitation following baloon valvuloplasty for pulmonary stenosis. *J Am Coll Cardiol* 2010; **55**(10): 1041–1047.

29 Al Habib H, Jacobs J, Mavroudis C, *et al.* Contemporary patterns of management of tetralogy of Fallot: data from the Society of Thoracic Surgeons Database. *Ann Thorac Surg* 2010; **90**: 813–820.

30 Stumper O, Ramchandani B, Noonan P, *et al.* Stenting of the right ventricular outflow tract. *Heart* 2013; **99**: 1603–1608.

31 Dohlen G, Chaturvedi RR, Benson LN, *et al.* Stenting of the right ventricular outflow tract in the symptomatic infant with tetralogy of Fallot. *Heart* 2008; **95**: 142–147.

32 Gedicke M, Morgan G, Parry A, *et al.* Risk factors for acute shunt blockage in children after modified Blalock–Taussig shunt operations. *Heart Vessel* 2010; **25**: 405–409.

33 Peters B, Ewert P, Berger F. The role of stents in the treatment of congenital heart disease: current status and future perspectives. *Ann Pediatr Cardiol* 2009; **2**(1): 3–23.

34 Tweddell JS, Pelech AN, Frommelt PC, *et al.* Factors affecting longevity of homograft valves used in right ventricular outflow tract reconstruction for congenital heart disease. *Circulation* 2000; **102**(Suppl 3): 130–135.

35 Zeevi B, Keane JF, Perry SB, Lock JE. Balloon dilation of postoperative right ventricular outflow obstructions. *J Am Coll Cardiol* 1989; **14**: 401–408.

36 Hosking MC, Benson LN, Nakanishi T, Burrows PE, Williams WG, Freedom RM. Intravascular stent prosthesis for right ventricular outflow obstruction. *J Am Coll Cardiol* 1992; **20**: 373–380.

37 Brown DW, McElhinney DB, Araoz PA, *et al.* Reliability and accuracy of echocardiographic right heart evaluation in the US Melody valve investigational trial. *J Am Soc Echocardiogr* 2012; **25**: 383–392.

38 Frigiola A, Tsang V, Bull C, *et al.* Biventricular response after pulmonary valve replacement for right ventricular outflow tract dysfunction: is age a predictor of outcome? *Circulation* 2008; **118**(Suppl): S182–S190.

39 Gatzoulis MA, Balaji S, Webber SA, *et al.* Risk factors for arrhythmia and sudden cardiac death late after repair of tetralogy of Fallot: a multicentre study. *Lancet* 2000; **356**(9234): 975–981.

40 Plymen CM, Bolger AP, Lurz P, *et al.* Electrical remodeling following percutaneous pulmonary valve implantation. *Am J Cardiol* 2011; **107**(2): 309–314.

41 Meadows J, Moore P, Berman D, *et al.* Use and performance of the Melody Transcatheter Pulmonary Valve in native and postsurgical, nonconduit right ventricular outflow tracts. *Circ Cardiovasc Interv* 2014; **7**(3): 374–380.

42 Nordmeyer J, Lurz P, Khambadkone S, *et al.* Pre-stenting with a bare metal stent before percutaneous pulmonary valve implantation: acute and 1-year outcomes. *Heart* 2011; **97**(2): 118–123.

43 Simpson KE, Huddleston CB, Foerster S, Nicholas R, Balzer D. Successful sub-xyphoid hybrid approach for placement of a Melody percutaneous pulmonary valve. *Catheter Cardiovasc Interv* 2011; **78**(1): 108–111.

44 Lurz P, Coats L, Khambadkone S, *et al.* Percutaneous pulmonary valve implantation: impact of evolving technology and learning curve on clinical outcome. *Circulation* 2008; **117**: 1964–1972.

45 Sosnowski C, Kenny D, Hijazi ZM. Bail out use of the Gore Excluder following pulmonary conduit rupture during transcatheter pulmonary valve replacement. *Catheter Cardiovasc Interv* 2013; **81**(2): 331–334.

46 Cubeddu RJ1, Hijazi ZM. Bailout perventricular pulmonary valve implantation following failed percutaneous attempt using the Edwards SAPIEN transcatheter heart valve. *Catheter Cardiovasc Interv* 2011; **77**(2): 276–280.

47 McElhinney DB, Hellenbrand WE, Zahn EM, *et al.* Short- and medium-term outcomes after transcatheter pulmonary valve placement in the expanded multicenter US melody valve trial. *Circulation* 2010; **122**: 507–516.

48 Eicken A, Ewert P, Hager A, *et al.* Percutaneous pulmonary valve implantation: two-centre experience with more than 100 patients. *Eur Heart J* 2011; **32**: 1260–1265.

49 Kenny D, Hijazi ZM, Kar S, *et al.* Percutaneous implantation of the Edwards SAPIEN transcatheter heart valve for conduit failure in the pulmonary position: early phase 1 results from an international multicenter clinical trial. *J Am Coll Cardiol* 2011; **58**: 594–598.

50 Lurz P, Nordmeyer J, Giardini A, *et al.* Early versus late functional outcome after successful percutaneous pulmonary valve implantation: are the acute effects of altered right ventricular loading all we can expect? *J Am Coll Cardiol* 2011; **57**: 724–731.

51 Ferraz Cavalcanti P, Sa M, Santos C, *et al.* Pulmonary valve replacement after operative repair of tetralogy of Fallot: meta-analysis and meta-regression of 3,118 patients from 48 studies. *J Am Coll Cardiol* 2013; **62**(23): 2227–2243.

52 McElhinney D, Cheatham J, Jones T, *et al.* Stent fracture, valve dysfunction, and right ventricular outflow tract reintervention after transcatheter pulmonary valve implantation: patient-related and procedural risk factors in the US Melody Valve Trial. *Circ Cardiovasc Interv* 2011; **4**: 602–614.

53 Law K, Phillips K, Butany J. Pulmonary valve-in-valve implants: how long do they prolong reintervention and what causes them to fail? *Cardiovasc Pathol* 2012; **21**: 519–521.

54 Nordmeyer J, Coats L, Lurz P, *et al.* Percutaneous pulmonary valve-in-valve implantation: a successful treatment concept for early device failure. *Eur Heart J* 2008; **29**: 810-815.

55 Raikou M, McGuire A, Lurz P, *et al.* An assessment of the cost of percutaneous pulmonary valve implantation (PPVI) versus surgical pulmonary valve replacement

(PVR) in patients with right ventricular outflow tract dysfunction. *J Med Econ* 2011; **14**: 47–52.

56 Gatlin S, Kim D, Mahle W. Cost analysis of percutaneous pulmonary valve replacement. *Am J Cardiol* 2011; **108**: 572–574.

57 Guccione P, Milanei O, Hijazi ZM. Transcatheter pulmonary valve implantation in native pulmonary outflow tract using the Edwards SAPIEN™ transcatheter heart valve. *Eur J Cardiothorac Surg* 2012; **41**(5): 1192–1194.

58 Schievano S, Taylor A, Capelli C, *et al.* First-in-man implantation of a novel percutaneous valve: a new approach to medical device development. *Euro Intervention* 2010; **5**: 745–750.

59 Nordmeyer J, Tsang V, Gaudin R, *et al.* Quantitative assessment of homograft function 1 year after insertion into the pulmonary position: impact of in situ homograft geometry on valve competence. *Eur Heart J* 2009; **30**: 2147–2154.

60 Cao Q, Kenny D, Zhou D, *et al.* Early clinical experience with a novel self-expanding percutaneous stent-valve in the native right ventricular outflow tract. *Catheter Cardiovasc Interv* 2014; **84**: 1131–1137.

61 Butera G, Milanesi O, Spadoni I, *et al.* Melody transcatheter pulmonary valve implantation: results from the registry of the Italian Society of Pediatric Cardiology (SICP). *Catheter Cardiovasc Interv* 2013; **81**: 310–316.

CHAPTER 67

Imaging for Planning and Guidance for Structural Heart Interventions

Ankit Parikh and Stamatios Lerakis

Emory University School of Medicine, Atlanta, GA, USA

The field of structural heart interventions is one that is expanding at an exponential pace. The role of the interventional echocardiographer and/or cardiac imaging specialist has become increasingly important to assist with the planning and guidance of these interventions. This chapter discusses the general role of imaging and specific role of echocardiography as an adjunct for selected structural heart interventions. As more types of interventions and devices become available, the role of the imager will continue to grow and develop. While imaging technology continues to improve in parallel with interventional techniques, it remains crucially important to understand the limitations of available imaging modalities. The interventional echocardiographer and imaging specialist have an important role in anticipating when imaging may be suboptimal and communicating this information to the interventional team.

Transcatheter aortic valve replacement

Transcatheter aortic valve replacement (TAVR) has become an alternative to surgery in patients with severe aortic stenosis (AS) who are inoperable or at high risk for surgical aortic valve replacement. Imaging is important to support TAVR procedures and assess potential complications. The determination of AS severity and the indications for intervention are discussed in recent guidelines [1,2]. Several excellent comprehensive reviews on the role of imaging during TAVR have also been recently published [3–7].

Knowing the planned procedural access site is an important initial consideration for the imager. Potential access sites include transfemoral, transapical, transcaval, transaortic, or transcarotid approaches. Basic knowledge about these approaches is important and can help the imager anticipate some of the information that will be needed during the procedure. For example, if a transapical approach is chosen, the imager can be asked to assist with localization of an optimal apical site for access and identification of any abnormalities such as apical thrombi that can result in significant complications.

Another important initial consideration involves the type of valve. The role of the imager may be different during cases in which a balloon-expandable valve is chosen compared to cases in which a self-expanding valve is chosen. Additionally, the anticipated complications are different for different types of valves. The current balloon-expandable valves include the second-generation SAPIEN XT and the third-generation SAPIEN 3 (Edwards Lifesicences, Irvine, CA, USA) [3,4]. The SAPIEN XT is composed of three bovine pericardial leaflets mounted on a cobalt chromium stent. The valve is deployed by delivering it to the desired site crimped over a balloon, and the balloon is then inflated to expand the valve (Figure 67.1). A fabric skirt mounted inside of the valve stent below the leaflets allows the valve to seal at the aortic annulus. There are three available sizes: 23, 26, and 29 mm. It is important to note that not all aortic annuli come in three sizes, and cases will often be encountered in which the annular size falls outside of the ideal range. Important aspects of valve sizing are discussed further later. The SAPIEN 3 requires a smaller delivery system and also has an outer skirt designed to attempt to reduce paravalvular leak (PVL), which remains one of the major complications of TAVR. The evaluation of PVL is also discussed later. The SAPIEN 3 also has a 20 mm valve size that allows for a wider range of annular dimensions to be considered for intervention. The CoreValve (Medtronic, Minneapolis, MN, USA) is a porcine pericardial valve mounted within a self-expanding nitinol frame [3,4]. A skirt is also mounted within the frame. As the valve is unsheathed, it deploys on its own, and the outflow end of the valve sits in the ascending aorta (Figure 67.2). It is available in four sizes: 23, 26, 29, and 31 mm.

When choosing the appropriate valve size, the most important measurement is the annular plane at the level of the hinge points (the lowest point of attachment of the three native aortic valve cusps) [4]. Because the annulus is often asymmetric and oval, echocardiographic measurement is challenging. The standard two-dimensional (2D) transthoracic echocardiographic (TTE) parasternal long-axis view is used to measure left ventricular outflow tract (LVOT) dimension for the calculation of aortic valve area by the continuity equation. However, this view is insufficient on its own for TAVR valve sizing. It is currently recommended to use either three-dimensional (3D) transesophageal echocardiography (TEE), computed tomography (CT), or both. With 3D TEE, annular sizing can be accomplished by rotating the planar views to cut through the aortic valve hinge points at the widest orthogonal dimensions of the aortic annulus. The resulting short-axis image can be used to either directly planimeter annular dimensions and area or indirectly obtain this information by marking off the annular hinge points on the corresponding long-axis planes at end-systole

Interventional Cardiology: Principles and Practice, Second Edition. Edited by George D. Dangas, Carlo Di Mario, and Nicholas N. Kipshidze.
© 2017 John Wiley & Sons, Ltd. Published 2017 by John Wiley & Sons, Ltd.

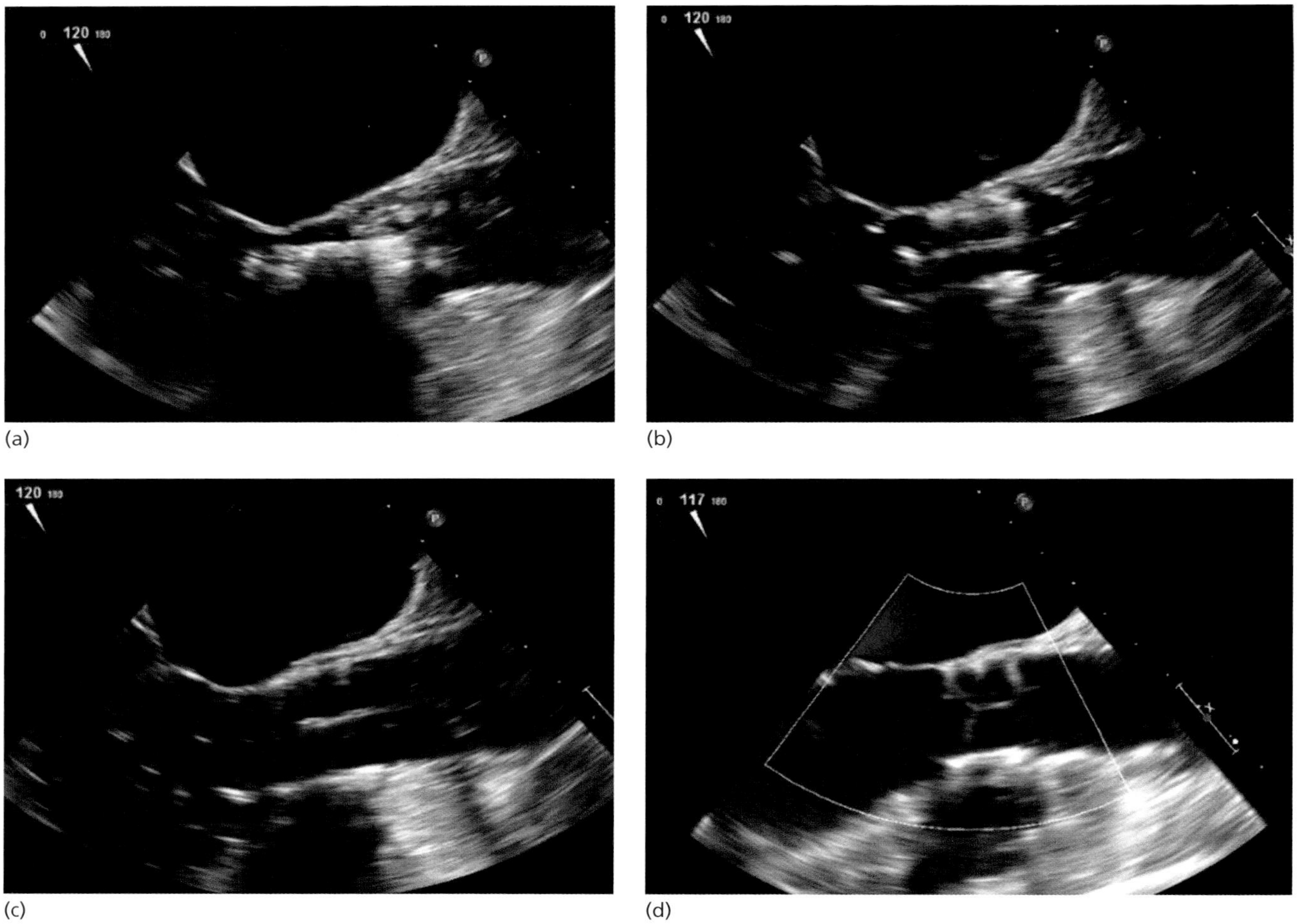

Figure 67.1 Two-dimensional transesophageal echocardiographic views demonstrating deployment of a balloon-expandable valve. (a) The stent frame crimped around the balloon. (b) The balloon in the process of expansion. (c) The balloon fully expanded. (d) The final result, with the balloon pulled back and the valve fully deployed.

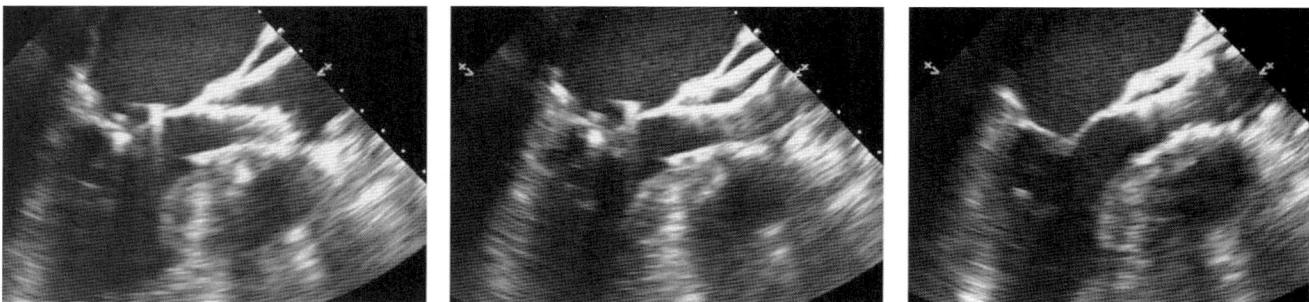

Figure 67.2 Two-dimensional transesophageal echocardiographic views demonstrating deployment of a self-expanding valve; the valve frame expands on its own (from left to right) as it is unsheathed.

[4]. If the indirect method is used, the points along the annulus are marked off and the echocardiographic software package then calculates annular dimensions and area (Figure 67.3). Because of the lower frame rate of 3D imaging than 2D imaging, it can be challenging to determine the occurrence of end-systole; the exact instant of end-systole often falls between two consecutive frames. In part because of this limitation, and because of the more invasive nature of TEE, CT has been used at many centers as an alternate method to calculate annular dimensions and area. With CT, the annular plane is identified in a similar fashion, by identifying the hinge points and then identifying the appropriate transaxial slice. Annular sizing with indirect planimetry on 3D TEE closely approximates that of CT and predicts mild or greater PVL with equivalent accuracy [8].

Ranges of annular area that correspond to available valve sizes have been published for both balloon-expandable and self-expanding

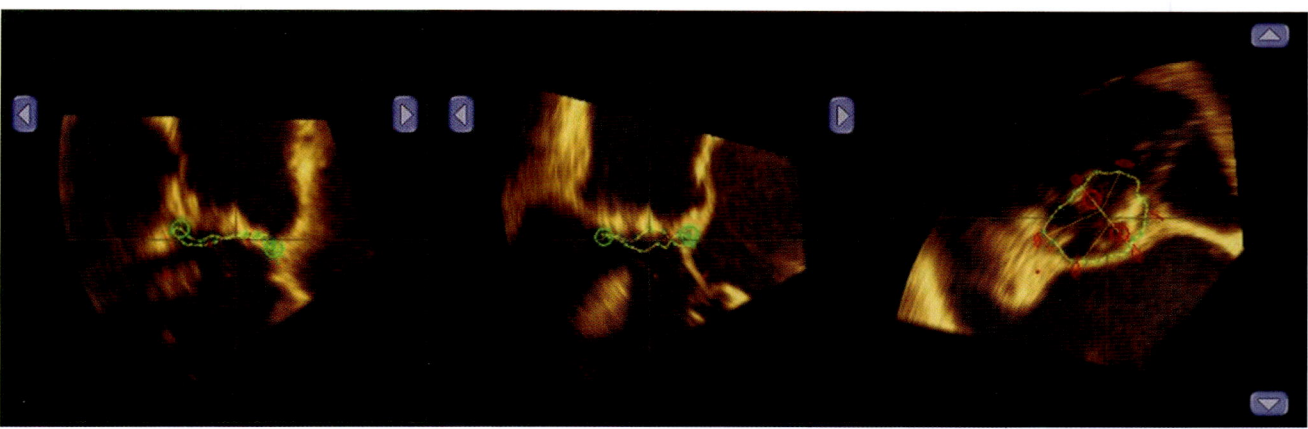

Figure 67.3 With three-dimensional transesophageal echocardiographic imaging, two orthogonal long-axis planes can be identified after a full volume is obtained (green and red panels). The hinge points are marked off on these two panels and the results are shown on the short-axis image (blue panel). The software then calculates annular dimensions and area.

valves [4]. Valves can be oversized compared to the native aortic annulus to ensure stable seating and minimize PVL. However, oversizing by >20% of aortic annular area is associated with a greater risk of rupture [9]. In contrast, valve undersizing can impact both PVL severity and transvalvular hemodynamic performance. In some cases, when the annular size falls in between two of the available valve size ranges, the interventionalist needs to consider intentional under-expansion of a larger valve, although again this can impact valve hemodynamics and performance.

Additional important observations must be made during the initial work-up to determine TAVR candidacy. These observations are made at each anatomic level, from the LVOT to the aortic sinotubular junction and beyond [4]. When assessing the LVOT, the imager should note the presence of marked basal septal hypertrophy. This is related to compensatory hypertrophy secondary to pressure overload in AS. Additionally, a sigmoid-shaped septum is often observed in older individuals. Marked basal septal hypertrophy can complicate the TAVR procedure by impeding the ability of the interventionalist to maintain coaxiality of the valve delivery system. As discussed further later, maintenance of coaxiality of the valve delivery system is an important component of valve positioning and deployment. Another important complication that can be observed during cases in which the septum is hypertrophied and hyperdynamic is post-procedural LVOT obstruction and mitral regurgitation (MR) from systolic anterior motion of the anterior mitral valve (MV) leaflet. In contrast, a thin septum can increase the risk of iatrogenic ventricular septal defect, and a calcified septum can increase the risk of post-deployment PVL and of annular rupture [4].

The native aortic valve leaflets must also be assessed for bulky calcification [4]. Not only can significant calcification impact valve deployment and seating, it can also lead to complications such as PVL, coronary occlusion (by displacement of calcium into the ostium of a coronary artery), or aortic trauma (annular or root perforation, rupture, hematoma, or dissection). Procedural results can be worse in patients with native bicuspid aortic valve disease, although this remains an area of active research [4].

Above the aortic valve, it is important to assess the sinuses of Valsalva, sinotubular junction, and the positions of the coronary ostia [4]. Occlusion of the left main coronary artery is more common than occlusion of the right coronary artery, and this is usually caused by displacement of a calcified nodule or a calcified native valve leaflet. Both TEE and CT can be used to measure coronary height above the annulus, and coronary patency can be monitored during the procedure both echocardiographically and angiographically [4]. It is also important to note the presence of plaques in the aortic arch and descending aorta, as these can impact the procedural approach, particularly if catheters will be directed retrogradely up the aorta.

After determining that a patient is a reasonable candidate for TAVR, it is important to consider the most appropriate intraprocedural imaging modality. While fluoroscopy and angiography remain the primary imaging tools used by the interventional cardiologist during the procedure, echocardiography has a very important adjunctive role in monitoring valve delivery and deployment as well as assessing for post-deployment complications. The choice of TTE versus TEE as the main echocardiographic adjunct to intraprocedural fluoroscopy and angiography remains an area of intense debate [10]. While TEE is most commonly used as the complementary imaging modality to fluoroscopy and angiography during the procedure, TTE is an acceptable alternative in transfemoral cases when the use of conscious sedation is planned as opposed to general anesthesia [11]. When deciding whether to choose TTE over TEE for intraprocedural guidance, it is important to consider the adequacy and quality of pre-procedural TTE images. Difficulties with obtaining adequate acoustic windows are likely to be exacerbated during the procedure, as are difficulties with visualization bcause of acoustic shadowing or artifacts. It is important for the interventional echocardiographer or advanced cardiac imaging specialist to convey to the interventionalist when imaging difficulties and suboptimal image quality are anticipated intraprocedurally based on the pre-procedural assessment. Useful TTE views include the parasternal long-axis and short-axis views as well as the apical five-chamber and three-chamber views. Useful TEE views include the mid-esophageal long-axis (110–130°) and short-axis (30–50°) views as well as the deep transgastric view (120°) looking upward at the LVOT and aortic prosthesis from a more inferior position.

Balloon aortic valvuloplasty (BAV) can be performed prior to TAVR to increase cusp exertion and to confirm annular sizing (Figure 67.4) [4]. BAV can also be useful to predict calcium displacement during final valve deployment and assure adequate coronary artery perfusion during balloon inflation [4]. Complications

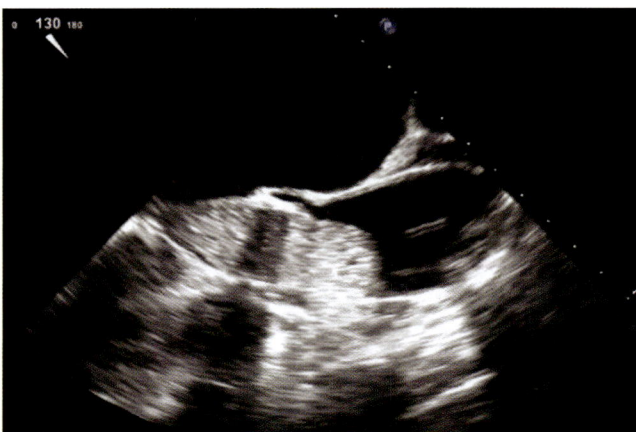

Figure 67.4 Two-dimensional transesophageal echocardiographic view of a balloon being inflated during balloon aortic valvuloplasty.

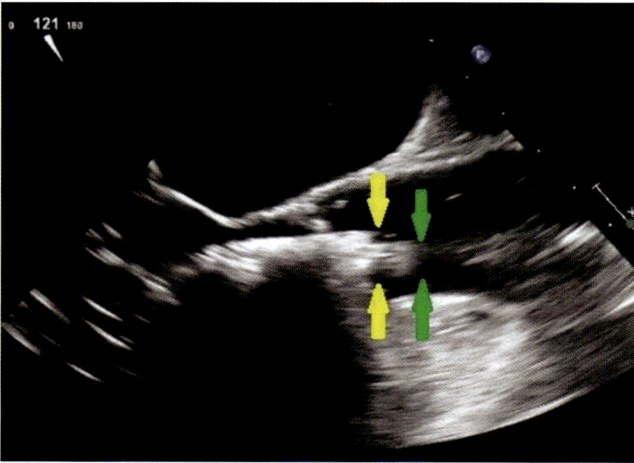

Figure 67.5 Two-dimensional transesophageal echocardiographic view of a valve stent frame that has been crimped around a balloon and is in the process of being positioned. The yellow arrows mark the edge of the stent frame, while the green arrows mark the edge of the balloon. Sometimes it can be difficult to differentiate the stent frame from the balloon.

of BAV include acute coronary occlusion, severe aortic regurgitation, or aortic trauma with the possibility of resultant cardiac tamponade.

Prior to deployment of a balloon-expandable valve, the echocardiographer must consider the coaxiality of the stent frame with the aortic annulus as well as the position of the edges of the stent frame with the aortic leaflets [4]. While maintaining coaxiality is very important, it is often difficult for the interventional cardiologist to obtain a perfect alignment. However, small deviations from a perfectly coaxial alignment will often correct themselves as the valve is being expanded. Prior to balloon expansion, the distal edge of the stent frame should cover the native leaflets but remain below the sinotubular junction and coronary ostia (Figure 67.5). Differentiation of the crimped stent from the underlying balloon can sometimes be difficult despite concerted efforts to tilt and rotate the ultrasound probe, especially in cases with poor acoustic

windows or significant acoustic shadowing. Options for better differentiation include reducing the echocardiographic gain or using live 3D imaging, if available [4]. Correlation with fluoroscopy and angiography can also increase confidence in appropriate stent frame positioning prior to valve deployment. Compared with the deployment of a balloon-expandable valve, the deployment of a self-expanding valve is a more gradual procedure, and fluoroscopy plays the primary part during procedural deployment as the valve is unsheathed. Echocardiography can assist in the diagnosis of deployment-related complications, such as PVL.

Echocardiography perhaps has its most critical role in assessing procedural complications after valve deployment. There are a number of observations that must be made to provide the interventional team with an integrated and comprehensive determination of procedural success. Many of these post-deployment observations rely on a combination of 2D and color Doppler imaging. Spectral Doppler can also be employed to assess valve hemodynamic function and gradients. It is often useful to correlate this information with invasive hemodynamic measurements obtained by the interventional cardiologist.

Initial observations include stent positioning, shape, and leaflet motion [4]. Leaflets that appear to open completely are unlikely to be associated with hemodynamically significant prosthetic valve stenosis. However, this qualitative information on valve opening and closing can be compared with quantitative determination of gradients by continuous wave Doppler. It can be more difficult to measure gradients across the valve with TEE than with TTE, as it is often more difficult to obtain adequate the deep transgastric views on TEE compared to the apical views obtained from the transthoracic approach. The ultrasound beam should be aligned as parallel as possible to the direction of blood flow to obtain the most accurate assessment of gradients across the valve.

A global assessment of left and right ventricular function should be made post-deployment, and new regional wall motion abnormalities should be noted [4]. A change in cardiac function can reflect consequences of rapid pacing used during balloon inflation, which can result in low forward cardiac output, with resultant hypotension and ischemia. A change in ventricular function can also result from coronary occlusion, and thus it is also important to assess for coronary patency post-deployment, as discussed earlier [4]. Coronary patency can be assessed with 2D imaging, and coronary arterial flow can be confirmed using color Doppler. This information can be correlated to that observed with post-deployment angiography, with power injection of contrast into the aortic root.

Other important observations include assessing the LVOT for obstruction, evaluating the function of the other cardiac valves, assessing the aortic annulus and root for signs of iatrogenic trauma, and evaluating for any rapidly accumulating pericardial effusion. LVOT obstruction can be seen in cases of basal septal hypertrophy and can be exacerbated by increased circulating catecholamines and relative hypovolemia [4]. Worsening MR can be a result of systolic anterior motion of the anterior mitral valve leaflet, or it could reflect damage to the mitral valve apparatus during the procedure [4]. If iatrogenic, the MR may be associated with chordal rupture or a flail MV leaflet. Additionally, the possibility of ischemic MR must be considered if the MR is observed in conjunction with new wall motion abnormalities after rapid pacing or after coronary occlusion. Iatrogenic ventricular septal defect can also be seen if the septum is perforated by the delivery apparatus. Dreaded aortic complications include rupture, dissection, and hematoma. Aortic trauma can be related to deployment itself or can be related to the displacement of sharp, bulky calcium into the aortic root during the procedure. If there is concern for aortic pathology post-deployment, it is important to correlate the appearance of the aortic root with that observed on pre-deployment images. Pericardial effusion can be caused by aortic perforation or rupture, or it can be related to cardiac chamber perforation from the right ventricular pacing wire or from the valve deployment apparatus. A rapidly accumulating pericardial effusion in a pericardial sac unaccustomed to such an effusion can result in potentially fatal cardiac tamponade. Comparison to pre-deployment images is critically important when assessing for progression of a pericardial effusion, especially if an effusion was present at the start of the procedure.

Echocardiography also has a major role in assessing the presence and severity of post-deployment PVL (Figures 67.6 and 67.7). In many cases this ends up being the primary component of the post-deployment assessment. Moderate or severe PVL is common after TAVR, with an incidence of approximately 14% at 30 days in the PARTNER trial [12]. This complication was far more common than

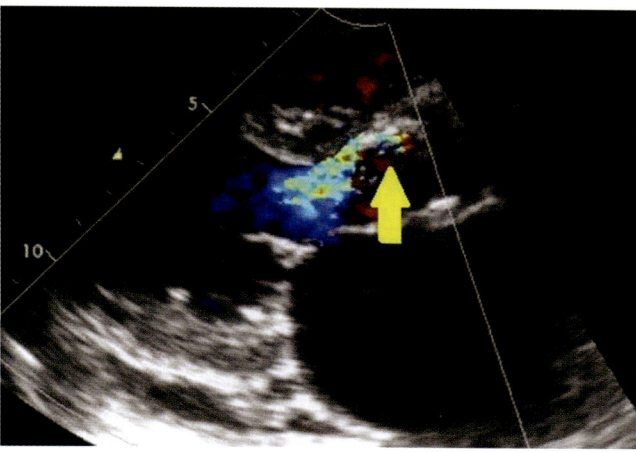

Figure 67.6 Two-dimensional transthoracic echocardiographic view demonstrating significant paravalvular leak after balloon-expandable valve deployment (yellow arrow).

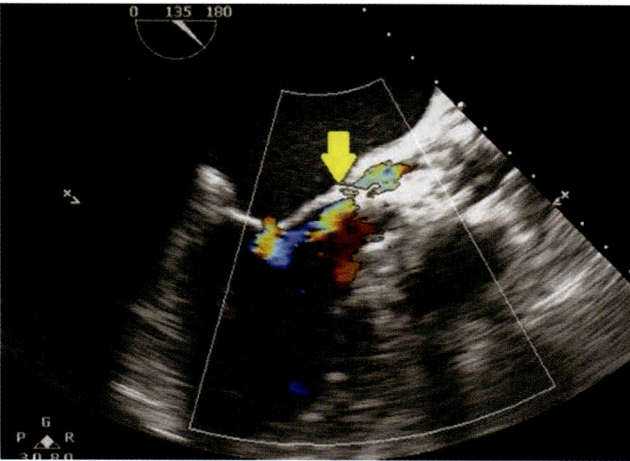

Figure 67.7 Two-dimensional transesophageal echocardiographic view demonstrating significant paravalvular leak after self-expandable valve deployment (yellow arrow).

similar degrees of PVL after surgical aortic valve replacement. PVL has been shown to be an independent predictor of mortality after the procedure, and even mild PVL was associated with an increased risk of mortality in the PARTNER trial [12,13], though this finding remains controversial, as other studies have not found a similar association between mild or trace PVL and mortality [14]. The development of PVL after TAVR can be related to annular issues, such as significant calcification, or it may be related technical and device-related issues, such as valve undersizing or maldeployment [14,15]. While valve oversizing can reduce the risk of significant PVL, it can increase the risk of annular rupture, coronary artery occlusion, and arrhythmic complications [14,16].

The assessment of PVL severity is not straightforward. Shielding and reverberations from the valvular frame or from the native calcified root that can obscure visualization can occur. In addition, the regurgitant orifices tend to be crescentic and irregular, leading to eccentric regurgitant jets that can be difficult to quantify [14,15]. Several guidelines regarding the grading of PVL severity have been published [1,3,7,17,18]. Semi-quantitative parameters include regurgitant jet width as a percentage of LVOT width and diastolic flow reversal in the proximal descending aorta. Quantitative parameters include regurgitant volume, regurgitant fraction, and effective regurgitant orifice area. A criterion about which there has been some disagreement has been the circumferential extent of the regurgitant jet expressed as a percentage of the aortic annular circumference on the short-axis view (either the transthoracic parasternal short-axis view or the transesophageal mid-esophageal short-axis view at 30–50°; Figure 67.8). While earlier publications endorse using a cut-off of >20% for severe PVL [3,18], more recent publications suggest a cut-off of >30% for severe PVL [7,17]. There is acknowledgment that this criterion is not well-validated and may overestimate PVL severity compared to quantitative Doppler echocardiography [17]. Because of the difficulty in characterizing PVL severity solely based on echocardiographic assessment, cardiovascular magnetic resonance (CMR) imaging has emerged as an alternate option [19]. Compared with CMR, the circumferential extent of PVL visualized echocardiographically in short-axis tends to overestimate PVL severity [20]. A regurgitant fraction >20%, as calculated by CMR, has been associated with a higher incidence of adverse events after TAVR [21].

While there are no universally established guidelines for the management of PVL after TAVR, potential intraprocedural options include balloon post-dilatation, valve repositioning by snaring, valve-in-valve replacement, or surgical conversion [14,15,22–24]. In patients with chronic PVL after TAVR, transcatheter device closure is an option [25,26]. Echocardiography is an important adjunct to these percutaneous closure procedures. TEE is generally the preferred imaging modality in this setting [3], although the use of intracardiac echocardiography has also been reported [27]. 3D TEE can also be used to demonstrate the irregular crescentric shape of the defect or defects and assist with accurate defect sizing [3]. The interventional echocardiographer must be cautious to avoid over-diagnosing areas of echocardiographic dropout as paravalvular defects; the addition of color Doppler can be helpful in avoiding this pitfall. The echocardiographer can assist the interventional cardiologist in following the passage of the guidewire and catheter through the defect [3], although the interventional cardiologist can also be use hemodynamic, fluoroscopic, and contrast-based angiographic data for this purpose. Subsequently, the echocardiographer can assure proper positioning of the selected closure device, proper seating of the device, and assess for residual regurgitation after device

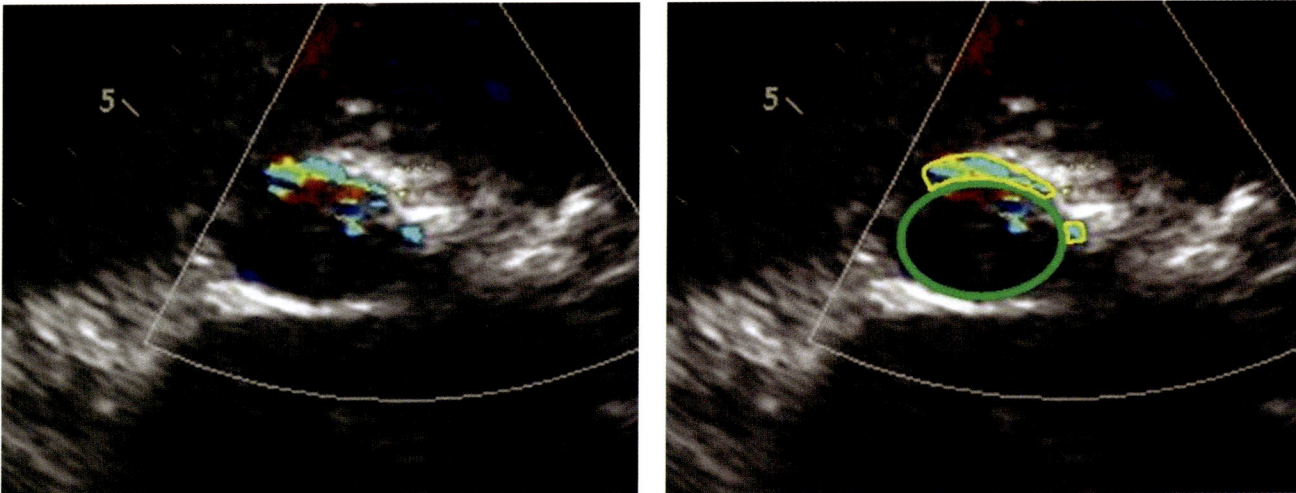

Figure 67.8 The left panel demonstrates severe paravalvular regurgitation visualized in short-axis. In the right panel, the left ventricular outflow tract area is traced in green and the regurgitant flow is traced in yellow. Note that the yellow tracings cover >30% of the circumferential extent of the left ventricular outflow tract. Also note the presence of multiple jets as well as the irregular crescentic shape of the regurgitant orifices.

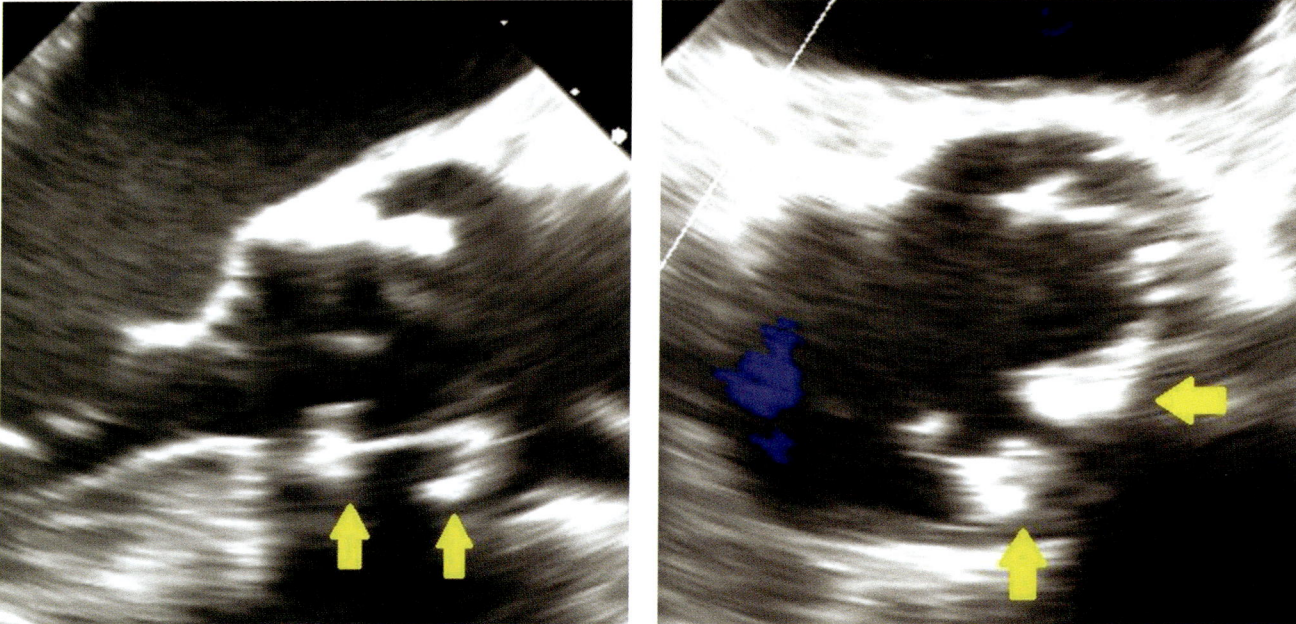

Figure 67.9 Deployment of two vascular plugs for correction of paravalvular leak (yellow arrows).

closure (Figure 67.9). It is important to ensure that device closure of a defect does not result in deterioration of prosthetic valve function; this undesired outcome would most commonly be caused by hindering of prosthetic leaflet motion by the closure device. When the defect is large or multiple defects exist, multiple closure devices may be required. Even when device closure results in hemodynamic improvement of the degree of regurgitation, it is possible for small amounts of residual regurgitation to result in significant hemolysis [3]. As with the index TAVR procedure, the echocardiographer must remain aware of the litany of potential complications that occur during repeat aortic valve intervention, as previously discussed.

Percutaneous mitral valve repair

Percutaneous MV repair has emerged as a therapeutic option for patients with significant symptomatic MR who are deemed to be too high risk for surgery or who have had previous cardiac surgeries. The current device used for percutaneous MV repair is the MitraClip (Abbott Vascular, Santa Clara, CA, USA). The preferred imaging modality to support percutaneous MV repair is TEE using a combination of 2D and 3D imaging; the procedure is typically performed under general anesthesia with endotracheal intubation, obviating the discomfort to the patient associated with prolonged TEE imaging. The role of the echocardiographer in pre-procedural planning, intraprocedural guidance, and post-procedural follow-up of percutaneous MV repair cannot be understated. While the following discussion is centered on percutaneous MV repair, it is important to note that the echocardiographic techniques used for procedural guidance can also be applied to other MV interventions, such as percutaneous closure of a paraprosthetic defect to correct significant paraprosthetic regurgitation (Figure 67.10).

The MitraClip is a polyester fabric-covered cobalt-chromium implant which has two arms that can be opened and closed, as well as a steerable guiding mechanism [3]. The design of the MitraClip is intended to replicate the double MV orifice created using the surgical Aliferi edge-to-edge repair [28]. The device is delivered to the right atrium via a femoral venous approach and then across the interatrial septum to the left atrium via transseptal puncture. By

aligning the device perpendicular to the line of coaptation between the involved leaflet segments, the goal is to grasp the involved leaflets and cinch them together with the clip mechanism, thus apposing the leaflets and reducing the degree of MR. The device has been used successfully in selected patients with either degenerative or functional MR [29]. In patients with flail MR, the flail gap, or gap between the flail leaflet and normal leaflet, should ideally be <10 mm wide, and the width of the flail segment or scallop should ideally be <15 mm [3]. Measurement of the flail gap is usually easily performed with 2D TEE imaging, while measurement of the flail width sometimes requires 3D imaging of the involved scallop. In functional MR that is secondary to left ventricular dysfunction, the length of leaflet tissue available for coaptation should ideally

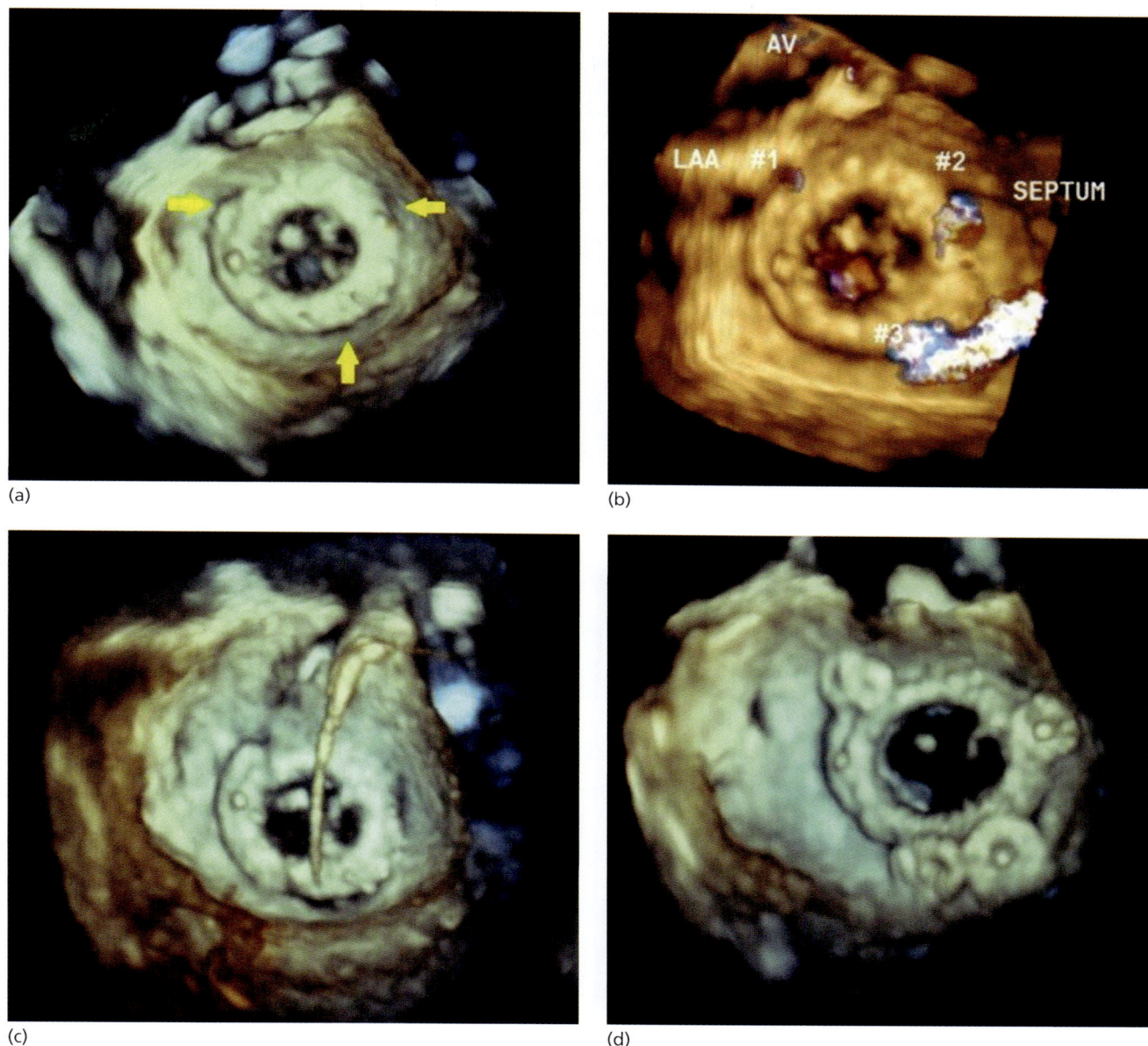

(a)

(b)

(c)

(d)

Figure 67.10 Three-dimensional transesophageal echocardiographic imaging of a bioprosthetic mitral valve in a patient with significant paraprosthetic regurgitation. (a) Three defects (yellow arrows), all of which are confirmed by the addition of color Doppler (b). The most prominent regurgitant jet originates from the defect at the 6 o'clock position. (c) A catheter crossing the largest defect after transseptal puncture. (d) The final result with deployment of four closure devices. AV, aortic valve; LAA, left atrial appendage.

be ≥2 mm in length and the depth from the mitral annular insertion points to the actual point of coaptation should ideally be ≤11 mm [3]. Determination of the severity of MR in the pre-procedural setting incorporates a number of observations, including the structure of the mitral apparatus, left atrial and left ventricular size and function, regurgitant jet area and vena contracta width by color Doppler, effective regurgitant orifice area (EROA) by the proximal isovelocity surface area (PISA) method, flow quantification by pulsed wave Doppler, jet profile by continuous wave Doppler, the peak mitral E velocity on the mitral inflow profile, and the pulmonary venous flow profiles by pulsed wave Doppler [1,30]. It is also useful to note the pre-procedural gradient across the mitral valve, as creation of the double orifice can increase the gradient across the valve significantly. It is important to understand that no single parameter in isolation can completely characterize MR severity, and a comprehensive evaluation is required in the pre-procedural setting in order to determine MR severity and procedural feasibility. It is also important to understand that the severity of MR can vary with loading conditions, and the assessment of severity can differ when the patient is ambulatory compared to when the patient is sedated under general anesthesia. As such, a focused re-evaluation is often warranted in the early procedural stages to determine if there have been any significant changes in perceived MR severity.

During transseptal puncture, the bicaval view at 90° can help the interventional cardiologist locate the tip of the transseptal catheter. The echocardiographer should assess for "tenting" of the interatrial septum to localize the point of planned septal puncture (Figure 67.11). The mid-esophageal short-axis (30–50°) and four-chamber (0°) views can be used to determine where the tenting point is in relation to other structures such as the aortic annulus and the mitral annular insertion points. Ideally, the tenting should be observed about 3.5–4.0 cm above the insertion point of the mitral valve leaflets prior to leaflet puncture [3].

After transseptal puncture, the echocardiographer assists the interventional cardiologist with proper delivery of the device [3].

This often requires a combination of 2D and 3D TEE imaging, and the echocardiographer must be prepared to quickly switch back and forth between 2D and 3D. It is often very helpful use biplane echocardiographic imaging to be able to simultaneously visualize the location of the device in two different orthogonal views (Figure 67.12). In the mid-esophageal bicomissural view (55–75°), the medial edge of the mitral annulus will typically be oriented on the left side of the echocardiographic image, in close proximity to the interventricular septum, while the lateral edge of the mitral annulus will typically be oriented on the right side of the image, in close proximity to the left atrial appendage. In the mid-esophageal long-axis view (110–130°), the posterior edge of the mitral annulus will typically be oriented on the left side of the image and the anterior edge will be oriented on the left side of the image, in close proximity to the aortic valve and annulus. The ridge of tissue between the aortic and mitral valves (the aortic–mitral curtain) is often a useful landmark on 3D TEE imaging, as it should be placed at the top of the screen in the "surgeon's view" looking down at the mitral valve from the left atrium (Figure 67.13). In this 3D view, the left atrial appendage will be on the left side of the screen at the 9 o'clock position and the aortic valve will be at the top of the screen at the 12 o'clock position. The anterior MV leaflet will be toward the top of the screen and posterior MV leaflet will be toward the bottom. The orientation of the scallops progresses from A1 to A3 or P1 to P3 in a left to right (lateral to medial) direction. By using a combination of 2D and 3D TEE imaging, the echocardiographer can facilitate guidance of the device into the proper position above the largest regurgitant orifice and perpendicular to the line of coaptation (Figure 67.14). Opening the arms of the device while in the left atrium can facilitate this alignment, but the arms should be closed when the MV is crossed and the device is situated in the left ventricle.

Leaflet grasping is performed in the "grasping view," which is essentially the mid-esophageal long-axis view between 110° and 130°; occasionally angles higher than 130° are required to adequately

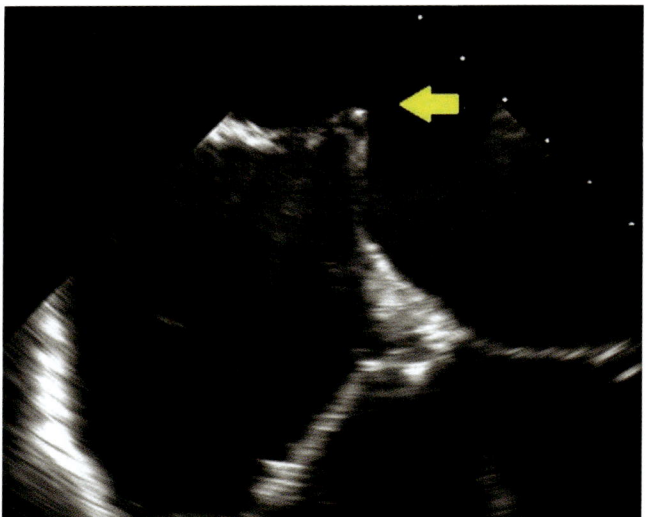
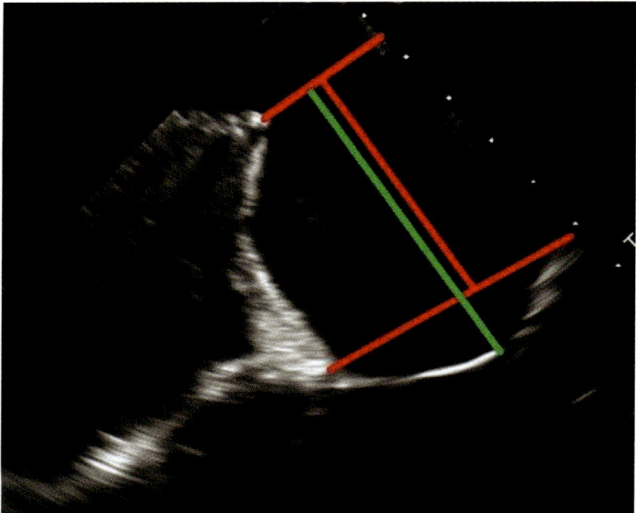

Figure 67.11 Two-dimensional transesophageal echocardiographic imaging of a transseptal puncture. The tenting of the interatrial septum is clearly visualized in the left panel (yellow arrow). The right panel demonstrates the measurement of the tenting height above the mitral annular insertion points. An imaginary line is drawn from the tenting point across the left atrium, parallel to the line connecting the mitral annular insertion points; a parallel line connecting these two is then drawn and measured (red lines). The green line shows the distance from the tenting point to the actual leaflet coaptation. The difference in distance between the green line and the red line represents the coaptation depth.

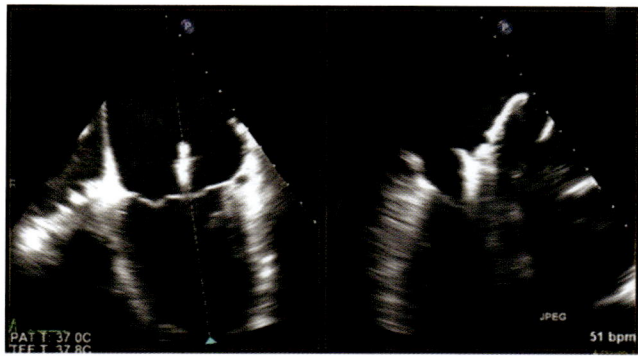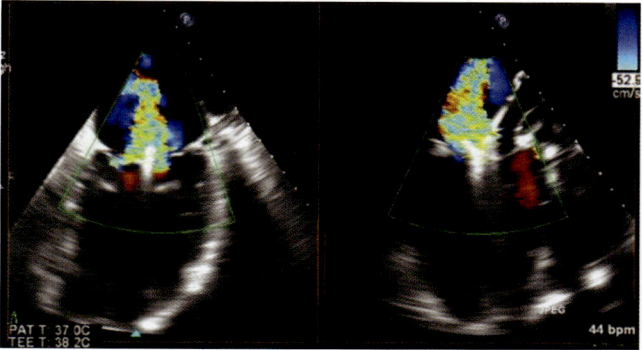

Figure 67.12 Biplane echocardiographic images without (left panel) and with (right panel) superimposed color Doppler, demonstrating the device in both the medial–lateral orientation (left side of both panels) and posterior–anterior orientation (right side of both panels). The right side of both panels demonstrates the mid-esophageal long-axis grasping view used to determine if the leaflets have been appropriately cinched by the device.

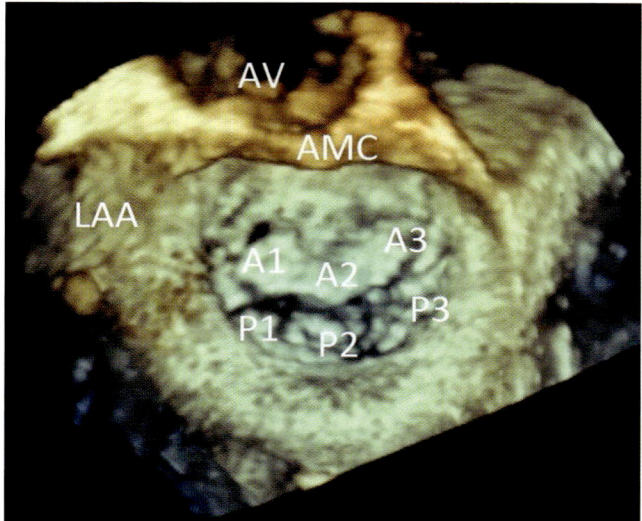

Figure 67.13 Three-dimensional transesophageal echocardiographic "surgeon's view" of the mitral valve as seen from the perspective of the left atrium. The aortic valve (AV) and aortic–mitral curtain (AMC) are aligned at the 12 o'clock position, and the left atrial appendage (LAA) is at the 9 o'clock position. The scallops of the anterior mitral leaflet are labeled A1–A3, and those of the posterior mitral leaflet are labeled P1–P3.

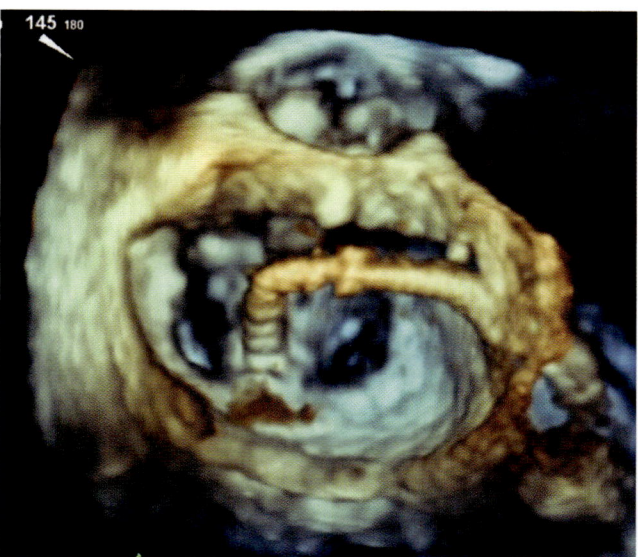

Figure 67.14 Three-dimensional transesophageal echocardiographic view of the device being aligned toward the mitral valve. Note that the device is perpendicular to the line of coaptation between the anterior and posterior leaflets.

visualize the MV leaflets in relation to the arms of the device, which have now been opened as the device is pulled back from the left ventricle toward the left atrium. Biplane echocardiographic imaging can be very useful at this point to ensure that the medial–lateral orientation of the device remains stable while the device is advanced. The key is to ensure that both leaflets have been grasped by the grippers of the device; this can often be one of the more challenging aspects of intraprocedural imaging (Figure 67.15). 3D imaging can be used to help determine if a double orifice has been formed (Figure 67.16). In the mid-esophageal bicommissural view, the medial orifice will be on the left and the lateral orifice will be on the right. If either leaflet has not been captured, or if it is unclear if both leaflets have been captured, the arms can be reopened and repeat grasps can be attempted. Once it is clear that both leaflets have been grasped, the

echocardiographer should perform a focused evaluation using color Doppler to determine residual MR severity, continuous wave Doppler to determine the medial and lateral gradients in order to exclude hemodynamically significant mitral stenosis, and pulsed wave Doppler of the pulmonary venous flow profiles to determine if there has been improvement in the degree of systolic flow reversal or blunting. Correlation with invasively obtained hemodynamics by the interventionalist can be useful; these include mean left atrial pressure and left atrial V-wave height pre- and post-deployment. If there is still significant residual MR, the decision must be made whether to deploy the first clip and prepare a second clip for deployment or to release the leaflets and attempt to regrasp at a more favorable position. It is not uncommon for a second clip to be required, and on occasion even a third clip is required. However, with each additional clip, it becomes increasingly important to exclude hemodynamically significant gradients across the valve.

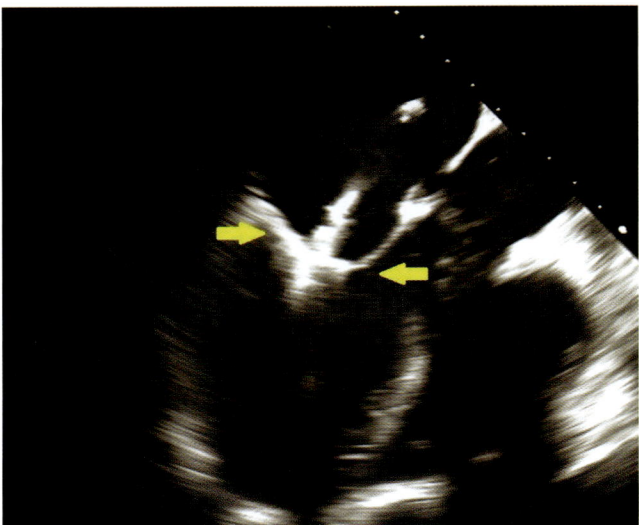

Figure 67.15 Two-dimensional transesophageal echocardiographic grasping view with the posterior leaflet on the left side of the image and the anterior leaflet on the right side of the image. Note the appearance of the mitral valve leaflets within the grippers of the device (yellow arrows).

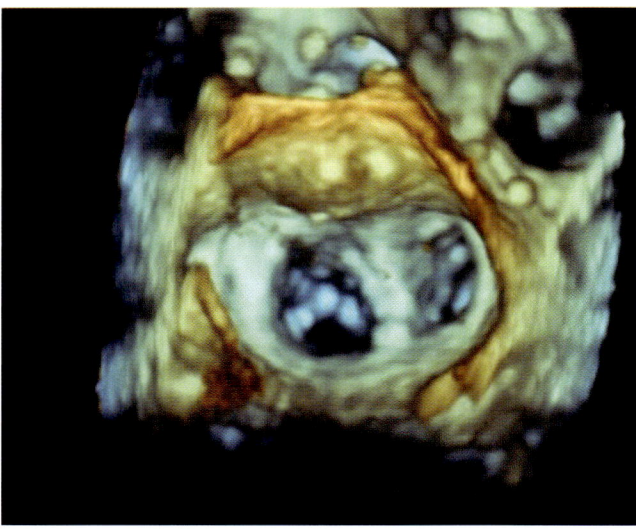

Figure 67.16 Double orifice seen at the conclusion of the procedure. The clip has apposed A2 and P2 in this case.

There are a number of potential complications of the procedure that can be imaged by TEE: chamber perforation with subsequent pericardial effusion formation; clip dehiscence after initial deployment; or leaflet or chordal trauma related to the device itself [3]. Post-procedural follow-up becomes challenging in that some of the traditional measurements described for quantifying native MR severity [1,30] are no longer validated for quantifying MR severity post-percutaneous MV repair. For example, flow quantification by pulsed wave Doppler becomes limited by the fact that there are now two pathways for flow to enter from the left atrium into the left ventricle [3]. Additionally, the calculation of EROA by the PISA method has not been validated in this setting, nor has it been

validated for the multiple regurgitant jets that can exist after clip deployment [3]. In this sense, pulmonary venous flow profiles take on added significance as surrogates for invasively measured hemodynamics.

Conclusions

The role of the structural imager in collaboration with the interventional cardiology team continues to grow and evolve. As imaging modalities continue to improve and new techniques become available, the structural imager will become even more integral to the function of the structural heart team. A thorough understanding of the views and techniques used will help the imager apply these principles to a number of novel interventions that become available in the future.

Interactive multiple choice questions are available for this chapter on www.wiley. com/go/dangas/cardiology

References

1 Nishimura RA, Otto CM, Bonow RO, *et al.* 2014 AHA/ACC guideline for the management of patients with valvular heart disease: a report of the American College of Cardiology/American Heart Association Task Force on Practice Guidelines. *J Am Coll Cardiol* 2014; **63**: e57–185.

2 Baumgartner H, Hung J, Bermejo J, *et al.* Echocardiographic assessment of valve stenosis: EAE/ASE recommendations for clinical practice. *J Am Soc Echocardiogr* 2009; **22**: 1–23.

3 Zamorano JL, Badano LP, Bruce C, *et al.* EAE/ASE recommendations for the use of echocardiography in new transcatheter interventions for valvular heart disease. *J Am Soc Echocardiogr* 2011; **24**: 937–965.

4 Hahn RT, Little SH, Monaghan MJ, *et al.* Recommendations for comprehensive intraprocedural echocardiographic imaging during TAVR. *J Am Coll Cardiol Imaging* 2015; **8**: 261–287.

5 Hahn RT, Kodali S, Tuzcu EM, *et al.* Echocardiographic imaging of procedural complications during balloon-expandable transcatheter aortic valve replacement. *J Am Coll Cardio! Imaging* 2015; **8**: 288–318.

6 Hahn RT, Gillam LD, Little SH. Echocardiographic imaging of procedural complications during self-expandable transcatheter aortic valve replacement. *J Am Coll Cardiol Imaging* 2015; **8**: 319–336.

7 Pibarot P, Hahn RT, Weissman NJ, Monaghan MJ. Assessment of paravalvular regurgitation following TAVR: a proposal of unifying grading scheme. *J Am Coll Cardiol Imaging* 2015; **8**: 340–360.

8 Khalique OK, Kodali SK, Paradis JM, *et al.* Aortic annular sizing using a novel 3-dimensional echocardiographic method: use and comparison with cardiac computed tomography. *Circ Cardiovasc Imaging* 2014; **7**: 155–163.

9 Barbanti M, Yang TH, Rodès Cabau J, *et al.* Anatomical and procedural features associated with aortic root rupture during balloon-expandable transcatheter aortic valve replacement. *Circulation* 2013; **128**: 244–253.

10 Kronzon I, Jelnin V, Ruiz CE, *et al.* Optimal imaging for guiding TAVR: transesophageal or transthoracic echocardiography, or just fluoroscopy? *J Am Coll Cardiol Imaging* 2015; **8**: 361–370.

11 Babaliaros V, Devireddy C, Lerakis S, *et al.* Comparison of transfemoral transcatheter aortic valve replacement performed in the catheterization laboratory (minimalist approach) versus hybrid operating room (standard approach): outcomes and cost analysis. *J Am Coll Cardiol Interv* 2014; **7**: 898–904.

12 Mack MJ, Leon MB, Smith CR, *et al.* 5-year outcomes of transcatheter aortic valve replacement or surgical aortic valve replacement for high risk surgical patients with aortic stenosis (PARTNER 1): a randomised controlled trial. *Lancet* 2015; **385**: 2477–2484.

13 Kodali SK, Williams MR, Smith CR, *et al.* Two-year outcomes after transcatheter or surgical aortic-valve replacement. *N Engl J Med* 2012; **366**: 1686–1695.

14 Lerakis S, Hayek SS, Douglas PS. Paravalvular aortic leak after transcatheter aortic valve replacement: current knowledge. *Circulation* 2013; **127**: 397–407.

15 Généreux P, Head SJ, Hahn R, *et al.* Paravalvular leak after transcatheter aortic valve replacement: the new Achilles' heel? A comprehensive review of the literature. *J Am Coll Cardiol* 2012; **59**: 1275–1286.

16 Wilson AB, Webb JG, Labounty TM, *et al.* 3-dimensional aortic annular assessment by multidetector computed tomography predicts moderate or severe paravalvular regurgitation after transcatheter aortic valve replacement: a multicenter retrospective analysis. *J Am Coll Cardiol* 2012; **59**: 1287–1294.

17 Kappetein AP, Head SJ, Généreux P, *et al.* Updated standardized endpoint definitions for transcatheter aortic valve implantation: the Valve Academic Research Consortium-2 consensus document. *Eur J Cardiothroac Surg* 2012; **42**: S45–60.

18 Zoghbi WA, Chambers JB. Dumesnil JG, *et al.* Recommendations for evaluation of prosthetic valves with echocardiography and Doppler ultrasound. *J Am Soc Echocardiogr* 2009; **22**: 975–1014.

19 Lerakis S, Hayek S, Arepalli CD, *et al.* Cardiac magnetic resonance for paravalvular leaks in post-transcatheter aortic valve replacement. *Circulation* 2014; **129**: e430–431.

20 Hayek S, Sawaya F, Oshinski J, *et al.* Multiparametric assessment of post-transcatheter aortic valve replacement paravalvular regurgitation grading by transthoracic echocardiography and cardiac magnetic resonance. *J Clin Exp Cardiolog* 2014; **5**: 291.

21 Hartlage GR, Babaliaros VC, Thourani VH, *et al.* The role of cardiovascular magnetic resonance in stratifying paravalvular leak severity after transcatheter aortic valve replacement: an observational outcome study. *J Cardiovasc Magn Reson* 2014; **16**: 93.

22 Nombela-Franco L, Rodés-Cabau J, DeLarochellière R, *et al.* Predictive factors, efficacy, and safety of balloon post-dilation after transcatheter aortic valve implantation with a balloon-expandable valve. *JACC Cardiovasc Interv* 2012; **5**: 499–512.

23 Vavouranakis M, Vrachatis DA, Toutouzas KP, *et al.* "Bail out" procedures for malpositioning of aortic valve prosthesis (CoreValve). *Int J Cardiol* 2010; **145**: 154–155.

24 Ussia GP, Barbanti M, Ramondo A, *et al.* The valve-in-valve technique for treatment of aortic bioprosthesis malposition an analysis of incidence and 1-year clinical outcomes from the Italian CoreValve registry. *J Am Coll Cardiol* 2011; **57**: 1062–1068.

25 Martinez CA, Singh V, O'Neill BP, *et al.* Management of paravalvular regurgitation after Edwards SAPIEN transcatheter aortic valve replacement: management of paravalvular regurgitation after TAVR. *Catheter Cardiovasc Interv* 2013; **82**: 300–311.

26 Reed GW, Tuzcu EM, Kapadia SR, *et al.* Catheter-based closure of paravalvular leak. *Expert Rev Cardiovasc Ther* 2014; **12**: 681–692.

27 Defterios S, Giannopoulos G, Raisakis K, Kaoukis K, Kossyvakis C. Intracardiac echocardiography imaging of periprosthetic valvular regurgitation. *Eur J Echocardiogr* 2010; **11**: E20.

28 Alfieri O, Maisano F, De Bonis M, *et al.* The double-orifice technique in mitral valve repair: a simple solution for complex problems. *J Thorac Cardiovasc Surg* 2001; **122**: 674–681.

29 Glower DD, Kar S, Trento A, *et al.* Percutaneous mitral valve repair for mitral regurgitation in high-risk patients: results of the EVEREST II study. *J Am Coll Cardiol* 2014; **64**: 172–181.

30 Zoghbi WA, Enriquez-Sarano M, Foster E, *et al.* Recommendations for evaluation of the severity of native valvular regurgitation with two-dimensional and Doppler echocardiography. *J Am Soc Echocardiogr* 2003; **16**: 777–802.

PART IV

Vascular Disease for the Interventionalist

CHAPTER 68

Acute Stroke Intervention

Stefan C. Bertog[1], Iris Q. Grunwald[2], Anna Luisa Kühn[3], Laura Vaskelyte[1], Ilona Hofmann[1], Sameer Gafoor[1,4], Markus Reinartz[1,5], Predrag Matic[1], and Horst Sievert[1,6]

[1]CardioVascular Center Frankfurt, Frankfurt, Germany

[2]Post Graduate Medical Institute, Anglia Ruskin University, Chelmsford, UK and Southend University Hospital, Southend-on-Sea, UK

[3]Department of Radiology, University of Massachusetts Medical School, Worcester, MA, USA

[4]Swedish Medical Center, Seattle, WA, USA

[5]Herz-Jesu-Krankenhaus, Dernbach, Germany

[6]Anglia Ruskin University, Chelmsford, UK

Background and evidence

Stroke remains the third leading cause of death and leading cause of disability in the USA and Europe [1]. Preventive and interventional strategies should be a high priority. In this context, interventional therapies for stroke prevention have gained momentum in the last two decades and become accepted treatment strategies in a number of countries. Carotid stenting has been demonstrated equivalent to carotid endarterectomy in suitable patients [2,3], patent foramen ovale closure has recently been shown to be effective for secondary prevention in patients with cryptogenic stroke [4], and left atrial appendage closure was superior to anticoagulation with warfarin at longer term follow-up in the largest randomized trial examining left atrial appendage closure published to date [5]. Moreover, to those involved in acute stroke intervention, based on personal experience of dramatic neurologic recovery (in selected patients) after timely culprit vessel revascularization, the merit of acute stroke intervention has been obvious. However, results of earlier randomized trials, with first generation devices, examining the efficacy of acute stroke intervention were mixed [6–8]. Importantly, with the publication of five recent randomized controlled acute stroke trials showing superiority of thromboembolectomy in addition to usual care (thrombolysis) versus usual care alone, interventional therapy has the potential to revolutionize acute stroke therapy in a similar manner as percutaneous coronary intervention has for treatment of acute myocardial infarction.

It is undisputed that thrombolysis significantly improves neurologic outcomes in acute stroke. It is widely available and can be administered rapidly in most hospitals. Based mainly on the National Institute of Neurological Disorders and Stroke (NINDS) recombinant tissue plasminogen activator (rt-PA) trial [9], in the absence of contraindications, rt-PA (0.9 mg/kg body weight; maximum 90 mg, with 10% administered as a bolus followed by the remainder over 60 minutes without concomitant antiplatelet or anticoagulant therapy) is a recommended treatment for patients who present less than 4.5 hours after stroke onset. In the NINDS trial, patients treated with thrombolysis within 3 hours of stroke

onset were 30% more likely to have minimal or no disability at 3-month follow-up than patients in the control group [9]. Subsequently, based on the results of the ECASS III randomized controlled trial [10], the therapeutic window for intravenous thrombolysis was extended to 4.5 hours. Nevertheless, thrombolysis is accompanied by a number of shortcomings. First, only a very small number (<5%) of patients are eligible for thrombolysis based on late presentation or contraindications. Second, culprit vessel recanalization rates are lower than those observed after thrombolysis in acute myocardial infarction. For example, acute vessel patency rates are ≥70% after thrombolysis for acute myocardial infarction with second-generation lytics [11] compared to 34% after thrombolysis for acute stroke [12]. The reason for the lower vessel patency rates may be the mechanism of initial vessel closure. Whereas in acute myocardial infarction the underlying mechanism is plaque rupture causing *in situ* thrombus formation, the overwhelming majority of strokes are caused by more heterogeneous embolic material from the carotid artery or aortic arch (including atherosclerotic debris with or without superimposed thrombus) or heart that may not respond well to thrombolysis. Moreover, the re-occlusion rate of intracerebral vessels is high. For example, in one study of patients who underwent thrombolysis in the setting of a middle cerebral artery (MCA) occlusion in the M1/M2 segment, the re-occlusion rate after initial recanalization was 34% [13]. Third, reperfusion into the injured brain tissue, in conjunction with a thrombolytic state, can lead to intracranial hemorrhage causing neurologic status deterioration in 6.8–8.8% of patients (treated with lytics) [9,14], thereby limiting the benefit of therapy. It is therefore not surprising that the likelihood of death and major disability remains high (>50%), despite administration of intravenous thrombolytic therapy [9,14,15].

In an effort to maximize thrombolytic effect in the culprit vessel while minimizing bleeding, intra-arterial thrombolysis with rt-PA was extensively studied.

In the Prolyse in Acute Cerebral Thromboembolism 1 (PROACT-1) (n=26) [16], PROACT-2 (n=180) [17], and the Middle Cerebral Artery Embolism Local Fibrinolytic Trial (MELT)

Interventional Cardiology: Principles and Practice, Second Edition. Edited by George D. Dangas, Carlo Di Mario, and Nicholas N. Kipshidze.
© 2017 John Wiley & Sons, Ltd. Published 2017 by John Wiley & Sons, Ltd.

(n = 114) [18], intra-arterial lytic therapy administered to patients with MCA occlusions in conjunction with intravenous heparin was compared with intravenous heparin only. Several observations are worth mentioning. Though the stroke vessel patency rates (defined as TIMI II–III in PROACT-1 and TIMI I–III in PROACT-2) were higher after intra-arterial lysis (58% vs. 14%, 66% vs. 18% in PROACT-1 and 2), brisk, TIMI III, flow was seen in a minority of patients (18% in PROACT-2). High doses of intravenous heparin (100 IU/kg loading dose followed by 1000 IU/hour) together with intra-arterial thrombolysis resulted in unacceptably high intracranial hemorrhage rates in PROACT-1 (70% in the lytic arm versus 20% in the control arm receiving intravenous heparin only) leading to heparin dose adjustment (2000 IU bolus followed by 500 IU/hour) for the remainder of PROACT-1 and 2. In PROACT-2, significantly more patients (40% vs. 25%; p = 0.045) achieved excellent neurologic outcomes (modified Rankin score ≤1) with no difference in mortality. Though in MELT there was no difference in the primary endpoint (modified Rankin score of ≤2), significantly more patients (42% vs. 23%) experienced an excellent neurologic recovery (defined as modified Rankin score of ≤1) after intra-arterial lysis (predefined endpoint) with no difference in mortality.

Data comparing intra-arterial with intravenous lytic therapy are limited. In a non-randomized study of 112 patients exhibiting a hyperdense media sign consistent with an MCA occlusion comparing intra-arterial lytic therapy (within 6 hours of symptom onset) with intravenous thrombolysis (within 3 hours of stroke onset), a favorable neurologic outcome was seen in significantly more patients after intra-arterial lysis (53% with modified Rankin score of ≤2 versus 23%; p <0.001) despite a shorter mean time to treatment administration with intravenous compared with intra-arterial thrombolysis (156 vs. 244 minutes) with significantly lower mortality (5% vs. 23%) in the group treated with intra-arterial thrombolysis [19]. In the Interventional Management of Stroke trial (IMS) I, 80 patients were assigned to reduced-dose intravenous lytic therapy (0.6 mg/kg bodyweight; maximum 60 mg) with 15% administered as a bolus followed by 85% over 60 minutes followed by cerebral angiography and intra-arterial lytic administration (up to 22 mg over a 2-hour period) if residual thromboembolic material was seen [20]. Results were compared with historical controls from the NINDS-rt-PA trial. With this strategy, 62% of patients received intra-arterial lytic therapy. At follow-up, 43% of patients were left with a favorable neurologic outcome (modified Ranking score of ≤2) compared with 39% and 28% in the historical NINDS trial population treated with and without lytics, respectively, with no difference in intracranial hemorrhage rates. Of note, similar to aforementioned studies, brisk, TIMI III occurred in only a minority of patients (11%). In IMS-II [21], a study with similar design as IMS-I, 81 patients received the same dose of intravenous lytics followed by angiography and intra-arterial lytics if residual thromboembolic material was seen in addition to low energy ultrasound application at the site of thromboembolic material via the EKOS (EKOS Corporation, Bothell, WA, USA) microinfusion catheter with favorable neurologic outcome in 46% of patients and no increase in intracranial hemorrhage.

In summary, though in selected patients intra-arterial lytic therapy appears to be superior to anticoagulation with heparin only, data are limited and virtually no data are available comparing a strategy using intravenous lytics with intra-arterial lytics as first line therapy. Even with intra-arterial lytic therapy, brisk, TIMI III flow is the exception rather than the rule. In an analogy to mechanical coronary reperfusion for acute ST-segment elevation myocardial infarction, an important observation appears to characterize most

studies. The degree of neurologic recovery and mortality correlates closely with infarct or stroke vessel patency. For example, in a meta-analysis of 53 studies examining data from 2066 patients who underwent cerebral angiography within 24 hours of therapy, spontaneous recanalization was observed in only 24%, 46% of patients after intravenous and 63% after intra-arterial thrombolysis [22]. Favorable neurologic recovery occurred in 58% of patients whose target vessel recanalized versus 25% when the target vessel remained occluded. Likewise, mortality was 42% in patients without and 12% in patients with successful target vessel recanalization. Furthermore, those vessels in which occlusion causes the most devastating neurologic consequences (internal carotid, carotid T, proximal MCA, or basilar artery) are typically least likely to recanalized after thrombolysis.

The recognition of the importance of early stroke vessel recanalization and the limitations encountered by thrombolytic therapy fostered the pursuit of mechanical thromboembolectomy. A number of thromboembolectomy devices have been studied. Initial enthusiasm was dampened by the announcement of the results of three trials in 2013, all of which did not show harm, but failed to demonstrate the expected benefit of mechanical thromboembolectomy compared to intravenous thrombolysis. The IMS-III trial was designed to randomize 900 patients to endovascular therapy in addition to conventional intravenous thrombolytic therapy versus conventional thrombolytic therapy alone but was stopped after enrollment of 656 patients demonstrated no additional benefit of endovascular therapy (primary endpoint of modified Rankin ≤2, 41% with endovascular therapy in addition to intravenous thrombolysis and 39% with conventional intravenous thrombolysis alone) [6]. There was also no difference in mortality or intracranial hemorrhage rates. Several shortcomings deserve attention. First, major (large) vessel occlusion was documented in less than 50% of patients. Second, the time delay from intravenous thrombolytic administration to percutaneous mechanical therapy was long (equal to or greater than 2 hours). Third, the rate of recanalization with brisk flow in the stroke related vessel (TICI IIb–III) was low (40%).

MR-RESCUE was a small (n = 68) randomized trial of endovascular therapy in addition to intravenous thrombolysis versus intravenous thrombolysis only [7]. The main goal of this trial was evaluation of endovascular therapy efficacy depending on the size of the penumbra assessed by pre-intervention imaging. At the conclusion of this trial there was no difference in neurologic outcome, death, or intracranial hemorrhage. The absence of efficacy was demonstrated regardless of the size of the penumbra. Though large vessel occlusion was documented prior to intervention by magnetic resonance tomography, similar to IMS-III, time to treatment was long (mean time from stroke symptom onset to therapy equal to or greater than 6 hours) and successful recanalization rate low (TICI IIb–III, 27%).

Finally, in SYNTHESIS Expansion, 362 patients were randomized to receive intravenous thrombolysis versus endovascular therapy (the overwhelming majority of whom received intra-arterial lytics) [8]. Compared with conventional intravenous thrombolysis, there was no difference in the rate of favorable neurologic outcome, death, or intracranial hemorrhage. Though the times to treatment were shorter than in the latter two trials (3.75 hours in the endovascular therapy group vs. 2.75 hours in the intravenous thrombolysis group), large vessel occlusion was again not confirmed prior to study inclusion. Of note, only 56 patients underwent mechanical thromboembolectomy. Hence, this trial should be considered mainly a comparison of intra-arterial versus intravenous thrombolysis rather than an evaluation of the merit of mechanical thrombectomy.

In summary, the aforementioned three trials should be interpreted keeping in mind the long treatment delays, inconsistent documentation of large vessel occlusion prior to inclusion, the lack of modern thrombectomy devices, the overall low recanalization rates, not to mention the small number of patients enrolled in each facility (0.8–3.6). The majority of devices used for thromboembolectomy in the mechanical arm were wire manipulation alone, the outdated first generation Merci Retriever (Stryker, Fremont, CA, USA) which worked by the principle of entrapment and retrieval via a Spiral and the Penumbra System (Penumbra, Alameda, CA, USA) using aspiration for thromboembolectomy. Though these devices have been shown to achieve recanalization rates superior to historical controls of conventional intravenous thrombolysis in small single-arm studies [23–26], their clinical efficacy has never been shown in randomized trials comparing the specific device with intravenous thrombolysis. Newer generation devices, particularly stent retrievers, were used in only 0–13% of patients in the interventional groups [6–8].

Stent retrievers are small, self-expanding stents with ultrafine stent struts delivered and expanded into the thrombus/embolus engulfing the thrombus/embolus within the stent struts. Deployment alone frequently establishes some degree of flow accompanied by improvement in neurologic status. The stent is non-detachable. Instead, in its expanded form, it is pulled back into the guide catheter or sheath while maintaining suction through the balloon-tipped guide catheter or sheath with the balloon inflated, preventing dislodgement of thromboembolic material into the cerebral circulation during retrieval. Removal of an expanded stent seems counterintuitive to operators accustomed to percutaneous coronary interventions during acute myocardial infarction. However, the main aspect (apart from the low profile and excellent flexibility) that allows safe retrieval of a deployed stent retriever from the intracranial circulation is the common absence of underlying atherosclerotic plaque or stenosis at the site of the cerebral vessel occlusion. Several registries and one randomized trial comparing results using a stent retriever (Solitaire, Medtronic, Dublin, Ireland) with prior older generation mechanical clot/embolus removal devices demonstrated more rapid reperfusion and higher vessel patency rates and better clinical outcomes after use of the stent retriever [27–30]. These findings promoted the conduction of a number of randomized trials that were recently published and are likely to change the landscape of acute stroke therapy.

The Multicenter Randomized Clinical Trial of Endovascular Treatment for Acute Ischemic Stroke in the Netherlands (MR CLEAN) was a multicenter trial randomizing patients (NIHSS score of ≥2, n = 500) with an acute distal internal carotid, MCA (M1/M2 segment) or anterior cerebral artery (A2/A2 segment) occlusion to endovascular therapy (mechanical thrombectomy, intra-arterial lysis or both) in addition to intravenous thrombolysis or intravenous thrombolysis alone [31]. Importantly, the overwhelming majority (82%) of patients were treated using stent retrievers. Treatment was open label but endpoint evaluation was performed in a blinded manner. Duration from symptom onset to administration of intravenous thrombolysis was equivalent in both treatment groups (85 minutes in the control arm versus 87 minutes in the endovascular therapy group) and median time from stroke onset to access site puncture was 260 minutes. The primary endpoint, modified Rankin score of ≤2 at 90 days, was achieved in 33% of patients in the endovascular therapy group versus 19% in the control group (significant 13% absolute difference in favorable outcome, adjusted OR 2.2, 05% CI 1.39–3.38). All other endpoints favored endovascular therapy. The 5–7 day NIHSS score was 2.9

points lower in the endovascular therapy as was the infarct volume (by 19 mL). Importantly, no residual occlusion was seen in 75% of patients on computed tomography (CT) angiography 24 hours after treatment in patients treated endovascularly compared with only 33% in patients treated conventionally. There was no significant difference in mortality or rate of intracranial hemorrhage. It was noted that, at 90 days' follow-up, 5.6% of patients who underwent endovascular therapy had exhibited signs of stroke in a different cerebral vascular territory than the initial stroke compared with only 0.4% in the control group. In summary, MR CLEAN demonstrated superiority of endovascular therapy in addition to conventional therapy compared with conventional therapy alone when administered within 6 hours of stroke onset without causing excess mortality or intracranial hemorrhage.

The design of the Endovascular Treatment for Small Core and Anterior Circulation Proximal Occlusion with Emphasis on Minimizing CT to Recanalization Times (ESCAPE) trial [32] was similar to MR CLEAN. Patients with acute stroke in the carotid T, M1, or M1 equivalent distribution confirmed on CT angiography and small infarct core based on the Alberta Stroke Early Computed Tomography (ASPECT) score of 6–10 were assigned randomly to endovascular therapy (intra-arterial lytic therapy, mechanical thrombectomy with stent-retrievers, or both) in addition to intravenous thrombolysis or thrombolysis alone. The planned enrollment was 500 patients but the trial was terminated early (after 316 patients) as a result of demonstrated efficacy. In the endovascular treatment group stent retrievers were used in 86% of patients. The primary endpoint, odds ratio of improving the modified Rankin score by 1 point at 90 days favored endovascular therapy (OR 2.5, 95% CI 1.7–3.8). In addition, the median 90-day modified Ranking score was 2 after endovascular therapy compared with 4 after conventional therapy, the likelihood of functional independence 53% versus 29%, and the 90-day mortality was significantly lower favoring intervention with no difference in intracranial hemorrhage. The median duration from CT scan and stroke symptom onset to reperfusion was very short (84 and 241 minutes, respectively). These results confirmed findings described by MR CLEAN trial investigators and emphasized the possibility and importance of short symptom onset to recanalization times.

The Extending the Time for Thrombolysis in Emergency Neurological Deficits—Intra-Arterial (EXTEND-IA) trial randomized acute stroke patients to intravenous thrombolysis or endovascular therapy using the Solitaire Flow Restoration Stent Retriever in addition to intravenous thrombolysis [33]. Intravenous therapy needed to be administered within 4.5 hours of stroke onset. Vascular access needed to be established within 6 hours of symptom onset and an infarct core of <70 mL with residual salvageable brain tissue on CT angiography was required for inclusion. Enrollment of 100 patients was planned, but the trial was stopped early (after 70 patients) due to efficacy. Similar to ESCAPE, the median time from symptom onset to vascular access was short (210 minutes). Three-day neurologic recovery was significantly more common after endovascular therapy (80% vs. 37%). Ninety-day functional independence (modified Rankin ≤2) occurred in 71% of patients in the endovascular therapy group compared with 40% in the conventional therapy group (p = 0.01). There was no difference in mortality or symptomatic intracranial hemorrhage. Though embolization into a territory different from the initial stroke was observed in 6% patients, this was not clinically apparent.

The Solitaire with the Intention for Thrombectomy as Primary Endovascular Treatment (SWIFT PRIME) [34] trial was also stopped prior to planned enrollment because of proof of efficacy.

At trial termination, 196 patients with acute stroke in the anterior circulation (internal carotid, T-occlusion or MCA occlusion) were randomized to conventional intravenous thrombolysis or mechanical thrombectomy using the Solitaire stent retriever (Medtronic, Dublin, Ireland) (successfully deployed in 89%) in addition to intravenous thrombolysis. Time from stroke onset to groin puncture (224 minutes) and from stroke onset to stent deployment (252 minutes) was very short. Substantial or complete reperfusion occurred in 88% of patients treated with the stent retriever and clinical efficacy was superior in patients who underwent endovascular therapy in addition to thrombolysis compared with patients who were treated with conventional thrombolysis only, reflected by lower modified Rankin scores in the interventional group as well as a higher percentage of patients who reached a low modified Ranking score of ≤ 2 (60% versus 35%; p <0.001). There was no difference in mortality or symptomatic intracranial hemorrhage.

In the Randomized Trial of Revascularization with Solitaire FR Device versus Best Medical Therapy in the Treatment of Acute Stroke Due to Anterior Circulation Large Vessel Occlusion Presenting within Eight Hours of Symptom Onset (REVASCAT), 206 patients with acute anterior circulation stroke were randomized to undergo intravenous thrombolysis alone (when eligible) versus mechanical thrombectomy with the Solitaire stent retriever in addition to venous thrombolysis if treatment was feasible within 8 hours of symptom onset and infarct area not large by neuroimaging [35]. The trial was stopped early given the superior neurologic outcome with endovascular therapy and publication of aforementioned trials demonstrating superiority of endovascular therapy in addition to intravenous thrombolysis over conventional intravenous thrombolysis alone. Stroke onset to reperfusion time in the group undergoing endovascular therapy was 355 minutes. Stent retrievers were used in 95% of the interventional group. Significantly more patients (44%) experienced a favorable neurologic outcome in the endovascular treatment group than the control group (28%). Similar to all four other trials, there was no difference in intracranial hemorrhage or mortality.

A recent meta-analysis of eight randomized trials, totaling 2423 patients, showed that endovascular thrombectomy was associated with improved functional outcomes (modified Rankin Scale 0–2, odds ratio 1.56, 95% CI 1.32–1.85; p < 0.00001). There was a tendency toward decreased mortality (odds ratio 0.84, 95% CI 0.67–1.05; p = 0.12), and symptomatic intracerebral hemorrhage was not increased (odds ratio 1.03, 95% CI 0.71–1.49; p = 0.88) compared with best medical management alone. The odds ratio for a favorable functional outcome increased to 2.23 (95% CI 1.77–2.81; p < 0.00001) when newer generation thrombectomy devices were used in greater than 50% of the cases in each trial. The meta-analysis demonstrates clear evidence for improvement in functional independence with endovascular thrombectomy, compared with standard medical care, suggesting that endovascular thrombectomy should be considered the standard effective treatment alongside thombolysis in eligible patients [36].

Acute stroke therapy: practical aspects
Clinical examination
A neurologic examination should be performed according to the National Institute of Health Stroke Scale (NIHSS). Precise and fast assessment of the NIHSS score requires experience and should be

> **Box 68.1** Contraindications for systemic lytic therapy
>
> - Intracerebral hemorrhage suspected or present on CT or MR imaging
> - Initial CT demonstrates evidence for tissue necrosis in more than one-third of the middle cerebral artery territory
> - History of intracranial hemorrhage
> - Presence of an arteriovenous malformation or large partially thrombosed aneurysm
> - Uncontrolled hypertension (BP >185/110 mmHg)
> - Profound hyperglycemia
> - History of Alzheimer's dementia
> - Unknown stroke duration (e.g., patient woke up with symptoms)
> - Stroke symptom onset >6 hours (relative contraindication)
> - Recent stroke (within 3 months)
> - Recent major surgery (<4 weeks)
> - Recent gastrointestinal bleeding (<4 weeks)
> - INR >1.7
> - Thrombocytopenia (<100,000 cells/mL)

practiced under non-acute circumstances. An excellent resource for demonstration of NIHSS stroke scale assessment is found at the following link: https://www.youtube.com/watch?v=x4bjXqtfn6k (NIH stroke scale training parts 1–4). The presence of a severe headache is rare in ischemic strokes [37] and should alert one to the possibility of intracranial hemorrhage. Similarly, neck pain in conjunction with a neurologic deficit should raise suspicion for carotid or vertebral artery dissection. Severe back pain, particularly if accompanied by a pulse deficit, can be a symptom of acute aortic dissection. Involvement of cranial vessels by the dissection can cause neurologic deficits by hypoperfusion. In the latter case, thrombolytic therapy or anticoagulation is contraindicated. Heart murmurs, fever, and constitutional symptoms in the setting of a neurologic defect can be symptoms of infectious endocarditis under which circumstances the administration of anticoagulation or thrombolysis can lead to neurologic deterioration because of hemorrhagic transformation of embolic strokes. Importantly, for the purpose of intravenous lytic administration, a brief history focusing on contraindications to lytic therapy (Box 68.1) should be performed. It is important to note that the presence of contraindications to lytic therapy does not preclude performance of endovascular therapy. Though the clinical benefit of stent retrievers has been demonstrated mainly in patients treated with intravenous thrombolysis, some stroke centers perform mechanical thromboembolectomy without prior lytic therapy and in the absence of systemic anticoagulation, provided continuous flush solution maintains clot-free catheters and sheaths.

Imaging
At the minimum, a non-contrast CT-scan should be performed to rule out intracerebral hemorrhage and stroke mimics (e.g., space occupying lesions). The Alberta stroke program early CT score (ASPECTS) quantitatively evaluates the core of ischemia on CT scans. ASPECTS is a topographic scoring system that divides the MCA territory of the brain that is affected by ischemic damage into 10 areas of interest. It is a strong predictor of both functional outcome and adverse events following treatment. Recently, the CE marked e-ASPECTS software has been developed to automate the ASPECTS scoring system for ischemic stroke patients. In a meta-analysis of the four studies that presented stratified ASPECTS data for mRS (ESCAPE, MR CLEAN, REVASCAT, and SWIFT PRIME), it was demonstrated that endovascular stroke treatment improved

functional independence compared with best medical treatment in patients with high baseline ASPECTS (OR 2.10, 95% CI 1.61–2.73; p <0.00001) [36]. Mechanical thrombectomy also improved functional independence with moderate baseline ASPECTS (OR 2.04, 95% CI 1.25–3.32; p = 0.004). There was no evidence of benefit of endovascular stroke treatment in patients with low baseline ASPECTS (OR 1.09, 95% CI 0.14–8.46; p = 0.93) but only 28 patients were included in this analysis because MR CLEAN was the only study that incorporated this group of patients in their trial. Overall, these results suggest that patients with baseline ASPECTS >4 benefit from endovascular stroke treatment. ASPECTS is recommended by the American Society of Neuroradiology, American Heart Association/American Stroke Association, European Stroke Organization, and the Canadian Stroke best practice.

Most centers have the capability of performing CT angiography, requiring minimal additional time. This allows localization of the occluded vessel and can facilitate the intervention by obviating the need for cerebral angiography of non-target vessels. Moreover, it can identify collateral circulation and clot length. Assessment of the presence and size of cerebral parenchymal damage guides candidacy for intravenous or intra-arterial therapy. MR or CT perfusion imaging allows the identification and quantification of the ischemic penumbra (ischemic, yet viable tissue at risk that may be salvaged by timely reperfusion) guiding further therapy, especially in wake-up strokes or presentations with onset of symptoms >4.5 hours. Mobile CT scanners or flat panel CT in the catheterization laboratory and intensive care units (or even ambulance) accelerates treatment decisions [38,39].

Laboratory tests

A complete blood count, partial thromboplastin time (pTT), prothrombin time, serum creatinine, electrolytes and glucose levels should be obtained upon patient arrival in the emergency department. To shorten potential delays, portable point of care laboratory systems that allow measurement of these parameters at the site of imaging or in the emergency department have been shown to be useful [40].

Cerebral angiography

Considerable debate surrounds the topic of whether the patient should be sedated or undergo general anesthesia. This depends on cooperation of the patient and comfort level of the operator. Absence of sedation or general anesthesia allows continued neurologic assessment during the intervention but occasionally makes invasive imaging and maneuvering of equipment more challenging because of patient movement. In addition, the patient can experience severe pain during clot extraction. In any case, stroke should be treated as "cerebral resuscitation" and an anesthetic team should be instantly available. Importantly, any drop in blood pressure during intubation should be avoided to optimize the reserve of collaterals.

With rare exceptions, femoral access is obtained. Use of a micropuncture system and fluoroscopic or ultrasound guidance facilitates single front wall common femoral artery puncture. Though a 6 Fr sheath can be used, in most cases a long 8 Fr balloon guide, allowing extra support, is preferable. Arch aortography using a 5 or 6 Fr pigtail catheter in 40° left anterior oblique angulation (10–15 mL contrast with digital subtraction imaging) is usually not necessary. A type I arch is the most favorable configuration with all cranial vessels (the innominate artery, left common carotid, and left subclavian artery) originating from the arch in one single plane with the outer curvature of the aortic arch. Type II (the innominate artery originates

between the outer and inner curvature of the aortic arch) and III (the innominate artery originates below the inner curvature of the aortic arch) arches are more difficult to navigate.

Attention should also be directed to the ostia, tortuosity, and presence of disease in the proximal arch vessels. The most common arch configuration is a separate take-off (from right to left) of the innominate artery, left common carotid and left subclavian artery (~70%) followed by a common origin of the innominate and left common carotid artery (~20%), origin of the left common carotid from the innominate artery ("bovine arch") (~7%), separate take-off of the left vertebral artery from the aortic arch and (0.5%), and separate take-off of the right subclavian artery from the arch distal to the left subclavian artery coursing posterior to the esophagus toward the right upper extremity (rare). With a straightforward arch configuration, all arch vessels can usually be engaged with a 5 Fr SIMS, H1, or vertebral catheter. A road map can be superimposed on fluoroscopic imaging to help direct the wire and catheter. A hydrophilic (0.035-inch) guidewire (e.g., angled Glide wire, Terumo, Tokyo, Japan) is advanced into the desired location to help track the diagnostic catheter. For angiography of the anterior circulation, the wire is advanced into the internal carotid artery, provided this vessel is not stenosed or occluded. Alternatively, it can be left in the distal common carotid artery and the diagnostic catheter advanced over the wire into the common carotid artery for angiography. First, angiography of the carotid bifurcation and proximal internal carotid artery is performed in a 30° ipsilateral oblique and lateral views (additional views; for example with caudal angulation or contralateral oblique views, can be obtained if initial images do not adequately demonstrate the proximal internal carotid). Cerebral angiography of the anterior circulation is performed in lateral and postero-anterior cranial (10–15°) views. Usually, injection of 2–4 mL contrast is sufficient for opacification. The stump of large vessel occlusions can usually be identified without difficulty (Video 68.1; Figure 68.1). However, in some cases, rotational angiography can be useful to identify vessel cut-off otherwise masked by overlapping branches (Video 68.7). Visualization of the cerebral veins and collaterals is important and this requires prolonged imaging and inclusion of the entire skull. For the posterior circulation, the wire can be positioned into the axillary artery and the diagnostic catheter advanced over the wire proximal to the vertebral artery ostium and non-selective angiography of the proximal vertebral artery can then be performed. Subsequently, the wire can be directed into the vertebral artery and the catheter tracked for engagement and angiography. It is often easier to cannulate the left vertebral artery first as this is the easier one to negotiate. The best views for the vertebral circulation are contralateral oblique for the segment from the origin to the location where the vertebral artery enters the first transverse foramen of C5 or C6 (V1 segment), ipsilateral oblique (alternatively, posteroanterior and lateral) for the segment between the first and last transverse foramen (V2 segment) as well as for the segment between the last transverse foramen and the foramen magnum (V3 segment), and lateral and postero-anterior cranial (~40°) for the intracranial vertebral segment (V4 segment), basilar artery, and posterior cerebral arteries. When encountering a difficult arch, arch vessel cannulation requires the use of a Simmons or Vitek catheter. These catheters are shaped such that, after delivery over a J-tipped 0.035-inch guidewire into the ascending thoracic aorta and withdrawal of the wire, the catheter is configured in the aortic arch and the vessel is cannulated by catheter withdrawal and rotation. Only when the

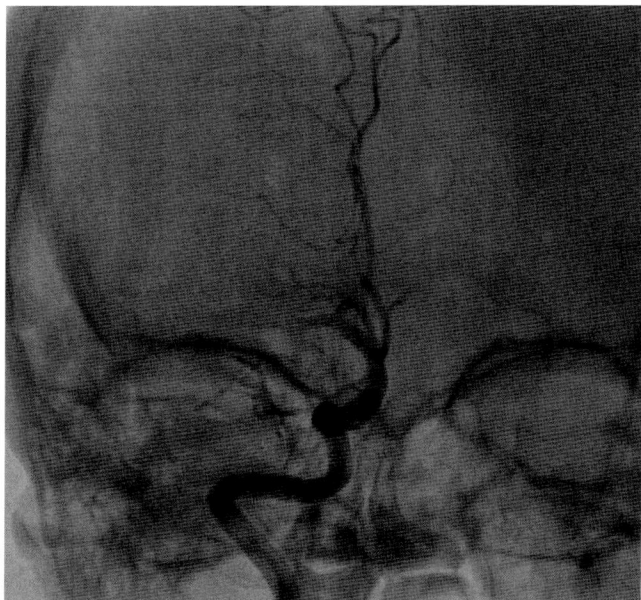

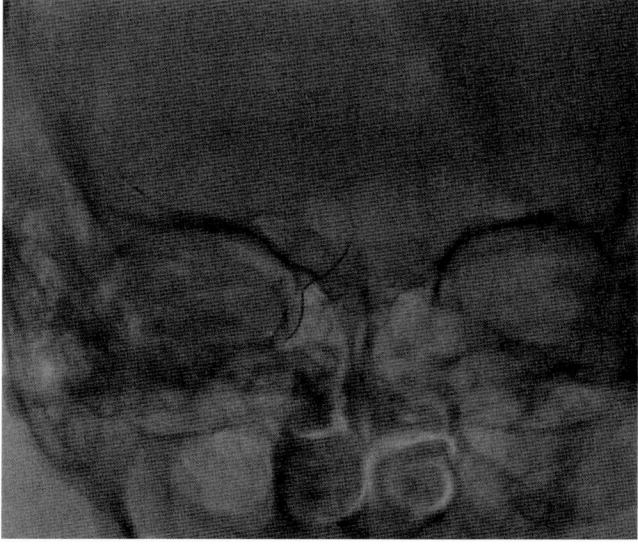

Figure 68.2 The microcatheter has been advanced over the 0.14-inch wire into the inferior branch of the right middle cerebral artery distal to the distal end of the occlusion, followed by a microcatheter. Subsequently, the wire has been removed and a Solitaire stent retriever (Medtronic, Dublin, Ireland) advanced into the microcatheter with the distal markers at the tip of the microcatheter.

Figure 68.1 Angiography demonstrating an acute thromboembolic occlusion of the right middle cerebral artery (see also Video 68.1).

catheter is straightened will it be possible to advance a 0.035-inch hydrophilic guidewire into the respective vessels. Even if the occluded vessel is known from CT angiography, it may be important to have information on the contralateral flow and anterior and posterior circulation, as there might be collaterals via the circle of Willis. This can have favorable prognostic value.

Intervention (example of an acute middle cerebral artery occlusion intervention illustrated in Videos 68.1–68.13 and Figures 68.1–68.11)

For clot extraction, currently, a stent retriever is most commonly used. Within the diagnostic catheter, a hydrophilic guidewire (e.g., angled Glide wire) is advanced into the carotid artery and the diagnostic catheter tracked over the wire. If necessary, the Glide wire is then exchanged for a stiffer (e.g., Amplatz Stiff, Cook Medical, Bloomington, IN, USA) wire, providing sufficient support to advance the sheath and guide catheter into the common carotid artery. If there is no significant carotid stenosis, the sheath or, preferably, balloon-tipped guide catheter (e.g., Cello balloon guide catheter, eV3, Irvine, CA, USA) can be advanced (over a guidewire) into the internal carotid artery to allow closer position to the thrombus or embolus. If a balloon-tipped guide catheter is not available it becomes even more important to generously aspirate through the guide catheter/sheath during stent retriever retraction into the guide or sheath. A long distal access catheter (Neuron, Penumbra Inc., Alameda, CA, USA; DAC, Concentric Medical, Mountain View, CA, USA; Fargo, Balt, Montmorency, France) can give extra stability. For interventions in the vertebrobasilar or posterior cerebral circulation a 6 Fr sheath is positioned into the vertebral artery using a hydrophilic 0.035-inch wire.

When advancing a microwire into the cerebral vessels, it is important to respect and avoid small branches (e.g., lenticostriate arteries). Some operators prefer off-label use of a coronary 0.014-inch guidewire (e.g., Whisper wire, Abbott Vascular, Redwood City, CA, USA; or ChoicePT wire, Boston Scientific, Marlborough, MA,

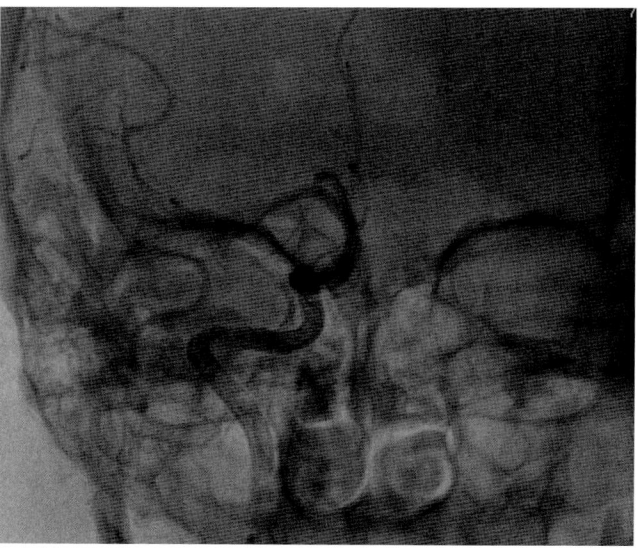

Figure 68.3 The Solitaire stent retriever (Medtronic, Dublin, Ireland) has been deployed (see also Video 68.2) by microcatheter retraction while maintaining Solitaire position. This causes partial flow restoration (see also Video 68.3).

USA), others prefer dedicated wires for the cerebral circulation (e.g., 0.014-inch Synchro microwire, Stryker, Kalamazoo, MI, USA; or Transcend wire, Boston Scientific, or 0.014-inch). An attempt should be made to position the distal wire tip beyond the occlusion as far as safely possible and, optimally, in a larger segment or branch (Video 68.8; Figure 68.8). Advancing the wire in the tortuous cerebral vasculature can be challenging. Tracking the wire with a microcatheter (e.g., Rebar 18 or 27™, Covidien, Dublin, Ireland, Prowler select plus Cordis, Hialeah, FL, USA; or Excelsior XT 27, Stryker)

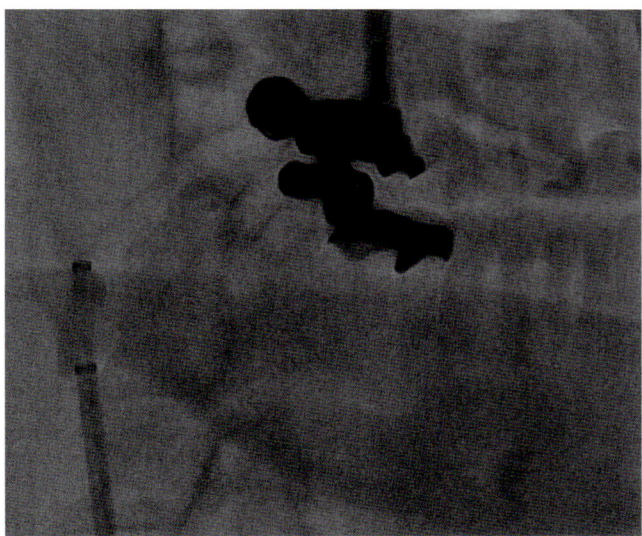

Figure 68.4 The balloon of the balloon-tipped guide catheter has been inflated (see also Video 68.4).

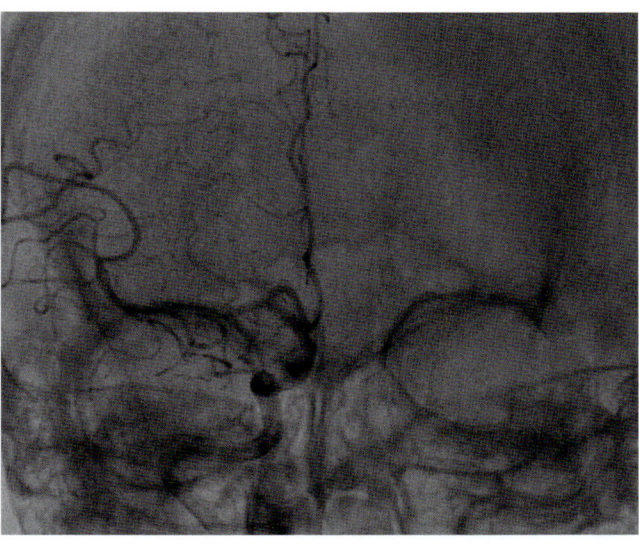

Figure 68.6 Angiography demonstrates flow restoration in the inferior branch of the right middle cerebral artery (see also Video 68.6).

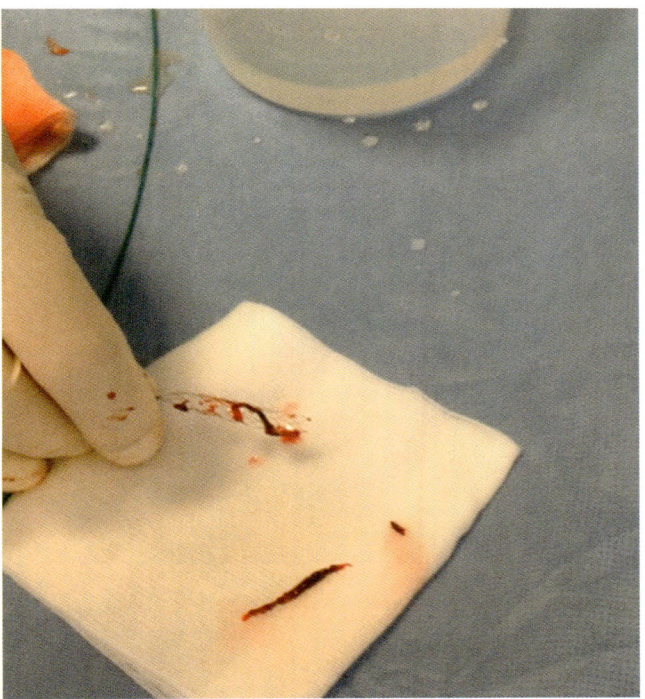

Figure 68.5 During balloon inflation and while applying continuous suction via the guide catheter, the Solitaire stent retriever (Medtronic, Dublin, Ireland) in its deployed state and the microcatheter are removed as a unit (see also Video 68.5). The captured thromboembolic material can be seen entrapped in the stent retriever after removal from the guide catheter.

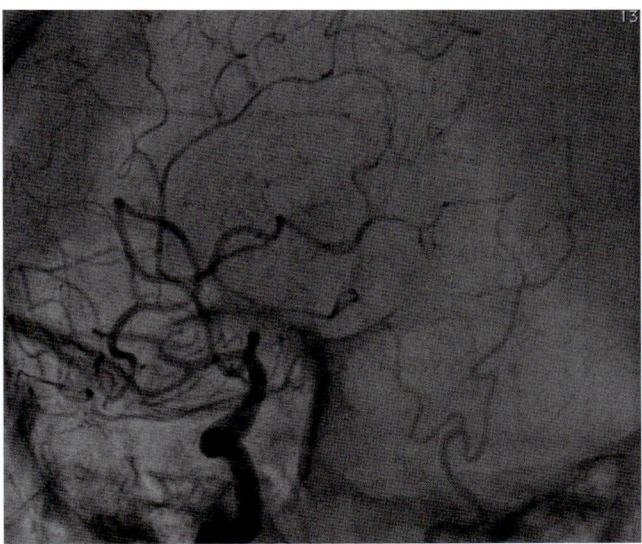

Figure 68.7 There is residual thrombus in the superior branch of the right middle cerebral artery (see also Video 68.7).

can provide better support and torque transmission. Occasionally, crossing the occlusion with the wire alone causes some improvement in flow. The microcatheter should be positioned with the tip distal (preferably 1–1.5 cm) to the thrombus or embolus (Video 68.9; Figure 68.9). Some operators proceed with removal of the wire and

gentle injection of a very small amount (0.5–1.0 mL) of contrast via the microcatheter to assure intravascular position and to outline the cerebral vasculature distal to the occlusion (Video 68.9; Figure 68.9); however, this carries the risk of dislodgement of distal fragments of the clot. Once intravascular position is confirmed, a Solitaire stent retriever is advanced through the microcatheter into the culprit vessel such that the distal marker aligns with the distal tip of the microcatheter (Video 68.10). The Solitaire stent retriever is available in four sizes: 4X15, 4X20, 6X20, and 6X30 mm. The 4 mm Solitaire can be used for 2.0–4.0 mm vessel diameters and the 6 mm device for 3.0–5.5 mm vessel diameters. If a Rebar microcatheter is used, the Rebar 18 is recommended for deployment of the 4 mm and the 27 (slightly larger inner diameter; 0.027 vs. 0.021 inch) for deployment of the 6 mm device. The microcatheter is

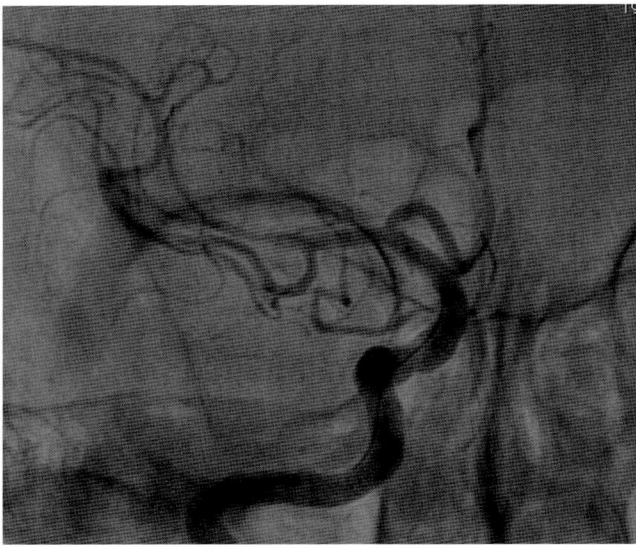

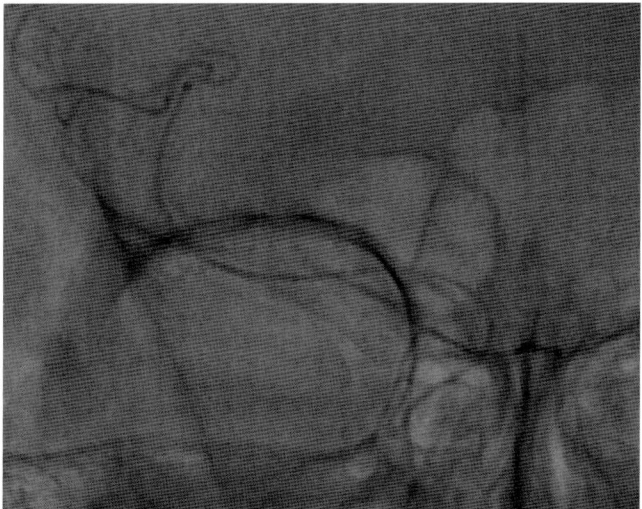

Figure 68.8 The superior branch of the right middle cerebral artery is wired (see also Video 68.8) and a microcatheter advanced over the wire into the superior branch of the right middle cerebral artery.

Figure 68.10 The Solitaire stent retriever (Medtronic, Dublin, Ireland) has been advanced to the tip of the microcatheter (see also Video 68.10) and is deployed by removal of the microcatheter while maintaining Solitaire position (see also Video 68.11). Deployment causes restoration of flow in the superior branch of the right middle cerebral artery (see also Video 68.12).

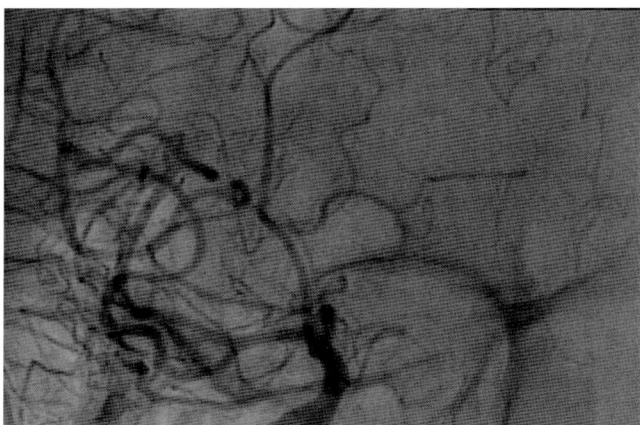

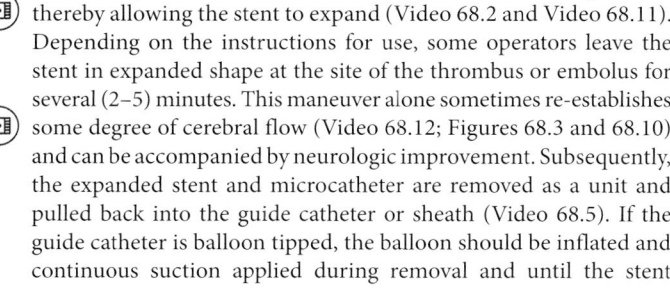

Figure 68.9 The wire has been removed and a small amount of contrast is injected into the superior branch of the right middle cerebral artery confirming intraluminal position of the microcatheter (see also Video 68.9).

Figure 68.11 The stent retriever has been removed and angiography now demonstrates brisk flow in both inferior and superior branch of the right middle cerebral artery (see also Video 68.13).

then slowly removed while maintaining stent retriever position, thereby allowing the stent to expand (Video 68.2 and Video 68.11). Depending on the instructions for use, some operators leave the stent in expanded shape at the site of the thrombus or embolus for several (2–5) minutes. This maneuver alone sometimes re-establishes some degree of cerebral flow (Video 68.12; Figures 68.3 and 68.10) and can be accompanied by neurologic improvement. Subsequently, the expanded stent and microcatheter are removed as a unit and pulled back into the guide catheter or sheath (Video 68.5). If the guide catheter is balloon tipped, the balloon should be inflated and continuous suction applied during removal and until the stent

retriever exits the proximal end of the catheter (Video 68.4; Figure 68.4). If a balloon-tipped guide cannot be used, carotid flow can be interrupted by external manual compression during stent retriever removal while applying suction to the guide or catheter. Angiography is repeated to assess whether reperfusion has occurred. If not, or incomplete (Video 68.7; Figure 68.7), the culprit vessel is rewired, a microcatheter advanced with the distal tip distal to the thrombus, and the previously used stent retriever can be re-advanced and deployed in the thrombus in a similar fashion as described earlier.

The optimal antiplatelet, anticoagulant, or thrombolytic strategy remains to be determined. It is worth mentioning that in all randomized trials demonstrating the efficacy of stent retrievers in acute stroke therapy, intravenous thrombolytic therapy had been initiated in most patients prior to proceeding with endovascular therapy. Some centers do not use thrombolytic therapy when the patient can be transferred directly the catheterization laboratory from the emergency department or CT scanner without delay once a stroke with sufficient deficit is identified that warrants endovascular therapy. However, the merit and safety of this approach remain to be determined. If thrombolytic therapy was not administered immediately before endovascular therapy, administration of low dose intravenous heparin (e.g., 25–40 IU/kg) can be considered.

Regardless of the thrombolytic strategy, given that routine intravenous heparin may not be used or used at low dose and/or antiplatelet therapy are not administered before or during the procedure, meticulous attention to continuous heparinized saline flush via the side arm of a Y-connector attached to the microcatheter and the side arm of the guide catheter is of paramount importance to avoid catheter-associated thrombus formation. Purposeful omission of intraprocedural intravenous heparin or oral/intravenous antiplatelet agents is counterintuitive to those performing coronary interventions but reduces the risk of intracranial hemorrhage.

Complications

Intracranial hemorrhage is, by far, the most devastating complication. Risk factors include age, delayed reperfusion, use of anticoagulant or antiplatelet therapy in addition to lytics, lytic dosage, hyperglycemia, and size of the perfusion defect [41]. The incidence of intracerebral hemorrhage after endovascular stroke therapy is often overestimated because of the misinterpretation of contrast used for the intervention. Symptomatic intracranial hemorrhage occurs in approximately 10% of patients in most larger trials using intra-arterial thrombolysis [42–45]. However, in most recent trials using stent retrievers for mechanical reperfusion, the incidence of symptomatic intracranial hemorrhage is lower at 1–7.7%. In case of intracranial hemorrhage it should be known that most thrombolytic agents are not reversible but relatively short acting. If concomitant heparin is used, the administration of protamine is recommended (1 mg/100 IU heparin administered, maximal dose 50 mg). If glycoprotein IIb/IIIa inhibitors are used, platelet transfusions can be considered. Meticulous technique during wiring avoiding small perforator branches and careful attention to blood pressure control after reperfusion may help reduce the likelihood of hemorrhagic complication. Nevertheless, hemorrhagic transformation can occur even in the absence of any endovascular, thrombolytic, or anticoagulant therapy and can be related to breakdown of the blood–brain barrier caused by parenchymal necrosis. Hence, it should be recognized that the occurrence of intracerebral hemorrhage does not necessarily imply a problem with procedural technique or patient management.

Conclusions

In the past 20 years two important milestones have been reached in the treatment of acute stroke, intravenous thrombolysis and, more recently, mechanical thrombectomy using stent retrievers. Intravenous thrombolysis, though proven effective in large randomized controlled trials, has a number of shortcomings, most importantly, the low rate of stroke vessel recanalization and functional neurologic recovery particularly in large vessel occlusions that cause the most dramatic neurologic deficits. Routine mechanical thrombectomy with stent retrievers, in addition to intravenous thrombolysis, if performed in a timely manner by experienced operators, has the advantage of substantially improving stroke vessel patency and neurologic outcome in large vessel occlusions of the anterior circulation without increasing the rate of intracranial hemorrhage or mortality. Under optimal conditions, this should be available to patients at most locations 24/7, similar to systems offering prompt percutaneous coronary interventions to patients with acute ST-segment elevation myocardial infarctions. To accomplish this, a sufficient number of centers with acute stroke management systems in place with an adequate number of well-trained physicians capable of cerebral thromboembolectomy are needed.

Interactive multiple choice questions are available for this chapter on www.wiley.com/go/dangas/cardiology

References

1 Sacco RL, Benjamin EJ, Broderick JP, et al. American Heart Association Prevention Conference. IV. Prevention and rehabilitation of stroke: risk factors. *Stroke* 1997; **28**: 1507–1517.

2 Yadav JS, Wholey MH, Kuntz RE, et al. Protected carotid-artery stenting versus endarterectomy in high-risk patients. *N Engl J Med* 2004; **351**: 1493–501.

3 Brott TG, Hobson RW 2nd, Howard G, et al. Stenting versus endarterectomy for treatment of carotid-artery stenosis. *N Engl J Med* 2010; **363**: 11–23.

4 Carroll J. RESPECT: Extended follow-up results. In: *Transcatheter Therapeutics (TCT)*. San Francisco: 2015.

5 Reddy VY, Sievert H, Halperin J, et al. Percutaneous left atrial appendage closure vs warfarin for atrial fibrillation: a randomized clinical trial. *JAMA* 2014; **312**: 1988–1998.

6 Broderick JP, Palesch YY, Demchuk AM, et al. Endovascular therapy after intravenous t-PA versus t-PA alone for stroke. *N Engl J Med* 2013; **368**: 893–903.

7 Kidwell CS, Jahan R, Gornbein J, et al. A trial of imaging selection and endovascular treatment for ischemic stroke. *N Engl J Med* 2013; **368**: 914–923.

8 Ciccone A, Valvassori L, Nichelatti M, et al. Endovascular treatment for acute ischemic stroke. *N Engl J Med* 2013; **368**: 904–913.

9 The National Institute of Neurological Disorders and Stroke rt-PA Stroke Study Group. Tissue plasminogen activator for acute ischemic stroke. *N Engl J Med* 1995; **333**: 1581–1587.

10 Hacke W, Kaste M, Bluhmki E, et al. Thrombolysis with alteplase 3 to 4.5 hours after acute ischemic stroke. *N Engl J Med* 2008; **359**: 1317–1329.

11 Granger CB, White HD, Bates ER, Ohman EM, Califf RM. A pooled analysis of coronary arterial patency and left ventricular function after intravenous thrombolysis for acute myocardial infarction. *Am J Cardiol* 1994; **74**: 1220–1228.

12 Wolpert SM, Bruckmann H, Greenlee R, Wechsler L, Pessin MS, del Zoppo GJ. Neuroradiologic evaluation of patients with acute stroke treated with recombinant tissue plasminogen activator. The rt-PA Acute Stroke Study Group. *AJNR Am J Neuroradiol* 1993; **14**: 3–13.

13 Alexandrov AV, Grotta JC. Arterial reocclusion in stroke patients treated with intravenous tissue plasminogen activator. *Neurology* 2002; **59**: 862–867.

14 Hacke W, Kaste M, Fieschi C, et al. Randomised double-blind placebo-controlled trial of thrombolytic therapy with intravenous alteplase in acute ischaemic stroke (ECASS II). Second European-Australasian Acute Stroke Study Investigators. *Lancet* 1998; **352**: 1245–1251.

15 Albers GW, Bates VE, Clark WM, Bell R, Verro P, Hamilton SA. Intravenous tissue-type plasminogen activator for treatment of acute stroke: the Standard Treatment with Alteplase to Reverse Stroke (STARS) study. *JAMA* 2000; **283**: 1145–1150.

16 del Zoppo GJ, Higashida RT, Furlan AJ, Pessin MS, Rowley HA, Gent M. PROACT: a phase II randomized trial of recombinant pro-urokinase by direct arterial delivery in acute middle cerebral artery stroke. PROACT Investigators. *Prolyse in Acute Cerebral Thromboembolism. Stroke* 1998; **29**: 4–11.

17 Furlan A, Higashida R, Wechsler L, et al. Intra-arterial prourokinase for acute ischemic stroke. The PROACT II study: a randomized controlled trial. *Prolyse in Acute Cerebral Thromboembolism. JAMA* 1999; **282**: 2003–2011.

18 Ogawa A, Mori E, Minematsu K, et al. Randomized trial of intraarterial infusion of urokinase within 6 hours of middle cerebral artery stroke: the middle cerebral artery embolism local fibrinolytic intervention trial (MELT) Japan. *Stroke* 2007; **38**: 2633–2639.

19 Mattle HP, Arnold M, Georgiadis D, *et al.* Comparison of intraarterial and intravenous thrombolysis for ischemic stroke with hyperdense middle cerebral artery sign. *Stroke* 2008; **39**: 379–383.

20 Interventional Management of Stroke Study Investigators. Combined intravenous and intra-arterial recanalization for acute ischemic stroke: the Interventional Management of Stroke Study. *Stroke* 2004; **35**: 904–911.

21 Tomsick T, Broderick J, Carrozella J, *et al.* Revascularization results in the Interventional Management of Stroke II trial. *AJNR Am J Neuroradiol* 2008; **29**: 582–587.

22 Rha JH, Saver JL. The impact of recanalization on ischemic stroke outcome: a meta-analysis. *Stroke* 2007; **38**: 967–973.

23 Gobin YP, Starkman S, Duckwiler GR, *et al.* MERCI 1: a phase 1 study of Mechanical Embolus Removal in Cerebral Ischemia. *Stroke* 2004; **35**: 2848–2854.

24 Smith WS, Sung G, Starkman S, *et al.* Safety and efficacy of mechanical embolectomy in acute ischemic stroke: results of the MERCI trial. *Stroke* 2005; **36**: 1432–1438.

25 Smith WS, Sung G, Saver J, *et al.* Mechanical thrombectomy for acute ischemic stroke: final results of the Multi MERCI trial. *Stroke* 2008; **39**: 1205–1212.

26 Penumbra Pivotal Stroke Trial I. The penumbra pivotal stroke trial: safety and effectiveness of a new generation of mechanical devices for clot removal in intracranial large vessel occlusive disease. *Stroke* 2009; **40**: 2761–2768.

27 Pereira VM, Gralla J, Davalos A, *et al.* Prospective, multicenter, single-arm study of mechanical thrombectomy using Solitaire Flow Restoration in acute ischemic stroke. *Stroke* 2013; **44**: 2802–2807.

28 Abou-Chebl A, Zaidat OO, Castonguay AC, *et al.* North American SOLITAIRE Stent-Retriever Acute Stroke Registry: choice of anesthesia and outcomes. *Stroke* 2014; **45**: 1396–1401.

29 Mokin M, Dumont TM, Veznedaroglu E, *et al.* Solitaire Flow Restoration thrombectomy for acute ischemic stroke: retrospective multicenter analysis of early postmarket experience after FDA approval. *Neurosurgery* 2013; **73**: 19–25; discussion 25–26.

30 Davalos A, Pereira VM, Chapot R, *et al.* Retrospective multicenter study of Solitaire FR for revascularization in the treatment of acute ischemic stroke. *Stroke* 2012; **43**: 2699–2705.

31 Berkhemer OA, Fransen PS, Beumer D, *et al.* A randomized trial of intraarterial treatment for acute ischemic stroke. *N Engl J Med* 2015; **372**: 11–20.

32 Goyal M, Demchuk AM, Menon BK, *et al.* Randomized assessment of rapid endovascular treatment of ischemic stroke. *N Engl J Med* 2015; **372**: 1019–1030.

33 Campbell BC, Mitchell PJ, Kleinig TJ, *et al.* Endovascular therapy for ischemic stroke with perfusion-imaging selection. *N Engl J Med* 2015; **372**: 1009–1018.

34 Saver JL, Goyal M, Bonafe A, *et al.* Stent-retriever thrombectomy after intravenous t-PA vs. t-PA alone in stroke. *N Engl J Med* 2015; **372**: 2285–2295.

35 Jovin TG, Chamorro A, Cobo E, *et al.* Thrombectomy within 8 hours after symptom onset in ischemic stroke. *N Engl J Med* 2015; **372**: 2296–2306.

36 Balami JS, Sutherland BA, Edmunds LD, *et al.* A systematic review and meta-analysis of randomized controlled trials of endovascular thrombectomy compared with best medical treatment for acute ischemic stroke. *Int J Stroke* 2015; **10**: 1168–1178.

37 Bogousslavsky J, Van Melle G, Regli F. The Lausanne Stroke Registry: analysis of 1,000 consecutive patients with first stroke. *Stroke* 1988; **19**: 1083–1092.

38 Fassbender K, Walter S, Liu Y, *et al.* "Mobile stroke unit" for hyperacute stroke treatment. *Stroke* 2003; **34**: e44.

39 Walter S, Kostopoulos P, Haass A, *et al.* Diagnosis and treatment of patients with stroke in a mobile stroke unit versus in hospital: a randomised controlled trial. *Lancet Neurol* 2012; **11**: 397–404.

40 Walter S, Kostopoulos P, Haass A, *et al.* Point-of-care laboratory halves door-to-therapy-decision time in acute stroke. *Ann Neurol* 2011; **69**: 581–586.

41 Lansberg MG, Thijs VN, Bammer R, *et al.* Risk factors of symptomatic intracerebral hemorrhage after tPA therapy for acute stroke. *Stroke* 2007; **38**: 2275–2278.

42 Furlan A, Higashida R, Wechsler L, *et al.* Intra-arterial prourokinase for acute ischemic stroke. The PROACT II study: a randomized controlled trial. *Prolyse in Acute Cerebral Thromboembolism. JAMA* 1999; **282**: 2003–2011.

43 Smith WS, Sung G, Starkman S, *et al.* Safety and efficacy of mechanical embolectomy in acute ischemic stroke: results of the MERCI trial. *Stroke* 2005; **36**: 1432–1438.

44 Smith WS, Sung G, Saver J, *et al.* Mechanical thrombectomy for acute ischemic stroke: final results of the Multi MERCI trial. *Stroke* 2008; **39**: 1205–1212.

45 Penumbra Pivotal Stroke Trial Investigators. The penumbra pivotal stroke trial: safety and effectiveness of a new generation of mechanical devices for clot removal in intracranial large vessel occlusive disease. *Stroke* 2009; **40**: 2761–2768.

CHAPTER 69

Carotid Artery Angioplasty and Stenting

Alberto Cremonesi, Shane Gieowarsingh, and Fausto Castriota
Maria Cecilia Hospital, GVM Care and Research, Cotignola, Italy

Stroke has been acknowledged as the third leading cause of death, subsequent to heart disease and cancer, in industrialized nations [1]. In the last decades, there has been unprecedented investment at national levels to develop the quality of services for heart disease and cancer leading to an improvement in patient survival. Recently, the focus has changed toward advancing the management of stroke patients, as it is recognized with an aging population the burden of this disease because of its high mortality, major disability, and dependence [2]. For this reason, it is vital that the more mature approach to the prevention and treatment at different levels in the pathogenesis and manifestation of this disease is pursued further by all concerned.

Ten to fifteen percent of all ischemic strokes originate from an atherosclerotic plaque at the level of the internal carotid artery (ICA). Carotid endarterectomy (CEA) has been shown to be efficacious in the long-term prevention of stroke for both symptomatic and asymptomatic patients with severe obstructive carotid disease [3–6]. Despite the controversial design and results of randomized trials comparing it with CEA, carotid angioplasty and stenting (CAS) is still a promising field because of its potential as a complementary therapy for patients who are considered high risk for CEA; and as an alternative, less invasive and effective revascularization procedure for a large subset of patients.

Background

The main goal of carotid intervention is the prevention of stroke, in particular disabling stroke. Following the application of surgical endarterectomy for treating carotid bifurcation disease in the 1950s, it was not until 40 years later that level 1 evidence from large randomized trials for its efficacy was established. Although there have been significant developments in pharmacotherapy for vascular disease over the last 30 years, the stroke prevention benefit has not been established specifically for patients with high-grade carotid stenosis [7,8]. CAS was developed to meet a need for a less-invasive revascularization strategy for patients considered high risk for surgical revascularization. The rapid advancement in endovascular technologies and techniques has resulted in the evolution of CAS to a refined technique with great potential to be applied to routine carotid revascularization practice.

Currently, controversy exists as to whether CAS should be accepted as an alternative to CEA. To answer this question there have been a few randomized trials comparing the therapies [9–15]; however, some have been hampered by difficulties with enrollment, results have been conflicting, many criticisms have been levied against trial designs and the required level of operator endovascular experience, and hence a clear consensus cannot be established. It is to be hoped that ongoing large randomized trials (SPACE-2; ACST-2; CREST-2; and ACT-1) [16,17] will address this uncertainty. Over the last decade single-center and multicenter case series and registry data have been published providing valuable evidence for the effectiveness of this therapy in both the short and medium term. Nonetheless, arising from these discussions and debates one thing is clear: to move forward toward the goal of stroke prevention, these procedures must be performed by high level and well-trained operators, preferable at high-volume CAS centers.

Important concepts and considerations
Tailored approach
To achieve a high level of procedural success the multifactorial CAS strategy involves a *tailored approach* in the application of endovascular devices and techniques to specific patients with specific lesions and vascular anatomies. This requires an in-depth knowledge of neuroassessment, carotid plaque characteristics, vascular anatomy, and technical features of endovascular materials: guiding catheters and sheaths, guidewires, embolic protection devices (EPDs), balloons and carotid stents. Following the experience gained in this field since 1997, with over 3000 procedures, our group strongly believes that each device has special characteristics and should be used in predefined indications.

Stent intrinsic antiembolic property
The major source of complications is distal embolization, either intraprocedural or post-procedural. For effective reduction of intraprocedural risk great emphasis is placed on the use of EPDs. An important concept to consider is the view that in the presence of an EPD, the type of stent implanted may not significantly impact on the risk of intraprocedural complications but subsequently plays a vital part in preventing neurologic events resulting from plaque

Interventional Cardiology: Principles and Practice, Second Edition. Edited by George D. Dangas, Carlo Di Mario, and Nicholas N. Kipshidze.
© 2017 John Wiley & Sons, Ltd. Published 2017 by John Wiley & Sons, Ltd.

prolapse. It is appreciated that whereas in open surgical techniques the atheroma and thrombus burden are excised, the stent-protected angioplasty technique compacts this material to the wall, retaining it with its supporting scaffolding and wall-coverage properties. The stent cell geometry thus has an *intrinsic antiembolic property* influencing the risk of plaque prolapse and distal embolization during the 24-hour post-procedural and recuperative period until re-endothelializaton is complete.

Safe CAS and protected procedure

The interventionalist *safe CAS and protected procedure* concept should encompass the idea that two protection positions should be implemented in practice. In addition to the use of high-tech devices to contain plaque (stents) or capture and remove embolic debris (EPDs), the implementation of the tailored philosophy to the entire management strategy from appropriate patient and lesion selection to meticulous device choice and interventional techniques is essential. An important element of this concept is the recognition of high-risk cases for CAS dependent primarily on the skill of the interventional vascular specialist. This is considerably more relevant in this field than other areas of percutaneous interventions.

Clinical governance and regulation

Establishment of standard operating procedures is critical to a successful CAS program. This is based on informed consent and patient choice, and effective clinical governance including consideration of setting up a prospective registry as a measure of quality assurance. This approach should be performed as part of a local institutional review board approved protocol with dispassionate oversight and assessment by an independent neurologist. This *regulation* must be emphasized because of the need to always be critical of our management to improve patient care.

Measurement of early outcomes and complications

In order to determine the safety of what we do in our clinical practice, *early outcomes and complications* should be analyzed in a focused manner. Several factors influence the 30-day risk of transient ischemic attack (TIA), stroke, and death: patient characteristics such as age and neurologic symptom status; and operational variables such as operator experience, aortic arch and carotid anatomy, plaque characteristics, stent technology, and type of EPD employed. If complications are recorded with no discrimination of time distribution, analysis of this cumulative data may not be useful to determine in detail the relevance of specified variables and can be misleading because of the heavy weight of confounding variables. Hence, we recommend documentation and analysis of adverse events within specified time periods: the intraprocedural period (those occurring after the beginning of the procedure to the time point when the patient leave the procedure room); the 24-hour post-procedural period (from the time point when the patient leaves the procedure room to 24-hours post-procedure); and the subsequent recuperative period of up to 30 days [18]. For a complete register of each adverse event, it should also be categorized according to its distribution: (i) access site complications; (ii) confined to the target vessel complications (arterial occlusion, severe vasospasm, dissection); (iii) organ-specfic complications (neurologic, cardiovascular, respiratory, gastrointestinal, renal, and liver); and (iv) systemic complications (allergic and anaphylactoid reaction, septicemia, idiosyncratic reaction to drugs). These tools allow prospective and retrospective analyses of each event [18].

Table 69.1 High surgical risk criteria.

Clinical criteria	Anatomic criteria
1　Age >75 years	1　High cervical lesion
2　CCS Class 3–4 or unstable angina	2　Tandem lesions >70%
3　NYHA Class III–IV	3　CEA restenosis
4　LVEF <35%	4　Contralateral ICA occlusion
5　MI <6 weeks	5　Hostile neck (prior irradiation, tracheostomy, radical neck dissection)
6　Multivessel coronary artery disease	6　Cervical immobility
7　Severe pulmonary disease	
8　Severe renal impairment	
9　Contralateral cranial nerve injury	

CCS, Canadian Cardiovascular Society; CEA, carotid endarterectomy; ICA, internal carotid artery; LVEF, left ventricular ejection fraction; MI, myocardial infarction; NYHA, New York Heart Association.

Box 69.1 Challenges for carotid angioplasty and stenting (CAS)

1　Tortuous iliac vessels
2　Bovine or type III aortic arch
3　Calcified and irregular aortic arch
4　Tortuous supra-aortic vessels
5　Long irregular dishomogeneous plaque
6　Highly calcified carotid lesions

Indications and contraindications

The indication for carotid intervention includes a symptomatic patient with an angiographic stenosis of ≥50% (i.e., a lesion-related neurologic event in the preceding 66 months), and an asymptomatic patient with an angiographic stenosis of ≥80%. The specific absolute contraindication for elective CAS is floating thrombus in the carotid artery. Standard relative contraindications to endovascular techniques would apply. The potential factors for considering a patient high risk for CEA, because of medical comorbidities or anatomic factors, thus indicating an endovascular approach, are shown in Table 69.1. Box 69.1 provides some insight into the issues that can prove challenging or increase the risk of the stenting procedure.

Carotid plaque characteristics

The evaluation of carotid plaque profile should describe, in addition to degree stenosis and vessel dimensions, both the length of disease and the morphologic features that predict plaque complexity and embolization risk ("vulnerable plaque").

Both long lesions and clinically unstable plaques (i.e., recurrent TIAs) define a high-risk lesion subset, because of high plaque burden and inflammatory activation, respectively. Indeed, Krapf *et al.* [19] reported, using diffusion-weighted MRI, that the risk of new cerebral ischemic lesions after CAS was related to the length of the lesion, and Aronow *et al.* [20] described preprocedural leukocyte count to be associated with increased microembolization during CAS.

A study analyzing 200 CEA specimens showed that plaque phenotype correlated with embolization risk, where "vulnerable plaques" characterized by a large lipid pool covered by a thin fibrous cap were more prone to perioperative microembolization than fibrous plaques [21]. These vulnerable plaques are less echogenic, described as "soft-lesions," and this pattern can be quantified by the Grey scale median (GSM) method. In the ICAROS study [22], the risk of CAS-related stroke was 7.1% in lesions with GSM <25 and 1.5% in lesions with GSM >25.

Therefore clinical, biochemical, and morphologic data should be assessed and integrated to predict the embolic risk of a specific carotid lesion in order to plan the tailored approach to intervention.

Vascular anatomy

Complete and standardized assessment of the patient's vascular profile is achieved by evaluating all vascular beds involved in CAS procedure according to the Five Arterial Zones classification. The angiographic analyses of the "aortic arch," "proximal vessel," "stenting segment," "distal vessel," and "cerebral vessel" zones predicts the procedural technical difficulties allowing the operator to chose suitable techniques and materials according to the most relevant anatomic aspects [23–25]. The Five Arterial Zones procedural anatomic classification is shown in Figure 69.1 and the theoretical correlation between each zone and the basic procedural steps of CAS procedure is described in Figure 69.2. This classification stresses the need for a

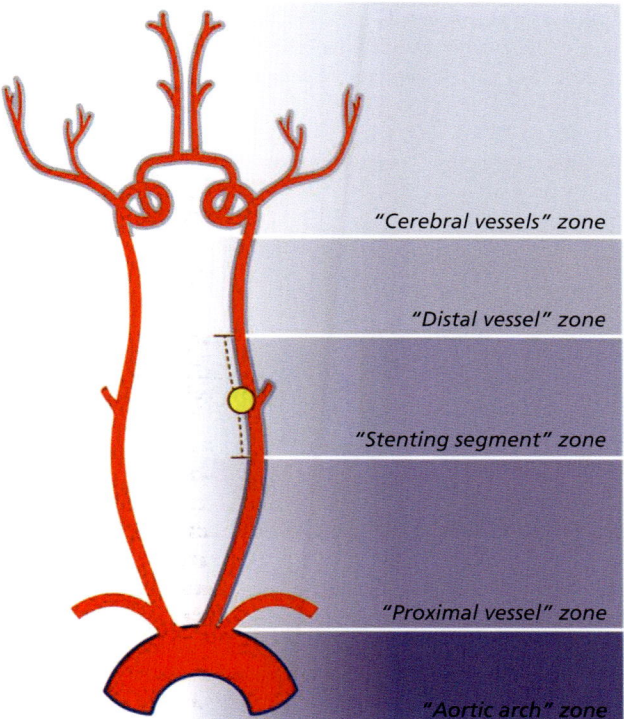

Figure 69.1 Schematic application of the "five arterial zones" classification system. The carotid lesion is represented by the yellow ball and the "stenting segment" limits by the red dashes. Source: de Campos Martins EC, *et al.* 2012 [24], p. 612. Reproduced with permission of Europa Digital & Publishing.

full anatomic evaluation, from the traditional aortic arch type (Figure 69.3) to the cerebral vessels pattern (Figure 69.4).

Cerebral protection devices

Carotid lesions contain friable, ulcerated plaque and thrombotic material that can embolize during an intervention as shown in histopathologic analysis [26] and transcranial Doppler studies [27]. Embolic particles can be classified as either macroemboli (>100 μm) or microemboli (<100 μm). Macroemboli, especially >200 μm, are usually associated with clinical events; however, the effects of microembolization are not well known and can include subtle changes in neurocognitive function. Despite advanced stenting techniques and dual antiplatelet therapy, embolization invariably occurs. A reduction of the Doppler-defined embolic load by an EPD has been shown [28], and preliminary results indicate that with the routine use of such devices the results of CAS are comparable with the best surgical series [29,30].

Protected CAS: clinical results

There has been no randomized trial comparing the efficacy of protected with unprotected CAS and it is difficult to imagine that such a study will ever be conducted on a significant number of patients. Recent literature data shed some light:

- Visible debris was documented in 60% of cases of filter-protected CAS by Sprouse *et al.* [31], and in 66.8% by our group [32].
- In the German registry [33], protected CAS was associated with a significantly lower rate of ipsilateral stroke (1.7% vs. 4.1%; p = 0.007).
- Our group reported a 79% reduction in the rate of embolic complications with protected CAS [34].
- In the early phase of the EVA-3S study, unprotected CAS was associated with a 3.9 times higher stroke rate at 30 days than protected CAS [35].
- A 2003 review of the global registry found that the rates of stroke and death were 5.2% for unprotected CAS and 2.2% for protected CAS [36].
- Kastrup *et al.* [29], in a systematic review of the literature regarding the early outcome of CAS with and without EPD, analyzed studies published between 1990 and 2002 (2537 unprotected CAS and 896 protected CAS procedures); the combined 30-day stroke and death rates were 5.5% and 1.8%, respectively (p <0.001).

On the basis of this review, EPDs appear to reduce thromboembolic complications during CAS.

Distal protection devices

Distal protection devices work by interrupting or filtering blood flow by positioning the device distal to the lesion in a straight portion of the ICA (landing zone). The first system utilized an occlusion balloon, but nowadays filters are usually employed because they are less complex and perhaps more intuitive to use. Filters entrap debris of medium to large size, generally particles >100 μm. Filter performance can be summed up in crossing profile and capturing capability. Crossing profile is an important characteristic justified by the fact that the wire and the filter, constrained in the delivery system, must pass the lesion without detaching friable material. Capturing capability is dependent on membrane pore size and adequate wall apposition of the filter.

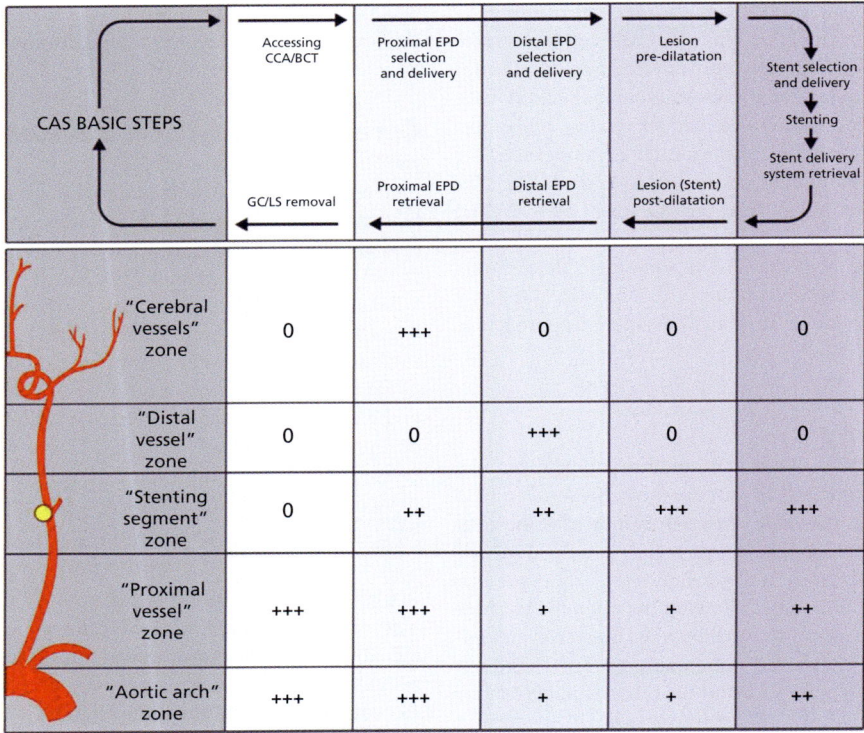

CAS BASIC STEPS	Accessing CCA/BCT	Proximal EPD selection and delivery	Distal EPD selection and delivery	Lesion pre-dilatation	Stent selection and delivery / Stenting / Stent delivery system retrieval
	GC/LS removal	Proximal EPD retrieval	Distal EPD retrieval	Lesion (Stent) post-dilatation	
"Cerebral vessels" zone	0	+++	0	0	0
"Distal vessel" zone	0	0	+++	0	0
"Stenting segment" zone	0	++	++	+++	+++
"Proximal vessel" zone	+++	+++	+	+	++
"Aortic arch" zone	+++	+++	+	+	++

Figure 69.2 Theoretical impact of the "five arterial zones" classification system on the technical evaluation of the basic carotid angioplasty and stenting (CAS) steps. The technical evaluation of CAS was divided into: (1) accessing and stabilising the system (guiding catheter, long-sheath or proximal EPD) in the CCA/BCT; (2) selection, deployment, and retrieval of proximal EPD; (3) selection, deployment, and retrieval of distal EPD; (4) lesion pre- and post-dilatation; and (5) stent selection, delivery, and deployment. 0: no influence; +: little influence; ++: moderate influence; +++: strong influence; BCT: brachiocephalic trunk; CAS: carotid artery stenting; CCA: common carotid artery; EPD: embolic protection devices; GC: guiding catheter; LS: long-sheath. Source: de Campos Martins EC, *et al.* 2012 [24], p. 614. Reproduced with permission of Europa Digital & Publishing.

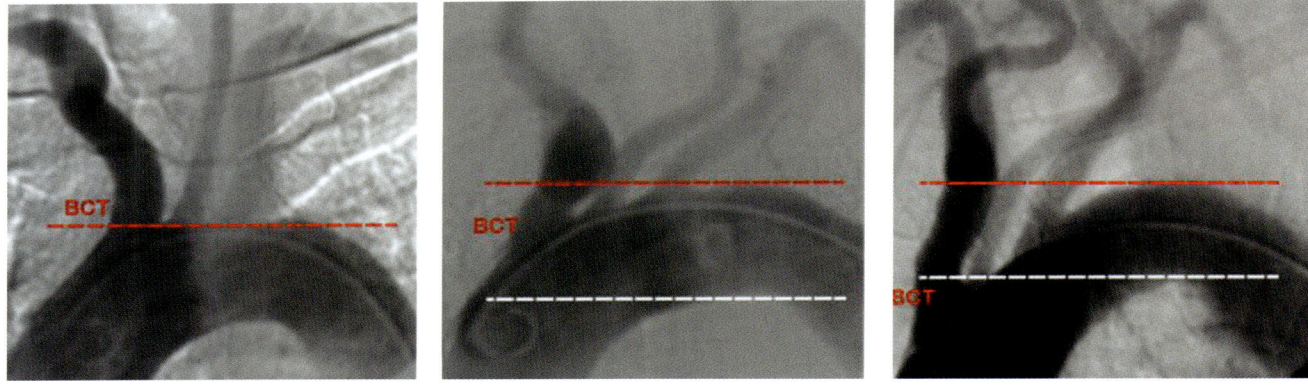

Figure 69.3 Aortic arch anatomy classified as types 1, 2, and 3 with increasing levels of complexity for catheter engagement and provision of support for intervention. The red and white dashed lines point the outer and inner aortic arch curvatures, respectively. The brachycephalic trunk origin (BCT) is represented in each figure. In aortic arch type 1 the origin of the BCT is at the level of the outer curve of the aortic arch; in type 2 the BCT originates between the levels of the outer and inner curve of the aortic arch, and in type 3 the BCT originates bellow the level of the inner curve of the aortic arch.

Limitations of distal protection devices

The distal occlusion balloon shares with filters, especially in tight stenoses, the limitation of unprotected crossing of the lesion in order to deploy the device. Filters are not effective in trapping microemboli, as they are limited by pore size. In tortuous or large distal ICA anatomy, incomplete wall apposition can allow even macroemboli to bypass the system. In addition, debris can be dislodged during the recapture phase (squeezing effect). The distal occlusion balloon, despite being able to block microemboli by occluding the ICA, can lead to embolization via collaterals from the external carotid artery

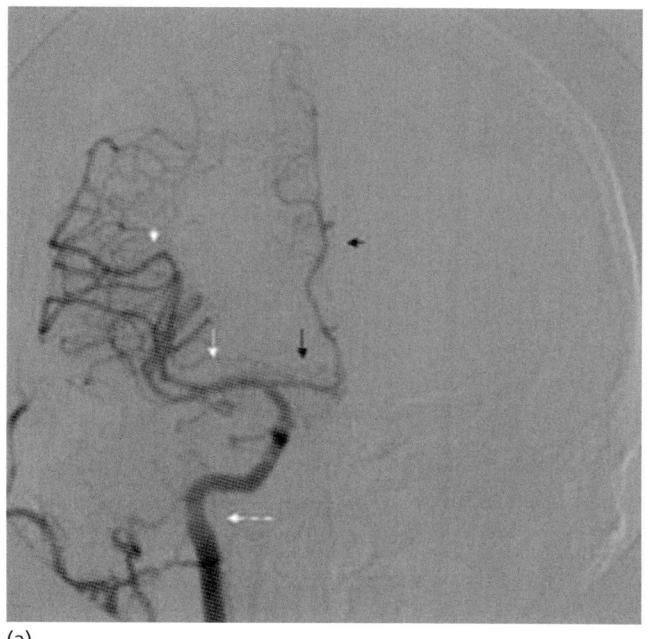

(a)

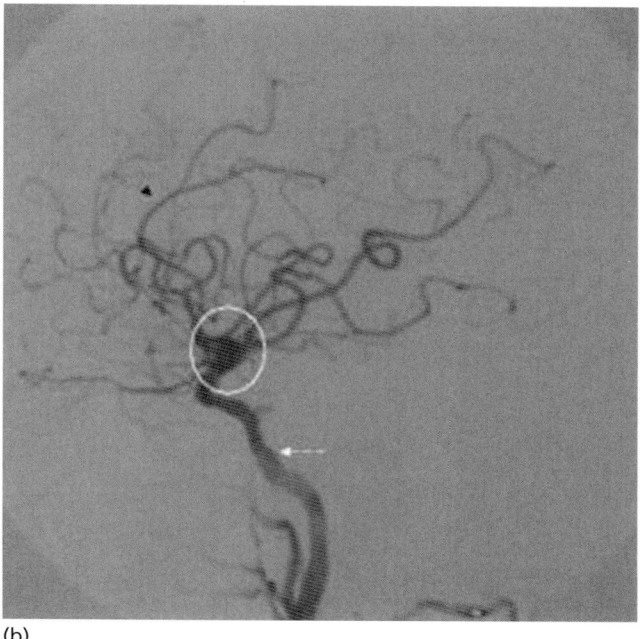

(b)

Figure 69.4 (a) Right AP intracranial angiogram. The outlined arrow shows the right internal carotid artery (ICA). The black arrow points to the anterior cerebral artery leading to the pericallosal artery (black arrowhead). The middle cerebral artery is showed by the white arrow and its branches (white arrowhead). (b) Right lateral intracranial angiogram. The outlined arrow shows the right ICA. The black arrowhead shows the pericallosal artery. The middle cerebral and anterior cerebral arteries are not well individualized in this projection.

(ECA) to the middle cerebral artery. Moreover, about 5–8% of patients develop clamping intolerance to the interruption of cerebral perfusion [37]. Additionally, both systems can be a source of embolism because of intimal damage at the landing zone.

Proximal protection devices

Proximal protection devices work by interrupting or reversing blood flow in the ICA. They offer the advantage of crossing the lesion under protection and blocking both macro- and micro-emboli. Moreover, navigation of the device in the distal ICA is not required, thus reducing the risk of intimal damage, spasm, or dissection. There are two such devices: the Mo.Ma and NeuroProtection systems.

Mo.Ma™ (Medtronic)

The Mo.Ma system consists of a 9 Fr sheath (8 Fr in the new system) with an effective working channel of 6 and 5 Fr, respectively, and two independently inflatable balloons placed at a distance of 7.2 cm. The distal balloon occludes the ECA up to a diameter of 6 mm and the proximal balloon occludes the common carotid artery (CCA) up to a diameter of 13 mm, thus preventing antegrade flow from the CCA and retrograde flow from the ECA. The lesion can be crossed and treated under protection. Following post-dilatation, three 20-mL syringes of blood are actively aspirated and checked for debris before deflating the balloons. Insertion of the system via a 9–10 Fr sheath is advisable in order to allow arterial pressure monitoring via the femoral sheath side-arm throughout the procedure.

NeuroProtection System™ (NPS) (Gore)

The NeuroProtection System, derived from the Parodi antiembolic system (PAES) (ArteriA), allows continuous passive ICA flow reversal through endovascular clamping of the CCA by inflating a balloon located at the tip of a 9 Fr compatible delivery system/sheath and of the ECA by inflating an independent balloon catheter advanced into the ECA via the sheath. The system allows connection to the contralateral femoral vein, and flow reversal of blood from the contralateral cerebral circulation via the circle of Willis, down the ICA, and through the sheath into the venous system. A filter (pore size 180 μm) collects debris before the blood re-enters the venous system. Then the lesion can be crossed and treated under protection. After each stage, particularly those associated with the greatest risk of embolization, 10 mL blood is actively aspirated and at the end of the procedure balloons are deflated while active suction is applied to retrieve any particle contiguous to the balloon occluder. The effective working channel of the assembled system is 6 Fr. Manufacturing of this particular system has ceased during the past 2 years, owing to the global limitation of carotid stenting procedures.

Proximal protection during CAS: clinical data

The available clinical experience is from five multicenter registries: EMPiRE trial (354 patients – including lead-in and continued access patients with the use of GORE flow reversal system) [38]; ARMOUR trial (262 pivotal plus lead-in patients with the use of MO.MA system) [39]; multicenter single-arm European trial (121 patients with the use of GORE flow reversal system) [40]; two prospective registries (157 patients with the MO.MA system and 233 patients using MO.MA and GORE flow reversal system) [41,42]; and one large-scale single center registry (1270 patients with the MO.MA system) [43], which have been summarized in a meta-analysis [44]. Among 2397 patients, the 30-day rate of composite stroke, myocardial infarction (MI), or death was 2.25%. Stroke, MI, and death were encountered in 1.71%, 0.02%, and 0.40%, respectively. Age and diabetic status were found to be the only significant independent risk predictors; however, total stroke rates remained below 2.6% in all subgroups, including symptomatic octogenarians. Other variables including gender, symptomatic status and contralateral carotid occlusion, were not found to be independent risk predictors. The authors speculate the potential benefits of proximal occlusion devices over distal protection devices were the result of two main factors: first, proximal protection allows neuroprotection throughout all phases of the procedure, transcranial Doppler studies have demonstrated that proximal protection is associated with fewer micro embolic signals (MES) during initial wire crossing when compared with distal protection [45,46], and, second, proximal protection devices are able to capture particulate debris with high efficiency [47]. Distal filter are known to face difficulty in capturing small particles (40–120 mL) [48,49]. Because of limitations in broad expansion of CAS, innovation in the area of proximal protection equipment has ceased.

New developments in cerebral protection
ENROUTE Neuroprotection System (Silk Road Medical)

The ENROUTE Neuroprotection System is a novel flow reversal system consisting of two sheaths, one surgically placed in the CCA (initial portion) via a transcarotid approach connected to a transfemoral percutaneous venous line. The procedure represents a combined surgical and endovascular approach to carotid revascularization. An in-line flow regulator allows the operator to modify the flow through the circuit from high flow up to temporary flow cessation. The carotid sheath is placed in the ipsilateral CCA via a surgical incision above the clavicle. The venous sheath is inserted percutaneously into the femoral vein. The arterial and venous return sheaths are connected by the flow line, which creates an arteriovenous shunt. Following the proximal protection concept, the flow reversal is induced prior to any lesion manipulation by occluding the carotid artery proximally to the carotid sheath resulting in pressure gradient. The ipsilateral ECA does not need to be occluded with this system, as it is the case with other proximal embolic protection devices. The main advantage of this system is the avoidance of aortic arch manipulation associated to robust proximal embolic protection. Disadvantages of the system include the requirement of a disease-free portion of CCA at the site of surgical incision.

The PROOF study was a first-in-man, single-arm feasibility study using the ENROUTE™ Neuroprotection System in 44 patients who were candidates for carotid artery revascularization. The primary endpoints were major stroke, MI, or death from the index procedure up to 30 days. Procedural microembolization was studied in a subgroup by performing diffusion-weighted magnetic resonance imaging (DW-MRI) pre and post-procedure. One minor contralateral stroke was reported at 30 days in a patient who was free of lesions on pre and post-procedural DW-MRI scans. There were no MIs or cranial nerve injuries [50]. A subset of 31 patients underwent DW-MRI of brain within 72 hours preprocedure and 24–48 hours post-procedure. Five patients had new white lesions (16.1%). This represents the lowest DW-MRI rate of any carotid stenting strategy to date.

The ROADSTER trial is an ongoing prospective, single-arm, multicenter investigational device exemption clinical trial of the ENROUTE Neuroprotection System (Silk Road Medical Inc. Sunnyvale, CA, USA) in conjunction with all commercially available carotid artery stents, approved by the Food and Drug Administration (FDA), used for revascularization in patients with carotid artery disease who were considered to represent a high risk for carotid endarterectomy. The trial has recently completed enrollment to target with 141 pivotal patients. The primary endpoint, a composite of stroke, death, and MI will be compared with an objective performance criterion based on the results from the CREATE trial and will be presented to the FDA for device approval.

Limitations of proximal protection devices

The drawbacks of proximal protection devices include their large size, clamping intolerance, and the impossibility of their use with severe disease of the ECA or CCA. Contralateral ICA occlusion is not necessarily a contraindication in the presence of a functional circle of Willis with adequate flow from the vertebral system.

The need for large femoral sheaths can preclude use in patients with severe peripheral disease and could be associated with an increase in access site complications. Nevertheless, with the first version of the Mo.Ma device (10 Fr), in the PRIAMUS registry, the rate of local complications was 4.1%, none requiring surgical repair or blood transfusions. Higher complication rates were reported by Rabe et al. [51] with the PAES, but, given the current availability of 8–9 Fr size for the Mo.Ma and 9 Fr for the NPS device, it is reasonable to expect a low rate of clinically significant access site complications.

Clamping intolerance occurs in up to 8% of patients and is generally associated with severe contralateral disease or poorly developed cerebral collateral circulation. An intraprocedural parameter predictive of intolerance is represented by a backpressure <40 mmHg occlusion [44]. Another key factor is overall clamping time, which has progressively shortened with increased experience (for the Mo.Ma system from 10 minutes in the study of Diederich et al. [52] to 5 minutes in the PRIAMUS registry [53], with a parallel decline in the rate of clamping intolerance from 12% to about 6%). The same holds true for the PAES/NPS device, as the rate of clamping intolerance dropped from 8% in 2001 to 3% in 2005 [54]. However, clamping intolerance has not been associated with higher major adverse coronary and cardiac events (MACCE), even in the presence of contralateral occlusion [44], and it does not represent an absolute contraindication to carry on the procedure. Indeed, three strategies can be adopted: hurry up in order to restore perfusion as soon as possible; positioning under protection a distal filter and then deflating the balloons ("seatbelt and airbag" technique); perform a step-by-step procedure in which the balloons are inflated and deflated at each procedural step.

When to use proximal or distal protection and potential complications

Large studies comparing proximal with distal protection are lacking, so device selection should be based on the tailored approach. In challenging anatomies, with angulated ICA-CCA take-off and/or lack of a suitable ICA landing zone, proximal protection should be strongly recommended. The same holds true for lesions with high embolic risk, because proximal protection devices seem to be more effective than filter systems in avoiding distal embolization. The most frequent complications with distal protection devices are spasm and slow flow with an incidence of up to 3.6% and 7.2%, respectively [55]. In our experience a gentle approach as well as the use of a soft-tipped filter wire minimized the frequency of this problem. Slow flow occurs when the filter pores are partially or completely occluded with debris and disappears following removal of the filter. Dissections at the landing zone have been described in 0.5–0.9% of cases [30,56]. Device retrieval occasionally poses a problem and it is here that the torqueability of a guiding catheter can help change the attitude of the system allowing the retrieval sheath to cross the stent. Other maneuvers include turning the patient's head or using a buddy wire. Complications related to proximal protection devices are mostly related to intolerance. In the recently completed Mo.Ma registry [57], intolerance was observed in 7.1% of patients; in 1.9% intermittent balloon deflation was necessary to complete the procedure, and in 0.6% a distal filter was positioned. All patients completed the procedure without in-hospital or 30-day neurologic complications.

Self-expanding carotid stents
Structural and functional characteristics
Braided-mesh stent
The first self-expanding stent dedicated to carotid application was the cobalt alloy braided-mesh frame which is highly flexible with acceptable radial strength. The frame is compressible and constrained within a sheath: a spring-like action allows it to expand as the sheath is withdrawn during deployment. Advantages include a small and flexible delivery system, a small free-cell area with high scaffolding and wall-coverage properties (plaque covering) and adaptability to the changing diameter across the bifurcation. However, it tends to straighten the vessel and has an unpredictable foreshortening during deployment.

Nitinol stents
The second group of self-expanding stents is represented by a nitinol structure (nickel-titanium alloy). The thermal expansion properties of nitinol characterize these devices and when exposed to body temperature they expand to the predetermined shape and size. Most are obtained from a tube of nitinol which is laser-cut to create a frame comprised of sequential aligned annular rings interconnected in a helical fashion. Another frame is the flat-sheet nitinol-roll closed-cell design. An advantage of the nitinol stents is minimal foreshortening on deployment.

Nitinol stents, for simplicity, can be categorized as an open cell, closed cell, and hybrid designs, with either a cylindrical or tapered shape. The open-cell designs tend to have a larger free-cell area than the closed-cell designs. The advantages of open-cell stents include high conformability and flexibility, and high vessel-wall adaptability. Disadvantages include moderate scaffolding and wall-coverage properties, and stent–strut malalignment in complex carotid lesions. The closed-cell stents have high scaffolding and wall-coverage properties but are disadvantaged by stiffness with poor conformability and flexibility. The semi-quantitative comparison of functional differences among stent designs are shown in Table 69.2. Hybrid nitinol stents can be characterized by a hybrid solution of open cells in the distal and proximal segments in order to enhance flexibility and adaptability, and a closed-cell design in the middle to obtain the appropriate scaffolding and wall coverage to prevent plaque prolapse (Figure 69.5). No study has definitively determined if an open, closed, or hybrid stent has a definite superiority in all lesions. Closed-cell design stents allow less plaque protrusion but also cause more arterial straightening and distal vessel kinking. The opposite effects are evident with open-cell design stents. Stent choice in a specific patient should be based on clinical judgment regarding which of the two concerns is more applicable in the individual case.

Is there a logical scheme for stent selection?
Different stent designs demonstrate functional equivalence when used in uncomplicated scenarios: simple supra-aortic anatomies, straight carotid bifurcations, and stable fibrous plaques. However, frequently the operator has to face challenging situations requiring a move toward a tailored approach. Table 69.3 shows a functional categorization where cobalt-alloy braided-mesh stents are the first choice when the greatest need is to achieve reliable plaque coverage and long-acting plaque prolapse prevention because of the constant radial force property (soft and long non-homogeneous lesions are very prone to distal embolization). Bosiers *et al* [58] demonstrated a clear benefit in favor of stent scaffolding and wall coverage for reducing post-procedural neurologic complications for symptomatic patients (unstable risky plaque). When the main technical challenge is represented by the carotid bifurcation and

Table 69.2 Semi-quantitative comparison of functional differences amongst stents.

Stent technical features	Braided mesh	Nitinol OCG*	Nitinol CCG†
(a) Foreshortening	TS	TI	TI
(b) Conformability/flexibility	+	++	−
(c) Vessel wall adaptability	+	++	+
(d) Scaffolding	++	+	++
(e) Radial strength	+	++	++
(f) Radial stiffness	+	+	+
(g) Wall coverage	++	−	++

Technically Insignificant (TI): <15%
Technically significant (TS): >15%
Worse than others (−)
Comparable with others (+)
Better than others (++)
* OCG, segmented crown, open cell geometry.
† CCG, closed cell geometry (including flat rolled sheath frame).

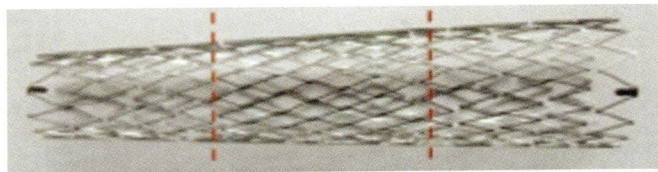

	Distal	Middle	Proximal
Flexibility	High	Appropriate	High
Radial force	Low	Appropriate	Low
Scaffolding	Low	High	Low
M/A ratio	Low	Appropriate	Low

(a)

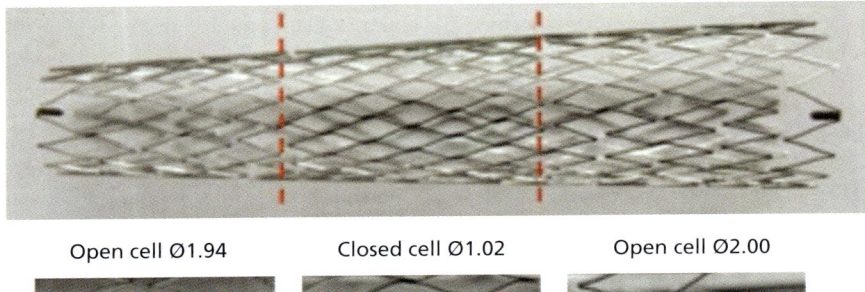

Open cell Ø1.94	Closed cell Ø1.02	Open cell Ø2.00

(b)

Figure 69.5 (a) Functional characteristics of the hybrid carotid stent. The closed-cell mid portion and two open-cell portions at both edges provide adequate scaffolding to the plaque while assuring high flexibility and vessel wall adaptability, respectively. (b) Comparison of free cell area (mm²) in the three segments of the hybrid carotid stent.

Table 69.3 Functional categorization of stents.

Carotid lesion/bifurcation profile	Type of stent
1 Medium to long lesions (15–25 mm)	Cobalt-alloy
2 Soft dishomogeneous lesions	braided mesh stent
3 Straight carotid bifurcations	
4 Carotid bifurcation lesions with ICA/ CCA diameter mismatch	Nitinol open-cell stents
5 Angled carotid bifurcation	
6 Short lesions (<15 mm)	Nitinol closed-cell stents
7 Highly calcified lesions	
8 Straight carotid bifurcation	

CCA, common carotid artery; ICA, internal carotid artery.

plaque complexity (severely angled lesions, plaque ulceration), or the main goal is to maintain the original anatomy/course of a very tortuous vessel, the in-vessel flexibility and the wall–plaque conformability of nitinol open-cell stents are unmatched. Nitinol closed-cell stents represent a great technical solution for focal concentric lesions, especially if resistant or calcified: in such a clinical subset the functional key point is the outward radial force exerted by the stent over time.

New developments in carotid stents
Double-layer mesh stent technology
The RoadSaver™ carotid stent (Terumo, Japan) is a self-expanding, double layer, micromesh scaffold compatible with a 0.014-inch guide wire and 7 Fr guiding catheter/6 Fr long sheath (Figure 69.6). The external nitinol mesh layer enables a flexible scaffold that can accommodate tortuous anatomy and allow for adequate strut apposition while the internal nitinol micromesh—the cell size is extremely small (0.381 mm²)—allows an increased plaque coverage, a characteristic that should be beneficial in terms of post-procedural embolic protection by very tight plaque coverage (Figure 69.7). The stent diameter currently available is in the range 5–10 mm while the length cover ranges from 20 up to 50 mm in 10-mm intervals. The promise of this technology is to achieve improved plaque coverage thanks to the internal micromesh that captures the prolapsing tissue, while the flexible external layer provides great adaptation to the vessel anatomy, thus reducing the rate of acute malapposition. It remains to be demonstrated whether this interesting concept will translate into a reduction of ischemic neurologic events associated with CAS; no such study can provide definitive evidence thus far.

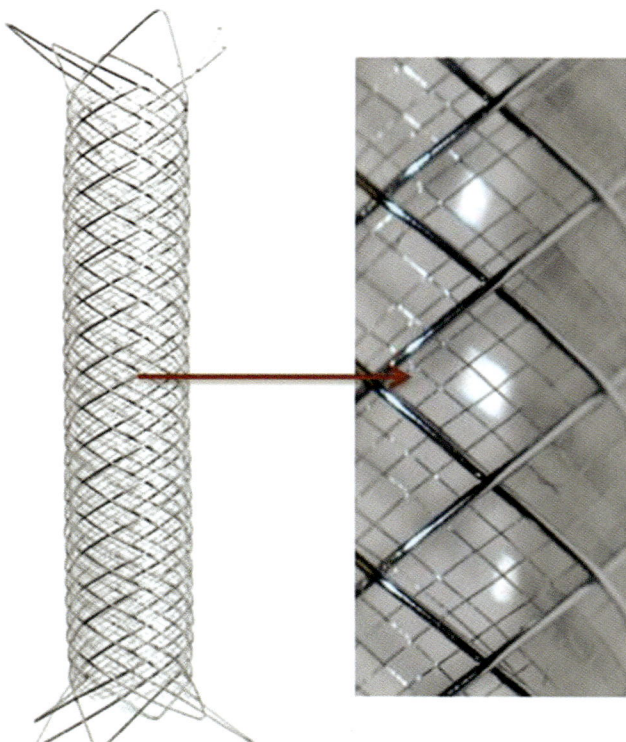

Figure 69.6 RoadSaver™ carotid stent (Terumo, Japan), a self-expanding double-layer micromesh scaffold. Source: Reproduced with permission of Terumo Europe NV.

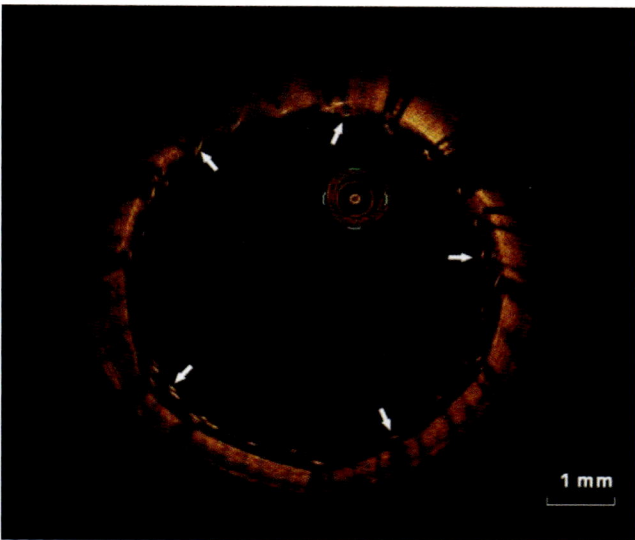

Figure 69.7 Optimal coherence tomography assessment of a RoadSaver™ stent showing no significant prolapse of plaque and good wall apposition. The white arrows point to the stent meshes.

Step-by-step technique of carotid stenting

Clinical protocol

Pre-medication

Dual antiplatelet therapy with aspirin and clopidogrel, ideally initiated 5 days before the procedure; and continued for at least 30 days, at which time clopidogrel is usually discontinued.

Pre-procedure investigations

- Carotid duplex scan, CTA/MRA scan.
- Independent neurologic evaluation.

General procedural measures

- Head restraint and no sedation, with neuroevaluation during procedure by simple communication and movement parameters.
- Standard monitoring of vital parameters.
- Heparin IV 70 IU/Kg (activated clotting time 250–300 seconds).

Technique

Vascular access

Femoral access is recommended, but in the presence of extreme tortuosity or occlusion of the iliac arteries the radial or brachial approach is feasible; however, consideration needs to be given to the compatibility of the materials in planning the intervention. Generally, the right CCA is approached from the left arm and vice versa, but in reality it is determined by the distance between the origins of the supra-aortic trunks.

Baseline angiographic evaluation

In the absence of a CTA/MRA scan, aortic arch angiography is undertaken with a pigtail catheter (30–45° LAO) to visualize the origin of the supra-aortic vessels. Selective cannulation of the target vessel is performed to evaluate the carotid bifurcation in at least two orthogonal projections, demonstrating the maximum severity of the lesion and adequate separation of the ICA from the ECA, in both digitally subtracted and regular formats. The RAO view is helpful to separate the division of the brachiocephalic trunk into the subclavian artery and CCA. It is mandatory to perform an intracranial angiogram which may reveal an unexpected arteriovenous malformation or for comparative assessment with the post-intervention angiogram in the event of embolization. Four-vessel angiography is indicated only where the complexity of the case recommends it as mandatory, such as establishing the adequacy of the collateral circulation and the function of the circle of Willis when considering endovascular clamping in the presence of contralateral ICA occlusion.

Common carotid engagement

Obtaining a safe and stable engagement of the CCA is one of the most important technical aspects to the CAS procedure. Two standard techniques are described outlining the most commonly used materials in our laboratory.

Guiding-catheter engagement

- A 90–100 cm 8 Fr guiding catheter is chosen according to the aortic arch configuration:
- For simple anatomy, a 40° angled soft-tip catheter is advanced to the mid-CCA over a soft-angled 0.035-inch standard hydrophilic wire positioned just below the bifurcation.
- For complex anatomy an angulated guide such as a "hockey stick" curve catheter is advanced into the proximal CCA.
- The introduction of two, or possibly three, 0.035-inch wires in order to advance the catheter in the presence of an unstable situation is feasible. Another option is the placement of a 0.014-inch wire in the ECA for increased stability during the intervention.

- The great advantage of this technique is steerability but it is critical to be cognizant of the risk of scraping the aortic arch during manipulation with the attendant risk of embolization. This can be avoided by meticulous technique, executed by gentle, small, and slow movements; always advancing under rotation and with the right orientation of the catheter using the wire to engage the artery. Of course, a drawback of this strategy is the large femoral access with the attendant risk of complications.

Sheath placement

- A 100 cm 5 Fr JR4 guiding-catheter is advanced over a soft-angled 0.035-inch standard hydrophilic wire into the CCA. The use of a guiding catheter allows contrast injection with a 0.035-inch wire. The same can be achieved with a 6 Fr Vitek or Berenstein type catheter according to anatomic suitability.
- Following an angiogram delineating the bifurcation, the hydrophilic wire is advanced into the ECA and positioned in a distal branch avoiding the lingual artery. The guiding catheter is then advanced deeply into the ECA in a stable position, and if added support is needed a 0.018-inch wire may also be accommodated. The standard 0.035-inch wire is exchanged for a long 260–300 cm 0.035-inch support wire.
- The guiding catheter is then withdrawn and a guiding sheath is advanced to the mid-CCA over the support wire. In our practice the Mo.Ma device, which incorporates the functional aspect of a proximal protection device into a shuttle sheath, is applied and its respective aspects are advanced into the ECA and CCA.
- The advantage of this technique is its safety but it is less steerable and with a tortuous CCA kinks can result or existing tortuous loops can be exaggerated and displaced cephalad. In addition, with significant disease in the proximal CCA or an occluded ECA this technique is not feasible.

EPD management

Managing the EPD in a safe and expeditious manner is one of the key points to successful CAS and several issues are discussed in the relevant sections.

Pre-dilatation

Pre-dilatation is reserved for very tight lesions, heavily calcified lesions, or stenoses with a high tendency to recoil such as long fibrotic lesions. This is usually undertaken with a low profile coronary balloon in the range of 2.5–4.0 mm diameter and 20–30 mm length, and inflated at nominal pressure to minimize the risk of embolization. Consideration should be given to using a cutting balloon for heavily calcified lesions, usually with a diameter of 3.5–4.0 mm and inflated at moderate pressure (8 atm). Our group reported on the use of this application in 111 patients with severe highly calcific *de novo* disease with a procedural technical success rate of 100% [59,60]. The combined all stroke and death rate at 30 days follow-up was 0.9%, with one major stroke. Pretreatment with 0.5–1 mg intravenous atropine is required at this stage and/or post-dilatation phase. Large doses of atropine are avoided in the elderly, as this can result in confusion and make accurate neurologic assessment difficult.

Stent deployment

The unconstrained diameter of the self-expanding stent should be 1–2 mm larger than the reference vessel diameter in order to obtain a stable position and a reliable wall apposition. Usually, we recom-

mend to stent from "angiographically normal-to-normal" vessel. In the presence of challenging anatomy it is helpful when bringing up materials across the arch is to view the stability of the guide in an LAO view. When deploying the stent, release at least 5 mm of the stent distally and wait for it to expand and stabilize against the wall before releasing the remainder of the stent. If the distal edge lands into a tortuous segment injury can result. It is prudent to be aware that tortuous segments are not straightened by a stent but are simply displaced cephalad and can be exaggerated. Speed and minimum use of devices across the lesion are not negligible keys for successful CAS.

Post-dilatation

Post-dilatation is always a critical step as the greatest amounts of emboli are released in this phase. To minimize the embolic load we recommend:

- Balloons no larger than 5.5 mm in diameter;
- Inflating to nominal pressure;
- Accepting a 10–15% residual stenosis;
- Persistent flow via the struts into an ulcer does not require further dilatation; and
- If the ECA becomes occluded, recanalization should be attempted only if the patient is symptomatic (jaw or facial pain) and in such a case it may be sufficient to restore only TIMI II flow.

Final angiographic evaluation

Following EPD removal, final angiograms are acquired in the same baseline projections. If a distal protection device was used the landing zone has to checked carefully, particularly if the ICA is tortuous, to exclude any spasm or dissection. Ipsilateral intracranial angiography should be routinely acquired.

Vascular access site management

General access site management should apply and take into account that an early ambulation and discharge can counteract the activated carotid sinus reflex and the occasionally observed post-procedural hypotension.

Case histories

The following cases were selected to illustrate the tailored approach to CAS.

Case 1: Technical issues related to the stenting segment: short and soft plaque associated with complex anatomy (Figure 69.8)
Technical issues
- Vessel tortuosity is challenging for distal EPDs and necessitates a stent with good conformability to respect the original vessel anatomy; and the mismatch between the ICA and CCA requires a tapered design.
- Soft, highly embologenic plaque needs a stent with high scaffolding properties.

"Tailored" CAS strategy
- Proximal EPDs avoid the risk of unprotected crossing of the lesion and tortuous segment with a distal device.
- The stent provides good conformability because of the open cells at the distal and proximal parts; the closed cells in the middle part afford adequate scaffolding and the tapered design suitably adjusts to the vessel mismatch.

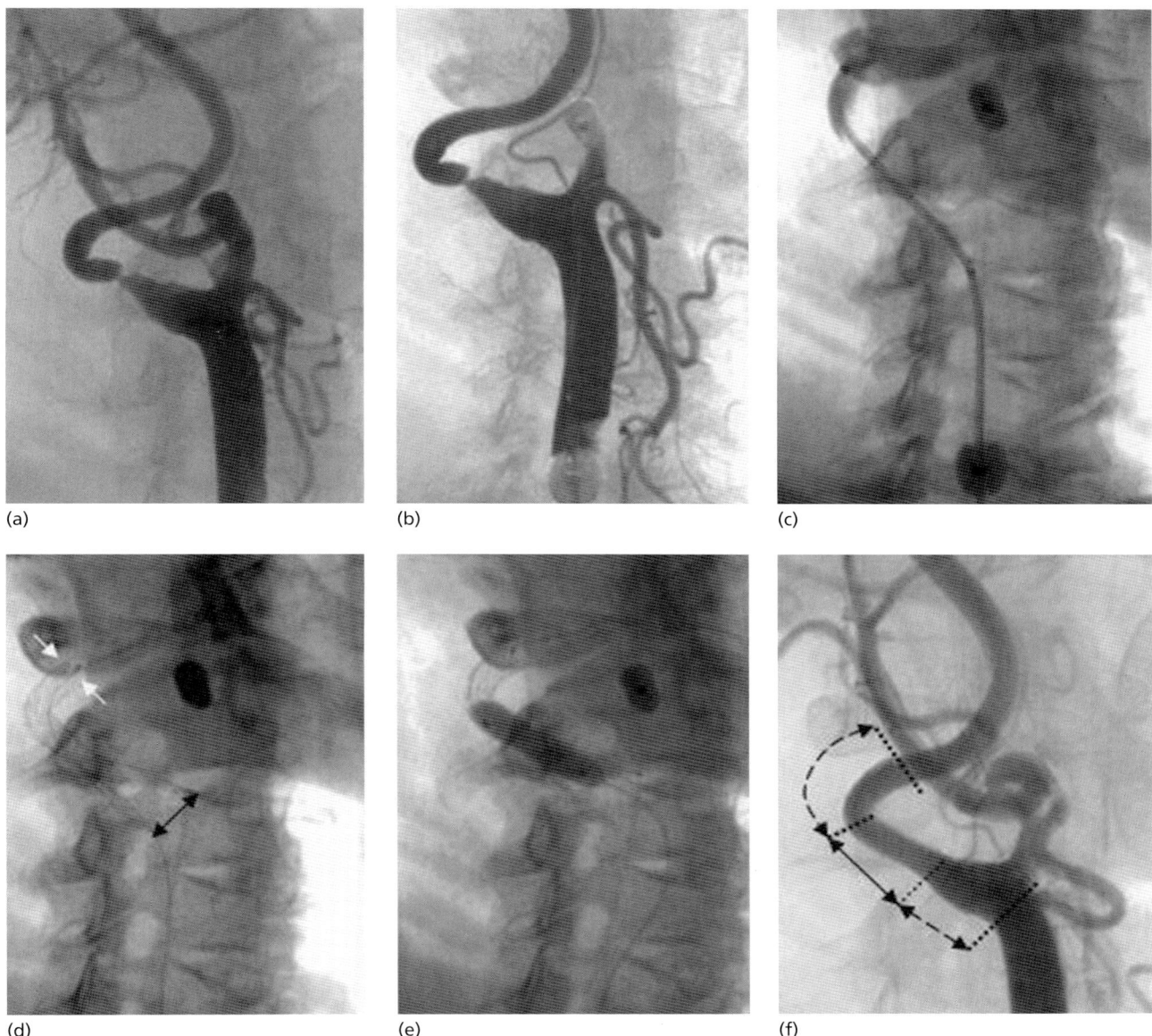

Figure 69.8 Stenting segment complexity: (a) Short and high-grade lesion in right ICA with significant "soft" component identified by duplex scan. (b) Contrast injection through the Mo.Ma device after flow blockage "roadmap." (c) Stent 7/10 x 40 mm positioning. (d) Stent deployed: distal edge diameter showed by white arrows, proximal edge diameter showed by black arrow. (e) Post-dilatation with a 5.5/20 mm balloon. (f) Final result: the closed-cell segment is shown by the full arrow and the outline arrows show the open-cell segments.

Case 2: Technical issues related to the proximal vessel zone: challenging supra-aortic anatomy (Figure 69.9)
Technical issues
- Marked tortuosity of the brachiocephalic trunk and CCA, in addition to posing a challenge to engagement makes it difficult to establish good support to complete the intervention.

"Tailored" CAS strategy
- Use of multiple wires to engage the CCA and maintain stability; in addition to the use of a soft-tip guiding catheter are key strategies.
- Also, the choice of a highly deliverable stent is crucial.

Case 3: Technical issues related to stenting segment: long ulcerated lesion (Figure 69.10)
Technical issues
- A long irregular lesion with severe ulcerations poses a high embologenic risk. In addition, crossing of the lesion with a wire affixed to a filter is risky.

"Tailored" CAS strategy
- The Spider filter (eV3) allows the choice of an independent 0.014-inch wire to gently cross the lesion.
- Carotid stent provides high scaffolding and long-acting plaque prolapse prevention until the ulcerations are obliterated. As the

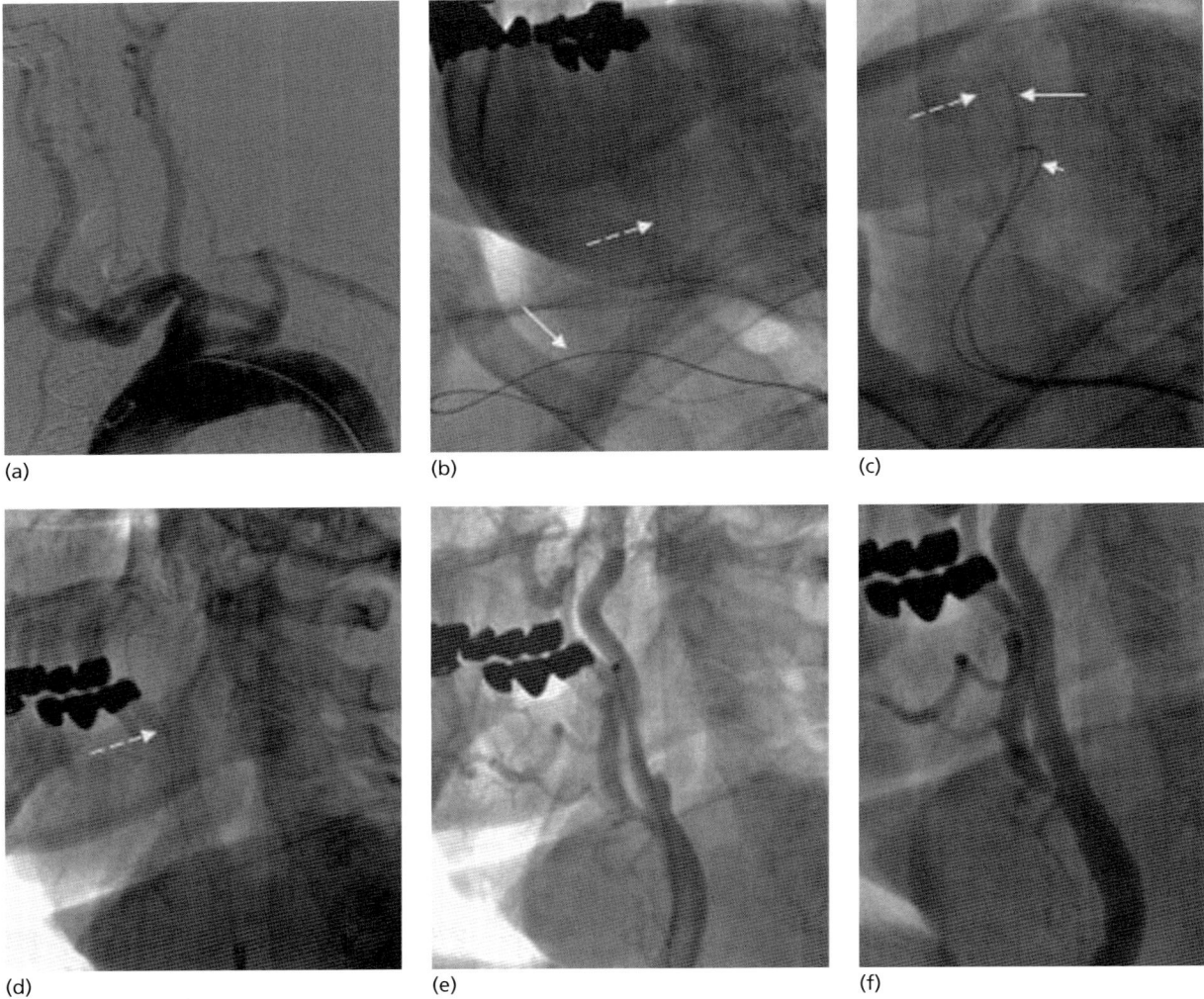

Figure 69.9 Proximal vessel zone complexity: (a) Arch angiogram shows marked tortuosity of the supra-aortic vessels. (b) A 0.035-inch hydrophilic wire placed in the right subclavian artery (full arrow) stabilizes the 40° 8 Fr guide in order to advance a 0.014-inch wire to the external carotid artery (ECA; outline arrow). (c) Then the 0.035-inch wire is brought up into the common carotid artery (CCA) followed by another 0.035-inch wire (arrowhead). With this support the guide can be safely advanced into the CCA. (d) A filter is positioned in the distal ICA with the 0.014-inch wire in the ECA providing extra support. (e) Carotid Wallstent (Boston Scientific) positioning. (f) Final result after post-dilatation.

ICA is aligned to the CCA the tendency of this stent to straighten the vessel does not pose a problem in this case.

Case 4: Technical issues related to the proximal vessel zone: very large CCA > 10 mm and consequent vessel mismatch (Figure 69.11)
Technical issues and "tailored" CAS strategy
The very large CCA and vessel mismatch requires the right stent, which can be sized 12 mm in diameter. In addition, availability in a tapered shape would be suitable for the vessel size mismatch.

Case 5: Technical issues related to the cerebral vessel zone: arteriovenus malformation (Figure 69.12)
A patient awaiting aortic valve surgery attended for intervention to an asymptomatic right ICA stenosis. Unexpectedly, intracranial angiography revealed an arteriovenous malformation (AVM)

feeding off from the right anterior cerebral circulation. Our neurosurgical colleagues were consulted and, based on the possibility that stenting will increase the perfusion pressure to the AVM thus risking a hemorrhagic complication, a decision was made to manage the patient conservatively until further assessment and treatment of the AVM. This case illustrates the value of obtaining an intracranial angiogram when planning CAS, and emphasizes the importance of teamwork and consultation of colleagues in a safe CAS practice.

Carotid stenting complications
Bradycardia and hypotension
Transient sinus bradycardia or asystole are relatively common responses during balloon dilatation at the carotid bifurcation and pretreatment with atropine is preventative. This is less commonly observed in treating restenosis after CEA where the receptors have

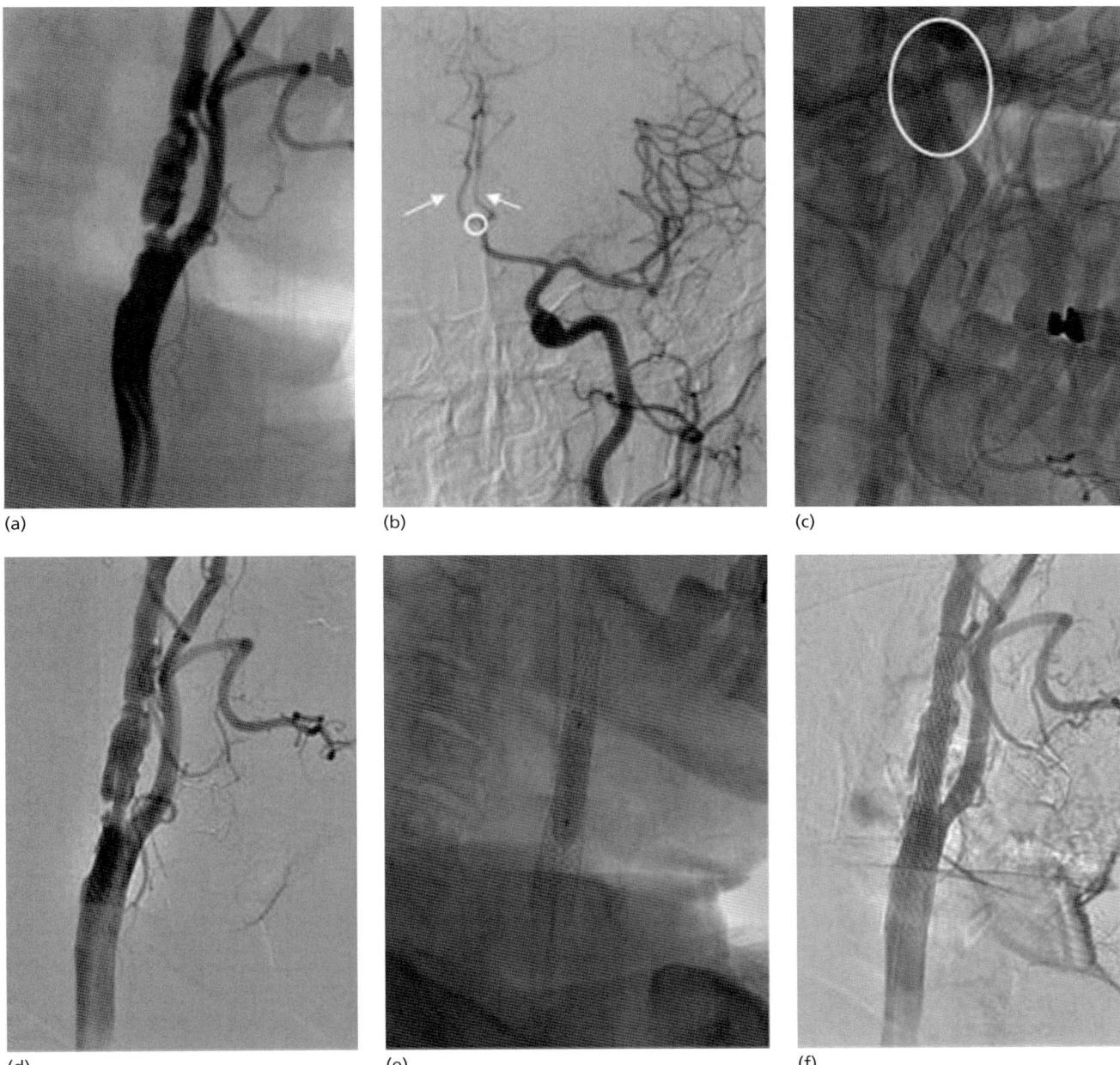

Figure 69.10 Stenting segment zone complexity. (a) Long ulcerated lesion involving the left ICA and distal CCA. (b) Cerebral angiogram shows a dominant left hemisphere with visualization of both anterior cerebral arteries (full arrows) and the anterior communicating artery (circle). (c) Confirmation of good wall apposition of filter (circle). (d) Suboptimal wall apposition of 9/40 mm stent. (e) Post-dilatation with a 5.5/20 mm balloon. (f) Final result showing good stent expansion. The concept to cover from angiographically normal-to-normal segments is illustrated. The persistent ulcerations will be excluded by in 2–3 weeks.

been denervated by surgical dissection. Hypotension from stimulation of the baroreceptors from both balloon dilatation and the persisting stretch of the self-expanding stent is not uncommon and is usually managed by adequate intravascular volume expansion, but with heavily calcified lesions can be more pronounced and require small doses of intravenous vasopressors such as 0.5 mg metaraminol. Continued hemodynamic monitoring in the 24-hour post-procedural period is crucial. Severe sustained hypotension can require dopamine infusion, but it is important not to overlook other potential causes of

hypotension such as retroperitoneal hemorrhage. Hypotension should be corrected expeditiously in the presence of contralateral ICA occlusion, intracranial stenoses, vertebrobasilar disease, and periprocedural cerebral ischemia secondary to an embolic event.

Carotid artery spasm

Spasm of the distal ICA following filter deployment usually resolves spontaneously within several minutes after removal. A flow-limiting spasm could be a potential hazard in the presence of contralateral

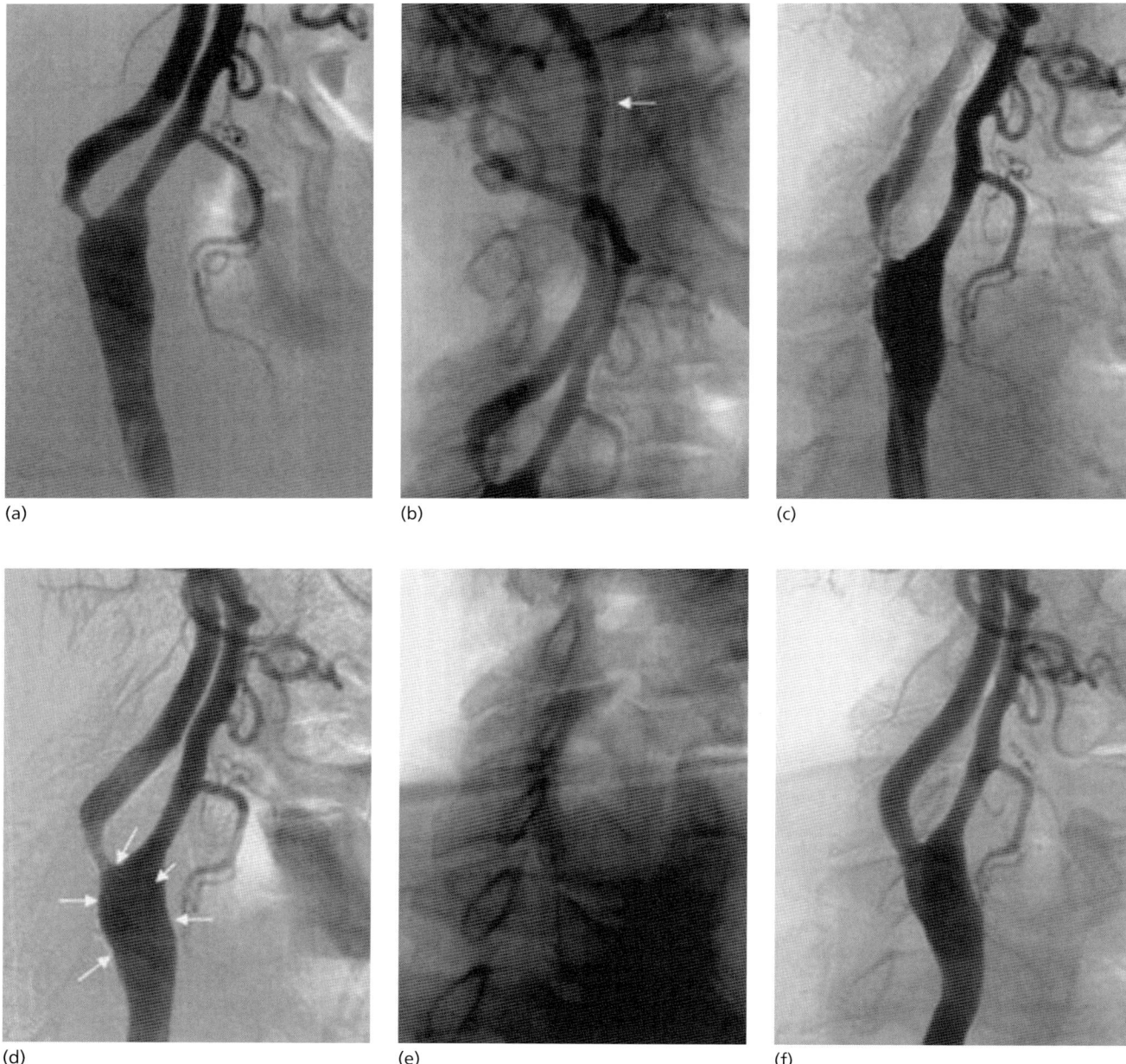

Figure 69.11 Stenting segment zone complexity. (a) Short and severe lesion of right ICA with an enormous CCA. (b) Confirmation of good filter wall apposition. (c) Stent positioning 8/12 x 40 mm. (d) Stent aspect after deployment, noting the struts in the CCA. (e) Post-dilatation with 5.5/20 mm balloon. (f) Final result.

ICA occlusion and/or incomplete circle of Willis. Intra-arterial administration of 100–400 µg nitroglycerin, once blood pressure allows, through the guiding catheter generally aids in resolution of the spasm. Recalcitrant spasm usually responds to low-pressure balloon angioplasty (≤2 atm).

Distal embolization

Symptomatic distal embolization is the most important complication but the extensive use of EPDs has reduced this to a rare event (0.4–1.5%). The predisposing factors are shown in Box 69.2. It is essential to monitor the patient's neurologic status after every step of the procedure. If a significant change appears and persists, gen-

eral patient care should be instituted with emphasis on maintaining normal blood pressure and intravascular volume status, stabilizing heart rate, and maintaining a viable airway with oxygen administration. If the patient becomes agitated and especially if the airway is compromised, the assistance of an anesthesiologist should be utilized. Whenever possible the procedure should be concluded quickly and intracranial angiography undertaken. The most likely sites are the distal ICA and the middle cerebral artery including its branches. Large vessel occlusion is easy to detect, but embolism in the smaller branches requires careful scrutiny utilizing the preprocedural angiogram. An attempt should be made to recanalize an occluded large vessel as soon as possible (balloon angioplasty,

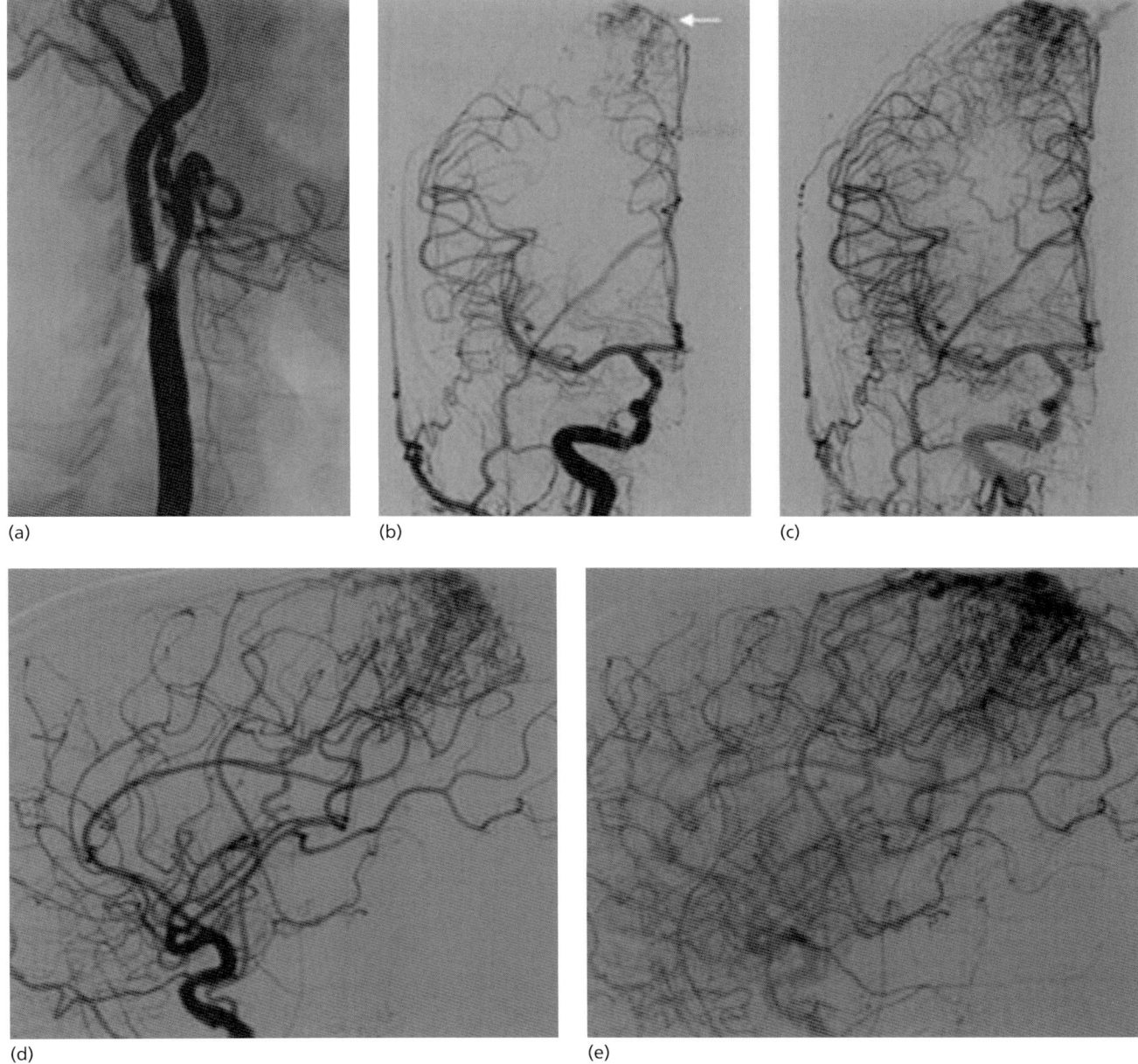

Figure 69.12 Cerebral vessel zone complexity. (a) Focal right ICA stenosis. (b–e) show the intracranial angiogram revealing an arteriovenous malformation.

thrombolytic agents, IIb/IIIa inhibitors). For a symptomatic small branch occlusion, adequate hydration, blood pressure, and anticoagulation should be ensured.

Intracranial hemorrhage
Cerebral hemorrhage is a life-threatening complication, though rare. Sudden loss of consciousness preceded by severe headache in the absence of vessel occlusion should alert the operator. A more subtle feature is signs of a localized expanding phenomenon on angiography. Once suspected, anticoagulation should be reversed and an emergency CT scan performed. Cerebral hemorrhage has been associated with a combination of excessive anticoagulation, poorly controlled hypertension, aggressive attempts at intracranial

neurovascular rescue, presence of a vulnerable berry aneurysm, or CAS in the presence of a recent ischemic stroke (less than 3 weeks).

Hyperperfusion syndrome
The hyperperfusion syndrome is related to long-standing hypoperfusion that results in impaired autoregulation of the microcirculation; thus following revascularization the increased perfusion pressure overwhelms the ability of the dilated arterioles to constrict. This is a rare complication manifested as ipsilateral headache, nausea, confusion, neurologic deficits, focal seizures, and intracranial hemorrhage; typically occurring in patients with severe carotid stenosis and poor collateral circulation, such as with occlusion of the contralateral ICA or underdeveloped circle of Willis. In addition,

Box 69.2 Considered factors increasing risk of embolization.

1 Inadequate pre-treatment with antiplatelet therapy
2 Inadequate anticoagulation
3 Prolonged attempts to engage common carotid artery in challenging anatomies
4 Soft plaque
5 Aggressive guidewire manipulation
6 Aggressive balloon dilatation pre- or post-stent implantation
7 Forceful crossing of a heavily calcified plaque with a high-profile stent

bilateral carotid stenting during the same sitting can contribute. Contrary to the surgical hyperperfusion syndrome where symptoms develop within a few days, the endovascular hyperperfusion syndrome develops during or in the immediate post-procedural period. This is likely related to heparin administration, dual antiplatelet agents, and the previous use of glycoprotein IIb/IIIa antagonists which is no longer recommended. Meticulous control of anticoagulation and blood pressure in predisposed patients is critical to prevention.

Contrast encephalopathy

Contrast encephalopathy is very rare and is a transient neurologic syndrome mostly related to a prolonged procedure where a large volume of contrast is used. Neurologic deficit with marked contrast enhancement "staining" in the basal ganglion and the cortex can develop, but without brain abnormalities on CT. No abnormalities on intracranial angiography are detected. Because the contrast medium does not cross the blood–brain barrier, this phenomenon can be caused by both a fine particulate embolization and excessive local contrast. Patients typically recover completely within 24 hours without permanent neurologic deficit.

Carotid dissection

Carotid dissection is a rare complication, predisposed by severe tortuosity and poor control of filter position or use of a distal balloon occlusion device. Post-dilatation of the distal stent edge within the ICA and aggressive manipulation of the guiding catheter in the CCA are also risky. Management options include balloon angioplasty, additional stent implantation, or a conservative strategy dependent on severity and flow.

Carotid perforation

Carotid perforation is an extremely rare event predisposed by oversizing the post-dilatation balloon or aggressive dilatation. Prolonged balloon inflation or a covered stent can be considered to manage the situation.

Acute stent thrombosis

Acute stent thrombosis is a remarkably rare event. Dual antiplatelet therapy has been demonstrated to lower the rate of stent thrombosis and peri-procedural embolic events. In addition, good stenting techniques can have a positive role. As a general rule, based mostly on common sense, we treat patients referred for non-atherosclerotic lesions or with suboptimal results with dual antiplatelet agents indefinitely.

Restenosis

The restenosis rate after CAS is remarkably low. Recently, Setacci *et al.* [61] reported on one of the largest assessments undertaken which showed an intrastent restenosis (>70%) rate of 2.7%.

Tailored approach to CAS: scientific evidence

Only a few published data are available regarding the potential impact of technical features of stents and EPDs on CAS clinical outcome. In 2009, our group published the tailored CASE Registry [62], which involved 1380 patients (1523 procedures) from April 1999 to September 2007 who were managed with mandatory neuroprotection and a tailored approach to intervention. A wide range of stents and EPDs were used. The primary endpoint was the cumulative incidence of all strokes and deaths at 30 days. The secondary endpoint was a composite of the primary endpoint plus cumulative incidence of all strokes or stroke-related deaths up to September 30, 2007. CAS success was 99.6% and the 30-day all-stroke/death rate was 1.5% (minor stroke 11, 0.7%; major stroke 8, 0.5%; death 5, 0.3%). Regarding symptomatic patients this risk was 2.7% versus 1.2% for asymptomatic patients (p = 0.042). Symptomatic octogenarians had a higher risk than other groups (OR 3.9, 95% CI 1.06–14.0): asymptomatic ≤79 1.2%, asymptomatic ≥80 1.2%, symptomatic ≤79 2.3%, and symptomatic ≥80 4.5%. The results from this large cohort demonstrate that carotid stenting for all-comers in a "real-world" setting, based on the tripod of expert operators, "tailored approach" and mandatory neuroprotection, is safe and efficacious, and durable in the long-term prevention of stroke.

In a previous study [32], we analyzed the embolic events in depth with regard to their temporal distribution during and after the procedure (Figure 69.13). It was clear that with a tailored approach procedural embolic complications were limited to TIAs, and embolic neurologic events (minor and major strokes) occurred invariably within the 24-hour post-procedural and recuperative periods up to 30 days' follow-up. It is a reasonable hypothesis that there was a partial stent-frame failure: despite the routine application of selected stents, advanced protection techniques, and combined antiplatelet therapy, we were able to protect the procedure but not the patient over time.

Owing to the early identification of high risk anatomy for carotid endarterectomy [63], the level of carotid lesion with respect to bony "obstacles" to surgical access for proximal and distal vessel control has been used for case selection for carotid stenting. High carotid bifurcation above the mandibular angle is a reason to avoid surgery, as is a high petrous segment lesion (most appropriately treated by neuroradiology techniques) and the proximal common carotid location. The latter can at times also preclude any type of embolic protection device because of the absence of an adequate landing zone and the risk versus benefit of its performance should be carefully evaluated.

Early clinical evidence also substantiated that balloon expandable stents are unsuitable for the treatment of carotid bifurcation disease [64]. Finally, contrast media-specific reactions that simulate neurologic injury should also be considered [65].

Future directions

Carotid stenting, although it has become a mature technique regularly applied with excellent outcomes in high volume centers by expert operators, is still struggling to find the consensus of the scientific community. Inadequate requirements in terms of operator endovascular experience, potentially leading to an increased adverse event rate related to both insufficient technical skills and inadequate patient selection, has been proposed as the central reason for the unfavorable outcomes related to CAS. In this scenario,

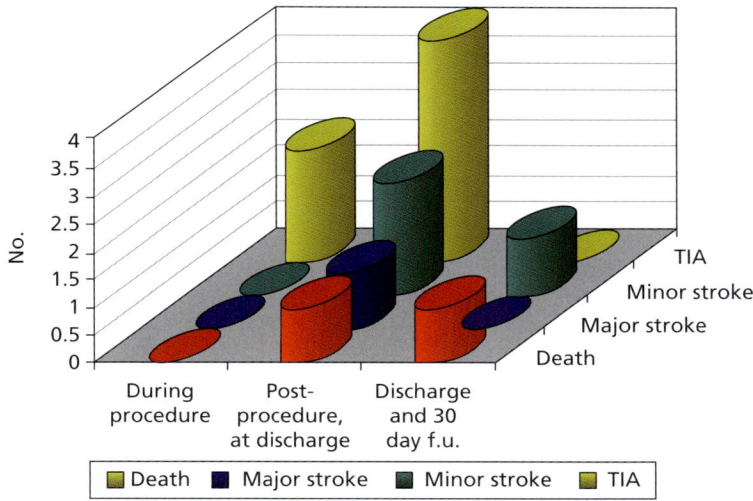

Figure 69.13 Temporal-distribution of CAS adverse embolic events.

one thing is clear: the need for highly trained operators. The *tailored approach* has been emphasized as the key to achieving a safe practice, a concept that, in its essence, requires from the operators a solid theoretical and practical learning curve on dedicated endovascular materials and techniques. Emerging technologies and further innovations pursuing stroke prevention will probably allow operators to address safer carotid endovascular revascularization only in the more general context of serious research protocols and formal training programs.

The entire field of carotid revascularization (via stenting or endarterectomy) for asymptomatic, highly stenotic disease has received heavy criticism from the clinical neurology community because of the tremendous progress of medical therapy in this area, in comparison to the era of the original randomized trials. In other words, neurologists question the window of clinical benefit with revascularization can be sufficiently large to justify the procedure when compared with state-of-the-art therapy with thienopyridine antiplatelet treatment (e.g., clopidogrel), plus high intensity statins (e.g., rosuvastatin, atorvastatin) and improved systemic arterial pressure control over time. At the same time, improved techniques have rendered both stenting and endarterectomy safer than in earlier eras. Accordingly, a prospective randomized trial (with NIH funding support) is underway to compare revascularization (either stent or endarterectomy) or not on a common background of state-of-the-art intense medical therapy in patients with asymptomatic highly stenotic carotid bifurcation disease.

Acknowledgments

We thank the entire organization of Maria Cecilia Hospital and Gruppo Villa Maria Care and Research for their support in the development of the carotid stenting program. Special thanks to Dr. Estêvão Carvalho de Campos Martins and Dr. Caterina Cavazza for their contribution to this chapter.

Interactive multiple choice questions are available for this chapter on www.wiley.com/go/dangas/cardiology

References

1 Rosamond W, Flegal K, Furie K, *et al.* Heart disease and stroke statistics—2008 update: a report from the American Heart Association Statistics Committee and Stroke Statistics Subcommittee. *Circulation* 2008; **117**: e25–146.

2 Department of Health. *Vascular Programme/Stroke*. National Stroke Strategy. Department of Health, London, 2007.

3 North American Symptomatic Carotid Endarterectomy Trial Collaborators. Beneficial effect of carotid endarterectomy in symptomatic patients with high-grade carotid stenosis. *N Engl J Med* 1991; **325**: 445–453.

4 European Carotid Surgery Trialists' Collaborative Group. MRC European Carotid Surgery Trial: interim results for symptomatic patients with severe (70–99%) or with mild (0–29%) carotid stenosis. *Lancet* 1991; **337**: 1235–1243.

5 Executive Committee for the Asymptomatic Carotid Atherosclerosis Study. Endarterectomy for asymptomatic carotid artery stenosis. *JAMA* 1995; **273**: 1421–1428.

6 Halliday A, Mansfield A, Marro J, *et al.* MRC Asymptomatic Carotid Surgery Trial (ACST) Collaborative Group. Prevention of disabling and fatal strokes by successful carotid endarterectomy in patients without recent neurological symptoms: randomised controlled trial. *Lancet* 2004; **363**: 1491–1502.

7 Yusuf S, Sleight P, Pogue J, *et al.* Effects of an angiotensin-converting-enzyme inhibitor, ramipril, on cardiovascular events in high-risk patients. The Heart Outcomes Prevention Evaluation Study Investigators. *N Engl J Med* 2000; **342**: 145–153.

8 Collins R, Armitage J, Parish S, *et al.* Heart Protection Study Collaborative Group. Effects of cholesterol-lowering with simvastatin on stroke and other major vascular events in 20536 people with cerebrovascular disease or other high-risk conditions. *Lancet* 2004; **363**: 757–767.

9 Endovascular versus surgical treatment in patients with carotid stenosis in the Carotid and Vertebral Artery Transluminal Angioplasty Study (CAVATAS): a randomised trial. *Lancet* 2001; **357**: 1729–1737.

10 Yadav JS, Wholey MH, Kuntz RE, *et al.* Stenting and Angioplasty with Protection in Patients at High Risk for Endarterectomy Investigators. Protected carotid-artery stenting versus endarterectomy in high-risk patients. *N Engl J Med* 2004; **351**: 1493–1501.

11 Mas JL, Chatellier G, Beyssen B, *et al.* EVA-3S Investigators. Endarterectomy versus stenting in patients with symptomatic severe carotid stenosis. *N Engl J Med* 2006; **355**: 1660–1671.

12 Mas JL, Trinquart L, Leys D, *et al.* EVA-3S Investigators. Endarterectomy Versus Angioplasty in Patients with Symptomatic Severe Carotid Stenosis (EVA-3S) trial: results up to 4 years from a randomised, multicentre trial. *Lancet Neurol* 2008; **7**: 885–892.

13 Ringleb PA, Allenberg J, Brückmann H, *et al.* SPACE Collaborative Group. 30 day results from the SPACE trial of stent-protected angioplasty versus carotid endarterectomy in symptomatic patients: a randomised non-inferiority trial. *Lancet* 2006; **368**: 1239–1247.

14 Ederle J, Dobson J, Featherstone RL, *et al.* International Carotid Stenting Study investigators. Carotid artery stenting compared with endarterectomy in patients with symptomatic carotid stenosis (International Carotid Stenting Study): an interim analysis of a randomised controlled trial. *Lancet* 2010; **375**: 985–997.

15 Brott TG, Hobson RW 2nd, Howard G, *et al.* CREST Investigators. Stenting versus endarterectomy for treatment of carotid-artery stenosis. *N Engl J Med* 2010; **363**: 11–23.

16 Reiff T, Eckstein HH, Amiri H, et al. SPACE-2 Study Group. Modification of SPACE-2 study design. *Int J Stroke* 2014; **9**: E12–13.

17 Halliday A, Bulbulia R, Gray W, et al. ACST-2 Collaborative Group. Status update and interim results from the asymptomatic carotid surgery trial-2 (ACST-2). *Eur J Vasc Endovasc Surg* 2013; **46**: 510–518.

18 Nedeltchev K, Pattynama PM, Biaminoo G, et al. DEFINE Group. Standardized definitions and clinical endpoints in carotid artery and supra-aortic trunk revascularization trials. *Catheter Cardiovasc Interv* 2010; **76**: 333–344.

19 Krapf H, Nägele T, Kastrup A, et al. Risk factors for periprocedural complications in carotid artery stenting without filter protection: a serial diffusion-weighted MRI study. *J Neurol* 2006; **253**: 364–371.

20 Aronow HD, Shishehbor M, Davis DA, et al. Leukocyte count predicts microembolic Doppler signals during carotid stenting: a link between inflammation and embolization. *Stroke* 2005; **36**: 1910–1914.

21 Verhoeven BA, de Vries JP, Pasterkamp G, et al. Carotid atherosclerotic plaque characteristics are associated with microembolization during carotid endarterectomy and procedural outcome. *Stroke* 2005; **36**: 1735–1740.

22 Biasi GM, Froio A, Diethrich EB, et al. Carotid plaque echolucency increases the risk of stroke in carotid stenting: the Imaging in Carotid Angioplasty and Risk of Stroke (ICAROS) study. *Circulation* 2004; **110**: 756–762.

23 Carvalho de Campos Martins E, Cremonesi A, Castriota F. Proposal of an anatomical-procedural classification for evaluating carotid angioplasty and stenting: latest aspect on carotid artery stenting. *Eurointervention* 2011; 7(suppl M): 269.

24 de Campos Martins EC, Cremonesi A, Castriota F. Proposed practical anatomical-procedural classification systems for evaluating carotid lesions and carotid artery stenting. *EuroIntervention* 2012; **8**: 607–616.

25 Cremonesi A, Roffi M, Carvalho de Campos Martins E, et al. Carotid artery stenting. In: Serruys PW, Wijns W, Vahanian A, et al. (ed). *Percutaneous Interventional Cardiovascular Medicine: The PCR-EAPCI Textbook*. PCR Publishing: 2012; Part III.

26 Angelini A, Reimers B, Della Barbera M, et al. Cerebral protection during carotid artery stenting: collection and histopathologic analysis of embolized debris. *Stroke* 2002; **33**: 456–461.

27 Crawley F, Clifton A, Buckenham T, et al. Comparison of hemodynamic cerebral ischemia and microembolic signals detected during carotid endarterectomy and carotid angioplasty. *Stroke* 1997; **28**: 2460–2464.

28 Al-Mubarak N, Roubin GS, Vitek JJ, et al. Effect of the distal-balloon protection system on microembolization during carotid stenting. *Circulation* 2001; **104**: 1999–2002.

29 Kastrup A, Gröschel K, Krapf H, et al. Early outcome of carotid angioplasty and stenting with and without cerebral protection devices: a systematic review of the literature. *Stroke* 2003; **34**: 813–819.

30 Reimers B, Schlüter M, Castriota F, et al. Routine use of cerebral protection during carotid artery stenting: results of a multicenter registry of 753 patients. *Am J Med* 2004; **116**: 217–222.

31 Sprouse LR 2nd, Peeters P, Bosiers M. The capture of visible debris by distal cerebral protection filters during carotid artery stenting: Is it predictable? *J Vasc Surg* 2005; **41**: 950–955.

32 Cremonesi A, Setacci C, Manetti R, et al. Carotid angioplasty and stenting: lesion related treatment strategies. *EuroIntervention* 2005; **1**: 289–295.

33 Zahn R, Mark B, Niedermaier N, et al. Arbeitsgemeinschaft Leitende Kardiologische Krankenhausärzte (ALKK). Embolic protection devices for carotid artery stenting: better results than stenting without protection? *Eur Heart J* 2004; **25**: 1550–1558.

34 Castriota F, Cremonesi A, Manetti R, et al. Impact of cerebral protection devices on early outcome of carotid stenting. *J Endovasc Ther* 2002; **9**: 786–792.

35 Mas JL, Chatellier G, Beyssen B; EVA-3S Investigators. Carotid angioplasty and stenting with and without cerebral protection: clinical alert from the Endarterectomy Versus Angioplasty in Patients With Symptomatic Severe Carotid Stenosis (EVA-3S) trial. *Stroke* 2004; **35**: e18–20.

36 Wholey MH, Al-Mubarek N, Wholey MH. Updated review of the global carotid artery stent registry. *Catheter Cardiovasc Interv* 2003; **60**: 259–266.

37 Whitlow PL, Lylyk P, Londero H, et al. Carotid artery stenting protected with an emboli containment system. *Stroke* 2002; **33**: 1308–1314.

38 Clair DG, Hopkins LN, Mehta M, et al. EMPiRE Clinical Study Investigators. Neuroprotection during carotid artery stenting using the GORE flow reversal system: 30-day outcomes in the EMPiRE Clinical Study. *Catheter Cardiovasc Interv* 2011; **77**: 420–429.

39 Ansel GM, Hopkins LN, Jaff MR, et al. Investigators for the ARMOUR Pivotal Trial. Safety and effectiveness of the INVATEC MO.MA proximal cerebral protection device during carotid artery stenting: results from the ARMOUR pivotal trial. *Catheter Cardiovasc Interv* 2010; **76**(1): 1–8.

40 Nikas D, Reith W, Schmidt A, et al. Prospective, multicenter European study of the GORE flow reversal system for providing neuroprotection during carotid artery stenting. *Catheter Cardiovasc Interv* 2012; **80**: 1060–1068.

41 Reimers B, Sievert H, Schuler GC, et al. Proximal endovascular flow blockage for cerebral protection during carotid artery stenting: results from a prospective multicenter registry. *J Endovasc Ther* 2005; **12**: 156–165.

42 Stabile E, Garg P, Cremonesi A, et al. European Registry of Carotid Artery Stenting: results from a prospective registry of eight high volume EUROPEAN institutions. *Catheter Cardiovasc Interv* 2012; **80**: 329–334.

43 Stabile E, Salemme L, Sorropago G, et al. Proximal endovascular occlusion for carotid artery stenting: results from a prospective registry of 1,300 patients. *J Am Coll Cardiol* 2010; **55**: 1661–1667.

44 Bersin RM, Stabile E, Ansel GM, et al. A meta-analysis of proximal occlusion device outcomes in carotid artery stenting. *Catheter Cardiovasc Interv* 2012; **80**: 1072–1078.

45 Schmidt A, Diederich KW, Scheinert S, et al. Effect of two different neuroprotection systems on microembolization during carotid artery stenting. *J Am Coll Cardiol* 2004; **44**: 1966–1969.

46 Garami ZF, Bismuth J, Charlton-Ouw KM, et al. Feasibility of simultaneous pre- and postfilter transcranial Doppler monitoring during carotid artery stenting. *J Vasc Surg* 2009; **49**: 340–344.

47 Ohki T, Parodi J, Veith FJ, et al. Efficacy of a proximal occlusion catheter with reversal of flow in the prevention of embolic events during carotid artery stenting: an experimental analysis. *J Vasc Surg* 2001; **33**: 504–509.

48 Müller-Hülsbeck S, Jahnke T, Liess C, et al. Comparison of various cerebral protection devices used for carotid artery stent placement: an in vitro experiment. *J Vasc Interv Radiol* 2003; **14**: 613–620.

49 Siewiorek GM, Wholey MH, Finol EA. In vitro performance assessment of distal protection filters: pulsatile flow conditions. *J Endovasc Ther* 2009; **16**: 735–743.

50 Pinter L, Ribo M, Loh C, et al. Safety and feasibility of a novel transcervical access neuroprotection system for carotid artery stenting in the PROOF Study. *J Vasc Surg* 2011; **54**: 1317–1323.

51 Rabe K, Sugita J, Gödel H, et al. Flow-reversal device for cerebral protection during carotid artery stenting: acute and long-term results. *J Interv Cardiol* 2006; **19**: 55–62.

52 Diederich KW, Scheinert D, Schmidt A, et al. First clinical experiences with an endovascular clamping system for neuroprotection during carotid stenting. *Eur J Vasc Endovasc Surg* 2004; **28**: 629–633.

53 Coppi G, Moratto R, Silingardi R, et al. PRIAMUS--proximal flow blockage cerebral protection during carotid stenting: results from a multicenter Italian registry. *J Cardiovasc Surg (Torino)* 2005; **46**: 219–227.

54 Parodi JC, Ferriera LM, Lamura R, et al. Results of the first 200 cases of carotid stents using the ArteriA device. Presented at International Congress of Endovascular Interventions XVII; February 13–17, 2005; Scottsdale, AZ.

55 Reimers B, Corvaja N, Moshiri S, et al. Cerebral protection with filter devices during carotid artery stenting. *Circulation* 2001; **104**: 12–15.

56 Cremonesi A, Manetti R, Setacci F, et al. Protected carotid stenting: clinical advantages and complications of embolic protection devices in 442 consecutive patients. *Stroke* 2003; **34**: 1936–1941.

57 Reimers B, Sievert H, Schuler GC, et al. Proximal endovascular flow blockage for cerebral protection during carotid artery stenting: results from a prospective multicenter registry. *J Endovasc Ther* 2005; **12**: 156–165.

58 Bosiers M, de Donato G, Deloose K, et al. Does free cell area influence the outcome in carotid artery stenting? *Eur J Vasc Endovasc Surg* 2007; **33**: 135–141.

59 Gieowarsingh S, Castriota F, Spagnolo B, et al. Carotid percutaneous interventions for both restenosis and calcified lesions: success and safety with cutting balloon angioplasty. presented at cardiovascular revascularization therapies; February 11–13, 2008; Washington, DC.

60 Castriota F, de Campos Martins EC, Setacci C, et al. Cutting balloon angioplasty in percutaneous carotid interventions. *J Endovasc Ther* 2008; **15**: 655–662.

61 Setacci C, Chisci E, Setacci F, et al. Grading carotid intrastent restenosis: a 6-year follow-up study. *Stroke* 2008; **39**: 1189–1196.

62 Cremonesi A, Gieowarsingh S, Spagnolo B, et al. Safety, efficacy and long-term durability of endovascular therapy for carotid artery disease: the tailored-Carotid Artery Stenting Experience of a single high-volume centre (tailored-CASE Registry). *EuroIntervention* 2009; **5**: 589–598.

63 Dangas G, Laird JR Jr, Mehran R, et al. Carotid artery stenting in patients with high-risk anatomy for carotid endarterectomy. *J Endovasc Ther* 2001; **8**(1): 39–43.

64 Dangas G, Laird JR Jr, Satler LF, et al. Postprocedural hypotension after carotid artery stent placement: predictors and short- and long-term clinical outcomes. *Radiology* 2000; **215**(3): 677–683.

65 Dangas G, Monsein LH, Laureno R, et al. Transient contrast encephalopathy after carotid artery stenting. *J Endovasc Ther* 2001; **8**(2): 111–113.

CHAPTER 70

Cerebral Aneurysms: Diagnosis, Indications, and Strategies for Endovascular Treatment

Gyula Gál

Odense University Hospital, Odense, Denmark

Cerebral aneurysms are located under the arachnoid membrane, and can be classified as ruptured, causing life-threatening hemorrhage, or unruptured (elective). The latter can be further classified as symptomatic, mainly due to the mass effect, or asymptomatic, also called incidental. The diagnosis of a ruptured aneurysm is an emergency angiography in the acute phase, as soon as possible after the bleeding, followed by the treatment, surgical or endovascular. If the latter, it should be carried out in the same session, if possible, to prevent rebleeding, which can have disastrous consequences.

The indication for treatment of a ruptured aneurysm is absolute, because it is a life-saving procedure. According to the results of the ISAT [1], endovascular treatment had significant lower risk for adverse effects than surgical clipping, which is why this has become the method of choice since the publication of the results in *The Lancet, 2002.*

There is a wide variety of indications and treatment strategies for elective aneurysms, depending on factors like size, shape, location, age, and whether they are symptomatic.

Intracranial aneurysms are located outside of the arachnoid membrane, intra-, or extradural, mainly on the cavernous portion of the internal carotid artery (ICA), in the cavernous sinus (CS), and rarely on the petrous portion of the ICA. If asymptomatic, there are no indications to treat them, because they cannot bleed into the subarachnoid space, but if large they can cause cranial nerve palsy (III, IV, or VI) beginning with diplopia, hearing loss (VIII), or—if ruptured—a direct carotico-cavernous fistula (CCF) with similar symptoms, plus bruit. In these cases, endovascular treatment is indicated.

Diagnosis
Ruptured aneurysms

The first and most important step in the diagnosis of a ruptured aneurysm is the correct evaluation of the clinical signs and symptoms, which start with sudden, intense headache, often followed by nausea and vomiting. The pain can be so intense that the patient becomes unconscious for a short period or longer. Clinical examination can reveal nuchal rigidity. The next step in the diagnosis is a cranial computed tomography (CT) scan, which can detect the hemorrhage, which is most often subarachnoid, but can be intraventricular, intracerebral, and rarely even subdural, or a combination of these. CT shows the thickness of the clot, which is one of the predictors of clinical outcome. The blood distribution can localize the likely source of the bleeding, especially if a hematoma surrounds the aneurysm. With negative CT findings, lumbar puncture (LP) should then be performed, to confirm or rule out small intrathecal bleeding, so-called warning leak that can be undetected on CT, or—when several days have passed after the ictus—to evaluate blood degradation products in the cerebrospinal fluid, which can confirm subacute bleeding up to 3 weeks prior to the examination. If subarachnoid hemorrhage (SAH) has been confirmed, "four-vessel" digital subtraction angiography (DSA) should be the next step, ideally under general anesthesia, to evaluate the cerebral circulation, in order to reveal the bleeding source, further classify its shape and configuration, and assess the collateral circulation. Rotational angiography with three-dimensional reconstruction (3DRA) of the aneurysm is essential, in order to obtain accurate measurements and define the exact anatomy of the sack and the neck in relation to the parent artery and to decide the best therapeutic option. In significant bleed but negative angiogram, the patient should be kept in hospital and DSA repeated after 10–14 days, to reveal aneurysm that might been thrombosed or a blood blister-like aneurysm, which were undetectable at the time of the initial angiogram.

Elective aneurysms

Following intravenous injection of iodine-based contrast material, CT can readily visualize the intracranial vessels. As the method is quick, cheap, and can accurately demonstrate intracranial space-occupying processes, a large number of these examinations are performed in every X-ray unit equipped with a CT scanner, for many different indications, often including headache, even without neurologic symptoms, because it can rule out severe pathologic processes, like tumors. The vast majority of these examinations do not demonstrate any pathologic findings, but can reveal cerebral aneurysms as incidental findings. As every physician—and also many patients—is aware of how dangerous these aneurysms can be if ruptured, many of these findings will lead to referrals to neurosurgical centers, to evaluate whether that particular aneurysm needs further medical attention. In the author's praxis, serving a catchment area of approximately 2 million people, the evaluation of these incidental

Interventional Cardiology: Principles and Practice, Second Edition. Edited by George D. Dangas, Carlo Di Mario, and Nicholas N. Kipshidze.

© 2017 John Wiley & Sons, Ltd. Published 2017 by John Wiley & Sons, Ltd.

aneurysms takes a couple of hours every week, within a frame of a neurovascular conference, involving one senior interventional neuroradiologist, and at least one senior and some younger vascular neurosurgeons.

With the evolving development of technology, like the introduction of spiral and multislice CT, examination time has decreased significantly, and a complete examination of the cerebral vessels, CT angiography (CTA), can nowadays be performed in 10–15 seconds. As this is a non-invasive method, it is routinely used to evaluate the cerebral circulation if an incidental aneurysm has been detected. Also, in a patient with a ruptured aneurysm associated with a hematoma that requires surgical evacuation, a good quality CTA can replace the DSA, giving the neurosurgeon immediate information to be able to clip the aneurysm safely during evacuation, without waiting for DSA to be performed, to minimize the time the brain tissue is subjected to high intracranial pressure.

Everything that has been mentioned about CT and CTA is also valid for magnetic resonance imaging (MRI, or nowadays just MR) and magnetic resonance angiography (MRA). This technology can distinguish the intracranial tissues even more accurately than CT, without the need for ionizing radiation. Imaging of the cerebral vessels with MRA is easy if the patient can cooperate (i.e., keep still for several minutes). It can be performed without intravenous contrast, which is why it has become the method of choice as a screening procedure for cerebral aneurysms during the last two decades. Both CTA and MRA can depict aneurysms in the range of 1 mm, which is sufficient for the diagnosis of unruptured aneurysms. MRA is also utilized as follow-up examination of aneurysms treated by endovascular means, and as serial follow-up of untreated aneurysms to detect progress of their size.

Indications for endovascular treatment
Ruptured aneurysms

This is a very serious condition that kills 30% of patients before they reach the hospital. All patients surviving the first bleed have a significant risk for early rebleeding that is highest in the first hours following the initial bleed, successively diminishing over the weeks. According to the natural history, rebleeding would kill an additional 10–15% of untreated patients within the first months. According to Kassell *et al.* [2], based on the clinical outcome of 3521 patients with ruptured cerebral aneurysms, early surgery is no more hazardous than delayed surgery, and eliminates the risk of rebleeding, which is the major cause of mortality. This result prompted neurosurgeons to perform surgical intervention—clipping—as soon as possible following the bleeding. The same conclusion is valid for endovascular treatment as well. In the author's institution, endovascular treatment of eligible patients with ruptured aneurysm is performed on the day of admission, if the procedure can be started before 8 pm at latest, unless there is evidence of rebleeding. In case of the latter, the treatment is performed during the night as well, to prevent repeated rebleeding, which can be fatal.

Elective aneurysms
Incidental aneurysms <7 mm in the anterior circulation

Following the publication of the ISUIA [3], which assessed 4060 patients, stating that the risk for rupture of an incidental cerebral aneurysm located in the anterior circulation, measuring less than 7 mm is very low, while treatment of elective aneurysms carries a significant risk, which often exceeds the risk of rupture according to the natural history, a scientific debate among neurologists,

neurosurgeons, and interventional neuroradiologists has taken place, questioning the validity of the conclusions in the era of modern endovascular therapy, because the risk–benefit calculation of the treatment was based mostly on surgical clipping: 1917 versus 451 endovascular procedures. Worldwide clinical experience could not verify the low rupture risk of these aneurysms, which is why the results of the study have not been fully implemented into clinical practice. The established clinical routine in most of the high volume institutions, where both neurosurgical clipping and endovascular treatment are available—including the author's—is that all referred cases are discussed in scheduled neurovascular conferences, where the decision whether or not the treatment—be it surgical or endovascular—should be offered to a patient is made, taking into consideration the patient's age, general health condition, and following a careful analysis of the location and configuration of the aneurysm.

Incidental aneurysms >7 mm in the anterior and all sizes in the posterior circulation

According to the same study [3], the natural history of these aneurysms showed that the risk of rupture was significantly higher in the posterior circulation, including posterior communicating aneurysms, and increased with size. However, the risk associated with the repair in the study—again, mainly based on surgical clipping—often equalled or exceeded these rates. As the study was published in 2003, analyzing the data based mainly on surgical clipping performed roughly 20 years ago has no relevance for current practice, in the author's opinion. The indication for endovascular treatment of these aneurysms with the tools available now is valid, because it can eliminate the risk of bleeding, with a reasonably low risk associated with the treatment.

Coincidental aneurysms

This is a special group of aneurysms, discovered during DSA of a patient with bleeding from another aneurysm or arteriovenous malformation (AVM). Clinical experience shows that aneurysms associated with other ruptured aneurysms have higher risk for bleeding than "pure" incidental aneurysms, which is why the indication for endovascular treatment of them is also stronger. For that reason, in the author's institution, these aneurysms are treated, either in the same session as the presumed ruptured one, if the patient is in good clinical condition and the treatment is technically easy to perform without the need for platelet inhibitors, or at the scheduled follow-up of the ruptured aneurysm, usually 9 months after treatment, or earlier, depending on clinical judgment.

Unruptured aneurysms associated with AVMs—flow-related aneurysms—have a different natural history, with a similar or lower rupture rate to pure incidental aneurysms, which is why the indication for and optimal timing of endovascular treatment is dependent on the strategy regarding the AVM. If the AVM is ruptured, and the patient is eligible for the treatment, it has to be treated first. Following successful treatment of that—by endovascular, surgical or radiation therapy, or the combination of these—the aneurysm(s) may shrink or disappear. Follow-up angiography 2 years after completed treatment (5 years after radiation therapy) can usually give relevant information about these flow-related aneurysms to decide whether they need further medical attention.

Symptomatic aneurysms

These aneurysms are usually large (15–25 mm) or giant (>25 mm), and patients can present with pain caused by their mass effect, compressing the dura mater, cranial nerves and other neural structures, and they can cause visual disturbances, motor weakness/hemiparesis, sensory loss, and epileptic seizures. The symptoms are mainly related to the location of the aneurysm, but because of their size, they can be partially thrombosed, and patients can also present with transient ischemic attack(s) (TIA) in the vascular territory downstream of the aneurysm. As a result of these disabling symptoms, endovascular treatment is indicated even if the aneurysm is outside of the subarachnoid space, but if it is within, the indication is very strong, because the risk for rupture of these aneurysms in the subarachnoid space is high, and, if ruptured, the treatment—endovascular or surgical—is technically difficult and associated with high risk, which is why subacute, prophylactic endovascular treatment is strongly recommended to prevent rupture.

Strategies for endovascular treatment
Historical background
The first surgical clipping of an intracranial aneurysm was performed by Dandy in 1937. With this operation, he set the direction for aneurysm surgery for the following 70 years.

The first report of endovascular treatment of intracranial aneurysms was published in 1974, by Serbinenko [4], who described navigation of balloon-tipped microcatheters in the intracranial vessels, performing temporary and— by detachment of the balloon—permanent occlusion and subsequently the application of the same technique also for intracranial aneurysms. This was a sensational scientific communication, and the method was taken up within a short time by several highly skilled interventional neuroradiologists worldwide. During the following 17 years, balloon occlusion of the aneurysmal sac or the parent artery to redirect the flow from the aneurysm was the only endovascular therapeutic option for aneurysms unsuitable for clipping. However, the results were disappointing, with high morbidity and mortality rates.

In 1991, a report describing a totally new concept was published by Guglielmi et al. [5], who introduced a detachable, soft platinum coil, Guglielmi Detachable Coil (GDC) into 15 experimental saccular aneurysms, created on the carotid artery in a swine model. The platinum coil was soldered to a stainless steel wire. Applying low positive direct current on the wire thrombosed the aneurysms, which was interpreted by the authors as happening due to the attraction of the negatively charged white and red blood cells, platelets, and fibrinogen to the positively charged coil, which was subsequently detached by the electric current (electrolysis). Follow-up angiograms obtained 2–6 months post-embolization confirmed permanent occlusion of the aneurysms as well as patency of the parent artery in all cases. This experimental work is considered to be the starting point of modern endovascular treatment of intracranial aneurysms.

The first human experience with this new device, published by the same group from the UCLA [6], in the same issue of the same journal, described successful endovascular occlusion of 15 intracranial, saccular aneurysms, 8 of them ruptured, all of them considered as having high risk for surgical clipping. Following this initial success, endovascular treatment of intracranial aneurysms with detachable coils soon became an important part of interventional neuroradiology, and after the publication of the results of the ISAT [1], it was considered as the first line treatment option for ruptured aneurysms.

During the following 24 years, many new devices and techniques were developed to improve the angiographic and clinical results of patients with intracranial aneurysms, treated by endovascular means. The most important was probably the remodeling technique, introduced by Moret et al. [7]. Utilizing this technique, aneurysms with an unfavorable neck to dome ratio can also be treated with coils that are placed while a non-detachable balloon is temporarily inflated in front of the neck of the aneurysm, to force the coil to remain in the sac. A new technique that has been developed in the late 1990s is stent-assisted coiling, utilizing first balloon-expandable coronary stents, later self-expandable "neuro" stents that act as a scaffold to support the coils at the neck of the aneurysm.

The first self-expandable, braided intracranial stent with a tight mesh, the Leo (Balt) was developed in 2002. Based on this technology, the first flow diverter, the SILK (Balt) was introduced in 2007. The next step in the same direction was the introduction of intrasaccular flow diverters in 2010 (Luna, Nfocus Medical, Palo Alto, CA, USA and WEB, Sequent Medical, Aliso Viejo, CA, USA) utilizing similar technology. In 2013, a new neck-bridging device, the PulseRider (Pulsar Vascular, San Jose, CA, USA) was introduced, for the treatment of wide neck aneurysms at a bifurcation. This is a self-expanding nitinol implant, which acts as a scaffold, supporting the coils at the neck.

General considerations
Placement of foreign bodies, like catheters, guidewires, or any kind of embolic agent into a blood vessel will induce platelet aggregation on its surface, which can cause thromboembolic complications, which can have severe consequences in the cerebral vessels. To prevent neurologic deficit, the use of drugs with anticoagulant effects, like heparin or platelet inhibitors, is mandatory in most interventional neuroradiology procedures. On the other hand, ruptured aneurysms are prone to rebleed, which is why premedication with platelet inhibitors is contraindicated in the acute phase following the rupture. This means that some of the recently developed tools, like stents and flow diverters, should only be utilized if adequate treatment cannot be performed with other adjunctive devices or methods, such as surgery.

In the following section, the currently available devices are briefly introduced, highlighting the pros and cons of their use, followed by treatment strategies for ruptured and elective aneurysms. As a comprehensive description of all available tools and methods is beyond the scope of this chapter, focus is placed on the most frequently used devices, based on the author's experience with endovascular treatment of >3000 cerebral aneurysms during the last 20 years.

Tools
To reach aneurysms located on the intracranial vessels, it is necessary to use *guiding catheters*, (sometimes also long sheaths), to support the navigation and placement of *microcatheters* steered by *microguidewires*. To occlude them, we need embolic agents, like *detachable coils*; adjunctive devices, like *balloons*, *stents*, and *intraluminal* or *intrasaccular flow diverters*.

Guiding catheters In the majority of cases, endovascular treatment of cerebral aneurysm can be performed with a microcatheter—and a balloon, if necessary—through an ordinary 6 Fr (1 Fr = 1/3 mm) 100 cm long, multipurpose tip, guiding catheter, like the Envoy (Codman Neuro, Raynham, MA, USA) which can be navigated via a short femoral sheath, over a Terumo 0.035-inch guidewire with hydrophilic coating (Terumo, Tokyo, Japan) into the ICA or vertebral artery, and its tip placed at the desired level (highest possible without provoking vasospasm or intimal lesion). The tip is soft enough to be placed up to the petrous portion of the ICA, while the shaft is stiff enough to support the navigation of a microcatheter and a balloon with moderate tortuosity distal to the tip. In case of significant tortuosity, a 6 Fr, long femoral sheath—NeuronMax 80/90 cm (Penumbra, Alameda, CA, USA), IVA 80 (Balt), Destination 90 cm (Terumo)—is placed over a 0.035-inch, stiff exchange-guidewire (Terumo) to the proximal ICA or vertebral artery, and a 6 Fr, 105–115 cm long, soft-tip, guiding catheter—Fargomax (Balt), Benchmark (Penumbra)—is navigated over the guidewire or the microcatheter/microguidewire up to the highest possible level the tortuosity permits, up to the cavernous portion of the ICA or to the intracranial portion of the vertebral artery, followed by careful coaxial navigation of the long sheath to a higher position, if necessary, to get enough support for the microcatheter and the balloon, if chosen.

Microcatheters The majority of coils can be delivered through the 0.010-inch microcatheters, which actually have an inner diameter of 0.0165-inch. These are 150 cm long, braided with hydrophilic coating to diminish the friction between the microcatheter and the microguidewire or coil. They have different degrees of suppleness, with a more rigid proximal and an extra soft distal portion, with radio-opaque markers at the tip and 3 cm proximal to that, to match the detachment marker on the coil, in order to be able to safely detach the coils in the sac, even if the detachment point is obscured by the previously placed coils. The tip should be shaped under steam or hot air, according to the anatomy of that particular aneurysm and the parent artery. Alternatively, pre-shaped microcatheters can be used. The author's preferred microcatheter is the Excelsior SL 10 (Stryker, Kalamazoo, MI, USA) with straight tip, due to its shapeability, trackability over 0.014-inch microguidewires, stability of the tip in the sac and the microcatheter in the parent artery, and support to the coil during the packing of the sac. All sizes of coils, manufactured by other companies too, can be delivered through this microcatheter, except one, recently introduced, the Penumbra (Penumbra), which has a diameter that is double that of the other coils, thus a volume that is four times greater than the others of the same length, and consequently needs a larger microcatheter, the PX Slim (Penumbra), with an inner diameter of 0.025-inch. Using this microcatheter and a remodeling balloon in the same guiding catheter requires a larger inner diameter, which is why, in the author's institution, it is usually performed through a NeuronMax (Penumbra), which has softer tip than the other long sheaths, which is why it can be placed higher. Flow diverters, some intracranial stents, and neck-bridging devices also need larger microcatheters, in the range of 0.021–0.035-inch, and consequently stronger support, which is why utilizing long sheaths is essential.

Microguidewires Most microcatheters used in the cerebral vessels can be navigated on 0.014-inch microguidewires. These are 200 cm long. Their tip should be easily shapeable–and reshapeable—to facilitate the navigation and placement of the microcatheter into the aneurysm, and they should ideally retain this shape. Furthermore, the distal portion, especially the tip, should be very soft, so as not to rupture the wall of the aneurysm or the parent artery. One of the most valuable 0.014-inch microguidewires is the Traxcess (Microvention, Tustin, CA, USA), which has a 40 cm long, 0.012-inch distal portion, with a 3 cm long radio-opaque tip that is extra soft, and can help to detect the position of the tip of the microcatheter between the previously placed coils. Another great advantage of this microguidewire is that it can easily be extended at the

proximal end, which is why exchange of microcatheters can easily be done leaving the tip in the same position.

Coils Since the introduction of the GDC in 1991, when only two groups of coils with different thickness from the same company were available, the market has been continuously growing, and nowadays there are a plethora of coils to choose from, produced by many companies. This does not mean that all endovascular therapists have to have detailed knowledge of, and experience with all of them. However, it is essential to know some basic properties.

All types of coils used in the endovascular treatment of cerebral aneurysms should be soft enough not to provoke rupture of the aneurysm while packing them, because they obviously have to touch the wall of the sac during treatment. To achieve that, they are made of platinum, a very soft metal, with a thin primary wire as the basic component which builds up a secondary wire that has two-, or three-dimensional memory shape, and different degrees of softness. They are chosen according to the size and the shape of the aneurysm. They are retrievable, thus can be repositioned in the sac, to fit its shape, and also replaced should the size be wrong. For small aneurysms, <3 mm, the softest available small sizes should be chosen, while the larger ones can be packed with coils of successively incremental thickness, diameters, and lengths, according to the physician's choice and experience. There are hundreds of different types of coils, with lengths from 1 to 70 cm, diameters from 1 to 25 mm, and thicknesses of 0.010 to 0.020-inch. Interestingly, a thick coil is not necessarily more rigid than a thin one, because of its complex structure. Some coils have firm three-dimensional memory shape, making them suitable to place in aneurysms with wide necks, even without adjunctive devices.

Use of remodeling balloons This has several advantages and practically no disadvantages, which is why its regular use, especially treating ruptured aneurysms, is beneficial for the patient. Aneurysms are vulnerable, especially the ruptured ones. Touching their wall with a microguidewire and/or a microcatheter or coil can provoke bleeding, which is why the procedure should be carried out very carefully. Should a rupture occur, inflating the balloon at the neck of the aneurysm can be life-saving, because it can seal the sac, and give at least 5 minutes to reverse the effect of the heparin with IV protamine sulfate—usually slow injection of 50 mg is sufficient—and quickly packing the aneurysm with coils, until the rupture site is occluded. The other advantage is that the inflated balloon can keep the tip of the microcatheter in the desired position, which can add to the safety of the procedure, especially when treating small aneurysms, where the tip should be at the neck, or just outside of it, to avoid direct contact with the wall of the aneurysm. Furthermore, the balloon can help to achieve higher packing density, which is the most important factor to avoid recurrence [8].

The following balloons are the most frequently used: Hyperglide, Hyperform (Medtronic, Dublin, Ireland), Copernic, Eclipse (Balt, Montmorency, France), Transform (Stryker), Scepter (Microvention, Tustin, CA, USA). The first five have a single lumen, and their tips are sealed by the microguidewire when it is pushed through that, so that they can be inflated via a rotatory valve, with a mixture of contrast material— containing 300 mg iodine/mL—and saline, 2 : 1. In the Medtronic balloons, a 0.010-inch microguidewire will fit, in the Balt balloons a 0.012-inch, while in the Transform and Scepter a 0.014-inch, making navigation easier and the position of the balloon more steady for working with the larger wires. Furthermore, the Scepter has a double lumen, making it unique, because having reached the desired position, the microguidewire can be removed, and embolic tools like coils, small stents, and also fluid embolic agents or spasmolytic drugs can be delivered, while the balloon remains inflated. The same balloons can be used in the endovascular treatment of vasospasm, which is, next to rebleeding, the most devastating complication of SAH.

Stents All modern intracranial stents are self-expandable. The main purpose of their use is to support coils treating wide necked aneurysms, but sometimes also to slowly dilate stenotic vessels. There are two major groups.

1 Laser-cut stents, made of nitinol, with two different designs:
   a *Open-cell:* Neuroform EZ (Stryker), available in diameters of 2.5–4.5 mm (in increments of 0.5 mm), and lengths of 10–30 mm; and
   b *Closed-cell:* Enterprise (Codman), available in diameter 4.5 mm, which can be placed in vessels 2–4.5 mm diameter, and lengths of 14, 22, 28, and 37 mm.

The Neuroform needs a 0.027-inch microcatheter while the Enterprise can be delivered through a 0.021-inch, thus can reach more distal targets. Both have radio-opaque markers at the ends, low metal surface coverage (MSC), high porosity, and low pore density, thus no significant flow diverting -effect, but have been able to assist in the treatment of wide necked aneurysms for >10 years, and still have a role in endovascular treatment of aneurysms that need double stenting.

2 Braided stents, woven of nitinol wires that are loosely connected to each other, which allows for optimal vessel wall apposition and easy passage of the microcatheter through the stent mesh. Four devices are available: the LVIS & LVIS Jr. (Microvention), which can be placed in vessels of 2.5–5.5 mm in diameter and lengths of 14–34 mm, and the Leo + & Leo + Baby (Balt), which can be placed in vessels of 1.5–6.5 mm in diameter, and lengths of 8–80 mm. The Jr. and the Baby can be delivered through 0.0165-inch microcatheters, while the larger ones need from 0.021 up to 0.028-inch for the largest Leo. The LVIS has markers at the ends, while the Leo has two platinum filaments along the stent, for enhanced visibility on fluoroscopy. All have flared ends, for improved stability in the vessel. The Balt stents have a significant flow diverting effect, which, in the author's experience, has contributed to excellent long-term angiographic results in >100 cerebral aneurysms.

Flow diverters These are tightly woven devices, with high MSC, pore density, and low porosity. The aim is to achieve reduction and stagnation of the intra-aneurysmal flow, which will promote thrombosis and aneurysm occlusion without the need for coils. They can be divided into two groups:

1 Intraluminal flow diverters, deployed in the parent artery. These are stent-like devices, braided of wires of nitinol, (SILK, Balt; p64, Phenox, Bochum, Germany; FRED, Microvention); or cobalt-chromium (PED, Medtronic; Surpass, Stryker). They represent a paradigm shift in endovascular treatment of cerebral aneurysms, replacing coil embolization of aneurysms with endovascular repair, which is a fundamentally different approach. All of them are highly thrombogenic, which is why premedication with platelet inhibitors is mandatory. The SILK covers 1.5–5.8 mm diameter vessels, and can, up to 4.5 mm diameter be delivered through a 0.021-inch microcatheter, while the two largest sizes need a 0.025-inch microcatheter. The PED covers 2–5 mm diameter, the FRED 3–5.5 mm diameter, the Surpass 2–5 mm diameter, with appropriate lengths, and all of these need a 0.027-inch microcatheter for delivery. Currently, all of them are partially retrievable, and one, the p64, can be fully deployed and then detached at the discretion of the treating physician. The clinical experience with the SILK and PED is significant, with more than 10,000 patients treated with each, including long-term follow-up. The results are excellent, with a complication rate <5%. The author's medium-term experience with the FRED is excellent, with the p64 is good, and with the Surpass is limited.

2 Intrasaccular flow diverters are deployed into the aneurysm. These are spherical implants, braided of nitinol wires, and, due to the microbraid technique, have higher MSC and pore density than the intraluminal flow diverters, thus can induce rapid thrombosis of the aneurysm. As these devices are placed in the aneurysm, platelet inhibition is not mandatory, which is why they can be also used in ruptured aneurysms. Currently, only one of the initially introduced two devices is available, the Woven EndoBridge, WEB (Sequent Medical, Aliso Viejo, CA, USA). The original version was double layered, while the latest two versions are monolayered. The available devices are 4–11 mm in diameter, delivered through the VIA microcatheter, with an inner diameter of 0.021–0.033-inch. The large size of the microcatheter is a disadvantage of the system. Several initial clinical reports were promising, but a recently published paper [9] showed 36% residual aneurysms and 57% neck remnants at mid-term follow-up, which is why the long-term efficacy and safety of the device needs to be further analyzed.

PulseRider Utilizing this new neck-bridging device, wide necked—up to 10 mm—aneurysms can be treated with coils. It has an open cell frame, with significant less metal in the parent artery than double stenting. It can be deployed through a 0.021-inch microcatheter, followed by placement of a coil-delivery microcatheter into the sac through its mesh at the neck, and coil occlusion of the sac. The author has treated 15 cases, and the initial results are promising, but the overall clinical experience with this device is still limited.

Treatment strategies

Ruptured aneurysm approach Occlusion of ruptured aneurysms has to happen quickly and safely. The goal of the treatment is to prevent rebleeding, which is the most feared complication in the acute phase. In the author's institution, following the evaluation of the angiographic findings of a ruptured aneurysm, including the 3DRA, a short neurovascular conference between a senior interventional neuroradiologist and neurosurgeon, or a neurosurgeon on call is organized, to discuss the best treatment option for the patient. Based on the relevant information about the patient's clinical status, and the analysis of the angiographic findings, the decision for surgical or endovascular treatment is taken in consensus. If endovascular treatment is chosen, the senior interventional neuroradiologist decides the strategy for the procedure, which must include the following steps:

1 Analysis of the access route, tortuosity, to assess whether high placement of a guiding catheter, possibly supported by a long sheath, is necessary to reach the target.

2 Further analysis of the angiography, to assess whether the remodeling technique is necessary or feasible to occlude the aneurysm safely. The optimal working projection should visualize the neck and its relation to the parent artery, allowing safe occlusion of the sac, without interfering with the flow in the parent artery. If biplane equipment is available, the other working projection should be perpendicular to the first, to fully exploit the advantage of this technology.

Independently from the above decisions, a bolus dose of intravenous (IV) heparin should be given at the start of the procedure, to protect the patient from thromboembolic complications. In the author's praxis, 5000 International Unit (IU) is the average bolus dose, which can be higher or lower, depending on the patient's body weight. Both the guiding catheter and the microcatheter should be flushed with isotonic NaCl solution, which is ideally heparinized. In the author's experience, 5000 IU/L in all flushing fluids is usually enough to keep the activated clotting time (ACT) at the desired level: 250–300 seconds. The ACT should be measured 15–20 minutes after the bolus dose was given, and regularly once per hour during the whole procedure.

Aneurysms with reasonable dôme : neck ratio can be occluded with coils, without balloon remodeling, depending on the physician's experience. Coil placement should be performed on a high quality road-map. The first coil should have the largest possible diameter the sac can accommodate, to fill the peripheral portion of that, covering also the neck area. The following coils should be smaller and shorter, depending on the remaining space in the sac, which can readily be visualized with a short DSA if or when necessary. All coils should be delivered carefully, but the first and the last are the most critical ones for the risk of peri-procedural rupture. Ruptured aneurysms should be fully occluded, to avoid rebleeding. However, it is better to accept a small neck remnant than to provoke bleeding or thromboembolic complications with aggressive packing. Following the finishing DSA in the working projection(s), a final angiogram in standard projections should be performed and compared with the initial one, to detect early signs of thromboembolic complications.

Elective aneurysm approach According to existing experience with the currently available tools described earlier, endovascular treatment of elective aneurysms is feasible, safe, and the results are predictable. Utilizing flow diverters and braided stents, alone or in combination with coils, makes the procedure safer, because tight packing of the sac is no longer necessary, and has been made easier, knowing that these potent tools will facilitate endovascular repair after the completed treatment. Thromboembolic complications can be prevented by platelet inhibitors. However, rigorous routines regarding the measurement of the effect of these drugs must be established, because >25% of the population is a non- or low responder to clopidogrel, which has to be addressed. On the other hand, utilizing these drugs is potentially dangerous for the patient, because a periprocedural rupture can cause life-threatening bleeding. For that reason, endovascular treatment of these aneurysms should only be performed by specialists properly trained in neuro-interventional procedures, with significant experience to handle both expected and unforeseen complications. The risk : benefit ratio associated with the endovascular treatment of each patient with elective aneurysm has to be individually analyzed with the neurovascular team, followed by careful selection of the best treatment option, based on the experience of the endovascular therapist.

Interactive multiple choice questions are available for this chapter on www.wiley. com/go/dangas/cardiology

References

1 Molyneux A, Kerr R, Stratton I, *et al.* International Subarachnoid Aneurysm Trial (ISAT) of neurosurgical clipping versus endovascular coiling in 2143 patients with ruptured intracranial aneurysms: a randomised trial. *Lancet* 2002; **360**(9342): 1267–1274.

2 Kassell NF, Torner JC, Jane JA, *et al.* The International Cooperative Study on the Timing of Aneurysm Surgery. Part 2: Surgical results. *J Neurosurg* 1990; **73**(1): 37–47.

3 Wiebers DO, Whisnant JP, Huston J 3rd, *et al.* Unruptured intracranial aneurysms: natural history, clinical outcome, and risks of surgical and endovascular treatment. *Lancet* 2003; **362**(9378): 103–110.

4 Serbinenko FA. Balloon catheterization and occlusion of major cerebral vessels. *J Neurosurg* 1974; **41**(2): 125–145.

5 Guglielmi G, Viñuela F, Sepetka I, Macellari V. Electrothrombosis of saccular aneurysms via endovascular approach. Part 1: Electrochemical basis, technique, and experimental results. *J Neurosurg* 1991; **75**(1): 1–7.

6 Guglielmi G, Viñuela F, Dion J, Duckwiler G. Electrothrombosis of saccular aneurysms via endovascular approach. Part 2: Preliminary clinical experience. *J Neurosurg* 1991; **75**(1): 8–14.

7 Moret J, Cognard C, Weill A, *et al.* Reconstruction technic in the treatment of wide-neck intracranial aneurysms. Long-term angiographic and clinical results: a propos of 56 cases. *J Neuroradiol* 1997; **24**(1): 30–44.

8 Slob MJ, Sluzewski M, van Rooij WJ. The relation between packing and reopening in coiled intracranial aneurysms: a prospective study. *Neuroradiology* 2005; **47**(12): 942–945.

9 Cognard C, Januel AC. Remnants and recurrences after the use of the WEB intrasaccular device in large-neck bifurcation aneurysms. *Neurosurgery* 2015; **76**(5): 522–530.

CHAPTER 71

Management of Acute Aortic Syndromes

Christoph A. Nienaber and Rachel E. Clough

University Heart Center Rostock, Rostock, Germany

The concept of an acute aortic syndrome (AAS) summarizes conditions with high risk of rupture, identification of patients with aortic pain, and expedites early implementation of definitive treatment. These conditions include acute aortic dissection, intramural hematoma (IMH), and penetrating aortic ulcer (PAU), with a common denominator of a disrupted media layer (Figure 71.1). Aortic dissection has the highest incidence (62–88%) followed by IMH (10–30%) and PAU (2–8%) [1–3]. AAS is also an important differential to be considered along with acute coronary syndrome (ACS), pulmonary embolism (PE), and pneumothorax. AAS has a relatively low annual incidence compared with acute coronary syndrome, but a high rate of mortality [4]. It is the most frequently fatal condition in the spectrum of patients presenting with chest pain [5]. Besides clinical symptoms contemporary imaging techniques have contributed to understanding of the evolution, natural history, and diagnosis of AAS.

Epidemiology

The estimated incidence of aortic dissection of 2.6–3.5 cases per 100,000 persons per year [6] is likely to be underestimated as it is underreported because of death prior to hospital admission; 22% of thoracic aneurysm and dissection are diagnosed at autopsy [7] and frequently missed *in vivo* [8]. Approximately 65% of patients are male, with an average age of 65 years [9]. Systemic hypertension is most common and found in 72%; other risk factors include atherosclerosis, a history of prior cardiac surgery, known aortic aneurysm, and a family history of AAS [3]. The epidemiology of aortic dissection is different in young patients (<40 years of age) frequently including Marfan's syndrome and other connective tissue diseases. Recent data suggest an increasing incidence to 4.3 cases per 100,000 persons per year as a result of improved diagnostic testing. There is overlap within AAS, with PAU acting as an entry site for dissection, or IMH evolving to aortic dissection and increasing incidence with age [10].

Conditions in the context of AAS
Gender and age

Men are at higher risk for dissection with an age-adjusted incidence of 5.2 per 100,000 per year and 2.2 per 100,000 per year in women [7]. Two-thirds of dissection patients are males consistent in both

Stanford type A and B [9–13]. The ratio is similar for IMH whereas the proportion of men with PAU appears to be slightly lower than women [14,15].

A sex-based comparison suggests that women are older than men at the onset of aortic dissection (mean age 67 years for women and 60 years for men) [12]. A greater proportion of women have delayed diagnosis and treatment, with 40% hospitalized more than 24 hours after dissection onset. Interestingly, clinical signs at onset seem to differ between men and women; altered consciousness and congestive heart failure, as well as periaortic hematoma and pericardial or pleural effusions, are more common in women, whereas abrupt onset of pain, pulse deficits, and a widened mediastinum are more common in men [12]. The average age at onset of dissection type A and B is 61 years and 66 years, respectively [4,9,10,16]. However, it is important to keep in mind that AAS occurs at a much younger age in patients with connective tissue disorders than in sporadic cases.

Pregnancy

Pregnancy has been considered a risk factor for thoracic aortic disease (TAD) while considered an artifact of "selective reporting" and "markedly overstated" [17]. Subsequently, data from the International Registry of Aortic Dissection (IRAD) showed a substantial proportion of women develop TAD during the first four decades during or shortly after pregnancy [12,18]. Whereas 0.6% of women with TAD were pregnant when their dissection occurred, nearly 13% of TAD in women aged <40 years occurred peripartum. By striking contrast, the Swedish national birth registry from 1987 to 2007 reported that 62% of female patients with TAD who were aged ≤40 years were pregnant [19]. The incidence of TAD among pregnant women under 40 years was 1.39 per 100,000 women per year, compared to 0.06 per 100,000 women per year under 40 who were not pregnant [19]. These estimates translated to a 23-fold greater risk of TAD for pregnant women than for non-pregnant women in this age group. However, this study did not account for the potential impact of other risk factors, such as Marfan's syndrome, and so this is inconclusive.

A recent expert consensus document recommended that women with Marfan's syndrome and an aortic root diameter >4 cm carry a 10% risk of TAD during pregnancy, versus a 1% risk of TAD or other major cardiac complications for women with Marfan's

Interventional Cardiology: Principles and Practice, Second Edition. Edited by George D. Dangas, Carlo Di Mario, and Nicholas N. Kipshidze.
© 2017 John Wiley & Sons, Ltd. Published 2017 by John Wiley & Sons, Ltd.

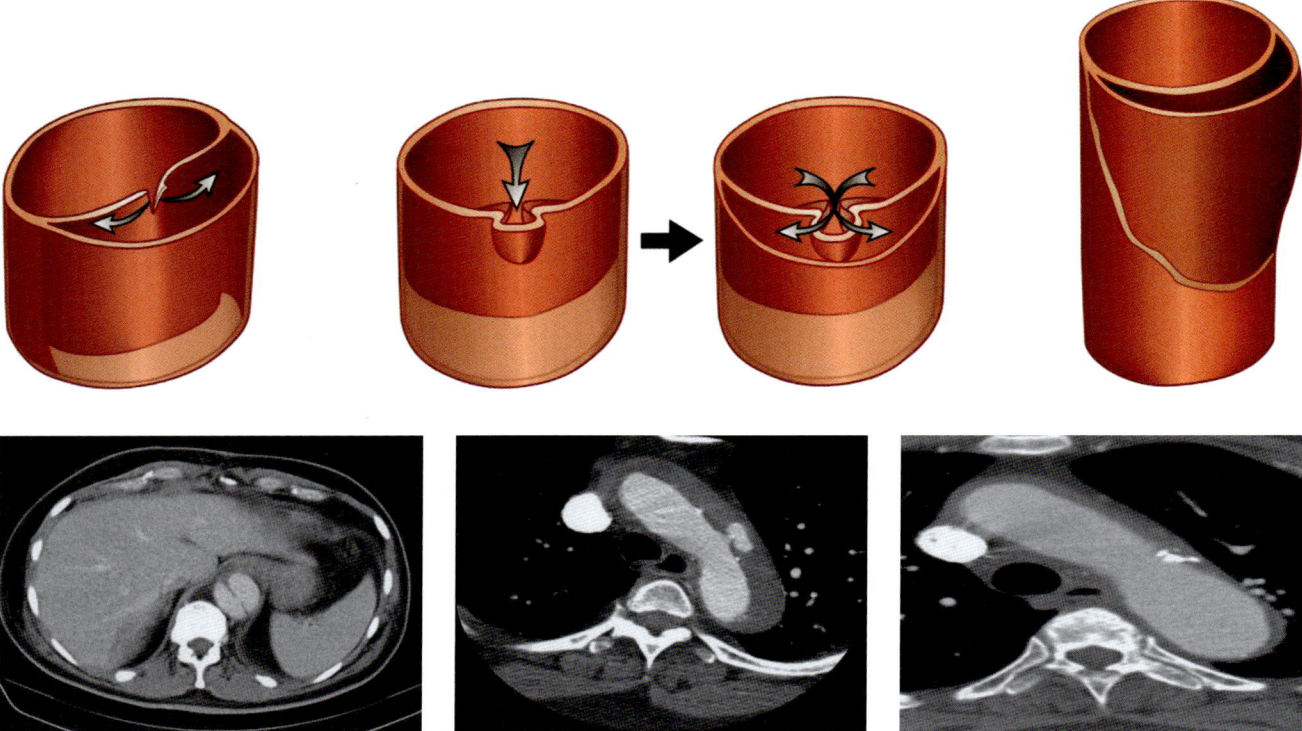

Figure 71.1 Schematic illustration and tomographic imaging display of all constituents of acute aortic syndrome with full dissection, penetrating aortic ulcer, and intramural hematoma (from left to right).

syndrome and an aortic root diameter <4 cm; in women with aortic root diameters ≥4.5 cm, elective aortic root replacement before pregnancy lowers the risk of TAD in pregnancy [20]. In pregnant women who develop TAD, more than two-thirds have type A TAD, and fewer than one-third have type B TAD [21–23]. Of pregnancy-related cases of TAD, ≥60% occur prepartum, usually after 24 weeks' gestation, whereas ≤40% occur after delivery [23]. Aortic complications during pregnancy are associated with maternal mortality of up to 11%, and the incidence of maternal death is 0.4 per 100,000 women per year [19,22,24]. Fetal mortality tends to be around 33% [22].

Drug use

US centers have reported that 10% of TAD is related to cocaine use [25,26]. However, only five individuals in IRAD, equivalent to <0.5%, have used cocaine before dissection [26–28]. Eary mortality associated with cocaine-related TAD is similar to non-cocaine-related TAD, although late mortality appears to be higher in cocaine users [25–27]. Amphetamine use is also associated with an 3.3-fold risk of TAD [29]; sildenafil could also be associated with TAD [30,31]. However, although a temporal relationship might exist, other risk factors such as hypertension, smoking, or bicuspid aortic valve could have caused both of these TAD cases.

Genetics and clinical manifestations of AAS

Congenital cardiovascular defects (bicuspid aortic valve, aortic coarctation, and annuloaortic ectasia), syndromic conditions (Marfan's syndrome, Loeys–Dietz syndrome, Ehlers–Danlos syndrome), non-syndromic conditions (ACTA2), and genetic variants such as single nucleotide polymorphisms have been linked to development of AAS and acute aortic dissection [32,33]. Marfan's syndrome is an autosomal dominant connective tissue disorder caused by mutations in the fibrillin 1 (*FBN1*) gene. Loeys–Dietz syndrome is caused by mutations in the genes that encode the TGF-β type 1 and 2 receptors (*TGFBR1* and *TGFBR2),* which can lead to an increase in TGF-β signaling. Both syndromes frequently present with acute aortic symptoms [34,35]. Differential expression of elastin assembly genes predispose to structural failure in aortic dissection; such changes were associated with diminished fibulin-1 and enhanced MMP-9 levels [36]. Fibulin-1 exhibits distinct interactions with collagen IV which is down-regulated in aortic dissection (Table 71.1) [37].

The symptoms of an IMH and PAU are similar to classic aortic dissection (Table 71.2) and differentiation between these aortic conditions is difficult. The differential exclusion of cardiac and pulmonary causes of chest pain by myocardial enzyme and D-dimer blood tests, electrocardiogram (ECG), and imaging is essential; but 20% of patients with AAS show non-specific ST-T segment changes [3], prompting urgent CT and transesophageal echocardiographic (TEE) imaging [38,39]. Pain is the most common presenting symptom in 84%, independent of age, sex, or other associated clinical features [6,40]. Pain radiating to the neck, throat, and/or jaw indicates the involvement of the ascending aorta, particularly when associated with the murmur of aortic regurgitation, pulse differentials, or signs of tamponade; conversely, pain in the back or abdomen indicates dissection of the descending aorta. Pericardial effusion occurs in 8%, syncope in 4%, and circulatory shock in 3% [3,41–43].

Table 71.1 Human monogenic disorders in acute aortic dissection (see also http://www.ncbi.nlm.nih.gov/omim).

Site	Gene	Function	Clinical manifestation
Ascending aorta	FBN1	Microfibrils, elastogenesis, TGF-β bioavailability and SMC phenotype	Marfan's syndrome (OMIM #154700)
	EFEMP2	Fibulin-4, elastic fibres	Cutis laxa autosomal recessive IIA (OMIM #219200)
Thoracic aorta	FBN1	Microfibrils, elastogenesis, TGF-β bioavailability	Marfan's syndrome (OMIM #154700)
	TGFBR1/2, TGFB	Signaling domain of TGF-β receptor	Loeys–Dietz syndrome (OMIM #609192)
	MYH11	SMC contraction	Familial thoracic aortic aneurysm with patent ductus arteriosus (OMIM #132900)
	ACTA2	SMC contraction	Familial thoracic aortic aneurysm (OMIM #611788)
	COL3A1	Type III collagen, altered ECM fibres	Ehlers–Danlos vascular type IV (OMIM #130050)
Aorta and other arteries	SLC2A10	Decreased GLUT10 protein in TG-β pathway	Arterial tortuosity syndrome
Aorta	SMAD3	Impaired TFG-β signal transmission	Syndromic form of aortic aneurysm and dissection

ECM, extracellular matrix. OMIM, Online Mendelian Inheritance in Man.
Gene symbols: ACTA2, actin alpha 2; COL3A1, collagen type III alpha; EFEMP2, EGF-containing fibulin-like extracellular matrix protein 2; FBN1, fibrillin 1; MYH11, myosin heavy chain 11 for SMC; PKD1/2, polycystic kidney disease 1 and 2; SLC2A10, solute carrier family 2 GLUT10; SMAD3, mothers against DPP homologs; TAAD, thoracoabdominal aortic dissection; TGFBR1/2, transforming growth factor beta receptors 1 and 2.

Table 71.2 Clinical symptoms associated with acute aortic syndromes.

Acute syndrome arising from	Presenting features	Other characteristics
Type A dissection	Syncope Tamponade Severe chest pain	Aortic insufficiency Collapse Pulse differential Myocardial ischemia Neurological signs
Type B dissection	Severe chest or back pain Migrating pain Distal pulse differential	High blood pressure Renal insufficiency Claudication Distal malperfusion
Leaking thoracic aneurysm	Diffuse pain in back or chest Rapid deterioration of hemodynamics Paleness Exsanguination	Rapidly increasing diameter of TAA Sudden death within 1 hour
Intramural hematoma	Chest or back pain Tamponade*	High blood pressure Rarely any malperfusion
Penetrating ulcer	Painless or low intensity pain Pain located in back or abdomen	High blood pressure Collapse with perforation
Traumatic dissection or rupture	Deceleration trauma Severe pain Pulse differential Syncope Exsanguination Tamponade*	Stable at low blood pressure Rapid pulse prior to exsanguination

* Rare in proximal intramural hematoma.

Diagnostic pathways

Non-invasive imaging in emergency department ensures early diagnosis of even subtle forms of AAS; half of patients with clinical suspicion of AAS have normal findings on chest X-ray, and only 30% have a widened mediastinum. CT echocardiography and magnetic resonance (MR) imaging all have excellent accuracy and have become preferred diagnostic options (Table 71.2). The hemodynamic instability and local expertise often determine the

Table 71.3 Comparative diagnostic utility of imaging techniques in aortic dissection.

	TEE	CT	MRI	Aortography
Sensitivity	++	++	+++	++
Specificity	+++	++	+++	++
Classification	+++	++	++	+
Intimal flap	+++	–	++	+
Aortic regurgitation	+++	–	++	++
Pericardial effusion	+++	++	++	–
Branch vessel involvement	+	++	++	+++
Coronary artery involvement	++	+	+	+++

CT, computed tomography; MRI, magnetic resonance imaging; TEE, transesophageal echocardiography.

Table 71.4 Biomarkers in aortic dissection.

Marker	Elevated for	Sensitivity	Specificity	In clinical use
D-dimer	hours – days	++	+	+
Elevated CRP	hours – weeks	++	–	+
SM myosin heavy chain	hours – day 2	+++	(+)	–
Soluble elastin fragments	hours – days	++ (type A)	(+)	–
S 100 A 12	hours	+ (type I)	(+)	–

CRP, C-reactive protein; SM, serologic marker.

primary modality with computed tomography (CT) in 62%; TEE in 32%, and MRI in 1%.

Computed tomography

The investigation of choice for the presence of AAS is CT scanning. Unenhanced scans should be included to provide information regarding the presence of IMH or any mediastinal bleeding [44]. A combined unenhanced and contrast-enhanced CT has a sensitivity of 95% and specificity of 87–100% for detection of AAS [45]. Triple rule-out CT protocols are being used to differentiate between different causes of chest pain such a AAS, ACS, and PE. Post-acquisition reformatting of images by multiplanar reconstruction and maximum intensity projection are useful to improve detection and characterization of AAS [46]. Disadvantages are nephrotoxic contrast medium and exposure to ionizing radiation.

Surface echocardiography

The sensitivity and specificity for type A and B dissection is 78–100% and 31–55%, respectively [47]. Moreover, tamponade, aortic regurgitation, and wall motion abnormalities are clearly identified. In contrast to both CT and MR technology, modern ultrasound equipment is mobile and TEE acquisition can be performed at the bedside for unstable cases with sensitivity and specificity of 99% and 89%, respectively, and a negative predictive accuracy of 99% for AAS [45,48,49]. It does not provide any information below the diaphragm and has limited views of the proximal arch because of interposition of the air-filled trachea and main bronchus. While it detects valve regurgitation and pericardial effusion, it is not suited for surveillance. During thoracic endovascular aortic repair (TEVAR), TEE emerged as a powerful tool to quality control the TEVAR procedure [50–52]. Yet, intravascular ultrasound may emerge as a useful adjunct to guide endovascular procedures.

Magnetic resonance imaging

MR imaging is a highly accurate, non-invasive imaging modality, with a sensitivity and specificity in the range of 95–88% and 94–98%, respectively [53]. However, the MR environment is not compatible with life support and monitoring equipment required for critically ill patients. Thus, MRI is reserved for serial follow-up studies in patients with an anticipated long surveillance. Contrast-enhanced MR imaging with intravenous gadolinium has emerged as a standard (Table 71.3) [54].

Serologic markers

Currently, there are no reliable biomarkers diagnostic of AAS, although a number of markers have been suggested: smooth muscle proteins, soluble elastin fragments, fibrin degradation products, myosin heavy chain, and creatine kinase BB isoforms [36,39,55]. Elevated D-dimers in the clinical context of suspected AAS should prompt urgent further investigation. S100A12 has also been recently proposed as a marker of thoracic aortic dissection [56]. Myocardial markers of ischemia should be requested to help in the differential diagnosis. Elevated C-reactive protein (CRP) has been associated with adverse outcomes in patients with aortic dissection and IMH [57,58]. While a series of conceptually promising biomarkers are under study, only a few have been shown to be useful (Table 71.4).

Initial medical management of aortic dissection

Initial management of AAS is directed at limiting propagation by control of blood pressure over time. Reduction in pulse pressure with a target systolic pressure of 100–120 mmHg and a heart rate of 60–80 beats per minute to maintain sufficient end-organ perfusion is a priority. Intravenous beta-blockade is suggested as first-line therapy, although often multiple agents are required, Appropriate triage and image sharing is important if transfer to a specialized aortic center is considered [59].

Acute aortic dissection

The proximal aorta has highest risk of dissection because of steepest fluctuations in pressure. The proximal entry tear can occur at any point although it is frequently found in the ascending aorta (an area of great hydraulic stress) or in the proximal segment of descending thoracic aorta. It is not uncommon to find one or more re-entry tears allowing communication between the true and false lumen throughout the descending thoracic aorta and abdominal aorta. Over time, the false lumen of the dissection can undergo expansion with aneurysmal degeneration, which can eventually lead to aortic rupture.

Classification systems

Acute aortic dissection can be classified *anatomically* according to either the site of the intimal tear and extent of the dissection, or the part of the aorta affected (Figure 71.2). Dissections can also be classified *temporally* into acute and chronic phases; the acute phase with

higher inherent mortality is defined as <14 days from the onset of symptoms and chronic beyond this period [60]. This classification system has recently been redesigned into four time domains: hyperacute (<24 hours); acute (2–7 days); subacute (8–30 days); and chronic (>30 days) (Figure 71.3) [61]. Additionally, dissections are typically classified as *complicated* or *uncomplicated*. Complicated dissections involve those with malperfusion, rupture or impending rupture, refractory hypertension, continued pain, expansion >1 cm/year, or an overall aortic diameter of >5.5 cm [62]. Approximately 30% of type B dissections are considered complicated at initial presentation and are associated with an increased early risk of death [63]. Despite advances in non-invasive diagnosis of aortic dissection and in therapy, up to 28-55% of patients die without an *in vivo* diagnosis. The incidence of in-hospital complications is higher with type A than type B dissection with a mortality of nearly 24% at day 1, 29% at day 2, 44% at day 7, and 50% after 2 weeks [4]. Less than 10% of untreated patients with proximal aortic dissection live for 1 year, and almost all die within 10 years. Acute aortic dissection of the descending aorta is less frequently lethal. In the absence of obvious complications, survival rates are 89% at 1 month, 84% at 1 year, and 80% at 5 years [4,64].

Predictors of outcome

Among patients with type B aortic dissection, >60% of deaths are caused by rupture of the false lumen. Continued patency of the false lumen leads to aneurysmal dilatation while false lumen thrombosis is predictor of false lumen stability [65]. However, false lumen thrombosis has shown an inconsistent association with survival; partial thrombosis tends to predict post-discharge mortality compared with complete thrombosis or no thrombosis. It was suggested that thrombus in the distal false lumen could impede outflow, resulting in aneurysmal expansion and rupture [66,67].

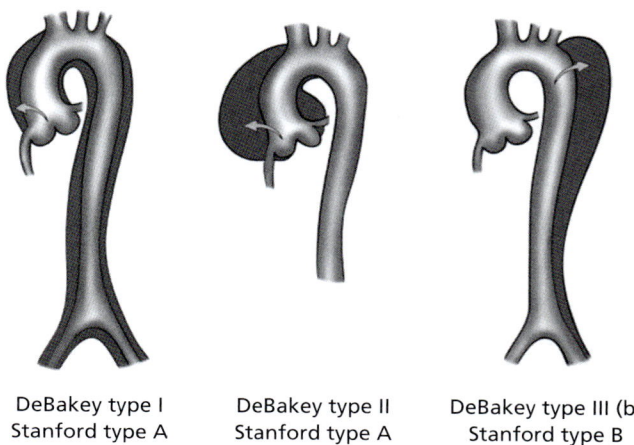

| DeBakey type I | DeBakey type II | DeBakey type III (b) |
| Stanford type A | Stanford type A | Stanford type B |

Figure 71.2 Standard classification system of aortic dissection with focus on anatomic involvement and prognosis.

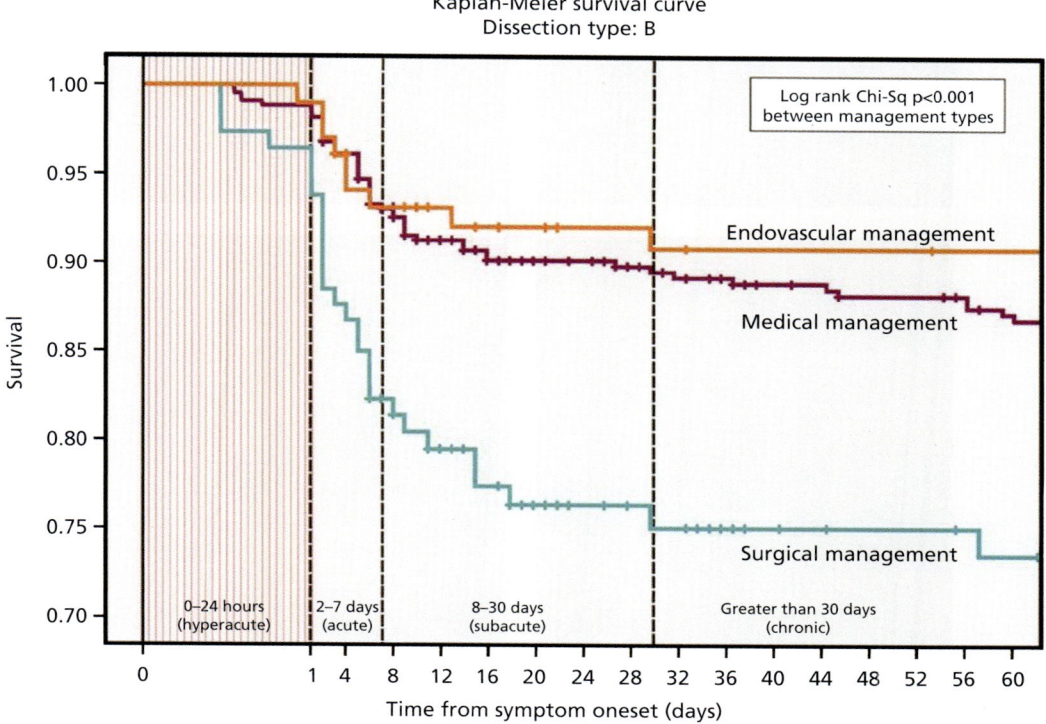

Figure 71.3 The International Registry of Aortic Dissection (IRAD) classification system of aortic dissection with focus on the time domain. Survival in the early phase is lowest with open surgical management.

Visceral branches which arise from the false lumen, re-entry tears and a maximum diameter of the false lumen in the abdominal aorta are risk factors for incomplete thrombosis of the false lumen [68]. In addition, refractory pain or hypertension, and age ≥70 years were predictors of in-hospital mortality (OR 3.3 and 5.1, respectively) [69], while a large proximal entry tear identifies high risk patients [70]. Patient-specific simulation tools are being developed to analyze hemodynamics in aortic dissection with focus on velocity, stroke volume, and helicity of blood flow by four-dimensional phase contrast MR (4D PC-MR) imaging (Figure 71.4) [71,72].

Treatment of type A dissection

The mainstay of treatment in acute type A aortic dissection is open resection preventing lethal complications such as aortic rupture, stroke, visceral ischemia, cardiac tamponade, and circulatory failure. During surgery the aorta is reconstructed with interposition of synthetic graft and reimplantation of the coronary arteries and restoration of aortic valve competence. Operative mortality for ascending aortic dissections varies widely between 10% and 35%, but clearly below the mortality of medical therapy [73]. Endovascular treatment for type A dissection has been reported in highly selected cases and remains under development [74–76].

Treatment of type B dissection

Recent data suggest significant differences with respect to in-hospital death stratified by type of treatment for patients with acute type B aortic dissection. IRAD reported an in-hospital mortality of 32% for those treated with surgery, and 10% for patients managed with medical therapy alone [4]. With 90% of patients surviving to hospital discharge, medical management constitutes the current standard of care for stable, clinically silent patients [77]. Conversely, open surgical replacement of dissected aorta has recently been abandoned because of the risk of left posterolateral thoracotomy in conjunction with single-lung ventilation, full heparinization, cardiopulmonary bypass, profound hypothermia, cerebrospinal fluid drainage, and circulatory arrest [78,79]. Data from IRAD, however, suggest a significant mortality rate for complicated type B dissection over the last 5 years, and an in-hospital mortality of 17% with open surgery [4], or even higher in presence of renal or mesenteric ischemia at 50–88%, respectively [80,81].

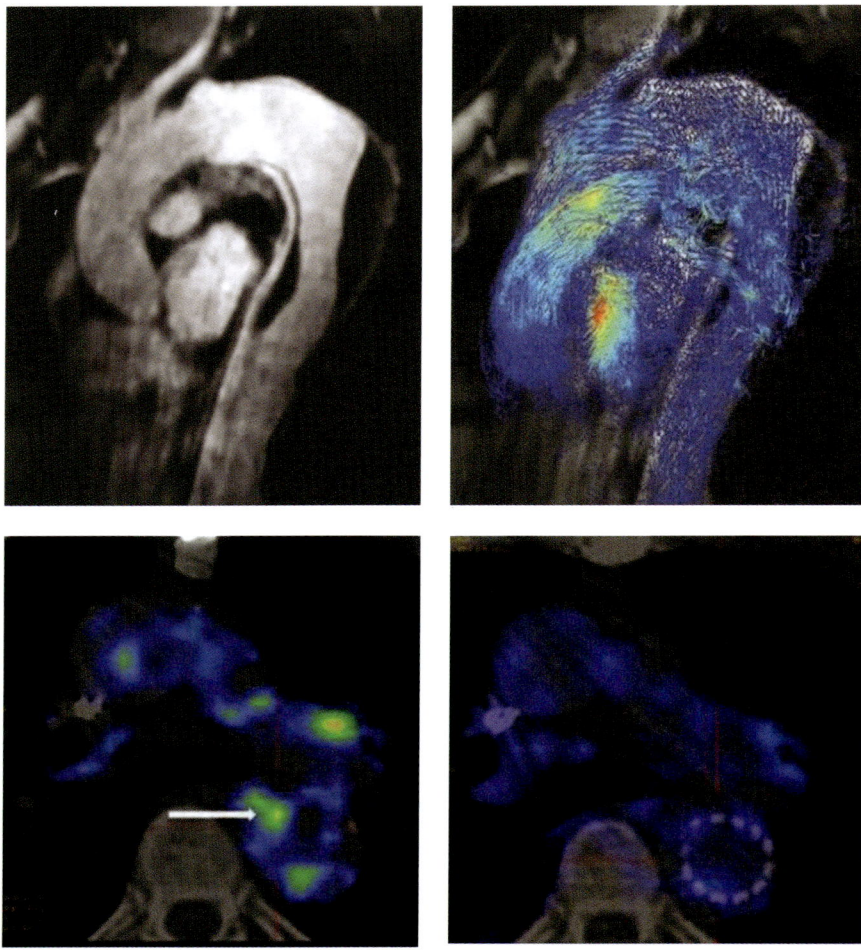

Figure 71.4 Functional imaging in aortic dissection; the upper row shows a two-dimensional magnetic resonance (MR) image after injection of gadolinium (left) with compromised true lumen and an expanded false lumen with partial thrombosis in the setting of chronic type B aortic dissection; the corresponding four-dimensional MR image identifies areas of highest flow turbulence and pulse pressure (right). The lower row reveals on transactional positron emission tomography (PET) image enhanced local ¹⁸FDG-uptake in areas of inflammation and impending rupture (left) that can be stabilized by thoracic endovascular aortic repair (TEVAR) and induced remodeling of the dissected aorta.

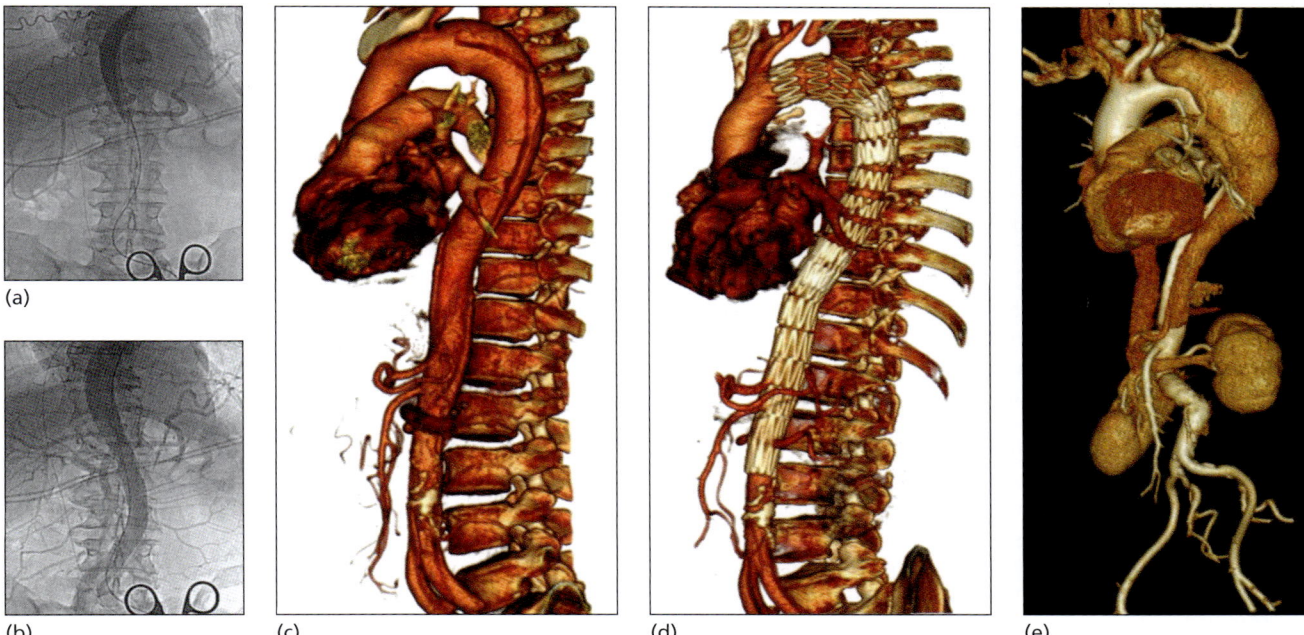

Figure 71.5 Angiographic documentation of distal malperfusion before (a) and after TEVAR (b) of the proximal descending thoracic aorta in complicated type B dissection; three-dimensional CT reconstruction of the same dissection before (c) and after PETTICOAT TEVAR (d) to prevent an evolution to irreversible changes and false lumen expansion in the chronic state of 3 years post-dissection (e).

Endovascular management

The feasibility of TEVAR for aortic dissection has been established since 1999 as an alternative to high-risk open surgical treatment in patients with complicated type B aortic dissection. A recent report using Medicare data suggests that 25% of type B dissection repairs are now treated endovascularly, with lower mortality and morbidity rates compared with open repair [82]. A meta-analysis revealed an in-hospital mortality of 9%, stroke in 3.1%, paraplegia in 1.9%, conversion to type A dissection in 2%, bowel infarction in 0.9%, and major amputation in 0.2% [83].

The INSTEAD and ADSORB trials were designed to investigate the role of TEVAR in uncomplicated type B aortic dissection; 5-year results of INSTEAD-XL trial showed a reduction in aortic-related death and disease progression with endovascular repair and optimum medical therapy compared with optimum medical therapy alone [84], while ADSORB demonstrated better aortic remodeling in the TEVAR group. If further remodeling of the aorta is required a bare metal stent can help, known as the PETTICOAT concept (Figure 71.5) [85]. Patients treated in the acute setting are prone to aortic growth, particularly of the abdominal aorta [86,87].

Intramural hematoma

IMH is identified as a contained intramural hemorrhage in absence of a detectable intimal tear (Figure 71.1) [45]. IMH also occurs as a result of blunt trauma [88]. Complications of IMH are common, with progression to complete dissection in 28–47%, and aneurysm or rupture in 20–45% of patients [88,89]. IMH of the ascending aorta is often complicated by pericardial effusion, pleural effusion, and aortic insufficiency and needs surgical repair. Patients with IMH tend to be older and there is a higher incidence in male patients [45]. Similar to Stanford, type A IMH involves the ascending aorta and Stanford B IMH does not involve the ascending aorta

[3,90]. There is controversy regarding the natural history of IMH in North America and Europe compared with Japan and Korea. The incidence of IMH from Western centers was 6% (58/1010), versus an incidence in Eastern series of 28.3% and 29% [45,91,92]. While in Western populations IMH is similar to dissection, oriental patients seem to be more stable [93,94]. In a recent Japanese series, early and late progression was 30% and 10%, respectively [91]; in a Korean registry ≥80% of patients were treated medically [3] and survived [95,96].

Treatment

Western centers reported early mortality with surgery of 8% versus 55% with medical treatment and recommend open repair in proximal IMH [44,97–99]. Conversely, type A patients from Asia showed no difference in early mortality between surgical (10.1%) and medical strategies (14.4%) [100]. Other Asian studies have found high rates of progression in patients treated medically, with a mortality rate of 32%, prompting these authors to recommend surgical resection for these patients [101]. Immediate surgery resulted in a 14.3% mortality, whereas mortality was 7.1% in those undergoing delayed surgery; in those awaiting surgery, 33% of type A IMHs converted to aortic dissection (none within the first 72 hours) [102].

Predictors of disease progression

Development of ulcer-like projections during follow-up of IMH has been reported to be a predictor of poor prognosis [103,104]. These lesions can progress to both localized dissection and aneurysmal dilatation, with complications occurring more commonly in proximal than in distal IMH. Other predictors of disease progression in IMH include age >70 years, cardiac tamponade, maximum hematoma thickness of ≥10 mm, and an aortic diameter ≥50 mm for type A [91,103].

Penetrating aortic ulcer

PAU is a painful ulceration in the aortic wall caused by rupture of the intima allowing blood through the internal elastic lamina, with pseudoaneurysm formation over time or rupture [89]. Patients are at risk of rupture, even at a normal aortic diameter. PAU has the highest incidence of rupture of all constituents of AAS with rates of up to 42% [105], and occurs in older men with lesions of 4–30 mm in depth and 2–25 mm in diameter [106]. PAU occurs more frequently in the descending, but rarely in the ascending aorta [107,108]. The typical patient is elderly, hypertensive, with a history of tobacco abuse, presenting with chest or back pain, but no signs of aortic regurgitation or malperfusion; asymptomatic patients can also be found and 27.8% of cases were associated with a saccular aneurysm, while 14% were associated with IMH [109].

Predictors of disease progression

Recurrent or refractory pain is considered to be one of the most important clinical symptoms in determining the appropriateness of intervention. Predictors of progression include sustained or recurrent pain (p <0.0001), increasing pleural effusion (p = 0.0003), and both the diameter (p = 0.004) and depth (p = 0.003). PAU involving the ascending aorta is considered to be associated with a high risk of rupture and requires emergency or urgent intervention. Computational fluid-structure analysis may demonstrate structural fragility of the PAU wall [110].

Treatment

Urgent surgical repair is recommended for type A lesions although the majority of patients with PAU may not be suitable for conventional surgery. Type B PAU represents an ideal target for TEVAR due to segmental and well-localized wall pathology, particularly in a patient population with multiple comorbidities [106,111].

Outlook and conclusions

Survival of patients with AAS is 81% at 1 year and 63% at 5 years [112]. Medical therapy including beta-blockers is needed to minimize aortic wall stress in all patients, and serial imaging to detect signs of progression should be performed annually. Each case should be referred and discussed at a multidisciplinary meeting to consider patient age, general life expectancy, and fitness for either open surgery or TEVAR. After TEVAR, secondary aortic interventions are common and should prompt long-term surveillance [113]. Grouping various aortic conditions into the entity of AAS offers a structured early identification of patients at risk [114–116]. Nonetheless, optimal management of patients with AAS remains challenging. The advent of minimally invasive endovascular techniques has shifted the treatment paradigm with treatment no longer limited to open surgery or best medical therapy alone. The current challenge is to determine the patient population best suited for active (open or endovascular) treatment rather than just best medical therapy to ensure individualized optimal care.

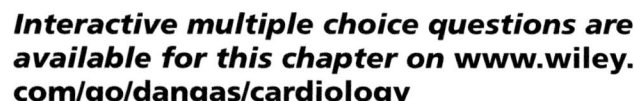

Interactive multiple choice questions are available for this chapter on www.wiley. com/go/dangas/cardiology

References

1 Patel PJ, Grande W, Hieb RA. Endovascular management of acute aortic syndromes. *Semin Interv Radiol* 2011; **28**: 10–23.

2 Brinster DR. Endovascular repair of the descending thoracic aorta for penetrating atherosclerotic ulcer disease. *J Card Surg* 2009; **24**: 203–208.

3 Cho JR, Shin S, Kim JS, et al. Clinical characteristics of acute aortic syndrome in Korean patients: from the Korean multi-center registry of acute aortic syndrome. *Korean Circ J* 2012; **42**: 528–537.

4 Hagan PG, Nienaber CA, Isselbacher EM, et al. The International Registry of Acute Aortic Dissection (IRAD): new insights into an old disease. *JAMA* 2000; **283**: 897–903.

5 Kouchoukos NT, Dougenis D. Surgery of the thoracic aorta. *N Engl J Med* 1997; **336**: 1876–1888.

6 Tsai TT, Nienaber CA, Eagle KA. Acute aortic syndromes. *Circulation* 2005; **112**: 3802–3813.

7 Olsson C, Thelin S, Stähle E, et al. Thoracic aortic aneurysm and dissection: increasing prevalence and improved outcomes reported in a nationwide population-based study of more than 14,000 cases from 1987 to 2002. *Circulation* 2006; **114**: 2611–2618.

8 Elefteriades JA, Barrett PW, Kopf GS. Litigation in nontraumatic aortic diseases: a tempest in the malpractice maelstrom. *Cardiology* 2008; **109**: 263–272.

9 Clouse WD, Hallett JW Jr, Schaff HV, et al. Acute aortic dissection: population-based incidence compared with degenerative aortic aneurysm rupture. *Mayo Clin Proc* 2004; **79**: 176–180.

10 Mészáros I, Mórocz J, Szlávi J, et al. Epidemiology and clinicopathology of aortic dissection. *Chest* 2000; **117**: 1271–1278.

11 Sato F, Kitamura T, Kongo M, et al. Newly diagnosed acute aortic dissection: characteristics, treatment modifications, and outcomes. *Int Heart J* 2005; **46**: 1083–1098.

12 Nienaber CA, Fattori R, Mehta RH, et al. Gender-related differences in acute aortic dissection. *Circulation* 2004; **109**: 3014–3021.

13 Olsson C, Eriksson N, Stähle E, Thelin S. Surgical and long-term mortality in 2,634 consecutive patients operated on the proximal thoracic aorta. *Eur J Cardiothorac Surg* 2007; **31**: 963–969.

14 Evangelista A, Mukherjee D, Mehta RH, et al. Acute intramural hematoma of the aorta: a mystery in evolution. *Circulation* 2005; **111**: 1063–1070.

15 Brinster DR, Wheatley GH 3rd, Williams J, et al. Are penetrating aortic ulcers best treated using an endovascular approach? *Ann Thorac Surg* 2006; **82**: 1688–1691.

16 Wu IH, Yu HY, Liu CH, et al. Is old age a contraindication for surgical treatment in acute aortic dissection? A demographic study of national database registry in Taiwan. *Card Surg* 2008; **23**: 133–139.

17 Oskoui R, Lindsay J Jr. Aortic dissection in women <40 years of age and the unimportance of pregnancy. *Am J Cardiol* 1994; **73**: 821–823.

18 Januzzi JL, Isselbacher EM, Fattori R, et al. Characterizing the young patient with aortic dissection: results from the International Registry of Aortic Dissection (IRAD). *J Am Coll Cardiol* 2004; **43**: 665–669.

19 Nasiell J, Lindsay PG. Aortic dissection in pregnancy; the incidence of a life-threatening disease. *Eur J Obstet Gynecol Reprod Biol* 2010; **149**: 120–121.

20 Task Force on the Mangement of Cardiovascular Diseases During Pregnancy of the European Society of Cardiology. Expert consensus document on management of cardiovascular diseases during pregnancy. *Eur Heart J* 2003; **24**: 761–781.

21 Pacini L, Digne F, Boumendil A, et al. Maternal complication of pregnancy in Marfan syndrome. *Int J Cardiol* 2009; **136**: 156–161.

22 Immer FF, Bansi AG, Immer-Bansi AS, et al. Aortic dissection in pregnancy: analysis of risk factors and outcome. *Ann Thorac Surg* 2003; **76**: 309–3014.

23 Goland S, Barakat M, Khatri N, Elkayam U. Pregnancy in Marfan syndrome: maternal and fetal risk and recommendations for patient assessment and management. *Cardiol Rev* 2009; **17**: 253–262.

24 Beauchesne LM, Connolly HM, Ammash NM, Warnes CA. Coarctation of the aorta: outcome of pregnancy. *J Am Coll Cardiol* 2001; **37**: 1728–1733.

25 Daniel JC, Huynh TT, Zhou W, et al. Acute aortic dissection associated with use of cocaine. *J Vasc Surg* 2007; **46**: 427–433.

26 Singh S, Trivedi A, Adhikari T, et al. Cocaine-related acute aortic dissection: patient demographics and clinical outcomes. *Can J Cardiol* 2007; **23**: 1131–1134.

27 Eagle KA, Isselbacher EM, DeSanctis RW. Cocaine-related aortic dissection in perspective. *Circulation* 2002; **105**: 1529–1530.

28 Hsue PY, Salinas CL, Bolger AF, Benowitz NL, Waters DD. Acute aortic dissection related to crack cocaine. *Circulation* 2002; **105**: 1592–1595.

29 Westover AN, Nakonezny PA. Aortic dissection in young adults who abuse amphetamines. *Am Heart J* 2010; **160**: 315–321.

30 Tiryakioglu SK, Tiryakioglu O, Turan T, Kumbay E. Aortic dissection due to sildenafil abuse. *Interact Cardiovasc Thorac Surg* 2009; **9**: 141–143.

31 Nachtnebel A, Stöllberger C, Ehrlich M, Finsterer J. Aortic dissection after sildenafil-induced erection. *South Med J* 2006; **99**: 1151–1152.

32 Oliver JM, Gallego P, Gonzalez A, et al. Risk factors for aortic complications in adults with coarctation of the aorta. *J Am Coll Cardiol* 2004; **44**: 1641–1647.

33 Ando M, Okita Y, Morota T, Takamoto S. Thoracic aortic aneurysm associated with congenital bicuspid aortic valve. *Cardiovasc Surg* 1998; **6**: 629–634.

34 Attias D, Stheneur C, Roy C, et al. Comparison of clinical presentations and outcomes between patients with TGFBR2 and FBN1 mutations in Marfan syndrome and related disorders. *Circulation* 2009; **120**: 2541–2549.

35 Nienaber CA, von Kodolitsch Y. Therapeutic management of patients with Marfan syndrome: focus on cardiovascular involvement. *Cardiol Rev* 1999; **7**: 332–341.

36 Cheuk BL, Cheng SW. Differential expression of elastin assembly genes in patients with Stanford Type A aortic dissection using microarray analysis. *J Vasc Surg* 2011; **53**: 1071–1078.

37 Kobayashi N, Kostka G, Garbe JH, et al. A comparative analysis of the fibulin protein family. Biochemical characterization, binding interactions, and tissue localization. *J Biol Chem* 2007; **282**: 11805–11816.

38 Eggebrecht H, Naber CK, Bruch C, et al. Value of plasma fibrin D-dimers for detection of acute aortic dissection. *J Am Coll Cardiol* 2004; **44**: 804–809.

39 Suzuki T, et al. Diagnosis of acute aortic dissection by D-dimer: the International Registry of Acute Aortic Dissection Substudy on Biomarkers (IRAD-Bio) experience. *Circulation* 2009; **119**: 2702–2707.

40 Suzuki T, Metha RH, Ince H, et al. Clinical profiles and outcomes of acute type B aortic dissection in the current era: lessons from the International Registry of Aortic Dissection (IRAD). *Circulation* 2003; **108**: 312–317.

41 von Kodolitsch Y, Schwartz AG, Nienaber CA. Clinical prediction of acute aortic dissection. *Arch Intern Med* 2000; **160**: 2977–2982.

42 Klompas M. Does this patient have an acute thoracic aortic dissection? *JAMA* 2002; **287**: 2262–2272.

43 von Kodolitsch Y, Nienaber CA, Dieckmann C, et al. Chest radiography for the diagnosis of acute aortic syndrome. *Am J Med* 2004; **116**: 73–77.

44 Nienaber CA, von Kodolitsch Y, Petersen B, et al. Intramural hemorrhage of the thoracic aorta: diagnostic and therapeutic implications. *Circulation* 1995; **92**: 1465–1472.

45 Evangelista A, Mukherjee D, Mehta RH, et al. Acute intramural hematoma of the aorta: a mystery in evolution. *Circulation* 2005; **111**: 1063–1070.

46 Troxler M, Mavor AI, Homer-Vanniasinkam S. Penetrating atherosclerotic ulcers of the aorta. *Br J Surg* 2001; **88**: 1169–1177.

47 Baliga RR, Nienaber CA, Bossone E, et al. The role of imaging in aortic dissection and related syndromes. *JACC Cardiovasc Imaging* 2014; **7**: 406–424.

48 Nienaber CA, von Kodolitsch Y, Nicolas V, et al. The diagnosis of thoracic aortic dissection by noninvasive imaging procedures. *N Engl J Med* 1993; **328**: 1–9.

49 Erbel R, Alfonso F, Boileau C, et al. Diagnosis and management of aortic dissection. *Eur Heart J* 2001; **22**: 1642–1681.

50 Sommer T, Fehske W, Holzknecht N, et al. Aortic dissection: a comparative study of diagnosis with spiral CT, multiplanar transesophageal echocardiography, and MR imaging. *Radiology* 1996; **199**: 347–352.

51 Evangelista A, Garcia-del-Castillo H, Gonzalez-Alujas T, et al. Diagnosis of ascending aortic dissection by transesophageal echocardiography: utility of M-mode in recognizing artifacts. *J Am Coll Cardiol* 1996; **27**: 102–107.

52 Penco M, Paparoni S, Dagianti A, et al. Usefulness of transesophageal echocardiography in the assessment of aortic dissection. *Am J Cardiol* 2000; **86**: 53–56.

53 Shiga T, Wajima Z, Apfel CC, Inoue T, Ohe Y. Diagnostic accuracy of transesophageal echocardiography, helical computed tomography, and magnetic resonance imaging for suspected thoracic aortic dissection: systematic review and meta-analysis. *Arch Intern Med* 2006; **166**: 1350–1356.

54 Murray JG, Manisali M, Flamm SD, et al. Intramural hematoma of the thoracic aorta: MR image findings and their prognostic implications. *Radiology* 1997; **204**: 349–355.

55 van Bogerijen GH, Tolenaar JL, Rampoldi V, et al. Predictors of aortic growth in uncomplicated type B aortic dissection. *J Vasc Surg* 2014; **59**: 1134–1143.

56 Jiang W, Wang Z, Hu Z, et al. Highly expressed S100A12 in aortic wall of patients with DeBakey type I aortic dissection could be a promising marker to predict perioperative complications. *Ann Vasc Surg* 2014; **28**: 1556–1562.

57 Sakakura K, Kubo N, Ako J, et al. Peak C-reactive protein level predicts long-term outcomes in type B acute aortic dissection. *Hypertension* 2010; **55**: 422–429.

58 Kitai T, Kaji S, Kim K, et al. Prognostic value of sustained elevated C-reactive protein levels in patients with acute aortic intramural hematoma. *J Thorac Cardiovasc Surg* 2014; **147**: 326–331.

59 Raymond CE, Aggarwal B, Schoenhagen P, et al. Prevalence and factors associated with false positive suspicion of acute aortic syndrome: experience in a patient population transferred to a specialized aortic treatment center. *Cardiovasc Diagn Ther* 2013; **3**: 196–204.

60 Hirst AE jr, Johns VJ jr, Kime SW Jr. Dissecting aneurysm of the aorta: a review of 505 cases. *Medicine (Baltimore)* 1958; **37**: 217–279.

61 Booher AM, Isselbacher EM, Nienaber CA, et al. The IRAD classification system for characterizing survival after aortic dissection. *Am J Med* 2013; **126**: 730 e19–24.

62 Fattori R, Cao P, De Rango P, et al. Interdisciplinary expert consensus document on management of type B aortic dissection. *J Am Coll Cardiol* 2013; **61**: 1661–178.

63 Fattori R, Tsai TT, Myrmel T, et al. Complicated acute type B dissection: is surgery still the best option?: a report from the International Registry of Acute Aortic Dissection. *JACC Cardiovasc Interv* 2008; **1**: 395–402.

64 Estrera AL, Miller CC 3rd, Safi HJ, et al. Outcomes of medical management of acute type B aortic dissection. *Circulation* 2006; **114**: 384–389.

65 Onitsuka S, Akashi H, Tayamar K, et al. Long-term outcome and prognostic predictors of medically treated acute type B aortic dissections. *Ann Thorac Surg* 2004; **78**: 1268–1273.

66 Tsai TT, Evangelista A, Nienaber CA, et al. Partial thrombosis of the false lumen in patients with acute type B aortic dissection. *N Engl J Med* 2007; **357**: 349–359.

67 Clough RE, Hussain T, Uribe S, et al. A new method for quantification of false lumen thrombosis in aortic dissection using magnetic resonance imaging and a blood pool contrast agent. *J Vasc Surg* 2011; **54**: 1251–1258.

68 Qin YL, Deng G, Li TX, Jing RW, Teng GJ. Risk factors of incomplete thrombosis in the false lumen after endovascular treatment of extensive acute type B aortic dissection. *J Vasc Surg* 2012; **56**: 1232–1238.

69 Trimarchi S, Eagle KA, Nienaber CA, et al. Importance of refractory pain and hypertension in acute type B aortic dissection: insights from the International Registry of Acute Aortic Dissection (IRAD). *Circulation* 2010; **122**: 1283–1289.

70 Evangelista A, Salas A, Ribera A, et al. Long-term outcome of aortic dissection with patent false lumen: predictive role of entry tear size and location. *Circulation* 2012; **125**: 3133–3141.

71 Alimohammadi M, Agu O, Balabani S, Diaz-Zuccarini V. Development of a patient-specific simulation tool to analyse aortic dissections: assessment of mixed patient-specific flow and pressure boundary conditions. *Med Eng Phys* 2014; **36**: 275–284.

72 Clough RE, Waltham M, Giese D, Taylor PR, Schaeffter T. A new imaging method for assessment of aortic dissection using four-dimensional phase contrast magnetic resonance imaging. *J Vasc Surg* 2012; **55**: 914–923.

73 Sabik JF, Lytle BW, Blackstone EH, et al. Long-term effectiveness of operations for ascending aortic dissections. *J Thorac Cardiovasc Surg* 2000; **119**: 946–962.

74 Metcalfe MJ, Karthikesalingam A, Black SA, et al. The first endovascular repair of an acute type A dissection using an endograft designed for the ascending aorta. *J Vasc Surg* 2012; **55**: 220–222.

75 Sobocinski J, O'Brien N, Maurel B, et al. Endovascular approaches to acute aortic type A dissection: a CT-based feasibility study. *Eur J Vasc Endovasc Surg* 2011; **42**: 442–427.

76 Lyons O, Clough R, Patel A, et al. Endovascular management of Stanford type a dissection or intramural hematoma with a distal primary entry tear. *J Endovasc Ther* 2011; **18**: 591–600.

77 Acosta S, Blomstrand D, Gottsater A. Epidemiology and long-term prognostic factors in acute type B aortic dissection. *Ann Vasc Surg* 2007; **21**: 415–422.

78 Estrera AL, Miller CC 3rd, Huynth TT, et al. Preoperative and operative predictors of delayed neurologic deficit following repair of thoracoabdominal aortic aneurysm. *J Thorac Cardiovasc Surg* 2003; **126**: 1288–1294.

79 Safi HJ, Estrera AL, Miller CC, et al. Evolution of risk for neurologic deficit after descending and thoracoabdominal aortic repair. *Ann Thorac Surg* 2005; **80**: 2173–2179; discussion 2179.

80 Tsai TT, Fattori R, Trimarchi S, et al. Long-term survival in patients presenting with type B acute aortic dissection: insights from the International Registry of Acute Aortic Dissection. *Circulation* 2006; **114**: 2226–2231.

81 Svensson LG, Kouchoukos NT, Miller DC, et al. Expert consensus document on the treatment of descending thoracic aortic disease using endovascular stent-grafts. *Ann Thorac Surg* 2008; **85**: 1–41.

82 Jones DW, Goodney PP, Nolan BW, et al. National trends in utilization, mortality, and survival after repair of type B aortic dissection in the Medicare population. *J Vasc Surg* 2014; **60**: 11–19.

83 Parker JD, Golledge J. Outcome of endovascular treatment of acute type B aortic dissection. *Ann Thorac Surg* 2008; **86**: 1707–1712.

84 Nienaber CA, Kische S, Rousseau H, et al. Endovascular repair of type B aortic dissection: long-term results of the randomized investigation of stent grafts in aortic dissection trial. *Circ Cardiovasc Interv* 2013; **6**: 407–416.

85 Lombardi JV, Cambria RP, Nienaber CA, et al. Prospective multicenter clinical trial (STABLE) on the endovascular treatment of complicated type B aortic dissection using a composite device design. *J Vasc Surg* 2012; **55**: 629–640.

86 Lombardi JV, Cambria RP, Nienaber CA, et al. Aortic remodeling after endovascular treatment of complicated type B aortic dissection with the use of a composite device design. *J Vasc Surg* 2014; **59**: 1544–1554.

87 Ruddy JM, Reisenman P, Priestley J, et al. Stent-graft therapy for False lumen Aneurysmal Degeneration in Established Type B aortic Dissection (FADED) results in differential volumetric remodeling of the thoracic versus abdominal aortic segments. *Ann Vasc Surg* 2014; **28**: 1602–1609.

88 Vilacosta I, Aragoncillo P, Canadas V, et al. Acute aortic syndrome: a new look at an old conundrum. *Heart* 2009; **95**: 1130–1139.

89 Ganaha F, Miller DC, Sugimoto K, et al. Prognosis of aortic intramural hematoma with and without penetrating atherosclerotic ulcer: a clinical and radiological analysis. *Circulation* 2002; **106**: 342–348.

90 Harris KM, Braverman AC, Eagle KA, *et al*. Acute aortic intramural hematoma: an analysis from the International Registry of Acute Aortic Dissection. *Circulation* 2012; **126**: 91–96.

91 Kitai T, Kaji S, Yamamuro A, *et al*. Clinical outcomes of medical therapy and timely operation in initially diagnosed type a aortic intramural hematoma: a 20-year experience. *Circulation* 2009; **120**: 292–298.

92 Song JK, Yim JH, Ahn JM, *et al*. Outcomes of patients with acute type a aortic intramural hematoma. *Circulation* 2009; **120**: 2046–2052.

93 Tittle SL, Lynch RJ, Cole PE, *et al*. Midterm follow-up of penetrating ulcer and intramural hematoma of the aorta. *J Thorac Cardiovasc Surg* 2002; **123**: 1051–1059.

94 Song JK, Kim HS, Song JM, *et al*. Outcomes of medically treated patients with aortic intramural hematoma. *Am J Med* 2002; **113**: 181–187.

95 Knollmann FD, Lacomis JM, Ocak I, Gleason T. The role of aortic wall CT attenuation measurements for the diagnosis of acute aortic syndromes. *Eur J Radiol* 2013; **82**: 2392–2398.

96 Kitai T, Kaji S, Yamamuro A, *et al*. Detection of intimal defect by 64-row multidetector computed tomography in patients with acute aortic intramural hematoma. *Circulation* 2011; **124**: 174–178.

97 Robbins RC, McManus RP, Mitchell RS, *et al*. Management of patients with intramural hematoma of the thoracic aorta. *Circulation* 1993; **88**: 1–10.

98 Maraj R, Rerkpattanapipat P, Jacobs LE, Makornwattana P, Kotler MN. Meta-analysis of 143 reported cases of aortic intramural hematoma. *Am J Cardiol* 2000; **86**: 664–668.

99 von Kodolitsch Y, Csösz SK, Koschyk DH, *et al*. Intramural hematoma of the aorta: predictors of progression to dissection and rupture. *Circulation* 2003; **107**: 1158–1163.

100 Kan CB, Chang RY, Chang JP. Optimal initial treatment and clinical outcome of type A aortic intramural hematoma: a clinical review. *Eur J Cardiothorac Surg* 2008; **33**: 1002–1006.

101 Ho HH, Cheung CW, Jim MH, *et al*. Type A aortic intramural hematoma: clinical features and outcomes in Chinese patients. *Clin Cardiol* 2011; **34**: 1–5.

102 Estrera A, Miller C 3rd, Lee TY, *et al*. Acute type A intramural hematoma: analysis of current management strategy. *Circulation* 2009; **120**: 287–291.

103 Kaji S, Akasaka T, Katayama M, et al. Long-term prognosis of patients with type B aortic intramural hematoma. *Circulation* 2003; **108**: 307–311.

104 Sueyoshi E, Matsuoka Y, Imada T, *et al*. New development of an ulcerlike projection in aortic intramural hematoma: CT evaluation. *Radiology* 2002; **224**: 536–541.

105 Coady MA, Rizzo JA, Elefteriades JA. Pathologic variants of thoracic aortic dissections. Penetrating atherosclerotic ulcers and intramural hematomas. *Cardiol Clin* 1999; **17**: 637–657.

106 Botta L, Buttazzi K, Russo V, *et al*. Endovascular repair for penetrating atherosclerotic ulcers of the descending thoracic aorta: early and mid-term results. *Ann Thorac Surg* 2008; **85**: 987–992.

107 Stanson AW, Kazmier FJ, Hollier LH, *et al*. Penetrating atherosclerotic ulcers of the thoracic aorta: natural history and clinicopathologic correlations. *Ann Vasc Surg* 1986; **1**: 15–23.

108 Quint LE, Williams DM, Francis IR, *et al*. Ulcerlike lesions of the aorta: imaging features and natural history. *Radiology* 2001; **218**: 719–723.

109 Nathan DP, Boonn W, Lai E, *et al*. Presentation, complications, and natural history of penetrating atherosclerotic ulcer disease. *J Vasc Surg* 2012; **55**: 10–15.

110 D'Ancona G, Amaducci A, Rinaudo A, *et al*. Haemodynamic predictors of a penetrating atherosclerotic ulcer rupture using fluid–structure interaction analysis. *Interact Cardiovasc Thorac Surg* 2013; **17**: 576–578.

111 Eggebrecht H, Herold U, Schmermund A, *et al*. Endovascular stent-graft treatment of penetrating aortic ulcer: results over a median follow-up of 27 months. *Am Heart J* 2006; **151**: 530–536.

112 Clough RE, Mani K, Lyons OT, *et al*. Endovascular treatment of acute aortic syndrome. *J Vasc Surg* 2011; **54**: 1580–1587.

113 Scali ST, Beck AW, Butler K, *et al*. Pathology-specific secondary aortic interventions after thoracic endovascular aortic repair. *J Vasc Surg* 2014; **59**: 599–607.

114 Alpert JS, Thygesen K, Antman E. Bassand JP. Myocardial infarction redefined: a consensus document of The Joint European Society of Cardiology/American College of Cardiology Committee for the redefinition of myocardial infarction. *J Am Coll Cardiol* 2000; **36**: 959–969.

115 Amsterdam EA, Kirk JD, Bluemke DA, *et al*. Testing of low-risk patients presenting to the emergency department with chest pain: a scientific statement from the American Heart Association. *Circulation* 2010; **122**: 1756–1776.

116 O'Connor RE, Brady W, Brooks SC, *et al*. Part 10: acute coronary syndromes: 2010 American Heart Association Guidelines for Cardiopulmonary Resuscitation and Emergency Cardiovascular Care. *Circulation* 2010; **122**: 787–817.

Thoracic Endovascular Aortic Aneurysm Repair

Paul S. Lajos and Michael L. Marin

Icahn School of Medicine at Mount Sinai, New York, NY, USA

Thoracic aortic aneurysms and their complications have been noted since antiquity [1–3] with Paré in 1572 speculating on a direct link with syphilis [2]. The principle of proximal ligation of aneurysms was originally described by Anel in 1710 [4] and surgical replacement of descending thoracic aortic aneurysms using an aortic homograft was reported by Lam and Aram in 1951 with the patient expiring three months later [5]. In 1953, Bahnson presented his series of repairs by lateral resection and aortorrhaphy [6] and later the same year DeBakey and Cooley described the first successful replacement of a descending thoracic aortic aneurysm using a prosthetic graft [7]. In 1951, Cooley performed what appeared to be the first open repair of an aortic arch aneurysm by cross-clamping and oversewing [8].

Today, open thoracic aortic aneurysm (TAA) repair while highly studied and optimized [11] still remains a more morbid repair than its open abdominal counterpart. Open repair of TAAs has been associated with significant morbidity and mortality according to Stevens and Farber [9], who reviewed 1600 patients undergoing elective open repair for descending TAAs with mean 30-day mortality of 9.2% and a range of 4.4–31%. The National Inpatient Sample Administrative Database reports an operative mortality of 10% for all descending TAAs [10]. From Baylor, a high volume center, a series reports 387 patients undergoing repair of TAAs with a paraplegia rate of 2.6%, stroke rate of 1.8%, renal failure 7.5%, and mortality 4.4% [11].

Dake performed the first thoracic endovascular aortic aneurysm repair (TEVAR) in 1994 [12]. TEVAR has revolutionized the treatment of this highly morbid condition into a durable and minimally invasive treatment. The Food and Drug Administration (FDA) approved the first commercially available stent graft for thoracic aortic aneurysms in 2005, the W.L. Gore TAG endograft (Flagstaff, AZ, USA), and in 2008 both the Cook Zenith TX2 (Bloomington, IN, USA) [13] and Medtronic Talent (Santa Rosa, CA, USA) became commercially available. Currently, there are four thoracic grafts commercially available in the USA: W.L. Gore C-TAG (Flagstaff, AZ, USA); Medtronic Valiant (Santa Rosa, CA, USA); Cook TX2 (Bloomington, IN, USA); and Bolton Relay (Sunrise, FL, USA).

TEVAR remains a preferred technique because of its minimally invasive approach, ease of application and deployment, shorter operating times, reduced blood loss, and decreased morbidity and mortality, and length of stay. Devices have continued to evolve since the introduction of smaller access sheaths, hydrophilic coatings, and smaller delivery and deployment systems. TEVAR is a safe and effective therapy for different aortic pathologies leading to promising long-term results, with patients with acute type B aortic dissections, aneurysms, and traumatic ruptures seeming to benefit the most [14].

Demographics

Among all aortic aneurysms, 60% are located in the abdominal aorta and 20% in the thoracic or thoracoabdominal aorta. Of those 20%, 40% are confined to the ascending aorta, 15% to the arch, 35% to the upper thoracic, and 10% to the lower distal thoracic aorta [15].

TAAs have an incidence of 6 per 100,000 patient-years with a rupture risk of 3.5–5 per 100,000 patient-years with an overall 5-year rupture risk of 20% [16]. The natural history of TAAs is progressive expansion leading to rupture, which is usually fatal. Aneurysm growth is strongly related to maximal diameter and this increases exponentially with aneurysm size [16–18]. Risk of rupture is seven times higher in women than men and is directly related to diameter >6 cm [19]. Thoracoabdominal aortic aneurysms, on the other hand, have an 80% 1-year risk of rupture when ≥8 cm [20].

Etiology

The majority of TAAs are the result of medial degeneration within the wall of the aorta. Medial degeneration or previously cystic medial necrosis is a complex combination of hemodynamic forces, genetic factors, and matrix metalloproteinases (MMPs). The end product is breakdown of extracellular matrix and smooth muscle within the aortic wall. While the majority of TAAs are secondary to medial degeneration, 20–50% are believed to have arisen from an area of previous aortic dissection [15–18].

TAAs and thoracic aortic dissections are classified as syndromic, familial, or sporadic. Syndromic consist of less than 5% and arise from a collection of clinical manifestations of Marfan's, Ehler–Danlos type IV, or Loeys–Dietz syndromes. Endografting is generally not recommended in this group due to continued aortic dilation.

Marfan's syndrome (MFS) is a connective tissue disorder with an autosomal dominant inheritance pattern with an incidence of 1 in 10,000 individuals. MFS displays varying physical traits including dolichostenomelia, arachnodactyly, ectopia lentis, and thoracic

Interventional Cardiology: Principles and Practice, Second Edition. Edited by George D. Dangas, Carlo Di Mario, and Nicholas N. Kipshidze.
© 2017 John Wiley & Sons, Ltd. Published 2017 by John Wiley & Sons, Ltd.

aortic aneurysm and dissection. The defect is in the fibrillin (*FBN1*) gene [21,22].

Loeys–Dietz syndrome (LDS) manifests in very young patients with bifid uvula or cleft palate, hypertelorism, craniosynostosis, and as aneurysms or dissections in abdominal or thoracic aorta with missense mutations in transforming growth factor B1 and B2 receptors and in *TGFBR2* or *TGFBR1* genes [23].

Ehler–Danlos IV (EDS) manifests as tissue fragility of skin and joints, internal organs, and blood vessels with type IV as rupture or dissection in medium-sized vessels of chest and abdomen as opposed to the aorta, which is in contradistinction to MFS. Its incidence is 1 in 50,000 individuals with a mutation in the *COL3A1* gene, which encodes for type III collagen.

Familial TAAs comprise roughly 15–20% and roughly 80% are sporadic in etiology and about 15–20% have a first degree relative with a TAA [17]. These cluster in families but do not have an association with a connective tissue disorder like MFS, EDS, or LDS. The Familial TAAs are inherited as an autosomal dominant disorder and patients generally present at a younger age than with the sporadic form and have an association with a bicuspid aortic valve or patent ductus arteriosus. Primary genes associated with this are *ACTA2, TGFBR2,* and *MYH11.*

Indications

Surgical intervention is advised in the presence of symptoms, rapid dilatation, and compression of adjacent thoracic or abdominal structures, rupture, and diameter ranging 5–7 cm depending on age, associated risks, and medical comorbidities.

Open repair of TAA and thoracoabdominal aortic aneurysm (TAAA) confers significant morbidity and measureable mortality, potential blood loss, and physiologic stresses to heart and lungs. TEVAR offers less potential blood loss, preservation of forward blood flow, avoidance or aortic cross-clamping and cardiac stress; and avoidance of potential morbidity as related to thoracotomy and laparotomy. Advances in stent graft technology and newer generation devices, debranching techniques to extend landing zones, and percutaneous access have increased potential cases suitable for TEVAR to 70–80%. Anesthesia can performed under local, regional, or general anesthetic. Cardiac stability is improved and spinal chord ischemia, length of stay, and duration of postoperative recovery all are diminished.

Diagnostic imaging
Duplex ultrasound
Duplex ultrasound is not routinely useful because of air in the thoracic cavity generating poor image quality. However, it is important in assessing size and quality of access vessels, such as iliac, femoral, carotid, and left subclavian arteries.

Computed tomography
Computed tomography remains the gold standard for preoperative imaging. Post-imaging processing using specific vascular protocols allows three-dimensional rendering and simulations or angiography for accurate measurements in graft sizing useful for case planning. Utilizing large numbers of axial slices and combination with multiplanar reconstructions can provide computed tomographic angiography. Extent and nature of aortic disease and iliac disease, location and size diameters, and quality can be obtained and measured for stent graft repair. CT scan can delineate calcifications, intramural thrombus, access vessel sizing, and architecture. Potential disadvantages for CT include contrast load and radiation exposure.

Angiography
Conventional diagnostic angiography has been largely replaced by CT angiography but may be appropriate for the measurement of questionable landing zones and assessment of potential side branches. Three-dimensional angiography is also helpful as rotational angiography on newer fixed mounted units. Angiography has the disadvantage of being invasive and requiring intra-arterial contrast.

Magnetic resonance
MR angiography is performed with intravenously injected paramagnetic contrast (i.e., gadolinium) or has the advantage of being performed without contrast in some scanners. High performance systems can chase a single contrast bolus throughout the body for MRA but generally requires a long period of time (e.g., 45 minutes) for image acquisition. MRA may not be possible in some patients because of the extended period of time needed and images are affected by motion artifact.

Transesophogeal echocardiography
Transesophogeal echocardiography can provide short and long-axis images of the descending thoracic aorta to the level of the stomach to assess aortic atherosclerosis. It can be helpful especially in dissections for locating intimal re-entry tears in the dissected TAA. Benefits include lack of contrast load; quality of imaging is operator dependent and is not readily available in some centers.

Anatomic requirements
Thoracic stent grafts were originally designed as modified designs of abdominal endografts. Thoracic pathology requires significant constraints and challenges including the requirement to conform to the curve of the aortic arch to gain accurate and secure fixation. These requirements have led to significant challenges including tortuous aortas, limited proximal and distal landing zones, and pathologies.

Successful anatomic requirements for successful TEVAR include proximal landing zone diameter needing to be <40 mm; adequate proximal landing zone length of 20 mm on the lesser curve of the aortic arch; at least 15 mm of normal aorta required for distal landing zone; landing zone cannot potentially have an acutely angled arch and cannot form a tight circumferential seal. The proximal stent graft can cover the left subclavian artery with arm ischemia reported to be quite low [24]. The role of subclavian artery transposition or common carotid to subclavian bypass is controversial with some evidence of spinal chord ischemia and posterior circulation compromise being higher in patients who do not undergo prior revascularization [25]. Tortuosity of the descending thoracic aorta can cause difficulties with endograft placement and fixation although newer generation devices have improved tracking and flexibility and less kinking possibilities [26]. If distally more landing zone is required it may necessitate taking the TEVAR graft to the abdominal aorta and potentially cover or snorkel some of the larger visceral vessels (i.e., celiac, superior mesenteric artery, and/ or renals) or perform surgical debranching. There are reports of covering the celiac artery to increase distal landing zones; however, this must be carried out in the setting of adequate superior mesenteric artery perfusion [27]. Access vessels remain an important consideration as calcified and tortuous iliac arteries can be a contraindication with a minimum iliac diameter of 7 mm being the necessary to accommodate most commercially available devices (Box 72.1).

Evidence to support TEVAR

TEVAR has been used successfully in all aortic pathologies, both emergent and elective including aortic transection, aneurysmal disease, and dissection.

The European Collaborators on Stent/Graft Techniques for Aortic Aneurysm (EUROSTAR) and UK Thoracic Registries reported a multicenter series of 443 patients undergoing TEVAR for degenerative aneurysm, dissection, false aneurysm, and traumatic injuries [28]. Technical success was 87%. Left subclavian artery coverage occurred in 17% with 50% undergoing revascularization. Thirty-day mortality was 10% in TAA group (5.7% for elective and 27.9% for emergent procedures). Cumulative survival was 80% with a 1% late rupture rate.

In a study by Bavaria *et al.* [29], the randomized trial that led to the approval of the Gore TAG device showed that with good anatomy TEVAR can be performed with lower mortality than open surgery (2.1% vs. 11.7%); less spinal chord ischemia (3% vs. 14%); less renal failure (1% vs. 13%); and less respiratory insufficiency (4% vs. 20%). However, access-related complications were more common in the TEVAR group.

The INSTEAD XL trial (INvestigation of STEnt grafts in patients with type B aortic dissection), a randomized clinical trial completed in Europe, in uncomplicated type B aortic dissections, initially at 1 year did not show a mortality benefit to TEVAR [30]. Their 5-year follow-up showed an aorta-specific survival benefit in patients treated with TEVAR versus medical therapy of 6.9% versus 19.3%, respectively in risk of aorta-specific mortality, as well as less progression of disease of 27.0% versus 46.1%, respectively [30].

In a complicated aortic dissection trial (branch vessel malperfusion, impending rupture, aortic diameter ≥40 mm, rapid aortic expansion, and persistent pain or hypertension despite maximum medical therapy) using Cook proximal TX2 thoracic stent grafts and distal bare metal dissection stents (Zenith Dissection Endovascular System; Cook Medical, Bloomington, IN, USA), 10 centers enrolled 40 patients in acute, subacute, and chronic aortic dissections. The overall mean time from symptom onset to treatment was 20 days (range 0–78 days). Seven combinations of stent grafts and dissection stents were used, and all devices were successfully deployed and patent. The 30-day mortality rate was 5% (2 of 40) with two deaths occurring after 30 days, leading to a 1-year survival rate of 90%. Thirty-day morbidity included stroke in 7.5%; transient ischemic attack in 2.5%; paraplegia in 2.5%; retrograde dissection in 5%; and renal failure in 12.5%. Four patients (10%) underwent secondary interventions within 1 year. Favorable aortic remodeling was observed during the course of follow-up, indicated by an increase in the

---

Box 72.1 Indications for operation

- Penetrating aortic ulcer
- Rapid dilatation
- Compression
- Rupture
- Dissection
- Blunt thoracic trauma
- Twice size of distal aortic arch
- Size 5–7 cm

Source: Adapted from Howard A. Loftus I. Thoracic aneurysms (endovascular repair). In Thompson M. *Endovascular Intervention for Vascular Disease*. New York, NY: CRC Press: 2008; 221–233.

📖 Case study

A 73-year-old male presented to an outside hospital with acute sudden back and chest pain. He had a history of coronary artery disease with prior placed stents and hypertension. Chest CT angiogram revealed a focal penetrating ulcer at distal transverse aortic arch with aneurysmal dilatation at the aortopulmonary window and intramural aortic hematoma extending into the arch and descending thoracic aorta (Figure 72.1). He was started on beta-blocker therapy with control of his blood pressure;

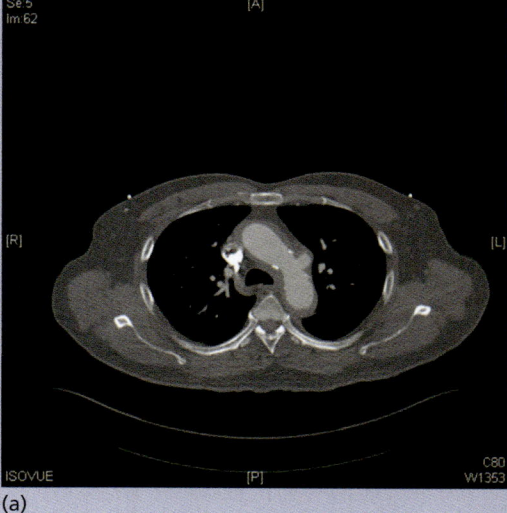
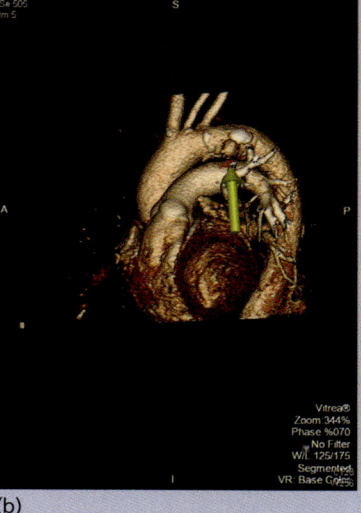

(a) (b)

Figure 72.1 (a) Preoperative CT scan showing aneurysmal dilatation (arrow) with intra aortic hematoma. (b) Three-dimensional rendering of thoracic arch showing intramural hematoma at aortopulmonary window (arrow).

however, his back pain persisted despite optimal medical therapy. On day 7 he underwent repeat imaging which revealed unchanged intramural aortic hematoma with penetrating ulcer and aneurysmal dilatation (Figure 72.1).

Due to the close proximity of the left subclavian artery with a questionable proximal landing zone, he underwent thoracic

arch aortogram. Diagnostic arch aortogram confirmed location of aneurysm exactly 2 cm from the distal left subclavian artery to the arch aneurysm (Figure 72.2).

The following day he underwent an ultrasound-assisted left transfemoral placement of percutaneous conformable Gore TAG endoprosthesis (W.L. Gore, Flagstaff, AZ, USA) through the left groin via the Preclose Proglide (Abbott Laboratories, Redwood City, CA, USA). The patient had resolution of his back pain and follow up CT scan revealed complete exclusion of his penetrating ulcer (Figure 72.3).

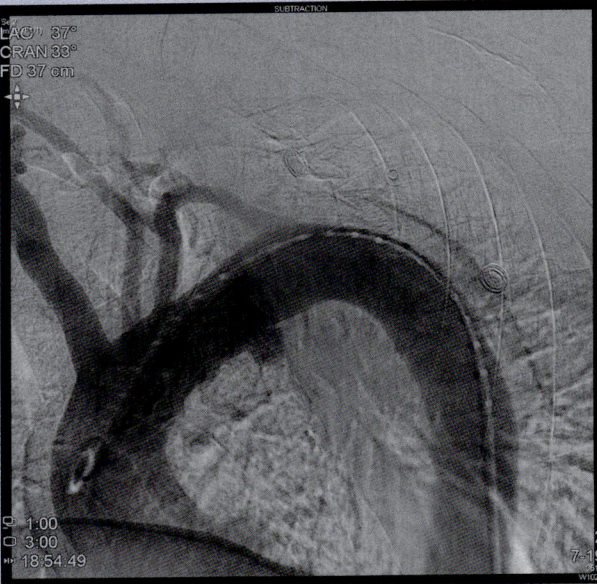

Figure 72.2 Preoperative thoracic aortogram demonstrating aneurysmal dilatation at the distal transverse aortic arch with an exact 2 cm proximal landing zone in a relatively straight segment of the distal arch.

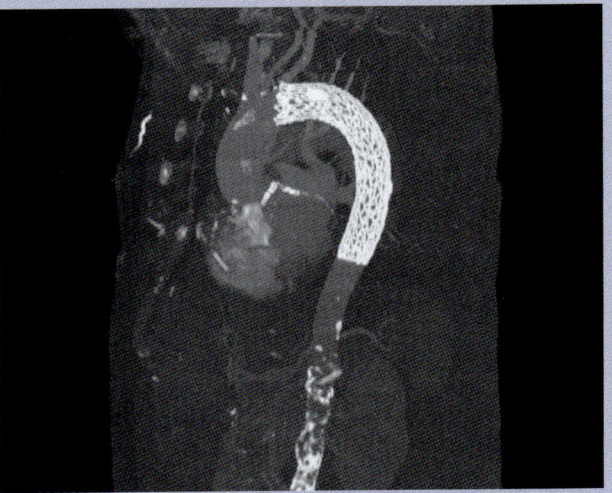

Figure 72.3 Postoperative time resolved MRA showing placement of thoracic endograft with complete exclusion of aortic aneurysm.

true lumen size and a decrease in the false lumen size along the dissected aorta, with completely thrombosed thoracic false lumen observed in 31% of patients at 12 months as compared to 0% at baseline [31].

In an aortic transection meta-analysis, Tang *et al.* [32] reviewed 370 patients treated with TEVAR and 329 patients managed with open surgery. Technical success rates were similar between groups; however, mortality was significantly lower in the TEVAR group (7.6% vs. 15.2%) as were rates of paraplegia (0% vs. 5.6%) and stroke (0.85% vs. 5.3%). The most common procedure-related complications for each technique were iliac artery injury during TEVAR and recurrent laryngeal nerve injury after open surgery. Their study showed a significant reduction in mortality, paraplegia, and stroke rates in patients who undergo TEVAR versus open repair.

Conclusions

In closing, TEVAR can be performed safely and effectively in appropriate patients. Attention to access vessel size and quality and appropriate proximal and distal landing zones in the thoracic aorta are paramount to successful long-term outcomes. Strong reliance on preoperative high-quality CT scan will help aid in diagnostic workup and appropriate case planning.

Interactive multiple choice questions are available for this chapter on www.wiley. com/go/dangas/cardiology

References

1 Kampmeier RH. Saccular aneurysm of the thoracic aorta: a clinical study of 633 cases. *Ann Intern Med* 1938; **12**(5): 624–651.
2 Malgaigne JF. *Oeuvres complètes d'Ambroise Paré. Livre V: Des tumeurs en générale.* JB Baillière, Paris, 1840.
3 Boyd LJ. A study of four thousand reported cases of aneurysm of the thoracic aorta. *Am J Med Sci* 1924; **168**: 654–668.
4 Sloffer CA, Lanzino G. Historical vignette. Dominique Anel: father of the Hunterian ligation? *J Neurosurg* 2006; **104**(4): 626–629.
5 Lam CR, Aram HH. Resection of the descending thoracic aorta for aneurysm; a report of the use of a homograft in a case and an experimental study. *Ann Surg* 1951; **134**(4): 743–752.
6 Bahnson HT. Definitive treatment of saccular aneurysms of the aorta with excision of sac and aortic suture. *Surg Gynecol Obstet* 1953; **96**(4): 383–402.
7 DeBakey ME, Cooley DA. Successful resection of aneurysm of thoracic aorta and replacement by graft. *JAMA* 1953; **152**: 673–676.
8 Cooley DA, DeBakey MA. Surgical considerations of intrathoracic aneurysms of the aorta and great vessels. *Ann Surg* 1952; **135**(5): 660–680.
9 Stevens SL, Farber MA (eds). *Thoracic Endovascular Aorta.* Knoxville, TN: Tennessee Valley Publishing: 2008; 181–194.
10 Schermerhorn ML, Giles KA, Hamdan AD, *et al.* Population-based outcomes of open descending thoracic aortic aneurysm repair. *J Vasc Surg* 2008; **48**(4): 821–827.

11 Coselli JS, LeMaire SA, Conklin LD, *et al.* Left heart bypass during descending thoracic aortic aneurysm repair does not reduce the incidence of paraplegia. *Ann Thorac Surg* 2004; 77(4): 1298–1303; discussion 1303.

12 Dake MD, Miller DC, Semba CP, *et al.* Transluminal placement of endovascular stent-grafts for the treatment of descending thoracic aortic aneurysms. *N Engl J Med* 1994; 331(26): 1729–1734.

13 Torsello GF, Torsello GB, Austermann M. Zenith TX2 LowProfile TAA Endovascular Graft: a next generation thoracic stent-graft. *J Cardiovasc Surg (Torino)* 2012; 53(2): 153–159.

14 Wiedemann D, Mahr S, Vadehra A, *et al.* Thoracic endovascular aortic repair in 300 patients: long-term results. *Ann Thorac Surg* 2013; 95(5): 1577–1583.

15 Bickerstaff LK, Pairolero PC, Hollier LH, *et al.* Thoracic aortic aneurysms: a population-based study. *Surgery* 1982; 92(6): 1103–1108.

16 Johansson G, Markstrom U, Swedenborg J. Ruptured thoracic aortic aneurysms: a study of incidence and mortality rates. *J Vasc Surg* 1995; 21(6); 985–988.

17 Coady MA, Davies RR, Roberts M *et al.* Familial patterns of thoracic aortic aneurysms. *Arch Surg* 1999 Apr; 134(4): 361–367.

18 McNamara JJ, Pressler VM. Natural history of arteriosclerotic thoracic aortic aneurysms. *Ann Thorac Surg* 1978; 26(5): 468–473.

19 Clouse WD, Hallett JW Jr, Schaff HV, *et al.* Improved prognosis of thoracic aortic aneurysms: a population-based study. *JAMA* 1998; 280(22): 1926–1929.

20 Davies RR, Goldstein LJ, Coady MA, *et al.* Yearly rupture or dissection rates for thoracic aortic aneurysms: simple prediction based on size. *Ann Thorac Surg* 2002; 73(1): 17–27; discussion 27–28.

21 Dapunt OE, Galla JD, Sadeghi AM, *et al.* The natural history of thoracic aortic aneurysms. *J Thorac Cardiovasc Surg* 1994; 107(5): 1323–1332; discussion 1332–1333.

22 Lee B, Godfrey M, Vitale E, *et al.* Linkage of Marfan syndrome and a phenotypically related disorder to two different fibrillin genes. *Nature* 1991; 352(6333): 330–334.

23 Pannu H, Tran-Fadulu V, Milewicz DM. Genetic basis of thoracic aortic aneurysms and aortic dissections. *Am J Med Genet C Semin Med Genet* 2005; 139C(1): 10–16.

24 Braverman AC. Heritable thoracic aortic aneurysm disease: recognizing phenotypes, exploring genotypes. *J Am Coll Cardiol* 2015; 65(13): 1337–1339.

25 Klocker J, Koell A, Erlmeier M, *et al.* Ischemia and functional status of the left arm and quality of life after left subclavian artery coverage during stent grafting of thoracic aortic diseases. *J Vasc Surg* 2014; 60(1): 64–69.

26 Gravereaux EC, Faries PL, Burks JA, *et al.* Risk of spinal cord ischemia after endograft repair of thoracic aortic aneurysms. *J Vasc Surg* 2001; 34(6): 997–1003.

27 Makaroun MS, Dillavou ED, Kee ST, *et al.* Endovascular treatment of thoracic aortic aneurysms: results of the phase II multicenter trial of the GORE TAG thoracic endoprosthesis. *J Vasc Surg* 2005; 41(1): 1–9.

28 Vaddineni SK, Taylor SM, Patterson MA, Jordan WD Jr. Outcome after celiac artery coverage during endovascular thoracic aortic aneurysm repair: preliminary results. *J Vasc Surg* 2007; 45(3): 467–471.

29 Leurs LJ, Bell R, Degrieck Y, *et al.* Endovascular treatment of thoracic aortic diseases: combined experience from the EUROSTAR and United Kingdom Thoracic Endograft registries. *J Vasc Surg* 2004; 40(4): 670–679; discussion 679–680.

30 Bavaria JE, Appoo JJ, Makaroun MS, *et al.* Endovascular stent grafting versus open surgical repair of descending thoracic aortic aneurysms in low-risk patients: a multicenter comparative trial. *J Thorac Cardiovasc Surg* 2007; 133(2): 369–377.

31 Nienaber CA, Kische S, Rousseau H, *et al.* Endovascular repair of type B aortic dissection: long-term results of the randomized investigation of stent grafts in aortic dissection trial. *Circ Cardiovasc Interv* 2013; 6(4): 407–416.

32 Tang GL, Tehrani HY, Usman A, *et al.* Reduced mortality, paraplegia, and stroke with stent graft repair of blunt aortic transections: a modern meta-analysis. *J Vasc Surg* 2008; 47(3): 671–675.

CHAPTER 73

Endovascular Aortic Aneurysm Repair

William Beckerman, Paul S. Lajos, and Peter L. Faries
Icahn School of Medicine at Mount Sinai, New York, NY, USA

The first open repair of an abdominal aortic aneurysm (AAA) was performed by Charles Dubost in 1951 at the Hôpital Broussais in Paris using a cadaveric arterial graft, a technique later brought to the USA by Cooley and DeBakey [1,2]. Another major advancement occurred in 1978 when Cooley developed a double-velour Dacron graft that quickly became the standard graft for open AAA repair [3]. Despite decades of experience with open aneurysm repair that continue to this day, open surgical repair has meant longer recovery times, even with decreased perioperative mortality rates that have fallen to between 1% and 7% [4,5].

In 1991, Parodi's placement of a balloon-expandable stent graft delivered endovascularly under fluoroscopy to treat AAA ushered in a new era in vascular surgery [6]. This technology was soon adopted worldwide and the first two endovascular devices, Guidant's Ancure and Medtronic's AneuRx, gained regulatory approval from the US Food and Drug Administration (FDA) in 1999 [7]. By 2006, endovascular aneurysm repair (EVAR) overtook open repair as the most common elective treatment for AAA [8]. At the time of this publication, there are currently six FDA-approved abdominal aortic stent grafts commercially available in the USA: Cook Zenith (Bloomington, IN, USA); Endologix AFX (Irvine, CA, USA); Gore Excluder (Flagstaff, AZ, USA); Lombard Aorfix (Irvine, CA, USA); Medtronic Endurant (Santa Rosa, CA, USA); and the Trivascular Ovation (Santa Rosa, CA, USA).

Since its initial use over two decades ago, the prevalence of EVAR to treat AAA has been increasing steadily, validated by a number of randomized controlled studies showing decreased perioperative mortality and non-inferior long-term mortality versus traditional open surgery in addition to obvious benefits including decreased length of stay [9–11]. Smaller delivery sizes and access sheaths have evolved in EVARs now being able to be performed entirely percutaneously (PEVAR), expanding the scope of interventionalists who can perform the procedure.

Demographics

AAAs are responsible for approximately 13,000 deaths annually in the USA and are the fifteenth leading cause of death overall and the tenth leading cause of death in men above the age of 55 [12,13]. AAA primarily affects adults over the age of 50 (and increases with increasing age), with men affected 2–6 times more frequently than women and 5 times more commonly in patients with a smoking history. Other risk factors for AAA include Caucasian race, a family history of AAA, the presence of other large aneurysms, and atherosclerosis [14,15]. The incidence of AAA is 3.5–6.5 per 1000 person-years in males with a reported incidence of rupture of 1–21 per 100,000 person-years [16–18]. Aneurysm rupture carries a particularly poor prognosis, with an overall mortality of 78%, with the majority of those deaths occurring before the patient presents to a medical center. Incidence of rupture increases exponentially with increasing aneurysm diameter, with an estimated rupture risk of approximately 30–50% per year for those aneurysms >8 cm. Among all aortic aneurysms, 60% are distributed in the abdominal aorta with the vast majority involving the infrarenal aorta and only 5–15% involving the aorta above the renal arteries [19].

Etiology

AAAs are typically the result of chronic loss of vascular structural proteins and subsequent decrease in aortic wall strength [20]. While atherosclerosis is a risk factor for AAA, atherosclerosis alone does not cause AAA. Atherosclerosis is limited to changes in the inner layers of the aorta whereas AAA is transmural involving loss of elastin and smooth muscle and abnormal collagen remodeling. Circulating markers of inflammation including C-reactive protein (CRP) and interleukins (especially interleukin-6) are both associated with aneurysm formation. This chronic inflammation is thought to degrade elastin and collagen in the aortic wall through the work of proteases, including plasmin, matrix metalloproteinases (MMPs), and cathepsins S and K from endothelial and smooth muscle cells and inflammatory cells in the media and adventitia.

Connective tissue disorders, including Marfan's syndrome, Loeys–Dietz syndrome, and Ehler–Danlos type IV have all been implicated in AAA formation. Inflammatory aneurysms, which comprise approximately 5% of all AAAs, are a distinct entity involving notable aortic wall thickening with increased vascularity and elevated erythrocyte sedimentation levels [21].

The natural history of AAA typically involves an increase in AAA diameter of approximately 0.3 cm/year, with larger aneurysms tending to grow faster than smaller ones, and active smoking increasing aneurysm growth as well as risk of rupture [22].

Interventional Cardiology: Principles and Practice, Second Edition. Edited by George D. Dangas, Carlo Di Mario, and Nicholas N. Kipshidze.
© 2017 John Wiley & Sons, Ltd. Published 2017 by John Wiley & Sons, Ltd.

Indications

EVAR is indicated as treatment for symptomatic AAA (e.g., limb ischemia, thromboembolic events, abdominal, back or flank pain), inflammatory AAA (characterized by chronic abdominal pain, weight loss, and elevated erythrocyte sedimentation rate), or ruptured AAA. EVAR is also indicated as prophylactic treatment to prevent aneurysm rupture in the case of rapidly expanding AAA (generally described as aneurysm growth >0.5 cm in 6 months or >1 cm in 1 year), or for AAA greater than 5.5 cm in maximum diameter (with some proposing >5 cm in low operative risk females) [23,24]. Coexisting AAA in association with aneurysms of the iliac arteries would also prompt EVAR.

In the preoperative evaluation of a patient for elective EVAR, risk of aneurysm rupture and associated morbidity and mortality must be weighed against operative risk. Perioperative mortality from EVAR ranges from 4% in some population studies to less than 1% at centers of excellence [25]. While a thorough workup involving cardiovascular testing should be performed for all elective cases, the decreased blood loss, avoidance of aortic cross-clamping, decreased procedure time and postoperative recovery and increased options for anesthesia (including general, local, moderate sedation, and spinal anesthesia) all increase the range of patients who can be successfully treated at lower perioperative risk than conventional open operative repair [26].

Ruptured AAA

EVAR is increasingly being used to treat ruptured AAA [27]. The largest randomized clinical trial, Immediate Management of the Patient with Rupture: Open versus Endovascular Repair (IMPROVE), was a multicenter trial out of the UK and Canada that attempted to examine this treatment in real-world conditions [28]. A total of 613 patients with suspicion of ruptured AAA but prior to imaging were randomized into endovascular or open repair groups. While there was no difference in 30-day mortality between the two groups as initially randomized, of the patients treated with the different modalities, mortality was significantly lower in the EVAR group (25%) than the open repair group (38%). Additionally, more patients were discharged directly to home in the EVAR group (94% vs. 77%). It is also interesting to note that of the 266 patients starting out in the endovascular arm of the study, 174 (64%) were deemed to have suitable anatomy for EVAR.

Ideally, a patient being considered for EVAR for ruptured AAA should be hemodynamically stable with preoperative CT imaging to determine suitability for EVAR [28]. If not feasible, an aortic occlusion balloon can be inflated to stabilize the patient. The same basic anatomic criteria for elective EVAR hold true for ruptured EVAR. Absolute contraindications are an infrarenal aortic neck diameter >32 mm (as the largest diameter device on the market is 36 mm and approximately 10% oversizing needs to be considered) or an infrarenal aortic neck length <7 mm (to avoid covering the renal arteries while maintaining aortic wall apposition). Heavily calcified or thrombus-filled aortic necks, angulated aortic necks (>60°), small iliac arteries (<7 mm) are all relative contraindications [29,30].

Special preoperative considerations for ruptured EVAR versus elective EVAR include permissive hypotension (aiming for goal systolic blood pressure of 80–100 mmHg), resuscitation with blood products as opposed to crystalloid fluids (as well as alerting the blood bank to the potential need for massive transfusion protocol), and avoidance of spinal or epidural anesthesia both for time considerations as well as their effect on blood pressure [28,31].

Diagnostic imaging
Duplex ultrasound

Abdominal B-mode ultrasound is the most frequently used screening modality to look for AAA. Indeed, for patients in the USA, Medicare covers a one-time screening for those with a family history of AAA and men aged 65–75 years who have smoked at least 100 cigarettes in their lifetime [32]. Ultrasound is both inexpensive as well as non-invasive; however, it may be associated with decreased accuracy and higher interobserver variability [33]. Visualization of the suprarenal aorta and iliac arteries is often difficult, especially in patients with larger body habitus, and the ability to predict impending rupture is not usually possible. It is the preferred method to diagnose and monitor AAA until they become suitably sized for operative treatment as well as for postoperative monitoring for endoleaks.

Computed tomography angiography

Computed tomographic angiography (CTA) requires exposure to radiation as well as intravenous contrast material; however, in spite of this it remains the primary imaging modality for diagnosis as well as for pre-operative planning. It has greater accuracy and less interobserver variability when compared with ultrasound [34]. Three-dimensional reconstruction of CTA with centerline measurements has been valuable for greater accuracy in measurements and for visualizing the complete vasculature from the aortic arch down to the access vessels. It is also the best modality for defining the quality of the patient's vessels including thrombus and calcifications. Given the rapid image acquisition speed of CTA, stable patients presenting with ruptured AAA can be considered for immediate preoperative case planning to treat these patients endovascularly (REVAR).

Rotational angiography

Conventional diagnostic angiography has been largely replaced by CT angiography; however, the use of on-table rotational angiography as a primary imaging modality in the event of ruptures is being studied. It appears to be limited in clarity as well as field size (when attempting to visualize both iliac arteries and access vessels) when compared with CTA but can be effective in detecting endoleaks intraoperatively. Angiography also has the disadvantage of being invasive and requiring intra-arterial contrast [35].

Magnetic resonance

Magnetic resonance imaging (MRI) and magnetic resonance angiography (MRA) both offer radiation-free alternatives to CT and conventional angiography for AAA imaging. Disadvantages include high cost, long acquisition time (making it less tolerated in claustrophobic patients), poor visualization of calcified plaque and lower spatial resolution, and sensitivity to motion artifact. While use of gadolinium paramagnetic contrast makes it a reasonable imaging modality for patients with allergies to traditional intravenous contrast, it is not a benign alternative for patients with renal insufficiency because of increased risk of potentially fatal nephrogenic sclerosing fibrosis [36].

Anatomic requirements

Standard EVAR has a number of anatomic requirements that are roughly similar amongst the various stent-graft devices. That being said, each stent-graft model has its own instructions for use (IFU) outlining more specific device detail about the exact anatomic parameters and limitations that should be met for optimal outcomes. Traditionally, however, EVAR requires healthy points of apposition (known as landing zones) at the proximal and distal fixation points of the stent-graft as well as healthy access vessels to deliver the device safely into the aorta [29]. Furthermore, excessive tortuosity, especially of the infrarenal aorta has been associated with poorer outcomes with associated graft failure and endoleaks. As a rough guide, IFU for most EVAR devices specify an infrarenal aortic neck diameter between 16 and 32 mm and a landing zone of at least 10 mm of healthy infrarenal aorta with less than 60° of angulation. The iliac arteries should have >10 mm of length to land the distal aspect of the device with a diameter between 8 and 25 mm to accommodate most commercially available grafts. Heavily calcified vessels or vessels with extensive thrombus both make device apposition more challenging [30].

For patients with suboptimal anatomy or aneurysms encroaching on or involving the visceral or renal arteries, a number of methods and device modifications have been developed to ensure adequate graft fixation. Utilizing smaller parallel stent grafts into visceral or renal arteries, it is possible to maintain perfusion in these vessels in a technique known as snorkeling (or chimneying) [37]. More recently, fenestrated EVAR (FEVAR), a preordered and patient-specific manufactured aortic stent graft with cutouts for visceral and renal vessels, is being used as a newer alternative to snorkeling in patients with more difficult anatomy [38]. Branched devices, with a smaller stent-graft sutured onto the main device to preserve flow to a branch artery (such as a renal or hypogastric artery) are also in development and being used at select centers in the USA at time of publication.

It is common for the aneurysmal disease in the aorta to extend into the iliac arteries. In cases where it is not possible to find healthy landing zone proximal to the takeoff of the hypogastric artery, it may be necessary to embolize one, or even both (in a staged fashion) hypogastric arteries in order to extend the iliac artery landing zone distally beyond the hypogastric artery. This can be accomplished in a retrograde fashion from the ipsilateral femoral side or an antegrade fashion from either the contralateral femoral side or from superiorly via brachial or even radial artery access. These larger vessels usually require either embolization plugs such as the St. Jude Amplatzer (Saint Paul, MN, USA), embolization coils, or a combination of the two [39]. Often, the inferior mesenteric artery (IMA) is not visualized on pre-operative imaging because of thrombosis from the aneurysm sac. When the IMA is patent and visualized on flush angiography, some centers report decreased endoleak rates and increased sac shrinkage with embolization prior to stent graft placement [40]. Similar to the hypogastric artery, the IMA is a fairly large vessel, and embolization coils or microcoils are typically needed to achieve complete thrombosis of the artery. The rationale behind these embolizations is to prevent endoleaks, discussed later in this chapter.

Access vessels remain an important consideration as calcified and tortuous iliac arteries may be a contraindication and a minimum iliac diameter of 7 mm necessary to accommodate most commercially available devices

EVAR devices

The initial aortic stent grafts were simple tubular devices, constructed by marrying available stents to a Dacron tube graft [6]. This was soon followed by the 1993 development of the bifurcated aortobiiliac stent graft which became the prototype for most devices

Table 73.1 FDA-approved endovascular aneurysm repair (EVAR) devices.

Device	Device diameter (mm)	Main body sheath size (Fr)	Fixation
Cook Zenith	22–36	18–22	Suprarenal barbed stents
Endologix AFX	22–34	17	Suprarenal stents, anatomic seating at aortic bifurcation
Gore Excluder	23–31	18–20	Infrarenal barbs
Lombard Aorfix	24–31	22	Infrarenal barbs
Medtronic Endurant	23–36	18–20	Suprarenal barbed stents
Trivascular Ovation	20–34	14–15	Suprarenal barbed stents, infrarenal polymer-filled rings

that followed [41]. The current FDA-approved devices all fit this basic bifurcated design; however, differences do exist between approved devices (Table 73.1). The Cook Zenith, Gore Excluder, Lombard Aorfix, and Medtronic Endurant are all modular devices with woven polyester (Zenith, Aorfix, Endurant) or ePTFE (Excluder) graft material supported by the stent. Infrarenal fixation is accomplished by means of either suprarenal barbed stents in the case of the Zenith and Endurant or by barbs or hooks at the infrarenal edge of the stent graft in the case of the Aorfix and Excluder. The Ovation is unique in eschewing a traditional stent material for most of the main body, using polymer-sealing rings to create wall apposition but maintaining traditional iliac limbs. The Endologix AFX is unique in two ways: both in its passive fixation with its flow divider seated at the aortic bifurcation as well as its graft fabric lying on the outside surface of the stents. These latter two devices both utilize suprarenal fixation stents for additional protection against migration. Selection of device is at the discretion of the operator; to date there have been no randomized controlled trials comparing EVAR devices with each other [42].

Endoleaks

Blood flow in the aneurysm sac after stent graft deployment is known as an endoleak. This continued filling of the aneurysm sac can lead to aneurysm rupture in the post-EVAR patient. There are five distinct types of endoleaks that will be discussed in brief here [43].

A type I endoleak is defined as persistent blood flow into the aneurysm sac from around the stent graft proximally (type IA, typically around the main body) or distally (type IB, typically around an iliac limb). As these are considered antegrade, high-pressure leaks, type I endoleaks are usually repaired whenever discovered, be it on post-EVAR completion angiogram or surveillance CTA. This usually entails extension of the graft with either a cuff proximally or iliac extension limb distally. Type II endoleaks involve persistent filling of the aneurysm sac from retrograde blood flow of side branches, typically the inferior mesenteric artery or lumbar branches. These are considered low pressure, and frequently resolve up to 80% of the time without any need for intervention. As such, these are typically only treated (often making use of microcatheters, embolization coils and/or N-butyl cyanoacrylate glue) when there is enlargement of the aneurysm sac on surveillance CTA [44].

Type III endoleaks describe blood flow into the aneurysm sac through a tear in the graft fabric or from component separation. Similar to the type I endoleak, these are considered high-pressure antegrade leaks and are treated whenever seen, usually by stent graft re-lining.

Type IV endoleaks involve filling of the aneurysm sac through the graft fabric caused by porosity, not rips or tears. These are sometimes noted within the first 30 days of graft implantation before resolution, but are seen less frequently with newer stent grafts compared with earlier models.

Finally, type V endoleaks are due to "endotension," described as elevated sac pressure or sac enlargement without a demonstrated leak. The cause is thought to be either an undetected type I–IV endoleak or by pressure transmitted through thrombus. Re-lining with proximal or distal extension is the most common intervention for this endoleak, with complete operative explant being reserved for the most recalcitrant cases.

Evidence to support EVAR

EVAR has been validated as an effective treatment for abdominal aortic aneurysms in a number of randomized controlled trials, including the DREAM, the OVER, and EVAR 1 trials.

The Dutch Randomized Endovascular Aneurysm Management (DREAM) trial was a 2004 study that randomly assigned 351 patients with >5 cm AAA and suitable anatomy to either open or endovascular aneurysm repair. Thirty-day and 2-year aneurysm-related mortality were both significantly lower in the EVAR group (1.2% vs. 4.6% and 2.1% vs. 5.7%, respectively), the difference entirely a result of increased perioperative mortality in the open repair. All-cause mortality, however, equalized at 1 year postoperatively and stayed equivalent until the longest follow-up of 6 years (68.9% in the EVAR group vs. 69.9% in the open group). There were greater rates of reintervention (29.6% in EVAR vs. 18.1% in open) but fewer moderate and severe systemic complications (11.7% vs. 26.4%) for EVAR compared with open repair, respectively [10].

The Endovascular Aneurysm Repair Versus Open Repair in Patients With AAA (EVAR 1) trial was a randomized controlled trial involving 1252 patients, with exactly half (n = 626) divided to receive open repair and half to receive EVAR. The perioperative (30-day) mortality was significantly less for EVAR (1.8% vs. 4.3%), but no significant differences were seen in overall mortality. Similar to DREAM, graft-related complications and rates of reintervention occurred more frequently with EVAR [9].

The Open Versus Endovascular Repair (OVER) trial was a Veterans Affairs multicenter study involving 881 veterans with AAA >5.0 cm, AAA with iliac aneurysm of diameter ≥3.0 cm, or a AAA diameter of ≥4.5 cm with rapid enlargement (>0.5 cm growth over 6 months or 1.0 cm in 1 year) randomized to either open AAA repair or EVAR. Overall mortality was similar between groups over 9 years of follow-up (7.0% EVAR vs. 9.8% open repair) with an increased but not statistically significant difference in aneurysm rupture in the EVAR group. Not surprisingly, EVAR was also associated with shorter procedure times (2.9 vs. 3.7 hours), shorter intensive care unit stay (1 vs. 4 days), and shorter hospital lengths of stay (3 vs. 7 days) [11].

While there have been no randomized controlled trials in the USA comparing EVAR with open repair for ruptured or symptomatic AAA, a systematic review of 23 observational studies involving 7040 patients with symptomatic or ruptured AAA was performed including 6300 open and 740 endovascular repairs, all on an urgent or emergent basis. Emergent EVAR was associated with a significantly reduced perioperative (30-day) mortality risk relative to open repair (pooled odds ratio [OR] 0.62, 95% CI 0.52–0.75) [45].

Conclusions

EVAR has proven to be a safe and effective procedure for treating AAAs in appropriate patients. All-cause perioperative mortality, as well as AAA-related mortality at short- and intermediate-term follow-up, are lower in patients undergoing endovascular stent graft placement versus open surgery in randomized trials. However, this was associated with higher repeat intervention rate in the endovascular group noted at intermediate follow-up. Long-term survival appears to converge between the two groups, as it is dominated by the natural history of severe cardiovascular disease [46,47].

As in all procedures, patient selection is paramount and preoperative case planning with CT angiography is mandatory for successful outcomes. Advancements in EVAR technology including lower device profiles and increasing use of parallel grafts and fenestrated EVAR should increase the potential candidates for EVAR in the future.

📖 Case study

A 50-year-old male presented with known infrarenal AAA incidentally revealed on screening ultrasound. He had a strong family history for aneurysm as his father died of a ruptured AAA. Serial CT scan showed progression to 5 cm over the course of 6 months. He was electively sized for repair (Figure 73.1).

He was sized for Endologix AFX bifurcated main body and suprarenal proximal aortic extension cuff lying below the lowest renal artery (left). He underwent percutaneous placement of the device utilizing the Abbott Perclose Proglide (Abbott Laboratories, Abbott Park, IL, USA) for his femoral access.

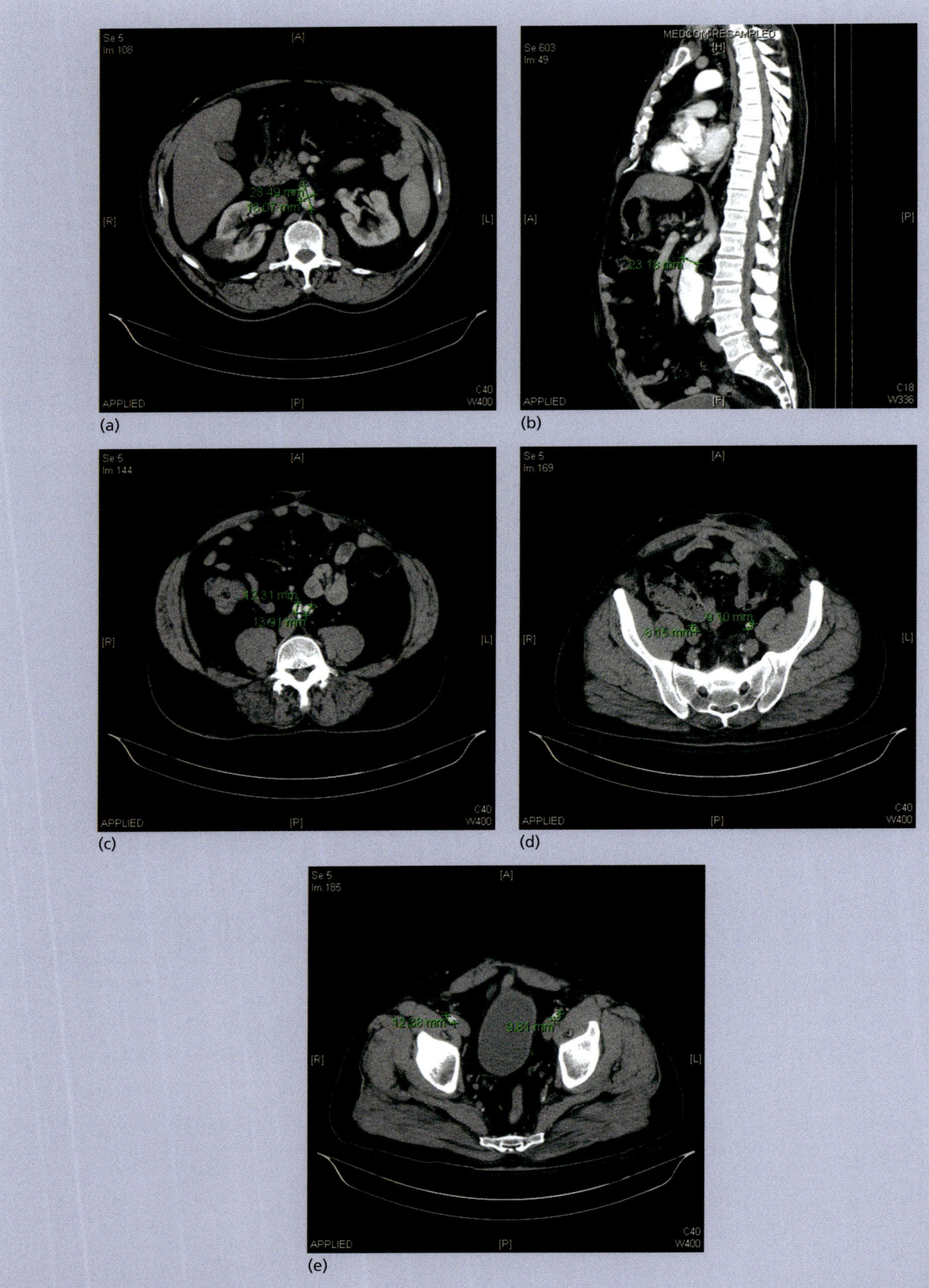

Figure 73.1 (a) Cross-sectional and (b) sagittal CT scan views showing adequate iliac arteries with appropriate vessel diameters and favorable anatomy for endovascular aneurysm repair (EVAR). (c,d,e) Sizing of common and mid and distal external iliac arteries showing adequate access vessels to accommodate EVAR device.

(icon) *Interactive multiple choice questions are available for this chapter on www.wiley.com/go/dangas/cardiology*

References

1 Dubost C, Allary M, Oeconomos N. Resection of an aneurysm of the abdominal aorta: reestablishment of the continuity by a preserved human arterial graft, with result after five months. *Arch Surg* 1952; **64**(3): 405.

2 Barker WF. *Clio Chirurgica: The Arteries*. RG Landes, Austin, TX: 1992; **273**.

3 Wukasch DC, Cooley DA, Bennett JG, *et al*. Results of a new Meadox-Cooley double velour dacron graft for arterial reconstruction. *J Cardiovasc Surg* 1978; **20**(3): 249–260.

4 Sarac TP, Bannazadeh M, Rowan AF, *et al*. Comparative predictors of mortality for endovascular and open repair of ruptured infrarenal abdominal aortic aneurysms. *Ann Vas Surg* 2011; **25**(4): 461–468.

5 Martin MC, Giles KA, Pomposelli FB, *et al*. National outcomes after open repair of abdominal aortic aneurysms with visceral or renal bypass. *Ann Vas Surg* 2010; **24**(1): 106–112.

6 Parodi JC, Palmaz JC, Barone HD. Transfemoral intraluminal graft implantation for abdominal aortic aneurysms. *Ann Vasc Surg* 1991; **5**: 491–499.

7 Marin ML, Veith FJ. Images in clinical medicine: transfemoral repair of abdominal aortic aneurysm. *N Engl J Med* 1994; **331**: 1751.

8 Schwarze ML, Shen Y, Hemmerich J, *et al*. Age-related trends in utilization and outcome of open and endovascular repair for abdominal aortic aneurysm in the United States, 2001–2006. *J Vasc Surg* 2009; **50**: 722–729.

9 Greenhalgh RM, Brown LC, Kwong GP, Powell JT, Thompson SG; EVAR trial participants. Comparison of endovascular aneurysm repair with open repair in patients with abdominal aortic aneurysm (EVAR trial 1), 30-day operative mortality results: randomised controlled trial. *Lancet* 2004; **364**(9437): 843–848.

10 Prinssen M, Verhoeven EL, Buth J, *et al*. Dutch Randomized Endovascular Aneurysm Management (DREAM) Trial Group. A randomized trial comparing conventional and endovascular repair of abdominal aortic aneurysms. *N Engl J Med* 2004; **351**(16): 1607–1618.

11 Lederle FA, Freischlag JA, Kyriakides TC, *et al*. Outcomes following endovascular vs open repair of abdominal aortic aneurysm: a randomized trial. *JAMA* 2009; **302**(14): 1535–1542.

12 Heron M. Deaths: leading causes for 2007. *Natl Vital Stat Rep* 2011; **59**: 1–95.

13 Silverberg E, Boring CC, Squires TS. Cancer statistics, 1990. *CA: Cancer J Clin* 1990; **40**(1): 9–26.

14 Gillum RF. Epidemiology of aortic aneurysm in the United States. *J Clin Epidemiol* 1995; **48**: 1289–1298.

15 Blanchard JF. Epidemiology of abdominal aortic aneurysms. *Epidemiol Rev* 1999; **21**: 207–221.

16 Wilmink ABM, Hubbard CS, Day NE, *et al*. The incidence of small abdominal aortic aneurysms and the change in normal infrarenal aortic diameter: implications for screening. *Eur J Vasc Endovasc Surg* 2001; **21**(2): 165–170.

17 Lederle FA, Johnson GR, Wilson SE, *et al*. Yield of repeated screening for abdominal aortic aneurysm after a 4-year interval. *Arch Intern Med* 2000; **160**(8): 1117–1121.

18 Wilmink ABM, Quick CRG. Epidemiology and potential for prevention of abdominal aortic aneurysm. *Br J Surg* 1998; **85**(2): 155–162.

19 Olsen PS, Schroeder T, Agerskov K. Surgery for abdominal aortic aneurysms: a survey of 656 patients. *J Cardiovasc Surg* 1990; **32**(5:636–642.

20 Wassef M, Baxter BT, Chisholm RL, *et al*. Pathogenesis of abdominal aortic aneurysms: a multidisciplinary research program supported by the National Heart, Lung, and Blood Institute. *J Vasc Surg* 2001; **34**(4): 730–738.

21 Eagleton MJ. Inflammation in abdominal aortic aneurysms: cellular infiltrate and cytokine profiles. *Vascular* 2012; **20**(5): 278–283.

22 Brady AR, Thompson SG, Fowkes FGR, *et al*. Abdominal aortic aneurysm expansion risk factors and time intervals for surveillance. *Circulation* 2004; **110**(1): 16–21.

23 UK Small Aneurysm Trial Participants. Mortality results for randomised controlled trial of early elective surgery or ultrasonographic surveillance for small abdominal aortic aneurysms. *Lancet* 1998; **352**(9141): 1649–1655.

24 Brewster DC, Cronenwett JL, Hallett JW, *et al*. Guidelines for the treatment of abdominal aortic aneurysms: report of a subcommittee of the Joint Council of the American Association for Vascular Surgery and Society for Vascular Surgery. *J Vasc Surg* 2003; **37**(5): 1106–1117.

25 Landon BE, O'Malley AJ, Giles K, *et al*. Volume-outcome relationships and abdominal aortic aneurysm repair. *Circulation* 2010; **122**(13): 1290–1297.

26 Elisha S, Nagelhout J, Heiner J, *et al*. Anesthesia case management for endovascular aortic aneurysm repair. *AANA J* 2014; **82**(2): 145–152.

27 Lesperance K, Andersen C, Singh N, Starnes B, Martin MJ. Expanding use of emergency endovascular repair for ruptured abdominal aortic aneurysms: disparities in outcomes from a nationwide perspective. *J Vasc Surg* 2008; **47**(6): 1165–1171.

28 IMPROVE Trial Investigators. Endovascular or open repair strategy for ruptured abdominal aortic aneurysm: 30 day outcomes from IMPROVE randomised trial. *BMJ* 2014; **348**: f7661.

29 Howell M, Villareal R, Krajcer Z. Percutaneous access and closure of femoral artery access sites associated with endoluminal repair of abdominal aortic aneurysms. *J Endovascular Ther* 2001; **8**(1): 68–74.

30 Schanzer A, Greenberg RK, Hevelone N, *et al*. Predictors of abdominal aortic aneurysm sac enlargement after endovascular repair. *Circulation* 2011; **123**(24): 2848–2855.

31 Reimerink JJ, Hoornweg LL, Vahl AC, Wisselink W, Balm R. Controlled hypotension in patients suspected of a ruptured abdominal aortic aneurysm: feasibility during transport by ambulance services and possible harm. *Eur J Vasc Endovasc Surg* 2010; **40**(1): 54–59.

32 Your Medicare Coverage. Abdominal Aortic Aneurysm Screening. https://www.medicare.gov/coverage/ab-aortic-aneurysm-screening.html (accessed May 25, 2016).

33 Jaakkola P, Hippeläinen M, Farin P, *et al*. Interobserver variability in measuring the dimensions of the abdominal aorta: comparison of ultrasound and computed tomography. *Eur J Vasc Endovasc Surg* 1996; **12**(2): 230–237.

34 Lederle FA, Wilson SE, Johnson GR, *et al*. Variability in measurement of abdominal aortic aneurysms. *J Vasc Surg* 1995; **21**(6): 945–952.

35 Nordon IM, Hinchliffe RJ, Malkawi AH, *et al*. Validation of DynaCT in the morphological assessment of abdominal aortic aneurysm for endovascular repair. *J Endovasc Ther* 2010; **17**(2): 183–189.

36 Wiginton CD, Kelly B, Oto A, *et al*. Gadolinium-based contrast exposure, nephrogenic systemic fibrosis, and gadolinium detection in tissue. *AJR Am J Roentgenol* 2008; **190**(4): 1060–1068.

37 Coscas R, Kobeiter H, Desgranges P, *et al*. Technical aspects, current indications, and results of chimney grafts for juxtarenal aortic aneurysms. *J Vasc Surg* 2011; **53**(6): 1520–1527.

38 Greenberg RK, Sternbergh WC, Makaroun M, *et al*. Intermediate results of a United States multicenter trial of fenestrated endograft repair for juxtarenal abdominal aortic aneurysms. *J Vasc Surg* 2009; **50**(4): 730–737.

39 Vandy F, Criado E, Upchurch GR, *et al*. Transluminal hypogastric artery occlusion with an Amplatzer vascular plug during endovascular aortic aneurysm repair. *J Vasc Surg* 2008; **48**(5): 1121–1124.

40 Axelrod DJ, Lookstein RA, Guller J, *et al*. Inferior mesenteric artery embolization before endovascular aneurysm repair: technique and initial results. *J Vasc Interv Radiol* 2004; **15**(11): 1263–1267.

41 Chuter TA, Donayre C, Wendt G. Bifurcated stent-grafts for endovascular repair of abdominal aortic aneurysm. *Surg Endosc* 1994; **8**(7): 800–802.

42 Duffy JM, Rolph R, Waltham M. Stent graft types for endovascular repair of abdominal aortic aneurysms. *Cochrane Database Syst Rev* 2015; **9**: CD008447.

43 White GH, Yu W, May J, Chaufour X, Stephen MS. Endoleak as a complication of endoluminal grafting of abdominal aortic aneurysms: classification, incidence, diagnosis, and management. *J Endovasc Surg* 1997; **4**(2): 152–168.

44 Brewster DC, Jones JE, Chung TK, *et al*. Long-term outcomes after endovascular abdominal aortic aneurysm repair: the first decade. *Ann Surg* 2006; **244**(3): 426.

45 Sadat U, Boyle JR, Walsh SR, *et al*. Endovascular vs open repair of acute abdominal aortic aneurysms—a systematic review and meta-analysis. *J Vasc Surg* 2008; **48**(1): 227–236.

46 Dangas G, O'Connor D, Firwana B, *et al*. Open versus endovascular stent graft repair of abdominal aortic aneurysms: a meta-analysis of randomized trials. *JACC Cardiovasc Interv* 2012; **5**(10): 1071–1080.

47 Firwana B, Ferwana M, Hasan R, *et al*. Open versus endovascular stent graft repair of abdominal aortic aneurysms: do we need more randomized clinical trials? *Angiology* 2014; **65**(8): 677–682.

CHAPTER 74

Acute and Chronic Mesenteric Ischemia

Robert J. Rosen, Amit Jain, and Jennifer Drury

Lenox Hill Heart and Vascular Institute, New York, NY, USA

Mesenteric ischemia is a relatively uncommon but potentially catastrophic clinical problem [1]. Acute mesenteric ischemia (AMI) is a true emergency which can rapidly progress to fatal intestinal gangrene if there is a delay in its diagnosis and subsequent management [2,3]. Chronic mesenteric ischemia (CMI) has more insidious presentation and is usually encountered in patients with widespread atherosclerotic vascular disease. The classic presentation of CMI, abdominal angina, is characterized by postprandial abdominal pain and weight loss secondary to "food fear" [4]. In spite of the similar anatomic location of the pathophysiology in both acute and chronic forms of mesenteric ischemia, the difference in their clinical presentation and management mandate separate consideration of these conditions.

Acute mesenteric ischemia

AMI is most commonly associated with acute occlusion of the superior mesenteric artery, either embolic or thrombotic (Figure 74.1). Most emboli originate in the heart secondary to atrial fibrillation, myocardial ischemia, valvular heart disease, left ventricular aneurysm, or extensive atherosclerotic aortic disease. Acute obstruction can also be seen in the setting of aortic dissection or as a complication of aortic surgery or endovascular interventions. While embolic disease is generally considered the most frequent cause of acute ischemia, in situ mesenteric thrombosis was actually found to be a more frequent cause of AMI in several recent reviews [2,5–7]. The sudden onset of generalized abdominal pain with pre-existing symptoms of CMI (intestinal angina, weight loss) suggests acute thrombosis of advanced atherosclerotic lesions in the mesenteric vasculature. Cholesterol crystal embolization can also cause AMI and should be suspected in an elderly person with widespread atherosclerotic vascular disease who has severe abdominal pain, out of proportion to their physical examination, hours after a recent diagnostic or therapeutic catheter-based vascular intervention [8]. Cutaneous mottling of the trunk and lower extremities often accompanies this scenario.

As mortality secondary to AMI increases exponentially once transmural necrosis of bowel sets in, it is of paramount importance to make the correct diagnosis early and intervene as quickly as possible [2]. Irreversible transmural necrosis of the bowel wall can

develop in 6–12 hours, depending on the level of arterial occlusion, the presence of collateral flow, and the patient's overall circulatory status. A high clinical suspicion is the key, as diagnosis is often delayed because of non-specific clinical findings. Abdominal pain is of sudden onset and severe but is generally not localized early on. Localization of this pain with peritoneal signs suggests transmural necrosis of bowel. Physical examination is usually unremarkable with occasional abdominal distension and diarrhea, which may become bloody as time progresses secondary to mucosal sloughing. Laboratory findings are non-specific and include an elevated white blood cell (WBC) count, lactic acidosis (highly sensitive but relatively non-specific), and increased serum amylase levels in about half of these patients [2,3,5,9]. More recent experimental studies have suggested the possible value of tests including serum alpha-glutathione S-transferase (alpha-GST) and cobalt albumin binding assay (CABA) [10,11].

Imaging studies should include plain films of the abdomen which can demonstrate an ileus or gasless abdomen. When findings such as air in the bowel wall (pneumatosis intestinalis), mucosal edema ("thumbprinting"), free air under the diaphragm or air in the portal system are identified, the ischemia is well advanced and the mortality rate is very high. Computed tomography (CT) scans will show these findings at a much earlier stage, while CT angiography will often demonstrate the actual site of vascular compromise as well as revealing any associated pathology such as aortic dissection [12]. A recent study evaluating the accuracy of biphasic mesenteric multidetector CT angiography in mesenteric ischemia showed a positive predictive value of 100% and a negative predictive value of 94% [13].

In spite of the accuracy of CT imaging techniques, selective angiography remains the gold standard for making the diagnosis of acute intestinal ischemia, providing specific information on the location of the obstruction as well as the presence of residual flow through either the superior mesenteric artery (SMA) or collateral pathways. The angiographic study should be started by performing flush aortography in the anteroposterior (AP) and lateral projections, as it is essential to evaluate the origins of the celiac and mesenteric arteries, the most frequent sites of atherosclerotic disease. The aortogram can also show other sites of embolization (especially in the spleen or kidneys), as well as demonstrating the

Interventional Cardiology: Principles and Practice, Second Edition. Edited by George D. Dangas, Carlo Di Mario, and Nicholas N. Kipshidze.
© 2017 John Wiley & Sons, Ltd. Published 2017 by John Wiley & Sons, Ltd.

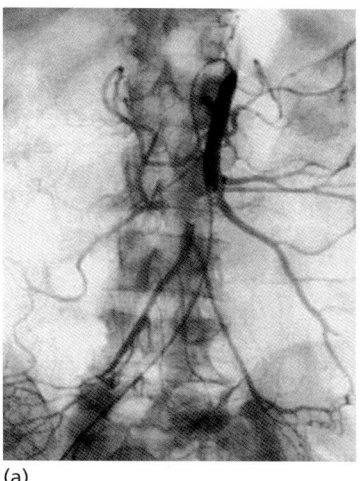 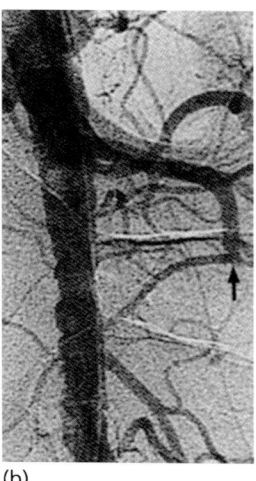

(a) **(b)**

Figure 74.1 AP selective superior mesenteric artery (SMA) study (a) and lateral (b) aortogram demonstrating acute embolic occlusion (arrow) of SMA with distal reconstitution of branches. Lateral aortogram should be performed initially to visualize the SMA origin and prevent distal embolization.

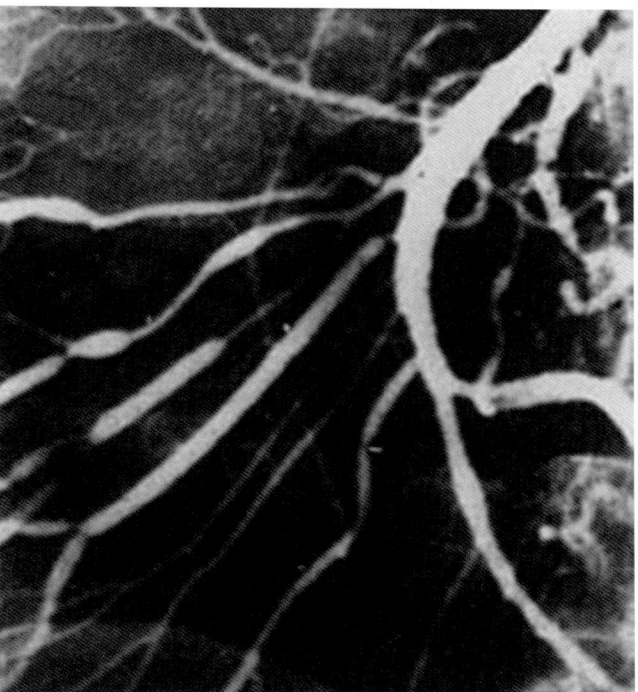

Figure 74.2 SMA angiogram in non-occlusive mesenteric ischemia (NOMI) associated with shock state. Note the irregular areas of segmental vasoconstriction.

status of the inferior mesenteric and hypogastric arteries. Selective studies are then performed, using prolonged injections of contrast with imaging of the arterial, mucosal, and portal phases. Having a catheter in place also provides access for initiating endovascular treatment, including thrombolysis, vasodilator infusions, and stenting. Previously, catheter-based intervention has been infrequently used to treat AMI, as reflected in the American Gastroenterological Association (AGA) guidelines which generally recommended laparotomy after the diagnosis was confirmed [14].

Thrombolysis, both pharmacologic and mechanical, has been reported in some series when there has been early diagnosis [15,16]. The time required for complete lysis may not always be available, as the window for restoring the blood flow is limited and the potential risk of distal embolization is high. Thrombolytic therapy should only be considered when the diagnosis has been made within 8 hours of the onset of abdominal pain, and should not be used when there is evidence of gastrointestinal bleeding or transmural infarction. The most common lytic agent used is tissue plaminigen activator (tPA), which is infused selectively into the occluded artery (nearly always the SMA) with or without an initial bolus of the drug. If, after 4 hours of initiating the infusion, there is no evidence of significant clot lysis, or if there is evidence of thrombus progression or clinical deterioration, the infusion should be stopped and an open surgical approach initiated. The use of endovascular interventions for AMI is on the rise [5,7,17] and has been even proposed by some authors to be the primary treatment modality given its reduced complications and improved outcomes [12].

In the setting of acute thrombosis of an atherosclerotic plaque, Wyers *et al.* [18] recently reported a hybrid approach to retrograde open SMA stenting (ROMS) in AMI during the emergency laparotomy to assess and resect non-viable bowel if necessary. They proposed local thromboendarterectomy of the SMA inferior to the transverse colon mesentery and a patch angioplasty. This was followed by a retrograde cannulation of the SMA and stenting of the proximal lesion.

Non-occlusive mesenteric ischemia (NOMI) is sometimes encountered in critically ill patients as one of the manifestations of

a shock state. The patient may be so ill that diagnosis is delayed until it is too late for treatment. The patient is generally in a low flow state secondary to cardiogenic shock or septic shock and is often on a high dose vasopressor agent. A high index of suspicion in any patient who develops abdominal pain in the suggested clinical settings leads to the diagnosis which is most often confirmed by endoscopy and contrast angiography. Angiography will typically show diffuse or irregular vasoconstriction (Figure 74.2) in the mesenteric circulation and the treatment is primarily directed at improving the overall hemodynamic status of the patient. Catheter directed intra-arterial infusion of vasodilator drugs into the SMA, particularly papaverine, has been used to improve flow to the intestine in this setting [19,20].

Mesenteric venous thrombosis (MVT), particularly of the superior mesenteric vein (SMV), is a rare cause of bowel ischemia. Presentation is similar to other causes of AMI but with a more insidious onset of diffuse abdominal pain progressing over a few days with or without nausea, vomiting or diarrhea and can progress to signs of localized peritonitis with eventual transmural bowel necrosis [21]. Direct injury, hypercoagulable states (particularly factor V Leiden, protein C, protein S, antiphospholipid antibodies, prothrombin gene mutation), dehydration, sepsis, laparoscopic surgery, and portal venous congestion secondary to cirrhosis or congestive heart failure (CHF) are the usual risk factors [22,23]. An increasing number of MVT have been recently reported after laparoscopic bariatric surgeries [24,25]. Diagnosis is usually made by the radiologist on the contrast CT scan performed for abdominal pain or by the surgeon intraoperatively at the time of bowel resection. MVT usually extends into the portal and splenic venous trunks. Systemic anticoagulation with bowel rest and parenteral nutrition is treatment of choice for patients without peritonitis.

Patients with persistent symptoms or deterioration while on anti-coagulation benefit from endovascular thrombolysis with or without stenting of the portomesenteric axis to maintain flow [26,27]. Compared with systemic anticoagulation, early mechanical or pharmacologic thrombolysis of acute porto-mesenteric venous thrombosis via transjugular or percutaneous transhepatic approach prevents progression of bowel ischemia in the short term and in the long term prevents development of portal hypertension [27].

Acute aortic dissection involving the abdominal aorta can cause malperfusion syndrome and AMI when the dissection flap causes either a dynamic or static obstruction of the visceral arterial origins. CT or magnetic resonance (MR) angiograms are crucial in making a diagnosis. Surgical repair of the proximal intimal tear is the most effective treatment for type A dissection [28]. Endovascular treatment of acute complicated type B dissection with malperfusion syndrome has a low morbidity and mortality compared to open repair and can now be considered the therapy of choice [28–30]. This involves covering the proximal site of aortic intimal tear via stent graft, re-expansion of true aortic lumen with or without a stent, obliteration of false lumen, and restoration of flow to the distal aorta and all its branches. In some cases of aortic dissection, distal reperfusion involves stenting of the visceral branches and endovascular fenestration of the aortic septum. Percutaneous fenestration can be achieved with either a re-entry needle or the stiff end of the 0.014-inch wire followed by balloon angioplasty to 12–15 mm. Open surgical approach to malperfusion syndrome is by direct resection of the dissecting septum with direct repair of the ostia of visceral vessels.

Vasculitis affecting small and medium size vessels is a rare cause of mesenteric ischemia [31]. Polyarteritis nodosa, Buerger's disease, systemic lupus erythematosus, and Behçet's disease can involve mesenteric vessels, causing small bowel ischemia leading to mucosal sloughing, bleeding, or transmural necrosis and gangrene. Takayasu's disease affects the visceral aorta and causes narrowing of major branches with eventual fibrosis and scaring which can lead to thrombosis and extensive mesenteric ischemia.

Chronic mesenteric ischemia

CMI is nearly always the result of atherosclerotic stenosis or occlusion of the SMA. The prevalence of asymptomatic mesenteric artery stenosis—peak systolic velocity (PSV) >200 cm/s for celiac and >270 cm/s for SMA—can be as high as 17.5 % in the elderly population [32]. The typical presentation consists of postprandial abdominal pain, progressing to "food fear," and eventually leading to weight loss, which is often dramatic [4]. These patients very often go through a prolonged series of diagnostic studies to rule out other common gastrointestinal disorders before the correct diagnosis of CMI is considered, as the initial symptoms are non-specific and can mimic so many other disorders. CMI is more common in women, and there is invariably a history of extensive atherosclerotic vascular disease. While the gastrointestinal tract is normally supplied by three vascular trunks (celiac, SMA, and inferior mesenteric artery; IMA), extensive collateralization between them allows the body to compensate for a significant degree of occlusive disease. Occlusion or stenosis of the celiac trunk is actually fairly common, either caused by atherosclerosis or extrinsic compression by the arcuate ligament of the diaphragm (median arcuate ligament syndrome, discussed later). Isolated celiac arterial disease, either stenosis or occlusion, is nearly always asymptomatic because of extensive collateralization from the SMA, primarily via the gastroduodenal

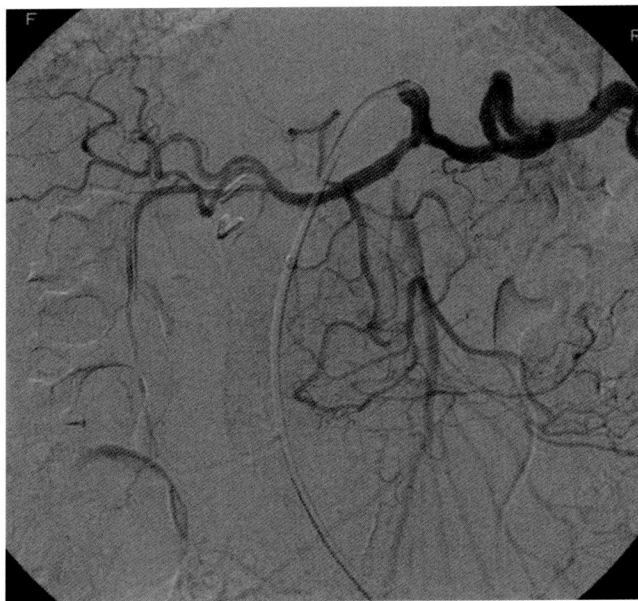

Figure 74.3 Celiac arteriogram shows occlusion of SMA at its origin with reconstitution via gastroduodenal artery collaterals. Celiac occlusions are common and usually asymptomatic. SMA occlusions are much more likely to be associated with visceral ischemia.

arcade [32]. Similarly, the much smaller IMA commonly becomes occluded as a result of infrarenal aortic atherosclerosic disease or aneurysm formation and this is also generally asymptomatic because of the collaterals from the SMA and hypogastric circulation. The SMA, conversely, is the critical vessel for maintaining visceral flow and its occlusion is nearly always clinically significant (Figure 74.3).

Aside from the history and obvious cachexia, there are few specific clinical findings to suggest the diagnosis. Abdominal bruits, while considered a classic physical finding, are often appreciated retrospectively after the diagnosis has been made. With the widespread availability of CT and MR angiography, the diagnosis can now be made earlier than in the past, when angiography was required [33]. Color flow Doppler imaging is now being used increasingly as a cost-effective and non-invasive modality to diagnose mesenteric arterial stenosis. Currently, catheter angiography is performed primarily to confirm the diagnosis, allow treatment planning, and in selected cases to carry out endovascular intervention. Involvement of the SMA by atherosclerosis is fairly stereotypical and is nearly always confined to its origin and proximal few centimeters of the vessel with normal distal anatomy. The involvement resembles that found in the renal artery in that the process is an extension of the aortic wall disease into the ostium of the vessel. This localized nature of the disease makes it suitable for both surgical and endovascular treatments. The choice of treatment is somewhat controversial at present, with each approach having strong advocates.

Median arcuate ligament (MAL) syndrome, the existence of which is still challenged by several authors, is the postprandial pain complex, weight loss and abdominal bruit associated with dynamic obstruction of celiac artery trunk by the fibers of median arcuate ligament. Elevated PSV at end expiration on duplex ultrasound may point to a diagnosis [34]. CT angiography can show the relationship of the narrow portion of the celiac artery to the diaphragm and also highlight post-stenotic dilation [35]. Recently, minimally invasive combined modality of treatment via both laparoscopic release of MAL and endovascular treatment of the celiac artery have been proposed [36]. Late follow-up in one of the largest case series reported a 76% freedom from symptoms in those treated with both celiac decompression and revascularization versus only 53% in those treated with decompression alone [37]. Angioplasty alone as a treatment of MAL syndrome has been associated with failures [38–40]. It has also been theorized that the symptoms may be secondary to compression of the celiac ganglion, which is located on top of the celiac artery, and relief of symptoms can occur with celiac ganglion block [41].

The primary issues in the treatment of CMI concern the morbidity and mortality of the initial procedure and durability of the results. Traditionally, open surgical repair has been the standard for CMI. Open revascularizations are durable with a 81–92% symptom-free survival at 3–5 year follow-up [42–46]. The disadvantages of open repair are higher morbidity (20–30%) and mortality (4–15%) with prolonged hospitalization [42–44,46].

The last two decades have seen an increasing trend toward endovascular management of CMI (Figure 74.4) as the first line of intervention [47,48]. Several retrospective studies from high volume centers comparing their open with endovascular results for CMI have shown a similar incidence of in-hospital morbidity and mortality [17,49,50]. However, a few others have noted similar mortality but higher morbidity with open repair [43]. In the analysis of the Nationwide Inpatient Sample, the mortality was lower after percutaneous transluminal angioplasty/stent compared to open bypass in CMI (3.7% vs. 13%; p <0.01) [48].

In a recent review of such retrospective studies comparing open with endovascular repair [45], overall results were comparable between the two modes of treatment in terms of technical success (100% vs. 95%) and immediate pain relief (93% vs. 88%). Endovascular repair has the advantage of decreased short-term morbidity but the disadvantage of decreased long-term primary patency compared with open repair (58% vs. 90% at 1 year [49]; 27% vs. 66% at 3 years [17]; and 41% vs. 88% at 5 years [43]).

Brown *et al.* [51] compared their mesenteric stenting group with an open surgical group and concluded that stent patients had lower perioperative major morbidity and shorter hospital and ICU length of stay; however, stent patients were 7 times more likely to develop restenosis, 4 times more likely to develop recurrent symptoms, and 15 times more likely to undergo reintervention.

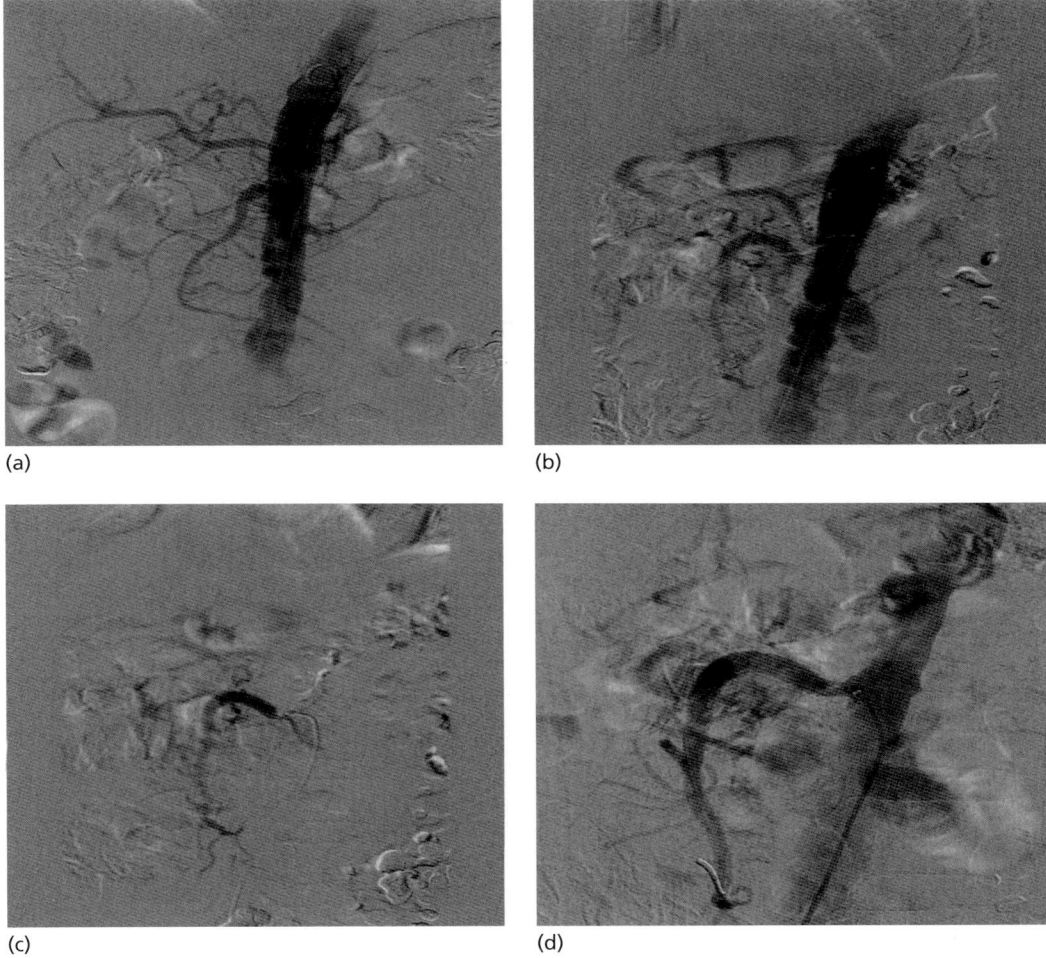

(a) (b)

(c) (d)

Figure 74.4 Patient with symptoms of chronic visceral ischemia. (a) AP aortogram shows what appears to be patent SMA. (b) Oblique view demonstrates severe ostial stenosis of SMA. (c) Selective SMA study shows the proximal stenosis more clearly. (d) Post placement of stent with resolution of stenosis. No effort is made to match the caliber of the post-stenotic dilatation.

Endovascular therapy for CMI offers the advantage of early recovery, less short-term morbidity and shorter length of stay in hospital; despite high recurrence and re-intervention rates it may be the ideal option in a patient with severe comorbidities and short life expectancy or poor functional status. Open repair, on the other hand, has excellent durability and should be considered the best treatment for a patient fit for surgery and with lesions not amenable to endovascular repair.

Technical considerations

Once the diagnosis of visceral ischemia is suspected, abdominal angiography should be performed. The SMA is by far the most critical of the three visceral trunks and because of its size and anatomic alignment with the aorta it is the vessel most frequently involved by embolus. The study should begin with a flush aortogram using a pigtail catheter in AP and lateral projections to identify the origins and proximal segments of the celiac and superior mesenteric arteries. Starting with selective catheterizations risks showering proximal emboli distally, which might turn a simple embolectomy into a case of multiple distal occlusions that cannot be salvaged. As a rule, acute thrombosis of a pre-existing stenosis of the SMA will present as an ostial or proximal occlusion, as the plaque is usually an aortic process extending into the origin of the vessel. An acute embolus, on the contrary, is typically cardiac in origin and more often lodges in the SMA beyond a few centimeters from its ostium, usually at the origin of the middle colic artery. Even in the presence of an acute embolic occlusion, angiography will nearly always demonstrate some distal reconstitution of mesenteric branches. Once it has been determined that the ostium is free of thrombus, a selective catheter (Cobra 2 or Sos) can be used to study the SMA in order to demonstrate the extent of occlusion, the site of reconstitution, as well as evidence of any other process such as a low-flow state (non-occlusive mesenteric ischemia), or mesenteric venous thrombosis. In general, if the patient is an operative candidate, operative embolectomy should be carried out immediately and the viability of the bowel can be assessed at the same time.

However, if the lesion is deemed amenable to endovascular treatment, the short sheath is then replaced by a long sheath (Shuttle, Raabe, Ansel) and advanced as close to the lesion as possible. The diseased segment of the artery is crossed with a steerable but atraumatic wire which is then exchanged for a more supportive wire which will enable balloon and stent placement. There has been a general trend toward the use of coronary type wires (0.016 or 0.018 diameter), balloons, and stents instead of standard guidewires (0.035 or 0.038) because of decreased trauma and better tracking. In terms of stent selection, precise placement and superior radial strength have favored the use of balloon expandable rather than self-expanding stents in the visceral circulation. As these are generally ostial lesions, it is important to extend the stent slightly into the aortic lumen in order to prevent plaque progression and stent occlusion. Embolic protection devices have been recommended by some authors but are not at present used in most institutions performing visceral stenting. They are somewhat problematic to use in ostial lesions, and if they are positioned in the hepatic artery there is a risk of spasm or dissection of this unusually delicate vessel.

Some authors routinely use an upper extremity approach (radial, brachial, axillary) for visceral stenting because of the acute angle of take-off of the visceral trunks. In our institution, we generally start with a femoral approach, which provides more catheter control and shorter systems. Only on occasion is a change to an upper extremity approach necessary.

In a review of endovascular treatment of CMI from the Cleveland Clinic [52], most of the stents placed in mesenteric vessels were balloon expandable (91.5%) and had a mean diameter of 6.5 ± 2.2 mm, and the average length was 18.8 ± 6.4 mm. No difference was noted in the patency rates irrespective of the stent type, size, number, or the vessel treated. Oderich et al. [53], in their experience from the Mayo Clinic, used balloon-expandable stent in 98% of patients with a large profile system in 52% and femoral access in 68% versus brachial approach in 32% of patients.

Drug-eluting stents (DES) can prove useful by blocking cellular proliferation and reducing intimal hyperplasia in the treated vessel. The stent diameter of currently available DES is generally too small (<5 mm) for use in the mesenteric arteries.

Tallarita et al. [54], from the Mayo Clinic, used covered stents in four patients to treat in-stent restenosis and reported no restenosis in any of these patients as compared with a 50% second restenosis rate in those treated with PTA or bare metal stents. Erdoes et al. [55] recently reported a superior primary patency for covered stent versus bare metal stent at 18 months as 86% vs. 34%.

Controversy persists as to whether a single vessel intervention is better than multivessel treatment. While a few studies have shown equivalent outcomes after single and multiple vessel revascularization [42,46], better long-term patency and symptom-free survival of open revascularization has been attributed to a multivessel intervention. Van Petersen et al. [45] summarized the outcomes from eight recent studies comparing open with endovascular repair showing that both primary patency and freedom from recurrent symptoms were better with open surgical interventions than endovascular interventions. Similar differences have been observed in other studies [17] with proposal to improve durability of endovascular treatment by two-vessel revascularization.

Post-procedure follow-up

There are no established guidelines for follow-up of patients who had endovascular repair of their mesenteric circulation. Given the high restenosis rate and reasonable success of repeat interventions it is imperative that a close follow-up is maintained. Although duplex ultrasound is not as accurate in stented vessels as in native arteries it does offer an inexpensive and easily available non-invasive objective tool to follow these patients. At our institution we routinely study patients with duplex ultrasound at 1, 3, and 6 month intervals. Duplex ultrasound velocity criteria for detecting native SMA and celiac arterial stenosis or occlusion are highly variable. Various authors have different criteria ranging from a PSV $\leq$275 cm/s to 400 cm/s in the SMA for >70% stenosis and $\leq$200 cm/s to 320 cm/s in the celiac artery for >70% stenosis [56,57]. A few others rely on end diastolic velocities of >45 cm/s for a >50% stenosis of the SMA and >55 cm/s for a >50% stenosis of the celiac artery [58,59]. There is a tendency toward higher velocities in stented celiac artery/SMAs in comparison to native arteries [60] and these criteria of the native SMAs cannot be applied to a previously stented SMAs as they overestimate the lesions [61]. Any significant change in the PSV is then followed up with a contrast imaging study to assess the situation and plan further interventions if needed (Figure 74.5). Sudden recurrence of abdominal pain can be the earliest sign of stent thrombosis. Hence, patient education is of paramount importance and they are explicitly instructed to seek urgent medical care if they experience any abdominal symptoms.

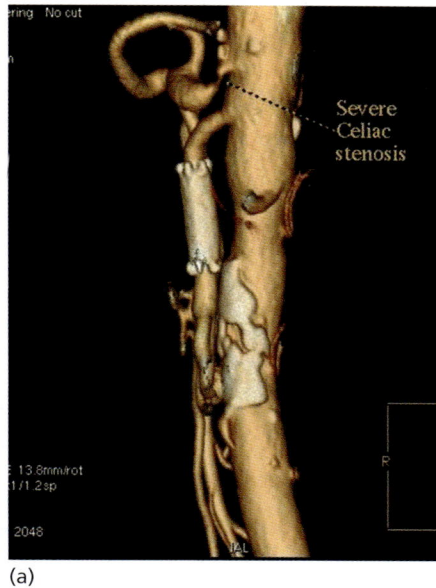
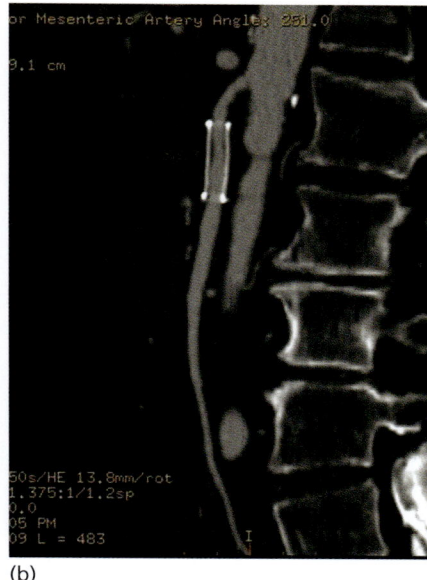

(a)   (b)

Figure 74.5 Follow-up CT angiogram 6 months after SMA stent demonstrates early intimal hyperplasia, a frequent problem in visceral stenting. Note that the celiac is severely stenotic at its origin.

Complications

Mesenteric vascular interventions can potentially cause mesenteric arterial dissection, thrombosis, distal embolization, stent dislodgment, or vessel perforation with resulting bowel ischemia or bleeding with mesenteric hematoma. Oderich et al. [53], in a review of 156 patients and 173 mesenteric stents, reported an overall morbidity of 15% and mortality of 2.5% with a 7% incidence of mesenteric artery complications during angioplasty and stent placement. They noted that factors associated with complications were use of large profile devices, non-visualization of the wire tip in the main SMA trunk, mesenteric occlusion, severe calcification, and lesion length >30 mm. Use of an embolic protection device was recommended for high risk lesions [62]. Antiplatelet therapy started before the procedure also decreased the risk of embolization and thrombosis. A recent analysis of the national inpatient sample by Schermerhorn et al. [48] showed a mortality of 3.7% for the percutaneous interventions compared to 13% after open repairs. On a mean follow-up of 29 months, Tallarita et al. [54] reported a 36% in-stent restenosis rate defined by duplex PSV >330 cm/s and angiographic stenosis of >60%.

Conclusions

Mesenteric ischemia is a relatively uncommon condition, but one where delayed diagnosis and intervention can be deadly. The condition is clearly divided into acute and chronic presentations. AMI is an extreme emergency, as delayed diagnosis and treatment will rapidly lead to intestinal infarction and high mortality. The most common cause of AMI is embolization from a cardiac source, while less commonly it can occur in the setting of acute thrombosis of a chronic atherosclerotic lesion, acute aortic dissection, or iatrogenically. Most embolic occlusions are handled surgically, as the window for restoration of mesenteric flow is short and embolectomy is a fairly straightforward undertaking. There has been an increasing use of endovascular techniques, but their role in the acute setting remains unclear.

CMI can present insidiously, and its manifestations frequently mimic other abdominal conditions so that diagnosis is often delayed. The hallmarks of the condition include postprandial pain, weight loss, and "food fear," and it is generally encountered in patients with known widespread atherosclerotic disease. The diagnosis can usually be made by CT or MR angiography and confirmed by catheter angiography. The optimal type of intervention remains controversial, with advocates of both endovascular and open surgical revascularization. Stenting can be performed safely with minimal morbidity; however, open surgical reconstruction has indisputably better long-term patency, at least at present.

Interactive multiple choice questions are available for this chapter on www.wiley.com/go/dangas/cardiology

References

1 Thomas JH, Blake K, Pierce GE, et al. The clinical course of asymptomatic mesenteric arterial stenosis. *J Vasc Surg* 1998; **27**(5): 840–844.

2 Kougias P, Lau D, El Sayed HF, et al. Determinants of mortality and treatment outcome following surgical interventions for acute mesenteric ischemia. *J Vasc Surg* 2007; **46**(3): 467–474.

3 Park VM, Gloviczki P, Cherry KJ Jr, et al. Contemporary management of acute mesenteric ischemia: factors associated with survival. *J Vasc Surg* 2002; **35**(3): 445–52.

4 Moawad J, Gewertz BL. Chronic mesenteric ischemia: clinical presentation and diagnosis. *Surg Clin North Am* 1997; **77**(2): 357–369.

5 Ryer EJ, Kalra M, Oderich GS, et al. Contemporary results of revascularization for acute mesenteric ischemia. *J Vasc Surg* 2012; **55**(6): 1682–1689.

6 Park VM, Gloviczki P, Cherry KJ Jr, et al. Contemporary management of acute mesenteric ischemia: factors associated with survival. *J Vasc Surg* 2002; **35**: 445–452.

7 Arthurs ZM, Titus J, Bannazadeh M, et al. A comparison of endovascular revascularization with traditional therapy for the treatment of acute mesenteric ischemia. *J Vasc Surg* 2011; **53**(3): 698–705.

8 Kronzon I, Saric M. Reviews in cardiovascular medicine cholesterol embolization syndrome. *Circulation* 2010; **122**: 631–641.

9 Oldenburg WA, Lau LL, Rodenberg, TJ, *et al.* Acute mesenteric ischemia: a clinical review. *Arch Intern Med* 2004; **164**(10): 1054–1062.

10 Gearhart SL, Delaney CP, Senagore AJ, *et al.* Prospective assessment of the predictive value of alpha-glutathione S-transferase for intestinal ischemia. *Am Surg* 2003; **69**: 324.

11 Polk JD, Rael LT, Craun ML, *et al.* Clinical utility of the cobalt-albumin binding assay in the diagnosis of intestinal ischemia. *J Trauma* 2008; **64**: 42.

12 Menke J. Diagnostic accuracy of multidetector CT in acute mesenteric ischemia: systematic review and meta-analysis. *Radiology* 2010; **256**(1): 93–101.

13 Aschoff AJ, Stuber G, Becker BW, *et al.* Evaluation of acute mesenteric ischemia: accuracy of biphasic mesenteric multi-detector CT angiography. *Abdom Imaging* 2009; **34**: 345.

14 Brandt LJ, Boley SJ. American Gastroenterological Association. *Gastroenterology* 2000; **118**: 951.

15 Schoots IG, Levi MM, Reekers JA, *et al.* Thrombolytic therapy for acute superior mesenteric artery occlusion. *J Vasc Interv Radiol* 2005; **16**(3): 317–329.

16 Hollingshead M, Burke CT, Mauro MA, *et al.* Transcatheter thrombolytic therapy for acute mesenteric and portal vein thrombosis. *J Vasc Interv Radiol* 2005; **16**(5): 651–661.

17 Kougias P, Huynh TT, Lin PH, *et al.* Clinical outcomes of mesenteric artery stenting versus surgical revascularization in chronic mesenteric ischemia. *Int Angiol* 2009; **28**(2): 132–137.

18 Wyers MC, Powell RJ, Nolan BW, *et al.* Retrograde mesenteric stenting during laparotomy for acute occlusive mesenteric ischemia. *J Vasc Surg* 2007; **45**: 269–275.

19 Boley SJ, Brandt LJ, Sammartano RJ. History of mesenteric ischemia: the evolution of a diagnosis and management. *Surg Clin North Am* 1997; **77**: 275.

20 Björck M, Wanhainen A. Nonocclusive mesenteric hypoperfusion syndromes: recognition and treatment. *Semin Vasc Surg* 2010; **23**(1): 54–64.

21 Rhee Ry, Gloviczki P, Mendonca CT, *et al.* Mesenteric venous thrombosis: still a lethal disease in the 1990s. *J Vasc Surg* 1994; **20**(5): 688–697.

22 Acosta S, Alhadad A, Svensson P, *et al.* Epidemiology, risk and prognosis factors in mesenteric venous thrombosis. *Br J Surg* 2008; **95**: 1245–1251.

23 James AW, Rabl C, Westphalen AC, *et al.* Portomesenteric venous thrombosis after laparoscopic surgery: a systematic literature review. *Arch Surg* 2009; **144**(6): 520–526.

24 Bellanger DE, Hargroder AG, Greenway FL. Mesenteric venous thrombosis after laparoscopic sleeve gastrectomy. *Surg Obes Relat Dis* 2010; **6**(1): 109–111.

25 DeMaria EJ, Pate V, Warthen M, *et al.* Baseline data from American Society for Metabolic and Bariatric Surgery: designated bariatric surgery centers of excellence using the bariatric outcomes longitudinal database. *Surg Obes Relat Dis* 2010; **6**(4): 347–355.

26 Suplee R, Nassiri N, Sung R, *et al.* Acute mesenteric venous thrombosis after laparoscopic duodenal switch: successful treatment using percutaneous transhepatic mechanical thrombectomy with stenting. *J Vasc Surg* 2011; **54**(3): 926.

27 DiMinno MN, Milone F, Milone M, *et al.* Endovascular thrombolysis in acute mesenteric vein thrombosis: a 3-year follow-up with the rate of short and long-term sequelae in 32 patients. *Thromb Res* 2010; **126**(4): 295–298.

28 Tsai TT, Trimarchi S, Nienaber CA. Acute aortic dissection: perspectives from the Interventional Registry of Acute Aortic Dissection (IRAD). *Eur J Vasc Endovasc Surg* 2009; **37**(2): 149–159.

29 Szeto WY, McGarvey M, Pochettino A, *et al.* Results of a new surgical paradigm: endovascular repair for acute complicated type B aortic dissection. *Ann Thorac Surg* 2008; **86**(1): 87–94.

30 Fattori R, Tsai TT, Myrmel T, *et al.* Complicated acute type B dissection: is surgery still the best option? A report from the International Registry of Acute Aortic Dissection (IRAD). *JACC Cardiovasc Interv* 2008; **1**(4): 395–402.

31 Krupski WC, Selzman CH, Whitehill TA. Unusual causes of mesenteric ischemia. *Surg Clin North Am* 1997; **77**(2): 471–502.

32 Hansen KJ, Wilson DB, Craven TE, *et al.* Mesenteric artery disease in the elderly. *J Vasc Surg* 2004; **40**(1): 45–52.

33 Horton KM, Fishman EK. Multidetector CT angiography in the diagnosis of mesenteric ischemia. *Radiol Clin North Am* 2007; **45**(2): 275–288.

34 Erden A, Yurdakul M, Cumhur T. Marked increase in flow velocities during deep expiration: a duplex Doppler sign of celiac artery compression syndrome. *Cardiovasc Interv Radiol* 1999; **22**(4): 331–332.

35 Horton KM, Talamini MA, Fishman EK. Median arcuate ligament syndrome: evaluation with CT angiography. *Radiographics* 2005; **25**(5): 1177–1182.

36 Duffy AJ, Panait L, Eisenberg D, *et al.* Management of median arcuate ligament syndrome: a new paradigm. *Ann Vasc Surg* 2009; **23**(6): 778–784.

37 Reilly LM, Ammar AD, Stoney RJ, *et al.* Late results following operative repair for celiac artery compression syndrome. *J Vasc Surg* 1985; **2**(1): 79–91.

38 Delis KT, Gloviczki P, Altuwaijri M. Median arcuate ligament syndrome: open celiac artery reconstruction and ligament division after endovascular failure. *J Vasc Surg* 2007; **46**(4): 799–802.

39 Wang X, Impeduglia T, Dubin Z, *et al.* Celiac revascularization as a requisite for treating the median arcuate ligament syndrome. *Ann Vasc Surg* 2008; **22**(4): 571–574.

40 Matsumoto AH, Angle JF, Spinosa DJ, *et al.* Percutaneous transluminal angioplasty and stenting in the treatment of chronic mesenteric ischemia: results and longterm follow-up. *J Am Coll Surg* 2002; **194**(1 Suppl): S22–S31.

41 Skiek N, Cooper LT, Duncan AA, *et al.* Median arcuate ligament syndrome: a nonvascular, vascular diagnosis. *Vasc Endovasc Surg* 2011; **45**(5): 433–437.

42 Park WM, Cherry KJ Jr, Chua HK, *et al.* Current results of open revascularization for chronic mesenteric ischemia: a standard for comparison. *J Vasc Surg* 2002; **35**(5): 853–859.

43 Oderich GS, Bower TC, Sullivan TM, *et al.* Open versus endovascular revascularization for chronic mesenteric ischemia: risk-stratified outcomes. *J Vasc Surg* 2009; **49**(6): 1472–1479.e3.

44 Mateo RB, O'Hara PJ, Hertzer NR, *et al.* Elective surgical treatment of symptomatic chronic mesenteric occlusive disease: early results and late outcomes. *J Vasc Surg* 1999; **29**(5): 821–831.

45 Van Petersen AS, Kolkman JJ, Beuk RJ, *et al.* Open or percutaneous recascularization for chronic splanchnic syndrome. *J Vasc Surg* 2010; **51**(5): 1309–1316.

46 Foley MI, Moneta GL, Abou-Zamzam AM Jr, *et al.* Revascularization of the superior mesenteric artery alone for treatment of intestinal ischemia. *J Vasc Surg* 2000; **32**(1): 37–47.

47 White CJ. Chronic mesenteric ischemia: diagnosis and management. *Prog Cardiovasc Dis* 2011; **54**(1): 36–40.

48 Schermerhorn ML, Giles KA, Hamdan AD, *et al.* Mesenteric revascularization: management and outcomes in the United States, 1988–2006. *J Vasc Surg* 2009; **50**(2): 341–348.e1.

49 Atkins MD, Kwolek CJ, LaMuraglia GM, *et al.* Surgical revascularization versus endovascular therapy for chronic mesenteric ischemia: a comparative experience. *J Vasc Surg* 2007; **45**(6): 1162–1171.

50 Kasirajan K, O'Hara PJ, Gray BH, *et al.* Chronic mesenteric ischemia: open surgery versus percutaneous angioplasty and stenting. *J Vasc Surg* 2001; **33**(1): 63–71.

51 Brown DJ, Schermerhorn ML, Powell RJ, *et al.* Mesenteric stenting for chronic mesenteric ischemia. *J Vasc Surg* 2005; **42**: 268–274.

52 Sarac TP, Altinel O, Kashyap V, *et al.* Endovascular treatment of stenotic and occluded visceral arteries for chronic mesenteric ischemia. *J Vasc Surg* 2008; **47**(3): 485–491.

53 Oderich GS, Tallarita T, Gloviczki P, *et al.* Mesenteric artery complications during angioplasty and stent placement for atherosclerotic chronic mesenteric ischemia. *J Vasc Surg* 2012; **55**(4): 1063–1071.

54 Tallarita T, Oderich GS, Macedo TA, *et al.* Reinterventions for stent restenosis in patients treated for atherosclerotic mesenteric artery disease. *J Vasc Surg* 2011; **54**(5): 1422–1429.

55 Erdoes L, Mixon H, Lesar C, *et al. Superior patency of covered stents over bare metal stents in patients with chronic mesenteric ischemia.* Orlando, FL: 2011 Society for Clinical Vascular Surgery annual meeting.

56 Moneta GL, Yeager RA, Dalman R, *et al.* Duplex ultrasound criteria for diagnosis of splanchnic artery stenosis or occlusion. *J Vasc Surg* 1991; **14**(4): 511–518.

57 AbuRahma AF, Stone PA, Srivastava M, *et al.* Mesenteric/celiac duplex ultrasound interpretation criteria revisited. *J Vasc Surg* 2012; **55**(2): 428–436.

58 Bowersox JC, Zwolak RM, Walsh DB, *et al.* Duplex ultrasonography in the diagnosis of celiac and mesenteric artery occlusive disease. *J Vasc Surg* 1991; **14**(6): 780–786.

59 Zwolak RM, Fillinger MF, Walsh DB, *et al.* Mesenteric and celiac duplex scanning: a validation study. *J Vasc Surg* 1998; **27**(6): 1078–1088.

60 AbuRahma AF, Mousa AY, Stone PA, *et al.* Duplex velocity criteria for native celiac/superior mesenteric artery stenosis vs in-stent stenosis. *J Vasc Surg* 2012; **55**(3): 730–738.

61 Mitchell EL, Chang EY, Landry GJ, *et al.* Duplex criteria for native superior mesenteric artery stenosis overestimate stenosis in stented superior mesenteric arteries. *J Vasc Surg* 2009; **50**(2): 335–340.

62 Tallarita T, Gustavo S, Oderich MD, *et al.* Embolic protection in mesenteric artery stenting. *J Vasc Surg* 2011; **54**(5): 1422–1429.

CHAPTER 75

Renal Artery Interventions

Mark Shipeng Yu, Kun Xiang, Steven T. Haller, and Christopher J. Cooper
University of Toledo, Toledo, OH, USA

Renal artery stenosis

Renal artery stenosis (RAS) is narrowing of the renal arteries, most often occurring in the main renal artery. Many etiologies are responsible for RAS, including atherosclerosis, fibromuscular dysplasia (FMD), vasculitis, congenital abnormalities, aneurysm, William's syndrome, trauma, arteriovenous malformations or fistulas, thromboemboli, extrinsic compression, radiation, and neurofibromatosis. Atherosclerosis, which accounts for approximately 90% of cases, and FMD, which is present in up to 10% of cases, are the most common etiologies. Atherosclerotic renal artery stenosis (ARAS) is caused by atherosclerotic plaque in the renal artery wall and is a chronic inflammatory process affected by multiple factors. In many individuals with ARAS, the plaques appear to be extension of aortic plaque into the ostium of the renal artery. In contrast, FMD is a non-inflammatory arterial wall dysplasia causing RAS.

RAS has been underrecognized clinically in the past. With the increasing use of non-invasive diagnostic imaging techniques such as duplex ultrasonography, computed tomography (CT) angiography, and magnetic resonance angiography [1] and increased awareness of ischemic renal disease, the diagnosis of RAS has become increasingly common. ARAS was found in about 7% of the general population older than 65 years of age when a very liberal duplex peak systolic velocity threshold of 1.8 m/s was used during community screening [2]. The prevalence of ARAS in patients with comorbidities is even higher, reaching 20% in patients with hypertension and diabetes, 25% in patients with peripheral vascular disease, and has been reported to be as high as 54% in those with congestive heart failure [3].

Natural history and clinical outcomes

ARAS can progress anatomically at the atherosclerotic lesion or in association with declining kidney function in a minority of individuals. In the pre-statin era, progression to occlusion occurred in 6% [2] to 39% [3] in patients with stenosis >60% [2] to >75% [3]; however, with appropriate medical therapy this risk is likely overstated. Several conditions have been associated with renal artery disease progression, including severity of disease and comorbid conditions such as diabetes and hypertension [4].

ARAS causes ischemic nephropathy in some individuals. Ischemic nephropathy is defined as renal dysfunction resulting from stenosis of a main renal artery [4]. ARAS has been estimated to be the cause of end-stage renal disease (ESRD) in approximately 15% of patients over age 50 who begin dialysis [5]. Chronic ischemia produces inflammation, tubulosclerosis, fibrosis, thickening of Bowman's capsule, intrarenal arterial medial thickening, and atrophy in the kidney [6]. The possible mechanisms of renal fibrosis caused by a hemodynamically significant RAS include microvascular damage, endothelial and epithelial factors, activation of renin–angiotensin–aldosterone system with subsequent vasoconstriction [7], and CD40 signaling within the proximal tubule leading to interstitial fibrosis [8].

RAS is also a potential cause of secondary hypertension, and can be present in as many as 5% of individuals with hypertension. Activation of renin–angiotensin–aldosterone systems and increased sympathetic nerve output contribute to the elevated blood pressure [9]. Patients with RAS and hypertension can be resistant to medical therapy and some develop early complications including left ventricular hypertrophy, heart failure, and renal failure.

Patients with ARAS are at high risk for fatal and non-fatal cardiovascular and renal events. It was found that ARAS is an independent predictor for mortality in patients undergoing diagnostic coronary angiography [10] and in patients with peripheral arterial disease [11]. The risk ratio (versus age-matched controls) was 3.3 for overall mortality and 5.7 for cardiovascular mortality in a cohort of patients with RAS lesions exceeding 50% [12]. The annual mortality rate in patients with ARAS was 16.3% in a Medicare analysis and was three times higher than Medicare patients without ARAS [13]. However, it is not apparent whether this relationship is attributable to the RAS per se, or whether RAS is simply a marker for more diffuse atherosclerosis.

Additionally, a strong relationship has been identified between chronic kidney disease and mortality in patients undergoing stent revascularization [14]. Patients with ARAS are 6–28 times more likely to die of a cardiovascular event than ESRD [1,15]. However, if a patient with ARAS develops ESRD and requires dialysis, the annual mortality rate approaches 36% [16]. The underlying mechanisms connecting loss of kidney function with increased mortality and non-fatal cardiovascular and renal events are not fully clear.

Interventional Cardiology: Principles and Practice, Second Edition. Edited by George D. Dangas, Carlo Di Mario, and Nicholas N. Kipshidze.
© 2017 John Wiley & Sons, Ltd. Published 2017 by John Wiley & Sons, Ltd.

The possible answers are activation of the renin–angiotensin–aldosterone and sympathetic nervous systems, associated renal insufficiency, concomitant atherosclerosis in other vascular beds, and activation/alteration of other neuroendocrine systems [17].

FMD occurs mainly in middle-aged females and involves the mid to distal renal artery and other arterial vasculatures (e.g., carotid arteries, external iliac arteries, coronary arteries, and mesenteric arteries). Most patients with FMD are asymptomatic, but resistant secondary hypertension in young patients is the most common clinical presentation. FMD can cause loss of renal mass in up to 63% of patients [18], but it rarely causes loss of renal function. Stenosis progression occurs in a minority of patients with FMD [18]; however, progression to occlusion is rare. FMD predisposes to dissection and aneurysm because of the dysplasia of arterial walls.

Indications for screening

Currently, there is controversy regarding the appropriate use of screening for the detection of RAS. In younger individuals with unexplained hypertension, screening for FMD is often warranted as identification of FMD can lead to a hypertension cure with balloon angioplasty. However, in older individuals who might be suspected as having ARAS, the value of screening is less certain. With several convincingly negative trials for revascularization of ARAS, the role for screening is under debate. The most recent American College of Cardiology/American Heart Association (ACC/AHA) guideline on peripheral arterial diseases published in 2013 suggested screening renal arterial disease with diagnostic studies for several clinical situations [19]. However, these recommendations predate the results of the CORAL study. As a result it may be reasonable to limit screening for ARAS to patients with suspected RAS who have clearly failed management with aggressive medical therapy.

Class I indications:
- Onset of hypertension with age <30 years old (level of evidence B);
- Onset of severe hypertension after the age of 55 years (level of evidence B);
- Certain clinical characteristics: (i) accelerated hypertension (sudden and persistent worsening of previously controlled hypertension); (ii) resistant hypertension; and (iii) malignant hypertension (hypertension with acute end-organ damage) (level of evidence C);
- New azotemia or worsening renal function after the administration of an angiotensin-converting enzyme (ACE) inhibitor or an angiotensin receptor blocker (ARB) (level of evidence B);
- Unexplained atrophic kidney or a discrepancy in size between two kidneys of >1.5 cm (level of evidence B);
- Sudden unexplained pulmonary edema, especially with azotemia (level of evidence B).

Class IIa indications Unexplained renal failure, including starting dialysis or renal transplantation (level of evidence B).

Class IIb indications Multiple vessel coronary artery disease without evidence of peripheral arterial disease at the time or unexplained congestive heart failure or refractory angina (level of evidence C).

Diagnosis

Duplex ultrasonography, computed tomographic angiography (CT angiography, or CTA), and magnetic resonance angiography (MRA) are recommended by guideline as screening tests to establish the diagnosis of RAS [19]. When these tests are inconclusive and clinical suspicion is high, catheter angiography is the next step [19]. Captopril test, captopril renal scintigraphy, and selective renal vein renin measurement are not recommended as screening tests to establish the diagnosis [19]. Duplex ultrasonography is the most cost-effective study, although it is dependent on the technician's proficiency and experience in the procedure. In a high-volume and experienced center, duplex ultrasonography is the preferred method of screening. CTA has better resolution than MRA, but CTA carries risk of contrast nephrotoxicity and ionizing radiation. MRA with gadolinium contrast cannot be used in patients with advanced chronic kidney disease and patients with certain devices, because of electromagnetic interference.

Duplex ultrasonography
Duplex ultrasonography has a sensitivity of 75–98% and specificity of 87–100% for RAS, and 67% sensitivity in identifying accessory renal arteries [20]. Duplex can evaluate the artery anatomy, blood flow velocity and waveform, and kidney size. The peak systolic velocity (PSV) should be measured at the origin, proximal portion, at the mid aspect, near the helium, and at any site of color aliasing or suspected stenosis [21]. Doppler waveforms should be recorded within the stenosis and distal to the stenosis. If there are accessory renal arteries, the PSV should be measured. The aortic PSV is used to calculate the ratio of the PSV in the renal artery to the aorta at the level of renal artery. Many Doppler velocity criteria have been proposed to diagnose RAS. The most commonly accepted diagnostic criteria for RAS by duplex ultrasound are listed in Table 75.1 [2,20]. In clinical practice a PSV of 180 cm/s is sensitive at the expense of poor specificity. This high sensitivity threshold is appropriate for the purpose of screening but because of poor specificity it should not be used to confirm the diagnosis. For confirmation, a velocity of >300 cm/s is more useful [22].

Color Doppler interrogation of the segmental or interlobar arteries within the kidney can provide additional clues of RAS. A significant stenosis delays the systolic rise in the arteries distal to the stenosis, shown as tardus parvus waveform [23]. The significant stenosis (e.g., >60%) will also cause slowing (<3 m/s²) or absence of the early systolic peak or notch at the beginning of systole in the intrarenal segmental and interlobar arteries [23]. The time from the start of the systolic upstroke to the first peak is the systolic acceleration time, with >0.07 s indicating main RAS >60%. The renal arterial resistive index (RI) is calculated with the following formula:

$$RI = \left(\text{peak systolic velocity} - \text{end diastolic velocity} \right) / \text{peak systolic velocity}.$$

Duplex ultrasound evaluation after a renal artery stent procedure should include recording a PSV in the proximal renal artery, within the stent, and distal to the stent [21]. The diagnostic criteria for in-stent restenosis vary among clinicians, from criteria same as native RAS in Table 75.1, to a higher velocity (e.g., >225 cm/s [24], >280 cm/s [25]), or a renal : aortic ratio >4.5 [25]).

Computed tomographic angiography
CTA has a sensitivity of 94% and specificity of 60–90% in detection of ARAS [26,27]. The better spatial resolution of CTA than MRA enables it to detect small accessory renal arteries. The specificity of CTA is not as efficient as MRA. However, CTA can be used in patients who are claustrophobic, intolerant of long time positioning, and have a non-MRI-friendly implanted device. Because CTA

Table 75.1 Diagnosis criteria of renal artery stenosis by duplex ultrasound.

Stenosis severity percentage	Peak systolic velocity (PSV)	Renal : aortic ratio (RAR)	Post-stenotic turbulence
<60%	>180 cm/s	<3.5	No
>60%	>180 cm/s	>3.5	Yes
Total occlusion	None	Not available	Not available

sees the thickness of the vessel wall, and positive remodeling occurs commonly in atherosclerosis, simply measuring the degree of narrowing at the stenosis can overestimate the severity of the lesion. A more reliable strategy is to compare the degree of narrowing at the stenosis to the caliber of the more distal renal artery, after any post-stenotic dilatation. Extensive calcification in the renal artery and adjacent aorta can be a challenge for CTA image interpretation. CTA also cannot be used in patients with significantly impaired kidney function because of the risk of contrast-induced nephropathy, unless the benefit outweighs the risk.

Magnetic resonance angiography

MRA has a sensitivity of 93% and specificity of 91% for ARAS [26]. MRA has better specificity than CTA. MRA also offers the benefit of avoiding iodinated contrast and radiation exposure. But MRA cannot be used in advanced chronic kidney disease because of the risk of systemic fibrosis from accumulated gadolinium-based contrast medium used in MRA. It is also not used in patients with non-MRI-friendly devices and who are claustrophobic.

Catheter angiography

Renal angiography, typically using the digital subtraction technique, provides the most accurate diagnosis when non-invasive studies are inconclusive and clinical suspicion is high. With angiography, the visual estimation of diameter reduction compared to the reference vessel is used for stenosis severity evaluation (e.g., 60%, 70%, and 80% stenosis, etc.). Angiography can also evaluate the anatomy of the renal vasculature including the intrarenal vessels and accessory renal arteries, and the gross anatomy of the kidney. While ARAS most often (about 90% cases) presents as ostial stenosis, FMD often presents uniquely on angiography as a "string of beads."

However, of concern has been the practice of performing selective catheter angiography for the detection of RAS using preformed catheters to engage the renal artery. Often excellent image quality can be obtained with aortography, performed at the level of the renal arteries, using modest volumes of contrast (10–15 mL per injection). This strategy is superior to selective angiography for the following reasons:
- Avoids aortic scraping that can lead to atheroembolization;
- More often identifies origins of renal arteries, when multiple arteries are present;
- Permits thoughtful catheter selection if selective angiography becomes necessary; and
- Oftent results in lower total contrast dosing.

Translesional pressure gradient, pressure ratio of distal renal artery to aorta, and renal fractional flow reserve

Several additional parameters can be measured at the time of angiography. The translesional pressure gradient can be measured across the stenosis, comparing aortic pressure with pressure in the renal artery after the stenosis. The most reliable method uses an 0.014-inch pressure sensing guidewire as catheter-based gradients can grossly overestimate lesion severity [28].

Most stenoses that are truly >80% stenosis by angiography will have a pressure gradient [1]. For 60–80% lesions, it is considered hemodynamically significant if the peak systolic translesional pressure gradient is >20 mmHg [1]. The ratio of peak systolic pressure distal to the lesion over peak systolic aortic pressure at the renal artery level is called renal : aorta pressure ratio. A ratio of <0.9 is associated with increased renin production and the stenosis of this type is considered as hemodynamically significant [21,29]; however, these data were derived from acute ischemia experiments and may not be as relevant in the setting of chronic ischemia. The renal fractional flow reserve (FFR) has been studied during angiography using intrarenal papaverine and an FFR <0.8 is considered as severe stenosis [29]. Recently, the renal FFR has been correlated with residual plaque volume and clinical outcome [30]. These parameters (e.g., visual estimation of stenosis severity, translesional pressure gradient, and FFR) were shown to correlate with each other in some studies [29], but not in others [30].

In individuals with FMD, translesional pressure gradients are often extremely helpful in clinically differentiating "cosmetic" FMD (stenosis without hemodynamic significance) from those that are functionally significant. Furthermore, repeating pressure gradients after each balloon angioplasty provides an objective tool to indicate when the lesion has been adequately dilated and the webs are sufficiently disrupted to allow normal blood flow and pressure. Importantly, though, there are no trials that show whether treatment of patients with ARAS with some threshold for stenosis severity (pressure gradient, angiographic percent stenosis, renal FFR) results in improved clinical outcome when comparing patients managed medically with those undergoing revascularization.

Treatment options for ARAS

While balloon angioplasty is the standard interventional treatment for FMD, for ARAS there has been considerable debate over the past several decades about which treatment modality is better when considering medical therapy versus stenting. Fortunately, several recent clinical trials provide more evidence about this choice.

Three randomized trials have been completed that directly compared medical therapy alone with medical therapy with stenting: the Cardiovascular Outcomes in Renal Atherosclerotic Lesions (CORAL) trial, the trial of STent placement and blood pressure and lipid-lowering for the prevention of progression of renal dysfunction caused by Atherosclerotic ostial stenosis of the Renal artery (STAR), and the Angioplasty and Stenting for Renal Artery Lesions (ASTRAL) trial [1,31,32]. The STAR trial [32] was a randomized study that tested whether stenting could reduce by 50% the proportion of patients that experienced a 20% decline in GFR. The authors of STAR concluded that "confidence bounds are compatible with both efficacy and harm, so the finding is inconclusive."

The ASTRAL trial [31] enrolled 806 patients but failed to demonstrate an improvement in the primary endpoint, slope of reciprocal creatinine (-0.0713×10^{-3} vs. -0.13×10^{-3} μm/L/year; p = 0.06). This difference was neither statistically nor clinically significant, as were the findings of the secondary analyses from ASTRAL.

The most recent trial, Cardiovascular Outcomes in Renal Atherosclerotic Lesions trial (CORAL) [1] published in 2014, was designed to compare optimal medical therapy alone with stenting with optimal medical therapy, with a primary endpoint of the occurrence of major cardiovascular or renal events. This was defined as a composite of death from cardiovascular or renal causes, stroke, myocardial infarction, hospitalization for congestive heart failure, progressive renal insufficiency, or the need for permanent renal replacement therapy. In CORAL, 947 patients with ARAS and either hypertension or chronic kidney disease were randomized into two groups: optimal medical therapy (ARB, atorvastatin, and an antiplatelet agent, with or without thiazide or amlodipine), or optimal medical therapy with stenting. There was no significant difference in the occurrence of the primary composite endpoint, or any of its individual components, between the stent group and medical therapy-only group, and no difference in all-cause mortality. Systolic blood pressure was modestly lower in the stent group than in the medical therapy-only group (-2.3 mmHg; 95% CI -4.4 to -0.2 mmHg; p = 0.03), and the difference persisted throughout the follow-up period. The CORAL study showed that, when added to a background of high-quality medical therapy, contemporary renal artery stenting provides no incremental benefit for patients with ARAS. Thus, it is clear that optimal medical therapy without stenting is the preferred management strategy for the majority of people with ARAS.

Stenting in specific populations with ARAS

Several studies suggest that stenting can improve kidney function in patients with stenosis affecting all of the kidney parenchyma; however, CORAL showed no clinical advantage in this subgroup with global renal ischemia. A study by Watson et al. [33] focused on patients with progressive, but not severe, chronic renal insufficiency and with global high-grade stenosis. Renal artery stenting was performed in 33 patients who displayed a serum creatinine >1.5 mg/dL (mean 2.1 mg/dL), and found an improvement in the rate of loss of GFR, when compared with the rate of loss prior to the procedure. An additional study found favorable responses to revascularization for patients with ARAS and rapidly declining kidney function [34]. However, as stated earlier, when compared with a contemporary group of individuals managed medically, there is no evidence that stenting improves kidney function more than medical therapy alone.

In a single center, observational study in patients with ARAS presenting with "flash pulmonary edema," a term for acute heart failure, revascularization reduced mortality (HR 0.4, 95% CI 0.2–0.9; p = 0.01), but did not affect cardiovascular event or ESRD rates [35]. This observation is confounded significantly though by significant age differences between the medical therapy and revascularized subjects. The small observational studies have described cohorts of patients with RAS with acute heart failure that appeared to benefit from renal artery revascularization [36,37]. In general terms these cohorts demonstrated that 75% of subjects undergoing revascularization had no further episodes after treatment [36,37]. Whether similar results would be seen with medical therapy is not known.

There have been efforts in developing predictors that can identify subgroups of patients who will benefit from revascularization.

As assessed by MRI, a high ratio of renal parenchymal volume to single-kidney GFR was reported to be an indicator of improvement in GFR after revascularization in a study of 50 patients [38]. High blood oxygen level-dependent (BOLD) MRI signal to single kidney isotopic GFR has been shown to be a predictor for improvement of renal function after revascularization in a clinical study of 28 patients [39]. Pre-intervention brain natriuretic peptide (BNP) levels of >80 pg/mL were reported to be predictive of a response to revascularization in a study of 27 patients [40]; however, this finding was not replicated when it was tested in a larger cohort of individuals [41]. On the other hand, a renal resistance index of more than 80 by duplex Doppler ultrasound was reported to be an indicator of unresponsiveness to revascularization [42]; yet again the finding was not replicated in subsequent studies [43,44]. More data are needed to draw a convincing conclusion.

Medical therapy of ARAS

The ultimate goal of ARAS treatment is the reduction of mortality (mainly cardiovascular and renal mortality) and morbidity (adverse cardiovascular and renal events), and prevention of complications. Medical therapy is the cornerstone of care for patients with ARAS. There are unfortunately few comparative data between different regimens of medical therapy. Clearly, anti-atherosclerotic therapies are indicated, such as lipid-lowering agents, especially statins. Antiplatelet therapy, diabetes management, and hypertension medications are all indicated in patients with ARAS. Lifestyle modification is also important such as smoking cessation, exercise, and weight reduction. Previously it was advised that ACE/ARBs should be avoided in this setting; however, data suggest the risk to be low [45,46]. ACEI/ARB treatment in observational studies is associated with a significant mortality and morbidity benefit in patients with ARAS [47]; however, it is also associated with a slightly elevated risk of acute renal failure. The usage of ACEI/ARB should be considered for all patients with ARAS. Smoking is not only a cardiovascular risk factor, it is also a risk factor for chronic kidney disease and can increase the risk of nephropathy progression [48]. All patients with cardiovascular disease or cardiovascular disease equivalents are high-risk for adverse cardiovascular events. Importantly, with optimal medical treatment of ARAS, the mortality rate can be decreased, at least in the setting of cohorts selected for participation in clinical trials, as shown by the ASTRAL trial (average annual mortality rate of 8%) [31] and the more recent CORAL trial (average annual mortality rate of 4%) [1]. Details of medical therapy can be found in a recent review [49].

Indications for endovascular intervention (revascularization)

Recently published guidelines for renal artery revascularization, according to current AHA/ACC guidelines published in 2013, are listed here [19]. As more evidence becomes available, the guidelines will be modified as many of these subgroups of patients with ARAS were not benefited in the recently completed randomized trials. We believe that the strongest rationale for revascularization in the atherosclerotic patient is for those infrequent individuals with severe renal stenosis and advanced chronic kidney disease who are faced with the choice of an attempt at revascularization or instituting renal replacement therapy in the near future. However, this is not an evidence-based recommendation but is grounded in clinical experience.

- Asymptomatic patients with bilateral or solitary kidney with a hemodynamically significant RAS (level of evidence C);
- Resistant, accelerated, or malignant hypertension with hemodynamically significant RAS, or hypertension with unilateral

unexplained small kidney or intolerance to medications (level of evidence B);

- Progressive chronic kidney disease with bilateral or solitary functioning kidney and with RAS (level of evidence B), or with unilateral RAS (level of evidence C);
- Recurrent, unexplained congestive heart failure or sudden, unexplained pulmonary edema in patients with hemodynamically significant RAS (level of evidence B);
- Unstable angina in patients with hemodynamically significant RAS (level of evidence B).

Contraindications for endovascular intervention

The commonly accepted contraindications for percutaneous transluminal renal angioplasty include the following:

- A non-functioning kidney, generally <8 cm pole-to-pole length;
- Limited life expectancy;
- Generally poor surgical or endovascular intervention candidate;
- Pregnancy; and
- Non-compliance with medical therapy.

Technical aspects of renal endovascular intervention for renal artery stenosis

The direct goal of renal artery intervention is to obtain the optimal patency of the artery while minimizing the risk of atheroembolization, renal artery dissection, and other complications. We first describe the techniques for stenting ostial ARAS, as these are the most common. This type of lesion involves the ostium of renal artery at its origin from the aorta.

Arterial access

Common femoral arterial access site is most commonly used. Radial or brachial artery access site should be considered for antegrade approach if the takeoff of the renal artery is sharply downward angulated or in the presence of severe bilateral aortoiliac disease and/or tortuosity. In the presence of an aortic aneurysm, the angulation of the renal artery could favor upper or lower extremity access. Similarly, if a renal artery has been covered by a stent during an aortic procedure, careful selection of access and willingness to change access sites may be the difference between a successful and unsuccessful procedure. A longer sheath (e.g., 23 cm rather than 11 cm) should be considered for tortuous arteries.

Renal artery angiography

Abdominal aortography prior to stenting should be performed to identify the local anatomy, including the severity and location of aortic pathology, location of the renal ostia, the extent of the ostial stenosis, the angulation of the renal artery takeoff from the abdominal aorta, accessory renal arteries, and the presence of aneurysms and calcification. A shallow left anterior oblique projection is often the best angle view for identifying both the right and left renal ostia. If CTA or MRA images are available the angulation of the ostia can be more precisely estimated. Prior to the first selective renal angiography, active aspiration of 10 mL blood via a Y-connector or passive back-bleeding can be performed to clean debris from the guiding catheter to reduce the risk of embolism.

Engagement of guide catheter

Anticoagulation should be started after sheath insertion. Indirect engagement of the renal artery ostium using the guide catheter is preferred over direct engagement of the renal ostium because of the higher risk of renal artery complications associated with direct engagement (e.g., dissection, atheroembolism, artery abrupt closure, and aortic injury). Indirect engagement of the renal ostium can be achieved through two kinds of approaches: the "exchange technique" or the "no touch" technique.

For the exchange technique, after renal angiography a 4-Fr diagnostic catheter is inserted through the sheath and used to engage the renal ostium gently. The soft small diagnostic catheter carries a lower risk of atheroembolization and dissection than the stiffer guiding catheter. After engagement of the diagnostic catheter in the renal artery ostium, a guidewire, 0.014 or 0.018 inch, is introduced into the main renal artery through the diagnostic catheter. The guide is then advanced over the wire and diagnostic catheter, after which the diagnostic catheter is removed leaving the guidewire in place.

For the "no touch technique", a 0.035-inch J-tip guidewire is placed above the ostium and the guide catheter is introduced in close proximity to the renal artery ostium over the J-tip guidewire. Then the guidewire is retracted to allow the guide catheter to assume its angled shape. The tip of the guidewire is against the aortic wall above the renal artery ostium. The opening of the guide catheter is then adjusted gently to align the opening of the guide catheter with the ostium of renal artery. A 0.014-inch wire is introduced through the guide catheter and engaged into the distal renal artery, after which the J-tip guidewire is removed, leaving 0.014-inch wire in the renal artery. An 0.014-inch wire is compatible with most stent platforms and distal protection devices. Hydrophilic wires should generally be avoided because of the higher risk of renal parenchymal perforation.

A 6-Fr guiding catheter is most often used and its shape should reflect the angle between renal artery and the aorta with consideration of other characteristics of local anatomy. A variety of guiding catheter configurations are available (e.g., "hockey stick," renal double curve, internal mammary artery, right Judkins, and right Amplatz). Our current "workhorse" shape for most renal interventions is the IMA or internal mammary shape. The "hockey stick" guide catheter can be used for radial or brachial approach.

Percutaneous renal transluminal angioplasty

Balloon angioplasty is the treatment of choice for FMD and can be used for predilation and sizing of the renal artery prior to stent placement. With FMD, balloon angioplasty is the treatment of choice and the goal is to tear the webs in the renal artery thus minimizing the pressure drop-off across the area of involvement. Balloon angioplasty can be performed with a 0.014 inch pressure-sensing guidewire in place that allows the success of each dilatation to be ascertained. Generally, the balloon size in FMD is matched to vessel size; however, at times it may be necessary to slightly oversize the balloon to achieve the desired result. When this is done great care should be taken for symptoms of pending arterial rupture or dissection, heralded as back pain, at which time the balloon is gently deflated. Generally, stenting should be avoided, if at all possible, when treating FMD. The stent is an unnecessary expense and young patients especially can suffer from the consequence of metal stent fatigue or corrosion over the patient's lifetime, resulting in device fracture and restenosis. In atherosclerotic stenoses, predilatation is achieved through a balloon with a slightly smaller diameter than the reference vessel.

Percutaneous renal stenting

The atherosclerotic renal artery often recoils after angioplasty resulting in restenosis, so stenting is a better approach to maintain the patency of the artery. Balloon expandable stents are favored over self-expanding stents because of the lack of precision associated with the latter stents. Balloon expandable stents are sized 1:1 with the reference vessel diameter, not the post-stenotic dilated segment. Stent length should be as short as possible while being long enough to completely cover the entire lesion. Using the shortest stent possible that allows complete lesion coverage can be helpful because the renal artery displaces dynamically during the respirophasic cycle and longer stents are subject to greater stress and potentially fracture risk.

The stent should be positioned with 1 mm protruding into the aorta, in order to completely cover the arterial ostium. An ostial stent, the ArchStent™ (Ostial Corporation, Mountainview, CA, USA), enables rapid and precise placement of the stent for ostial lesions. It uses a dual-balloon delivery system, with a locator balloon stopping at the ostium for visually confirming the right position. The second balloon inflation results in stent placement. Further inflation of the locator balloon results in flaring of the proximal stent end and full ostial coverage. Another stent device developed to help stenting ostial lesions is the Ostial Pro stent positioning system (Ostial Solutions, Kalamazoo, MI, USA).

After proper positioning of the stent, the balloon is inflated to its nominal diameter to achieve a 1 : 1 ratio with the diameter of the reference vessel. Inadequate stent expansion results in high rates of restenosis; thus, it is important to further dilate the stent if it appears to be underdeployed initially. Larger balloons with higher inflation pressure can be utilized to further dilate an underexpanded stent. Caution, though, should be exercised in trying to maximize stent diameter. Specifically, when the patient experiences back pain during balloon inflation, this can be the only warning sign before main renal artery rupture or perforation. Should this complication occur, placement of a covered stent is clearly indicated if the perforation of the renal artery is not promptly sealed with balloon inflation. Importantly, in order to adequately stabilize the patient it may be necessary to place a larger diameter balloon, inflated to low pressure (1–2 atmospheres), to adequately seal the vessel. A final selective angiogram should be performed to assess the stent position, exclude dissection, perforation and spasm, and the renal parenchymal blush to exclude atheroembolism.

The "kissing balloon technique" can be utilized for the renal arteries with same origin without a common trunk or in the presence of a short main trunk. This technique can be carried out in two ways. The first utilizes a single guiding catheter through which two wires and two balloons are introduced by femoral access route. However, this technique is limited by the relatively large diameter of the stents and their delivery balloons, making this impractical for lesions of the main renal arteries that require stents of 5 mm diameter or larger. The other strategy utilizes two guiding catheters, two wires, and two balloons with one guiding catheter through femoral access and the other guiding catheter through radial or brachial access. In the latter approach, it is far easier if ipsilateral vascular access is used (i.e., right arm and right leg as an example).

For a short common renal trunk, two balloons can be placed in the trunk, extending into each renal artery branch respectively. After predilation, a stent with appropriate length is placed in the trunk over one of the wires and then two balloons are inflated within the stent to deploy the stent within the trunk and into two renal artery branches. When this is done caution should be used in selecting balloon size.

Stenting other types of renal artery stenosis

Atherosclerotic plaques not involving the ostium cause RAS within the trunk, or distal RAS. The optimum intervention on these lesions is not as clear. Angioplasty is preferred by some interventional physicians and angioplasty with stenting is preferred by others. If angioplasty results in suboptimal result, stenting is then needed. Self-expanding stents oversized by 1 mm over the reference vessel can be useful because of their flexibility and better fracture resistance compared with balloon-expandable stents, as there is significant bending stress on the stent within the mid renal artery during cardiorespiratory motion [50,51].

For vasculitis-caused RAS, the actual technical procedure is the same as the procedure for ARAS. However, there is no conclusive preference for angioplasty or stenting if endovascular intervention is warranted. A recent retrospective study suggested superiority of angioplasty over stenting for Takayasu's disease [52]. Regardless of which endovascular procedure is chosen, perioperative appropriate medical treatment of the underlying pathophysiologic disease process (e.g., immunosuppression) is required for better clinical outcome [53].

Distal protection devices to prevent atheroembolization

The atherosclerotic plaque burden associated with ARAS is quite high, although much of this risk resides in the aorta. It is intuitive to imagine the debris shattered from the fractured plaques going distally in the renal artery resulting in parenchymal inflammation and impaired kidney function. The debris is often observed when an embolic protection device is used [54]. These devices are unlikely to catch 100% of the debris but decrease the debris burden. The question to ask is the risk–benefit ratio. The distal protection device was shown to be beneficial in improving or stabilizing the renal function by several authors [55,56]. The combination of a distal filter protection device and abciximab was shown to protect kidney function after atherosclerotic renal artery stenting [54]. The risks of using these devices include increased case complexity and time, renal artery spasm, and dissection. Use of a distal protection device is sometimes not feasible for short renal arteries simply because there is no room to deploy the protection device.

Peri-interventional care

Aspirin (81–325 mg) should be started at least 1 day before the intervention and continued for life. Clopidogrel (75 mg) is used for at least 4 weeks after stenting by most interventional physicians, although there has been no study yet to validate the benefit. Anticoagulation is not needed after intervention. As described earlier, abciximab was shown to protect kidney function after atherosclerotic renal artery stenting over the short term when used in combination with an embolic protection device [54]. Blood pressure medications should not be held on the day of the procedure and should be continued after the procedure. Overnight observation is suggested for monitoring blood pressure, adjusting blood pressure medications, and monitoring for complications. Intravenous hydration can be used prior to and after the contrast exposure to prevent contrast-induced acute kidney injury.

Duplex ultrasound is useful 1 month after discharge to establish the baseline characteristics for comparison with later imaging. Follow-up by duplex ultrasound is recommended at 6 and 12 months, or if kidney function declines, to evaluate renal stent patency.

Complications and management

The most common complications in renal artery intervention are vascular access-related, including local hematoma (~5%), retroperitoneal hematoma, pseudoaneurysm, ateriovenous fistula, blood vessel and nerve injury.

Atheroemboli can happen during catheter manipulations in the aorta, resulting from disruption of plaques or thrombi on the aortic wall. This risk can be heightened in the presence of highly atheromatous aortas or with aneurysms. Every effort should be made to minimize the manipulation, and especially scraping, of catheters along the aortic wall. Embolism can also occur because of plaque disruption during predilatation, stenting, and post-dilatation within the renal artery. Distal embolic protection devices can be utilized; however, their utility is still uncertain.

Renal artery dissection can occur during the procedure, especially during catheter engagement or during stenting. The "exchange technique" and "no touch technique" are useful. In all cases, gentle engagement is preferred. Bailout stent placement can be used to treat the dissection. Aortic wall dissection can also occur. Stenting and conservative treatment are the usual modality of treatment.

Renal artery perforation is a severe complication that is somewhat unpredictable. It can be associated with guidewire injury or over expansion of a lesion. Some patients have back pain as their warning sign; when this is experienced the balloon should be deflated and repeat imaging performed. When the patient experiences acute back pain during balloon inflation it is safer to err on the side of underexpansion and risk of restenosis than it is to err on the side of a "perfect result" and vessel rupture. Hemodynamic instability may or may not occur. Prolonged balloon inflation, use of covered stent, or, rarely, surgical intervention are required.

Wire perforation of the renal parenchyma also occurs at low frequency and, if not addressed, can result in severe hemorrhage and loss of the kidney. The kidney is more sensitive to perforation than the heart or lower extremity, especially when hydrophilic guidewires are used. To avoid perforation, meticulously track the distal position of the wire during the entirety of the procedure. Should perforation occur, immediate treatment using an embolic strategy (coils, foam, glue, etc.) is likely required.

In-stent restenosis and management

The restenosis rate after renal artery stenting ranges from 10% to 40% [57–60], with higher rates in smaller diameter renal arteries (<4.5 mm) [61] and lower rates in larger diameter arteries (5–7 mm) [60]. Risk factors for atherosclerosis, including smoking and diabetes, contribute to the development of in-stent restenosis [62]. Duplex ultrasound monitoring after initial stent placement can be useful to monitor for the development of restenosis, especially if patients have recurrent clinical problems such as resistant hypertension or worsening kidney function. In-stent stenosis is suspected when the duplex ultrasonography demonstrates an in-stent velocity >200 cm/s and a peak systolic velocity ratio (renal : aortic) >3.5 [63].

Various methods have been used to treat renal artery in-stent stenosis successfully, including balloon angioplasty [59,64], bare-metal [57,59] or drug (paclitaxel) eluting stent placement [59,65,66], covered stent [65], or endovascular brachytherapy [67]. However, the optimum strategy to prevent recurrent restenosis remains unknown [59]. Although sirolimus-eluting stent was suggested to be effective in maintaining long-term patency by one study [68], a subsequent study suggested that use of a sirolimus-eluting stent is associated with a high restenosis rate in treating renal artery in-stent restenosis [69]. Aggressive risk factor management including diabetes control, smoke cessation, hypertension control, and use of aspirin and statins is recommended [49].

Interactive multiple choice questions are available for this chapter on **www.wiley. com/go/dangas/cardiology**

References

1 Cooper CJ, Murphy TP, Cutlip DE, *et al*. Stenting and medical therapy for atherosclerotic renal-artery stenosis. *N Engl J Med* 2014; **370**(1): 13–22.

2 Caps MT, Perissinotto C, Zierler RE, *et al*. Prospective study of atherosclerotic disease progression in the renal artery. *Circulation* 1998; **98**(25): 2866–2872.

3 Schreiber MJ, Pohl MA, Novick AC. The natural history of atherosclerotic and fibrous renal artery disease. *Urol Clin North Am* 1984; **11**(3): 383–392.

4 Weber BR, Dieter RS. Renal artery stenosis: epidemiology and treatment. *Int J Nephrol Renovasc Dis* 2014; **7**: 169–181.

5 Mailloux LU, Napolitano B, Bellucci AG, Vernace M, Wilkes BM, Mossey RT. Renal vascular disease causing end-stage renal disease, incidence, clinical correlates, and outcomes: a 20-year clinical experience. *Am J Kidney Dis* 1994; **24**(4): 622–629.

6 Haller ST, Evans KL, Folt DA, Drummond CA, Cooper CJ. Mechanisms and treatments for renal artery stenosis. *Discov Med* 2013; **16**(90): 255–260.

7 Textor SC. Ischemic nephropathy: where are we now? *J Am Soc Nephrol* 2004; **15**(8): 1974–1982.

8 Haller ST, Kalra PA, Ritchie JP, *et al*. Effect of CD40 and sCD40L on renal function and survival in patients with renal artery stenosis. *Hypertension* 2013; **61**(4): 894–900.

9 Gottam N, Nanjundappa A, Dieter RS. Renal artery stenosis: pathophysiology and treatment. *Exp Rev Cardiovasc Ther* 2009; **7**(11): 1413–1420.

10 Conlon PJ, Little MA, Pieper K, Mark DB. Severity of renal vascular disease predicts mortality in patients undergoing coronary angiography. *Kidney Int* 2001; **60**(4): 1490–1497.

11 Mui K-W, Sleeswijk M, van den Hout H, van Baal J, Navis G, Woittiez AJ. Incidental renal artery stenosis is an independent predictor of mortality in patients with peripheral vascular disease. *J Am Soc Nephrol* 2006; **17**(7): 2069–2074.

12 Johansson M, Herlitz H, Jensen G, Rundqvist B, Friberg P. Increased cardiovascular mortality in hypertensive patients with renal artery stenosis: relation to sympathetic activation, renal function and treatment regimens. *J Hypertens* 1999; **17**(12 Pt 1): 1743–1750.

13 Kalra PA, Guo H, Kausz AT, *et al*. Atherosclerotic renovascular disease in United States patients aged 67 years or older: risk factors, revascularization, and prognosis. *Kidney Int* 2005; **68**(1): 293–301.

14 Dorros G, Jaff M, Mathiak L, *et al*. Four-year follow-up of Palmaz-Schatz stent revascularization as treatment for atherosclerotic renal artery stenosis. *Circulation* 1998; **98**(7): 642–647.

15 Alderson HV, Ritchie JP, Kalra PA. Revascularization as a treatment to improve renal function. *Int J Nephrol Renovasc Dis* 2014; **7**: 89–99.

16 Guo H, Kalra PA, Gilbertson DT, *et al*. Atherosclerotic renovascular disease in older US patients starting dialysis, 1996 to 2001. *Circulation* 2007; **115**(1): 50–58.

17 Dworkin LD, Cooper CJ. Clinical practice: Renal-artery stenosis. *N Engl J Med* 2009; **361**(20): 1972–1978.

18 Slovut DP, Olin JW. Fibromuscular dysplasia. *N Engl J Med* 2004; **350**(18): 1862–1871.

19 Anderson JL, Halperin JL, Albert NM, *et al*. Management of patients with peripheral artery disease (compilation of 2005 and 2011 ACCF/AHA guideline recommendations): a report of the American College of Cardiology Foundation/American Heart Association Task Force on Practice Guidelines. *Circulation* 2013; **127**(13): 1425–1443.

20 Olin JW, Piedmonte MR, Young JR, DeAnna S, Grubb M, Childs MB. The utility of duplex ultrasound scanning of the renal arteries for diagnosing significant renal artery stenosis. *Ann Intern Med* 1995; **122**(11): 833–838.

21 American Institute of Ultrasound in Medicine practice guideline for the performance of native renal artery duplex sonography. *J Ultrasound Med* 2013; **32**(7): 1331–1340.

22 Soares GM, Murphy TP, Singha MS, Parada A, Jaff M. Renal artery duplex ultrasonography as a screening and surveillance tool to detect renal artery stenosis: a comparison with current reference standard imaging. *J Ultrasound Med* 2006; **25**(3): 293–298.

23 Stavros AT, Parker SH, Yakes WF, *et al*. Segmental stenosis of the renal artery: pattern recognition of tardus and parvus abnormalities with duplex sonography. *Radiology* 1992; **184**(2): 487–492.

24 Rocha-Singh K, Jaff MR, Lynne Kelley E. Renal artery stenting with noninvasive duplex ultrasound follow-up: 3-year results from the RENAISSANCE renal stent trial. *Catheter Cardiovasc Interv* 2008; **72**(6): 853–862.

25 Mohabbat W, Greenberg RK, Mastracci TM, Cury M, Morales JP, Hernandez AV. Revised duplex criteria and outcomes for renal stents and stent grafts following endovascular repair of juxtarenal and thoracoabdominal aneurysms. *J Vasc Surg* 2009; **49**(4): 827–837; discussion 837.

26 Eklof H, Ahlstrom H, Magnusson A, *et al.* A prospective comparison of duplex ultrasonography, captopril renography, MRA, and CTA in assessing renal artery stenosis. *Acta Radiol* 2006; **47**(8): 764–774.

27 Rountas C, Vlychou M, Vassiou K, *et al.* Imaging modalities for renal artery stenosis in suspected renovascular hypertension: prospective intraindividual comparison of color Doppler US, CT angiography, GD-enhanced MR angiography, and digital substraction angiography. *Renal Fail* 2007; **29**(3): 295–302.

28 Colyer WR Jr, Cooper CJ, Burket MW, Thomas WJ. Utility of a 0.014″ pressure-sensing guidewire to assess renal artery translesional systolic pressure gradients. *Catheter Cardiovasc Interv* 2003; **59**(3): 372–377.

29 Kadziela J, Witkowski A, Januszewicz A, *et al.* Assessment of renal artery stenosis using both resting pressures ratio and fractional flow reserve: relationship to angiography and ultrasonography. *Blood Pressure* 2011; **20**(4): 211–217.

30 Ito T, Tani T, Fujita H, Ohte N. Relationship between fractional flow reserve and residual plaque volume and clinical outcomes after optimal drug-eluting stent implantation: insight from intravascular ultrasound volumetric analysis. *Int J Cardiol* 2014; **176**(2): 399–404.

31 Wheatley K, Ives N, Gray R, *et al.* Revascularization versus medical therapy for renal-artery stenosis. *N Engl J Med* 2009; **361**(20): 1953–1962.

32 Bax L, Woittiez AJ, Kouwenberg HJ, *et al.* Stent placement in patients with atherosclerotic renal artery stenosis and impaired renal function: a randomized trial. *Ann Intern Med* 2009; **150**(12): 840–848.

33 Watson PS, Hadjipetrou P, Cox SV, Piemonte TC, Eisenhauer AC. Effect of renal artery stenting on renal function and size in patients with atherosclerotic renovascular disease. *Circulation* 2000; **102**(14): 1671–1677.

34 Muray S, Martin M, Amoedo ML, *et al.* Rapid decline in renal function reflects reversibility and predicts the outcome after angioplasty in renal artery stenosis. *Am J Kidney Dis* 2002; **39**(1): 60–66.

35 Ritchie J, Green D, Chrysochou C, Chalmers N, Foley RN, Kalra PA. High-risk clinical presentations in atherosclerotic renovascular disease: prognosis and response to renal artery revascularization. *Am J Kidney Dis* 2014; **63**(2): 186–197.

36 Bloch MJ, Trost DW, Pickering TG, Sos TA, August P. Prevention of recurrent pulmonary edema in patients with bilateral renovascular disease through renal artery stent placement. *Am J Hypertens* 1999; **12**(1 Pt 1): 1–7.

37 Pelta A, Andersen UB, Just S, Baekgaard N. Flash pulmonary edema in patients with renal artery stenosis: the Pickering Syndrome. *Blood Pressure* 2011; **20**(1): 15–19.

38 Cheung CM, Chrysochou C, Shurrab AE, Buckley DL, Cowie A, Kalra PA. Effects of renal volume and single-kidney glomerular filtration rate on renal functional outcome in atherosclerotic renal artery stenosis. *Nephrol Dial Transplant* 2010; **25**(4): 1133–1140.

39 Chrysochou C, Mendichovszky IA, Buckley DL, Cheung CM, Jackson A, Kalra PA. BOLD imaging: a potential predictive biomarker of renal functional outcome following revascularization in atheromatous renovascular disease. *Nephrol Dial Transplant* 2012; **27**(3): 1013–1019.

40 Silva JA, Chan AW, White CJ, *et al.* Elevated brain natriuretic peptide predicts blood pressure response after stent revascularization in patients with renal artery stenosis. *Circulation* 2005; **111**(3): 328–333.

41 Jaff MR, Bates M, Sullivan T, *et al.* Significant reduction in systolic blood pressure following renal artery stenting in patients with uncontrolled hypertension: results from the HERCULES trial. *Catheter Cardiovasc Interv* 2012; **80**(3): 343–350.

42 Radermacher J, Chavan A, Bleck J, *et al.* Use of Doppler ultrasonography to predict the outcome of therapy for renal-artery stenosis. *N Engl J Med* 2001; **344**(6): 410–417.

43 Crutchley TA, Pearce JD, Craven TE, Stafford JM, Edwards MS, Hansen KJ. Clinical utility of the resistive index in atherosclerotic renovascular disease. *J Vasc Surg* 2009; **49**(1): 148–155, 55 e1–3; discussion 155.

44 Bruno RM, Daghini E, Versari D, *et al.* Predictive role of renal resistive index for clinical outcome after revascularization in hypertensive patients with atherosclerotic renal artery stenosis: a monocentric observational study. *Cardiovasc Ultrasound* 2014; **12**: 9.

45 Hodsman GP, Brown JJ, Cumming AM, *et al.* Enalapril (MK421) in the treatment of hypertension with renal artery stenosis. *J Hypertens Suppl* 1983; **1**(1): 109–117.

46 Karlberg BE, Fyhrquist F, Gronhagen-Riska C, Tikkanen I, Ohman KP. Enalapril and lisinopril in renovascular hypertension: antihypertensive and hormonal effects of two new angiotensin-converting-enzyme (ACE) inhibitors. A preliminary report. *Scand J Urol Nephrol Suppl* 1984; **79**: 103–106.

47 Chrysochou C, Foley RN, Young JF, Khavandi K, Cheung CM, Kalra PA. Dispelling the myth: the use of renin-angiotensin blockade in atheromatous renovascular disease. *Nephrol Dial Transplant* 2012; **27**(4): 1403–1409.

48 Orth SR, Hallan SI. Smoking: a risk factor for progression of chronic kidney disease and for cardiovascular morbidity and mortality in renal patients—absence of evidence or evidence of absence? *Clin J Am Soc Nephrol* 2008; **3**(1): 226–236.

49 Yu MS, Folt DA, Drummond CA, *et al.* Endovascular versus medical therapy for atherosclerotic renovascular disease. *Curr Atheroscler Rep* 2014; **16**(12): 459.

50 Wang LC, Scott DJ, Clemens MS, Hislop SJ, Arthurs ZM. Mechanism of stent failure in a patient with fibromuscular dysplasia following renal artery stenting. *Ann Vasc Surg* 2015; **29**(1): e19–21.

51 Tanaka A, Takahashi S, Saito S. Migration of fractured renal artery stent. *Catheter Cardiovasc Interv* 2011; **77**(2): 305–307.

52 Park HS, Do YS, Park KB, *et al.* Long term results of endovascular treatment in renal arterial stenosis from Takayasu arteritis: angioplasty versus stent placement. *Eur J Radiol* 2013; **82**(11): 1913–1918.

53 Perera AH, Youngstein T, Gibbs RG, Jackson JE, Wolfe JH, Mason JC. Optimizing the outcome of vascular intervention for Takayasu arteritis. *Br J Surg* 2014; **101**(2): 43–50.

54 Cooper CJ, Haller ST, Colyer W, *et al.* Embolic protection and platelet inhibition during renal artery stenting. *Circulation* 2008; **117**(21): 2752–2760.

55 Henry M, Klonaris C, Henry I, *et al.* Protected renal stenting with the PercuSurge GuardWire device: a pilot study. *J Endovasc Ther* 2001; **8**(3): 227–237.

56 Holden A, Hill A, Jaff MR, Pilmore H. Renal artery stent revascularization with embolic protection in patients with ischemic nephropathy. *Kidney Int* 2006; **70**(5): 948–955.

57 Bax L, Mali WP, Van De Ven PJ, Beek FJ, Vos JA, Beutler JJ. Repeated intervention for in-stent restenosis of the renal arteries. *J Vasc Interv Radiol* 2002; **13**(12): 1219–1224.

58 N'Dandu ZM, Badawi RA, White CJ, *et al.* Optimal treatment of renal artery in-stent restenosis: repeat stent placement versus angioplasty alone. *Catheter Cardiovasc Interv* 2008; **71**(5): 701–705.

59 Stone PA, Campbell JE, Aburahma AF, *et al.* Ten-year experience with renal artery in-stent restenosis. *J Vasc Surg* 2011; **53**(4): 1026–1031.

60 Gray BH. Intervention for renal artery stenosis: endovascular and surgical roles. *J Hypertens Suppl* 2005; **23**(3): S23–29.

61 Lederman RJ, Mendelsohn FO, Santos R, Phillips HR, Stack RS, Crowley JJ. Primary renal artery stenting: characteristics and outcomes after 363 procedures. *Am Heart J* 2001; **142**(2): 314–323.

62 Shammas NW, Kapalis MJ, Dippel EJ, *et al.* Clinical and angiographic predictors of restenosis following renal artery stenting. *J Invasive Cardiol* 2004; **16**(1): 10–13.

63 Chi YW, White CJ, Thornton S, Milani RV. Ultrasound velocity criteria for renal in-stent restenosis. *J Vasc Surg* 2009; **50**(1): 119–123.

64 Otah KE, Alhaddad IA. Intravascular ultrasound-guided cutting balloon angioplasty for renal artery stent restenosis. *Clin Cardiol* 2004; **27**(10): 581–583.

65 Kakkar AK, Fischi M, Narins CR. Drug-eluting stent implantation for treatment of recurrent renal artery in-stent restenosis. *Catheter Cardiovasc Interv* 2006; **68**(1): 118–122; discussion 123–124.

66 Douis H, Shabir S, Lipkin G, Riley P. Drug-eluting stent insertion in the treatment of in-stent renal artery restenosis in three renal transplant recipients. *J Vasc Interv Radiol* 2008; **19**(12): 1757–1760.

67 Silverman SH, Exline JB, Silverman LN, Samson RH. Endovascular brachytherapy for renal artery in-stent restenosis. *J Vasc Surg* 2014; **60**(6): 1599–1604.

68 Lookstein RA, Talenfeld AD, Raju R, Vorchheimer DA, Olin JW, Marin ML. Sirolimus-eluting stent placement for refractory renal artery in-stent restenosis: sustained patency and clinical benefit at 24 months. *Vasc Med* 2009; **14**(4): 361–364.

69 Kiernan TJ, Yan BP, Eisenberg JD, *et al.* Treatment of renal artery in-stent restenosis with sirolimus-eluting stents. *Vasc Med* 2010; **15**(1): 3–7.

CHAPTER 76

Revascularization for Arteries in the Pelvis

Femi Philip and Jason H. Rogers

University of California, Davis Medical Center, Sacramento, CA, USA

Normal erectile function is a complex neurovascular event that requires neurochemical stimulation and end-organ response for the initiation and maintenance of erection. Erectile dysfunction (ED) is a common medical problem affecting over 50% of men between the ages of 45–75 years [1]. There are currently over 150 million men worldwide with ED and this number is projected to increase to 322 million by 2025, the majority of the increase being in developing countries mirroring the increase in cardiovascular risk factors in these societies [2]. The etiology of ED is multifactorial but a vasculogenic cause either coexists with or has a dominant role underlying this disorder in over 40% of cases. Vasculogenic etiologies include endothelial dysfunction with impaired smooth muscle relaxation, arterial insufficiency caused by proximal atherosclerotic stenosis, or venous insufficiency because of inability to trap blood in the corpus cavernosa because of venous leak. The exact frequency distribution of these etiologies in patients with ED remains poorly defined. Coronary artery disease and ED share many cardiovascular risk factors such as age, diabetes, hypertension, hyperlipidemia, and tobacco use [3]. Erectile dysfunction is also an emerging risk factor for the development of antecedent symptomatic coronary artery disease and adverse cardiovascular events [4].

The current therapy for ED uses pharmacologic agents such as phosphodiesterase-5 inhibitors (PDE5i) that increase penile arterial blood flow and improve endothelial function. However, a large proportion of patients (~50%) have a poor response to these agents or have a contraindication to their use and are relegated to the use of vacuum constrictor devices, intrapenile injection of prostaglandins, or implantation of a penile prosthesis [5,6]. There is currently evidence documenting the presence of angiographically severe penile arterial inflow (PAI) disease in a significant proportion of older patients with ED [7]. Clinical trials have reported some limited efficacy in erectile function after percutaneous intervention on vascular stenosis related to PAI. Despite these data, penile arterial revascularization remains investigational to date and is currently not recommended by the American Urological Association [6].

A novel minimally invasive approach targeting PAI disease may prove to be a safe and effective treatment strategy for ED related to impaired arterial inflow. This chapter reviews the normal penile arterial blood supply, describes the angiographic anatomy in ED, and critically discusses the available literature on microsurgical and endovascular techniques to treat vasculogenic ED.

Penile arterial blood supply and anatomy
Normal penile vascular anatomy

The abdominal aorta bifurcates into the right and left common iliac artery. The common iliac bifurcates into the internal and external iliac arteries. The internal iliac artery passes downward to the upper margin of the greater sciatic foramen where it divides into anterior and posterior branches. The anterior division provides the majority of blood supply to the pelvic and reproductive organs including the internal pudendal artery. The posterior division provides arterial supply to the gluteal and lumbosacral musculoskeleton via the ilio-lumbar, lateral sacral, and superior gluteal arteries (Figure 76.1). Any artery proximal to the internal pudendal artery (IPA) can be considered an erectile-related artery (ERA) and stenosis could lead to ED because of arterial insufficiency. As the vast majority of penile inflow is normally carried through the bilateral IPAs, the focus of discussion will be on the IPA and its anatomic variations.

The IPA is the smaller of the two terminal branches of the anterior trunk of the internal iliac artery. This artery passes outward along the lower border of the greater sciatic foramen, and emerges from the pelvis across the ischial spine and re-enters the perineum through the lesser sciatic foramen. The artery then passes along the lateral wall of the ischiorectal fossa and in between the fascial layers of the urogenital diaphragm along with the pudendal nerve (Alcock's canal) and terminates by forming the common penile artery which then divides into the bulbocavernosal, deep cavernosal, and dorsal arteries of the penis. The IPA has multiple branches: inferior rectal artery, perineal artery, artery of the urethral bulb, urethral arteries, and the cavernosal and dorsal arteries in the penis (Figure 76.2). The inferior rectal artery arises above the ischial tuberosity and supplies the muscles and integument of the anal region. The perineal artery provides several posterior scrotal branches that are distributed to the skin. The artery of the urethral bulb and the urethral artery are short blood vessels that supply the urethral bulb, the posterior part of the corpus cavernosum, and the glans penis. The cavernosal arteries of the penis run bilaterally forward in the center of the corpus cavernosa, to which its branches are distributed and there are communicating branches between the cavernosal arteries. The dorsal artery of the penis ascends between the crus penis and the pubic symphysis and runs

Interventional Cardiology: Principles and Practice, Second Edition. Edited by George D. Dangas, Carlo Di Mario, and Nicholas N. Kipshidze.
© 2017 John Wiley & Sons, Ltd. Published 2017 by John Wiley & Sons, Ltd.

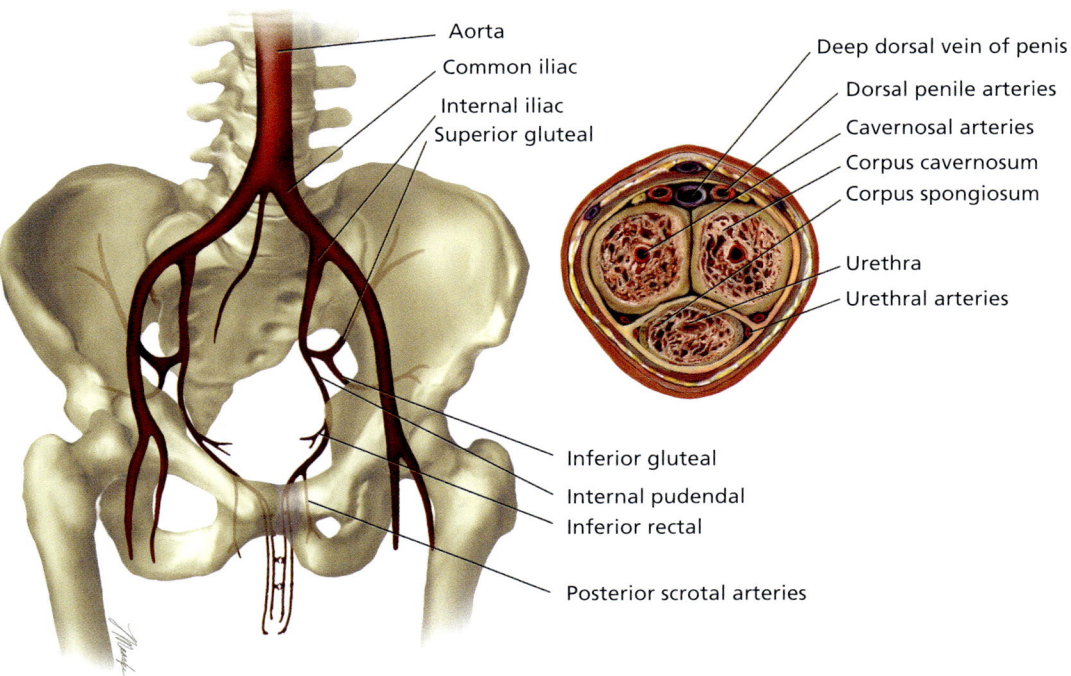

Figure 76.1 Normal pelvic arterial blood supply. A schematic view of the pelvis showing the most common arterial anatomy.

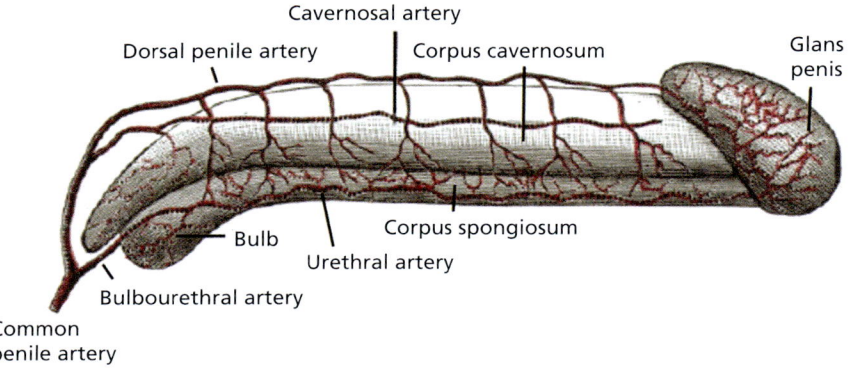

Figure 76.2 Penile arterial blood supply.

forward on the dorsum of the penis to the glans, where it divides into two branches, which supply the glans and prepuce.

Common anatomic variations in penile arterial anatomy

The most frequent anatomic variation occurs when the IPA ends as the artery of the urethral bulb or less frequently the perineal artery. In these cases, the dorsal and deep arteries of the penis are derived from an accessory pudendal artery. These accessory arteries originate from the external iliac, obturator, vesical, and femoral arteries, and in some men constitute the dominant or only arterial supply to the corpus cavernosum. Accessory pudendal arteries are identified in up to 70% of cadaveric studies, and 7–14% by radiographic studies. These anatomic aspects are essential to consider when planning an endovascular strategy. Yamaki *et al.* [7] studied 645 pelvic halves from Japanese cadavers and proposed a classification for the branching patterns of the internal iliac artery consisting of four groups (detailed in

Figure 76.3). The most common branching patterns involve the IPA originating either as the first branch, terminal branch, or trifurcating branch of the inferior division of the internal iliac artery.

Angiographic studies in erectile dysfunction

Leriche [8] first described the association between ED and occlusive disease in the aorta in 1923. This was caused by the presence of aorto-iliac occlusion resulting in lower extremity ischemia and PAI insufficiency. This association remained unexplored until 1969 when it was noted that 70% of the men with aorto-iliac occlusion had impotence [9]. In the same year, relief of impotence after bilateral endarterectomy of occluded internal iliac arteries was reported [10]. There was still no firm evidence that organic disease was responsible for impotence until 1973 when

Modified adachi classification

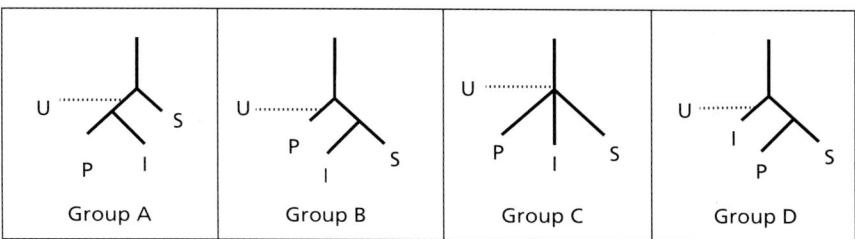

Figure 76.3 The branching pattern of the internal iliac artery, as classified by Adachi and modified by Yamaki. Group A: The internal pudendal artery is a terminal branch of the inferior division of the internal iliac artery after the inferior gluteal and superior gluteal arteries. Group B: The internal pudendal artery is the first branch of the inferior division of the internal iliac artery. Group C: The inferior division of the internal iliac artery trifurcates into internal pudendal artery, superior and inferior gluteal arteries. Group D: The internal pudendal artery is the second branch after the inferior gluteal artery is given off. I, inferior guteal artery; S, superior gluteal artery; P, internal pudendal artery; U, umbilical artery.

angiographic and histologic data suggested the coexistence of severe arterial disease in patients with impotence [11]. This was again confirmed in 1978 with the angiographic demonstration of the presence of arterial inflow disease in patients with ED [12]. These observations came in parallel with the evolution of conventional angiography. At the time, angiography was limited to visualization of the aorta and iliac vessels and more selective techniques to visualize smaller caliber vessels like the internal pudendal and penile arteries were not possible. Visualization of the smaller caliber penile vessels was possible with the use of retrograde phallo-arteriography. With this technique, 30 males with ED had translumbar aortography followed by puncture of the dorsal artery of the penis and contrast administration followed by radiographic image acquisition [13]. This technique was the first study to demonstrate severe disease or occlusion of the vessels supplying the cavernosal bodies in patients with ED.

To date there have been 10 studies assessing penile arterial blood flow in 629 patients with ED (Table 76.1) [14–23]. Collectively, these studies show a high incidence of PAI disease that ranges between 37–79% with an average incidence of 76%. The proportion of patients with arterial inflow disease may be overestimated as the majority of patients included in these studies have concurrent symptomatic coronary or peripheral vascular disease as opposed to the larger majority of patients without such comorbidities with ED. The atherosclerotic process affecting the IPA is diffuse and often involves the ostial or proximal segments of the vessels in 56% of cases and the distal segments of the vessel (small penile vessels) in over 60% [19,24]. There is also multisegment disease and this feature is often seen in older patients or those with diabetes mellitus although the numbers of patients studied in the literature are small and poorly documented.

Previous studies have also identified a considerable anatomic variation with the IPA. The IPA arises as a gluteopudendal trunk from the inferior gluteal artery in 70% of patients or as an independent branch from the anterior division of the internal iliac artery in 30% [17]. While this makes identification of the vessel more challenging, the location and origin of the IPA relative to the internal iliac artery can also influence erectile function, as there is some evidence that in Japanese men this plays a part as a cause for ED but the broader implications of this recent finding is currently unknown [25]. Accessory pudendal arteries arise in up to 21% of patients and originate as an independent branch from the obturator artery, remnant of the urachal artery, and superior division of

the internal iliac artery [19]. It is therefore critical to consider angiography as the current gold standard for evaluation of penile arterial blood supply.

The angiographer must perform a quality angiogram, otherwise angiography can be misleading, resulting in both false positive and false negative diagnosis. Important considerations include: inclusion of both the large pelvic and the distal vessels, location of the source of blood flow to cavernosal arteries using direct cannulation of the pudendal or accessory pudendal artery, and recognizing variant arterial anatomy. Finally, it is essential to place the anatomic information obtained during angiography within the context of functional assessments of penile blood flow obtained via Doppler ultrasound examination during pharmacologic induction of erection to exclude venous leak. It is not known if arterial revascularization of patients with venous leak will result in improvement of erectile function, but venous leak should theoretically limit the efficacy of any improvement in arterial inflow.

Penile arterial revascularization: surgical and endovascular approaches
Surgical approach to penile arterial revascularization

Michal *et al.* [26] reported the first penile arterial revascularization in 1973, by anastomosis of the inferior epigastric artery (IEGA) to the corpus cavernosum which was successful in the short term but resulted in cavernosal smooth muscle fibrosis leading to thrombosis of the graft in the long term. The Michal II procedure was then popularized, where the IEGA was anastomosed in an end-to-side fashion to the dorsal penile artery [27]. Hauri [28] proposed direct arterial anastomosis of the IEGA to the dorsal artery but, in addition, incorporating the deep dorsal vein into the anastomosis (arterialization). In principle, arterialization of the dorsal vein would improve arterial flow to the corpora cavernosa in a retrograde manner via the emissary veins. Virag *et al.* [29] described a procedure in which the IEGA was anastomosed directly to the deep dorsal vein, introducing the concept of venous arterialization. In theory, these modifications improve inflow while reducing venous outflow. In concept, these procedures can be attractive not only in men with pure arteriogenic ED, but also those with a venogenic component. However, these procedures are rarely performed given the limited experience and the associated morbidity and mortality from the operation.

Thirty-one studies have been performed to evaluate these surgical techniques and those included in the American Urologic

Table 76.1 Penile arterial inflow studies in erectile dysfunction.

Study	n	Anatomic variations of internal pudendal and accessory arteries	Location of stenosis
Michal 1978 [11]	30	N/A	100% cavernosal arteries
Herman 1978 [15]	35	N/A	100% IPA disease
Struyven 1979 [16]	14	N/A	50% IPA disease
Huguet 1981 [17]	200	85% from ILA, 65% from gluteopudendal artery	Not described
Buvat 1981 [18]	29	N/A	37% proximal IPA 48% distal disease (perineal and cavernous arteries)
Bruhllman 1981 [19]	24	Accessory pudendal artery from superior vesical, urachal and obturator arteries	71% IPA 24% mid-segment of the IPA 59% bilateral IPA 100% deep and dorsal arteries of the penis
Gary 1982 [21]	73	21% had accessory pudendal arteries, of these 14% were unilateral and 7% were bilateral	44% ILA or proximal IPA 44% distal IPA or cavernosal arteries
Nessi 1987 [20]	44	N/A	79% IPA 20% occlusion of the IPA or bilateral disease 52% with single vessel occlusion or multiple lesions in a single vessel
Valji 1988 [22]	57	N/A	19% ILA 70% IPA 40% distal disease 56% intrapenile disease
Rosen 1990 [23]	170	N/A	Cavernosal arteries in the majority
Rogers 2010 [14]	10	N/A	90% IPA
Total*	629		IPA disease: 144/259 (56%) Small vessel disease: 274/459 (59%)

ED, erectile dysfunction; ILA, internal iliac artery; IPA, internal pudendal artery; N/A, not available.

*Patients from Huguet *et al.* and Rosen *et al.* studies were excluded from the total numbers due to lack of data regarding degree and location of stenosis of the IPA and cavernosal arteries.

Association (AUA) position statement are listed in Table 76.2. One of the largest contemporary retrospective series is that of Kawanishi where 51 men with vasculogenic ED had comprehensive assessments of ED which included intracavernosal pharmacologic erection tests, penile duplex Doppler, and digital subtraction angiography [30]. The etiology of the arterial lesions was blunt perineal trauma in 33 and unknown in 35. Either the Hauri or Furlow–Fischer procedure (IEGA to deep dorsal vein but circumflex collaterals are preserved and dorsal venous valves are not disrupted) was used for penile revascularization. The patency of the neoarterial blood flow was assessed objectively by color flow duplex Doppler. A significant improvement in penile blood flow was noted and was sustained in approximately 70% of the patients [31]. Of the 31 publications on penile revascularization surgery reviewed by the AUA, only four reports for a total of 50 patients met the peer review criteria set by these guidelines. These reports document a success rate of 36–91% [5]. The most important limitation of the current surgical literature is that patients who underwent these operations generally had blunt trauma without atherosclerosis. Furthermore, surgery was associated with a wide range of complications that included penile parasthesia and retrograde ejaculation (a reflection of the pelvic nerve damage). Because of these findings, the AUA considers vascular reconstructive approaches to ED experimental, with revascularization reserved for patients with trauma who have focal lesions without any evidence of vascular disease. These procedures provided a conceptual framework for consideration of endovascular therapies in treating this problem.

Table 76.2 Outcomes of penile revascularization surgery.

Study	n	Procedure	Follow-up (months)	Overall intercourse success rates (%)
Jarow 1997 [36]	11	DDVA	50	92
Lukkarinen 1997 [37]	24	Hauri F-F	Not described	72
Manning 1998 [38]	62	Virag Hauri	41	54
Manning 1998 [38]	42	DDVA	Not described	57
Kawanishi 2000 [30]	18	DA Hauri F-F	32	94
Sarramon 1997 [39]	114	DA DDVA	17	63
Sarramon 2001 [40]	38	DDVA	61	N/A
Vardi 2002 [5]	61	N/A	60	N/A
Kawanishi 2004 [31]	51	Hauri	36–60	85.6

DA, dorsal arterialization; DDVA, dorsal artery to deep vein anastomosis; F-F, Furlow–Fisher technique, arterialization of a dorsal vein segment (after ligating its proximal and distal ends including its circumflex branches); Hauri, three-vessel anastomosis with side-to-side between the dorsal artery and vein, covered by a spatulated inferior epigastric artery; Virag, deep dorsal vein arterialization using the retrograde approach from the emissary veins.

Endovascular approach to penile arterial revascularization

The current experience with transluminal angioplasty or stenting for the treatment of ED is very limited and detailed in Table 76.3. Almost all endovascular studies to date focused on large vessel inflow disease (common and internal iliac arteries). There are only limited case reports of transcatheter means of excluding pelvic venous insufficiency but not venous leak related to the penile emissary veins. Additionally, the duration of follow-up and methods in many of the published literature are lacking.

More recently, the ZEN trial (Zotarolimus-Eluting Peripheral Stent System for the Treatment of Erectile Dysfunction in Males with Suboptimal Response to PDE5 Inhibitors) has evaluated the role of endovascular intervention in patients with drug refractory ED. The study addressed many of the limitations associated with previous literature. A total of 30 patients (out of 383 subjects screened) with ED were enrolled. Procedural success was 100% with no major adverse events through follow-up. The primary feasibility endpoint at 6 months was achieved by 59.3% of intention-to-treat subjects and 69.6% of per-protocol subjects. Duplex ultrasound peak systolic velocity of the cavernosal arteries increased from baseline by 14.4 ± 10.7 cm/s at 30 days and 22.5 ± 23.7 cm/s at 6 months. Angiographic binary restenosis was reported in 11 (34.4%) of 32 lesions.

The ZEN trial clearly demonstrated the feasibility and safety of stenting atherosclerotic IPA lesions in highly selected subjects. Many subjects (but not all) reported subjective improvement in erectile function after these procedures, and there were concomitant increases in penile flow as determined by duplex ultrasound. Angiographic follow-up demonstrated no stent fractures and

reasonable binary patency considering the first-in-man use of a drug-eluting stent (DES) in a new vascular bed. Although the ZEN trial demonstrated safe and feasible stenting of the IPA in selected patients, most patients screened for this trial did not qualify and the main reasons for exclusion were: (i) excessive or insufficient angiographic disease; (ii) lack of arterial insufficiency by duplex; or (iii) venous leak. Additionally, a higher binary restenosis rate at 6 months (34%) highlights the unknowns in applying DES to the pelvic vasculature. Furthermore, the mechanism by which clinical improvement in erectile function persisted at 6 months despite angiographic binary restenosis in one-third of subjects remains unknown. Given these considerations, the authors concluded that the results of the ZEN trial precluded widespread use for the treatment of PAI [47].

Given the anatomic variations and the degree of diffuse disease noted in the ZEN Trial, Wang *et al.* performed the PElvic Revascularisation For arteriogenic EreCTile dysfunction (PERFECT-1) study. They used CT angiography to assess the safety and feasibility of catheter-based therapy for isolated penile artery stenoses in patients with erectile dysfunction. Twenty-five patients with ED and isolated penile artery stenoses (unilateral stenosis $\geq 70\%$ or bilateral stenoses $\geq 50\%$) identified by pelvic computed tomographic angiography were enrolled. A total of 20 patients (mean age 61 years; range 48–79 years) underwent balloon angioplasty. Three patients had bilateral penile artery stenoses. Procedural success was achieved in all 23 penile arteries, with an average balloon size of 1.6 mm (range 1.00–2.25 mm). The average International Index for Erectile Function-5 (IIEF-5) score improved from 10.0 ± 5.2 at baseline to 15.2 ± 6.7 (p <0.001) at 1 month and 15.2 ± 6.3 (p <0.001) at 6 months. Clinical success

Table 76.3 Endovascular treatment of erectile dysfunction.

Study	n	Angiographic stenosis	Technique	Follow-up	Success rate
Castaneda-Zunga 1982 [41]	2	Internal iliac	PTA	18 months	2/2 (100%)
Van Unnik 1984 [42]	1	External iliac	PTA	N/A	1/1 (100%)
Goldwasser 1985 [43]	1	Internal iliac	N/A	N/A	1/1 (100%)
Dewar 1985 [44]	30	70% aorto-iliac 47% internal iliac	PTA	N/A	10/33 (33%)
Angelini 1985 [45]	5	100% internal iliac	PTA	2–18 months	4/5 (80%)
Valji 1988 [22]	3	N/A	PTA	N/A	N/A
Urigo 1994 [46]*	23	65% internal iliac 13% internal pudendal	N/A	N/A	15/23 (65%) 3/3 (100%)
Rogers 2011 [47]	30	100% internal pudendal	PTA and drug-eluting stents	3 months	68.2% had improvement in IIEF score >4 points

IIEF, International Index on Erectile Function; N/A, not available; PTA, percutaneous transluminal balloon angioplasty.

* In this study, 65% of patients with internal iliac artery had improvement in erectile function, while all patients with pudendal artery disease had successful outcomes.

(change in the IIEF-5 score ≥4 or normalization of erectile function; IIEF-5 ≥ 22) was achieved in 15 (75%), 13 (65%), and 12 (60%) patients at 1, 3, and 6 months, respectively. Despite lack of angiographic follow-up or the use of a control group in this study, the authors concluded that penile artery angioplasty is safe and can achieve clinically significant improvement in erectile function in 60% of patients with ED and isolated penile artery stenosis [48].

Endovascular therapy for PAI is currently limited to a few studies showing modest benefit. This therapy should be reserved for a very select population of patients who have been evaluated by a multidisciplinary team for all potential causes of ED, and who have true PAI with anatomically suitable vessels for interventions after both functional assessment and invasive angiographic or computed tomographic imaging.

Patient selection and work-up

Patients at risk for atherosclerosis or with established coronary artery disease or peripheral vascular disease can be screened for the presence of vascular ED using a five-question subset of the IIEF questionnaire [32]. This is a validated, multidimensional, self-administered questionnaire used for the assessment of ED and treatment outcomes in clinical studies. The whole questionnaire consists of five separate response domains of sexual function: erectile function (questions 1–5, with a possible score of 25); orgasmic function (questions 9 and 10; possible score of 0–10), sexual desire (questions 11 and 12; possible score of 0–10); intercourse satisfaction (questions 6–8; possible score of 0–15); and overall satisfaction (questions 13 and 14; possible score of 2–10). A subset of five

questions are the Sexual Health Inventory for Men (SHIM, or IIEF-5) which assesses erectile function by rating each question on a scale of 1 (almost never or never) to 5 (almost always or always). A score of 0 indicates no attempt at sexual intercourse [33]. A score of less then 17 is considered consistent with severe ED. These patients should be referred to an urologist who specializes in ED who can perform a focused examination to exclude other causes such as Peyronie's disease (distortion of the architecture of the penis that does not allow intercourse irrespective of arterial supply). Additional blood tests such as testosterone levels, thyroid stimulating hormone (TSH), and prostate specific antigen (PSA) should also be obtained. If these are normal, the patient should be referred for duplex ultrasonography with cavernosal injection for measurements of systolic and diastolic penile blood flow. A peak systolic velocity (PSV) consistently exceeding 25 cm/s within 5 minutes of intracavernous injection will rule out PAI disease, while a PSV less than 25 cm/s has a sensitivity of 100% and a specificity of 95% in patients with abnormal pudendal angiography [34,35]. A persistent end-diastolic flow velocity (EDV) (>5 cm/s) accompanied by quick detumescence after stimulation is consistent with venogenic impotence (venous leak through the emissary veins) and the patient is unlikely to benefit from restoration of arterial inflow. Venogenic impotence occurs when there is incompetence of the venous drainage of the penis resulting in failure of engorgement of the cavernosal bodies leading to impotence. Patients with ED should be referred to urology or sexual medicine clinics and a duplex ultrasound should be considered to assess for PAI. If they fail current medical therapy and have evidence of PAI with no venous leak then they may be considered suitable candidates for PAI restoration.

Angiographic technique

Various unpublished methods are used for angiographic evaluation of the pelvic penile blood flow. We propose the following step-by-step angiographic guide for adequate visualization of PAI.

1 A Foley catheter is placed in the bladder and the penis is stretched and taped to the contralateral thigh when selective angiography of internal iliac and pudendal artery is performed. Consider gonadal shielding as per institutional radiation safety standards.

2 Femoral arterial access is obtained. An AP conventional pelvic angiography is performed after placement of a pigtail catheter above the aortic bifurcation and digital subtraction angiography with iliofemoral run-off is conducted (Figure 76.4). This allows an assessment of distal aorta, common and proximal internal iliac arteries. Additionally, it serves as a roadmap to locate the origin of the IPA or accessory vessels.

3 A 4 or 5 Fr diagnostic low profile catheter is then placed in the ostium of the internal iliac artery and selective angiography is performed. The origin of the vessel is best seen in the ipsilateral cranial oblique projection (20–30°). The mid and distal aspect of the vessel is best seen in ipsilateral oblique (20–30°) with mild caudal angulation 10–20° as shown in Figure 76.5a. The penis is positioned pointing to the contralateral side of injection to allow visualization of run-off into the penile vessels.

4 Penile vasodilatation may be necessary prior to angiography and can be accomplished by intracavernosal injection of 15 μg prostagladin E1. This serves to relax the cavernosal musculature and augments blood flow, vessel caliber, and markedly improves angiographic quality. This is especially useful when the anatomy is not clearly demarcated and the functional significance of a stenosis is uncertain.

5 Interventional therapy is frequently performed using 0.014-inch wires and coronary balloons and DES. It is important to have one-to-one sizing of the vessel with no oversizing of the vessel (Figure 76.5b).

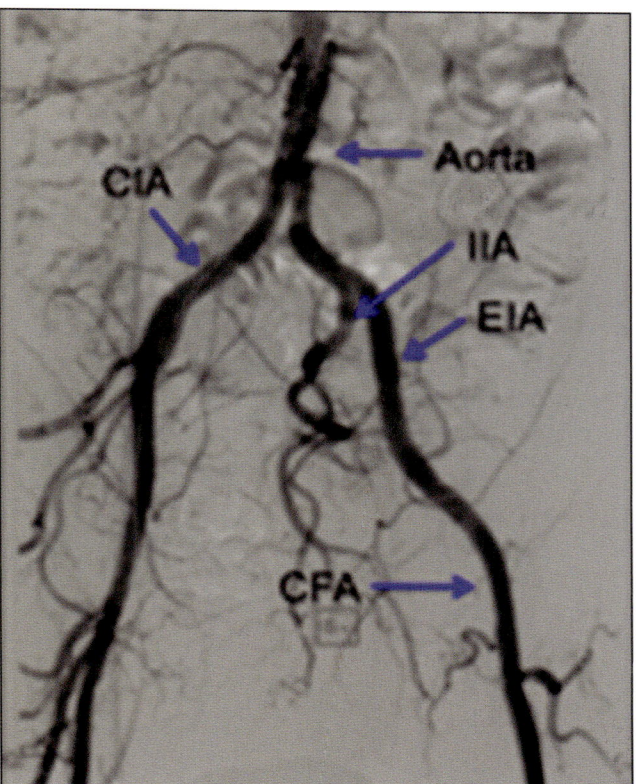

Figure 76.4 Aortogram in the AP projection showing the aorta, common iliac (CIA), external iliac (EIA), internal iliac (ILA), and common femoral arteries (CFA).

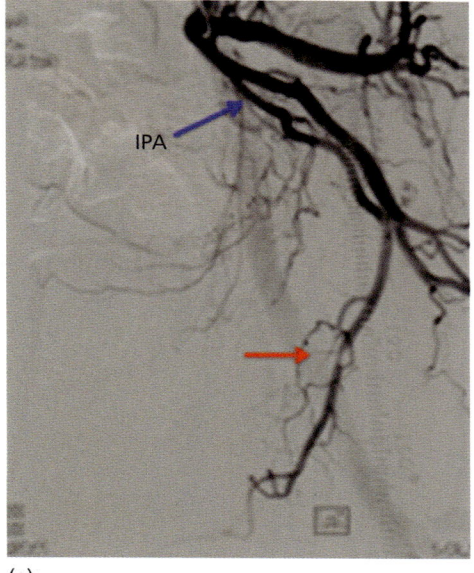

(a)

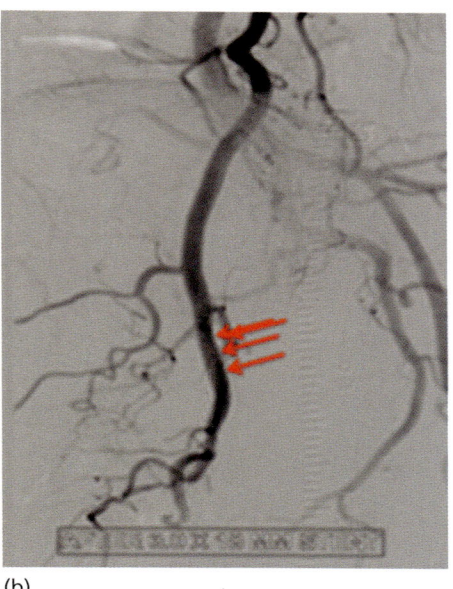

(b)

Figure 76.5 (a) Left ipsilateral cranial oblique projection looking at the inferior division of the internal iliac artery showing a stenosis in the distal internal pudendal artery (IPA). (b) The IPA after placement of a Resolute stent in the distal segment. Red arrow shows a stenotic segment.

Conclusions

ED and PAI disease coexists with a high frequency (~76%). Patients who have ED without psychogenic or organic cause should be referred for Doppler ultrasound examinations in collaboration with a urologist. While there is limited experience using contemporary endovascular therapies for this indication, this avenue promises to be an exciting and evolving field that is slowing gaining momentum in the context of the recent emerging evidence for benefit with minimal risk. Future randomized trials should fully evaluate the role of endovascular therapy for ED.

 Interactive multiple choice questions are available for this chapter on www.wiley.com/go/dangas/cardiology

References

1 Bhatt DL, Steg PG, Ohman EM. International prevalence, recognition, and treatment of cardiovascular risk factors in outpatients with atherothrombosis. *JAMA* 2006; **295**: 180–189.

2 Ayta IA, McKinlay JB, Krane RJ. The likely worldwide increase in erectile dysfunction between 1995 and 2025 and some possible policy consequences. *BJU Int* 1999; **84**: 50–56.

3 Thompson IM, Tangen CM, Goodman PJ. Erectile dysfunction and subsequent cardiovascular disease. *JAMA* 2005; **294**: 2996–3002.

4 Gazzaruso C, Giordanetti S, De Amici E. Relationship between erectile dysfunction and silent myocardial ischemia in apparently uncomplicated type 2 diabetic patients. *Circulation* 2004; **110**: 22–26.

5 Wespes E, Amar E, Hatzichristou D. Guidelines on erectile dysfunction. *Eur Urol* 2002; **41**: 1–5.

6 Montague DK, Jarow JP, Broderick GA. Chapter 1: The management of erectile dysfunction: an AUA update. *J Urol* 2005; **174**: 230–239.

7 Yamaki KI, Tsuyoshi S, Yoshiaki D. A statistical study of the branching of the human internal iliac artery. *Kurume Med J* 1998; **45**: 333–340.

8 Leriche R. *La Presse medicale*. 1949; **57**: 906.

9 May AG, DeWeese JA, Rob CG. Changes in sexual function following operation on the abdominal aorta. *Surgery* 1969; **65**: 41–47.

10 Carstensen G. [Treatment of impotentia coeundi by reconstructing the circulation in the internal iliac artery]. *Langenbecks Archiv Chir* 1969; **325**: 885–888.

11 Michal V, Kramar R, Pospichal J. [Direct arterial anastomosis on corpora cavernosa penis in the therapy of erective impotence]. *Rozhledy v chirurgii : mesicnik Ceskoslovenske chirurgicke spolecnosti*. 1973; **52**: 587–590.

12 Zorgniotti AW, Padula G, Rossi G. Impotence caused by pudendal arteriovenous fistula. *Urology* 1979; **14**: 161–162.

13 Michal V, Pospichal J. Phalloarteriography in the diagnosis of erectile impotence. *World J Surg* 1978; **2**: 239–248.

14 Rogers JH, Karimi H, Kao J. Internal pudendal artery stenoses and erectile dysfunction: correlation with angiographic coronary artery disease. *Catheter Cardiovasc Interv* 2010; **76**: 882–887.

15 Herman A, Adar R, Rubinstein Z. Vascular lesions associated with impotence in diabetic and nondiabetic arterial occlusive disease. *Diabetes* 1978; **27**: 975–981.

16 Struyven J, Gregoir W, Giannakopoulos X. Selective pudendal arteriography. *Eur Urol* 1979; **5**: 233–242.

17 Huguet JF, Clerissi J, Juhan C. Radiologic anatomy of pudendal artery. *Eur J Radiol* 1981; **1**: 278–284.

18 Buvat J, Lemaire A, Buvat-Herbaut M. Comparative investigations in 26 impotent and 26 nonimpotent diabetic patients. *J Urol* 1985; **133**: 34–38.

19 Bruhlmann W, Pouliadis G, Zollikofer C. Arteriography of the penis in secondary impotence. *Urologic Radiol* 1982; **4**: 243–249.

20 Nessi R, De Flaviis L, Bellinzoni G. Digital angiography of erectile failure. *Br J Urol* 1987; **59**: 584–589.

21 Gray RR, Keresteci AG, St Louis EL. Investigation of impotence by internal pudendal angiography: experience with 73 cases. *Radiology* 1982; **144**: 773–780.

22 Valji K, Bookstein JJ. Transluminal angioplasty in the treatment of arteriogenic impotence. *Cardiovasc Interv Radiol* 1988; **11**: 245–252.

23 Rosen MP, Greenfield AJ, Walker TG. Arteriogenic impotence: findings in 195 impotent men examined with selective internal pudendal angiography. *Radiology* 1990; **174**: 1043–1048.

24 Buvat J, Lemaire A, Besson P. Lack of correlations between penile thermography and pelvic arteriography in 29 cases of erectile impotence. *J Urol* 1982; **128**: 298–299.

25 Kawanishi Y, Muguruma H, Sugiyama H. Variations of the internal pudendal artery as a congenital contributing factor to age at onset of erectile dysfunction in Japanese. *BJU Int* 2008; **101**: 581–587.

26 Michal V, Kramar R, Hejhal L. [Tactics of reconstruction interventions in the aortoiliac area from the viewpoint of erectivity disorders in men]. *Rozhledy v chirurgii: mesicnik Ceskoslovenske chirurgicke spolecnosti*. 1973; **52**: 591–595.

27 Michal V, Kramar R, Pospichal J, Hejhal L. Direct arterial anastomosis on corpora cavernosal penis in the therapy of erectile impotence. *J Sex Med* 2008; **5**: 1062–1065.

28 Hauri D. [Surgical possibilities in treatment of vascular-induced erectile impotence]. *Der Urologe Ausg A* 1989; **28**: 260–265.

29 Virag R, Saltiel H, Floresco J. [Surgical treatment of vascular impotence by arterialization of the dorsal vein of the penis: experience of 292 cases]. *Chirurgie; memoires de l'Academie de chirurgie* 1988; **114**: 703–714.

30 Kawanishi Y, Kimura K, Yamaguchi K et al. [Microsurgical penile revascularization in patients with pure arteriogenic erectile dysfunction]. *Japanese J Urol* 2000; **91**: 62–68.

31 Kawanishi Y, Kimura K, Nakanishi R. Penile revascularization surgery for arteriogenic erectile dysfunction: the long-term efficacy rate calculated by survival analysis. *BJU Int* 2004; **94**: 361–368.

32 Rosen RC, Cappelleri JC, Smith MD. Development and evaluation of an abridged, 5-item version of the International Index of Erectile Function (IIEF-5) as a diagnostic tool for erectile dysfunction. *Int J Impotence Res* 1999; **11**: 319–326.

33 Heruti RJ, Yossef M, Shochat T. Screening for erectile dysfunction as part of periodic examination programs: concept and implementation. *Int J Impotence Res* 2004; **16**: 341–345.

34 Valji K, Bookstein JJ. Diagnosis of arteriogenic impotence: efficacy of duplex sonography as a screening tool. *Am J Roentgenol* 1993; **160**: 65–69.

35 Quam JP, King BF, James EM. Duplex and color Doppler sonographic evaluation of vasculogenic impotence. *Am J Roentgenol* 1989; **153**: 1141–1147.

36 Jarow JP, Oates RD, Buch JP. Effect of level of anastomosis and quality of intra-epididymal sperm on the outcome of end-to-side epididymovasostomy. *Urology* 1997; **49**: 590–595.

37 Lukkarinen O, Tonttila P, Hellstrom P. Non-prosthetic surgery in the treatment of erectile dysfunction: a retrospective study of 45 impotent patients in the University of Oulu. *Scand J Urol Nephrol* 1998; **32**: 42–46.

38 Manning M, Spahn M, Junemann KP. [Vascular surgery, implant surgery and vacuum erectile aids: review-overview-prospects of 3 therapy options in erectile dysfunction]. *Der Urologe Ausg A* 1998; **37**: 509–515.

39 Sarramon JP, Bertrand N, Malavaud B. [Surgical treatments of erectile impotence]. *Rev Med Interne* 1997; **18**(Suppl 1): 36s–40s.

40 Sarramon JP, Malavaud B, Braud F. Evaluation of male sexual function by the International Index of Erectile Function after deep dorsal vein arterialization of the penis. *J Urol* 2001; **166**: 576–580.

41 Castaneda-Zuniga WR, Smith A, Kaye K. Transluminal angioplasty for treatment of vasculogenic impotence. *Am J Roentgenol* 1982; **139**: 371–373.

42 Van Unnik JG, Marsman JW. Impotence due to the external iliac steal syndrome treated by percutaneous transluminal angioplasty. *J Urol* 1984; **131**: 544–545.

43 Goldwasser B, Carson CC 3rd, Braun SD. Impotence due to the pelvic steal syndrome: treatment by iliac transluminal angioplasty. *J Urol* 1985; **133**: 860–861.

44 Dewar ML, Blundell PE, Lidstone D. Effects of abdominal aneurysmectomy, aortoiliac bypass grafting and angioplasty on male sexual potency: a prospective study. *Can J Surg* 1985; **28**: 154–156, 159.

45 Angelini G, Pezzini F, Mucci P. [Arteriosclerosis and impotence]. *Minerva Psichiatr* 1985; **26**: 353–417.

46 Urigo F, Pischedda A, Maiore M. [Role of arteriography and percutaneous transluminal angioplasty in the diagnosis and treatment of arterial vasculogenic impotence]. *Radiol Med* 1994; **88**: 86–92.

47 Rogers J, Goldstein I and Kandzari D. Drug eluting stents for the treatment of erectile dysfunction – results of the ZEN trial. *J Am Coll Cardiol* 2012; **60**: 2618–2627.

48 Wang TD, Wen-Jeng L, Shao-Chi Y. Safety and six-month durability of angioplasty for isolated penile artery stenoses in patients with erectile dysfunction: a first-in-man study. *EuroIntervention* 2014; **10**: 147–156.

CHAPTER 77

Iliac Interventions

Manish Taneja[1] and Apoorva Gogna[2]

[1] Interventional Radiology, Raffles Hospital, Singapore

[2] Interventional Radiology Centre, Department of Diagnostic Radiology, Singapore General Hospital, Singapore

Approximately one-third of peripheral arterial occlusive disease (PAOD) affects the aorto-iliac segment in Western populations [1]. The prevalence of PAOD is reported to be 16% in patients aged 60–69, rising to 34% in those aged over 70 years [2]. While the TransAtlantic Inter-Society Consensus (TASC-II) guidelines [3], published in 2007, recommend endovascular treatment for type A and B lesions, the accumulation of experience, and improvements in equipment (lower profile wires and balloons, re-entry devices) and imaging have rapidly allowed TASC-II C and even D lesions to be successfully treated using endovascular means.

There is evidence for percutaneous coronary intervention (PCI) to be considered first line therapy even for complex and long aorto-iliac stenoses and occlusions [4] and hence many authors now advise a far more aggressive PCI approach than the original TASC-II treatment recommendations. In fact, the March 2015 Society of Vascular Surgery guidelines [5] recommend PCI as first line treatment in all aorto-iliac occlusive disease (AIOD) classes, and reserve surgery only for failed PCI and severe disease in presence of aortic aneurysms. This recommendation is further strengthened by studies showing that PCI does not preclude further surgical options in AIOD [6].

In a diseased vessel that is not completely occluded, the true lumen is still visible, hence there is usually no need to cross a blind segment and usually no acute blood clots are present. The TASC-II D subtype comprises lesions of greatly varying technical complexity for PCI because both long segment occlusions and multifocal stenoses are included. In practical terms, it is more useful to separate chronic total occlusions (CTO), acute occlusions, and stenoses because they each present unique challenges for PCI. Here we discuss the current recommended treatment guidelines for these categories and other special subsets.

Clinical presentation and diagnosis

Patients with AIOD typically present with symptoms of chronic limb ischemia although acute on chronic presentations are also occasionally seen.

Acute limb ischemia (ALI) is defined as sudden reduction of limb perfusion, usually within 14 days, which threatens limb viability. In the AIOD territory, acute presentations usually relate to graft or stent thrombosis, *in situ* thrombosis of a diseased segment, and,

less likely, occlusion by an acute embolus. Acute and subacute (less than 30 days) occlusions should first be considered for surgical treatment, although pharmacomechanical lysis options are available. Caution is needed because of the large amount of thrombus load which increases the risk of distal embolization, and, concurrently, the treatment chosen should be expedient to prevent irreversible tissue necrosis and reperfusion syndrome. ALI is covered in greater detail elsewhere in the book.

Chronic limb ischemia (CLI) tends to present in an insidious fashion but is far more common than ALI. Severity can be classified using the Rutherford [7] and Fontaine scales, and ranges from asymptomatic subclinical disease to gangrene.

Claudication caused by stenosis results from the inability of the vessel segment to increase demand-related blood flow to the muscle during times of increased activity (e.g., walking). Patients report pain or fatigue during walking which is relieved with rest, gait disturbances, and reductions in walking speed. This can greatly impair patients' quality of life. Conservative treatment with supervised progressive walking programs and medial therapy (e.g., cilostazol) should be attempted first for several months. Endovascular treatment can be offered to patients who fail or are unsuitable for conservative therapy.

Critical limb ischemia refers to rest pain and tissue loss (ulceration, gangrene) when blood flow is insufficient to even meet the resting metabolic tissue requirement. Typically, rest pain is relieved partially by gravity dependent positioning of the limb below the level of the heart (e.g., sitting position or hanging the leg over the side of the bed).

On physical examination, a bruit over the lower abdomen and/or a weak or absent femoral pulse can be detected. The lower extremities should be examined for signs of ischemia. The ankle-brachial index (ABI) is a quick measurement of the overall perfusion at the level of the distal extremity but is unable to quantify the extent and severity of disease in each segment of the lower limb.

Arterial imaging can be performed using non-invasive (ultrasound, CT, or MR angiography) or invasive (catheter angiography, pressure gradients, intravascular ultrasound) methods; the latter usually combined with treatment.

Ultrasound remains the cornerstone of preoperative imaging because it offers cheap, high resolution, real-time information

Interventional Cardiology: Principles and Practice, Second Edition. Edited by George D. Dangas, Carlo Di Mario, and Nicholas N. Kipshidze.
© 2017 John Wiley & Sons, Ltd. Published 2017 by John Wiley & Sons, Ltd.

about the anatomy and flow dynamics of the vessel segment. However, imaging of the aorto-iliac segments is difficult with ultrasound alone because of interference by overlying bowel loops and reduced signal with increasing depth. Abnormal waveforms (i.e., loss of the normal triphasic waveform) at the groin does raise suspicion of inflow disease in the AIOD, but can also result from distal disease. We find preoperative imaging of this segment with CT or MR angiography very useful to define the extent and nature of the occlusion. Non-contrast MR angiography techniques are possible for patients with contraindications to intravenous gadolinium-based contrast (typically, patients with advanced renal failure).

Percutaneous intervention

AIOD lesions can be approached using one or more of four main access ports: ipsilateral common femoral artery, contralateral common femoral artery (CFA), upper limb artery (e.g., brachial or radial), or ipsilateral distal artery (e.g., popliteal). The choice depends on the location of the primary lesion, associated lesions en route to the lesion, and size of instruments desired to be conveyed to the treatment site. In practical terms, the femoral retrograde access is most commonly used. Ipsilateral approaches offer better vis-a-tergo and torque hence improving maneuverability of the catheter or wire. Conversely, the contralateral antegrade access allows crossing in the direction of flow, and allows better imaging to be performed showing the proximal and distal reconstituted segments. Realistically, both groins should be prepared for every intervention to allow change of access site if needed.

For non-CTO lesions, a single contralateral CFA access can be sufficient to treat the aorto-iliac and infra-inguinal disease. For origin or bifurcation lesions, bilateral access is often required (see section on bifurcation lesions). For CTOs, ipsilateral and contralateral or arm access facilitates definition of extent of disease and lesion crossing. In rare cases, popliteal access is chosen to traverse long contiguous CTOs of the iliac and femoral segments.

Premedication with oral aspirin is normally given, with some authors adding oral clopidogrel. Intravenous heparin is typically given according to body weight (70 units/kg), to achieve activated clotting times of 220–250 s. Post-stenting, aspirin should be continued lifelong, while thienopyridines such as clopidogrel or prasugrel are given for at least 1 month [8].

The choice of wire platform and balloon for angioplasty is very much operator dependent, and no consensus exists as to the ideal strategy. We tend to use the 0.014-inch platform for most cases because it allows larger 0.018-inch platform and even 0.035-inch platform balloons to advance over the wire. When more support is needed, we then exchange for larger platform wires after initial dilatation.

Some authors recommend predilatation with a balloon sized about 2 mm smaller than the native vessel diameter [9,10], to prevent distal embolization; others recommend primary stenting for the same purpose.

Aorto-iliac stenoses

The Cardiovascular and Interventional Radiological Society of Europe (CIRSE) guidelines [4] on AIOD, published in 2012, recommend PCI as first line for TASC-II A–C due to low morbidity and mortality, and over 90% technical success (class 1 recommendation, level of evidence C).

Studies comparing PCI with open surgical treatments for AIOD have shown approximately equivalent patency, limb salvage, and overall survival rates, yet lower morbidity and mortality than surgical reconstruction [6,10,11].

Kashyap et al. [6] provided a detailed comparison of PCI versus open surgery. They observed worse post-PCI patency rates in younger patients. Conversely, worse post-surgery patency was noted in diabetics and presence of poor runoff to the lower extremity. A small diameter aorta also appears to perform poorly post open bypass [12].

Indes et al. [2] reviewed all patients who underwent open and endovascular procedures within the HCUP-NIS (a large American inpatient database of over 8 million hospital stays per year) within the 2004–2007 period, and reported an overall inpatient complication rate of 16% in the PCI group compared to 25% in the open surgical group (p <0.001). Further, average length of stay was 2.2 days versus 5.8 days, while total inpatient cost was $13,661 versus $17,161, both in favor of PCI (p <0.05).

Sachwani et al. [10] reviewed patients (January 2000 to December 2011) with symptomatic (intermittent claudication 69%; rest pain 19%; and toe gangrene 15%) iliac occlusions who underwent PCI (n = 100 patients) or aorto-bifemoral graft bypass (n = 101 patients). Open bypass was preferred for patients with long segment common iliac artery (CIA) or external iliac artery (EIA) occlusions with heavy calcifications and infra-inguinal disease and also patients with previous failed PCI/stent interventions, and small diameter vessels. While the primary patency rate after 72 months was higher in the surgical group (91% vs. 73%; p = 0.01), the secondary patency rate was not significantly different. Target lesion revascularization (TLR) in the PCI group involved catheter-directed thrombolysis, restenting, and balloon angioplasty. TLR in the bypass group required open thrombectomy or catheter-directed thrombolysis. The authors also observed a trend favoring PCI over bypass toward the latter half of their study period, attributed to increasing experience and availability of technical aids.

Chronic totally occlusive lesions

The PCI procedure in a chronic total occlusion can be technically challenging. Ultrasound, fluoroscopic, or roadmap guidance can be helpful to puncture a pulseless femoral artery [10]. Bilateral femoral artery, and in some cases brachial access may be needed to provide both antegrade and retrograde imaging and wiring. The tram-track calcifications of an occluded vessel are often very helpful during wire crossing, and should be viewed in orthogonal planes on high quality angiography equipment.

Many authors recommend the use of an angled catheter (e.g., 5 Fr Kumpe, Cook Inc., Bloomington, IN, USA) and a 0.035-inch hydrophilic wire (Glidewire, Terumo Medical, Japan). Alternatively, low profile support microcatheters (CXI, Cook Inc.) and 0.014-inch weighted CTO wires (e.g., Winn 40, 80, Abbott Medical) can be used. A combined antegrade and retrograde approach can be very useful in limiting the subintimal dissection to the affected segment, and assisting in re-entry. Often, the catheter can be "selected" from the contralateral access, thereby alleviating the need for an expensive snare device.

Re-entry devices such as Outback (Cordis Johnson & Johnson), Frontrunner (Cordis), and Pioneer IVUS catheter (Medtronic) have been used in only a minority of cases in several large series [10], suggesting that the simple and cost-effective wire and catheter technique suffices in the majority of patients. This has also been our experience, where re-entry devices are required in less than 5% of cases (unpublished data). The re-entry device serves to direct a wire in the subintimal plane back into the patent true lumen beyond the distal cap of the occlusion.

Jongkind et al. [13] published a systematic review of PCI for TASC C and D subtype AIOD in 2010 based on 19 studies (n = 1711 patients) published between the years 2000 and 2009 which fit the systematic review criteria. PCI with or without combined surgical techniques for the aorto-iliac and outflow were used, and primary stenting with bare metal stents (BMS) or stent grafts performed in most studies. Technical success was 86–100%, improvement in clinical outcome 83–100%, morbidity 3–45% (comprising access site hematoma, distal embolization, arterial dissection, pseudo-aneurysms, or rupture). Primary and assisted patency rates were 70–97%, 88–100% at 1 year, respectively and 60–86%, 80–98% at 4 or 5 years, respectively.

Stents: covered and uncovered

Overall primary patency of stents is 85–95% at 1 year, 70–85% at 3 years, and 55–75% at 5 years [10,14–16]. The CFA is an area of high biomechanical stress, considered by many as a "no-stent area," and is traditionally a surgical lesion. This is contributed by a relatively easy surgical exposure of the EIA for endarterectomy, compared to the aorto-iliac and infra-inguinal segments. Lesions extending from the EIA into the CFA have hence been approached in a combined fashion (e.g., stent implantation with femoral patch plasty).

The severity of AIOD has a bearing on stent selection. Kudo et al. reported worse outcomes (increased risk for recurrent disease) after stenting for TASC-II C and D compared to A and B [17]; however, Sixt et al. [18] reported comparable primary patency rates at 1 year of 98–100% irrespective of TASC-II lesion type.

Suero et al. [19] performed a retrospective analysis of 99 consecutive patients with claudication (n = 70) and critical limb ischemia (n = 29) treated for occlusive EIA disease. The mean lesion length was 42.2 mm. Balloon angioplasty alone was used in seven limbs and stenting with self-expanding (n = 65), balloon expandable (n = 24), or covered stents (n = 12) in 101 lesions.

The recent STAG trial [15] (stents vs. angioplasty for the treatment of iliac artery occlusions) compared primary stenting and balloon angioplasty for symptomatic iliac artery occlusions of up to 8 cm in length (n = 112 patients). It showed no difference between the two groups in primary and secondary patency of the iliac segment; however, stenting was associated with improved technical success and reduced procedure complications.

Lesion length also appears to correlate to stent patency. While there is no universal definition of a long AIOD lesion, 100 mm appears to be the cut-off favored by most authors. A 2014 study (for TASC B–D lesions) by Benetis et al. showed a significant difference in patency rates for stents greater versus those less than 61 mm: 1 and 2 year patency rates of 90.6% and 86.6% versus 67.7% and 60.2%, respectively, in favour of the shorter stents [20].

Primary stenting (without predilatation) versus stenting after initial balloon angioplasty remains an unresolved issue. Primary stenting of the affected segment (without predilatation) has been considered by several authors as a strategy to reduce embolization, by trapping clot/atheroma between the stent and vessel wall. Further, primary stenting can result in less neointimal hyperplasia.

The issue of primary versus selective stenting for iliac stenoses has been much debated. In 1998, Tetteroo et al. [21] published results of a randomized trial comparing primary stenting (n = 143 patients) with angioplasty with selective stenting (n = 136 patients) for patients presenting with intermittent claudication. They found no difference in short- and long-term outcomes between the groups, including technical success, quality of life, 2-year patency, and reintervention rates. They concluded that the latter option (selective stenting) should be used because of its lower overall cost. However, note that this trial mainly focused on TASC A and B lesions.

Conversely, Bosiers et al. [22] reported subgroup analysis of TASC A and B lesions treated under the BRAVISSIMO study and concluded that primary stenting is the preferred option for TASC A/B lesions, with a 12 month primary patency of 94% for TASC A, and 96.5% for TASC B lesions (p = ns).

Ye et al. [14] performed a meta-analysis of studies reported between 2000 and 2010 (16 articles, n = 958 patients) for TASC C and D lesions, and demonstrated 1-year primary patency rates of 92.1% for primary stenting and 82.9% for selective stenting although not statistically significant.

Bechter-Hugl et al. [1] studied outcomes of primary stenting for symptomatic iliac occlusions, and found 1, 3, 5, and 7 year primary patency rates of 90.3%, 77.2%, 60.2%, and 46.4% for women, and 89.9%, 71.%, 63.6%, and 59.7% for men, respectively (p = ns). However, on subgroup analysis, younger age was found to adversely affect outcomes: restenosis rates were 23.9% in men and 22.1% in women older than 63.5 years, and 32.1% in men and 49.1% in women younger than 63.5 years, respectively (p <0.05).

Other factors limiting stent patency are the quality of the distal runoff, critical limb ischemia (as opposed to claudication), diabetes, and subintimal recanalization [14].

Balloon expandable stents are made of cobalt-chromium or stainless steel. In the iliac segment, the patency of both types of stents appears equivalent; however, there are some practical differences. Balloon expandable stents tend to be more difficult to maneuver through tortuous or calcified vessels as they are much stiffer. Their maximum available length is also about 8 cm for this reason. When advanced without a long sheath ("bare-back"), there is a tendency for the stent to get caught on calcific plaque and slip off the balloon. However, the balloon stent deployment is very accurate as there is no tendency for the stent to "jump" during deployment— hence these are good for placement "flush" with the origin of the contralateral common iliac, or the internal iliac artery.

Self-expandable stents are usually made of nickel-titanium alloy (nitinol). The available lengths are much longer (up to 150 cm) in diameters of 6–10 mm. As the stent is much more flexible, it can be advanced through calcified or tortuous vessels more easily. As it comes constrained within a sheath, there is no tendency for the stent to dislodge. However, it does tend to "jump" forward during initial deployment, although improvements in delivery systems have minimized this.

COBEST [23] was a prospective, randomized, multicenter, controlled trial in severe AIOD (n = 125 patients, 168 iliac arteries), with patients randomly assigned to receive balloon-expandable BMS (varied) or balloon-expandable stent grafts (Advanta V12, Atrium Medical). The covered stent group was more likely to remain free of binary restenosis and occlusions, particularly for TASC C and D lesions. The ongoing randomized, prospective, double-blind DISCOVER trial [24] should provide further guidance in this issue.

Our preference is to use self-expanding stents, generally 7–10 mm diameter in the common iliac segment, and 5–8 mm in the EIA, depending on the native diameter of the vessel. Others have reported preference for balloon expanded stents in the CIA segment, because of more accurate placement. We always review the patient's previous cross-sectional imaging (CT, MRI) as this can be very useful in estimating the native diameter of the diseased vessel prior to angiography for accurate stent sizing.

Bifurcation lesions

Reconstruction of the aorto-iliac bifurcation with "kissing" angioplasty and/or stenting represents a special category because of the added complexity. Bilateral femoral, and sometimes brachial, access is required for simultaneous antegrade/retrograde access, and placement of balloons and stents. Both self-expanding or balloon expandable stents can be used, but the same type should be implanted in bilateral ostial iliac locations. However, certain lesions can be heavily calcific or heavily fibrotic in a way that may obviate the use of self-expanding stents because of their lower radial force; such cases are better targeted with balloon expandable stents. When a deep dissection or localized perforation is feared, a covered stent should be utilized.

Kissing stents should be deployed simultaneously, and extended 0.5–1.5 cm into the distal aorta. The covered endovascular reconstruction of aortic bifurcation (CERAB) technique uses three balloon expanded covered stents to reconstruct the aortic bifurcation for TASC-II C and D lesions.

Complications

Complication rate from the literature is 7–20% overall [9,10,15,25], with expectedly worse outcomes for more severe cases. A meta-analysis [14] reported overall mortality rate of 2.9% and morbidity rate of 15.3% for AIOD PCI (for TASC C and D lesions). Typical complications include groin hematomas, arteriovenous fistulas, pseudoaneurysms, and acute stent thrombosis (about 3% overall). Distal embolization from fragmentation of clot and atheroma occurs in up to 5% [9,10] and can be treated in most cases with aspiration thrombectomy using a long guiding catheter.

The most feared complication of AIOD PCI is iliac artery rupture, reported in 1.73% (range 0.2–3.4%) of patients [4,10]. Because of the high volume flow in the iliac segment (over 200 mL/minute at rest) and the surrounding potential space which can accommodate a large blood volume, catastrophic bleeding can occur rapidly if undiagnosed. Maintaining wire access and early detection is critical. A range of stent grafts should be maintained in the procedure suite for this purpose. In the interim, balloon tamponade should be performed using low pressure inflation of an angioplasty balloon, typically the same balloon that was used for angioplasty prior to rupture. Reversal of heparin with intravenous protamine sulfate (typically, 10 mg for every 1000 units heparin given, up to maximum of 50 mg protamine), blood transfusion, and ICU monitoring may be indicated.

For stent thrombosis, anticoagulant therapy regimens are essential, and comprise combinations of low molecular weight heparin until discharge from hospital, lifelong oral aspirin (81–325 mg/day), and clopidogrel 75 mg/day.

Open surgical repair studies report significantly higher rates of cardiac arrest, hematoma, blood transfusion requirements, respiratory complications, post operative infections, and seroma formation [2].

Conclusions

There is little doubt that in this day and age, AIOD can be managed through an endovascular approach because of comparable long-term results, a relatively low barrier to re-treatment even for recurrent disease, and preservation of surgical option if all else fails. Primary stenting remains an area of some controversy because although medium-term results are good and somewhat better than angioplasty alone, the downside of leaving permanent metal behind should be weighed, especially for younger, active patients.

Interactive multiple choice questions are available for this chapter on www.wiley.com/go/dangas/cardiology

References

1 Bechter-Hugl B, Falkensammer J, Gorny O, Greiner A, Chemelli A, Fraedrich G. The influence of gender on patency rates after iliac artery stenting. *J Vasc Surg* 2014; **59**(6): 1588–1596. doi.org/10.1016/j.jvs.2014.01.010

2 Indes JE, Mandawat A, Tuggle CT, Muhs B, Sosa J. Endovascular procedures for aorto-iliac occlusive disease are associated with superior short-term clinical and economic outcomes compared with open surgery in the inpatient population. *J Vasc Surg* 2010; **52**(5): 1173–9.e1. doi.org/10.1016/j.jvs.2010.05.100

3 Norgren L, Hiatt WR, Dormandy JA, *et al.* Inter-Society Consensus for the management of peripheral arterial disease (TASC II). *J Vasc Surg* 2007; **45**(1): S5–S67.

4 Rossi M, Iezzi R. Cardiovascular and interventional Radiological Society of Europe guidelines on endovascular treatment in aortoiliac arterial disease. *Cardiovasc Interv Radiol* 2014; **37**(1): 13–25.

5 Conte MS, Pomposelli FB, Clair DG, *et al.* Society for Vascular Surgery practice guidelines for atherosclerotic occlusive disease of the lower extremities: management of asymptomatic disease and claudication. *J Vasc Surg* 2015; **61**(3): 2S–41S.

6 Kashyap VS, Pavkov ML, Bena JF, *et al.* The management of severe aortoiliac occlusive disease: endovascular therapy rivals open reconstruction. *J Vasc Surg* 2008; **48**(6): 1451–1457.

7 Rutherford RB, Baker JD, Ernst C, *et al.* Recommended standards for reports dealing with lower extremity ischemia: revised version. *J Vasc Surg* 1997; **26**(3): 517–538.

8 Robertson L, Ghouri M, Kovacs F. Antiplatelet and anticoagulant drugs for prevention of restenosis/reocclusion following peripheral endovascular treatment. *Cochrane Database Syst Rev* 2012; **8**: CD002071.

9 Ko YG, Shin S, Kim KJ, *et al.* Efficacy of stent-supported subintimal angioplasty in the treatment of long iliac artery occlusions. *J Vasc Surg* 2011; **54**(1): 116–122.

10 Sachwani GR, Hans SS, Khoury MD, *et al.* Results of iliac stenting and aortofemoral grafting for iliac artery occlusions. *J Vasc Surg* 2013; **57**(4): 1030–1037. doi.org/10.1016/j.jvs.2012.09.038

11 Tewksbury R, Taumoepeau L, Cartmill A, Butcher A, Cohen T. Outcomes of covered expandable stents for the treatment of TASC D aorto-iliac occlusive lesions. *Vascular* 2015; **23**(6): 630–636.

12 Reed AB, Conte MS, Donaldson MC, Mannick JA, Whittemore AD, Belkin M. The impact of patient age and aortic size on the results of aortobifemoral bypass grafting. *J Vasc Surg* 2003; **37**(6): 1219–1225.

13 Jongkind V, Akkersdijk GJM, Yeung KK, Wisselink W. A systematic review of endovascular treatment of extensive aortoiliac occlusive disease. *J Vasc Surg* 2010; **52**(5): 1376–83. doi.org/10.1016/j.jvs.2010.04.080

14 Ye W, Liu CW, Ricco JB, Mani K, Zeng R, Jiang J. Early and late outcomes of percutaneous treatment of TransAtlantic Inter-Society Consensus class C and D aorto-iliac lesions. *J Vasc Surg* 2011; **53**(6): 1728–1737.

15 Goode SD, Cleveland TJ, Gaines PA. Randomized clinical trial of stents versus angioplasty for the treatment of iliac artery occlusions (STAG trial). *Br J Surg* 2013; **100**(9): 1148–1153.

16 Bekken J, Jongsma H, Ayez N, Hoogewerf CJ, Van Weel V, Fioole B. Angioplasty versus stenting for iliac artery lesions. *Cochrane Database Syst Rev* 2015; **5**: CD007561.

17 Kudo T, Chandra FA, Ahn SS. Long-term outcomes and predictors of iliac angioplasty with selective stenting. *J Vasc Surg* 2005; **42**(3): 466–475.

18 Sixt S, Alawied AK, Rastan A, *et al.* Acute and long-term outcome of endovascular therapy for aortoiliac occlusive lesions stratified according to the TASC classification: a single-center experience. *J Endovasc Ther* 2008; **15**(4): 408–416.

19 Suero RS, López MI, Rydings HM, *et al.* Endovascular treatment of external iliac artery occlusive disease: midterm results. *J Endovasc Ther* 2014; **21**(2): 223–229.

20 Benetis R, Kavaliauskiene Z, Antusevas A, Kaupas RS, Inciura D, Kinduris S. Comparison of results of endovascular stenting and bypass grafting for TransAtlantic Inter-Society (TASC II) type B, C and D iliac occlusive disease. *Arch Med Sci* 2016; **12**(2): 353–359. doi: 10.5114/aoms.2016.59261

21 Tetteroo E, van der Graaf Y, Bosch JL, *et al.* Randomised comparison of primary stent placement versus primary angioplasty followed by selective stent placement in patients with iliac-artery occlusive disease. Dutch Iliac Stent Trial Study Group. *Lancet* 1998; **351**(9110): 1153–1159.

22 Bosiers M, Deloose K, Callaert J, Verbist J, Keirse K, Peeters P. BRAVISSIMO study: 12-month results from the TASC A/B subgroup. *J Cardiovasc Surg* 2012; **53**(1): 91–99.

23 Mwipatayi BP, Surg M, Sa FCS, *et al.* A comparison of covered vs bare expandable stents for the treatment of aortoiliac occlusive disease. *J Vasc Surg* 2011; **54**(6): 1561–1570.e1. doi.org/10.1016/j.jvs.2011.06.097

24 Bekken JA, Vos JA, Aarts RA, de Vries JPM, Fioole B. DISCOVER: Dutch Iliac Stent trial: COVERed balloon-expandable versus uncovered balloon-expandable stents in the common iliac artery: study protocol for a randomized controlled trial. *Trials* 2012; **13**(1): 215.

25 Klein WM, van der Graaf Y, Seegers J, Moll FL, Mali WPTM. Long-term cardiovascular morbidity, mortality, and reintervention after endovascular treatment in patients with iliac artery disease: The Dutch Iliac Stent Trial Study. *Radiology* 2004; **232**(2): 491–498.

CHAPTER 78

Superficial Femoral Artery Interventions

Cristina Sanina[1], Pedro R. Cox-Alomar[2], Prakash Krishnan[3], and Jose M. Wiley[4]

[1] University of Miami Miller School of Medicine, Miami, FL, USA
[2] University of Florida College of Medicine, Jacksonville, FL, USA
[3] The Zena and Michael A. Weiner Cardiovascular Institute, Icahn School of Medicine at Mount Sinai, New York, NY, USA
[4] Albert Einstein College of Medicine; Montefiore Einstein Center for Heart & Vascular Care, Bronx, NY, USA

In the USA, peripheral arterial disease (PAD) affects 8–12 million people. Almost 20% of the population older than 70 years of age has signs or symptoms of PAD [1–3]. Intermittent claudication (IC), defined as pain in the muscles of the leg with ambulation, is the earliest and most frequent presenting symptom in patients with lower extremity PAD. As the disease progresses in severity patients experience pain at rest, especially when the legs are elevated in bed at night, which is relieved by dependency. Although claudication symptoms are typically localized in the calf or the thigh, "rest pain" is characteristically present in the foot. In the late stages of PAD, tissue hypoperfusion progresses to ischemic ulceration and gangrene, and major amputation is eventually required in more than one-third of these patients [4]. For patients with IC, approximately 20% have progressive symptoms and 1–2% develop critical limb ischemia (CLI) within 5 years with a 1-year mortality rate of about 20% in several series [5–7].

The femoral-popliteal segment is the most commonly involved compartment among atherosclerotic PAD [8] comprising around 60% of PAD lesions [9,10]. Femoral-popliteal lesions are usually long and have varying degrees of calcification with most of these lesions being TransAtlantic Inter-Society Consensus (TASC) C and D lesions [11,12]. Endovascular techniques and strategies have rapidly evolved over the past decade and have become the initial strategy for most femoral-popliteal lesions. Even in complex lesions, such as in patients who present with CLI, the endovascular approach is the preferred choice in most cases.

Endovascular interventions

The last few years have seen an increase in the use of percutaneous interventions for superficial femoral artery disease in the setting of symptomatic PAD. Proponents of endovascular therapy cite two contentions to justify continued use of these modalities. The first is that the decrease in durability is offset by the less invasive nature of endovascular interventions and resultant decrease in morbidity. The second reason is that it is infrequent for a patient to have clinical or angiographic worsening upon failure of an endovascular intervention and so interventions can be repeated if they fail [7].

The following endovascular techniques have been used for recanalization of the superficial femoral arteries:
- Balloon angioplasty (percutaneous transluminal angioplasty; PTA);
- Bare metal stents;
- Drug-eluting stent placement;
- Drug-eluting balloon angioplasty;
- Cryotherapy;
- Atherectomy.

Balloon angioplasty

The main advantages of balloon angioplasty (PTA) are its low complication rate of 0.5–4%, high technical success rates approaching 90% even in long occlusions (Figure 78.1a–d), and good clinical outcomes [11,13]. Conventionally, PTA has been the mainstay therapy for revascularization in aorto-iliac, femoro-popliteal, and below-the-knee arteries, and in many interventional centers PTA still is the first and most frequently used endovascular therapy [14].

Several trials have compared medical therapy, endovascular intervention, and surgery in symptomatic patients with disease in the superficial femoral artery (SFA). A meta-analysis that compared exercise therapy with PTA in patients with IC reported at 3 months' follow-up, the ankle-brachial index (ABI) was significantly improved in the angioplasty group but not in the exercise group with similar quality of life outcomes [15]. A cost-effective analysis between endovascular therapy, PTA, surgery, and exercise alone showed that endovascular therapies were more effective than exercise alone, and the cost-effectiveness ratio was within the generally accepted range [16].

Despite advances in endovascular technologies, long-term patency rates of femoral-popliteal interventions are poor when compared with iliac interventions [17,18]. PTA of the SFA has a high rate of technical success, but target lesion revascularization (TLR) and target vessel revascularization (TVR) remains high at 30–80% at 6 months [19], especially in total occlusions and longer diseased segments. Failure rates can be as high as 70% at 1 year in long lesions [20,21].

Interventional Cardiology: Principles and Practice, Second Edition. Edited by George D. Dangas, Carlo Di Mario, and Nicholas N. Kipshidze.
© 2017 John Wiley & Sons, Ltd. Published 2017 by John Wiley & Sons, Ltd.

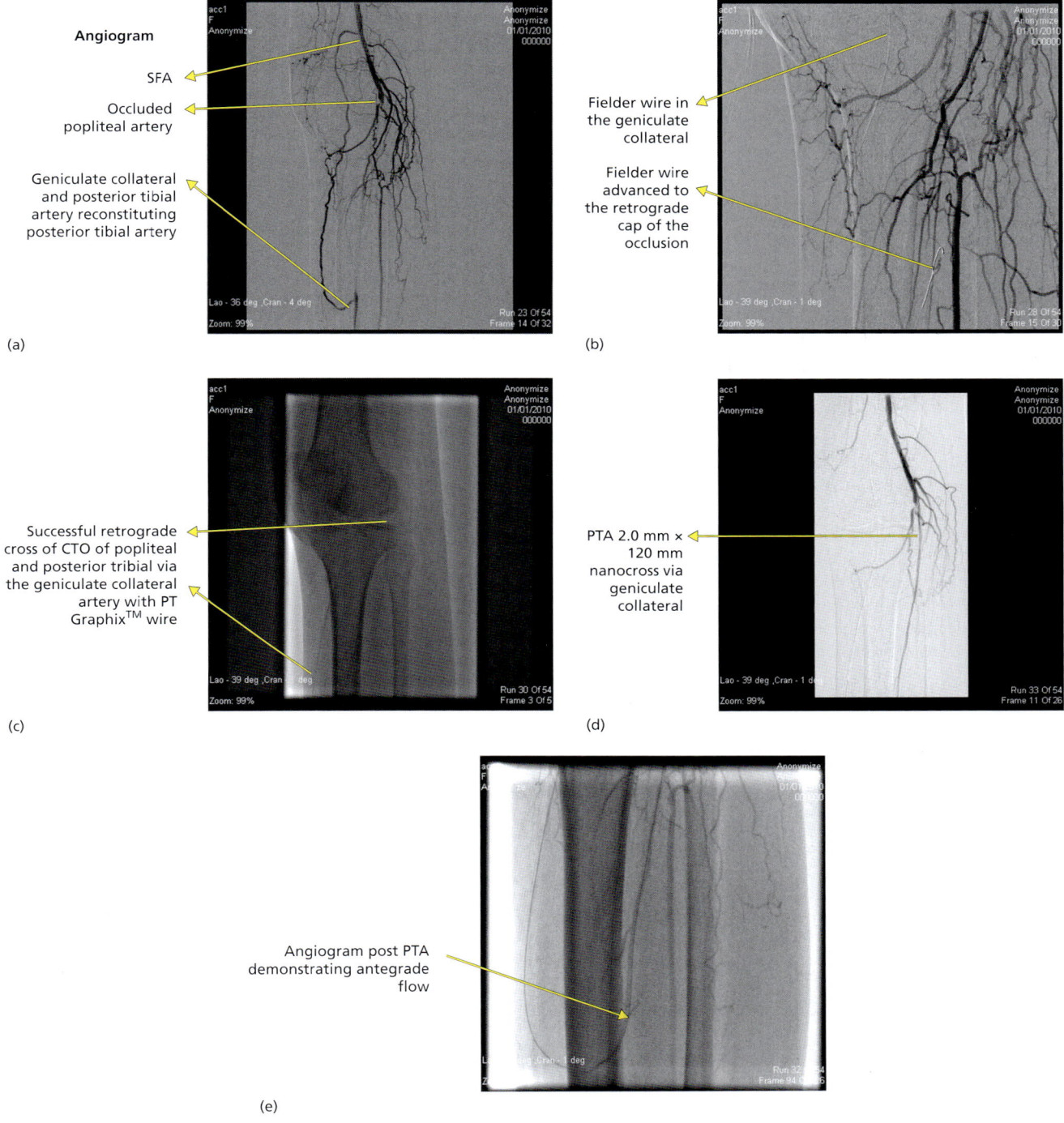

Figure 78.1 Percutaneous transluminal angioplasty (PTA) of occluded distal popliteal artery via infrapopliteal retrograde transcollateral approach: (a) occluded distal popliteal artery with reconstitution in the posterior tibialis artery; (b) 0.014-inch wire in the posterior tibialis artery via geniculate collaterals; (c) retrograde recanalization of distal popliteal artery; (d) PTA distal popliteal artery via retrograde approach; (e) post-PTA angiogram.

Moreover, there is no evidence to support the superiority of endovascular treatment over saphenous vein bypass for SFA disease. However, there is a single multicenter prospective randomized study, the Bypass Versus Angioplasty in Severe Ischemia of the Leg (BASIL) trial, which investigated the difference between angioplasty and open surgical repair for infrainguinal PAD and CLI in 452 patients and concluded that there was no difference in the primary outcome of 6-month amputation-free survival between the two treatment modalities [22]. However, the updated results with 3- to 7-year follow-up showed that while bypass surgery using veins as conduits offered the best long-term amputation-free survival, balloon angioplasty appeared to be superior to a polytetrafluoroethylene bypass procedure [23].

Bare metal stents

Stent placement for femoral popliteal disease has gained progressive attention. However, there is no level 1 evidence for primary stenting in this segment. Several studies have shown mixed results, although the preponderance of the data do not support primary stenting in all cases. Stents avoid the problems of early elastic recoil, residual stenosis, and flow-limiting dissection after PTA and can thus be used for the treatment of long and complex lesions, even in heavily calcified arteries [17].

Several randomized controlled trials have compared PTA with self-expanding nitinol stents in femoral-popliteal segment. The Femoral Artery Stenting Trial (FAST) compared PTA with primary stenting in short superficial femoral lesions (<50 mm) and showed no statistically significant difference between the two treatment modalities in the primary endpoint of ultrasound-assessed binary restenosis at 12 months [18]. Moreover, no statistically significant differences were seen in TLR, improvement in resting ABI, and improvement by at least 1 Rutherford category of peripheral arterial disease.

For longer lesions (>50 mm) randomized trials of PTA versus primary stenting have shown the benefit of stenting over PTA. In the ABSOLUTE trial [17], 104 patients with severe claudication or chronic limb ischemia caused by stenosis or occlusion of the superficial femoral artery were randomly assigned to undergo primary stent implantation or angioplasty. The results revealed that at 6 months the rate of restenosis on angiography was 24% in the stent group and 43% in the angioplasty group (p = 0.05); at 12 months the rates on duplex ultrasonography were 37% and 63%, respectively (p = 0.01). Patients in the stent group were able to walk significantly further on a treadmill at 6 and 12 months than those in the angioplasty group. Data reported after 2 years sustained the morphologic benefit and showed a trend toward clinical benefit of stents for longer lesions [24]. In the RESILIENT trial, a total of 206 patients from 24 centers in the USA and Europe with obstructive lesions of the superficial femoral artery and proximal popliteal artery presenting with intermittent claudication were randomized to implantation of nitinol stents or PTA [25]. The mean total lesion length was 71 mm for the stent group and 64 mm for the angioplasty group. At 12 months, freedom from TLV was 87.3% for the stent group and 45.1% for the angioplasty group (p <0.0001). Duplex ultrasound-derived primary patency at 12 months was better for the stent group (81.3% vs. 36.7%; p <0.0001). In the 3-year follow-up, freedom from TLR at 3 years was significantly better in the stent group (75.5% vs. 41.8%; p <0.0001), as was clinical success (63.2% vs. 17.9%; p <0.0001) [26].

Drug-eluting stents

The proven efficacy of drug-coated stents in the treatment of coronary artery disease gave rise to the notion that they might have a better patency than bare-metal stent (BMS) in patients with PAD. Metallic stents with good radial strength obliterate recoil and manage dissections, but in-stent restenosis remains the Achilles heel, especially in patients with CLI and those with poor infrapopliteal arterial run-off [27,28]. The 12-month primary patency rates of BMS in the SFA range between 50% and 65% [29,30]. Other factors contributing to poor patency are stent fracture and vessel kinking at the adductor's canal and popliteal segment. The former is caused by internal and external rotation, compression and expansion; the latter is secondary to high flexion forces. With the advent of drug-eluting stents (DES) the panorama appears to be changing, although

the first multicenter randomized double blind trial of DES versus BMS, the Sirolimus-Coated Cordis Self-expandable Stent (SIROCCO), did not yield positive results, showing lack of significant difference in restenosis between groups [31]. The most recent Zilver PTX study demonstrated appreciable clinical efficacy in symptomatic femoropopliteal disease patients [32]. This study was a prospective, multinational, randomized controlled trial that compared the Zilver PTX stent with PTA and provisional BMS placement. Results showed that the primary DES group demonstrated significantly superior 2-year event-free survival (86.6% vs. 77.9%; p = 0.02) and primary patency (74.8% vs. 26.5%; p <0.01). In addition, the provisional DES group exhibited superior 2-year primary patency compared with the provisional BMS group (83.4% vs. 64.1%; p <0.01) and achieved higher sustained clinical benefit (83.9% vs. 68.4%; p = 0.05). Two-year freedom from TLR with primary DES placement was 80.5% in the single-arm study and 86.6% in the randomized controlled trial. However, the trial was criticized for treating only short lesions, thus not representing real-world experience.

Drug-eluting balloons

Drug-coated balloons (DCBs) are an attractive alternative to DES as they can deliver an antiproliferative agent, which ameliorates the process of neointimal proliferation and leaves no stent behind. There are three key features in the use of DCBs [33]. First, vessel preparation (PTA utilizing a non-coated undersized balloon) followed with a DCB to facilitate even distribution of the drug. Second, the antiproliferative preferred agent is paclitaxel, as it tends to stay in the local microenvironment, thus increasing its inhibitory effects on intimal cell proliferation. Third, the preferred delivery system is a hydrophilic spacer, which can deliver the drug in a very short time frame with minimal loss into the systemic circulation. Prolonged drug elution is not necessary to obtain sustained inhibition of intimal hyperplasia [34]. Nonetheless, delivery of the antiproliferative drug during the most active phase of neointimal proliferation should be enough to decrease restenosis.

Several trials have paved the way for the use of DCBs in PAD. The THUNDER trial (Local Taxane with Short Exposure for Reduction of Restenosis in Distal Arteries) was the first human trial of DCB in non-coronary arteries [35]. It was a multicenter study with a three-way randomization protocol consisting of 154 patients with severe disease or total occlusion of the femoropopliteal segment. The first group was treated with a paclitaxel-coated balloon, the second group was treated with a standard uncoated balloon and the third group was treated with an uncoated balloon with paclitaxel dissolved in iopromide contrast medium. The mean lesion length was 7.4 cm. The primary endpoint was 6-month angiographic late lumen loss (LLL). The paclitaxel-coated balloon group had a marked reduction in LLL (0.4 ± 1.2 mm vs. 1.7 ± 1.8 mm vs. 2.2 ± 1.6 mm; p <0.001) when compared with the other two groups. TLR at 6 months was reduced in the paclitaxel-coated balloon when compared with the standard uncoated balloon (4% vs. 29%; p = 0.001). These favorable DCB effects were sustained at 24-month follow-up. Also, at 5 years, the decrease in LLL persisted [36]. However, TLR rates were not statistically different from the group of uncoated balloon with paclitaxel dissolved in contrast medium (4% vs. 29%; p = 0.41).

The FEMPAC (femoral paclitaxel) trial [37] randomized 87 patients in a 1 : 1 fashion between standard uncoated balloon and paclitaxel-coated balloon. Femoropopliteal lesions were short in length (5.7 vs. 6.1 cm). Results were similar to THUNDER trial. At 6-month follow-up, the primary endpoint of LLL was significantly lower in the DCB group (0.5 ± 1.1 mm versus 1.0 ± 1.1 mm; $p = 0.031$). Similarly, TLR rates were lower in the DCB group (6.7% vs. 33%; $p = 0.002$). These results were sustained at 18 months. There was significant improvement in Rutherford class, but there was no significant difference in ABI. These multicenter trials were limited to relatively short, non-complex femoropopliteal lesions, heterogeneous study subjects, unconventional endpoints, angiographic follow-up limited to only 6 months, and small sample sizes.

The Lutonix Paclitaxel-Coated Balloon for the Prevention of Femoropopliteal Restenosis (LEVANT 1) trial [38] was a prospective, multicenter, randomized study, which evaluated the safety of paclitaxel-coated MOXY balloon. A total of 101 patients with de novo and restenotic femoropopliteal lesions with CLI were randomized to paclitaxel-coated balloon (49 patients) or standard uncoated balloon (52 patients). The lesion lengths were 80.8 and 80.2 mm (varied from 4 to 15 cm). The primary endpoint of LLL at 6 months was significantly lower in the DCB group (0.46 vs. 1.09 mm; $p = 0.016$). In subgroup analysis, the DCB group showed significant reduction in LLL when compared with those patients who underwent PTA with an uncoated balloon. Also, the DCB group continued to demonstrate a reduction in LLL when compared with those patients who underwent stenting (26 patients) because of failed PTA (however, the trial was underpowered to conclude that there is a statistical difference between the stent and DCB groups). Composite 24-month major adverse events were lower in the DCB group (39%) than the non-DCB group (46%). These trials demonstrated that incomplete balloon expansion and geographic miss resulted in a significant decrease in primary patency and TLR rates at 12 months [39].

The Paclitaxel-coated Balloons in Femoral Indication to Defeat Restenosis (PACIFIER) trial [40] was a prospective, multicenter, randomized controlled single-blinded study, which enrolled 85 patients with 91 femoropopliteal lesions (44 were treated with the In.Pact Pacific DCB and 47 with standard uncoated balloon). The mean lesion length was 70 mm in the DCB group and 66 mm in the standard uncoated balloon group. The study met its primary endpoint (reduction in LLL at 6 months) where the In.Pact Pacific DCB balloon group had significant reduction in LLL at 6 months (−0.01 vs. 0.65 mm; $p = 0.0014$). Also, the DCB group had better TLR rates at 6 months (7.3% versus 22%; $p = 0.06$). In a subgroup analysis, the benefits of DCB with regards to LLL were seen irrespective of the lesion type or its length. At 12 months, the DCB group had fewer adverse events (death, amputation, or TLR) than the standard uncoated balloon group (7.1% vs. 34.9%; $p = 0.003$). A meta-analysis [41] of the THUNDER, FEMPAC, LEVANT I, and PACIFIER trials showed improved results with DCBs at a median follow-up of 10.3 months (significant reduction in TLR, LLL, and angiographic restenosis without an increase in adverse events).

Some of the more recent trials such as IN.PACT SFA I (European arm) and II (US arm) [42] are ongoing multicenter randomized studies. These trials intend to assess the safety and efficacy of the Admiral DCB in femoropopliteal lesions. Preliminary 12 month results of 331 patients randomized in a 2 : 1 fashion (220 in the DCB group and 111 in the standard balloon PTA group) across Europe (150 patients) and the USA (181 patients) showed that the DCB group did better ($p < 0.001$) than the standard uncoated balloon group in terms of primary patency (82.2% vs. 52.4%; primary endpoint), clinically driven TLR (2.4% vs. 20.6%), primary sustained clinical improvement (upgrade in Rutherford classification ≥1 class

in amputation- and TVR-free surviving patients), primary safety endpoint (freedom from 30-day device- and procedure-related death, target limb major amputation, and clinically driven TVR through 12 months), and MACE (death, clinically driven TVR, target limb major amputation, and thrombosis). The Drug-Eluting Balloon Evaluation for Lower Limb Multilevel Treatment (DEBELLUM) study [43] was a prospective, randomized, single center study that enrolled 50 patients with femoropopliteal (75.4%) and below-the-knee lesions. Twenty-five patients were randomized to be treated with the In.Pact Admiral DCB and 25 patients to be treated with a standard uncoated balloon. LLL at 6 months was better in the DCB group than in the standard uncoated balloon group. BIOLUX P-I was an international, multicenter, randomized controlled trial [44] that evaluated the safety and efficacy of the Passeo-18 Lux paclitaxel-coated balloon (30 patients) compared with standard uncoated balloon (30 patients). The DCB group showed a significant reduction in LLL when compared with the standard uncoated balloon group at 6 months. The overall major adverse event rate did not differ in both groups. The DCB group showed a slightly better outcome with regards to Rutherford class. The DEFINITIVE AR study was a European multicenter, prospective, randomized trial that evaluated the effectiveness of DCBs in heavily calcified lesions. Patients were randomized to directional atherectomy followed by paclitaxel-coated Cotavance balloon versus paclitaxel-coated Cotavance balloon alone. The 30-day preliminary results [45] showed significant higher technical success in the directional atherectomy followed by paclitaxel-coated Cotavance balloon arm than the paclitaxel-coated Cotavance balloon alone.

Cryotherapy

Cryoplasty therapy (cold balloon angioplasty) has been used as an effective primary strategy for limiting the incidence of dissection, vessel recoil, and subsequent intimal hyperplasia and restenosis associated with the endovascular dilatation of atherosclerotic lesions in the peripheral vasculature [46–50]. Specialized cryoplasty balloon catheters, approved by the US Food and Drug Administration (FDA), are inflated not with the standard mixture of saline solution and contrast medium but rather with nitrous oxide, which causes the plaque in the artery to freeze at −10 °C. Previous scientific studies have shown that this process results in weakening of the plaque, uniform vessel dilatation, alteration of elastin fibers to reduce vessel wall recoil while collagen fibers remain unperturbed and capable of maintaining architectural integrity [51,52], and induction of smooth muscle cell apoptosis which is associated with reduced neointima formation and reduced subsequent restenosis [53].

Studies involving cryoplasty have conflicting results with patency rates and need for re-intervention. Diaz *et al.* [54], in a 3-year analysis of re-intervention-free survival between cryoplasty versus conventional angioplasty in femoropopliteal arterial recanalization, demonstrated good immediate success rates with lower stent placement rates. However, during the 3-year follow-up, patency rates tended to equalize between the two modalities. A multicenter registry of 102 patients demonstrated a high degree of acute angiographic success with a low frequency of TLR. The patency rate observed compared favorably with that previously documented with conventional angioplasty [50]. The COBRA trial was a prospective, multicenter, randomized controlled clinical trial of diabetic patients to investigate whether post-dilatation of superficial femoral artery nitinol self-expanding stents using a cryoplasty balloon reduces restenosis compared to a conventional balloon. The key finding of this study was that, for patients with diabetes mellitus who underwent SFA stenting using self-expanding stents, post-dilatation using cryoplasty significantly reduced the 12-month in-stent restenosis rates compared to post-dilatation using a conventional balloon [55]. However, the benefit of cryoplasty over conventional angioplasty cannot be established, as the number of randomized controlled trials is small.

Atherectomy

Atherectomy devices are designed to debulk and remove atherosclerotic plaque by cutting, pulverizing, or shaving with catheter-deliverable blades. The development of the SilverHawk excisional atherectomy catheter (EV3, Minneapolis, MN, USA) has renewed interest in directional atherectomy, a technique that has historically been associated with high restenosis rates in the coronary and peripheral vasculature [56,57]. Like the excimer laser, excisional atherectomy offers the theoretical advantage, compared to PTA and stent implantation, of eliminating stretch injury on arterial walls, limiting acute dissection (and the need for adjunctive stenting) and elastic recoil, and thereby potentially reducing post-procedure inflammation and the rate of restenosis. Both rotational and orbital atherectomy share a niche on calcific lesions. Excimer laser has gained FDA approval for femoropopliteal in-stent restenosis (ISR) [58].

Directional atherectomy

Directional atherectomy involves the resection of the atherosclerotic plaque with a cutting device in the longitudinal plane [59]. Two devices are approved by the FDA for directional atherectomy: the SilverHawk™ (Covidien, Plymouth MN, USA) and the TurboHawk™ (Covidien, Plymouth MN, USA). The recent published DEFINITIVE LE trial is the largest multicenter study that evaluated the intermediate and long-term effectiveness of stand-alone SilverHawk™/TurboHawk™ Plaque Excision Systems for endovascular treatment of PAD in the femoropopliteal and tibial–peroneal arteries [60]. Its primary endpoints were patency at 1 year in claudicants and freedom of unplanned amputation at 1 year in CLI patients. A total of 800 patients were studied. More than half were diabetic and 66% of the lesions were located in the femoropopliteal segment. Final results revealed 78% patency rate in all claudicants and 71% in CLI patients with a 95% of freedom of amputation. The major limitations of the trial were lack of randomization and follow-up after 12 months.

Rotational atherectomy

The Pathway PV system (Pathway Medical, Kirkland, WA, USA) has a unique feature compared to other rotational atherectomy devices. The ability to remove the atherectomized plaque material through aspiration ports reduces the risk of obstructing the microvasculature and avoids increasing erythrocyte degradation products, especially in patients with impaired renal function. High-speed rotational devices without aspiration capabilities increase these degradation products, such as haptoglobin and potassium, which can result in life-threatening cardiac arrhythmias [61]. Additionally, the aspiration feature of the catheter allows the device to be used in lesions containing both occlusive material, including solid, even calcified plaque and fresh thrombus. Potentially, the Pathway PV can be used as a thrombectomy device in subacute and acute vessel occlusions.

Zeller *et al.* [62] reported results on a prospective non-randomized multicenter trial using a rotational atherectomy system with aspiration capabilities. In this study, a 99% technical success rate was achieved using the Pathway PV Atherectomy System in 210 infra-inguinal cases. Adjunctive balloon angioplasty was performed in 59% and stenting in 7%. Primary and secondary patency rates at 1 year were 61.8% and 81.3%. The 1-year limb salvage rate was 100%. These patency rates are similar to SilverHawk study cohorts.

Orbital atherectomy

The Diamondback 360° Orbital atherectomy System (CSI, St. Paul, MN, USA) uses a plaque ablation catheter. This has an abrasive eccentrically shaped crown with a diamond-coated surface which rotates and creates lumen enlargement by plaque abrasion. Orbital atherectomy appears to have some similarities to mechanical rotational atherectomy (Rotablator) (Boston Scientific, Natick, MA, USA).

Analysis of the CONFIRM registries found that high rates of success in subjects with PAD were equally favorable in men and women. Overall final residual stenosis in the CONFIRM registries was 10% and was actually lower in female patients than in male patients. These findings are in agreement with the OASIS trial, a multicenter, prospective, non-randomized registry of 124 patients (33% women) who underwent orbital atherectomy for the treatment of infrapopliteal lesions. The OASIS trial demonstrated a high success rate (90.1% patients had final diameter stenosis ≤30%) and a low rate of major adverse events at 6 months (10.4%) [63]. Korabathina *et al.* [64] enrolled 98 patients (54% women) in a single-arm registry database of patients with infra-inguinal lesions treated with OAS. They showed a low rate of major adverse events at 30 days (2.2%) and an overall favorable safety profile.

Excimer laser-assisted angioplasty

Continuous wave laser were evaluated and abandoned for peripheral interventions in the late 1980s because of the high complication rate caused by thermal damage to surrounding tissue [65]. In contrast, excimer laser angioplasty (ELA) of the leg arteries has been used commercially in Europe since 1994 [66]. The 308 nm excimer laser utilizes flexible fiber optic catheters to deliver intense short duration pulses of ultraviolet (UV) energy. The advantages of pulsed UV energy lies in the short penetration depth of 50 μm and its ability to break molecular bonds directly by a photochemical process, instead of a thermal one. Excimer laser catheters remove a tissue layer of about 10 μm with each pulse of energy. Tissue is vaporized only on contact without a consequent rise in temperature to surrounding tissue.

The multicenter Laser Atherectomy for Critical Ischemia (LACI) trial of excimer laser-assisted angioplasty treated 423 lesions (41% SFA, 15% popliteal, 41% infrapopliteal) in 155 limbs (91% with at least one occlusion) of 145 patients with CLI (Rutherford categories 4–6, 69% with tissue loss, 66% diabetics) who were determined to be poor candidates for surgical revascularization. Procedural success (defined as <50% residual stenosis in all treated lesions) was achieved in 85% of the treated limbs [67,68]. The median total length of treated artery per limb was 11.0 cm. Procedural complications in 12% of the treated limbs included major dissection (4%), acute thrombus formation (3%), distal embolization (3%), and perforation (2%). The excimer procedure was followed with adjunctive balloon angioplasty in 96% of the limbs. Stents (mainly bare nitinol) were placed adjunctively in 61% of the SFA lesions, 38% of the popliteal lesions, and 16% of the tibial lesions. Mean lesion stenosis (by visual estimate) was decreased from 92% at baseline to 55% after laser debulking and to 18% at final assessment. At 6-month follow-up, limb salvage was achieved in 110 (92%) of 119 surviving patients

(118 of 127 limbs; 93%); 56% of ischemic ulcers had healed completely [67]. Despite treating a very unfavorable patient cohort, excimer laser assisted angioplasty achieved limb salvage comparable to the gold standard of bypass surgery. Following the LACI protocol, a single-center US registry and a five-center Belgian trial achieved comparable outcomes with the device [69,70].

More recently, the EXCITE ISR study is the first trial conducted under an IDE to support to gain FDA indication for femoropopliteal ISR. The trial was stopped at 250 enrolled patients after successful primary endpoint analysis. ELA + PTA demonstrated better procedural success with a significant reduction in procedural complications and post-treatment stenosis than PTA alone. The primary safety and efficacy endpoints established superiority of ELA + PTA compared to PTA alone [58].

The future

Finally, the concept of biodegradable stents is promising and enticing. The fact that we can achieve the delivery of the antiproliferative drug, prevent acute recoil and negative remodeling with the disappearance of the stent when the process of neointimal proliferation halts is an attractive concept. Recently, a multicenter, non-randomized registry evaluating the efficacy and safety of a biodegradable (REMEDY) stent demonstrated a primary patency of 71% and TLR of 22% [71].

 Interactive multiple choice questions are available for this chapter on www.wiley. com/go/dangas/cardiology

References

1 Shammas NW. Epidemiology, classification, and modifiable risk factors of peripheral arterial disease. *Vasc Health Risk Manag* 2007; **3**(2): 229–234.

2 Aronow H. Peripheral arterial disease in the elderly: recognition and management. *Am J Cardiovasc Drugs* 2008; **8**(6): 353–364.

3 Hirsch AT, Criqui MH, Treat-Jacobson D, et al. Peripheral arterial disease detection, awareness, and treatment in primary care. *JAMA* 2001; **286**(11): 1317–1324.

4 Luther M, Lepantalo M, Alback A, Matzke S. Amputation rates as a measure of vascular surgical results. *Br J Surg* 1996; **83**(2): 241–244.

5 Hirsch AT, Haskal ZJ, Hertzer NR, et al. ACC/AHA 2005 Practice Guidelines for the management of patients with peripheral arterial disease (lower extremity, renal, mesenteric, and abdominal aortic): a collaborative report from the American Association for Vascular Surgery/Society for Vascular Surgery, Society for Cardiovascular Angiography and Interventions, Society for Vascular Medicine and Biology, Society of Interventional Radiology, and the ACC/AHA Task Force on Practice Guidelines (Writing Committee to Develop Guidelines for the Management of Patients With Peripheral Arterial Disease): endorsed by the American Association of Cardiovascular and Pulmonary Rehabilitation; National Heart, Lung, and Blood Institute; Society for Vascular Nursing; TransAtlantic Inter-Society Consensus; and Vascular Disease Foundation. *Circulation* 2006; **113**(11): e463–654.

6 ICAI Group (Gruppo di Studio dell'Ischemia Cronica Critica degli Arti Inferiori). The Study Group of Criticial Chronic Ischemia of the Lower Exremities. Long-term mortality and its predictors in patients with critical leg ischaemia. *Eur J Vasc Endovasc Surg* 1997; **14**(2): 91–95.

7 Ouriel K. Peripheral arterial disease. *Lancet* 2001; **358**(9289): 1257–1264.

8 Brodmann M. Prime time for drug eluting balloons in SFA interventions? *J Cardiovasc Surg* 2014; **55**(4): 461–464.

9 Kasapis C, Gurm HS. Current approach to the diagnosis and treatment of femoral-popliteal arterial disease: a systematic review. *Curr Cardiol Rev* 2009; **5**(4): 296–311.

10 Zeller T, Schmitmeier S, Tepe G, Rastan A. Drug-coated balloons in the lower limb. *J Cardiovasc Surg* 2011; **52**(2): 235–243.

11 Dormandy JA, Rutherford RB. Management of peripheral arterial disease (PAD). TASC Working Group. TransAtlantic Inter-Society Consensus (TASC). *J Vasc Surg* 2000; **31**(1 Pt 2): S1–S296.

12 Norgren L, Hiatt WR, Dormandy JA, et al. Inter-Society Consensus for the management of peripheral arterial disease (TASC II). *Eur J Vasc Endovasc Surg* 2007; **33**(Suppl 1): S1–75.

13 Norgren L, Hiatt WR, Dormandy JA, et al. Inter-Society Consensus for the management of peripheral arterial disease (TASC II). *J Vasc Surg* 2007; **45**(Suppl S): S5–67.

14 Schillinger M, Minar E. Percutaneous treatment of peripheral artery disease: novel techniques. *Circulation* 2012; **126**(20): 2433–2440.

15 Spronk S, Bosch JL, Veen HF, den Hoed PT, Hunink MG. Intermittent claudication: functional capacity and quality of life after exercise training or percutaneous transluminal angioplasty—systematic review. *Radiology* 2005; **235**(3): 833–842.

16 de Vries SO, Visser K, de Vries JA, Wong JB, Donaldson MC, Hunink MG. Intermittent claudication: cost-effectiveness of revascularization versus exercise therapy. *Radiology* 2002; **222**(1): 25–36.

17 Schillinger M, Sabeti S, Loewe C, et al. Balloon angioplasty versus implantation of nitinol stents in the superficial femoral artery. *N Engl J Med* 2006; **354**(18): 1879–1888.

18 Krankenberg H, Schluter M, Steinkamp HJ, et al. Nitinol stent implantation versus percutaneous transluminal angioplasty in superficial femoral artery lesions up to 10 cm in length: the femoral artery stenting trial (FAST). *Circulation* 2007; **116**(3): 285–292.

19 Matsi PJ, Manninen HI, Vanninen RL, et al. Femoropopliteal angioplasty in patients with claudication: primary and secondary patency in 140 limbs with 1–3-year follow-up. *Radiology* 1994; **191**(3): 727–733.

20 Capek P, McLean GK, Berkowitz HD. Femoropopliteal angioplasty: factors influencing long-term success. *Circulation* 1991; **83**(2 Suppl): 170–180.

21 Laird JR. Limitations of percutaneous transluminal angioplasty and stenting for the treatment of disease of the superficial femoral and popliteal arteries. *J Endovasc Ther* 2006; **13**(Suppl 2): 30–40.

22 Conrad MF, Crawford RS, Hackney LA, et al. Endovascular management of patients with critical limb ischemia. *J Vasc Surg* 2011; **53**(4): 1020–1025.

23 Rana MA, Gloviczki P. Endovascular interventions for infrapopliteal arterial disease: an update. *Semin Vasc Surg* 2012; **25**(1): 29–34.

24 Schillinger M, Sabeti S, Dick P, et al. Sustained benefit at 2 years of primary femoropopliteal stenting compared with balloon angioplasty with optional stenting. *Circulation* 2007; **115**(21): 2745–2749.

25 Laird JR, Katzen BT, Scheinert D, et al. Nitinol stent implantation versus balloon angioplasty for lesions in the superficial femoral artery and proximal popliteal artery: twelve-month results from the RESILIENT randomized trial. *Circ Cardiovasc Interv* 2010; **3**(3): 267–276.

26 Laird JR, Katzen BT, Scheinert D, et al. Nitinol stent implantation vs. balloon angioplasty for lesions in the superficial femoral and proximal popliteal arteries of patients with claudication: three-year follow-up from the RESILIENT randomized trial. *J Endovasc Ther* 2012; **19**(1): 1–9.

27 Muradin GS, Bosch JL, Stijnen T, Hunink MG. Balloon dilation and stent implantation for treatment of femoropopliteal arterial disease: meta-analysis. *Radiology* 2001; **221**(1): 137–145.

28 Grimm J, Muller-Hulsbeck S, Jahnke T, Hilbert C, Brossmann J, Heller M. Randomized study to compare PTA alone versus PTA with Palmaz stent placement for femoropopliteal lesions. *J Vasc Interv Radiol* 2001; **12**(8): 935–942.

29 Moses JW, Kipshidze N, Leon MB. Perspectives of drug-eluting stents: the next revolution. *Am J Cardiovasc Drugs* 2002; **2**(3): 163–172.

30 Rocha-Singh KJ, Jaff MR, Crabtree TR, Bloch DA, Ansel G, Viva Physicians I. Performance goals and endpoint assessments for clinical trials of femoropopliteal bare nitinol stents in patients with symptomatic peripheral arterial disease. *Catheter Cardiovasc Interv* 2007; **69**(6): 910–919.

31 Duda SH, Bosiers M, Lammer J, et al. Drug-eluting and bare nitinol stents for the treatment of atherosclerotic lesions in the superficial femoral artery: long-term results from the SIROCCO trial. *J Endovasc Ther* 2006; **13**(6): 701–710.

32 Dake MD, Ansel GM, Jaff MR, et al. Sustained safety and effectiveness of paclitaxel-eluting stents for femoropopliteal lesions: 2-year follow-up from the Zilver PTX randomized and single-arm clinical studies. *J Am Coll Cardiol* 2013; **61**(24): 2417–2427.

33 De Vries JP, Karimi A, Fioole B, Van Leersum M, Werson DA, Van Den Heuvel DA. First- and second-generation drug-eluting balloons for femoro-popliteal arterial obstructions: update of technique and results. *J Cardiovasc Surg* 2013; **54**(3): 327–332.

34 Deloose K, Lauwers K, Callaert J, et al. Drug-eluting technologies in femoral artery lesions. *J Cardiovasc Surg* 2013; **54**(2): 217–224.

35 Tepe G, Zeller T, Albrecht T, et al. Local delivery of paclitaxel to inhibit restenosis during angioplasty of the leg. *N Engl J Med* 2008; **358**(7): 689–699.

36 Minar E, Schillinger M. Innovative technologies for SFA occlusions: drug coated balloons in SFA lesions. *J Cardiovasc Surg* 2012; **53**(4): 481–486.

37 Werk M, Langner S, Reinkensmeier B, et al. Inhibition of restenosis in femoro-popliteal arteries: paclitaxel-coated versus uncoated balloon: femoral paclitaxel randomized pilot trial. *Circulation* 2008; **118**(13): 1358–1365.

38 Scheinert D, Duda S, Zeller T, *et al.* The LEVANT I (Lutonix paclitaxel-coated balloon for the prevention of femoropopliteal restenosis) trial for femoropopliteal revascularization: first-in-human randomized trial of low-dose drug-coated balloon versus uncoated balloon angioplasty. *JACC Cardiovasc Interv* 2014; **7**(1): 10–19.

39 Scheinert D. *Lessons learned from LEVANT 1 First-in-man study: 12 month analysis.* Presented at Leipzig Interventional Course, Leipzig, Germany, 2012.

40 Werk M, Albrecht T, Meyer DR, *et al.* Paclitaxel-coated balloons reduce restenosis after femoro-popliteal angioplasty: evidence from the randomized PACIFIER trial. *Circ Cardiovasc interv* 2012; **5**(6): 831–840.

41 Cassese S, Byrne RA, Ott I, *et al.* Paclitaxel-coated versus uncoated balloon angioplasty reduces target lesion revascularization in patients with femoropopliteal arterial disease: a meta-analysis of randomized trials. *Circ CardiovasC interv* 2012; **5**(4): 582–589.

42 http://clinicaltrials.gov/show/NCT01566461

43 Fanelli F, Cannavale A, Boatta E, *et al.* Lower limb multilevel treatment with drug-eluting balloons: 6-month results from the DEBELLUM randomized trial. *J Endovasc Ther* 2012; **19**(5): 571–580.

44 Scheinert D, Karl-Ludwig S, Thomas Z, *et al.* TCT-585 Six month results of the BIOLUX P-I first in man study comparing a paclitaxel releasing balloon catheter versus an uncoated balloon catheter in femoropopliteal lesions. *J Am Coll Cardiol* 2012; **60** (17 Suppl).

45 http://evtoday.com/2013/09/definitive-ar-30-day-results-presented-on-directional-atherectomy-plus-dcb

46 Das T, McNamara T, Gray B, *et al.* Cryoplasty therapy for limb salvage in patients with critical limb ischemia. *J Endovasc Ther* 2007; **14**(6): 753–762.

47 Das TS, McNamara T, Gray B, *et al.* Primary cryoplasty therapy provides durable support for limb salvage in critical limb ischemia patients with infrapopliteal lesions: 12-month follow-up results from the BTK Chill Trial. *J Endovasc Ther* 2009; **16**(2 Suppl 2): 19–30.

48 Fava M, Loyola S, Polydorou A, *et al.* Cryoplasty for femoropopliteal arterial disease: late angiographic results of initial human experience. *J Vasc Interv Radiol* 2004; **15**(11): 1239–1243.

49 Laird JR, Biamino G, McNamara T, *et al.* Cryoplasty for the treatment of femoropopliteal arterial disease: extended follow-up results. *J Endovasc Ther* 2006; **13**(Suppl 2): 52–59.

50 Laird J, Jaff MR, Biamino G, *et al.* Cryoplasty for the treatment of femoropopliteal arterial disease: results of a prospective, multicenter registry. *J Vasc Interv Radiol* 2005; **16**(8): 1067–1073.

51 Gage AA, Fazekas G, Riley EE Jr. Freezing injury to large blood vessels in dogs: with comments on the effect of experimental freezing of bile ducts. *Surgery* 1967; **61**(5): 748–754.

52 Mandeville AF, McCabe BF. Some observations on the cryobiology of blood vessels. *Laryngoscope* 1967; **77**(8): 1328–1350.

53 Tatsutani KN, Joye JD, Virmani R, Taylor MJ. In vitro evaluation of vascular endothelial and smooth muscle cell survival and apoptosis in response to hypothermia and freezing. *Cryo Lett* 2005; **26**(1): 55–64.

54 Diaz ML, Urtasun F, Barberena J, Aranzadi C, Guillen-Grima F, Bilbao JI. Cryoplasty versus conventional angioplasty in femoropopliteal arterial recanalization: 3-year analysis of reintervention-free survival by treatment received. *Cardiovasc Interv Radiol* 2011; **34**(5): 911–917.

55 Banerjee S, Das TS, Abu-Fadel MS, *et al.* Pilot trial of cryoplasty or conventional balloon post-dilation of nitinol stents for revascularization of peripheral arterial segments: the COBRA trial. *J Am Coll Cardiol* 2012; **60**(15): 1352–1359.

56 Tielbeek AV, Vroegindeweij D, Buth J, Landman GH. Comparison of balloon angioplasty and Simpson atherectomy for lesions in the femoropopliteal artery: angiographic and clinical results of a prospective randomized trial. *J Vasc Interv Radiol* 1996; **7**(6): 837–844.

57 Garcia LA, Lyden SP. Atherectomy for infrainguinal peripheral artery disease. *J Endovasc Ther* 2009; **16**(2 Suppl 2): 105–115.

58 Dippel EJ, Makam P, Kovach R, *et al.* Randomized controlled study of excimer laser atherectomy for treatment of femoropopliteal in-stent restenosis: initial results from the EXCITE ISR trial (EXCImer Laser Randomized Controlled Study for Treatment of FemoropopliTEal In-Stent Restenosis). *JACC Cardiovasc Interv* 2015; **8**(1 Pt A): 92–101.

59 Al Khoury G, Chaer R. Evolution of atherectomy devices. *J Cardiovasc Surg* 2011; **52**(4): 493–505.

60 McKinsey JF, Zeller T, Rocha-Singh KJ, Jaff MR, Garcia LA. Lower extremity revascularization using directional atherectomy: 12-month prospective results of the DEFINITIVE LE Study. *JACC Cardiovasc Interv* 2014; **7**(8): 923–933.

61 Mehta SK, Laster SB. Hemolysis induced pancreatitis after orbital atherectomy in a heavily calcified superficial femoral artery. *Catheter Cardiovasc Interv* 2008; **72**(7): 1009–1011.

62 Zeller T, Krankenberg H, Steinkamp H, *et al.* One-year outcome of percutaneous rotational atherectomy with aspiration in infrainguinal peripheral arterial occlusive disease: the multicenter pathway PVD trial. *J Endovasc Ther* 2009; **16**(6): 653–662.

63 Lee MS, Canan T, Rha SW, Mustapha J, Adams GL. Pooled analysis of the CONFIRM registries: impact of gender on procedure and angiographic outcomes in patients undergoing orbital atherectomy for peripheral artery disease. *J Endovasc Ther* 2015; **22**(1): 57–62.

64 Korabathina R, Mody KP, Yu J, Han SY, Patel R, Staniloae CS. Orbital atherectomy for symptomatic lower extremity disease. *Catheter Cardiovasc Interv* 2010; **76**(3): 326–332.

65 White RA, White GH, Mehringer MC, Chaing FL, Wilson SE. A clinical trial of laser thermal angioplasty in patients with advanced peripheral vascular disease. *Ann Surg* 1990; **212**(3): 257–265.

66 Visona A, Perissinotto C, Lusiani L, *et al.* Percutaneous excimer laser angioplasty of lower limb vessels: results of a prospective 24-month follow-up. *Angiology* 1998; **49**(2): 91–98.

67 Laird JR, Zeller T, Gray BH, *et al.* Limb salvage following laser-assisted angioplasty for critical limb ischemia: results of the LACI multicenter trial. *J Endovasc Ther* 2006; **13**(1): 1–11.

68 Laird JR Jr, Reiser C, Biamino G, Zeller T. Excimer laser assisted angioplasty for the treatment of critical limb ischemia. *J Cardiovasc Surg* 2004; **45**(3): 239–248.

69 Bosiers M, Peeters P, Elst FV, *et al.* Excimer laser assisted angioplasty for critical limb ischemia: results of the LACI Belgium Study. *Eur J Vasc Endovasc Surg* 2005; **29**(6): 613–619.

70 Biamino G. The excimer laser: science fiction fantasy or practical tool? *J Endovasc Ther* 2004; **11**(Suppl 2): 207–222.

71 Vermassen F, Bouckenooghe I, Moreels N, Goverde P, Schroe H. Role of bioresorbable stents in the superficial femoral artery. *J Cardiovasc Surg* 2013; **54**(2): 225–234.

CHAPTER 79

Popliteal Artery Interventions

Karthik Gujja[1], Gopi Punukollu[2], Vishal Kapur[1], and Prakash Krishnan[1]

[1] The Zena and Michael A. Weiner Cardiovascular Institute, Icahn School of Medicine at Mount Sinai, New York, NY, USA
[2] Lenox Hill Hospital (North Shore LIJ), New York, NY, USA

Peripheral arterial disease (PAD) is defined as an obstructive arterial disease of the lower extremities that reduces arterial flow during exercise or, in advanced stages, at rest [1]. It affects 8–12 million people in the USA with many of these cases related to popliteal artery (PA) occlusive disease. As superficial femoral artery (SFA) and PA diseases are often grouped together in medical literature, the number of PAD cases involving just the PA is unknown [2]. PAD is one of the major manifestations of systemic atherosclerosis, advancing to critical limb ischemia (CLI) in 1–2% of patients with PAD who are 50 years of age or older [3]. CLI is a complex, multifactorial disease leading to a high risk of morbidity and mortality. The American College of Cardiology/American Heart Association (ACC/AHA) practice guidelines suggest that patients with CLI have a 25% 1-year cardiovascular mortality, a 25% 1-year amputation rate, and a 50% rate of being alive with two limbs 1 year after diagnosis [3]. Duplex ultrasound is valuable in determining candidates for intervention with the ankle-brachial systolic pressure index (ABI) being 95% sensitive and almost 100% specific for PAD [1]. An ABI of less than 0.4 correlates to a 5-year survival of only 44% compared with 90% for those patients with an ABI greater than 0.85 [1]. CLI involving the PA is a situation that requires prompt diagnosis and treatment to preserve the ischemic limb by establishing inflow to the tibial and the pedal vessels. More than 100,000 peripheral arterial reconstructive operations and 50,000 lower limb amputations for lower extremity ischemia are performed in the USA each year [3,4].

Interventions for popliteal artery disease

Patients with PAD often have multiple medical comorbidities requiring an array of drugs, conservative management, and invasive therapies. If the patient is a surgical candidate and there is sufficient venous conduit, surgical bypass with autogenous veins has historically been the first-line revascularization therapy involving the middle and the distal PA [2]. According to the most recently released TASC II recommendations, lesions involving either the PA or common femoral artery are classified as class D lesions and are strongly recommended for surgery [5]. However, open surgery is not always possible because of prohibiting comorbidities, unsuitable venous conduit, or lack of an adequate distal artery for revascularization [6]. The use of "minimally" invasive endovascular therapies as surgical alternatives has opened up a new realm of treatments for PA lesions and the patency and long-term clinical outcomes from these endovascular treatments must be considered [2].

Balloon angioplasty

Several options exist for minimally invasive therapy of arterial lesions with balloon angioplasty (PTA), with or without stenting, being the most widely accepted endovascular option with high patency rates and low levels of restenosis [7]. PTA of PA lesions is effective at acutely restoring flow but restenosis occurs in 40–60% of patients within 1 year, leading to therapeutic failure and reintervention [8]. Drug-coated balloon (DCB) have been developed to increase the patency of PA angioplasty and reduce restenosis, thereby decreasing the need for reintervention in comparison with traditional PTA [9]. The IN.PACT SFA trial was a prospective, multicenter, single-blinded, randomized controlled trial assessing the safety and efficacy of the IN.PACT Admiral DCB. It showed significantly better patency (82.2%) at 12 months when compared with traditional PTA (52.4%) [9]. These outcomes are in concordance with multiple other trials showing a favorable primary patency of DCB versus PTA at 1 and 2 years [8,10,11]. The Micari et al. [10] multicenter registry showed a patency of 83.7% at 1 year and 72.4% at 2 years. The LEVANT 1 trial showed a DBC primary patency of 67% at 1 year and 57% at 2 years when compared with PTA [8]. The ILLUMINATE trial showed the Stellarex DCB primary potency of 89.5% at 1 year and 80.3% at 2 years (Figure 79.1) [11].

Stenting

Overall, stenting is not routinely performed in PA PAD because of the anatomic location of the PA and the fact that it is not contained within a muscular compartment which leaves it exposed to compression, torsion, and elongation [4,12]. The mobility of the knee joint further presents the potential for external stent fractures, which are associated with stent restenosis or re-occlusions in about two-thirds of cases [12,13]. Stenting was first introduced to femoropopliteal occlusive therapy when balloon expandable stainless steel stents were used to treat short lesions [14]. Then the application of self-expanding nitinol technology added to treatment options with better patency rates in longer lesions compared with

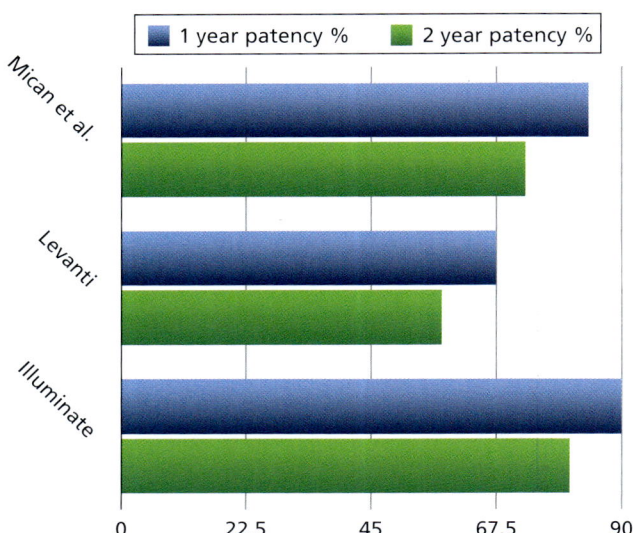

Figure 79.1 The 1- and 2-year primary patency rates reported in first-in-human studies for various paclitaxel drug-coated balloons [8,10,11].

earlier metal stents but restenosis remained a major issue [14]. A meta-analysis review was completed by Mwipatayi *et al.* [15] to compare the short- and long-term results of primary stenting and angioplasty of femoropopliteal occlusive disease. In the stent implantation group, the 12 month primary patency rates varied from 63% to 90%, and 24 month primary patency ranged from 46% to 87% [15]. The 12 month primary patency rates following balloon angioplasty alone ranged from 45% to 84.2% and at 24 months it varied from 25% to 77.2% [15]. These results and that of various other trials suggest that stent placement in the femoropopliteal occlusive disease has some limitations and more research needs to be done to determine the patency rate when compared with angioplasty alone [14–18]. A recent randomized, multicenter trial, the Endovascular Treatment of Atherosclerotic Popliteal Artery Lesions–Balloon Angioplasty Versus Primary Stenting (ETAP) study, investigated the 1- and 2-year results of primary nitinol stent placement in comparison with PTA in true PA lesions beyond the proximal (P1) segment [19,20]. ETAP revealed equivalent patency at 1 year and possibility of a shift toward higher patency rates in favor of primary stenting at 2 years [18–20].

More promising results have been seen with the development of the Supera helical interwoven nitinol stent which has superior radial strength, fracture resistance, and flexibility when compared with the traditional laser-cut nitinol stents [13]. In a single-center study PA stenting with the Supera@ system proved to be safe and effective, with high patency rates and no stent fractures [13,21]. The primary stent patency rates at 6 and 12 months were 94.6±2.3% and 87.7±3.7%, respectively [21]. Despite the challenging clinical conditions of PA occlusive disease, a good clinical effect of treatment with the Supera@ stent has also been demonstrated with the ABI increasing from 0.58±0.16 preoperative to 0.87±0.14 postoperative [21,22].

Stent placement still remains controversial; however, as drug-eluting technology is becoming more popular the potential for successful use of drug-eluting stents (DES) in the treatment of femoropopliteal artery disease exists although data are limited regarding this. In the Zilver PTX randomized trial DES were

suggested to increase the patency of lesions and reduce the risk of restenosis [2]. The Zilver PTX trial has added to our knowledge of DES with the outcome being a 83.1% primary patency at 12 months with the use of paclitaxel-eluting stents in comparison with standard balloon angioplasty and bare metal stents in femoropopliteal disease [23]. The 2-year follow-up from the Silver PTX trial further supported the safety and effectiveness of paclitaxel-eluting stents in patients with femoropopliteal artery disease, including the long-term superiority of the DES to PTA and to provisional BMS placement [24]. The 2-year primary patency rate was 74.8% for the primary DES group and 26.5% for the long-term PTA subgroup [24]. These data are encouraging and have shown great potential with the opportunity for more studies comparing endovascular interventions in the treatment of PAD.

Adjunctive endovascular technologies

Emerging adjunctive therapies or alternatives to traditional PTA aim to prevent restenosis and include atherectomy to remove atherosclerotic plaque by debulking; brachytherapy to inhibit cellular proliferation by using ionizing radiation; and cryoplasty to induce smooth cell apoptosis and reduce intimal dissection/damage by cold-induced alteration of the arteriosclerotic plaque [4,25]. These and other technologic advancements are rapidly emerging and outpacing clinical trial data to support their efficacy [4]. These technologies may prove a potential solution to the problem of long-term patency and restenosis of femoropopliteal disease following PTA. The 3-year primary patency rates have been reported as a low 50% for PTA and first-generation stents [26].

Atherectomy

The mechanical atherectomy devices are designed to improve the vessel lumen and flow by debulking and removing atherosclerotic plaque with a rotating blade that captures the plaque in a catheter housing and requires intermittent emptying [2]. Currently available technologies for this therapy include orbital, laser, directional, and rotational atherectomy. The benefit of these atherectomy devices is potential avoidance of trauma to the vessel wall such as tears and stretches caused by popliteal artery PTA [27]. The study by Semaan *et al.* [28] compared atherectomy with angioplasty alone in the popliteal artery lesions and found a higher technical success rate with atherectomy. However, there are complications with all these debunking technologies including an increased distal embolization rate when compared with traditional PTA, which has the low rate of less than 1% embolization [26]. A large prospective registry of 1029 patients evaluated the embolization rate during percutaneous lower extremity interventions of 2137 lesions and found the overall embolization rate to be 1.6% with the Jetstream and Diamondback atherectomy devices having a 22% rate, the Silverhawk atherectomy device having a 1.9% rate, and laser atherectomy having a 3.6% embolic rate [26]. More large randomized controlled trials are needed to identify if atherectomy will be a benefit over standard PTA with or without stenting (Figure 79.2) [4].

Popliteal aneurysms

A popliteal aneurysm is the dilatation of the popliteal artery to a diameter of 1.5 cm or 1.5 times the size of the normal proximal artery which results in weakness of the artery [29,30]. The aneurysm progressively dilates and if left untreated it increases the risk

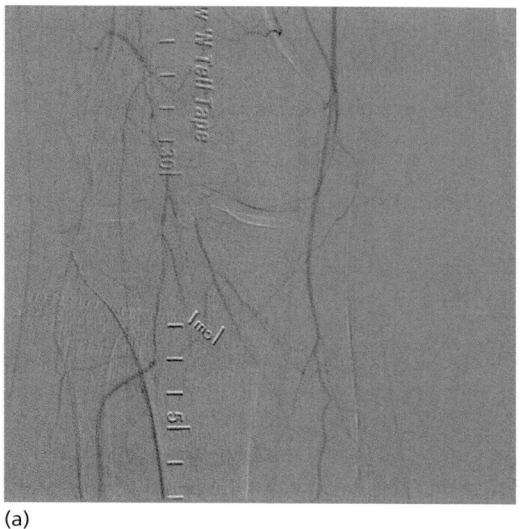 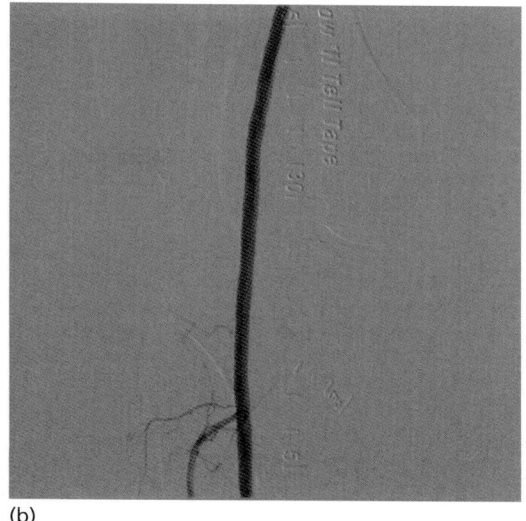

(a)   (b)

Figure 79.2 (a) Left popliteal artery chronic total occlusion. (b) Left popliteal artery post-intervention (post-atherectomy and PTA).

of thrombosis or embolization leading to CLI with an amputation rate of around 15% [31,32]. Although rare in the general population, occurring at an incidence of less than 0.1%, they are the second most common peripheral aneurysm at about 70% [33]. Popliteal artery aneurysms (PAAs) are more common in men than women (20 : 1 ratio), the incidence increases with age, and approximately half are bilateral [30].

The goal of PAA repair is to eliminate the aneurysm from the circulation to maintain perfusion to the lower extremity. Symptomatic patients can present with claudication and the consensus is that all symptomatic PAAs should be repaired regardless of size [30]. Asymptomatic PAAs are recommended to be treated if the aneurysm diameter is greater than 2 cm, mural thrombus is present, or the patent has poor runoff [30]. The current gold standard of PAA repair is saphenous vein bypass grafting either via open surgery or endovascular approach [30,32]. Open surgical repair is by various operation techniques with the two most popular approaches being the medial approach where the patient is supine and the posterior approach where the patient is in prone position [30]. Both approaches provide comparable results concerning primary patency rates and open surgical repair delivers reproducible therapeutic success [32]. Open surgery for PAAs is marked by low perioperative mortality and morbidity and provides excellent long-term results [34].

Endovascular techniques have been increasingly used with the rational of low complication rates, shortened length of hospital stay, and long-term patency rates presumed similar to those following open surgical repair; however, current evidence is lacking prospective randomized trials [35–39]. A high standard for endovascular popliteal aneurysm repair (EPAR) has been found to match open popliteal aneurysm repair (OPAR) procedures in which the primary patency rate was 90% with a freedom from reintervention rate of 70% at 10 postoperative years (Figure 79.3) [34]. However, a nonrandomized multicentered study found relatively equivalent primary patency rates (73% for EPAR, 64% for OPAR) and freedom from reintervention rates (75% and 72%, respectively) at a mean

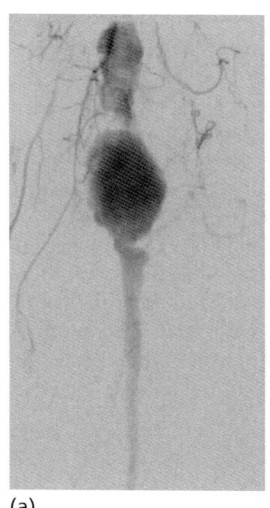 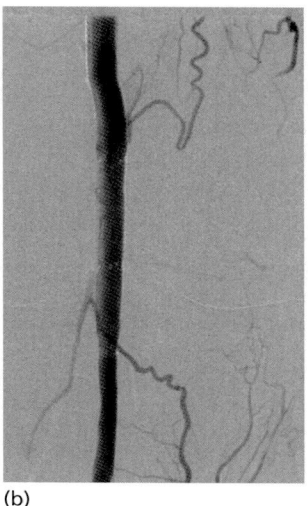

(a)   (b)

Figure 79.3 (a) Left popliteal artery aneurysm. (b) Left popliteal artery stent (resolved aneurysm post-stent).

surveillance period of 31 ± 28 months [38]. Further, the largest meta-analysis on this topic to date is based on 652 cases and the results suggest that patient outcomes after endovascular repair are equal to open surgical repair, and that endovascular technique appears to be a viable alternative to open surgery [39]. EPAR appears to be safe and efficient when compared with OPAR; nevertheless, current evidence on endovascular repair is limited and further research is necessary to draw firm conclusions [39]. The greatest benefit of endovascular stent grafting is for patients with high preoperative risk for surgery and multiple medical comorbidities [37]. The definitive evidence on the comparison of endovascular repair with open surgical repair of popliteal artery aneurysms remains inconclusive (Figure 79.4) [34–39].

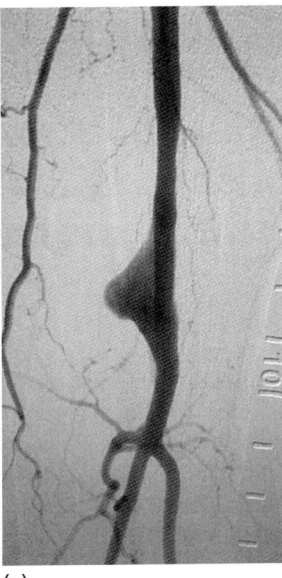
(a)

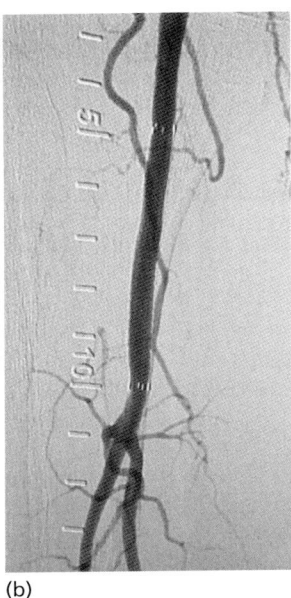
(b)

Figure 79.4 (a) Left popliteal artery focal aneurysm (prior vein patch aneurysm). (b) Left popliteal artery stent (resolved aneurysm post-stent).

Conclusions

As the population ages, it is anticipated that the prevalence of peripheral vascular disease will increase. Endovascular therapies are improving the safety and effectiveness of percutaneous revascularization in the treatment of PAD with a high success rate; however, long femoropopliteal lesions still represent one of the major challenges of endovascular therapy [6]. The use of endovascular repair increased more than threefold, bypass surgery decreased 42%, and the amputation rate decreased by 29% [18]. Today, most interventionists treat PA disease with PTA when there is clear indication and, when possible, surgical bypass as the gold standard [2]. Percutaneous procedures and new technologic advancements such as DEB, DES, and atherectomy devices continue to replace open surgery with the challenge being to ensure relevant studies are being carried out to collect definitive data to support these therapeutic measures in the treatment and prevention of PAD [2]. Further, cost-effectiveness data must be considered to accommodate economic considerations and provide cost conscious care while avoiding limb amputation and mortality.

Interactive multiple choice questions are available for this chapter on www.wiley. com/go/dangas/cardiology

References

1 Shamoun F, Sural N, Abela G. Peripheral artery disease: therapeutic advances. *Exp Rev Cardiovasc Ther* 2008; **6**(4): 539–553.

2 Hirsch AT, Haskal ZJ, Hertzer NR, *et al.* ACC/AHA 2005 Practice Guidelines for the management of patients with peripheral arterial disease (lower extremity, renal, mesenteric, and abdominal aortic): a collaborative report from the American Association for Vascular Surgery/Society for Vascular Surgery, Society for Cardiovascular Angiography and Interventions, Society for Vascular Medicine and Biology, Society of Interventional Radiology, and the ACC/AHA Task Force on Practice Guidelines (Writing Committee to Develop Guidelines for the Management of Patients With Peripheral Arterial Disease): Endorsed by the American Association of Cardiovascular and Pulmonary Rehabilitation; National Heart Lung,

and Blood Institute; Society for Vascular Nursing; TransAtlantic Inter-Society Consensus; and Vascular Disease Foundation. *Circulation* 2006; **113**: e463–e654.

3 Hirsch A, Haskal Z. ACC/AHA 2005 Practice guidelines for the management of patients with peripheral arterial disease (lower extremity, renal, mesenteric, and abdominal aortic): a collaborative report from the American Association for Vascular Surgery/Society for Vascular Surgery, Society for Cardiovascular Angiography and Interventions, Society for Vascular Medicine and Biology, Society of Interventional Radiology, and the ACC/AHA Task Force on Practice Guidelines. *Circulation* 2006; **113**: e463–654.

4 Shortell C, Rowe V. Popliteal artery occlusive disease. Medscape. http://emedicine. medscape.com/article/461910-overview (accessed May 29, 2016).

5 Norgren L, Hiatt WR, Dormandy JA, Nehler MR, Harris KA, Fowkes F; GTASC II Working Group. Inter-society consensus for the management of peripheral arterial disease (TASC II). *J Vasc Surg.* 2007; **45**(Suppl S): 5–67.

6 Zeller T, Rastan A, Macharzina R, *et al.* Drug-coated balloons vs. drug-eluting stents for treatment of long femoropopliteal lesions. *J Endovasc Ther* 2014; **21**: 359–368.

7 Malas M, Enwerem N, Qazi U, *et al.* Comparison of surgical bypass with angioplasty and stenting of superficial femoral artery disease. *J Vasc Surg* 2014; **59**(1): 129–135.

8 Scheinert D, Duda S, Zeller T, *et al.* The LEVANT I (Lutonix paclitaxel-coated balloon for the prevention of femoropopliteal restenosis) trial for femoropopliteal revascularization: first-in-human randomized trial of low-dose drug-coated balloon versus uncoated balloon angioplasty. *JACC Cardiovasc Interv* 2014; **7**(1): 10–19.

9 Gunner T, Laird J, Schneider P, *et al.* Drug-coated balloon versus standard percutaneous transluminal angioplasty for the treatment of superficial femoral and popliteal peripheral artery disease 12-month results from the IN.PACT SFA Randomized Trial. *Circulation* 2015; **131**: 495–502.

10 Micari A, Cioppa A, Vadalà G, *et al.* 2-year results of paclitaxel-eluting balloons for femoropopliteal artery disease: evidence from a multicenter registry. *JACC Cardiovasc Interv* 2013; **6**: 282–289.

11 Schroeder H, Meyer DR, Lux B, Ruecker F, Martorana M, Duda S. Two-year results of a low-dose drug-coated balloon for revascularization of the femoropopliteal artery: outcomes from the ILLUMENATE first-in-human study. *Catheter Cardiovasc Interv* 2015; **86**(2): 278–286.

12 Scheinert D, Scheinert S, Sax J, *et al.* Prevalence and clinical impact of stent fractures after femoropopliteal stenting. *J Am Coll Cardiol.* 2005; **45**(2): 312–315.

13 León J, Dieter R, Pacanowski J, *et al.* Clinical research study: preliminary results of the initial United States experience with the Supera woven nitinol stent in the popliteal artery. *J Vasc Surg* 2013; **57**: 1014–1022.

14 Schillinger M, Minar E. Past, present and future of femoropopliteal stenting. *J Endovasc Ther* 2009; **16**(Suppl I): 147–152.

15 Mwipatayi B, Hockings A, Hofmann M, Garbowski M, Sieunarine K. Balloon angioplasty compared with stenting for treatment of femoropopliteal occlusive disease: a meta-analysis. *J Vasc Surg* 2008; **47**: 461–469.

16 Laird JR. Limitations of percutaneous transluminal angioplasty and stenting for the treatment of disease of the superficial femoral and popliteal arteries. *J Endovasc Ther* 2006; **13**(Suppl 2): 30–40.

17 Geronemus AR, Peña CS. Endovascular treatment of femoral-popliteal disease. *Semin Interv Radiol* 2009; **26**(4): 303–314.

18 Slovut D, Lipsitz E. Surgical technique and peripheral artery disease. *Circulation* 2012; **126**: 1127–1138.

19 Semaan E, Hamburg N, Nasr W, *et al.* Endovascular management of the popliteal artery: comparison of atherectomy and angioplasty. *Vasc Endovasc Surg* 2010; **44**: 25–31.

20 Rastan A, Krankenber H, Baumgartner I, *et al.* Stent placement versus balloon angioplasty for the treatment of obstructive lesions of the popliteal artery: a prospective, multicenter, randomized trial. *Circulation* 2013; **127**: 2535–2541.

21 Chan Y, Cheng S, Ting A, Cheung G. Primary stenting of femoropopliteal atherosclerotic lesions using new helical interwoven nitinol stents. *J Vasc Surg* 2014; **59**(2): 384–391.

22 Scheinert D, Werner M, Scheinert S, *et al.* Treatment of complex atherosclerotic popliteal artery disease with a new self-expanding interwoven nitinol stent: 12-month results of the Leipzig SUPERA popliteal artery stent registry. *JACC Cardiovasc Interv* 2013; **6**(1): 65–71.

23 Dake MD, Ansel GM, Jaff MR, *et al.* Paclitaxel-eluting stents show superiority to balloon angioplasty and bare metal stents in femoropopliteal disease: twelve-month Zilver PTX randomized study results. *Circ Cardiovasc Interv* 2011; **4**: 495–504.

24 Dake MD, Ansel GM, Jaff MR, *et al.* Sustained safety and effectiveness of paclitaxel-eluting stents for femoropopliteal lesions: 2-year follow-up from the Zilver PTX randomized and single-arm clinical studies. *J Am Coll Cardiol* 2013; **61**: 2417–2427.

25 Jahnke T, Mueller-Huelsbeck S, Charalambous N, *et al.* Prospective, Randomized single-center trial to compare cryoplasty versus conventional angioplasty in the popliteal artery: midterm results of the COLD Study. *J Vasc Interv Radiol* 2010; **21**: 186–194.

26 Samson R, Showalter, D, Lepore M, Ames S. CryoPlasty therapy of the superficial femoral and popliteal arteries: a single center experience. *Vasc Endovasc Surg* 2007; **40**(6): 446–450.

27 Zeller T, Rastan A, Sixt S, *et al.* Long-term results after directional atherectomy of femoro-popliteal lesions. *J Am Coll Cardiol* 2006; **48**(8): 1573–1578.

28 Semaan E, Hamburg N, Nasr W, *et al.* Endovascular management of the popliteal artery: comparison of atherectomy and angioplasty. *Vasc Endovasc Surg* 2010; **44**: 25–31.

29 Wright L, Matchett J, Cruz C, *et al.* Popliteal artery disease: diagnosis and treatment. *RadioGraphics* 2004; **24**(2): 467–479.

30 Wissgott C, Lüdtke C, Vieweg H, *et al.* Endovascular treatment of aneurysms of the popliteal artery by a covered endoprosthesis. *Clin Med Insights Cardiol* 2014; **8**(Suppl 2): 15–21.

31 Joshi D, James RL, Jones L. Endovascular versus open repair of asymptomatic popliteal artery aneurysm. *Cochrane Database Syst Rev* 2014; **8**: CD010149.

32 Wagenhäuser M, Herma K, Sagban T, *et al.* Long-term results of open repair of popliteal artery aneurysm. *Ann Med Surg (Lond)* 2015; **4**(1): 58–63.

33 Antonello M, Frigatti P, Battocchio P, *et al.* Endovascular treatment of asymptomatic popliteal aneurysms: 8-year concurrent comparison with open repair. *J Cardiovasc Surg (Torino)* 2007; **48**: 267.

34 Dorweiler B, Gemechu A, Doemland M, *et al.* Durability of open popliteal artery aneurysm repair. *J Vasc Surg* 2014; **60**: 951.

35 Ying H, Gloviczki P. Popliteal artery aneurysms: rationale, technique, and results of endovascular treatment. *Perspect Vasc Surg Endovasc Ther* 2008; **20**(2): 201–213.

36 Eslami MH, Rybin D, Doros G, Farber A. Open repair of asymptomatic popliteal artery aneurysm is associated with better outcomes than endovascular repair. *J Vasc Surg* 2015; **61**: 663.

37 Huang Y, Gloviczki P, Oderich GS, *et al.* Outcomes of endovascular and contemporary open surgical repairs of popliteal artery aneurysm. *J Vasc Surg* 2014; **60**: 631.

38 Pulli R, Dorigo W, Castelli P, *et al.* A Multicentric experience with open surgical repair and endovascular exclusion of popliteal artery aneurysms. *Eur J Vasc Endovasc Surg* 2013; **45**(4): 357–363.

39 Von Stumm M, Teufelsbauer H, Reichenspurnera H, Debusc E.S. Two decades of endovascular repair of popliteal artery aneurysm: a meta-analysis. *Eur J Vasc Endovasc Surg* 2015; **50**(3): 351–359.

CHAPTER 80

Below the Knee Interventions in Critical Limb Ischemia

Karthik Gujja, Katarzyna Nasiadko, Arthur Tarricone, and Prakash Krishnan
Icahn School of Medicine at Mount Sinai, New York, NY, USA

Background

Peripheral arterial disease (PAD) of the lower extremities is one of the major manifestations of systemic atherosclerosis affecting 8–12 million people. The disorder affects both men and women equally with the risk of PAD increasing two- to threefold for every 10-year increase in age after 40 years and is highly associated with cardiovascular risk factors such as cigarette smoking, diabetes mellitus, hyperlipidemia, and hypertension [1]. The two most important risk factors are diabetes mellitus and smoking, each being associated with a three- to fourfold increase in the risk for PAD [1].

The Rutherford classification is the current industry standard for reports dealing with severity of PAD with categories 4–6 characterizing critical limb ischemia (CLI) on the basis of persistent rest pain with or without ongoing degree of tissue loss in the presence of PAD (Table 80.1) [2].

CLI represents the most severe clinical manifestation of lower extremity PAD and is defined as "greater than 2 weeks of rest pain, ulcers, or tissue loss attributed to arterial occlusive disease" [3]. CLI occurs when arterial lesions impair blood flow to such an extent that the nutritive requirements of the tissues cannot be met. Multiple tests have been devised to confirm the diagnosis of CLI, assess foot perfusion, and predict wound healing (Box 80.1) [3]. The diagnosis of CLI can be confirmed with measurement of an ankle-brachial index (ABI) or toe systolic pressure, with an ankle pressure of ≤50 mmHg or a toe pressure of ≤30 mmHg suggesting CLI.

CLI develops in approximately 1% of patients with PAD each year and is expected to grow in developed countries as the prevalence of diabetes increases with the World Health Organization (WHO) projecting that diabetes will be the seventh leading cause of death by 2030. Patients diagnosed with CLI have a high cardiovascular morbidity and mortality, high risk of major amputation, and experience poor physical function and quality of life [4]. The goals of treatment for CLI are relieving ischemic pain, healing ulcers, preventing limb loss, improving patient function and quality of life, and prolonging survival [4]. Prompt surgical or endovascular revascularization to achieve a straight-line flow to the foot to promote wound healing is currently recommended for limb salvage in CLI, as "nearly 40% of patients with CLI will progress to amputation within 6 months in the absence of revascularization" [5]. Partial revascularization of iliac or femoropopliteal arteries alone is usually insufficient to heal advanced leg ulcers or gangrene.

Evaluation of the lower extremity arterial system

To assess the lower extremity arteries, it is necessary to understand the arterial anatomy of the lower extremity. The clinician must know the branches of the lower extremity arterial system and the areas of the limb they supply. The angiosome concept highlights five distinct three-dimensional blocks of tissue fed by source arteries and that guiding revascularization to the wound site by restoring flow to the corresponding ischemic angiosome improves wound healing and higher amputation-free rates (Figure 80.1) [6].

To identify the ischemic area and anatomically characterize the disease, non-invasive imaging with duplex ultrasonography, computed tomography angiography (CTA), or magnetic resonance angiography (MRA) can be utilized to help determine the interventional options [5]. Further, potency of the iliac and common femoral arteries is of practical importance because it will determine whether the optimal strategy is via an ipsilateral anterograde or contralateral retrograde common femoral approach [7].

The choice of preprocedural imaging depends on the patient and is based on the advantages and disadvantages of each particular method. The evaluating physician should be fully aware of all revascularization options to select the most appropriate intervention that takes into consideration the goals of therapy, risk–benefits ratios, patient comorbidities, and life expectancy [8]. Box 80.2 lists indications and contraindications of endovascular management for below-the-knee (BTK) arterial occlusive disease [7]. For some patients, primary amputation is the only option.

Approach to BTK intervention

To standardize evaluation of the extent of disease in the lower extremity vessels, a working group was created to devise a classification scheme based on anatomic extent, morphologic assessment, and location of lesions within the vascular system. This group, comprising experts from the USA and Europe, developed the Transatlantic Inter-Society Consensus (TASC) classification strategy and made recommendations regarding appropriate management and therapy for different lesions [1]. The recommendations vary by the location and extent of the lesion (Box 80.3) [7].

Generally, in BTK or infrapopliteal (IP) lesions classified as TASC A or B, endovascular revascularization is preferred, while in

---

Interventional Cardiology: Principles and Practice, Second Edition. Edited by George D. Dangas, Carlo Di Mario, and Nicholas N. Kipshidze.
© 2017 John Wiley & Sons, Ltd. Published 2017 by John Wiley & Sons, Ltd.

Table 80.1 Rutherford classification of peripheral artery disease and critical limb ischemia [2].

Grade	Category	Clinical description	Objective description
	0	Asymptomatic	Normal treadmill or reactive hyperemia test
I	1	Mild intermittent claudication	Treadmill exercise limited to 5 min; ankle pressure after exercise >50 mmHg but at least 20 mmHg lower than at rest
I	2	Moderate intermittent claudication	Between Rutherford 1 and 3 disease
I	3	Severe intermittent claudication	Treadmill exercise limited to <5 min; ankle pressure after exercise <50 mmHg
II	4	Ischemic rest pain	Resting ankle pressure <40 mmHg and/or great toe pressure <30 mmHg; pulse volume recording barely pulsatile or flat
III	5	Minor tissue loss: non healing ulcer, focal gangrene with diffuse pedal ischemia	Resting ankle pressure <60 mmHg and/or great toe pressure <30 mmHg; pulse volume recording barely pulsatile or flat
III	6	Major tissue loss: extending above transmetatarsal level, functional foot no longer salvageable	Resting ankle pressure <60 mmHg and/or great toe pressure <30 mmHg; pulse volume recording barely pulsatile or flat

---

Box 80.1 Features of critical limb ischemia [3]

Physical examination
- Dry skin, thickened nails, loss of hair, loss of subcutaneous fat or muscle atrophy
- Coolness to palpation
- Decreased or absent pulses
- Elevation pallor or dependent rubor
- Non-healing wound or ulcer, especially over bony prominences, distally, and on the plantar surface of the foot

Non-invasive vascular laboratory
- Ankle-brachial index ≤0.4
- Ankle systolic pressure ≤50 mmHg
- Toe systolic pressure ≤30 mmHg
- Measures of skin microcirculation
- Capillary density ≤20 mm²
- Absent reactive hyperemia on capillary microscopy
- TcPO2 <10 mmHg

TASC D lesions, surgical vein bypass is recommended. In TASC C lesions, surgical revascularization is the preferred treatment in good-risk patients while considering the patient's comorbidities and preferences, as well as the operator's success rates. However, in the absence of a suitable vein and/or adequate distal runoff vessels, and in high-risk surgical patients, endovascular treatment represents the only valid therapeutic option of CLI [7].

There is no level I evidence to support the superiority of endovascular treatment over saphenous vein bypass for infrainguinal or IP disease. However, a multicenter prospective randomized study, the Bypass Versus Angioplasty in Severe Ischemia of the Leg (BASIL) trial, investigated the difference between endovascular (balloon angioplasty) and open surgical treatment for infrainguinal PAD and CLI. The study randomized 452 patients with severe limb ischemia to surgical bypass first or angioplasty-first strategy. The BASIL trial indicated that patients presenting with CLI caused by infrainguinal atherosclerosis who are suitable for both treatments could be treated with either method with no difference in the primary outcome of

6-month amputation-free survival between the two treatment modalities [9]. Angioplasty alone was clinically equivalent to the "gold standard" of surgical bypass in the treatment of CLI, unless the individual's life expectancy was greater than 2 years [10]. The updated results with 3–7 year follow-up concluded that bypass surgery with vein offers the best long-term amputation-free survival, but balloon angioplasty appears to be superior to a polytetrafluoroethylene bypass procedure (Figure 80.2). The most recent American College of Cardiology/American Heart Association (ACC/AHA) guidelines for the management of PAD are consistent with recommendations made by the BASIL trial investigators (Box 80.4) [11]. Overall, an individualized approach is the best treatment strategy and most specialists initially pursue an endovascular intervention if it seems feasible. This is because bypass surgery is associated with greater mortality and morbidity, with the potential for hospital readmission, prolonged ulcer healing, wound complications, and graft failure leading to reoperation [2]. In a study that used the National Surgical Quality Improvement Program database, the 30-day composite mortality/major morbidity rate of infrainguinal bypass surgery was as high as 19.5%, which made the authors conclude that "stringent indications for infra-inguinal bypass surgery should be maintained when considering the method of lower extremity revascularization" [12].

Endovascular management of below the knee critical limb ischemia

Infrainguinal distal bypass surgery has long been considered the gold standard treatment for CLI but a great number of patients are not eligible because of various underlying comorbidities commonly present in the CLI population or the absence of suitable vein conduits and/or patent non-diseased distal run-off vessels [13]. Moreover, there has been a push in modern CLI treatment towards a more "endovascular first" rationale, especially in patients with a life expectancy of <2 years [13]. Several options exist for endovascular therapy of arterial lesions BTK (Table 80.2) [11]. The minimally invasive nature of these endovascular procedures results in very low morbidity, mortality, and complication rates.

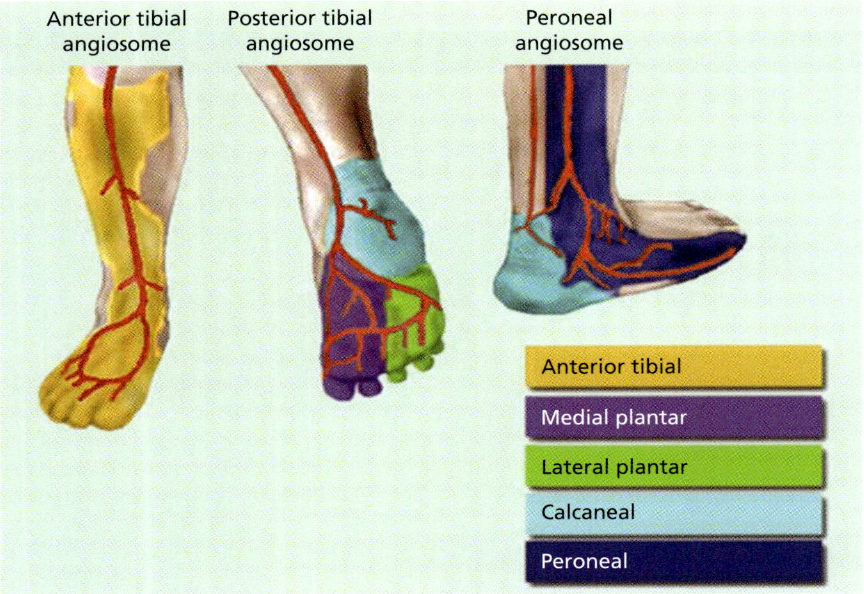

Figure 80.1 The angiosome concept. Five territories supplied by three arteries and their branches [6].

Box 80.2 Indications and contraindications of endovascular management for below-the-knee arterial occlusive disease [7]

Indications
- Critical limb ischemia: rest pain (Rutherford category 4) or non-healing ulcer/gangrene
- Significant flow-limiting stenosis of the anatomizes or outflow vessels in failing below-the-knee femoropopliteal or distal tibial bypass grafts

Absolute contraindications
- Medically unstable patients
- Life-threatening infected (wet) gangrene or/and life-threatening osteomyelitis of the target limb unless it is used to enable a more limited amputation
- Uncorrectable bleeding disorders
- Absent runoff vessels to and in the distal foot

Relative contraindications
- Pregnancy
- Inability of the patient to lie flat and immobile
- Critically ill elderly patients with impaired mobility and dementia
- Buerger disease
- Impaired renal function (EGFR <30 mL/min/1.73 m²)

Box 80.3 Transatlantic Inter-Society Consensus (TASC) classification of morphologic stratification of below the knee lesions

TASC type A
- Single stenosis shorter than 1 cm in the tibial or peroneal vessels

TASC type B
- Multiple focal stenosis of the tibial or perennial vessel, each less than 1 cm in length
- One or two focal stenosis, each less than 1 cm long at the tibial trifurcation
- Short tibial or perennial stenosis in conjunction with femoropopliteal PTA

TASC type C
- Stenosis 1–4 cm in length
- Occlusions 1–2 cm in length of the tibial or perennial vessels
- Extensive stenosis of the tibial trifurcation

TASC type D
- Tibial or peroneal occlusions longer than 2 cm
- Diffusely diseased tibial or peroneal vessels

Percutaneous transluminal angioplasty

At present, balloon angioplasty, also known as percutaneous transluminal angioplasty (PTA), is the primary technique to consider in endovascular treatment of BTK occlusive disease with success rates of IP PTA reported to be as high as 80–100% [7]. Procedural success is defined as the re-establishment of direct "in-line" pulsatile flow to the foot through at least one IP artery [13]. An example of a successful PTA is seen in Figure 80.3.

PTA access

The site and direction of the arterial access depend on the inflow status [7]. In non-obese patients without iliac, common femoral artery (CFA), or very proximal superficial femoral artery (SFA)

lesions, a direct antegrade puncture is preferable because it offers superior agility and trackability of the materials to cross hard, calcified distal occlusions, while it allows easier catheter and guidewire maneuvers [7]. With the standard anterograde percutaneous approach, procedural failure can be up to 20% often relating to long chronic total occlusions (CTOs), wall calcifications, and diffuse involvement of the pedal arteries, compromising distal run-off at the foot level, after trivial recanalization [14].

In patients where the antegrade approach has failed, various retrograde techniques can be used as the ultimate resort for limb salvage. The options for retrograde pedal approach are different, such as retrograde–antegrade recanalization (pedal-plantar loop

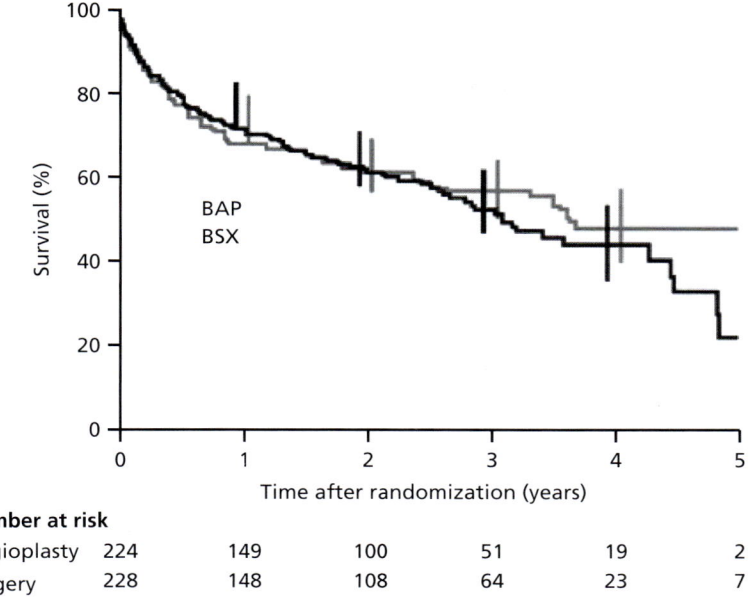

Figure 80.2 Results of Bypass Versus Angioplasty in Severe Ischemia of the Leg (BASIL) trial [9].

Number at risk

Angioplasty	224	149	100	51	19	2
Surgery	228	148	108	64	23	7

Box 80.4 Recommendations for critical limb ischemia: endovascular and open surgical treatment for limb salvage [11]

- The recommendations for CLI for patients with limb-threatening lower extremity ischemia and an estimated life expectancy of 2 years or less or in patients in whom an autogenous vein conduit is not available, balloon angioplasty is reasonable to perform when possible as the initial procedure to improve distal blood flow (level of evidence B)
- The recommendations for CLI for patients with limb-threatening ischemia and an estimated life expectancy of more than 2 years, bypass surgery, when possible and when an autogenous vein conduit is available, is reasonable to perform as the initial treatment to improve distal blood flow (level of evidence B)

Table 80.2 Options for interventional treatment of lower extremity arterial disease [11].

Treatment	12 month patency (%)	Notes
Angioplasty with critical limb ischemia	40–60	TASC A and B lesions
Cryoplasty	70	Lesions <8 cm and minimal calcification
Cutting balloon angioplasty	No data	
Laser	60–80	Assisted angioplasty
Mechanical atherectomy	80	30% assisted angioplasty
Stent	60–80	TASC A and B lesions
Drug-eluting stent	80–100	Decreases to 60% at 2 years
Covered stent	60–80	TASC A and B lesions
Brachytherapy	60–80	Difficult application

technique or transcollateral recanalization), which combines retrograde and integrate arterial recanalization using a single entry site, retrograde percutaneous distal access at different locations (pedal or plantar arteries), or advanced access (tarsal branches, transplanter arch, or digital access) [14]. The SAFARI technique, originally described by Spinosa et al. [15], involves a "combination" approach of antegrade and retrograde access in patients whose lesions cannot be addressed in standard fashion. Each approach has advantages and disadvantages, and the success rate is largely dependent upon physician experience (Box 80.5).

Pedal access technique

Transpedal access also requires operator experience but the technique can have a short learning curve.

Ultrasound guided

Using handheld duplex ultrasound can help to locate the tibiopedal vessels. The pedal vessels are usually accessed under local anesthesia with a 4 or 5 Fr microaccess needle. The most commonly accessed pedal arteries are the dorsalis pedis artery, followed by the

posterior tibial artery and peroneal artery. However, the peroneal artery's course lies on the interosseous ligament, and manual pressure for hemostasis can prove cumbersome. Operator familiarity with the ultrasound is important and is a short learning curve. Usually, pedal arteries are accompanied by dual pedal veins, which make accessing the vein much easier, and make the arterial access cumbersome. Compressing the pedal access site with the ultrasound probe slightly will collapse the veins thereby making arterial access easier and precise. A handheld duplex ultrasound can

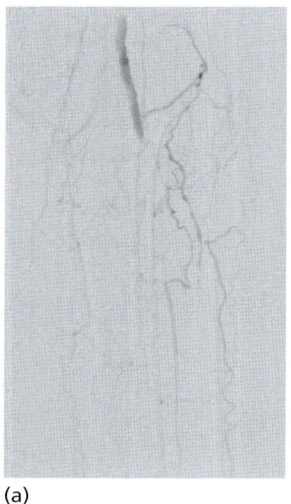
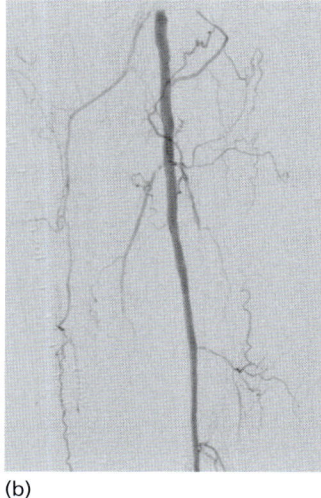

(a)   (b)

Figure 80.3 An example of a successful percutaneous transluminal angioplasty (PTA): (a) before PTA; (b) after PTA.

Box 80.5 Summary of percutaneous transluminal angioplasty (PTA) access methods

Contralateral access
• Can be obtained but balloon's shaft length and catheter length can limit the ability to reaching distal tibiopedal lesions
• Loss of ability of the crossing wire to carry torque, which affects pushability
• Device deliverability can pose a challenge because of tortuosity and length limit

Antegrade femoral access
• Increases the ability to cross tibiopedal lesions because of the ability for pushability, deliverability, and availability of catheters, wires with adequate support for catheter crossing
• Antegrade femoral access requires operator experience because the risk of multiple punctures resulting in hematoma is high
• Antegrade puncture can also cause difficulty in access management, especially in obese patients

Retrograde pedal access
• By this method you can attain optimal result especially when combined with a contralateral approach (SAFARI technique)
• Limitations are dissection during access and possible vessel closure

---

provide an image of the pedal artery in both short and long axis; short axis is easy to puncture with the needle and changing to the long-axis view to introduce the wire is the preferred approach.

Fluoroscopy guided

Approach to transpedal access includes road mapping or image overlay especially with orthogonal angles. However, this method can be difficult if the patient moves or if there is table movement, and it also requires the use of additional contrast. This method requires operator expertise because the puncture must be made at a 90° angle to the flow. Exposure of fingers to radiation is also a concern here.

Access site procedure

An attempt must be made to achieve access with the first puncture to prevent spasm, and if the puncture is through and through, slow withdrawal of the needle will facilitate access with a micropuncture

guidewire. The access wire should be advanced only to the occluded segment of the pedal artery to prevent vessel dissection. Dilator placement over the wire will facilitate placement of a micropuncture sheath or a catheter directly. Regular access sheaths should not be introduced into the vessel as this can cause spasm and occlusion of the vessel.

To prevent clotting and vessel spasm use nitroglycerin, a small dose of heparin, and verapamil. A 0.014–0.018 inch wire can be advanced via micropuncture sheath. Additional support can be achieved with a 0.018-inch support catheter. This method allows crossing of lesions and subsequent insertion of the wire into a sheath from femoral access or the snaring of the pedal wire from the top. Further delivery of balloons and stents can be performed via the femoral approach (SAFARI technique). The pedal sheath and the catheters can be removed and manual pressure held. Dedicated micropuncture pedal access sets are available in 4 and 5 Fr outer diameters. We recommend no sheaths be placed via pedal access site except micropuncture sheath.

Access site hemostasis

Usually, manual compression is the preferred approach and can achieve adequate hemostasis without hematoma unless the puncture is high. Use of transradial band has been adopted by certain operators but patient discomfort, outflow obstruction, and band misfit in obese patients especially are drawbacks.

Modified angioplasty techniques

Among the drawbacks of balloon angioplasty remains the potential of a suboptimal acute outcome because of elastic recoil and/or flow-limiting dissection resulting in technical failure and/or progressive vascular restenosis with relapse of clinical symptomatology [13]. In order to cope with the imminent technical failure of balloon angioplasty, modified angioplasty techniques have been used [13].

Stents

BTK stent placement has been historically used in limited fashion and mostly for failed initial angioplasty although primary stenting is being heavily evaluated as a first-line consideration [16]. In 2004, the first study to investigate primary below-knee stent-supported angioplasty (BKSSA) for restoring straight in-line arterial flow in patients with CLI demonstrated its clinical and hemodynamic efficacy and safety [17]. The study found that BKSSA is associated with a high rate of angiographic success, minimal major adverse events (MAEs; defined as death, stroke, myocardial infarction (MI), renal failure, retroperitoneal bleed, unplanned tibial/pedal bypass, major infection, compartment syndrome, acute renal failure, or need for procedure-related transfusion), and short hospital stay, even in the elderly patient with multiple comorbidities [17].

Bare metal stents

Stent placement for IP disease has gained progressive attention. However, there is no level I evidence for primary stenting in IP arterial disease. Several studies have shown mixed results, although the preponderance of the data do not support primary stenting in all cases of CLI. Randon *et al.* [18] reported on a prospective randomized trial that compared PTA alone with primary stenting for IP lesions. The authors randomized a total of 38 limbs in 35 patients to PTA (n = 22) or stenting (n = 16). Thirty-six limbs had occlusions and 20 had stenosis. They found no statistically significant difference in primary or secondary patency, limb salvage, or survival between the two groups at 12 months. This study was limited by small sample size, but is the setter for the trend with no worse outcomes reported for primary stenting.

On the same theme, Brodmann et al. [19] performed a randomized trial in patients with CLI in the setting of IP disease. They randomized 54 patients; 33 to PTA, and 21 to primary stenting with balloon-expandable bare metal stents (BMS). Seventy-five percent of patients had clinical improvement (81% in the PTA group and 65% in the stent group). Primary patency at 12 months was 48.1% with PTA and 35.3% with stents, with a secondary patency of 70% and 53%, respectively [19]. None of the differences were statistically significant. This study was also limited by the small size and failed to show a benefit of primary stenting over PTA alone.

Donas et al. [20] reported on a series of 53 high-risk patients with CLI treated with IP arterial stent placements as bailout after suboptimal angioplasty. The authors used self-expanding nitinol stents for all interventions. They treated 30 stenoses and 23 occlusions with a mean lesion length of 5.5 ± 1.9 cm. Their mean follow-up was 24.1 months. They reported 98.1% technical success with 75.5% 2-year cumulative primary patency. Freedom from amputation was reported at 88.7% with secondary patency of 88%. They also showed that proximal lesions had significantly better patency than distal crural lesions (83.3% vs. 65.2%) and that there was no difference in patency between stenosis and occlusions [20]. Their conclusion was that IP stent placement is a durable bailout treatment option in high-risk CLI patients with suboptimal angioplasty.

Drug-eluting stents

The proven efficacy of drug-coated stents in the treatment of coronary artery disease gave rise to the notion that they might have a better patency than BMS in small IP vessels. Siablis et al. [21] conducted a non-randomized, prospective, single-center study of the Cypher sirolimus-eluting balloon-expandable coronary stent (SES) versus a conventional balloon-expandable BMS (Evolution, Spiral Force, Tsunami, or Zeus) employed for bailout after IP PTA (65 lesions in 41 IP arteries) for CLI (Rutherford categories 4–6). Indications for bailout stenting (29 patients in each treatment group) were elastic recoil, flow-limiting dissection, or residual stenosis >30% after the initial PTA. Technical success was 96.6% in the BMS group versus 100.0% in the SES group. At 1 year, primary patency by intra-arterial DSA (86.4% vs. 40.5%) was still significantly higher and binary in-stent restenosis (36.7% vs. 78.6%) and in-segment restenosis (59.1% vs. 9%) were still significantly lower for the SES group. The SES was associated with significantly fewer cumulative target lesion revascularization (TLR) at 6 months (4.0% vs. 17.0%) and at 1 year (9.1% vs. 26.2%). At 1 year, the differences between the two groups in rates of mortality (13.8% for SES vs. 10.3% for BMS), minor amputations (10.3% for SES vs. 17.2% for BMS), and limb salvage (100% for SES vs. 96% for BMS) were not significant.

Scheinert et al. [22] treated 60 consecutive patients with IP artery obstructions under a protocol of primary implantation of SES or BMS into tibial and peroneal arteries. Inclusion criteria for this prospective registry were Rutherford category 3–6 and >70% diameter stenosis of the target lesion; maximum allowable lesion length was 30 mm, and only patients with lesions treatable with a single stent could be enrolled. Thirty patients (83.3% diabetics)

received balloon-expandable Cypher stents, while 30 other patients (76.6% diabetics) received uncoated BMS (Bx Sonic). In 21 cases, inflow lesions in the femoral and/or popliteal arteries required treatment prior to the BTK intervention. At follow-up (mean 9.3 months for the SES patients, mean 9.8 months for the BMS patients), the cumulative rate of MAEs was 10.0% for the SES patients versus 46.6% for the BMS patients. The rates of major amputation, bypass surgery, and TLR were all 0% for the SES patients and 10.0%, 0%, and 23.3%, respectively, for the BMS patients. There were three deaths in the SES group and four deaths in the BMS group. On angiographic follow-up of 24 SES patients, no relevant obstructions were seen, while in the BMS group, the rate of binary restenosis was 39.1%; the mean degree of in-stent restenosis was $1.8\% \pm 4.8\%$ for the SES patients versus $53.0\% \pm 40.9\%$ for the BMS patients. Hence, drug-coated stents achieve significantly higher primary and secondary patency than BMS for focal IP artery lesions.

In the PReventing Amputations using Drug eluting Stents (PaRADISE) trial 106 patients (118 limbs) were treated with 228 DES. The number of stents per limb was 1.9 ± 0.9, and 35% of limbs received overlapping DES (length of 60 ± 13 mm). There were no procedural deaths, and 96% of patients were discharged within 24 hours. The 3-year cumulative incidence of amputation was $6\% \pm 2\%$, survival was $71\% \pm 5\%$, and amputation-free-survival was $68\% \pm 5\%$. TLR occurred in 15% of patients, and repeat angiography in 35% of patients revealed a binary restenosis in 12% [17]. In the YUKON Drug-Eluting Stent Below the Knee-Randomized Double-Blind Study, the trial included 161 patients with mean target lesion length of 31 ± 9 mm. Thirty-five (23.3%) patients died during a mean follow-up period of 1016 ± 132 days. The event-free survival rate was 65.8% in the SES group and 44.6% in the BMS group (log-rank p = 0.02). Amputation rates were 2.6% and 12.2% (p = 0.03), and target vessel revascularization rates were 9.2% and 20% (p = 0.06), respectively [21]. The Destiny trial and Achilles study showed similar results as the prior two studies and showed the importance of DES in IP lesions for patency rates. Advances in DES could be field changing [23].

The use of balloon-expandable BMS as well as drug-eluting stents (DES) in BTK lesions are endovascular technologies with the promise of significant inhibition of vessel restenosis and improved clinical outcomes [16]. Patency and limb salvage rates are all quite similar in the short term, with limb salvage rates higher in general versus vessel patency rates (70–100% vs. 60–80% at 1 year) [16]. However, bailout DES achieves superior long-term primary patency rates compared with bailout BMS. Balloon expandable BMS were found to improve the initial technical success rates of BTK endovascular treatment but did not result in satisfactory long-term results mainly because of the phenomenon of in-stent restenosis [13]. Restenosis remains the leading unresolved issue following every kind of endovascular treatment and is mainly attributed to the continuous mechanical irritation caused by the metal stent mesh, resulting in the inflammatory–proliferative response of the vessel wall, subsequent intimal hyperplasia, negative remodeling, and finally restenosis [13].

Drug-coated balloons

Drug-coated balloon (DCB) technology has emerged as a potential answer to the limitations presented by the utilization of DES and is based on the combination of balloon angioplasty and local, single-dose, cytostatic drug delivery, without the permanent implantation of an endovascular device, with the aim to lower restenosis rates

[13]. An advantage of DCB technology is the superior drug dose fixed on the balloon's surface compared with the dose on the surface of DES, potentially resulting in higher dose delivery to the target vessel [13]. There are a variety of diverse DCB catheters available for IP use and although they all use the same type of drug (paclitaxel) and dosage (3 µg/mm), the coating technology is completely different [24]. More recently, bioabsorbable variations are being investigated and short-term results are anticipated in the near future [16].

Cryoplasty, peripheral cutting balloon, and AngioSculpt Scoring Balloon

Studies investigating the use of PTA with adjunctive therapies such as cryoplasty, peripheral cutting balloon, and AngioSculpt Scoring Balloon provide more meaningful and current information regarding the role of PTA.

Cryoplasty

Cryoplasty (cold balloon angioplasty) combines the pressure of angioplasty with cold energy by delivering nitrous oxide to inflate a non-compliant balloon [1]. Cryoplasty using the PolarCath Peripheral Dilatation System (Boston Scientific Corporation) has an FDA indication for treating stenotic lesions in the peripheral vasculature (iliac, femoral, popliteal, IP, renal, and subclavian arteries) among other indications [16]. During inflation of the balloon, within a separate lumen in the balloon catheter, liquid nitrous oxide is converted to gas thereby cooling the surface of the balloon to –10°C [16]. The theoretical mechanisms of action involve altered plaque response, reduced elastic recoil, and induction of apoptosis within the endothelium, thereby reducing the rate of restenosis. Cryoplasty has been used as an effective primary strategy for limiting the incidence of dissection, vessel recoil, and subsequent intimal hyperplasia and restenosis associated with the endovascular dilatation of atherosclerotic lesions in the peripheral vasculature [25].

The BTK Chill Trial, examining the use of primary cryoplasty for BTK occlusive disease in patients with CLI, included 108 patients involving 111 limbs with 115 target IP lesions. The primary endpoints were acute technical success (ability to achieve ≤50% residual stenosis and continuous inline flow to the foot) and absence of major amputation of the target limb in 6 months. Acute technical success was achieved in 108 (97.3%) of treated limbs, and major amputation at 6 months was avoided in 85 of 91 patients (93.4%) [25]. The study group concluded that cryoplasty therapy was safe and effective in treating IP disease, providing excellent results and a high rate of limb salvage in patients with CLI [26].

Peripheral cutting balloon

In cutting balloon angioplasty, the balloon contains three or four sharp microtomes fixed longitudinally about the outer surface of a non-compliant balloon [1]. Radial expansion of the balloon results in longitudinal incisions in the plaque, thereby relieving hoop stress in the arterial wall [1]. Use of the peripheral cutting balloon for BTK intervention has been described as an effective alternative for IP lesions with significant calcification and/or resistance to standard PTA [16]. A single institution study of its use in the IP segment found the technical success rate was 80% which improved to 100% when adjunctive stenting was included [1].

AngioSculpt Scoring Balloon

The AngioSculpt Scoring Balloon is a semicompliant balloon with a flexible nitinol-scoring element that scores the target lesion with the intended effect of a more uniform and precise outcome [16].

Atherectomy

The mechanical atherectomy device removes plaque with a rotating blade and captures the plaque in a catheter housing which requires intermittent emptying [1]. The use of atherectomy in the IP segment has been largely based on the idea that "debulking" or "lesion prep" will provide a more acceptable acute and more durable angioplasty or stenting result. Numerous registries and single-center studies have been published, but these have the inherent weaknesses of studies of this design, namely, there are no randomized or comparative data.

Most physicians use atherectomy as an adjunct to PTA or stenting and it has become more widespread in the last several years with the development of devices such as the Silver Hawk Plaque Excision System (Plymouth, MN, USA), the Diamondback 360 Orbital Atherectomy System (St. Paul, MN, USA), the CLiRPath Turbo Elite laser catheter (Colorado Springs, CO, USA), and the Jetstream Atherectomy Catheter (Kirkland, WA, USA) [13]. The Silver Hawk Plaque Excision System is an excisional atherectomy device with a rotating carbide atherotome that is able to capture the plaque in the nose cone of the device and remove it. The Diamondback 360 Orbital Atherectomy System is based on the idea of differential "sanding" of complex and calcified plaque, using centrifugal force to orbit a diamond-encrusted crown within the vessel to create a more compliant vessel for adjunctive PTA or stenting. The OASIS trial was a multicenter, non-randomized, prospective registry evaluating the safety and efficacy of the Diamondback device. The CLiRPath Turbo Elite laser catheter uses an excimer (excited dimer) laser that generates 308-nm pulsed ultraviolet light to "photoablate" plaque, thereby creating a channel to perform additional intervention [16].

Excisional atherectomy

Atherectomy devices are designed to debulk and remove atherosclerotic plaque by cutting, pulverizing, or shaving with catheter-deliverable blades. The development of the Silver Hawk excisional atherectomy catheter (Minneapolis, MN, USA) has occasioned some renewed interest in directional atherectomy, a technique that has historically been associated with high restenosis rates in the coronary and peripheral vasculature [27]. Like the excimer laser, excisional atherectomy offers the theoretical advantage, compared to PTA and stent implantation, of eliminating stretch injury on arterial walls, limiting acute dissection (and the need for adjunctive stenting) and elastic recoil, and thereby potentially reducing post-procedure inflammation and the rate of restenosis. Kandzari et al. [28] used the device to treat 160 lesions (40% IP, mean length ATK 74 mm, mean length BTK 51 mm; 34% total occlusions, 80% moderate to severe calcification) in 69 patients with severe CLI (Rutherford categories 5–6, 78% diabetics, 55% with ≤1 patent run-off vessel) at seven different sites. Residual diameter stenosis after the procedure was <50% in all but one of the procedures; adjunctive angioplasty was employed without stent placement in 11% of the procedures, and stents were placed in 6%. There were no reported instances of perforation or embolization and only one instance of abrupt closure. The 6-month rate of major adverse events was 23%, reflecting the significant comorbidity of the patient group. There was no morphologic measurement of restenosis reported; the rate of TLR was 4%. Through 6-month follow-up, there were no unplanned amputations; in 82% of patients amputation was either less extensive than initially planned or avoided altogether.

Zeller *et al.* [29] reported outcomes through 2 years for SilverHawk treatment of 49 BTK lesions (mean length 46 mm, mean diameter stenosis 89%; 22% total occlusions, 18% in-stent restenosis) in 36 patients (53% with CLI, 61% diabetics). Predilatation was required for 33% of the lesions. Post-atherectomy angioplasty was performed for 38% of the lesions, and 4% required stent implantation as a result of dissection. Mean residual stenosis, which was 12% following the atherectomy, was reduced to 8% following any adjunctive therapy; residual stenosis ≤30% was achieved in 98% of lesions. The mean ABI increased significantly from 0.48 ± 0.39 to 0.81 ± 0.10 (p <0.05) before discharge and remained improved during follow-up. Primary and secondary patency rates (<70% restenosis by duplex ultrasound and/or angiography) were 67% and 91% after 1 year and 60% and 80% after 24 months. The rate of restenosis was significantly lower for lesions <50 mm in length versus those ≥50 mm (25.8% vs. 44.4%; p <0.05).

Many have suggested that stenosis in the IP arteries can be treated by atherectomy without predilatation, while occlusions should be predilated with an undersized balloon to ensure that the wire crosses the occlusion intraluminally. It is strongly advised against the use of atherectomy in cases in which the occlusion was crossed subintimally because of the potential for perforation.

Excimer laser-assisted angioplasty

Continuous wave laser were evaluated and abandoned for peripheral interventions in the late 1980s because of the high complication rate caused by thermal damage to surrounding tissue [30]. In contrast, excimer laser angioplasty of the leg arteries has been practiced commercially in Europe since 1994 [31]. The 308 nm excimer laser utilizes flexible fiberoptic catheters to deliver intense, short duration pulses of ultraviolet (UV) energy. The advantages of pulsed UV energy lies in the short penetration depth of 50 μm and its ability to break molecular bonds directly, by a photochemical instead of thermal process. Excimer laser catheters remove a tissue layer of about 10 μm with each pulse of energy. Tissue is vaporized only on contact without a consequent rise in temperature to surrounding tissue.

The multicenter Laser Atherectomy for Critical Ischemia (LACI) trial of excimer laser-assisted angioplasty treated 423 lesions (41% SFA, 15% popliteal, 41% IP) in 155 limbs (91% with at least one occlusion) of 145 patients with CLI (Rutherford categories 4–6, 69% with tissue loss, 66% diabetics) who were determined to be poor candidates for surgical revascularization. Procedural success (defined as <50% residual stenosis in all treated lesions) was achieved in 85% of the treated limbs [32]. The median total length of treated artery per limb was 11.0 cm. Procedural complications, occurring in 12% of the treated limbs, included major dissection (4%), acute thrombus formation (3%), distal embolization (3%), and perforation (2%). The excimer procedure was followed with adjunctive balloon angioplasty in 96% of the limbs. Stents (mainly bare nitinol) were placed adjunctively in 61% of the SFA lesions, 38% of the popliteal lesions, and 16% of the tibial lesions. Mean lesion stenosis (by visual estimate) was decreased from 92% at baseline to 55% after laser debulking and to 18% at final assessment. At 6-month follow-up, limb salvage was achieved in 110 of 119 (92%) surviving patients (118 of 127 limbs; 93%); 56% of

ischemic ulcers had healed completely [33]. Despite treating a very unfavorable patient cohort, excimer laser-assisted angioplasty achieved limb salvage comparable to the gold standard of bypass surgery. Following the LACI protocol, a single-center US registry and a five-center Belgian trial achieved comparable outcomes with the device [34,35].

Rotational atherectomy with aspiration

The Pathway PV system (Kirkland, WA, USA) has a unique feature compared to other rotational atherectomy devices. The ability to remove the atherectomized plaque material through aspiration ports reduces the risk of obstructing the microvasculature and avoids increasing erythrocyte degradation products, especially in patients with impaired renal function. High-speed rotational devices without aspiration capabilities increase these degradation products, such as haptoglobin and potassium, which can result in life-threatening cardiac arrhythmias [36]. Additionally, the aspiration feature of the catheter allows the device to be used in lesions containing both occlusive material, including solid, even calcified plaque and fresh thrombus. Potentially, the Pathway PV can be used as a thrombectomy device in subacute and acute vessel occlusions.

Zeller *et al.* [29] reported results on a prospective non-randomized multicenter trial using a rotational atherectomy system with aspiration capabilities. In this study, a 99% technical success rate was achieved using the Pathway PV Atherectomy System in 210 infrainguinal cases. Adjunctive balloon angioplasty was performed in 59% and stenting in 7%. Primary and secondary patency rates at 1 year were 61.8% and 81.3%, respectively. The 1-year limb salvage rate was 100%. These patency rates are similar to the Silver Hawk study cohorts.

Orbital atherectomy

The Diamondback 360Orbital Atherectomy System (St. Paul, MN, USA) uses a plaque ablation catheter. This has an abrasive eccentrically shaped crown with a diamond-coated surface, which rotates and creates lumen enlargement by plaque abrasion. Orbital atherectomy appears to have some similarities to mechanical rotational atherectomy (Rotablator, Natick, MA, USA). However, the Rotablator has greater limitations with respect to device size and lumen enlargement. Although the efficiency of lumen enlargement is 92% for Rotablator (a 2-mm burr will create a lumen diameter of 1.8 mm) [37], it is greater than 175% for orbital atherectomy.

A prospective, non-randomized, multicenter registry examined the safety and 6-month outcomes of 124 patients IP disease and either CLI or claudication. A total of 90.1% of patients achieved the primary outcome of <30% final diameter stenosis and no major amputations at 6 months (2.4% minor amputations). Adjunctive angioplasty was performed in 39.3% and stenting in 2.5% of lesions [38].

Complications of endovascular procedures

As with open vascular surgery procedures, the potential for life and limb-threatening complications can occur with endovascular procedures. The number of endovascular procedures being performed is increasing rapidly and so complications of procedures are being encountered with increasing frequency [1]. Immediate complications occurring during or shortly after IP endovascular procedures are reported in 2–10% of cases [8]. As all vascular punctures cause injury to a vessel access site, complications can occur including chronic pain, hematoma, pseudoaneurysms, AV fistula, vessels thrombosis, vessel rupture, embolization, and dissection. Up to 1% of all patients revascularized will develop a graft infection secondarily to wound breakdown with a 15% mortality rate and 40% incidence of major limb loss [39]. Postoperative lymphedema is considered an important factor in prolonging incisional healing and patient discomfort [39]. To help limit complications constant technologic advancements are being made in catheter and wire construction so the best selection of specific tools is used. Imaging technology is optimized to improve diagnostic accuracy and therapeutic precision.

Conclusions

CLI is a complex multifactorial disease and encompasses the most extreme end of the PAD spectrum leading to significant morbidity and mortality [24]. Preventing amputation in CLI is arguably the most important goal and is predicated on the ability to restore and maintain straight line tibial arterial flow to the foot. Favorably, as the management of patient with CLI evolves, the number of major limb amputation rates will continue to decline significantly.

Historically, bypass surgery with autogenous veins for flow restoration has been the first-line revascularization therapy for CLI; however, advances in endovascular techniques and device technology has changed the treatment paradigm [40]. Angioplasty has become the first-line intervention for patients with BTK CLI with lower morbidity and mortality than surgical treatments, which should be considered for more complex anatomic lesions of BTK vessels or in patients with endovascular failure and persisting clinical symptoms of CLI [41]. Despite extensive research into interventional modalities for treatment of lower extremity atherosclerotic disease, all treatments are associated with some degree of recurrence and an inability to achieve long-term patency [1]. Things to look out for in the future of BTK interventions include bioabsorbable platforms as better biocompatibility is important to reduce the need for long-term antiplatelet therapy and reduce the risk of thrombosis [23].

Interactive multiple choice questions are available for this chapter on www.wiley.com/go/dangas/cardiology

References

1 Rooke T, Sullivan T, Jaff M. *Vascular Medicine and Endovascular Interventions.* Columbia, MD: Society for Vascular Medicine and Biology; 2007.

2 Lumsden AB, Davies MG, Peden EK. Medical and endovascular management of critical limb ischemia. *J Endovasc Ther* 2009; **16**(Suppl 2): 31–62.

3 Slovut DP, Sullivan TM. Critical limb ischemia: medical and surgical management. *Vasc Med* 2008; **13**(3): 281–291.

4 Mangiafico RA, Mangiafico M. Medical treatment of critical limb ischemia: current state and future directions. *Curr Vasc Pharmacol* 2011; **9**(6): 658–676.

5 Gahtan V, Costanza M. *Essentials of Vascular Surgery for the General Surgeon.* Syracuse, NY: Springer-Verlag; 2015.

6 Dominguez A, Bahadorani J, Reeves R, Mahmud E, Patel M. Endovascular therapy for critical limb ischemia. *Expert Rev Cardiovasc Ther* 2015; **13**(4): 1–16.

7 Van Overhagen H, Spiliopoulos S, Tsetis D. Below-the-knee interventions. *Cardiovasc Interv Radiol* 2013; **36**(2): 302–311.

8 Baumann F, Bloesch S, Engelberger RP, et al. Clinically driven need for secondary interventions after endovascular revascularization of tibial arteries in patients with critical limb ischemia. *J Endovasc Ther* 2013; **20**(5): 707–713.

9 Adam DJ, Beard JD, Cleveland T, et al. Bypass versus angioplasty in severe ischaemia of the leg (BASIL): multicenter randomized controlled trial. *Lancet* 2005; **366**(9501): 1925–1934.

10 Quevedo H, Arain S, Ali G, Rafeh N. A critical view of the peripheral atherectomy data in the treatment of infrainguinal arterial disease. *J Invasive Cardiol* 2014; **26**(1): 22–29.

11 Rooke TW, Hirsch AT, Misra S, et al. 2011 ACCF/AHA focused update of the guideline for the management of patients with peripheral artery disease (updating the 2005 guideline). *Vasc Med* 2011; **16**(6): 452–476.

12 LaMuraglia GM, Conrad MF, Chung T, et al. Significant perioperative morbidity accompanies contemporary infrainguinal bypass surgery: an NSQIP report. *J Vasc Surg* 2009; **50**:299–304.

13 Karnabatidis D, Spiliopoulos S, Katsanos K, Siablis D. Below-the-knee drug-eluting stents and drug-coated balloons. *Expert Rev Med Devices* 2012; **9**(1): 85–94.

14 Palena L, Manzi M. Retrograde pedal approach for below-the-ankle revascularization in patients with critical limb ischemia. *Vasc Dis Manag* 2014; **11**(9): E180–E190.

15 Spinosa DJ, Harthun NL, Bissonette EA, et al. Subintimal arterial flossing with antegrade-retrograde intervention (SAFARI) for subintimal recanalization to treat chronic critical limb ischemia. *J Vasc Interv Radiol* 2005; **16**(1): 37–44.

16 Wiechmann B. Tibial intervention for critical limb ischemia. *Semin Intervent Radiol* 2009; **26**(4): 315–323.

17 Feiring AJ, Wesolowski AA, Lade S. Primary stent-supported angioplasty for treatment of below-knee critical limb ischemia and severe claudication. *J Am Coll Cardiol* 2004; **44**(12): 2307–2314.

18 Randon C, Jacobs B, De Ryck F, Vermassen F. Angioplasty or primary stenting for infrapopliteal lesions: results of a prospective randomized trial. *Cardiovasc Intervent Radiol* 2010; **33**(2), 260–269.

19 Brodmann M, Froehlich H, Dorr A, et al. Percutaneous transluminal angioplasty versus primary stenting in infrapopliteal arteries in critical limb ischemia. *Vasa* 2011; **40**(6), 482–490.

20 Donas KP, Torsello G, Schwindt A, Schonefeld E, Boldt O, Pitoulias GA. Below knee bare nitinol stent placement in high-risk patients with critical limb ischemia is still durable after 24 months of follow-up. *J Vasc Surg* 2010; **52**(2), 356–361.

21 Siablis D, Karnabatidis D, Katsanos K, Ravazoula P, Kraniotis P, Kagadis GC. Outflow protection filters during percutaneous recanalization of lower extremities' arterial occlusions: a pilot study. *Eur J Radiol* 2005; **55**(2): 243–249.

22 Scheinert D, Ulrich M, Scheinert S, Sax J, Braunlich S, Biamino G. Comparison of sirolimus-eluting vs. bare-metal stents for the treatment of infrapopliteal obstructions. *EuroIntervention* 2006; **2**(2): 169–174.

23 Dieter RS, Nanjundappa A. Ask the experts: a focus on stenting for lower extremity peripheral arterial disease. *Clin Pract* 2012; **9**(5): 499–501.

24 Gulati A, Botnaru I, Garcia LA. Critical limb ischemia and its treatments: a review. *J Cardiovasc Surg* 2015; **56**(5): 775–785.

25 Das TS, McNamara T, Gray B, et al. Cryoplasty therapy for limb salvage in patients with critical limb ischemia. *J Endovasc Ther* 2007; **14**(6): 753–762.

26 Das TS, McNamara T, Gray B, et al. Primary cryoplasty therapy provides durable support for limb salvage in critical limb ischemia patients with infrapopliteal lesions: 12-month follow-up results from the BTK Chill Trial. *J Endovasc Ther* 2009; **16**(2 Suppl 2): 19–30.

27 Garcia LA, Lyden SP. Atherectomy for infrainguinal peripheral artery disease. *J Endovasc Ther* 2009; **16**(2 Suppl 2): 105–115.

28 Kandzari DE, Kiesz RS, Allie D, et al. Procedural and clinical outcomes with catheter-based plaque excision in critical limb ischemia. *J Endovasc Ther* 2006; **13**(1): 12–22.

29 Zeller T, Sixt S, Schwarzwalder U, et al. Two-year results after directional atherectomy of infrapopliteal arteries with the SilverHawk device. *J Endovasc Ther* 2007; **14**(2): 232–240.

30 White RA, White GH, Mehringer MC, Chaing FL, Wilson SE. A clinical trial of laser thermal angioplasty in patients with advanced peripheral vascular disease. *Ann Surg* 1990; **212**(3): 257–265.

31 Visona A, Perissinotto C, Lusiani L, et al. Percutaneous excimer laser angioplasty of lower limb vessels: results of a prospective 24-month follow-up. *Angiology* 1998; **49**(2): 91–98.

32 Laird JR, Reiser C, Biamino G, Zeller T. Excimer laser assisted angioplasty for the treatment of critical limb ischemia. *J Cardiovasc Surg (Torino)* 2004; **45**(3): 239–248.

33 Laird JR, Zeller T, Gray BH, et al. Limb salvage following laser-assisted angioplasty for critical limb ischemia: results of the LACI multicenter trial. *J Endovasc Ther* 2006; **13**(1): 1–11.

34 Biamino G. The excimer laser: science fiction fantasy or practical tool? *J Endovasc Ther* 2004; **11**(Suppl 2): 207–222.

35 Bosiers M, Peeters P, Elst FV, *et al.* Excimer laser assisted angioplasty for critical limb ischemia: results of the LACI Belgium Study. *Eur J Vasc Endovasc Surg* 2005; **29**(6): 613–619.

36 Mehta SK, Laster SB. Hemolysis induced pancreatitis after orbital atherectomy in a heavily calcified superficial femoral artery. *Catheter Cardiovasc Interv* 2008; **72**(7): 1009–1011.

37 Safian RD, Freed M, Reddy V, *et al.* Do excimer laser angioplasty and rotational atherectomy facilitate balloon angioplasty? Implications for lesion-specific coronary intervention. *J Am Coll Cardiol* 1996; **27**(3): 552–559.

38 Safian RD, Niazi K, Runyon J, *et al.* Orbital atherectomy for infrapopliteal disease: device concept and outcome data for the OASIS trial. *Catheter Cardiovasc Interv* 2009; **73**(3): 406–412.

39 Nehler MR, Peyton BD. Is revascularization and limb salvage always the treatment for critical limb ischemia? *J Cardiovasc Surg* 2004; **45**(3): 177–184.

40 Dominguez A, Bahadorani J, Reeves R, Mahmud E, Patel M. Endovascular therapy for critical limb ischemia. *Expert Rev Cardiovasc Ther* 2015; **13**(4): 429–444.

41 Setacci C, de Donato G, Teraa M, *et al.* Treatment of critical limb ischaemia. *Eur J Vasc Endovasc Surg* 2011; **42**(Suppl 2): 43–59.

CHAPTER 81

Subclavian, Vertebral, and Upper Extremity Vascular Disease

Ian Del Conde[1], Cristina Sanina[2], and Jose M. Wiley[3]

[1] Miami Cardiac and Vascular Institute, Miami, FL, USA
[2] University of Miami Miller School of Medicine, Miami, FL, USA
[3] Albert Einstein College of Medicine; Montefiore Einstein Center for Heart & Vascular Care, Bronx, NY, USA

Subclavian and upper extremity arterial disease

Epidemiology

Upper extremity vascular diseases are significantly less common than those involving the lower extremities. Nevertheless, they are important because of the potentially disabling effects on arm and hand function. Upper extremity vascular disease can be conceptually divided into "large-artery" disease involving the inflow arteries, such as the subclavian and axillary arteries, or "small-artery" disease involving the arteries distal to the wrist. While the list of occupational factors and medical conditions associated with small-artery disease is long and heterogeneous [1], the causes of upper extremity large-artery disease is more limited and includes atherosclerosis of the subclavian artery; arteritis (giant cell or Takayasu's arteritis); thoracic outlet syndrome; and radiation arteritis. Fibromuscular dysplasia (FMD) rarely occurs in the inflow arteries of the upper extremity and causes occlusive disease [2]. Use of drugs causing vasospasm, such as ergotamine, cocaine, and amphetamines, can cause intense upper extremity arterial vasospasm. Embolism from a proximal source, including the ascending aorta and cardiac sources of embolism, must be considered in patients presenting with acute thrombotic occlusion on the arteries in the upper extremity, especially if the disease in unilateral.

Causes of subclavian and upper extremity arterial disease

Atherosclerosis

Hemodynamically significant atherosclerosis is 20 times less common in the upper extremities than the lower extremities. When atherosclerosis causes a hemodynamically significant stenosis in the upper extremity, it is almost always localized to the proximal subclavian artery; atherosclerosis distal to the subclavian artery is very uncommon [3].

Takayasu's arteritis and giant cell arteritis

Takayasu's arteritis (TA) and giant cell arteritis (GCA) are granulomatous arteritides that can involve the aorta and its major branches [4].

Takayasu's arteritis has higher prevalence rates in Asian countries, including Japan, Korea, India, and China, than in Western countries [5]. Most patients present in their third decade, and are usually female. Constitutional symptoms, such as fatigue or low-grade fevers, are present in up to 40% of patients [6]. However, TA can be an incidental finding given that up to 20% of patients are asymptomatic. The most common vascular symptom in TA is arm claudication, occurring in 60% of patients, reflecting disease predilection for the aortic arch vessels [7,8]. TA should be suspected in any young (age <40 years) patient presenting with evidence of arterial stenosis or occlusion despite the absence of traditional cardiovascular risk factors, with no history of drug abuse (especially cocaine and amphetamines), and who have no evidence of an underlying prothrombotic state (e.g., antiphospholipid antibody syndrome) or causes of accelerated atherosclerosis. Importantly, serum markers of systemic inflammation, such as erythrocyte sedimentation rate (ESR) and C-reactive protein (CRP), can be normal in up to 50% of patients, even in those with active disease.

Elevated plasma levels of interleukin-6 have been found to closely correlate with disease activity, and can be useful clinically for monitoring and treatment adjustments in patients with TA [9]. In TA, vessel wall inflammation results in stenosis, occlusion, and potentially secondary thrombosis in involved arteries. The innominate and subclavian arteries are most frequently involved, followed by the aorta, common carotids, and renal arteries. Aneurysms develop as a long-term sequela of TA, with higher prevalence rates in Asian countries. In terms of treatment, glucocorticoids are the mainstay of treatment in TA, with resolution of symptoms in 25–100% of patients.

Giant cell arteritis is a relatively common arteritis that usually affects individuals older than 50 years, with a mean age of 70 years, and a female : male ratio of 2 : 1 [10]. Constitutional symptoms are common, and are often the reason why patients seek medical attention. Polymyalgia rheumatic (PMR), which is closely linked to GCA, is seen in up to 40% of patients with GCA and is characterized by symmetrical, proximal aching; morning stiffness, bursitis, and tenosynovitis. Headache is common in GCA, and tends to be localized to the temporal areas, where the temporal arteries can be quite tender. Vision loss is one of the most feared complications of CGA, and is caused by ischemia of the optic nerve. Approximately 15% of patients develop arterial occlusive disease of the large arteries of the upper extremities. Although upper extremity stenoses typically occur in the subclavian and axillary arteries, brachial artery stenoses also occur. Exclusion of atherosclerotic disease, which is also common in this patient population, is an essential step

Interventional Cardiology: Principles and Practice, Second Edition. Edited by George D. Dangas, Carlo Di Mario, and Nicholas N. Kipshidze.
© 2017 John Wiley & Sons, Ltd. Published 2017 by John Wiley & Sons, Ltd.

in the management of these patients. Similar to TA, a normal ESR or CRP does not rule out the possibility of GCA. However, the diagnosis should ideally be confirmed by temporal artery biopsy. In terms of treatment, GCA is extremely sensitive to steroids.

Thoracic outlet syndrome

Thoracic outlet syndrome (TOS) refers to the extrinsic compression of the subclavian artery, subclavian vein, and/or brachial plexus, as these course through the *scalene triangle*, formed by the first rib, the clavicle, the scalenus medius muscle, and the costoclavicular ligament. The type of TOS depends on the structure that is compressed: arterial TOS results from compression of the subclavian artery, venous TOS from compression of the subclavian vein, and neurogenic TOS from compression of the brachial plexus. Neurogenic TOS is by far the most common form of TOS; patients typically present with paresthesias, weakness, or pain in the hand, arm, or shoulder. Raynaud's phenomenon and cold hands are often seen. Patients with venous or arterial TOS usually have a history of repetitive physical exertion using their upper extremities (e.g., baseball pitcher, weightlifting). Patients with venous TOS (also called Paget–Schroetter syndrome) present with arm swelling. Patients with arterial TOS (the least common form of TOS) present with arm claudication, or hand/digit ischemia from distal embolization.

The evaluation of patients with suspected TOS includes measurement of bilateral brachial blood pressures, as well as pulse examination or pulse volume recordings with provocative maneuvers, such as the Adson and EAST (external rotation and abduction stress test) maneuver. Plain X-rays are useful for the evaluation of cervical ribs. Cross-sectional imaging studies, such as CT angiography or MR angiography, are often used, as well as electromyography and nerve conduction tests for the evaluation of neurogenic TOS.

Radiation

Although overall uncommon, radiation-induced arterial injury is a well-documented complication in patients with a history of previous head and neck or mediastinal radiation. The pattern of radiation arteritis depends on the time period elapsed since radiation therapy. Early disease (<5 years since irradiation) is often caused by endothelial injury and mural thrombus. Late disease (usually 10 years or more following irradiation) is caused by fibrotic occlusion of the artery or accelerated atherosclerosis. In radiation-induced arteritis, stenoses or occlusions tend to be caused by smooth vessel narrowing. Calcification and fibrosis often predominates in the wall of the artery that was in closest proximity to the radiation source.

Diagnostic evaluation
History and physical examination

All patients with upper extremity arterial disease should have a detailed cardiovascular history taken. Especially important aspects that should be covered in the patient's history include:

- Description of the symptoms, whether their onset was insidious or acute, unilateral or bilateral, persistent or intermittent, history of Raynaud's, and the presence of ulceration;
- Relevant comorbidities, such as autoimmune disorders, cardiovascular risk factors, prothrombotic states;
- Tobacco use;
- Drugs and medications, especially argot alkaloids, chemotherapeutic agents, cocaine, amphetamines;
- Occupational exposures, including those associated with TOS, vibration injury; and

- Relevant review of symptoms, especially those suggestive of an underlying rheumatologic or autoimmune disorder, or a prothrombotic state.

The upper extremity exam should focus on:

- Inspection: changes that may uncover an underlying connective tissue disorder (e.g., CREST syndrome), distal embolization to a digit (e.g., digit pallor, or discoloration), and the presence of ulceration.
- The subclavian, axillary, brachial ulnar, and radial pulses should all be carefully noted and compared with the contralateral side. An Allen's test should be performed. If TOS is suspected, provocative maneuvers should be elicited while palpating the radial pulse.

Non-invasive and invasive studies

Non-invasive vascular testing can be broadly classified as: (i) functional (or physiologic) studies that provide information on the hemodynamic effects of arterial occlusive disease in the upper extremity, and (ii) anatomic studies that provide detailed information about the location and other physical characteristics related to the occlusive disease. The presence and extent of upper extremity ischemia can be gauged through physiologic studies, which include the wrist-brachial index (WBI), pulse volume recordings (PVRs), and digit photoplethysmography (PPG). CT and MR angiography provide anatomic data. Duplex ultrasonography provides anatomic as well as hemodynamic information.

The WBI is the ratio of the systolic blood pressure measured at the wrist to the pressure measured at the brachial artery, and indicates the presence of occlusive lesions between the brachial arteries and distal radial and ulnar arteries. A WBI is reported for each arm. A WBI <0.7 is considered abnormal. Instead of measuring the pressure at the wrist (i.e., distal radial or ulnar artery), the ratio can be obtained between the finger pressure and the brachial pressure, resulting in a finger-to-brachial pressure index (FIBI). An FIBI <0.7 is considered abnormal.

Similar to the lower extremities, PVR tracings can be obtained in the upper extremities [11]. Cuffs are placed in the upper arms, forearms, and wrists. Systolic blood pressures are obtained by Doppler at each level (Figure 81.1a). Systolic pressures are compared with adjoining levels in the ipsilateral limb, as well as with the contralateral one. A blood pressure differential that exceeds 15–20 mmHg is suggestive of the presence of significant occlusive disease proximal to that level. PVRs depict changes in the volume of the limb during arterial pulsations. A normal PVR waveform is similar to the waveform seen with intra-arterial blood pressure tracings, and consists of a rapid systolic upstroke, a rapid initial downstroke, a prominent dicrotic notch, and smooth late equalization in the remainder of diastole. When a PVR waveform is deteriorated (or blunted), occlusive disease in a proximal segment should be suspected. With severe disease, the waveforms ultimately become flat or non-pulsatile. If PVR waveforms in both upper arms are severely dampened, a cardiac etiology, including severe aortic stenosis, should be considered.

Ten-digit PPG should be part of a complete upper extremity non-invasive arterial evaluation. PPGs are performed by placing a strapped sensor in the distal end of each finger to measure changes in blood flow. Finger PPG tracings showed be obtained with the patient as warm as possible. A normal finger PPG tracing consists of a rapid upstroke, sharp systolic peak with reflected wave. With decreased blood flow, for example as seen with a proximal severe stenosis or vasospasm, the waveforms become dampened, with low amplitude, and may even flatline (Figure 81.1b).

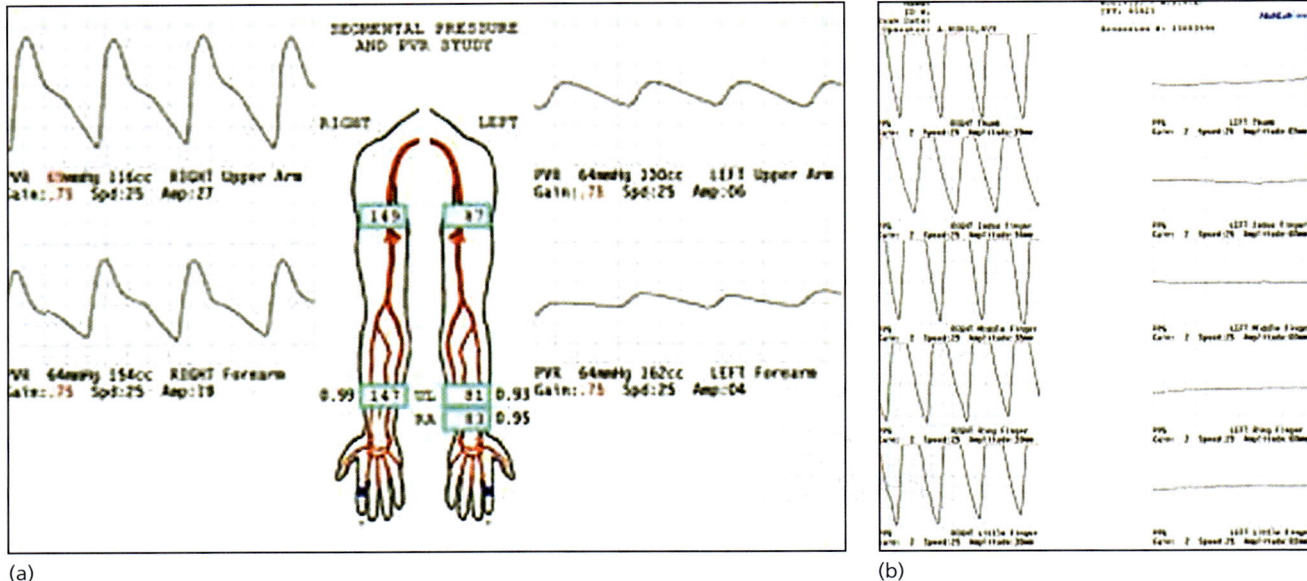

(a)   (b)

Figure 81.1 (a) Bilateral upper extremity wrist-brachial indices, pulse volume recordings (PVR), and segmental pressures. A significant brachial pressure differential is noted. PVR waveforms on the right are normal, with brisk upstrokes and dichrotic notches. Left upper and lower arm PVR waveforms are markedly blunted, suggesting disease proximal to the brachial artery. (b) Finger photoplethysmography (PPG) tracings are normal on the right, and severely blunted on the left.

Maneuvers for the thoracic outlet syndrome

These maneuvers are used to evaluate patients suspected of having arterial TOS. In each of the maneuvers, the radial artery is palpated. With a positive test, the amplitude of the pulse is decreased. It should be mentioned that there are a significant number of false positive results, as occlusion of the subclavian artery can be elicited by forceful TOS maneuvers, even in healthy individuals without TOS.

- *Adson's test*: the patient sits upright, takes a deep breath in, looks upward, and turns his head to the affected side.
- *EAST maneuver*: The patient is asked to extend his/her arms, externally rotated and behind the head. The patient makes fists repeatedly for 3 minutes. Radial pulses are felt at the end of the test.
- *Military position*: shoulders are thrust downward and backwards maximally.

Duplex ultrasonography

Normal Doppler signals in the upper extremity should be triphasic. A change from triphasic to biphasic can be significant; however, in some patients biphasic flow patterns are normal. Monophasic waveforms with prominent diastolic flow are always abnormal and are usually seen distal to severe stenosis or occlusion. Waveforms in areas of severe stenosis often demonstrate high velocities and spectral broadening, reflecting turbulent blood flow. If the ratio between the velocity at the area of stenosis and the velocity in the proximal arterial segment is >4, a 75–99% stenosis is suspected (Figure 81.2).

Computer tomography and magnetic resonance angiography

CT angiography (CTA) and magnetic resonance angiography (MRA) have become among the most valuable non-invasive imaging modalities for the assessment of upper extremity vascular diseases. The vessel wall can be well visualized, aiding in the diagnosis of large-vessel vasculitis, such as TA. Modern reconstruction packages allow the three-dimensional presentation of volumetric information, which can be of significant value in vascular interpretation. These modalities are most useful for the visualization of the proximal larger arteries of the upper extremities. Their value is more limited in the visualization of the small distal arteries of the arm and hand. PVRs can be measured instead of feeling the radial pulsations by physical examination alone.

Catheter-based angiography

Catheter-based angiography should be reserved for patients who may require an endovascular intervention, or to those in whom the architecture and morphology of the distal arm, hand, and digit arteries must be investigated, for example, in a case of small-vessel arterial occlusive disease (Figure 81.3).

Treatment
Medical management

The treatment of GCA is often initiated on the basis of clinical suspicion. Most patients respond to prednisone 60 mg/day within 3–5 days. Patients with immediately threatening symptoms, such as visual loss, should be treated with pulsed intravenous methylprednisolone 1000 mg/day for 3 days. Low dose aspirin should be started, provided that there are no contraindications, to reduce the risk of associated ischemic complications such as vision loss.

Most patients with TA require immunosuppressive agents, initially begun as prednisone 1 mg/kg/day for 1–3 months [12]. If remission and improvement of the disease is not evident, the addition of cytotoxic agents such as methotrexate, azathioprine, cyclophosphamide, or mycophenolate mofetil can be effective. The latter is shown to achieve 90% clinical resolution of symptoms in patients for whom conventional medical therapy has failed [13].

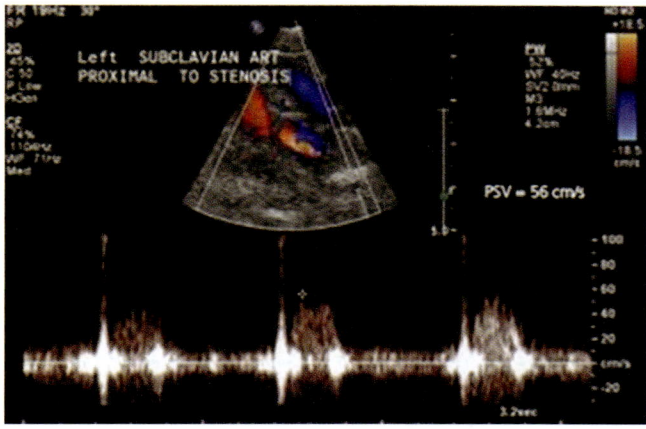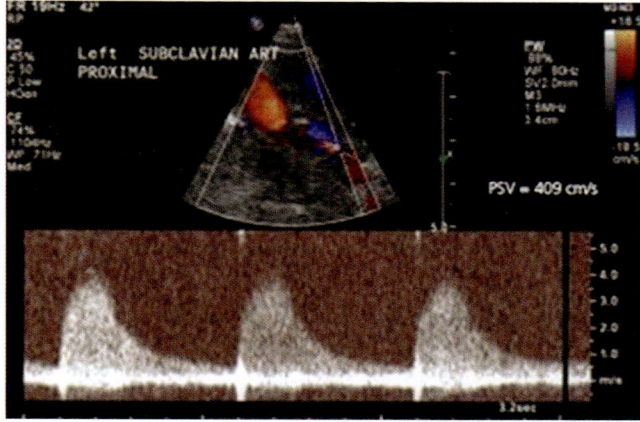

Figure 81.2 Same patient as Figure 81.1. A significant velocity shift is seen in the left subclavian vein, associated with monophasic waveforms. These findings indicate the presence of a severe (75–99%) stenosis.

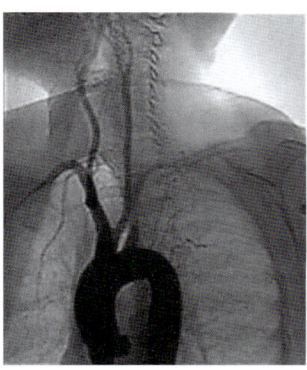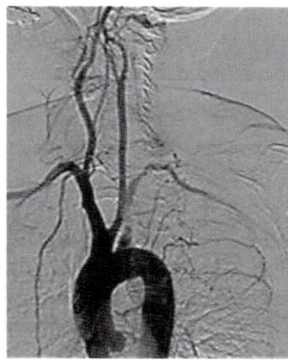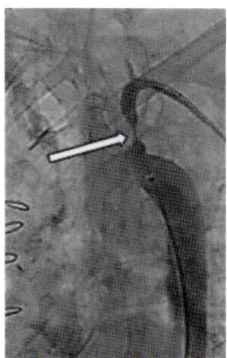

Figure 81.3 Same patient as Figure 81.1. Angiogram of the aortic arch and its branches shows severe stenosis in the proximal left subclavian artery.

Surgical management

Surgical management of GCA and TA is reserved for when the disease is quiescent. Indications for arterial reconstruction include lesions that produce hemispheric cerebral symptoms, rest pain, effort fatigue, embolism, vertebral–subclavian steal syndrome, or coronary ischemia as a result of subclavian–coronary steal syndrome in patients who have undergone internal mammary to coronary bypass.

Surgical options can be performed through the chest or neck for patients with subclavian and upper extremity occlusive disease. Selection of surgical option depends on the location, extent, presenting symptoms, and patient comorbidities. The three most common reconstruction procedures are carotid–subclavian bypass, carotid–subclavian transposition, and aorto-innominate/aorto-carotid bypass.

In patients with venous TOS, surgical decompression of the thoracic outlet is indicated; however, the timing of surgical decompression is controversial. Some groups use decompression within 3–6 months with interim use of oral anticoagulation [14]. The surgical treatment of arterial TOS is indicated in all symptomatic patients with ischemia and in those who are asymptomatic but have aneurysmal degeneration. Surgical decompression consists of resection of a cervical rib followed by either primary repair of the diseased subclavian artery or replacement bypass with a prosthetic conduit. In patients with neurogenic TOS, 70% will respond to physical therapy for

8 weeks. Patients who fail to achieve symptomatic improvement may require surgical management [15].

Endovascular management

Percutaneous repair of the subclavian artery has shown excellent initial success in comparison with surgical options. However, long-term durability favors surgical revascularization. A femoral approach is usually adequate. Unfractionated heparin should be administered prior to selective catheter engagement to prevent thrombus from forming and embolization. Non-selective angiography in a 45° left anterior oblique (LAO) projection is usually performed with a pigtail catheter in the ascending aorta. Selective catheterization of the supra-aortic vessels is usually achieved with a JR4, Headhunter, or angled Glide catheter. The diseased vessel is commonly crossed with either a non-hydrophilic or a hydrophilic 0.035-inch wire. In the case of crossing the lesion with a hydrophilic wire, it is then exchanged for a 0.035-inch non-hydrophilic wire. The diagnostic catheter is then exchanged for a long 6–7 Fr 90 cm sheath, or alternatively can be telescoped over the diagnostic catheter until it reaches the subclavian artery proximal to the diseased segment. Selective angiography with a non-inflated predilatation balloon matched to the reference vessel size is performed in two views: LAO 40° to position the balloon in the ostium, and a contralateral cranial view to determine the proximity of the distal end of the balloon to the origin of the vertebral artery. After predilatation, the sheath is telescoped over the balloon and exchanged for a balloon expandable or self-expandable stent for ostial or non-ostial lesions, respectively. The stent is unsheathed and deployment is carried out using the two views previously described. Post-angioplasty angiography is performed, after which the equipment is removed.

In the case of TOS, those presenting with acute subclavian–axillary venous thrombosis, catheter-directed thrombolysis is the preferred initial management strategy. If started within 14 days of symptom onset, the likelihood of success is good when combined with thoracic outlet decompression [16].

Vertebral artery disease
Epidemiology and clinical presentation

Approximately 80% of strokes are ischemic in origin. However, one in four ischemic strokes occur in the posterior circulation [17]. Patients with symptomatic vertebrobasilar insufficiency (VBI) have a 25–40% incidence of vertebral artery stenosis (VAS) [18]. However, symptoms of vertebrobasilar ischemia such as dizziness, ataxia, visual disturbances, and motor sensory deficit are rare. It is well known that ligature of one of two vertebral arteries is well tolerated in humans [19,20]. Even though atherosclerotic occlusive disease of both vertebral arteries is the most common culprit, other combinations of innominate, carotid, or subclavian artery stenosis can compromise the posterior circulation and elicit symptoms of vertebrobasilar insufficiency.

The prognosis for patients with atherosclerotic occlusion of the VBS is poor, with 80–100% mortality [21]. Symptomatic VBI carries a 5–11% incidence of stroke or death at 1 year [22,23]. Transient ischemic attacks (TIA) resulting from extracranial VAS are associated with a stroke rate of 30% at 5 years [24].

Treatment

The initial treatment consists of antithrombotic and antiplatelet therapy. However, there is lack of evidence supporting the use of these drugs for this disease or comparing these drugs with other treatment options [25,26]. If symptoms continue despite maximal medical therapy, an arch and four-vessel angiography, CTA or magnetic MRA is indicated [24].

Three surgical techniques to revascularize one vertebral artery in bilateral symptomatic disease have been described: transection of the vertebral artery above the stenosis and re-implantation into the ipsilateral subclavian or carotid artery; vertebral artery endarterectomy; or vein patch angioplasty. These approaches carry significant morbidity [27]. In one series by Berguer *et al.* [28], 174 patients undergoing proximal vertebral artery reconstruction had no in-hospital death but reported complications: recurrent laryngeal nerve palsy 2%; Horner's syndrome 15%; lymphocele 4%; chylothorax 0.5%; and acute thrombosis 1%. Secondary patency rates were 95% and 91% at 5 and 10 years, respectively. Seventy-five patients undergoing reconstruction of the distal vertebral artery had a mortality of 4% and an immediate graft thrombosis rate of 8%. Secondary patency rates for distal vertebral reconstruction were 87% and 82% at 5 and 10 years, respectively. Other reports quote a combined morbidity and mortality rate of VAS of 10–20% and have dampened enthusiasm for this option [29].

The first reported successful treatment of the vertebrobasilar system by intraoperative percutaneous transluminal angioplasty (PTA) was by Sundt *et al.* in 1980 [30]. As the most common location for VAS is at or near its origin from the subclavian artery, considerable recoil often accompanies PTA alone. Endoluminal stenting of the vertebral artery lesion is an attractive approach,

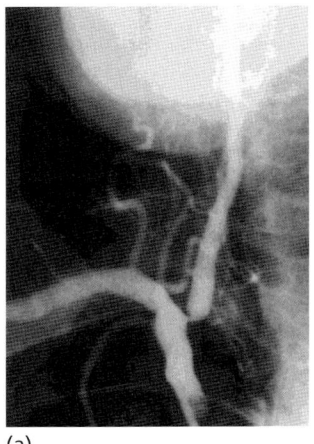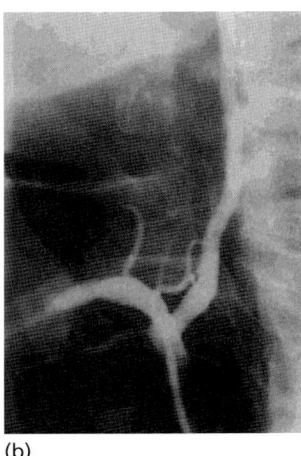

(a)   (b)

Figure 81.4 (a) Right vertebral artery angiogram demonstrates severe ostial stenosis (95%). (b) After balloon angioplasty and stent placement, there is a 0% residual stenosis when compared with the reference vessel diameter.

which has proven safety, efficacy, and durability as evidenced by low recurrence rates (Figure 81.4).

Endovascular technique

The femoral approach is the most common access site. Patients should receive aspirin 325 mg/day and clopidogrel 75 mg/day. After arterial access they should receive of anticoagulation with 5000–10,000 units unfractionated heparin. Selective catheterization of the vertebral artery is performed using a 6 Fr Judkins Right-4, internal mammary artery or multipurpose catheter. The diagnostic catheter is then exchanged for a 6–8 Fr multipurpose guide catheter, or a long 6–7 Fr 90 cm sheath can be telescoped over the diagnostic catheter until it reaches close to the ostium of the vertebral artery. A 0.014-inch wire is then advanced into the artery and advanced distally, avoiding advancing past the end of the distal portion (V4) of the vertebral artery (Figure 81.5). Distal embolic protection devices are seldom used because of severe spasm of the vertebral artery. A balloon matched to the reference size is then advanced to the lesion for predilatation, followed by a balloon expandable stent. Post-deployment angiography is performed to include the posterior intracranial circulation. No sedation is used during the procedure and continuous neurologic monitoring is performed.

Vertebral artery trauma and dissection

Over 80% of unilateral vertebral artery traumatic injuries are asymptomatic. Patients may present with VBI, posterior headache, or neck pain. Those with bilateral vertebral artery injuries may present with more severe symptoms. The grade of injury to the vertebral injury does not correlate with its associated risk of stroke or death, which remains at approximately 20% and 8%, respectively.

All patients with traumatic vertebral artery injury, regardless of their symptomatic status, should undergo anticoagulation with unfractionated heparin followed by warfarin, if there are no contraindications, and serial neurologic examination to monitor for progression. Embolic stroke is the major cause of morbidity and mortality in patients with vertebral artery dissection. The treatment of dissection is for the most part conservative. Most dissections heal spontaneously and the associated aneurysms never rupture and only rarely cause delayed ischemic symptoms. Surgical treatment of

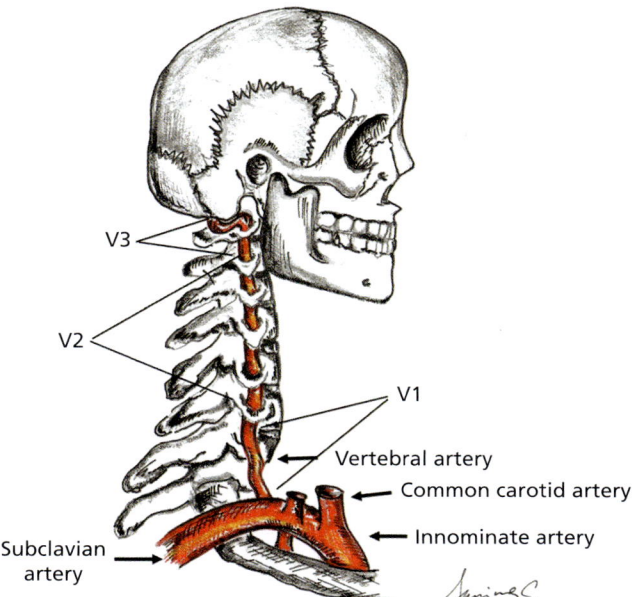

Figure 81.5 Vertebral artery segments: V1 is the most proximal segment prior to entering its bony canal at the C6 transverse process; V2 is the segment within the intraosseous canal; V3 is the extracranial segment between C2 and the base of the skull; and V4 is intracranial. Source: Image courtesy of Dr. Christina Sanina.

dissections consisting of an *in situ* interposition graft of extracranial–intracranial bypass is indicated only for those patients with persistent symptoms refractory to maximal medical therapy who are not candidates for endovascular treatment.

Interactive multiple choice questions are available for this chapter on www.wiley.com/go/dangas/cardiology

References

1 Jst Y. Upper extremity occlusive disease. In Greenfield LJ, Mulholland M, Oldham KT, Zelenock GB, Lillemoe KD (eds) *Greenfield's Surgery: Scientific Principles and Practice*, 3rd edn. Philadelphia, PA: Lippincott Williams & Wilkins; 2001: 1684–1691.

2 Olin JW, Froehlich J, Gu X, *et al.* The United States Registry for Fibromuscular Dysplasia: results in the first 447 patients. *Circulation* 2012; **125**(25): 3182–3190. PubMed PMID: 22615343.

3 Greenfield LJ, Rajagopalan S, Olin JW. Upper extremity arterial disease. *Cardiol Clin* 2002; **20**(4): 623–631. PubMed PMID: 12472048.

4 Maksimowicz-McKinnon K, Clark TM, Hoffman GS. Takayasu arteritis and giant cell arteritis: a spectrum within the same disease? *Medicine (Baltimore)*. 2009; **88**(4): 221–226. PubMed PMID: 19593227.

5 Arend WP, Michel BA, Bloch DA, *et al.* The American College of Rheumatology 1990 criteria for the classification of Takayasu arteritis. *Arthritis Rheuma* 1990; **33**(8): 1129–1134. PubMed PMID: 1975175.

6 Numano F (ed.) *Takayasu's Arteritis.* New York: Marcel Dekker; 2002.

7 Moriwaki R, Noda M, Yajima M, Sharma BK, Numano F. Clinical manifestations of Takayasu arteritis in India and Japan: new classification of angiographic findings. *Angiology* 1997; **48**(5): 369–379. PubMed PMID: 9158381.

8 Kerr GS, Hallahan CW, Giordano J, et al. Takayasu arteritis. *Ann Intern Med* 1994; **120**(11): 919–929. PubMed PMID: 7909656.

9 Noris M, Daina E, Gamba S, Bonazzola S, Remuzzi G. Interleukin-6 and RANTES in Takayasu arteritis: a guide for therapeutic decisions? *Circulation* 1999; **100**(1): 55–60. PubMed PMID: 10393681.

10 Cid MC, Merkel PA. Giant cell arteritis. In: Creager MA, Beckman JA, Loscalzo J, (eds). *Vascular Medicine.* Philadelphia: Elsevier; 2013: 525–532.

11 Ouriel K. Noninvasive diagnosis of upper extremity vascular disease. *Semin Vasc Surg* 1998; **11**(2): 54–59. PubMed PMID: 9671234.

12 Hoffman GS, Leavitt RY, Kerr GS, Rottem M, Sneller MC, Fauci AS. Treatment of glucocorticoid-resistant or relapsing Takayasu arteritis with methotrexate. *Arthritis Rheum* 1994; **37**(4): 578–582. PubMed PMID: 7908520.

13 Daina E, Schieppati A, Remuzzi G. Mycophenolate mofetil for the treatment of Takayasu arteritis: report of three cases. *Ann Intern Med* 1999; **130**(5): 422–426. PubMed PMID: 10068416.

14 Machleder HI. Evaluation of a new treatment strategy for Paget–Schroetter syndrome: spontaneous thrombosis of the axillary–subclavian vein. *J Vasc Surg* 1993; **17**(2): 305–315; discussion 16–7. PubMed PMID: 8433426.

15 Brooke BS, Freischlag JA. Contemporary management of thoracic outlet syndrome. *Curr Opin Cardiol* 2010; **25**(6): 535–540. PubMed PMID: 20838336.

16 Molina JE, Hunter DW, Dietz CA. Paget–Schroetter syndrome treated with thrombolytics and immediate surgery. *J Vasc Surg* 2007; **45**(2): 328–334. PubMed PMID: 17264012.

17 Bamford J, Sandercock P, Dennis M, Burn J, Warlow C. Classification and natural history of clinically identifiable subtypes of cerebral infarction. *Lancet* 1991; **337**(8756): 1521–1526. PubMed PMID: 1675378.

18 Wityk RJ, Chang HM, Rosengart A, *et al.* Proximal extracranial vertebral artery disease in the New England Medical Center Posterior Circulation Registry. *Arch Neurol* 1998; **55**(4): 470–478. PubMed PMID: 9561974.

19 Weber W, Mayer TE, Henkes H, *et al.* Efficacy of stent angioplasty for symptomatic stenoses of the proximal vertebral artery. *Eur J Radiol* 2005; **56**(2): 240–247. PubMed PMID: 15961267.

20 Alexander W. The treatment of epilepsy by ligature of the vertibral artery. *Brain* 1942; **5**: 170–180.

21 Levy EI, Horowitz MB, Koebbe CJ, *et al.* Transluminal stent-assisted angiplasty of the intracranial vertebrobasilar system for medically refractory, posterior circulation ischemia: early results. *Neurosurgery* 2001; **48**(6): 1215–1221; discussion 1221–1223. PubMed PMID: 11383722.

22 Ausman JI, Diaz FG, Sadasivan B, Dujovny M. Intracranial vertebral endarterectomy. *Neurosurgery* 1990; **26**(3): 465–471. PubMed PMID: 2320215.

23 Chimowitz MI, Kokkinos J, Strong J, *et al.* The warfarin-aspirin symptomatic intracranial disease study. *Neurology* 1995; **45**(8): 1488–1493. PubMed PMID: 7644046.

24 Fields WS, North RR, Hass WK, *et al.* Joint study of extracranial arterial occlusion as a cause of stroke. I. Organization of study and survey of patient population. *JAMA* 1968; **203**(11): 955–960. PubMed PMID: 5694317.

25 Hass WK, Easton JD, Adams HP Jr, *et al.* A randomized trial comparing ticlopidine hydrochloride with aspirin for the prevention of stroke in high-risk patients. Ticlopidine Aspirin Stroke Study Group. *N Engl J Med* 1989; **321**(8): 501–507. PubMed PMID: 2761587.

26 Gent M, Blakely JA, Easton JD, *et al.* The Canadian American Ticlopidine Study (CATS) in thromboembolic stroke. *Lancet* 1989; **1**(8649): 1215–1220. PubMed PMID: 2566778.

27 Smith RBI. The surgical treatment of peripheral vascular disease. In: Hurst JW, Schlant RC, Rackley CZ, Sonnenblick EH, Wenger NK (eds.) *The Heart*, 7th edn. New York: McGraw-Hill; 1992: 2235–2236.

28 Berguer R. Long-term results of vertebral artery reconstruction In: Yao JST, Pearce WH (eds.) *Long-term Results in Vascular Surgery.* Norwalk, CT: Appleton and Lange; 1993: 69.

29 Imparato AM. Vertebral arterial reconstruction: a nineteen-year experience. *J Vasc Surg* 1985; **2**(4): 626–634. PubMed PMID: 4009848.

30 Sundt TM Jr, Smith HC, Campbell JK, Vlietstra RE, Cucchiara RF, Stanson AW. Transluminal angioplasty for basilar artery stenosis. *Mayo Clinic Proc* 1980; **55**(11): 673–680. PubMed PMID: 7442321.

CHAPTER 82

Antithrombotic Strategies in Endovascular Interventions: Current Status and Future Directions

Mehdi H. Shishehbor
Heart & Vascular Institute, Cleveland Clinic, Cleveland, OH, USA

Peripheral artery disease (PAD) affects the cerebral circulation and extracranial vessels, the aorta, great vessels, mesenteric and renal arteries, and the lower extremities. In recent years the number of endovascular procedures to treat this condition have significantly increased; however, despite this, little level 1 evidence is available regarding the role of antithrombotic therapy in patients undergoing these endovascular procedures. The current practice in this regard is heterogeneous and has been mainly driven by data from coronary artery disease and percutaneous coronary intervention (PCI). This chapter discusses the role of antithrombotic agents for endovascular intervention.

Pathophysiology

Thrombosis has a significant role in morbidity and mortality associated with cardiovascular, cerebrovascular, and peripheral artery disease. In addition to inflammation and atherosclerosis, hemostatic factors also have a role in the pathogenesis of PAD. For example, plasma fibrinogen and cross-linked fibrin degradation products have been shown to be elevated in patients with claudication compared to controls [1–4]. Furthermore, individuals with PAD have elevated levels of thrombin–antithrombin III complex, D-dimer, von Willebrand factor (vWF), tissue plasminogen activator antigen, plasminogen activator inhibitor-1 levels, C-reactive protein, and prothrombin fragments 1 and 2 [1–4]. It has been suggested that these hemostatic factors are associated with PAD, its progression, and clinical events such as restenosis.

Endovascular intervention has been shown to activate platelets and the inflammatory cascade, possibly resulting in thrombosis and restenosis. Thrombin has been linked to restenosis by activation of thrombin receptors on the smooth muscle cells, macrophages, fibroblasts, and endothelial cells [5–9]. For example, among patients with severe in-stent restenosis, thrombelastometry-derived value coagulation time was significantly shorter than that of patients without restenosis [10]. Furthermore, high levels of plasma heparin factor II, an inhibitor of thrombin action, has been associated with reduced incidence of in-stent restenosis [11].

Platelets are important mediators of atherosclerosis and thrombosis [12]. During endovascular intervention platelets are activated and exposured to collagen and vWF [13]. Through activation of

integrin receptors an array of inflammatory and prothrombotic mediators such as ADP, thromboxane A_2 (TxA_2), and thrombin are released [13], which will then result in further platelet activation [14]. Ultimately, rapid recruitment and activation of platelets leads to thrombus formation manifesting as stoke, acute limb ischemia, restenosis, and graft failure.

Aspirin

Aspirin is an irreversible inhibitor of prostaglandin H-synthase, which inhibits the actions of thromboxane [15]. It is a cyclo-oxygenase 1 (COX-1) selective inhibitor resulting in impaired synthesis of TxA_2. The role of aspirin in cardiovascular disease has been well established; however, controversy exists as to whether aspirin could have a net clinical benefit in patients with peripheral vascular disease. A recent meta-analysis of 18 trials with 5269 patients with PAD revealed a reduction in cardiovascular events (adjusted hazard ratio 0.88, 95% CI 0.76–1.04); however, this was not statistically significant [16]. Importantly, no significant reduction in all-cause or cardiovascular mortality was identified [16]. The current American College of Cardiology/American Heart Association (ACC/AHA) guidelines have give a class I indication for the use of aspirin in patients with PAD [17]. Limited data are available on the impact of aspirin post-endovascular intervention; however, the combination of aspirin and dipyridamole has been shown to reduce recurrent obstruction after endovascular angioplasty for up to 12 months [18–20]. Importantly, high dose aspirin had no advantage over low dose therapy in these trials and was associated with significant gastrointestinal symptoms [18–20].

While the current guidelines continue to support the use of aspirin for prevention of cardiovascular endpoints in patients with PAD, few studies have shown benefit with low dose aspirin and the combination of aspirin and dipyridamole has failed to show a significant reduction in reocclusion after lower extremity percutaneous transluminal angioplasty (PTA) [18–20]. Early epidemiologic studies such as the Physicians' Health Study revealed a significant reduction in the rate of lower extremity revascularization with the use of low dose aspirin in men [21]. However, in the current era of stents and other advanced therapies there is no level 1 evidence that chronic aspirin therapy results in better patency, lower rates of

Interventional Cardiology: Principles and Practice, Second Edition. Edited by George D. Dangas, Carlo Di Mario, and Nicholas N. Kipshidze.
© 2017 John Wiley & Sons, Ltd. Published 2017 by John Wiley & Sons, Ltd.

in-stent restenosis, or better limb-associated outcomes. However, it is likely that aspirin has cardiovascular advantages in patients with PAD.

Ticlopidine

A first generation ADP receptor antagonist, ticlopidine is no longer available in the USA. This ADP receptor antagonist inhibitor is of P2Y$_{12}$ subtype. The two main drugs in this class are ticlopidine and clopidogrel. Early data in patients undergoing PCI showed encouraging results with ticlopidine; however, the Clopidogrel ASpirin Stent International Cooperative Study (CLASSIC) trial compared ticlopidine with clopidogrel and showed much better safety and efficacy profiles with clopidogrel [22].

There are no data from randomized trials with ticlopidine in patients undergoing endovascular intervention. However, ticlopidine has been shown to be superior to aspirin for maintaining vein graft patency [23] but the combination of aspirin plus ticlopidine was not shown to be superior to aspirin alone in maintaining graft patency in the CASPAR trial [24].

Clopidogrel

An ADP receptor antagonist, clopidogrel has the most clinical data for prevention of thrombosis after aspirin. There is a significant body of evidence supporting the use of clopidogrel in patients undergoing PCI and in those presenting with acute coronary syndrome [25–28]. However, the data for the use of clopidogrel in patients with PAD to prevent cardiovascular endpoint remain controversial. The first signal showing potential benefit with clopidogrel in patients with PAD was derived from the Clopidogrel versus Aspirin in Patients at Risk of Ischemic Events (CAPRIE) study (Figure 82.1) [29,30]. In this study, an 8.7% relative risk reduction was seen with clopidogrel compared to aspirin alone and the benefit was mostly seen in those with symptomatic PAD (Figure 82.2). Unfortunately, the Clopidogrel and Aspirin in the Management of Peripheral Endovascular Revascularization (CAMPER) trial was withdrawn because of lack of enrollment. Another trial that evaluated the role of clopidogrel for primary and secondary prevention was Clopidogrel for High Atherothrombotic Risk and Ischemic

Stabilization Management and Avoidance (CHARISMA) trial [31]. A total of 15,063 patients were randomized to clopidogrel plus aspirin or aspirin alone. In the overall population, dual antiplatelet therapy was not superior to aspirin alone for preventing cardiovascular death, stroke, and myocardial infarction (MI) [31]. However, in a subgroup analysis, in those with established cardiovascular disease, dual antiplatelet therapy resulted in a 12.5% significant relative risk reduction. Importantly, dual antiplatelet therapy was associated with a higher risk of bleeding compared to aspirin alone (Table 82.1). Despite the overwhelming data in support of dual antiplatelet therapy for acute coronary syndrome and PCI, currently there are few data to support its use for endovascular intervention. The current ACC/AHA guidelines recommend clopidogrel as monotherapy for those individuals who cannot tolerate aspirin; however, dual antiplatelet therapy is not recommended [17].

Despite these recommendations there are variable treatment approaches for patients undergoing endovascular intervention. A recent survey revealed variable treatment duration and a mix of approaches [32]. Most operators treat patients with dual antiplatelet after most endovascular interventions; however, the duration of dual antiplatelet therapy is variable [32].

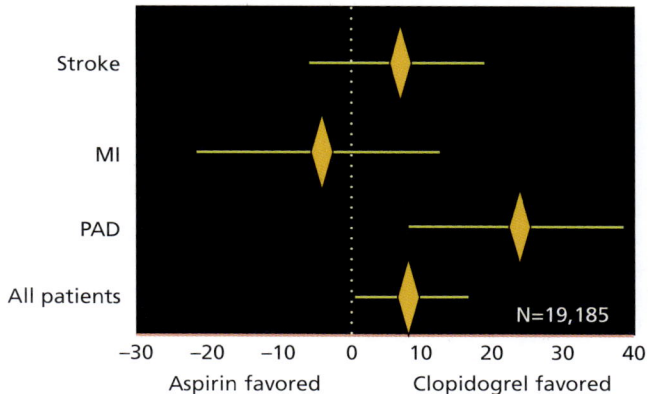

Figure 82.2 Subgroup analysis of CAPRIE trial showing a significant benefit in patients with peripheral artery disease. Source: CAPRIE Steering Committee 1996 [30]. Copyright 1996 Elsevier.

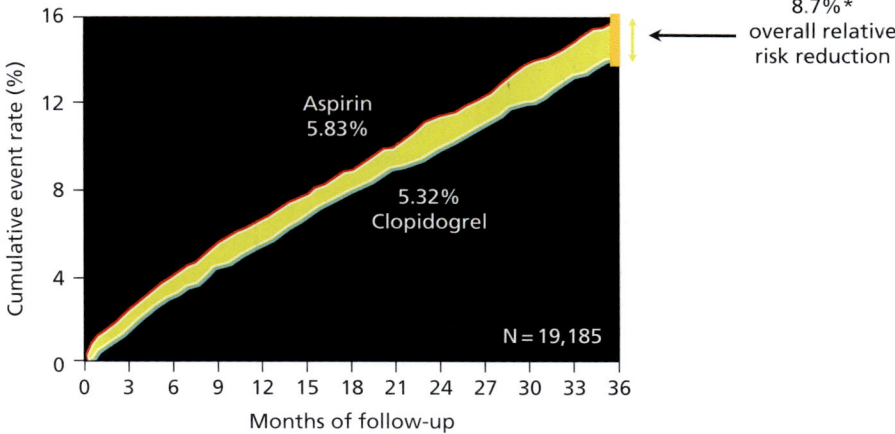

Figure 82.1 Efficacy of clopidogrel versus aspirin in reducing MI, ischemic stroke, or vascular death in the CAPRIE trial. Source: CAPRIE Steering Committee 1996 [30]. Copyright 1996 Elsevier.

Table 82.1 Risk of bleeding among the two treatment arms in the CHARISMA trial.

	Clopidogrel + ASA	Placebo + ASA	RR (95% CI)
Safety outcome adjudicated by ITT analysis	(n = 7802)	(n = 7801)	
GUSTO severe bleeding	130 (1.7%)	104 (1.3%)	1.25 (0.97–1.61)
Fatal bleed	26 (0.3%)	17 (0.2%)	1.53 (0.83–2.82)
Intracranial hemorrhage	26 (0.3%)	27 (0.3%)	0.96 (0.56–1.65)
GUSTO moderate bleeding	164 (2.1%)	101 (1.3%)	1.62 (1.27–2.08)

ASA, aspirin; CI, confidence interval; ITT, intention to treat; RR, relative rate.
Source: Data from Bhatt DL, *et al.* 2006 [31].

Other ADP receptor antagonists

Newer antiplatelet therapies have recently been developed to address some of the limitations of clopidogrel: platelet resistance, longer onset of action, and modest degree of platelet inhibition [12]. Of these, ticagrelor and prasugrel have received US Food and Drug Administration (FDA) approval for PCI. Ticagrelor is a cyclopentyl triazolopyrimidine that directly and reversibly inhibits the $P2Y_{12}$ receptor. Prasugrel is a prodrug whose active metabolites irreversibly bind to $P2Y_{12}$ receptors. However, few data are available for their use in patients with PAD or in those undergoing endovascular intervention. The EUCLID trial will examine the role of ticagrelor versus clopidogrel monotherapy for patients with PAD. This trial allows enrollment of patients who are 30 days post-endovascular or surgical revascularization; therefore, data from this trial should help guide antiplatelet therapy for patients with PAD with or without revascularization. The trial has reached full enrollment and the results are anticipated to be released in 2016.

Dipyridamole

Dipyridamole is an inhibitor of the cAMP phosphodiesterase and cyclic GMP phosphodiesterase type V enzyme. It is also a potent inhibitor of adenosine deaminase resulting in increased concentrations of adenosine. In a recent Cochrane meta-analysis of six randomized trials with a total of 356 patients, the combination therapy failed to prevent 6 month reocclusion (fixed effect odds ratio 0.69, 95% CI 0.44–1.10; p = 0.12) [33].

Vorapaxar

Vorapaxar is a novel antiplatelet agent that selectively inhibits the cellular action of thrombin through antagonism of PAR-1. It has been evaluated for use for secondary prevention in patients with prior history of MI, ischemic stroke, or PAD; however, after 2 years those with ischemic stroke were excluded because of increased risk of intracranial hemorrhage. The study showed some benefit for the composite endpoint of cardiovascular death, MI, stroke, or recurrent ischemia leading to revascularization; however, this was associated with increased risk of bleeding. A subgroup analysis of 3787 patients with PAD did show a reduction in acute limb ischemia and peripheral revascularization; however, no difference in cardiovascular death, MI, or stroke was observed [34]. Given the limited data with this agent, its use is currently limited in the USA.

Low molecular weight heparins

Peri-interventional treatment with low molecular weight heparin (LMWH) has been shown to be superior to unfractionated heparin in femoropopliteal obstructions [35]. However, long-term therapy (for 3 months) with dalteparin failed to reduce femoropopliteal occlusions after PTA [36]. LMWH is used as a bridge in those requiring endovascular procedures but also have a strong indication for anticoagulation.

Glycoprotein IIb/IIIa receptor antagonists

Glycoprotein IIb/IIIa receptor antagonists prevent binding of fibrinogen to the platelet and hence prevent fibrinogen cross-linking. A significant body of literature for their use in the setting of PCI is available; however, over time their use has declined significantly. They have a very limited role during endovascular intervention and are rarely used.

Three clinical trials compared the rates of patency for abciximab with placebo and one trial compared abciximab plus urokinase with urokinase alone [37–40]. The results from these trials were mixed. Duda *et al.* [40] showed no significant advantage with abciximab at 24 hours and 3 months; however, another trial found better patency at 24 hours and 3 months [39]. Overall, there appeared to be higher rates of bleeding with abciximab. Because of limited efficacy, potential cost, and risk of bleeding, abciximab is rarely used as an adjunct to endovascular procedures.

Vitamin K antagonist

Vitamin K antagonist (VKA) has been compared with aspirin plus dipyridamole for better patency. A pooled comparison of two trials showed no benefit with VKA at 1, 3, 6, and 12 months [41,42]. Tan *et al.* [43] conducted a randomized trial comparing clopidogrel plus aspirin with LMWK and coumadin. No statistically significant differences were noted between the two groups at 1, 6, and 12 months for patency. As expected, those treated with LMWH followed by warfarin had higher bleeding complications [43]. The combination of VKA and suloctidil also was not superior to VKA alone [44]. Similarly, VKA was compared with ticlopidine in 197 patients. VKA was not superior to ticlopidine in preventing primary occlusion; however, it was associated with more side effects. Overall, the use of VKA is reserved for select patients with clinical events and hypercoagulable state and in those with recurrent lower extremity graft occlusion.

Cilostazol

Cilostazol is a phosphodiesterase inhibitor with therapeutic focus on cAMP. It is a potent inhibitor of platelet aggregation and is a direct arterial vasodilator. It is the only approved pharmacologic therapy to increase walking distance in patients with claudication. There is also some evidence to support its use for prevention of restenosis in patients undergoing coronary stenting; however, data for use in the lower extremities are less conviencing [45–47]. Iida *et al.* [48] conducted a randomized clinical trial of 127 patients with de novo femoropopliteal lesions in which cilostazol plus aspirin showed a high rate of patency at 12, 24, and 36 months compared with ticlopidine plus aspirin. Similarly, in a retrospective analysis, cilostazol therapy showed better primary patency rates than the ticlopidine group [49].

Bivalirudin

Bilalirudin is a thrombin-specific anticoagulant mainly used to treat patients with heparin-induced thrombocytopenia (HIT) and in those undergoing PCI and has been considered for selective endovascular procedures [50]. It can be associated with fewer bleeding and vascular complications than heparin; however, no level 1 data in this regard are available. In a small registry from four institutions no adverse events were reported, with 100% procedural success rate. Bivalirudin has also been evaluated in the setting of endovascular abdominal aneurysm repair (EVAR). Overall, bivalirudin was found to be a safe and feasible alternative to unfractionated heparin in patients undergoing EVAR [51]. In retrospective studies bivalirudin has also been shown to be safe and effective compared to heparin alone in patients undergoing carotid artery stenting [52]. A number of other smaller registries and single-center studies have evaluated the role of bivalirudin in different endovascular settings. These reports have been presented at various national and international meetings but they have yet to be published in peer reviewed journals. However, given the cost and lack of level 1 evidence for better safety and efficacy compared with unfractionated heparin, its use has been limited to select centers and in those with allergic reaction to heparin (HIT).

Conclusions

Despite technical advances and increasing rates of endovascular procedures, limited level 1 evidence is available with regards to antithrombotic therapy in this setting. Most operators use some form of anticoagulation during the procedure and continue antiplatelet therapy thereafter; however, little evidence exists to support this approach. Luckily, the field of antiplatelet and anticoagulant therapies is evolving rapidly with newer agents such as vorapaxar, novel antiplatelet drugs like ticagrelor and prasugrel, and antithrombotic agents like rivaroxaban, eliquis, and dabigatran. In the future, specific therapies for patients with PAD and critical limb ischemia should become available.

🔲 ***Interactive multiple choice questions are available for this chapter on www.wiley. com/go/dangas/cardiology***

References

1 Lassila R, Peltonen S, Lepantalo M, Saarinen O, Kauhanen P, Manninen V. Severity of peripheral atherosclerosis is associated with fibrinogen and degradation of cross-linked fibrin. *Arterioscler Thromb* 1993; **13**(12): 1738–1742.

2 Lee AJ, Fowkes FG, Rattray A, Rumley A, Lowe GD. Haemostatic and rheological factors in intermittent claudication: the influence of smoking and extent of arterial disease. *Br J Haematol* 1996; **92**(1): 226–230.

3 Lowe GD, Fowkes FG, Dawes J, Donnan PT, Lennie SE, Housley E. Blood viscosity, fibrinogen, and activation of coagulation and leukocytes in peripheral arterial disease and the normal population in the Edinburgh Artery Study. *Circulation* 1993; **87**(6): 1915–1920.

4 Smith FB, Lowe GD, Fowkes FG, *et al.* Smoking, haemostatic factors and lipid peroxides in a population case control study of peripheral arterial disease. *Atherosclerosis* 1993; **102**(2): 155–162.

5 Aihara K, Azuma H, Akaike M, *et al.* Heparin cofactor II is an independent protective factor against peripheral arterial disease in elderly subjects with cardiovascular risk factors. *J Atheroscler Thromb* 2009; **16**(2): 127–134.

6 Hasenstab D, Lea H, Hart CE, Lok S, Clowes AW. Tissue factor overexpression in rat arterial neointima models thrombosis and progression of advanced atherosclerosis. *Circulation* 2000; **101**(22): 2651–2657.

7 Hering J, Amann B, Angelkort B, Rottmann M. Thrombin–antithrombin complex and the prothrombin fragment in arterial and venous blood of patients with peripheral arterial disease. *Vasa* 2003; **32**(4): 193–197.

8 Patterson C, Stouffer GA, Madamanchi N, Runge MS. New tricks for old dogs: nonthrombotic effects of thrombin in vessel wall biology. *Circ Res* 2001; **88**(10): 987–997.

9 Wilensky RL, Pyles JM, Fineberg N. Increased thrombin activity correlates with increased ischemic event rate after percutaneous transluminal coronary angioplasty: lack of efficacy of locally delivered urokinase. *Am Heart J* 1999; **138**(2 Pt 1): 319–325.

10 Cvirn G, Hoerl G, Schlagenhauf A, *et al.* Stent implantation in the superficial femoral artery: short thrombelastometry-derived coagulation times identify patients with late in-stent restenosis. *Thromb Res* 2012; **130**(3): 485–490.

11 Takamori N, Azuma H, Kato M, *et al.* High plasma heparin cofactor II activity is associated with reduced incidence of in-stent restenosis after percutaneous coronary intervention. *Circulation* 2004; **109**(4): 481–486.

12 Meadows TA, Bhatt DL. Clinical aspects of platelet inhibitors and thrombus formation. *Circ Res* 2007; **100**(9): 1261–1275.

13 Ruggeri ZM. Platelets in atherothrombosis. *Nat Med* 2002; **8**(11): 1227–1234.

14 Offermanns S. Activation of platelet function through G protein-coupled receptors. *Circ Res* 2006; **99**(12): 1293–1304.

15 Weiss HJ, Aledort LM. Impaired platelet-connective-tissue reaction in man after aspirin ingestion. *Lancet* 1967; **2**(7514): 495–497.

16 Berger JS, Krantz MJ, Kittelson JM, Hiatt WR. Aspirin for the prevention of cardiovascular events in patients with peripheral artery disease: a meta-analysis of randomized trials. *JAMA* 2009; **301**(18): 1909–1919.

17 Hirsch AT, Haskal ZJ, Hertzer NR, *et al.* ACC/AHA 2005 Practice Guidelines for the management of patients with peripheral arterial disease (lower extremity, renal, mesenteric, and abdominal aortic): a collaborative report from the American Association for Vascular Surgery/Society for Vascular Surgery, Society for Cardiovascular Angiography and Interventions, Society for Vascular Medicine and Biology, Society of Interventional Radiology, and the ACC/AHA Task Force on Practice Guidelines (Writing Committee to Develop Guidelines for the Management of Patients With Peripheral Arterial Disease): endorsed by the American Association of Cardiovascular and Pulmonary Rehabilitation; National Heart, Lung, and Blood Institute; Society for Vascular Nursing; TransAtlantic Inter-Society Consensus; and Vascular Disease Foundation. *Circulation* 2006; **113**(11): e463–654.

18 Weichert W, Meents H, Abt K, *et al.* Acetylsalicylic acid–reocclusion–prophylaxis after angioplasty (ARPA-study). A randomized double-blind trial of two different dosages of ASA in patients with peripheral occlusive arterial disease. *Vasa* 1994; **23**(1): 57–65.

19 Minar E, Ahmadi A, Koppensteiner R, *et al.* Comparison of effects of high-dose and low-dose aspirin on restenosis after femoropopliteal percutaneous transluminal angioplasty. *Circulation* 1995; **91**(8): 2167–2173.

20 Ranke C, Creutzig A, Luska G, *et al.* Controlled trial of high- versus low-dose aspirin treatment after percutaneous transluminal angioplasty in patients with peripheral vascular disease. *Clin Investig* 1994; **72**(9): 673–680.

21 Goldhaber SZ, Manson JE, Stampfer MJ, *et al.* Low-dose aspirin and subsequent peripheral arterial surgery in the Physicians' Health Study. *Lancet* 1992; **340**(8812): 143–145.

22 Theroux P, Ouimet H, McCans J, *et al.* Aspirin, heparin, or both to treat acute unstable angina. *N Engl J Med* 1988; **319**(17): 1105–1111.

23 Becquemin JP. Effect of ticlopidine on the long-term patency of saphenous-vein bypass grafts in the legs. Etude de la Ticlopidine apres Pontage Femoro-Poplite and the Association Universitaire de Recherche en Chirurgie. *N Engl J Med* 1997; **337**(24): 1726–1731.

24 Belch JJ, Dormandy J, Biasi GM, *et al.* Results of the randomized, placebo-controlled clopidogrel and acetylsalicylic acid in bypass surgery for peripheral arterial disease (CASPAR) trial. *J Vasc Surg* 2010; **52**(4): 825–833.

25 Thompson PD, Zimet R, Forbes WP, Zhang P. Meta-analysis of results from eight randomized, placebo-controlled trials on the effect of cilostazol on patients with intermittent claudication. *Am J Cardiol* 2002; **90**(12): 1314–1319.

26 Randomised trial of intravenous streptokinase, oral aspirin, both, or neither among 17,187 cases of suspected acute myocardial infarction: ISIS-2. ISIS-2 (Second International Study of Infarct Survival) Collaborative Group. *Lancet* 1988; **2**(8607): 349–360.

27 Baigent C, Collins R, Appleby P, Parish S, Sleight P, Peto R. ISIS-2: 10 year survival among patients with suspected acute myocardial infarction in randomised comparison of intravenous streptokinase, oral aspirin, both, or neither. The ISIS-2 (Second International Study of Infarct Survival) Collaborative Group. *BMJ* 1998; **316**(7141): 1337–1343.

28 Roux S, Christeller S, Ludin E. Effects of aspirin on coronary reocclusion and recurrent ischemia after thrombolysis: a meta-analysis. *J Am Coll Cardiol* 1992; **19**(3): 671–677.

29 Collaborative overview of randomised trials of antiplatelet therapy. I: Prevention of death, myocardial infarction, and stroke by prolonged antiplatelet therapy in various categories of patients. Antiplatelet Trialists' Collaboration. *BMJ* 1994; **308**(6921): 81–106.

30 CAPRIE Steering Committee. A randomised, blinded, trial of clopidogrel versus aspirin in patients at risk of ischaemic events (CAPRIE). *Lancet* 1996; **348**(9038): 1329–1339.

31 Bhatt DL, Fox KA, Hacke W, *et al.* Clopidogrel and aspirin versus aspirin alone for the prevention of atherothrombotic events. *N Engl J Med* 2006; **354**(16): 1706–1717.

32 Allemang MT, Rajani RR, Nelson PR, Hingorani A, Kashyap VS. Prescribing patterns of antiplatelet agents are highly variable after lower extremity endovascular procedures. *Ann Vasc Surg* 2013; **27**(1): 62–67.

33 Robertson L, Ghouri MA, Kovacs F. Antiplatelet and anticoagulant drugs for prevention of restenosis/reocclusion following peripheral endovascular treatment. *Cochrane Database Syst Rev* 2012; **8**: CD002071.

34 Bonaca MP, Creager MA. Pharmacological treatment and current management of peripheral artery disease. *Circ Res* 2015; **116**(9): 1579–1598.

35 Schweizer J, Muller A, Forkmann L, Hellner G, Kirch W. Potential use of a low-molecular-weight heparin to prevent restenosis in patients with extensive wall damage following peripheral angioplasty. *Angiology* 2001; **52**(10): 659–669.

36 Koppensteiner R, Spring S, Amann-Vesti BR, *et al.* Low-molecular-weight heparin for prevention of restenosis after femoropopliteal percutaneous transluminal angioplasty: a randomized controlled trial. *J Vasc Surg* 2006; **44**(6): 1247–1253.

37 Ansel GM, Silver MJ, Botti CF Jr, *et al.* Functional and clinical outcomes of nitinol stenting with and without abciximab for complex superficial femoral artery disease: a randomized trial. *Catheter Cardiovasc Interv* 2006; **67**(2): 288–297.

38 Baumgartner DA Jr. A time to say no. *Ohio Med* 1988; **84**(10): 783–784.

39 Dorffler-Melly J, Mahler F, Do DD, Triller J, Baumgartner I. Adjunctive abciximab improves patency and functional outcome in endovascular treatment of femoropopliteal occlusions: initial experience. *Radiology* 2005; **237**(3): 1103–1109.

40 Duda SH, Tepe G, Luz O, *et al.* Peripheral artery occlusion: treatment with abciximab plus urokinase versus with urokinase alone: a randomized pilot trial (the PROMPT Study). Platelet Receptor Antibodies in Order to Manage Peripheral Artery Thrombosis. *Radiology* 2001; **221**(3): 689–696.

41 Do DD, Mahler F. Low-dose aspirin combined with dipyridamole versus anticoagulants after femoropopliteal percutaneous transluminal angioplasty. *Radiology* 1994; **193**(2): 567–571.

42 Pilger E, Lammer J, Bertuch H, *et al.* Nd:YAG laser with sapphire tip combined with balloon angioplasty in peripheral arterial occlusions: long-term results. *Circulation* 1991; **83**(1): 141–147.

43 Tan JY, Shi WH, He J, Zhu L, Wang TP, Yu B. [A clinical trial of using antiplatelet therapy to prevent restenosis following peripheral artery angioplasty and stenting]. *Zhonghua Yi Xue Za Zhi* 2008; **88**(12): 812–815.

44 Mahler F, Schneider E, Gallino A, Bollinger A. Combination of suloctidil and anticoagulation in the prevention of reocclusion after femoro-popliteal PTA. *Vasa* 1987; **16**(4): 381–385.

45 Ge J, Han Y, Jiang H, *et al.* RACTS: a prospective randomized antiplatelet trial of cilostazol versus ticlopidine in patients undergoing coronary stenting: long-term clinical and angiographic outcome. *J Cardiovasc Pharmacol* 2005; **46**(2): 162–166.

46 Kozuma K, Hara K, Yamasaki M, *et al.* Effects of cilostazol on late lumen loss and repeat revascularization after Palmaz–Schatz coronary stent implantation. *Am Heart J* 2001; **141**(1): 124–130.

47 Park SW, Lee CW, Kim HS, *et al.* Effects of cilostazol on angiographic restenosis after coronary stent placement. *Am J Cardiol* 2000; **86**(5): 499–503.

48 Iida O, Nanto S, Uematsu M, Morozumi T, Kitakaze M, Nagata S. Cilostazol reduces restenosis after endovascular therapy in patients with femoropopliteal lesions. *J Vasc Surg* 2008; **48**(1): 144–149.

49 Ikushima I, Yonenaga K, Iwakiri H, Nagoshi H, Kumagai H, Yamashita Y. A better effect of cilostazol for reducing in-stent restenosis after femoropopliteal artery stent placement in comparison with ticlopidine. *Med Devices (Auckl)* 2011; **4**: 83–89.

50 Bittl JA, Chaitman BR, Feit F, Kimball W, Topol EJ. Bivalirudin versus heparin during coronary angioplasty for unstable or postinfarction angina: final report reanalysis of the Bivalirudin Angioplasty Study. *Am Heart J* 2001; **142**(6): 952–959.

51 Stamler S, Katzen BT, Tsoukas AI, Baum SZ, Diehm N. Clinical experience with the use of bivalirudin in a large population undergoing endovascular abdominal aortic aneurysm repair. *J Vasc Interv Radiol* 2009; **20**(1): 17–21.

52 Stabile E, Sorropago G, Tesorio T, *et al.* Heparin versus bivalirudin for carotid artery stenting using proximal endovascular clamping for neuroprotection: results from a prospective randomized study. *J Vasc Surg* 2010; **52**(6): 1505–1510.

CHAPTER 83

Chronic Venous Insufficiency

Karthik Gujja[1], Cristina Sanina[2], and Jose M. Wiley[3]

[1] The Zeta and Michael A. Weiner Cardiovascular Institute, Icahn School of Medicine at Mount Sinai, New York, NY, USA

[2] University of Miami Miller School of Medicine, Miami, FL, USA

[3] Albert Einstein College of Medicine; Montefiore Einstein Center for Heart & Vascular Care, Bronx, NY, USA

Chronic venous disease is an important source of morbidity in Western Europe and the USA. Varicose veins are a common manifestation of chronic venous insufficiency and affect approximately 25% of adults in the Western hemisphere, where prevalence varies greatly by geographic area. The reported incidence of chronic venous insufficiency varies from around 1–40% in women and around 1–17% in men. Estimates for varicose veins are higher; around 1–73% in women and 2–56% in men [1]. These reported ranges reflect differences in the population distribution of risk factors, accuracy in the application of diagnostic criteria, and the quality and availability of medical diagnostic and treatment resources. Various risk factors are responsible for these incidences: older age, pregnancy (especially multiple), family history of venous disease, female gender, obesity, and occupations that result in significant orthostasis from prolonged standing [2]. Venous insufficiency is most often associated with great saphenous vein (GSV) reflux, but can also be present in the small saphenous vein (SSV) or perforator veins.

Historically, the treatment has been surgery, with high ligation and stripping, combined with phlebectomies. Such treatment efficiently reduces symptoms, improves quality of life (QOL), and reduces the rate of reoperation. However, the operation can occasionally be associated with significant postoperative morbidity, including bleeding, groin infection, thrombophlebitis, and saphenous nerve damage. However, major complications are rare based on the current available data. Conventional surgery is expensive as it is often performed in hospital using general or regional anesthesia.

In the past decade, alternative treatments such as endovenous laser ablation (EVLA), radiofrequency ablation (RFA), and ultrasonography-guided foam sclerotherapy have gained popularity. Performed as office-based procedures using tumescent local anesthesia, the new minimally invasive techniques have been shown in numerous studies to obliterate the affected vein, eliminate reflux, and improve symptoms safely and effectively [3].

Predisposing factors

Age and gender

The prevalence of varicose veins in women is approximately twice that in men [4]. Advanced age has also been determined to be a risk factor [5]. Varicose veins have an estimated prevalence of 5–30% in the adult population, with a female to male predominance of 3 : 1, although a more recent study supports a higher male prevalence [6]. The Edinburgh Vein Study screened 1566 subjects for venous reflux and found chronic venous insufficiency (CVI) in 9.4% of men and 6.6% of women. After age adjustment, the prevalence increased with age (21.2% in men >50 years old, and 12.0% in women >50 years old) [7]. The Tampere study investigated a large cohort of 3284 men and 3590 women with varicose veins and showed a prevalence of 18% and 42%, respectively. The overall prevalence of varicose veins at ages 40, 50, and 60 years was 22%, 35%, and 41%, respectively [8].

Pregnancy

Multiparity has been shown to be a major predisposing factor for development of varicose veins and part of its increase in prevalence has been attributed to female gender. In the Tampere study, the prevalence of varicose veins in women with 0, 1, 2, 3, and 4 or more pregnancies was 32%, 38%, 43%, 48%, and 59%, respectively [8]. The exact mechanism of pregnancy-induced venous insufficiency is not fully understood. It has been attributed to both hydrostatic and hormonal effects. Pressure of the gravid uterus on the pelvic vasculature is associated with lower extremity venous hypertension, venous distention, and valve rupture. High serum estradiol levels have been shown by Ciardullo et al. [9] to increase venous distensibility and varicose vein formation in menopausal women. The saphenous veins have been shown to contain estrogen and progesterone receptors that may enable the estradiol-rich hormonal state of pregnancy to exert a similar effect.

Hereditary

A positive family history of varicose veins is associated with a significantly increased risk of development of varicose veins. A study conducted in Japan showed that 42% of women with varicose veins reported a positive family history compared with 14% without the disease [10]. Various genetic predispositions have been linked to development of varicose veins. Downregulation of the desmuslin gene affecting the smooth muscle cells in the saphenous vein wall, thrombomodulin mutation (1208/1209 TT deletion) caused by varicose vein formation via deep vein thrombosis, expression of structural genes regulating the extracellular matrix (ECM), cytoskeletal proteins, and myofibroblasts have all been shown to be

Interventional Cardiology: Principles and Practice, Second Edition. Edited by George D. Dangas, Carlo Di Mario, and Nicholas N. Kipshidze.
© 2017 John Wiley & Sons, Ltd. Published 2017 by John Wiley & Sons, Ltd.

associated with increased risk. Certain mutations have been linked to a variety of syndromes, including Klippel–Trenaunay syndrome (translocation involving chromosome 8q22.3 and 14q13; cutaneous capillary malformations, t tissues), lymphedema distichiasis syndrome (*FOXC2* mutation; extra eyelashes from meibomian glands, varicose veins, congenital heart defects, vertebral anomalies, extradural cysts, ptosis, and cleft palate), cerebral autosomal dominant arteriopathy with subcortical infarcts and leukoencephalopathy (CADASIL; heterozygous mutation, −1279G>T), Chuvash polycythemia (autosomal recessive disorder caused by homozygous mutation of the von Hippel–Lindau gene [598>T] on chromosome 3p25), and other genes have been associated with poor wound healing causing venous ulceration (*F13A1* gene: factor XIII deficiency, *HFE* gene mutation, *FGFR-2* [SNP 2451AG] mRNA instability, *MMP-12* [SNP 82AA]; functional change predisposing to ulcer) [11].

Lifestyle
Sedentary work and prolonged standing at work are independent risk factors for development of venous insufficiency [12]. In the Tampere study, the prevalence of varicose veins in standing versus sitting workers was 36% and 27%, respectively. The Edinburgh Vein Study has also shown predisposition of varicose veins in patients whose work involved prolonged standing.

Body habitus
Epidemiologic studies have shown that varicose veins are more common in female patients with increased body mass index (BMI) (especially >30 kg/m²). It has been assumed that subcutaneous deposition of adipose and fibrous tissue disrupts the cutaneous venous network, impairs drainage, and promotes stasis. The Edinburgh Vein Study supported the findings that increased BMI in women is a risk factor. Callam *et al.* [2], in his epidemiologic review series, reached similar conclusions.

Pathogenesis
Several theories have been proposed for the causal basis of CVI. There are two universally accepted theories: (i) primary valvular incompetence and (ii) primary congenital vein wall weakness.

Primary valvular incompetence is the oldest theory and was postulated by Sir William Harvey in 1628. It states that varicose veins develop as a sequela of central valvular incompetence related to paucity or atrophy of its valves. It causes venous hypertension in the vein segment below, which in turn damages adjacent peripheral valves and propagates varicose transformation in a centralto-peripheral direction. This theory conflicts with the fact that valves are strong structures capable of withstanding pressures of 200 mmHg without leakage or degenerative changes in leaflets and that varicose veins can occur below or between competent valves [13]. The primary vein wall weakness theory states that varicose veins develop from a defect in vein wall integrity rather than from a problem within the valves. The components of a normal vein wall include collagen matrix that provides strength, elastic fibers that provide compliance, and three smooth muscle layers (circular media surrounded by longitudinal intimal and adventitial layers) that control vascular tone. Histologic studies show that compared with normal veins, varicose veins show proliferation of the collagen matrix with disruption and distortion of the muscle fiber layers. In the most diseased areas, the muscle layer is completely disrupted, leaving only elastic tissue and collagen as the sole components of the vein wall. This histologic alteration in turn causes loss of

contractility, sagging of the muscular grid, and vessel dilatation in response to venous hypertension. The characteristic serpiginous appearance of varicose veins reflects segments of dilatation interspersed between segments of normal vein [14].

Various factors influence the development of CVI: venous stasis, venous hypertension, fibrin cuff, water hammer effect, and leukocyte trapping.

Venous stasis
This concept suggests that stagnant accumulation of blood in tortuous, non-functioning, dilated skin veins results in subsequent tissue anoxia and cell death leading to skin changes and ulceration. Arteriovenous fistulae in limbs with varicosities have also been attributed to low oxygen content and CVI skin changes [15].

Venous hypertension
This concept has been attributed to muscle pump dysfunction and venous ulceration. It has been hypothesized that venous hydrostatic pressure is equal in the deep and superficial venous systems both at rest and in the erect position. During calf muscle contraction, the pressure in the deep veins increases more than in the superficial veins. However, valve closure prevents the pressure from being transmitted to the superficial veins. In contrast, pump dysfunction or valvular incompetence causes venous pressure to be transmitted to the superficial veins leading to CVI symptoms and ulceration [16–19].

Fibrin cuff
Pericapillary fibrin cuff has been associated with restriction of oxygen diffusion across the vessel wall leading to edema and dermatosclerotic skin changes. Pericapillary fibrin cuffs may act as a barrier, a marker for endothelial cell damage, or as part of an overall mechanism of macromolecular leakage and trapping [20].

Water hammer effect
This theory is the most widespread pathogenesis of CVI. It contends that reflux is mainly transmitted to the superficial veins through perforators. Studies by Raju and Fredericks have shown that this effect explains and correlates with most venous ulceration cases. At rest 20–25% of patients might have normal ambulatory venous pressure; nonetheless, Valsalva-induced venous hypertension transmits pressure, resulting in skin changes and ulceration [18,21].

Leukocyte trapping
The concept of leukocyte trapping was described very early and explains most of the CVI symptoms. Because of stasis and venous pressure changes, margination of the white cells occurs resulting in capillary plugging with further tissue hypoxia and damage. These cells also activate free radicals and cytokine (interleukin-1, tumor necrosis factor) release, resulting in tissue damage and apoptosis [22]. Unifying concepts of leukocyte trapping and venous hypertension have also been proposed [16].

Clinical manifestations
CVI manifests at different stages. At first it can present as telangiectasia or reticular veins and advance to more complicated stages such as skin fibrosis and venous ulceration. The main clinical features of CVI are leg pain, leg edema, varicose veins, and cutaneous changes. Various pathogenic mechanisms produce different clinical manifestations (incompetent valves as varicose veins, venous obstruction as

leg edema, and pump dysfunction as either symptom). Varicose veins are dilated superficial veins that become progressively more tortuous and large. They are prone to develop bouts of superficial thrombophlebitis. Edema begins in the perimalleolar region but later ascends causing leg edema with dependent accumulation of fluid. The leg pain or discomfort is described as heaviness or aching after prolonged standing and is relieved by elevation of the leg. Edema produces pain by increasing intracompartmental and subcutaneous volume and pressure. Tenderness along varicose veins is in the result of venous distention. Obstruction of the deep venous system can lead to venous claudication, or intense leg cramping with ambulation. Cutaneous changes include skin hyperpigmentation with hemosiderin deposition and eczematous dermatitis. Fibrosis also develops in the dermis and subcutaneous tissue (lipodermatosclerosis).

There is an increased risk of cellulitis, leg ulceration, and delayed wound healing. Longstanding CVI can also lead to the development of lymphedema, representing a combined disease process [23]. Several tools have been described to assess the severity of CVI and also monitor the effects of therapy. The CEAP (clinical, etiology, anatomic, pathophysiology) classification was the initial module developed by an international consensus conference to provide a basis for uniformity in reporting, diagnosing, and treating CVI. The CEAP classification takes into account all the diagnostic variables of CVI. In 2004, the CEAP revised consensus refined the class definitions and improved reproducibility of physician observations (Box 83.1; Table 83.1) [24–26]. Because of limitations of the CEAP clinical classification in delineating categories, a venous severity score was developed to complement the CEAP classification. The venous clinical severity score consists of 10 attributes (pain, varicose veins, venous edema, skin pigmentation, inflammation, induration, number of ulcers, duration of ulcers, size of ulcers, and compressive therapy) with four grades (absent, mild, moderate,

---

Box 83.1 Advanced CEAP classification

Superficial veins
1 Telangiectasias/reticular veins
2 GSV above knee
3 GSV below knee
4 Lesser saphenous vein
5 Non-saphenous veins

Deep veins
6 Inferior vena cava
7 Common iliac vein
8 Internal iliac vein
9 External iliac vein
10 Pelvic: gonadal, broad ligament veins, other
11 Common femoral vein
12 Deep femoral vein
13 Femoral vein
14 Popliteal vein
15 Crural: anterior tibial, posterior tibial, peroneal veins (all paired)
16 Muscular: gastrocnemial, soleal veins, other

Perforating veins
17 Thigh
18 Calf

This classification is the same as the basic classification with the addition that any of 18 named venous segments can be used as locators for venous disorders.

Source: Eklof B, *et al.* 2004 [25]. Copyright 2004 Elsevier.

Table 83.1 CEAP classification for chronic venous disorders

Clinical classification	
C0	No visible or palpable signs of venous disease
C1	Telangiectasias, reticular veins, malleolar flares
C2	Varicose veins
C3	Edema without skin changes
C4	Skin changes attribute to venous disease (e.g., pigmentation, venous eczema, lipodermatosclerosis)
C4a	Pigmentation or eczema
C4b	Lipodermatosclerosis or atrophie blanche
C5	Skin changes as defined earlier with healed ulceration
C6	Skin changes as defined earlier with active ulceration
S	Symptomatic, including ache, pain, tightness, skin irritation, heaviness, and muscle cramps, and other complaints attributable to venous dysfunction
A	Asymptomatic
Causal classification	
Ec	Congenital
Ep	Primary
Es	Secondary (post-thrombotic)
En	No venous cause identified
Anatomic classification	
As	Superficial veins
Ap	Perforator veins
Ad	Deep veins
An	No venous location identified
Pathophysiologic classification	
Pr	Reflux
Po	Obstruction
Pr,o	Reflux and obstruction
Pn	No venous pathophysiology identifiable

Therapy can alter the clinical category of chronic venous disease. Limbs should therefore be reclassified after any form of medical or surgical treatment.
Source: Adapted from Eklof B, *et al.* 2004 [25]. Copyright 2004 Elsevier.

severe). The venous anatomic segmental score assigns a numerical value to segments of the venous system in the lower extremity that account for both reflux and obstruction (Table 83.2) [27,28].

The venous disability score comes from the ability to perform normal activities of daily living with or without compressive stockings. The venous severity score has been mainly shown to be useful in evaluating the response to treatment [29]. The REVAS classification identifies patients with recurrent varices after surgery. In conjugation with the CEAP classification, it adds valuable information in evaluating patients with chronic venous disease after surgery [30].

QOL and economic impact

The impact of venous insufficiency on QOL was investigated by the Venous Insufficiency Epidemiologic and Economical Study (VEINES), an international survey. In VEINES, 65.2% of subjects with varicose veins had additional venous disease processes (edema, skin changes, ulceration), and both physical and mental QOL scores concomitant with the severity of their venous disease [31]. In the most severe cases, those in which venous ulceration was present, the QOL rating was worse than with chronic lung disease, back pain, or arthritis [32]. The VEINES study has two components: a QOL assessment (VEINES-QOL), which

Table 83.2 Revised venous clinical severity score.

Attribute	None: 0	Mild: 1	Moderate: 2	Severe: 3
Pain or other discomfort (i.e., aching, heaviness, fatigue, soreness, burning) Presumes venous origin	N/A	Occasional pain or other discomfort (not restricting regular daily activities)	Daily pain or other discomfort (interfering with but not preventing regular daily activities)	Daily pain or discomfort (limits most regular daily activities)
Varicose veins Varicose veins must be ≥3 mm in diameter to qualify in the standing position	N/A	Few: scattered (i.e., isolated branch varicosities or clusters) Also includes corona phlebectatica (ankle flare)	Confined to calf or thigh	Involves calf and thigh
Venous edema Presumes venous origin	N/A	Limited to foot and ankle area	Extends above ankle but below knee	Extends to knee and above
Skin pigmentation Presumes venous origin Does not include focal pigmentation over varicose veins or pigmentation caused by other chronic diseases (i.e., vasculitis purpura)	None or focal	Limited to perimalleolar area	Diffuse over lower third of calf	Wider distribution above lower third of calf
Inflammation More than just recent pigmentation (i.e., erythema, cellulitis, venous eczema, dermatitis)	N/A	Limited to perimalleolar area	Diffuse over lower third of calf	Wider distribution above lower third of calf
Induration Presumes venous origin of secondary skin and subcutaneous changes (i.e., chronic edema with fibrosis, hypodermitis). Includes white atrophy and lipodermatosclerosis	N/A	Limited to perimalleolar area	Diffuse over lower third of calf	Wider distribution above lower third of calf
Active ulcer number	0	1	2	3
Active ulcer duration (longest active)	N/A	<3 months	>3 months but <1 year	Not healed for >1 year
Active ulcer size (largest active)	N/A	Diameter <2 cm	Diameter 2–6 cm	Diameter >6 cm
Use of compression therapy	Not used	Intermittent use of stockings	Wears stockings most days	Full compliance: stockings

N/A, not applicable.
Source: Vasquez MA, et al.; American Venous Forum Ad Hoc Outcomes Working Group 2010 [28]. Copyright 2010 Elsevier.

estimates disease effect; and a symptoms questionnaire, which measures symptoms prevalence (VEINES-Sym). Other assessment programs used in clinical practice to assess the impact of CVI on QOL are the Aberdeen Varicose Vein Questionnaire (AVVQ), Charing Cross Venous Ulcer Questionnaire (CXVUQ), and Specific Quality of Life and Outcomes Response–Venous (SQOR-V) questionnaire [33,34].

Diagnosis

Multiple modalities have shown benefit in diagnosing the cause of CVI. Physical examination is the most important one. A thorough physical examination is usually enough to diagnose CVI. It also provides guidance during therapy.

Physical examination

Physical examination involves inspection of the skin for signs of CVI. Skin changes such as hyperpigmentation, stasis dermatitis, atrophic blanche (white scarring at the site of previous ulcerations with a paucity of capillaries), or lipodermatosclerosis are frequently seen. Varicose veins follow the path of superficial vein insufficiency [23]. Tenderness is almost always observed along the varicose veins. Skin edema is usually pitting, unless chronic edema makes the skin brawny and difficult to examine. Venous ulcerations are most common along the medial supramalleolar area at the site of a major perforator vein of high hydrostatic pressure. The classic tourniquet or Trendelenburg test can be performed at the bedside to help distinguish between deep and superficial reflux. The test is performed with the patient lying down to empty the lower extremity veins. The upright posture is then resumed after applying a tourniquet or using manual compression at various levels. In the presence of superficial disease the varicose veins remain collapsed if compression is distal to the point of reflux. With deep (or combined) venous insufficiency, the varicose veins appear despite the use of the tourniquet or manual compression. Although useful to help determine the distribution of venous insufficiency, this test does not help to determine the extent or severity of disease or to provide information about the cause [35].

Duplex imaging

Doppler is an important tool in diagnosing CVI and monitoring therapy. The goal of duplex imaging is to identify any obstruction or reflux in the deep veins, look for any presence of deep vein thrombosis, diagnose reflux in the superficial veins (great saphenous vein, perforator vein, and small saphenous vein), and localize branch varicose veins and perforator veins. Low-frequency transducers (2–3 MHz) are usually used to evaluate the iliac veins and inferior vena cava. High-frequency transducers (5–10 MHz) are used to evaluate lower extremity veins. Reflux thresholds for deep veins are greater than 1000 ms, superficial veins greater than 500 ms, and for perforators greater than 350 ms [36,37]. The most common site for reflux is the confluence of the GSV and common femoral vein, contributing to 65% of all cases, in a review of 2036 patients [38]. However, duplex has a weak correlation with the severity of the disease. Physical examination and duplex scan can guide most therapy. Venous compressibility complemented with flow characteristics are key elements in excluding thrombosis. The use of a cuff inflation deflation method with rapid cuff deflation in the standing position is preferred to induce reflux [39].

Plethysmography

Photoplethysmography (PPG) can be used to establish a diagnosis of CVI [38]. Relative changes in blood volume in the dermis of the limb can be determined by measuring the backscatter of light emitted from a diode with a photosensor. The venous refill time is the time required for the PPG tracing to return to 90% of the baseline after cessation of calf contraction. A venous refill time less than 18–20 s, depending on the patient's position during the study, indicates CVI. A venous refill time greater than 20 s suggests normal venous filling. The use of a tourniquet or low-pressure cuff allows superficial disease to be distinguished from deep venous disease. Refill time depends on several factors, including the volume of reflux and the vessel diameter. This technique has been used to assess emptying of the venous system during calf muscle contraction and venous outflow. PPG can provide an assessment of the overall physiologic function of the venous system, but is most useful in determining the absence or presence of disease [40,41].

Air plethysmography (APG) has the ability to measure each potential component of the pathophysiologic mechanisms of CVI: reflux, obstruction, and muscle pump dysfunction. Venous outflow is assessed during rapid cuff deflation on an elevated limb that has a proximal venous occlusion cuff applied. The outflow fraction at 1 s (or venous outflow at 1 s expressed as a percentage of the total venous volume) is the primary parameter used to evaluate the adequacy of outflow. A normal venous filling index is less than 2 mL/s, whereas higher levels (>4–7 mL/s) have been found to correlate with the severity of CVI. Complications of CVI, such as ulceration, have been shown to correlate with the severity of reflux assessed with the venous filling index and ejection capacity [42,43].

Computed tomography and magnetic resonance venography

Used in identifying more rare and complex causes of CVI, computed tomography (CT) is an important tool in recognizing thromboembolic disease in the proximal veins, whereas magnetic resonance venography has a major role in determining the age of thrombus. CVI syndromes such as May–Thurner syndrome, Paget–Schroetter syndrome, nutcracker syndrome, pelvic congestion syndrome, venous malformations, and atrioventricular malformations can be diagnosed effectively with these advanced imaging techniques [44,45].

Treatment
Initial treatment: behavioral measures and compression garments

Conservative measures have been proposed to reduce symptoms caused by CVI and prevent secondary complications and progression of disease. Behavioral measures such as elevating the legs to minimize edema and reducing intra-abdominal pressure should be advocated. The use of compressive stockings is the mainstay of conservative management. The Bisgaard regimen has been proposed for the healing of venous ulcers. This regimen has four components: patient education, foot elevation, elastic compression garments, and evaluation subsequently with CEAP classification. Non-elastic ambulatory below-knee compression aggressively counters the impact of reflux from venous pump failure.

Compression therapy is used for venous leg ulcers and can decrease blood vessel diameter and pressure, preventing blood from flowing backwards [46,47]. Compression is also used to decrease release of inflammatory cytokines, reduce capillary leak, prevent swelling, and delay clotting by decreasing activation of thrombin and increasing that of plasmin. Compression is applied using elastic bandages or boots specifically designed for the purpose. It is not clear whether non-elastic systems are better than multilayer elastic ones. Patients should wear as much compression as it is comfortable. The type of dressing applied beneath the compression does not seem to matter, and hydrocolloid has not been shown to be superior to simple low-adherent dressings. The use of graded elastic compressive stockings (with 20–50 mmHg of tension) is well established in the treatment of CVI. Treatment with 30–40 mmHg compression stockings results in significant improvement in pain, swelling, skin pigmentation, activity, and overall well-being as long as a compliance of 70–80% is achieved [48]. In patients with venous ulcers, graded compression stockings and other compressive bandage modalities are effective in both healing and preventing recurrences of ulcers. With a structured regimen of compression therapy, 93% of patients with venous ulcers can achieve complete healing at a mean of 5.3 months. Compression stockings have been shown to reduce residual volume fraction, an indicator of improvement in the calf muscle pump function, and to reduce reflux in vein segments [49].

Failure of conservative therapy

Symptomatic patients who fail conservative therapy should be followed closely. These patients should have venous duplex studies and/or APG if conservative therapy fails or if there is any progression of symptoms in CEAP class. Further treatment is based on the results of non-invasive studies and specific treatment is based on severity of disease, with CEAP clinical classes 4–6 often requiring invasive treatment. Referral to a vascular specialist should be made for patients with CEAP classes 4–6 (and probably for CEAP class 3 with extensive edema). These patients with uncorrected advanced CVI are at risk for ulceration, recurrent ulceration, and non-healing venous ulcers with progression to infection and lymphedema.

Non-invasive study: venous reflux disease
Superficial venous reflux

Various therapies have been used for superficial venous reflux including cool-touch laser, RFA ablation, venous sclerotherapy, ligation, and phlebectomy.

Cool-touch laser

The first procedure to replace ligation and stripping of the GSV was radiofrequency-mediated thermal ablation. Long-term experience with cool-touch endovenous laser ablation showed that tissue water within the vein wall has a specific target chromophore of 1320-nm laser and the presence or absence of red blood cells within the vessels is unimportant. Water is the main component in the walls of a vein; they are composed mainly of water and collagen. The chromophore for the 1.32-mm or 1320-nm wavelength laser is water. This wavelength penetrates as deep as 500 mm in tissue. This provides a safety margin by reducing the risks of penetration of laser energy beyond the vein wall. For even greater control of energy distribution, the 1320-nm CTEV is coupled with an automatic pullback device that can retract the fiber at a rate of 0.5, 1, or 2 mm/s [50]. Endovenous laser treatments at 810, 940, and 980 nm are designed to produce endothelial and vein wall shrinkage by non-specific heating of the vessel [51]. This non-specific heating is accomplished by creating a superheated coagulum at the fiber tip or by the heating of hemoglobin within

red blood cells to create steam bubbles at extremely high temperatures. Without the presence of blood in the vein, such as an experimental situation in which the vein is filled with saline, laser-induced vessel wall injury is confined to the site of direct laser impact. By contrast, blood-filled veins show extensive thermal damage even in remote areas from the laser fiber, including the vein wall opposite to the laser impact. In the absence of blood, the situation is even worse; the areas of vein wall injury or burning result in intense postoperative pain and early recanalization of the treated vein. More importantly, superheating of hemoglobin leads to high temperatures (often higher than 1200 °C), which results in vein perforations, hematoma, and postoperative pain [52].

RFA therapy

Few studies have shown the superiority of RFA compared with EVLA in terms of pain, bruising, and postprocedure recovery, with GSV occlusion rates being comparable. The LARA study was a randomized control trial conducted to determine whether RFA of the GSV is associated with less pain and bruising than EVLA in 87 leg interventions [53]. In the bilateral group, RFA resulted in significantly less pain than EVLA on days 2–11 after surgery. RFA also resulted in significantly less bruising than EVLA on days 3–9. There were no significant differences in mean postoperative pain, bruising, and activity scores in the unilateral group. Both RFA and EVLA resulted in occlusion rates of 95% at 10 days after surgery [54]. The RECOVERY study randomized 87 veins in 69 patients to Closure FAST or 980-nm EVLA treatment of the GSV. It was a multicenter, prospective, randomized, single-blinded trial, performed at five American sites and one European site. All scores referable to pain, ecchymosis, and tenderness were statistically lower in the Closure FAST group at 48 hours, 1 week, and 2 weeks. Minor complications were more prevalent in the EVLA group (p <0.0210); there were no major complications. Venous clinical severity scores and QOL measures were statistically lower in the Closure FAST group at 48 hours, 1 week, and 2 weeks. Radiofrequency thermal ablation was significantly superior to EVLA as measured by a comprehensive array of postprocedure recovery and QOL parameters [55]. The EVOLVeS trial studied the clinical outcomes of rates of recurrent varicosities, neovascularization, ultrasonography changes of the GSV, and QOL changes in patients undergoing RFA, ligation, or vein stripping. Two-year clinical results of radiofrequency obliteration are at least equal to those after high ligation and stripping of the GSV [56].

Venous sclerotherapy

This treatment modality is used for obliterating telangiectasias, varicose veins, and venous segments with reflux. Sclerotherapy can be used as a primary treatment or in conjunction with surgical procedures in the correction of CVI. Sclerotherapy is indicated for a variety of conditions including spider veins (<1 mm), venous lakes, varicose veins of 1–4 mm in diameter, bleeding varicosities, and small cavernous hemangiomas (vascular malformation). The terminal interruption of reflux source technique involves blocking off the veins that drain the ulcer bedusing Sotradecol or Polidocanol foam, administered under ultrasonography guidance [57]. Patients with CVI need to be evaluated for surgical treatment if they have a non-healing ulcer refractory to conservative and minimally invasive therapy resulting in delayed healing, recurrent varicose veins, CVI with disabling symptoms, persistent discomfort refractory to other therapy, non-compliant patients with conservative therapy, and to complement therapy with conservative measures.

Ligation and venous phlebectomy

Surgical ligation of the GSV has been shown to improve symptoms in patient with CEAP classes 2–6. GSV removal with high ligation of the sapheno-femoral junction has long been considered the standard treatment for patients with significant venous reflux, non-healing ulcers, and symptomatic patients with concomitant deep venous reflux [58]. Transilluminated power phlebectomy (or TriVex) is a new surgical technique that uses tumescent dissection, transillumination, and powered phlebectomy. A prospective randomized controlled trial of 141 patients comparing conventional with powered phlebectomy has shown a trend toward reduced operating time in extensive varicosities, and significantly fewer incisions. There was no difference in nerve injury, bruising, and cosmetic score during follow-up [59]. The ESCHAR study evaluated around 500 patients with venous ulcer and reflux of superficial and deep venous systems and randomized them to either conventional saphenous vein surgery with compression or to compression alone. The study showed a significant reduction in ulcer recurrence at 12 months in favor of surgery with compression compared with compression alone (12% vs. 28%) [60]. A follow-up study to observe the improvement in perforating vein incompetence included 261 patients from the ESCHAR trial. Surgical correction of superficial reflux was shown to abolish incompetence in some calf perforators but also helped wound healing and reflux symptoms by preventing development of new perforator incompetence [61].

Deep venous reflux
Valve reconstruction surgery and valvuloplasty

CVI has been shown to be partially attributable to venous valve injury and incompetence. Venous valve reconstruction of the deep vein valves has been performed in selected patients with advanced CVI who have recurrent ulceration with severe and disabling symptoms [62]. Open valve surgery was initially performed to repair the femoral vein valve but subsequently transcommissural valvuloplasty was developed for venous repair. Venous valvuloplasty has been shown to provide 59% competency and 63% ulcer-free recurrence at 30 months. Complications from valvuloplasty include bleeding (because patients need to remain anticoagulated), deep venous thrombosis, pulmonary embolism, ulcer recurrence, and wound infections [63]. This procedure is reserved for selected patients refractory to other therapies. Valve replacements and transposition procedures have been attempted successfully when native valves have post-thrombotic valve destruction (not amenable to valvuloplasty). Valve transposition has been performed with the axillary vein valve, profunda femoris valve, or cryopreserved valve allografts. Cryopreserved vein valve allografts have also been shown to have early thrombosis, poor patency and competency, as well as high patient morbidity, precluding their use as a primary intervention [64].

Perforator reflux
Subfascial endoscopic perforator surgery

Perforator vein incompetence has been proposed as a cause for CVI. Some surgical options have been proposed for the treatment of incompetent perforators, including subfascial endoscopic perforator surgery (SEPS). This procedure involves ligation of the incompetent perforator veins by gaining access from a remote site on the leg that is away from the treatment area and is free of lipodermatosclerosis or ulcers. The North American Study Group performed a study with 146 patients showing cumulative ulcer healing at 1 year of 88% (median time to healing was 54 days). Ablation of superficial venous

reflux combined with lack of deep venous obstruction predicted ulcer healing (p <0.05). Clinical score improved from 8.93 to 3.98 at the last follow-up (p <0.0001). Cumulative ulcer recurrence at 1 year was 16% and at 2 years was 28% (standard error, <10%). Post-thrombotic limbs had a higher 2-year cumulative recurrence rate (46%) than did those limbs with primary valvular incompetence (20%; p <0.05) [65]. The interruption of perforators with ablation of superficial venous reflux is effective in decreasing the symptoms of CVI and in earlier healing of ulcers. SEPS in conjunction with vein ablation showed better ulcer healing and improvement in clinical severity score [66].

Non-invasive study: chronic venous flow obstruction
May–Thurner syndrome

Endovascular therapy in the treatment of CVI has become increasingly important to restore outflow of the venous system and provide relief of obstruction. Approximately 10–30% of patients with severe CVI can be diagnosed with a significant abnormality in venous outflow involving iliac vein segments that contributes to persistent symptoms. Before endovascular therapy, iliac vein stenosis and obstruction causing CVI was treated with surgical procedures such as cross-femoral venous bypass or iliac vein reconstructions with prosthetic materials. Because of the success of venous stenting, surgical venous bypass is infrequently performed. In a large single-center series of 429 patients with CVI and outflow obstruction, iliac vein stenting resulted in significant clinical improvement: 50% of patients were completely relieved of pain and 33% experienced complete resolution of edema. Furthermore, 55% of patients with venous ulcers experienced complete healing of their ulcers. Patency of iliac vein stents is good, with a primary patency of 75% at 3 years. Close follow-up is mandatory to ensure that stent patency is maintained. Also early intervention is necessary in patients with recurrent symptoms that indicate in-stent restenosis, which occurs in approximately 23% of patients [67,68].

Chronic axillary–subclavian vein thrombosis or Paget–Schroetter syndrome

The pathogenesis of chronic axillary–subclavian thrombosis is associated with anatomic abnormalities at the thoracic outlet (cervical rib, congenital bands, hypertrophy of scalenus tendons, and abnormal insertion of the costoclavicular ligament) and repetitive trauma of the endothelium of the subclavian vein during activity of the upper extremities. The narrow costoclavicular space leads to compression and restricted mobility of the vein resulting in venous stasis. The repetitive endothelial trauma leads to intimal hyperplasia, inflammation, and fibrosis, resulting in venous webs, extensive collateral formation, and perivenular fibrosis worsening the stasis and costoclavicular crowding. Clinically, axillary–subclavian thrombosis preferentially involves the dominant arm and presents with swelling and discomfort of the arm. Other symptoms include heaviness and rubor of the arm with cyanotic, dilated, and visible veins across the shoulder and upper arm. The onset is usually acute or subacute but rarely can present with chronic symptoms. Most patients associate the onset with activities that involve vigorous and sustained upper extremity movements as well as outstretched arm. Complications include pulmonary embolism, post-thrombotic syndrome, and recurrent thrombosis. Despite the classic clinical presentation, the diagnosis of axillary–subclavian thrombosis should be confirmed initially with compression duplex ultrasonography followed, as needed, with more specific and sensitive tests (e.g., radionucleotide, magnetic resonance, computed tomographic venography, or invasive contrast venography). Management of axillary–subclavian thrombosis primarily includes catheter-directed thrombolysis and thoracic outlet decompression (resection of the first rib, division of the scalenus muscles and the costoclavicular ligament) with or without venoplasty/venous bypass. The best surgical approach to achieve thoracic outlet decompression is still debatable and excellent results are reported with both transaxillary and anterior, or sub-clavicular, approaches. Early and aggressive treatment includes optimal surgical strategy to prevent recurrent thrombosis and patient disability. Long-term anticoagulation can be reasonable in patients with coexistent thrombophilia and suboptimal surgical results [69].

Non-invasive study: muscle pump dysfunction

Abnormalities in the calf and foot muscle pumps have a significant role in the pathophysiology of CVI. Graded exercise programs have been used in an effort to rehabilitate the muscle pump and improve CVI symptoms. In a small controlled study, 31 patients with CEAP class 4–6 CVI were randomized to structured calf muscle exercise or routine daily activities. Venous hemodynamics were assessed with duplex ultrasonography, APG, and muscle strength assessed with a dynamometer. After 6 months, patients receiving a calf muscle exercise regimen had normalized their calf muscle pump function parameters but experienced no change in the amount of reflux or severity scores. Padberg et al. [70] concluded that structured exercise to re-establish calf muscle pump function in CVI can prove beneficial as a supplemental therapy to medical and surgical treatment in advanced disease.

Interactive multiple choice questions are available for this chapter on www.wiley. com/go/dangas/cardiology

References

1 Beebe-Dimmer JL, Pfeifer JR, Engle JS, Schottenfeld D. The epidemiology of chronic venous insufficiency and varicose veins. *Ann Epidemiol* 2005; **15**(3): 175–184.

2 Callam MJ. Epidemiology of varicose veins. *Br J Surg* 1994; **81**(2): 167–173.

3 Dwerryhouse S, Davies B, Harradine K, Earnshaw JJ. Stripping the long saphenous vein reduces the rate of reoperation for recurrent varicose veins: five-year results of a randomized trial. *J Vasc Surg* 1999; **29**(4): 589–592.

4 Brand FN, Dannenberg AL, Abbott RD, Kannel WB. The epidemiology of varicose veins: the Framingham Study. *Am J Prevent Med* 1988; **4**(2): 96–101.

5 Sisto T, Reunanen A, Laurikka J, et al. Prevalence and risk factors of varicose veins in lower extremities: mini-Finland health survey. *Eur J Surg* 1995; **161**(6): 405–414.

6 Evans CJ, Fowkes FG, Ruckley CV, Lee AJ. Prevalence of varicose veins and chronic venous insufficiency in men and women in the general population: Edinburgh Vein Study. *J Epidemiol Community Health* 1999; **53**(3): 149–153.

7 Ruckley CV, Evans CJ, Allan PL, Lee AJ, Fowkes FG. Chronic venous insufficiency: clinical and duplex correlations. The Edinburgh Vein Study of venous disorders in the general population. *J Vasc Surg* 2002; **36**(3): 520–525.

8 Laurikka JO, Sisto T, Tarkka MR, Auvinen O, Hakama M. Risk indicators for varicose veins in forty- to sixty-year-olds in the Tampere varicose vein study. *World J Surg* 2002; **26**(6): 648–651.

9 Ciardullo AV, Panico S, Bellati C, et al. High endogenous estradiol is associated with increased venous distensibility and clinical evidence of varicose veins in menopausal women. *J Vasc Surg* 2000; **32**(3): 544–549.

10 Hirai M, Naiki K, Nakayama R. Prevalence and risk factors of varicose veins in Japanese women. *Angiology* 1990; **41**(3): 228–232.

11 Anwar MA, Georgiadis KA, Shalhoub J, Lim CS, Gohel MS, Davies AH. A review of familial, genetic, and congenital aspects of primary varicose vein disease. *Circ Cardiovasc Genet* 2012; **5**(4): 460–466.

12 Hobson J. Venous insufficiency at work. *Angiology* 1997; **48**(7): 577–582.

13 Rose SS, Ahmed A. Some thoughts on the etiology of varicose-veins. *J Cardiovasc Surg* 1986; **27**(5): 534–543.

14 Lim CS, Davies AH. Pathogenesis of primary varicose veins. *Br J Surg* 2009; **96**(11): 1231–1242.

15 Gourdin FW, Smith JG, Jr. Etiology of venous ulceration. *South Med J* 1993; **86**(10): 1142–1146.

16 Mustoe T. Understanding chronic wounds: a unifying hypothesis on their pathogenesis and implications for therapy. *Am J Surg* 2004; **187**(5A): 65S–70S.

17 Recek C. Calf pump activity influencing venous hemodynamics in the lower extremity. *Int J Angiol* 2013; **22**(1): 23–30.

18 Recek C. Impact of the calf perforators on the venous hemodynamics in primary varicose veins. *J Cardiovasc Surg* 2006; **47**(6): 629–635.

19 Stanley AC, Lounsbury KM, Corrow K, et al. Pressure elevation slows the fibroblast response to wound healing. *J Vasc Surg* 2005; **42**(3): 546–551.

20 Van de Scheur M, Falanga V. Pericapillary fibrin cuffs in venous disease: a reappraisal. *Dermatol Surg* 1997; **23**(10): 955–959.

21 Raju S, Fredericks R. Evaluation of methods for detecting venous reflux: perspectives in venous insufficiency. *Arch Surg* 1990; **125**(11): 1463–1467.

22 Hahn TL, Unthank JL, Lalka SG. Increased hindlimb leukocyte concentration in a chronic rodent model of venous hypertension. *J Surg Res* 1999; **81**(1): 38–41.

23 Eberhardt RT, Raffetto JD. Chronic venous insufficiency. *Circulation* 2005; **111**(18): 2398–2409.

24 Porter JM, Moneta GL. Reporting standards in venous disease: an update. International Consensus Committee on Chronic Venous Disease. *J Vasc Surg* 1995; **21**(4): 635–645.

25 Eklof B, Rutherford RB, Bergan JJ, et al. Revision of the CEAP classification for chronic venous disorders: consensus statement. *J Vasc Surg* 2004; **40**(6): 1248–1252.

26 Carpentier PH, Cornu-Thenard A, Uhl JF, Partsch H, Antignani PL, Societe Francaise de Medecine Vasculaire, et al. Appraisal of the information content of the C classes of CEAP clinical classification of chronic venous disorders: a multicenter evaluation of 872 patients. *J Vasc Surg* 2003; **37**(4): 827–833.

27 Rutherford RB, Padberg FT Jr, Comerota AJ, Kistner RL, Meissner MH, Moneta GL. Venous severity scoring: an adjunct to venous outcome assessment. *J Vasc Surg* 2000; **31**(6): 1307–1312.

28 Vasquez MA, Rabe E, McLafferty RB, et al. Revision of the venous clinical severity score: venous outcomes consensus statement: special communication of the American Venous Forum Ad Hoc Outcomes Working Group. *J Vasc Surg* 2010; **52**(5): 1387–1396.

29 Kakkos SK, Rivera MA, Matsagas MI, et al. Validation of the new venous severity scoring system in varicose vein surgery. *J Vasc Surg* 2003; **38**(2): 224–228.

30 Perrin MR, Labropoulos N, Leon LR Jr. Presentation of the patient with recurrent varices after surgery (REVAS). *J Vasc Surg* 2006; **43**(2): 327–334; discussion 334.

31 Abenhaim L, Kurz X. The VEINES study (VEnous Insufficiency Epidemiologic and Economic Study): an international cohort study on chronic venous disorders of the leg. *VEINES Group. Angiology* 1997; **48**(1): 59–66.

32 Kurz X, Lamping DL, Kahn SR, et al. Do varicose veins affect quality of life? Results of an international population-based study. *J Vasc Surg* 2001; **34**(4): 641–648.

33 Lamping DL, Schroter S, Kurz X, Kahn SR, Abenhaim L. Evaluation of outcomes in chronic venous disorders of the leg: development of a scientifically rigorous, patient-reported measure of symptoms and quality of life. *J Vasc Surg* 2003; **37**(2): 410–419.

34 Kahn SR, Lamping DL, Ducruet T, et al. VEINES-QOL/Sym questionnaire was a reliable and valid disease-specific quality of life measure for deep venous thrombosis. *J Clin Epidemiol* 2006; **59**(10): 1049–1056.

35 Bradbury A, Ruckley CV. Clinical assessment of patients with venous disease. In Gloviczki P, Yao J (eds). *Handbook of Venous Disorders: Guidelines of the American Venous Forum*, 2nd edn. New York, NY: Arnold; 2001: 71–83.

36 van Bemmelen PS, Bedford G, Beach K, Strandness DE. Quantitative segmental evaluation of venous valvular reflux with duplex ultrasound scanning. *J Vasc Surg* 1989; **10**(4): 425–431.

37 Malgor RD, Labropoulos N. Diagnosis of venous disease with duplex ultrasound. *Phlebology* 2013; **28**(Suppl 1): 158–161.

38 Garcia-Gimeno M, Rodriguez-Camarero S, Tagarro-Villalba S, et al. Duplex mapping of 2036 primary varicose veins. *J Vasc Surg* 2009; **49**(3): 681–689.

39 Markel A, Meissner MH, Manzo RA, Bergelin RO, Strandness DE Jr. A comparison of the cuff deflation method with Valsalva's maneuver and limb compression in detecting venous valvular reflux. *Arch Surg* 1994; **129**(7): 701–705.

40 Nicolaides AN, Cardiovascular Disease Educational and Research Trust, European Society of Vascular Surgery, The International Angiology Scientific Activity Congress Organization, International Union of Angiology, et al. Investigation of

chronic venous insufficiency: a consensus statement (France, March 5–9, 1997). *Circulation 2000*; **102**(20): E126–163.

41 Abramowitz HB, Queral LA, Finn WR, *et al.* The use of photoplethysmography in the assessment of venous insufficiency: a comparison to venous pressure measurements. *Surgery* 1979; **86**(3): 434–441.

42 Owens LV, Farber MA, Young ML, *et al.* The value of air plethysmography in predicting clinical outcome after surgical treatment of chronic venous insufficiency. *J Vasc Surg* 2000; **32**(5): 961–968.

43 Gillespie DL, Cordts PR, Hartono C, *et al.* The role of air plethysmography in monitoring results of venous surgery. *J Vasc Surg* 1992; **16**(5): 674–678.

44 Meissner MH, Moneta G, Burnand K, *et al.* The hemodynamics and diagnosis of venous disease. *J Vasc Surg* 2007; **46**(Suppl S): 4S–24S.

45 Davies MG, Lumsden AB (eds). *Chronic Venous Insufficiency*, 2011.

46 van Gent WB, Wilschut ED, Wittens C. Management of venous ulcer disease. *BMJ* 2010; **341**: c6045.

47 Motykie GD, Caprini JA, Arcelus JI, Reyna JJ, Overom E, Mokhtee D. Evaluation of therapeutic compression stockings in the treatment of chronic venous insufficiency. *Dermatol Surg* 1999; **25**(2): 116–120.

48 Mayberry JC, Moneta GL, Taylor LM Jr, Porter JM. Fifteen-year results of ambulatory compression therapy for chronic venous ulcers. *Surgery* 1991; **109**(5): 575–581.

49 Ibegbuna V, Delis KT, Nicolaides AN, Aina O. Effect of elastic compression stockings on venous hemodynamics during walking. *J Vasc Surg* 2003; **37**(2): 420–425.

50 Goldman MP, Mauricio M, Rao J. Intravascular 1320-nm laser closure of the great saphenous vein: a 6- to 12-month follow-up study. *Dermatol Surg* 2004; **30**(11): 1380–1385.

51 Weiss RA. Comparison of endovenous radiofrequency versus 810 nm diode laser occlusion of large veins in an animal model. *Dermatol Surg* 2002; **28**(1): 56–61.

52 Proebstle TM, Sandhofer M, Kargl A, *et al.* Thermal damage of the inner vein wall during endovenous laser treatment: key role of energy absorption by intravascular blood. *Dermatol Surg* 2002; **28**(7): 596–600.

53 Goode SD, Chowdhury A, Crockett M, *et al.* Laser and radiofrequency ablation study (LARA study): a randomised study comparing radiofrequency ablation and endovenous laser ablation (810 nm). *Eur J Vasc Endovasc Surg* 2010; **40**(2): 246–253.

54 Nordon IM, Hinchliffe RJ, Brar R, *et al.* A prospective double-blind randomized controlled trial of radiofrequency versus laser treatment of the great saphenous vein in patients with varicose veins. *Ann Surg* 2011; **254**(6): 876–881.

55 Lurie F, Creton D, Eklof B, *et al.* Prospective randomized study of endovenous radiofrequency obliteration (closure procedure) versus ligation and stripping in a selected patient population (EVOLVeS Study). *J Vasc Surg* 2003; **38**(2): 207–214.

56 Almeida JI, Kaufman J, Gockeritz O, *et al.* Radiofrequency endovenous ClosureFAST versus laser ablation for the treatment of great saphenous reflux: a multicenter, single-blinded, randomized study (RECOVERY study). *J Vasc Interv Radiol* 2009; **20**(6): 752–759.

57 Bush RG. New technique to heal venous ulcers: terminal interruption of the reflux source (TIRS). *Perspect Vasc Surg Endovasc Ther* 2010; **22**(3): 194–199.

58 Sarin S, Scurr JH, Coleridge Smith PD. Stripping of the long saphenous vein in the treatment of primary varicose veins. *Br J Surg* 1994; **81**(10): 1455–1458.

59 Aremu MA, Mahendran B, Butcher W, *et al.* Prospective randomized controlled trial: conventional versus powered phlebectomy. *J Vasc Surg* 2004; **39**(1): 88–94.

60 Barwell JR, Davies CE, Deacon J, *et al.* Comparison of surgery and compression with compression alone in chronic venous ulceration (ESCHAR study): randomised controlled trial. *Lancet* 2004; **363**(9424): 1854–1859.

61 Gohel MS, Barwell JR, Wakely C, *et al.* The influence of superficial venous surgery and compression on incompetent calf perforators in chronic venous leg ulceration. *Eur J Vasc Endovasc Surg* 2005; **29**(1): 78–82.

62 Kistner RL. Surgical repair of the incompetent femoral vein valve. *Arch Surg* 1975; **110**(11): 1336–1342.

63 Raju S, Berry MA, Neglen P. Transcommissural valvuloplasty: technique and results. *J Vasc Surg* 2000; **32**(5): 969–976.

64 Neglen P, Raju S. Venous reflux repair with cryopreserved vein valves. *J Vasc Surg* 2003; **37**(3): 552–557.

65 Gloviczki P, Bergan JJ, Rhodes JM, Canton LG, Harmsen S, Ilstrup DM. Mid-term results of endoscopic perforator vein interruption for chronic venous insufficiency: lessons learned from the North American subfascial endoscopic perforator surgery registry. The North American Study Group. *J Vasc Surg* 1999; **29**(3): 489–502.

66 Bianchi C, Ballard JL, Abou-Zamzam AM, Teruya TH. Subfascial endoscopic perforator vein surgery combined with saphenous vein ablation: results and critical analysis. *J Vasc Surg* 2003; **38**(1): 67–71.

67 Danza R, Navarro T, Baldizan J. Reconstructive surgery in chronic venous obstruction of the lower limbs. *J Cardiovasc Surg* 1991; **32**(1): 98–103.

68 Neglen P, Raju S. Intravascular ultrasound scan evaluation of the obstructed vein. *J Vasc Surg* 2002; **35**(4): 694–700.

69 Alla VM, Natarajan N, Kaushik M, Warrier R, Nair CK. Paget–Schroetter syndrome: review of pathogenesis and treatment of effort thrombosis. *West J Emerg Med* 2010; **11**(4): 358–362.

70 Padberg FT Jr, Johnston MV, Sisto SA. Structured exercise improves calf muscle pump function in chronic venous insufficiency: a randomized trial. *J Vasc Surg* 2004; **39**(1): 79–87.

CHAPTER 84

Cardiac Vein Anatomy and Transcoronary Sinus Catheter Interventions in Myocardial Ischemia

Werner Mohl[1], Levente Molnár[2], and Béla Merkely[2]

[1]Department of Cardiac Surgery, Medical University of Vienna, Vienna, Austria
[2]Semmelweis University, Budapest, Hungary

Aims of transcoronary sinus interventions

There is no better way to reach compromised ischemic microcirculation or no reflow zones after initial reperfusion in primary percutaneous coronary intervention (PCI) than with transcoronary sinus interventions (trans-CSI). Since the historical clinical series from Claude Beck reversing flow in the coronary circulation, at least partially, as a means to treat diffuse coronary artery disease, several therapeutic concepts have been formulated to use the "back door of the heart" to effectively reduce disease burden. Demographic changes in coronary artery disease, but also in heart failure, with more complex lesions, advanced comorbidities, and state of the art interventional technologies increase the need for trans-CSI.

In cardiac surgery, the ease of inserting catheters transatrially, the acceptance of retrograde cardioplegia, decades ago allowed cardioprotection for more than 2 hours of complex cardiac surgery without interfering with the surgical approach and undoing the tight relationship between the duration of global ischemic arrest and patient outcome. A different success story is resynchronization therapy enabled by using cardiac veins to reach left ventricular myocardium to adapt contractility dynamics and reduce dyssynchony and therefore the burden of heart failure.

For today's interventional cardiologist the advent of more complex lesions and the inherent invisible barrier of current treatment options in coronary artery disease demand innovative alternatives to reduce the amount of compromised microcirculation in acute coronary syndromes (ACS). But trans-CSI span their potential from preventing ischemia in elective cases (i.e., total coronary occlusion) to treating high risk patients with diffuse coronary artery disease and ischemic cardiomyopathies. Even the clinical potential of retro-infusion cardioprotective molecules and regenerative cells are currently under clinical scrutiny [1].

For the interventional cardiologist, trans-CSI became more important for the treatment of microvascular obstruction, no reflow zones, and to enhance and support the healing process of myocardial infarcts. From the many historical concepts of retrograde coronary sinus procedures this chapter focuses on a short overview of procedures that became clinically relevant or are still in clinical use. In addition, the following chapter highlights the clinical potential of a particular coronary sinus intervention, pressure controlled intermittent coronary sinus occlusion (PICSO),

which has proven validity in inducing myocardial salvage and apparently has the potential to regenerate the failing heart.

Anatomy of cardiac veins

To understand the clinical potential of trans-CSI one has to study the special features of the anatomy and pathophysiology of the cardiac venous system. Unlike the coronary arteries and the plethora of knowledge in the field of coronary circulation, cardiac veins are relatively neglected and knowledge about their role in structure and function is sparse. The anatomy of cardiac veins and their nomenclature was described by von Lüdinghausen [2]. Seventy-five percent of venous drainage is collected in the coronary sinus. Most parts of the left ventricle, excluding the upper septum, drain into the coronary sinus; however, most parts of the right ventricle drain via so-called lesser veins into both atria and ventricles. Thebesian veins or direct connections of the venous vasculature into the ventricles were described several centuries ago [3,4]. Although controversial, it stimulated knowledge of the anatomy of cardiac veins and their importance for the coronary circulation. In fact, the venous circulation outnumbers coronary arteries by far and creates a dense meshwork of interconnected channels allowing perfect access to the most important functional parts (i.e., anterior and lateral aspects of the left heart). The proximity between cardiac veins accessible for transcoronary sinus catheter interventions and coronary arteries, as well as the distance between mitral annulus and the great cardiac vein, shows the limitations to some of the methods used to correct structural and functional heart disease. Good reviews of the clinical assessment using CT scans of cardiac veins and their relationship to other anatomic landmarks have recently been published [5–7].

In contrast to trans-CSI for treating structural heart disease as transcoronary sinus mitral annuloplasty, functional modifications such as electrode deployment and radiofrequency ablation also involve the limiting factor of the proximity of the circumflex artery and the importance of reaching left ventricular excitable myocardium to fully explore the potential of resynchronization therapy.

For the use of trans-CSI in interventional cardiology, especially the deployment of catheters, the "silent zone" of the great cardiac vein is important [8]. "Silent zone" means that no additional branching veins enter the collecting chamber of the coronary sinus. Studies on the nomenclature of cardiac veins as well as all important parameters such as distances, angles, and landmarks of the coronary sinus

Interventional Cardiology: Principles and Practice, Second Edition. Edited by George D. Dangas, Carlo Di Mario, and Nicholas N. Kipshidze.
© 2017 John Wiley & Sons, Ltd. Published 2017 by John Wiley & Sons, Ltd.

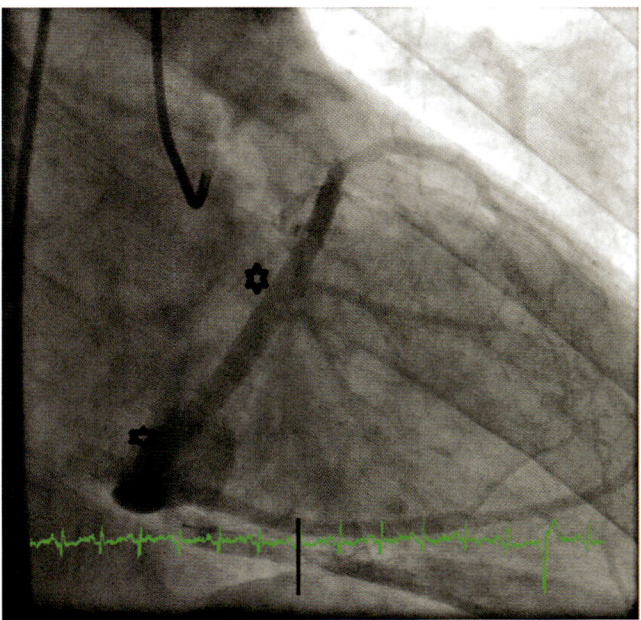 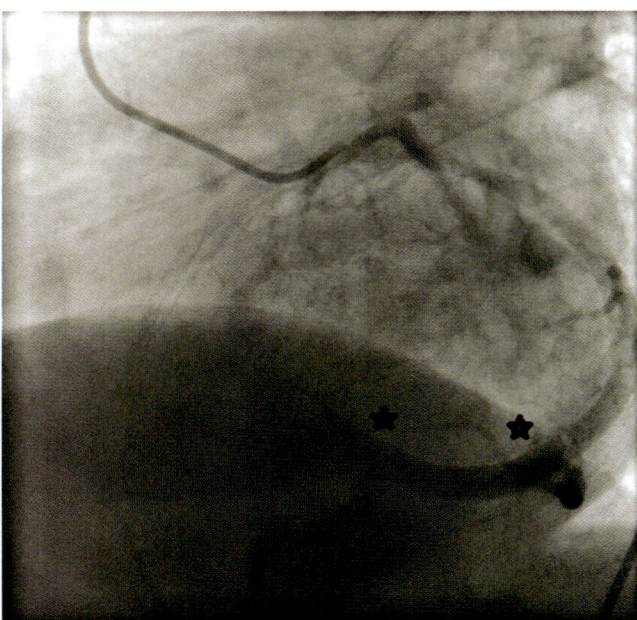

Figure 84.1 Late phase of a normal coronary arteriogram in two plans. Note the silent zone of the coronary sinus (great cardiac vein). This is the portion the catheter for transcoronary sinus interventions has to be positioned to achieve optimal redistribution of flow toward the deprived myocardium.

anatomy to catheterize the coronary sinus successfully are collected in the Coronary Sinus Library (www.coronarysinus.com), which contains the reprinted versions of proceedings of several seminars and symposia on myocardial protection via the coronary sinus held in the late 1980s [9–11].

The silent zone of the coronary sinus visualized in the late phase of the coronary arteriogram is depicted in Figure 84.1. The ideal place for a therapeutic catheter such as a PICSO catheter is between the stars in the angiogram. Stability of the catheter might be difficult because there is an enormous outward back pressure of venous blood and it requires special catheter technology to hold the catheter in place and to reduce the risk of catheter dislodgement.

In the majority of cases the coronary sinus is a tapered structure of about 4 cm in length from its entrance into the right atrium. The "silent zone" begins after inflow of the posterior interventricular vein until the first branches of the marginal veins. A variable structure of venous valves can hinder the catheterization of the coronary sinus. The width of the coronary sinus varies in patients with normal pressures in the right atrium from 6 to 18 mm² with a median of about 8–10 mm². In patients with increased prohormone of brain natriuretic peptide (proBNP) and manifest right heart failure, diameters can even increase in size. Unlike the coronary sinus orifice with its endocardial quality and embedded nerve endings, the great cardiac vein's surface is covered with endothelial layers. Reflexes such as hypotension and bradycardia have been described in the past by Muers and Sleight [12] as potential hazards of coronary sinus occlusion techniques.

Pathophysiologic background of transcoronary sinus interventions
Microvasculature and salvage

Allowing basal metabolism in deprived zones during ischemia and reopening "no reflow" zones in the center of reperfused myocardium remains an important challenge in today's treatment of acute coronary artery syndromes. For this purpose it is important to redistribute venous flow like a sloughing wavefront into underperfused microcirculation, expand the vasculature, and by reverting this flow entraining toxic metabolites and cellular debris, thus reopening avenues for arterial inflow via collaterals in border zones [13–15]. PICSO, as it reverses venous flow during coronary sinus occlusion and washes out edema during the release phase, is a feasible intervention accessing the deprived microcirculation [16].

In a series of experimental and clinical studies, myocardial salvage was established as a dose-dependent treatment during pressure controlled intermittent obstruction of coronary venous outflow. In a meta-analysis, Syeda [17] was able to substantiate significant myocardial salvage in different experimental settings and animal models of about 30%. About the same magnitude of myocardial salvage was found in experimental infarction by Jacobs in the early reperfusion period and this has been corroborated in a few clinical series even using primary PCI and modern technology showing the same potential in reducing infarct size [18–20].

The first application of PICSO in ACS was in combination with lysis therapy and, although now outdated and not today's standard of care, showed the way to important discoveries. As already shown in experiments by Miyazaki et al. [21], the duration between onset of intravenous lysis and culprit lesion reopening through clot lysis was significantly shorter in the PICSO group [20]. The second important conclusion is based on the 5-year follow-up of these patients. Even after correction for differences in residual stenosis 30 days after treatment with PICSO in ACS and also correcting for differences in the duration of pain onset to reperfusion, there was a significant 96% reduction for reinfarction and 86% reduction in major adverse coronary events (MACE) over the 5 year follow-up in the PICSO-treated group, which heralded a paradigm change in the perception of trans-CSI and the beginning of an alternative in regeneration research [20].

Resynchronization therapy

The breakthrough in trans-CSI occurred at the advent of resynchronization therapy. The ability to improve heart failure with a relatively simple intervention and the chance to reach the left ventricle via a venous access was attractive. Biventricular pacing when applied to current guidelines show superiority in survival and quality of life and has been accepted by clinicians as well as patients [21,22]. Although coronary sinus catheterization is similar to interventional cardiology, the majority of cases are performed via the left subclavian vein. The ability to find an excitable myocardial space in the vicinity of a penetrable coronary vein correcting dyssynchrony is sometimes difficult and requires additional technology [23,24]. In spite of unquestionable successes of this therapy there is still room for innovations and to improve patient groups as non-responders. For this purpose, biomarkers sampled from the coronary sinus as well as other parameters are currently under investigation to improve outcome [25–27].

Mitral annulus modifications

In the quest to find minimal invasive techniques to improve heart failure and mitral insufficiency, the assumed proximity between coronary sinus and mitral valve annulus stimulated the development of several percutaneous cinching devices positioned into the coronary sinus. Enthusiasm for these devices have been hampered recently by lack of clinical efficiency. The obvious distance between the coronary sinus and the mitral valve, especially near the posteromedial commissure where most valve pathologies develop, as well as difficulties in device development and safety, reduced early enthusiasm for this procedure. In addition, cinching devices are in danger of compressing the crossing circumflex branch of the left coronary artery, thus generating iatrogenic myocardial infarction [28–32]. Today, these procedures are less often used clinically and will soon vanish from the clinical arena.

Regenerative potential of transcoronary sinus interventions

The vast meshwork of coronary venous microcirculation is not only important for revascularization procedures using the transcoronary sinus access to deprived myocardial perfusion zones, but also for substance exchange and recently encountered stimulation of innate developmental pathways to initiate structural regeneration. Long-term follow-up in patients treated with PICSO prompted a paradigm change in trans-CSI. Puzzled by the obvious long-term effect of PICSO inexplicable by myocardial salvage and its confounding parameters, several experimental fundamental studies have been performed. Weigel et al. [33] showed in a porcine model that according to the clinical findings a causative gene expression was enhanced in the tissue of treated animals. Two important molecules—HO-hemoxygenase and vascular endothelial growth factor (VEGF) gene expression—increased significantly in remote and also partly in border and infarct zones. As HO-hemoxygenase is not only a vasoactive substance that might act during the acute collateralization of the border zone, but also an anti-atherosclerotic and cardioprotective molecule supposed to be a causative element in preventing restenosis and in risk reduction of MACE and reinfarction. The observed absolute risk reduction resulting from PICSO was 29% (95% confidence interval 10.1–73.7%; $p = 0.001$). This means, in 100 patient-years, an estimated number of at least 10 events (obtained from the lower confidence limit) can be prevented by PICSO. The number needed to treat was 3.4 (95% CI 1.38–9.90), or, put another way, treating 3.4 patients by PICSO would on average save one MACE per year. Recalculation

counting MACE events only during the first year of follow-up resulted in a higher absolute rate reduction of 51.2%, but at the same time in a wider confidence interval (−1.2% to +131%; $p = 0.059$), caused by the considerably lower number of events. This result indicates that PICSO may be more beneficial during the first year of follow-up than afterwards. Because of these unexpected results we went back to the drawing board and tried to envision the cause of long-term effects and decipher changes in the molecular healing cascade after myocardial infarction. We therefore looked at the similarities between cardiac development and innate regenerative processes in the adult heart and formulated the hypothesis of "embryonic recall" [34–36]. Miyasaka found that micro-RNA are expressed in rodents during and after the first heart beat, meaning that the hemodynamic force of the flowing blood and actual pulsations are acting via mechanotransduction on the endocardium, producing a burst of developmental signals. There is an obvious analogy here to PICSO acting on venous endothelium (Figure 84.2). Ongoing analysis of PICSO in adult patients with severe heart failure and cardiac resynchronization therapy (CRT) plus/minus PICSO is evidently supporting the hypothetical considerations. Deciphering the clinical potential of PICSO in heart failure patients will open up completely new horizons in cardiac regeneration beyond cellular therapy.

How to access jeopardized myocardium
Expertise necessary to use transcoronary sinus catheter interventions

The anatomy of the coronary sinus in regard to venous access needs special requirements of catheter systems as well as the expertise of the interventionist. Wang et al. [24] recently reported on a steerable catheter system facilitating coronary sinus cannulation under ECG guidance reducing access and procedure time. As the orifice of the coronary sinus is not in the same plane as the inferior cava, one has to rotate the tip back and to the right upwards to obtain good access via the femoral vein.

The ultimate goal in considering the potential success of transcoronary sinus interventions, one may ask when the device manufacturer will come up with a low profile, steerable, and blind (i.e., ECG guidance) catheter system allowing access via brachial veins or at least uncomplicated subclavian, jugular access. Figure 84.3 shows that even in patients with ACS, access as well as adjunct therapy like PICSO can be applied without losing procedure time.

Current transcoronary sinus catheter interventions in myocardial jeopardy
PICSO

Transcoronary sinus catheter interventions developed from historic arterial retroperfusion techniques. A comprehensive review on past and present procedures and their background and clinical potential show the uniqueness of PICSO among trans-CSI with two independent principles. The first is the redistribution of flow and subsequent washout with its dose-dependent salvage potential. The second is its threshold dependent mode of action based on the developed pulsatility and backflow of venous blood in cardiac veins initiating molecular responses through mechanotransduction in venous endothelium reiterating developmental processes [37–39]. First-in-man study of PICSO dates back to the 1980s and was performed during the early reperfusion period in patients undergoing

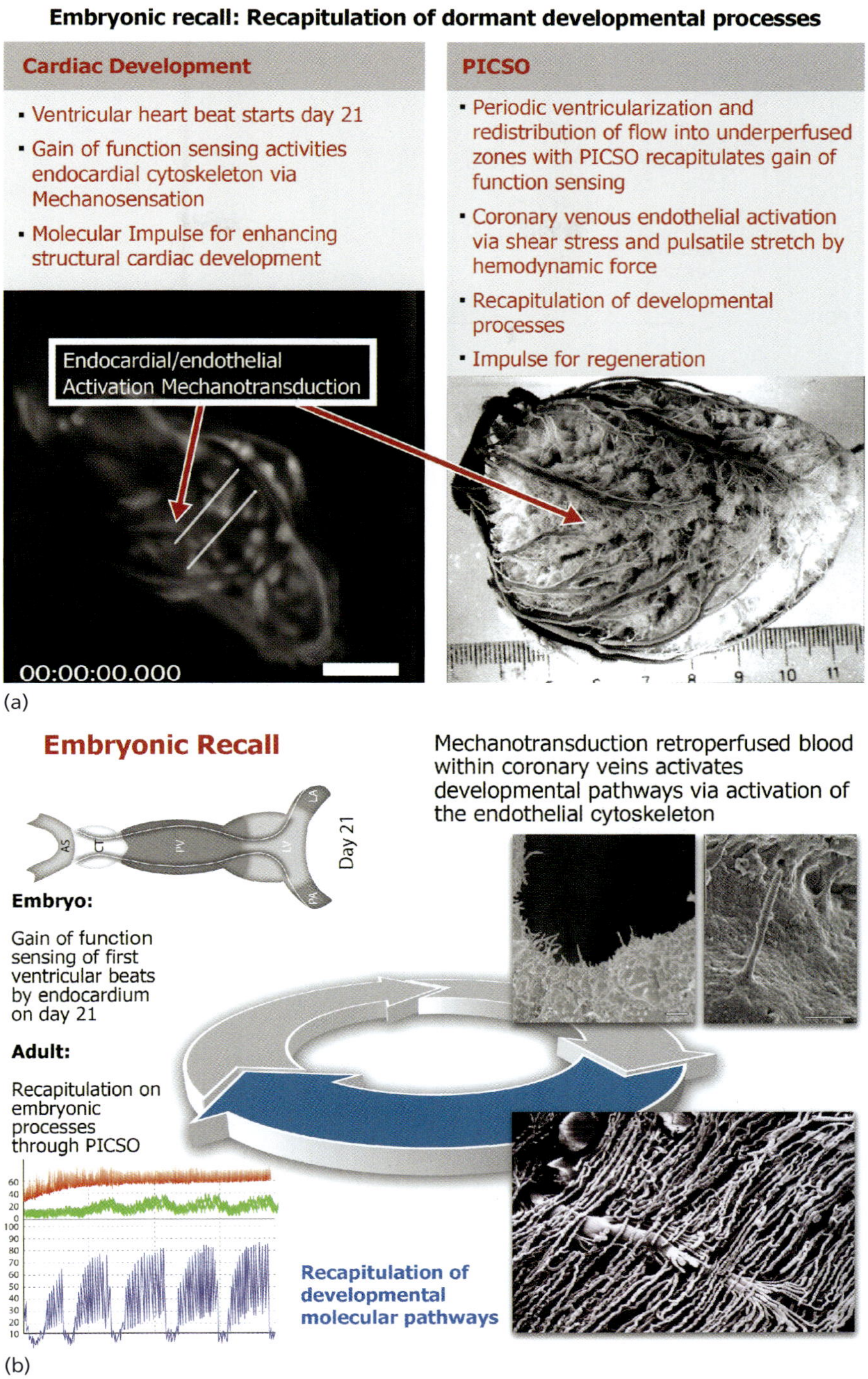

Embryonic recall: Recapitulation of dormant developmental processes

(a)

(b)

Figure 84.2 The hypothesis of "embryonic recall." Note the analogy of pressure and flow activating endocardium during development as soon as the heart tube starts to beat with the pulsations in the microcirculation during pressure controlled intermittent coronary sinus occlusion (PICSO) (a). The PICSO tracing with temporarily increased pressures in cardiac veins are depicted (b).

coronary artery bypass grafting. Results showed an improvement in regional wall motion in severely depressed myocardium as well as a trend toward, but an insignificant, improvement in clinical outcomes after 30 days (fewer catecholamines, fewer postoperative infections, shorter intubation time, etc.) [40].

In interventional cardiology, relief of ischemic burden and consequences of reperfusion injury are of outmost importance. PICSO in

ACS has recently been applied in ST-segment elevation myocardial infarction (STEMI) as well as non-STEMI (NSTEMI) patients using the new technology. Noteworthy, however, is the effect that the hemodynamic sloughing blood wave reduces the no reflow zone, the obstructed microcirculation after primary PCI, and induces washout and apparently enhances even decomposition of occluding clots in coronary arteries thus improving prognosis in this patient group [19,20].

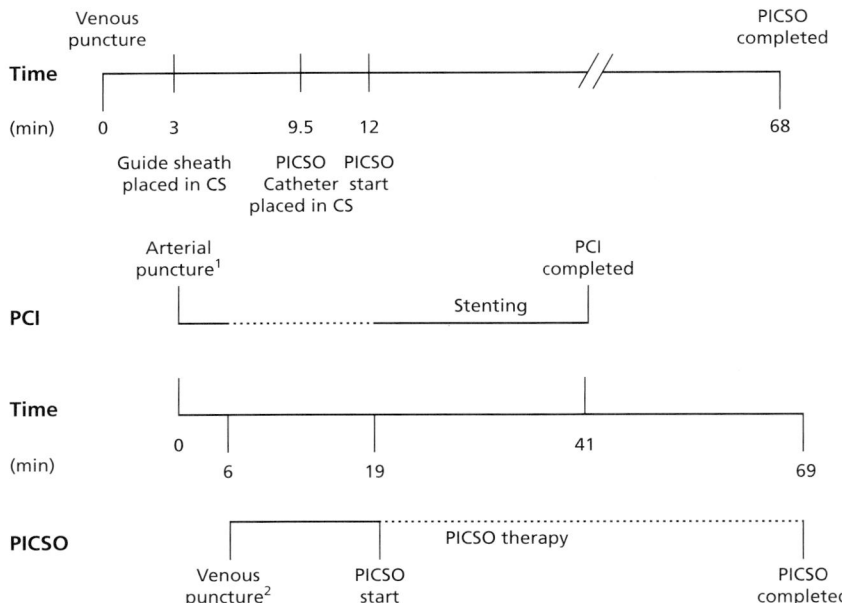

Figure 84.3 Timetable of a typical PICSO study in a patient. Note that the timing of catheterization does not interfere with arterial reopening. PICSO application is timed according to the PICSO quantity an empiric parameter claiming to fully evolve the PICSO benefit.

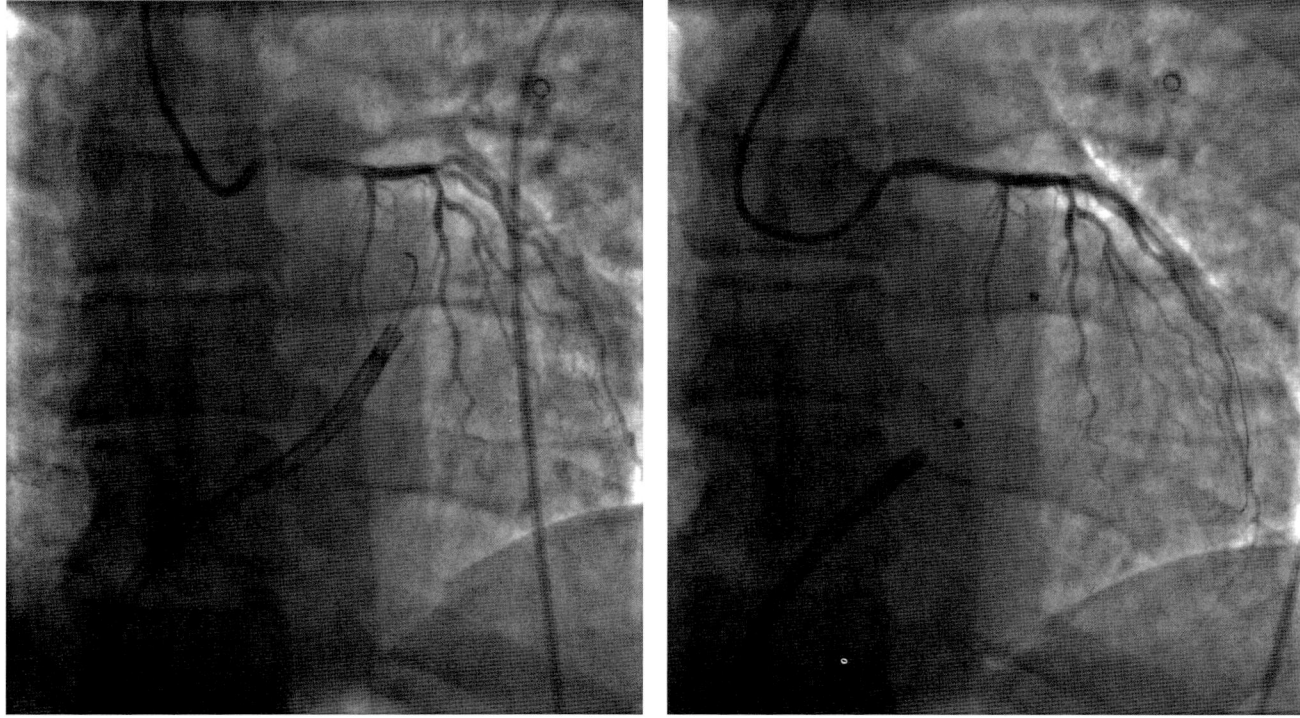

Figure 84.4 PICSO catheter in place in a patient undergoing PCI and PICSO (see also Videos 84.1, 84.2, and 84.3).

A first-in-man study using state of the art technology and automated pressure control was performed by Van de Hoef *et al.* [41] and showed feasibility and anti-ischemic effects in elective patients undergoing PCI. Present state-of-the-art application of PICSO in patients with ACS and primary PCI (PPCI) show the feasibility of this method. As seen in Video 84.1, the catheter is positioned in the silent zone of the coronary sinus and temporary occlusion there-fore enables redistribution of flow into the reperfused zone. In Video 84.2, the screen of the PICSO controller/pump system is shown illustrating the pressure increase in the venous circulation according to PICSO. Video 84.3 shows the balloon inflation during the PICSO procedure and PPCI (Figures 84.3 and 84.4; Videos 84.1, 84.2, and 84.3). Of importance is the pressure control which is based on an algorithm tested in a series of experiments analyzing the amount of blood retroperfused during balloon occlusion and the forward flow during balloon deflation showing a net washout phenomenon implying that more fluid and potentially edema is transported out of the myocardium [16,42]. Pressure control is also important because we found in our first-in-man studies a direct relationship between rise time of coronary sinus pressure increase and coronary flow (i.e., there is a sharp increase in pressure amplitudes and a shortening of the rise time when coronary artery bypass grafts are opened). It becomes evident that unphysiologic obstruction of venous circulation beyond the plateau of pressure peaks can increase impedance to arterial inflow. This effect underscores the necessity of present automatic pressure control as depicted in the video (Videos 84.2 and 84.3).

What can be expected from PICSO application in ACS in PPCI? Although current data analysis relies only on one historic clinical study and an additional trial with only a small number of treated patients using new technology and automated pressure control, there are anti-ischemic effects and almost certainly the same salvage potential as in experimental infarction, which however have to be proven by a large propensity-matched trial to establish clinical significance. Using the gold standard for salvage imaging, however, has one severe confounding factor in addition when studying PICSO patients. In experimental infarction, the area at risk is measured before the start of the therapy, which is impracticable in patients with ACS. Therefore the area at risk is measured on day 3 or 4 using the area with increased water content. As PICSO not only induces washout, but also reduces the perfusion deficit by supporting vasodilatation in border zones, the area at risk in PICSO patients will be smaller and therefore also the calculable salvage effect. In our opinion, evidence on the clinical significance of PICSO has to take this into account and it will be necessary to develop a special algorithm between PICSO quantity, or dose, and ultimate infarct size as well as microvascular obstruction, which also can be measured with MRI [14–17]. Another important effect is the coronary sinus pressure dynamics over the time of PICSO application. In our experience, during myocardial infarction and ischemia, coronary sinus pressure increases over time, because of improvement of nutritive flow and subsequently myocardial performance. However, this is not the case in early reperfusion with its temporal hyperemic flow response. Coronary sinus pressure dynamics during early reperfusion after primary PCI in patients show a gradual decline in amplitudes as well as an increase in rise time. This might be caused, as Khattab et al. [43] showed in porcine experiments, by two independent factors: first, the effect of opening up the obstructed microcirculation as additional space to fill retrogradely (and therefore longer rise times); and, second, the temporary hyperemic response in early reperfusion reducing the pressure amplitude at the end of the application. Especially in patients with low ejection fraction and large infarcts with low mean arterial pressure, coronary sinus pressure might even fail to increase substantially because of the reduced driving force of myocardial contraction and low coronary venous flow (which is predictive for outcome) which may limit the efficiency of PICSO [44]. However, in a case report on a PICSO application in acute shock patients presented by A. Colombo and his group, myocardial contraction was markedly improved within hours in no-option patients with otherwise failed cardiac support (personal communication and report at EuroPCR 2016).

In all therapies aiming to reduce infarct size and to induce salvage, clinical endpoints and outcome are of enormous importance. Long-term 5-year follow-up in PICSO studies is only available for historic data and their positive interaction on restenosis, reinfarction, and MACE have to be corroborated with modern technology in primary PCI and analyzed in larger propensity-matched trials, but one can also expect interesting results in registries of PICSO in STEMI and NSTEMI and even heart failure patients [20]. Recently another important application of PICSO has shown promising results: patients with elective PCI in need of cardiac support may benefit from PICSO since this intervention reduces the ischemic burden and clears the microcirculation from debris produced by the coronary intervention.

Banai stent

A different approach is the Banai stent as permanent throttle in the great cardiac vein as a means to reduce chronic angina in high risk patients with diffuse coronary artery disease. There are clinical data supporting this notion in a limited number of patients and Konigstein recently published long-term follow-up data on this intervention. However, there is controversy between the Banai stent concept and scientific considerations on temporal or permanent pressure elevation in cardiac veins [45–48]. The ease of the concept and the potential benefit may develop the application of this technology.

Retroinfusion (cells and gene therapy)

Retroinfusion of cells and molecules have been tried by several groups with high efficacy. Tuma et al. [1] showed that even in clinical studies the retrograde access is superior to other more sophisticated or invasive methods like transcoronary artery and myocardial delivery. First, the access to deprived myocardium and diffuse coronaries is an attractive alternative and principles of substrate exchange and the role of venous endothelium might be of importance for success [49–52].

Conclusions and future directions

Demographic changes in patients with more and more complex comorbidities and older age are the imperative to develop new standards in patient care. Based on the special anatomy and pathophysiology of cardiac veins, the options for trans-CSI to develop into a standard of care are enormous. There are several facts supporting the rise of these procedures. In the past, coronary sinus access was troubled by the lack of expertise of interventionists, the paucity of supporting clinical evidence, and shortcomings in interventional technology. Especially in the emergency settings of acute ischemia, the unquestioned evidence of time-dependent myocardial salvage in coronary revascularization procedures made it almost impossible to apply these methods clinically despite supporting evidence of improved long-term outcome. Today the situation has changed drastically. Modern imaging techniques have shown that for all trials to achieve timely reperfusion microcirculatory obstruction persists and that additional methods beyond salvage appear essential. Stem cell transplantation reopened the window of adjunct therapies even days after the acute event. This stimulated research on reperfusion injury and infarct healing as well as therapeutic concepts. Concomitantly, the formation of heart teams for engaging structural heart disease and the success story of resynchronization therapy increased the expertise to catheterize the coronary sinus. Dedicated knowledge focusing on transcoronary sinus catheter interventions are currently supplying the necessary technology and equipment. It is therefore plausible that technologies like PICSO ameliorating the ischemic burden and claiming to regenerate and recover the heart will develop into a standard of care procedure.

 ### *Interactive multiple choice questions are available for this chapter on www.wiley. com/go/dangas/cardiology*

References

1 Tuma J, Fernandez-Vina R, Carrasco A, *et al.* Safety and feasibility of percutaneous retrograde coronary sinus delivery of autologous bone marrow mononuclear cell transplantation in patients with chronic refractory angina. *J Transl Med* 2011; **9**: 183.

2 von Lüdinghausen M. The venous drainage of the human myocardium. *Adv Anat Embryol Cell Biol* 2003; **168**: 1–104.

3 Pratt FH. The circulation through the veins of Thebesius. *J Boston Soc Med Sci* 1897; **1**(15): 29–34.

4 Zanoschi C. [Controversies about the Vieussens-Thebesius veins]. *Rev Med Chir Soc Med Nat Iasi* 1988; **92**(4): 776–778.

5 Sun C, Pan Y, Wang H, *et al.* Assessment of the coronary venous system using 256-slice computed tomography. *PLoS ONE* 2014; **9**(8): e104246. doi:10.1371/journal. pone.0104246

6 Nakamura K, Funabashi N, Naito S, *et al.* Anatomical relationship of coronary sinus/great cardiac vein and left circumflex coronary artery along mitral annulus in atrial fibrillation before radiofrequency catheter ablation using 320-slice CT. *Int J Cardiol* 2013; **168**(6): 5174–5181.

7 Del Valle-Fernández R, Jelnin V, Panagopoulos G, Ruiz CE. Insight into the dynamics of the coronary sinus/great cardiac vein and the mitral annulus: implications for percutaneous mitral annuloplasty techniques. *Circ Cardiovasc Interv* 2009; **2**(6): 557–564.

8 Tschabitscher M. The so called "silent zone" of the coronary sinus. In W. Mohl (ed.) The Coronary Sinus Library, Vol 1: Anatomy and Pathophysiology of the Coronary Venous Circulation. Reprinted from the Proceedings of the Society of Coronary Sinus Interventions, 1989, reprinted 2002; 49–52.

9 Tschabitscher M. Anatomy of coronary veins. In W. Mohl (ed.) The Coronary Sinus Library, Vol 1: Anatomy and Pathophysiology of the Coronary Venous Circulation. Reprinted from the Proceedings of the Society of Coronary Sinus Interventions, 1989, reprinted 2002; 30–47.

10 von Ludinghausen M; v. Ratajczyk-Pakalska E, Tschabitscher M, Maurer G, Glogar D, Mohl W. Nomenclature: Venae cardiacae-cardiac veins. W. Mohl (ed.) The Coronary Sinus Library, Vol 1: Anatomy and Pathophysiology of the Coronary Venous Circulation. Reprinted from the Proceedings of the Society of Coronary Sinus Interventions, 1989, reprinted 2002; 3–7.

11 von Lüdinghausen M. Nomenclature and distribution pattern of cardiac veins in man. In the W. Mohl (ed.) The Coronary Sinus Library, Vol 1: Anatomy and Pathophysiology of the Coronary Venous Circulation. Reprinted from the Proceedings of the Society of Coronary Sinus Interventions, 1989, reprinted 2002; 7–26.

12 Muers MF, Sleight P. The reflex cardiovascular depression caused by occlusion of the coronary sinus in the dog. *J Physiol* 1972; **221**: 259–282.

13 Mohl W. The momentum of coronary sinus interventions clinically. *Circulation* 1988; **77**(1): 6–12.

14 Schopf M, Schuster M, Müller M, *et al.* Effects of PICSO on purine nucleotides in ischemic canine and reperfused human hearts. In W. Mohl (ed.) The Coronary Sinus Library, Vol 1: Anatomy and Pathophysiology of the Coronary Venous Circulation. Reprinted from the Proceedings of the Society of Coronary Sinus Interventions, 1989, reprinted 2002; 124–131.

15 Mayr H, Glogar D, Mohl W, *et al.* Effect of PICSO treatment on arrhythmias during early myocardial ischemia. In W. Mohl (ed.) The Coronary Sinus Library, Vol 1: Anatomy and Pathophysiology of the Coronary Venous Circulation. Reprinted from the Proceedings of the Society of Coronary Sinus Interventions, 1989, reprinted 2002; 39–43.

16 Kenner T, Moser M, Mohl W. Arteriovenous difference of the blood density in the coronary circulation. *J Biomech Eng* 1985; **107**(1): 34–40.

17 Syeda B. The salvage potential of coronary sinus interventions: meta-analysis and pathophysiologic consequences. *J Thorac Cardiovasc Surg* 2004; **127**: 1703–1212.

18 Jacobs AK, Faxon D, Coats D, *et al.* The effect of pressure controlled intermittent coronary sinus occlusion during reperfusio. In W. Mohl (ed.) The Coronary Sinus Library, Vol 1: Anatomy and Pathophysiology of the Coronary Venous Circulation.

Reprinted from the Proceedings of the Society of Coronary Sinus Interventions, 1989, reprinted 2002; 35–37.

19 van den Hoef TP, Nijveldt R, van der Ent M, *et al.* Pressure-controlled Intermittent coronary sinus occlusion (PICSO) in acute ST-segment elevation myocardial infarction: results of the prepare RAMSES safety and feasibility study. *EuroIntervention* 2014; **11**: 37–44.

20 Mohl W, Komamura K, Kasahara H, *et al.* Myocardial protection via the coronary sinus. *Circ J* 2008; **72**: 526–533.

21 Miyazaki A, Hatori N, Tadokoro H, RydÉN L, Corday E, Drury J. More rapid thrombolysis with coronary venous retroinfusion of streptokinase compared with intravenous administration: an experimental study in canines. *Eur Heart J* 1990; **11**(10): 936–944.

22 Wilcox JE, Fonarow GC, Zhang Y, *et al.* Clinical effectiveness of cardiac resynchronization and implantable cardioverter-defibrillator therapy in men and women with heart failure: findings from IMPROVE HF. *Circ Heart Fail* 2014; **7**(1): 146–153.

23 Hai OY, Mentz RJ, Zannad F, *et al.* Cardiac resynchronization therapy in heart failure patients with less severe left ventricular dysfunction. *Eur J Heart Fail* 2015; **17**: 135–143.

24 Wang L, Yuan S, Borgquist R, Hoijer CJ, Brandt J. Coronary sinus cannulation with a steerable catheter during biventricular device implantation. *Scand Cardiovasc J* 2014; **48**(1): 41–46.

25 Zhou W, Hou X, Piccinelli M, *et al.* 3D fusion of LV venous anatomy on fluoroscopy venograms with epicardial surface on SPECT myocardial perfusion images for guiding CRT LV lead placement. *JACC Cardiovasc Imaging* 2014; **7**: 1239–1248

26 Truong QA, Januzzi JL, Szymonifka J, *et al.* Coronary sinus biomarker sampling compared to peripheral venous blood for predicting outcomes in patients with severe heart failure undergoing cardiac resynchronization therapy: The BIOCRT study. *Heart Rhythm* 2014; **11**(12): 2167–2175.

27 Vernooy K, van Deursen CJ, Strik M, Prinzen FW. Strategies to improve cardiac resynchronization therapy. *Nat Rev Cardiol* 2014; **11**(8): 481–493.

28 Wang J, Su Y, Bai J, Wang W, Qin S, Ge J. Elevated pulmonary artery pressure predicts poor outcome after cardiac resynchronization therapy. *J Interv Cardiac Electrophysiol* 2014; **40**(2): 171–178.

29 Feldman T, Young A. Percutaneous approaches to valve repair for mitral regurgitation. *J Am Coll Cardiol* 2014; **63**(20): 2057–2068.

30 Machaalany J, Bilodeau L, Hoffmann R, *et al.* Treatment of functional mitral valve regurgitation with the permanent percutaneous transvenous mitral annuloplasty system: results of the multicenter international percutaneous transvenous mitral annuloplasty system to reduce mitral valve regurgitation in patients with heart failure trial. *Am Heart J* 2013; **165**(5): 761–769.

31 Degen H, Schneider T, Wilke J, Haude M. [Coronary sinus devices for treatment of functional mitral valve regurgitation. Solution or dead end?]. *Herz* 2013; **38**(5): 490–500.

32 Machaalany J, St-Pierre A, Senechal M, *et al.* Fatal late migration of viacor percutaneous transvenous mitral annuloplasty device resulting in distal coronary venous perforation. *Can J Cardiol* 2013; **29**(1): 130 e1–4.

33 Weigel G, Kajgana I, Bergmeister H, *et al.* Beck and back: a paradigm change in coronary sinus interventions—pulsatile stretch on intact coronary venous endothelium. *J Thorac Cardiovasc Surg* 2007; **133**: 1581–1587.

34 Mohl W, Embryonic recall: myocardial regeneration beyond stem cell transplantation. *Wien Klin Wochenschr* 2007; **119**: 333–336.

35 Mohl W, Milasinovic D, Aschacher T, *et al.* The hypothesis of "embryonic recall": mechanotransduction as common denominator linking normal cardiogenesis to recovery in adult failing hearts. *J Cardiovasc Dev Dis* 2014; **1**: 73–82.

36 Miyasaka KY, Kida YS, Banjo T, *et al.* Heartbeat regulates cardiogenesis by suppressing retinoic acid signaling via expression of miR-143. *Mech Dev* 2011; **128**: 18–28.

37 Mohl W, Mina S, Milasinovic D, *et al.* Is activation of coronary venous cells the key to cardiac regeneration? *Nat Clin Pract Cardiovasc Med* 2008; **5**: 528–530.

38 Khatami N, Wadowski P, Wagh V, *et al.* Pressure-controlled intermittent coronary sinus occlusion (PICSO) study on mechanical control of cardiac tissue morphogenesis. *Cardiovasc Res* 2012; **93**(Suppl. 1): S56.

39 Mohl W, Mina S, Milasinovic D, *et al.* The legacy of coronary sinus interventions: endogenous cardioprotection and regeneration beyond stem cell research. *J Thorac Cardiovasc Surg* 2008; **136**: 1131–1135.

40 Mohl W, Simon P, Neumann F, Schreiner W, Punzengruber C. Clinical evaluation of pressure-controlled intermittent coronary sinus occlusion: randomized trial during coronary artery surgery. *Ann Thorac Surg* 1988; **46**(2): 192–201.

41 Van de Hoef TP, Nolte F, Delewi R, *et al.* Intracoronary hemodynamic effects of pressure-controlled intermittent coronary sinus occlusion (PICSO): results from the first-in-man prepare PICSO study. *J Interv Cardiol* 2012; **25**: 549–556. doi: 10.1111/j.1540-8183.2012.00768.

42 Mohl W, Kajgana I, Bergmeister H, Rattay F. Intermittent pressure elevation of the coronary venous system as a method to protect ischemic myocardium. *Interact Cardiovasc Thorac Surg* 2005; **4**(1): 66–69.

43 Khattab AA, Stieger S, Kamat PJ, *et al.* Effect of pressure-controlled intermittent coronary sinus occlusion (PICSO) on myocardial ischaemia and reperfusion in a closed-chest porcine model. *EuroIntervention* 2013; **9**(3): 398–406.

44 Mohl W. Coronary sinus interventions: from concept to clinics. *J Card Surg* 1987; **2**: 467–493.

45 Banai S, Ben Muvhar S, Parikh KH, *et al.* Coronary sinus reducer stent for the treatment of chronic refractory angina pectoris: a prospective, open-label, multicenter, safety feasibility first-in-man study. *J Am Coll Cardiol* 2007; **49**(17): 1783–1789.

46 Konigstein M, Meyten N, Verheye S, Schwartz M, Banai S. Transcatheter treatment for refractory angina with the coronary sinus reducer. *EuroIntervention* 2014; **9**(10): 1158–1164.

47 Paz Y, Shinfeld A. Mild increase in coronary sinus pressure with coronary sinus reducer stent for treatment of refractory angina. *Nat Clin Pract Cardiovasc Med* 2009; **6**(3): E3.

48 Mohl W, Milasinovic D, Steurer G. Coronary venous pressure elevation "risks and benefit". *Nat Clin Pract Cardiovasc Med* 2009; **6**(3): E4.

49 Hinkel R, Lebherz C, Fydanaki M, *et al.* Angiogenetic potential of Ad2/Hif-1alpha/VP16 after regional application in a preclinical pig model of chronic ischemia. *Curr Vasc Pharmacol* 2013; **11**(1): 29–37.

50 Hinkel R, Lebherz C, Fydanaki M, *et al.* Angiogenetic potential of Ad2/Hif-1alpha/VP16 after regional application in a preclinical pig model of chronic ischemia. *Curr Vasc Pharmacol* 2013; **11**(1): 29–37.

51 Kupatt C, Hinkel R, Pfosser A, *et al.* Cotransfection of vascular endothelial growth factor-A and platelet-derived growth factor-B via recombinant adeno-associated virus resolves chronic ischemic malperfusion role of vessel maturation. *J Am Coll Cardiol* 2010; **56**(5): 414–422.

52 Hinkel R, Bock-Marquette I, Hatzopoulos AK, Kupatt C. Thymosin beta4: a key factor for protective effects of eEPCs in acute and chronic ischemia. *Ann N Y Acad Sci* 2010; **1194**: 105–111.

Index

Notes:

Clinical trial names are given in the abbreviated form only

Page numbers in *italics* indicate figures and those in **bold** denote tables and boxes

---

Interventional Cardiology: Principles and Practice, Second Edition. Edited by George D. Dangas, Carlo Di Mario, and Nicholas N. Kipshidze.
© 2017 John Wiley & Sons, Ltd. Published 2017 by John Wiley & Sons, Ltd.

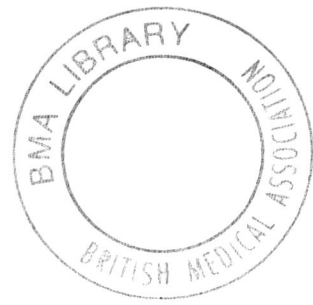